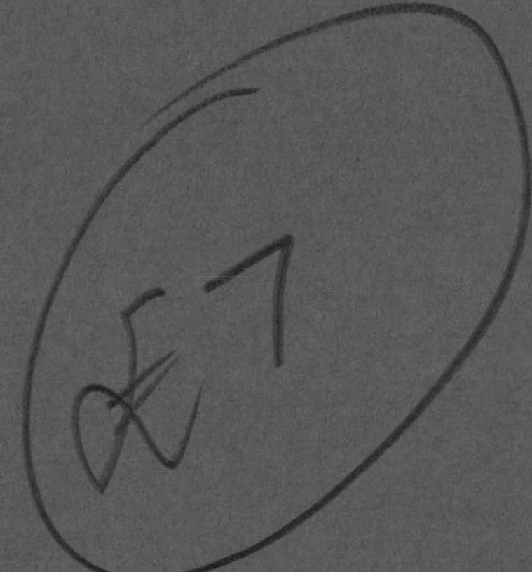
£7

D1294077

Editorial Offices:
Osney Mead, Oxford OX2 0EL
25 John Street, London WC1N 2BL
23 Ainslie Place, Edinburgh EH3 6AJ
350 Main Street, Malden
MA 02148 5018, USA
54 University Street, Carlton
Victoria 3053, Australia

Other Editorial Offices:

Blackwell Wissenschafts-Verlag GmbH
Kurfürstendamm 57
10707 Berlin, Germany

Blackwell Science KK
MG Kodenmacho Building
7–10 Kodenmacho Nihombashi
Chuo-Ku, Tokyo 104, Japan

First published 1992
Second edition 1998

Set by Setrite Typesetters, Hong Kong
Printed and bound in Great Britain by
MPG Books Ltd, Bodmin, Cornwall

A catalogue record for this title
is available from the British Library

ISBN 0-86542-629-5

Library of Congress
Cataloging-in-publication Data

Clinical endocrinology/ edited by
Ashley Grossman. — 2nd ed.
p. cm.
Includes bibiiographical references
and index.
ISBN 0–86542–629–5
1. Endocrinology. 2. Endocrine glands—
Diseases. I. Grossman, Ashley.
[DNLM: 1 Endocrine Diseases.
WK 140 C6414 1997]
RC648.C5633 1997
616.4—DC21
DNLM/DLC
for Library of Congress 97-7266
CIP

DISTRIBUTORS

Marston Book Services Ltd
PO Box 269
Abingdon
Oxon OX14 4YN
(*Orders*: Tel: 01235 465500
Fax: 01235 465555)

USA
Blackwell Science, Inc.
Commerce Place
350 Main Street
Malden, MA 02148 5018
(*Orders*: Tel: 800 759 6102
617 388 8250
Fax: 617 388 8255)

Canada
Copp Clark Professional
200 Adelaide St West, 3rd Floor
Toronto, Ontario M5H 1W7
(*Orders*: Tel: 416 597-1616
800 815-9417
Fax: 416 597-1617)

Australia
Blackwell Science Pty Ltd
54 University Street
Carlton, Victoria 3053
(*Orders*: Tel: 3 9347 0300
Fax: 3 9347 5001)

SECOND EDITION

Clinical Endocrinology

Edited by
Ashley Grossman
BA, BSc, MD, FRCP
Professor of Neuroendocrinology
Department of Endocrinology
St Bartholomew's Hospital
London

Foreword by
Shlomo Melmed MD

b
Blackwell
Science

CLINICAL ENDOCRINOLOGY

Contents

Part 16: The Hyperlipidaemias: Diagnosis and Management

Part 17: The Endocrinology of Cancer

Part 18: Endocrine Manifestations of Systemic Disease

Part 19: Protocols for Common Endocrine Tests

Part 20: History of Endocrinology

List of contributors

C.B.T. Adams MChir, FRCS, *Department of Neurological Surgery, Radcliffe Infirmary, Oxford, OX2 6HE*

E.M. Alstead MD, FRCP, *The Digestive Diseases Research Centre, St Bartholomew's and Royal London School of Medicine and Dentistry, 2 Newark Street, London, E1 2AD*

B. Ambrosi MD, *Institute of Endocrine Sciences, University of Milan, Ospedale Maggiore IRCCS, 35 via Francesco Sforza, 20122 Milan, Italy*

D.C. Anderson MD, FRCP, *1417, Princes Building, Hong Kong*

P. Armstrong MB BS, FRCR, *Academic Department of Radiology, St Bartholomew's Hospital, London, ECIA 7BE*

S.L. Atkin BSc, PhD, MRCP, *Michael White Diabetes Centre, Brocklehurst Building, 220–236 Anlaby Road, Hull, HU3 2RW*

P.H. Baylis BSc, MD, FRCP, *Endocrine Unit, Royal Victoria Infirmary, Queen Victoria Road, Newcastle Upon Tyne, NE1 4LP*

M.G. Baroni MD, PhD, *Clinica Medica, University La Sapienza, Rome, Italy*

P. Belchetz MD, MSc, FRCP, *Department of Endocrinology, Leeds General Infirmary, Great George Street, Leeds, LS1 3EX*

G.M. Besser MD, DSc, FRCP, *Departments of Medicine and Endocrinology, St Bartholomew's Hospital, London, EC1A 7BE*

L.C. Best BSc, PhD, *Multipurpose Building, Manchester Royal Infirmary, Oxford Road, Manchester, M13 9WL*

J.S. Bevan MD, FRCP(Edin), *Department of Endocrinology, Aberdeen Royal Infirmary, Foresterhill, Aberdeen, AB25 2ZN*

S.P. Bidey BSc, PhD, *Endocrine Sciences Research Group, University of Manchester, Stopford Building, Oxford Road, Manchester, M13 9PT*

S.R. Bloom MA, MD, DSc, FRCP, *Department of Medicine, Hammersmith Hospital, Du Cane Road, London, W12 0HS*

P.-M.G. Bouloux BSc, MD, FRCP, *Centre for Neuroendocrinology, The Royal Free Hospital, Pond Street, London, NW3 2QG*

J.-P. Bourguignon MD, PhD, *Department of Paediatrics, CHU Sart Tilman, B-4000 Liège, Belgium*

M.-L. Brandi MD, PhD, *Department of Clinical Physiopathology, University of Florence Medical School, Viale Pieraccini 6, 50139 Florence, Italy*

N.A. Bridges DM, MRCP, *Chelsea and Westminster Hospital, Fulham Road, London, SW10 9NH*

C.G.D. Brook MD, FRCP, FRCPCH, *London Centre for Paediatric Endocrinology and Metabolism, The Middlesex Hospital, Mortimer Street, London, W1N 8AA*

F. Camanni MD, *Department of Internal Medicine, Division of Endocrinology, University of Turin, Corso Dogliotti 14, 10126 Turin, Italy*

F.F. Casanueva MD, PhD, *Department of Medicine, Division of Endocrinology, C.H.U.S. University of Santiago Hospital Complex, PO Box 563, E-15780, Santiago de Compostela, Spain*

J.D. Challis BSc, SRD, *19 Keswick Close, Tilehurst, Reading, RG30 4SD*

S.L. Chew BSc, MD, *Department of Endocrinology, St Bartholomew's Hospital, London, EC1A 7BE*

E. Ciccarelli MD, *Department of Internal Medicine, Division of Endocrinology, University of Turin, C.so Dogliotti 14, 10126 Turin, Italy*

A.J.L. Clark DSc, FRCP, *Molecular Endocrinology Section, Department of Endocrinology, St Bartholomew's Hospital, London, EC1 7BE*

J. Compston BSc, MB BS, MD, FRCPath, FRCP, *Department of Medicine, University of Cambridge Clinical School, Addenbrooke's Hospital, Hills Road, Cambridge CB2 2QQ*

J.R.E. Davis MD, PhD, FRCP, *Endocrine Sciences Research Group, University of Manchester, Stopford Building, Oxford Road, Manchester, M13 9PT*

L.J. De Groot MD, *Department of Medicine, The University of Chicago Medical Center, Thyroid Study Unit, 5841 South Maryland Avenue, Chicago IL 60637, USA*

V. De Sanctis MD, *Department of Paediatrics and Adolescent Medicine, Arcispedale S. Anna, Corso Giovecca 203, 44100 Ferrara, Italy*

G. Delitala MD, *Istituto di Patologia Medica, Via San Pietro 8, 07100 Sassari, Italy*

C. Dieguez MD, Department of Physiology, University of Santiago de Compostela, PO Box 563, E-15780, Santiago de Compostela, Spain

C.R.W. Edwards MD, MB, BChir, FRCP FRCP(Ed) FRSE, *Sherfield Building, Imperial College School of Medicine, Exhibition Road, London, SW7 2AZ*

C. Eng MD, *PhD, Dana-Farber Cancer Institute, Harvard Medical School, 44 Binney Street, Boston, MA 02115–6084, USA*

G. Faglia MD, *Institute of Endocrine Sciences, University of Milan, Ospedale Maggiore IRCCS, 35 via Francesco Sforza, 20122 Milan, Italy*

A. Falchetti MD, *Department of Clinical Physiopathology, University of Florence Medical School, Viale Pieraccini 6, 50139 Florence, Italy*

M.J.G. Farthing MD, FRCP, *The Digestive Diseases Research Centre, St Bartholomew's and Royal London School of Medicine and Dentistry, 2 Newark Street, London, E1 2AD*

J.A. Franklyn MD, PhD, FRCP, *Department of Medicine, University of Birmingham, Queen Elizabeth Hospital, Birmingham, B15 2TH*

S. Franks MD, FRCP, Hon MD (Uppsala), Department of Obstetrics and Gynaecology, Imperial College School of Medicine at St Mary's, St Mary's Hospital, London, W2 1PG

D.J. Galton DSc, FRCP, *Department of Human Metabolism and Genetics, St Bartholomew's Hospital, London, EC1A 7BE*

J.S. Garrow MD, PhD, FRCP, *The Dial House, 93 Uxbridge Road, Rickmansworth, Herts, WD3 2DQ*

J.Girard MD, Department of Endocrinology, University Children's Hospital, Romergasse 8, CH-4005 Basel, Switzerland

V. Grill MB BS, FRACP, *Department of Medicine, St Vincent's Hospital, 41 Victoria Parade, Fitzroy, Victoria 3065, Australia*

R.J. Hart MB BS, MRCOG, *Minimally Invasive Therapy Unit, University Department of Obstetrics and Gynaecology, The Royal Free Hospital, Pond Street, London, NW3 2QG*

D.A. Heath MB, ChB, FRCP, *Department of Medicine, University of Birmingham, Selly Oak Hospital, Raddlebarn Road, Selly Oak, Birmingham, B29 6JD*

D.J. Hemrika MD, PhD, *O L Vrouwe Gasthuis, Department of Obstetrics and Gynaecology, PO Box 95500, 1090 HM Amsterdam, The Netherlands*

W.F. Hendry MD, ChM, FRCS, *149 Harley Street, London, W1N 2DE*

M. Hewison PhD, *Department of Medicine, University of Birmingham, Queen Elizabeth Hospital, Birmingham, B15 2TH*

P.C. Hindmarsh MD, FRCP, *London Centre for Paediatric Endocrinology and Metabolism, The Middlesex Hospital, Mortimer Street, London, W1N 8AA*

J.P. Hinson PhD, *Department of Biochemistry, Faculty of Basic Medical Sciences, Queen Mary and Westfield College, Mile End Road, London, E1 4NS*

F. Holsboer MD, PhD, *Max Planck Institute of Psychiatry, Kraepelinstrasse 2–10, 80804 Munich, Germany*

R. Howell MB BS, FRCOG, *Fertility Unit, Homerton Hospital, Homerton Row, London E9 6SR*

P.D. Hollett MD, FRCPC, *Division of Nuclear Medicine, Medical Imaging Program, 300 Prince Phillip Drive, St John's, NF A1B 3V6, Canada*

T.A. Howlett MD, FRCP, *Department of Diabetes and Endocrinology, Leicester Royal Infirmary, Leicester, LE1 5WW*

I.A. Hughes MD, FRCP, FRCP(C), FRCPCH, *Department of Paediatrics, University of Cambridge School of Clinical Medicine, Level 8 Addenbrooke's Hospital, Hills Road, Cambridge, CB2 2QQ*

C. Irwin MB BS, MRCP, FRCR, Department of Radiotherapy, Walsgrave Hospital, Clifford Bridge Road, Coventry, CV2 2DX

P.J. Jenkins MA, MRCP, *Department of Endocrinology, St Bartholomew's Hospital, London, EC1A 7BE*

R.C. Jenkins MB BS, BMedSci, *Department of Medicine, Clinical Sciences Centre, Northern General Hospital, Sheffield, S5 7AU*

D.G. Johnston PhD, FRCPath, FRCP, *Unit of Metabolic Medicine, Imperial College School of Medicine at St Mary's, Norfolk Place, London, W2 1PG*

N. Josso MD, *Unité de Recherches sur l'Endocrinologie du Développement, INSERM U.293 Ecole Normale Supérieure, Département de Biologie, 1 rue Maurice Arnoux, 92120 Montrouge, France*

N. Joughin MBBChir, MRCPsych, MPhil, *Marchwood Priory Hospital, Hythe Road, Marchwood, Southampton, Hants, S040 4WU*

R.T. Jung MA, MD, FRCP(Edin), FRCP(London), *The Diabetes Centre, Ninewells Hospital and Medical School, Dundee, DD1 9SY*

P. Kendall-Taylor MD, FRCP, *Endocrine Unit, Royal Victoria Infirmary, Queen Victoria Road, Newcastle UponTyne, NE1 4LP*

P.G. Kopelman MD, FRCP, *Medical Unit, St Bartholomew's and Royal London School of Medicine and Dentistry, Queen Mary and Westfield College, Turner Street, London E1 2AD*

A.C.Nieuwenhuijzen Kruseman MD, PhD, *Department of Medicine and Endocrinology, University of Maastricht, PO Box 616, 6200 MD Maastricht, The Netherlands*

S.W.J. Lamberts MD, PhD, *Department of Medicine, University Hospital Rotterdam, 3015 GD Rotterdam, The Netherlands*

I.G. Lawrence MRCP, *Department of Diabetes and Endocrinology, Leicester, LE1 5WW*

J.H. Lazarus MA, MD, FRCP, *Department of Medicine, University of Wales College of Medicine, Heath Park, Cardiff, CF4 4XN*

S.L. Lightman MB BCh, PhD, FRCP, *Department of Medicine, University of Bristol, Bristol Royal Infirmary, Marlborough Street, Bristol, BS2 8HW*

D.G. Lowe MD, FRCS, FRCPath, FIBiol, *Department of Histopathology, St Bartholomew's Hospital, London, EC1A 7BE*

P.J. Lowry DSc, *School of Animal and Microbial Sciences, University of Reading, Whiteknights, Reading, RG6 6AJ*

E.A. MacGregor MB BS, *26 Waubrey Walk, London, W8 7JG*

A.L. Magos MB BS, MRCOG, *Minimally Invasive Therapy Unit, The University Department of Obstetrics and Gynaecology, The Royal Free Hospital, Pond Street, London, NW3 2QG*

M.N. Maisey BSc, MD, FRCP, FRCR, *Radiological Sciences, UMDS Guy's and St Thomas's Hospital, London, SE1 9RT*

V. Marks MA, MD, FRCP(Lond & Edin), FRCPath, MAE, *Office of the Dean of Medicine, University of Surrey EIHMS, Stirling House Campus, Surrey Research Park, Guildford, Surrey, GU2 5RF*

T.J. Martin MD, DSc, FRACP, FRCPA, *St Vincent's Institute of Medical Research, St Vincent's Hospital, 41 Victoria Parade, Fitzroy, Victoria 3065, Australia*

L. Masi MD, PhD, *Department of Clinical Physiopathology, University of Florence Medical School, Viale Pieraccini 6, 50139 Florence, Italy*

A.F. Massoud MB BS, MRCP, *London Centre for Paediatric Endocrinology and Metabolism, The Middlesex Hospital, Mortimer Street, London, WIN 8AA*

P.L. Matson PhD, *Concept Fertility Centre, King Edward Memorial Hospital, 374 Bagot Road, Subiaco, WA 6008, Australia*

T.J. McKenna MD, FRCP (Irl, Lond and Edin), *Department of Endocrinology and Diabetes Mellitus, St Vincent's Hospital, Elm Park, Dublin 4, Ireland*

V.C. Medvei CBE, MD, FRCP, *38 Westmoreland Terrace, London, SW1V 3HL*

M.E. Molitch MD, *Center for Endocrinology, Metabolism and Molecular Medicine, Northwestern University Medical School, 303 E Chicago Avenue, Chicago, IL 60611, USA*

J.P. Monson MD, FRCP, *Departments of Medicine and Endocrinology, St Bartholomew's Hospital, London, EC1A 7BE*

J.C. Moore-Gillon MA, MD, FRCP, *Department of Respiratory Medicine, St Bartholomew's Hospital, London, EC1A 7BE*

O.A. Müller MD, *Department of Medicine, Rotkreuz-Krankenhaus, Nymphenburgher Str. 163, 80634 München, Germany*

J. Newell-Price MA, MB BChir, MRCP, *Department of Endocrinology, St Bartholomew's Hospital, London, ECIA 7BE*

K. Öberg MD, PhD, *Department of Internal Medicine Endocrine Oncology Unit, University Hospital, S-751 85 Uppsala, Sweden*

D. O'Shea MD, MRCPI, *Department of Endocrinology, Charing Cross Hospital, Hammersmith Hospitals NHS Trust Fulham Palace Road, London W6 8RF*

F. Pacini MD, *Institute of Endocrinology, University of Pisa, Via Paradisa 2, 56124 Pisa, Italy*

N. Panay BSc, MRCOG, MFFP, Department of Obstetrics and Gynaecology, Chelsea and Westminster Hospital, 369 Fulham Road, London, SWIO 9MH

P. Perros MD, MB BS, MRCP, *Freeman Hospital NHS Trust, Freeman Road, Newcastle Upon Tyne, NE7 7DN*

P.N. Plowman MA, MD, FRCP, FRCR, *Department of Clinical Oncology, St Bartholomew's Hospital, London, EC1A 7BE*

B.A.J. Ponder PhD, FRCP, *CRC Human Cancer Genetics Research Group, Addenbrooke's Hospital, Hills Road, Cambridge, CB2 2QQ*

M.A. Preece MD, MSc, FRCP, *Division of Medicine, Institute of Child Health, University College London Medical School, 30 Guildford Street, London, WC1N 1EH*

P.A. Price MB, BSc, FRCP, *Department of Medicine, Princess Margaret Hospital, Swindon, SN1 4JU*

A.E.G. Raine DPhil, FRCP, (Deceased)

D.W. Ray PhD, MRCP, *Endocrine Sciences Research Group, University of Manchester, Stopford Building, Oxford Road, Manchester, M13 9PT*

R. Rey MD, PhD, *Unité de Recherches sur l'Endocrinologie du Développment, INSERM U.293 Ecole Normale Supérieure, Département de Biologie, 1 rue Maurice Arnoux, 92120 Montrouge, France*

R.H. Reznek MBChB, FRCR, FRCP, *Department of Radiology, St Bartholomew's Hospital, London, EC1A 7BE*

P.C. Richardson BMedSci, BM BS(Hons), MRCP, *Novartis Pharmaceuticals, Wimblehurst Road, Horsham, RH12 4AB*

R.J.M. Ross MB BS, MD, FRCP, *Clinical Sciences Centre, Northern General Hospital, Sheffield; S5 7AU*

W.G. Rossmanith MD, PhD, *Department of Obstetrics and Gynaecology, University of Ulm, Prittwitzstr. 43, D-89075 Ulm, Germany*

M.O. Savage MD, FRCP, *Department of Paediatric Endocrinology, St Bartholomew's Hospital, London, EC1A 7BE*

P. Savage PhD, MRCP, *Department of Clinical Oncology, Royal Postgraduate Medical School, Hammersmith Hospital, Du Cane Road, London, W12 0NN*

M.F. Scanlon MD, FRCP, *University of Wales College of Medicine, Heath Park, Cardiff, CF4 4XN*

J. Schoemaker MD, PhD, *Free University Hospital, Department of Obstetrics & Gynaecology, PO Box 7057, 1007 MB Amsterdam, The Netherlands*

D. Sebag-Montefiore MRCP, FRCP, Cookridge Hospital, Yorkshire Regional Centre for Cancer Treatment, Cookridge, West Yorkshire, LS16 6QB

S.M. Shalet MD, FRCP, *Department of Endocrinology, Christie Hospital, Wilmslow Road, Withington, Manchester M20 4BX*

P.S. Sharp MD, FRCP, *Department of Diabetes and Endocrinology, Northwick Park Hospital, Watford Road, Harrow, Middlesex, HA1 3UJ*

M.C. Sheppard PhD, FRCP, *Department of Medicine, University of Birmingham, Queen Elizabeth Hospital, Birmingham, B15 2TH*

P.C. Sizonenko MD, MSc, *Division of Biology of Growth & Reproduction, Department of Paediatrics, Hospital Cantonal Universitaire, 1211 Geneva 14, Switzerland*

T.C.B. Stamp MD, FRCP, *Metabolic Unit, Royal National Orthopaedic Hospital, Brockley Hill, Stanmore, Middlesex, HA7 4LP*

J.W.W. Studd DSc, MD, FRCOG, *Department of Obstetrics and Gynaecology, Chelsea and Westminster Hospital, Fulham Road, Chelsea, London, SW10 9NH*

C. Sultan MD, PhD, *Unite d'Endocrinologie, Service de Pédiatrie I, Hôpital A. de Villeneuve, 34295 Montpellier, France*

R.V. Thakker MD, FRCP, *MRC Molecular Endocrinology Group, Royal Postgraduate Medical School, Hammersmith Hospital, Du Cane Road, London, W12 0NN*

R.C. Thuraisingham MB BS, MRCP, *Department of Nephrology, St Bartholomew's Hospital, London, EC1A 7BE*

A.D. Toft CBE, BSc, MD, FRCP(Edin), *Endocrine Clinic, Royal Infirmary, Edinburgh, EH3 9YW*

P.J. Trainer MD, MRCP, *Departments of Medicine and Endocrinology, St Bartholomew's Hospital, London, EC1A 7BE*

S. Tsagarakis MD, PhD, *Department of Endocrinology, Diabetes and Metabolism, Evangelismos Hospital, Athens, Greece*

E. Ur MB, MRCP, *Department of Endocrinology, Dalhousie University, Victoria General Hospital, Halifax, Nova Scotia, B3H 2Y9, Canada*

A.G. Vagenakis MD, *University of Patras, Department of Medicine, University Hospital, Patras 26500, Greece*

M. Vallejo MD, PhD, *Reproductive Endocrine Unit, Massachusetts General Hospital, Bartlett Hall Extension, 511 Boston, MA 02114, USA*

G.P. Vinson PhD, DSc, *Department of Biochemistry, Faculty of Basic Medical Sciences, Queen Mary and Westfield College, Mile End Road, London, E1 4NS*

N.R. Watson MB BS, MRCOG, *Department of Obstetrics and Gynaecology, Hillingdon Hospital, Pield Heath Road, Uxbridge, Middlesex, UB8 3NN*

K. von Werder MD, FRCP, *Schlosspark Klinik, Humboldt University of Berlin, Heubnerweg 2, 14059 Berlin, Germany*

J. Waxman BSc, MD, MB BS, FRCP, *Department of Clinical Oncology, Royal Postgraduate Medical School, Hammersmith Hospital, Du Cane Road, London, W12 0NN*

S.M. Webb MD, *Endocrinology Section, San Pablo Hospital, Autonomous University Hospital of Barcelona, Avda. SA Maria Claret 167, 08025 Barcelona, Spain*

A.P. Weetman MD, DSc, FRCP, *Department of Medicine, University of Sheffield Clinical Sciences Centre, Northern General Hospital, Sheffield, S5 7AU*

M.C. White MD, FRCP, (Deceased)

B.J. Whitehouse PhD, *Biomedical Sciences Division, King's College London, Campden Hill Road, London, W8 7AH*

B. Wonke MD, FRCP, MRCP, *Department of Haematology, Whittington Hospital, Highgate Hill, London, N19 5NFR*

D.F. Wood MD, FRCP, *Department of Endocrinology, St Bartholomew's and the Royal London School of Medicine, Royal London Hospital, London E1 1BB*

R.J. Woods MSc, PhD, *School of Animal and Microbial Sciences, University of Reading, Whiteknights, Reading, RG6 6AJ*

D. Wynick MD, MRCP, *Department of Endocrinology, Bristol Royal Infirmary, Marlborough Street, Bristol, BS2 8HW*

M.C. Young MB BS, MRCP, Department of Pediatrics, Tulane University Medical Center, 1430 Tulane Avenue, New Orleans, Louisiana 70112, USA

J.L. Yovich MB BS, FRCOG, FRACOG, *PIVET Medical Centre, 166–8 Cambridge Street, Leederville, Perth WA 6007, Australia*

Foreword

The educational challenge of system-based medical disciplines is to 'transcend the organ' and to integrate a strong knowledge base into a body of clinically relevant text. The expert authors of this edition of *Clinical Endocrinology* have succeeded in providing the authoritative educational tool for the student and practitioner encountering patients with hormonal disorders.

Building on the sub-cellular fundamentals of hormone synthesis, secretion and action, the authors provide a unique opportunity for the clinician to learn how molecular techniques are applied to unravelling mechanisms for pathophysiologic principles. The systematic neuro-endocrine, thyroid, adrenal, pancreas, parathyroid, bone and reproductive disorders are each introduced by cutting-edge scientific background followed by crisp descriptions of clinical approach, diagnosis and management of these classic endocrine syndromes. However, a further strength of this comprehensive textbook resides in the ensuing chapters integrating systemic disorders of growth, obesity, cancer endocrinology and the endocrine manifestations of systemic disease. These superb chapters serve to bring the true definition of endocrinology as a discipline of multi-tissue communication to the reality of patient-based bedside medicine.

Furthermore, cutting-edge techniques for hormone assays, imaging, radioreceptor imaging and endocrine test protocols provide the reader with the required tools to diagnose both structural and functional endocrine disorders.

Finally, in recognition of the tremendous basic advances in our understanding of mechanisms of clinical hormone disorders, this volume provides a fitting and appropriate recognition of our forebears' early genius in recognising endocrine syndromes prior to the availability of scientific tools to assist the observational skills of the physician.

Thus, *Clinical Endocrinology* eminently succeeds in integrating a strong subspecialty knowledge base into a comprehensive text encompassing all aspects of endocrine-based patient care. This volume will be of invaluable use to medical students, graduate trainees, clinicians and scientists seeking both a strong scientific base for disease pathogenesis, and state-of-the art diagnosis and management.

SHLOMO MELMED
August 1997
Cedars-Sinai Medical Center
Los Angeles

Preface to the second edition

What use is a textbook in clinical medicine? It might be thought that, with the explosion of information technology, the rapid pace of biological research and the concomitant massive expansion in journal numbers, any book attempting to incorporate a subject as vast as endocrinology is bound to be redundant. However, it should be remembered that the first encyclopaedias of the Enlightenment were produced by the French *philosophes*, such as Diderot, to allow the intelligent layman to be at least aware of the extent of all knowledge. This was thought to allow the citizens to be in a better position to organise and plan their lives. We may have abandoned the idea that any one person can resonably incorporate a knowledge of all that is known, even in a general sense, or even that the extent of knowledge is indeed finite. But once you get into a practical discipline such as clinical medicine, there is undoubtedly a need for a handbook rather than a textbook which produces a broad overview within a clinical discipline. This was fundamentally the aim of the first edition of *Clinical Endocrinology*, and I am very pleased that its success has now allowed us to produce this, the second edition, some five years on. To quote from the preface to the first edition, we hope that this will serve as a pragmatic guide to the best of current clinical practice in endocrinology, and to this end the text has been designed to be intelligible, informative and, above all, practical. As previously, this book is aimed at both the non-endocrinologist who needs to deal with endocrine problems as well as the super-specialist in contact with more general endocrine orders outside of their own area of particular expertise. The patient coming to see the endocrinologist does not readily have a sign pointing out a particular endocrinopathy, and the clinician needs to be aware of the broad sweep of endocrine knowledge and practice, often quite outside their own limited sub-specialty. Every chapter has either been revised by their original authors or completely rewritten, while around 10% of this edition is completely new. I am especially grateful to Dr Shern Chew for integrating the opening sections on molecular biology and basic endocrine mechanisms. We have also extended the range of our contributors beyond Europe and Australia to include North America, such that this is now truly an international volume. The French encyclopaedists were also keen to produce practical guides as much as reference works, and were indeed much criticised for their opinions. Our hopes persist that this will also be a truly useful guide to the practising endocrinologist, and that few clinical problems within endocrinology cannot be answered, at least initally, from within its pages.

Once again, I am most grateful to all the contributors for the massive amount of effort required to produce this edition, and for the great care and attention they have given to this project. It remains one of the mysteries of clinical and academic life as to why busy clinicians and academics should be prepared to devote so much of their time and energy to producing this type of textbook, as the rewards are certainly not financial. However, I do hope that the reader will agree with me that none of this effort has been wasted.

It is particularly sad to record that two of the major contributors to this volume, Professor Michael White and Professor Tony Raine, died during the production of this edition. They were both good colleagues and fine friends, and it is a matter of great sadness that their highly productive and creative lives were cut so unnecessarily short. I should also like to take the opportunity to mourn the passing of another old endocrine friend, Dr Harvey Besterman, who was one of the very first endocrinologists to initiate me into this fascinating field.

I am grateful once again to Rita Simpson for co-ordinating this massive project, and to Andrew Robinson and Jonathan Rowley of Blackwell Science for keeping me on the straight and narrow. This book is dedicated to a series of most important people in my life: Rose, Debbie, Emily, Sophie, Annabel, Camilla and Cordelia.

ASHLEY GROSSMAN
London, 1997

Preface to the first edition

Clinical endocrinology has rapidly expanded from a minor field devoted to a small group of ductless glands to embrace a whole variety of clinical entities, and seems ever ready to incorporate very much more. At least part of the reason for this impressive growth is that endocrinology has been more firmly established in scientific, and especially biochemical, principles than many other clinical disciplines. Thus, epochal advances in our understanding of molecular mechanisms have carried forward the clinical science of endocrinology. Our conceptual framework has also been transformed, as specifically endocrine secretions have become incorporated as one aspect of general cell-to-cell communications; this now forms an autocrine–paracrine–neurocrine–endocrine continuum. This progress has not been without casualties. Many now find that modern clinical endocrinology has become increasingly subspecialised, and other non-endocrine specialists are often wary of entering these fast-flowing waters.

Because of these recent changes, as well as the increasing fragmentation of the subject, it now appears to be an appropriate time to introduce a new textbook of clinical endocrinology; one which emphasises pragmatic clinical practice, but takes the reader from basic science to clinical decision making in clear steps. Thus, this book is aimed at both the non-endocrinologist who needs to deal with endocrine problems, as well as the super-specialist who may encounter more general endocrine disorders which are not within his/her specialised practice. For these reasons, we have included many areas which, while not classically 'endocrine', may be brought to the attention of the physician with an endocrine interest. Such areas, including obesity, anorexia nervosa, lipid disorders, hypothalamic tumours, *in vitro* fertilisation, premenstrual and menopausal syndromes, are often put the way of endocrinologists as probably 'hormonal', although their relationship to the classical 'ductless glands' may be considered as rather tangential. It is to the many physicians who deal with this plethora of associated disorders that this book is dedicated, and to whom we hope it will serve as a pragmatic guide to the best of current clinical practice.

The text is designed to be intelligible, informative and, above all, practical. With this in mind, the book includes considerably more detail than is to be found in most basic primers, although formulated in a more concise and readable manner than the totally comprehensive reference manual. The references are provided more for guidance than as complete surveys of the literature, while the reader requiring more exhaustive information will find directions to the relevant sources and reviews. Some chapters, for example those on molecular mechanisms or the pathogenesis of ectopic hormone production, or the neuroendocrinology of mental disease, have been included as they encompass many of the exciting growth points in endocrinology, of which the practising endocrinologist should be aware. Others, such as those concerning *in vitro* fertilization or the menopause, are particular areas where patients are likely to require detailed information from endocrinologists acting in the capacity of an adviser. By contrast, the chapters relating to anorexia nervosa are designed to provide highly practical information in defined situations, while detailed protocols for common endocrine tests are assigned to their own section. Each section includes a résumé of the basic anatomy and physiology, while each chapter has been written by an international expert with practical clinical experience. I have been particularly assisted by many of my colleagues at St Bartholomew's Hospital, but the majority of chapters have been contributed by British and continental European authorities, extending to Australia. All diagrams and illustrations have been specifically drawn for this volume. Above all, it is hoped that endocrinologists and non-endocrinologists alike will actively enjoy reading and browsing through this volume, and that answers to all but the most recherché clinical problem will be found here. However, errors of omission and areas inadequately covered remain the responsibility of the editor.

I am most grateful for all the help I have received throughout the preparation of this book by the staff of Blackwell Scientific Publications, and in particular Peter Saugman and, more recently, Andrew Robinson. I am also greatly indebted to Rita Simpson of the Department of Endocrinology at St Bartholomew's Hospital, who has undertaken the massive task of secretarial assistance essential to a volume of this magnitude.

Endocrinology is the science of molecular communication systems, so this book is dedicated to those who have taught me most about the importance of communication: to Debbie, Emily, Sophie and Annabel.

ASHLEY GROSSMAN
January 1992
St Bartholomew's Hospital
London

Part 1
Molecular Biology of Endocrine Systems

CHAPTER 1

Basic principles

M. Vallejo and S.L. Lightman

Introduction

Proteins are the fundamental components of cells. They are responsible for most biological activity, including cell maintenance, growth and development, and intercellular communications. The particular roles that they play are enormously varied: these include enzymes that catalyse an extraordinary number of chemical reactions; structural components that shape cell morphology and promote cell movement; surface receptors that recognise external signals, allowing cells to respond to their environment; molecular switches for the activation or repression of gene expression; and chemical pumps and ion channels that maintain the electrolytic balance and transport of required nutrients. The function of each protein is determined by its sequence, i.e. the linear order of amino acids that constitute the protein molecule. Therefore, protein synthesis and its regulation is a biological process of paramount importance for cell function.

All the information required for protein synthesis is stored in the DNA within the cell nucleus and is delivered by RNA to the cytoplasm, where the synthesis actually occurs. Both nucleic acids are polymers whose basic units are nucleotides. These are compounds that consist of a pentose sugar (deoxyribose in DNA and ribose in RNA), a phosphate group and an organic base (Fig. 1.1). There are two types of bases in nucleic acids, purines (adenine and guanine) and pyrimidines (cytosine, thymine and uracil). Adenine (A), guanine (G) and cytosine (C) are found in both DNA and RNA, whereas thymine (T) is only found in DNA. RNA contains uracil (U) instead of thymine.

Nucleotides are linked together through their phosphate groups, which join the 5′ carbon of one pentose sugar with the 3′ carbon of the next. This gives rise to a chain which can have any one of the four bases at each position. It is this linear arrangement which determines the sequence of amino acids in a protein. Amino acids are encoded by groups of three nucleotides that are known as codons (Fig. 1.2). There are 64 possible codons that can be formed with four bases (4^3). Three of them encode 'stop' signals which indicate where the synthesis of the peptide chain must end, whereas the other 61 encode amino acids. Since there are only 20 amino acids, each one of them may be encoded by more than one codon.

From a structural point of view, the DNA molecule is a double-stranded helix (Fig. 1.3). Each adenine and guanine on one strand is always paired with thymine and cytosine, respectively, on the other strand. This base-pairing configuration renders the two strands complementary, so that the sequence of either of them determines that of the other. Complementarity is of crucial importance for RNA synthesis. During this process, the DNA helix unwinds and the sequence of the coding strand is copied into RNA using the other strand as a template. The resulting messenger RNA (mRNA), encoding a particular polypeptide chain, migrates to the cytoplasm where protein synthesis is carried out.

Two additional types of RNA are required for protein synthesis: transfer RNA (tRNA) and ribosomal RNA (rRNA). Prior to its polymerisation into polypeptide chains, each amino acid is covalently attached to a molecule of tRNA in the cytoplasm (Fig. 1.4). These deliver the amino acids to the mRNA template, where they are able to recognise specific codons. Transfer RNA is therefore an adaptor molecule which decodes the sequence information stored in the mRNA. This process, in which the nucleotide sequence of mRNA dictates the linear order of amino acids resulting in the synthesis of a polypeptide, is called *translation*. Ribosomal RNA is a major component of ribosomes. These are complex particles composed of RNA and proteins organised in two different subunits. They contain binding sites for both mRNA and tRNA, providing a structural support that allows translation to take place.

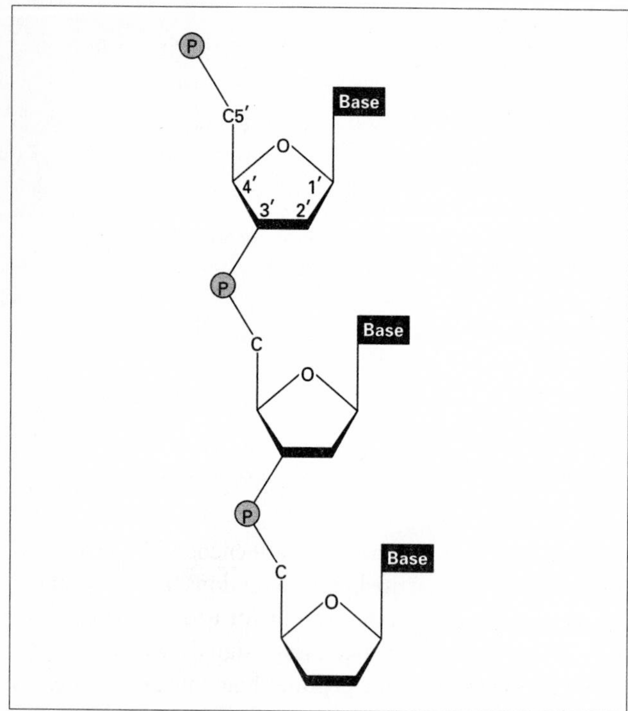

Fig. 1.1 Nucleic acid structure, consisting of polymers of nucleotides, each of which contains a pentose sugar, a phosphate group and an organic base.

AUG	UGU	CGA	GAA	CUU	UAC
Met	Cys	Arg	Glu	Leu	Tyr

Fig. 1.2 Groups of three nucleotides (codons) encode each amino acid.

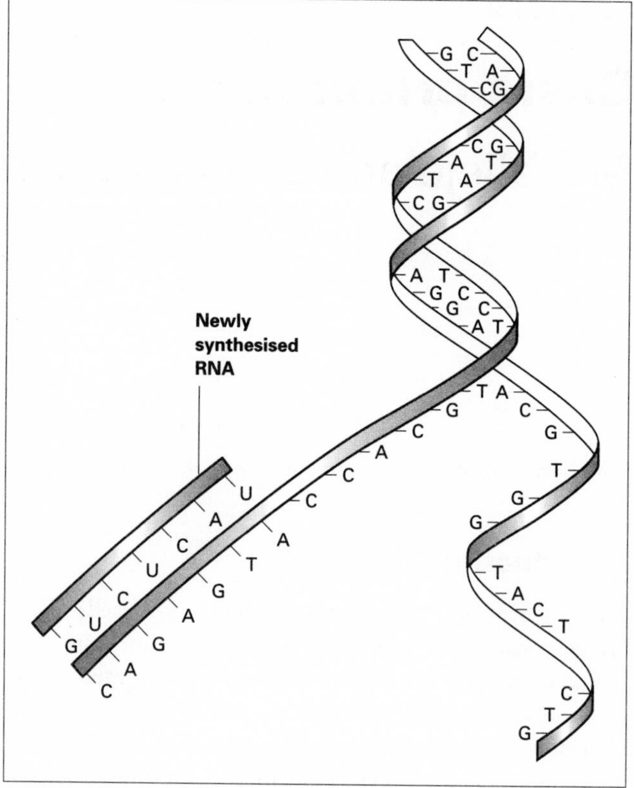

Fig. 1.3 Transcription of RNA from DNA template.

Gene organisation and expression

A gene can be defined as a region of the genome that contains both structural and regulatory sequences required for the synthesis of a functional RNA (Fig. 1.5). This synthetic process is called *transcription*, and involves the copying of

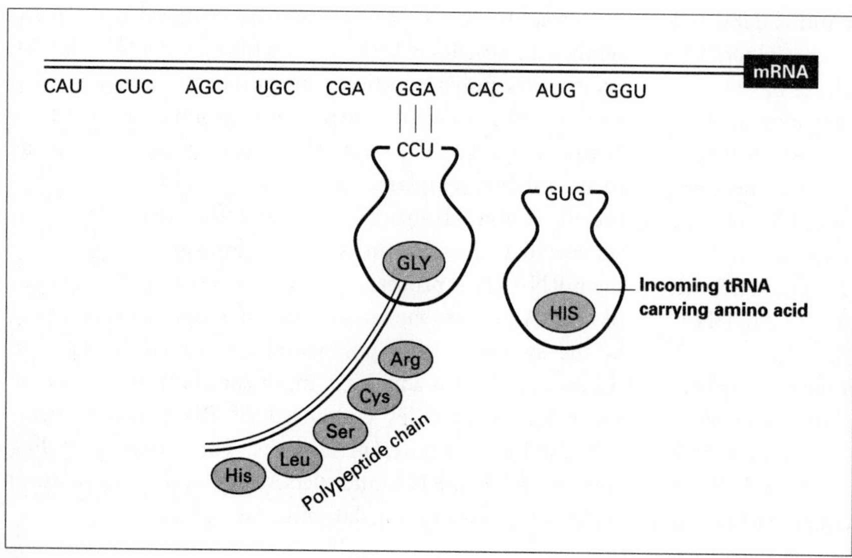

Fig. 1.4 Translation of messenger RNA (mRNA) nucleotide sequence into the amino acids which make up the nascent polypeptide.

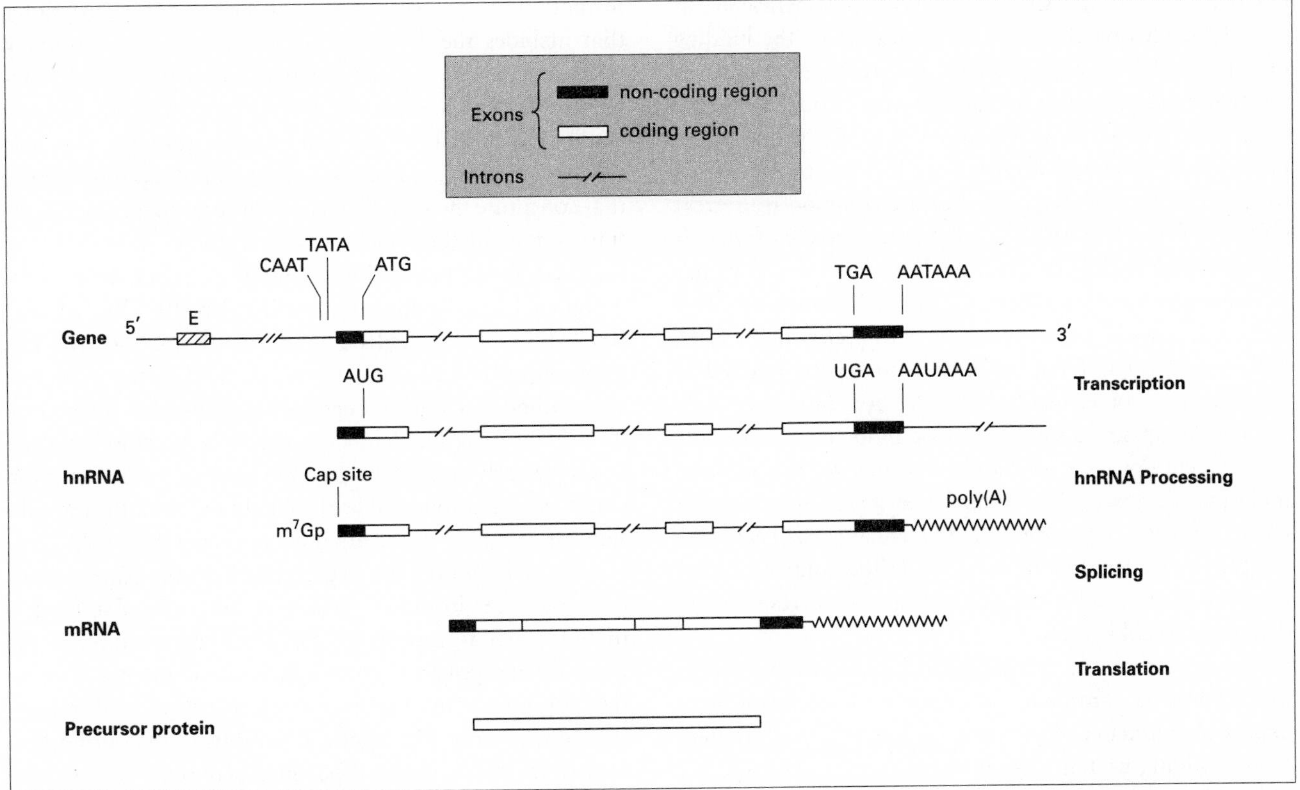

Fig. 1.5 The organisation of a eukaryotic gene, its transcription and subsequent RNA processing. E, enhancer.

the DNA template into RNA by a set of enzymes called RNA polymerases. There are three different types of these enzymes, each one responsible for the production of a different kind of RNA. RNA polymerase I synthesises ribosomal RNA; RNA polymerase II synthesises messenger RNA; and RNA polymerase III synthesises transfer RNA and other small nuclear RNAs. In this section, attention will be focused on the regulation of the expression of genes transcribed by RNA polymerase II, i.e. genes that encode proteins.

The sequences responsible for the regulation of the expression of the transcriptional unit are usually located

Fig. 1.6 Schematic representation of binding sites for 5′ upstream regulatory elements.

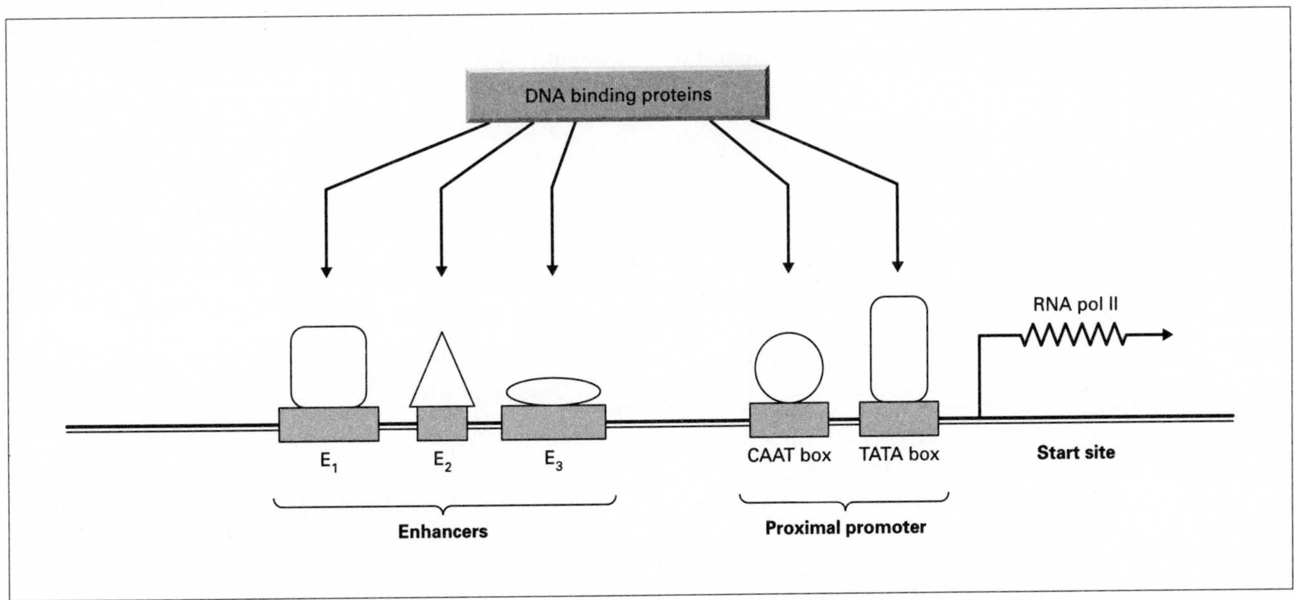

upstream (5′) to the site where RNA polymerase binds (Fig. 1.6). This regulation is accomplished by the binding of a particular class of proteins, generally referred to as transcription factors, that recognise short nucleotide sequences in the DNA known as *cis*-regulatory elements. The so-called proximal or promoter elements are located in the vicinity to the transcription start site and are common to a great number of type II genes. The most characteristic of them is the TATA or Goldberg–Hogness box, located 25–30 nucleotides upstream from the transcription initiation site. This element is essential for the initiation of transcription by RNA polymerase II. The TATA box is sometimes accompanied by another upstream element, the CAAT box. Situated 70–90 nucleotides upstream from the transcriptional initiation site, this element does not seem to be essential for the accurate initiation of transcription. A third type of regulatory element located further upstream are the enhancers. These are typically considered to be involved in the control of gene expression in specific cell populations or in response to defined external stimuli.

The regulation of transcriptional changes that occur in response to physiological stimuli to modulate gene expression ultimately depends on the interaction of different DNA-building proteins (*trans*-acting factors) with specific *cis*-regulatory elements on the DNA. The number, type and spatial distribution of these elements is different in each gene, allowing the organisation of protein–DNA complexes arranged in unique configurations. In this way, specific patterns of regulation are conferred to each gene by providing a molecular scaffolding for the integration of distinct biochemical pathways that relay signals triggered by hormones, growth factors or other stimuli.

Basic machinery for transcription initiation

Accurate initiation of transcription is dependent upon the formation of a protein complex on a region of the promoter that includes the TATA box. This complex is absolutely necessary for binding and enzymatic activity of RNA polymerase II. Chromatographic fractionation and biochemical studies using mammalian cell extracts revealed that this complex is composed of a set of several ubiquitous factors that constitute the so-called basic transcriptional machinery. Interactions of these factors with RNA polymerase II are required for transcriptional initiation. They have been designated transcription factors IIA, IIB, IID, IIE, IIF and IIH (TFIIA, TFIIB, TFIID, TFIIE, TFIIF and TFIIH). The most important of these factors is TFIID, the only one able to bind DNA in a sequence-specific manner interacting directly with the TATA box element. It is therefore involved at a very early step in the reaction leading to the initiation complex formation, and is absolutely required for the subsequent assembly of the other components (Fig. 1.7).

The elucidation of the structure and detailed interactions of these core promoter factors at the molecular level is of fundamental importance for our understanding of the mechanisms governing the synthesis of mRNA and its regulation by transcription factors that bind to distal upstream sequences. The precise identification and purification of these factors, as well as the cloning of the genes that encode them, has revealed a degree of complexity that had not been anticipated. At least 20 proteins must be assembled at the promoter, and complex interactions with transcription factors bound on DNA at a distance are being elucidated. An important breakthrough in the study of the basic transcriptional machinery was the discovery that a TFIID activity isolated from yeast, the simplest eukaryotic organism, could substitute for the human factor in a reconstituted *in vitro* transcription system [1], indicating a high degree of evolutionary conservation of the mechanisms of transcription initiation in eukaryotic cells. This finding led to the discovery that TFIID, a pivotal component for the assembly of the transcription initiation complex, is in fact

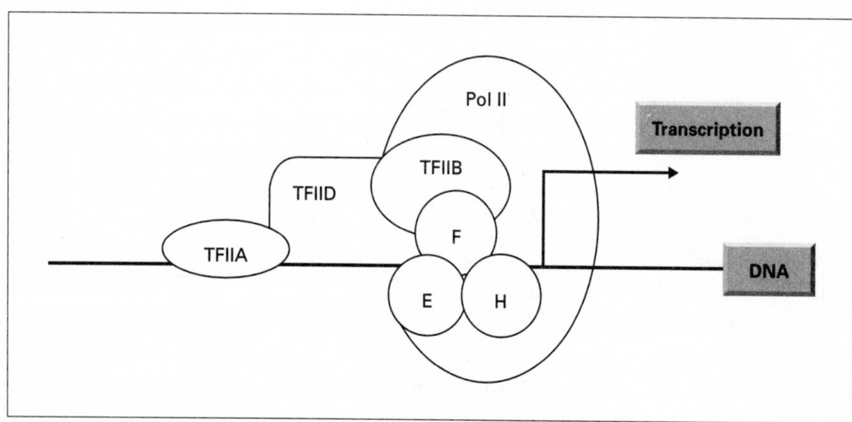

Fig. 1.7 Transcription initiation complex necessary for the enzymatic activity of RNA polymerase II.

composed of several proteins: a TATA-binding protein (TBP) and several TBP-associated factors (TAFs). Isolation of the complementary DNA (cDNA) encoding TBP from a wide variety of species from plants to humans revealed that this protein is one of the most highly conserved in eukaryotic cell evolution.

The assembly of the different components of the initiation complex (Fig. 1.7) takes place through the stepwise formation of hierarchically organised intermediate complexes [2]. The first step in the initiation reaction is, as indicated above, the recognition of the TATA element by TFIID, which is able to bind DNA independently and in the absence of other factors. A higher complex is formed by the interaction of TFIIA and TFIID. Although TFIIA lacks DNA-binding affinity of its own, it greatly increases the binding affinity of TFIID to the TATA element, and seems to play an important role in establishing and maintaining a transcriptionally committed complex on the promoter. A yet higher order of complex is formed by the addition of TFIIB. This factor, which is able to bind RNA polymerase II directly, is absolutely required for the interaction of this enzyme with the TFIID–TATA element complex. TFIIB is thought to be important for 'measuring' the distance between the TATA element and the transcription initiation site by bridging between the TATA-bound TFIID and RNA polymerase II.

The TFIID–TATA complex can also recruit TFIIF, which is composed of two subunits that bind tightly to RNA polymerase II. Biochemical studies indicate that TFIIF is similar or identical to RNA-activating protein (RAP) 30/74. Recruitment by RNA polymerase II seems to involve the small subunit, possibly via interaction with TFIIB. In turn, the large subunit (RAP 74) seems to be required for transcription initiation and elongation. Finally, TFIIE (probably a tetramer composed of two different subunits) and TFIIH are added to the complex. TFIIH, one of the last factors to be assembled (it is in fact a multisubunit protein), is particularly interesting due to the different array of biochemical activities associated with it. For example, it has kinase activity to phosphorylate RNA polymerase II, it exhibits DNA-dependent adenosine triphosphatase (ATPase) and helicase activities, and it appears to be involved in nucleotide excision and repair of DNA [3]. The helicase activity is responsible for the unwinding of the DNA helix, making the template strand accessible to the polymerase, and the ATPase activity of this complex explains the energy requirement required for the transcriptional activation process.

As mentioned earlier, TFIID is a multiprotein complex composed of TBP and TBP-associated factors (TAFs). Structural studies that led to the elucidation of the crystal structure of TBP revealed that this protein is shaped like a saddle that is predicted to straddle the DNA. That configuration leaves the outer larger surface available for interactions with TAFs, of which about 10 have so far been described ranging in size from 30 kDa to 250 kDa. This configuration is of great functional importance, inasmuch as TAFs serve as direct contacts with transcriptional transactivator proteins bound to DNA in other regions of the promoter. In this regard, TAFs are considered as transcriptional coactivator proteins required for the activity of transcription factors [4].

Structural features of transcription factors

A central problem in the study of the regulation of gene expression has been the elucidation of the precise mechanisms through which specific DNA–protein interactions result in the stimulation or repression of transcriptional activity. A great deal of information about the structural determinants that are related to the function of DNA-binding proteins has been gathered in the last few years. A generalised notion that has emerged as a consequence of these studies is that transcription factors are *modular* proteins: i.e. they have well-defined domains responsible for binding to DNA that are functionally distinct and independent of the *trans*-activating region, which is required for transcriptional activity.

DNA-binding domains

The region responsible for binding to specific DNA sequences is usually 60–100 amino acids in length, and contains a high proportion of basically charged residues. This domain is necessary, but not sufficient, for transcriptional activation. Depending on the structures determined by their amino-acid sequences, the DNA-binding domains of transcription factors can be classified in different groups including zinc fingers, leucine zippers, helix-turn-helix, helix-loop-helix and winged helix.

Zinc fingers are structures in which an atom of zinc is tetrahedrically coordinated to spatially conserved cysteines and histidines (Fig. 1.8). The basic motif that gives rise to this structure has the consensus sequence Cys-N_2-Cys-N_{12}-His-N_3-His, where N denotes non-specified amino acids. The 12 residues intervening between the cysteine and the histidine doublets, which are predominantly basic, are thought to loop out forming a finger-like structure. Usually, there are several zinc fingers in the same protein arranged in tandems of two to 10 units. In a number of proteins the histidine doublet is substituted by a second cysteine doublet, generating a slightly different type of zinc finger. Although the cysteines, histidines and the zinc atom are absolutely required for binding to DNA, they are not capable of conferring sequence specificity. This depends, in turn, on non-conserved amino acids that lie outside the tetrahedrically coordinated structure. Zinc

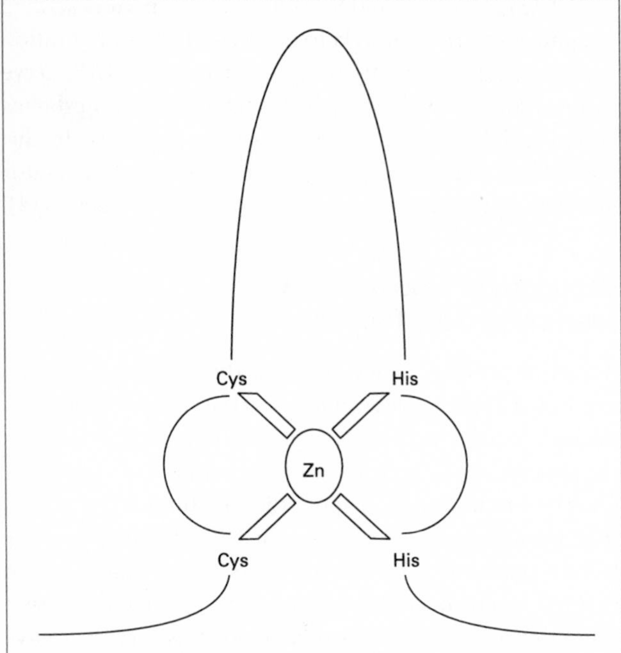

Fig. 1.8 Zinc finger structure.

fingers are therefore thought to provide a structural framework necessary for DNA-sequence recognition. Examples of DNA-binding proteins that belong in this group are the steroid and thyroid hormone receptors.

A number of transcription factors have been identified with the common feature of sharing a region containing four or five leucine residues spaced from each other by exactly seven amino acids. This domain, known as the leucine zipper, is adjacent to another highly conserved region of about 30 amino acids whose main characteristic is its basic charge (Fig. 1.9). The leucine zipper, which has been shown to be required for dimerisation, has a structure that results in the alignment of the leucine residues every two turns of an α-helix. In this particular case the α-helix is amphipathic, i.e. it is hydrophobic on one side, where the leucines are located, and hydrophilic on the other side. The leucines from two protein molecules have been proposed to interdigitate in such a way that they form a very stable complex responsible for protein dimerisation. This structure is common to a group of transcription factors including those mediating transcriptional responses to the second messengers cyclic adenosine monophosphate (cAMP) and diacylglycerol.

The leucine zipper is required for binding to DNA. However, it is the adjacent basic region that is responsible for making direct contacts with the nucleic acid and for dictating sequence specificity. Thus, dimerisation results in a unique structural arrangement of two basic regions that recognise specific DNA sequences. The leucine zipper motif can also

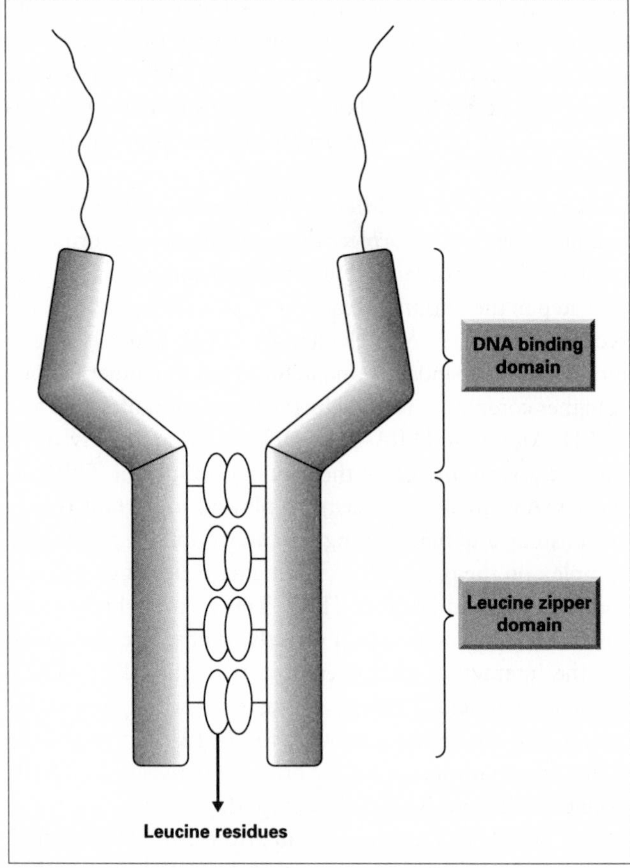

Fig. 1.9 Leucine zipper structure.

mediate the formation of heterodimers between two different proteins of the same family. The reciprocal recognition of two leucine zippers is highly specific, probably due to the particular sequences in each helix, so that only some of the proteins of this group can heterodimerise with one another. In this way, the specificity and versatility of transcriptional regulatory mechanisms is greatly increased by protein–protein interactions.

A third type of DNA-binding motif is the so called helix-turn-helix motif (Fig. 1.10). This is shared by many DNA regulatory proteins present in organisms from bacteria to mammals, and was the first one to be characterised. X-ray crystallographic analysis of these proteins and of DNA–protein complexes has provided a great deal of detailed information about their spatial arrangement, and functionally important interactions have been confirmed by mutational analysis of specific amino acids and DNA sequences. This motif consists of two successive α-helices separated by a β-turn. The helix located in the more carboxy-terminal position is termed the recognition helix, since it is the one directly involved in the interactions with the target DNA. This helix lies in the major groove of the DNA, where critically positioned amino acids make direct contacts with exposed

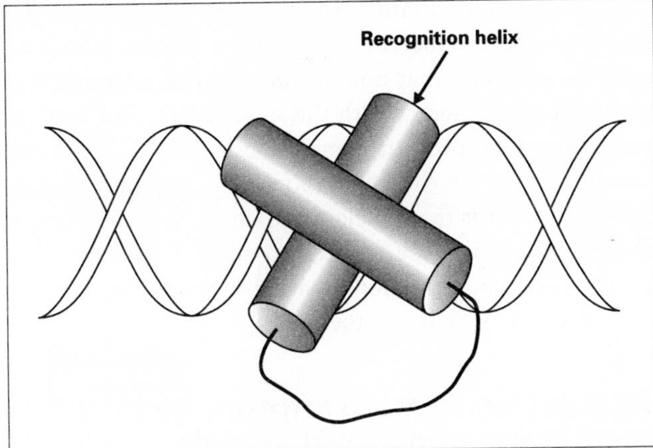

Fig. 1.10 Helix-turn-helix structure.

bases. The other helix lies across the major groove, and contributes to the stabilisation of the complex by non-specific contacts.

The helix-turn-helix motif is typical of some prokaryotic repressors, but it also occurs in eukaryotic transcription factors such as homeodomain proteins. These constitute a large family of developmentally regulated proteins, originally described as regulators of body form in *Drosophila,* characterised by the existence of a common DNA-binding structure known as the homeodomain that contains three highly conserved α-helices. Nuclear magnetic resonance spectroscopy and X-ray crystallography have been used to elucidate the three-dimensional structure of the homeodomain bound to DNA. Helix 3 is the so-called recognition helix that is positioned in the major groove of the DNA, where most intermolecular contacts occur. The stretch of amino acids between helices 2 and 3 forms the 'turn' of the helix-turn-helix motif. Finally, helices 1 and 2 adopt an antiparallel configuration above the DNA, roughly perpendicular to helix 3, to stabilise the protein–DNA complex [5].

Analysis of the amino-acid sequences of a group of cloned DNA-binding proteins involved in the regulation of immunoglobulin genes led to the discovery of another type of binding and dimerisation motif termed helix-loop-helix. It consists of two amphipathic α-helices linked by a stretch of 6–10 amino acids that form a loop, a secondary structure with the shape of the Greek letter omega (Ω) [6]. This motif is typical of proteins of the *myc* family of transcription factors.

Finally, a distinct group of transcription factors whose prototype is the hepatocyte nuclear factor 3 (HNF-3) has been the object of intense study over the last few years [7]. Some of the proteins in this group are thought to play important roles during embryonic development [8]. The three-dimensional structure of the highly conserved DNA-binding domain of HNF-3γ bound to DNA was determined

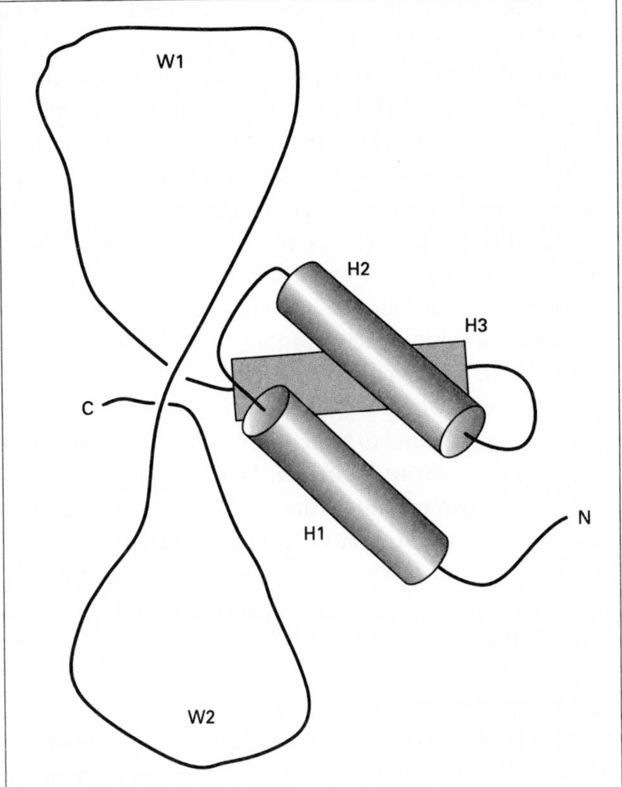

Fig. 1.11 Winged helix structure.

by X-ray crystallographic studies. The DNA-binding domain of HNF-3γ, which binds DNA as a monomer, is a complex structure composed of three α-helices and three β-strands interconnected by loops of different sizes. The motif defining this structure is known as a 'winged helix' because it resembles a butterfly (Fig. 1.11). Two amino-acid loops (W1 and W2) correspond to the wings, whereas the three α-helices (H1, H2 and H3) correspond to the thorax. H3 is the recognition helix that contacts the major groove of the DNA.

Trans-activation domains

These are domains that are responsible for the *trans*-activating activity of transcription factors on DNA. In fact, DNA-binding domains may be thought of as devices to recruit *trans*-activation domains to DNA, where interactions with proteins of the basal transcription apparatus result in the activation of RNA polymerase II. In contrast to the well-defined DNA-binding domains described above, the activation domains of transcription factors have for the most part ill-defined sequences that make it difficult to group them in different types. There are, however, general features that are shared by some of them. For example, the *trans*-activation domains of some DNA-binding proteins are very rich in glutamine residues, whereas others are characterised by their high content of prolines.

One of the most studied types of *trans*-activation domains is found in proteins that can actually function in a way almost irrespective of their particular sequence, provided that there is a high excess of acidic residues [9]. The modular nature of transcription factors has been of great importance for designing the experiments that led to this conclusion. Perhaps one of the most elegant of these experiments consisted of the construction of chimaeric proteins with a known binding domain fused to random polypeptides encoded by fragments of genomic DNA from the bacteria *Escherichia coli*. Some of these proteins were able to activate transcription in eukaryotes. These were found to share a common feature, the excess of acidic residues in their random activating sequences. Further experiments demonstrated that an amphipathic α-helix was also required, so that the negative charges lie on one side of the helix. It has been hypothesised that this may be of importance for promoting direct interactions with some of the proteins forming the transcription-initiation complex.

The mechanisms by which acidic, glutamine-rich and proline-rich domains activate transcription remain unknown, although direct interactions with coactivator proteins in the transcription-initiation complex are being described for an increasing number of transcription factors. However, evidence indicates that not all *trans*-activation domains of a specific type interact with the same target, and thus the mechanisms of specificity remain obscure [10]. A possible interpretation of the relatively small amount of data gathered so far is that, in close proximity with their target, these domains may be induced to adopt a specific three-dimensional conformation creating hydrophobic surfaces that recognise specific partners.

Regulation of transcription by membrane-generated signals

A number of peptide hormones, neurotransmitters and growth factors utilise a signalling mechanism to relay information to the cell nucleus which involves the production of intracellular second-messenger molecules (Fig. 1.12). These second messengers activate specific protein kinases that in turn are responsible for the phosphorylation of transcription factors that modulate gene activity. A common feature of these kinases is that they phosphorylate their substrates at serine or theronine residues. Cyclic AMP and diacylglycerol serve as two commonly used second-messenger

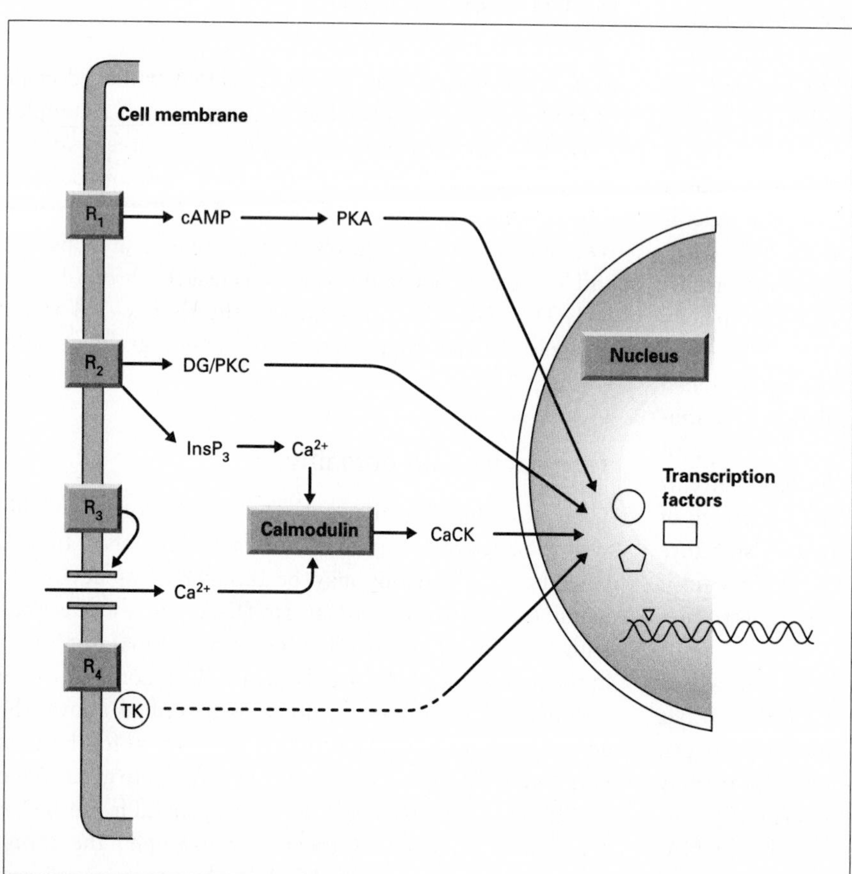

Fig. 1.12 Intracellular second messenger transduction pathways. R_1–R_4, receptors for extracellular signals; PKA, cyclic AMP-dependent protein kinase A; DG/PKC, diacylglycerol/protein kinase C; $InsP_3$, inositol trisphosphate; CaCK, calcium/calmodulin-dependent protein kinase; TK, receptor-associated tyrosine kinase.

molecules. Also, Ca^{2+} is an important intracellular signal transducer through its interaction with calmodulin. This is a ubiquitous protein that functions as an intracellular receptor which undergoes a conformational change when it binds Ca^{2+}. This allosteric transition allows the interaction of the complex with so-called calcium–calmodulin-dependent protein kinases [11], which in turn phosphorylate a set of specific substrates that mediate the particular biological effects. These will be considered in more detail in Chapter 4 (see also [12] and [13]).

Protein kinase C-dependent transcription

Upon binding with their specific receptors, some extracellular ligands activate the enzyme phospholipase C, that leads to the hydrolysis of membrane polyphosphoinositides. This results in the generation of two second-messenger molecules: inositol trisphosphate, which is released into the cytoplasm to increase the levels of intracellular Ca^{2+} from the endoplasmic reticulum, and diacylglycerol, which remains in the membrane to activate protein kinase C (PKC) [14].

Activation of PKC results in an increase in the transcriptional activity of several genes. Studies to investigate these effects of PKC have been greatly facilitated by the use of a set of tumour-promoter drugs known as phorbol esters, which have the property of directly activating this enzyme. The most commonly used of these drugs is 12-O-tetradecanoyl-phorbol-13-acetate, usually referred to as TPA. For this reason, the DNA sequences that mediate the PKC-dependent transcriptional activation are known as TPA-responsive elements (TREs). These *cis*-regulatory elements are strikingly similar to cAMP-responsive elements, differing only by the absence of one guanosine residue (TGACTCA). Initial studies indicated that this DNA sequence is recognised by a transcription factor known as activating protein 1 (AP-1), but this is now thought to be a complex comprising a heterologous group of transcriptionally active proteins.

The sequence of the TRE is also closely related to that of the binding site for GCN4, a yeast transcriptional activator which regulates the expression of genes involved in amino-acid synthesis. Similarities between the DNA-binding domain of GCN4 and the carboxyl-terminal portion of the product of the viral oncogene v-*jun* led to the hypothesis that its cellular counterpart, the proto-oncogene c-*jun*, might encode a protein that would bind the TRE. This was indeed demonstrated after the cloning of c-*jun*, identifying its product as one of the components of AP-1 [15,16].

Independently, studies on v-*fos*, another viral oncogene, revealed that the product of its cellular counterpart, c-*fos*, aggregates in a complex with a set of antigenically related proteins referred to as Fos-related antigens (FRAs). One of these proteins was identified as c-Jun, indicating therefore that c-Fos is also a component of the AP-1 family. However, although Fos had been shown to alter gene activity, no direct binding to DNA could be demonstrated. This apparent paradox was solved by the indication that dimer formation is essential for DNA binding, and that c-Fos would only bind the TRE in the presence of c-Jun. Thus, it was demonstrated that Fos and Jun are leucine-zipper proteins able to form heterodimers that bind the TRE with high affinity and are strong transcriptional activators; Jun homodimers are less stable so that they behave as weaker *trans*-activators; the Fos protein does not form homodimers and does not bind DNA. The Fos-Jun heterodimers, therefore, play a key role in the PKC-dependent activation of gene transcription.

Other members of the Fos family of transcription factors have also been identified. Thus, *fos*-B and *fra*-1 and *fra*-2 have been cloned, and their products have been shown to heterodimerise with Jun [17,18]. In addition, two other members of the Jun family, Jun-B and Jun-D, also form heterodimers with Fos. An important concept that has emerged in the last few years is that heterodimerisation among members of leucine zipper proteins is specific but not restricted to one partner. Instead, one of these proteins can interact with several others, so that different heterodimer combinations are generated with distinct DNA-binding affinities and specificities.

Regulatory elements different from the TRE also confer TPA responsivity to genes. The best characterised one has the consensus sequence CCCCAGGC, and is recognised by a transcription factor designated AP-2. The AP-2-binding site was originally recognised in the promoters of the simian virus 40 and the human metallothionein II_A genes, and shown to mediate the responses to activation of PKC by phorbol esters. In contrast to AP-1, AP-2 is a single transcription factor, as demonstrated by the cloning of its encoding cDNA, which predicts a protein with a molecular weight of 43 kDa.

Cyclic AMP-dependent transcription

The second messenger cAMP is generated as a result of the activation of the enzyme adenylate cyclase after ligand–receptor interactions at the cell surface. Most, if not all, of the intracellular effects of cAMP are mediated by a cAMP-dependent kinase, known as protein kinase A (PKA). This enzyme exists in the cytoplasm as an inactive tetramer of two regulatory and two catalytic subunits. Cyclic AMP binding to the regulatory subunits results in the dissociation of the catalytic subunits, that in this way become active to phosphorylate specific substrates at serine residues. Some of these substrates are nuclear proteins involved in mediating the transcriptional effects of cAMP. They are subjected to the action of PKA after translocation of the enzyme to the nucleus, which occurs quickly after dissociation from the regulatory subunit (see Chapter 4).

Cyclic AMP regulates the activity of a variety of genes including those encoding somatostatin, vasointestinal peptide (VIP) and the α-subunit of the glycoprotein hormones. Studies to identify the DNA sequences mediating the cAMP-dependent activation of transcription revealed the existence of *cis* elements with the common core consensus sequence TGACGTCA, which was designated cAMP response element (CRE).

At least three highly homologous CRE-binding transcription factors that act as nuclear substrates for PKA have been identified. These are the leucine zipper-containing proteins cAMP response element binding protein (CREB), cAMP response element modulator τ (CREMτ) and activating transcription factor 1 (ATF-1), which share with the members of the Fos/Jun family significant amino-acid similarity in the regions responsible for DNA binding and dimerisation. CREB, CREMτ and ATF-1 share a common amino-acid motif, Arg-Arg-Pro-Ser-Tyr, which contains the phosphoacceptor serine residue phosphorylated by PKA.

CREB was the first member of the group to be identified and cloned [19]. Its phosphoacceptor serine resides in the *trans*-activation domain on the amino-terminal portion of the protein, within a stretch of 60 amino acids known as the kinase inducible domain (KID). The KID also contains additional serine residues that serve as substrate of processive protein kinases such as casein kinase II and glycogen synthase kinase III, although the possible functional significance of these phosphorylation events remains unclear.

Flanking the KID, the *trans*-activation domain of CREB contains two glutamine-rich regions termed Q1 and Q2. Integrity of these regions is required for basal and full transcriptional activity by CREB. It has been proposed that they serve as constitutive *trans*-activation domains that become exposed upon PKA phosphorylation of the KID for interactions with target effector proteins of the TFIID complex [20]. It seems, however, that CREB interacts with more than one coactivator protein to gain access to the basal transcription apparatus assembled on the promoter of target genes. Thus, a large coactivator known as CREB-binding protein (CBP) has been identified [21]. CBP is required, and mediates, CREB-dependent responses induced by cAMP, and it interacts with CREB only after phosphorylation of the serine residue present in the KID. The target protein of the CREB/CBP complex appears to be TFIIB, one of the constitutive proteins of the basal transcription apparatus.

The other protein of this group of CRE-binding transcription factors is CREM. Several protein isoforms of CREM, arising from alternative RNA splicing, have been described. The isoform corresponding to the full-length protein is CREMτ, and acts as an activator of cAMP-dependent transcriptional responses. The other isoforms consist of proteins containing a truncated *trans*-activation domain and an intact leucine zipper/DNA-binding domain, and therefore act as repressors of cAMP-dependent transcription. Two additional repressor isoforms, S-CREM and ICER (inducible cAMP early repressor), are generated by use of an internal translational initiation codon, or by transcription from a second alternative promoter, respectively. Interestingly, generation of ICER by this promoter is dependent on cAMP stimulation, thus generating a negative autoregulatory loop that involves activation followed by repression of target cAMP-inducible genes (for an example of this, see Chapters 3 and 4).

CREB acts as a common target where several distinct signal transduction pathways converge. Thus, in addition to PKA, the serine residue of the KID is phosphorylated by calcium–calmodulin-dependent kinase. In this manner, CREB mediates transcriptional responses induced by membrane depolarisation and Ca^{2+} influx into cells. In addition, CREB is also the target for phosphorylation by another kinase, known as CREB kinase (CREBK), that is activated upon stimulation of the Ras signalling pathway. CREBK appears to be important for the rapid activation of immediate early gene expression induced by growth factors.

In genes lacking CRE motifs, cAMP responsivity may be conferred by a different kind of *cis*-regulatory elements. Thus, the AP-2-binding site previously mentioned to mediate TPA-dependent stimulation can be responsive to cAMP [22]. This provides the basis for a mechanism of convergence of both signal transduction pathways. The AP-2 *cis*-regulatory element confers cAMP responsivity to genes such as the one encoding proenkephalin. However, its presence does not seem to be necessarily sufficient for induction by this second-messenger pathway. For example, the AP-2-binding sites in the promoters of the growth hormone and prolactin genes are not required for regulation by cAMP. Since these genes lack CRE motifs, this raises the possibility that novel CREs exist that have yet to be identified. The transcription factor AP-2 is absent in some undifferentiated cell types, but its expression can be induced by differentiating agents such as retinoic acid. It is therefore likely that AP-2 may be part of a developmental switch able to alter the pattern of gene expression by providing a mechanism that determines the commitment to cAMP and PKC inducibility of a particular gene network [23].

The JAK-STAT signalling pathway

The recent discovery of the JAK-STAT signalling system has revealed a previously unknown paradigm regarding molecular mechanisms for the delivery of signals from the cell membrane to the nucleus. This system was initially found to be associated with interferon receptors, but it is now clear that a wide variety of polypeptide ligands interacting with a large number of membrane receptors use this system [12]. Receptors that utilize the JAK-STAT signalling pathway can be grouped into different families whose prototypes are those recognising interleukin-2 (IL-2), IL-3, IL-6, interferon and growth hormone, respectively.

With the exception of the single-chained growth hormone and prolactin receptors, these receptors are composed of at least two chains. The ligand interacts with one of these components, the ligand-binding chain or α-subunit, located on the cell surface, that is in turn able to interact with another subunit, known as the signal transducing or β chain, which contains a transmembrane and a cytoplasmic domain. When this tripartite complex is formed (ligand, α-subunit and β-subunit), one of the members of the Janus kinase (JAK) family of proteins which is associated with the cytoplasmic domain of the β-subunit is activated. In turn, this kinase phosphorylates a cytoplasmic protein known as STAT (Signal Transducer and Activators of Transcription), which is then translocated to the nucleus to act as a transcription factor on specific target genes. At least four members of the JAK and six members of the STAT families of proteins have been described. The close association of the JAK kinase with the receptor even in the inactive state provides an explanation for the rapid induction of responses upon ligand binding.

Receptors of the IL-2 family are composed of three chains, and recognise IL-2, IL-4, IL-7, IL-9, IL-13 and IL-15. Binding of the ligand to a specific α-subunit results in its interaction with the other two chains, the β-subunit and the γC subunit, which is common for all members of this group. Dimerisation of the β and γC subunits is necessary for signal transduction. These receptors interact with Jak-1 and Jak-3.

The IL-3 family is composed of IL-3, IL-5 and granulocyte-macrophage stimulating factor (GM-CSF). Receptors for these ligands consist of a specific α-subunit and a common β chain which interacts with Jak-2. In addition, the distal domain of the β chain interacts with cellular components that are involved in the activation of the Ras-related signalling pathway.

Members of the IL-6 family include IL-6, IL-11, Oncostatin M (OnM), Leukaemia inhibitory factor (LIF) and Ciliary neurotrophic factor (CNTF). Receptors for these ligands are found in a wide range of tissues and all share a common signal transducing β-chain known as gp130 that assembles in different ways with other receptor components. Thus IL-6 recognises a ligand-binding α-chain that associates with gp130. This interaction promotes gp130 dimerisation, which is required for receptor activity. In contrast, LIF does not interact with an α-chain, but rather with a signal transducer chain known as LIFRβ. Dimerisation of LIFRβ with gp130 upon LIF binding results in receptor activation.

Yet another variation in this group is that of the CNTF receptor (Fig. 1.13). CNTF interacts with a specific α-chain that lacks transmembrane and cytoplasmic domains, anchored to the outer surface of the cell membrane by a glycosyl phosphatidylinositol linkage. According to a model based on recent studies [24], binding of CNTF to its specific α-chain results in the recruitment of gp130 to the complex. In this case, however, gp130 homodimerisation does not occur. Instead, the CNTF-gp130 complex interacts with LIFRβ. Therefore, the heterodimerisation of gp130 and LIFRβ is the event that results in receptor activation.

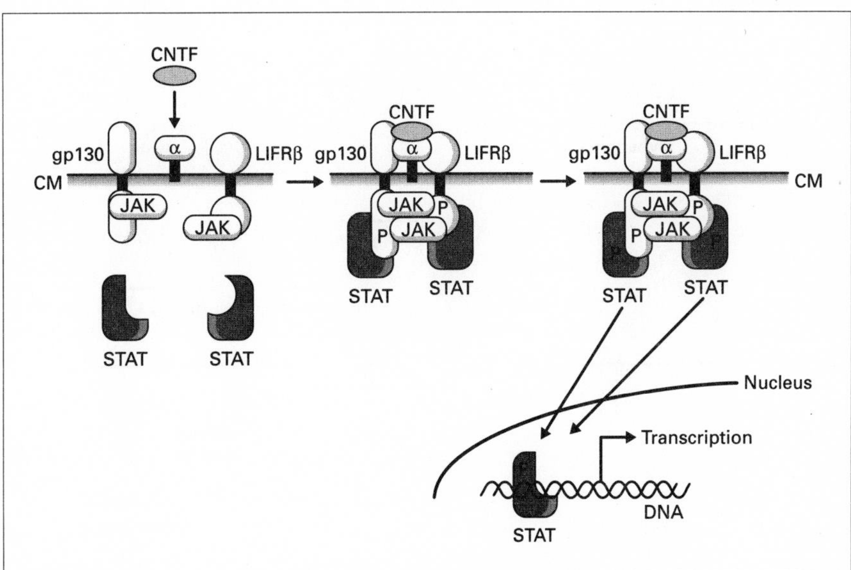

Fig. 1.13 CNTF receptor signalling via the JAK-STAT pathway. CM, cellular membrane.

Finally, the growth hormone receptor consists of a single chain that contains both the ligand-binding and the intracellular signal-transducing domains. Binding of growth hormone promotes receptor dimerisation and activation of Jak-2, which results in phosphorylation of STAT proteins including STAT1 and STAT3.

A key and unique feature of STAT proteins is that they act as signal transducers in the cytoplasm and transcriptional *trans*-activators in the nucleus. They recognise specific DNA *cis*-regulatory elements with the loose consensus sequence TTNNNNNAA, located in the promoters of target genes (although *in vitro* experiments indicate that the palindromic sequence TTCCNGGAA is a high-affinity binding site). Some STAT proteins can form homodimers or heterodimers with other members of this family, although the exact number of possible combinations and their functional significance in activating gene expression remains to be determined.

Other aspects of the JAK/STAT pathway are discussed in Chapter 4.

Regulation of transcription by nuclear receptors

Unlike membrane-bound receptors, receptors of the nuclear receptor superfamily are small intracellular lipophilic molecules which have evolved to mediate responses to extracellular signals by direct control of target genes. Nuclear receptors actually represent the largest group of transcription factors found in eukaryotic cells. These include two subgroups of receptors: (i) the steroid receptor family—glucocorticoid receptor (GR), mineralocorticoid receptor (MR), oestrogen receptor (ER), progesterone receptor (PR), androgen receptor (AR); and (ii) the non-steroid nuclear receptors—thyroid hormone receptor (THR), vitamin D receptor (VDR), retinoic acid receptor (RAR), 9-*cis*-retinoic acid receptor (RXR), peroxisome proliferator activated receptor (PPAR), and the insect receptor for ecdysone (EcR). Cloning procedures have now isolated over 150 members of this superfamily, many of which have been shown to bind to signalling molecules *in vitro*. Comparisons with *Drosophila* homologues suggest that they are all derived from a single ancestor gene which predates the differentiation of the vertebrate and invertebrate phyla.

Similarities in the amino-acid sequences of some regions of these proteins indicate a common structure which demonstrates shared functional domains (Fig. 1.14). The one that shows the highest degree of conservation lies in the central core of the molecule, and is responsible for DNA binding. This region contains a high proportion of basic amino acids and a series of cysteine residues which are responsible for the formation of two zinc fingers, in which a zinc atom is tetrahedrically coordinated to four cysteines; this region also seems to contribute to *trans*-activation functions.

The region located on the N-terminal side of the DNA-binding domain is hypervariable in size and amino-acid composition. Its function is not fully understood, but it seems to be important for *trans*-activation. However, the sequence of this region is not conserved among the different members of the receptor superfamily, and different mechanisms of regulation must exist.

Adjacent to the C-terminal end of the DNA-binding domain is a short sequence responsible for the nuclear localisation of the receptor, and next to it the hormone-binding region. This region, responsible for ligand specificity of each receptor, is perhaps the most complex one within the molecule, since different overlapping subdomains can be identified. Thus, it contains an additional nuclear localisation signal, and is also involved in *trans*-activation. Interaction of the receptors with heat-shock protein 90 (Hsp 90) and with other receptors to form dimers also occurs through this region.

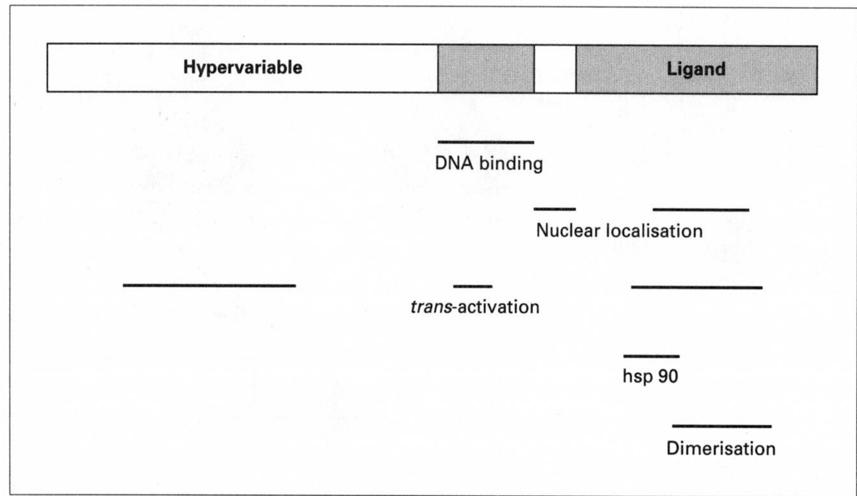

Fig. 1.14 Common structure and functional domains of the steroid hormone receptor family.

Steroid-hormone receptors

Steroid-hormone receptors (SHRs) bind to specific DNA sequences called hormone-response elements (HREs) which contain two hexanucleotide half-sites, AGAACA, orientated as palindromes and spaced by three nucleotides [25]. The oestrogen receptor is the single exception to this rule, having an HRE similar to that of the non-steroid hormone receptors—AGGTCA.

SHRs are associated with large multiprotein complexes which include the 90-kDa chaperone, Hsp 90 and the immunophilin Hsp 56, which keep the receptor in an inactive form which is readily available for binding to its ligand. These and other chaperones are also important in the expression of normal SHR function [26].

Binding of the cognate hormonal ligand induces a conformational change which triggers the dissociation of the Hsp 90 and refolding and activation of the receptor. The changes that take place during this process are part of what is known as receptor transformation. In the course of these events a nuclear localisation signal normally repressed by the hormone-binding region, and responsible for the translocation of the ligand–receptor complex, is relieved. However, experimental evidence shows that although nuclear localisation is necessary, it alone is not sufficient for transcriptional activity, since receptor binding to DNA is also dependent on the presence of the hormone.

SHRs have a direct interaction with the components of the transcription-initiation complex, and recent data suggest that there are additional coactivators which act to bridge between the transcriptional activation domain AF-2 SHRs and the transcription-initiation complex [27]. RIP140, for instance, is a coactivator that only binds to transcriptionally active oestrogen receptors [28], while transcriptional intermediary factor 1 (TIF-1) belongs to a family of 'RING' (really interesting new gene) proteins and interacts with oestrogen, progesterone and retinoid X receptor [29]. Suppressor of Gal 1 (SUG-1) is another AF-2-binding protein which is actually part of the RNA polymerase II holoenzyme and binds with several SHRs, suggesting a possible route for the regulation of hormone-receptor-dependent transcription [30].

In neuroendocrine systems in particular, SHRs can be powerful transcriptional repressors as well as stimulators. Although this may occur through competition for the DNA-binding sites, or by competition for common mediators to the transcription-initiation complex, more information is being obtained for an action via sequestration of AP-1 and nuclear factor - κB(NF-κB) transcription factors into inactive forms. Thus, gluco-corticoid receptors act synergistically with Jun homodimers but antagonise Fos-Jun heterodimers [31]. This suggests that protein–protein interactions result in conformational changes which in turn alter activity. GRs can also block NF-κB DNA binding *in vitro*, but in addition to this they induce IκBa synthesis [32,33] which in turn traps NF-κB in the cytoplasm.

One final area of SHR regulation is that of interactions or 'cross-talk' with other signalling pathways. This is best exemplified in the ER system where the ligand-induced transcriptional activity of ER can be enhanced by growth factors such as epidermal growth factor (EGF) and insulin-like growth factor (IGF) [34]. Recent evidence suggests that this synergy takes place by activation of membrane-associated protein kinases and the Ras-MAPK cascade to phosphorylate the transcriptional activation domain AF-1 in the NH_2-terminal region of the ER. Phosphorylation at this site is required for full activation of the ER.

Non-steroid nuclear receptors

This is an extremely broad family of receptors with known ligands as diverse as the thyroid hormones, vitamin D, the retinoids and products of metabolism such as the prostanoids. The activated receptors associate with HREs which have a minimum consensus sequence AGGTCA in different motifs [35]. Unlike the SHRs, which only bind as homodimers to palindromes separated by three nucleotides, the non-steroid receptors can bind as homodimers, heterodimers or monomers.

Each receptor recognises a unique HRE and the most potent HREs are direct repeats (DRs) of the AGGTCA half-site. The HREs for: (i) the RXR and the PPAR; (ii) a second retinoic acid response element; (iii) the VDR; (iv) the TR; and (v) the first RAR are actually composed of DRs spaced by 1, 2, 3, 4, 5 nucleotides, respectively. With the exception of a few orphan receptors that bind as monomers, all the receptors bind to DNA as either hetero- or homodimers. The VDR, TR and RAR can only bind in high affinity in the presence of RXR which is clearly needed for heterodimer formation. Surprisingly, however, the transcriptional activity of RXR itself is suppressed when complexed with VDR, TR or RAR—the heterodimer preventing RXR from binding its ligand, and thus 9-*cis*-retinoic acid responsiveness is not an obligatory consequence of heterodimerisation with RXR.

The response to thyroid hormones illustrates the potential flexibility and complexity of this type of signalling system. In the absence of hormone the homo- and heterodimeric receptor complexes exert an inhibitory effect via intermediary corepressor proteins resulting in the repression of basal cell transcription [36]. Binding of thyroid hormone to the carboxy-terminal region of the receptor produces conformational changes which initiate homodimer dissociation and relief of repression. The TR-RXR heterodimer, however, remains stable after ligand binding, and can now activate gene transcription by recruitment of other intermediary proteins or coactivators [37]. This is just one example of RXR as a critical component of heterodimer formation which is absolutely vital for a large number of both hormonal and non-hormonal responses.

Finally, it is important to emphasize that it is not only extracellular signals that can act on nuclear receptors. A particularly good example of the ability of intermediary metabolites to act on nuclear receptors is seen in lipid homeostasis and adipocyte differentiation. Prostaglandins are derived from fatty acids, primarily arachidonic acid, by the action of phospholipases. Prostaglandin D_2 (PGD_2) is converted to the biologically active PGJ_2 series which have many major effects including differentiation of fibroblasts into cells of the adipose lineage. It now appears that the action of PGJ_2 occurs via the binding of a metabolite to the orphan nuclear receptor PPARg and the activation of PPAR response elements [38]. This suggests an important role for PPARg and its endogenous ligand in adipocyte development. Since this receptor is also activated by the antidiabetic thiazolidinediones, it may additionally function as a mediator of insulin action. There are many new avenues to be explored in this area, but it is already clear that it will provide a major insight into our understanding of endocrine and metabolic regulation.

Cell-specific transcriptional regulation

The differentiation of a cellular phenotype depends on the selective expression of a particular set of tissue specific genes. This specificity is determined by the interplay of multiple ubiquitous transcription factors, together with more restricted tissue-specific factors, to create a molecular code responsible for the positive or negative regulation of selected gene networks. This is a key concept that underscores the importance of combinatorial interactions of distinct signalling pathways with transcription factors present in different cell types.

Several transcription factors have been discovered whose expression is associated with the acquisition of tissue-specific phenotypic features during some stages of embryonic development. MyoD1, pancreatic transcription factor-1 (PTF-1) and GATA factor-1 (GF-1) provide three examples in non-endocrine tissues. Expression of MyoD1 is important for muscle determination and differentiation [39]; PTF-1 is a heteromeric oligomer containing two DNA-binding proteins whose presence is required for acinar pancreas-specific gene expression [40]; and GF-1 is involved in the regulation of genes that are specifically expressed in the erythroid cell lineage [41].

One of the first transcription factors whose expression could be associated with differentiation of specific cellular phenotypes in endocrine tissues was Pit-1, which appears to be involved in the determination of a pituitary phenotype [42]. This factor is responsible for the cell-specific expression of the genes encoding growth hormone, prolactin and thyroid-stimulating hormone β (TSH-β). Pit-1 contains a homeobox domain, which is present in a group of proteins encoded by a multigene family implicated in the regulation of early development events in organisms as divergent as insects and mammals; it also has an adjacent region of 75 residues which shares homology with two mammalian transcription factors, Oct-1 and Oct-2, and with the product of *unc-86*, a gene that regulates neuronal cell fate during the development of the nematode *Caenorhabditis elegans*. These regions have therefore been designated POU (Pit, Oct, unc) homeodomain and POU-specific domain, respectively, and are collectively referred to as POU domain [43]. The POU homeodomain is directly responsible for sequence-specific DNA binding, and has a helix-turn-helix structure typical of the homeobox proteins. The adjacent POU-specific region does not make direct contact with the DNA, but seems to be important for the stability and specificity of binding.

From a clinical perspective, the discovery of mutations in the gene encoding Pit-1 has provided an answer for the aetiology of different endocrine disorders due to a deficient pituitary function. Thus, in a patient with combined pituitary hormone deficiency a heterozygous mutation was found resulting in the production of a mutant Pit-1 that binds DNA but acts as a dominant inhibitor of the wild-type Pit-1 encoded by the normal allele [44]. In another case, a homozygotic mutation in the Pit-1 gene was found in a patient with combined pituitary hormone deficiency and cretinism [45].

Additional proteins containing a conserved POU domain have been identified. Their expression in different areas of the developing nervous system, testis and skin suggests that they are encoded by a large family of genes that appear to play an important role in the determination of tissue-specific phenotypes in different regions of the developing organism. One of these proteins, known as Brn-2, has been shown to be necessary for the differentiation of neurons in the hypothalamic paraventricular and supraoptic nuclei [46].

Another example with important endocrinological implications is that of the pancreas-specific transcription factor IDX-1 (also known as STF-1 and IPF-1) [47]. Islet and duodenum homeobox-1 (IDX-1) is a homeodomain transcription factor which is expressed in pancreatic islets and duodenum, and is thought to regulate the cell-specific expression of the insulin and somatostatin genes. Its expression in the duodenum during early devel-opment, in a region which corresponds to the pancreatic *anlagen*, suggested that IDX-1 could participate in pancreatic development, acting at early determination or differentiation of the pancreas. This seems indeed to be the case, as indicated by experiments in which both alleles of the IDX-1 gene were mutated by homologous recombination in mice. These animals develop normally but selectively lack a pancreas, and die shortly after birth [48].

RNA processing and splicing

It had been thought for a long time that the region comprising the structural sequences in a gene was defined by a continuous stretch of DNA encoding a given polypeptide chain throughout its length. Indeed, this seems to be the case in bacterial cells. In the late 1970s, however, it became clear that eukaryotic genes are generally split into several segments, such that the coding sequences are interrupted by non-coding fragments of DNA with no apparent function (Fig. 1.5). These fragments were designated as intervening sequences, or introns, whereas the coding fragments were named as exons [49].

Both exons and introns are copied into RNA by the action of RNA polymerase II. They therefore constitute what is known as a transcriptional unit. The resultant RNA, known as primary transcript or heterogeneous nuclear RNA (hnRNA) is of an immature form which contains both coding and non-coding regions (Fig. 1.5). The mature mRNA is then generated by removal of the intron regions of this transcript and splicing of the exons [50]. The first exon also generates a region which will not be translated into protein, and is important for the binding of the mature mRNA to the ribosome. Likewise, there is also a 3′ untranslated region corresponding to the last exon.

Before transcription is finished, the hnRNA is 'capped' at its 5′ end with a guanosine residue methylated at position 7 (m7Gp). The cap site indicates the beginning of the 5′ untranslated region of the first exon, which is also known as the leader sequence. The 3′ end of this region is always followed by the initiation codon AUG, encoding methionine, the first amino acid in all newly synthesized proteins. In turn, the end of the protein-coding region is signalled by a so-called stop codon (UGA, UAA or UAG), after which a 3′ non-coding region is located. This untranslated region contains the sequence AAUAAA, which is considered to be the signal for the addition, approximately 20 bases downstream, of a polyA tail 100–200 nucleotides long. These modifications of the hnRNA are important for the stability and transport of the mature mRNA.

The splicing of the exon transcripts of the hnRNA and the removal of the intron transcripts is the final step towards the production of the mature mRNA. Exon and intron transcripts meet at the so-called splice sites, which are conserved sequences defining intron–exon boundaries. A typical characteristic of these sequences is the presence of GU at the beginning of the intron transcript, and AG at the end.

A very abundant species of RNA comprising a group of molecules collectively known as small nuclear RNAs (snRNAs) play a central role in the splicing mechanism. They were first detected by Weinberg and Penman [51] and extensively characterised biochemically by Ro-Choi and Busch [52], and by Zieve and Penman [53]. These molecules, which are different from the RNAs described in previous sections, are complexed with one or several proteins to form small nuclear ribonucleoproteins (snRNPs). Their function was still unknown when Lerner and Steitz [54] discovered that antibodies from patients with the autoimmune disease systemic lupus erythematosus reacted with protein components of the snRNPs, named U_{1a}, U_{1b} and U_2, because of their high content of the pyrimidine base uracil. In addition, they identified three new species, U_4, U_5 and U_6, which were also associated with similar antigens. It was shortly after this that it was first proposed that some snRNPs may be involved in RNA splicing [55,56]. It is now known that the above-mentioned snRNPs are part of a multicomponent complex, termed the 'spliceosome', where the splicing reaction takes place.

The formation of the spliceosome and the mechanism of the splicing reaction can be seen in Fig. 1.13. U_1 particles bind to a sequence of about 17 nucleotides in the intron at the 5′ (upstream) splice site. U_2 binds to a 40-nucleotide intron fragment surrounding the branch point of the intron (see below), while the U_5 particle binds to about 15 nucleotides at the downstream splice site. Whether U_4 and U_6 interact with the primary RNA sequence or interact with other snRNA particles is unknown, but the presence of all of these components is necessary for splicing to occur.

Splicing involves two consecutive steps. First, the RNA is cleaved at the 5′ splice site and a 2′–5′ phosphodiester bond is formed between the 5′ end of the intron and the 2′-OH group of a specific acceptor adenosine at the so-called 'branch point' in the intron. The second step consists of cleavage of the 3′ splice point releasing the noose-shaped (lariat) intron, and the two exons are ligated together (Fig. 1.15).

The lariat branch point is specified by the sequence surrounding the branch point and an adjacent downstream polypyrimidine tract [57]. The 3′ splice point is not necessary for spliceosome assembly or cleavage at the 5′ splice site.

Differential RNA splicing of hormone genes

Alternative splicing of pre-mRNA can generate different polyproteins by the inclusion or exclusion of specific exons of a given transcriptional unit. For example, it has been suggested that two different forms of human gastrin-releasing peptide are encoded by two mRNAs generated by alternative

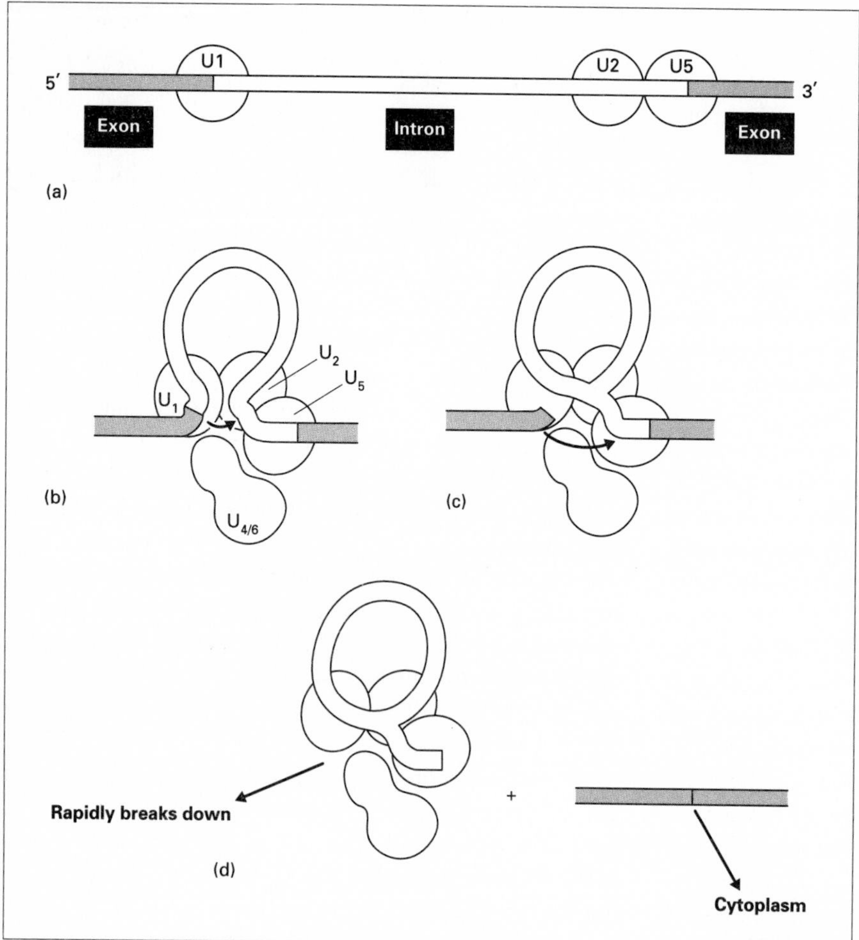

Fig. 1.15 Stages of RNA splicing: (a) and (b) small nuclear RNAs (snRNAs) bind to intron, forming spliceosome complex; (c) upstream splice site is cut and attached to U_2 binding site, and finally (d) the exons join and the intron is released.

processing of the primary transcript of the same gene. In addition, alternative RNA splicing allows the synthesis of precursors encoding different peptides such as substance P and substance K (also called neurokinin A) or calcitonin and calcitonin gene-related peptide (CGRP).

The tachykinins, substance P and substance K, are derived from three different precursors (and therefore three different mRNAs) arising from the same gene. The transcriptional unit of this gene contains seven exons. Exon 3 contains the sequence encoding substance P, whereas exon 6 encodes substance K. The different mRNAs generated by the alternative splicing of the primary transcript are as follows.

1 α-Preprotachykinin (α-PPT) mRNA, which contains the sequence of all the exons except exon 6. It therefore encodes a protein including the substance P sequence, but not substance K. Post-translational processing of this protein generates the peptide substance P.

2 β-Preprotachykinin (β-PPT) mRNA contains all the exons, and therefore encodes a common precursor for both substance P and substance K.

3 γ-Preprotachykinin (γ-PPT) mRNA, which lacks the sequence corresponding to exon 4. It therefore also encodes a common precursor for substance P and substance K, but it is shorter than the one encoded by β-PPT mRNA.

The relative amounts of α-, β- and γ-PPT vary significantly in the several different tissues that have been analysed, including a number of areas of the central nervous system. This suggests that the mechanisms regulating RNA-splicing events are tissue specific. The nature of the regulatory machinery dictating the tissue specificity of the processing of the PPT primary transcript is currently unknown.

The manner in which the calcitonin–CGRP primary transcript is spliced seems to differ from that of PPT (Fig. 1.16). The gene encoding these peptides contains six exons. The fragment encoding calcitonin is within exon 4, whereas CGRP is encoded by exon 5 [58]. Two mRNAs are derived from the primary transcript encoded by this gene: the calcitonin mRNA is generated by the splicing of the first four exons in thyroid C cells; in the nervous system, on the other hand, the first three exons are spliced to the fifth and sixth, generating the CGRP mRNA. Therefore, either the fifth and sixth, or the fourth exon, respectively, are

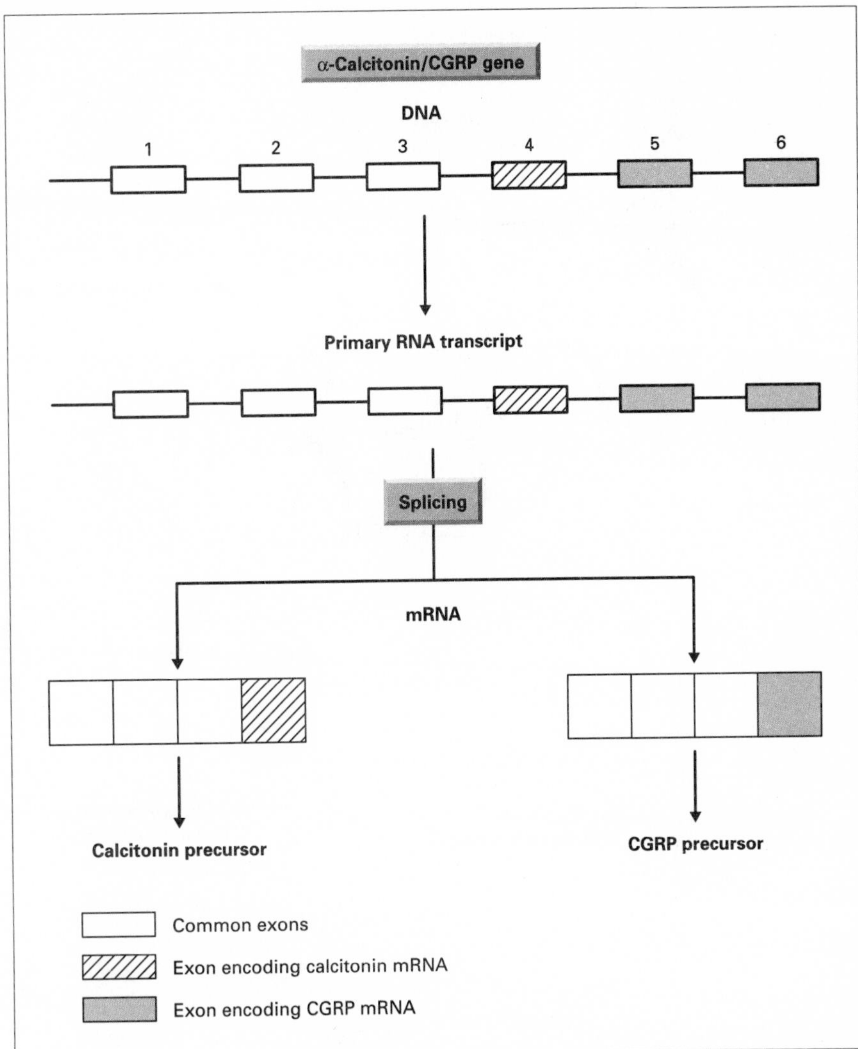

Fig. 1.16 Alternative splicing of the human α-calcitonin/calcitonin gene-related peptide (CGPR) gene.

removed in a tissue-specific manner. It has been suggested that the production of each one of these different mRNAs is due to the selective utilisation of two different polyadenylation sites [59], although other splice choice signals may be used. Li *et al.* [60] have recently reported the proteins which may be involved in determining the tissue-specific splicing of the calcitonin–CGRP transcript.

It is also of considerable potential importance to realise that as well as the hormones or neurotransmitters, receptors may also be regulated by differential RNA splicing. This is well illustrated by the D_2 dopamine receptor which has now been described in two forms which differ by a sequence of 29 amino acids in the third cytoplasmic loop (Fig. 1.17). Because this part of the receptor is involved in activation of G-proteins, differential splicing may result in different G-protein responses.

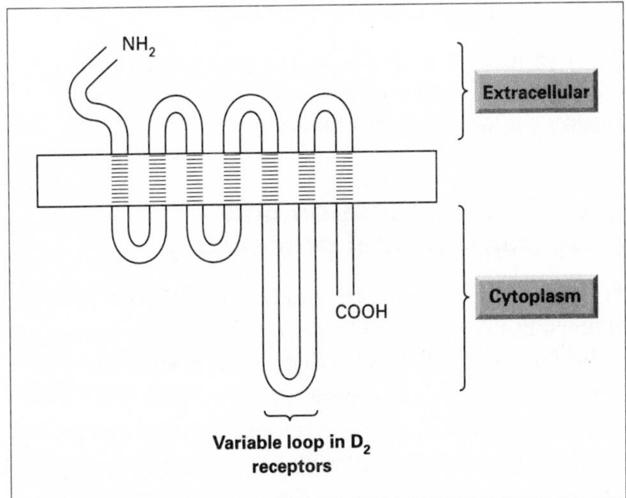

Fig. 1.17 Location of the additional 29 amino acids in the third cytoplasmic loop of one of the isoforms of the rat D_2 dopamine receptor. (Further details in three independent papers in *Nature*, 21 December 1989.)

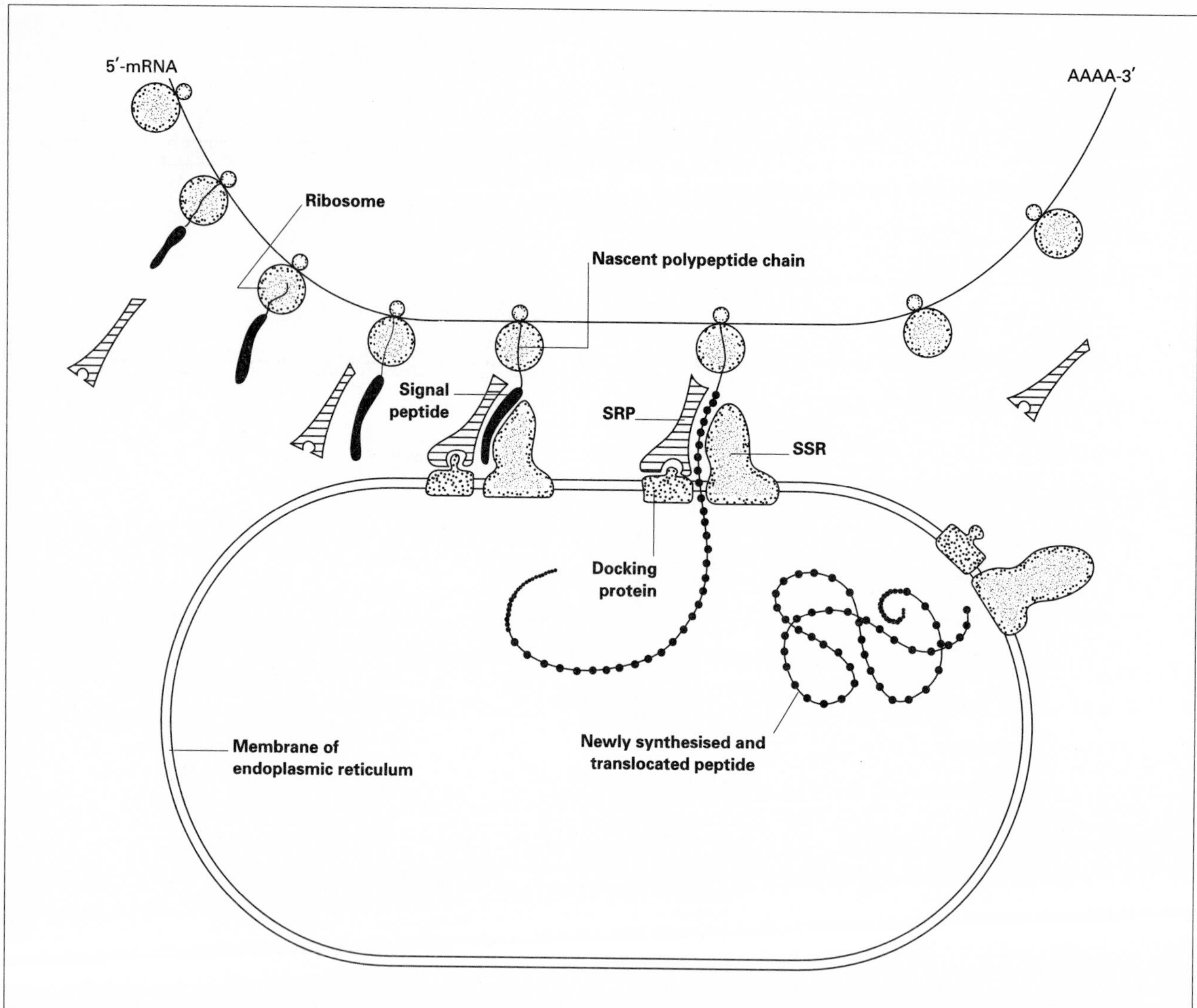

Fig. 1.18 Role of the signal recognition particle (SRP) and signal sequence receptor (SSR) in the synthesis and translocation of peptides into the endoplasmic reticulum.

Protein translocation and post-translational processing

Polypeptide hormones are synthesised as part of large precursors, usually 90–250 amino acids in length, considered to be devoid of biological activity. Such precursors contain a hydrophobic signal peptide at the N-terminus (15–30 amino acids long) which directs the newly synthesised protein through the rough endoplasmic reticulum membrane into the cisternae. The mechanism by which this occurs is unclear, but some components have been identified [61]. The most important is the signal recognition particle (SRP), a constitutive component of all cells. This consists of one RNA molecule of about 300 nucleotides and six non-identical polypeptide chains. SRP binds to the ribosome and to the signal peptide emerging from it: translation is then arrested. This complex is then recognised by a membrane protein in the endoplasmic reticulum known as the SRP receptor or docking protein (Fig. 1.18). This allows the interaction of the signal peptide with an integral protein of the endoplasmic reticulum (ER) membrane known as the signal sequence receptor [62] which engages the nascent polypeptide through the membrane. The SRP and its receptor are then released from the complex, leaving the ribosome membrane bound by means of the nascent polypeptide chain, and the translation arrest is lifted.

It is now becoming increasingly clear that this whole system is amenable to rapid regulatory control. In basal states, for instance, build-up of ribosomes has been demonstrated at specific hold-up points in preprolactin mRNA. Stimulation of secretion can result in decreased hold-up of these ribosomes with more regular spacing along the mRNA and presumably increased peptide translation. This is likely

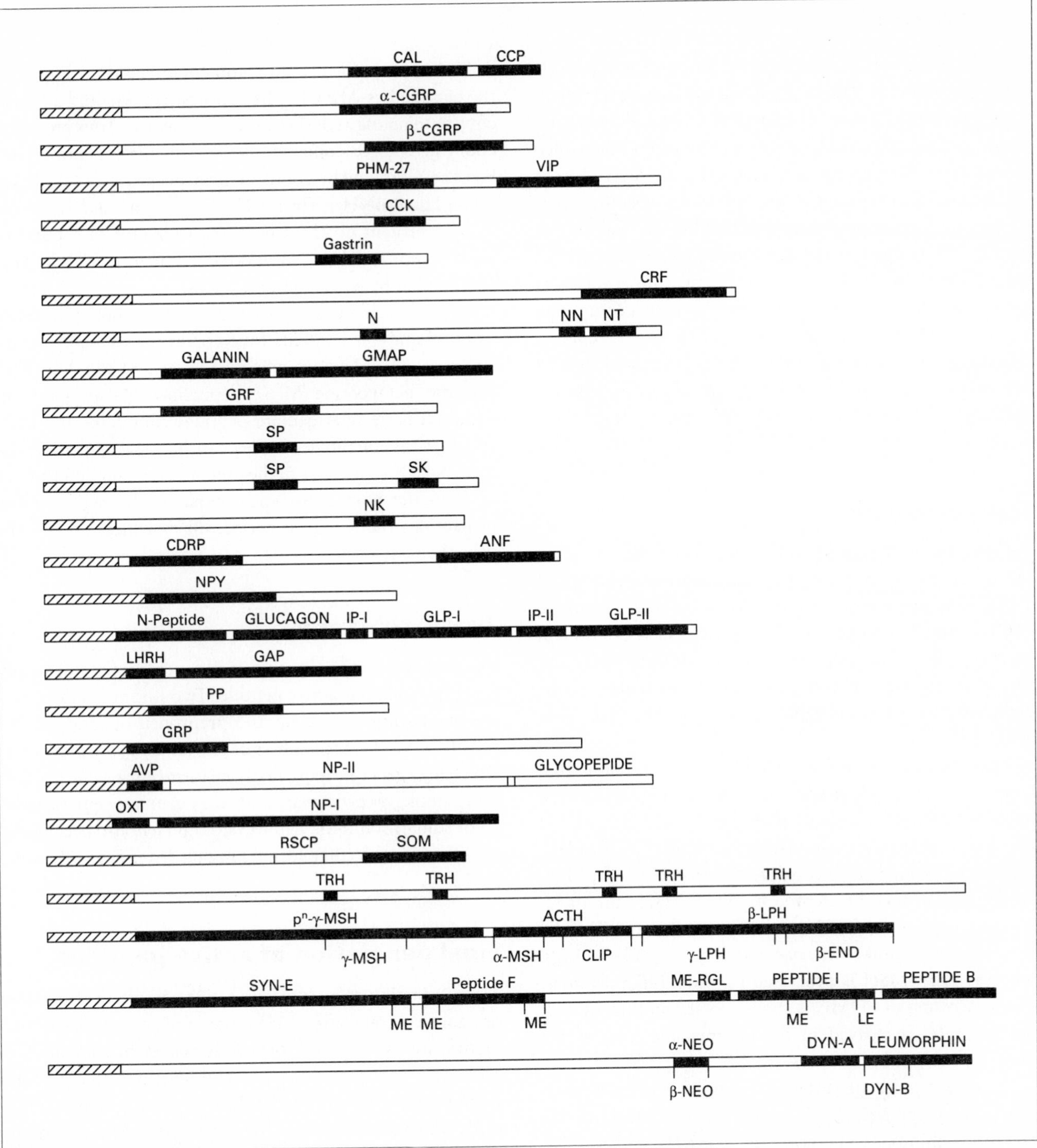

Fig. 1.19 Examples of polyprotein precursors of polypeptide hormones. Note that biological activities of some of these peptides (such as CCP, IP, RSCP etc.) have not been demonstrated. CAL, calcitonin; CCP, calcitonin cleavage product; α-CGRP, β-CGRP, calcitonin gene-related peptide; PHM-27, peptide histidine-methionine; VIP, vasoactive intestinal peptide; CCK, cholecystokinin; CRF, corticotrophin releasing factor; N, neuromedin N-like peptide; NN, neuromedin N; NT, neurotensin; GMAP, galanin message-associated peptide; GRF, growth hormone-releasing factor; SP, substance P; SK, substance K; NK, neuromedin K; CDRP, cardiodilatin-related peptide; ANF, atrial natriuretic factor; NPY, neuropeptide Y; IP, intervening peptide; GLP, glucagon-like peptide; LHRH, luteinising hormone-releasing hormone; GAP, GnRH (gonadotrophin-releasing hormone) associated peptide; PP, pancreatic polypeptide; GRP, gastrin-releasing peptide; AVP, arginine vasopressin; NP, neurophysin; OXT, oxytocin; RSCP, (rat) somatostatin cryptic peptide; SOM, somatostatin; TRH, thyrotrophin releasing hormone; MSH, melanocyte-stimulating hormone; ACTH, adrenocorticotrophic hormone; CLIP, corticotrophin-like intermediate lobe peptide; LPH, lipotrophin; β-END, β-endorphin; ME-RGL, Met-enkephalin-arg-gly-leu; ME, Met-enkephalin; LE, Leu-enkephalin; α-NEO, β-NEO, neoendophin; DYN-A, DYN-B, dynorphin A, B.

to prove an important mechanism in the control of peptide hormone synthesis, translocation and subsequent secretion.

As mentioned above, all known polypeptide hormones are synthesised as part of larger precursors generically named polyproteins. Biologically active peptides are derived from the high-molecular-weight precursors by specific post-translational processing carried out within the cisternae of the ER. An analysis of the distribution of peptides within these precursors allows one to distinguish three different types of polyprotein family: type I are precursors containing a number of different peptides; type II are precursors containing several copies of the same peptide; and type III are precursors containing only one copy of a given peptide. Individual precursors representative of each one of these families are depicted in Fig. 1.19.

Type I polyprotein

Perhaps the most representative member of this family is pro-opiomelanocortin (POMC). Although the existence of a common precursor for adrenocorticotrophic hormone (ACTH) and β-endorphin had been established by classical biochemical methods, the actual complexity of POMC was first observed after its complete amino-acid sequence was deducted from a bovine cDNA clone isolated by Nakanishi *et al.* [63].

Apart from the signal peptide in the N-terminal region common to all peptide precursors, POMC is initially cleaved into three different fragments, β-lipotrophin (β-LPH), ACTH and pro-γ melanocyte-stimulating hormone (pro-γ-MSH). β-LPH can be further processed to β-endorphin and γ-LPH, which may in turn be cleaved to give β-MSH and an N-terminal peptide. ACTH is cleaved to produce α-MSH and a corticotrophin-like intermediate-lobe peptide (CLIP), whereas pro-γ-MSH is processed to γ-MSH-like peptides. The processing of POMC is tissue specific so that ACTH, for example, is cleaved in the intermediate lobe of the pituitary but not in the anterior lobe.

Other examples of different peptides generated from the same precursor are substance P and substance K, gonadotrophin-releasing hormone (GnRH) and GnRH-associated peptide (GAP), and several opioid peptides from prodynorphin.

Type II polyproteins

The prototype of this family is given by the thyrotrophin-releasing hormone (TRH) precursor. This was first cloned from the frog *Xenopus laevis*, taking advantage of the high abundance of this peptide in the skin of this animal. The deduced TRH precursor from the cloned cDNA was found to be 123 amino acids long, and contained three copies of the peptide Lys-Arg-Glu-His-Pro-Lys/Arg-Arg and a fourth copy terminating at the Pro residue. Cleavage of this precursor could give three copies of the intermediate peptide Glu-His-Pro-Gly, which would in turn be processed to TRH (pGlu-His-ProNH_2). The rat TRH precursor was later found to be a protein of 255 amino acids containing a putative signal peptide and five copies of the sequence Glu-His-Pro-Gly flanked by paired basic residues.

Preproenkephalin can also be considered another member of this family. It contains four copies of Met-enkephalin, and one copy of Leu-enkephalin, Met-enkephalin-Arg^6-Phe^7 and the octapeptide Met-enkephalin-Arg^6-Gly^7-Leu^8. In addition, large intermediate peptides containing the Met- and Leu-enkephalin sequences can be generated from the precursor. The large size of the preproenkephalin (263 amino acids in the bovine sequence) explains the high number of peptides that it can generate, all of which contain the enkephalin sequence.

Type III polyproteins

The post-translational processing of members of this family generates only one active peptide. Two hormonal examples are preprocholecystokinin and preproneuropeptide Y. We can also consider as members of this family those precursors which may generate more than one form of the same peptide; for example, preprosomatostatin may generate somatostatin-28 or somatostatin-14. Cholecystokinin has also been found in different molecular forms ranging from 8 to 58 amino acids.

Final generation of active peptides

The production of biologically active peptides is dependent on correct translation, cleavage and post-translational modifications. The signal peptide is cleaved by a membrane-associated endopeptidase. The biologically active peptides within the precursors are flanked by pairs of basic amino acids which are recognized by carboxypeptidase-processing enzymes in the ER. The presence of a glycine residue preceding these pairs is also important for the donation of amide groups at the C-terminus of peptides such as vasopressin, whilst other post-translational modifications including the formation of disulphide bridges (as in vasopressin, oxytocin and insulin) or asparagine-linked glycosylation (as in the glycopeptide hormones, luteinising hormone, follicle-stimulating hormone, chorionic gonadotrophin and thyroid-stimulating hormone) are needed for the final generation of the mature peptide.

References

1 Horikoshi M, Wang CK, Fujii H, Cromlish JA, Weil PA, Roeder RG. Purification of a yeast TATA box-binding protein that exhibits human transcription factor IID activity. *Proc Natl Acad Sci USA* 1989; **86**: 4843–7.

2 Buratowski S. The basics of basal transcription by RNA polymerase II. *Cell* 1994; **77**: 1–3.

3 Drapkin R, Sancar A, Reinberg D. Where transcription meets repair. *Cell* 1994; **77**: 9–12.

4 Sauer F, Hansen SK, Tjian R. Multiple TAF_{II}s directing synergistic activation of transcription. *Science* 1995; **270**: 1783–8.

5 Gehring WJ, Qian YQ, Billeter M *et al.* Homeodomain-DNA recognition. *Cell* 1994; **78**: 211–23.

6 Murre C, McCaw PS, Baltimore D. A new binding and dimerization motif in immunoglobulin enhancer binding, *daughterless, MyoD* and *myc* proteins. *Cell* 1989; **56**: 777–83.

7 Lai E, Clark KL, Burley SK, Darnell JE. Hepatocyte nuclear factor 3/fork head of "winged helix" proteins: a family of transcription factors of diverse biological function. *Proc Natl Acad Sci USA* 1993; **90**: 10421–3.

8 Xuan S, Baptista CA, Balas G, Tao W, Soares VC, Lai E. Winged helix transcription factor BF-1 is essential for the development of the cerebral hemispheres. *Cell* 1995; **14**: 1141–52.

9 Ptashne M. How eukaryotic transcriptional activators work. *Nature* 1988; **335**: 683–9.

10 Gill G, Pascal E, Tseng Z, Tjian R. A glutamine-rich hydrophobic patch in transcription factor Sp1 contacts the $dTAF_{II}110$ component of the Drosophila TFIID complex and mediated transcriptional activation. *Proc Natl Acad Sci USA* 1994; **91**: 192–6.

11 Lukas TJ, Haiech J, Lau W *et al.* Calmodulin and calmodulin regulated protein kinases as transducers of intracellular calcium signals. In: *Molecular Biology of Signal Transduction,Cold Spring Harbor Symposia on Quantitative Biology* Vol. LIII. New York: Cold Spring Harbor Laboratory Press, 1988: 185–93.

12 Schindler C, Darnell JE. Transcriptional responses to polypeptide ligands: the JAK-STAT pathway. *Ann Rev Biochem* 1995; **64**: 621–51.

13 Hill S, Trisman R. Transcriptional regulation by extracellular signals: mechanisms and specificity. *Cell* 1995; **80**: 199–211.

14 Berridge MJ. Inositol triphosphates and calcium signalling. *Nature* 1993; **361**: 315–25.

15 Bohmann D, Bos TJ, Admon A, Nishimura T, Vogt PK, Tjian R. Human proto-oncogene c-*jun* encodes a DNA binding protein with structural and functional properties of transcription factor AP-1. *Science* 1987; **238**: 1386–92.

16 Angel P, Allegretto EA, Okino ST *et al.* Oncogene *jun* encodes a sequence-specific *trans*-activator similar to AP-1. *Nature* 1988; **332**: 166–71.

17 Cohen D, Ferreira P, Gentz R, Franza R, Curran T. The product of *fos*-related gene, *fra*-1, binds cooperatively to the AP-1 site with Jun: transcription factor AP-1 is comprised of multiple protein complexes. *Genes Dev* 1989; **3**: 173–84.

18 Zerial M, Toschi L, Rysek R, Schuermann M, Muller R, Bravo R. The product of a novel growth factor activated gene, fos-B, interacts with JUN proteins enhancing their DNA binding activity. *EMBO J* 1989; **8**: 805–13.

19 Hoeffler JP, Meyer TE, Yun Y, Jameson JL, Habener JF. Cyclic AMP-responsive DNA binding protein: structure based on a cloned placental cDNA. *Science* 1988; **242**: 1430–3.

20 Ferreri K, Gill G, Montminy MR. The cAMP regulated transcription factor CREB interacts with a component of the TFIID complex. *Proc Natl Acad Sci USA* 1994; **91**: 1210–13.

21 Chrivia JC, Kwok RPS, Lamb N, Hagiwara, Montminy M, Goodman RH. Phosphorylated CREB binds specifically to the nuclear protein CBP. *Nature* 1993; **365**: 855–9.

22 Park K, Kim KH. The site of cAMP action in the insulin induction of gene expression of acetyl-CoA carboxylase is AP-2. *J Biol Chem* 1993; **268**: 17811–19.

23 Williams T, Admon A, Luscher B, Tjian R. Cloning and expression of AP-2, a cell-type specific transcription factor that activates inducible enhancer elements. *Genes Dev* 1988; **2**: 1557–69.

24 Ip N, Yancopoulos GD. The neurotrophins and CNTF: two families of collaborative neurotrophic factors. *Annu Rev Neurosci* 1996; **19**: 491–515.

25 Freedman LP, Luisi BF. On the mechanism of DNA binding by nuclear hormone receptors: a structural and functional perspective. *J Cell Biochem* 1993; **5**: 140–50.

26 Pratt WB. The role of heat shock proteins in regulating the function, folding and trafficking of the glucocorticoid receptor. *J Biol Chem* 1993; **268**: 21455–8.

27 Tsai MJ, O'Malley BW. Molecular mechanisms of action of steroid/thyroid receptor superfamily members. *Ann Rev Biochem* 1994; **63**: 451–486.

28 Cavailles V, Dauvois S, L'Illorset F, Lopez G, Hoare S, Kushner PJ, Parker MG. Nuclear factor RIP140 modulates transcriptional activation by the estrogen receptor. *EMBO J* 1995; **14**: 3741–51.

29 Le Douarin, Zechel C, Garnier JM *et al.* The N-terminal part of TIF1, a putative mediator of the ligand-dependent activation function (AF-2) of nuclear receptors, is fused to B-raf in the oncogenic protein T18. *EMBO J* 1995; **14**: 2020–33.

30 Mangelsdorf DJ, Evans RM. The RXR heterodimers and orphan receptors. *Cell* 1995; **83**: 841–9.

31 Yamamoto KR, Pearce D, Thomas J, Miner JN. Combinatorial regulation at a mammalian composite element. In: McKnight SL, Yamamoto KR, eds. *Transcriptional Regulation*. New York: Cold Spring Harbor Laboratory Press, 1993: 3–32.

32 Scheinman RI, Cogswell PC, Lofquist AK, Baldwin AS, Jr. Role of transcriptional activation of IkBa in mediation of immunosuppression by glucocorticoids. *Science* 1995; **270**: 283–6.

33 Auphan N, Didonato J, Rosette C, Hemberg A, Karin M. Immunosuppression by glucocorticoids: inhibition of NF-kB activity through induction of IkB synthesis. *Science* 1995; **270**: 286–90.

34 Aronica SM, Katzenellenbogen BS. Stimulation of Estrogen receptor-mediated transcription and alteration in the phosphorylation state of the rat uterine estrogen receptor by estrogen, cyclic adenosine monophosphate, and insulin-like growth factor-1. *Mol Endocrinol* 1993; **7**: 743–52.

35 Glass CK. Differential recognition of target genes by nuclear receptor monomers, dimers, and heterodimers. *Endocrinol Rev* 1994; **15**: 391–407.

36 Horlein A, Naar AM, Heinzel T *et al.* Ligand-independent repression by the thyroid hormone receptor mediated by a nuclear receptor co-repressor. *Nature* 1995; **377**: 397–404.

37 Lee JW, Ryan F, Swaffield JC, Johnson SA, Moore DD. Interaction of thyroid hormone receptor with a conserved transcriptional mediator. *Nature* 1995; **374**: 91–4.

38 Forman BM, Tontonoz P, Chen J, Brun RP, Spiegelman BM, Evans RM. 15-Deoxy-D12,14-Prostaglandin J2 is a ligand for the adipocyte determination factor PPARg. *Cell* 1995; **83**: 803–12.

39 Tapscott H, Davis RL, Thayer MJ, Cheng PF, Weintraub H, Lassar AB. MyoD1: a nuclear phosphoprotein requiring a Myc homology region to convert fibroblasts to myoblasts. *Science* 1988; **242**: 405–11.

40 Roux E, Strubin M, Hagenbuchle O, Wellauer PK. The cell-specific transcription factor PTF-1 contains two different subunits that interact with the DNA. *Genes Dev* 1989; 3: 1613–24.
41 Tsai SF, Martin DIC, Zon LI, D'Andrea AD, Wong GG, Orkin SH. Cloning of cDNA for the major DNA-binding protein of the erythroid lineage through expression in mammalian cells. *Nature* 1989; **339**: 446–51.
42 Ingraham HA, Chen R, Mangalam HJ *et al.* A tissue-specific transcription factor containing a homeodomain specifies a pituitary phenotype. *Cell* 1988; **55**: 519–29.
43 Herr W, Sturm RA, Clerc RG *et al.* The POU-domain: a large conserved region in the mammalian *pit-1*, *oct-1*, *oct-2* and *C. elegans unc-86* gene products. *Genes Dev* 1988; **2**: 1513–16.
44 Radovick S, Nations M, Du Y, Berg LA, Weintraub BD, Wondisford FE. A mutation in the POU-homeodomain of Pit-1 responsible for combined pituitary hormone deficiency. *Science* 1992; **257**: 1115–17.
45 Tatsumi K, Miyai K, Notomi T, Kaibe K, Amino N, Mizuno Y, Kohno H. Cretinism with combined hormone deficiency caused by a mutation in the PIT1 gene. *Nature Genet* 1992; **1**: 56–8.
46 Schonemann MD, Ryan AK, McEvilly RJ *et al.* Development and survival of the endocrine hypothalamus and posterior pituitary gland requires the neuronal POU domain factor Brn-2. *Genes Dev* 1995; **9**: 3122–35.
47 Miller CP, McGehee RE, Habener JF. IDX-1: a new homeodomain transcription factor expressed in rat pancreatic islets and duodenum that transactivates the somatostatin gene. *EMBO J* 1994; **13**: 1145–56.
48 Jonsson J, Carlsson L, Edlund T, Edlund E. Insulin-promoter factor 1 is required for pancreas development in mice. *Nature* 1994; **371**: 606–9.
49 Gilbert W. Why genes in pieces? *Nature* 1978; **271**: 501.
50 Sharp PA. Split genes and RNA splicing. *Cell* 1994; **77**: 805–15.
51 Weinberg R, Penman S. Small molecular weight monodisperse nuclear RNA. *J Mol Biol* 1968; **38**: 289–304.
52 Ro-Choi TS, Busch H. Low molecular weight nuclear RNA. In: Busch H, ed. *The Cell Nucleus*. New York: Academic Press, 1974: 151–208.
53 Zieve G, Penman S. Small RNA species of the Hela cells: metabolism and subcellular localisation. *Cell* 1976; **8**: 19–31.
54 Lerner MR, Steitz JA. Antibodies to small nuclear RNAs complexed with proteins are produced by patients with systemic lupus erythematosus. *Proc Natl Acad Sci USA* 1979; **76**: 5495–9.
55 Lerner MR, Boyle JA, Mount SM, Solin SL, Steitz JA. Are snRNPs involved in splicing? *Nature* 1980; **283**: 220–4.
56 Rogers J, Wall R. A mechanism for RNA splicing. *Proc Natl Acad Sci USA* 1980; **77**: 1877–9.
57 Smith CWJ, Poro EB, Patton JG, Nadal-Ginard B. Scanning from an independently specified branch point defines the 3′ splice site of mammalian introns. *Nature* 1989; **343**: 243–7.
58 Rosenfeld MG, Mermod J-J, Amara SG *et al.* Production of a novel neuropeptide encoded by the calcitonin gene via tissue-specific RNA processing. *Nature* 1983; **304**: 129–35.
59 Amara SG, Evans RM, Rosenfield MG. Calcitonin/calcitonin-gene related peptide transcription unit: tissue-specific expression involves selective use of alternative polyadenylation sites. *Mol Cell Biol* 1984; **4**: 2151–60.
60 Li S, Klein ES, Russo AI, Simmonds DM, Rosenfelt MG. Isolation of cDNA clones encoding small nuclear ribonucleoparticle-associated proteins with different tissue specificities. *Proc Natl Acad Sci USA* 1989; **86**: 9778–82.
61 Siegel V, Walter P. The affinity of signal recognition particle for presecretory proteins is dependent on nascent chain length. *EMBO J* 1988; **7**: 1769–75.
62 Wiedmann M, Kurzchalia TV, Hartmann E, Rapoport TA. A signal sequence receptor in the endoplasive reticulum membrane. *Nature* 1987; **328**: 830–3.
63 Nakanishi S, Teranishi Y, Watanabe Y *et al.* Isolation and characterisation of the bovine corticotropin/β-lipoprotein gene. *Eur J Biochem* 1981; **115**: 429–38.

CHAPTER 2

Methods of investigation

M. Hewison, J.A. Franklyn and M.C. Sheppard

Introduction

Over the last few years, continuing developments in molecular biology have greatly expanded the availability of methods used in endocrine investigation. Analysis of the expression of target genes is now routine in many laboratories, but advances in gene cloning have meant that isolation and identification of new gene sequences can now be approached with similar ease. This has, in part, been due to the advent of 'convenience' kits, allowing most laboratory workers to carry out genetic manipulations previously considered to be relatively complex. Techniques such as complementary DNA (cDNA) library synthesis can now be carried out efficiently and with minimum loss of time for optimisation of protocols. The continued evolution of polymerase chain reaction (PCR)-based methods has also contributed to the accessibility of technology for assessing and manipulating gene expression. This chapter highlights some of the new molecular approaches available to the clinical investigator, particularly in endocrinology, whilst detailing the fundamentals of molecular biology as applied to these techniques.

Restriction enzymes and other enzymes used in recombinant DNA technology

The most important tools available to the molecular biologist for manipulating nucleic acids are restriction enzymes or endonucleases, as well as other enzymes which modify the structure of DNA and RNA. These tools, which have been termed 'molecular scissors', are critical to cloning of eukaryotic DNA, to production and labelling of DNA and RNA probes, and to the analysis of DNA and RNA structure.

Restriction enzymes, which are found naturally in a large number of bacterial strains, have the important property of cleaving double-stranded DNA (dsDNA) at specific sites within or adjacent to a particular sequence (a recognition sequence). A vast array of such enzymes has been characterized and made available for use in recombinant DNA studies. The majority of these enzymes recognise specific DNA sequences which are 4, 5 or 6 nucleotides in length (Fig. 2.1), but a few enzymes specifically recognise longer sequences or sequences which are degenerate.

This property of cleaving DNA at specific sites to produce fragments with particular characteristics is fundamental to the ability to insert or clone pieces of foreign DNA into plasmid and phage vectors such as those described below. A vector containing a selected gene sequence can then be grown or amplified in host bacteria and large amounts of DNA containing the inserted gene of interest isolated. In addition, restriction enzymes play a fundamental role in the investigation of human disease by their ability to produce 'restriction maps', or specific patterns of DNA fragments resulting from the digestion of genomic DNA. For this purpose, DNA is usually prepared from circulating lymphocytes; the DNA fragments produced by restriction digestion are then separated by agarose gel electrophoresis, the rate at which fragments move through the gel being a function of their size. Since individual variations in DNA structure may give rise to changes in the number and position of restriction enzyme sites in human DNA, naturally occurring DNA polymorphisms can give rise to 'restriction fragment length polymorphisms' described below, an occurrence which has considerable implications for the investigation of inherited endocrine diseases.

Many enzymes in addition to restriction endonucleases, or modifying enzymes, are used routinely in molecular cloning. These include the DNA polymerases which are critical to the synthesis of DNA *in vitro*. Such enzymes require a template upon which to act; this template is usually another fragment of DNA, and enzyme action results in the synthesis

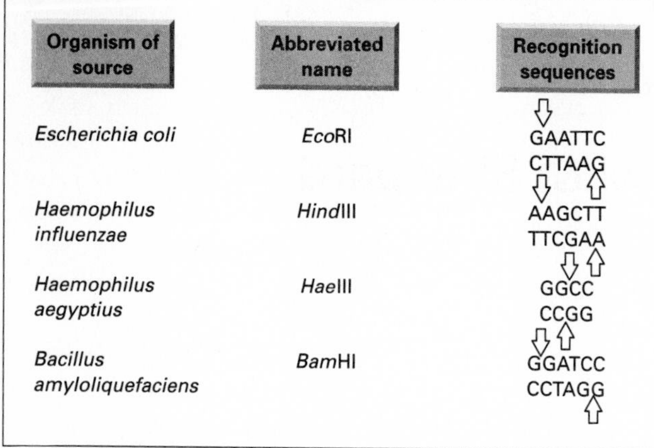

Fig. 2.1 Examples of restriction enzymes and the sequences they cleave.

of a DNA product whose sequence is complementary to that of the original DNA template. Examples of these enzymes are DNA polymerase I (DNA Pol I) and the Klenow fragment of DNA polymerase I (Klenow). DNA Pol I will add a nucleotide to the 3′ hydroxyl end of one strand of a dsDNA providing the strand is 'nicked' (see DNase 1 below), whilst simultaneously it will remove nucleotides from the adjacent 5′ terminus. This is known as 5′→3′ exonuclease activity and forms the basis of nick translation labelling of DNA described below and in Fig. 2.2a. The Klenow fragment was originally produced by proteolytic digestion of DNA Pol I, although it is now available as a pure recombinant enzyme. The enzyme lacks 5′→3′ exonuclease activity but is able to copy single-stranded cDNA in a 5′→3′ direction from the 3′ end of a primer annealed to the cDNA (Fig. 2.2b). Synthesis of DNA from primers annealed to a template forms the basis of PCR amplification of DNA. A major breakthrough leading to widespread application of this technique has been the purification of a DNA polymerase capable of withstanding repeated incubation at 95°C. This was achieved after purification of a thermostable *Taq* polymerase from the thermophilic bacterium, *Thermus aquaticus*. PCR applications of this enzyme and more recent modifications of its polymerase activity are detailed below.

Another DNA polymerase, termed terminal transferase, has the specific property of adding nucleotides to the termini of existing DNA molecules, while reverse transcriptase has the property of producing DNA molecules from RNA templates, a property which is fundamental to the production of cDNA molecules from molecules of messenger RNA (mRNA). Reverse transcriptase is used principally to transcribe mRNA into double-stranded cDNA, which in turn can be inserted into the cloning vectors described below. In addition, this variant of DNA polymerase may be used in the labelling of probes and in DNA sequencing.

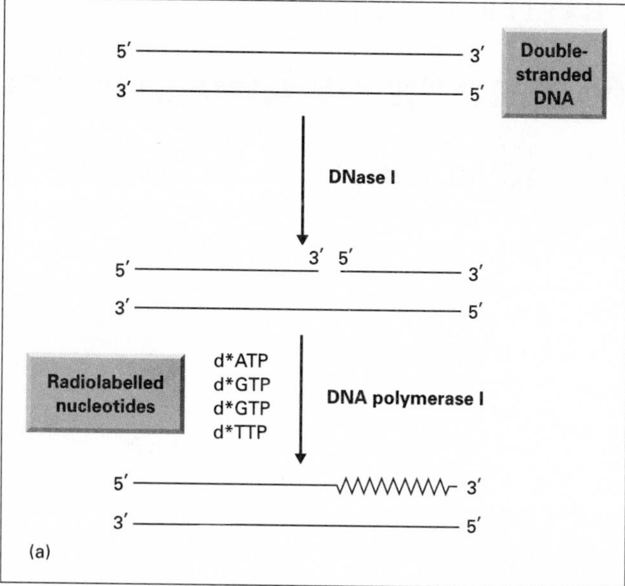

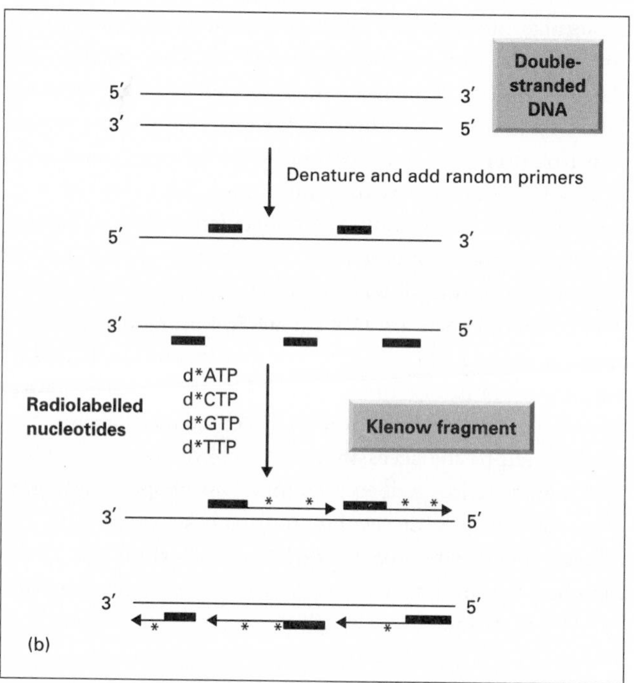

Fig. 2.2 (a) Nick translation labelling of double-stranded DNA by the enzyme DNA polymerase I. 'Nicks' or breaks in the DNA are produced by treatment with DNase I. These nicks then serve as primers for new DNA synthesis catalysed by DNA polymerase I. During synthesis radiolabelled nucleotide precursors are incorporated so that the resulting product can be used as a hybridisation probe. (b) Random primer labelling of double-stranded DNA by the Klenow fragment of DNA polymerase I. After denaturation of the DNA short random oligonucleotides anneal to single-stranded DNA and act as primers for Klenow enzyme. During extension of the primers radiolabelled nucleotide precursors are incorporated to produce a labelled hybridisation probe.

Specific products of the bacterial viruses, bacteriophages, represent further varieties of enzyme which are widely used, for example in transcription of RNA *in vitro* from DNA templates that include specific bacteriophage promoter sequences. The *in vitro* synthesis of RNA molecules is used for the production of specific RNA probes for hybridisation studies or to express cloned eukaryotic genes in bacteria. A further series of enzymes used to join together two pieces of DNA are termed DNA ligases; again, these enzymes are used in the labelling of DNA probes for hybridisation assays and in cloning strategies prior to insertion of foreign DNA into vector molecules (see Fig. 2.4, p. 30).

In contrast to the activity of the enzymes described above which share the property of synthesising or extending molecules of DNA or RNA, *nucleases* represent a class of enzyme which digest or destroy specific DNA or RNA sequences. An example of such an enzyme is S1 nuclease which degrades single-stranded DNA or RNA while double-stranded molecules or DNA–RNA hybrids are relatively resistant to its action. This property has proved useful in carrying out genomic mapping with cDNA clones. The endonuclease deoxynuclease 1 (DNase 1) is commonly used in nick translation labelling of DNA (Fig. 2.2a). However, its ability to 'nick' dsDNA means that under carefully controlled conditions it can digest single base pairs to give a complete base-pair ladder. DNA specifically bound to a protein is protected against this activity. This effect has been utilised in the technique known as 'DNase footprinting', which was developed to identify protein-binding sequences in the promoter regions of genes. RNA-specific nucleases are now also commonly used in standard molecular biology techniques. Ribonuclease (RNase) A and RNase T1 are single-stranded nucleases which can be used to degrade RNA which is not hybridised to another strand of RNA or DNA. This forms the basis of the 'RNase protection assay' in which a labelled cDNA or RNA probe is added to sample RNA and then subjected to RNase digestion. Target RNA which hybridises to the probe is protected from enzyme action and can then be detected following gel electrophoresis. In contrast, RNase H is specific for the RNA component of an RNA–DNA hybrid. The enzyme can thus be used to eliminate template RNA from cDNA preparations following reverse transcription of mRNA, and features in several methods for cDNA library preparation.

Vectors for cloning and production of eukaryotic DNA

A fundamental requirement for cloning of eukaryotic sequences of DNA such as those encoding hormones or hormone-regulated products is the availability of vectors which can be used to carry such foreign DNA, as well as bacteria in which to propagate such vectors. Bacterial plasmids represent the vectors which have been used in cloning strategies most commonly; such plasmids are double-stranded, circular DNA molecules which vary in size from 1000 bases to 200 000 bases (200 kb) and are found naturally in many bacteria. Plasmid DNA is not integrated into host bacterial DNA but, none the less, plasmids have the ability to replicate within the bacterial host, making use of enzymes and proteins produced by the host organism.

Specific properties of several plasmids make them ideal for use in cloning, the most important of these being the ability to confer antibiotic resistance upon host bacteria. This property determines that if plasmid DNA is introduced into bacteria in the laboratory by the process of transformation, such transformed colonies can then be selected. Brief exposure to divalent cations will make them permeable to DNA whilst with electroporation passing a current across the bacteria forms pores which allow the entry of DNA. Bacteria which have been successfully transformed can be selected by treatment of the bacterial culture with the appropriate antibiotic (Fig. 2.3). An example of such a plasmid in common use is pBR322, which carries genes for resistance to both ampicillin and tetracycline. In addition, restriction enzyme sites may be present within these antibiotic-resistance coding sequences in plasmid DNA so that when foreign DNA is recombined into one of these sites, resistance to that antibiotic is lost, while resistance to the other antibiotic is retained, and insertion of foreign DNA can be readily detected.

Since the development of the plasmid vector pBR322, there have been considerable advances in plasmid technology which have facilitated cloning of larger fragments of DNA as well as fragments which have been produced by cleavage of eukaryotic DNA sequences with a wide range of restriction enzymes. Smaller plasmid vectors than pBR322 have been developed since these can accommodate larger pieces of foreign DNA without impairing the efficiency of transformation of bacteria, since transformation efficiency is inversely related to vector size. In addition, smaller plasmids replicate with greater efficiency than larger plasmids. Examples of these include the pUC, pGEM and pcDNA series of vectors, all of which are approximately 3 kb in size. A feature which has been essential to the evolution of these plasmids has been the incorporation of multiple cloning or 'polylinker' sequences. These synthetic cloning sites consist of short stretches of DNA containing unique sites for a variety of restriction enzymes not found elsewhere in the plasmid. The availability of these polylinker sequences means that such vectors can be used to clone DNA produced by cleavage with a large array of restriction enzymes.

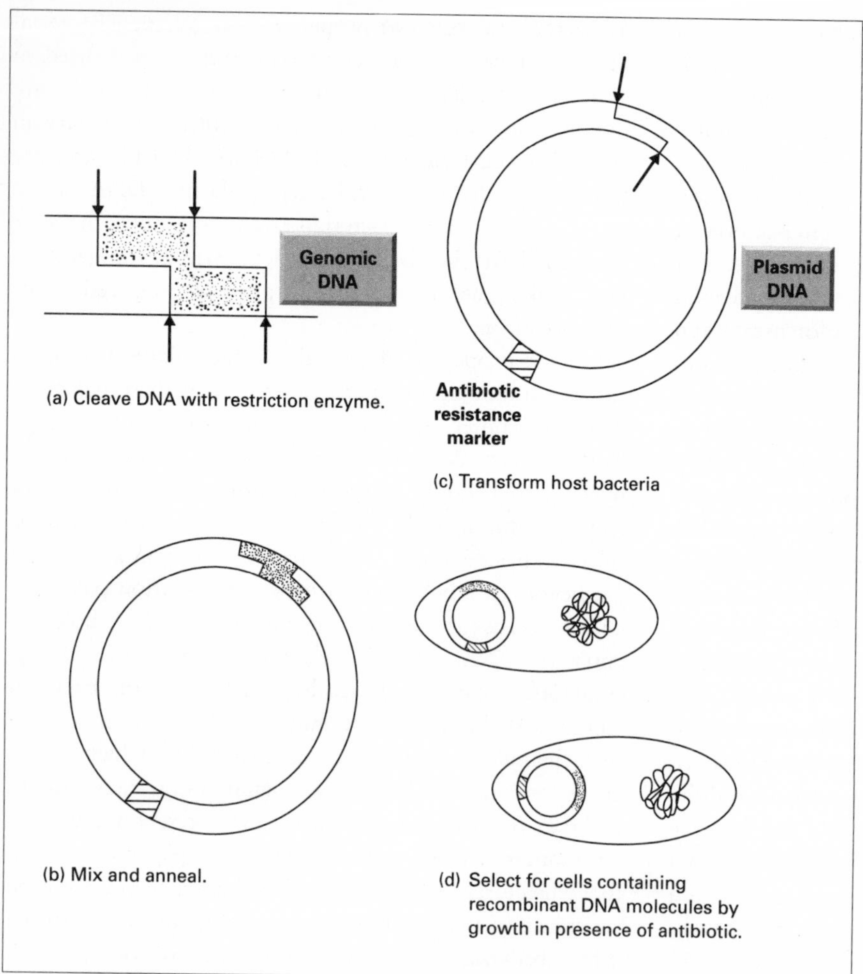

Fig. 2.3 The cloning of DNA in a plasmid.

Other developments in plasmid technology include the production of plasmid sequences which allow the direct identification of recombinant clones using histochemical techniques. The most common example of this is incorporation of a polylinker sequence within a specially adapted gene for the *lacZ* α-peptide. In the absence of cloned DNA within the cloning site, a *lac* promoter upstream of the *lacZ* gene induces transcription of this protein. In tandem with another protein from the host cell (*lacZ*ΔM15) the α-peptide produces a functional β-galactosidase protein. The resulting enzyme drives conversion of a colourless compound, 5-bromo-4-chloro-3-indolyl-β-D-galactoside (Xgal) to a deep blue substance, 5-bromo-4-chloroindigo. Thus, by addition of Xgal to agar plates it is possible to identify bacteria *without* insert-containing plasmids as blue colonies. However, successful DNA cloning leads to disruption of the α-peptide and, as a consequence, positive recombinants remain as *colourless* colonies. Bacteria without any plasmids will not survive because of the antibiotic in the agar gel.

Expression vectors which allow *in vitro* transcription of foreign DNA usually contain promoter sequences from bacteriophages such as T3, T7 or SP6: thus, if recombinant plasmid DNA is linearised and incubated with the appropriate RNA polymerase enzyme, as well as ribonucleotide precursors, then foreign DNA can be transcribed into mRNA *in vitro* (see below). The RNA molecules made *in vitro* can then be used as hybridisation probes or translated in cell-free systems to their protein products. Yet further plasmid vectors have been developed which contain powerful promoters of viral origin: these allow transcription of large quantities of mRNA from cloned foreign DNA sequences and expression of foreign proteins in bacterial cells. Likewise, a series of larger vectors have been developed for expression of cloned DNA in eukaryotic cells. High-level expression of recombinant protein is driven by a viral promoter such as the cytomegalovirus (CMV) promoter. Examples of these vectors include the pCMV series of eukaryotic expression vectors, which have been widely used in transient transfection, either in expression cloning experiments (see below) or in conjunction with gene reporter systems. The latter has been an essential feature of studies of the interaction of steroid-hormone receptors with target gene promoters

[1]. Eukaryotic expression vectors containing receptor cDNA are cotransfected with plasmids incorporating small fragments of the 'upstream' or regulatory part of a specific gene promoter. The cotransfected plasmid is known as a reporter plasmid because the upstream promoter fragment is cloned into a polylinker connected to a sequence for a reporter gene. Examples include the pCAT series of vectors which incorporate a chloramphenicol acetyl transferase (CAT) gene and the pGL series of vectors which utilise a luciferase gene. Functional activity of both of these enzymes is dependent on induction by the cloned upstream promoter, which is itself usually dependent on binding by regulatory proteins such as the steroid-hormone receptors. Induction of promoter activity can then be quantified by measuring the conversion of substrate to product. In particular, the luciferase system has proved to be a very rapid and simple system for analysing gene promoter activity. The luciferase protein catalyses the oxidation of firefly beetle luciferin, releasing a photon of light which can then be measured using a luminometer following cell extraction. The relative ease of this assay can be contrasted with CAT assays which require thin-layer chromatography and autoradiography to resolve the mono- and di-acetylated products of the substrate. Further eukaryotic expression vectors have been developed which allow stable transfection of cloned DNA. As with the transient expression vectors, these plasmids have CMV or Rous sarcoma virus promoters but also include a gene sequence to enable selection of successfully transfected cells. Resistance to treatment with hygromycin is a common selection gene, and plasmids incorporating this sequence can be maintained in cells over several months of culture.

In addition to the use of plasmid vectors in cloning strategies, other cloning vehicles have been developed. These include bacteriophage lambda and cosmid vectors, both of which may have practical advantages over plasmid vectors depending on the specific aim of the cloning process. Bacteriophages are viruses which multiply in bacteria and have the property of rapid multiplication within the bacterial host. In contrast to plasmid DNA, bacteriophage DNA has the ability to integrate into host chromosomal DNA and to accommodate within its structure large fragments of foreign DNA (up to 15 kb in length). This means that an entire 'library' of eukaryotic DNA can be inserted into a bacteriophage vector and screened for the foreign DNA insert of interest with relative ease. Improvements to this technology include the introduction of 'phagmid' vectors such as λZAP. This phage vector can incorporate up to 10-kb DNA inserts which can then be excised and inserted into other vectors, such as eukaryotic expression plasmids. Still larger fragments of DNA can be inserted into cosmid vectors. This allows the cloning of entire genes within a single recombinant rather than cloning of a gene as several fragments in plasmid or bacteriophage lambda vectors. In their simplest form, cosmid vectors represent modified plasmids containing DNA sequences ('cos' sequences) required for packaging DNA into bacteriophage lambda particles. Such vectors, like plasmids, contain antibiotic-resistance sequences, can be introduced into bacteria using standard transformation techniques and can be propagated in the same way as plasmids. Cosmid vectors may be used to clone 40–50 kb of DNA, but recently developed yeast artificial chromosomes (YACs) have extended the range of possible insert sizes to over 100 kb. YAC DNA libraries are now an important feature of the analysis of genes causing inherited diseases (see below).

Strategies for cloning of eukaryotic genes

By using restriction enzymes and prokaryotic vectors described above, it is possible to prepare DNA from a human tissue such as circulating lymphocytes, cut the DNA into fragments, insert or recombine those fragments into a suitable vector and introduce the recombinant DNA vectors into bacteria in which they can be propagated. If total genomic DNA is packaged in such a way, then the resulting transformed bacteria carry what can be termed a 'genomic' library. Likewise, if complementary or cDNA molecules (molecules complementary to the total mRNAs expressed in a given tissue or cell line) are packaged in a similar way, a 'cDNA library' may be produced. The problem faced after production of such libraries is to separate or isolate the DNA sequences of interest from the overwhelming number of sequences which remain. Several strategies have evolved for tackling this problem, the most commonly used of which employ specific DNA probes which will hybridise to complementary sequences of DNA.

Strategies for the preparation of genomic and complementary DNA libraries and screening of such libraries with labelled nucleic acid probes, as well as by other methods, are described briefly below.

Construction and analysis of cDNA libraries

The production of double-stranded cDNA by enzymatic conversion from mRNA templates and insertion of this DNA into prokaryotic vectors has become one of the most fundamental procedures of molecular biology. The production of cDNA depends in part on the observation that the vast majority of mRNA molecules have at their 3′ ends a series of adenine nucleotide residues termed a polyA tail. The existence of this tail, which is specific to mRNAs, allows the relative purification of mRNAs from other RNA molecules by the use of synthetic strands of oligo-dT residues which are complementary to polyA sequences, allowing the production of 'polyA+' mRNA.

The first step in the cDNA cloning process is purification of such polyA+ mRNA. The higher the concentration of the mRNA sequences of interest in polyA+ mRNA, the template for cDNA production, the easier the task of isolating relevant cDNA clones from a cDNA library. The simplest strategy for ensuring a high concentration of relevant mRNAs is to prepare mRNA from a cell line or tissue which is known to express the relevant gene product in abundance. Thus, in the synthesis of pituitary-hormone cDNAs, the construction of a cDNA library from mRNA prepared from pituitary tissues represents the obvious choice [2]. Initially, the ability to clone cDNAs was confined to mRNAs produced in great abundance by specific tissues, such as globin production by bone marrow cells. In this example, the mRNA species of interest represents up to 90% of total polyA+ RNA within that tissue, so that no further purification of mRNA is required before proceeding to synthesis of cDNA [3]. The relevant cDNA can in turn be identified easily by hybridisation of recombinant plasmid clones to radiolabelled single-stranded cDNA produced *in vitro* from mRNA by the action of reverse transcriptase; there is a high probability that any hybridising colony will contain the cDNA sequences of interest. Unfortunately, this cloning strategy is relevant to only a handful of abundant mRNAs, with more sophisticated techniques being required for the preparation of other cDNAs.

A typical mammalian cell contains approximately 20 000 different mRNA species, so that account has to be taken of the size of the cDNA library required to ensure that the mRNA of interest is represented in the library and then great care taken to identify and isolate the relevant clone. If attempts are made to isolate a cDNA whose corresponding mRNA is of very low abundance, then steps have to be taken to enrich the mRNA from which cDNA is prepared. One such method of enrichment is fractionation of mRNA by size. This strategy works most efficiently if the size of the mRNA of interest is clearly different from the bulk of the mRNA species within the cell. In such cases, the mRNA can be enriched approximately 10-fold by density gradient centrifugation carried out under denaturing conditions. This method of enrichment depends upon estimation of likely mRNA size from an estimation of the size of its protein product, but it has to be noted that there is considerable variation in the relationship between mRNA and protein product size due to variation in lengths of 3′ and 5′ untranslated regions of mRNA molecules. After fractionation of mRNA species according to size, each fraction can be investigated for the presence of the relevant mRNA by the efficiency of production of its specific protein or polypeptide product. Typically, separate fractions of mRNA can be translated *in vitro* and resulting protein products immunoprecipitated in order to identify the fraction directing the greatest amount of synthesis of the relevant product. Alternatively, cDNA molecules, rather than mRNA molecules, can be fractionated according to size. This method has the advantage that cDNA molecules are less susceptible to degradation by nucleases than mRNAs, and the molecules of cDNA can be separated according to size more accurately by using agarose gels. A further method of enrichment involves the use of specific antibodies to concentrate polysomes which are synthesizing the protein or polypeptide of interest.

All methods for the synthesis of cDNA from mRNA employ the enzyme reverse transcriptase described above to catalyse the reaction. Like other polymerases, reverse transcriptase requires a primer to initiate its action; the most frequently used primer is synthetic oligo-dT which binds to the polyA tails of mRNA molecules and allows efficient catalysis of cDNA synthesis (Fig. 2.4). At the end of this

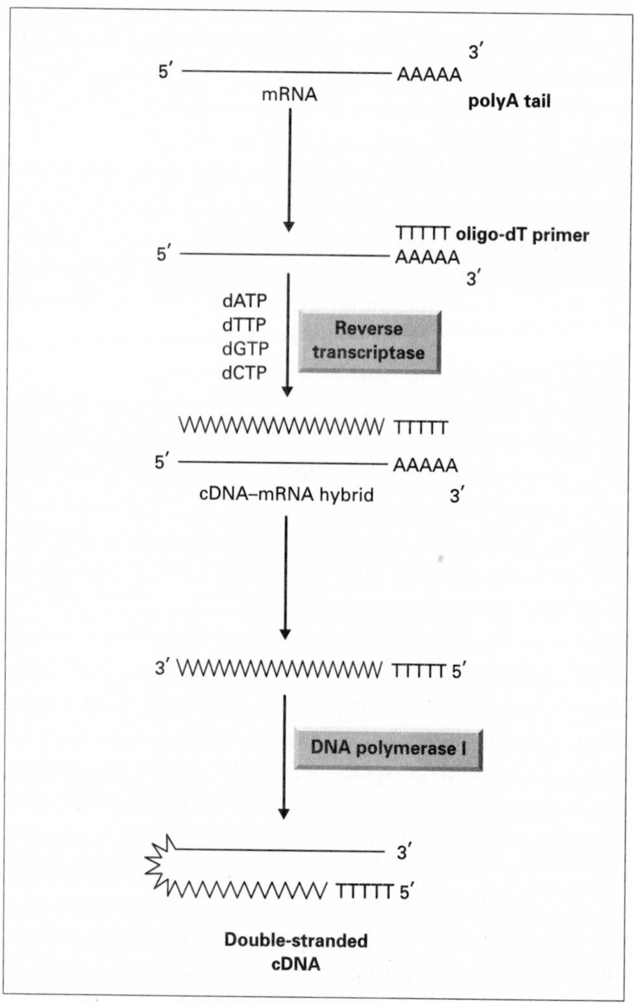

Fig. 2.4 Synthesis of cDNA from mRNA.

reaction a cDNA–mRNA hybrid is formed, the next step in the cDNA cloning process being to denature this hybrid to produce single-stranded cDNA. Several strategies have been developed for the production of double-stranded cDNA molecules from single-stranded templates, the most straightforward of which is illustrated in Fig. 2.4. This method involves the synthesis of the second strand of cDNA from the first strand by use of a DNA polymerase. In an alternative strategy, the mRNA–cDNA hybrid is used as a template for a 'nick translation' reaction (Fig. 2.2a), the mRNA strand of the hybrid being replaced by the second strand of the cDNA molecule. The resulting cDNA molecules are then inserted into prokaryotic vectors as described above, and various methods are employed to screen the resulting cDNA library for clones of interest.

After construction of a cDNA library, recombinant clones may be screened with either antibodies or nucleic acid probes. Nucleic acid hybridisation represents the most commonly used method of screening libraries since this technique allows large numbers of clones to be examined simultaneously and does not necessitate the synthesis of a biologically or immunologically active peptide or protein product. Homologous DNA probes are used when an incomplete cDNA is already available and can be used as a probe to screen a library for a clone containing a full-length cDNA, while partially homologous probes can be used to detect cDNAs which are closely related structurally to the available probe, such as a cDNA encoding the same protein product but in a different species. Examples of these approaches in endocrine research include the cloning of a full-length cDNA for the rat glycoprotein hormone α-subunit [4], and the cloning of the human cDNA for the thyrotrophin receptor using a canine cDNA encoding the same receptor [5].

An alternative strategy is termed differential hybridization, an approach which is used to detect a cDNA corresponding to an mRNA which is transcriptionally regulated by factors such as hormones. Labelled single-stranded cDNAs are synthesized *in vitro* from sets of mRNAs prepared from cells or tissues which have either been treated by the known regulatory factor or are untreated controls. The two sets of cDNA probes are then used to screen replicas of a cDNA library prepared from treated cells or tissues (if searching for a gene product which is induced by treatment) or untreated cells (if searching for a gene product which is repressed), and clones that hybridise preferentially to one of the cDNA probes are chosen for further analysis. This approach was used successfully to clone the cDNA for rat malic enzyme, an enzyme induced by the thyroid hormone triiodothyronine [6].

An alternative method for screening cDNA libraries for clones of interest involves the use of synthetic oligonucleotide probes, i.e. short nucleotide sequences of known structure which are produced *in vitro*. This method is used increasingly and depends upon the availability of limited sequence information regarding the clone of interest; information is usually based upon the partial amino-acid structure of its gene product, or partial sequence information from cDNAs which have already been cloned. Because of degeneracy of the genetic code, it is impossible to predict with certainty the oligonucleotide sequence giving rise to a particular amino-acid sequence, but one solution to this problem is to synthesise a group of oligonucleotides containing all of the theoretical sequences that will code for a given group of amino acids. A variation on this method is to carry out hybridisation under conditions of low stringency (i.e. high salt) which will allow probe–cDNA association under conditions of less than 100% base-pair matching. Another approach to library screening aimed at identifying novel genes which are related to previously isolated genes is the use of degenerate oligonucleotide-primed PCR (see below).

Complementary DNA libraries which have been constructed in expression vectors, i.e. vectors which direct the *in vitro* transcription and translation of cloned sequences, can alternatively be screened with antibody directed against the protein of interest. Using this approach, transformed bacteria are lysed, their intracellular proteins transferred to a hybridisation membrane and the membrane soaked in a solution of antibody. Hybridisation of antibody to a specific protein product of the host bacterial colony is then detected by reaction with a second antibody or *Staphylococcus aureus* protein A. Screening with antibodies for specific protein products synthesized *in vitro* from recombinant sequences in expression vectors has been used successfully in the cloning of several important endocrine-related cDNAs including the DNA-binding COUP (chicken ovalbumin upstream promoter) transcription factor [7]. The potential success of this approach has been enhanced by a recent modification to DNA library protocols which increases the number of clones capable of producing functional protein. Directional cloning produces cDNA species which are orientated 5′–3′ with respect to the plasmid promoter and are thus able to produce a functional transcript. This is achieved by adding a specific restriction enzyme site to the 3′ end of the oligo-dT sequence used to reverse transcribe each mRNA. By cutting with the enzyme specific for this site, together with another enzyme to cut at the 5′ end, it is possible to correctly orientate the cDNA clone with respect to plasmid transcription. Directionally cloned cDNA libraries have been essential in the development of the technique of 'expression cloning'. This method is dependent on the cDNA library being divided into large numbers of 'pools', each containing 1000–3000 clones. These are then transfected and expressed in eukaryotic cells so that pools containing a cDNA of interest can be detected using a functional assay for the target protein. Positive pools can then be further divided until a single clone remains. Expression cloning has enabled the isolation of a variety of genes including cell-surface antigens detected using antibody-binding assays. However, in endocrinology this approach has been particularly successful in enabling the identification of steroidogenic enzymes such as 17β-hydroxysteroid dehydrogenase type 2, each cDNA pool being screened by simple 'substrate–product' reactions [8].

Despite promising hybridisation of cDNA clones within a library to a DNA or oligonucleotide probe, or hybridisation of the protein product of those clones to a relevant antibody, several steps have to be taken to ensure that the identified cDNAs include the sequences of interest. These steps include: (i) the identification of cloned cDNA sequences appropriate to the known amino-acid sequence of the protein product; (ii) immunoprecipitation of polypeptide or protein synthesized *in vitro* from the cDNA by antibodies to the authentic polypeptide or protein gene product; or (iii) expression from the full-length cDNA of a protein with appropriate biological activity. Despite these methods of verification, it is still possible to draw the wrong conclusions from analysis of the structure and properties of cloned cDNAs.

Construction of genomic libraries

Similar principles are used in the construction of genomic DNA libraries to those used in the construction of cDNA libraries described above. Initially, production of such libraries involved the complete digestion of genomic DNA with a restriction enzyme such as EcoRI, but since such an enzyme is capable of digesting DNA into multiple small fragments of approximately 4 kb in size, a huge number of recombinants is required to ensure inclusion of the sequences of interest. The solution to this and other problems related to the small size of DNA fragments is the cloning of larger fragments of DNA produced by partial enzyme digestion or mechanical shearing. The resulting DNA fragments are then fractionated by density centrifugation to select those of appropriate size, and cloned into vectors which will accommodate larger fragments of DNA. Such vectors include bacteriophage lambda, cosmids or YACs described above. Random cleavage of DNA by partial digestion with restriction endonucleases has several advantages over complete digestion including: (i) reduction in size of the library required to ensure incorporation of the sequences of interest; (ii) the ability to clone sequences of DNA without prior knowledge of the restriction sites close to the gene under investigation; (iii) the ability to generate overlapping DNA clones from each chromosome. The latter facilitates identification of the entire DNA sequence of an individual chromosome, information which is likely to prove valuable in the characterisation of 'disease' genes specific to that chromosome. Another potential use for genomic libraries is in the cloning of genomic sequences of specific hormone or hormone-regulated genes. Availability of genomic sequences, rather than cDNA sequences, allows investigation of the mechanisms determining the control of gene expression, in particular investigation of the structure and function of 5′ flanking DNA sequences [9] which are intimately involved in the control of gene transcription as described above.

Preparation of radiolabelled DNA, RNA and oligonucleotide probes

The hybridisation of one molecule of nucleic acid to another represents a fundamentally important reaction in recombinant DNA technology, with every aspect of gene cloning and analysis involving the hybridization or binding of nucleic acids to each other. These aspects include the identification of clones of interest in cDNA and genomic libraries by hybridisation to DNA or oligonucleotide probes as described above, and analysis of DNA and RNA structure by Southern and Northern hybridisation to DNA and oligonucleotide probes as described below. The feasibility of these techniques depends upon the ability to radioactively label fragments of DNA or RNA copies of such fragments. Standard methods for radioactive labelling of probes are described in this section.

Two methods initially found wide acceptance in the production of labelled probes for use in hybridisation experiments: (i) the 'end-labelling' of DNA or RNA by transfer of the γ-phosphate of adenosine triphosphate (ATP) to the 5′ hydroxyl-terminus of DNA or RNA; and (ii) the labelling of dsDNA by 'nick translation'. Application of the former technique is limited by the ability to introduce only one radioactive atom into a molecule of nucleic acid at its 5′ end, while nick translation results in the production of fragmented probes containing sequences of both strands of DNA which may bind to each other in competition for binding to target sequences. To avoid these problems and to achieve probes of high specific activity, methods have been developed more recently for the production of single-stranded RNA probes complementary to cloned DNA sequences. This method, as well as nick translation and random primer labelling methods, are described briefly below.

The principle of nick translation of dsDNA probes has been illustrated in Fig. 2.2a. This labelling reaction depends on the property of *Escherichia coli* DNA polymerase I to add nucleotide residues to the 3′ hydroxyl end that is created when one strand of a dsDNA molecule is 'nicked' and at the same time to remove nucleotides from the 5′ end of the nick. Thus, by incubating a dsDNA template with the 'nicking' enzyme DNase I and radioactively labelled nucleotides, pre-existing non-labelled nucleotides are replaced by their labelled counterparts as DNA polymerase I results in propagation of 'nicks' along the molecules of DNA.

Another method in widespread use in the production of DNA probes is that of labelling using random oligonucleotide primers. It has been clearly established that polymerases can initiate DNA synthesis in the presence of appropriate primers and DNA or RNA templates. If small oligonucleotides of heterogeneous structure are used as primers in this reaction, they will hybridise at multiple sites on the DNA or RNA template and initiate the synthesis of a complete complementary product under the influence of RNA-dependent DNA polymerase (reverse transcriptase), in the case of a single-stranded RNA template, or Klenow enzyme/reverse transcriptase when the template is single-stranded DNA. By using radioactive nucleotides as precursors for DNA synthesis in this reaction, probes of high specific activity can be produced (Fig. 2.2b).

Nick translation and random primer methods have similar efficiencies when used to label approximately 50 ng of template. However, if larger amounts of labelled cDNA are required (approximately 1 μg) then nick translation is the preferred approach. Random primer labelling is the preferred technique when non-radioactive nucleotides are used to produce a probe. Fluorescent nucleotides are increasingly being used as an alternative to radioactive labelling, particularly with techniques such as *in situ* hybridisation. In addition to obvious safety aspects, fluorescent nucleotides produce labelled DNA which is much more stable than radioactively labelled DNA although the resulting hybridisations can be detected using similar autoradiographic methods. This approach, known as 'direct labelling', can also be used in conjunction with single-stranded RNA labelling (see below and Fig. 2.5). Other non-radioactive methods include 'indirect labelling' techniques which utilise digoxigenin or biotin-labelled DNA which is then detected by an antibody (or streptavidin in the case of biotin) complex containing an enzyme such as horseradish peroxidase. The enzyme can then be used to produce a colour change or, by catalysis of luminol oxidation, to generate light which can then be visualised using photographic film.

Single-stranded probes, comprising only one strand of a specific sequence of nucleic acid, have certain advantages over the use of the double-stranded probes described above, particularly the elimination of competitive hybridisation of complementary sequences of double-stranded probes to each other. However, the higher tissue binding may be complicated by an increase in non-specific binding. Single-stranded probes can be easily prepared using two methods: firstly, the production of labelled DNA complementary to

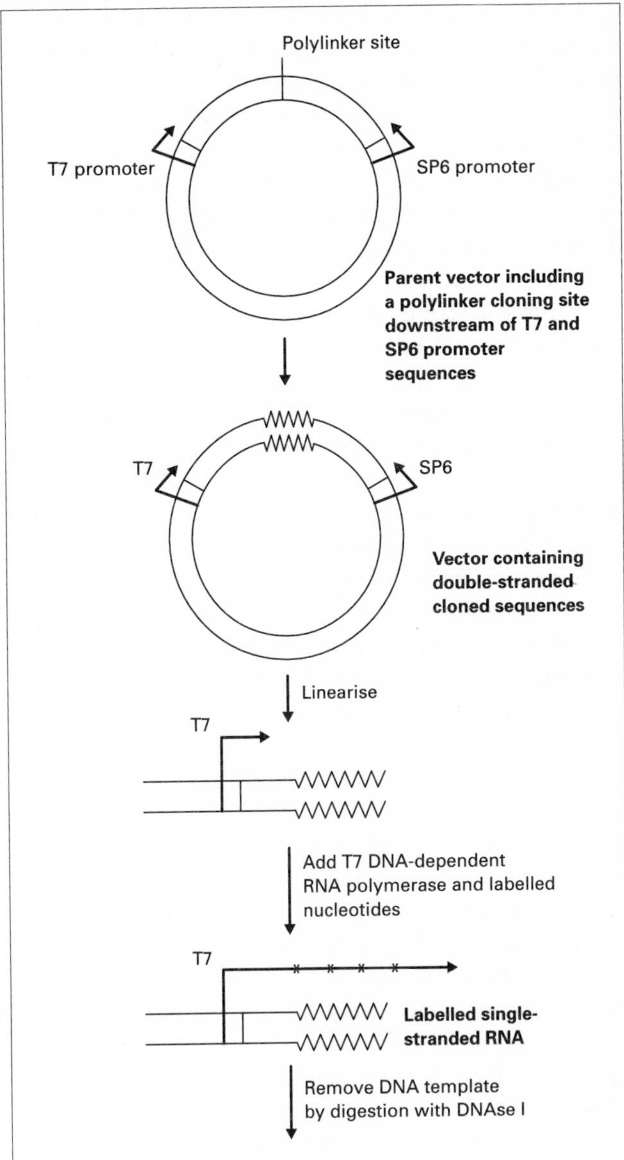

Fig. 2.5 Production of single-stranded RNA probes *in vitro*.

sequences cloned into certain bacteriophage vectors, and secondly, transcription of labelled RNA probes from DNA templates cloned into vectors which include bacteriophage RNA polymerase-dependent promoter sequences. Since the latter method does not necessitate the use of cumbersome methods of separation of labelled probe from template, it is now finding increasing application in the production of probes for use in hybridisation reactions.

The advances in vector technology that made it possible to synthesise single-stranded RNA of high specific activity *in vitro* included the development of vectors including synthetic polylinker sites described above and the location of such sites downstream of specific bacteriophage promoters such as SP6, T7 and T3, which are recognised specifically by DNA-dependent RNA polymerases encoded by their respective bacteriophages. This property of these bacteriophage promoters determines that when a linearised plasmid containing relevant sequences of cloned DNA is incubated in the presence of the appropriate RNA polymerase and radiolabelled nucleotide precursors, then synthesis of a single-stranded RNA molecule with incorporated labelled nucleotides is initiated at the bacteriophage promoter and terminates at the end of the linear molecule of DNA (Fig. 2.5). The transcripts produced from such a reaction are complementary to only one strand of the template and, by using specific RNA polymerases, it is possible to generate strand-specific probes for use in a number of hybridisation reactions described below. Single-stranded RNA probes share some of the advantages of single-stranded DNA probes, but in addition hybridise with greater affinity to target molecules of DNA because of the inherently greater stability of RNA–DNA hybrids over DNA–DNA hybrids.

Another group of probes used in hybridisation reactions is synthetic oligonucleotides. Usually these probes are single oligonucleotide strands of defined sequence which are synthesised *in vitro* according to the known amino-acid structure of the polypeptide or protein of interest, or match part of the sequence of a previously cloned cDNA. Such probes, which are generally between 20 and 40 nucleotides in length to allow specific hybridisation to complementary sequences, are used to screen cDNA or genomic libraries, as well as in Southern and Northern blot hybridisation assays described below. In addition, they have a part to play in the detection of specific mutations resulting from site-directed mutagenesis of cloned genes. Oligonucleotide probes used for these purposes are usually labelled as described above by end-labelling by transfer of the γ-phosphate of ATP to the 5′ hydroxyl-terminus of the oligonucleotide molecule.

In the preceding sections the basic tools of the molecular biologist have been described, namely the enzymes, prokaryotic vectors, nucleic acid probes and methods of labelling of such probes which are used in the investigation of gene structure and function. In the sections which follow, the application of these basic tools of recombinant DNA technology to endocrinology will be described, beginning with their role in the investigation of DNA structure and function and proceeding to their role in the investigation of RNA structure and function.

DNA extraction, purification and analysis

The basic technique which is used in the localization of specific sequences of DNA within genomic DNA is that of Southern blotting, described originally by Southern [10]. Briefly, genomic DNA is digested with one or more restriction enzymes and the resulting fragments of DNA are separated according to size by agarose gel electrophoresis. The DNA is then denatured and transferred by capillary or osmotic transfer from the agarose gel to a hybridisation membrane which is constructed from nitrocellulose or nylon. A replica of the DNA fragments on the gel is thus created on the membrane and immobilised DNA can be hybridised to an appropriate radiolabelled probe. Autoradiography of the membrane gives rise to a precise pattern of bands representing the fragment or fragments of DNA which contain sequences complementary to the probe employed (Fig. 2.6).

Southern blotting or Southern transfer is an important tool applied widely in the investigation of endocrine disease. Given the existence of a suitable cDNA or oligonucleotide probe, the structure of specific genes encoding hormones or other ‘candidate’ genes implicated in the aetiology of endocrine diseases can be analysed using this technique without the necessity for cloning of the complete hormone or candidate gene. The technique of Southern blotting is particularly applicable to investigation of endocrine diseases since the inherited nature of many endocrine disorders is well established, as illustrated in Table 2.1. These include single gene disorders inherited in both Mendelian dominant and recessive fashions, for which deletions or mutations in specific genes have been defined, and disorders for which the precise genetic basis of the disease has not been determined but in which linkage to a particular gene or chromosome locus has been found [11]. In addition to these single gene disorders, many common endocrine problems such as autoimmune thyroid disease and diabetes mellitus have a clear genetic component, albeit a polygenic component, and Southern blotting with analysis of restriction

Table 2.1 Examples of endocrine disorders with a genetic basis.

Disease	Affected gene or its localisation
Congenital adrenal hypoplasia	DAX-1
Congenital adrenal hyperplasia	21-hydroxylase β
GH deficiency type 1A	GH
Thyroid hormone resistance	β T3 receptor
Vitamin D resistant rickets type II	Vitamin D receptor
Testicular feminisation	Androgen receptor
Pseudohypoparathyroidism	G-protein α-subunit
Laron dwarfism	GH receptor
Insulin resistance	Insulin receptor
MEN 1	Chromosome 11
MEN 2	Chromosome 10 (RET proto-oncogene?)

DAX, dosage-sensitive sex, adrenal hypoplasia congenita critical region on the X-chromosome, gene 1; GH, growth hormone; MEN, multiple endocrine neoplasia; RET, receptor with tyrosine kinase activity.

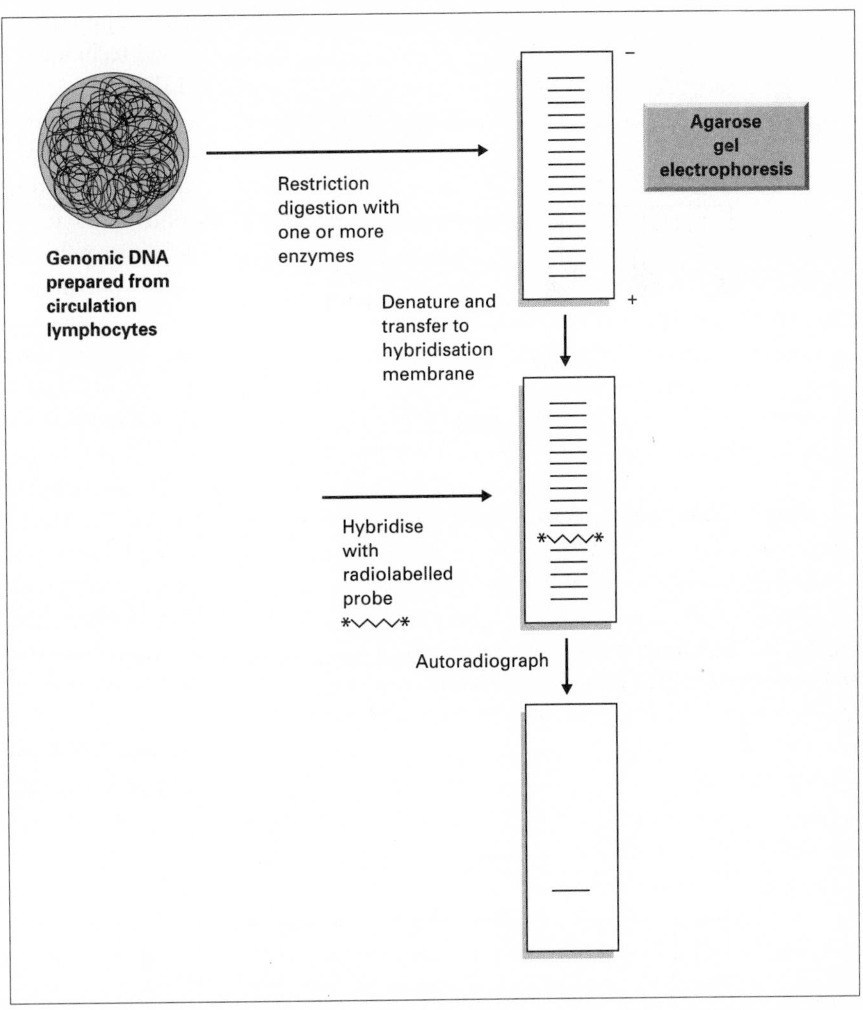

Fig. 2.6 Southern blotting of human genomic DNA.

fragment length polymorphisms has provided clues to the genetic basis of these disorders.

One of the first endocrine disorders to be investigated using the technique of Southern blotting was that of isolated growth hormone (GH) deficiency [12]. Several single gene disorders with different modes of inheritance have been found to result in isolated GH deficiency. In type IA deficiency, GH secretion is entirely absent, a problem which has been shown to be related to a large deletion of chromosome 17 which includes one of a cluster of GH genes found in the human genome. An example of a Southern blot from a kindred with type IA GH deficiency is illustrated in Fig. 2.7. In these studies, total genomic DNA was prepared from circulating white blood cells, digested with a specific restriction enzyme chosen to cut the GH gene into fragments of defined length and at the same time to digest the rest of the DNA into fragments of differing sizes, prior to fractionation of these fragments by gel electrophoresis, Southern transfer to a hybridisation membrane and hybridisation to a radiolabelled GH cDNA probe. In the example shown, a different pattern of hybridisation of the GH probe to DNA fragments is seen in the parents who are heterozygous for the disorder to that seen in the affected offspring, who exhibit homozygous deletion of the critical GH gene sequences.

Another endocrine disorder with a similar genetic basis to type IA GH deficiency is deficiency of the enzyme 21-hydroxylase which results in congenital adrenal hyperplasia. This enzyme defect results in 90–95% of cases of congenital adrenal hyperplasia, and is inherited as an autosomal recessive trait closely linked to the human leucocyte antigen (HLA) major histocompatability complex on the short arm of chromosome 6. Prenatal detection of congenital adrenal hyperplasia is essential for genetic counselling as well as for treatment of affected females. This has been addressed, in part, by Southern blot analysis of DNA isolated from chorionic villi. However, it is now evident that 21-hydroxylase deficiency results from a complex series of mutations; approximately 95% of these resulting in recombinations between the 21-hydroxylase gene (CYP21) and a linked homologous gene, CYP21P. In view of this, more

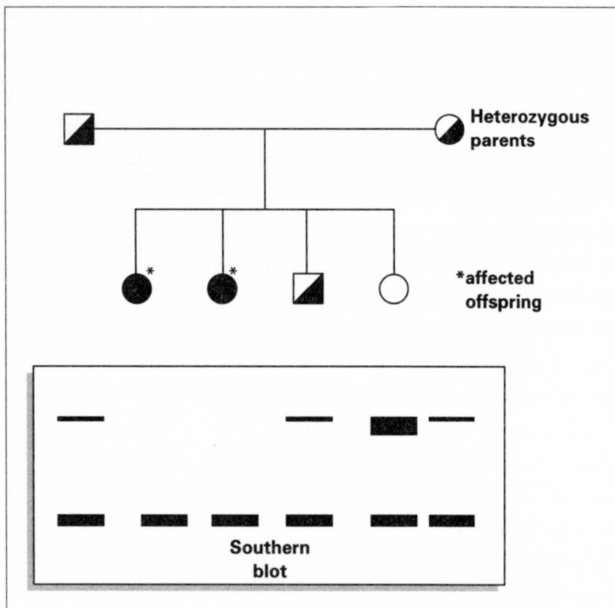

Fig. 2.7 Southern blotting of genomic DNA prepared from a family affected by type IA growth hormone deficiency and hybridisation to a radiolabelled growth hormone cDNA probe.

recent approaches to prenatal diagnosis have utilised PCR-based techniques to identify recipients of a defective gene [13].

Unlike isolated GH deficiency and 21-hydroxylase deficiency, the precise basis of some inherited disorders is far from obvious. None the less, Southern blotting has contributed to our understanding of these disorders by defining a pattern of inheritance through restriction fragment length polymorphisms (RFLPs) and by determination of more precise chromosomal locations for disease loci. This has, in turn, allowed more detailed analysis of candidate regions of chromosomes. Perhaps the best examples of this are the multiple endocrine neoplasia (MEN) syndromes type I and II (see below and Chapters 45 and 46).

RFLPs reflect individual variations in DNA sequence which are due to deletions, additions or base substitutions. These variations in DNA structure are common, especially in non-coding sequences, and usually do not affect gene function. None the less, they may result in the presence or absence of specific restriction sites, so that a DNA polymorphism may result in the production of an RFLP. The exact number and size of restriction fragments resulting from digestion of genomic DNA will vary between individuals in relation to the number of restriction sites for a specific enzyme present.

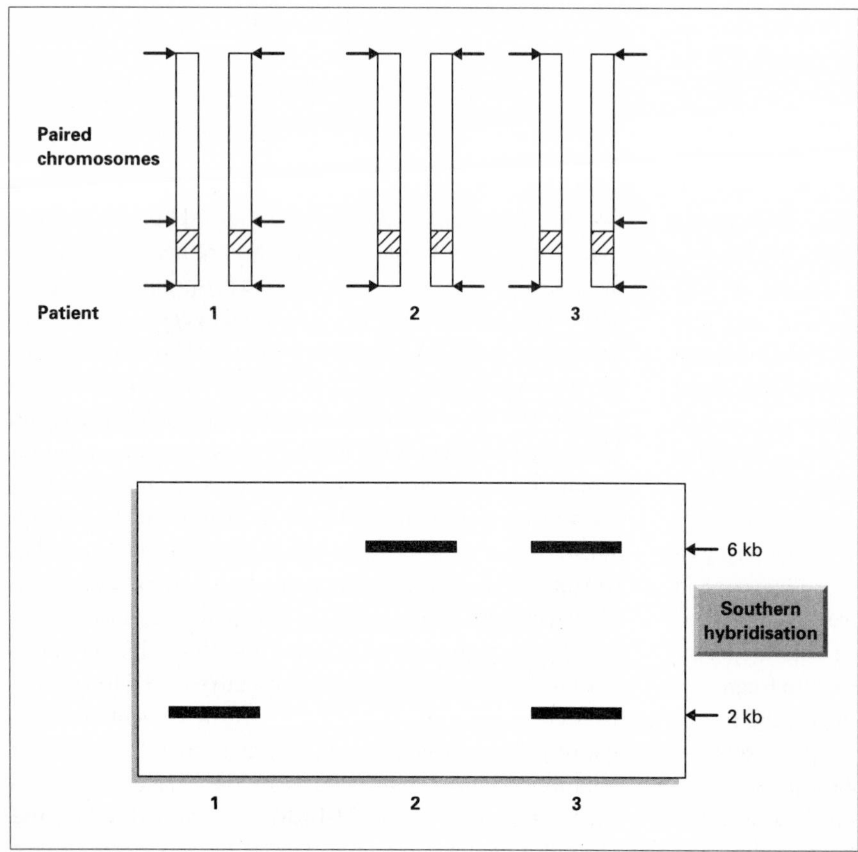

Fig. 2.8 Diagrammatic representation of restriction fragment length polymorphisms arising from changes in DNA structure giving variations in the number of restriction sites. Arrows indicate the presence of restriction sites and shaded areas the sequences complementary to the radiolabelled probe.

An example of such a polymorphism is shown in Fig. 2.8. In this example, one individual has three enzyme cleavage sites in the region of DNA under investigation so that digestion of DNA results in fragments of 2 and 4 kb in size. Only one of these fragments contains sequences complementary to the labelled probe so that hybridization with the probe results in the presence of a 2-kb band visible on the autoradiogram. In contrast, the second individual has lost one of these restriction sites through a minor change in DNA structure so that enzyme digestion results in the presence of only a 6-kb DNA fragment; this fragment contains the sequences within the 2-kb band visualised in the first case so that in this instance a 6-kb band is visible on the autoradiogram. In the third example shown, this subject is heterozygous for the presence and absence of the restriction enzyme site described in the second case, so that hybridisation with the probe in this instance reveals two DNA fragments of 2 and 6 kb in size. These RFLPs, which are inherited in a Mendelian fashion, can be used as markers of disease in families with inherited endocrine disorder such as MEN syndromes and can be used to follow the pattern of inheritance through the family.

The consistent inheritance of a specific RFLP allelle with a particular disease indicates that the locations of the restriction enzyme site and the disease gene are close. RFLP alleles which are close to a disease gene will consistently be co-inherited with the disease, whereas alleles that are further away will not cosegregate, except due to chance crossing-over or recombination of DNA occurring at meiosis. By investigating these recombination events in families affected with particular disorders such as MEN syndromes, it has proved possible to define the distance between one gene and a second (the disease gene) and ascertain the likelihood that they are linked. Through examination of RFLP linkages arising from use of a large number of chromosome marker probes in affected families it has been demonstrated that the gene for MEN syndrome type 1 resides in the pericentromeric region of the long arm of chromosome 11 [14]. Using a similar approach, MEN type 2 was initially localized to the centromeric region of chromosome 10 (see also Chapters 46 and 47). Further RFLP analysis has mapped the MEN 2 disease locus to a 500 kb region within chromosome 10 and the probable causative gene has been proposed (RET proto-oncogene) [15]. While this approach has a lot to offer to our knowledge of single gene disorders, it has also added to our understanding of endocrine disorders inherited in a more complex fashion. Much attention currently focuses on the genetic basis of common autoimmune endocrine disorders such as Graves' disease and insulin-dependent diabetes mellitus.

This type of work has been expanded even more by the realisation that there are large numbers of non-coding areas of the genome in which there are repeating regions of, typically, a pair of nucleotides, the number of repeats in any given region being highly variable. These variable-number tandem repeats (VNTRs) are also highly polymorphic, i.e. they vary considerably between individuals. Furthermore, a specific VNTR can be rapidly identified using PCR amplification technology (see below), and thus a VNTR of a known number of repeats associated with a nearby gene of interest. Thus, a given gene can be tracked through families in terms of its associated VNTR. In addition, the highly polymorphic nature of the VNTRs is the basis of the fingerprinting of genomic DNA, which has become an essential tool in forensic medicine.

While the methods of DNA analysis described in this section have resulted in major advances in our understanding of the genetic basis of endocrine disease, determination of the precise genetic nature of these disorders requires complete understanding of DNA structure and hence deduction of gene structure and function. This in turn demands the application of methods for the sequencing of DNA.

DNA sequencing

The most common method of DNA sequencing currently in use is the enzymatic method of Sanger [16]. In this method, specific terminators of DNA chain elongation, i.e. 2′, 3′ dideoxynucleotide triphosphates (ddNTPs), are used. These molecules differ from normal dNTPs in that they lack a hydroxyl residue at the 3′ position of deoxyribose. Like other deoxynucleotides, they can be incorporated into a growing chain of DNA produced by the action of DNA polymerases through binding of their 5′ triphosphate groups but they cannot form phosphodiester bonds with the next dNTP molecule. Thus, when a ddNTP such as ^{35}S-ddATP is included in the reaction mix for new DNA synthesis along with a DNA polymerase and an appropriate template, the products of a series of DNA chains are terminated at the dideoxy residue (Fig. 2.9). If four separate reactions, each containing a different ddNTP, are completed then the products of each reaction will be a series of oligonucleotide chains whose lengths are determined by the distance between the terminus of the primer used to initiate DNA synthesis and the sites of premature termination of DNA production. If these oligonucleotide products are separated by polyacrylamide gel electrophoresis, then the exact nucleotide sequence of a given fragment of DNA can be determined since populations of oligonucleotides will have been generated which terminate at positions occupied by every A, C, G, or T in the template strand of DNA.

In recent years increased demand for convenient DNA sequencing has led to a rapid evolution of protocols. Adaptations to the Sanger and Coulson method have allowed

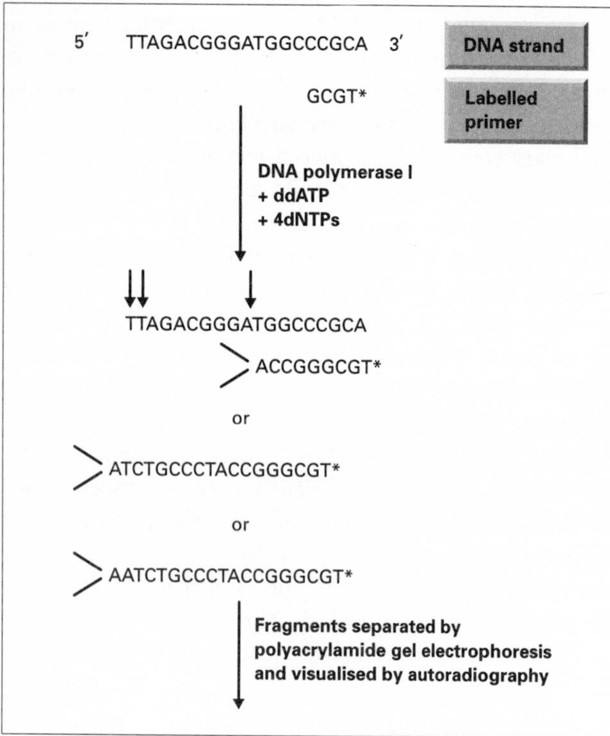

Fig. 2.9 Sequencing of DNA by the Sanger method. Arrows indicate the sites of termination of DNA synthesis by incorporation of ddATP.

DNA sequencing to become a routine laboratory technique, and access to automated DNA sequencers is now common for many laboratories. The advances which have enabled this include the use of variable DNA templates, additional sequencing enzymes and fluorescent labelling systems. However, recombinant plasmids can also be sequenced directly without the need for isolation of single-stranded DNA. Likewise, with the advent of PCR amplification of DNA products, direct sequencing of PCR fragments is now possible. In all of these cases a prerequisite is that the DNA template is relatively pure, either isolated on caesium chloride density gradients or by careful purification after separation on agarose gels. The size of the DNA template which can be sequenced varies according to the type of DNA and the sequencing enzyme, but is likely to be in the range of 200–500 bp. More recent advances in automated DNA sequencing have extended this capacity so that up to 1000 bp may be resolved using more expensive equipment.

Initial dideoxy sequencing involved the use of Klenow fragment DNA polymerase activity (Fig. 2.9) and, in some cases, reverse transcriptase. Each of these enzymes may have difficulty 'reading' certain DNA sequences and so they are frequently used in tandem. More recent protocols have employed *Taq* DNA polymerase and a modified T7 polymerase often referred to by its trademark, 'Sequenase'. Both of these enzymes have a higher rate of nucleotide incorporation than Klenow or reverse transcriptase and produce bands with consistent intensity and a high degree of accuracy. *Taq* polymerase is particularly useful because it has a high reaction temperature (70–80°C) which allows any secondary structures within the DNA to be melted out, thus permitting more efficient sequencing of certain DNA sequences. Visualisation of sequencing products is usually achieved by the incorporation of radiolabelled nucleotides and autoradiography. In Fig. 2.9 the sequencing reaction is illustrated by the use of a primer end-labelled with ^{32}P-ATP. However, labelling may also be carried out by incorporating a radiolabelled nucleotide into the mixture of dNTPs which extend the primer.

DNA sequencing has now become a common technique in many laboratories, particularly as more recent approaches to DNA sequencing have utilised the basic Sanger method whilst incorporating automated detection systems for analysis of sequencing products. A crucial feature of automated sequencing has been the development of fluorescent dyes as an alternative to radiolabelling. In addition to improving the ease of handling, fluorescent dyes allow rapid and efficient analysis of sequencing products. Basic sequencing is carried out using the above Sanger method with each of four reaction tubes receiving ddCTP, ddGTP, ddTTP or ddATP, together with either a blue, yellow, red or green fluorescent labelled primer. At the end of the reaction all four tubes are combined and separated in a single lane of a conventional sequencing gel which is housed in the automated sequencer. As the dye-labelled DNA bands migrate through the gel they pass a detection window which identifies the specific fluorescent colours. Thus, a blue band followed by a red and then a green would represent a DNA fragment ending in the sequence CTA. This method is known as 'dye-priming', but sequencing can also be carried out using a technique known as 'dye-termination' in which fluorescent dideoxynucleotides are used. Both *Taq* and modified T7 polymerase can be used with the above methods.

The advent of automated DNA sequencing has greatly expanded the scope for gene sequencing in endocrinology. This has, in part, been due to the characterisation of newly cloned genes but also reflects increased interest in identification of the specific gene defects which cause inherited hormone-related diseases. The latter include the afore-mentioned 21-hydroxylase defects [13], as well as more recently identified mutations in the gene for 11β-hydroxysteroid dehydrogenase [17,18]. Advances in gene sequencing have enabled extensive characterisation of abnormalities in the receptors for hormones. For example, identification of point mutations in the genes for proteins such as the androgen receptor [19], vitamin D receptor [20] and thyroid hormone receptor have now made it possible to analyse diseases of hormone resistance at the level of the nanometre. The widespread use of DNA sequencing in molecular endocrinology has been greatly facilitated by improvements in associated techniques, prominent amongst which are the advances in methods for DNA amplification.

Amplification of DNA by PCR

PCR is used to amplify a fragment of DNA that lies between two regions of DNA of known sequence. A pair of oligonucleotide molecules with structures complementary to the sequences flanking a particular region of interest are used as primers, and the reaction involves DNA polymerase directed synthesis of overlapping fragments of DNA which occurs in opposite directions. The template DNA is first denatured by heating in the presence of a molar excess of the oligonucleotide primers to be used and four specific dNTPs. The reaction mixture is then cooled so that single-stranded primers anneal to the denatured single-stranded DNA; under the influence of DNA polymerase I, DNA synthesis proceeds in a 5′→3′ direction. After further heat denaturation, the newly synthesised molecules, as well as the original template DNA, can reassociate with the primer and act as templates for further rounds of DNA synthesis. The cycle of denaturation, annealing and DNA synthesis is then repeated many times and theoretically amplification of the sequence of interest will increase exponentially to 2^n, where n is the number of cycles (Fig. 2.10). In practice, amplification levels of 10^9 to 10^{10} can be achieved with approximately 60 sequential cycles of denaturation, annealing and primer extension.

A major breakthrough leading to widespread application of this technique of DNA amplification was the purification of a thermostable *Taq* polymerase (isolated from the thermophilic bacterium *Thermus aquaticus*). This enzyme, which can survive incubation at 95°C, is not inactivated by the heat denaturation step in the PCR cycle and does not therefore need to be replaced with each new

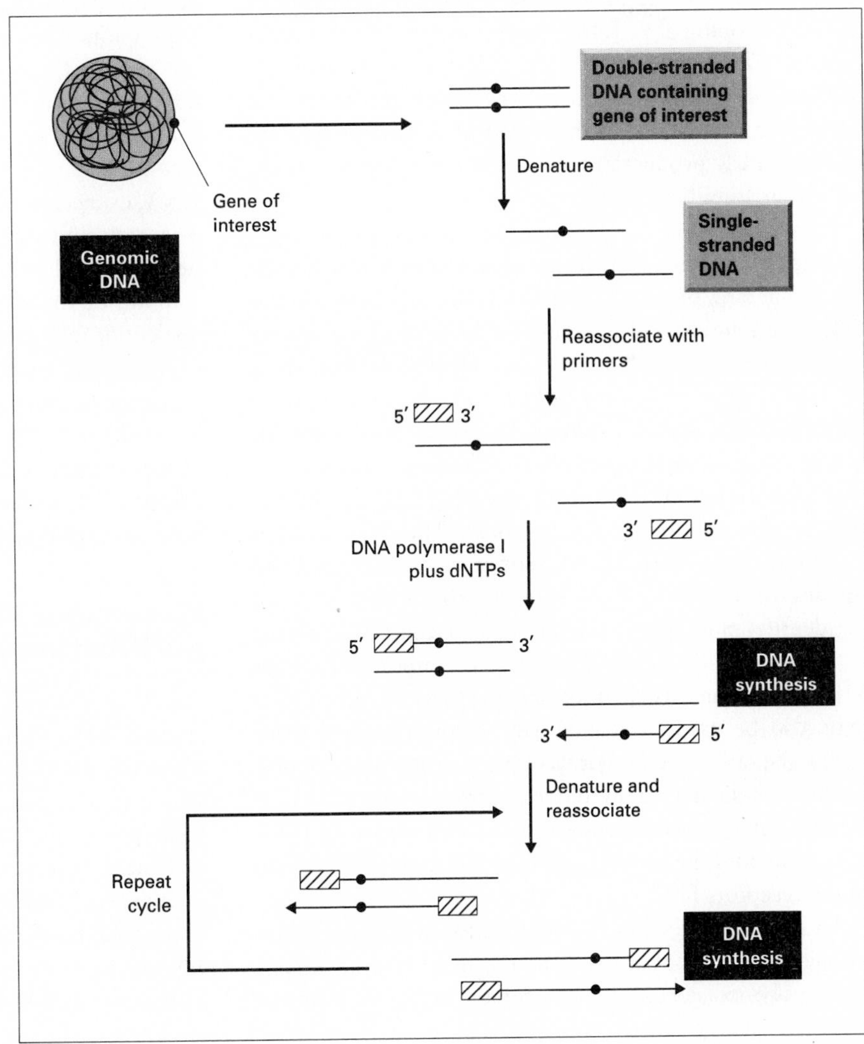

Fig. 2.10 Polymerase chain reaction amplification of specific sequences of human DNA.

cycle, leading to improvements in yield and specificity of the technique.

PCR amplification has found extensive application in the investigation of the genetic basis of human disease, including endocrine disorders, in the forensic analysis of DNA samples extracted from very small samples of DNA and in the identification of viral pathogens. More generally, the technique is finding application in the production of specific sequences of cloned cDNA for use as hybridisation probes, generation of large quantities of DNA for sequencing and for construction of libraries and in the analysis of point mutations. Rapid cloning of DNA using PCR methods has been improved following the observation that some preparations of *Taq* polymerase add an extraneous nucleotide (usually A) to the 3′ end of the amplified DNA fragment. As a result, several plasmid vectors have been designed which have a 'T overhang', thereby allowing direct cloning of the PCR fragment into the vector. PCR products can also be cloned into conventional vectors by 'blunt ending' the DNA using an enzyme such as T4 polymerase, the resulting DNA being ligated into a similarly blunt-ended plasmid. Cloning of PCR fragments into restriction enzyme-digested sites (see above and Fig. 2.3) can also be achieved using modified PCR primers. Sequences for restriction enzymes can be added to the 5′ end of primers so that the resulting PCR product automatically has a restriction site following amplification.

Primer variation has become the cornerstone of many new applications of PCR technology. In particular, the use of 'degenerate' primers to amplify DNA sequences similar to known gene sequences has greatly accelerated the cloning of novel genes. The basis of this method is that short oligonucleotides will prime DNA for PCR even when there is not a 100% match between the primer and target. At low annealing temperatures oligonucleotides may have several mismatches in relation to the target DNA and yet still be able to amplify the fragment. Thus, novel DNA similar to genes with known sequences can be amplified by 'degenerate primer PCR'. This approach has been used to identify interspecies similarities/variations for specific genes, such as the recent cloning of the mouse cDNA for 11β-hydroxysteroid dehydrogenase [21]. Degenerate primers may also be used to isolate cDNAs for related proteins within the same species. For example, recent cloning of new members of the steroid/thyroid receptor superfamily has been carried out using degenerate primers to a region of DNA which encodes the highly conserved DNA-binding domain of the receptors [22].

Another feature of PCR amplification which has revolutionised gene cloning concerns the development of new DNA polymerase enzymes which have improved both the fidelity of amplification and the size of templates which can be amplified. Basic *Taq* polymerase enzymes have a high capacity for DNA amplification over the variable temperature ranges required for PCR. However, depending on reaction conditions, the use of *Taq* may result in the incorporation of incorrect nucleotides to an amplified strand. This is because, unlike enzymes such as T4 and T7 polymerase, *Taq* does not have any 3′→5′ 'proof-reading' exonuclease activity. This may not be particularly important for many PCR applications but is crucial when PCR is used as part of a DNA-sequencing protocol. New thermostable DNA polymerase preparations (such as *pfu* and Vent) have been developed which include a mixture of 5′→3′ polymerase activity at high temperatures as well as proof-reading 3′→5′ activity, allowing PCR amplification of high-fidelity DNA fragments in excess of 20 kb in size. This so-called 'long-range' PCR has been important in the amplification and analysis of large fragments of genomic DNA so that complete exons or introns can be isolated.

PCR was originally used to directly amplify fragments of genomic DNA but is now frequently used to study RNA expression. This has many applications in cDNA cloning but reverse transcriptase PCR (RT-PCR) can now also be considered as an alternative to Northern blotting as a method for assessing expression of a particular mRNA species. The technique is dependent on reverse transcription of target RNA, using either oligo-dT or random hexamers as primers. The resulting cDNA can then be amplified by specific primers and detected on a gel directly by ethidium bromide staining of the DNA or by incorporating a radiolabelled nucleotide into the PCR mixture. RT-PCR has the advantage of requiring much smaller amounts of RNA than for Northern blotting (usually less than 1 μg) and may therefore be preferable when analysing small amounts of tissue. Disadvantages of RT-PCR include the relatively poor quantification of product, although several new methods have been developed which may solve this problem.

Messenger RNA extraction, purification and analysis

Preceding sections have described the major techniques applied in the analysis of DNA, i.e. in the analysis of gene structure in health and disease. Direct examination of the structure and hence function of the specific products of these genes, including both normal and abnormal gene products, demands analysis of the mRNA transcripts of such genes. Messenger RNA comprises approximately 5% of the total RNA present in a eukaryotic cell, the remaining RNA being made up of ribosomal RNA and small molecules of transfer RNA. Messenger RNA molecules which are transcribed from structural genes vary considerably in size from a few hundred bases to several kilobases and together encode all of the polypeptide or protein products of a given tissue or cell.

A critical step in the purification of mRNA from tissues or cells is inactivation of RNases liberated by cell lysis since mRNAs are especially susceptible to degradation by such enzymes. This involves treatment of all glassware by heating to destroy exogenous RNases and the use of specific chemical inhibitors of RNase actions. One of the most widely applied methods of RNA preparation which involves the use of an RNase inhibitor has been described by Chirgwin [23]; in this procedure the RNase inhibitor guanadinium isothiocyanate is used to disrupt cells or tissues, additional mechanical homogenisation being used as necessary. In the past RNA has then been separated from other nucleic acids by centrifugation of the homogenate through a caesium chloride density gradient [24]. Alternative methods of RNA preparation involve the separation of nuclear and cytoplasmic fractions of cells or tissues by tissue disruption with a detergent, centrifugation to produce a nuclear pellet and extraction of RNA from the cytoplasmic fraction using a mixture of phenol and chloroform. These latter techniques have been optimised such that routine extraction of RNA from tissue can now be readily accomplished in an hour or two.

A number of methods have been developed to quantify RNA production and to investigate the size of specific mRNAs, to map their 3′ and 5′ termini and to localise their production to specific cells or tissues.

Northern blot hybridisation represents one of the most widely applied techniques in RNA analysis. It involves separation, according to size, of total mRNA molecules prepared from a specific tissue by denaturing agarose gel electrophoresis. The mRNA is then transferred to a hybridisation membrane (using a similar method described in Southern blotting) and hybridised to radiolabelled DNA, RNA or oligonucleotide probes in order to locate the complementary mRNA species of interest. This technique is used to determine the size of specific mRNA transcripts of genes for which DNA, RNA or oligonucleotide probes are available, and to determine factors which regulate the degree of transcription of that gene and hence alter the level of mRNA in a given tissue [25].

A simpler technique which does not involve gel electrophoresis in the size separation of mRNAs is that of dot hybridisation described by White and Bancroft [26]. This technique allows analysis of mRNA levels in multiple tissue or cell samples and can therefore be used in studies of regulation of gene transcription since levels of specific mRNAs in treated or untreated samples can be quantified. In this method, samples of RNA are applied directly to a hybridisation membrane, which is usually held in a manifold to allow precise immobilisation of the RNA samples in 'dots' or 'slots', and hybridisation to a radiolabelled cDNA or oligonucleotide probe as before. Densitometric tracings of resulting autoradiograms allow comparative estimates of the amount of target mRNAs in different tissue or cell samples; this technique, like that of Northern blotting, has been widely applied in endocrinology in the investigation of regulation of hormone gene expression by other hormones, growth factors, etc. and in studies of hormonal regulation of other target genes [27]. From such studies it has been possible to deduce the importance of transcriptional regulation of hormone genes and hormonal regulatory effects on other genes in cell physiology and endocrine disease, and for the first time has allowed sensitive examination of the factors that control hormone synthesis.

Alternative techniques for measurement of RNA expression include RT-PCR (see above) and RNase protection assays. The latter utilises the ability of RNase enzymes such as RNase A or S1 nuclease to degrade single-stranded RNA. Specific mRNAs can therefore be detected by adding a radiolabelled complementary probe (transcribed *in vitro*) which anneals to the target message. The resulting double-stranded mRNA is protected against ribonuclease activity and can be detected by gel separation and autoradiography. RNase protection assays are much more sensitive than Northern blots as they eliminate the inefficiencies which occur during the transfer of RNA to nitrocellulose membranes. This approach has been particularly successful in the mapping of the transcription-initiation sites of genes.

While all of the techniques described in this section have found widespread application in the investigation of endocrine physiology and pathology, they all harbour the limitation that they do not provide information regarding *which* cell within a given tissue is expressing the mRNA product of interest. Addressing this question demanded the development of the technique of *in situ* hybridisation, which is related to the technique of immunocytochemistry. *In situ* hybridisation involves the hybridisation of radiolabelled RNA or DNA probes complementary to the mRNA under investigation in frozen or paraffin embedded fixed tissue sections. After hybridisation the sections are dipped in photographic emulsion and stained. Cells which express the gene under investigation are then identified by the presence of silver grains localised over the cell. This technique has proved invaluable in a number of endocrine systems, such as the localisation of somatostatin in different tissues and cell types [28] and in the investigation of cell-specific expression of parathyroid hormone-related peptide [29].

Future applications of recombinant DNA technology to endocrinology

As outlined above, advances in recombinant DNA technology have revolutionised our approach to the understanding of the molecular basis of endocrine physiology and endocrine diseases. Some examples of specific areas in which recombinant DNA technology has contributed are illustrated in Table 2.2. Clinical endocrinology has benefited greatly from advances in molecular biology, not only because the inheritance patterns of a large number of endocrine disorders have been well characterised, but also because a large number of hormone and target genes have been cloned, providing unique information regarding the structure and function of these gene products. The availability of detailed sequence information for certain hormone genes, including those encoding insulin and growth hormone, is already exerting a major therapeutic impact through production of recombinant hormones *in vitro*. In addition, the precise chromosomal location of the 'disease' genes which cause various endocrine disorders has led to the prenatal diagnosis of some of these disorders and, in cases such as congenital adrenal hyperplasia, is leading to prenatal treatment.

Developments for the future are likely to involve increasing sophistication of recombinant DNA techniques, allowing improved sensitivity and specificity of the results of hybridisation methods, identification of the specific DNA sequences in coding and non-coding regions of the genome which result in expression of inherited endocrine disorders, and precise characterisation of the abnormal gene products which account for the phenotypic expression of such disorders. The continuing evolution of PCR-based methods is likely to play a prominent role in the development of new approaches to endocrine analysis. Techniques such as 'differential display PCR' (DD-PCR) have greatly expanded the scope for identifying new target genes for hormone action [30]. DD-PCR is also known as 'RNA fingerprinting' and is based on the concept that, by using particular combinations of reverse transcriptase primers and PCR primers, it is possible to amplify a known percentage of mRNAs for a given tissue under specific conditions. Like many of the other methods described above, DD-PCR can now be carried out using convenience kits. Another approach to gene cloning which may become more accessible in future is that of so-called 'reverse genetics'. Many inherited disorders are likely to occur as the result of defects in, as yet, unknown genes. Reverse genetics seeks to identify these genes by mapping the gene locus to a specific area of a particular chromosome. This requires large numbers of patient samples for initial analysis of RFLPs (see above), which enables the gene locus to be more precisely located and which may then allow the appropriate piece of genomic DNA to be cloned into a vector. This fragment of DNA may consist of more than 100 000 bp and a variety of complex procedures are then required to precisely localise the target gene within this fragment. At present this approach to gene cloning is extremely demanding but has led to some important discoveries in the field of inherited endocrine disorders [31].

The technological advances so far achieved are beginning to make it worthwhile to consider new remedies for endocrine disorders with a genetic basis, as well as some hormone deficiency states which are not strictly genetic in origin.

Table 2.2 Advances in endocrine physiology and disease which have resulted from application of recombinant DNA technology.

Physiology	Disease
Plasma membrane receptors—TSH, insulin	Insulin resistance
Intracellular signalling systems—G-proteins, protein kinases	Pseudohypoparathyroidism
Nuclear hormone receptors—thyroid and steroid hormones	Thyroid, androgen and vitamin D resistance
Hormone response elements—thyroid and steroid hormones	
Hormone gene structure—growth hormone, insulin	Growth hormone, insulin deficiency
Transcriptional regulation of hormone genes—insulin, pituitary hormones	
Hormone processing and secretion—insulin	
Hormone transport proteins—thyroid hormone binding proteins	Transthyretin, thyroxine-binding globulin and serum thyroid hormone levels
Steroid hormone metabolism—glucocorticoid androgen and oestrogen metabolism	Apparent mineralocorticoid excess, congenital adrenal hyperplasia, polycystic ovary syndrome

TSH, thyroid-stimulating hormone.

Correction of insulin deficiency has recently become a practical proposition [32]. Several proposals for this have been put forward including the production of 'foreign' insulin from transgenic animals expressing the human insulin gene or by using 'surrogate islets'—intraperitoneal injection of cells transfected with a glucose-sensitive insulin gene expression vector. Further developments in gene therapy are likely to arise from the direct incorporation of engineered genes into embryonic stem cells, allowing the integration and expression of this gene into the developing embryo [33,34].

Endocrinology is traditionally a field of medicine which is based upon sound cell biology and physiology, and it is in our general understanding of endocrine physiology and more broadly in our understanding of the impact of hormone action on cell function in areas such as oncogenesis, ageing and reproduction that the application of molecular biology is likely to exert its greatest impact.

References

1 Carlberg C, Bendik I, Wyss A *et al.* Two nuclear signalling pathways for vitamin D. *Nature* 1993; **361**: 657–60.

2 Chin WW, Kronenburg HM, Dee PC, Maloof F, Habener JF. Nucleotide sequence of the mRNA encoding the pre-α subunit of mouse thyrotrophin. *Proc Natl Acad Sci USA* 1981; **78**: 5329–31.

3 Rougeon F, Kourilsky P, Mach B. Insertion of a rabbit β globin gene sequence into an E coli plasmid. *Nucleic Acids Res* 1975; **2**: 2365–9.

4 Godine JC, Chin WW, Habener JF. α Subunit of the rat pituitary glycoprotein hormones. *J Biol Chem* 1982; **257**: 8368–71.

5 Libert F, Lefort A, Gerard C *et al.* Cloning, sequencing and expression of the human TSH receptor: evidence for binding of autoantibody. *Biochem Biophys Res Commun* 1989; **165**: 1250–5.

6 Magnuson MA, Nikodem VM. Molecular cloning of a cDNA sequence for rat malic enzyme. *J Biol Chem* 1983; **258**: 12712–17.

7 Wang L-H, Tsai SY, Cook RG, Beattie WG, Tsai M-J, O'Malley BW. COUP transcription factor is a member of the steroid receptor superfamily. *Nature* 1989; **340**: 163–6.

8 Wu L, Einstein M, Geissler WM, Chan HK, Elliston KO, Andersson S. Expression cloning and characterization of human 17β-hydroxysteroid dehydrogenase type 2, a microsomal enzyme possessing 20α-hydroxysteroid dehydrogenase activity. *J Biol Chem* 1993; **268**: 12964–9.

9 Balfour NJ, Franklyn JA, Gurr JA, Sheppard MC. Multiple DNA elements determine basal and thyroid hormone regulated expression of the human glycoprotein α subunit gene in pituitary cells. *J Endocrinol* 1990; **4**: 187–90.

10 Southern EM. Detection of specific sequences among DNA fragments separated by gel electrophoresis. *J Mol Biol* 1975; **98**: 503–17.

11 Jameson JL, Arnold A. Recombinant DNA strategies for determining the molecular basis of endocrine disorders. *J Clin Endocrinol Metab* 1990; **70**: 301–7.

12 Vnencak-Jones CL, Phillips JA, Chen EY, Seeburg PH. Molecular basis of human growth hormone deletions. *Proc Natl Acad Sci USA* 1988; **85**: 5615–19.

13 Owerbach D, Draznin MB, Carpenter RJ, Greenberg F. Prenatal diagnosis of 21-hydroxylase deficiency congenital adrenal hyperplasia using the polymerase chain reaction. *Human Genet* 1992; **89**: 109–10.

14 Petty EM, Green JS, Marx SJ, Taggart RT, Farid N, Bale AE. Mapping the gene for hereditary hyperparathyroidism and prolactinoma (MEN1Burin) to chromosome 11q: evidence for a founder effect in patients from Newfoundland. *Am J Hum Gen* 1994; **54**: 1060–1066.

15 Mulligan LM, Kwok JBJ, Healey CS *et al.* Germ-line mutations of the RET proto-oncogene in multiple endocrine neoplasia type 2a (MEN2A). *Nature* 1993; **363**: 458–69.

16 Sanger F, Coulson AR. A rapid method for determining sequences in DNA by primed synthesis with DNA polymerase. *J Mol Biol* 1975; **94**: 441–8.

17 Mune T, Rogerson FM, Nikkila H, Agarwal AK, White PC. Human hypertension caused by mutations in the kidney isoenzyme of 11β-hydroxysteroid dehydrogenase. *Nature Genet* 1995; **10**: 394–9.

18 Stewart PM, Krozowski ZS, Gupta A Milford DV, Howie AJ, Sheppard MC, Whorwood CB. Hypertension in the syndrome of apparent mineralocorticoid excess due to a mutation of the 11β-hydroxysteroid dehydrogenase type 2 gene. *Lancet* 1995; **347**: 88–91.

19 Patterson MN, McPhaul MJ, Hughes IA. Androgen insensitivity syndrome. *Baillière's Clin Endocrinol Metab* 1994; **8**: 379–404.

20 Hewison M, O'Riordan JL. Vitamin D resistance. *Baillière's Clin Endocrinol Metab* 1994; **8**: 305–15.

21 Cole TJ. Cloning of the mouse 11β-hydroxysteroid dehydrogenase type 2 gene: tissue specific expression and localization in distal con-voluted tubules and collecting ducts of the kidney. *Endocrinology* 1995; **136**: 4693–6.

22 Carlberg C, Hooft van Huijsduijnen R, Staple JK, DeLamarter JF, Becker-Andre M. RZRs, a new family of retinoid-related orphan receptors that function as both monomers and homodimers. *Mol Endocrinol* 1994; **8**: 757–70.

23 Chirgwin MJ, Przybyla AE, MacDonald RJ, Rutter WJ. Isolation of biologically active ribonucleic acid from sources enriched in ribonuclease. *Biochemistry* 1979; **18**: 5294–9.

24 Glisin V, Crkvenjakov R, Byus C. Ribonucleic acid isolated by cesium chloride centrifugation. *Biochemistry* 1974; **13**: 2633–7.

25 Franklyn JA, Wood DF, Balfour NJ, Ramsden DB, Docherty K, Chin WW, Sheppard MC. Effect of hypothyroidism and thyroid hormone replacement in vivo on pituitary cytoplasmic concentrations of TSH β and α subunit mRNAs. *Endocrinology* 1987; **120**: 2279–88.

26 White BA, Bancroft FC. Cytoplasmic dot hybridization. Simple analysis of relative mRNA levels in multiple small cell or tissue samples. *J Biol Chem* 1982; **257**: 8569–72.

27 Franklyn JA, Sheppard MC. Hormonal control of gene expression. *Clin Endocrinol* 1988; **29**: 337–48.

28 Hoefler H, Childers H, Montminy MR, Lechan RM, Goodman RH, Wolfe HJ. In situ hybridization methods for the detection of somatostatin mRNA in tissue sections using antisense RNA probes. *Histochem J* 1986; **18**: 597–604.

29 Heath DA, Senior PV, Varley JM, Beck F. Parathyroid-hormone-related protein in tumours associated with hypercalcaemia. *Lancet* 1990; i: 66–9.

30 Liang P, Pardee AB. Differential display of eukaryotic messenger RNA by means of the polymerase chain reaction. *Science* 1992; **257**: 967–71.

31 Zanarla E, Muscatelli F, Bardoni B *et al.* An unusual member of the nuclear hormone receptor superfamily responsible for X-linked

adrenal hypoplasia congenita. *Nature* 1994; **372**: 635–41.
32 Newgard CB. Cellular engineering and gene therapy strategies for insulin replacement in diabetes. *Diabetes* 1994; **43**: 341–50.
33 Dillon M. Regulating gene expression in gene therapy. *Trends Biotechnol* 1993; **11**: 167–73.
34 Evans M, Affara N, Lever AML. Gene therapy—future prospects and the consequences. *Br Med Bull* 1995; **51**: 226–34.

CHAPTER 3

Molecular aspects of hormonal regulation

S.L. Chew

Introduction

The hormone response is specific and dynamic. The differences between stimulated and unstimulated (control) states in tissues and cells have been exploited by molecular biologists to open a detailed view of hormonal regulation. The response to hormones involves the nucleus, the cytoplasm and areas outside the cell (Fig. 3.1). The rapid advances began with radioimmunoassay 20 years ago and now involve combinations of genetic and biochemical techniques, permitting study of interactions between macromolecules (DNA, RNA and protein). In this chapter, several themes are explored:

1 endocrine regulation by RNA processing and splicing;
2 regulation of the circadian rhythm—the molecular clock;
3 localisation and targeting of proteins;
4 control of the development of endocrine organs.

RNA processing and splicing

There are many opportunities for regulation in the processing of messenger RNA (mRNA). Gene transcription and the interaction between hormonal signals and transcription factors are discussed in Chapter 4. The first product of gene transcription is a copy of the gene in the form of RNA (pre-mRNA) (see Fig. 3.2). Once the pre-mRNA has been transcribed, a 'cap' (7-methyl guanosine) is added to the 5′ end of the molecule, the introns are removed and a 'tail' (poly-adenosine or polyA) is added. The end-product is mature mRNA which then leaves the nucleus to be translated into protein in the cell cytoplasm. The removal of introns from the pre-mRNA is a process known as splicing (see Chapter 1) and is very accurate. Exons are spliced to-gether with great fidelity and speed, even if they are separated by up to 200 000 bases of intronic sequence [1,2]. Fidelity of pre-mRNA splicing is achieved by a combination of *cis* elements (i.e. the sequence information on the pre-mRNA) and *trans*-acting factors (proteins or other factors interacting with the pre-mRNA). Although the biochemical mechanisms of intron cleavage and exon ligation are to some extent understood, one of the main difficulties is how splice sites are selected. This is a problem both for constitutive splicing and alternative splicing (alternative splicing occurs because the nuclear splicing apparatus may change the splice site). Thus, the consensus sequence for a 5′ splice site is a loose one, and a large number of variants have been catalogued as active splice sites. Conversely, many sequences that match the consensus are never used as splice sites. The problem of splice site selection is even more difficult when a splice site is used only under certain conditions, as in alternative splicing.

The best characterised example of the regulation of alternative splicing is the sex-determining pathway of the fruit fly, *Drosophila* (Fig. 3.3). This pathway is a cascade of alternative splicing events of three genes: sex-lethal, transformer and double-sex [3]. The example is somewhat complex, but is worth following because it illustrates both positive and negative regulation of splice-site usage. At the top of the cascade is sex-lethal, which has two splicing patterns (exon 2 to exon 3 or exon 2 to exon 4). In the male embryo, sex-lethal mRNA has a splicing pattern (exon 2 to exon 3) which results in a truncated, non-functional, sex-lethal protein because of a stop codon in exon 3. In female embryos exon 2 is spliced to exon 4 instead and this results in a full-length sex-lethal protein. The full-length sex-lethal product is itself a splicing protein which influences 3′ splice site selection of its own gene by blocking splicing to exon 3 (the male-specific exon) and splicing occurs to exon 4 (and thus more full-length protein).

The functional (female) sex-lethal protein also regulates the splicing of the next gene in the cascade (transformer). The choice between functional (female) and non-functional (male) transformer protein is also one of alternative splicing,

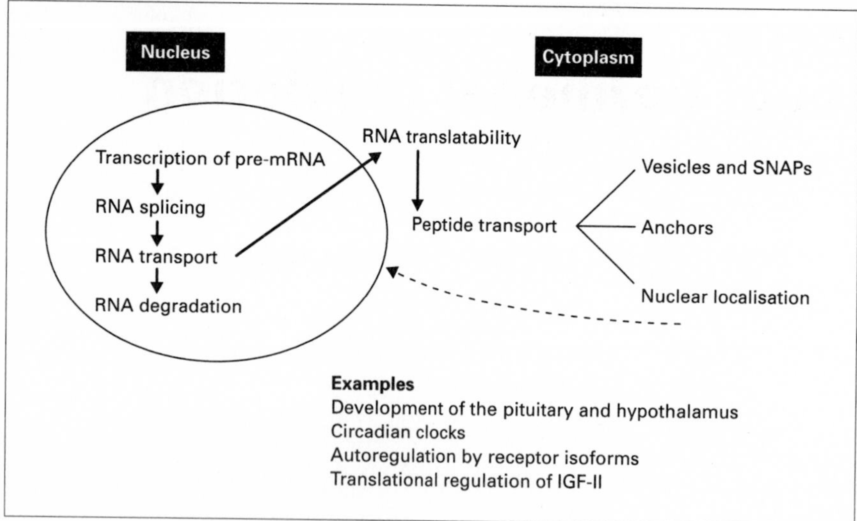

Fig. 3.1 Molecular aspects to the hormone response. The illustration shows a cell with nucleus and cytoplasm and the areas vital to hormone production and secretion, or where hormones may have regulatory function. For details about the examples given, see text.

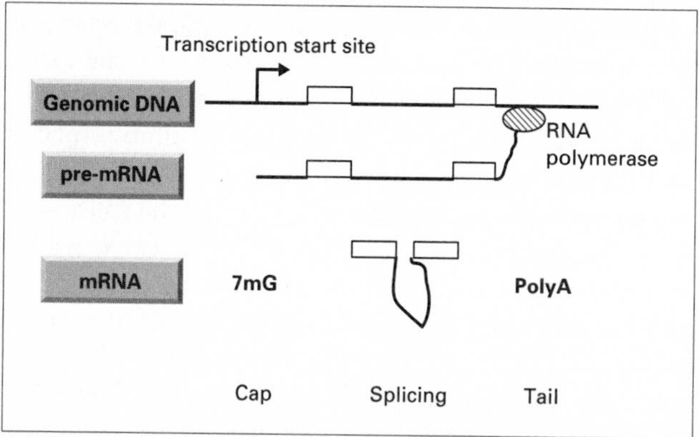

Fig. 3.2 Messenger RNA processing. The steps in mRNA processing are shown. Genomic DNA is transcribed by RNA polymerase II from the transcription start site (arrow). The boxes represent the exons and the lines are introns. The pre-mRNA contains introns and the post-transcriptional events include capping of the mRNA, splicing out of the introns and addition of a polyA tail.

by a choice of two 3′ splice sites (exon 1 to exon 2 or exon 1 to exon 3). The exon 1 to exon 2 splice is the default splice (occuring when there is no regulation). There is no functional transformer product from exon 2, again because of an in-frame stop codon. In the female embryo the full-length functional sex-lethal protein blocks the splicing of transformer mRNA to exon 2, so that exon 1 splices to exon 3, generating a full-length functional transformer protein.

Finally, the functional (female) transformer protein and another splicing factor (transformer 2) activate the use of the female-specific exon 4 (by binding to regulatory sequences in exon 4), to give female-specific splicing of the double-sex gene. In males, the lack of transformer protein causes exon 4 to be skipped because it has a poor 3′ acceptor splice site. The product of the double-sex gene which includes exon 4 results in the female phenotype.

Both transformer and transformer-2 proteins have serine–arginine repeats (SR) which are important in interactions between the splicing proteins [4,5]. Thus, two mRNAs from the same gene have very different functions, vital to the determination of sex in *Drosophila.*

In *Drosophila*, proteins which regulate the usage of splice sites (such as the SR proteins) interact with sequences on the pre-mRNA. The nature of the sequences in the sex-determining cascade is well understood. Progress has also been made in understanding the sequence elements on endocrine genes which regulate alternative splicing, and in some cases these have been shown to interact with SR splicing proteins [6–8].

Many hormone-related genes are subject to alternative splicing which is tissue specific (e.g. calcitonin/calcitonin gene-related peptide (CGRP), see Chapter 1). There has been much progress in understanding the RNA sequence elements and proteins responsible for use of the alternative or tissue-specific splice sites. However, one problem is that the proteins responsible are found ubiquitously [9]. Thus, there is a contrast between tissue-specific transcription (where the regulating transcription factor is present only in the given tissue, as in the examples given later in this chapter), and tissue-specific alternative splicing (where the effect may be due to changes in the relative levels of several splicing proteins [10]).

Hormonal stimuli have been found to influence RNA splicing and processing in a few examples [11,14,71,72] (Table 3.1). The best studied is the insulin receptor gene where exon 11 of the 22 exon gene may be included or skipped from the mature mRNA. The two insulin-receptor protein

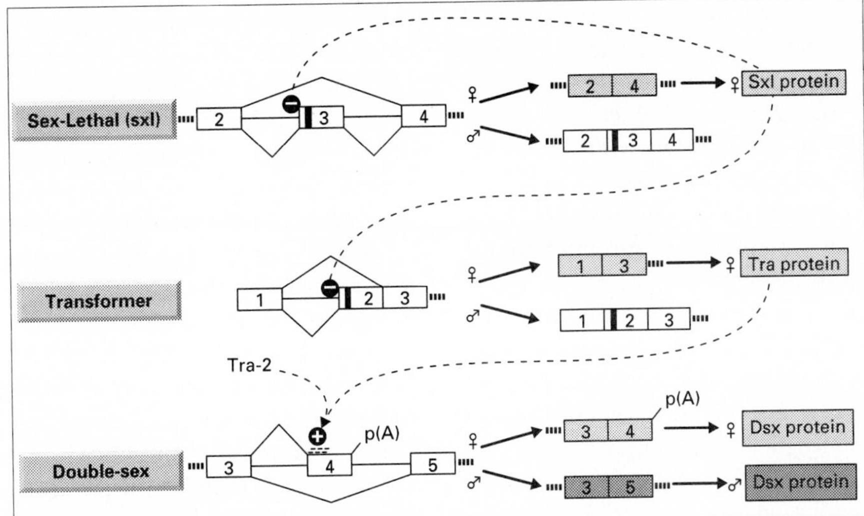

Fig. 3.3 The alternative splicing cascade of the sex-determining pathway of *Drosophila*. The full-length (female, shaded) product of the sex-lethal (*sxl*) gene regulates splicing of its own gene by binding and blocking (⊖) the 3′ acceptor splice site of exon 3, resulting in exon 2 splicing to exon 4. In the absence of full-length sex-lethal, exon 3 is included and a truncated non-functional sex-lethal product results because there is an in-frame stop codon (bar). Full-length sex-lethal also blocks the splicing to exon 2 of transformer (*tra*) mRNA and the resultant exon 2 to exon 4 splicing gives a full-length (female) Tra protein. Tra and Tra-2 enhance (⊕) splicing to exon 4 of double-sex (*dsx*) which give the female phenotype. Redrawn from [3].

Table 3.1 Hormonal regulation of alternative mRNA splicing.

Alternatively spliced mRNA	Stimulus
Insulin receptor	Dexamethasone Glucose Insulin
Protein kinase Cβ	Insulin
PTB-1B	Growth factors
Insulin-like growth factor 1	Growth hormone

isoforms have different activities [12,13]. Dexamethasone can alter the splice choice and increases inclusion of exon 11 in the mature mRNA [14,15], thereby increasing the less insulin-sensitive receptor isoform.

Some genes of the cytokine family are regulated by altering the rate at which unspliced pre-mRNA is spliced to mature mRNA and hence influencing gene expression. Thus, the rate of gene transcription remains unchanged, but unspliced mRNA accumulates at the expense of mature mRNA in response to inflammatory signals, and splicing becomes the rate-limiting regulatory step. This appears to occur with tumour-necrosis factor-α, interleukin-1β and interleukin-2. This regulation may involve the action of a kinase in a phosphorylation–dephosphorylation mechanism [16]. Kinase and phosphatase mechanisms certainly exist to control the localisation and assembly of the spliceosome (the splicing apparatus) [17–20].

Although there are some data on the mechanisms and effects of RNA transcription and splicing on the endocrine system, less is known about other important regulatory steps in RNA processing such as processing of the cap and polyA tail, and the mechanisms of RNA degradation and transport.

RNA degradation is a regulated process, and the rate of decay of an RNA species can vary over two orders of magnitude [21]. The polyA tail of mRNA is the most important determinant of mRNA degradation and also interacts with the cytoskeleton to mediate transport. PolyA tail degradation can be the first step in mRNA decay and the rate of decay of an mRNA can be related to the rate of degradation of the tail [22]. Once the tail is degraded, the RNA is decapped at the 5′ end and also subjected to 3′ → 5′ exonuclease activity. The rate of decay of the polyA tail may be increased by nucleotide sequences (e.g. the AU-rich regions in mRNAs of highly inducible proteins) in the 3′ untranslated region of the transcript [23]. Some mRNAs may also be degraded by de-adenylation-independent pathways, involving direct decapping or endonucleolytic cleavage (e.g. insulin-like growth factor 2 (IGF-2), see below).

There are examples of hormones changing the use of the polyadenylation signal. If a hormone alters the polyadenylation signal used, then the 3′ untranslated region of the mRNA will also be changed and this may have implications for the survival of the mRNA in question. For example, the cyclic adenosine monophosphate (cAMP) response element modulator τ (CREMτ) mRNA polyadenylation signal alters in response to follicle-stimulating hormone (FSH) and transcript stability increases [24], vital during the process of spermatogenesis (*CREM* gene knockout mice have absent spermatogenesis [25]).

In some cases regulation has been shown to affect the length of the polyA tail. Vasopressin post-transcriptional regulation has been well investigated. The polyA tail of vasopressin mRNA varies in length with osmolality [26]. Prolactin polyA tail length increases after pituitary explant, and this can be regulated by the dopamine agonist bromocriptine [27]. There are several other examples of regulation of polyA tail length (Table 3.2).

As another example of the effect of hormones on RNA stability, thyroid hormone, in the form of T3, induces acetylcholinesterase activity in primary rat neuronal cultures, while thyroidectomy reduces acetylcholinesterase activity in fetal rat brain. This change in activity relates to changes in stability of acetylcholinesterase mRNA levels. How T3 stabilises the acetylcholinesterase transcript is uncertain, but it may involve a serine/threonine protein kinase signalling pathway [28].

IGF-II mRNA has several transcripts by use of different promoter sites for transcription. The regulation of these transcripts is an example of de-adenylation-independent mRNA degradation. Thus, IGF-II mRNA undergoes endonucleolytic cleavage in the 3′ untranslated region, possibly in a manner dependent on the growth state of cultured liver cells, by a cytoplasmic binding protein of about 50 kDa [29]. Another form of regulation is that IGF-II mRNA variants have different stabilities [29] and different rates of translation once they are associated with the ribosomes [30].

In order to function, mRNA must be exported from the nucleus to the translational apparatus and the polyribosomes. This process is dependent on energy and a guanosine triphosphate (GTP)-exchange mechanism (Ran GTPase), and can be saturated [31]. RNA is exported bound to RNA-binding proteins and passes through nuclear pore complexes. There is some evidence for regulation of the RNA export mechanism during embryo development and by viral proteins [32]. This mechanism is probably fundamental to the dynamic response of the nucleus to hormonal stimulus, but there is no knowledge as to how hormones may influence the kinetics of RNA transport.

Table 3.2 Regulation of polyA tail length. Based on [27].

Messenger RNA	Regulator(s)
Growth hormone	Glucocorticoids, thyroid status
Insulin	Glucose
LH β-subunit	Ovariectomy, LHRH
Prolactin	Dopamine agonists
TSH β-subunit	Thyroid hormone
Vasopressin	Osmolality, circadian rhythm, gonadal steroids

LH, luteinising hormone; LHRH, luteinising hormone-releasing hormone; TSH, thyroid-stimulating hormone.

Little is known about the role of mRNA localisation in the hormone response. However, the localisation of mRNA to regions of the embryo where the translated product is required is well studied in embryo development [33]. Production of a protein only at the site where its action is needed would be a very efficient method of running a cell. There are examples of mRNAs whose products are involved in signalling (calmodulin-dependent protein kinase II in dendrites and a homologue of the transforming growth factor (TGF) TGF-α in oocytes) being localised and translated in subcompartments of the cell where their action is required [33]. Thus far, the specific signals that localise mRNA have been exclusively mapped to 3′ untranslated regions and are of the order of several hundred nucleotides in length: some of the proteins binding these RNA localisation signals have been identified [33].

Clocks

A major regulator of endocrine gene expression is circadian rhythm. Progress has been made in understanding how the circadian clock works in *Drosophila* and in rodents, but it is unknown how the clock regulates cell function including hormonal output. The strategy in *Drosophila* has usually been to generate flies with no (or aberrant) circadian rhythms and identify the mutated gene by positional cloning. Two genes are vital to the clock mechanism: period (*per*) and timeless (*tim*). The peptide products of these genes, Per and Tim, cycle up and down, high at night and low in the day: both proteins are needed. When the *tim* gene is mutated, Per protein accumulates in the cytoplasm and does not move to the nucleus, with consequent disruption of the clock. The Per protein regulates itself in that it enters the nucleus to switch off transcription of the *per* gene. Thus, at first light the levels of per and tim mRNA are low (Per and Tim proteins have switched off gene transcription of their own genes) and the protein levels fall. The fall in Per and Tim levels in the day releases gene transcription and the mRNA accumulates so that when night arrives the protein levels are high again. Light can influence this rhythm by destroying Tim protein (by an unknown mechanism) causing resynchronisation [34–36] (Fig. 3.4). Much less is understood about the human circadian clock, but there are two human expressed sequence tags (EST) similar to *Drosophila per* in the genome database.

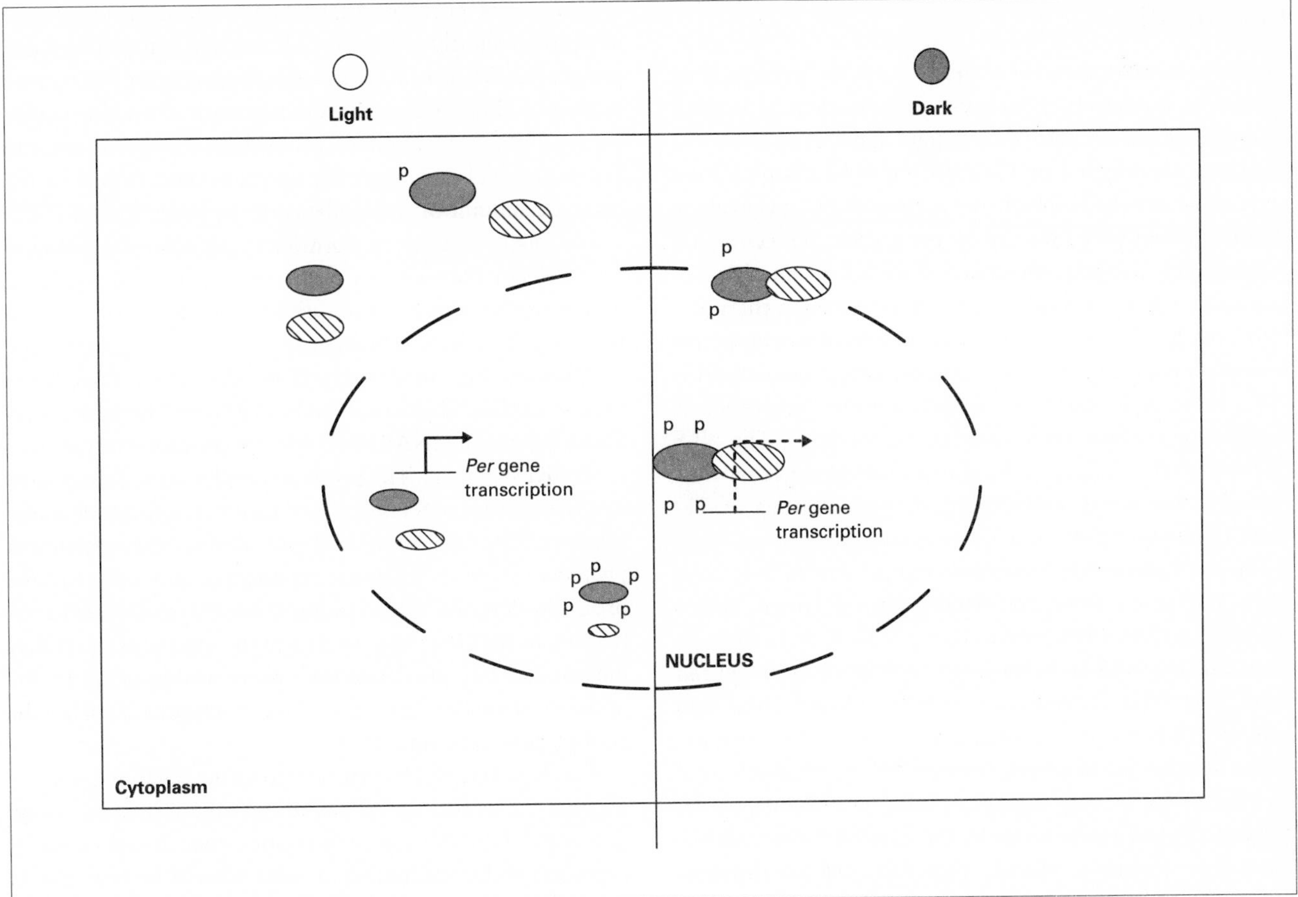

Fig. 3.4 The *Drosophila* clock. The rhythm of PER (closed ovals) and TIM (hatched) proteins is shown. Their cellular location is shown in the large rectangle, with the nucleus shown as a dashed oval. The light-dark rhythm is given above the rectangle; lights on (open circle) and lights off (closed circle). The proteins are high at night (larger ovals), phosphorylated (p) and they dimerise and pass into the nucleus to swith off transcription of their own genes (dotted arrow). By morning, both per and tim mRNA levels are low and PER and TIM protein levels are falling (smaller ovals). Light disrupts the PER-TIM dimer by degrading TIM. In the day, PER and TIM are low and *per* and *tim* gene transcription are high (heavy arrow). The figure is adapted from [36].

In mammals, the pineal gland produces melatonin, a major end-product of regulation by the circadian rhythm. Melatonin production is by the pineal enzyme serotonin *N*-acetyltransferase (NAT) whose mRNA is under circadian control [37]. The molecular mechanisms of the mammalian clock focus on the cAMP signalling system. The mammalian clock appears to lie in the hypothalamic suprachiasmatic nucleus and influences the pineal by noradrenergic pathways [38,39]. Noradrenergic signals (high at night) stimulate cAMP and thereby gene transcription via the intermediates CREB (cAMP response element binding protein) and CREM (see Chapter 1). CREB is not inducible and cAMP signalling through CREB is not dependent on new protein synthesis, but is a phosphorylation event (typical of the class of 'early response' genes). CREM has multiple isoforms generated by alternative splicing or use of an alternative promoter. The products of alternative splicing of CREM (α, β, γ and τ) are *not* induced by activation of the cAMP signalling pathway [40]. However, a product from the alternative promoter is induced by cAMP signalling (ICER, inducible cAMP early repressor). ICER lacks several domains seen in CREM isoforms, particularly the phosphorylation domain, but it has the DNA-binding domain, and it can feed back to switch off its own transcription. ICER is expressed predominantly in endocrine and neuroendocrine tissues. In the pineal gland ICER mRNA levels are high at night and low in the day [41], and changes in ICER regulate the circadian rhythm in rodents [42]. Thus, in rodents, as in *Drosophila*, an autoregulatory molecular mechanism underlies the circadian rhythm, and further work is likely to establish the relationship of these molecular processes to human circadian rhythmicity.

Localisation

The import and export of material from the nucleus is of interest to endocrinologists because the nucleus is a target of hormone action, and thus it may show how hormone responses are targeted, and because it may be a rate-limiting and regulated step. The nucleus is surrounded by an envelope which contains pores formed by the nuclear pore complex (NPC), with aqueous channels of about 10 nm. Macromolecules less than 40 kDa may diffuse through the pore. However, movement of larger macromolecules is an active process, mediated by NPC proteins, called nucleoporins [43]. Proteins destined for nuclear import have nuclear localisation signals (NLS) of basic amino acids. The NLS docks onto the NLS receptor which binds to nucleoporins: transport then occurs and is energy dependent, using a GTP/GDP (guanosine diphosphate) exchange mechanism (Ran GTPase) [44]. Several hormones and growth factors have NLS. The best studied are platelet-derived growth factor (PDGF) and fibroblast growth factor 3 (FGF-3). In the case of PDGF, the NLS is coded for by an alternatively spliced exon [45]. Thus, alternative mRNA splicing gives two isoforms of PDGF, one containing a functional C-terminal NLS, the other isoform being secreted. The encoding of either an NLS or a secretory signal can also be regulated at the level of protein translation. In the case of the androgen-dependent prostatic protein probasin, use of different translation initiation signals on one mRNA species gives isoforms with or without a secretory signal peptide; the isoform without the signal peptide is found in the nucleus [46]. In the case of FGF-3, however, there is both a secretory signal and an NLS on the single peptide. The secretory signal lies six amino-acid residues N-terminal to the NLS. The two signals on the same protein appear to compete. Thus, about half FGF-3 ends up in the nucleus, while the other 50% is secreted by interaction with the signal recognition particle and is found in the endoplasmic reticulum and Golgi apparatus. More FGF-3 ends up in the secretory pathway if the secretory signal is separated (by experimental mutagenesis) from the NLS. If the FGF-3 NLS is replaced by a consensus NLS, more FGF-3 is found in the nucleus than in the secretory apparatus [47].

Several hormones are subject to nuclear translocation after binding to receptors and internalisation, for example growth hormone [48]. This process appears to be receptor mediated, and is independent of cytoskeletal elements. The mechanism and function of this receptor-mediated nuclear translocation of hormones are unknown.

The export of macromolecules from the nucleus is also an active process. For example, export of mRNA requires many proteins and is also dependent on a GTP/GDP exchange mechanism (via Ran GTPase).

Heat-shock proteins and steroid receptors are examples of proteins shuttling between nucleus and cytoplasm. Some progress has been made in the understanding of the mechanism of protein shuttles with the identification of nuclear export signals [49]. A 14-amino-acid residue sequence in protein kinase inhibitor mediates the rapid nuclear export of the catalytic subunit of cAMP-dependent protein kinase [50].

The major export of hormones and neurotransmitters from cells by the secretory pathway is mediated by vesicles. A receptor system has been discovered that mediates and regulates the selective fusion of a vesicle to the appropriate membrane. Fusion events are mediated by membrane proteins called SNAREs. The SNAREs on the vesicles (v-SNAREs) bind to SNAREs on appropriate target membranes (t-SNAREs) [51,52]. The SNARE complex is then recognised by proteins that effect membrane fusion, *N*-ethylmaleimide-sensitive fusion protein (NSF) and soluble NSF attachment proteins (SNAPs). This system operates not only to take products destined for secretion from the endoplasmic reticulum to the Golgi apparatus and then to the extracellular membrane, but also functions to return proteins in the opposite direction from the Golgi apparatus back to the endoplasmic reticulum [53].

A protein may still be exported from the cell to the exterior without a classical signal peptide to take it into the Golgi apparatus. Fibroblast growth factor 1 (which lacks a signal peptide) can be released from cultured cells by heat shock, possibly by direct interaction with phospholipids in the plasma membrane [54].

Another important question is how large proteins and cells cross from the circulation into target tissues, and how they concentrate in a specific tissue. Organ-selective peptide sequences have been identified (by use of a phage expression and recovery system; phages are viruses which infect bacteria) that can concentrate phage particles or red cells in brain and kidney tissue. For example, peptides containing an SRL (Ser-Arg-Leu) motif mediate localisation of phage and red cells to the brain [55].

Phosphorylation and dephosphorylation mechanisms of signalling and regulation are common to all hormones. Where tyrosine kinases are concerned, localisation of signals can be accounted for partly by specificity of coupling to substrates with SH2 and SH3 domains such as Grb2 or insulin receptor substrate (IRS-1) [56]. For example, the mutation of the *ret* proto-oncogene causing multiple endocrine neoplasia type 2B [57] alters the substrate recognition pocket of the intracellular tyrosine kinase domain of the RET transmembrane receptor, thereby coupling to a different substrate (see Chapter 47 and [58]).

Specificity of signalling may also be achieved by localising substrates or enzymes to a particular part of the cell [59]. The concept of 'anchor' and 'scaffold' proteins has been

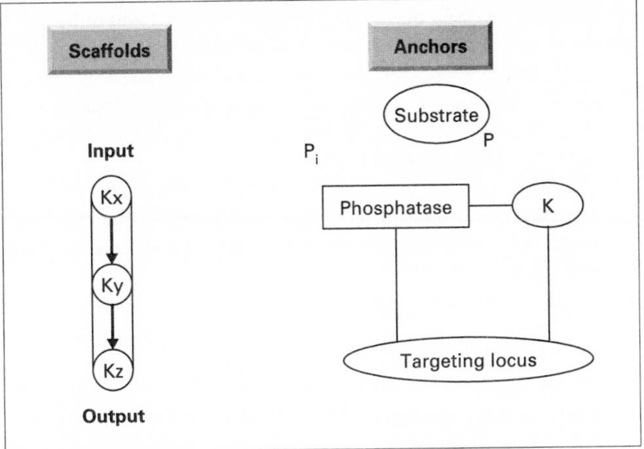

Fig. 3.5 Scaffold and anchor proteins. Scaffold proteins hold a series of kinases (K) in a chain to localise signal transduction from one part of the cell (input) to another (output). Anchor proteins, on the other hand, hold a number of kinases and phosphatases in a complex localised to one part of the cell. P, bound phosphate; P_i, free phosphate. Redrawn from [59].

suggested for signalling through serine/threonine kinases and phosphatases (Fig. 3.5). In the scaffolding model, a protein holds a series of kinases in line from the ligand-binding region (input) to the effector region (output). AKAP79 is the best studied of the 'anchor' proteins and anchors a complex of protein kinase A, phosphatase 2B and calcineurin at the post-synaptic density of cultured hippocampal neurons [60]).

Endocrine organ development

Rapid progress has been made in understanding the molecular biology of endocrine tissue development. This has partly been due to knockout experiments involving transcription factor genes in mice. The fate of endocrine tissues in embryo development appears to be linked to specific and dynamic expression of transcription factors. Table 3.3 lists some of the transcription factors important to the development and differentiation of the major endocrine organs.

POU (an acronym of Pit-1, Oct-1, Unc-86; three peptides containing a conserved DNA-binding domain of ~ 60 residues) domain-containing transcription factors are important in the development of the neuroendocrine system. The transcription factor Pit-1 contains a POU domain and is important to the growth of the pituitary and to the expression of growth hormone, prolactin and the growth hormone-releasing hormone (GHRH) receptor [61,62]. The number of POU domain-containing transcription factors has increased and there are currently six classes recognised. Class III POU-domain transcription factors (including Brn-1, Brn-2 and Brn-3) are interesting because they are the only POU-domain genes without introns and because they are important in the development of the hypothalamus and frontal brain. Brn-1 and Brn-3 are important to the initial development of the frontal neurons and hypothalamus [63], but Brn-2 is important later in hypothalamic development and particularly the paraventricular and supraoptic nuclei [64]. Brn-2 exerts its effects in the same developmental time frame as Pit-1 [63].

Another DNA-binding protein, T/ebp (thyroid-specific enhancer binding protein), is important in the development of the entire pituitary (as well as the thyroid and lung). This protein is so named because it was identified initially as a binding protein to an enhancer sequence upstream of the thyroid peroxidase gene [65]. In the mouse, the *Lhx3* gene is expressed in the pituitary throughout development and

Table 3.3 Transcription factors in endocrine tissue development and differentiation.

Organ	Factor	Functional correlates
Pituitary	Pit-1	Somato-/lacto-/thyrotroph secretion, pituitary development
	T/ebp	Whole pituitary gland development
	Lhx3	Anterior/intermediate lobes absent except corticotrophs
	Ptx1	Corticotroph specific, knockout mouse awaited
Adrenal	SF-1	Gonadal and adrenal agenesis
Testes/ovary	SF-1	Gonadal and adrenal agenesis
Endocrine hypothalamus	Brn-1 and Brn-3	Early hypothalamic development
	Brn-2	PVN and SON development
Posterior pituitary	Brn-2	Vasopressin/oxytocin levels reduced by 50% in +/– mice
Thyroid	T/ebp	Also effects pituitary and lung development

PVN, paraventricular nucleus; SON, supraoptic nucleus.

Lhx3 homozygous knockout mice have no anterior or intermediate lobes of the pituitary; however, there is sparing of the corticotroph cells [66]. *Lhx3*, like *Pit-1*, is a homeobox gene (i.e. it encodes a POU peptide domain with homology to DNA-binding motifs found in proteins controlling *Drosophila* segment development). Another homeobox gene, *Ptx-1*, may be important in the development of the corticotroph, and is certainly involved in transcription of the pro-opiomelanocortin gene [67].

Gene knockout experiments have also shown the importance of the *Ftz-F1* gene in adrenal, gonadal and ventromedial hypothalamus development [68,69]. The *Ftz-F1* gene has two products, SF-1 (steroidogenic factor 1) and an alternative splice (ELP). SF-1 is an orphan nuclear receptor which regulates the use of the Müllerian inhibiting substance gene, probably with a silencing mechanism similar to the action of the thyroid hormone receptor [70].

Conclusion

Endocrine systems and hormonal responses have been productive areas for molecular biologists. A complex and detailed view of the hormone response has been revealed. The major advances have been in understanding circadian clocks, macromolecule localisation and transport and the influence of RNA processing on gene expression.

References

1 Green MR. Biochemical mechanisms of constitutive and regulated pre-mRNA splicing. *Ann Rev Cell Biol* 1991; **7**: 559–99.

2 Maniatis T. Mechanisms of alternative pre-mRNA splicing. *Science* 1991; **251**: 33–4.

3 Moore MJ, Query CC, Sharp PA. Splicing of precursors to mRNA by the spliceosome. In: Gesteland RF, Atkins JF, eds. *The RNA World*. New York: Cold Spring Harbor Laboratory Press, 1993: 303–57.

4 Wu JY, Maniatis T. Specific interactions between proteins implicated in splice site selection and regulated alternative splicing. *Cell* 1993; **75**: 1061–70.

5 Amrein H, Hedley ML, Maniatis T. The role of specific protein–RNA and protein–protein interactions in positive and negative control of pre-mRNA splicing by *Transformer 2*. *Cell* 1994; **76**: 735–46.

6 Sun Q, Mayeda A, Hampson RK, Krainer A, Rottman FM. General splicing factor SF2/ASF promotes alternative splicing by binding to an exonic splicing enhancer. *Genes Dev* 1993; **7**: 2598–608.

7 van Oers CCM, Adema GJ, Zandberg H, Moen TC, Baas PD. Two different sequence elements within exon 4 are necessary for calcitonin-specific splicing of the human calcitonin/calcitonin gene-related peptide I pre-mRNA. *Mol Cell Biol* 1994; **14**: 951–60.

8 Del Gatto F, Breathnach R. Exon and intron sequences, respectively, repress and activate splicing of a fibroblast growth factor receptor 2 alternative exon. *Mol Cell Biol* 1995; **15**: 4825–34.

9 Min H, Chan RC, Black DL. The generally expressed hnRNP F is involved in a neural-specific pre-mRNA splicing event. *Genes Dev* 1995; **9**: 2659–71.

10 Caceres JF, Stamm S, Helfman DM, Krainer A. Regulation of alternative splicing *in vivo* by overexpression of antagonistic splicing factors. *Science* 1994; **265**: 1706–9.

11 Chew SL, Lavender P, Clark AJL, Ross RJM. An alternatively spliced human *IGF-I* transcript (*IGF-IEc*) with hepatic tissue expression that diverts away from the mitogenic IBE1 peptide. *Endocrinology* 1995; **136**: 1939–44.

12 Mosthaf L, Grako K, Dull TJ, Coussens L, Ullrich A, McClain DA. Functionally distinct insulin receptors generated by tissue-specific alternative splicing. *EMBO J* 1990; **9**: 2409–13.

13 Kosaki A, Pillay TS, Xu L, Webster NJG. The B isoform of the insulin receptor signals more efficiently than the A isoform in HepG2 cells. *J Biol Chem* 1995; **270**: 20816–23.

14 Kosaki A, Webster NJG. Effects of dexamethasone on the alternative splicing of the insulin receptor mRNA and insulin action in HepG2 hepatoma cells. *J Biol Chem* 1993; **268**: 21990–6.

15 Norgren S, Li L, Luthman H. Regulation of human insulin receptor RNA splicing in HepG2 cells: effects of glucocorticoid and low glucose concentration. *Biochem Biophys Res Commun* 1994; **199**: 277–84.

16 Jarrous N, Osman F, Kaempfer R. 2-aminopurine selectively inhibits splicing of tumor necrosis factor alpha mRNA. *Mol Cell Biol* 1996; **16**: 2814–22.

17 Gui J, Lane WS, Fu X. A serine kinase regulates intracellular localization of splicing factors in the cell cycle. *Nature* 1994; **369**: 678–82.

18 Mermoud JE, Cohen PTW, Lamond AI. Regulation of mammalian spliceosome assembly by a protein phosphorylation mechanism. *EMBO J* 1994; **13**: 5679–88.

19 Colwill K, Pawson T, Andrews B *et al.* The Clk/Sty protein kinase phosphorylates SR splicing factors and regulates their intranuclear distribution. *EMBO J* 1996; **15**: 265–75.

20 Rossi F, Labourier E, Forne T *et al.* Specific phosphorylation of SR proteins by mammalian DNA topoisomerase I. *Nature* 1996; **381**: 80–2.

21 Sachs AB, Wahle E. Poly(A) tail metabolism and function in eucaryotes. *J Biol Chem* 1993; **268**: 22955–8.

22 Beelman CA, Parker R. Degradation of mRNA in eukaryotes. *Cell* 1995; **81**: 179–83.

23 Asson-Batres MA, Spurgeon SL, Diaz J, DeLoughery TG, Bagby GC, Jr. Evolutionary conservation of the AU-rich 3′ untranslated region of messenger RNA. *Proc Natl Acad Sci USA* 1994; **91**: 1318–22.

24 Foulkes NS, Schlotter F, Pevet P, Sassone-Corsi P. Pituitary hormone FSH directs the CREM functional switch during spermatogenesis. *Nature* 1993; **362**: 264–7.

25 Nantel F, Monaco L, Foulkes NS *et al.* Spermiogenesis deficiency and germ-cell apoptosis in CREM-mutant mice. *Nature* 1996; **380**: 159–62.

26 Carrazana EJ, Pasieka KB, Majzoub JA. The vasopressin poly (A) tail is unusually long and increases during stimulation of vasopressin gene expression *in vivo*. *Mol Cell Biol* 1988; **8**: 2267–74.

27 Carter DA, Chew LJ, Murphy D. *In vitro* regulation of rat prolactin messenger ribonucleic acid poly(A) tail length: modulation by bromocriptine. *J Neuroendocrinol* 1993; **5**: 201–4.

28 Puymirat J, Etongue-Mayer P, Dussault JH. Thyroid hormones stabilize acetylcholinesterase mRNA in Neuro-2A cells that overexpress the beta1 thyroid receptor. *J Biol Chem* 1995; **270**:

30651–6.

29 Scheper W, Holthuizen PE, Sussenbach JS. The cis-acting elements involved in endonucleolytic cleavage of the 3′ UTR of human IGF-II mRNAs bind a 50 kDa protein. *Nucleic Acids Res* 1996; **24**: 1000–7.

30 Nielsen FC, Ostergaard L, Nielson J, Christiansen J. Growth-dependent translation of IGF-II mRNA by a rapamycin-sensitive pathway. *Nature* 1995; **377**: 358–62.

31 Cheng Y, Dahlberg JE, Lund E. Diverse effects of the guanine nucleotide exchange factor RCC1 on RNA transport. *Science* 1995; **267**: 1807–10.

32 Izaurralde E, Mattaj IW. RNA export. *Cell* 1995; **81**: 153–9.

33 St Johnson D. The intracellular localization of messenger RNAs. Cell 1995; **81**: 161–70.

34 Zeng H, Qian Z, Myers MP, Rosbash M. A light-entrainment mechanism for the Drosophila circadian clock. *Nature* 1996; **380**: 129–35.

35 Myers MP, Wager-Smith K, Rothenfluh-Hilfiker A, Young MW. Light-induced degradation of TIMELESS and entrainment of the Drosophila circadian clock. *Science* 1996; **271**: 1736–40.

36 Lee C, Parikh V, Itsukaichi T, Bae K, Edery I. Resetting the Drosophila clock by photic regulation of PER and a PER-TIM complex. *Science* 1996; **271**: 1740–4.

37 Borjigin J, Wang MW, Snyder SH. Diurnal variation in mRNA encoding serotonin N-acetyltransferase in pineal gland. *Nature* 1995; **378**: 783–5.

38 Takahashi JS. Circadian clocks a la CREM. *Nature* 1993; **365**: 299–300.

39 Hastings M. Circadian rhythms: peering into the molecular clock. *J Neuroendocrinol* 1995; **7**: 331–40.

40 Molina CA, Foulkes NS, Lalli E, Sassone-Corsi P. Inducibility and negative autoregulation of CREM: an alternative promotor directs the expression of ICER, an early response repressor. *Cell* 1993; **75**: 875–86.

41 Stehle JH, Foulkes NS, Molina CA, Simonneaux V, Pevet P, Sassone-Corsi P. Adrenergic signals direct rhythmic expression of transcriptional repressor CREM in the pineal gland. *Nature* 1993; **365**: 314–20.

42 Foulkes NS, Duval G, Sassone-Corsi P. Adaptive inducibility of CREM as transcriptional memory of circadian rhythms. *Nature* 1996; **381**: 83–5.

43 Rexach M, Blobel G. Protein import into nuclei: association and dissociation reactions involving transport substrate, transport factors, and nucleoporins. *Cell* 1995; **83**: 683–92.

44 Nehrbass U, Blobel G. Role of the nuclear transport factor p10 in nuclear import. *Science* 1996; **272**: 120–2.

45 Maher DW, Lee BA, Donoghue DJ. The alternatively spliced exon of the Platelet-Derived Growth Factor A chain encodes a nuclear targeting signal. *Mol Cell Biol* 1989; **9**: 2251–3.

46 Spence AM, Sheppard PC, Davie JR *et al.* Regulation of a bifunctional mRNA results in synthesis of secreted and nuclear probasin. *Proc Natl Acad Sci USA* 1989; **86**: 7843–7.

47 Kiefer P, Acland P, Pappin D, Peters G, Dickson C. Competition between nuclear localization and secretory signals determines the subcellular fate of a single CUG-initiated form of FGF3. *EMBO J* 1994; **13**: 4126–36.

48 Lobie PE, Mertani H, Morel G, Morales-Bustos O, Norstedt G, Waters MJ. Receptor-mediated nuclear translocation of growth hormone. *J Biol Chem* 1994; **269**: 21330–9.

49 Gerace L. Nuclear export signals and the fast track to the cytoplasm. *Cell* 1995; **82**: 341–4.

50 Wen W, Meinkoth JL, Tsien RY, Taylor SS. Identification of a signal for rapid export of proteins from the nucleus. *Cell* 1995; **82**: 463–73.

51 Ferro-Novick S, Jahn R. Vehicle fusion from yeast to man. *Nature* 1994; **370**: 191–3.

52 Rothman JE. Mechanisms of intracellular protein transport. *Nature* 1994; **372**: 55–63.

53 Lewis MJ, Pelham HRB. SNARE-mediated retrograde traffic from the Golgi complex to the endoplasmic reticulum. *Cell* 1996; **85**: 205–15.

54 Tarantini F, Gamble S, Jackson A, Maciag T. The cysteine residue responsible for the release of fibroblast growth factor-1 resides in a domain independent of the domain for phosphatidylserine binding. *J Biol Chem* 1995; **270**: 29039–42.

55 Pasqualini R, Ruoslahti E. Organ targeting in vivo using phage display peptide libraries. *Nature* 1996; **380**: 364–6.

56 Hill CS, Treisman R. Transcriptional regulation by extracellular signals: mechanisms and specificity. *Cell* 1995; **80**: 199–211.

57 Hofstra RMW, Landsvater RM, Ceccherini I *et al.* A mutation in the ret proto-oncogene associated with multiple endocrine neoplasia type 2B and sporadic medullary thyroid carcinoma. *Nature* 1994; **367**: 375–6.

58 Songyang Z, Carraway KLI, Eck MJ *et al.* Catalytic specificity of protein-tyrosine kinases is critical for selective signalling. *Nature* 1995; **373**: 536–9.

59 Faux MC, Scott JD. Molecular glue: kinase anchoring and scaffold proteins. *Cell* 1996; **85**: 9–12.

60 Coghlan VM, Perrino BA, Howard M *et al.* Association of protein kinase A and protein phosphatase 2B with a common anchoring protein. *Science* 1995; **267**: 108–11.

61 Bodner M, Castrillo JL, Theill LE, Deerinck M, Ellisman M, Karin M. The pituitary-specific transcription factor GHF-1 is a homeobox-containing protein. *Cell* 1988; **55**: 505–18.

62 Ingraham HA, Chen RP, Mangalam HJ *et al.* A tissue-specific transcription factor containing a homeodomain specifies a pituitary phenotype. *Cell* 1988; **55**: 519–29.

63 Schonemann MD, Ryan AK, McEvilly RJ *et al.* Development and survival of the endocrine hypothalamus and posterior pituitary gland requires the neuronal POU domain factor Brn-2. *Genes Dev* 1995; **9**: 3122–35.

64 Nakai S, Kawano H, Yudate T *et al.* The POU domain transcription factor Brn-2 is required for the determination of specific neuronal lineages in the hypothalamus of the mouse. *Genes Dev* 1995; **9**: 3109–21.

65 Kimura S, Hara Y, Pineau T *et al.* The T/ebp null mouse: thyroid-specific enhancer-binding protein is essential for the organogenesis of the thyroid, lung, ventral forebrain, and the pituitary. *Genes Dev* 1996; **10**: 60–9.

66 Sheng HZ, Zhadanov AB, Mosinger BJ *et al.* Specification of pituitary cell lineages by the LIM homeobox gene Lhx3. *Science* 1996; **272**: 1004–7.

67 Lamonerie T, Tremblay JJ, Lanctot C, Therrien M, Gauthier Y, Drouin J. Ptx1, a bicoid-related homeo box transcription factor involved in transcription of the pro-opiomelanocortin gene. *Genes Dev* 1996; **10**: 1284–95.

68 Luo XR, Ikeda Y, Parker KL. A cell-specific nuclear receptor is essential for adrenal and gonadal development and sexual differentiation. *Cell* 1994; **77**: 481–90.

69 Ikeda Y, Luo XR, Abbud R, Nilson JH, Parker KL. The nuclear receptor steroidogenic factor-1 is essential for the formation of the ventromedial hypothalamic nucleus. *Mol Endocrinol* 1995; **9**: 478–86.

70 Shen W, Moore CCD, Ikeda Y, Parker KL, Ingraham HA. Nuclear receptor steroidogenic factor 1 regulates the Mullerian inhibiting substance gene: a link to the sex determination cascade. *Cell* 1994; 77: 651–61.
71 Shifrin VI, Neel BG. Growth factor-inducible alternative splicing of nontransmembrane phosphotyrosine phosphate PTB-1B premessenger RNA. *J Biol Chem* 1993; **268**: 21990–6.
72 Sell SM, Reese D, Ossowski VM. Insulin-inducible changes in insulin-receptor mRNA splice variants. *J Biol Chem* 1994; **269**: 30769–72.

Part 2
Hormone Receptors and Intracellular Signalling

CHAPTER 4

Hormone receptors and intracellular signalling

S.P. Bidey, L.C. Best, D.W. Ray, and J.R.E. Davis

Introduction

The communication of hormonal signals to the interior of the cell can be achieved either by the generation of second messengers at the cell membrane or by hormones crossing the cell membrane, binding to intracellular receptors and in some way regulating the expression of specific genes. Sutherland *et al.* in 1965 [1] proposed that some hormones which themselves do not enter the cell mediate their effects through intracellular regulators or 'second messengers'. Sutherland and coworkers found that cyclic adenosine monophosphate (cAMP) played a key role in the response of the liver to adrenaline and to glucagon, and discovered the enzyme responsible for the formation of cAMP from adenosine triphosphate (ATP), adenylate cyclase. Many hormones have now been shown to stimulate adenylate cyclase in cell membranes, but it is now clear that the cAMP system is but one of a number of signalling pathways, and others include signalling by calcium, pH and tyrosine kinase cascades. In fact, a complex array of signalling systems allows for subtle cross-talk, such that a range of cellular responses are generated depending on the hormonal environment.

In this chapter, we will introduce current concepts regarding G-protein-coupled hormone receptors, nuclear hormone receptors and signal transduction pathways; we will outline the adenylate cyclase–cAMP signalling system and the Ca^{2+} signalling system, and also the recently described tyrosine kinase cascades typical of cytokine receptor and insulin-receptor activation.

Hormone receptors: general structure and function

The response of a target cell to a hormone depends on recognition of the ligand by receptor molecules on or within the cell. The binding reaction between hormone and receptor must therefore be highly specific and selective, with an affinity that corresponds to the physiological concentration range of the hormone. A number of hormones, notably the steroids and thyroid hormones, are lipophilic and are able to diffuse through the phospholipid bilayer of the plasma membrane, to interact with receptor proteins on the nuclear membrane or within the cytosol (Fig. 4.1). In contrast, most polypeptide hormones are lipid insoluble, and their effects are mediated through receptors located within the ionic environment of the outer cell membrane. Whether the receptor is on the cell surface or within the cytosol, however, the hormone interacts specifically with receptor, altering receptor conformation and thereby signalling its presence to the cell. In addition to a binding or 'recognition' component, the receptor complex for any given peptide hormone also encompasses a distinct catalytic component which translates hormone binding into a cellular response. This must be rapidly initiated, sensitive to small changes in the concentration of circulating hormone, and subject to immediate termination upon withdrawal of the hormone.

The ability of a cell to respond to a hormonal stimulus is determined by the hormone-binding properties, as well as the density and biological half-life of the receptor population. In turn, these parameters are influenced by a variety of factors, including age, cellular environment and prior exposure of the cell to hormones and drugs. Even under physiological conditions, the receptor population for any given hormone is not constant but varies widely according to the endocrine/paracrine environment. The synthesis, expression and degradation of a population of receptors thus imposes an ultimate control over the sensitivity of the cell to any given hormonal stimulus.

The hormone-binding site

The hormone recognition or 'binding' site recognises and

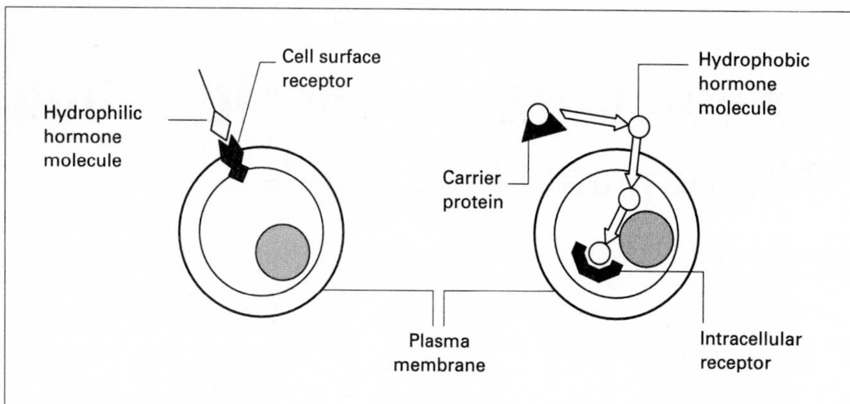

Fig. 4.1 Mechanisms of interaction of hydrophilic and hydrophobic hormones with their target cells. Hydrophilic hormones are unable to cross the plasma membrane, and interact with receptors on the surface of the target cell. Hydrophobic hormones are lipid soluble, and cross the plasma membrane to bind to intracellular receptors. Hydrophobic hormones are presented to their target cells in association with specific carrier proteins, from which they dissociate before crossing the plasma membrane.

interacts specifically with hormone, and this may involve discrimination between a number of closely similar molecular structures and conformations. The high level of selectivity demanded for effective hormone interaction is well illustrated by the similarity between the pituitary glycoprotein hormones thyroid-stimulating hormone (TSH), follicle-stimulating hormone (FSH) and luteinising hormone (LH), all of which possess identical α-subunits and show highly homologous β-subunits.

Binding of the hormone to its receptor involves the same type of weak interactions that characterise the binding of an enzyme to its substrate, including ionic and van der Waals' bonds and hydrophobic interactions. Hormone–receptor binding can thus be described by the simple equation R + H = [RH] and K_m = [R][H]/[RH] where [R] and [H] represent the concentrations of free receptor and hormone, respectively; [RH] is the concentration of the receptor–hormone complex, and K_m is a measure of the affinity of the receptor for the hormone. The K_m values for hormone receptors approximate to the concentration of hormone in the circulation. Accordingly, changes in hormone level will be reflected in proportional adjustments in the fraction of the receptor population that is occupied. Cells are frequently required to respond maximally to small changes in circulating hormone, and one mechanism by which this is achieved involves the binding of two or more hormone molecules to each receptor. Under such conditions, the cell's response depends upon the simultaneous binding of two hormone molecules:

$$\mathrm{R} + \mathrm{H} \underset{}{\overset{K_{m1}}{\rightleftharpoons}} [\mathrm{RH}]$$

then

$$[\mathrm{RH}] + [\mathrm{H}] \overset{K_{m2}}{\rightleftharpoons} [\mathrm{RH2}] \rightarrow \text{response.}$$

Although the simultaneous binding of two hormone molecules can be non-cooperative, such that the interaction of the first hormone molecule does not affect that of the second (i.e. $K_{m1} = K_{m2}$), the binding of more than one molecule of hormone to a receptor often demonstrates positive cooperativity (i.e. $K_{m1} > K_{m2}$, a lower K_m value indicating higher affinity), thereby enhancing the target-cell sensitivity to small increases in hormone concentration.

Various types of membrane receptors have been identified that transmit the response to hormone–receptor interaction through the lipid-rich cell membrane. All such receptors so far characterised have apparent molecular masses ranging from 30 000 to 300 000 kDa, and three principal structural forms may be identified (Fig. 4.2). In the simplest of these, the hormone-binding subunit resides at the outer end of a transmembrane polypeptide chain where it is exposed to the aqueous extracellular environment. The inner region of the chain lies within the cell membrane, close to the regulatory and catalytic subunits of the receptor.

One large family of receptors is characterised by seven transmembrane segments connected by three extra- and three intracellular loops, for example the TSH receptor [2] and the dopamine D2 receptor. In common with the receptors for the other glycoprotein hormones (i.e. LH/CG and FSH [3]), the TSH receptor has an extended amino-terminal domain that encodes the specificity for hormone recognition and binding (Fig. 4.2a).

Another form of receptor is that of a single transmembrane peptide which, while containing a hormone-binding site at its outer extremity, is devoid of intrinsic catalytic activity. The activity of this form of receptor is dependent on this hormone-binding peptide being covalently linked to further peptide chains with effector activity, such as a protein kinase. Some members of the cytokine receptor superfamily have this structure (Fig. 4.2b).

A third form of receptor involves association of a non-membrane-permeating subunit which contains the hormone-binding site together with a further subunit which traverses the membrane bilayer to interact with the regulatory and catalytic subunits (Fig. 4.2c). Examples of this structure

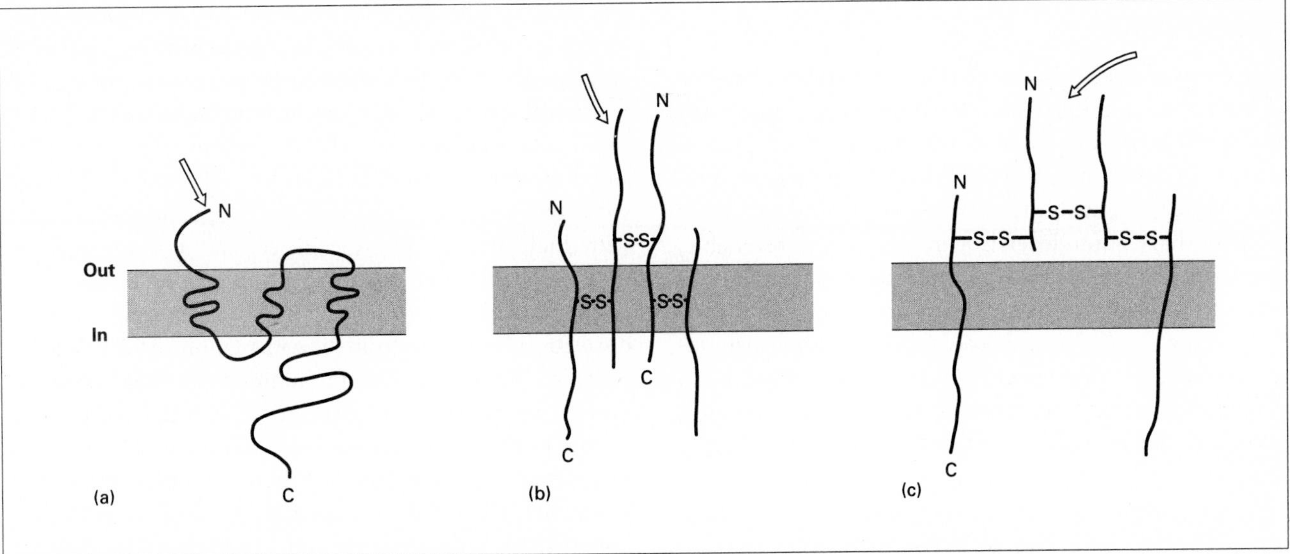

Fig. 4.2 Models of plasma membrane receptors for polypeptide hormones. (a) A single, transmembrane polypeptide chain. The hormone-binding site is associated with the amino-terminal end, there may be one or more transmembrane domains, while the carboxy-terminal region of the chain may interact with the regulatory and catalytic subunits of the receptor. (b) A series of covalently linked transmembrane polypeptides. The hormone-binding site may reside on the amino-terminal region of a single chain, as shown, or within a complex formed by two or more chains. (c) Pairs of peptide chains, one of which may be entirely extracellular, linked by disulphide bridges. Conformational changes induced by a hormone in one of the subunits may perturb the second, transmembrane, chain whose intracellular domain effects the signalling response.

include the receptors for insulin and insulin-like growth factor 1.

Regulation of receptor availability

At the surface of any hormone-responsive cell, the population of hormone-binding sites reflects a dynamic equilibrium between synthesis and degradation of receptors. Receptor availability for any given hormone may be increased ('up-regulation') or decreased ('down-regulation') under physiological conditions. This both allows for responsiveness to small variations in hormone level, and also provides the ability to cope with sudden large alterations in circulating hormone level.

Endocytosis

Many peptide hormones, including insulin and glucagon, bind to receptor and are then internalised by receptor-mediated endocytosis. The resulting endocytotic vesicles are hydrolysed and degraded by lysosomal enzymes. The internalisation process not only terminates the hormonal signal, but also regulates the availability of hormone-binding subunits at the cell surface. Under normal conditions, receptor degradation and regeneration occur simultaneously and continually, and in the absence of hormonal internalisation the receptor may have a half-life of a few days. Although some internalised receptors eventually recycle back to the cell surface, a number of agonists, including epidermal growth factor, increase the rate of degradation of their receptors so that the net receptor density at the cell surface is progressively reduced. Some ingested hormone molecules are further translocated within the cell and may accumulate at the Golgi region. Once the internalised hormone has entered a particular organelle, it may subsequently interact with specific receptors and directly influence the function of that organelle through membrane-mediated actions, in the same way that hormonal effects are mediated at the plasma membrane.

Conformation change

Instead of inducing down-regulation through internalisation and degradation of receptors, some hormones, including adrenaline, reversibly inactivate their receptors after interaction. This results from a prolonged but reversible alteration in receptor protein conformation, effectively preventing the receptor from responding to a further hormone molecule for a considerable period following dissociation of the original agonist molecule. This reversible inactivation of cell-surface receptors may reduce either the hormone-binding ability or the catalytic activity of the receptor.

Phosphorylation

Some forms of desensitisation of receptor-coupled adenylate cyclase involve specific phosphorylation events, which may involve the actions of both protein kinase A and protein kinase C [4]. Although phosphorylated receptors can bind hormone, they are unable to activate adenylate cyclase. Since this phosphorylation-dependent inactivation is reversible, removal of the agonist is followed by a progressive reactivation of the cell-surface receptor population. Accordingly, cells which show this form of receptor desensitisation demonstrate a feedback loop system in which raised cAMP leads to phosphorylation and densensitisation of the receptor, decreasing the subsequent response to the extracellular hormone.

Hormone-receptor families and signalling cascades

A number of families of receptors have now been well characterised, and each has distinctive associated signalling pathways. The signalling pathways will be described alongside the different classes of receptors in the following sections.

1 G-protein-coupled receptors located on the cell membrane; the cascade of cAMP, adenylate cyclase, protein kinase A (PKA) and cAMP response element binding protein (CREB) transcription factors; the Ca^{2+} signalling system, inositol phosphates, calmodulin, protein kinase C (PKC), and the AP-1 transcription factor; exocytotic mechanisms and ion channels.

2 Cytokine receptors and receptor tyrosine kinases such as the insulin receptor; cascades of protein phosphorylation through sets of intracellular kinases; JAK kinases and STAT transcription factors.

3 Intracellular hormone receptors—the steroid/thyroid/retinoid hormone-receptor superfamily and hormone receptors as transcription factors.

1 G-protein-coupled receptors

The receptor-binding sites for a large number of non-hydrophobic hormones are coupled to the catalytic subunit of the receptor complex through guanyl nucleotide-binding regulatory proteins, the so-called G-proteins [5]. The G-protein-associated receptor superfamily represents an extraordinarily versatile group of glycoproteins that transmit signals across the plasma membrane with a high degree of efficiency. The G-proteins are a group of closely related heterotrimeric proteins consisting of three subunits designated α (39–46 kDa), β (37 kDa) and γ (8 kDa), which are distinct gene products. They constitute part of the superfamily of guanosine triphosphatases (GTPases) that includes cytoskeletal proteins such as tubulin, soluble proteins (initiation and elongation factors involved in protein synthesis), and low-molecular-weight monomeric proteins such as the $p21^{ras}$ proto-oncogene and *ras*-related proteins. The G-protein subset of the superfamily shares several common features with other members. Thus, they all bind guanine nucleotides with high affinity and specificity, and possess intrinsic GTPase activity that modulates interactions between the G-protein and other elements. Other features, however, distinguish G-proteins from the wider family of GTP-binding proteins. These include, in addition to their common heterotrimeric structure, association with the cytoplasmic surface of the plasma membrane, and functional activity as receptor–effector couplers. Within the complex, the β- and γ-subunits are tightly complexed through non-covalent bonding, while the α-subunit (G_α) contributes the GTPase activity and has a high affinity for GTP. The α-subunit also confers the essential specificity to receptor–effector coupling, and directly modulates the activity of the effector. The receptors for a hormone which is dependent upon the actions of G-proteins may thus be considered as a multicomponent complex involving, at the very least, a binding subunit, a regulatory or G-protein complex, a catalytic subunit (e.g. adenylate cyclase) and associated regulatory enzymes.

Activation of adenylate cyclase: G_s

Historically, the earliest characterised G-protein-coupled receptor–effector system was β-adrenergic receptor-coupled adenylate cyclase [6], which has since been demonstrated to represent a wide variety of receptors utilising cAMP as their second messenger. Adenylate cyclase can be regarded as the effector protein which triggers a cascade of intracellular events as described later. There are now known to be at least six adenylate cyclase subtypes in mammalian cells, with different tissue-specific distribution. The 120 kDa adenylate cyclase enzyme consists of cytoplasmic and transmembrane α-helical domains.

As described below, specific and unique combinations of G-proteins enable diverse receptors to transduce the effects of a multitude of different ligands, and more than 100 G-protein-associated receptors have already been described. However, although the structures of G-protein-linked receptors show a high degree of heterogeneity, they share the general structure of a single polypeptide chain forming seven transmembrane sections, as depicted in Fig. 4.3. Agonists interact with the N-terminus or domains within the external loops, while the C-terminus of the receptor, or one or more of the intracellular loops, represent the presumed site(s) of G-protein interaction. The coordinated and tightly regulated interaction of the extracellular and intracellular domains,

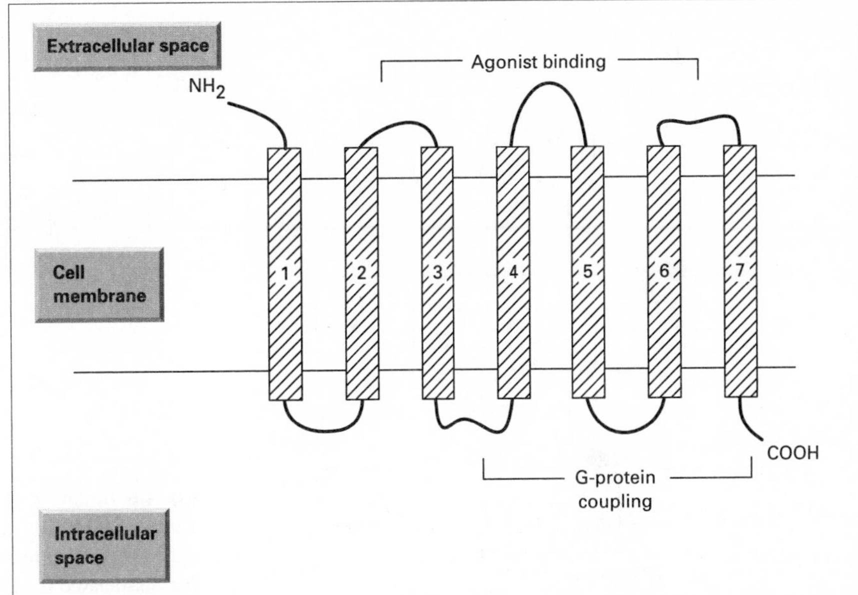

Fig. 4.3 Typical structure of a G-protein-coupled hormone receptor. Seven transmembrane α-helices span the cell membrane, and are connected by three extracellular and three intracellular loops. The N-terminal and external loop domains contain the recognition sites for agonist binding, and the intracellular domain is involved in G-protein coupling.

via the transmembrane portion of the receptor, is fundamental to generation of the appropriate intracellular response.

Hormone binding alters the conformation of receptor subunit in such a way that it binds to the G-protein. The resultant allosteric change displaces guanosine diphosphate (GDP) from the G_α-subunit, in turn binding GTP (Figs 4.3 and 4.4). Upon binding of GTP to G_α, the G_α-subunit dissociates from the βγ complex. The G_α–GTP complex, after dissociation from the receptor, undergoes a conformational change to enable it to activate a catalytic subunit (e.g. adenylate cyclase). GTP is then hydrolysed to GDP, activating the catalytic subunit, and the now inactive G_α–GDP complex is able to return to the receptor and reassociate with the βγ complex. Simultaneously with this transfer of G_α–GDP, the catalytic subunit (adenylate cyclase) is inactivated (Fig. 4.4). An effective GTP–GDP recycling system is, therefore, a fundamental requirement for the hormone-dependent activation and inactivation of adenylate cyclase (Fig. 4.5). Confirmation of the importance of the GTP–GDP recycling system to the hormonal activation of adenylate cyclase has been obtained in studies using cholera toxin, which irreversibly modifies the α-subunit of the G-protein through ADP ribosylation. While activating adenylate cyclase normally, this modified subunit is unable to hydrolyse bound GTP to GDP. Accordingly, GTP remains bound to the G_α-subunit which therefore, together with adenylate cyclase, remains permanently active, and thus continues to generate cAMP.

Within the G-protein complex, G_α may in effect be considered as a link between the hormone-binding site and the catalytic subunit, although it also functions as a signal transducer, relaying the hormone-induced conformational change in the receptor to an eventual alteration in the activity of the catalytic subunit. Since the G_α–GTP complex interacts with both the hormone-binding and catalytic subunits, it plays a crucial role in terminating the intracellular response to the hormone. Thus, replacement of the GDP bound to G_α by GTP results in a decreased affinity of the receptor for the hormone, a shift in the receptor–hormone equilibrium in favour of dissociation, and consequently to inactivation of the catalytic subunit. Until recently, the βγ dimer had no recognised role in signal transduction other than to attenuate G_α function. However, a number of direct catalytic effects of the dissociated βγ-subunit have now been identified and characterised; recognised targets include phospholipase C [7].

Prominent among the hormones acting through G-protein-coupled receptors are the majority of the hypothalamic releasing hormones and the anterior and posterior pituitary hormones, albeit with the notable exceptions of growth hormone and prolactin, and many other peptide hormones, monoamines and prostaglandins. Although the classic model for the study of G-proteins has been the activation of adenylate cyclase and the generation of cAMP, it is now apparent that several different hormones may, in any given cell, operate through distinct G-protein-coupled pathways to regulate a single physiological action (Fig. 4.6).

Inhibition of adenylate cyclase: G_i

There are a number of instances in which hormone–receptor interaction leads to a *decrease* rather than an increase in effector activity. For example, in the adipocyte, adrenaline, adrenocorticotrophic hormone (ACTH) and vasopressin stimulate adenylate cyclase whereas prostaglandin E inhibits

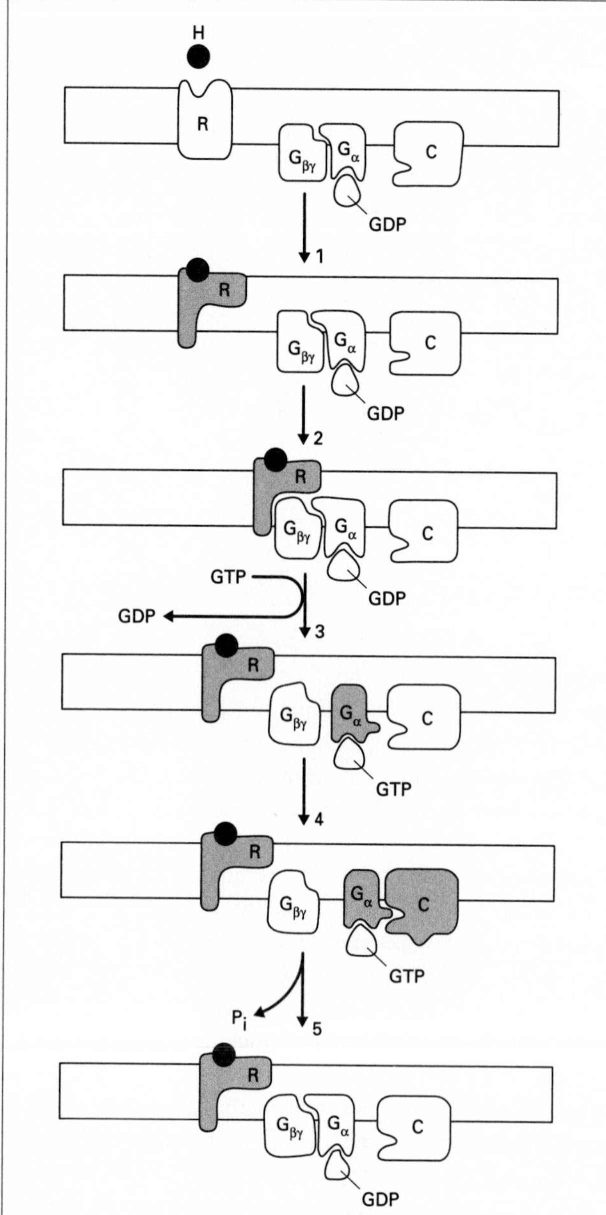

Fig. 4.4 Activation of adenylate cyclase by hormone–receptor interaction. The outer cell membrane contains a receptor protein (R) for a specified hormone (H). Adenylate cyclase (the catalytic subunit, C) together with the regulatory subunit or G-protein complex (G) are located on the inside surface of the membrane. In the non-activated cell, guanosine diphosphate (GDP) is bound to the α-subunit of G. Binding of a hormone induces conformational change in R (1). Activated R binds to G (2), releasing (GDP) and allowing guanosine triphosphate (GTP) to bind. In turn, this causes the G_α and the $G_{\beta\gamma}$ subunits to dissociate (3). Free G_α subunit then binds to C and activates it, catalysing the synthesis of cyclic adenosine monophosphate (cAMP) from adenosine triphosphate (ATP) (4). This step may involve a conformational change in G_α. After hydrolysis of GTP to GDP, G_α is no longer able to activate C (5), so that G_α and $G_{\beta\gamma}$ are able to reassociate. The hormone then dissociates from its receptor and the system returns to a resting state.

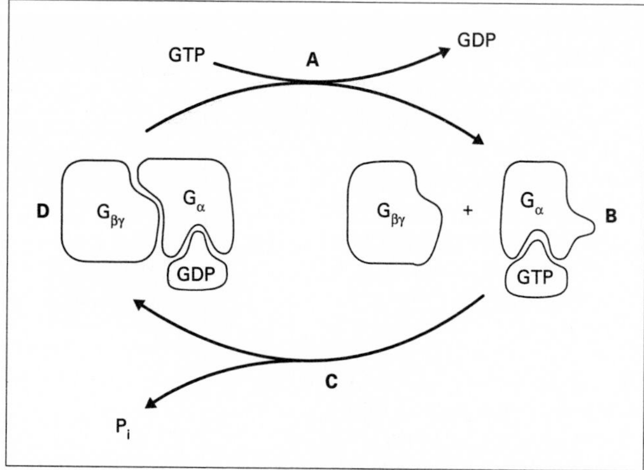

Fig. 4.5 Recycling of the G-protein complex between guanosine triphosphate (GTP) and guanosine diphosphate (GDP). (a) activation of GTP hydrolysis after hormone–receptor interaction. (b) The dissociated G_α–GTP complex activates adenylate cyclase. (c) Bound GTP is hydrolysed, resulting in inactivation of adenylate cyclase. This step is thought to be catalysed by the G_α subunit itself, and is inhibited by cholera toxin. (d) The G_α–GDP subunit reassociates with the $G_{\beta\gamma}$ subunit. This complex cannot stimulate adenylate cyclase.

it; in the pituitary, dopamine inhibits cAMP-mediated prolactin secretion. These inhibitory receptors are coupled to the catalytic subunit via an inhibitory G-protein (G_i) which, while containing the same β- and γ-subunits as the stimulatory G-protein, contains a different G_α ($G_{i\alpha}$). This subunit also binds GTP and GDP, and in response to hormone binding at the receptor, G_i binds GTP and this complex dissociates into $G_{i\alpha}$–GTP and $G_{\beta\gamma}$. Such dissociation, however, results in an inhibition rather than an activation of adenylate cyclase activity (Fig. 4.7). Although the precise mechanism of inhibition remains uncertain, the system allows the cell to maintain a very tight regulation of its cAMP level through integrating the response of several hormones, each of which binds to a specific cell-surface receptor. In an analogous manner to the effect of cholera toxin on the stimulatory subunit of the G-protein, pertussis toxin can irreversibly modify the α-subunit of G_i by adenosine diphosphate (ADP) ribosylation, preventing dissociation of the complex and resulting in failure of inhibition.

Heterogeneity and diversity of G-protein isotypes

The diverse nature of G-protein effects is made possible by the multitude of different isotypes of each subunit, and the family of known members continues to expand. Molecular cloning studies have revealed the existence of over 20 complementary DNAs (cDNAs) coding for G-protein α-subunits that are the products of at least 17 genes. The family of G_0,

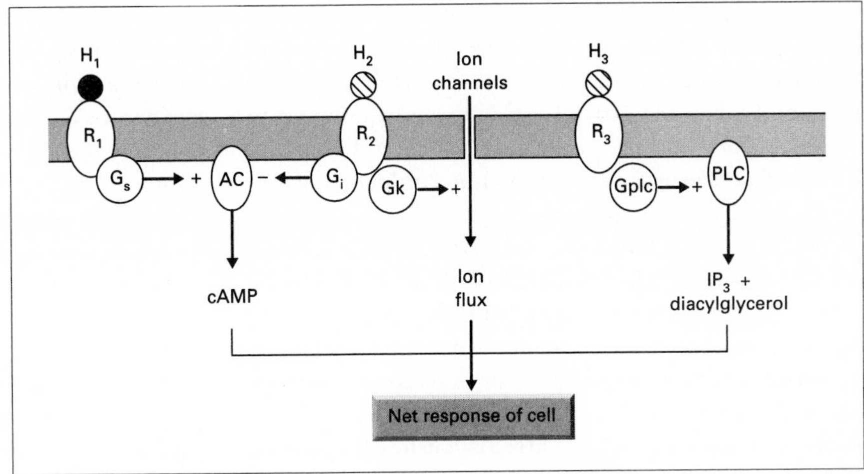

Fig. 4.6 Different G-proteins mediate the physiological actions of diverse hormones in a single cell type. As illustrated in this example, three distinct receptors (R_1, R_2, R_3) selectively interact with three different hormones (first messengers) (H_1, H_2, H_3). R_1 is linked to adenylate cyclase (AC) by G_s. R_2 is coupled to inhibition of adenylate cyclase by G_i, and to regulation of ion channels, by G_k (stimulation of K^+ channels) and G_o (inhibition of Ca^{2+} channels). R_3 is linked to phospholipase C. In any given cell, different pathways may predominate, but in some cells, each pathway may be responsive to distinct first messengers.

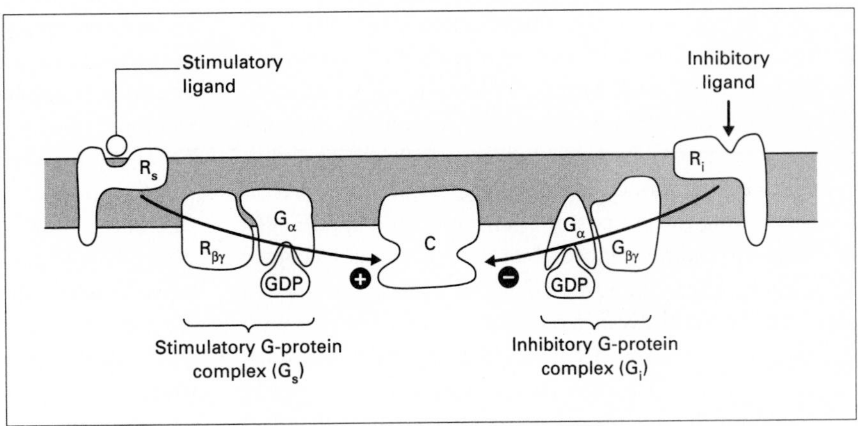

Fig. 4.7 The activation and inhibition of adenylate cyclase are mediated through different G-proteins. As shown in Fig. 4.3, hormone action is effected by a stimulatory G-protein, the G_α subunit of which, in association with guanosine triphosphate (GTP), binds to and activates the catalytic subunit of adenylate cyclase. Other hormone–receptor complexes interact with a different G-protein, the activated α-subunit of which inhibits, rather than stimulates, adenylate cyclase. The inhibitory G_α subunit and its receptor differ from those associated with cyclase activation, although the G_α and $G_{\beta\gamma}$ subunits are identical with those mediating the actions of stimulatory hormones.

G_S, G_{i1}, G_{i2}, G_{i3}, G_{t1}, G_{t2}, and $G_{x(z)}$, may be further subdivided into various isotypes generated as a result of alternative gene splicing events [8]. Such events have been shown, for example, to account for the expression of four forms of G_S. Expression of certain α-subunits is restricted to specific cell types, whereas others such as G_S and G_{12} are expressed ubiquitously. Other G-proteins show an intermediate pattern of tissue distribution.

In addition to the heterogeneity of G_α, two distinct genes exist for each of the β- and γ-subunits, leading to further possible permutations in structure of the G-protein complex. The β-subunits demonstrate approximately 80% homology and are anchored to the cell membrane by prenyl groups. Specificity has been demonstrated in the ability of β- and γ-subunits to interact: while the β1-subunit can associate with γ1 and γ2, β2 can only dimerise with γ2, while β3 cannot dimerise with either γ1 or γ2.

Although much is known of the structure and interactions of individual G-protein subunits, the specificity of interaction between G-proteins, receptors and effectors has been defined in relatively few cases. However, studies utilising G-proteins and purified receptors in phospholipid vesicles have shown that β-adrenergic receptors couple, in decreasing order of efficiency, to $G_S > G_i >> G_t$. Many G-protein-coupled receptors, together with a variety of effectors, including adenylate cyclase, certain Ca^{2+} and K^+ channels, and phospholipase C, are subject to regulation by one or more pertussis-toxin-sensitive G-proteins. Similarly, studies of G-protein–effector interactions have demonstrated that while $G_{\alpha s}$ alone can serve as an activator of adenylate cyclase, G_t alone activates cyclic guanosine monophosphate (cGMP) phosphodiesterase [9]. Other G_α subunits have been associated with activation of the phospholipase C family [10]. The nature of the endogenous G-proteins responsible for coupling most other receptors and effectors, however, remains to be elucidated.

Despite the apparent complexity of the interactions of G-proteins with both receptor-binding sites and the catalytic subunit of adenylate cyclase, the design of this system confers several major advantages upon the cellular response to hormone–receptor interaction. Since several G-complexes are converted to the active G_α–GTP form in response to the binding of a single hormone molecule, several adenylate cyclase molecules are also activated. Accordingly, each of the activated catalytic subunits generates a large number of cAMP molecules as long as G_α–GTP is bound, and in many instances several hundred molecules of cAMP can be formed before the hormone dissociates from the binding site of the receptor. Amplification of the extracellular signal is facilitated both by the capacity of a single receptor to activate multiple G-protein units, and also by the fact that the α-subunit remains active for several seconds before hydrolysing its bound GTP, even though the activating hormone has become dissociated from the membrane-bound receptor [10–12]. In addition to this amplification effect, the intervention of the G-protein family provides the cell with a means of rapidly terminating its response on withdrawal of hormone. By the same token, the continuous presence of hormone is required for full activation of adenylate cyclase to be maintained. The involvement of three proteins in transmitting the actions of a hormone on a specific cell function also allows more than one hormone–receptor complex to affect the same adenylate cyclase enzyme. In such cases, several distinct receptor proteins interact with the same G-protein and convert the inactive G-complex to the active G_α–GTP form. Accordingly, both the level of G_α–GTP and the activity of adenylate cyclase will reflect the additive effect of the individual hormones binding to their own specific receptors.

On account of their critical position in the pathway of hormone action, G-protein mutations profoundly influence the signal transduction process. Thus, changes that lead to the loss of G-protein function are frequently associated with hormone resistance, while changes involving constitutive G-protein activation lead to hormone-independent transmission of second-messenger signals. For example, 40% of the somatotroph adenomas that give rise to acromegaly, together with a small number of functioning thyroid adenomas, display constitutive activation of adenylate cyclase due to several possible mutations in the $G_{S\alpha}$ subunit, collectively known as the *gsp* oncogene [13,14].

The cAMP signalling system, protein kinase A and CREB

Cyclic AMP regulates a wide variety of intracellular processes in all endocrine cell types, and indeed in all nucleated eukaryotic cells. Its intracellular concentration is tightly controlled as a function of its production and its degradation, both of which are regulated by a variety of hormones in different endocrine cells. Much of our understanding of the cAMP signalling system in endocrine cells has relied on the use of pharmacological tools which affect its production or degradation at a variety of different levels, for example forskolin (which stimulates the catalytic subunit of adenylate cyclase) and cholera toxin (ADP-ribosylates $G_{S\alpha}$ subunit and so prevents GTP hydrolysis and therefore stimulates adenylate cyclase).

Most hormones whose effects are primarily mediated by cAMP act by increasing or reducing its production from ATP (with magnesium as a cofactor) by adenylate cyclase. The action of a hormone in stimulating adenylate cyclase causes rapid changes in cAMP concentration, with manifold increases occurring over a few seconds. However, tightly regulated and rapid changes in cAMP concentration can occur only because it is also removed rapidly by cAMP phosphodiesterases which hydrolyse cAMP to adenosine 5′-monophosphase (5′-AMP). The activity of one of these enzymes is modulated by intracellular calcium and calmodulin (see below), and hence it is affected by other hormones for which calcium is the primary second messenger substance; thus, the kinetics of the cAMP response to one hormone may be markedly altered by the calcium response to another signal. This is one example of several ways in which interactions may occur between intracellular signalling systems allowing subtle integration of the final cellular response to a series of different hormonal signals.

Cyclic AMP and protein kinases

Cyclic AMP activates cAMP-dependent protein kinase, PKA, which phosphorylates many potential substrate proteins. In many cases the substrate proteins are enzymes and this phosphorylation increases or decreases their activity. PKA consists of an inactive complex containing two regulatory and two catalytic subunits (Fig. 4.8). The regulatory subunit varies amongst different cell types, but the catalytic subunit structure is conserved. Cyclic AMP binds to the regulatory subunits to cause dissociation of free catalytic subunits with enhanced kinase activity. These subunits are able to diffuse within the cell to phosphorylate several target proteins (including the regulatory subunit itself), and may enter organelles such as the cell nucleus.

Activated PKA can phosphorylate both serine and threonine residues of proteins that contain the phosphorylation consensus sequence Arg-Arg-X-Ser/Thr-X, where X represents another amino acid. The three-dimensional crystal structure of PKA has shown that ATP and substrate protein are bound in a cleft between two lobes, allowing the transfer of the γ-phosphate from ATP to the serine or threonine residue of the target protein.

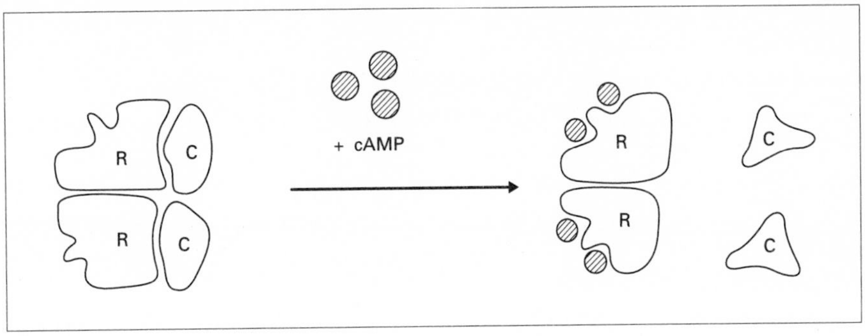

Fig. 4.8 Protein kinase A is a heterotetramer comprising regulatory (R) and catalytic (C) subunits. Free active C subunits dissociate after cyclic adenosine monophosphate (cAMP) binding to the R subunits.

The cAMP stimulation of protein kinases is not permanent, and the termination of the cAMP signal involves both the removal of cAMP itself by phosphodiesterase and also the inactivation of phosphorylated substrate proteins by phosphoprotein phosphatases, which remove the newly added phosphate groups. These phosphatases may themselves be activated by cAMP or by the calcium–calmodulin system. However, a phosphatase inhibitor protein is among the substrate proteins activated by the catalytic subunit of cAMP-dependent protein kinase, and this temporarily inhibits the phosphatase enzyme. As cAMP levels fall, the phosphatase is activated, and the initial kinase-induced phosphorylation is reversed, terminating the signal. This cycle of protein phosphorylation ensures that a short-lived cAMP signal induced by receptor activation produces only a transient cellular response.

In many cases the substrates for cAMP-dependent protein kinases are not yet known, but they clearly differ widely and are found in specific cell types to give a variety of cAMP responses. One effect of the cAMP–kinase system may be to allow amplification of the initial signal at the plasma membrane with a series of kinases, resulting in a magnified cellular response, but in some cases the effects may be much simpler. One case where cAMP effects have now been studied in some detail is that of cAMP-regulated gene transcription.

The effects of cAMP on gene transcription

As an example of a complete signalling cascade, the cAMP–kinase system has direct effects on gene regulation within the nucleus, resulting in altered synthesis of proteins; the mechanisms for this effect at the level of the gene are becoming very much clearer [15]. The identification of cAMP responsive elements (CREs) within promoter regions of certain genes allowed the purification of DNA-binding proteins. One such protein (CREB) is a 43-kDa protein, which is phosphorylated by purified catalytic subunit of PKA. CREB phosphorylation promotes dimerisation to enhance its activity as a transcription factor [16]. In this case, at least, activation of a substrate protein is a *direct* consequence of cAMP-dependent protein kinase, rather than the end result of a more complex cascade (Fig. 4.9).

A large family of CREB-related proteins has emerged, including CREB splice variants, activating transcription factor proteins (ATFs 1–8) and a series of CRE modulators (CREMs). CREB itself, the best characterised member of the CREB/ATF family, comprises two major structural elements, a C-terminal DNA-binding domain (including a leucine zipper that allows dimerisation), and a highly acidic N-terminal *trans*-activation region which includes the phosphorylation site. CREB may form both CREB–CREB homodimers and CREB–ATF1 heterodimers, although other CREB family members show a wide variety of potential heterodimers with other leucine-zipper transcription factors. CREB activity is modulated not only by PKA phosphorylation, but also by other kinases including PKC, and by interaction with inhibitory CREM proteins and inducible cAMP response element repressor (ICER) proteins. Thus, with a ramifying network of related DNA-binding proteins, there is scope for great complexity and subtlety of response even at this last stage of this particular receptor–effector–kinase–substrate signalling cascade [17].

The Ca^{2+} signalling system

A large number of hormones and neutrotransmitters such as vasopressin, TSH, acetylcholine and noradrenaline exert their effects on the target cell by raising the intracellular concentration of cytosolic free Ca^{2+} ($[Ca^{2+}]i$). In mammalian cells $[Ca^{2+}]i$ is maintained within close limits of approximately 10^{-7} mol/l in the unstimulated cell. Since extracellular $[Ca^{2+}]i$ is in the millimolar range (10^{-3} mol/l), there is clearly an extremely large (of the order of 10 000-fold) Ca^{2+} gradient across the plasma membrane. A considerable proportion of the cell's energy expenditure is coupled directly or indirectly to the maintenance of this Ca^{2+} gradient, the existence of which is crucial to the life and functioning of the cell [18].

A number of processes are collectively responsible for the maintenance of low $[Ca^{2+}]i$. These can be divided into two groups: those involved in pumping Ca^{2+} from the cytosol

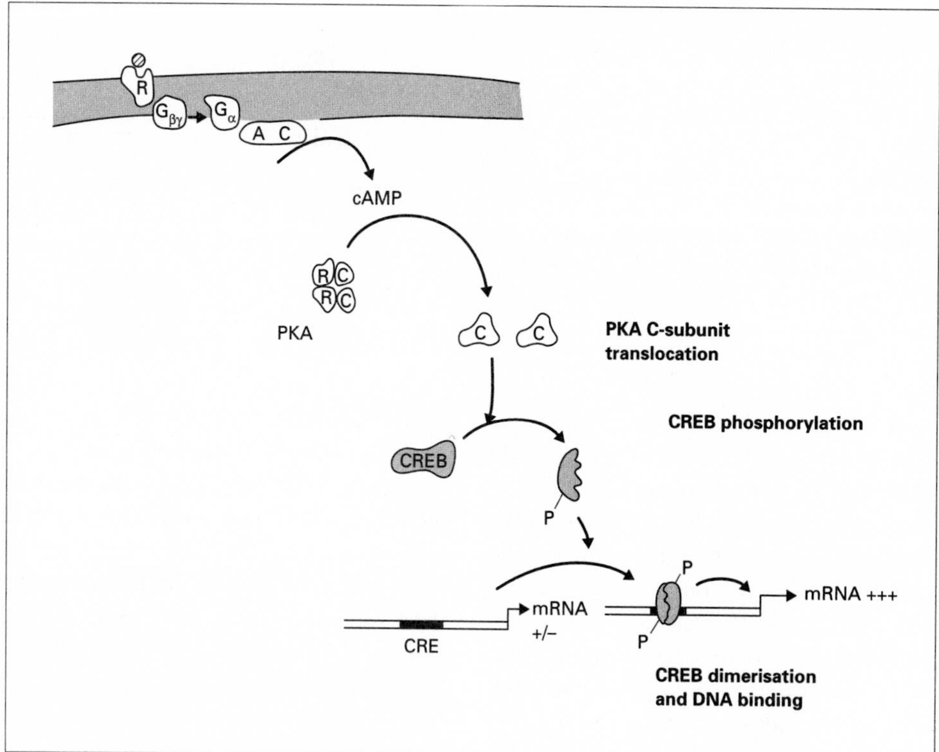

Fig. 4.9 Simplified diagram of the signalling cascade leading from activation of adenylate cyclase (AC) to protein kinase A (PKA) activation and cyclic adenosine monophosphate (cAMP) response element binding protein (CREB) phosphorylation. Phosphorylated CREB binds to the cAMP response element (CRE) as a dimer to activate gene transcription.

into the extracellular medium and those responsible for sequestering Ca^{2+} into intracellular organelles (Fig. 4.10a). The plasma membrane has two principal mechanisms for extruding Ca^{2+} from the cell: a Ca^{2+} ATPase which pumps Ca^{2+} out of the cell using energy released from the hydrolysis of intracellular ATP, and a Na^+/Ca^{2+} exchange system which couples the entry of Na^+ into the cell, down its concentration gradient, with Ca^{2+} extrusion. This latter system is driven both by the inwardly directed Na^+ gradient and, since the system is electrogenic ($3Na^+/1Ca^{2+}$), by the inside-negative membrane potential of the cell. A number of intracellular organelles including smooth endoplasmic reticulum and secretory granules also accumulate Ca^{2+} via ATP-driven Ca^{2+} pumps. Ca^{2+} is also sequestered from the cytosol into mitochondria, a process depending upon the inside-negative mitochondrial membrane potential and hence mitochondrial metabolism.

Modulation of $[Ca^{2+}]i$:

As stated above, the actions of several hormones, neurotransmitters and other agonists depend on their ability to cause a rise in $[Ca^{2+}]i$ in the target cell. There are several mechanisms by which such an effect may be brought about depending on the agonists and, to a certain extent, the target cell in question [19].

Depolarisation

First, stimulation of some types of excitable cell with certain agonists causes depolarisation of the plasma membrane, either by activating Na^+ channels, thus allowing Na^+ to enter the cell (e.g. acetycholine binding to nicotinic receptors in neurons), or by inhibiting K^+ channels, thus restricting the efflux of K^+ ions from the cell (e.g. glucose stimulation of the pancreatic β-cell). In either case, this depolarisation results in the opening of a specific type of plasma membrane Ca^{2+} channel known as the voltage-sensitive Ca^{2+} channel (VSCC). The opening of the VSCCs will allow Ca^{2+} to enter the cell, down the inwardly directed Ca^{2+} gradient, thus causing a rise in $[Ca^{2+}]i$ (Fig. 4.10b).

Receptor-operated Ca^{2+} channels

A second, more direct, route of agonist-induced Ca^{2+} entry occurs via receptor-operated Ca^{2+} channels (ROCC) [20]. In this case, the receptor is in direct functional association with the Ca^{2+} channel such that the binding of an agonist results in opening of the channel (Fig. 4.10b). The stimulation

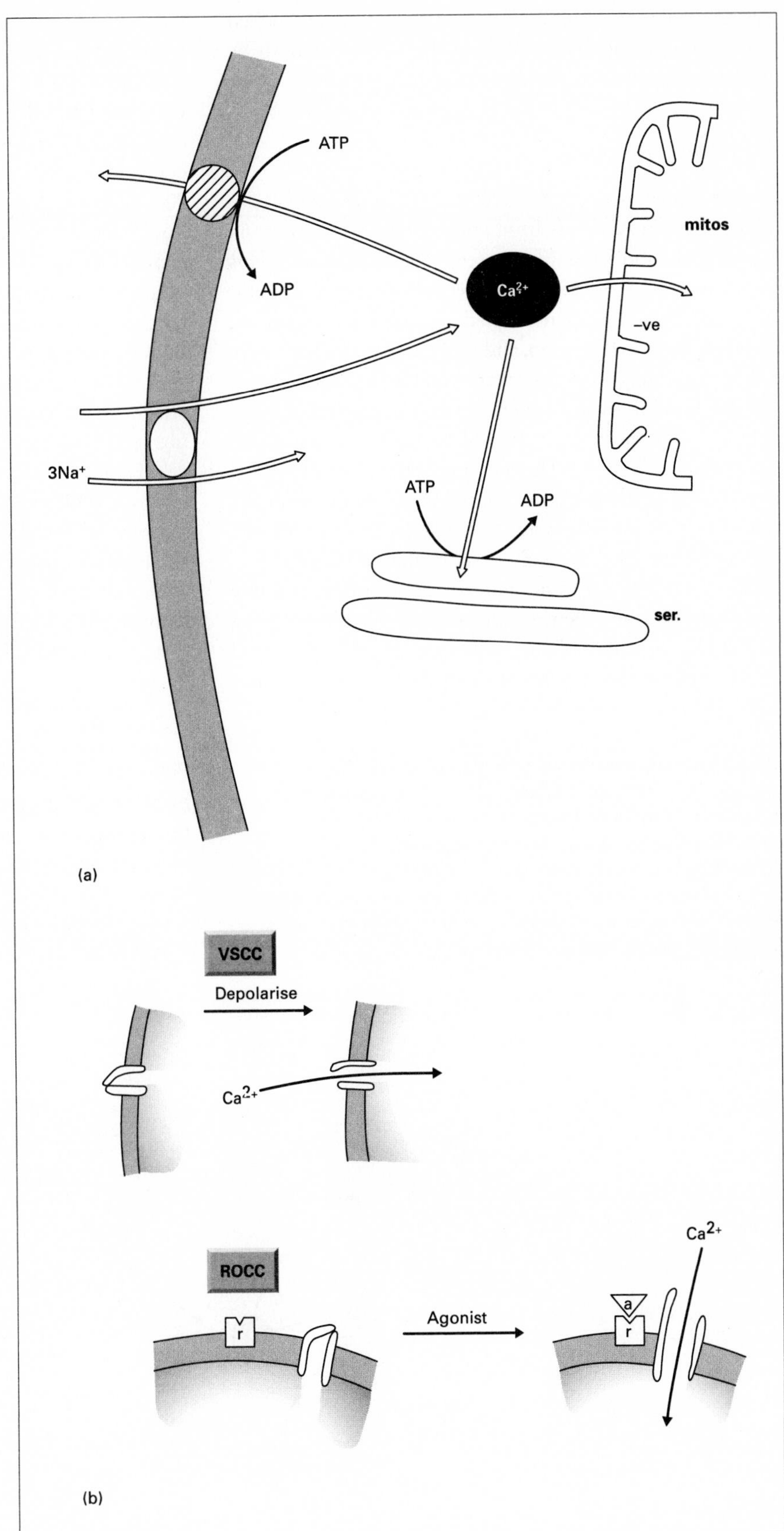

Fig. 4.10 (a) Principal mechanisms for extrusion of Ca^{2+} from the cytosol into the extracellular fluid and into intracellular organelles, smooth endoplasmic reticulum (ser) and mitochondria (mitos). (b) Two distinct classes of Ca^{2+} channel exist in the plasma membrane: voltage-sensitive (VSCC) and receptor-operated (ROCC) Ca^{2+} channels. a, agonist; r, receptor.

of certain cell types (e.g. smooth muscle and blood platelets) by purine nucleotides (ATP and ADP) is thought to be mediated via this type of channel.

Inositol–lipid signalling

A third mechanism whereby certain types of agonist can induce a rise in $[Ca^{2+}]i$ is from intracellular Ca^{2+} stores via the inositol–lipid signalling system [21] (Fig. 4.11). This system is one of the best-characterised signalling systems activated by G-protein-coupled membrane receptors, alongside the cAMP system, and is of particular importance in Ca^{2+} signalling in non-excitable endocrine cells. In this case the binding of the agonist to its receptor on the cell surface results in the activation of a membrane-associated phospholipase C (PLC). The coupling of the receptor to PLC involves the participation of specific G-proteins, or in the case of certain growth factor receptors, a tyrosine kinase. The activated PLC hydrolyses phosphatidylinositol-4,5-bisphosphate (PIP_2), a minor but critical inositol-containing phospholipid component of the plasma membrane. The breakdown products of this hydrolysis are diacylglycerol (DAG) and inositol-1,4,5-trisphosphate (IP_3). IP_3 is water soluble and hence is able to diffuse into the cytosol, bind to a specific receptor on the smooth endoplasmic reticulum, and cause the release of Ca^{2+} from this organelle into the cytosol. The release of Ca^{2+} from IP_3-sensitive stores is coupled, in some way, to enhanced entry of Ca^{2+} into the cell, a process known as capacitative Ca^{2+} entry (Fig. 4.11). The exact mechanism underlying this process is unknown but could involve a so-called 'Ca^{2+} release-activated Ca^{2+} channel' (I_{CRAC}) in the plasma membrane. It has also been suggested that inositol 1,3,4,5-tetrakisphosphate (IP_4), formed by phosphorylation of IP_3, could be involved in capacitative Ca^{2+} entry (Fig. 4.11).

In recent years, another putative intracellular signal, cyclic ADP–ribose, has been implicated in Ca^{2+} mobilisation from intracellular pools [19]. This compound is synthesised from cellular nicotinamide adenine dinucleotide (NAD^+) by the enzyme ADP–ribosyl cyclase, and has been suggested to be the physiological agonist for the ryanodine receptor. This receptor controls Ca^{2+} release from intracellular stores in some cell types (especially excitable cells), and can also be activated by a local rise in $[Ca^{2+}]i$, thus giving rise to a process of Ca^{2+}-induced Ca^{2+} release (see below) [19].

Fig. 4.11 Certain receptors are linked, via a specific G-protein complex, to phospholipase C (PLC). This enzyme hydrolyses phosphatidyl-inositol 4,5-bisphosphate (PIP_2) to form two intracellular signals: *inositol 1,4,5-trisphosphate (IP_3)* binds to receptors on the smooth endoplasmic reticulum (ser) and mobilises Ca^{2+}; *diacylglycerol* (DAG) binds to and activates protein kinase C (PKC). IP_4 may be involved in refilling of intracellular Ca^{2+} stores through Ca^{2+}-release-activated channels (I_{CRAC}).

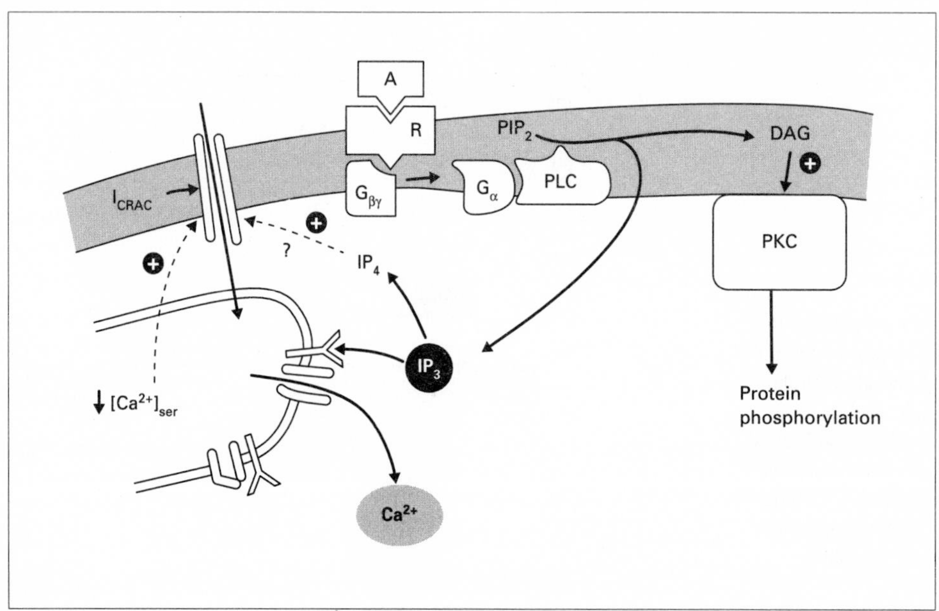

Ca^{2+} oscillations

Following the development of techniques for the measurement of $[Ca^{2+}]i$, particularly at the single-cell level, it has become apparent that agonist-stimulated increases in $[Ca^{2+}]i$ in many cell types occur as a pattern of oscillations, or transients, rather than a sustained rise in $[Ca^{2+}]i$ [22] (Fig. 4.12a) . In such cases, the frequency of the Ca^{2+} oscillations is modulated by the concentration of agonist. An additional

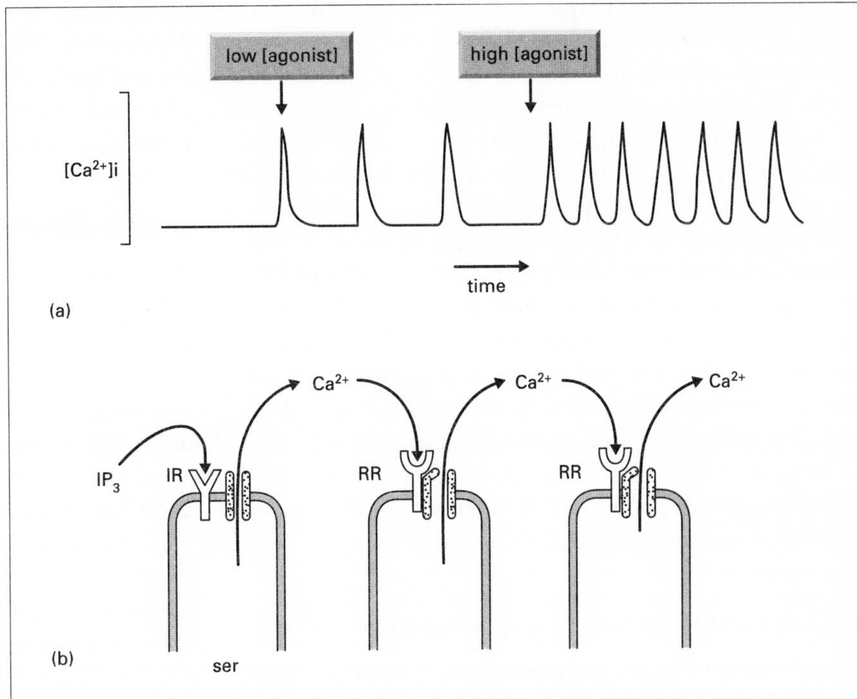

Fig. 4.12 (a) Frequency modulation of Ca^{2+} oscillations by varying concentrations of hormone agonist. (b) Proposed mechanism for Ca^{2+}-induced release of further Ca^{2+} from intracellular stores: inositol 1,4,5-trisphosphate (IP_3) activates IP_3 receptors on smooth endoplasmic reticulum (ser), to release stored Ca^{2+}; this in turn activates ryanodine receptors (RR) on other intracellular organelles, and a positive-feedback cascade is set up giving a rapid local accumulation of free cytosolic Ca^{2+} in a 'hot spot' within the cell.

feature of Ca^{2+} signalling which has become evident from 'imaging' $[Ca^{2+}]$i in a single cell is that changes in $[Ca^{2+}]$i do not occur uniformly throughout the cytosol, but rather as 'hot spots' in certain specific areas of the cell. These localised increases in $[Ca^{2+}]$i can often be seen to propagate through the cytosol as a wave of Ca^{2+}, a process which could involve IP_3-induced and Ca^{2+}-induced Ca^{2+} release from intracellular stores (Fig. 4.12b). These spatio-temporal aspects of Ca^{2+} signalling, whilst clearly complex, potentially enable more information to be transmitted though the cell and are probably important in providing an integrated control of cellular physiology.

Calmodulin

Changes in $[Ca^{2+}]$i form a key part of a ubiquitous signalling system found in all endocrine cells. Ca^{2+} can exert effects on a large number of cellular enzymes, either directly or, more commonly, via an intracellular Ca^{2+}-binding protein such as calmodulin [23,24]. Calmodulin is found in all eukaryotic cells, and is highly conserved throughout evolution. It is a single-chain polypeptide molecule which contains four interacting binding sites for Ca^{2+} and two sites which bind either Ca^{2+} or Mg^{2+} ions. It is activated by a rise in $[Ca^{2+}]$i to a level high enough to cause Ca^{2+} binding (approximately 10^{-6} mol/L). Calmodulin appears to function as a subunit of several enzymes and cytoskeletal complexes, and is known to regulate the activity of many enzymes including myosin light-chain kinase, a specific Ca^{2+}/calmodulin-dependent protein kinase, cAMP phosphodiesterase and adenylate cyclase, emphasising the interrelationships between the Ca^{2+} and cAMP signalling systems. The phosphorylated substrate proteins of the specific calmodulin-dependent kinase generally differ from those phosphorylated by the cAMP-dependent protein kinase A (although there may be some substrates phosphorylated by both kinases at different sites), and interactions between the activated proteins are thought to allow synergistic effects of dual messenger system activation.

Diacylglycerol and PKC

The Ca^{2+} mobilisation induced by IP_3 is just one arm of the bifurcating inositol–lipid signalling pathway. Apart from IP_3, the other major product of PIP_2 hydrolysis by PLC is DAG, which directly activates another cellular enzyme, PKC. PKC is a phospholipid-dependent Ca^{2+} activated kinase, and exists in two forms, a cytosolic form which is relatively inactive and a membrane-associated form. Association of the kinase with DAG in the plasma membrane dramatically increases its affinity for Ca^{2+} to make it a highly active kinase, and this activation may be mimicked pharmacologically by DAG analogues or by the tumour-promoting phorbol ester 12-O-tetradecanoyl-phorbol-14-acetate (TPA). There are now known to be several members of a family of PKC molecules, all of which consist of a single polypeptide chain [25]. Interestingly, the structure of these kinases includes a cysteine-rich sequence which is able to coordinate the binding of zinc ions to form a 'zinc finger' such as is found in many DNA-binding proteins. Although this conservation of structure suggests an important functional role, there is so far no evidence of the kinase itself binding to DNA.

A wide range of functions has been assigned to PKC including regulation of hormone secretion, modulation of ion channels, gene regulation and cell proliferation. Hormone secretory responses have been analysed in some detail and, in general, pharmacological activation of PKC gives rise to sustained secretory responses whereas rises in $[Ca^{2+}]i$; alone result in transient responses. The simultaneous activation of PKC and mobilisation of intracellular calcium (see above) frequently results in an integrated synergistic response many times greater than the sum of the individual components. This may allow amplification of the final cellular response to a signal at the plasma membrane, as has been proposed for the cAMP kinase system.

PKC and activating protein 1 in gene regulation

The promoter regions for many peptide hormone genes contain 7-bp DNA sequences which mediate the transcriptional response to PKC activation by the phorbol ester TPA (TPA response elements or TREs). Recently, DNA-binding proteins have been identified which are specifically involved in PKC signalling at the level of the gene. One of these, known as activating protein 1 (AP-1), has been identified as a 44–47 kDa DNA-binding protein complex. A major constituent of AP-1 is the product of the c-*jun* proto-oncogene, the normal cellular counterpart of the avian v-*jun* oncogene found in avian sarcoma virus, ASV-17. Jun, like CREB, is a transcription factor with a clearly defined C-terminal DNA-binding domain, a leucine-zipper dimerisation domain, and an N-terminal *trans*-activation domain [26]. Jun activation may involve C-terminal *dep*hosphorylation by a PKC-activated phosphatase, together with N-terminal phosphorylation.

It has been proposed that the Jun protein interacts with other proteins such as Fos (another proto-oncogene product which is cAMP inducible) or CREB to form heterodimers which interact with the promoter sequences to regulate gene expression; thus, the AP-1 complex bound to a phorbol ester response element may comprise Jun–Jun, Jun–Fos or other heterodimers. The precise mechanism whereby these phosphoprotein complexes regulate gene transcription is still not clearly established [17,27].

Interestingly, the cAMP–PKA–CREB system and the PKC–Jun system may interact at the level of DNA itself. The consensus TRE sequence differs by only 1 bp from the CREs described above, and cAMP can synergise with phorbol esters in transcription of genes containing a TRE. In addition, a separate DNA-binding protein has been identified (AP-2) which appears to mediate responses to both cAMP and phorbol ester. Thus, distinct messenger pathways may converge at the level of protein–DNA binding with a network of related DNA elements regulated by a series of related DNA-binding proteins [17].

Other phospholipases and membrane lipids

The membrane lipid DAG may be derived not only from PIP_2, but also from phosphatidylcholine, as a result of hydrolysis by phospholipase D (PLD). PLD [28] is activated by PKC, and it is thought that hormone–receptor binding may therefore activate both phospholipases C and D sequentially, resulting in initial (transient), and later (sustained), elevations of DAG content in membrane lipids. One other significant enzyme in phospholipid signalling is phospholipase A2 [29], again activated by PKC, which cleaves DAG to release arachidonic acid, a major precursor of further intracellular signalling molecules, including leukotrienes, thromboxanes and prostaglandins.

Cytosolic pH in stimulus–response coupling

The measured values for intracellular pH (pHi) are considerably more alkaline than would be the case if the distribution of protons across the plasma membrane were determined solely by their electrochemical gradient. For example, a membrane potential of –60 mV would result in a pHi of approximately 6.4, a value that would be toxic to the cell. In fact, the cell has a number of mechanisms for maintaining pHi at considerably higher values and within closely defined limits [30]. These mechanisms can be divided into the buffering capacity provided by intracellular bicarbonate and proteins, and mechanisms for controlling proton fluxes across the cell membrane. The latter are probably the most important, both in terms of capacity and regulation.

The most widespread mechanism for pHi regulation is the plasma membrane Na^+/H^+ antiporter. This exchange system responds to a fall in pHi by extruding protons from the cell in exchange for Na^+, and is driven by the large inward Na^+ gradient. Na^+/H^+ exchange is found universally in eukaryotic cells, and is blocked by the diuretic amiloride and its derivatives.

Two types of HCO_3^-/Cl^- exchange system have also been described to play a role in pHi regulation in a large number of cell types. One of these takes HCO_3^- into the cell in exchange for Cl^- efflux. This system is Na^+ dependent and provides a mechanism for disposal of an intracellular acid load. The other type of HCO_3^-/Cl^- antiport is Na^+ independent and may be reversible depending on the transmembrane HCO_3^- (H^+) and Cl^- gradients.

A large number of enzymes, and consequently cellular processes such as muscle contraction and oxidative metabolism, are highly pH dependent. Consequently, pHi regulation could be viewed as playing an important permissive function. Changes in pHi may constitute an intracellular signalling system in stimulus–response coupling, and have also been implicated in cell–cycle control, but the significance of these effects remains subject to conjecture.

Exocytosis, stimulus–response coupling and intracellular signalling

Secreted proteins are synthesized on ribosomes attached to the rough endoplasmic reticulum, entering the lumen of the endoplasmic reticulum by virtue of the hydrophobic leader sequence of amino acids comprising the 'pre-region'. The proteins are transported via transport vesicles to the Golgi complex where they are modified (post-translational modification) and concentrated before being packaged into storage/secretory vesicles which pinch off from the Golgi. The process whereby the contents of these granules are released into the extracellular fluid is exocytosis.

In recent years, it has become evident that exocytosis is a complex, highly ordered process involving a number of 'docking' or attachment proteins (e.g. Soluble NSF attachment proteins (SNAPs), and SNAP receptors (SNAREs)) and other regulatory factors responsible for the physical association and subsequent fusion of the vesicle with the plasma membrane [31]. These docking and regulatory proteins are likely sites of action of Ca^{2+}/calmodulin and protein kinases/phosphatases, although the precise details of this mechanism remain to be established.

Continued secretion must also depend upon the mobilisation of vesicles and their transport towards the cell surface. This process has been suggested to involve participation of a microtubular–microfilamentous system. Microtubules are the polymerised form of the protein tubulin and it appears that enhanced secretory activity is accompanied by a Ca^{2+}-dependent increase in tubulin polymerisation involving Ca^{2+}/calmodulin- and cAMP-dependent phosphorylation of microtubular proteins. Microfilaments form a network or cytoskeleton beneath the plasma membrane and are comprised of at least two proteins, the predominant ones being actin and myosin. As is the case with tubulin, actin appears to exist in secretory cells in a dynamic equilibrium between the depolymerised and polymerised forms. Again, the degree of polymerisation of actin appears to be increased in cells actively undergoing exocytosis. By analogy with smooth-muscle contraction, a rise in $[Ca^{2+}]i$ could result in calmodulin-dependent phosphorylation of myosin, its association with filamentous actin and ATP-dependent contractile activity. Microfilament contraction could provide a physical driving force for the transport of secretory vesicles.

2 Cytokine and growth-factor receptors

A surprisingly diverse group of ligands, comprising classical hormones, cytokines and growth factors, have been recently shown to utilise a group of receptors without obvious intracellular signalling potential [32]. These receptors require dimerisation within the cell membrane as a prerequisite for signal induction, and share a number of structural features (Fig. 4.13). The extracellular portion of the receptors share a series of common motifs, and apparently are derived from an ancestral fibronectin receptor. These include conserved cysteine residues, and a Trp–Ser sequence (the WSXWS motif) close to the membrane [33]. The intracellular portion of these receptors is highly variable, ranging from the long tail of the interleukin 4 (IL-4) receptor to the IL-6 and ciliary neurotrophic factor (CNTF) receptors which do not have any significant intracellular component. Two regions within the intracellular portion of the receptors have, however, been

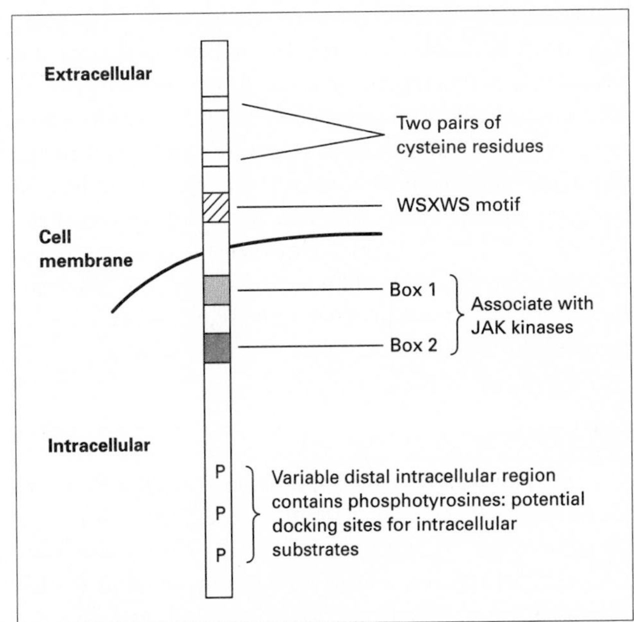

Fig. 4.13 Schematic representation of a cytokine receptor. The extracellular domain is variable, reflecting the diverse group of ligands this family serves, but two pairs of cysteine residues are conserved, and are thought to impart structural stability to the molecule. In addition, a WSXWS motif is found in the membrane proximal portion of the receptor. The intracellular portion of the receptor is highly variable, and may be absent, as in the case of the interleukin-6 (IL-6) receptor, the ciliary neurotrophic factor (CNTF) receptor, and the soluble form of the leukaemia inhibitory factor (LIF) receptor. There are two conserved motifs close to the membrane, boxes 1 and 2, which associate with JAK kinase family members, and distal tyrosine residues which can be phosphorylated to provide docking sites for kinase substrates such as the STAT molecules.

found to be conserved between members of this family. These have been named 'box 1' and 'box 2' and reside close to the transmembrane region. The different family members have all been found to be associated with one or more members of the Janus kinase (JAK) family of soluble tyrosine kinases. These kinases are thought to couple receptor activation to intracellular signalling [34,35].

The principal function of the extracellular portion of these receptors appears to be recognition of ligand, after which the receptor chains are brought together, either as homodimers as in the case of the growth-hormone receptor or heterodimers as in the case of the interleukin receptors. The crystal structure of the growth-hormone receptor conjugated with its ligand has been solved and has shown two separate regions of the hormone to contact respectively the initial receptor chain encountered and the subsequent, second receptor chain [36]. A series of altered growth-hormone molecules have been generated and these have shown that increases in ligand–receptor affinity are possible, but these 'superligands' fail to induce receptor dimerisation and so are functional growth hormone *antagonists*. It is likely that small molecule superagonists will be developed for possible use as therapeutic agents in the future. Further work with the leukaemia inhibitory factor (LIF) receptor, which usually heterodimerises with the IL-6 signal transducing chain gp130, has shown that by introducing additional cysteine residues in the membrane-proximal portion of the extracellular domain it is possible to generate a homodimeric receptor. This receptor will not bind ligand, but is constitutively 'on' and transduces the same signal as the liganded gp130–LIFR complex.

JAK kinases

The JAK family of tyrosine kinases comprises Jak-1, -2 and -3, as well as Tyk-2 (for *ty*rosine *k*inase). They all have a molecular mass of approximately 120–130 kDa and have a C-terminal tyrosine kinase domain. In addition to this functional kinase they all also have a pseudo-kinase domain, which led to them being thought of as two-faced, as the Roman god Janus (Fig. 4.14). There are no other recognised functional protein domains. The JAKs are found in all tissues, with the exception of Jak-3 which is restricted to haemopoietic cells. A JAK homologous gene has been identified in *Drosophila* attesting to the early expression of this family in evolution of multicellular organisms.

JAK kinases associate with receptors in one of three ways. Jak-2 associates with single-chain receptors using their conserved membrane proximal region. Receptor dimerisation brings two Jak-2 molecules into close apposition which permits each kinase to tyrosyl phosphorylate its neighbour at a KEYY site. This change markedly enhances the kinase activity of the Jak-2 molecule, and probably leads to tyrosyl phosphorylation of the receptor, the kinase, and one or several substrate molecules [34,35].

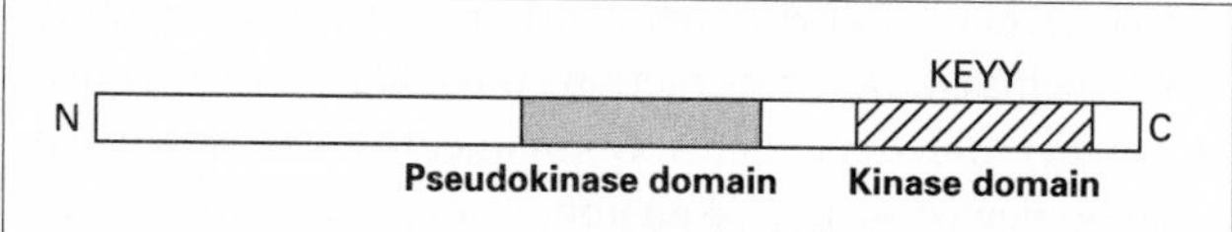

Fig. 4.14 Schematic representation of the JAK family of kinases. The N-terminal domain is variable and does not contain any recognisable protein motifs. The C-terminus contains two kinase domains, of which only one appears functional, the other referred to as the pseudokinase domain. The true kinase domain contains a KEYY amino-acid sequence which is tyrosyl *trans*-phosphorylated by other JAK molecules.

The receptors for IL-3 and IL-6 work differently. The functional receptor consists of a ligand-binding α-chain and a shared β-chain. The receptors for IL-3, IL-5 and granulocyte/macrophage colony-stimulating factor (GM-CSF) each have separate, specific chains and share a common β-subunit. Jak-2 is found in association with the β-unit and ligand-mediated receptor aggregation allows the kinase to transphosphorylate. The receptors for the cytokines IL-6, IL-11, oncostatin M (OSM), LIF and CNTF all have ligand-specific chains which bind ligand and then interact with the signalling molecules gp130 or LIFR-β. The gp130 molecule can associate with Jak-1, Jak-2 or Tyk-2, but activation of one Jak-1 is essential for signalling [34,35].

The third identified mechanism is exemplified by IL-2 and the interferon family of receptors. These require two chains for signalling. The IL-2 receptor consists of α-, β- and γ-chains, with the cytoplasmic domains of the latter two being absolutely required to allow signalling. The γ-chain is shared with receptors for IL-4, -7, -9, and -15. Jak-1 and Jak-3 are associated with the membrane proximal portions of the intracellular receptor domains and are brought together by ligand-induced dimerisation. The shared γ-subunit is encoded on the X chromosome and has been found to be mutated or deleted in the most common form of severe combined immunodeficiency syndrome (X-linked severe combined immunodeficiency (SCID)) [34]. The transphosphorylation of JAKs is critical to signal trans-mission, and in most cases different JAK family members are responsible for phosphorylating each other. Jak-2 appears to be the only member capable of efficiently phosphorylating an identical partner.

The importance of the JAKs was originally delineated in a series of classical genetic complementation experiments. Cell lines resistant to the effects of interferon were generated, and were found to be deficient in one or other of the JAKs. Fusion with cells replete with the missing kinase restored signalling. Furthermore, kinase-deficient JAKs have been shown to inhibit the action of erythropoeitin and IL-6.

JAK signalling

The cytokine receptors share with the receptor tyrosine kinase family of receptors (such as the insulin receptor, see below) the ability to activate a number of signalling cascades. Most cytokines activate Ras via phosphorylation of the *shc* protein, and other targets include phosphatidylinositol 3-OH kinase (PI(3)K) and more rarely PLC. These three signalling molecules are thought to interact directly with the intracellular portion of the cytokine receptor by recognition of *src* homology 2 (SH_2) domains for tyrosyl phosphate residues on the receptor. It has been shown that JAK kinase activity is essential for the initiation of these three cascades, but it is not clear whether JAKs phosphorylate the signalling molecules, or by phosphorylating the receptor permit association of the substrates with the receptor chain.

Additional convolutions in cytokine signalling complexity are suggested by recent reports that mitogen-activated protein kinase (MAP kinase, also termed ERK-2) activity is stimulated by interferon receptors, and that the MAP kinase associates closely with another JAK substrate molecule, STAT-1α. It seems likely that intimate association of signalling molecules at the receptor may allow subtle cross-talk between them to generate a cytokine-specific, cell-type-specific response.

Tyrosyl phosphorylation of the insulin-receptor substrate molecule IRS-1 and the related IRS-2 (previously identified as an IL-4 receptor tyrosyl phosphorylation substrate 4-PS) can be induced by IL-4 and IL-9, alone among the interleukins, and also by growth hormone, and the gp130-related cytokine LIF. However, it may be that cell-type-specific factors determine whether growth hormone and LIF are able to use the IRS pathway. How this specificity is achieved is uncertain at present.

STAT activation

The STAT family of transcription factors (*s*ignal *t*ransduction and *a*ctivation of *t*ranscription) were first identified in studies of how interferons changed the pattern of actively transcribed genes in target cells [37]. There are currently six cloned STAT family members, and it is likely that additional members of this group will be identified. These proteins exist in a quiescent form in cytoplasm, and are associated with the intracellular portion of cytokine receptors either constitutively or after tyrosyl phosphorylation of specific residues in the receptor by JAK kinases.

STATs contain a C-terminal *src* homology 2 (SH2) domain, an SH3-like domain and a single tyrosine which is the target for phosphorylation by JAK kinases. In addition to tyrosyl phosphorylation, STATs may also be phosphorylated on serine/threonine residues, possibly by MAP kinase, an event which appears to enhance their effectiveness in stimulating gene transcription. Indeed, immunoprecipitated STAT-1 has been shown to be bound to activated MAP kinases.

Analysis of cytokine-stimulated genes has revealed a core consensus sequence in the regulatory DNA which recognizes STAT proteins, originally recognised as a γ-interferon-activated site, or GAS, consisting of the inverted repeat TTnnnnnAA (Fig. 4.15). Each STAT can be shown

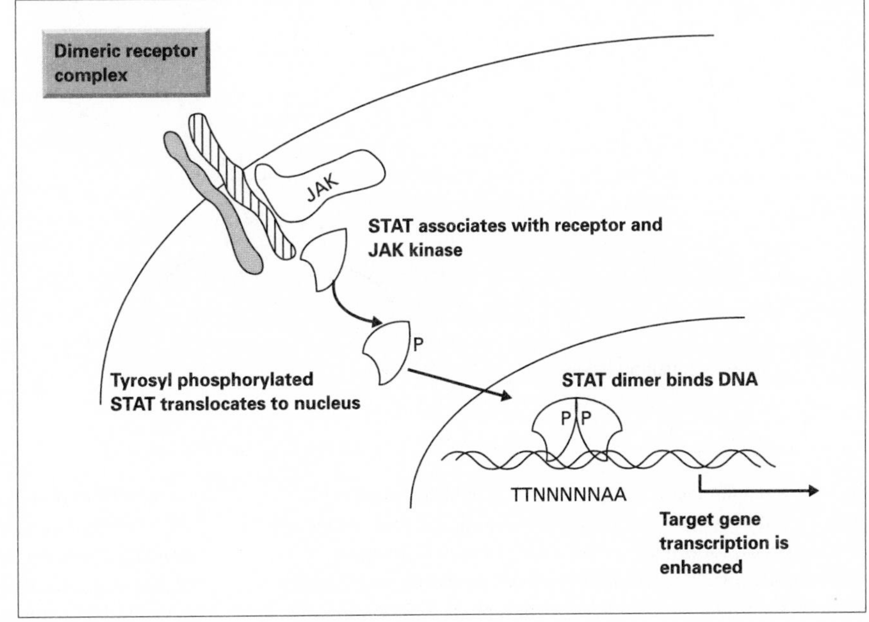

Fig. 4.15 Representation of the JAK–STAT signalling cascade. The receptor is dimerised after ligand binding and this brings JAK kinases into close apposition. The kinases transphosphorylate each other, the receptor and various substrates, in particular the STAT family. Tyrosyl phosphorylated STATs migrate to the nucleus and dimerise, either as homodimers as depicted here or heterodimeric complexes, to bind to DNA and stimulate transcription of target genes.

to bind *in vitro* to synthetic DNA, but *in vivo* it is clear that certain STATs prefer specific variations on this theme.

It is uncertain how such a diverse group of cytokines and hormones can act through such a small number of signalling molecules to elicit unique cellular responses. It is clear that the diversity within the intracellular portions of the cytokine receptors plays a role in 'selecting' which signalling molecules will be brought in contact with the receptor-associated kinases, and that the pattern of signalling pathway activation rather than the potential of each individual pathway has a key specificity-determining role.

The insulin receptor—a tyrosine kinase receptor

The insulin receptor (IR) is an example of a class of receptor tyrosine kinases, distinct from the cytokine receptor superfamily, but whose signalling pathway partly overlaps with that of the cytokine receptors. The receptor comprises two β-subunits and two α-subunits, which are covalently linked by intra- and intersubunit disulphide bridges. Thus, this particular receptor is a dimerised receptor, in contrast to other tyrosine kinase receptors which dimerise in response to ligand binding. Insulin binds to the extracellular α-subunits, while the transmembrane and intracellular β-subunits possess intrinsic tyrosine kinase activity [38]. Currently emerging evidence suggests that selective forms of insulin resistance may result from impairments in receptor function which result from modifications of individual domains within the β-subunit of the receptor [39].

The IR is similar in overall structure to the insulin-like growth factor 1 (IGF-1) receptor (IGFR), and indeed hybrid IR–IGFR receptors have been described, consisting of an IR αβ 'monomer' linked to a cognate IGFR 'monomer' [40]. The pathways of signalling for the IR are complex, and only recently becoming understood. Physiological substrates for the IR are now known to include IRS-1 [41] and IRS-2, which in turn interact through multiple phosphotyrosyl residues with a series of other signalling molecules that possess SH2 domains, including *Grb*-2 *Nck*, *Syp* and *p85*; additional substrates include *shc* and the IR β-subunit itself, and indirectly, PI(3)K [42] (Fig. 4.16). Many of the kinases in these ramifying pathways may be activated by more than one receptor in any given cell type, which poses the question of how receptor specificity occurs. This is still unresolved, but may be a function of spatial organisation within the cell.

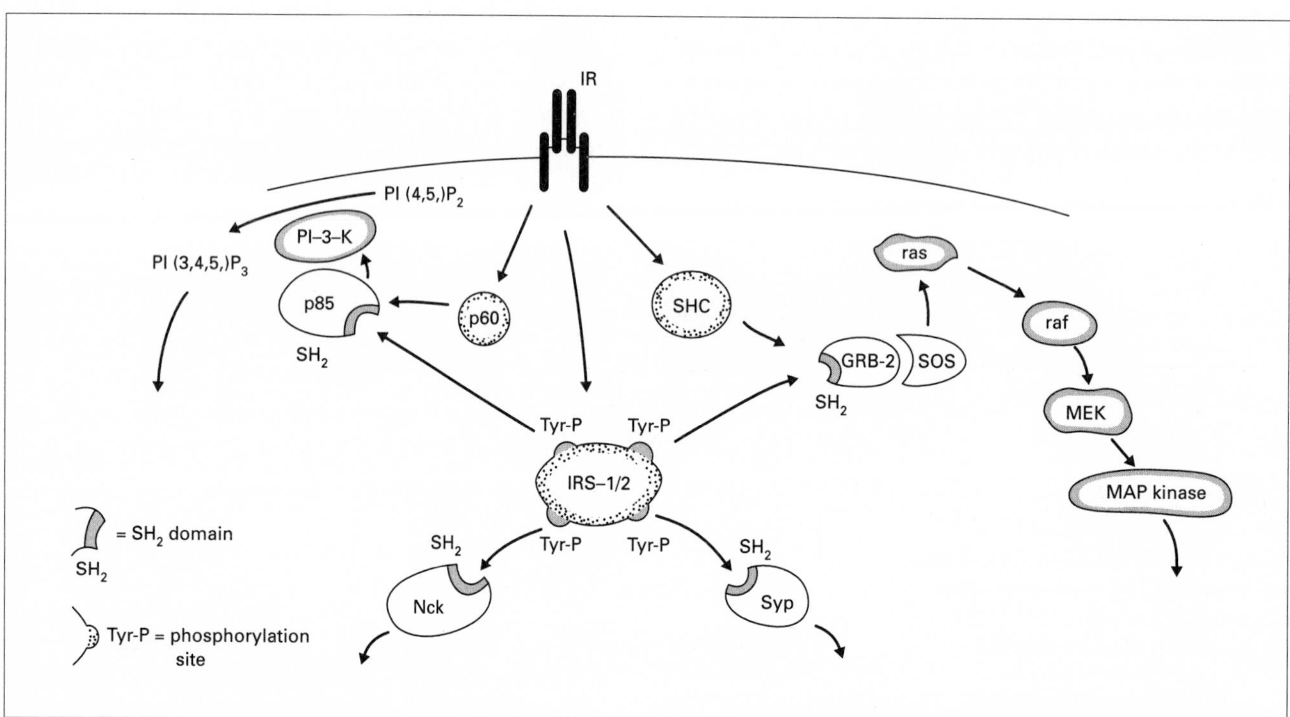

Fig. 4.16 Insulin receptor signalling. A simplified diagram of possible pathways of kinase phosphorylation cascades in response to insulin-receptor (IR) activation. Insulin-receptor substrate (IRS-1, and/or IRS-2) has multiple tyrosine kinase domains, which when phosphorylated, dock with *src*-homology 2 (SH2) domains on several further proteins, including *p85*, *GRB*-2, *Nck* and *Syp*. *GRB*-2 further interacts with *sos* to affect the *ras*-MAP kinase signalling pathway; *p85* interacts with phosphatidyl-inositol 3-kinase (PI3K) to phosphorylate PI-(4,5)-bisphosphate (PIP_2) to PI-(3,4,5)-trisphosphate (PIP_3).

3 Intracellular hormone receptors

While peptide hormones act at receptors in the plasma membrane, lipid-soluble hormones, particularly the steroids and the thyroid hormones, bind to specific receptors in the cell nucleus (Fig. 4.17). A superfamily of DNA-binding nuclear proteins is now recognised with over 30 members, including the receptors for steroid and thyroid hormones, vitamins A and D, glucocorticoids, and retinoids [43]. The superfamily includes a number of 'orphan' receptors, for which no ligands have been identified. In general, these intracellular receptors act as ligand-activated transcription factors, with direct effects to activate or repress gene transcription within the nucleus, with no intervening cascade of intracellular second-messenger molecules.

Control of gene transcription by nuclear hormone receptors involves the receptor binding to specific hormone responsive elements (HREs) [44] within the promoter regions of target genes. Identical ligand–receptor complexes activate different genes in different target cell types, and a given ligand may therefore initiate responses that differ from cell to cell. The selectivity of steroid hormone action in a particular case may differ according to the hormonal ligand, the cell type, and the nature of the target DNA [45,46].

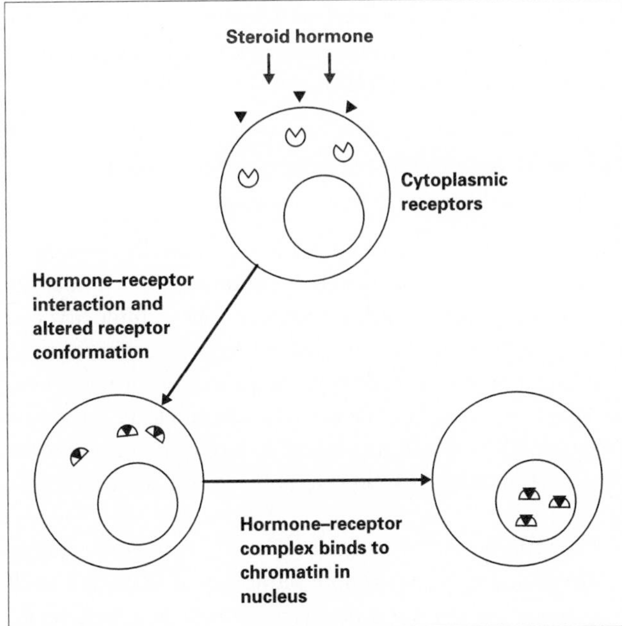

Fig. 4.17 Interaction of steroid hormones with the nucleus. Steroid hormone molecules diffuse across the plasma membrane of the target cell and interact with specific receptor proteins within the cytoplasm. This results in a conformational change in the receptor protein, allowing access of the hormone–receptor complexes to the nucleus, where they bind to DNA to regulate transcription of specific genes.

Most mammalian cells contain between 1000 and 10 000 steroid receptors, each of which binds a single steroid molecule. Molecular cloning studies have revealed conservation of structure throughout the steroid receptor superfamily, consisting of an N-terminal region, a cysteine-rich DNA-binding domain, and a C-terminal domain. The N-terminal region is poorly conserved and is involved in cell-specific gene expression through the hormone-independent transcription factor TAF-1 [43]. Although variable between different receptors, the C-terminal region is more conserved than the N-terminal region, and specifies ligand binding. The most conserved region within steroid hormone receptors is the DNA-binding domain. The DNA-binding domain contains globular 'zinc fingers' which are responsible for interaction with the HRE of the gene [47].

All steroid hormone receptors are phosphoproteins, and several are phosphorylated after hormone binding. Recent studies have suggested that receptor phosphorylation is progressive, occurring in different cellular compartments, and involves the coordinated activity of multiple kinases. One model of the phosphorylation process [48] proposes that receptors are phosphorylated cotranslationally prior to interaction with DNA, a process which continues as a post-translation event over 6–10 hours (Fig. 4.18). Allosteric changes resulting from ligand binding lead to a rapid further phosphorylation step, preceding receptor dimerisation and DNA binding. A final phosphorylation step is facilitated by conformational changes in the receptors after DNA binding, as further serine residues become accessible.

All nuclear receptors possess a nuclear localisation signal which is similar in different receptors [43]. However, the mechanism of receptor translocation to the nucleus differs for individual receptors. The receptors for oestrogens, androgens, glucocorticoids and mineralocorticoids interact with the 90-kDa heat shock protein, Hsp90 [49,50], which may be regarded as a protein transporter to which the steroid receptors are tightly bound as they translocate the cytoplasm, via the cytoskeletal components of the cell, to enter the nucleus [50]. In cells not exposed to hormone, Hsp90 suppresses the formation of protein aggregates and binding to target proteins [51]. On hormone binding, there is dissociation of receptor from Hsp90, and nuclear translocation and DNA binding can occur.

In contrast to those receptors associated with heat-shock proteins, the progesterone receptor is transported to the nucleus by an energy-dependent karyophilic mechanism [52] and is not dependent upon cytoskeletal components for translocation. *In vitro* mutagenesis studies have shown that deletion of the karyophilic signal leads to cytoplasmic accumulation of the progesterone receptor.

The 9S heterocomplex form of the steroid receptor also contains two additional heat-shock proteins, Hsp56 and

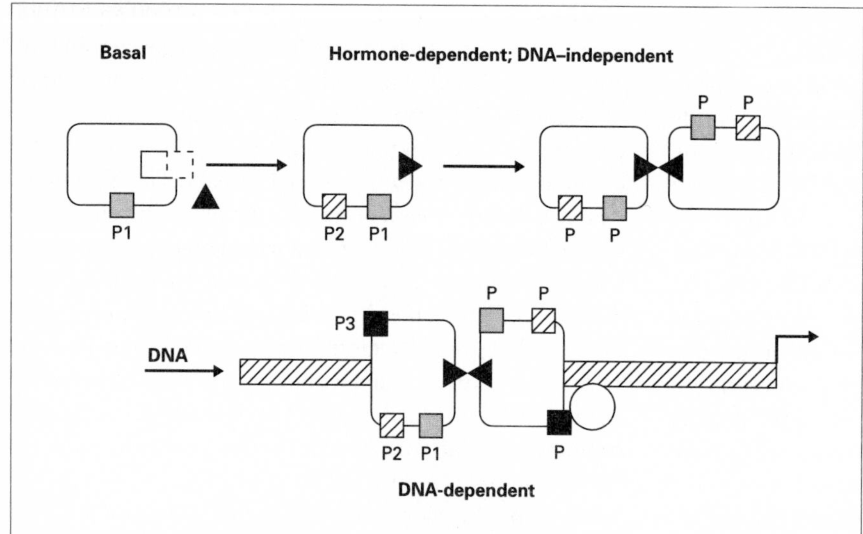

Fig. 4.18 Progressive phosphorylation of steroid receptors after ligand binding. Initially, receptors are basally phosphorylated (P1). After ligand binding, allosteric modifications in structure expose additional phosphorylation sites (P2). This rapid phosphorylation may precede the dimerisation of receptors. DNA binding is accompanied by further changes in receptor conformation, exposing new phosphorylation sites (P3). The DNA-associated, fully phosphorylated receptor dimers may then interact with adaptor proteins (shown as a circle) to regulate the transcriptional apparatus.

Hsp70, in addition to Hsp90, and a complex containing all three heat-shock proteins is present in cytosol independent of the presence of steroid receptors; Hsp70 and Hsp90 may regulate protein folding and movement in the cell. Association of the Hsps with steroid hormone receptors thus serves: (i) to mask the DNA-binding site, preventing binding to DNA in the absence of ligand; and (ii) to assist in the folding and transport of newly synthesised receptor following release from ribosomes. In the absence of hormone the receptors remain attached to the heat-shock protein complex; on exposure to steroid, receptors dissociate from Hsp90 and bind to target DNA sequences as homodimers or heterodimers to regulate transcription.

Thyroid hormone receptors

Like the steroids, the thyroid hormone triiodothyronine (T3) is a small lipophilic molecule which readily diffuses across the plasma membrane and binds to intracellular receptors. Several different T3 receptors have been identified, resulting from alternatively spliced mRNA products of two receptor genes (T3Rα and T3Rβ), which differ in their patterns of expression [53]. In contrast to steroid receptors, thyroid hormone receptors do not interact with Hsp90 and, in the absence of hormone, such receptors move directly to high-affinity T3 response elements within target gene promoters [53,54].

Unlike steroid hormone receptors, those for T3 are located on the nuclear membrane even when not complexed with hormone, while an additional population is found on the inner mitochondrial membrane. A variety of T3 response genes have been identified in diverse tissues. Thus, T3 regulates expression of mRNA for the TSH α- and β-subunits, as well as growth hormone and prolactin in the pituitary gland, ornithine aminotransferase in the kidney, and Na^+/K^+-dependent ATPase in skeletal muscle. A series of hepatic enzymes are transcriptionally regulated by T3, including malic enzyme, cytochrome C, α-glycerophosphate dehydrogenase and phosphoenolpyruvate carboxykinase.

While the predominant effects of T3 are direct transcriptional effects occurring within the nucleus, some 'non-genomic' rapid cellular responses (e.g. amino-acid transport) have been described. Effects of T3–receptor complexes on membrane-related phenomena are extremely rapid, and are not mediated through RNA or protein synthesis.

Nuclear hormone receptor dimerisation: retinoid receptors and thyroid hormone action

The nuclear hormone receptors were originally thought to bind to target DNA as simple homodimers, but in fact the situation is generally more complex. The complexity was first realised in the case of thyroid hormone receptors, in that they required a nuclear protein factor in order to bind to DNA *in vitro*. This factor was identified as a retinoid receptor, RXR, which was found to be required also for the action of vitamin D receptors and retinoic acid receptors [55,56].

The retinoids are lipid molecules, which include vitamin A (retinol), and its metabolite retinoic acid (RA); RA itself undergoes isomerisation between all-*trans* and 9-*cis* forms [57]. Receptors for retinoids are encoded by six different genes, and comprise the retinoic acid receptors (RAR α, β and γ), and the retinoid X receptors (RXR α, β and γ). RARs can bind both all-*trans*-RA and 9-*cis*-RA, while RXRs bind only the 9-*cis* isomer [58]. Additional RAR isoforms are generated through differential gene splicing and the use of multiple promoters. These receptors have highly conserved ligand- and DNA-binding domains but, interestingly, the RAR is even more closely related to the T3R in its ligand binding domain, despite the difference between the ligands themselves. The RXRs form heterodimers with RARs, T3Rs, the vitamin D receptors and the peroxisome proliferator activated receptor (PPAR), but can also form functional RXR–RXR homodimers.

Although individually RXR, T3R and RAR bind poorly to response elements, heterodimers bind strongly, and the RXR within the heterodimer is an essential prerequisite for this. Heterodimers of T3R and RAR are thus ineffective at interacting with DNA response elements. Each heterodimer has particular DNA target sequence specificity, and whereas RAR–RXR heterodimers interact strongly with a RARE, they do not bind to a TRE. It is likely that TR–RXR or TR–RAR heterodimers are the most physiologically active complexes on most characterised T3REs. The contribution of each activated receptor to the heterodimer-mediated transactivation is response-element specific [55,56]. Figure 4.19 summarises the essential features of our present state of understanding of the role of RXR heterodimers and RXR homodimers as mediators of thyroid hormone and retinoic acid signals.

Nine-*cis* retinoic acid induces the formation of RXR, but not RAR, homodimers [58], that activate a subset of RAREs, giving rise to a distinct retinoid response pathway (Fig. 4.20). Since the formation of RXR homodimers limits the availability of RXR molecules for heterodimerisation

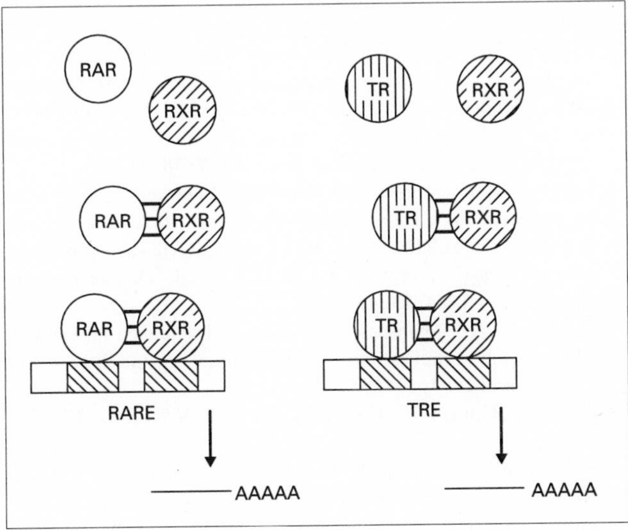

Fig. 4.19 Retinoid X receptors (RXR) heterodimerise with retinoic acid receptors (RAR) and thyroid hormone receptors (TR) to mediate thyroid hormone and retinoic acid action. TR–RXR complexes bind to T3 response elements (TREs), whereas RAR–RXR complexes interact with RA response elements (RAREs). Binding to DNA does not require hormone.

with other receptors, one of the important roles of 9-*cis*-RA and associated RXR homodimers may be to regulate cross-talk between specific hormonal pathways.

Heterodimerisation of transcription factors thus serves to generate a vast increase in the possibilities for regulatory control. It is clear that RARs and TRs require heterodimerisation for effective interaction with DNA, and that heterodimers are generally physiologically active forms of TRs and RARs. This may also be relevant to steroid receptors, as it has been found recently that the glucocorticoid receptor (GR) is able to interact with the mineralocorticoid receptor (MR), and that the heterodimer has different transcriptional properties from either GR or MR homodimers alone [59].

HREs: palindromes, direct repeats, composites

The nature of the target DNA is critical for binding of nuclear hormone receptors. HREs for the GR, the T3R and the oestrogen receptor (ER) generally have a palindromic structure, consisting of an inverted repeat of 'half-sites' of 5–6 bp (such as AGGTCA) separated by a spacer of 3 bp or none. However, other T3REs have been recognised which consist of direct repeats of half-sites, and here a variety of possible spacings dictate the specificity of the response element for different nuclear hormone receptor heterodimers. Thus, a tandem T3RE with a four-nucleotide spacing will bind a T3R–RXR heterodimer; however, it can be converted into a RARE (binding a RAR–RXR dimer) by increasing the spacing to four nucleotides, or into a vitamin D3 response element (binding a VDR–RXR dimer) with a spacing of three nucleotides [60].

In addition to tandem repeat HREs, some response elements act as composites. This has been best characterised for glucocorticoid action, where GR and MR are equally able to bind to a palindromic 'simple GRE', but only GR can act at a 'composite GRE'. A composite GRE comprises a low-affinity GRE together with a binding site for the AP-1 transcription factor: activated (i.e. hormone-bound) GR can block AP-1-enhanced transcription from this composite element, whereas MR cannot, hence providing a degree of specificity [61]. Similar overlap has been described in some genes where GR and CREB compete for DNA binding, with rival transcriptional effects.

Adaptor proteins and transcriptional control

The actual mechanism whereby nuclear hormone receptors activate (or repress) gene transcription is only recently starting to be understood. The retinoid receptors have been intensively studied, and possess two activation function domains, AF-1 and AF-2. AF-1 is located at the N-terminal

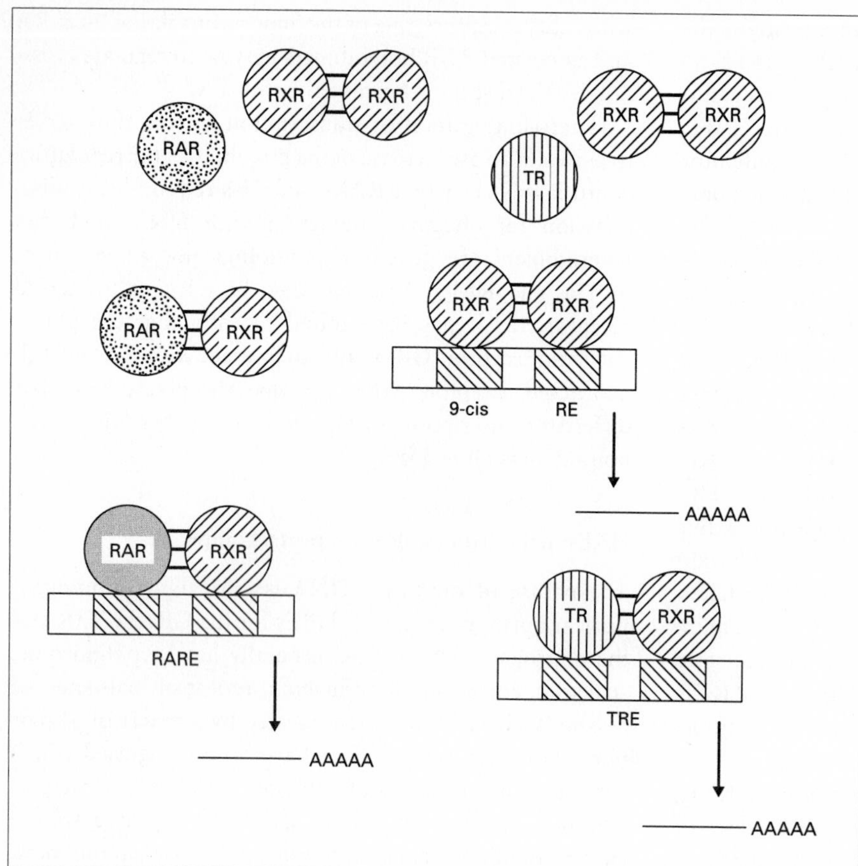

Fig. 4.20 Ligand-induced retinoid X-receptor (RXR) homodimer formation. In the absence of retinoic acid (RA), RXR monomers and RXR heterodimer complexes are in equilibrium, but the presence of 9-*cis* RA shifts this equilibrium towards the formation of RXR homodimers which bind and activate specific response elements. These may be distinct from the response elements activated by RAR–RXR or TR–RXR heterodimers.

of RARs and RXRs, while AF-2 is close to the ligand-binding domain, and its function depends upon binding of ligand. Crystallographic studies indicate that retinoic acid binding to a hydrophobic pocket within RAR-γ results in repositioning of the AF-2 domain allowing it to interact with an adaptor protein, or transcription intermediary factor, termed TIF-1 [62]. TIF-1 does not appear to interact directly with the apparatus of gene transcription, such as TATA-binding protein, or TFIIB, but may be involved in remodelling of the chromatin template to promote transcription indirectly. A series of other adaptor proteins have been identified that interact with other nuclear hormone receptors, including 'Trip-1' (or T3 receptor interacting protein), which is closely related to a yeast transcriptional mediator, Sug-1 [63], and 'ERAP160' (ER-associated protein, 160-kDa), which binds to ER in the presence of oestradiol but not anti-oestrogens such as tamoxifen [64]. For a recent review of nuclear receptor co-activator and co-repressor proteins see [65].

References

1 Sutherland EW, Øye I, Butcher RW. The action of epinephrin and the role of the adenyl cyclase system in hormone action. *Recent Prog Horm Res* 1965; **21**: 623–43.

2 Vassart G, Dumont JE. The thyrotropin receptor and the regulation of thyrocyte function and growth. *Endocr Rev* 1992; **13**: 596–611.

3 Ascoli M, Segaloff DL. On the structure of the luteinizing hormone/chorionic gonadotropin receptor. *Endocr Rev* 1989; **10**: 27–44.

4 Sibley DR, Benovic JL, Caron MG, Lefkovitz RJ. Phosphorylation of cell surface receptors: a mechanism for regulating signal transduction pathways. *Endocr Rev* 1988; **9**: 38–45.

5 Spiegel AM. Receptor–effector coupling by G-proteins: implications for endocrinology. *Trends Endocrinol Metab* 1989; **1**: 72–6.

6 Benovic JJ, Short REL, Caron MG, Lefkovitz RJ. The mammalian beta-adrenergic receptor; purification and characterisation. *Biochemistry* 1984; **23**: 4510–15.

7 Gordeladze JO, Johansen PW, Paulssen RH, Paulssen EI, Gautvik M. G-proteins: implications for pathophysiology and disease. *Eur J Endocrinol* 1994; **131**: 557–74.

8 Hepler JR, Gilman AG. G proteins. *Trends Biol Sci* 1992; **17**: 383–7.

9 Simonds WF, Goldsmith PK, Woodard CJ, Unson CG, Spiegel AM. Receptor and effector interactions of Gs: functional studies with antibodies to the carboxyl-terminal decapeptide. *FEBS Lett* 1989; **249**: 189–94.

10 Spiegel A, Carter A, Brann M *et al.* Signal transduction by guanine nucleotide-binding proteins. *Rec Prog Horm Res* 1988; **44**: 337–42.

11 Linder ME, Gilman AG. G-proteins. *Sci Am* 1992; **267**: 56–65.

12 Conklin BR, Bourne HR. Structural elements of G_α subunits

that interact with Gβγ, receptors, and effectors. *Cell* 1993; **73**: 631–41.

13 Landis CA, Masters SB, Spada A, Pace AM, Bourne HR, Vallar L. GTPase inhibiting mutations activate the α-chain of Gs and stimulate adenylate cyclase in human pituitary tumours. *Nature* 1989; **340**: 692–6.

14 Van Sande J, Parma J, Tonacchera M, Swillens S, Dumont J, Vassart G. Somatic and germline mutations of the TSH receptor gene in thyroid diseases. *J Clin Endocrinol Metab* 1995; 80: 2577–85.

15 Karin M. Complexities of gene regulation by cAMP. *Trends Genet* 1989; 5: 65–67.

16 Meyer TE, Habener JF. Cyclic adenosine 3′,5′-monophosphate response element binding protein (CREB) and related transcription-activating deoxyribonucleic acid-binding proteins. *Endocr Rev* 1993; **14**: 269–90.

17 Hoeffler JP, Deutsdh PJ, Lin J, Habener JF. Distinct adenosine 3′,5′-monophosphate and phorbol ester-responsive signal transduction pathways converge at the level of transcriptional activation by the interactions of DNA-binding proteins. *Mol Endocrinol* 1989; **3**: 868–80.

18 Clapham DE. Calcium signaling. *Cell* 1995; **80**: 259–68.

19 Clapham DE. Repleneshing the stores. *Nature* 1995; **375**: 634–5.

20 Hallam TJ, Rink TJ. Receptor-mediated calcium entry: diversity of function and mechanism. *Trends Pharmacol Sci* 1989; **10**: 8–11.

21 Berridge MJ. Inositol trisphosphate and calcium signalling. *Nature* 1993; **361**: 315–25.

22 Berridge MJ, Dupont G. Spatial and temporal signalling by calcium. *Curr Opinion Cell Biol* 1994; **6**: 267–74.

23 Cohen P, Klee CB, eds. *Calmodulin.* Oxford: Elsevier, 1988.

24 Heizmann CW, Hunziker W. Intracellular calcium binding proteins: more sight than insight. *Trends Biochem Sci* 1991; **16**: 98–103.

25 Nishizuka Y. Protein kinase C and lipid signaling for sustained cellular responses. *FASEB J* 1995; **9**: 484–96.

26 Pennypacker KR, Hong JS, McMillian MK. Pharmacological regulation of AP-1 transcription factor DNA binding activity. *FASEB J* 1994; **8**: 475–8.

27 Herrlich P, Ponta H. Mutual cross-modulation of steroid/retinoic acid receptor and AP-1 transcription factor activities: a novel property with practical implications. *Trends Endocrinol Metab* 1994; **5**: 341–6.

28 Billah MM. Phospholipase D and cell signaling. *Curr Opin Immunol* 1993; **5**: 114–23.

29 Axelrod J. Phospholipase A2 and G proteins. *Trends Neurosci* 1995; **18**: 64–5.

30 Frelin C, Vigne P, Ladoux A, Lazdunski M. The regulation of the intracellular pH in cells from vertebrates. *Eur J Biochem* 1988; **174**: 3–14.

31 Edwardson JM, Marciniak SJ. Molecular mechanisms in exocytosis. *J Membr Biol* 1995; **146**: 113–22.

32 Horseman ND, Yu-Lee L-Y. Transcriptional regulation by the helix bundle peptide hormones: growth hormone, prolactin and haemopoietic cytokines. *Endocr Rev* 1994; **15**: 627–49.

33 Bazan JF. Structural design and molecular evolution of a cytokine receptor superfamily. *Proc Natl Acad Sci USA* 1990; **87**: 6934–8.

34 Ihle JN. Cytokine receptor signalling. *Nature* 1995; **377**: 591–4.

35 Finidori J, Kelly PA. Cytokine receptor signalling through two novel families of transducer molecules: Janus kinases, and signal transducers and activators of transcription. *J Endocrinol* 1995; **147**: 11–23.

36 De Vos AM, Ultsch M, Kossakoff AA. Human growth hormone and extracellular domain of its receptor: crystal structure of the complex. *Science* 1992; **255**: 306–12.

37 Darnell JE, Jr, Kerr IM, Stark GR. JAK–STAT pathways and transcriptional activation in response to interferons and other extracellular signalling proteins. *Science* 1994; **264**: 1415–21.

38 Lee J, Pilch PF. The insulin receptor: structure, function and signaling. *Am J Physiol Cell Physiol* 1994; **266**: 35–2, C319–34.

39 Accili D. Molecular defects of the insulin receptor gene. *Diabetes Metab* Rev 1995; **11**: 47–62.

40 Siddle K, Soos MA, Field CE, Nave BT. Hybrid and atypical insulin/insulin-like growth factor-1 receptors. *Hormone Res* 1993; **41** (Suppl. 2): 56–64.

41 Sun X-J, Rothenberg PL, Kahn CR *et al.* Structure of the insulin receptor substrate IRS-1 defines a unique signal transduction protein. *Nature* 1991; **352**: 73–7.

42 Myers MG, Jr, White MF. New frontiers in insulin receptor substrate signaling. *Trends Endocrinol Metab* 1995; **6**: 209–15.

43 Tsai M-J, O'Malley BW. Molecular mechanisms of actions of steroid/thyroid receptor superfamily members. *Ann Rev Biochem* 1994; **63**: 451–6.

44 Evans RM. The steroid and thyroid hormone receptor superfamily. *Science* 1988; **240**: 889–95.

45 Katzenellenbogen JA, O'Malley BW, Katzenellenbogen BS. Tripartite steroid hormone receptor pharmacology: interaction with multiple effector sites as a basis for the cell- and promoter-specific action of these hormones. *Mol Endocrinol* 1996; **10**: 119–31.

46 Glass CK. Differential recognition of target genes by nuclear receptor monomers, dimers, and heterodimers. *Endocr Rev* 1994; **15**: 391–407.

47 Zilliacus J, Wright APH, Carlstedt-Duke J, Gustaffson J-Å. Structural determinants of DNA-binding specificity by steroid receptors. *Mol Endocrinol* 1995; **9**: 389–400.

48 Takimoto GS, Horwitz KB. Progesterone receptor phosphorylation: complexities in defining a functional role. *Trends Endocrinol Metab* 1993; **4**: 1–7.

49 Catelli MG, Binart N, Jung-Testas I *et al.* The common 90 kDa protein component of non-transformed '8S' steroid receptors is a heat-shock protein. *EMBO J* 1985; **4**: 3131–5.

50 Brinkman AO. Steroid hormone receptors: activators of gene transcription. *J Paed Endocrinol* 1994; **4**: 1–8.

51 Wiech H, Buchner J, Zimmerman R, Jacob V. Hsp90 chaperones protein folding *in vitro*. *Nature* 1992; **358**: 169–70.

52 Guichon-Mantel A, Lescop C, Christin-Maitre H, Loossefelt M, Perrot-Applanat M, Milgrom E. Nucleocytoplasmic shuttle of the progesterone receptor. *EMBO J* 1991; **10**: 3851–9.

53 Lazar MA. Thyroid hormone receptors: multiple forms, multiple possibilities. *Endocr Rev* 1993; **14**: 184–93.

54 Dalman FC, Koenig RJ, Perdew GH, Massa E, Pratt WB. In contrast to the glucocorticoid receptor, the thyroid hormone receptor is translated in the DNA-binding state and is not associated with hsp90. *J Biol Chem* 1990; **265**: 3615–18.

55 Hermann T, Hoffmann B, Zhang X-K, Tran P, Pfahl M. Heterodimeric receptor complexes determine 3,5,3′-triiodothyronine and retinoid signaling specificities. *Mol Endocrinol* 1992; **6**: 1153–62.

56 Zhang X-K, Pfahl M. Regulation of retinoid and thyroid hormone action through homodimeric and heterodimeric receptors. *Trends Endocrinol Metab* 1993; **4**: 156–62.

57 Giguère, V. Retinoic acid receptors and cellular retinoid binding proteins: complex interplay in retinoid signalling. *Endocr Rev* 1994;

15: 61–79.
58 Levin AA, Sturzenbecker LJ, Kazmer S *et al.* 9-*cis* retinoic acid stereoisomer binds and activates the nuclear receptor RXRα. *Nature* 1992; **355**: 359–61.
59 Trapp T, Rupprecht R, Castrén M, Reul JMHM, Holsboer F. Heterodimerization between mineralocorticoid and glucocorticoid receptor: a new principle of glucocorticoid action in the CNS. *Neuron* 1994; **13**: 1457–62.
60 Umesono K, Murakami KK, Thompson CC, Evans RM. Direct repeats as selective response elements for the thyroid hormone, retinoic acid, and vitamin D3 receptors. *Cell* 1991; **65**: 1255–66.
61 Funder JW. Mineralocorticoids, glucocorticoids, receptors and response elements. *Science* 1993; **259**: 1132–3.
62 Renaud J-P, Rochel N, Ruff M *et al.* Crystal structure of the RAR-γ ligand-binding domain bound to all-*trans* retinoic acid. *Nature* 1995; **378**: 681–9.
63 Lee JW, Ryan F, Swaffield JC, Johnston SA, Moore DD. Interaction of thyroid-hormone receptor with a conserved transcriptional mediator. *Nature* 1995; **374**: 91–4.
64 Halachmi S, Marden E, Martin G, MacKay H, Abbondanza C, Brown M. Estrogen receptor-associated proteins: possible mediators of hormone-induced transcription. *Science* 1994; **264**: 1455–8.
65 Horwitz KB, Jackson TA, Bain DL, Richer JK, Takimoto GS, Tung L. Nuclear receptor co-activators and co-repressors. *Mol Endocrinol* 1996; **10**: 1167–77.

Part 3
Neuroendocrinology

CHAPTER 5

Structure and function of the hypothalamus and pituitary

A.C. Nieuwenhuijzen Kruseman

History

Probably the first detailed description of neuroendocrine derangement was published at the beginning of this century, when Froelich reported on the history of a 14-year-old boy with headache, vomiting, partial visual loss, obesity and hypogonadism. A pituitary tumour was diagnosed and removed via the transsphenoidal route. However, as the existence of neurohormones and the hypothalamo-pituitary interaction was obviously unknown, the pathophysiological mechanism of genital dystrophy in this patient was not recognised. This was first studied about 30 years later when Harris demonstrated the significance of the hypophysial-portal blood supply as the necessary link connecting the innervation-poor anterior pituitary with the hypothalamus. Also at that time, Ernst and Bertha Scharrer recognised the ability of certain hypothalamic neurons to secrete neurohumoral agents and proposed the principles of neurosecretion, subsequently further defined as neuroendocrine secretion, which stands for the link between neural activity and endocrine and metabolic control.

The isolation and characterisation of hypothalamic hormones has been undertaken during the past four decades and has resulted in the identification of a variety of neurohypophysial and hypophysiotrophic peptides. Over the same period, immunohistochemical studies have contributed to a better understanding of the structure of the endocrine hypothalamus and pituitary, and the relation of these structures to other parts of the nervous system. It is now clear that the hypothalamus is one of the principal centres of regulation of an extensive and wide-ranging peptidergic neuron system, and can be considered as the final common pathway by which signals from a variety of centres from the brain reach the pituitary. A substantial number of peptides involved in this system can be found outside the nervous system as well, in particular in endocrine cells in derivatives of the primitive gut that exhibit amine precursor uptake and decarboxylation (APUD) characteristics. On the other hand, gastrointestinal APUD hormones and peptides such as angiotensin II and bradykinin are also found in the hypothalamus and in many other regions of the nervous system (Table 5.1), indicating a functional relationship between the nervous system and visceral organs in homeostasis, mediated through the activity of shared neuropeptides.

Types of neurosecretion

To characterise neurosecretory cells which possess endocrine functions, the term neuroendocrine transducers is used. Neuroendocrine transducers share the capacity to transform neuronal signals into hormonally mediated information. The neurosecretory cells in neuroendocrine transducer systems are neurosecretory cells which resemble typical neurons in their ability to be excited and to conduct action potentials, and are also able to synthesise, transport and release specific hormonal substances.

A variety of neurotransducer systems can be distinguished in the hypothalamo-pituitary unit and involve neurotransmitter or neuromodulator, neuroendocrine, paracrine and endocrine functions (Fig. 5.1). The hypothalamic neurotransmitters are simple amino acids, bioamines or peptides. The bioamines include dopamine, noradrenaline, adrenaline, serotonin, acetylcholine, γ-aminobutyric acid (GABA) and histamine. The neuropeptides include corticotrophin, growth hormone, thyrotrophin and gonadotrophin releasing hormones which stimulate, and somatostatin which inhibits, the secretion of anterior pituitary hormones, vasoactive intestinal peptide (VIP), substance P, neurotensin, components of the renin–angiotensin system, cholecystokinin, opioid peptides, atrial natriuretic peptides, galanin, endothelin and neuropeptide Y. Axons of the hypothalamic neurons, which synthesise and secrete hypophysiotrophic hormones, terminate

Table 5.1 Bioactive peptides in anterior pituitary cells. Modified from [5] and [7].

Brain–gut peptides	*Gonadal peptides*
Vasoactive intestinal peptide	Inhibin
Substance P	Activin
Galanin	Follistatin
Neuropeptide Y	
Neurotensin	*Posterior lobe peptides*
Bombesin	Oxytocin
Gastrin-releasing peptide	Vasopressin
Gastrin	Neurophysin
Cholecystokinin	
Motilin	*Hypothalamic releasing and inhibiting hormones*
Secretin	Growth hormone-releasing hormone
Neuromedin U	Gonadotrophin-releasing hormone
	Thyrotrophin-releasing hormone
Opioid peptides	Corticotrophin-releasing hormone
Prodynorphin products	Somatostatin
Proenkephalin A peptides	
Pro-opiomelanocortin products	*Other peptides*
	Chromogranin A and B
Peptides related to the salt–water balance or the cardiovascular system	Secretogranin
	Calcitonin
Atrial natriuretic factor	Calcitonin gene-related peptide
Renin–angiotensin	δ Sleep-inducing peptide
Endothelins	Kinins
	Lipocortin 1
Growth factors	
Basic and acidic fibroblast growth factor	
Transforming growth factor α and β	
Epidermal growth factor	
Insulin-like growth factor 1 and 2	
Vascular endothelial growth factor	
Interleukin	

directly in the perivascular zone surrounding the capillaries of the median eminence (Fig. 5.2). The hypophysiotrophic hormones are transported via this hypophysial portal vessel system to the trophic cells of the anterior pituitary. Neurosecretory neurons located in the supraoptic and paraventricular nuclei of the hypothalamus synthesise the neurohypophysial hormones oxytocin and vasopressin. The axons of these neurons terminate near to the venules in the infundibular process or posterior lobe of the pituitary, which is an extension of the hypothalamus and is composed mostly of neural tissue.

Apart from terminations in the median eminence and posterior pituitary, hypothalamic neurosecretory cells have synaptic contacts with homotypic and heterotypic neurons of hypothalamic nuclei and other parts of the central nervous system. This supports the supposition that the action of the hypothalamic hormones is not limited to the pituitary, but that they may also directly influence hypothalamic neurons via ultrashort feedback loops, and modulate brain function by the action of hormones as neurotransmitters or neuromodulators.

Anatomy of the hypothalamo-pituitary unit

The hypothalamo-pituitary unit is located at the base of the brain beneath the thalamus. The lower part of the third ventricle separates the hypothalamus into two identical parts containing a varity of semidiscrete nuclei. Anteroposteriorly, it extends from the level of the optic chiasm to just behind the mammillary bodies (Fig. 5.3). The basal part of the hypothalamus, located below the inferior portion of the third ventricle, is the median eminence, which is connected to the pituitary gland by the infundibular stem or pituitary stalk. These structures make up the contact zone between the endings of the hypophysiotrophic neurons and the capillaries of the hypophysial portal circulation (Fig. 5.4). These capillaries are termed gomitoli, and drain into the sinusoidal portal hypophysial vessels which have no outlet to the general circulation, but instead pass down through the stalk into the sinusoids of the anterior lobe of the pituitary. The axons of specific hypothalamic neurons terminate on equally specific and localised gomitoli, so favouring the concept of

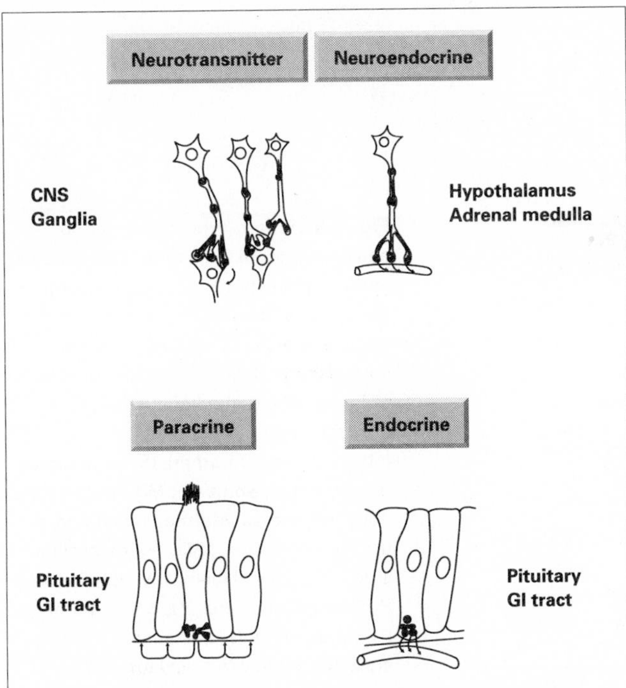

Fig. 5.1 Possible modes of peptide secretion. Peptides synthesised by neurons in the central nervous system or autonomic ganglia and released into the synaptic cleft through an axodendritic synapse or presynaptically through an axoaxonic synapse are termed neurotransmitters or neuromodulators. In neuroendocrine secretion the neuronal products are released into the bloodstream. In paracrine secretion, the peptide is secreted locally to affect a neighbouring cell. As a hormone, the peptides are secreted by endocrine cells into the bloodstream.

a regional distribution of portal blood within the anterior pituitary. There is probably also a retrograde blood flow between the pituitary and the hypothalamus, providing a means of direct feedback between pituitary hormones and their neuroendocrine control.

The pituitary can be divided into an anterior and posterior part. The anterior part or adenohypophysis can be subdivided into the pars distalis, the pars intermedia and the pars tuberalis. The pars distalis is the bulk of the gland in humans, and wraps superiorly around the pituitary stalk to form the pars tuberalis. The adenohypophysis originates from Rathke's pouch, an ectodermal evagination of the oropharynx, and migrates to join the posterior part of the pituitary or neurohypophysis. The portion of Rathke's pouch in contact with the neurohypophysis forms the intermediate zone. In humans, a distinct intermediate lobe cannot be distinguished, but colloid cysts and groups of epithelial cells extending into the neurohypophysis are found in the expected region. The colloid cysts are considered to be the remnants of the original lumen or cleft of Rathke's pouch. During the migration of Rathke's pouch, cells may persist beneath the sphenoid bone and form the pharyngeal pituitary. These cells have the potential to secrete hormones and can undergo adenomatous transformation. The posterior pituitary or neurohypophysis is derived from the diencephalon, and forms with the pituitary stalk and the infundibular process the contiguous link with the hypothalamus.

The pituitary gland, of which the anterior lobe constitutes two-thirds, weighs between 0.4 and 0.9 g and measures approximately 14 mm across, extends 10 mm anteroposteriorly and is 6 mm deep. It may double in size during pregnancy, and reduces in size at old age. The pituitary lies in the sella turcica, a depression of the sphenoid bone at the base of the skull, and is covered by a layer of dura mater attached to the clinoid processes of the sphenoid wings and dorsum sellae, the diaphragma sellae, through which the

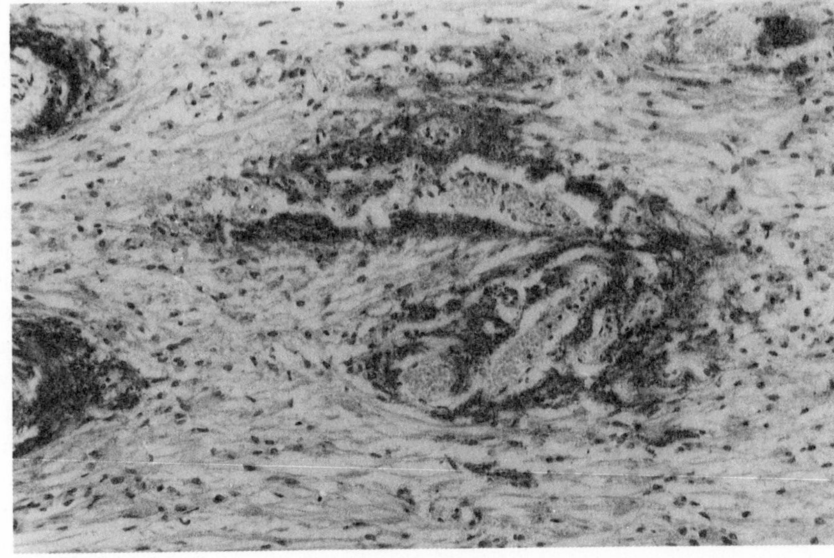

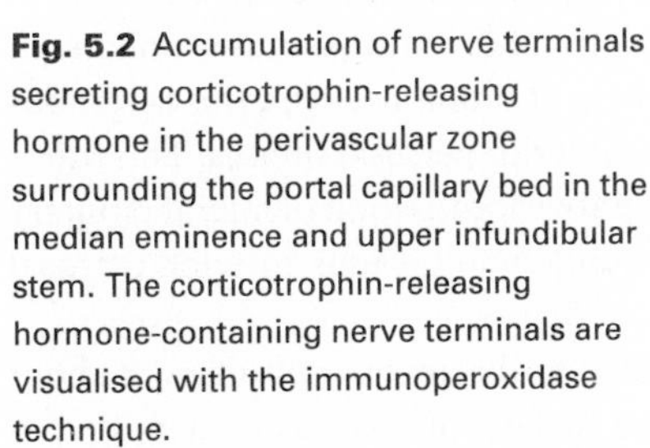

Fig. 5.2 Accumulation of nerve terminals secreting corticotrophin-releasing hormone in the perivascular zone surrounding the portal capillary bed in the median eminence and upper infundibular stem. The corticotrophin-releasing hormone-containing nerve terminals are visualised with the immunoperoxidase technique.

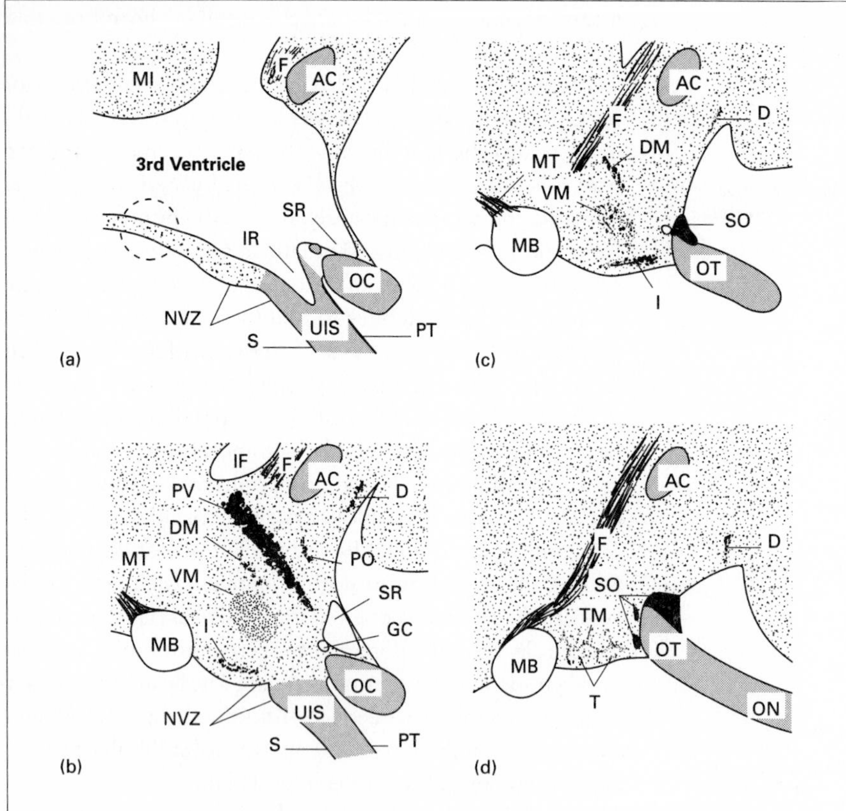

Fig. 5.3 Human hypothalamus and adjacent parts in the sagittal (longitudinal vertical) plane (anterior is to the right). Sequence of diagrams passing from the midline laterally (a)–(d). AC, anterior commissure; D, nucleus of diagonal band of Broca; DM, dorsodial nucleus; F, anterior column of fornix; IF, intraventricular foramen; IR, infundibular recess of third ventricle; MB, mammillary body; MI, massa intermedia and part of the hypothalamus; NVZ, neurovascular zone; OC, optic chiasm; ON, optic nerve; PO, preoptic nucleus; PT, pars tuberalis; PV, paraventricular nucleus; S, pituitary stalk; SO, supraoptic nucleus; SR, supraoptic recess of third ventricle; T, lateral tuberal nucleus; TM, tuberomammillary cells; UIS, upper infundibular stem; VM, ventromedial nucleus. From [1].

pituitary stalk passes. The lateral walls of the pituitary gland are in direct apposition of the cavernous sinuses and separated from them by dural folds. The optic chiasm lies 5–10 mm above the diaphragma sellae and anterior to the pituitary stalk. Since the sella turcica tends to conform to the shape and size of the gland, there is considerable variability in the contours of this bony structure.

Blood supply of the hypothalamo-pituitary unit

Apart from the median eminence and adjacent hypothalamic nuclei, the hypothalamus receives its arterial supply from the circle of Willis. The anterior suprachiasmatic part of the hypothalamus and the superior part of the chiasm are supplied by the anterior cerebral and anterior communicating arteries. The middle hypothalamus to the anterior part of the mammillary bodies receives blood from the posterior communicating arteries. The posterior hypothalamus and the posterior part of the mammillary bodies are supplied by the bifurcation of the basilar and posterior cerebral arteries. Venous blood draining from these areas enters the venous circle lying above the circle of Willis which, in turn, empties into the basal vein and the vena cerebri magna.

The arterial supply of the median eminence and upper infundibular stem is formed directly from branches of the superior hypophysial artery (Fig. 5.4), which arise from the internal carotid prior to its entry into the subarachnoid space. These arteries form the capillary network of the hypophysial portal circulation that recombines in the long portal veins that transport the hypothalamic hypophysiotrophic hormones through the pituitary stalk to the anterior pituitary. In addition, branches of the inferior hypophysial artery form a second capillary network in the lower infundibular stem draining via short portal veins to the anterior pituitary. The blood supply to the posterior pituitary is largely separated from that to the anterior pituitary, and is derived from branches of the inferior hypophysial artery as well. The venous drainage of the pituitary, through which adenohypophysial hormones reach the systemic circulation, is via intrasellar venous channels to the cavernous sinus, and then posteriorly into the superior and inferior petrosal sinuses to the jugular bulb and internal jugular vein. The drainage of each hemihypophysis into the ipsilateral cavernous sinus is unilateral, with insignificant mixture of blood between the cavernous sinuses and between the inferior petrosal sinuses. This offers the possibility of preoperative localisation of lateral pituitary adenomas by bilateral and simultaneous inferior petrosal sinus sampling.

The average blood flow to the anterior pituitary is about 0.8 ml/g/min, and is the highest of any tissue identified in

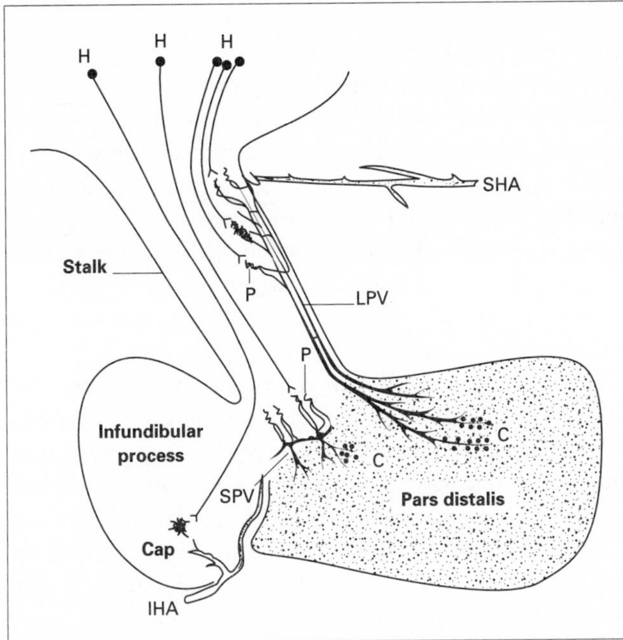

Fig. 5.4 Diagram of human pituitary gland in the sagittal plane to illustrate the neurovascular pathways by which nerve cells in certain hypothalamic nuclei (H) control the output of anterior and posterior pituitary hormones. The axon on the left ends on the capillary bed (Cap) in the infundibular process and represents the tract from the large nerve cells of the supraoptic and paraventricular nuclei which are concerned with posterior pituitary function. The other axons shown have their origin in the nerve cells in the so-called hypophysiotrophic area of the hypothalamus, and terminate on the capillary bed (P) feeding the portal vessels which supply the pars distalis. Here they transmit their neurohormones into the bloodstream and these are then carried through the long and the short portal vessels (LPV, SPV) to the epithelial cells (C) in a given area of the pars distalis to control the synthesis and secretion of hormones by these cells. From [1].

the mammal. This blood flow appears to be maintained at a relatively constant level under a variety of circumstances.

Microscopy of the hypothalamo-pituitary unit

The hypothalamus comprises nervous nuclei and nuclear groups with neuroendocrine and vegetative functions. The vegetative or autonomic functions involve regulation of sexual activity, body temperature, appetite, water and caloric balance, and circadian rhythms, and are concerned with nuclei predominantly located in the lateral zone of the hypothalamus. The neuroendocrine nuclei are situated in the zone of the hypothalamus near to the third ventricle (Fig. 5.3). The paraventricular nucleus occupies a crucial position in regulating hypothalamic function, and synthesises the majority of hypophysiotrophic and neurohypophysial hormones. This nucleus consists of a dense accumulation of large and small neurosecretory cells. The large cells form, with neurosecretory cells of the supraoptic nucleus, the magnocellular neurosecretory system. The small cells form, with the neurosecretory cells of the supraoptic and ventromedial nuclei, the parvocellular neurosecretory system. Axons of the magnocellular neurosecretory system containing vasopressin and oxytocin lead either directly to or through the supraopticohypophysial tract, which then descends through the infundibular stem to end in the neurohypophysis in the proximity of posterior pituitary venules; these then drain to the venous sinuses. Other neurosecretory axons containing hypophysiotrophic hormones lead from the paraventricular and ventromedial nuclei to the capillary networks in the median eminence and the infundibular stem.

Immunocytochemical studies have located the neurohypophysial and hypophysiotrophic hormones and other neuropeptides mentioned before in the hypothalamic nuclei, but also in the extrahypothalamic brain. Many of these peptides are found to be costored in the same neurons with other peptides or with more classical neurotransmitters such as dopamine, noradrenaline, acetylcholine, GABA and the enkephalins. Subcellular studies of hypothalamic and extrahypothalamic brain tissue have shown that these neuropeptides are concentrated in nerve terminals or the synaptic region, in line with the ideas of neurotransmitter and neuromodulator activities of these peptides. This might also imply that these peptides directly participate in the control of the pituitary. This has indeed been documented in *in vivo* and *in vitro* studies in which, for instance, VIP has been shown to stimulate the release of growth hormone, prolactin and adrenocorticotrophic hormone (ACTH), substance P stimulates prolactin and inhibits the corticotrophin-releasing hormone (CRH)-stimulated ACTH release, and calcitonin inhibits growth hormone-releasing hormone (GHRH)-stimulated growth hormone release.

The functional morphology of hypothalamic nuclei in humans is still poorly understood. There is probably a large overlap in functional areas, regulated according to physiological needs by the release of neuropeptides and biogenic amines. In particular, a subsystem of the dopaminergic neurons also regulates the activity of the anterior pituitary. Dopaminergic fibres of the tuberoinfundibular system end in the capillary networks of the median eminence and pituitary stalk, and inhibit prolactin release and probably also inhibit or facilitate release of other anterior pituitary hormones. Dopaminergic fibres also run via the supraopticohypophysial tract to the infundibular process and intermediate zone. In experimental animals, the dopaminergic neurons have an inhibitory effect on α-melanocyte stimulating hormone (α-MSH) release by intermediate lobe cells. In humans, such activity is uncertain as the human pituitary has no distinct functional intermediate lobe.

The anterior pituitary consists of a network of irregular lobules composed of secretory cells, surrounded by a continuous basement membrane and a thin layer of connective tissue which separates them from the interjacent sinusoids. The lobules are composed of a mixture of the different hormone-secreting cells and a few 'non-secreting' follicular or stellate cells; these latter have recently been shown to synthesise cytokines such as interleukins. These cytokines play a role in the response to infection and appear also to be involved in the regulation of the hypothalamo-pituitary–adrenal axis. The ultrastructure of the anterior pituitary cells exhibits all the characteristics of peptide synthesis and secretion, for example a rough-surfaced endoplasmic reticulum (RER), Golgi zone and secretory granules. It has been claimed that the different endocrine cells can be recognised by the density and size of the secretory granules. However, the granules grow by fusion during their transport to the cell surface, whereas the process of granule formation and release occurs in cycles. The granule size can therefore not be used for identification of the type of hormones stored. Ultrastructural studies may never the less give an impression of the secretory activity of the endocrine cells. An expanded RER and Golgi zone, together with sparse granulation along the cell membrane, indicates increased synthesis and release rather than storage, whereas the reverse is true for cells in a resting or storage phase.

The histological classification of anterior cells is based on the presence of secretory granules in the cytoplasm and the affinity of these granules for acidic and basic dyes. Simple staining techniques such as the haematoxylin and eosin method or more sophisticated trichrome methods serve to distinguish the granulated acidophil and basophil cells from unstained, and thus non-granulated, chromophobe cells. The acidophil cells secrete growth hormone and prolactin, the basophil cells secrete ACTH and other derivatives of the prohormone pro-opiomelanocortin (POMC) and the glycoprotein hormones follicle-stimulating hormone (FSH), luteinising hormone (LH) and thyroid-stimulating hormone (TSH). The basophil cells are also reactive with the periodic acid–Schiff (PAS) reagent, due to the carbohydrate moiety of the glycoprotein hormones and glycosylated POMC. However, because histological staining procedures are not specific for the nature of the hormone present in the cells, and the tinctorial properties of pituitary cells are strongly dependent on the modes of tissue preservation and staining techniques applied, histological techniques are not useful for a functional classification of anterior pituitary cells. This can only be done with either light- or electron-microscopic immunocytochemistry.

The topographical distribution of anterior pituitary cells is not random. The growth hormone and prolactin cells together represent the largest group of pituitary cells, and are in particular situated in the large lateral wings of the pituitary. During gestation, the prolactin cells show hyperplasia resulting in enlargement of the pituitary. In the fetal human pituitary, growth hormone and prolactin are localised within the same cell, which together with the observation of colocalisation of prolactin in pituitary adenomas of acromegalic patients confirms the view that growth hormone and prolactin cells are embryologically related.

The thyrotrophic cells are localised in the anteromedial part of the anterior pituitary and are the least numerous among the hypophysial cell types. In primary hypothyroidism these cells undergo hypertrophy, which may result in pituitary enlargement, sometimes with suprasellar extension.

The gonadotroph cells are found distributed throughout the human pituitary, but with an accumulation in the posteromedial portion immediately in front of the intermediate zone. Both FSH and LH are produced by these cells, although the concentration of these two hormones varies from cell to cell.

The corticotroph cells, comprising about one-fifth of the cell population of the anterior pituitary, are distributed in the mucoid wedge, in the anterior and anterolateral portions of the pituitary, around the borders of the posterolateral wings, and in the zona intermedia, and often extend into the adjacent neurohypophysis. In addition to ACTH, these cells produce derivatives of the prohormone as 1–28 N-terminal POMC, α-MSH and β-endorphin. A subset of the corticotroph cells in the anterior lobe, and of the intermedia zone cells extending into the neurohypophysis, processes a portion of its ACTH to des-acetyl-α-MSH and an 18–39 corticotrophin-like intermediate lobe peptide (CLIP). These cells are most abundant in pituitaries of human fetuses, but are also present in small numbers in the human pituitary. Because α-MSH cannot be detected in the human circulation, the functional significance of these cells is unknown. It has been suggested that they can give rise to dopamine-sensitive corticotroph adenomas found in some patients with Cushing's disease, but the evidence in favour of this suggestion is still minimal.

In addition to the well-known pituitary hormones, the anterior pituitary has been shown to contain a wide variety of bioactive peptides: brain–gut peptides, growth factors, hypothalamic releasing factors, posterior lobe peptides, opioids and various other peptides (Table 5.1). The localisation of most of these peptides was first established by immunocytochemical methods on animal tissues and some of the peptides were localised in identified cell types. Not all have been identified in human pituitary tissue. Although intracellular localisation of a peptide may be the consequence of internalisation from the plasma compartment, there is evidence for local synthesis of most of these peptides in the anterior pituitary based on the identification of their messenger RNA. Because the quantity of most of these peptides is very low (except for POMC peptides and galanin), endocrine functions are not expected. There is more evidence for paracrine, autocrine, or intracrine roles in growth, differentiation and regeneration, or in the control of hormone release.

Further reading

1 Daniel P, Prichard MML. Studies of the hypothalamus and the pituitary gland. *Acta Endocrinol* 1975; **80** (Suppl.): 201–24.

2 Doniach I. Histopathology of the pituitary. *Clin Endocrinol Metab* 1985; **14**: 765–89.

3 Froelich A. Ein Fall von Tumor der Hypophysis Cerebri ohne Akromegalie. *Wien Klin Rdsch* 1901; **15**: 883–6.

4 Green J, Harris GW. The neurovascular link between the neurohypophysis and the adenohypophysis. *J Endocrinol* 1947; **5**: 136–46.

5 Houben H, Denef C. Bioactive peptides in anterior pituitary cells. *Peptides* 1994; **15**: 547–82.

6 Kurosumi K. Ultrastructural immunocytochemistry of the adenohypophysis in the rat: a review. *J Electron Microsc Tech* 1991; **19**: 42–56.

7 Moore RM, Black PM. Neuropeptides. *Neurosurg Rev* 1991; **14**: 97–110.

8 Pelletier G. Anatomy of the hypothalamic–pituitary axis. *Methods Ach Exp Pathol* 1991; **14**: 1–22.

9 Scharrer E, Scharrer B. Hormones produced by neurosecretory cells. *Recent Prog Horm Res* 1954; **10**: 183–240.

10 Scheithauer BW, Horvath E, Kovacs K. Ultrastructure of the neurohypophysis. *Microsc Res Tech* 1992; **20**: 177–86.

11 Swaab DF, Hofman MA, Lucassen PJ, Purba JS, Raadsheer FC, van de Nes JA. Functional neuroanatomy and neuropathology of the human hypothalamus. *Anat Embryol* 1993; **187**: 317–30.

CHAPTER 6

Regulation of the hypothalamus and pituitary

J.S. Bevan and M.F. Scanlon

Introduction

The portal circulation enabling communication between the hypothalamus and anterior pituitary has already been described. This chapter deals primarily with the chemical mediators by which the hypothalamus exerts both stimulatory and inhibitory control over anterior pituitary hormone synthesis and release. These substances are mainly small peptides released from hypothalamic neurons into hypophysial portal blood; the five principal neuropeptides are summarised in Table 6.1. Other regulatory factors include biogenic amines (e.g. dopamine), neurotransmitters (e.g. acetylcholine) and other neuropeptides (e.g. vasoactive intestinal peptide (VIP), opioids, etc.). These act either directly on the anterior pituitary or indirectly by modulating the activity of other releasing-factor neurons within the hypothalamus. Intrahypothalamic regulation is complex and remains incompletely understood.

Most anterior pituitary hormones are released in a pulsatile fashion. For example, growth hormone (GH) is secreted in bursts lasting 1–2 hours, especially in the first half of the night during slow-wave sleep. Prolactin (PRL) is also secreted intermittently in pulses lasting about 90 minutes. The release of the gonadotrophins (follicle-stimulating hormone (FSH), luteinising hormone (LH)) is perhaps the best known example of pulsatile secretion and shows some concordance with the pulsatile secretion of thyroid-stimulating hormone (TSH), suggesting the presence of a common hypothalamic pulse generator. There are major physiological influences on anterior pituitary hormone release; some of these are shown in Table 6.2. The circadian rhythms for GH, PRL, adrenocorticotrophic hormone (ACTH) and TSH are well described, as is stress-related release of prolactin (PRL), GH and ACTH. These physiological factors will be mentioned together with their chemical mediators (where known) in subsequent sections on individual hormones. They illustrate the fact that inputs from higher neural centres can override (or amplify) the basic hypothalamo-pituitary regulatory mechanisms. The chapter concludes with the control of arginine vasopressin (AVP) and oxytocin neurosecretion.

Prolactin

Inhibition of PRL secretion

PRL, in contrast to the other anterior pituitary hormones, is under tonic inhibitory control by the hypothalamus. It was demonstrated in the early 1960s that PRL secretion is increased by pituitary stalk section, lesions of the median eminence or transplantation of the pituitary away from the hypothalamus. For several years there was considerable controversy as to the nature of the PRL inhibitory factor (PIF), but there is now general consensus that the most important regulator is dopamine, secreted by tuberoinfundibular neurons arising in the arcuate nucleus of the hypothalamus. The nanomolar concentrations of dopamine measured in hypophysial stalk plasma of rhesus monkeys are sufficient to inhibit PRL release from anterior pituitary cells *in vitro*. D_2 dopamine receptors are present in anterior pituitary cell membranes, particularly those of lactotrophs, and are negatively coupled with adenylate cyclase. Receptor activation leads to a fall in intracellular cyclic adenosine monophosphate (cAMP) concentration which reduces both PRL release and gene transcription. There is also inhibition of inositol phosphate metabolism producing similar effects on PRL secretion and synthesis. Administration of D_2 dopamine receptor antagonists, such as domperidone or metoclopramide, raises serum PRL concentrations *in vivo*. Conversely, dopamine and D_2-receptor agonists reduce PRL secretion from both normal and tumorous pituitary cells. Endogenous opioids have been implicated in the neural

Table 6.1 The principal hypothalamic neuropeptides.

Neuropeptide	Year of characterization	Amino-acid residues	Chromosomal location of human gene	Principal anterior pituitary actions
Thyrotrophin-releasing hormone (TRH)	1969	3	3	Releases TSH and prolactin
Gonadotrophin-releasing hormone (GnRH)	1971	10	8	Releases LH and FSH
Somatostatin (SS)	1973	14	3	Inhibits GH and TSH
Corticotrophin-releasing hormone (CRH)	1981	41	8	Releases ACTH and other POMC peptides
Growth hormone-releasing hormone (GHRH)	1982	44	20	Releases GH

TSH, thyroid-stimulating hormone; LH, luteinising hormone; FSH, follicle-stimulating hormone; GH, growth hormone; ACTH, adrenocorticotrophic hormone; POMC, pro-opiomelanocortin.

control of PRL secretion and may be the central mediators of stress-induced hyperprolactinaemia; there is evidence that this is due to inhibition of hypothalamic dopaminergic neurons, with subsequent reduction in inhibition of PRL secretion. However, the type of stress is important; naloxone suppresses the PRL response to exercise in trained athletes, but not that to insulin-induced hypoglycaemia or most other stimuli.

There is some doubt as to whether dopamine is the only hypothalamic inhibitor of PRL, since the concentration in hypophysial plasma does not suppress PRL release completely. This conclusion derives from studies in which hypothalamic inhibition was reduced by median eminence lesions or treatment with α-methyl-*p*-tyrosine (a dopamine-synthesis blocker), and the animals then infused with dopamine to reproduce levels measured in hypophysial stalk plasma. However, such experiments are subject to various criticisms, including the observation that endogenous dopamine secretion is highly variable; the pattern of dopamine release is an important determinant of PRL secretion.

Another proposed PIF is γ-aminobutyric acid (GABA).

Table 6.2 Physiological influences on anterior pituitary hormone release.

	Prolactin	GH	LH/FSH	ACTH	TSH
Circadian rhythm	(↑)	(↑)	– (↑Early puberty)	↑ (peak 0600–0900 hours)	↑ (peak 2300–0200 hours)
Sleep	↑	↑ (slow wave)	–	–	(↑)
Stress	↑	↑	↓	↑	–/↓
Exercise	↑	↑	↓	↑	–/↓
Food ingestion	– (↑ protein)	↓ (carbohydrate) ↑ (protein)			
Food deprivation	–	↑	↓	(↑)	–/↓
Pregnancy	↑	–	↓	↑	–
Suckling	↑				
Coitus	↑ (women)				

GH, growth hormone; LH, luteinising hormone; FSH, follicle-stimulating hormone; ACTH, adrenocorticotrophic hormone; TSH, thyroid-stimulating hormone.
↑ Increase.
– No change.
↓ Decrease.
( ) Minor influence.

The median eminence contains GABA neurons, and GABA receptors are found in anterior pituitary cell membranes, but in most studies GABA concentrations in hypophysial stalk plasma were lower than those required to inhibit PRL release from pituitary cells *in vitro*. There is a theoretical possibility that other factors may sensitise lactotrophs to GABA but, overall, its contribution to the inhibition of PRL appears to be small.

The 56-amino-acid peptide extension of the gonadotrophin-releasing hormone (GnRH) prohormone has been proposed as another PIF, and is known as GnRH-associated peptide (GAP). It has been suggested that its cosecretion with GnRH may provide a physiological mechanism by which the secretion of PRL and gonadotrophins is coordinated. GAP inhibits PRL release by rat and human anterior pituitary cells *in vitro* and has been shown by immunocytochemistry to be present in the median eminence. Immunisation of rabbits against various portions of the GAP molecule produces hyperprolactinaemia. Furthermore, administration of GAP to hypogonadal mice (hpg), which have a deletion of the GnRH gene, lowers serum PRL. For several reasons, however, the physiological relevance of GAP remains unclear. First, at the time of the preovulatory LH surge in the rat, there is a concurrent rise in serum PRL. Secondly, GAP and GnRH pulses are synchronised in sheep portal blood, yet in women there appears to be synchronous secretion of PRL and LH. Finally, basal serum PRL levels are lower in untreated hpg mice than in normal mice, not higher as one would predict. Further clarification of the role of GAP is awaited.

In summary, the present evidence suggests that, although dopamine may not be the only inhibitor of PRL, it is certainly the most important one.

PRL autoregulation

An important aspect of the control of PRL secretion is that of 'short-loop' feedback, whereby PRL—which is not, as far as is known, dependent on feedback inhibition from a target endocrine organ—regulates its own secretion. For example, dopamine levels in hypophysial portal blood are increased in hyperprolactinaemic rats with ectopically transplanted prolactinomas. Furthermore, specific PRL-binding sites have been identified in rat median eminence and several studies have shown a stimulatory effect of PRL on hypothalamic dopamine synthesis and release. In the human, too, there is much evidence to suggest that PRL enhances hypothalamic dopaminergic turnover. The administration of dopamine antagonists to patients with microprolactinomas produces an exaggerated release of TSH and LH (both these hormones are under inhibitory dopaminergic control), whilst the PRL response is reduced or absent. This probably indicates that, in this situation, the normal thyrotrophs and gonadotrophs are exposed to increased hypothalamic dopaminergic tone (Fig. 6.1).

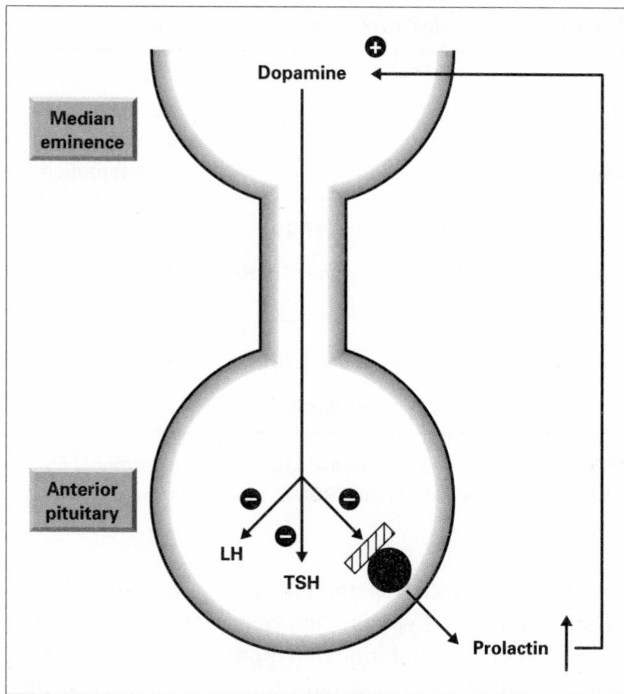

Fig. 6.1 Dopamine-mediated mechanisms between prolactin, thyroid-stimulating hormone (TSH) and luteinising hormone (LH) in the presence of an autonomous microprolactinoma.

Prolactin stimulates increased hypothalamic dopamine release which produces increased dopaminergic inhibition of TSH and LH secretion. The increased dopamine concentrations are unable to control prolactin release by the adenomatous cells because of either reduced sensitivity to dopamine, or defective vascular delivery of dopamine to the adenoma.

Stimulation of PRL secretion

Increased PRL secretion may result from either reduced inhibition or increased stimulation, and there is evidence for each of these mechanisms in the hypothalamic control of PRL secretion. Acute dopamine withdrawal, either *in vitro* or *in vivo*, produces a large rebound increase in PRL release. Suckling may produce transient decreases in hypothalamic dopamine release, but the evidence is conflicting and animals treated with dopamine synthesis inhibitors and given a constant infusion of dopamine still show suckling-induced PRL release. It is likely, however, that acute dopamine withdrawal increases lactotroph sensitivity to thyrotrophin-releasing hormone (TRH).

Besides the inhibitory control of PRL secretion, the existence of counterbalancing stimulatory mechanisms is widely accepted (Fig. 6.2). This stems from numerous reports of PRL-

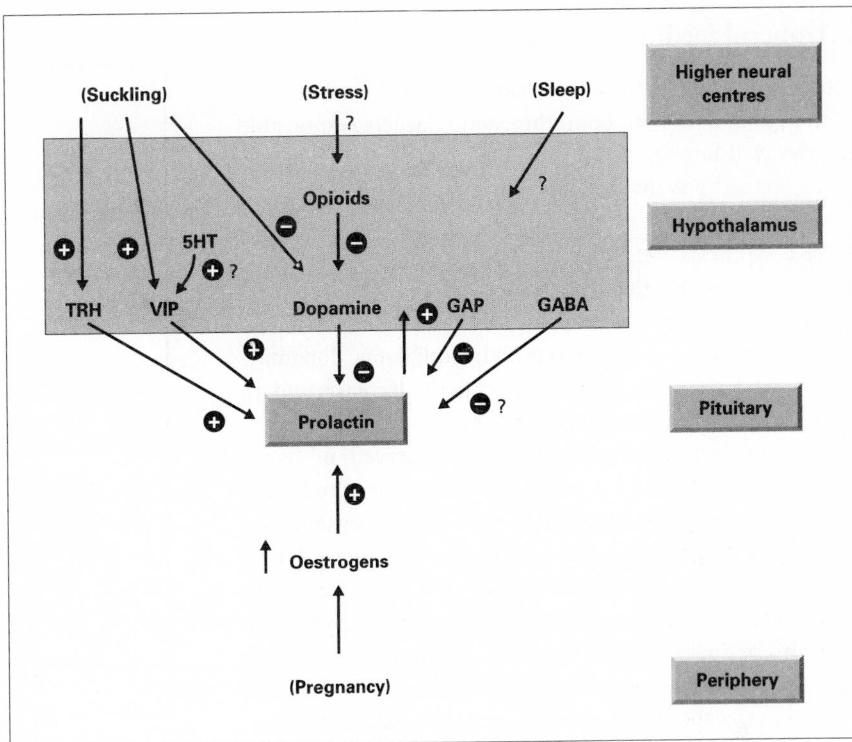

Fig. 6.2 Neuroendocrine control of prolactin secretion.

releasing factors (PRFs) in various purified hypothalamic extracts. A bewildering number of substances have been proposed as PRFs including TRH, VIP, serotonin, neurotensin, bombesin, angiotensin II, AVP, substance P and epidermal growth factor (EGF), to name but a few. Even though these substances are capable of releasing PRL *in vitro*, this fact alone does not prove their *in vivo* role as PRFs.

An important feature of a PRF might be the capacity to release PRL when its secretion is relatively restrained by dopamine. It has been noted already that suckling can induce PRL release in the presence of dopamine. Of the above list of possible PRFs, TRH and VIP seem the strongest candidates as physiological releasers of PRL. TRH induces PRL release by a direct pituitary action and its concentration in hypophysial stalk plasma is considerably higher than in peripheral plasma. TRH receptors are present on the membranes of normal and tumorous lactotrophs and post-receptor mechanisms involve intracellular Ca^{2+} mobilisation and activation of protein kinase C, which increase PRL release and gene transcription. In the rat, both suckling and TRH stimulate dual secretion of PRL and TSH. TRH levels in hypophysial stalk plasma are increased by mammary nerve stimulation and suckling. Some investigators have reported an attenuation of the PRL surge in pro-oestrus rats after immunisation with TRH antiserum. In sheep immunised against TRH, the PRL response to heat exposure is reduced. Pituitary superfusion studies have shown that combined treatment of TRH and a brief fall in dopamine stimulates greater PRL release than either treatment alone. Furthermore, oestradiol enhances this effect.

The amount of VIP in the human median eminence is higher than in any other brain area. In the rat, VIP concentrations in pituitary portal blood are very much greater than in peripheral samples. Intravenous administration of VIP provokes PRL release in the human and the rat. In the stalk-transected rhesus monkey, intravenous VIP causes a rise in serum PRL indicating that it acts, at least in part, directly on the pituitary. This has been confirmed by *in vitro* experiments using cultured pituitary cells from various species. Some workers have shown attenuation or delay in the PRL response to suckling in the rat following the administration of VIP antiserum. In some studies, VIP appears to be additive to, or synergistic with, the effects of TRH on PRL release. It is likely that serotonin-induced PRL release is mediated by VIP. At the pituitary level, VIP is associated almost exclusively with lactotrophs where its receptor is positively coupled with adenylate cyclase, and increased cAMP levels promote PRL release and gene transcription.

In addition to their effects on pituitary cell growth, locally produced growth factors may have effects on PRL synthesis and secretion. EGF increases PRL gene expression in rat pituitary tumour cells, whilst basic fibroblast growth factor (FGF) enhances lactotroph responsiveness to TRH.

Peripheral feedback signals

Oestradiol influences the secretion of PRL by actions on both hypothalamus and pituitary, and is largely responsible for the well-known rise in serum PRL during pregnancy, when lactotrophs increase in both number and functional capacity. The main direct pituitary action involves stimulation of PRL synthesis. Yet, in humans and monkeys, oestrogens appear to enhance the sensitivity of PRL to inhibition by dopamine and increase lactotroph responsiveness to TRH. Oestrogens have complex effects on hypothalamic dopamine release and have been reported to both decrease and to increase release of dopamine in the rat.

Hyperprolactinaemia is sometimes observed in hypothyroidism, and some have speculated that this may be due to increased hypothalamic TRH release as a consequence of reduced negative-feedback inhibition by thyroid hormones. Certainly, TRH gene transcription is increased in hypothyroidism. Hyperprolactinaemia in hypothyroidism may also be due to reduced hypothalamic dopamine activity; lactotrophs from hypothyroid rats also show reduced sensitivity to the inhibitory effects of dopamine which is probably secondary to reduced number rather than affinity of dopamine receptors. It should be noted that both the clearance and distribution volume of PRL are decreased in the hypothyroid rat which may contribute to the mild hyperprolactinaemia which can occur.

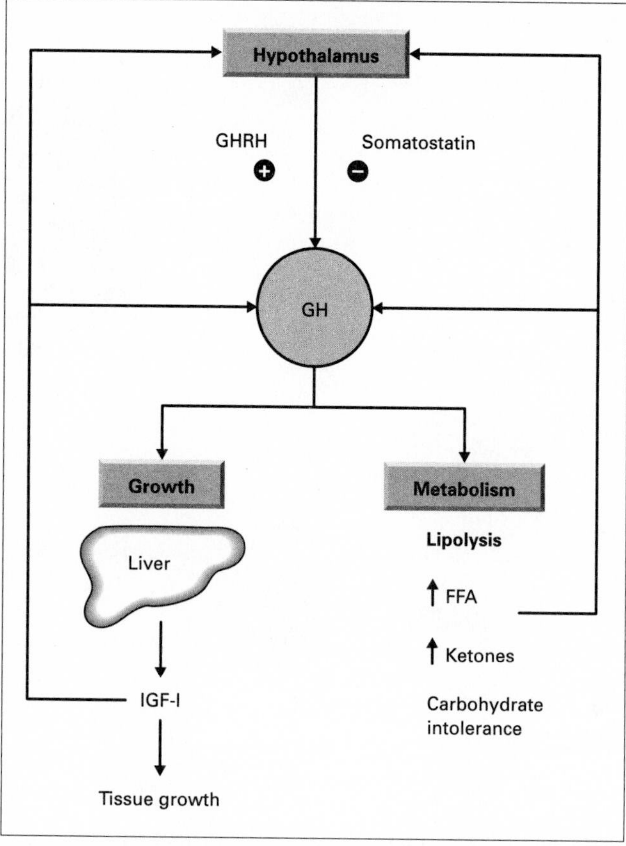

Fig. 6.3 A simple perspective of growth hormone (GH) regulation. FFA, free fatty acids.

Growth hormone

GH is regulated principally by interaction between the hypothalamic peptides somatostatin (SS) and growth hormone-releasing hormone (GHRH), and feedback by insulin-like growth factor 1(IGF-1) and GH itself. However, GH control is much more complex than this, and many other neuropeptides, neurotransmitters, peripheral hormones, growth factors and metabolites modulate its secretion. Some of the pathways involved in the regulation of GH are shown in Fig. 6.3.

Somatostatin

GH-release inhibiting activity in hypothalamic extracts was discovered in the 1960s and the 14-amino-acid cyclic peptide, SS, was eventually sequenced and characterised by Brazeau and coworkers in 1973. It was the first hypothalamic regulator to be identified outside that region, and is now known to have important actions elsewhere in the central nervous system and in the gastrointestinal tract. Several precursor forms of SS were found, and their identity was confirmed when the preprosomatostatin gene was sequenced in 1984. Prosomatostatin is processed post-translationally to C-terminal 28 (SS-28) and 14 (SS-14) amino acids. In the hypothalamus, somatostatinergic neurons are located within the periventricular and anterior zones, and cosecrete SS-14 and SS-28. There is strong conservation of the prosomatostatin sequence between species and the gene has been localised to chromosome 3 in humans. Somatostatin release is under complex control by hormones (GH and IGF-1), neurotransmitters (acetylcholine and catecholamines), nutrients and metabolites (glucose, free fatty acids (FFA), amino acids).

GH-releasing hormone

The existence of GH-releasing factor was established in the 1950s when Reichlin showed that bilateral hypothalamic lesions abolished linear growth in rats. However, it was not until 1982 that human GHRH was isolated as 44- and 40-amino-acid forms from two pancreatic tumours in patients with acromegaly due to ectopic GHRH production. Subsequent studies of the human hypothalamus have confirmed that GHRH(1–44) is the authentic hormone and GHRH(1–40) and (1–37), which are also fully active, represent processed versions of the larger molecule. This family of GHRHs derive from larger precursors (preproGHRH 107 and 108), and the human GHRH gene is located on chromosome 20. GHRH(1–44), (1–40) and (1–29) are equipotent on a molar basis in their capacity to stimulate GH release in humans. GHRH is rapidly inactivated by a plasma dipeptidyl aminopeptidase, producing the more stable metabolite GHRH(3–44), which is 1000 times less potent than GHRH(1–44); the biological half-life of GHRH(1–44) is around 7 minutes. Immunoreactive GHRH is present at highest concentration in neurons of the median eminence and arcuate nuclei, but is present also in anterior and other areas of the hypothalamus. Moreover, it has been identified in both the secretory granules and nuclei of pituitary somatotrophs, as well as in peripheral plasma, upper gastrointestinal tract and placenta.

Regulation of GH by neuropeptides

There is now comprehensive evidence that SS and GHRH play an important pivotal role in the regulation of GH secretion, and this is summarised in Table 6.3.

GHRH increases both GH synthesis and release after binding to specific receptors in somatotroph cell membranes

Table 6.3 Growth hormone-releasing hormone (GHRH) and somatostatin control of growth hormone (GH) secretion.

1 Acute administration of GHRH or somatostatin both *in vivo* and *in vitro* causes rapid, dose-related and specific release or inhibition of GH in a variety of mammalian and non-mammalian species

2 Rats treated with anti-GHRH antibodies or treated neonatally with monosodium glutamate (which reduces GHRH in the median eminence) show an abolition of pulsatile GH secretion and a decrease in somatic growth, whereas rats treated with antisomatostatin antibodies show an increase in basal and stimulated GH levels and increased body weight

3 GHRH and somatostatin are present in portal vessels at concentrations which stimulate or inhibit GH release and GH gene transcription. GHRH levels are increased whereas somatostatin levels are reduced at the time of the expected GH secretory episode

4 Chronic administration of GHRH to intact rats or humans leads to an increase in GH and IGF-1 levels as well as somatic growth. Chronic administration of somatostatin inhibits basal and stimulated GH release

5 Elevation of plasma GHRH levels (ectopic GHRH-secreting tumours or transgenic mice expressing the GHRH gene) elevates GH levels and increases somatic growth

6 Specific, high-affinity, low-capacity GHRH and somatostatin receptors are present in anterior pituitary membranes

which activate adenylate cyclase via the guanosine triphosphate (GTP) regulatory protein, G_s. Stimulation of GH release is cAMP and Ca^{2+} dependent, whilst stimulation of GH gene transcription is cAMP, but not Ca^{2+}, dependent. SS inhibits basal and GHRH-induced GH release after binding to specific transmembrane receptors on somatotrophs. At least five different subtypes of SS receptor have recently been cloned from different genes: the predominant anterior pituitary receptors are SSTR2 and 5 which are negatively linked to adenylate cyclase via the inhibitory subunit of the guanine nucleotide regulatory protein. However, SS also acts independently of cAMP by reducing Ca^{2+} influx and inducing hyperpolarisation of membranes through conventional G-protein linkage to Ca^{2+} and K^+ channels, respectively.

GH itself stimulates SS release from the hypothalamus *in vitro*. The administration of GH to normal subjects reduces the GH responses to GHRH; this effect can be observed within a few hours of GH administration, before any rise in IGF-1 levels. These data support the view that GH stimulates SS release from the hypothalamus *in vivo*, although direct feedback inhibition on the pituitary is also possible. Indeed, recent evidence suggests that GH induces local pituitary IGF-1 gene transcription and synthesis, thus providing possible short-loop autocrine or paracrine feedback control of its own secretion. IGF-1 acts in concert with IGF-2 to directly inhibit hypothalamic GHRH release. Finally, there is some evidence that GHRH and SS may regulate their own secretion by short-loop negative feedback at the hypothalamic level. Repeated or prolonged continuous administration of GHRH *in vitro* and *in vivo* leads to a reduction in GH release. Concomitant administration of SS reduces this desensitisation in response to GHRH, suggesting that depletion of a GHRH-sensitive releasable pool of GH may contribute to this phenomenon. Other mechanisms are also involved however since prior treatment with GHRH *in vitro*, in the presence or absence of SS, causes a decreased cAMP response to GHRH, as well as an increase in the ED_{50} for the stimulation of both cAMP and GH by GHRH. The physiological importance of such true desensitisation is unclear since GHRH pretreatment *in vitro* leads to a 50% fall in somatotroph GHRH receptor number, whereas a maximal GH response to GHRH is obtained at only 10–20% receptor occupancy. Certainly, GHRH desensitisation is much less important physiologically, both quantitatively and functionally, than GnRH desensitisation in relation to the gonadotrophins (see GnRH section). Furthermore, in clinical practice somatotroph desensitisation is relatively unimportant since persistent elevation of GH and IGF-1 levels follows chronic GHRH administration, and acromegaly occurs in situations of ectopic GHRH production.

In addition to GHRH and SS it is clear that opioids, TRH, GH-releasing peptide (GHRP) and other neuropeptides can

Table 6.4 Growth hormone responses to thyrotrophin-releasing hormone in various pathological conditions.

Endocrine
Acromegaly
Primary hypothyroidism
Diabetes mellitus
Neuropsychiatric
Anorexia nervosa
Depression
Schizophrenia
Metabolic
Cirrhosis
Chronic renal failure
Protein-calorie malnutrition

exert effects on GH secretion. In animals, opioids stimulate GH secretion by a GHRH-dependent mechanism, since pretreatment with GHRH antiserum abolishes the GH response. There is no direct evidence that endogenous opioids play a major role in the control of GH secretion in humans, though it is possible that they are responsible for the elevated GH levels seen in some forms of stress such as marathon running and calorie restriction. TRH stimulates GH secretion in some pathological situations (Table 6.4), but not in normal human subjects. In contrast, GH responses to L-dopa, arginine and insulin-induced hypoglycaemia are reduced or abolished during TRH administration. TRH stimulation of GH secretion in pathological states is due to a direct pituitary effect, whereas the inhibitory action of TRH is probably exerted at a hypothalamic level via enhanced SS release, since it is abolished in rats treated with SS antiserum.

Over the last 5–10 years the importance of additional GHRPs has become established following the initial synthesis of peptidic molecules based on the structure of Met-enkephalin, a known GH secretagogue. A range of peptides (GHRPs) have been derived from the initial hexapeptide, GHRP-6 (Hexarelin). They are all small peptides although a non-peptidic, orally active form is also now available. GHRPs mimic the action of an endogenous ligand (structure not yet published) for a membrane-bound receptor distinct from the GHRH receptor which has recently been cloned. *In vitro* GHRPs have a small action to release GH from anterior pituitary tissue which is additive to the action of GHRH indicating separate intracellular pathways. However, the most dramatic effect on GH release is seen when GHRPs are administered *in vivo* when they exert a potent, synergistic interaction with GHRH in the release of GH. This occurs even with doses of GHRH which are subthreshold for GH release. *In vivo* GHRPs activate hypothalamic GHRH neurons and their GH-releasing actions can be reduced but not abolished by antibodies to GHRH. The profound synergistic interaction between GHRPs and GHRH cannot be satisfactorily explained by direct actions of GHRPs on either GHRH or SS neurons; thus, although it is clear that GHRPs exert important hypothalamic actions, their full nature is hitherto unknown. The isolation of the putative endogenous peptide is still awaited.

Many other neuropeptides have been shown to influence GH secretion in a variety of experimental models and these include VIP (possibly via GHRH receptors in view of its sequence homology with GHRH), glucagon, galanin, α-melanocyte-stimulating hormone (α-MSH), bombesin and several others. Their relevance to normal physiology remains unclear.

Peripheral feedback signals

Growth factors

IGFs play a negative-feedback role in the control of GH release in addition to mediating the tissue effects of GH. This occurs at both hypothalamic and pituitary levels. IGF-1 is considerably more potent than IGF-2 and has greater affinity for the pituitary IGF receptor, which was characterised in 1984. Thyroid hormones play a permissive role in these actions since hypothyroid pituitary cells in culture are less sensitive than cells of euthyroid animals to IGF-1 negative feedback. EGF decreases triiodothyronine (T_3)-induced synthesis and secretion of GH *in vitro*, and EGF receptors are present in normal rat and human pituitary membranes. In contrast, acute exposure of normal rat pituitary cells in a superfusion system to EGF leads to increased GH secretion.

Thyroid hormones

Thyroid hormones play a critical role in the control of GH synthesis and secretion both *in vivo* and *in vitro*. GH gene transcription is increased by T_3 several-fold *in vitro* in rat pituitary cell lines and the c-*erb*-A proto-oncogene, which encodes the T_3 nuclear receptor, has been shown to induce GH gene expression. The DNA sequences of the rat GH gene which confer T_3 responsiveness contain a domain which binds the c-*erb*-A proto-oncogene product. GH responses to hypoglycaemia, arginine, GHRH and sleep are impaired in patients with hypothyroidism. In contrast, however, GH responses to TRH are increased in the hypothyroid state. The decreased GH responsiveness to GHRH in hypothyroidism is due to reduced GH synthesis, while the increased GH responsiveness to TRH could be explained by the well-known inhibitory effect of thyroid hormones on the expression of pituitary TRH receptors. In addition to their direct effects on GH secretion at the pituitary level, thyroid hormones can influence GHRH and SS production in the hypothalamus.

Metabolic feedback

Elevation of blood glucose and FFAs reduces basal and stimulated GH levels whereas hypoglycaemia stimulates GH release. Hypoglycaemia causes GH release by a mechanism which is independent of GHRH and may be due to reduced SS release, but the evidence for this is inconclusive. Administration of FFAs to normal subjects reduces the responses to hypoglycaemia, exercise, L-dopa, clonidine, arginine, sleep and GHRH. This effect is probably due to enhanced SS release since it does not occur in rats treated with anti-SS antibodies.

Gonadal hormones

Male rat pituitaries contain more GH than female glands and episodic GH secretion is greater in male than female rats. Treatment of rats *in vivo* with oestrogens and testosterone causes an increase and decrease, respectively, in GH responses to GHRH of the cultured pituitary cells *in vitro*, though the mechanism is unknown. Human females show greater GH responses to arginine than males, and such responses are greater at mid-cycle than in the early follicular phase. It is well established that sex-hormone priming of children with delayed puberty enhances the GH responses to hypoglycaemia, arginine and GHRH. Most evidence suggests that the sex differentiation of GH secretion is mediated via GHRH.

Glucocorticoids

Glucocorticoids are potent stimulators of pituitary GH synthesis and secretion *in vitro*. This is mediated by glucocorticoid receptor binding to a glucocorticoid response element in the first intron of the human GH gene. *In vivo*, however, a dominant inhibitory effect of glucocorticoids is usually observed following chronic administration of glucocorticoids or in hypercortisolism. This is probably exerted at a hypothalamic level via modulation of GHRH and/or SS release. This *chronic* effect of glucocorticoids should be distinguished from the *acute* action *in vivo* of glucocorticoids to cause acute release of GH over a 3–4 hour period. This has been proposed as another secretagogue test of GH release. The mechanism is unknown at present.

Neurotransmitter regulation

Cholinergic muscarinic pathways are important in the regulation of GH secretion. Cholinergic activation with pyridostigmine enhances basal GH and its response to GHRH whereas antagonists, such as atropine and pirenzepine, can abolish the GH responses to all physiological and pharmacological stimuli with the exception of the GH response to

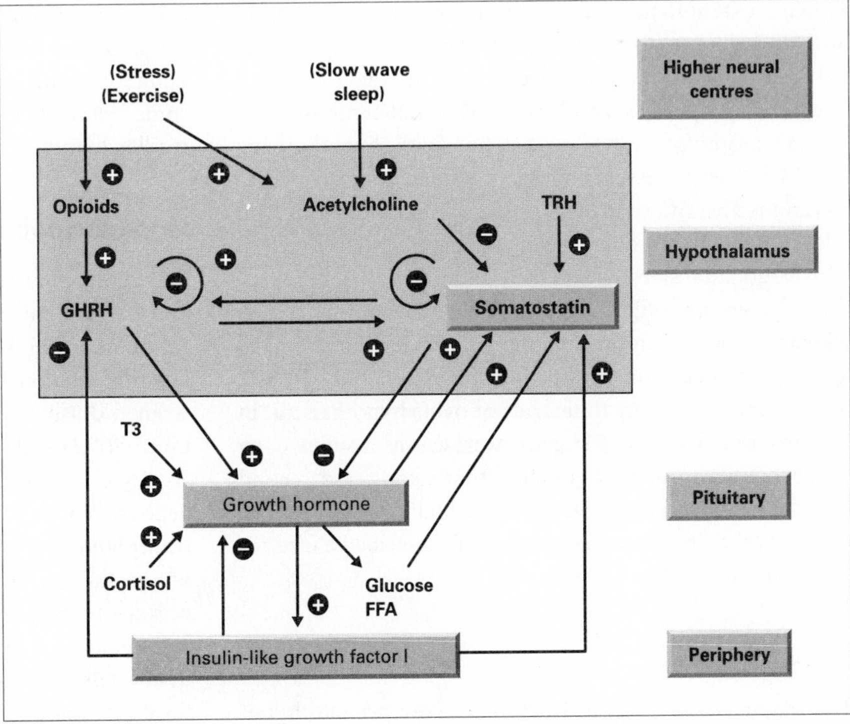

Fig. 6.4 Neuroendocrine control of growth hormone secretion.

insulin-induced hypoglycaemia (Fig. 6.4). For example, slow-wave sleep-related GH release is abolished by such treatment. Since antibodies to SS block the inhibition of GH secretion by muscarinic antagonists in rats, it is likely that these agents antagonise an inhibitory effect exerted by acetylcholine on SS release from the hypothalamus; this effect can clearly be overcome by hypoglycaemia-induced reduction in SS release which may be of importance teleologically. Dopamine and dopamine agonist drugs cause increased GH release in normal subjects, but the hypothalamic mechanism is unknown. β-Adrenergic pathways inhibit and α-noradrenergic pathways stimulate GH secretion *in vivo*; again, the precise mechanism and site of action are unclear. Although serotoninergic pathways are stimulatory to GH secretion in the rat, it is not possible to draw any firm conclusions on the role of these pathways in the control of GH secretion in humans. Likewise, the physiological relevance of melatonin, histamine and GABA to the control of GH in humans has still to be clarified, although there is some evidence for the involvement of each.

Gonadotrophins

Gonadotrophin-releasing hormone

Characterisation

The synthesis and secretion of the two gonadotrophins, LH and FSH, are principally under the control of the hypothalamic peptide GnRH. GnRH stimulates release of LH to a greater extent than FSH, and this relatively weaker action on FSH led some to postulate the existence of a separate FSH-releasing hormone. However, this is not now given much credence, as it has been clearly shown that appropriate administration of GnRH to patients with hypothalamic GnRH deficiency restores both fertility and gonadal steroid secretion. The differential action of GnRH on LH and FSH release is probably due to complex interactions between GnRH, gonadal steroids and the inhibin family of polypeptide hormones, as will be seen. GnRH is a linear decapeptide which is identical in all mammalian species. Its chemical identity was determined by Schally and Guillemin in 1971 using extracts of many thousands of ovine hypothalami. In humans, the neural GnRH gene is present as a single copy on chromosome 8, and contains four exons; the second encodes pro-GnRH and part of exon 2, all of 3 and part of 4 encode the 56-residue peptide, GAP, described earlier in this chapter.

Localisation

The major group of GnRH neurons in the primate hypothalamus is located in the medial basal hypothalamus and projects to the lateral area of the median eminence. Negative feedback of testosterone and oestrogens occurs on these neurons and pulsatile release of LH and FSH is not abolished if they are isolated from the rest of the central nervous system (CNS) by surgical division of connecting neural pathways. A second group of GnRH neurons is situated in the anterior hypothalamus and preoptic area; about half of these project to the median eminence and the remainder to other areas of the CNS including the limbic system. In the rat, these neurons are under positive oestrogen feedback and are responsible for the midcycle LH/FSH surge, whereas in primates this is not the case. In lower mammals, such as the rat, the anterior hypothalamus seems to be important in the integration of sexual behaviour and neuroendocrine responses. GnRH is also found within the CNS and has been found in ovary, testis, placenta and breast milk. Its functions in these sites are unknown.

Regulation of synthesis and release

The regulation of GnRH release is complex and poorly understood. Probable functional differences between subpopulations of GnRH neurons in close anatomical proximity within the hypothalamus increase the investigational difficulties. GnRH neurons in the preoptic area may be regulated positively by serotoninergic or negatively by corticotrophin-releasing hormone (CRH) neurons. GnRH neurons of the medial basal hypothalamus are stimulated by ascending α_1-adrenergic and inhibited by dopaminergic neurons, the latter action possibly mediated by intrahypothalamic endorphins. Pulsatility of GnRH secretion is an important feature of gonadotrophin secretion and this will now be considered in some detail, with particular reference to gonadal steroid feedback and neural mechanisms of pulsatility.

Gonadotrophin pulsatility

Gonadotrophin secretion is pulsatile in men and women and greater than 70% of FSH pulses coincide with LH pulses. In the ram, LH pulses are followed by testosterone pulses, but this relationship is not clearly seen in normal men. In women during the follicular phase of the menstrual cycle, up to 80% of LH pulses are followed by oestrogen pulses. A very clear relationship is evident in sheep when ovarian venous blood is sampled from animals with an ovary transplanted to the neck. During mid- and late-luteal phases of the human menstrual cycle large LH pulses stimulate pulses of progesterone secretion from the corpus luteum. The evidence is overwhelming from direct sampling studies in animals that pulses of LH secretion by the pituitary are the direct result of pulses of GnRH secreted from the median

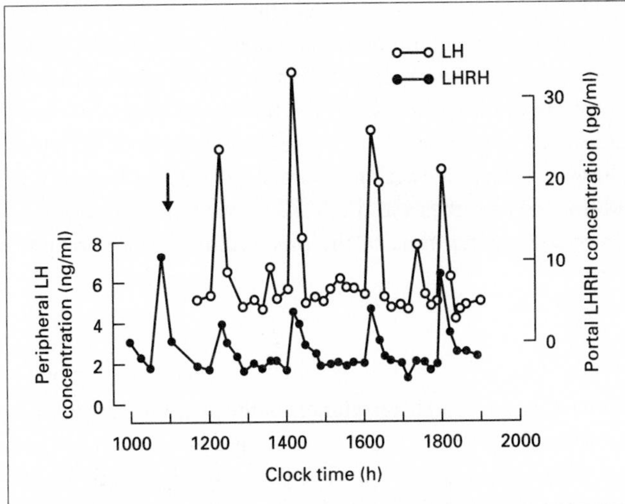

Fig. 6.5 Hypophysial portal luteinising hormone (LH)-releasing hormone (LHRH) and jugular venous LH concentrations in an ovariectomized ewe. From Clarke and Cummins (1982), with permission.

eminence into the hypophysial portal blood (Fig. 6.5). In men the pulse *pattern* of LH and FSH is variable between and within subjects. In women the LH pulse pattern depends on the stage of the menstrual cycle; in the follicular phase there is a marked increased in LH pulse frequency which is associated with increased oestrogen secretion from the developing ovarian follicle(s). Positive oestrogen feedback ultimately induces the preovulatory LH surge at which time there is a large increase in the frequency and size of LH pulses. In contrast, LH cycle frequency is relatively low during the luteal phase of the cycle.

Gonadal steroid feedback

Progesterone, acting synergistically with oestrogens, exerts negative feedback on the hypothalamus during the luteal phase, thus limiting GnRH pulsatility and slowing LH pulse frequency. The mechanism of positive oestrogen feedback at the time of the LH surge has been much debated. There is now evidence that enhancement of both hypothalamic GnRH pulse generator activity and pituitary responsiveness to GnRH are involved. All species so far studied have shown an increased 'self-priming' effect of GnRH on the pituitary during the preovulatory period. LH pulses are more frequent at the time of the LH surge than at any other time, and portal sampling experiments have confirmed a concurrent change in the pattern of GnRH release. In males, the situation is more straightforward. Since LH surges do not occur, only negative-feedback effects are relevant. Testosterone (and its active metabolite dihydrotestosterone, DHT) exerts major suppressive effects on both LH and FSH secretion, largely by inhibiting the GnRH pulse frequency generator, but possibly also by direct pituitary actions. Oestrogens in the male reduce pituitary responsiveness to GnRH.

Neural mechanisms of pulsatility

Electrophysiological studies of the medial basal hypothalamus have shown that neural activity can be correlated with pulses of LH release, although the nature and precise site of the neural pacemaker remains unknown. There is a large body of evidence which suggests that central ascending α_1-adrenergic pathways regulate GnRH pulsatility, but the observation that GnRH pulsatility was not abolished in the rhesus monkey by the surgical creation of mediobasal hypothalamic 'islands' suggested that the pacemaker was intrinsic to the hypothalamus. However, it is impossible to rule out the possibility that, under normal circumstances, afferent inputs are involved. It is probable that extra-hypothalamic inputs are important for the generation of the preovulatory LH surge, and are important in steroid hormone modulation of the pulse generator.

Neuropeptides and pulsatility

Several neuropeptides have been found to influence GnRH/LH pulsatility, most notably the opioids β-endorphin, Met-enkephalin and dynorphin. Opiate antagonists, such as naloxone, produce an increase in LH secretion in men, women, monkeys and other mammals. Such effects are gonadal steroid dependent. In women, naloxone responsiveness is most marked during the progesterone-dominated luteal phase, though effects have been found during the oestrogen-dominated follicular phase. In males, castration eliminates the naloxone response but gonadal steroids reinstate it. It is probable that endogenous opioids modulate aminergic inputs to the GnRH neurons, mainly at the cell-body level. Animal studies suggest that excitatory amino acids, substance P, neuropeptide Y (NPY) and VIP may also regulate GnRH release. Most importantly, there is increasing evidence for the involvement of excitatory amino-acids and NPY in the increase in GnRH during the oestrus surge and during puberty, possibly being mediated by nitric oxide or other gaseous neurotransmitters. Overall, the current hypothesis is that GnRH neurons possess intrinsic pulsatility that is regulated by aminergic input, with neuropeptides acting either in concert with the aminergic system (e.g. NPY) or by modulating the aminergic signal (e.g. opioids).

Mechanism of GnRH action

The binding of GnRH to gonadotrophs is different from

each of the other hypothalamic peptides in the sense that continuous GnRH exposure results in marked suppression of LH/FSH synthesis and secretion. This down-regulation or desensitisation is the basis for the use of long-acting GnRH agonists in the treatment of precocious puberty or gonadal steroid-sensitive malignancies such as prostatic carcinoma. Conversely, therapeutic interventions with GnRH to stimulate gonadotrophin secretion require pulsatile delivery every 60–120 minutes to mimic normal LH/FSH pulsation, which is presumed to reflect endogenous GnRH pulsation.

The extensively characterised GnRH receptor interacts predominantly with arginine at position 8 in the GnRH molecule, whereupon receptors dimerise by covalent cross-linking and become internalised and recycled. Long-term exposure to GnRH reduces the number of GnRH receptors available for binding. GnRH binding is associated with a rise in free intracellular Ca^{2+} and calmodulin antagonists will block GnRH-induced LH release. Second-messenger signalling involves activation of phospholipase C and phosphatidyl inositol hydrolysis. At least part of GnRH-induced desensitisation is due to depletion of protein kinase C. The well known 'self-priming' action of GnRH is mediated by activation of protein kinase C, while GnRH receptor number and affinity are also increased.

Inhibins and activins

Inhibins

The term 'inhibin' was chosen to describe a non-steroidal factor, derived from the gonads, which specifically reduces FSH secretion. In 1985 four groups of researchers purified inhibin in ovarian follicular fluid from several animal species, using cultured pituitary cells as the detecting bioassay. It was shown that basal and GnRH-stimulated FSH secretion were suppressed by inhibin, but LH was unaffected. Ultimately a protein of molecular weight 32 kDa was isolated and shown to be a glycoprotein heterodimer of two disulphide-linked subunits (α and β) of molecular size 18 and 14 kDa. It was then demonstrated that two types of β-subunits (β_A and β_B) exist in ovarian follicular fluid. There is >80% homology between the α-subunit of human, porcine, bovine and rodent inhibin, the β_A-subunits are identical and the β_B-subunits differ by only one to three amino acids. The precursor regions of these peptides are also highly conserved between species. There is also considerable homology between the inhibin β-subunits and transforming growth factor-β (TGF-β). TGF is a homodimer of two 12.5-kDa subunits whose biological actions include inhibition of mitogenesis and stimulation of FSH release from cultured pituitary cells. Inhibin also shares sequence homology with the C-terminal portion of Müllerian inhibiting hormone, a glycoprotein hormone produced by the developing testis to inhibit development of the female genital tract in male embryos. Inhibin is synthesised predominantly in ovarian granulosa cells in the female and Sertoli cells in the male. Inhibin levels increase during the late follicular phase, the hormone acting synergistically with oestradiol to inhibit FSH synthesis and release, though this inhibition is overridden at the time of the preovulatory gonadotrophin surge.

Activins

Both the homo- and heterodimers of the β-subunits of inhibin promote the release of FSH from cultured pituitary cells and have been termed activins. The $\beta_A\beta_A$ and $\beta_B\beta_B$ activins are equipotent and their FSH-releasing activity is antagonised by inhibin. Activins are more potent at releasing FSH than GnRH, but their maximal action is delayed until 24–48 hours of incubation, in contrast to GnRH which produces peak release within 1 hour. The physiological role of activin has still to be elucidated.

In addition to their effects on pituitary function it is becoming apparent that the inhibins and activins have intragonadal autocrine or paracrine actions which modulate steroidogenesis. It is possible that they provide a means of communication between Sertoli and Leydig cells in the testis, and the granulosa and theca cells in the ovary. The inhibin family of peptides is summarised in Fig. 6.6.

A glycopeptide with FSH inhibiting activity (follistatin) has been isolated from follicular fluid but shows no structural similarity to the inhibins or activins. Its inhibitory effects on pituitary secretion of FSH are additive to those of inhibin, and it also inhibits FSH stimulated oestrogen production from cultured granulosa cells. Like the activins, its physiological relevance is unclear at present.

Some of the inter-relationships between the hormones controlling gonadotrophin release in the female and the male are shown in Fig. 6.7 and 6.8.

Adrenocorticotrophic hormone

Corticotrophin-releasing hormone

Characterisation

CRH in hypothalamic extracts was identified and partially characterised in 1955, but biochemical characterisation of CRH took a further 25 years. It was eventually achieved by analysis of fractionated extracts of half a million sheep hypothalami, used previously to identify GnRH, and in 1981 Vale and colleagues reported a 41-amino-acid peptide which had potent ACTH and β-endorphin-releasing effects on

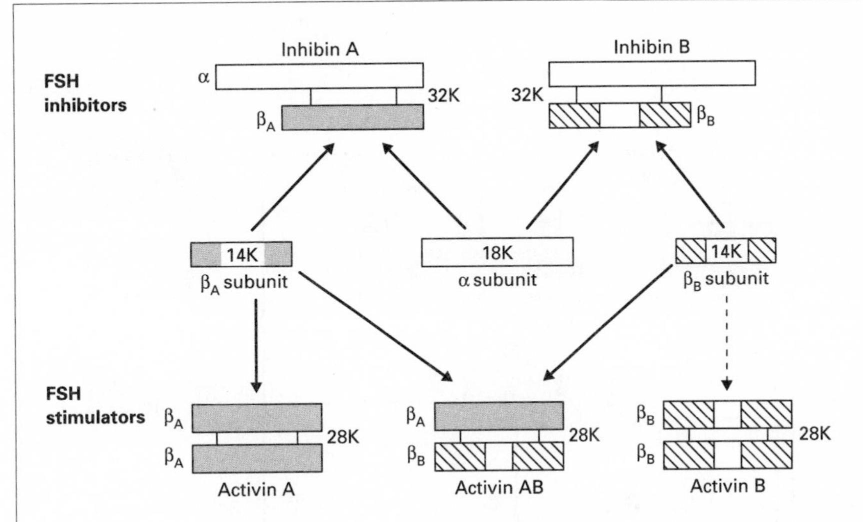

Fig. 6.6 Combinations of the inhibin subunits to form the dimers with follicle-stimulating hormone (FSH) stimulatory and inhibitory activity. Molecular sizes (kDa) are indicated beside and inside the dimers and monomers, respectively.

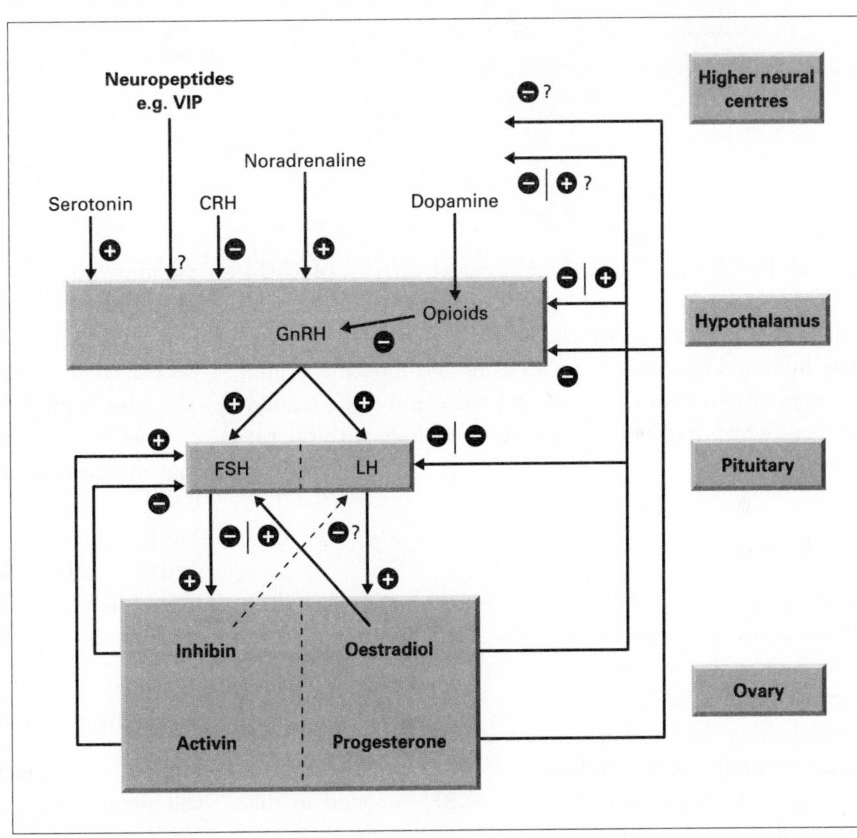

Fig. 6.7 Neuroendocrine control of the gonadotrophins in the female.

cultured anterior pituitary cells. *In vivo* studies using synthetic CRH and antisera against it confirmed that CRH is the dominant ACTH-releasing factor in animals and humans. It is several-fold more potent than the other two major ACTH-releasing factors, AVP and catecholamines. In 1983, Shibahara successfully sequenced the human CRH gene, from which the structure of human CRH (hCRH) could be deduced; hCRH also comprises 41 amino acids, seven of which differ from those in ovine CRH (oCRH). Rat CRH, however, is identical to the human hormone. Mammalian CRHs show homology with two peptides of potent ACTH-releasing activity found in lower animals: sauvagine, a 40-amino-acid peptide in frog skin, and urotensin II, secreted by the caudal gland of the fish. Human pro-CRH is a pep-

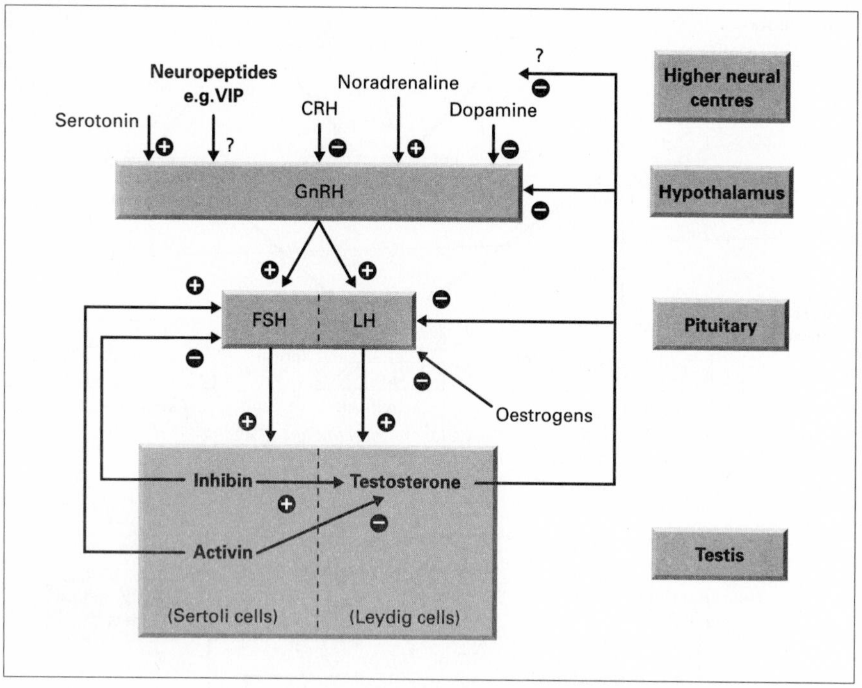

Fig. 6.8 Neuroendocrine control of the gonadotrophins in the male.

tide of 190 amino acids; the biological activity of CRH resides in its carboxy-terminus, with CRH(15–41) retaining full biological activity, though lower CRH-receptor binding. The human CRH gene is located on chromosome 8 and consists of two exons, CRH being encoded on the second of these which has 94% nucleotide homology with the rat gene.

Localisation

Many of the early CRH localisation studies used oCRH antisera which cross-reacted with hCRH. Immunoassay studies show that most CRH is present in the hypothalamus, though substantial amounts occur in cerebral cortex and several other nuclei where CRH is believed to act as a neurotransmitter coordinating the stress responses. Within the hypothalamus, immunoreactive CRH is found in the parvicellular neurons of the paraventricular nucleus and nerve fibres round the vascular plexus in the pituitary stalk. The localisation of CRH to the neurosecretory granules of these neurons has now been demonstrated immunocytochemically. CRH is therefore thought to be synthesised in the paraventricular nucleus, transported in nerve fibres to the median eminence and secreted into the portal system to induce release of ACTH from the anterior pituitary. Adrenalectomy and hypophysectomy increase the hypothalamic content of CRH. The concentration present in portal blood is sufficient to stimulate ACTH release from cultured pituitary cells, and is increased by stress and decreased by destruction of the paraventricular nucleus. The observation that CRH immunoneutralisation did not completely abolish stress-induced ACTH release suggested that additional factors were responsible for ACTH regulation. CRH has also been visualised in the posterior pituitary, but its function there is unknown. CRH immunoreactivity and pro-CRH messenger RNA (mRNA) have been found in several tissues outside the brain including spinal cord, adrenal medulla, liver, pancreas and placenta.

Mechanism of action

High-affinity CRH receptors are present in corticotroph cell membranes, as well as in many areas of the CNS where CRH acts as a neurotransmitter. Such receptors are present also in the preoptic and arcuate nuclei of the hypothalamus, at which sites CRH may influence release of GnRH and other neuropeptides. In all these areas, CRH receptors are linked to the GTP regulatory protein, G_s, in turn linked to adenylate cyclase. In the anterior pituitary, receptor activation leads to a rapid rise in cAMP, with subsequent ACTH secretion within minutes and pro-opiomelanocortin (POMC) synthesis within a few hours. These cAMP effects

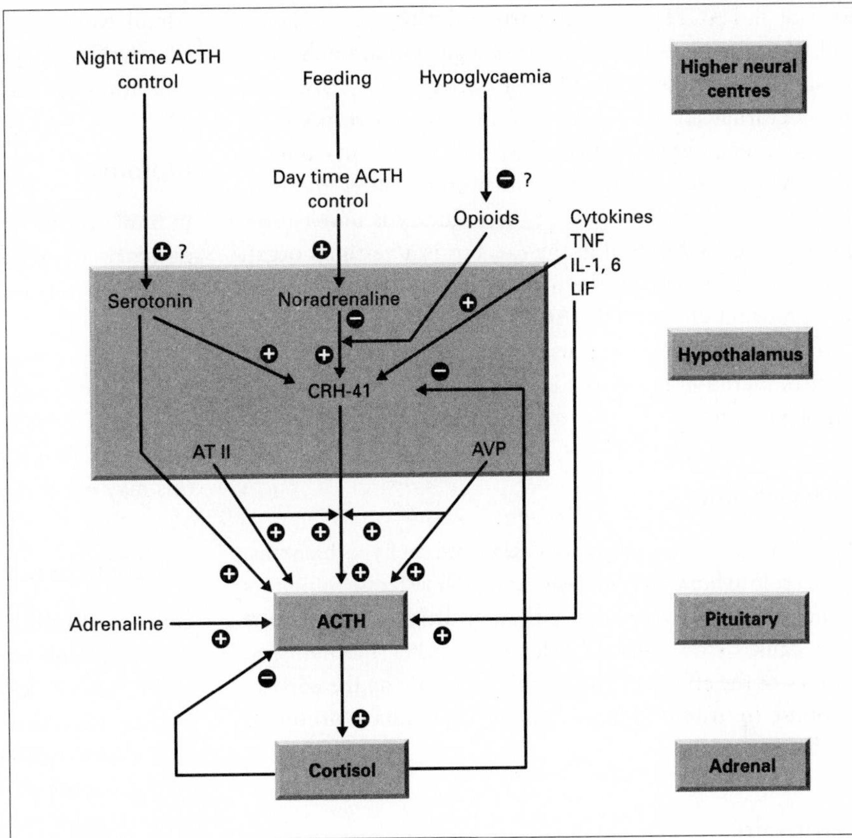

Fig. 6.9 Neuroendocrine control of adrenocorticotrophic hormone (ACTH) secretion.

are dependent on transmembrane Ca^{2+} flux, and one cAMP action may be to promote phosphorylation of Ca^{2+} channel proteins. Potentiators of CRH-induced ACTH release include vasopressin, which acts via the inositol phosphate system, and adrenaline and angiotensin II, which act also by cAMP-independent pathways. Although desensitisation of the pituitary to CRH has been shown *in vitro*, there is little evidence for this *in vivo*. Normal human subjects given CRH in the morning and in the evening show a greater response in the evening, when ACTH and cortisol levels are at their lowest. The major factor in humans which determines pituitary responsiveness to CRH is the prevailing cortisol level, glucocorticoids decreasing both ACTH release and POMC synthesis.

Regulation of CRH secretion and synthesis

The hypothalamo-pituitary–adrenal axis is regulated by a complex system of neuronal inputs to the paraventricular nucleus and median eminence from hypothalamic nuclei and other brain areas. The release of CRH and ACTH is also influenced by negative feedback by cortisol. The interactions between these various components have still to be fully elucidated (Fig. 6.9).

Catecholamines

In humans, intravenous infusions of lipid-soluble α_1-agonists and antagonists which cross the blood–brain barrier stimulate and inhibit ACTH release, respectively. In contrast, an equipotent dose of noradrenaline, which can reach both pituitary and median eminence but does not cross the blood–brain barrier, does not stimulate ACTH release. This suggests the presence of a stimulatory α_1-adrenergic pathway within the CNS. Lesioning experiments in animals suggest that this pathway ascends from the brainstem and abuts directly on the neurons of the paraventricular nucleus, thereby enhancing CRH release. High-dose noradrenaline infusion lowers plasma cortisol but the mechanism of this is obscure; it may be due to inhibition of vasopressin secretion. Adrenaline potentiates the direct effect of CRH on ACTH release by cultured rat anterior pituitary cells, but adrenaline infusion in humans—to elevate plasma adrenaline concentration to the level seen in most physiological and pathological situations—does not enhance CRH effects on ACTH and cortisol. There is no evidence in humans that circulating adrenaline plays a role in stimulating ACTH release. The stimulatory α_1-adrenergic pathway has been demonstrated in humans in two situations: the cortisol and ACTH secretory pattern during waking hours and the cortisol responses to food ingestion are enhanced by α_1-agonists and reduced by α_1-antagonists. However, the nocturnal cortisol surge and the cortisol response to hypoglycaemia are not affected by such treatments and are presumably mediated by other neurotransmitter mechanisms. The intermediate lobe of the pituitary is under tonic dopaminergic inhibition in the rat, but is a vestigial organ in the adult human. In the normal human, dopamine has no significant effect on the ACTH and cortisol response to CRH, and dopamine agonists and antagonists do not affect cortisol secretion basally or in response to insulin-induced hypoglycaemia.

Acetylcholine

Acetylcholine causes release of CRH from rat hypothalamus, but its role in humans is unclear. Anticholinesterase inhibitors stimulate ACTH secretion, although drug adverse effects may cause 'stress-related' release by other mechanisms. Studies of the effects of cholinergic blockade on the cortisol response to insulin-induced hypoglycaemia have produced conflicting results.

Serotonin

Serotonin may have both stimulatory and inhibitory effects on ACTH release. In animals, serotonin and drugs which potentiate its actions cause parallel increases in CRH in hypophysial portal blood and ACTH in peripheral plasma. In humans, serotonin precursors such as 5-hydroxytryptophan, and drugs such as fenfluramine which increase serotonin release, produce similar effects. The paraventricular nucleus receives fibres from the suprachiasmatic nucleus which is the circadian pacemaker responsible for diurnal variation in ACTH secretion. Cyproheptadine, a serotonin antagonist, inhibits the nocturnal rise in plasma cortisol, and thus the stimulatory effect of serotonin on CRH and ACTH release may be mediated by its effect on the suprachiasmatic nucleus. Furthermore, the presence of serotoninergic fibres has been demonstrated at the pituitary level, where serotonin stimulates ACTH release and may potentiate the action of vasopressin and CRH. The paraventricular nucleus also receives inputs from the limbic system but the neurochemistry has not been conclusively defined. It is possible, however, that at this site serotonin exerts inhibitory control on the subsequent release of ACTH.

γ-Aminobutyric acid

GABA inhibits CRH release induced by serotonin and acetylcholine *in vitro*. In contrast, GABA antagonists are powerful stimulators of ACTH release *in vivo*. There is some evidence that the GABA system is involved in glucocorticoid feedback inhibition of CRH activity.

Opioids

In humans, the opioids are inhibitory to the hypothalamo-pituitary–adrenal axis and naloxone administration produces a rise in plasma ACTH. Disinhibition of endogenous opioid tone may be responsible for the ACTH response to hypoglycaemic stress, and acts possibly on stimulatory α_1-adrenergic pathways. The opioids exert further inhibition of ACTH release at the pituitary level: Met-enkephalin analogues reduce the ACTH response to CRH, although this may occur via suppression of hypothalamic AVP.

Glucocorticoid feedback

Glucocorticoids exert negative-feedback inhibition on the hypothalamus to reduce CRH synthesis and secretion. CRH mRNA levels in the paraventricular nucleus and median eminence rise following adrenalectomy and fall after glucocorticoid replacement. The molecular mechanism of glucocorticoid-mediated down-regulation of the CRH gene is unknown; it is possible that the glucocorticoid-activated protein receptor may interfere with protein binding to the cAMP response element of the gene. Inhibitory glucocorticoid effects can, of course, be overridden by other neural pathways during stress, when cortisol levels are elevated.

Other factors affecting ACTH release

It has been seen already that not all ACTH-releasing activity is mediated by CRH itself. AVP augments the effects of CRH, whilst insulin-induced hypoglycaemia results in greater ACTH and cortisol release than CRH and AVP given together. Furthermore, the administration of a maximally stimulating dose of CRH fails to increase the ACTH and cortisol response to insulin-induced hypoglycaemia any further, suggesting maximal stimulation of endogenous CRH and the presence of additional releasing factors. Some such factors are likely to be the neurotransmitters described above but AVP, oxytocin and angiotensin II (ATII) deserve further mention.

Vasopressin

AVP was the first proposed as a CRF in 1955. However, AVP alone has modest effects on ACTH release and the Brattleboro rat—which lacks AVP—does not show any gross deficiency in pituitary–adrenal function. Two decades later, the idea that AVP is an important modulator of CRH action was reintroduced. Two main systems of AVP-containing neurons are present in the hypothalamus: one runs from the paraventricular nucleus and supraoptic nuclei to the posterior pituitary, while the other originates in the paraventricular nucleus and terminates in the median eminence. AVP and its mRNA in the latter system are increased after adrenalectomy, an effect prevented by glucocorticoids. AVP and CRH have been shown to coexist in median eminence nerve terminals, which suggests that they may be cosecreted under some circumstances. High levels of AVP are present in portal blood and synthetic AVP potentiates CRF activity in the Brattleboro rat. High-affinity AVP receptors are present in anterior pituitary membranes where they are pharmacologically different from V2 (antidiuretic) and V1 (vasopressor) AVP receptors: post-receptor mechanisms involve inositol phosphate hydrolysis. Recently, a distinct corticotroph vasopressin receptor, V_{1b} or V_3, has been cloned and sequenced, and shown to be a distinct entity.

Angiotensin II

ATII is present in the median eminence and has been shown to release ACTH *in vitro* and *in vivo* in the rat. In humans, however, its effect on ACTH secretion is controversial and most studies have shown no effect of exogenous ATII. It is possible that the role of ATII in humans is confined to the brain, rather than the peripheral renin–angiotensin system.

Oxytocin

Oxytocin is colocalized with CRH in the neuron of the paraventricular nucleus and supraoptic nuclei of normal and Brattleboro rats, and is found in large amounts in portal blood. Its relevance in humans is unclear, but the secretion of ACTH in response to hypoglycaemia has been reported in one study to be attenuated in the presence of oxytocin.

Cytokines and inflammatory mediators

Tumour-necrosis factor (TNF) is a peptide produced by macrophages that acts as an inflammatory mediator and can cause many of the clinical phenomena that accompany severe systemic illness. Interleukin 1 (IL-1α and β) is a cytokine produced by many cells, including monocytes and pituitary cells, that stimulates B- and T-lymphocytes to produce a range of other cytokines and lymphokines. TNF, IL-1 and IL-6 show synergistic interactions in the activation of the hypothalamo-pituitary–adrenal axis, probably via release of, and interaction with, CRH and probably AVP. Interferon-α, another inflammatory mediator, releases IL-6 (but not IL-1) which subsequently contributes to stimulation of ACTH and cortisol release. Expression of leukaemia inhibitory factor (LIF) and its receptor can be induced in the mouse pituitary and hypothalamus by the endotoxin, lipopolysaccharide. LIF activates POMC gene expression and acts synergistically with CRH in this respect. Synergistic interaction of some or all these pathways in acute and chronic illness contributes to the overall response to stress.

The CRF complex

Many of the above releasers of ACTH can act on the pituitary individually or in concert. Crude hypothalamic extracts are more potent than any ACTH secretagogue given alone. There is evidence from portal blood sampling studies in animals that factors are released differentially according to the type of stress applied. For example, AVP is preferentially released in severe forms of physical stress, whereas relatively more CRH is released in response to acute haemorrhage. Therefore, although CRH is a major hypothalamic releaser of ACTH, variations in the release of other hypothalamic hormones, cytokines and lymphokines in different forms of stress serve to modulate overall activity of the hypothalamo-pituitary–adrenal axis.

Thyrotrophin

The hypothalamus stimulates thyroid function via TSH since hypothyroidism occurs if the hypothalamus is lesioned or diseased or if the pituitary stalk is transected. This stimulatory hypothalamic control is exerted by the tripeptide TRH. Circulating thyroid hormones exert powerful negative-feedback inhibitory actions on the thyrotrophs and also on TRH-producing hypothalamic neurons. In addition, several secondary modulators exert lesser degrees of control over TSH secretion, the net result of which is the maintenance of a steady output of TSH and therefore of thyroid hormones. The most important secondary modulators are SS and dopamine, both of which inhibit the function of the thyrotrophs, and α-adrenergic pathways, which are, in general, stimulatory. Other modulators of thyroid function include glucocorticoid hormones, various cytokines, and other inflammatory mediators.

Negative-feedback action of thyroid hormones

Serum TSH is rapidly suppressed to 10% of pretreatment concentrations within a few hours of parenteral T_3 administration. About half of pituitary nuclear T_3 is derived from the intracellular 5′-monodeiodination of thyroxine (T_4), which is a greater fraction than in other tissues; this monodeiodination may be the mechanism by which the thyrotrophs respond to changes in serum T_4 concentrations.

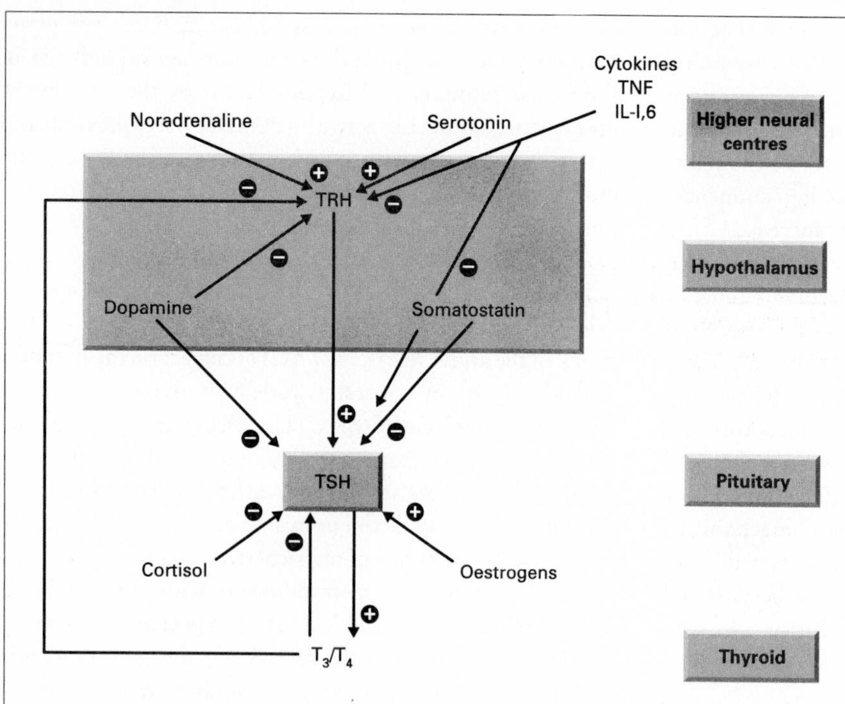

Fig. 6.10 Neuroendocrine control of thyroid-stimulating hormone (TSH) secretion.

The major actions of thyroid hormones are to regulate gene expression after binding to specific nuclear receptors. Thyroid hormone receptors are structurally related to the viral oncogene v-*erb* A and, together with steroid, vitamin D and retinoic acid receptors, form a family of receptor proteins with important structural similarities. Several complementary DNAs (cDNAs) that encode different thyroid hormone receptors (α and β) have been described. Binding of T_3 to a site on the carboxy-terminal end of the receptor activates the receptor so that the T_3-receptor complex binds to specific nucleotide sequences on target genes. In thyrotrophs, the activated T_3 receptor inhibits transcription of the α-subunit and TSH-β-subunit genes in proportion to nuclear T_3-receptor occupancy.

In addition to this action, thyroid hormones also modulate the expression of the TRH-receptor gene. The number of TRH receptors on thyrotrophs increases in hypothyroidism and can be reduced by thyroid hormone replacement. Conversely, in rat pituitary tumour cells, TRH itself reduces T_3-receptor gene expression, receptor number and T_3 responsiveness which may represent a further site of feedback interaction between T_3 and TRH at the level of the pituitary. Thyroid hormones exert negative-feedback actions on the hypothalamus. TRH mRNA increases in the paraventricular nuclei in hypothyroidism and is reduced by thyroid hormone treatment. Furthermore, rats with bilateral lesions of the paraventricular nuclei do not show a normal rise of serum TSH and TSH-subunit mRNA after induction of primary hypothyroidism, an effect that presumably reflects depletion of TRH. These results indicate that the paraventricular nuclei are a target for the action of thyroid hormones in the control of TRH gene expression and release, providing an additional mechanism for thyroidal regulation of TSH secretion (Fig. 6.10).

Structure and actions of TRH

TRH was the first hypothalamic hormone to be characterised and chemically identified as a weakly basic tripeptide, pyroglutamyl-histidyl-proline-amide, in 1969. Like other more complex peptides, it is derived from post-translational cleavage of a larger precursor molecule. The cDNA sequence of the TRH precursor (gene on human chromosome 3) encodes a protein with a molecular size of 29 000 Da that contains five copies of the sequence Glu-His-Pro-Gly. Rat pro-TRH is processed at paired basic residues to a family of peptides that include TRH and flanking and intervening sequences. These peptides may exert important intracellular or extracellular actions, in particular prepro-TRH(160–169), which stimulates TSH gene expression. There may be preferential processing of pro-TRH to produce different peptides in different brain regions.

TRH- and pro-TRH-positive cell bodies are present in the parvicellular division of the paraventricular nuclei of the hypothalamus and are the major site of origin of immunoreactive TRH in the median eminence, as opposed to other brain regions such as the tractus solitarius. The

TRH gene is also expressed in the anterior pituitary, and TRH-positive axons are present in posterior pituitary tissue. However, lesions of the paraventricular nuclei reduce the content of TRH in both anterior and posterior pituitary tissue, indicating that the hypothalamus is the source of most of the immunoreactive TRH in these areas.

The dominant stimulatory role of the hypothalamus in the control of the thyrotroph is mediated by TRH. The pituitary TRH receptor (gene on human chromosome 8) belongs to the family of seven-transmembrane-domain, G-protein-coupled receptors. TRH is present in hypophysial portal blood at physiologically relevant concentrations and administration of antibodies to TRH to animals can cause hypothyroidism. Intravenous administration of TRH to humans causes a dose-related release of TSH. In addition to stimulating TSH release, TRH also stimulates TSH synthesis by promoting transcription and translation of the TSH subunit genes, actions that involve Ca^{2+} influx, activation of phosphatidyl-inositol pathways and protein kinase C. These actions are modulated by cAMP and the pituitary-specific transcription factor, Pit-1.

TRH plays an important role in the post-translational processing of the oligosaccharide moieties of TSH and hence exerts an important influence on the biological activity of TSH. Full glycosylation of TSH is required for complete biological activity. This provides an explanation for the clinical observation that some patients with central hypothyroidism and slightly elevated basal serum TSH concentrations secrete TSH with reduced biological activity that increases after TRH administration. It is likely that alterations in both hypothalamic TRH secretion and in the response of thyrotrophs to TRH contribute to the variable biological activity of the TSH secreted by patients with different thyroid disorders and those with TSH-secreting pituitary adenomas.

Control of TSH by somatostatin

SS-14 and SS-28 are equipotent in the inhibition of basal and TRH-stimulated TSH release from rat anterior pituitary cells; the physiological relevance of this was established in studies using antisera against SS. Incubation of anterior pituitary cells with anti-SS serum causes increased secretion of TSH (as well as GH), and administration of antiserum to rats increases basal serum TSH levels and responses to both cold stress and TRH. In humans, SS administration reduces the elevated serum TSH in patients with primary hypothyroidism, reduces the serum TSH response to TRH, abolishes the nocturnal elevation in TSH secretion and prevents TSH release after administration of dopamine antagonist drugs. GH administration in humans decreases basal and TRH-stimulated TSH secretion, probably because of direct stimulatory effects of GH on hypothalamic SS release. In patients with pituitary disease, TSH secretory status correlates inversely with GH secretory status. Despite these potent acute inhibitory effects of SS on TSH secretion in humans, long-term treatment with SS or the long-acting analogue, octreotide, does not cause hypothyroidism, presumably because the great sensitivity of the thyrotrophs to any decrease in serum thyroid hormone concentrations overrides the inhibitory effect of SS in the long term.

Control of TSH by neurotransmitters

There is reasonable evidence that α-adrenergic and serotoninergic pathways have a stimulatory effect on TSH release, whereas dopaminergic pathways are inhibitory. For example, the TSH response to cold stress in rats can be abolished by either α-adrenergic blocking agents or anti-TRH antibodies, suggesting that α-adrenergic pathways stimulate TRH release in this model. However, *in vitro* studies of hypothalamic TRH release have produced a large amount of conflicting data and the precise intrahypothalamic actions of dopamine, noradrenaline, serotonin and histamine are unclear in relation to TRH and TSH release. SS has been shown to inhibit TRH release *in vitro*, but it is unclear whether this is physiologically important.

Although part of the action of catecholamines is undoubtedly mediated via hypothalamic mechanisms, there is now good evidence that dopamine and noradrenaline exert direct effects on TSH release at the pituitary level. Specific high-affinity dopamine (D_2) and α_1-adrenoreceptors are present on thyrotroph cell membranes, and dopamine and noradrenaline concentrations in portal blood are sufficient to cause inhibition and stimulation respectively of TSH release by cultured pituitary cells. Similarly, *in vivo* administration of D_2-receptor antagonists or α_1-adrenoreceptor agonist drugs cause a small, acute release of TSH, whereas D_2 agonists or α_1-adrenoreceptor antagonists can acutely inhibit basal TSH secretion. However, long-term treatment with such drugs does not affect thyroid function presumably because of the dominant sensitivity of the thyrotroph to the feedback actions of thyroid hormones. There is also evidence for the existence of an ultrashort-loop feedback control pathway of TSH on the thyrotroph itself by means of which TSH increases the number of dopamine receptors, enhancing the functional inhibition of TSH release by dopamine.

Actions of cytokines and inflammatory mediators

Both TNF and IL-1β, which activate the hypothalamo-pituitary–adrenal axis in inflammatory states, inhibit TSH secretion in rats and mice, and IL-1β causes a relative and inappropriate reduction in TRH gene expression in the paraventricular nucleus in the face of low thyroid hormone concentrations. These molecules each produce a biochemical pattern similar to that which occurs in patients with acute non-thyroidal illness (see Chapter 31). This family of molecules plays a crucial role in mediating and coordinating the thyroidal and adrenal responses to non-thyroidal illness. IL-1β is produced by rat anterior pituitary cells as well as many other cell types including monocytes, and its release from them can be stimulated by bacterial lipopolysaccharide (endotoxin). It colocalises with TSH in thyrotroph cells. Presumably, IL-1β subserves an important autocrine or paracrine role in anterior pituitary control, as has been suggested for the IL-1-dependent cytokine IL-6, which is also produced by rat anterior pituitary cells, particularly folliculostellate cells.

Oestrogens

Females show a greater TSH response to TRH than males and also show a greater response during the follicular phase than during the luteal phase of the menstrual cycle. This is probably oestrogen related since oestrogen administration to males leads to an enhancement of the TSH response to TRH, without alteration in basal TSH levels. Oestrogens have been shown to increase TRH receptor number on anterior pituitary cells. In the human, oestrogen administration increases the inhibitory effect of exogenous dopamine on TSH (and PRL) secretion, probably via an increase in pituitary dopamine receptor number.

Physiological and secondary TSH changes

TSH is secreted in a pulsatile manner with increases in pulse amplitude and frequency at night. The secretory pulses of TSH–α-subunit and the gonadotrophins are concordant, consistent with the operation of a common hypothalamic pulse generator. A clear circadian variation is evident in serum TSH levels which begin to rise several hours before the onset of sleep, reaching maximal concentrations between 2300 hours and 0400 hours and declining gradually thereafter, with the lowest concentrations occurring at about 1100 hours. The concentrations during the nocturnal surge are sometimes slightly above the normal range reported by most clinical laboratories. Sleep itself modulates TSH secretion, by reducing pulse amplitude rather than frequency, but the underlying mechanisms are not clear. Although there is some evidence that oestrogens can enhance and androgens reduce serum TSH responses to TRH, no sex-related difference in amplitude or frequency of circadian TSH changes has been found. Patients with severe primary hypothyroidism have increased pulse amplitude throughout the day but loss of the usual nocturnal increase in pulse amplitude. Also, circadian changes in serum TSH concentrations can be detected in some patients with mild thyrotoxicosis, suggesting that central mechanisms can override to some extent the powerful negative-feedback effects of thyroid hormones at the pituitary level.

The mechanisms underlying circadian and pulsatile changes in TSH secretion are not fully understood. They are not secondary to changes in catecholaminergic activity or peripheral factors, such as changes in serum T_4 and T_3 concentrations, haemoconcentration or changes in cortisol secretion, although the latter may modulate TSH rhythms. Basal serum TSH concentrations rise slightly after serum cortisol concentrations are lowered by 11β-hydroxylase inhibition with metyrapone, suggesting that cortisol exerts a small inhibitory influence on TSH secretion. Furthermore, pharmacological doses of glucocorticoids acutely inhibit basal TSH secretion and abolish the circadian variation in serum TSH concentrations. This mechanism may well explain the reduction in basal and TRH-stimulated serum TSH concentrations and in circadian TSH changes that occurs in patients with depression, after major surgery, in non-thyroidal illness and in hypercortisolism. Total abolition of the circadian rhythm of cortisol with metyrapone, however, did not cause disruption of overall circadian TSH changes, although a small but significant decrease did occur in the acrophase and amplitude of the TSH profile.

Cold exposure in rats causes an acute rise in serum TSH concentrations that is accompanied by an increase in hypothalamic TRH gene expression and increased TRH release. A similar phenomenon occurs in human neonates, but is unusual in adults; when it does occur the increase is very small. The cold-induced effect in rats can be abolished by either passive immunisation with anti-TRH antibodies or α-adrenergic blockade, indicating that adrenergic release of hypothalamic TRH mediates the phenomenon. Lesions that affect the temperature-regulating centre of the preoptic nucleus of the hypothalamus abolish the serum TSH response to cold stress but do not cause hypothyroidism.

Ageing itself causes a slight decrease in TSH secretion. Thyroid secretion, however, changes little, due to a resetting of the threshold of TSH inhibition by thyroid hormones as a result of increased pituitary conversion of T_4 to T_3, increased T_4 uptake by thyrotrophs, or decreased T_4 and T_3 clearance.

Caloric restriction also causes a small decrease in basal and TRH-stimulated serum TSH concentrations despite a decline in serum T_3 concentrations. In rats this is associated with reduced hypothalamic TRH gene expression. The components of the decrease in TSH secretion in humans are a reduction in the daytime serum TSH concentration and in the nocturnal increase in TSH secretion, with an overall decrease in TSH pulse amplitude. Passive immunisation with SS antiserum abolishes the starvation-induced decline in TSH secretion in rats, indicating a mediating role of hypothalamic somatostatinergic pathways secondary to unknown metabolic signals. There is no evidence of increased dopaminergic inhibition of TSH secretion during caloric restriction, and TRH administration does not reverse the acute decline in serum TSH concentrations during fasting.

In rats stress causes an acute decline in serum TSH concentrations. In humans, surgical stress causes transient acute lowering of serum TSH, despite a fall in serum free-T_3 concentrations, whereas serum free-T_4 concentrations do not change. In animals, both opioids and dopamine may play a role in this stress phenomenon, whereas in humans glucocorticoids and dopamine have been implicated. As with the effects of caloric restriction, these stress phenomena bear some resemblance to the altered neuroregulation of TSH that can occur in non-thyroidal illness and in certain neuropsychiatric disorders. Although basal serum TSH concentrations are usually normal in patients with both acute and chronic non-thyroidal illness, they may be either low or slightly raised. In addition to the frequent use of pharmacological agents such as glucocorticoids and dopamine that acutely inhibit TSH secretion, intrinsic central suppression of thyrotroph function is common, as illustrated by the abolition of the nocturnal increase in serum TSH concentrations in up to 60% of acutely ill patients in the presence of low serum free-T_3 concentrations. However, true central hypothyroidism is rare in these patients, who usually (although not always) have normal serum free-T_4 concentrations.

Abnormalities in TSH secretion also occur in patients with anorexia nervosa and endogenous depression. A common abnormality is a reduced serum TSH response to TRH. Even more common is loss of the nocturnal increase in TSH secretion which, together with the low serum free thyroid hormone, ferritin, and sex hormone-binding globulin concentrations may indicate central hypothyroidism. Once again, the mechanisms are unclear. Dopamine is not involved in central TSH suppression in anorexia nervosa but increased serum cortisol concentrations may contribute; both serum cortisol and body temperature changes have been implicated in depression.

It seems clear that, in addition to peripheral alterations in thyroid hormone economy usually manifest as low serum free T_3, high reverse T_3, and normal free-T_4 concentrations, there is central suppression of thyrotroph function in patients with severe non-thyroidal illness, for example with heart failure, infection, diabetes mellitus or chronic renal failure. The precise initiating signals and underlying mechanisms are unknown, although alterations in opioidergic, dopaminergic, and somatostatinergic activity may each contribute. Also, peripheral, glucocorticoid-mediated inhibitory feedback probably plays an important role, particularly in acutely ill patients. Finally, activation of the cytokine pathways involving TNF-α and IL-1β, each of which inhibit TSH and stimulate ACTH release in animals, may be a crucial mediating event in the coordination of the thyroidal and adrenal responses to stress and non-thyroidal illness.

Vasopressin

Characterisation, synthesis and localization

AVP is the antidiuretic hormone of most mammals, and its most important physiological action is the regulation of renal water excretion. AVP is a strongly basic nonapeptide containing disulphide linkage between the two cysteines at positions 1 and 6. It is structurally related to oxytocin; each comprises nine amino acids, seven of which are identical. AVP was identified and chemically synthesised in the mid-1950s and a variety of synthetic analogues with agonist or antagonist properties are now available. It was soon apparent that AVP is associated with larger polypeptides, called neurophysins, and these were thought originally to act as carrier proteins for the hormone. However, it is now known that the 145-amino-acid AVP precursor in the rat contains a signal peptide, AVP, a specific neurophysin and a small glycoprotein. The mid-portion of the AVP-specific neurophysin is markedly conserved between species. The genetic cause of diabetes insipidus in the Brattleboro rat has been defined as a deletion of a single guanine within the neurophysin coding region, although there is also evidence that the AVP gene may be abnormally regulated.

The AVP prohormone is synthesised within the cell bodies of the magnocellular neurons of the supraoptic and paraventricular nuclei, and then transported along the axons, many of which project to the posterior pituitary. Cleavage of the AVP precursor occurs during axonal transit, though both cleaved and uncleaved products are present within neurosecretory granules in the posterior pituitary. Exocytosis of these granules is Ca^{2+} dependent. AVP and its specific neurophysin are released in approximately equimolar amounts, but no biological role for circulating neurophysin is known. AVP has a short plasma half life of up to 15 minutes. The main vasopressinergic pathway projects from the supraoptic nucleus to the posterior lobe of the pituitary, which represents a direct extension of the forebrain. A separate smaller pathway runs from the paraventricular nucleus to the median eminence, as discussed in the above section on ACTH control. Vasopressinergic neurons are regulated by both osmoreceptors in the anterior hypothalamus and baroreceptor inputs relayed from the brainstem.

Control of AVP secretion

Central chemical mediators

Several monoamines and peptides have been proposed as central modulators of AVP release. Both noradrenaline and dopamine have been shown to promote AVP release but some of the evidence is conflicting. There is reasonable evidence that acetylcholine may also release AVP, though some of it is circumstantial. For example, large amounts of acetylcholine are found in both supraoptic and paraventricular nuclei and acetyl cholinesterase is present in the neurohypophysial tract. However, nicotinic cholinergic receptors seem to mediate the *in vitro* release of AVP from the hypothalamus and neurohypophysis in response to osmotic stimulation.

ATII also influences AVP secretion and may be important in the regulation of osmoreceptor function. Opioid peptides, particularly Leu-enkephalin, have been shown to inhibit AVP release following both osmotic and electrical stimulation.

Osmoregulation

Osmoregulation is the most important determinant of AVP secretion. In a series of classic experiments on dogs in the 1940s, Verney was the first to suggest that antidiuretic hormone secretion was regulated by the osmolality of body fluids. The advent of specific AVP radioimmunoassays confirmed the validity of this hypothesis; in healthy adults infused with hypertonic saline (855 mmol/l) there is a direct correlation between plasma osmolality and plasma AVP concentration. The plasma osmolality at which plasma AVP begins to increase in a normal human is 280 mmol/kg. Pregnancy causes slight lowering of this threshold for AVP secretion. A significant fall in plasma osmolality occurs during the luteal phase of the normal human menstrual cycle due to lowering of thirst and AVP release thresholds. Glucose fails to stimulate AVP release, urea is less potent than sodium chloride and alcohol inhibits AVP release. Thus, the response of the osmoreceptor to osmolality changes is in part determined by the type of solute. As plasma osmolality rises from 280 mmol/kg, AVP release progressively increases, as does urinary concentration. At a plasma osmolality of about 295 mmol/kg maximal antidiuresis is obtained at an AVP concentration of approximately 5 pmol/l. Further increases in osmolality, although releasing more AVP, do not lead to further conservation of renal water. Osmotic disequilibrium is presented in normal individuals by the stimulation of thirst osmoreceptors which induce drinking; the normal thirst threshold is about 295–298 mmol/kg. Subsequent fluid intake results in a lowering of plasma osmolality to the range in which changes in AVP secretion can again regulate renal water loss. The AVP and thirst osmoreceptors occur in the anterior and lateral hypothalamic regions, respectively, but their precise location and mechanism of action are still unknown.

Baroregulation

Reductions in blood volume and blood pressure both increase AVP release, but are less important factors under normal circumstances than changes in plasma osmolality. Changes in blood volume are mediated by low-pressure baroreceptors in the left atrium and great veins, whereas changes in blood pressure are mediated by high-pressure baroreceptors in the arch of the aorta and carotid arteries.

The vagus and glossopharyngeal nerves transmit baroreceptor information to the brainstem and it is then relayed to vasopressinergic neurons in the hypothalamus. There is some interrelation between osmoregulation and baroregulation of AVP secretion; as hypovolemia increases the osmotic threshold for AVP release is lowered and there is an increase in the sensitivity of the osmoreceptor/AVP releasing mechanism. This has the effect of preserving osmoregulation at lower plasma volumes. If hypovolemia is very severe, baroregulation overrides osmoregulation and plasma AVP concentrations rise to very high levels.

Other control mechanisms

Several other factors have been postulated to control AVP secretion, though many are now known to act through baroreceptor mechanisms. Nausea and emesis are potent stimuli of AVP release which seem to act independently of osmo- and baroregulatory mechanisms; dopamine is probably the central mediator. Hypoglycaemia also promotes AVP release but the mechanism is unknown; catecholamine release following hypoglycaemia does not completely account for the rise in AVP.

Oxytocin

Characterisation, synthesis and localization

The ability of posterior pituitary extracts to promote uterine muscle contraction and increase breast-milk flow in lactating animals has been known since the early part of this century. Oxytocin is the hormone responsible for these actions and, like AVP, is a nonapeptide. There are many close similarities between oxytocin and AVP with regard to gene structure, peptide precursors, hormonal structure, neuronal metabolism and transport, and exocytotic release of neurosecretory granules. Briefly, oxytocin is synthesised in the magnocellular neurons of the supraoptic and paraventricular hypothalamic nuclei but in separate cells from those synthesizing AVP. The oxytocin precursor comprises a signal peptide, oxytocin, oxytocin-specific neurophysin and a small non-glycosylated peptide. Cleavage of the prohormone occurs within the neurosecretory granules as they travel down axons projecting to the posterior pituitary. Exocytosis of neurosecretory granules is a Ca^{2+}-dependent process induced by a critical frequency of action potentials arriving at the nerve terminals. Oxytocinergic neurons are also present in the extrahypothalamic CNS where the hormone probably acts as a neurotransmitter or neuromodulator. Oxytocin occurs in both ovary and testis but its gonadal roles have yet to be determined.

Oxytocin and lactation

Milk-ejection reflex

The milk-ejection reflex is a classic neuroendocrine reflex arc. Stimulation of the nipple by the suckling infant leads to increased release of oxytocin which causes contraction of the myoepithelial cells surrounding the mammary alveoli and thus increases milk flow. The afferent limb of the reflex comprises somatic sensory neurons which probably travel in the spinothalamic tracts and eventually impinge on oxytocinergic neurons in the hypothalamus. Using microwire recording electrodes implanted into hypothalamic neurons of unanaesthetised rats, it has been shown that a burst of electrical activity occurs some 10–12 seconds before the rise in intramammary pressure. Suckling behaviour and oxytocin release varies considerably between species.

Neurotransmitters and oxytocin release

A number of neurotransmitters have been implicated in the release of oxytocin but the chemical involved at the final synapse with the oxytocinergic neuron remains unknown. α-Adrenergic agonists seem to be stimulatory and β-adrenergic agonists inhibitory with respect to oxytocin release. The site of action is somewhat difficult to define, however. For example, the intraventricular administration of isoproterenol, a β-adrenergic agonist, abolishes milk ejection but has no effect on electrical discharges within hypothalamic oxytocinergic neurons or mammary sensitivity to oxytocin. The administration of morphine by the same route has very similar effects. These results suggest that both β-adrenoceptor agonists and the opioids may have direct inhibitory effects on the nerve terminals releasing oxytocin. There is much immunocytochemical evidence for the presence of opioid peptides in the posterior pituitary, and there is increasing evidence that oxytocin and a Met-enkephalin-like peptide may coexist in the same neurosecretory granules. However, other investigators consider that the non-neuronal pituicyte cells in the posterior pituitary may be involved in opioid regulation of oxytocin release.

Oxytocin and parturition

There is still controversy about whether the uterine stimulant effect of oxytocin has physiological relevance to the initiation or maintenance of parturition, particularly in the human. Studies have been frustrated by several factors: pulsatile release of oxytocin, its short half-life and the presence in human blood of a pregnancy-related oxytocinase which causes rapid degradation of the hormone. Furthermore, distension of the uterine cervix causes oxytocin release which has made it impossible to define whether oxytocin is responsible for the *initiation* of parturition. Some workers have suggested that release of oxytocin by the fetus may be the initiator of parturition in the human. Most studies have shown an increase in plasma oxytocin during labour, and there is certainly a very large increase in the number of human myometrial oxytocin receptors during pregnancy. Furthermore, the uterine decidua contains large numbers of oxytocin receptors and their activation causes the release of the prostaglandin, $PGF_{2\alpha}$, which itself will bring about uterine contractions. Recent work suggests that changes in placental CRH and its receptors are also involved in this process.

Other effects of oxytocin

The factors controlling oxytocin secretion in the male and non-pregnant, non-lactating female remain unclear. Oxytocin is released following major haemorrhage but in much smaller amounts than AVP. Although oxytocin does not have a definite role in the male, there is some animal evidence that it enhances motility of the seminiferous tubules and seminal vesicles, and may underlie certain physiological changes during orgasm.

Further reading

General

Lechan RM. Neuroendocrinology of pituitary hormone regulation. *Endocrinol Metab Clin N Am* 1987; **16**: 475–501.

MacLean DB, Jackson IMD. Molecular biology and regulation of hypothalamic hormones. *Clin Endocrinol Metab* 1988; **2**: 835–68.

Prolactin

Ben-Jonathan N. Dopamine: a prolactin-inhibiting hormone. *Endocr Rev* 1985; **6**: 564–89.

de Greef WJ, van der Schoot P. Some recent developments in the study of prolactin in mammals. *Frontiers Horm Res* 1985; **14**: 70–99.

Dieguez C, Foord S, Peters J, Hall R, Scanlon MF. The neuroregulation of TSH and prolactin secretion. In: Medeiros-Neto G, Gaitan E, eds. *Frontiers in Thyroidology*, Vol. 1. New York: Plenum Medical Book Co., 1986: 49–55.

Leong DA, Frawley LS, Neill JD. Neuroendocrine control of prolactin secretion. *Ann Rev Physiol* 1993; **45**: 109–27.

Molitch M. Prolactin. In: Melmed S, ed. *The Pituitary*. Boston: Blackwell Science, 1995: 136–46.

Reichlin S. Neuroregulation of prolactin secretion. In: Landolt AM, Heitz PU, Zapf J, Girard J, del Pozo E, eds. *Advances in the Biosciences*, Vol. 69. Oxford: Pergamon Press, 1988: 277–92.

Growth hormone

Dieguez C, Page MD, Scanlon MF. Growth hormone neuroregulation and its alterations in disease states. *Clin Endocrinol* 1988; **28**: 109–43.

Guillemin R, Brazeau P, Bohlen P, Esch F, Ling N, Wehrenberg WB. Growth hormone releasing factor from a human pancreatic tumour that caused acromegaly. *Science* 1982; **218**: 585–7.

Lamberts SWJ. The role of somatostatin in the regulation of anterior pituitary hormone secretion and the use of its analogs in the treatment of human pituitary tumors. *Endocr Rev* 1988; **9**: 417–36.

Reisine T, Bell GI. Molecular biology of somatostatin receptors. *Endocr Rev* 1995; **16**: 427–40.

Rivier J, Spiess J, Thorner M, Vale W. Characterization of a growth hormone releasing factor from a human pancreatic islet tumour. *Nature* 1982; **300**: 276–8.

Adrenocorticotrophic hormone

Antoni FA. Hypothalamic control of adrenocorticotropin secretion: advances since the discovery of 41-residue corticotropin releasing factor. *Endocr Rev* 1986; **7**: 351–78.

Jones MT, Gillham B. Factors involved in the regulation of adrenocorticotropic hormone/β lipotropic hormone. *Physiol Rev* 1988; **68**: 743–818.

Linton EA, Lowry PJ. Corticotrophin releasing factor in man and its measurement: a review. *Clin Endocrinol* 1989; **31**: 225–49.

Ray DW, Ren SG, Melmed S. Leukaemia inhibitory factor (LIF) stimulates proopiomelanocortin (POMC) expression in a corticotroph cell line. Role of STAT pathway. *J Clin Invest* 1996; **97**: 1852–9.

Tsagarakis S, Grossman A. Corticotrophin releasing hormone: interaction with the immune system. *Neuroimmunomodulation* 1994; **1**: 329–34.

Vale W, Spiess J, Rivier C, Rivier J. Characterisation of a 41-residue ovine hypothalamic peptide that stimulates secretion of corticotropin and β-endorphin. *Science* 1981; **213**: 1394–7.

Gonadotrophins

Burger HG, ed. *Clinical Endocrinology and Metabolism*, Vol. 1, *Reproductive Endocrinology*. London: Balliere Tindall, 1987 (several relevant chapters).

Hazum E, Conn PM. Molecular mechanisms of gonadotropine releasing hormone (GnRH) action. I. The GnRH receptor. *Endocr Rev* 1988; **9**: 379–86.

McLachlan RI, Robertson DM, de Kretser DM, Burger HG. Advances in the physiology of inhibin and inhibin-related peptides. *Clin Endocrinol* 1988; **29**: 77–112.

Thyroid-stimulating hormone

Jackson IMD. Thyrotropin releasing hormone. *N Engl J Med* 1982; **306**: 145–55.

Peters JR, Foord SM, Dieguez C, Scanlon MF. TSH neuro-regulation and alteration in disease states. *Clin Endocrinol Metab* 1983; **12**: 669–94.

Scanlon MF, Hall R. Thyrotrophin-releasing hormone: basic and clinical aspects. deGroot LJ, ed. In: *Endocrinology*, Vol. 1, 3rd edn. Philadelphia: WB Saunders Co., 1995: 192–207.

Scanlon MF, Toft AD. Regulation of thyrotropin secretion. In: Braverman LE, Utiger RD, eds. *Werner and Ingbar's The Thyroid*, 7th edn. 1996. Philadelphia: Lippincott–Raven, 1966: 220– 40.

Schally AV, Bowers CY, Redding TW, Barrett JF. Isolation of thyrotropin releasing factor (TRF) from porcine hypothalamus. *Biochem Biophy Res Commun* 1966; **25**: 165–9.

Vasopressin

Baylis PH, Thompson CJ. Osmoregulation of vasopressin secretion and thirst in health and disease. *Clin Endocrinol* 1988; **29**: 549–76.

Oxytocin

Fuchs AR, Fuch F. Endocrinology of human parturition: a review. *Br J Obstet Gynaecol* 1984; **91**: 948–67.

Lincoln DW, Paisley AC. Neuroendocrine control of milk ejection. *J Repro Fertil* 1982; **65**: 571–86.

Russell JT, Brownstein MJ, Gainer H. Biosynthesis of vasopressin, oxytocin and neurophysins: isolation and characterization of two common precursors (propressophysin and prooxyphysin). *Endocrinology* 1980; **107**: 1880–91.

CHAPTER 7

Measurement of circulating hormones

R.J. Woods and P.J. Lowry

Bioassay

Before the advent of immunoassays in the late 1960s, circulating hormones and extracts from endocrine glands could be assayed only with biological systems which were all too laborious and costly for routine clinical use. Since the introduction of immunoassays, bioassay has assumed an essential role in their validation and improvement [1]. Bangham [2] has defined the term 'biological assay' as a system in which the measured response is derived from an alteration of some cellular function brought about in a cell or aggregate of cells which were metabolically active. This definition embraces *in vivo* bioassay (the use of whole animals) as well as *in vitro* bioassay (the use of isolated organs, tissues, cells or even organelles).

In vitro bioassays can recognise differences in the potency of the chemically related hormonal variants, termed 'isohormones', which are characteristic of some glycoprotein and peptide hormones, but they do not respond to differences in their *in vivo* half-life. In contrast, *in vivo* bioassays can measure complex physiological responses; they are affected by differences in the distribution, metabolism and half-life of isohormones [3]. *In vitro* bioassays usually take only hours to complete, while *in vivo* bioassays may take days or, for example where growth is measured, weeks. Interaction with other hormones may also contribute to the response. The bioassay for pituitary growth hormone (GH) in which measurements of the width of the proximal epiphyseal cartilage of hypophysectomised rats are made after 4 days of hormone treatment is affected by circulating thyroid hormones [4]. Having little effect themselves, they act synergistically with GH to produce the response upon which the assay depends.

Bioassays may be direct or indirect. Direct assays are those in which the amount of a test substance required to achieve a specific response, such as ovulation, is compared with a standard. Indirect assays are those in which several dilutions of standard and test preparations are employed to produce dose–response curves, and the relative potency of the test preparation is that dose which evokes the same biological response as a given dose of standard (Fig. 7.1). In these, the commonest type of bioassay, the ratio of the slopes of the two dose–response curves should not vary over the entire range of the response. In most indirect bioassays, the response bears a linear relationship to the logarithm of the dose. A distinct advantage of indirect bioassays is, therefore, the degree to which they provide internal evidence of their validity. Where the standard and test preparations contain the same hormone acting through the same receptor population the dose–response curves should be parallel; where they are not, and the potency ratio is not constant for all doses, the presence of other bioactive agents must be suspected. Bioassay offers the opportunity to assay a hormonal preparation in alternative systems and in different species in the knowledge that 'pure' standard and test preparations of the same hormone should exhibit identical potency ratios in each [5,6].

The discovery and characterisation of new hormones is closely associated with established bioassays, and, in order for it to be valid, routine measurement of hormones by immunoassay requires close correlation between their bioactivity and immunoactivity. For many hormones this correlation is poor and varies according to the particular bioassay and immunoassay involved. In both types of assay the hormone analyte is bound by specialised proteins, by target-cell receptors in the case of bioassays and by antibodies in immunoassays. The sites on the hormone to which they bind are rarely identical, and molecules that have no activity in a bioassay may produce a signal in an immunoassay. This distinction is particularly relevant for the measurement of those bioactive eicosanoids which are labile *in vitro* [7].

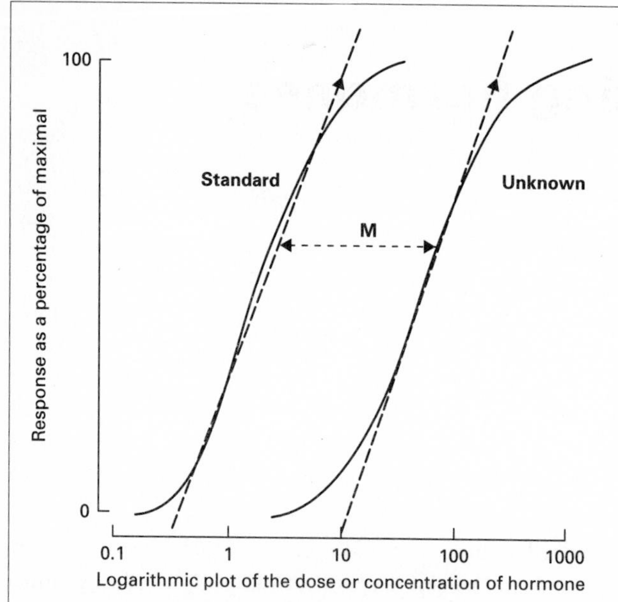

Fig. 7.1 The relative potency of an unknown preparation with respect to a standard preparation is determined from the ratio, M, of doses that evoke the same response.

Probably the most intractable cause of poor correlation between immunoassays and bioassays is the occurrence of many hormones in a variety of molecular forms. In 10% of circulating human growth hormone (hGH), 15 amino-acid residues in positions 32–46 are deleted. This 20-kDa form lacks the early insulin-like activity of the major 22-kDa form, and will not stimulate glucose uptake in a rat adipose tissue bioassay. Of two additional variants termed 'alkaline hGH', one stimulates weight gain in the pigeon crop sac bioassay to a greater degree than other forms of hGH [8]. The 22-kDa isohormone has a higher affinity for GH-binding protein than the 20-kDa form, which results in further modulation of their relative *in vivo* activity. Protein binding also prolongs the half-life of the bound hormone in plasma [9]. Although it is technically possible, these isohormones are not commonly distinguished by immunoassay.

The existence of isohormones represents a fundamental problem for the measurement of circulating hormones. Considerable difficulties have been encountered in the production of international reference preparations of human follicle-stimulating hormone (FSH), luteinising hormone (LH) and thyroid-stimulating hormone (TSH). These glycoproteins vary in their glycosyl moieties, especially in their sialic acid content [10]. The relevance of these variants, referred to as 'glycoforms', for hormone assay has been ably reviewed by Storring [11].

In an attempt to establish a new standard for human FSH, eight preparations were tested by 27 laboratories using *in vivo* and *in vitro* bioassays, receptor-binding assays and immunoassays [12]. The indirect *in vivo* bioassay based on weight gain by rat ovaries was consistent for all the laboratories involved; however, with reference to a previous standard, the new standards were twice as active in *in vivo* bioassay than in *in vitro* bioassays or receptor-based assays. Results with both one- and two-site immunoassays proved most variable and gave values which were much lower than the bioassays. The higher bioactivity of the new standards was attributed to the presence of more of the acidic forms of the hormone which have longer half-lives in the blood [13]. The low estimates of the new standard given by immunoassay were attributed to the presence of immunoreactive material devoid of biological activity in the old standard, thus rendering immunoassay alone inadequate for calibration purposes.

The consistency of *in vivo* bioassay has been previously demonstrated in a quest for a standard preparation of LH [14]. Twelve reference preparations were assessed by *in vitro* bioassays measuring testosterone production from Leydig cells and *in vivo* by measuring changes in seminal vesicle weight or ovarian ascorbic acid depletion in mice. In this case, *in vivo* bioassay did not correlate significantly with *in vitro* bioassay, and this was attributed to differences in the proportions of the more basic isohormones in each preparation: these are known to have the shortest half-life in the circulation.

Standards prepared by extracting naturally occurring hormones from tissues may have impurities which affect their behaviour in bioassays and immunoassays. The first international standard for porcine inhibin prepared from porcine ovarian follicular fluid was suspected to contain activin and follistatin which, being associated with inhibin, copurify with it [15]. In multicentre trials, *in vitro* bioassays involving the inhibition of release of FSH from dispersed rat anterior pituitary cells gave variable estimates of potency for this standard.

In order to overcome the problems posed by microheterogeneity and of impurities present in extracted hormone preparations, international standards have recently been produced using recombinant DNA technology. Erythropoietin (hEPO) [16] and GH [17] have both been expressed in eukaryotic cell cultures. In the case of hEPO, differences in purification and cell culture techniques resulted in preparations that differed from one another and from native hEPO when compared by isoelectric focusing, by *in vivo* and *in vitro* bioassays, and by immunoassay. It is apparent that a spectrum of glycoforms is secreted even by a single expression system [18]. Recombinant human FSH expressed by Chinese hamster ovary cells had isoform profiles that closely resemble those extracted from the human pituitary gland [19]. These are not, however, the same as the spectrum of isoforms found in the circulation, and more faithful standards may be prepared by expressing hFSH in embryonal kidney cells which produce more basic isoforms [20].

Individual components of a circulating hormone which consists of chemically related but distinct forms may give quite different values when measured by bioassay and immunoassay. In the human circulation, monomeric prolactin is present in glycosylated and non-glycosylated forms [21]. Glycosylation of prolactin modifies both bioactivity and immunoreactivity to different degrees [22]. Although correlation between bioassays and radioimmunoassay (RIA) in normal and hyperprolactinaemic states is usually quite good [23,24], more sophisticated tools for differential diagnosis might be obtained by raising monoclonal antibodies that are specific for individual variants.

A lack of correlation between bioassay and immunoassay has also been observed for circulating FSH [25], TSH [26], LH [27] and adrenocorticotrophic hormone (ACTH) [28]. The disparity may be influenced by clinical condition [26,29,30] or by age [27], or it may reflect an hereditary abnormality such as that reported to occur in the region of the bond between α- and β-subunits of LH [31]. It is now recognised that the epitopes on glycoprotein hormones that are important for immunoassay are confined to the peptide regions of the molecule and are usually unrelated to the receptor-binding site [32], whereas the glycosyl moieties are not antigenic but do influence bioactivity.

Even though immunological activities of highly purified glycoforms may be shown to correlate with their *in vitro* bioactivities [33], this may not be true for mixtures of glycoforms. Agreement may be sought by resorting to *in vitro* assays that detect similar structural features on each isoform such as the receptor-binding site. Receptor-binding assays have been introduced in order to improve upon the indirect estimates of potency obtained using antibodies. These may take the form of radioreceptor-binding assays [32,33] or assays for *in vitro* bioactivity that measure accumulation of cyclic AMP (cAMP) in transfected cell lines expressing the hormone receptor [34–36].

Measurement of isohormones poses a conceptual problem: a hormone may exert a multitude of physiological effects, some undiscovered, and the potency of its variants and metabolites may differ from bioassay to bioassay. The parameter measured in a bioassay may also be unrelated to any physiological effect of the hormone. This means that there cannot be an *absolute* measure of its bioactivity. The use of synthetic peptides and other molecules as immunogens for the development of 'two-site' immunoassays, as well as monoclonal antibodies directed against only bioactive forms, may increase the specificity of immunoassays, but even precise measurement of active species in peripheral blood would not reflect their activity at target tissues. Fortunately, these difficulties generally have little impact on the utility of immunoassay in the clinical measurement of circulating hormones, where absolute estimates are of less importance than well-defined indices such as the 'reference range'.

RIA and saturation analysis

The concept of RIA [37] combines the sensitivity of radioactivity measurements with the specificity of antibody–antigen reactions. An antibody raised against a given analyte is mixed with test samples of serum or plasma to which has been added a trace amount of radiolabelled analyte of known activity (Fig. 7.2). The samples are allowed to react with the antibody which is later separated from the mixture. Either free or antibody-bound radioactivity is then measured. The antibody binds both labelled and unlabelled antigen but, because analyte concentrations in samples are always in vast excess, only a small fraction of available analyte is bound. The concentration of unlabelled analyte is inversely related to bound radioactivity and is estimated by reference to known standards. 'Competitive' assays of this type rely upon the addition of only small amounts of antibody.

Although later technologies such as two-site immunoradiometric assay (IRMA) have somewhat superseded RIA for the measurement of peptide and protein hormones, these technologies cannot be applied to small hormone molecules such as steroids. Methods based on the principle of 'saturation analysis' are therefore likely to continue, but may be modified by the use of non-isotopic labels with their longer shelf-life and better reputation for safety. Alternatives include enzymic, fluorescent and chemiluminescent labels [38–41].

Because they are simple, quick to perform and are often more sensitive than contemporary bioassays, the 'labelled analyte' methods have had a very great impact on biology and medicine. Many of the theoretical and practical problems associated with all types of assays which use antibodies as reagents were first encountered with RIA. After initial difficulties in raising antibodies to small molecules had been overcome, the problem of antibodies 'cross-reacting' with substances of similar chemical structure remained. Cross-reactivity by both monoclonal and polyclonal antibodies has focused attention on the chemistry by which analytes are coupled to protein carriers for the purpose of making immunogens [42]. It may often be reduced by selecting coupling reactions which preserve epitopes peculiar to the antigen. Even if cross-reaction were slight it could invalidate an assay; for example that for triiodothyronine (T_3) which coexists in blood with a 100-fold molar excess of its analogue, thyroxine (T_4). Occasionally, cross-reactivity can be exploited to advantage where metabolic instability of the conjugated hapten has been overcome by immunising with a stable analogue [43].

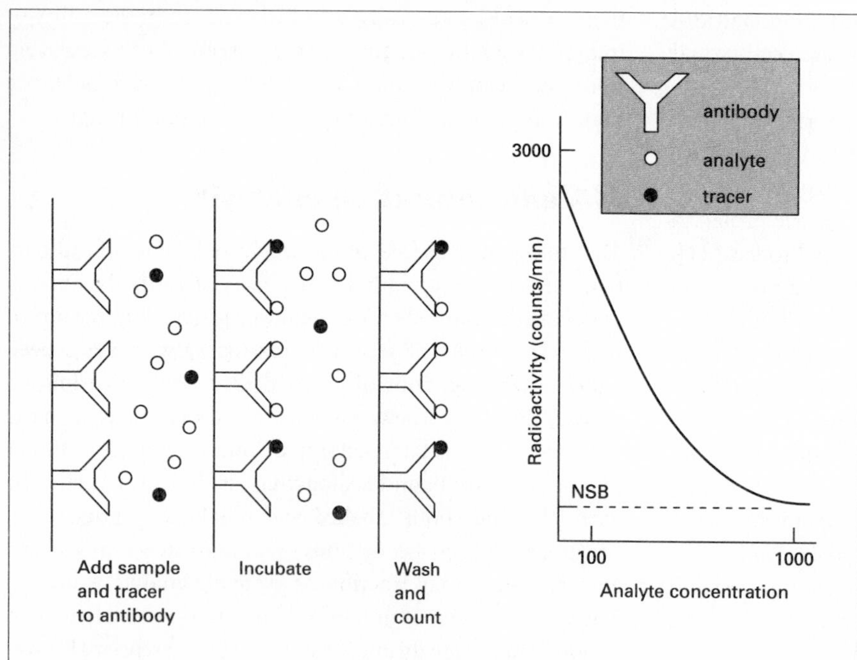

Fig. 7.2 Diagrammatic representation of the principal stages in a radioimmunoassay. Antibody, bound to a solid phase reacts with analyte and tracer. Bound radioactivity is inversely related to analyte concentration and tends at high analyte concentrations to equal the non-specific binding (NSB).

Choice of antigen may be critical in the development of an immunoassay. Much current research on the gonadal hormone, inhibin, in the circulation of humans and farm animals may be vitiated because most polyclonal antibodies raised against intact inhibin bind to the α-subunit but not to the β-subunit of the hormone and secretion from extragonadal sources of inactive, free α-subunit, has been demonstrated [44,45].

Furthermore, inhibin, which suppresses pituitary FSH secretion and activin which stimulates it share a common β-subunit (β_A or β_B) that cross-reacts in immunoassays. As activin is a dimer composed of two β-subunits, a panel of five specific assays would be required to measure each separately. This would best be achieved by 'two-site' immunoassays.

Antibodies used to measure peptide hormones by RIA can be raised by immunising with synthetic fragments of the hormone, often composed of fewer than 15 amino-acid residues. The choice of fragment can have profound consequences for the resulting RIA. Parathyroid hormone (PTH) is a peptide of 84 amino-acid residues which is metabolised partly in the parathyroid glands before secretion and partly in the liver; less than 10% of circulating material, only about 2 pmol/l, is intact PTH [46]. Most consists of a mid-molecule fragment and a short fragment from the carboxy-terminus. All the known biological activity resides in the first 34 residues constituting the amino-terminal fragment which circulates in concentrations too low to measure by immunoassay. Antibodies to this fragment have been used by some commercial RIAs to estimate intact PTH, but significant differences are observed in their reference ranges [47–49]. Intact PTH has a half-life of approximately 2 minutes [50] but carboxy-terminal and mid-molecule fragments have a much longer half-life. However, many of these problems can be avoided by the use of double-antibody immunometric assays [51,52].

Other problems associated with immunogens can be overcome by preparation and selection of appropriate monoclonal antibodies. Subjects with pituitary adenomas often have elevated serum levels of the α-subunit common to TSH, FSH and LH. These may be selectively determined by RIA with the aid of a monoclonal antibody which binds to a site which, in the intact hormone, is masked by the β-subunit [53].

Immunoassays, particularly RIAs, can suffer interference from factors present in serum or plasma which are unrelated to the analyte. The cause of these 'matrix effects' is ill defined, but has been attributed to plasma or serum proteins or sometimes to circulating antibodies [54]. They are revealed by comparing plots of the responses given by a high concentration of analyte in assay buffer and in biological fluid when both are serially diluted with assay buffer. Matrix effects result in curves which are non-parallel [55]. To compensate for matrix effects, standards may be prepared in protein solutions or in serum or plasma from which endogenous analyte has been removed. Due to matrix effects, assays for thyroid hormones in rat serum are best conducted with standards prepared in rat serum pretreated to remove endogenous thyroid hormones; standards prepared in human serum give artefactually high values [56]. In order to avoid matrix effects many RIA procedures are conducted after extraction of the analyte. Nearly all published RIA methods for atrial natriuretic peptide (ANP) require extraction with octadecasilyl-coated silica to separate ANP from an interfering serum protein of 70–90 kDa, as well as from proteases which attack the analyte [57].

Some hormones are now known to circulate in combination with specific binding proteins. They are recognised in RIA as interfering with the estimation of these hormones by competing with the antibody for analyte and radiolabelled analyte [58,59]. Measurements of true analyte concentrations can be made after extraction or addition of an agent capable of displacing analyte from the binding protein [60].

Activin-A may be released from its binding protein, follistatin, by introducing an analyte denaturation step into the assay procedure making it free to interact with antibody [61].

A binding protein present in human blood that is specific for corticotrophin-releasing hormone (CRH), interferes in CRH RIA but not in CRH IRMA because in IRMA both anti-CRH-antibodies are present in vast excess [62].

The physiological importance of binding proteins is not known, but it has been postulated that only unbound hormone is free to interact with target-tissue receptors. Measurements of the free hormone may therefore be of greater value to clinical diagnosis than total hormone [63]. This concept has added a new dimension to endocrinology, and attempts to measure free hormones have been made using a 'competitive' assay technique that resembles RIA. Commercial kits have been developed for direct measurement of free thyroid hormones (fT_3, fT_4) in serum. One such method depends on radiolabelled analogues which the manufacturers have claimed are incapable of binding to serum binding proteins yet bind to anti-T_3 or T_4 antibody [64]. Radiolabel bound to antibody is therefore inversely related to the concentration of free hormone in the sample.

It has been claimed, especially in non-thyroidal illness, that the performance of these assays may sometimes be affected by low but significant binding of the radiolabelled T_3 and T_4 analogues to proteins, particularly albumin [65,66]. One attempt to overcome this difficulty has been made using T_4 covalently linked to bovine immunoglobulin labelled with an arylacridinium ester. This 'analogue' competes with serum free T_4 for binding sites on a rabbit anti-T_4 antibody that is coupled to a solid phase; after incubation and washing a chemiluminescent signal is measured [67].

Modern innovations in RIA and 'saturation analysis' tend to concentrate on throughput, ease of performance, calculation of results and cost. Solid-phase antibody and coated tube technology have made easier the separation of bound and free label, but an interesting alternative, 'homogeneous' immunoassay, eliminates the need for separation and also facilitates automation. Most homogeneous assays use analyte coupled to an enzyme, a substrate or a fluorophor label, and measure the inactivation of the label when conjugated analyte binds to antibody. With a new technique called 'scintillation proximity RIA', only bound label produces a signal [68]. In this technique, antibody is covalently linked to microscopic beads containing a fluorophor. Test samples, analyte labelled with ^{125}I and beads are incubated together. Binding of radiolabelled analyte to the beads results in activation of the fluorophor by short-range electrons emitted by isotope decay. The light produced is measured by scintillation spectrometry; thus, with a range of fluorophors and antibodies, it may be possible to estimate several hormones simultaneously.

Immunoradiometric assay

'Labelled reagent' assays (IRMA), as distinct from 'labelled analyte' assays (RIA), are characterised by addition to test samples of radiolabelled antibody so that its concentration exceeds the concentration of endogenous analyte.

Early experiments with a 'one-site' assay have been superseded by 'two-site' procedures with antibodies which bind to two or more separate epitopes on the analyte. Typically, these 'sandwich' assays require the simultaneous reaction of all available analyte with radiolabelled antibody and with an excess of a second, unlabelled 'link' antibody added to facilitate separation of analyte-bound radiolabel (Fig. 7.3). Unlike RIA, bound radioactivity is directly related to the concentration of analyte [69]. Link antibodies may be immobilised or raised in a different animal species so that a third antibody raised against the link may be used to precipitate link and its immune complexes. The sensitivity of IRMA is, in theory, limited by the specific activity of radiolabel, the affinity of the antibody for analyte and the amount of radiolabel that is classified as 'bound' in the absence of analyte, termed non-specific binding [70]. The nature of the separation system has a significant effect on non-specific binding, and therefore upon sensitivity; hence, the use of polyethylene glycol to precipitate immune complexes in RIA is precluded from IRMA because it results in high levels of non-specific binding.

To obtain low levels of non-specific binding and high sensitivity, the antibodies that are to be radiolabelled must first be purified. This allows a suitably high specific activity to be achieved, and removes the impurities that tend to increase non-specific binding. Antigen-specific immunoglobulin fractions may be isolated from a polyclonal antiserum by affinity absorption to immobilised analyte [71]. Unfortunately, this may require large amounts of pure analyte. Alternatively, monoclonal antibodies may be recovered from ascites and from cultures by more conventional protein-enriching techniques without an affinity step.

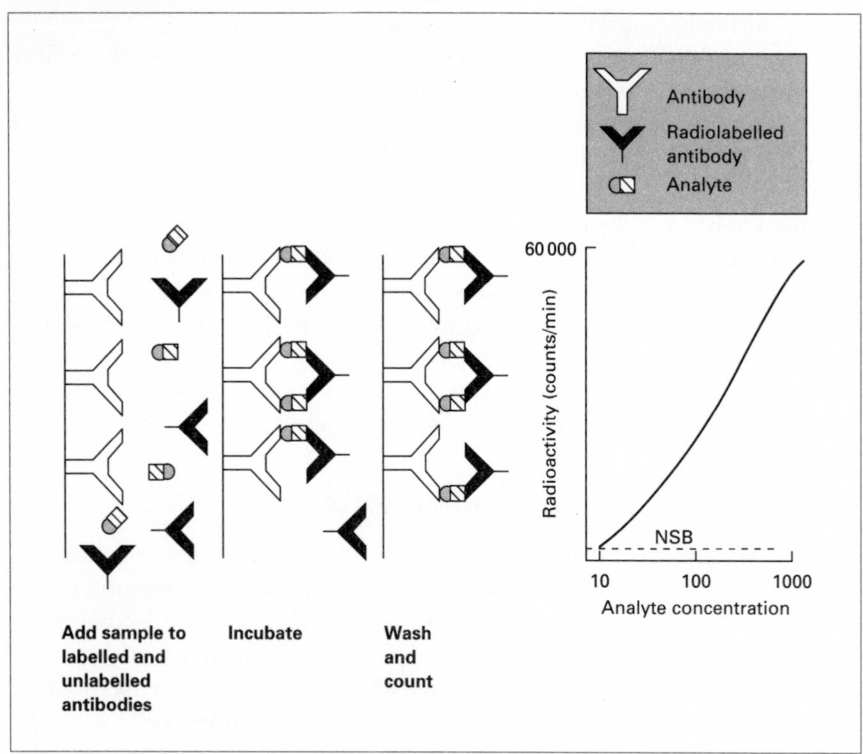

Fig. 7.3 Diagrammatic representation of the principal stages in a two-site immunoradiometric assay. An antibody bound to a solid phase and a radiolabelled antibody react with separate epitopes on an analyte. Bound radioactivity is directly related to analyte concentration. NSB, non-specific binding.

Because the concentration of specific antibody required for IRMA may be 50- or a 100-fold higher than that for a comparable RIA, it is commercially advantageous to invest in monoclonal antibodies which can, if necessary, be prepared in gram quantities.

The affinity of monoclonal antibodies for antigen is often lower than that of polyclonal antibodies, but this disadvantage may be offset by combining monoclonal antibodies so that the affinity of one antibody is increased by the binding of another antibody at an adjoining epitope [72]. Antibody cooperativity serves to stabilise the immune complex, achieving the same effect as cross-linking of analyte molecules by polyclonal antisera.

Apart from being more difficult to develop than RIA, two-site IRMA has the disadvantage of the 'high-dose hook effect'. In those IRMAs employing a single incubation step, analyte concentrations above a critical value can saturate both link and radiolabelled antibodies, such that the antibodies do not connect via analyte molecules (Fig. 7.4). As the concentration of the tripartite complexes formed from link, analyte and label decline, the assay response becomes inversely related to analyte concentration and the standard curve is inflected. This may have serious consequences for the diagnosis of tumours such as prolactinomas which can secrete prolactin in amounts sufficient to exceed the working range of an IRMA which is optimised with respect to the reference range. Levels of circulating prolactin may be so high that assay data may be misinterpreted as falling within the reference range. The problem may be solved by estimating prolactin before and after diluting sera, by removal of the sample before addition of radiolabelled antibody or, more conveniently, by RIA. Despite these reservations, two-site assays have many advantages [73]. Because antibodies are present in excess, pipetting errors in their addition are not critical and, furthermore, reaction rates are faster than in RIA; thus, assays may be completed in just a few hours.

Convenient methods for radiolabelling antibody with ^{125}I have been developed which can be universally applied to IRMA, whereas the chemistry of labelling diverse analytes for RIA can be difficult and may even reduce their antigenicity [74,75]. In addition, peptide hormone tracers of high specific activity are subject to chemical degradation due to radioactive decay which within 2–3 weeks adversely affects their performance in RIA. Radiolabelled antibodies are larger, more compact and more robust molecules, and their reactivity is much less affected by radiolysis. The working range of IRMA is typically three or four orders of magnitude of analyte concentration compared with two for RIA. Although all IRMAs have the potential to 'hook', their wide working range ensures that, in practice, this never occurs in the majority of assays.

It is difficult to assess theoretically the potential sensitivity of IRMA, but experience has shown that IRMA has

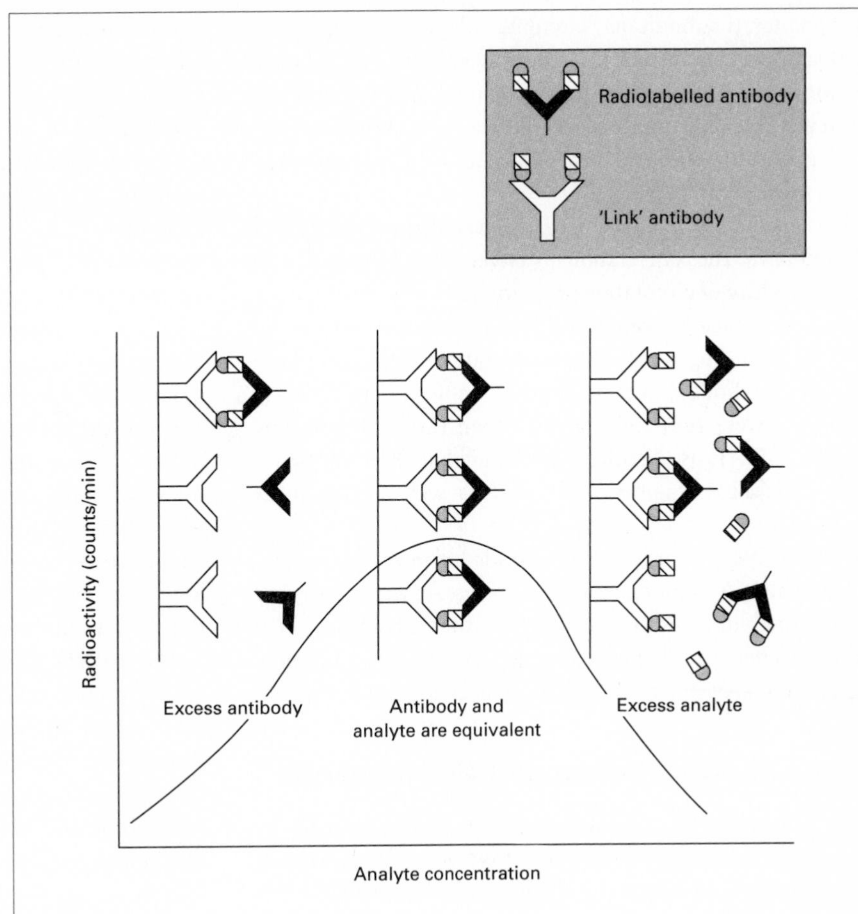

Fig. 7.4 Diagrammatic representation of the 'high-dose hook' effect. Immunoradiometric assays are carried out in the presence of excess antibodies. Excess analyte concentrations prevent radiolabelled antibody from binding to the complex formed with the solid phase 'link' antibody.

approximately 10 times more sensitivity than RIA when the same antibodies are used in both [62,76]. Improved assay sensitivity has made possible direct measurement of ACTH, CRH and intact PTH in plasma and serum without prior extraction [77–79]. In the cases of PTH and TSH, concentrations below the lower limit of the reference range can now be measured, thus adding to diagnostic capability [79–81].

Conventionally, 'two-site' immunoassays cannot be applied to the measurement of the concentration of small molecules that do not provide two sterically separate epitopes. It has now been reported that non-competitive immunometric assays using anti-idiotypic antibodies can be used to measure small molecules such as oestradiol [82], thus realising the advantages provided by non-competitive, two-site immunoassays. The first 'idiometric assay' to be published exploits the interaction of an immobilised, monoclonal antibody with its ligand such that new binding sites, recognised by a second labelled, antibody, are formed [83]. This type of assay, developed for the drug digoxin, may in principle be applied to other small analytes including eicosanoids, steroids and small peptides.

The labelled reagent format has the potential to increase assay sensitivity by exploiting the high affinity of the protein avidin, for its ligand biotin, a vitamin [84]. Purified immunoglobulin may be reacted with biotin derivatives forming sites for the attachment of several molar equivalents of avidin. Avidin, a protein present in egg white, or the more stable streptavidin, produced by *Streptomyces avidinii*, may be radiolabelled to a high specific activity without losing affinity for biotin. The specific activity of the complex may be 10-fold higher than that achieved by radiolabelling immunoglobulin. Assays incorporating labelled streptavidin tend to have low levels of non-specific binding and seem to be a flexible approach to the production of radiolabelled reagents for IRMA. Commercial exploitation of this principle is on the increase.

A singular advantage of two-site IRMA is the additional specificity for analytes conferred by the use of two antibodies. The estimation of human chorionic gonadotrophin (hCG) and gonadotrophin fragments affords a good example of this principle. hCG is composed of two subunits: the α-subunit, which is identical to that in LH, FSH and TSH, and a distinctive β-subunit. In cases of gynaecological malignancy, β-subunit may circulate independently together with a β-fragment which lacks a segment from the carboxy-terminus [85]. With pairs of monoclonal antibodies it has been possible to estimate separately the intact hormone and both gonadotrophin fragments when all were present in the same urine sample.

The specificity of two-site IRMA has also been reported to improve the correlation between the bioassay and immunoassay of circulating prolactin [24]. The discrepancy between published values for plasma concentrations of CRH in late pregnancy may be attributed to the difference in assay methods that were applied. Values obtained using RIA [86] were four times greater than those obtained by IRMA [87]. It is distinctly possible that RIA measurements included fragments of CRH as well as the intact peptide.

With respect to protein and peptide hormones, measurement by IRMA cannot guarantee complete structural integrity of the analytes, but considering its other advantages it is proving a better tool than RIA for both routine measurement and for research into the metabolism of circulating hormones.

Chemiluminescence and fluorescence

The sensitivity of all immunoassays is constrained by non-specific binding; the natural limit of antibody affinity is observed to be about 1×10^{12} l/mol. RIA and IRMA are further restricted by severe limitations to the specific activity of radiolabels [88]. The specific activity of ^{125}I, which has a half-life of 60 days, is such that, on average, only one atom in 7.5 million decays in a 1-s period. Raising specific activity has, therefore, the potential to increase assay sensitivity by several orders of magnitude. Enzymes as well as fluorescent and chemiluminescent compounds have been explored as alternatives to radioisotopes on the premise that every member of a population of these molecules may, when activated, generate at least one signal event within an acceptably short 'counting' period.

Fluorescence and chemiluminescence are examples of the phenomenon of luminescence. Luminescent substances are those which, if electronically excited, dissipate energy in the form of light. Fluorescent substances are capable of being excited by incident light of suitable wavelength to emit some part of that energy as light of a higher wavelength before returning to their ground state. This process may be repeated so that a fluorophor may amplify by generating more than one photon signal. In contrast, chemiluminescent molecules are excited by chemical oxidation to emit but one signal each during their conversion to an inactive product. That fraction of molecules in a potentially luminescent population which may be made to emit photons is termed the chemiluminescent quantum yield or quantum efficiency.

The advantage of signal amplification and high quantum efficiency offered by fluorescent labels is offset by endogenous fluorescence and quenching of incident light by some constituents of biological samples [89]. In addition, the detection apparatus is more expensive than the simpler luminometers required to measure chemiluminescence. The introduction in 1985 of time-resolved fluorescence has overcome the problem of background interference from nucleotides and other components of serum and plasma resulting in greater sensitivity than that attained by RIA. This technique uses chelated lanthanides, such as europium, as labels because they have exceptionally large Stokes' shifts and long decay times [90,91]. Samples are subjected to 1000 pulses of laser light per second, each a microsecond in duration. Fluorescence is measured between 400 and 800 microseconds after each pulse so that fluorescence from endogenous constituents, which is of short duration, will have subsided before measurement of light emitting from the chelate commences [92,93].

The first chemiluminescent labels to have been exploited are the aminophthalhydrazides, luminol and isoluminol [94]. The earliest applications of these chemiluminescent labels include homogeneous assays which exploit the enhancement of luminescence observed when analytes conjugated with isoluminol label bind to antibody [95,96]. The sensitivity of this system may be improved by introducing a fluorophor into the assay: one such homogeneous assay is based upon chemiluminescence energy transfer from analyte conjugated with an isoluminol analogue to an antibody conjugated with fluorescein [97]. The resulting shift in the wavelength of emitted light is used to measure analyte concentration. Despite the high specific activity of aminophthalhydrazide labels (aminobutylethylisoluminol is reported to emit 5.1×10^{18} photons per mole), homogeneous systems suffer the disadvantage that conjugates have lower quantum yields than the free labels. Homogeneous assays are also affected by variable quenching of the signal by bilirubin and other plasma components.

In heterogeneous assays the use of immobilised antibodies has permitted substances which interfere in signal detection to be removed by washing before activation of the chemiluminescent label [98,99]. Furthermore, for heterogeneous assays using analytes labelled with aminophthalhydrazides, an improved quantum yield is obtained by hydrolysing the conjugated analyte in the bound fraction with hot, strong alkali to release the label [100]. Light emission is then induced by addition of hydrogen peroxide and a catalyst such as transition metal ions or a peroxidase enzyme. Photodetector measurements must be made immediately after rapid injection of hydrogen peroxide, because light emission declines to half its maximum within seconds.

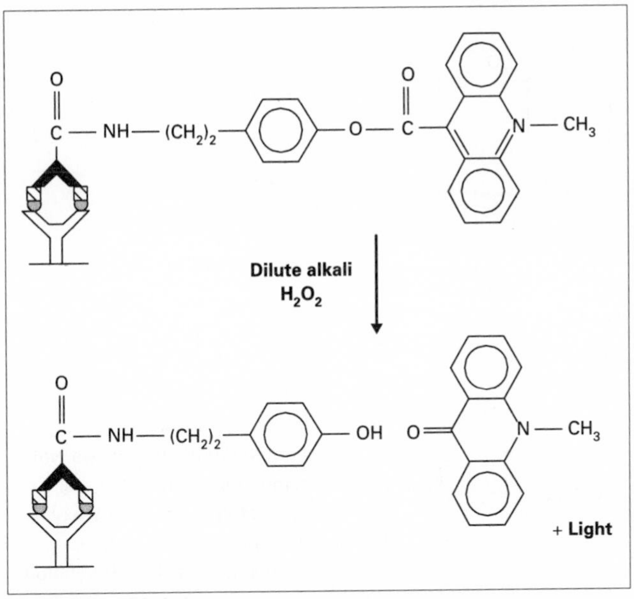

Fig. 7.5 In immunochemiluminometric assays using acridinium esters the chemiluminescent label is coupled to antibody. It is released by exposure to dilute alkali and activated by addition of hydrogen peroxide.

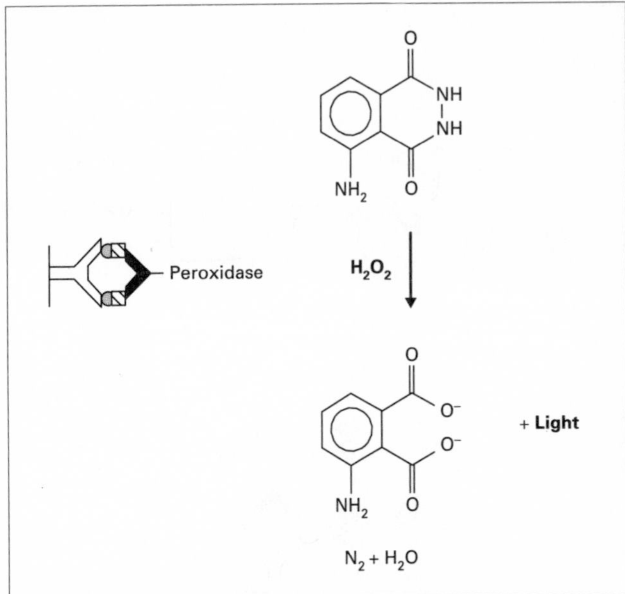

Fig. 7.6 In enzyme-linked immunochemiluminometric assays using the chemiluminescent substrate, luminol, peroxidase coupled to antibody acts as catalyst for the oxidation of luminol by hydrogen peroxide.

Some improvement in technique has resulted from the introduction of chemiluminescent acridinium esters which may be released from conjugates by brief exposure to cold, dilute alkali, and which require no catalyst for oxidation [101]. These have proved suitable for both labelled analyte [102] and for 'two-site' immunochemiluminometric assays (ICMA) [103–105] for which antibodies conjugated with arylacridinium esters can now be readily prepared [106] (Fig. 7.5). Quantum yields of isoluminol conjugates are approximately 1% [107] and those of acridinium esters are only between 2 and 5% [108], yet the performance of current heterogeneous chemiluminescent immunoassays (CIA) rivals that of RIA and IRMA [52,109–112]. Even further improvements in quantum yield and sensitivity may be expected from reactions in which reagents described as 'active oxylates' transfer energy during oxidation to fluorescent labels attached to antibodies [113].

The signal generated by labelled analytes and antibodies is limited by the quantity of label present in the bound fraction; however, great amplification can be obtained by conjugating antibodies with horseradish peroxidase instead of chemiluminescent compounds (Fig. 7.6). Peroxidase activity may be measured by absorptiometry using substrates that yield a coloured product, but measurements of signals generated by chemiluminescent substrates are even more sensitive [114]. In chemiluminescence enzyme immunoassay, peroxidase–antibody conjugates captured by solid phase are washed and luminol and hydrogen peroxide are added. Normally, the peroxidase would be rapidly inactivated by damaging oxidation products formed during the reaction but inclusion of substituted phenols such as *p*-iodophenol serves to protect the enzyme [115]. The intensity of emitted light is enhanced 1000-fold and continues at a stable rate for several minutes. It has therefore been possible commercially to develop high-throughput assays with analytes or link antibodies immobilised on microtitre plates allowing automated read-out of results. The introduction of 1,2-dioxetanes as chemiluminescent substrates for use with antibodies conjugated to alkaline phosphatase or β-D-galactosidase has further improved assay sensitivity. These substrates do not require the presence of an oxidising agent for chemiluminescence to occur, and therefore emission of light is more stable (Fig. 7.7). Using the substrate adamantyl dioxetane phenylphosphate, fewer than 1×10^{-15} moles of enzyme may be detected, which is about three orders of magnitude below that which can be achieved with luminol substrates [115].

Although CIA protocols may be more demanding and the predicted improvements in sensitivity have yet to be fully realised, the relative stability of chemiluminescent reagents and problems concerning the disposal of radioactivity are making CIA a popular alternative to RIA and IRMA. The detection of non-isotopic labels is currently less efficient than that of radioactivity, and improvements to CIA may be expected from refined instrumentation as well as from superior assay protocols [70,116].

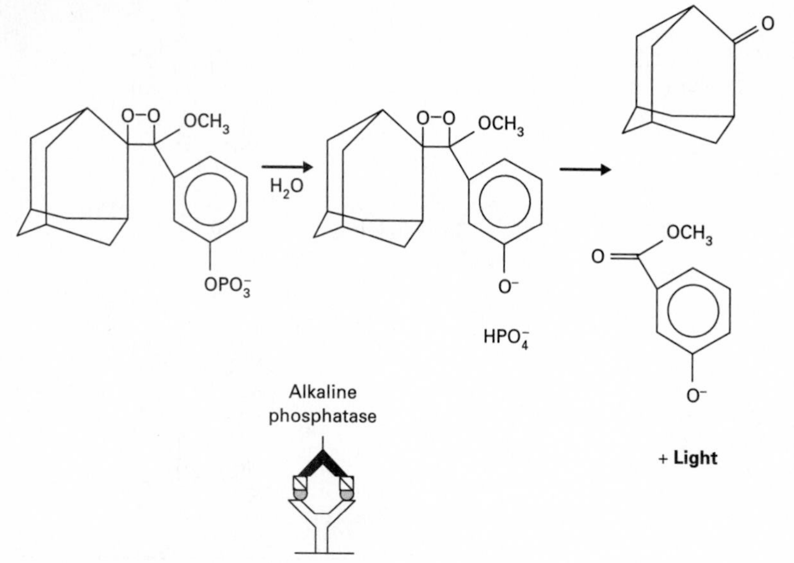

Fig. 7.7 In enzyme-linked immunochemiluminometric assays which use the chemiluminescent substrate, adamantane methoxy phosphoryloxy phenyl dioxetane (AMPPD), light is emitted as a result of dephosphorylation of the substrate. The presence of hydrogen peroxide is not required.

Chromatography

Several hormones circulate in a variety of chemically distinct but active forms (isohormones). Inactive precursors and metabolites may also be present [117]. Where specific antisera are not available, selective measurement of isohormones may be impossible and confusion with inactive forms may also occur. This problem is to some extent solved by extraction of biological samples and separation of the various hormonal components by chromatography. Extraction from plasma or serum is necessary in order to transfer analytes from their biological medium to buffers in which they may be separated by virtue of their differing physicochemical properties. The selection of a suitable protocol for sample extraction and prefractionation is as important for success as that chosen for chromatography [118]. In recent years, the most preferred technique for separating hormones has been high-pressure liquid chromatography (HPLC), referred to by equipment manufacturers as 'high-*performance* liquid chromatography'. Several excellent publications describe the theory and practice of HPLC and these are of help in the selection of appropriate column materials and solvents [119–121]. Many solid supports or stationary phases are manufactured for HPLC, all of which may be used with a wide range of mobile phases or eluants. Because silica-based stationary phases are not readily compressible, high perfusion rates and short columns result in most separations being completed in less than 30 min. Recoveries of analytes are high, and reproducibility and resolution are better than with paper or gel media. Furthermore, microprocessor control makes the use of sophisticated solvent gradients possible.

The most popular technique for the separation of catecholamines [122,123], steroid [124,125] and peptide hormones [123] is reversed-phase HPLC (RPC). This system depends on the partition of solutes or analytes between a non-polar, hydrophobic, stationary phase and an aqueous mobile phase containing an organic modifier such as methanol or, more commonly, acetonitrile or propanol. For peptides of 20–30 amino-acid residues, the best resolution is obtained by using columns coated with alkyl residues four or eight carbon-atoms long, but because the mobile phase remains the most influential factor many hormones have been separated using octadecasilyl coatings [126]. The selectivity of a column is not greatly affected by increasing the length of alkyl residues, but retention time is prolonged. Substitution of diphenyl residues for alkyl groups can profoundly affect separation of peptides containing aromatic amino acids because interaction due to Π cloud electrons may occur. Similarly, a coating with cyanopropyl residues permits interaction with the glycosyl moieties of glycopeptides, thus affecting separation. RPC protocols often involve gradients with increasing concentrations of organic solvents designed to displace the analytes from the hydrophobic stationary phase. Although peptides are unlikely to elute in order of chain length, physicochemical considerations do dictate the elution sequence of polymers: those with greater numbers of hydrophobic residues are more sensitive to smaller changes in the concentration of the organic modifier than those with fewer such residues [127].

The versatility of RPC can be extended by introducing into the mobile phase a hydrophobic acid before the separation of bases or a hydrophobic base before separating acid solutes. These counter-ions interact with polar analytes and improve their binding to hydrophobic stationary phases. This principle of ion-pair RPC has been applied to the isolation of circulating angiotensins [128] and to human growth hormone-releasing factor [129,130] which, due to interference by metabolites and precursors, cannot be estimated directly by RIA; gradient RPC was conducted in the presence of trifluoroacetic acid (TFA) as a counter-ion. A similar procedure has been published for separating fragments of cholecystokinin (CCK) using a stationary phase coated with octadecasilyl groups [131]. This separation is necessary because current CCK antisera all cross-react to some degree with gastrins [132].

Many protein hormones are denatured by the high concentrations of organic solvents and extremes of acidity associated with RPC, but they are amenable to the less rigorous conditions employed in ion exchange HPLC [118]. Some proteins, such as GH, can be purified by RPC [127–133], but hydrophobic interaction chromatography (HIC) using weakly hydrophobic supports together with purely aqueous eluants is now preferable [134]. Stationary phases for HIC consist of silica particles reacted at low density with alkyl or other hydrophobic groups [135], the object of which is to interact with hydrophobic regions of intact proteins without inducing them to unfold. Elution can be performed using conditions which are less harsh than those associated with RPC [136].

Analytes eluted from HPLC columns are commonly detected by their absorbance of ultraviolet (UV) light. The sensitivity of modern UV detectors is just adequate for measuring circulating levels of some steroids [124–137], but not for peptide or protein hormones. Although peptides in biological fluids may be detected after conversion to fluorescent derivatives [138], in most studies they are measured in eluate fractions by immunoassay [139–141].

The development of electrochemical detection, which is more sensitive for certain classes of compound than UV detection, has led to improved estimation of catecholamines. This technique has also been applied to steroids [142,143].

Separation of catecholamines and steroids by chromatography allows rapid comparison of the levels of hormones with their metabolites, which may be of more value than estimates of the hormones alone by immunoassay. In the context of peptide and protein hormones, the most significant application of chromatography to routine assay may be found in the preparation of pure standards and tracers.

Modern developments

Modern developments in the measurement of circulating hormones promised improved sensitivity as well as aiming at low-cost, high-throughput immunoassays. A novel approach to the improvement of assay sensitivity involves using the techniques of molecular biology to increase the affinity of antibodies for antigens [144]. In the future, difficulties associated with antibodies and their preparation may be obviated by a new development [145,146]. Binding sites formed by variable regions of the immunoglobulin G heavy chain have been cloned in *Escherichia coli*, and attempts have been made to increase their affinity for antigen by judicious point mutations [147].

An additional objective is to produce 'man-made antibodies' consisting of complementarity-determining regions (CDRs) from pairs of variable light- and heavy-chain peptides joined together by a short sequence [148]. Variable (*V*) genes encoding the CDRs can now be cloned from lymphocytes or from hybridomas producing monoclonal antibodies to the antigen of interest. By screening the bacterial clones and by introducing diversity through mutation it is possible to select those that secrete products having an increased affinity for the antigen.

In one promising new approach the initial selection, mutation and clonal expansion of *V* genes may be carried out in immunised mice. Subsequently, DNA recovered from antibody-expressing lymphocytes may be cloned in bacteriophage. Those phage with the *V* region suitably expressed on the surface can be selected using columns containing antigen bound to a solid phase. They are then eluted, propagated and again screened against antigen [149]. Elements of the heavy and light chains linked by a disulphide bridge have also been cloned as a single unit. In principle, these techniques may even dispense with the need to immunise animals [150,151]. If successful, this approach could revolutionise labelled-reagent assays.

In the diagnosis of endocrine disorders there is often a need to measure several related hormones or even isoforms simultaneously. In future this objective may be achieved by the 'multianalyte immunoassay' in which assays of antibody 'microspots' are arranged on a probe, each directed against a different analyte. The probe is incubated in test sample, washed and exposed to a second developing antibody, which may bind to free epitopes on large analyte molecules, captured by the 'sensor' antibodies on the probe or to epitopes on unoccupied 'sensor' antibodies in the case of small analytes. Thus, competitive and non-competitive assay formats may be used. Both 'developing' and 'sensor' antibodies may be labelled with different fluorophors such as fluorescein and Texas Red so that accurate estimates of occupied or unoccupied 'sensor' antibody may be made by measuring the ratio of the bound fluorescent markers. Bound fluorophors are activated by laser light and the signal is measured with the aid of a fluorescence microscope which automatically scans each spot [39].

Perhaps the most important technological innovation for the clinical measurement of circulating hormones is the introduction of an ever-expanding range of automated immunoassay systems. These machines are rapidly achieving a status equivalent to that of the clinical chemistry analysers. Although expensive, they reduce labour costs, require few handling skills, permit random access so that samples can be tested at any time, and are mostly designed to operate with chemiluminescent or even fluorescent labels [152–156]. Immunoanalysers have improved assay precision significantly and assay protocols are often more rapid than their non-automated counterparts. Advanced handling by sophisticated computer software worklists can itemise the tests required for each sample; one analyser model is capable of testing up to 100 samples for as many as 21 analytes in a single run.

References

1 Storring PL. Biological assays of peptide and protein hormones—the basis for their specificity and their role in improving the specificity of assays, such as immunoassays, and other assays which do not measure activity. *Scand J Clin Lab Invest* 1989; **49** (Suppl. 193): 34–42.

2 Bangham DR. Aspects by which assays may be characterized. *Scand J Clin Lab Invest* 1989; **49** (Suppl. 193): 11–19.

3 Robertson WR, Lambert A, Loveridge N. The role of modern bioassays in clinical endocrinology. *Clin Endocrinol* 1987; **27**: 259–78.

4 Li CH. Bioassay of pituitary growth hormone. In: Li CH, ed. *Hormonal Proteins and Peptides*, Vol. 4, *Growth Hormone and Related Proteins*. New York: Academic Press, 1977: 1–41.

5 Bangham DR. Assays and standards. In: Gray CH, James VHT, eds. *Hormones and Blood*, 3rd ed. London: Academic Press, 1983: 255–99.

6 Kirkwood TBL. Calibration and internal quality control. *Scand J Clin Lab Invest* 1989; **49** (Suppl. 193): 82–6.

7 Granström E, Kumlin M. Metabolism of prostaglandins and lipoxygenase products. Relevance for eicosanoid assay. In: Bennedetto C, McDonald-Gibson RG, Nigam S, Slater TF, eds. *Prostaglandins and Related Substances. A Practical Approach*. Oxford: IRL Press, 1987: 5–27.

8 Lewis UJ. Variants of growth hormone and prolactin and their posttranslational modifications. *Ann Rev Physiol* 1984: **46**: 33–42.

9 Baumann G, Amburn K, Buchanan TA. The effect of circulating growth hormone-binding protein on metabolic clearance, distribution and degradation of human growth hormone. *J Clin Endocrinol Metab* 1987; **64**: 657–60.

10 Pierce JG, Parsons TF. Glycoprotein hormones: structure and function. *Ann Rev Biochem* 1981; **50**: 465–95.

11 Storring PL. Assaying glycoprotein hormones—the influence of glycosylation on immunoreactivity. *Trends Biotechnol* 1992; **10**: 427–32.

12 Storring PL, Gaines Das RE. The international standard for pituitary FSH: collaborative study of the standard and of four other purified human FSH preparations of differing molecular composition by bioassays, receptor assays and different immunoassay systems. *J Endocrinol* 1989; **123**: 275–93.

13 Zaidi AA, Froysa B, Diczfalusy E. Biological and immunological properties of different molecular species of human follicle-stimulating hormone: electrofocusing profiles of eight highly purified preparations. *J Endocrinol* 1982; **27**: 1259–78.

14 Storring PL, Zaidi AA, Mistry YG, Lindberg M, Stenning BE, Diczfalusy E. A comparison of preparations of highly purified human pituitary luteinizing hormone: differences in the luteinizing hormone potencies as determined by *in vitro* bioassay and immunoassay. *Acta Endocrinol* 1982; **101**: 339–47.

15 Gaines Das RE, Rose M, Zanelli JM. International collaborative study by *in vitro* bioassays of the first international standard for porcine inhibin. *J Reprod Fertil* 1992; **96**: 803–14.

16 Storring PL, Gaines Das RE. The international standard for recombinant DNA-derived Erythropoietin: collaborative study of four recombinant DNA derived erythropoietins and two highly purified human urinary erythropoietins. *J Endocrinol* 1992; **134**: 459–84.

17 Bristow AF, Gaines Das R, Jeffcoate SL, Schulster D. The first international standard for somatotropin: report of an international collaborative study. *Growth Regul* 1995; **5**: 133–41.

18 Szkudlinski MW, Thotakura NR, Bucci I *et al.* Purification and characterization of recombinant human thyrotropin (TSH) isoforms produced by Chinese hamster ovary cells: the role of sialylation and sulfation in TSH bioactivity. *Endocrinology* 1993; **133**: 1490–503.

19 Cerpa-Poljak A, Bishop LA, Hort YJ *et al.* Isoelectric charge of recombinant human follicle stimulating hormone isoforms determines receptor affinity and *in vitro* bioactivity. *Endocrinology* 1993; **132**: 351–6.

20 Flack MR, Bennet AD, Froehlich J, Anasti JN, Nisula BC. Increased biological activity due to basic isoforms in recombinant human follicle-stimulating hormone produced in a human cell line. *J Endocrinol Metab* 1994; **79**: 756–60.

21 Markoff E, Lee DW. Glycosylated prolactin is a major circulating variant in human serum. *J Clin Endocrinol Metab* 1987; **65**: 1102–6.

22 Haro LS, Lee DW, Singh RNP, Bee G, Markoff E, Lewis UJ. Glycosylated human prolactin: alterations in glycosylation pattern modify affinity for lactogen receptor and values in prolactin radioimmunoassay. *J Clin Endocrinol Metab* 1990; **71**: 379–83.

23 Smith CR, Butler J, Hashim I, Norman MR. Serum prolactin bioactivity and immunoactivity in hyperprolactinaemic states. *Ann Clin Biochem* 1990; **27**: 3–8.

24 Maddox PR, Jones DL, Mansel RE. Bioactive and immunoactive prolactin levels after TRH-stimulation in the sera of normal women. *Horm Metab Res* 1992; **24**: 181–4.

25 Simoni M, Jockenhorel F, Nieschlag E. Polymorphism of human pituitary FSH: analysis of immunoreactivity and *in vitro* bioactivity of different molecular species. *J Endocrinol* 1994; **141**: 359–67.

26 Beck Peccoz P, Persani L. Variable biological activity of thyroid-stimulating hormone. *Eur J Endocrinol* 1994; **131**: 331–40.

27 Mitchell R, Hollis S, Rothwell C, Robertson WR. Age related changes in the pituitary–testicular axis in normal men; lower serum testosterone results from decreased bioactive LH drive. *Clin Endocrinol* 1995; **42**: 501–7.

28 Poland RE, Hamada K. Dissociation between plasma bioactive and immunoreactive ACTH concentrations in depressed patients. *Biol Psychiatry* 1994; **35**: 309–15.

29 Mechain C, Cedrin I, Pandrian C, Lemay A. Serum FSH bioactivity and response to acute gonadotrophin releasing hormone (GnRH) agonist stimulation in patients with polycystic ovary syndrome (PCOS) as compared to control groups. *Clin Endocrinol* 1993; **38**: 311–20.

30 Howanitz JH. Review of the influence of polypeptide hormone forms on immunoassay results. *Arch Pathol Lab Med* 1993; **117**: 369–72.

31 Okuda K, Takamatsu J, Okazaki T, Yamada T, Saeki M, Sugimoto O. Hereditary abnormality of luteinizing hormone resulting in discrepant serum concentration determined by different assays. *Endocr J* 1994; **41**: 639–44.

32 Dirnhofer S, Lechner O, Madersbacher S, Klieber R, de Leeuw R, Wick G, Berger P. Alpha subunit of human chorionic gonadotropin: molecular basis of immunologically and biologically active domains. *J Endocrinol* 1994; **140**: 145–54.

33 Burgon PG, Robertson DM, Stanton PG, Hearn MT. Immunological activities of highly purified isoforms of human FSH correlate with *in vitro* bioactivities. *J Endocrinol* 1993; **139**: 511–18.

34 Kelton CA, Cheng SV, Nugent NP *et al.* The cloning of the human follicle stimulating hormone receptor and its expression in COS-7, CHO and Y-1 cells. *Mol Cell Endocrinol* 1992; **89**: 141–51.

35 Gudermann T, Brockmann H, Simoni M, Gromoll J, Nieschlag E. *In vitro* bioassay for human serum follicle-stimulating hormone (FSH) based on L cells transfected with recombinant rat FSH receptor: validation of a model system. *Endocrinology* 1994; **135**: 2204–13.

36 Tano M, Minegishi T, Nakamura K, Karino S, Ibuki Y. Application of Chinese hamster ovary cells transfected with the recombinant human follicle stimulating hormone (FSH) receptor for measurement of serum FSH. *Fertil Steril* 1995; **64**: 1120–24.

37 Ekins RP. Basic principles and theory. *Br Med Bull* 1974; **30**: 3–11.

38 Ishikawa E, Hashida S, Kohno T, Hirota K. Ultrasensitive enzyme immunoassay. *Clin Chim Acta* 1990; **194**: 51–72.

39 Ekins R, Chu F, Biggart E. Fluorescence Spectroscopy and its application to a new generation of high sensitivity, multi-microspot, multianalyte, immunoassay. *Clin Chim Acta* 1990; **194**: 91–114.

40 Lüke F, Schlegel W. A time-resolved fluoroimmunoassay for the determination of prostaglandin $F_{2\alpha}$. *Clin Chim Acta* 1990; **189**: 257–66.

41 Diamandis EP. Analytical methodology for immunoassays and DNA hybridization assays—current status and selected systems—critical review. *Clin Chim Acta* 1990; **194**: 19–50.

42 Erlanger BF. The preparation of antigenic hapten-carrier conjugates: a survey. *Methods Enzymol* 1980; **70**: 85–104.

43 Wynalda MA, Brashler JR, Back MK, Morton DR, Fitzpatric FA. Determination of leukotriene C_4 by radioimmunoassay with a specific antiserum generated from a synthetic hapten mimic. *Anal Chem* 1984; **56**: 1862–65.

44 Knight PG, Beard AJ, Wrathall JHM, Castillo RJ. Evidence that the bovine ovary secretes large amounts of monomeric inhibin α-subunit and its isolation from bovine follicular fluid. *J Mol Endocrinol* 1989; **2**: 189–200.

45 Schneyer AL, Mason AJ, Burton LE, Ziegner JR, Crowley WF. Immunoreactive inhibin α-subunit in human serum: implications for radioimmunoassay. *J Clin Endocrinol Metab* 1990; **70**: 1208–12.

46 Goltzman D, Bennet HPJ, Koutsilieris M, Mitchell J, Rabbani SA, Rouleau MF. Studies of the multiple molecular forms of bioactive parathyroid hormone and parathyroid hormone-like substances. *Recent Prog Horm Res* 1986; **42**: 665–97.

47 Papapoulos SE, Manning RM, Hendy GN, Lewin IG, O'Riordan JLH. Studies of circulating parathyroid hormone in man using an homologous amino-terminal specific immunoradiometric assay. *Clin Endocrinol* 1980; **13**: 57–67.

48 Klee GG, Shikegawa J, Trainer TD. CAP survey of parathyroid hormone assays. *Arch Pathol Lab Med* 1986; **110**: 588–91.

49 Nisbet JA. Comparison of the parathyroid hormone assays. *Ann Clin Biochem* 1986; **23**: 429–33.

50 Martin KJ, Hruska KA, Freitag JJ, Klahr S, Slatopolsky E. The peripheral metabolism of parathyroid hormone. *N Engl J Med* 1979; **301**: 1092–8.

51 Nussbaum SR, Zahradnik RJ, Lavigne JR *et al.* Highly sensitive two site immunoradiometric assay of parathyrin and its clinical utility in evaluating patients with hypercalcaemia. *Clin Chem* 1987; **33**: 1364–7.

52 Klee GG, Preissner CM, Schryner PG, Taylor RL, Kao PC. Multisite immunochemiluminometric assay for simultaneously measuring whole-molecule and amino-terminal fragments of human parathyrin. *Clin Chem* 1992; **38**: 628–35.

53 Oppenheim DS, Kana AR, Sangha JS, Klibanski A. Prevalence of α-subunit hypersection in patients with pituitary tumours: clinically nonfunctioning and somatotroph adenomas. *J Endocrinol Metab* 1990; **70**: 859–64.

54 Boscato LM, Stuart MC. Heterophilic antibodies: a problem for all immunoassays. *Clin Chem* 1988; **34**: 27–33.

55 Feldkamp CS, Smith SW. Practical guide to immunoassay method evaluation. In: Chan DW, Derlstein MT, eds. *Immunoassay, a Practical Guide*. New York: Academic Press, 1987: 49–95.

56 Stringer BMJ, Wynford-Thomas D. Importance of maintaining species homology in thyroid, hormone radioimmunoassays: modification of 'human' radioimmunoassay kits for use with rat samples. *Horm Res* 1982; **16**: 392–7.

57 Richards AM, Tonolo G, McIntyre GD, Leckie BJ, Robertson JIS. Radioimmunoassay for plasma alpha human atrial natriuretic peptide: a comparison of direct and pre-extracted methods *J Hypertens* 1987; **5**: 227–36.

58 Ellis MJ, Livesey JH, Donald RA. Circulating plasma corticotrophin-releasing factor-like immunoreactivity. *J Endocrinol* 1988; **117**: 299–307.

59 Daughday WH, Kapadia M, Mariz I. Serum somatomedin binding proteins: physiological significance and interference in radioligand assay. *J Clin Endocrinol Metab* 1987; **109**: 355–63.

60 Fang VS, Refetoff S. Radioimmunoassay for serum triiodothyronine: evaluation of simple techniques to control interference from binding proteins. *Clin Chem* 1974; **20**: 1150–4.

61 Knight PG, Muttukrishna S, Groome NP. Development and application of a two-site immunoassay for the determination of total activin-A concentrations in serum and follicular fluid. *J Endocrinol* 1996; **148**: 267–79.

62 Linton EA, Lowry PJ. Comparison of a specific two-site immunoradiometric assay with radioimmunoassay for rat/human CRF-41. *Regul Pept* 1986; **14**: 69–84.

63 Ekins R. Measurement of free hormones in blood. *Endocr Rev* 1990; **11**: 5–46.

64 Wilkins TA, Midgley JEM, Barren N. Comprehensive study of a thyroxine-analog-based assay for free thyroxine ('Amerlex FT_4'). *Clin Chem* 1985; **31**: 1644–53.

65 Amino N, Nishi K, Nakatani K, Mizuta H, Ichihara K. Effect of albumin concentration on the assay of serum free thyroxine by equilibrium radioimmunoassay with labelled thyroxine analogue (Amerlex Free T_4). *Clin Chem* 1983; **29**: 321–5.

66 Byfield PGH, Lalloz MRA, Pearce CJ, Himsworth RL. Free thyroid hormone concentrations in subjects with various abnormalities of binding proteins: experience with Amerlex Free-T_4 and Free-T_3 assays. *Clin Endocrinol* 1983; **19**: 277–83.

67 Beaman J, Woodhead SJ, Liewendahl K, Mähönen H. The evaluation

of a chemiluminescent assay for free thyroxine by comparison with equilibrium dialysis in clinical samples. *Clin Chem Acta* 1989; **186**: 83–9.

68 Udenfriend S, Diekmann Gerber L, Brink L, Spector S. Scintillation proximity radioimmunoassay utilizing ^{125}I-labelled ligands. *Proc Natl Acad Sci USA* 1985; **82**: 8672–6.

69 Ekins RP. General principles of hormone assay. In: Loraine JA, Bell ET, eds. *Hormone Assays and their Clinical Application*. Edinburgh: Churchill Livingstone, 1976: 1–72.

70 Jackson TM, Marshall NJ, Ekins RP. Optimisation of immunoradiometric (labelled antibody) assays. In: Hunter WM, Carrie JET, eds. *Immunoassays for Clinical Chemistry*. Edinburgh: Churchill Livingstone, 1983: 557–75.

71 Hodgkinson SC, Lowry PJ. Selective elution of immunoadsorbed anti-(human prolactin) immunoglobulins with enhanced immunochemical properties. *Biochem J* 1982; **205**: 535–41.

72 Ehrlich PH, Moyle WR, Moustafa ZA, Canfield RE. Mixing two monoclonal antibodies yields enhanced affinity for antigen. *J Immunol* 1982; **128**: 2709–13.

73 Baker TS, Abbott SR, Daniel SG, Wright JF. Immunoradiometric assays. In: Collins WP, ed. *Alternative Immunoassays*. Chichester: John Wiley and Sons, 1984: 255–73.

74 Hunter WM, Bennie JG, Budd PS, van Heyningen V, James K, Micklem RI, Scott A. Immunoradiometric assays using monoclonal antibodies. In: Hunter WM, Carrie JET, eds. *Immunoassays for Clinical Chemistry*. Edinburgh: Churchill Livingstone, 1983: 531–44.

75 Salacinski PRP, Mclean C, Sykes JEC, Clement-Jones VV, Lowry PJ. Iodination of proteins, glycoproteins and peptides using a solid phase oxidising agent, 1,3,4,6-tetrachloro-3,6-diphenyl glycouril (Iodogen). *Anal Biochem* 1981; **117**: 136–46.

76 Hunter WM, Budd PS. Immunoradiometric versus radioimmunoassay: a comparison using alpha-fetoprotein as the model analyte. *J Immunol Methods* 1981; **45**: 225–73.

77 Hodgkinson SC, Allolio B, Landon J, Lowry PJ. Development of a non-extracted 'two-site' immunoradiometric assay for corticotropin utilizing extreme amino- and carboxy-terminally directed antibodies. *Biochem J* 1984; **218**: 703–11.

78 Linton EA, Mclean C, Nieuwenhuyzen Kruseman AC, Tilders FJ, van der Veen EA, Lowry PJ. Direct measurement of human plasma corticotropin-releasing hormone by 'two-site' immunoradiometric assay. *J Clin Endocrinol Metab* 1987; **64**: 1047–53.

79 Nussbaum SR, Zahradnik RJ, Lavigne JR *et al.* Highly sensitive two-site immunometric assay for parathyrin, and its clinical utility in evaluating patients with hypercalcemia. *Clin Chem* 1987; **33**: 1364–7.

80 Bassett F, Eastman CJ, Ma G, Maberly GF, Smith HC. Diagnostic value of thyrotropin concentrations in serum as measured by a sensitive immunoradiometric assay. *Clin Chem* 1986; **32**: 461–4.

81 Franklyn JA, Black EG, Betteridge D, Sheppard MC. Comparison of second and third generation methods for measurement of serum thyrotropin in patients with overt hyperthyroidism, patients receiving thyroxine therapy, and those with non-thyroidal illness. *J Clin Endocrinol Metab* 1994; **78**: 1368–71.

82 Mares A, De Boever J, Osher J, Quiroga S, Barnard G, Kohen F. A direct non-competitive idiometric enzyme immunoassay for serum oestradiol. *J Immunol Methods* 1995; **181**: 83–90.

83 Self CH, Dessi JL, Winger LA. High-performance assays of small molecules: enhanced sensitivity, rapidity, and convenience demonstrated with a non-competitive immunometric anti-immune complex assay system for digoxin. *Clin Chem* 1994; **40**: 2035–41.

84 Diamandis EP, Christopoulos TK. The biotin–(strept)avidin system: principles and applications in biotechnology. *Clin Chem* 1991; **37**: 625–36.

85 O'Connor JF, Schlatterer JP, Birken S *et al.* Development of highly sensitive immunoassays to measure human chorionic gonadotropin; its β-subunit and β core fragment in the urine: application to malignancies. *Cancer Res* 1988; **48**: 1361–6.

86 McLean M, Bisits A, Davies J, Woods R, Lowry P, Smith R. A placental clock controlling the length of human pregnancy. *Nature Med* 1995; **1**: 460–63.

87 Campbell EA, Linton EA, Wolfe CDA, Scraggs PR, Jones MT, Lowry PJ. Plasma corticotropin-releasing hormone concentrations during pregnancy and parturition. *J Clin Endocrinol Metab* 1987; **64**: 1054–9.

88 Ekins RP. An overview of present and future ultrasensitive non-isotopic immunoassay development. *Clin Biochem Rev* 1987; **8**: 12–23.

89 Hernmila I. Fluoroimmunoassays and immunofluorometric assays. *Clin Chem* 1985; **31**: 359–70.

90 Nikola H, Sundell AC, Hanninen E. Labelling of estradiol and testosterone alkoxime derivatives with a europium chelate for time-resolved fluoroimmunoassays. *Steroids* 1993; **58**: 330–4.

91 Markela E, Stahlberg TH, Hemmila I. Europium-labelled recombinant protein G. A fast and sensitive universal immunoreagent for time-resolved immunofluorometry. *J Immunol Methods* 1993; **161**: 1–6.

92 Storch MJ, Marbach P, Kerp L. A time-resolved fluoroimmunoassay for human insulin based on two monoclonal antibodies. *J Immunol Methods* 1993; **157**: 197–201.

93 Barnard G, Amir-Zaltsman Y, Lichter S, Gayer B, Kohan F. The measurement of oestrone-3-glucuronide in urine by non-competitive idiometric assay. *J Steroid Biochem Mol Biol* 1995; **55**: 107–14.

94 Messeri G, Martinazzo G, Tommasi A, Moneti G, Salemo R, Pazzagli M, Serio M. Chemiluminescent tracers for steroid measurement. In: Serio M, Pazzagli M, eds. *Luminescent Assays: Perspectives in Endocrinology and Clinical Chemistry*. New York: Raven Press, 1982: 207–14.

95 Kohen F, Kim JB, Barnard G, Lindner HR. An assay for urinary estriol-16α-glucuronide based on antibody-enhanced chemiluminescence. *Steroids* 1980; **36**: 405–19.

96 Messeri G, Caldini AL, Bolelli GF *et al.* Homogeneous luminescence immunoassay, for total estrogens in urine. *Clin Chem* 1984; **30**: 653–7.

97 Campbell AK, Patel A. A homogeneous immunoassay for cyclic nucleotides based on chemiluminescence energy transfer. *Biochem J* 1983; **216**: 185–94.

98 De Boever J, Kohen F, Vandekerckhore D, van Maele G. Solid-phase chemiluminescence immunoassay for progesterone in unextracted serum. *Clin Chem* 1984; **30**: 1637–41.

99 De Boever, Kohen F, Usanachitt C, Vandekerckhore D, Leyseele D, Vandewalle L. Direct chemiluminescence immunoassay for estradiol in serum. *Clin Chem* 1986; **32**: 1985–90.

100 Barnard GJ, Kim JB, Williams JL. Chemiluminescence immunoassay, and immunochemiluminometric assay. In: Collins WP, ed. *Alternative Immunoassays*. Chichester: John Wiley and Sons, 1984: 123–52.

101 Weeks I, Sturgess M, Brown RC, Woodhead JS. Immunoassays using acridinium esters. *Methods Enzymol* 1986; **133**: 366–87.

102 Richardson AP, Kim JB, Barnard GJ, Collins WP, McCapra F. Chemiluminescence immunoassay of plasma progesterone, with progesterone-acridinium ester used as the labelled antigen. *Clin Chem* 1985; **31**: 1664–8.

103 Weeks I, Woodhead JS. Measurements of human growth hormone (hGH) using a rapid immunochemiluminometric assay. *Clin Chim Acta* 1986; **159**: 139–45.

104 Bounaud MP, Bounaud JY, Bouin-Pineau MH, Orget L, Begon F. Chemiluminescence immunoassay of thyrotropin with acridinium-ester labelled antibody evaluated and compared with two other immunoassays. *Clin Chem* 1987; **33**: 2096–100.

105 Spencer CA, Lo Presti JS, Patel A *et al*. Applications of a new chemiluminometric thyrotropin assay to subnormal measurement. *J Clin Endocrinol Metab* 1990; **70**: 453–60.

106 Batmanghelich S, Brown RC, Woodhead JS, Weeks I, Smith K. Preparation of a chemiluminescent imidoester for the non-radioactive labelling of proteins. *J Photochem Photobiol B* 1992; **12**: 193–201.

107 Lee J, Seliger JJ. Absolute spectral sensitivity of phototubes and their application to the measurement of the absolute quantum yields of chemiluminescence and bioluminescence. *Photochem Photobiol* 1965; **4**: 1015–27.

108 Weeks I, Sturgess M, Brown RC, Woodhead JS. Immunoassays using acridinium esters. *Methods Enzymol* 1986; **133**: 366–87.

109 Kricka LJ. Ultrasensitive immunoassay techniques. *Clin Biochem* 1993; **26**: 325–331.

110 Wilkinson E, Rae PW, Thompson KJ, Toft AD, Spencer CA, Beckett GJ. Chemiluminescent third-generation assay (Amerlite TSH-30) of thyroid-stimulating hormone in serum or plasma assessed. *Clin Chem* 1993; **39**: 2167–73.

111 Pandrian MR, Odell WD, Carlton E, Fischer DA. Development of third-generation immunochemiluminometric assays of follitropin and lutropin and clinical application in determining pediatric reference ranges. *Clin Chem* 1993; **39**: 1815–19.

112 Rongen HA, Hoetelmans RM, Bult A, van-Bennekom WP. Chemiluminescence and immunoassays. *J Pharm Biomed Anal* 1994; **12**: 433–62.

113 Catherall CL, Palmer TF, Cundall RB. Determination of absolute chemiluminescence quantum yields for reactions of bis-(pentachlorophenyl) oxalate, hydrogen peroxide and fluorescent compounds. *J Biolumin Chemilumin* 1989; **3**: 147–54.

114 Pronovost AD, Baumgarten A. A comparison of chemiluminescence and absorptiometry in enzyme immunoassays for protein quantification. *Experientia* 1982; **38**: 304–6.

115 Thorpe GHG, Kricka LJ, Moseley SB, Whitehead TP. Phenols as enhancers of the chemiluminescent horseradish peroxidase-luminol-hydrogen peroxide reaction: application in luminescence monitored enzyme immunoassays. *Clin Chem* 1985; **31**: 1335–41.

116 Bronstein I, Kricka LJ. Clinical applications of luminescent assays for enzymes and enzyme labels. *J Clin Lab Anal* 1989; **3**: 315–22.

117 Frohman LA, Downs TR, Williams TC, Heimer EP, Pan YC, Felix AM. Rapid enzymatic degradation of growth hormone-releasing hormone by plasma *in vitro* and *in vivo* to a biologically inactive product cleaved at the NH_2 terminus. *J Clin Invest* 1986; **78**: 906–13.

118 Wehr CT. Sample preparation and column regeneration in biopolymer separations. *J Chromatogr* 1987; **418**: 27–50.

119 Fallon A, Booth RFG, Bell LD. Applications of HPLC in biochemistry. In: Burden RH, van Knippenberg PH, eds. *Laboratory Techniques in Biochemistry and Molecular Biology*. Amsterdam: Elsevier, 1987.

120 Patience RL, Penny ES. HPLC in endocrinology. *Adv Chromatogr* 1987; **27**: 37–72.

121 Oliver RWA, ed. *HPLC of Macromolecules. A Practical Approach*. Oxford: IRL Press, 1989.

122 Mefford IN, Caliguri EJ, Grady RK, Capella P, Durkin TA, Chevalier P. Microbore HPLC of biogenic amines in small biological samples. *Methods Enzymol* 1986; **124**: 402–12.

123 Kagedal B, Goldstein DS. Catecholamines and their metabolites. *J Chromatogr* 1988; **429**: 177–233.

124 Makin HL, Heftmann E. High performance liquid chromatography of steroid hormones. *Monogr Endocrinol* 1988; **30**: 183–234.

125 Erkoc FV, Ozsar S, Guven B, Kalkandelen G, Ugrar E. High-performance liquid chromatographic analysis of steroid hormones. *J Chromatogr Sci* 1989; **27**: 86–90.

126 Pearson JD, McCroskey MC, De Wald DB. Separation of protein hormones. *J Chromatogr* 1987; **418**: 245–76.

127 Corran PH. Reversed-phase chromatography of proteins. In: Oliver RWA, ed. *HPLC of Macromolecules. A Practical Approach*. Oxford: IRL Press, 1989: 127–56.

128 Reams GP, Souther M, Parisi M, van Stone JC, Bauer JH. Arterial-venous determinations of the 'immunoreactive' angiotensin peptides in human subjects. *J Lab Clin Med* 1989; **113**: 749–52.

129 Penny ES, Patience RL, Sopwith AM, Wass JA, Besser GM, Rees LH. Characterisation by high performance liquid chromatography of circulating growth hormone releasing factors in human plasma. *J Endocrinol* 1985; **105**(1): R_1–R_4.

130 Frohman LA, Downs TR. Measurement of growth hormone-releasing factor. *Methods Enzymol* 1986; **124**: 371–89.

131 Gaisano HY, Reilly W, Go VL, Olivero D, Miller LJ. Large forms of cholecystokinin circulating in humans. *Pancreas* 1986; **1**: 148–53.

132 Linden A, Carlquist M, Hansen S, Uvnas-Moberg K. Plasma concentrations of cholecystokinin, CCK-8, and CCK-33, 39 in rats, determined by a method based on digestion of gastrin before HPLC and RIA detection of CCK. *Gut* 1989; **30**: 213–22.

133 Patience RL, Rees LH. Comparison of reversed-phase and anion-exchange high-performance liquid chromatography for the analysis of human growth hormones. *J Chromatogr* 1986; **352**: 241–53.

134 Alpert AJ. Hydrophobic interaction chromatography of peptides as an alternative to reversed-phase chromatography. *J Chromatogr* 1988; **444**: 269–74.

135 Fausnaugh JL, Pfannkoch E, Gupta S, Regnier FE. High-performance hydrophobic interaction chromatography of proteins. *Annal Biochem* 1984; **137**: 464–72.

136 Heinitz ML, Kennedy L, Kopaciewicz W, Regnier FE. Chromatography of proteins on hydrophobic interaction and ion-exchange chromatographic matrices: mobile phase contributions to selectivity. *J Chromatogr* 1988; **443**: 173–82.

137 Oka K, Hirano T, Nogueki M. Changes in the concentration of testosterone in serum during the menstrual cycle, as determined by liquid chromatography. *Clin Chem* 1988; **34**: 557–60.

138 Vogt W, Egeler E, Sommer W, Eisenbeiss F, Meyer HD. High-performance liquid chromatographic determination of hormonal peptides and their fluorenylmethoxycarbonyl derivatives. *J Chromatogr* 1987; **400**: 83–9.

139 Schettler T, Kolk B, Atkinson MJ, Radeke H, Enters C, Hesch RD. Analysis of immunoreactive and biologically active human parathyroid hormone-peptides by high-performance liquid-chromatography. *Acta Endocrinol (Copenh)* 1984; **107**: 60–9.

140 Arendt RM, Stangl E, Zahringer J, Liebisch DC, Herz A. Demonstration and characterization of alpha-human atrial natriuetic factor in human plasma. *FEBS Lett* 1985; **189**: 57–61.
141 Venn RF. Combined high-performance liquid chromatographic-radioimmunoassay method for the analysis of endorphins, enkephalins and other neurotransmitter peptides. *J Chromatogr* 1987; **423**: 93–104.
142 Hayashi N, Hayata K, Sekiba K. Rapid and simultaneous measurement of estrone, estradiol, estriol and estertrol in serum by high-performance liquid chromatography with electrochemical detection. *Acta Med Okayama* 1985; **39**: 143–53.
143 Samaan GJ, Porquet D, Demelier JF, Biou D. Determination of cortisol and associated glucocorticoids in serum and urine by an automated liquid chromatographic assay. *Clin Biochem* 1993; **26**: 153–8.
144 Zola H, ed. *Monoclonal Antibodies. The Second Generation.* Oxford: BIOS, 1995.
145 Winter G, Milstein C. Man-made antibodies. *Nature* 1991; **349**: 293–9.
146 Geisow MJ. Improved selection systems for man-made antibodies. *Trends Biotech* 1992; **10**: 75–6.
147 Deng SJ, MacKenzie CR, Sadowska J *et al.* Selection of antibody single-chain variable fragments with improved carbohydrate binding by phage display. *J Biol Chem* 1994; **269**: 9533–8.
148 Holliger P, Prospero T, Winter G. 'Diabodies': Small bivalent and bispecific antibody fragments. *Proc Natl Acad Sci USA* 1993; **90**: 6444–8.
149 Chiswell D, McCafferty J. Phage antibodies: will new 'coliclonal' antibodies replace monoclonal antibodies? *Trends Biotechnol* 1992; **10**: 80–4.
150 Marks JD. By-passing immunization. Human antibodies from V-gene libraries displayed on phage. *J Mol Biol* 1991; **222**: 581–97.
151 Griffiths AD, Williams SC, Hartley O *et al.* Isolation of high affinity human antibodies directly from large synthetic repertoires. *EMBO J* 1994; **13**: 3245–60.
152 Romer M, Haeckel R, Capelli M, Rocipon J. The analytical performance of the Ciba Corning ACS: 180 automated immunoassay system: A multicentre evaluation. *Eur J Clin Chem Clin Biochem* 1994; **32**: 395–407.
153 Patterson W, Werness P, Payne WJ *et al.* Random and continuous-access immunoassays with chemiluminescent detection by Access automated analyser. *Clin Chem* 1994; **40**: 2042–45.
154 Costongs GM, van Oers RJ, Leerkens B, Hermans W, Janson PC. Evaluation of the Abbott automated random, immediate and continuous access immunoassay analyser, the Ax SYM. *Eur J Clin Chem Clin Biochem* 1995; **33**: 105–11.
155 Murthy JN, Hicks JM, Soldin SJ. Evaluation of the Technicon Immuno I random access immunoassay analyser and calculation of pediative reference ranges for endocrine tests, T-uptake and ferritin. *Clin Biochem* 1995; **28**: 181–5.
156 Vankrieken L, De Hertogh R. Rapid, automated quantification of total human chorionic gonadotropin in serum by a chemiluminescent enzyme immunometric assay. *Clin Chem* 1995; **41**: 36–40.

CHAPTER 8

Hypothalamic and pituitary tumours: general principles

M.E. Molitch

Introduction

Pituitary tumours are very common, occurring in about 11% of the population, as judged from some autopsy studies [1]. However, most of these are of little clinical significance. Small pituitary tumours may cause clinical syndromes due to their hormonal oversecretion but not due to mass effects. Larger pituitary tumours may also hypersecrete but can in addition give rise to a variety of problems due to their size; in particular, those with suprasellar extension may compress the optic chiasm or hypothalamic structures and the hypothalamo-pituitary stalk with resulting hypopituitarism. Similarly, tumours arising within the hypothalamus may also cause hypopituitarism and other clinical syndromes by compressing and distorting adjacent structures. Detailed hormonal evaluation coupled with magnetic resonance imaging (MRI) or computed tomography (CT) provides precise anatomical delineation of the extent of the lesion with considerable insight into the structural–functional relationships involved. The following summary is essentially an overview; detailed analysis of the lesions involved and their treatment can be found in subsequent chapters.

Classification

Hypothalamic tumours

Hypothalamic tumours are generally classified on the basis of their tissue of origin (Table 8.1). Craniopharyngiomas are the most common tumours affecting the hypothalamus after pituitary tumours. It is thought that they arise from remnants of Rathke's pouch. A variant or closely related lesion is the Rathke's cleft cyst, which develops from the space between the anterior and the rudimentary intermediate lobes. Clinically, the distinction is often impossible, although craniopharyngiomas are more commonly found in a suprasellar location while Rathke's cleft cysts are usually intrasellar [2,3].

Suprasellar dysgerminomas arise from primitive germ cells that have migrated to the central nervous system (CNS) during fetal life and structurally are identical to germ-cell tumours of the gonads. Other tumours and space-occupying lesions occurring in the suprasellar area include arachnoid cysts, meningiomas, gliomas, astrocytomas, chordomas, infundibulomas, cholesteatomas, neurofibromas, lipomas and metastatic cancer (particularly breast and lung). Other mass lesions that are not strictly tumours but must also be distinguished from pituitary and hypothalamic tumours include lymphocytic hypophysitis, Langerhans' cell histiocytosis, sarcoidosis, and infundibuloneurohypophysitis. Tumours are further classified as to malignancy, size, and invasiveness of surrounding structures with attention paid to the functional alteration of those surrounding structures, such as hypopituitarism [2,3].

Pituitary tumours

Pituitary tumours are generally classified clinically by:

1 the cell of origin, i.e. the hormones or subunits they produce;

2 size—whether they are microadenomas (< 10 mm in diameter), macroadenomas (> 10 mm in diameter), or macroadenomas with extrasellar extension (Fig. 8.1); and

3 invasiveness of surrounding structures (Table 8.2).

For most of the cell types, the degree of hormone overproduction dictates the severity of the clinical syndromes associated with the specific condition, for example acromegaly and Cushing's disease. However, for gonadotrophin-secreting adenomas symptoms relate primarily to the size of the lesion and not to the hormone overproduction.

Pituitary tumours are often further classified based on immunohistochemical and electron-microscopic characteristics.

Table 8.1 Classification of hypothalamic masses.

Cell rest tumours	Primitive germ-cell tumours
Craniopharyngioma	Germinoma
Rathke's cleft cyst	Dermoid
Epidermoid (cholesteatoma)	Teratoma
Infundibuloma	Atypical teratoma (germinoma)
Chordoma	Gliomas
Lipoma	Optic glioma
Arachnoid cyst	Oligodendroglioma
Hamartoma	Ependymoma
Gangliocytoma	Astrocytoma
Benign lesions	Granulomatous lesions
Meningioma	Sarcoidosis
Enchondroma	Mucocoele (sphenoid)
Arachnoid cyst	Giant-cell granuloma
Metastatic tumours	Langerhans´ cell histiocytosis
Aneurysms	Lymphocytic hypophysitis
Pituitary adenomas	Lymphocytic infundibuloneuro-hypophysitis

Thus, tumours may be sparsely or densely granulated, may show oncocytic characteristics [5], or may even have distant metastases and therefore be designated as being truly malignant. Over 40% of adenomas are invasive of surrounding tissue [6].

Epidemiology

Hypothalamic tumours

Craniopharyngiomas are the most common hypothalamic neoplasm, accounting for about 5–10% of brain tumours in childhood and 2.5% in all age groups. Although most tumours present during childhood with failure of normal growth being the primary finding, they may present at any age. Rathke's cleft cysts may be found in about 20% of normal pituitaries, but they are usually small and asymptomatic. Rarely they may be larger and present with

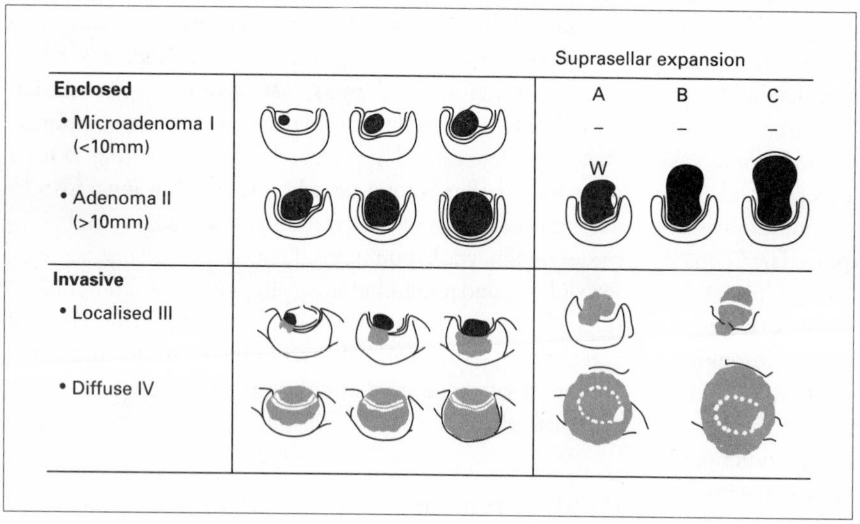

Fig. 8.1 Growth pattern of adenomas. From [4], with permission.

Table 8.2 Classification of pituitary tumours.

Hormone production	Size	Pathological characteristics
PRL producing	Microadenomas	Granulation (sparse, dense)
GH producing	Macroadenomas	Null cell (oncocytic/non-oncocytic)
ACTH producing	Macroadenomas with extrasellar extension	Hyperplasia
TSH producing	Invasive/non-invasive	Carcinoma
Gonadotrophin/subunit producing		
Plurihormonal		
Null cell		

PRL, prolactin; GH, growth hormone; ACTH, adrenocorticotrophic hormone; TSH, thyroid-stimulating hormone.

symptoms due to a mass lesion in the hypothalamo-pituitary area [2,3].

A hypothalamic hamartoma is a nodule of growth of hypothalamic neurons attached by a pedicle to the hypothalamus between the tuber cinereum and the mammillary bodies and extending into the basal cistern. Asymptomatic hamartomas may be present in up to 20% of random autopsies; rarely, these lesions may enlarge, causing disruption of hypothalamic function because of compression of adjacent tissue [2,3]. A variant of the hamartoma consisting of similar tissue present within the anterior pituitary but without a neural attachment to the hypothalamus is called a choristoma or gangliocytoma. These neuronal tumours are of particular endocrine interest because they can produce hypophysiotrophic hormones. A number of cases of hamartomas associated with precocious puberty have been reported in which the hamartomas produce gonadotrophin-releasing hormone (GnRH). Some gangliocytomas produce growth hormone (GH)-releasing hormone (GHRH) and acromegaly and others corticotrophin-releasing hormone (CRH) and Cushing's disease [7]. In some of these tumours, direct contact between the gangliocytoma GHRH-containing neuronal cells and the pituitary GH-secretory cells suggested a paracrine effect.

Dysgerminomas most commonly present in children and may account for up to 6.5% of brain tumours during childhood [8]. They usually cause a triad of hypopituitarism, diabetes insipidus and visual problems [9]. Hyperprolactinaemia occurs in over 50% and 10% have precocious puberty due to the production of chorionic gonadotrophin by the tumour [9]. About 10% are malignant and metastasize within and without the CNS [7].

Over 80% of optic gliomas present before the age of 10 with visual problems, diabetes insipidus and hypopituitarism. Overall, these tumours account for about 3% of brain tumours in childhood and 1% of intracranial tumours in adults [2,3]. About 20–25% of patients with such tumours have von Recklinghausen's neurofibromatosis [3]. Hypothalamic gliomas are much less common and, in young children, may be associated with the 'diencephalic syndrome', with failure to gain weight, a seeming 'hyperalert' appearance, diabetes insipidus, and visual disturbance [2].

Parasellar meningiomas are quite common and usually present between the ages of 40 and 50 years with women outnumbering men 4–10-fold. This parasellar location accounts for about 20% of all intracranial meningiomas. Visual disturbance, headache, diabetes insipidus and hypopituitarism are characteristic findings [2,3].

Metastatic disease to the sellar area occurs in 3–5% of malignancies, although 15–25% of patients with breast cancer may be found to have metastases to the pituitary. Lung and gastrointestinal malignancies are other frequent primary cancers for such metastases. Such lesions may be asymptomatic but may also cause hypopituitarism, diabetes insipidus and visual disturbance. Once detected because they had enlarged sufficiently to cause symptoms, they are usually found to grow much more quickly than other pituitary masses [10].

Granulomatous conditions such as sarcoidosis, Langerhans' cell histiocytosis or lymphocytic infundibuloneurohypophysitis usually present as infiltrative lesions but may present as mass lesions. The most common endocrine findings are varying degrees of hypopituitarism, diabetes insipidus and hyperprolactinaemia [2,3].

Lymphocytic hypophysitis virtually always presents as a mass lesion with extensive infiltration of the pituitary and extension into the suprasellar area. Direct pituitary destruction causes hypopituitarism with hyperprolactinaemia resulting from the stalk/hypothalamic disruption. Almost all present in the peripartum period and very few have been reported in men [11].

Pituitary tumours

The frequencies reported for any series of pituitary tumours are usually biased by the method of ascertainment. For example, surgical or pathology series usually under-report the frequency of prolactinomas, as most such are generally treated medically rather than surgically. Clinically non-functioning tumours and gonadotroph adenomas are usually reported as being macroadenomas, as they present with symptoms due to the size of the lesion rather than to hormone overproduction, so that microadenomas are not usually recognised during life.

Autopsy series report that pituitary adenomas may be found in about 11% of people but such adenomas are almost always microadenomas [1]. This suggests that virtually all macroadenomas come to clinical attention and therefore are not included in autopsy findings. Studies of CT or MRI scans in normal subjects show similar findings [12,13].

The number of pituitary adenomas that reach clinical significance because of hormone production or size is clearly smaller. Pituitary adenomas are estimated to comprise about 10% of all intracranial tumours [14]. In a surgical series in which all 1043 tumours were carefully immunostained, the following proportions of tumour types were found: prolactinomas, 27.2%; non-functioning tumours, 25.2%; GH-secreting adenomas, 14.0%; GH–PRL (prolactin)-secreting tumours, 8.4%; Cushing's disease, 8.0; gonadotroph adenomas, 6.4%; silent ACTH-producing adenomas, 6.0%; plurihormonal adenomas, 3.7%; and thyrotroph adenomas, 1% [5]. Over 90% of prolactinomas [15] and ACTH-secreting tumours [16] are microadenomas while only 25–50% of tumours in patients with acromegaly are microadenomas [17] and virtually no gonadotroph cell adenomas that come to clinical attention are microadenomas.

Pathogenesis of pituitary adenomas

The role of the hypothalamus in the pathogenesis of pituitary tumours is controversial. A primary defect in hypothalamic regulation of hormone secretion has been hypothesised to either cause or facilitate the growth of adenomas by some investigators (Fig. 8.2). Others hypothesise that most changes in hypothalamic function in patients with tumours are secondary to the tumours, the tumours arising *de novo* as intrinsic disorders of the pituitary [18].

Four lines of evidence point to the latter hypothesis as being correct:

1 there is no hyperplasia of the non-neoplastic hormone secretory cells in the non-neoplastic portions of the pituitary, as would be expected if hypothalamic dysfunction exists [18];

2 abnormal hormonal secretory dynamics resolve with pituitary-tumour resection implying that the abnormal dynamics are due to the tumour itself rather than due to underlying hypothalamic dysfunction [18];

3 most tumours can be permanently cured by pituitary tumour resection, and the fact that tumour recurrence generally happens early suggests that the recurrence is due to regrowth of tumour remnants rather than due to underlying hypothalamic dysfunction [18]; and

4 most pituitary tumours have been found to be monoclonal, as would be expected if they arise *de novo*, rather than polyclonal, as would be expected if hypothalamic dysfunction is primary [19].

However, these findings 'do not exclude a facilitory role for the hypothalamus in pituitary tumorigenesis, perhaps by inducing clonal expansion of a genomically altered cell [19].'

Somatic mutations that cause tumours have been investigated extensively. In about 40% of GH-secreting tumours a mutation has been identified, the *gsp* mutation that results in an amino-acid substitution at positions 201 or 227 in the α-subunit of the guanine nucleotide-binding stimulatory regulatory protein that couples the GHRH receptor to adenylyl cyclase, thereby causing unregulated, high activity of adenylyl cyclase coupled with excess secretion of GH. The *gsp* mutation results in tumours that tend to be smaller than tumours in which the mutation is not present but no other differences in biological activity are apparent [20,21]. Mutations have been sought without much success so far in genes for other proteins involved in hormone regulation or cell proliferation, such as hormone receptors, protein kinase C, *ras* and other proto-oncogenes, and transcription factors, such as Pit-1. How-ever, it is likely that additional pathogenetic mutations will be found with continued investigation.

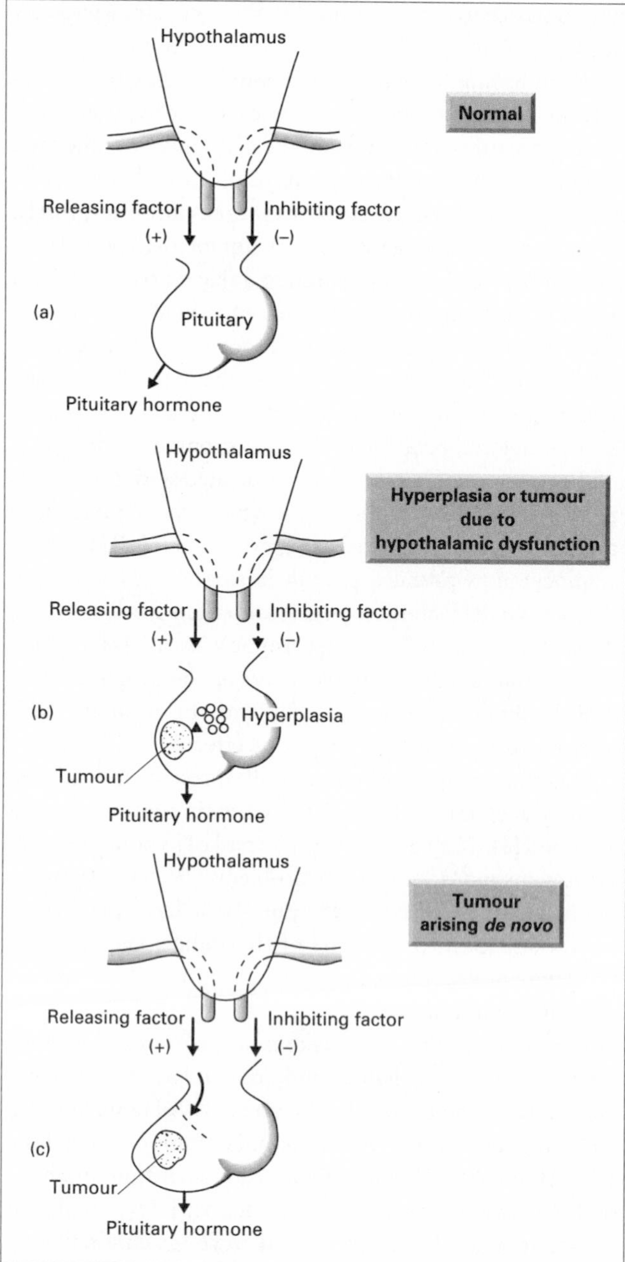

Fig. 8.2 Possible mechanisms leading to the formation of a hormone-secreting pituitary tumour. (a) Normal regulation by release and inhibiting factors. (b) Tumours could arise because of an increase in releasing factor or a decrease in inhibiting factor. (c) Tumours could arise *de novo* without hypothalamic influence, presumably as a result of a mutation occurring in a single cell with subsequent clonal proliferation. From [18], with permission.

Clinical manifestations

Hypothalamic tumours and pituitary macroadenomas extending superiorly to abut the hypothalamus may cause substantial disruption of hypothalamic function. The hypothalamic hypophysiotrophic neurons are concentrated in the area surrounding the third ventricle and their axonal pathways all come together in the medial basal hypothalamus as they converge on the median eminence. Thus, lesions located within this final common pathway might be expected to cause significant impairment of the hypothalamic regulation of pituitary function for all of the pituitary hormones. Other functions of the hypothalamus are more diffuse, such as the regulation of temperature which is located in a large region of the preoptic anterior hypothalamus. Hypothalamic dysfunction can be grouped into three major categories:

1 anterior pituitary dysfunction;
2 neurohypophyseal dysfunction; and
3 non-pituitary dysfunction, including disorders of temperature regulation, thirst, eating behaviour, sleep, autonomic nervous system regulation, memory, emotional behaviour and cognition.

Symptoms due to hypothalamic dysfunction are related to the size of the lesion and consequently the area of the hypothalamus involved, as well as the rapidity of increase in size of the lesion. Tumours in this area can often grow quite large (8–10 cm in diameter) over many years with little in the way of symptoms. Slowly growing lesions tend to cause problems of hormone dysregulation rather than to present with dramatic symptoms. However, a haemorrhage into even a small tumour of 1-cm diameter that causes it to increase rapidly to 2–3 cm diameter can cause major disruption of hypothalamic function, including decreased levels of consciousness, temperature dysregulation and disturbance of cardiovascular function. Large, slowly growing lesions can cause more acute problems, however, when a slight increment in growth results in eliminating remaining vestiges of vasopressin or ACTH secretion or completely occludes the aqueduct of Sylvius or the foramen of Monro causing hydrocephalus. Rarely, such tumours may cause mental dysfunction and symptoms and signs due to increased intracranial pressure, such as nausea, vomiting, headache and papilloedema.

Hypothalamic and pituitary tumours can cause varying degrees of hypopituitarism by either compressing the normal pituitary or, more commonly, by affecting the pituitary stalk and mediobasal hypothalamus, as discussed above. Although severe involvement can cause absolute deficiencies of the various hormones, more mild disease may cause a subtle alteration of feedback loops and timing such that, for example, the integration of signals necessary for menstrual cycling is lost, resulting in 'hypothalamic' amenorrhoea. Hyperprolactinaemia occurs commonly, due primarily to disinhibition by the hypothalamus, with decreased dopamine reaching the pituitary. PRL elevations due to such lesions are rarely greater than 10-fold that of normal, and usually are less than five-fold that of normal [22]. Hyperprolactinaemia occurring with hypothalamic dysfunction also causes a hypogonadotrophic hypogonadism that is reversible when the elevated PRL levels are brought down to normal. Evidence that hypopituitarism is from pituitary compression includes a low serum PRL level and a lack of thyroid-stimulating hormone (TSH) response to thyrotrophin-releasing hormone (TRH); pituitary function in such cases usually does not improve after treatment [23]. In patients with normal or elevated PRL levels, pituitary function often returns following tumour removal [23].

Precocious puberty is an uncommon manifestation of hypothalamic tumours. GnRH dependent precocious puberty represents a premature activation of the GnRH pulse generator by a variety of lesions or it may also be idiopathic. Boys tend to have more serious underlying disease, with hypothalamic hamartomas accounting for 38% of cases, other CNS lesions representing 31%, familial disease accounting for 23% and idiopathic disease accounting for only 8% [24]. The picture is quite different in girls, however, as hypothalamic hamartomas account for only 15% of cases, other CNS lesions represent 14%, the McCune–Albright syndrome (polyostotic fibrous dysplasia) accounts for 6% and fully 65% are idiopathic [24]. Germinomas in the suprasellar or pineal region can produce chorionic gonadotrophin (hCG) which acts like luteinising hormone (LH) in its stimulation of gonadal function. Usually such tumours cause increased sex steroid formation but fail to cause ovulation.

Diabetes insipidus can develop as a result of destructive lesions in the supraoptic and paraventricular nuclei or in the mediobasal hypothalamus in the path of the neural fibres containing vasopressin that are passing on to the posterior pituitary. Irritative lesions can trigger the release of vasopressin in an unregulated fashion, resulting in the syndrome of inappropriate ADH (vasopressin) secretion (SIADH).

Visual field defects due to chiasmal compression depend upon the amount of suprasellar extension for pituitary adenomas. Because of the great variation in how these tumours grow superiorly with respect to the location of the chiasm, visual field defects can range from the classical complete bitemporal hemianopia to small, partial quadrantic defects to scotomas [25]. Hypothalamic masses may cause similar visual field defects by compressing the optic chiasm against the sphenoid bone inferiorly [25].

Ophthalmoplegias are relatively uncommon, being due to invasion of the cavernous sinus with entrapment of cranial nerves III, IV and VI. The first and second divisions of the trigeminal nerve (V_1 and V_2) and the carotid artery are other major structures in the cavernous sinus that can be involved. In some patients a cavernous sinus syndrome may develop, consisting of ophthalmoplegia and pain or dysaesthesia in the distribution of V_1 [25].

Extensive invasion of the floor of the skull with massive destruction of bone occasionally occurs, occasionally causing problems by entrapping cranial nerves and compressing vital brain structures [26]. Erosion through the floor of the sella may cause cerebrospinal fluid (CSF) rhinorrhoea. Extrasellar extension in other directions may cause temporal lobe epilepsy and hydrocephalus [26]. These large, invasive tumours are uncommon but not rare and should be differentiated from true carcinomas; a demonstration of metastases distant from the primary tumour is necessary for the latter diagnosis [27].

Destruction of the ventromedial nucleus (VMN) inhibits satiety and results in hyperphagia and hypothalamic obesity [28]. The hyperphagia is due to destruction of noradrenergic fibres originating in the paraventricular nucleus and the hyperinsulinaemia that occurs with hypothalamic obesity is due to destruction of the VMN itself [29]. Hypothalamic anorexia is very rare, probably owing to the requirement for bilateral lesions. As opposed to a lesion in the mid-line which could easily damage both ventromedial nuclei, a single lesion damaging both sides of the hypothalamus in its lateral aspects would have to be very large and cause a great deal of other hypothalamic dysfunction. Similarly, because of the requirement for extensive hypothalamic damage, disturbances of temperature regulation are rare [30].

In addition to causing these mass effects, pituitary tumours may cause symptoms because of the hypersecretion of hormones. The specific clinical syndromes associated with PRL-, GH-, ACTH- and TSH-secreting tumours are detailed elsewhere. Gonadotrophin-producing tumours rarely cause symptoms related to the overproduction of the gonadotrophins or their subunits and usually present with mass effects.

Diagnosis

Patients generally come to clinical attention because of the symptoms described in the previous section. Once such a lesion is suspected, it is important to define it anatomically and then to characterise any hormone under- or oversecretion.

Anatomical evaluation

Conventional X-rays of the skull and polytomographic views of the sellar area lack sensitivity and specificity and are of little value nowadays. MRI with gadolinium enhancement currently represents the best way of discerning lesions affecting the hypothalamus and any consequent distortion of other hypothalamic structures. CT scanning with intravenous contrast and direct coronal thin sections (1.5 mm) is also quite good at delineating these lesions and may provide unique information regarding bone structure and distortion. In general, MRI creates better, artefact-free multiplanar images that may show the anatomical abnormality more clearly [31,32]. When assessing patients for anatomical evidence of secretory tumours, it is important to realise that with respect to microadenomas a number of other structures may give a similar appearance, including cysts, old infarcts and many of the lesions discussed above. In studies of normal subjects, CT and MRI scans of the sella reveal > 3 mm lesions in 4–20% [1].

Formal visual field testing may discern impingement of the optic nerves and chiasm by hypothalamic lesions, including the suprasellar extension of pituitary tumours. The lack of a visual field defect in no way excludes suprasellar disease, however, and very large lesions may be present which can be documented to distort the chiasm on MRI scan but may not cause visual field defects [25].

Hormonal evaluation

Detailed testing of hypothalamo-pituitary function may detect hormonal abnormalities with greater sensitivity and precision. Whenever hypothalamic lesions or pituitary macroadenomas are found, detailed evaluation of anterior and posterior hypothalamo-pituitary function is indicated. Often, however, dynamic testing of pituitary function will generally not differentiate between the hypothalamus and the pituitary as the specific primary locus of the defect. Hypopituitarism is very rare in patients with pituitary microadenomas and detailed testing is usually not warranted.

Testing for GH reserve is indicated clinically only in children who have not finished growing and therefore might be candidates for GH therapy. At present, GH therapy in adults is considered to be experimental and therefore testing for deficiency has no clear therapeutic consequences. There is no absolutely reliable test for GH reserve. The 'gold standard' of testing for GH deficiency is insulin-induced hypoglycaemia [33]. Other stimuli such as L-dopa, arginine, clonidine and exercise, alone or in combination, offer no increased reliability but because of ease of use, the relative unpleasantness of hypoglycaemic stimulation, and the limitation of hypoglycaemia in older individuals or those with CNS disorders, many groups use these alternative testing procedures. Insulin-like growth factor (IGF) binding protein 3 (BP3) functions as a reservoir for GH and is positively regulated by GH, being elevated in states of GH excess and decreased in states of GH deficiency. Some paediatricians measure IGF-1 and IGF-BP3 levels as a preliminary screen for GH deficiency [34]. Testing for GH deficiency with GHRH has not yet become a standard part of practice.

ACTH deficiency is the major, life-threatening hormone deficiency and must be tested for immediately when suspected. Most standardised tests have assessed ACTH secretion indirectly by measuring the cortisol response to stimuli, but recently the ACTH–IRMA assay allows precise estimates of ACTH release. Modalities of testing include the responses to insulin-induced hypoglycaemia, metyrapone and CRH

[35]. Metyrapone testing should never be carried out if basal cortisol levels are very low, as it may precipitate adrenal crisis.

Assessment for TSH deficiency simply requires measurement of TSH and thyroxine (T_4). When thyroid hormone levels are low, low or inappropriately normal or even mildly elevated TSH levels are found. Similar test results may also be found in patients with the euthyroid sick syndrome, although in the latter normal free-T_4 levels will usually be found. Testing with TRH is of little benefit, although patients with hypothalamic lesions tend to have TSH peaks delayed to 60–120 min instead of at 15–20 min [36]. In some patients, basal TSH levels may actually be mildly elevated to the 7–15 μU/ml range but this TSH is abnormally glycosylated, resulting in decreased biological activity [36].

The finding of low or normal gonadotrophins with low target-organ hormones (oestradiol or testosterone) points to the defect being in the pituitary or hypothalamus. Stimulation with GnRH is not reliable in distinguishing between a pituitary versus a hypothalamic site of the defect [37]. Intrinsic defects of this axis cannot readily be assessed while the patient is hyperprolactinaemic.

Vasopressin deficiency should be assessed by measuring the vasopressin response to an osmotic stimulus, obtained either by careful, observed dehydration or the administration of hypertonic saline, as long as the patient does not display baseline hyperosomolality. Dysregulated excessive vasopressin secretion (SIADH) can be documented by the finding of an inappropriately elevated urine osmolality at the time of plasma hypoosmolality or can be brought out with water loading.

Treatment

The goals of treatment of pituitary and hypothalamic tumours are:

1 to reduce or eliminate the mass effects due to the tumours;
2 to correct hypersecretion of hormones produced by pituitary tumours;
3 to preserve remaining pituitary function;
4 to prevent damage to other surrounding structures; and
5 to correct hormonal deficiencies and other sequelae of the tumour. Careful assessment of anatomical and functional aspects of the tumour, as outlined in the previous section, and the general clinical status of the patient will allow determination of the best therapeutic approach.

For all pituitary tumours except prolactinomas, transsphenoidal surgery remains the treatment of choice unless there are specific contraindications [38]. For microadenomas, initial cure rates of 70–80% with subsequent recurrence rates of 5–15% and virtually 100% preservation of remaining pituitary function may be expected in experienced neurosurgical hands [39]. Mortality rates for microadenomas approach those of anesthaesia alone and morbidity is generally under 2% (transient diabetes insipidus (DI), infection, CSF rhinorrhoea) [39]. In patients with macroadenomas, the cure rates fall and the complication rates rise with the size of the tumour [39]. With very large tumours, especially those with ex-tensive supra- or parasellar extension, craniotomy with a subfrontal approach may be necessary. Mortality rates from this approach are in the 1–10% range with concomitant marked increase in complications. For most patients with hypothalamic tumours, a craniotomy with a subfrontal approach is usually necessary. Panhypopituitarism and DI from cutting the hypothalamo-pituitary stalk and other hypothalamic damage are, unfortunately, fairly common sequelae of such surgery [40].

Conventional irradiation is of varying efficacy in reducing tumour size and decreasing hormone levels. It also carries substantial side-effects. Hypopituitarism resulting from surgery plus irradiation is very common [41] and is thought to be due to hypothalamic radiation damage [41]. By 8 years after surgery plus irradiation in one series, 100% were GH deficient, 96% were gonadotrophin deficient, 84% were ACTH deficient and 49% were TSH deficient [41]. Two recent series found a cumulative risk of 2–3% over 20 years of second brain tumours [42,43]. Other problems may also include an increased risk of stroke after pituitary irradiation [44] and, rarely, hypothalamic damage causing memory loss, temperature dysregulation, etc. There is a perception based on anecdotal experience that patients' memory, calculating ability and other critical thinking processes are commonly impaired by irradiation even with conventional doses but no prospective studies have confirmed this. Nevertheless, other centres have suggested that with a total radiation dose limited to 45 Gy, in low dose fractions via three fields, there is little or no risk of visual pathway or hypothalamic damage, with high cure rates (if delayed) and a low risk of hypopituitarism. However, because of the concerns raised above, irradiation is usually reserved for patients not cured by surgery and not responding to medical therapy. Similarly, patients with hypothalamic tumours generally are treated with radiotherapy when surgery has not been curative. One exception to this is the germinoma, which is exquisitely radiosensitive and, in some cases, may be treated with radiotherapy alone [9].

Specific medical therapies have been developed for various tumour types based primarily on what is known about basic hormone regulation. Thus, for prolactinomas, dopamine agonists such as bromocriptine have been used now for over 20 years, providing rates of normalisation of PRL (80–85% of patients) and tumour size reduction (75% of patients with macroadenomas) that are far better than that achieved by surgery. For this tumour type, medical therapy is widely regarded as primary therapy and surgery is generally carried out in those patients who do not respond to medical treatment [15]. Additional dopaminergic agents such as pergolide, quinagolide and cabergoline have also been developed that afford larger dosing intervals, but their safety experience during pregnancy limits their use when fertility is an issue, at least at present [15]. In women in whom fertility and tumour size reduction are not issues, replacement with oestrogen/progesterone may suffice [45].

Although dopaminergic agents paradoxically reduce GH levels in patients with acromegaly, only about 20% can achieve normal GH levels and an even smaller number can achieve normal IGF-1 levels [46]. The long-acting somatostatin analogue, octreotide, can cause a normalisation of GH and IGF-1 levels in over 50% of patients [47]. Octreotide has also been found to be extremely useful in patients with the more uncommon TSH-secreting tumours, reducing TSH and thyroid hormone levels to normal in 84% of patients treated for 3–61 months and reducing tumour size in 40% of patients [48].

In patients with Cushing's disease, therapeutic agents have been much less successful at reducing ACTH levels and corticotroph tumour size. Ketoconazole, an imidazole derivative which inhibits several enzymatic steps of steroid synthesis, lowers and maintains cortisol levels in the normal range with concomitant symptom relief in over 90% of patients [49]. Some groups have also had considerable success with the 11-hydroxylase inhibitor, metyrapone. Other medical therapies, including cyproheptadine, sodium valproate, bromocriptine and mitotane have had much lower degrees of success. Medical therapy of gonadotroph adenomas has been disappointing, dopamine agonists, GnRH antagonists and octreotide showing minimal if any tumour size reduction although hormone secretion can sometimes be decreased [38].

Medical therapy of hypothalamic tumours has generally not been carried out with the exception of hamartomas that produce GnRH. Successful treatment has been reported with the administration of a long-acting GnRH analogue which suppresses gonadotrophin secretion but does not affect the tumour itself. Medical therapy with the GnRH analogue may be the best choice as surgery can be non-curative or even fatal, if the hamartoma does not cause other problems from mass effects [50]. Other tumours that are unresectable, such as germinomas, may occasionally require treatment with more conventional forms of cancer chemotherapy.

When patients are found to have deficiencies of pituitary hormones, replacement therapy is usually indicated [35,38,51]. Glucocorticoids must always be replaced when deficits are demonstrated, prednisone being far cheaper than hydrocortisone. A replacement dose of 2.5–7.5 mg/day usually suffices and it is important to recognize the considerable variability in dose requirements. Such therapy will need to be increased in periods of stress such as infection, trauma or surgery. Patients also need to be informed about steroid cover during illness. Mineralocorticoid replacement is not necessary. L-Thyroxine must also be replaced but the dose cannot be titrated against the TSH level. Doses in the 0.075–0.2 mg/day range are usually necessary and the dose is adjusted according to clinical symptoms. Sex hormone replacement is strongly advised not only to permit normal libido and sexual function but also to prevent osteoporosis in both sexes and cardiovascular disease in women. As mentioned previously, GH treatment is, at present, indicated only in the child whose epiphyses have not closed. The use of GH in adults is still considered experimental and the benefit/risk ratio remains to be determined.

References

1 Molitch ME, Russell EJ. The pituitary "incidentaloma." *Ann Intern Med* 1990; **112**: 925–31.

2 Post KD, McCormick PC, Bellow JA. Differential diagnosis of pituitary tumours. *Endocrinol Metab Clin N Amer* 1987; **16**: 609–45.

3 Braunstein GD. The hypothalamus. In: Melmed S, ed. *The Pituitary*. Cambridge, MA: Blackwell Science, 1995: 309–40.

4 Hardy J. Transsphenoidal surgery of hypersecreting pituitary tumours. In: Kohler PO, Ross GT, eds. *Diagnosis and Treatment of Pituitary Tumours*. New York: Elsevier, 1973: 179–94.

5 Kovacs K, Horvath E. Pathology of pituitary tumours. *Endocrinol Metab Clin N Amer* 1987; **16**: 529–51.

6 Sautner D, Saeger W. Invasiveness of pituitary adenomas. *Path Res Pract* 1991; **187**: 632–6.

7 Saeger W, Puchner MJA, Lüdecke DK. Combined sellar gangliocytoma and pituitary adenoma in acromegaly or Cushing's disease. *Virchows Archiv* 1994; **425**: 93–9.

8 Jennings MT, Gelman R, Hochberg F. Intracranial germ-cell tumours: natural history and pathogenesis. *J Neurosurg* 1985; **63**: 155–67.

9 Sklar CA, Grumbach MM, Kaplan SL, Conte FA. Hormonal and metabolic abnomalities associated with central nervous system germinoma in children and adolescents and the effect of therapy: report of 10 patients. *J Clin Endocrinol Metab* 1981; **52**: 9–16.

10 Shubiger O, Haller D. Metastases to the pituitary–hypothalamic axis. An MR study of 7 symptomatic patients. *Neuroradiology* 1992; **34**: 131–4.

11 Powrie JK, Powell M, Ayers AB, Lowy C, Sönksen PH. Lymphocytic adenohypophysitis: magnetic resonance imaging features of two new cases and a review of the literature. *Clin Endocrinol* 1995; **42**: 315–22.

12 Chambers EF, Turski PA, LaMasters D, Newton TH. Regions of low density in the contrast-enhanced pituitary gland: normal and pathologic processes. *Radiology* 1982; **144**: 109–13.

13 Hall WA, Luciano MG, Doppman JL, Patronas NJ, Oldfield EH. Pituitary magnetic resonance imaging in normal human volunteers: occult adenomas in the general population. *Ann Intern Med* 1994; **120**: 817–20.

14 Gold EB: Epidemiology of pituitary adenomas. *Epidemiol Rev* 1981; **3**: 163–83.

15 Molitch ME. Prolactinoma. In: Melmed S, ed. *The Pituitary*. Cambridge, MA: Blackwell Science, 1995: 443–77.

16 Aron DC, Findling JW, Tyrrell JB. Cushing's disease. *Endocrinol Metab Clin N Amer* 1987; **16**: 705–30.

17 Nabarro JDN. Acromegaly. *Clin Endocrinol* 1987; **26**: 481–512.

18 Molitch ME. Pathogenesis of pituitary tumours. *Endocrinol Metab Clin N Amer* 1987; **16**: 503–27.

19 Herman V, Fagin J, Gonsky R, Kovacs K, Melmed S. Clonal origin of pituitary adenomas. *J Clin Endocrinol Metab* 1990; **71**: 1427–33.

20 Landis CA, Harsh G, Lyons J, Davis RL, McCormick F, Bourne HR.: Clinical characteristics of acromegalic patients whose pituitary tumours contain mutant G_s protein. *J Clin Endocrinol Metab* 1990; **71**: 1416–20.

21 Spada A, Arosio M, Bochicchio D *et al.* Clinical, biochemical and morphological correlates in patients bearing growth hormone-secreting pituitary tumours with or without constitutively active adenyl cyclase. *J Clin Endocrinol Metab* 1990; **71**: 1421–6.

22 Molitch ME, Reichlin S. Hypothalamic hyperprolactinemia: neuroendocrine regulation of prolactin secretion in patients with lesions of the hypothalamus and pituitary stalk. In: MacLeod RN, Thorner MO, Scapagnini U, eds. *Prolactin. Basic and Clinical Correlates. Proceedings of the IVth International Congress on Prolactin*. Padova, Italy: Liviana Press, 1985: 709–19.

23 Arafah BM. Reversible hypopituitarism in patients with large nonfunctioning pituitary adenomas. *J Clin Endocrinol Metab* 1986; **62**: 1173–9.

24 Stein DT. New developments in the diagnosis and treatment of sexual precocity. *Am J Med Sci* 1992; **303**: 53–71.

25 Melen O. Neuro-ophthalmologic features of pituitary tumours. *Endocrinol Metab Clin N Amer* 1987; **16**: 585–608.

26 Davis JRE, Sheppard MC, Heath DA. Giant invasive prolactinoma: a case report and review of nine further cases. *Quart J Med* 1990; **74**: 227–38.

27 Atienza DM, Vigersky RJ, Lack EE *et al.* Prolactin-producing pituitary carcinoma with pulmonary metastases. *Cancer* 1991; **63**: 1605–10.

28 Bray GA, Gallagher TF, Jr. Manifestations of hypothalamic obesity in man: a comprehensive investigation of eight patients and a review of the literature. *Medicine* 1975; **54**: 301–30.

29 Leibowitz SF. Brain monoamines and peptides: role in the control of eating behavior. *Fed Proc* 1986; **45**: 1396–403.

30 Boulant JA. Hypothalamic mechanisms in thermoregulation. *Fed Proc* 1981; **40**: 2843–50.

31 Elster AD. Modern imaging of the pituitary. *Radiology* 1993; **187**: 1–14.

32 Chong BW, Newton TH: Hypothalamic and pituitary pathology. *Radiol Clin N Amer* 1993; **31**: 1147–53.

33 Hoffman DM, O'Sullivan AJ, Baxter RC, Ho KKY. Diagnosis of growth-hormone deficiency in adults. *Lancet* 1994; **343**: 1064–8.

34 Blum WF, Albertsson-Wikland K, Rosberg S, Ranke MB. Serum levels of insulin-like growth factor I (IGF-1) and IGF binding protein 3 reflect spontaneous growth hormone secretion. *J Clin Endocrinol Metab* 1993; **76**: 1610–16.

35 Vance ML. Hypopituitarism. *N Engl J Med* 1994; **330**: 1651–62.

36 Samuels MH, Ridgway EC. Central hypothyroidism. *Endocrinol Metab Clin N Amer* 1992; **21**: 903–19.

37 Whitcomb RW, Crowley WF, Jr. Male hypogonadotropic hypogonadism. *Endocrinol Metab Clin N Amer* 1993; **22**: 125–43.

38 Klibanski Z, Zervas NT. Diagnosis and management of hormone-secreting pituitary adenomas. *N Engl J Med* 1991; **324**: 822–31.

39 Laws ER: Pituitary surgery. *Endocrinol Metab Clin N Amer* 1987; **16**: 647–65.

40 Fahlbusch R, Schrell U. Surgical therapy of lesions within the hypothalamic region. *Acta Neurochir* 1985; **75**: 125–35.

41 Littley MD, Shalet SM, Beardwell CG, Ahmed SR, Applegate G, Sutton ML. Hypopituitarism following external radiotherapy for pituitary tumours in adults. *Quart J Med* 1989; **262**: 145–60.

42 Brada M, Ford D, Ashley S *et al.* Risk of second brain tumour after conservative surgery and radiotherapy for pituitary adenoma. *Br Med J* 1992; **304**: 1343–6.

43 Tsang RW, Laperriere NJ, Simpson WJ, Brierley J, Panazrella T, Smyth HS. Glioma arising after radiation therapy for pituitary adenoma. *Cancer* 1993; **72**: 2227–33.

44 Bowen J, Paulsen CA. Stroke after pituitary irradiation. *Stroke* 1992; **23**: 908–11.

45 Corenblum B, Donovan L. The safety of physiological estrogen plus progestin replacement therapy and with oral contraceptive therapy in women with pathological hyperprolactinemia. *Fertil Steril* 1993; **59**: 671–3.

46 Jaffe CA, Barkan AL. Treatment of acromegaly with dopamine agonists. *Endocrinol Metab Clin N Amer* 1992; **21**: 713–35.

47 Ezzat S, Snyder PJ, Young WF *et al.* Octreotide treatment of acromegaly. A randomized, multicenter study. *Ann Intern Med* 1992; **117**: 711–18.

48 Chanson P, Weintraub BD, Harris AG. Octreotide therapy for thyroid-stimulating hormone-secreting pituitary adenomas. *Ann Intern Med* 1993; **119**: 236–40.

49 Sonino N, Boscaro M, Paoletta A, Manetero F, Ziliotto D. Ketoconazole treatment in Cushing's syndrome: experience in 34 patients. *Clin Endocrinol* 1991; **35**: 347–52.

50 Comite F, Pescovitz OH, Rieth KG *et al.* Luteinizing hormone-releasing hormone analog treatment of boys with hypothalamic hamartoma and true precocious puberty. *J Clin Endocrinol Metab* 1984; **59**: 888–92.

51 Molitch ME. Hypopituitarism. In: Rakel RE, ed. *Conn's Current Therapy, 1993*, 45th edn. Philadelphia: WB Saunders Co., 1993: 623–6.

CHAPTER 9

Hyperprolactinaemia: causes, biochemical diagnosis and tests of prolactin secretion

G. Delitala

Introduction

Although prolactin was first discovered in 1928, based upon its ability to cause lactation in pseudo-pregnant rabbits, it was not until 1971 that human prolactin was purified and verified to be distinct from human growth hormone. Since then the complementary DNA (cDNA) and gene for human prolactin have been cloned and sequenced and several forms of the prolactin receptors in a wide variety of tissues have been described in rodents. The multitude of tissues that bind prolactin, the diversity of the prolactin receptor isoforms and the structural overlap with the receptors of the hematopoietic receptor superfamily may partially explain the multiple biological activities attributed to prolactin in experimental animals [1].

So far only a single form of prolactin receptor has been identified in humans. Human prolactin consists of 199 amino-acid residues and circulates in more than one form owing to both post-transcriptional and post-translational modifications. About 80–90% of prolactin in serum is monomeric, 8–20% is dimeric and 1–5% is polymeric. Glycosylated prolactin represents 13–25% in the human pituitary gland, and circulates in the sera of men and women [2]. The larger-molecular-weight polymers and the glycosylated prolactin have decreased binding to receptors and biological activity, decreased serum clearance and are measured with different antisera. These facts may explain the syndrome of hyperprolactinaemia with normal reproductive function in the presence of markedly elevated proportions of polymeric prolactin.

Hyperprolactinaemia is the most common biochemical abnormality currently encountered in clinical endocrinology. However, the causes of hyperprolactinaemia are diverse and the diagnostic approach and treatment depend upon identification of the aetiological cause. Although prolactinomas represent approximately 30% of all surgically removed pituitary adenomas (about 40% of all subclinical pituitary adenomas incidentally discovered at autopsy are prolactinomas), they do not represent the principal cause of hyperprolactinaemia, since hypersecretion of prolactin occurs in various clinical and physiological conditions as well as during administration of certain drugs.

The clinical manifestations of patients with hyperprolactinaemia (reduced libido and impotence in men, menstrual disturbances and/or infertility in women) clearly result from the supraphysiological concentrations of the hormone, irrespective of its origin. Clinical signs of local compression such as headache and visual field defects are frequently found with large pituitary (and hypothalamic) tumours. However, they are usually absent with microprolactinomas, and the effects of hyperprolactinaemia usually represent the sole clinical abnormality. Since microadenomas may not all be identified yet by current radiographic techniques, the measurement of prolactin in plasma is still the best indicator of whether or not a prolactin-secreting tumour is present.

Since prolactin is secreted in a pulsatile fashion and is sensitive to stress and venepuncture, several determinations should be obtained, for example three samples on different mornings or three samples at 20-min intervals via an indwelling catheter, to establish a reliable diagnosis of hyperprolactinaemia. The upper range of normal in most laboratories is 20–25 ng/ml (400–500 mU/l), but it is lower (15–18 ng/ml; 300–360 mU/l) when prolactin is measured with monoclonal antibodies in immunoradiometric assays (IRMA). Pathological hyperprolactinaemia is currently defined as a consistently elevated serum prolactin level (>25 ng/ml; 500 mU/l) when the physiological causes of prolactin hypersecretion have been excluded.

Regulation of secretion

Prolactin is unique among the known pituitary hormones

since it increases following resection of the pituitary stalk. The connections between the median eminence (ME) and the anterior pituitary are critical in the maintenance of physiological secretion of prolactin. Thus, the hypothalamus exerts a predominantly inhibitory influence on this hormone through one or more prolactin-inhibiting factors (PIFs) that reach the pituitary by way of the hypothalamo-pituitary portal vessels [3]. Despite two decades of investigation, no potent PIF has been isolated with the exception of the neurotransmitter, dopamine [4]. The axons responsible for the release of dopamine into the ME originate in the arcuate and ventromedial nuclei of the hypothalamus (tubero-infundibular-dopaminergic (TIDA) system). Dopamine secreted by these neurons is transported into the anterior lobe via the long hypophysial portal vessels. Dopamine is also present in the posterior lobe of the pituitary and can reach the anterior pituitary via the short portal vessels. The inhibitory action of dopamine on lactotrophs is mediated by receptors of the D_2 type which are negatively coupled to adenylate cyclase [5]. The number of D_2 receptors are up-regulated by decreases in the concentrations of dopamine reaching the pituitary and down-regulated by oestrogens. Post-receptor events also include alterations in membrane phospholipid turnover and changes in intracellular levels of Ca^{2+}. Furthermore, dopamine inhibits prolactin synthesis at the level of transcription [6].

Dopamine synthetic processes are basically the same in TIDA and mesencephalic dopamine neurons; however, there are certain aspects that have important pathophysiological and pharmacological implications. First, TIDA neurons lack a high-affinity amine reuptake system: no presynaptic dopamine receptors in the ME have been documented. In addition, prolactin regulates the activity of TIDA neurons, since synthesis and turnover of dopamine in the ME is augmented by a sustained and prolonged hypersecretion of the hormone. Therefore, prolactin serves as its own inhibiting factor via a dopamine-mediated short-loop feedback [7].

Although of questionable physiological function in the human, additional regulating inhibitory factors have been suggested as modulators of prolactin secretion. γ-Aminobutyric acid (GABA) is secreted into the portal blood, receptors for GABA are present in the anterior pituitary and GABA inhibits prolactin *in vitro*. However, GABA potency is 100-fold lower than dopamine's [8]. Considerable PIF activity is exerted by a 56-amino-acid polypeptide that is present in the precursor to gonadotrophin-releasing hormone (Gn-RH), termed gonadotrophin-associated peptide (GAP). Other PIFs include somatostatin and α-melanocyte-stimulating hormone (α-MSH), although the physiological roles of these substances are incompletely defined in humans.

Although the major physiologic regulatory role of prolactin secretion appears to be inhibitory, several compounds stimulate the release of prolactin when administered acutely. Thyrotrophin-releasing hormone (TRH) induces a release of prolactin by a direct action of the pituitary gland and stimulates prolactin gene transcription via increases in intracellular Ca^{2+} [9]. Protein kinase C, known to be activated by TRH in pituitary cell lines, is apparently not involved in the prolactin response to TRH. In humans, TRH causes prolactin secretion even at the lowest doses capable of inducing a TSH response [10]. However, whether TRH has a physiological role in prolactin secretion appears to be unclear, particularly as TSH release does not increase in parallel with prolactin in physiological conditions, at least in humans.

Vasoactive intestinal peptide (VIP) has stimulatory effects that are selective for prolactin at concentrations found in hypothalamo-pituitary portal blood [11]. VIP and its cosynthesised peptide, peptide–histidine–isoleucine (PHI), act through a shared binding site to increase prolactin messenger RNA (mRNA) levels via the induction of cyclic adenosine monophosphate (cAMP). Since VIP can be synthesised from radiolabel precursors added to pituitary cell cultures, it has been suggested that VIP can function as an autocrine regulator of prolactin synthesis and release, at least in experimental animals.

In a variety of experimental studies, other peptides, including opioid peptides, substance P, neurotensin, angiotensin II, GHRH, vasopressin, galanin, cholecystokinin, gastrin, melatonin and others, have been shown to have prolactin-releasing properties. Their physiological significance, especially in humans, as endogenous prolactin-releasing factors (PRFs) still remains to be defined.

Serotonin and its precursors stimulate prolactin release through hypothalamic mechanisms involving stimulation of the release of PRF(s) and/or reduction in the activity of the TIDA neurons [12]. Histamine has also been shown to stimulate prolactin release through H_1-receptor mechanisms. Inhibition of prolactin release, however, occurs with activation of the H_2 receptors [13]. Acetylcholine generally is inhibitory, acting through muscarinic receptors, although the physiological role of this neurotransmitter in the control of human prolactin still remains controversial.

There is good evidence that the secretion of prolactin is pulsatile in humans. Studies performed in experimental animals (transplanted pituitary gland or pituitary stalk-sectioned animals) suggest that the pituitary lactotrophs possess an intrinsic capacity to secrete prolactin in a pulsatile fashion, which is probably modulated by paracrine and autocrine mechanisms [14]. Hypothalamic influences would regulate the amplitude, not the frequency, of this endogenous pulsatile secretion. On the contrary, hypothalamic neurogenic mechanisms are certainly involved in the other aspects of prolactin hypersecretion that occur in physiological states. Prolactin is secreted episodically, 13–14 peaks per day occurring in young subjects, with an interpulse interval of about 90 min. The release of prolactin is not controlled by a circadian rhythm, but is sleep dependent [15]. An increase in the amplitude of the prolactin secretory pulse begins about 60–90 min after sleep onset but is not associated with a specific sleep phase [16]. These sleep-dependent diurnal variations of prolactin also persist in situations of powerful physiological influences such as breast feeding [17]. Prolactin levels gradually decline during the morning, with minimal levels occurring around noon. Small rises in prolactin related to meals have been shown to be due to central stimulation by the amino acids generated from the protein component of the meals. However, these prolactin fluctuations during the day in non-stressed conditions are always within the limits of the normal range.

The physiological, pathological and pharmacological factors that influence prolactin secretion are listed in Table 9.1.

Table 9.1 Physiological and pathological causes of hyperprolactinaemia.

PHYSIOLOGICAL CAUSES

Neonatal, pregnancy, nursing, nipple stimulation, sleep, exercise, stress (surgery, hypoglycaemia, myocardial infarction, sexual intercourse, syncope, trauma)

PATHOLOGICAL CAUSES

Hypothalamic disease

Tumours (craniopharyngioma, hamartoma, glioma, germinoma, third-ventricle tumour, metastasis)

Infiltrative disease (eosinophilic granuloma, sarcoidosis, tuberculosis)

Others (cranial irradiation, pseudo-tumour cerebri, arteriovenous malformations, pituitary stalk transection)

Pituitary disease

Prolactinoma, acromegaly, Cushing's disease, craniopharyngioma, empty sella, lymphocytic hypophysitis, TSH-secreting adenoma, gonadotrophin-secreting adenoma, 'non secretory' adenoma, intrasellar cyst, Rathke's cleft cyst, intrasellar germinoma, intrasellar meningioma

Drugs

Dopamine blockers (neuroleptics, metoclopramide, sulpiride, domperidone), reserpine, α-methyl-dopa, carbidopa, benserazide, oestrogens, opiates, cimetidine (intravenous), antidepressants (imipramine, amitriptyline), verapamil, TRH, VIP

Other

Primary hypothyroidism, chronic renal failure, cirrhosis, chest-wall lesions, breast stimulation, polycystic ovary syndrome, pseudocyesis, adrenal insufficiency, ectopic prolactin secretion (renal cell carcinoma, gonadoblastoma, lung tumour), 'idiopathic'

TSH, thyroid-stimulating hormone; TRH, thyrotrophin-releasing hormone; VIP, vasointestinal peptide.

Physiological hyperprolactinaemia

Hyperprolactinaemia, probably oestrogen-induced, is a constant finding in newborns. Prolactin rises from the 20th week of gestation onward. After birth, prolactin levels progressively decrease reaching the normal range by 4–6 weeks. Serum prolactin levels are generally higher in fertile women than in men. This aspect reflects the effect of oestrogen on the lactotrophs.

During normal pregnancy serum prolactin rises progressively to levels of around 200–300 ng/ml (4000–6000 mU/l). This increase is considered to be due to rising oestrogen concentrations. Oestrogens are known to stimulate mitotic activity of the lactotrophs and to partially reduce the PIF activity of dopamine, thus leading to the lactotroph hyperplasia observed in pregnancy. Hyperprolactinaemia also occurs during lactation, particularly within the first 4–6 weeks post-partum [18]. The stimulus is entirely mechanical (it can be reproduced by a breast pump) and originates from the stimulation of the mammary nerve. The capacity of the breast to respond to stimulation appears to be oestrogen dependent and can be abolished in fertile women by the administration of anti-oestrogens. The same neural mechanism probably underlies the hyperprolactinaemia which is associated with chest-wall injury, such as trauma, burns and herpes zoster.

A variety of stresses, for example exercise, hypoglycaemia, myocardial infarction, sexual intercourse and surgery, cause significant elevation of prolactin in both sexes [19].

The prolactin rise that occurs during surgery depends on the type of surgical operation and is probably related to the stimuli of cutting and manipulation of tissues. Hyperprolactinaemia usually returns to normal values within 24 hours after abdominal or vaginal surgery, whereas prolactin levels may remain elevated for several weeks following thoracotomy or mastectomy. This different behaviour of prolactin is probably related to neural stimulation of the suckling reflex, particularly when tissues begin to heal. Elevated prolactin levels associated with chest injury or nipple stimulation can be normalised by intercostal nerve block [20]. Minor surgical manoeuvres such as gastroscopy or proctoscopy are also accompanied by a rise in prolactin. Naloxone has been reported to blunt the prolactin rise induced by abdominal surgery but not the prolactin rise induced by gastroscopy [21]. This would suggest different neuroendocrine mechanisms in the prolactin stimulation induced by different surgical manoeuvres.

Physical exercise is a potent stimulus to prolactin release. The relationship between the intensity of physical effort and hormone secretion demonstrates that prolactin rises only when the anaerobic threshold is reached [22]. The increase in lactic acid level, however, does not represent the causal factor for prolactin release. On the contrary, the participation of the opiate system has been suggested in this mechanism since naloxone suppressed prolactin secretion is induced by strenuous exercise in athletes [23]. Amenorrhoeic runners with a low oestradiol level often fail to increase prolactin response to a running test. This would suggest that oestrogen levels are an important variable in modulating the prolactin rise observed during exercise.

Although prolactin is often labelled as a stress hormone, a clear effect of mental and psychological stress on the release of this hormone has not been clearly demonstrated. Prolactin usually rises when stressors are accompanied by systemic symptoms, such as syncope or hypotension. These reactions are probably responsible for the prolactin rise observed following venesection.

Symptomatic hypoglycaemia is a potent stimulus for prolactin secretion in both sexes, but a teleologically satisfactory rationale for this phenomenon is not apparent in humans. Prolactin is mildly diabetogenic but does not play any role in the counter-regulatory control of blood glucose and/or in glucose homeostasis. Glycopenia is presumably the intracellular stimulus in the central nervous system, since the brain has negligible energy stores and obligatory aerobic metabolic pathways.

Pathological hyperprolactinaemia

Drugs

A variety of drugs can stimulate prolactin secretion. Since dopamine is the physiological PIF, the most common pharmacological causes of hyperprolactinaemia are centrally acting compounds that interact with hypothalamic dopamine system and/or pituitary dopamine receptors. Thus, all drugs that reduce central dopamine neurotransmission by blocking dopamine receptors (e.g. phenothiazines, butyrophenones, substituted benzamides), by depleting central catecholamine stores (e.g. reserpine), or by interfering in dopamine synthesis (e.g. α-methyl-dopa-decarboxylase inhibitors) cause hyperprolactinaemia. The mechanisms involved in the prolactin release induced by these compounds are different. Dopamine antagonists certainly act at the pituitary by blocking the action of endogenous dopamine on the lactotrophs [24]. Dopamine-depleting agents and inhibitors of catecholamine synthesis probably reduce the dopamine secreted from the ME into the portal capillary system, thereby allowing prolactin to rise.

The administration of high doses of oestrogens results in mild hyperprolactinaemia. However, low-dose oestrogen–progestogen oral contraceptives are unable to cause elevation of prolactin. The potential oestrogen-induced tumour formation during chronic oestrogen administration, although experimentally documented in animals, has not been demonstrated in humans.

H_2 antagonists, such as cimetidine, stimulate prolactin secretion only when given in large parenteral dosages, and this probably reflects the poor ability of the drug to cross the blood–brain barrier. The mechanisms involved in the prolactin-releasing activity of these compounds may be mediated through a reduction in dopamine tone in the hypothalamus since H_2 antagonists do not stimulate prolactin at the pituitary level [25]. Mild hyperprolactinaemia has been reported during therapy with monoaminoxidase inhibitors and Ca^{2+} blockers (e.g. verapamil). However, this is not the rule during chronic administration of these drugs.

Opiate alkaloids and agonists of opioid receptors are potent prolactin secretagogues in humans. The prolactin-releasing activity of opiates is probably mediated by a decrease in dopamine release in the ME, thus lowering dopamine levels in the pituitary stalk. Since opiates reduce gonadotrophin pulsatile secretion, hyperprolactinaemia together with reduced luteinising hormone (LH) levels are probably the pathogenetic causes of the hypogonadotrophic hypogonadal syndrome often associated with chronic opiate abuse [26]. This mechanism (e.g. enhanced hypothalamic opioid tone) has also been suggested in the pathogenesis of the reduced LH pulsatility observed in the majority of patients with chronic hyperprolactinaemia [27].

Primary hypothyroidism

Elevated prolactin levels and an exaggerated prolactin response to stimulation are often present in patients with primary hypothyroidism, but levels greater than 25 ng/ml (500/mU) are attained in less than 10%. Hyperprolactinaemia is commonly normalised by appropriate thyroid hormone replacement. Chronic primary hypothyroidism can occasionally present with marked hyperprolactinaemia and an enlarged sella turcica. This prolactin hypersecretion is probably secondary to local compression of the pituitary stalk by the 'feedback' tumour and can often (but not always) be reversed to normal with appropriate thyroxine therapy.

A reduced metabolic clearance rate may be the principal cause of hyperprolactinaemia in patients with chronic hypothyroidism, but increased secretion may also play a part.

Chronic renal failure

Hyperprolactinaemia occurs in about 30% of patients with

chronic renal failure and increases to 80% in patients during haemodialysis. Correction of the renal failure with transplantation causes a return of prolactin levels to normal. Hyperprolactinaemia is probably secondary to a reduction of about 30% of its metabolic clearance rate. However, the production rate of the hormone is also increased approximately threefold in chronic renal failure. This is due to a reduced ability of dopamine to inhibit prolactin secretion in these patients. The presence of non-dialysable substances that interfere with the binding of dopamine to its receptors on the lactotrophs or the development of post-receptor abnormalities has been suggested in uraemic patients.

Cirrhosis of the liver

Mild hyperprolactinaemia can occur in 5–15% of patients with cirrhosis of the liver. The mechanisms of this abnormality are not clear, but many factors may contribute to it (e.g. the increased production rate of oestrogens, the presence of a low-triiodothyronine (T_3) syndrome, an alteration in central monoamine metabolism, etc.).

Polycystic ovary syndrome

Mild hyperprolactinaemia can be observed in some patients with polycystic ovary syndrome. An exaggerated prolactin response to TRH and dopamine antagonists have also been reported in these obese patients. These aspects are probably due to the increased production rate of oestrogens via the peripheral conversion of ovarian and adrenal androgens. Some patients with prolactinomas, on the other hand, can have polycystic ovaries, and there is evidence that hyperprolactinaemia stimulates the adrenal production of androgens, particularly dihydroepiandrosterone-sulphate (DHEA-S) [28].

Pseudo-cyesis

This rare syndrome, commonly known as 'phantom pregnancy', is biochemically characterized by hypersecretion of LH and prolactin. Luteal function and galactorrhoea are maintained by an increased amplitude of pulsatile release of both hormones; this is probably secondary to reduced dopaminergic activity in the hypothalamus.

Hypothalamic disease

Hyperprolactinaemia may be a biochemical marker of disorders of the hypothalamus and pituitary stalk. Space-occupying lesions within the hypothalamus can destroy the hypothalamic TIDA neurons and/or interrupt dopamine delivery to the portal vessels. This category includes craniopharyngiomas, gliomas, inflammatory processes (eosinophilic granuloma, tuberculosis, sarcoidosis), distortion of the hypothalamus and stalk caused by such entities as the empty sella, and lymphocytic hypophysitis, metastases and arteriovenous malformations. Other causes include head injures with transection of the pituitary stalk, and external irradiation.

Non-prolactinoma pituitary tumours

Hyperprolactinaemia is demonstrated in approximately 40% of patients with acromegaly [29]. In some instances the modest hyperprolactinaemia is attributable to the effect of stalk section. However, in a significant proportion of patients, prolactin levels are elevated and caused by pituitary tumours with dual secretion of growth hormone and prolactin (mixed growth-hormone cell–prolactin cell adenoma, mammosomatotroph adenomas, and the acidophil stem-cell adenoma) [30]. Between 20 and 25% of patients with Cushing's disease and about 50% of those with Nelson's syndrome also have hyperprolactinaemia. Possible explanations of such prolactin hypersecretion include the coexpression of adrenocorticotrophic hormone (ACTH) and prolactin by the same tumour and/or tumour-associated distortion of the pituitary stalk. Similar mechanisms can be proposed for hyperprolactinaemia occurring with gonadotrophin and thyroid-stimulating hormone (TSH)-secreting adenomas. The majority of these plurihormonal pituitary adenomas are macroadenomas at presentation and invasive at the time of diagnosis.

Finally, hyperprolactinaemia due to compression of the pituitary stalk can occur with any other space-occupying lesions affecting the sella turcica.

Prolactinomas

Prolactinomas are diagnosed by radiological imaging when other causes have been excluded. They are classified clinically by size: microadenomas (< 10 mm in diameter) and macroprolactinoma (> 10 mm in diameter). They represent the most frequent autopsy findings in individuals with no history of pituitary disease; 25% of the general population have been found to harbour microadenomas, of which approximately half immunostained for prolactin [31]. However, the precise prevalence of prolactinoma is not known. Prolactinomas in men tend to be larger but are less frequent than in women. Gender-related differences aside, these tumours in men and women are immunohistochemically and ultrastructurally indistinguishable.

Usually, prolactin levels are extremely high (200 ng/ml; 4000 mU/l), with levels ranging from 40 to 25 000 ng/ml (800–500 000 mU/l). In general, serum prolactin levels parallel the size of the tumour. Although the levels of prolactin may suggest the presence of a pituitary adenoma (the higher the prolactin level, the more likely it is that the patient has an adenoma), exceptions to this rule are not infrequent, as prolactin levels lower than 100 ng/ml (2000 mU/l) may be found in patients with surgically proven prolactinomas.

The pathophysiology of the pituitary tumours is not clear and several potential mechanisms have been proposed. Since the majority of patients with proven prolactinoma show no prolactin response to dopamine receptor antagonists, the theory of defective hypothalamic neurotransmission has been applied to the pathogenesis of prolactinomas. Moreover, an impairment of L-dopa metabolism and/or a dopamine deficiency in the hypothalamus of these patients has been proposed, since the suppressive effect of L-dopa on prolactin in prolactinomas is blunted by the coadministration of carbidopa, a peripheral DOPA decarboxylase inhibitor [32]. However, other evidence suggests enhanced dopamine tone in the hypothalamus of patients harbouring a prolactinoma, probably due to the short-loop positive feedback action of prolactin on hypothalamic TIDA neurons. This is documented by the exaggerated TSH response to dopamine blockers in these patients [33] (Fig. 9.1). The hypothesis that lactotrophs in prolactinomas fail to express dopamine receptors, or the existence of a post-receptor defect, seems unlikely in view of the well-documented suppressive effect of dopamine and its agonists on prolactin secretion in the majority of patients with a proven prolactinoma. Moreover, the suppressive effect of dopamine is clearly blocked by dopamine antagonists either *in vivo* or *in vitro* [34]. On the other hand, a marked reduction in dopamine-binding sites has been demonstrated in prolactinomas removed from patients resistant to dopamine-like drugs. Moreover, in highly invasive prolactinomas, dopamine receptors have been shown to be uncoupled from adenyl cyclase inhibition [35]. Finally, reduced prolactin responsiveness to a threshold dose

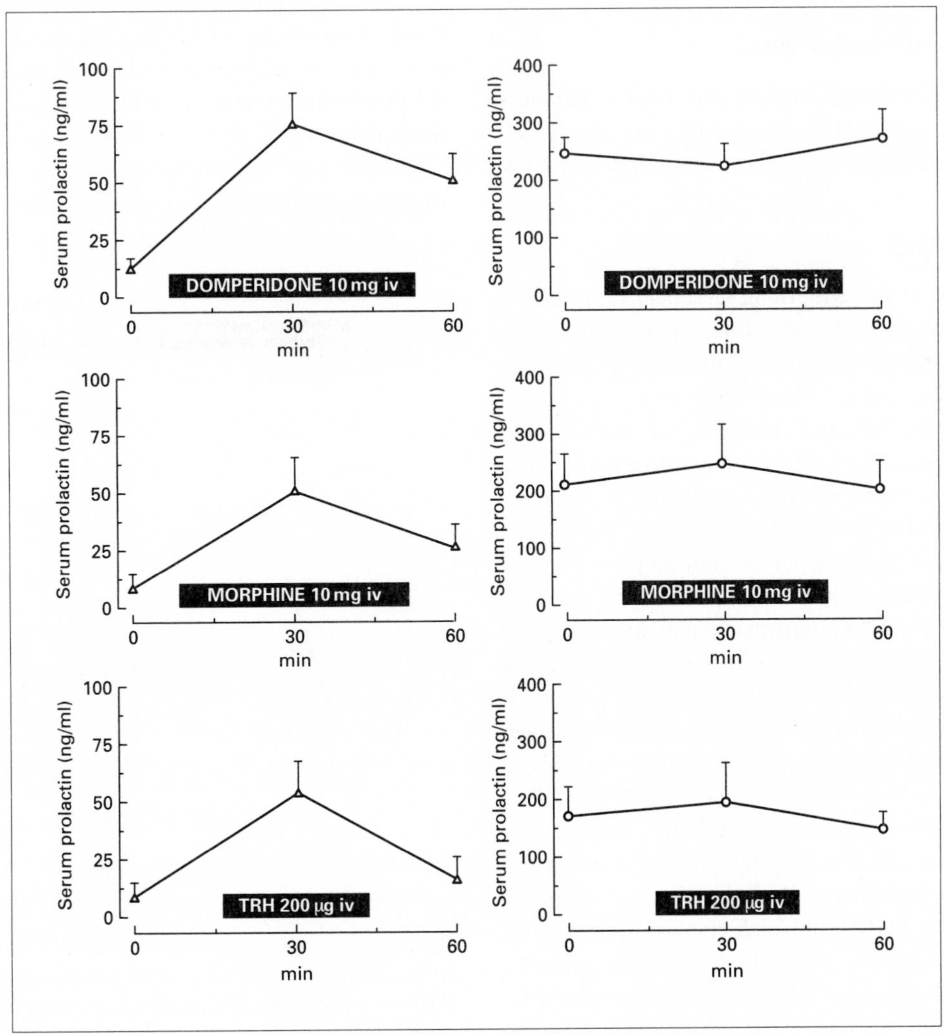

Fig. 9.1 Serum prolactin (mean ± SEM) following domperidone, morphine and thyrotrophin-releasing hormone (TRH) in normal women (left) and in patients with prolactinoma (right).

of dopamine infusion (0.02 μg/kg/min) has been reported in prolactinoma patients [36]. These findings, as well as the possible defective local delivery of hypothalamic dopamine to the adenomatous cells secondary to a vascular derangement, might account for some of the biochemical abnormalities associated with the presence of a prolactinoma.

Idiopathic hyperprolactinaemia

When no specific cause is found on evaluation, patients with mild hyperprolactinaemia, but without radiological evidence of a pituitary tumour and/or hypothalamic pathology, are often considered to have 'idiopathic' or 'functional' hyperprolactinaemia. In many such cases small prolactinomas may be present that cannot be detected by current radiological techniques since these small lesions may be below the limit of the resolution power of the radiographic methods currently used. Long-term follow-up of such patients reveals that a minority of these patients (< 15%) develop evidence of microadenomas.

Ectopic hyperprolactinaemia

Ectopic production of prolactin is extremely rare. Tumours that may secrete prolactin ectopically are renal cell carcinomas, gonadoblastoma and bronchogenic carcinomas.

Diagnostic testing

Although a single elevated morning level may be adequate to diagnose excess prolactin secretion, the pulsatile manner of prolactin release and its sensitivity to stress (e.g., venepuncture) suggests that it is prudent to obtain several samples before making the diagnosis of pathological hyperprolactinaemia [37]. This clinical approach is particularly important when patients with mildly elevated prolactin levels are investigated. It can easily be obtained by collecting the blood samples (on three separate mornings or via an indwelling cannula 30–45 min after cannulation) in a true basal state in the awake, unstressed patient. Once the diagnosis of hyperprolactinaemia has been confirmed, and the numerous causes of prolactin hypersecretion have been carefully considered (e.g. hypothyroidism, pregnancy, drugs, etc.), the precise hypothalamic and/or pituitary pathology requires further investigation. It is generally accepted that frankly enlarged pituitaries containing large adenomas do not require further dynamic testing for diagnosis of the origin of hyperprolactinaemia. With the advent of magnetic resonance imaging (MRI) and high-resolution computed tomography (CT) scanning, subtle alterations in the anatomy of the pituitary gland and surrounding sella turcica can be precisely visualised [38]. However, despite these technological advancements, imaging studies may not always demonstrate a tumour. For this reason, several dynamic tests have been proposed in clinical practice to attempt to differentiate hypothalamic from pituitary diseases and to determine if a pituitary microtumour is present.

Dopamine antagonists

These drugs were originally introduced in clinical practice on the premise that they act at the hypothalamic level, and therefore require the integrity of the central nervous system for the prolactin releasing effect. It is now clear that these compounds cannot differentiate between pituitary and hypothalamic causes of hyperprolactinaemia since dopamine blockers also act on the anterior pituitary, directly at the dopamine receptor of the lactotrophs [39]. Nevertheless, the majority of cases with a prolactinoma show no response to this stimulation (Fig. 9.1). Sulpiride (25–50 mg), metoclopramide (5–10 mg) or domperidone (5–10 mg) are administered orally or intravenously, and blood samples for prolactin measurements are taken before administration and then at intervals for 60–120 min. However, the practical use of these compounds in an attempt to distinguish the cause of hyperprolactinaemia is of little clinical use in diagnostic evaluation.

Patients with proven microprolactinoma usually show an exaggerated TSH elevation in response to administration

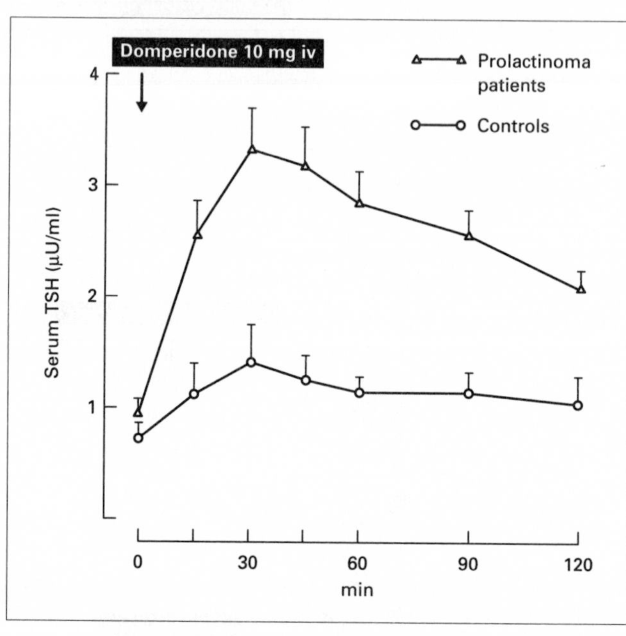

Fig. 9.2 Serum thyroid-stimulating hormone (TSH) response (mean ± SEM) to the intravenous administration of the dopamine blocker, domperidone, in women with microprolactinoma and in normal fertile women.

of dopamine blockers. This biochemical anomaly is due to the enhanced dopamine tone secondary to the short-loop feedback action of prolactin on the hypothalamic TIDA tract. This biochemical anomaly, although important from a pathophysiological point of view, does not have any practical role in the clinical diagnosis of these neoplasms (Fig. 9.2).

Thyrotrophin-releasing hormone

In normal subjects, the intravenous administration of TRH (200 µg) is followed by a rise in serum prolactin: the serum concentration of the hormone usually reaches a peak at 30 min. Absolute prolactin increases of 20–30 ng/ml (400–600 mU/l) for males and 50–100 ng/ml (1000–2000 mU/l) for fertile females are commonly observed in normal individuals.

The majority of patients harbouring a prolactinoma (about 80–90%) have a blunted or absent prolactin response to TRH. Again, a blunted prolactin response to TRH does not necessarily indicate the presence of a prolactinoma, since a reduced pituitary response to TRH may be observed in patients with suprasellar lesions (Fig. 9.1) [40].

Patients with ectopic hyperprolactinaemia usually do not respond to stimulation.

Arginine and cimetidine

These substances stimulate prolactin secretion in normal people. Although patients with hypothalamic and/or pituitary hyperprolactinaemia might be expected not to respond to these tests, arginine or cimetidine have no role in the clinical diagnosis of hyperprolactinaemia.

Insulin-induced hypoglycaemia

Symptomatic hypoglycaemia is usually achieved with the injection of regular insulin. The usual insulin dose is 0.15 U/kg, but may be less in patients with suspected hypopituitarism (0.05 U/kg). Blood is taken before insulin and then at intervals for 150–180 min. In normal subjects a clear prolactin rise is observed 45–60 min following insulin and only when clearly symptomatic hypoglycaemia is achieved (Fig. 9.3).

Although no prolactin rise in response to insulin is found in patients with hyperprolactinaemia of pituitary and hypothalamic origin, the practical use of this test in the diagnosis of hyperprolactinaemia is minimal. This procedure is currently used in patients with hypothalamic and/or pituitary lesions (with and without hyperprolactinaemia) in the assessment of hypothalamo-pituitary regulation of adrenocorticotrophic hormone and growth hormone.

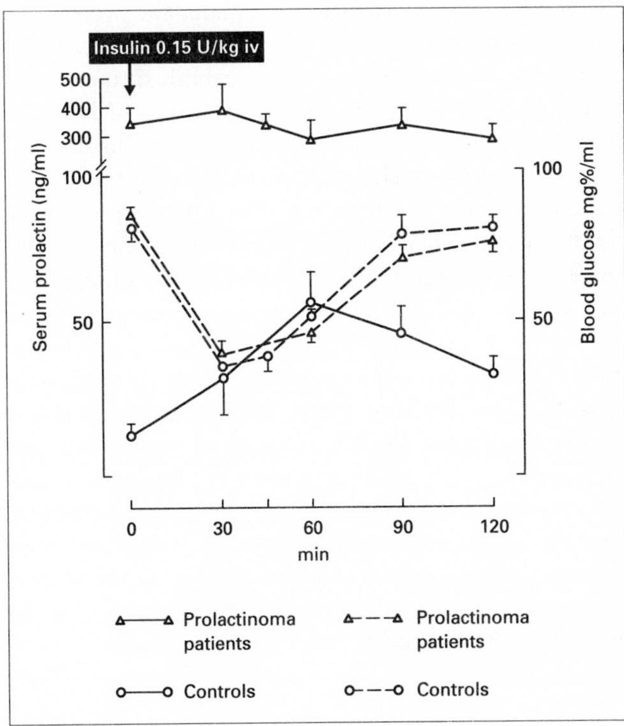

Fig. 9.3 Blood glucose and prolactin (PRL) response to insulin administration (0.15 U/kg) in normal women and in patients with prolactinoma.

Dopamine agonists

Indirect dopamine agonists (i.e. catecholamine reuptake inhibitors, such as amphetamine, nomifensine and amineptine) have no role in the clinical testing of hyperprolactinaemia in view of their poor ability to reduce prolactin in normal people. This is probably related to the lack of an effective catecholamine reuptake system in human hypothalamic TIDA neurons.

Dopamine and its direct agonist compounds (e.g. bromocriptine, lisuride, pergolide and cabergoline) act directly on the lactotrophs to suppress prolactin. Since they suppress all forms of prolactin hypersecretion, irrespective of the origin, the clinical use of these drugs for diagnostic purposes cannot add to the diagnosis of prolactinoma or other forms of hyperprolactinaemia [41].

Conclusions

Hyperprolactinaemic syndromes are a diverse group of disorders that are common in both men and women. Although hyperprolactinaemia is considered a biochemical marker of hypothalamo-pituitary dysfunction, true hyperprolactinaemia should be well documented with appropriate blood sampling. This will probably reduce the incidence of 'functional' or 'idiopathic' hyperprolactinaemia without the necessity of additional and expensive procedures. Once the diagnosis of hyperprolactinaemia has been established, the patient should be screened for the numerous causes of hormone hypersecretion; hence, an accurate medical history will help the clinician to eliminate the most frequent causes of hypersecretion of prolactin (e.g. drugs). In the presence of a tumour well defined by high-resolution CT scan or MRI, there is no need for further biochemical testing. When imaging does not demonstrate a lesion, the use of dynamic testing has been advocated to differentiate hypothalamic from pituitary causes of hyperprolactinaemia. Among these TRH has been the most widely used compound; a failure of the lactotrophs further to augment prolactin release is suggestive of a pituitary and/or hypothalamic lesion. Unfortunately, there are many false negatives and positives, and the tests are therefore of little use in the individual patient. Hence, accurate blood sampling in the awake, non-stressed patient is still the best 'functional test' in the great majority of patients with hyperprolactinaemia.

References

1 Kelly PA, Djiane J, Postel-Vinay MC, Edery M. The prolactin/growth hormone receptor family. *Endocr Rev* 1991; **12**: 235–51.

2 Lewis UJ, Singh RNP, Lewis LJ. Two forms of glycosylated human prolactin have different pigeon crop sac-stimulating activities. *Endocrinology* 1989; **124**: 1558–63.

3 Blackwell RE. Hyperprolactinaemia. Evaluation and management. *Endocrinol Metab Clin N Amer* 1992; **21**: 105–24.

4 Cooke NE. Prolactin: basic physiology. In: DeGroot LJ, ed. *Endocrinology*. Philadelphia: WB Saunders and Co., 1995: 368–93.

5 Awennen L, Denef C. Physiological concentrations of dopamine decrease adenosine 3′5′-monophosphate levels in cultured rat anterior pituitary cells and enriched populations of lactotrophs: evidence for a causal relationship to inhibition of prolactin release. *Endocrinology* 1982; **111**: 398–401.

6 Elsholtz HP, Lew AM, Albert PR, Sundmark VC. Inhibitory control of prolactin and Pit-1 gene promoter by dopamine. *J Biol Chem* 1991; **34**: 22919–25.

7 Gudelsky GA, Porter JC. Release of dopamine from tubero-infundibular neurons into pituitary stalk blood after prolactin and haloperidol administration. *Endocrinology*1980; **106**: 526–9.

8 Grossman A, Delitala G, Yeo T, Besser GM. GABA and muscimol inhibit the release of prolactin from dispersed rat anterior pituitary cells. *Neuroendocrinology* 1981; **32**: 145–9.

9 White BA, Bancroft FC. Epidermal growth factor and thyrotropin-releasing hormone interact synergistically with calcium to regulate prolactin mRNA levels. *J Biol Chem* 1983; **258**: 4618–22.

10 Noel GL, Dimond RC, Wartofsky L. Studies of prolactin and TSH secretion by continuous infusion of small amounts of thyrotropin releasing hormone (TRH). *J Clin Endocrinol Metab* 1974; **39**: 6–17.

11 Nagy G, Mulchahey JJ, Naill JD. Autocrine control of prolactin secretion by vasoactive intestinal peptide. *Endocrinology* 1988; **122**: 364–6.

12 Delitala G. Clinical neuropharmacology in the management of disorders of the pituitary and hypothalamus. In: DeGroot LJ, ed. *Endocrinology*. Philadelphia: WB Saunders and Co., 1989: 408–73.

13 Müller EE. Role of neurotransmitters and neuromodulators in the control of anterior pituitary hormone secretion. In: DeGroot LJ, ed. *Endocrinology*. Philadelphia: WB Saunders and Co., 1995: 178–91.

14 Denef C, Andries M. Evidence for paracrine interaction between gonadotrophs and lactotrophs in pituitary cell aggregates. *Endocrinology* 1983; **112**: 813–22.

15 Parker DC, Rossman LG, Vanderlaan EF. Relation of sleep-entrained human prolactin release to REM–nonREM Cycles. *J Clin Endocrinol Metab* 1973; **38**: 646–50.

16 Veldhuis JD, Johnson L. Operating characteristics of the hypothalamo-pituitary–gonadal axis in men. Circadian, ultradian, and pulsatile release of prolactin and its temporal coupling with luteinizing hormone. *J Clin Endocrinol Metab* 1988; **67**: 116–23.

17 Stern JM, Reichlin S. Prolactin circadian rhythm persists throughout lactation in women. *Neuroendocrinology* 1990; **51**: 31–35.

18 Johnston JM, Amico JA. A prospective longitudinal study of the release of oxytocin and prolactin in response to infant suckling in long term lactation. *J Clin Endocrinol Metab* 1986; **62**: 653–7.

19 Delitala G, Tomasi P, Virdis R. Growth hormone, prolactin, thyrotropin–thyroid hormone secretion during stress states in man. *Baillière's Clin Endocrinol Metab* 1987; **1**: 391–414.

20 Morley JE, Dawson M, Hodgkinson J, Kalk WJ. Galactorrhea and hyperprolactinaemia associated with chest wall injury. *J Clin Endocrinol Metab* 1977; **45**: 931–36.

21 Morley JE, Baranetsky NG, Wingert TD. Endocrine effects of naloxone–induced opiate receptor blockade. *J Clin Endocrinol Metab* 1980; **50**: 251–7.

22 De Meirleir KL, Baeyens L, L'Hermite-Baleriaux M. Exercise-induced prolactin release is related to anaerobiosis. *J Clin Endocrinol Metab* 1985; **60**: 1250–52.

23 Moretti C, Fabbri A, Gnessi L *et al.* Naloxone inhibits exercise-induced release of PRL and GH in athletes. *Clin Endocrinol* 1983; **18**: 135–8.

24 Neill JD. Prolactin secretion and its control. In: Knobil E, Neill LD, eds. *The Physiology of Reproduction*. New York: Raven Press, 1988: 1379–1401.

25 Delitala G, Stubbs WA, Yeo T, Grossman A, Besser GM. Failure of cimetidine to antagonise dopamine-induced suppression of prolactin *in vitro*. *Br J Clin Pharmacol* 1979; **7**: 117–19.

26 Grossman A, Moult PJA, McIntyre H *et al.* Opiate mediation of amenorrhoea in hyperprolactinaemia and weight-loss related amenorrhoea. *Clin Endocrinol* 1982; **17**: 379–84.

27 Delitala G. Opioid peptides and pituitary function. Basic and clinical aspects. In: Motta M, ed. *Brain Endocrinology*. New York: Raven Press, 1991: 217–44.

28 Luciano AA, Chapler FK, Sherman BM. Hyperprolactinaemia in polycystic ovary syndrome. *Fertil Steril* 1984; **41**: 719–25.

29 Vance ML, Thorner MO. Prolactin: hyperprolactinemic syndromes and management. In: DeGroot LJ, ed. *Endocrinology*. Philadelphia: WB Saunders and Co., 1995: 394–405.

30 Thapar K, Kovacs K, Muller PJ. Clinical–pathological correlations of pituitary tumours. *Baillière's Clin Endocrinol Metab* 1995; 243–70.

31 McComb DJ, Ryan N, Horvath E, Kovacs K. Subclinical adenomas of the human pituitary. New light on old problems. *Arch Path Lab Med* 1983; **107**: 488–91.

32 Fine SA, Frohman LA. Loss of central nervous system component of dopaminergic inhibition of prolactin secretion in patients with prolactin-secreting pituitary tumours. *J Clin Invest* 1978; **61**: 973–80.

33 Scanlon MF, Rodriguez-Arnao MD, McGregor AM. Altered dopaminergic regulation of thyrotropin release in patients with prolactinoma. Comparison with other tests of hypothalamic–

pituitary function. *Clin Endocrinol* 1981; **12**: 133–43.
34 Bression D, Le Dafniet M, Brandi AM, Racadot J, Peillon F. Dopamine receptors in human PRL- and GH-secreting adenomas. In: Camanni F, Müller EE, eds. *Pituitary Hyperfunction: Physiopathology and Clinical Aspects*. New York: Raven Press, 1984: 111–23.
35 Pellegrini I, Rasolonjanahary R, Gunz G. Resistance to bromocriptine in prolactinomas. *J Clin Endocrinol Metab* 1989; **69**: 500–505.
36 Serri O, Kueben O, Buu NT, Somla M. Differential effects of a low-dose dopamine infusion on prolactin secretion in normal and hyperprolactinaemic subjects. *J Clin Endocrinol Metab* 1983; **56**: 255–9.
37 Moult PJ, Dacie JE, Rees LH, Besser GM. Prolaction pulsatility in patients with gonadal dysfunction. *Clin Endocrinol* 1981; **14**: 387–94.
38 Witte RJ, Leighton PM, Daniels DL, Haughton VM. Radiographic evaluation of the pituitary and anterior hypothalamus. In: De Groot LJ, ed. *Endocrinology*. Philadelphia: WB Saunders and Co, 1995; 467–86.
39 Delitala G, Yeo T, Grossman A, Hathway NR, Besser GM. A comparison of the effects of four ergot derivatives on prolactin secretion by dispersed rat pituitary cells. *J Endocr* 1980; **87**: 95–102.
40 Klijn JGM, Lamberts SWJ, Dejong FH, Birkenhager JC. The value of the thyrotropin releasing hormone test in patients with prolactin-secreting pituitary tumors and suprasellar non-pituitary tumors. *Fertil Steril* 1981; **35(2)**: 155–61.
41 Vance ML, Evans WS, Thorner MO. Drugs five years later: Bromocriptine. *Ann Intern Med* 1984; **100**: 78–91.

CHAPTER 10

Prolactinomas

F. Camanni and E. Ciccarelli

Introduction

A prolactin-secreting pituitary adenoma represents the most frequent cause of chronic hyperprolactinaemia, and the most common pituitary tumour. In the past, it was usually included with the 'endocrinologically inactive chromophobe adenomas'. Rarely, the prolactin-secreting pituitary adenoma may be a component of the familial multiple endocrine neoplasia syndrome type 1, in association with parathyroid and pancreatic islet tumours [1]. Ectopic secretion of prolactin from malignant tumours is extremely rare [2].

It is well known in clinical practice that prolactinomas occur less frequently in men than in women, and may differ in terms of size, invasive growth and secretory activity [2–5]. At diagnosis, a higher proportion of prolactinomas in men than in women are macroadenomas (> 10 mm in diameter); microprolactinomas are particularly rare in the male population (Table 10.1). This may be due to a higher growth velocity or to a later diagnosis in men due to the lack of easily identifiable symptoms, but the precise reason remains unknown. Occasionally, prolactinomas may spontaneously infarct and be associated with a partially empty sella.

With conventional histological techniques, prolactin-secreting adenomas generally appear as chromophobes: only with electron microscopy can the characteristic specific secretory granules be shown in tumorous cells. Specific immunohistochemical stains prove the presence of prolactin. Adenomas composed of prolactin cells can be densely or sparsely granulated: the former correspond to the acidophilic adenoma and occur infrequently, while the latter are chromophobic and are the most common type of prolactin-secreting adenoma. Mixed prolactin and growth hormone tumours are not rare; most are made up of mixed cell types, but in some cases both hormones are secreted by the same cell [6].

Aetiology and pathogenesis

The pathogenesis of prolactin-secreting adenomas is essentially unknown. Similar to other active pituitary tumours (such as in Cushing's disease and acromegaly), the prolactin-secreting adenoma may be the result of autonomous tumorous lactotrophs or, alternatively, may be due to a primary abnormality of hypothalamic neuroregulation, particularly of dopaminergic neurotransmission. Histological and immunohistological quantitative analysis of the para-adenomatous normal pituitary gland suggests that some prolactinomas may originate from pre-existing prolactin-cell hyperplasia [7]. On the other hand, the results of many studies in patients with prolactin-secreting tumours appear to suggest the presence of an abnormal dopaminergic neurotransmission related to the control of prolactin secretion [8]. This abnormality may be responsible for the generation of an adenoma initially starting from lactotroph hyperplasia, similar to the situation in some experimental animal models. Whether the abnormality in dopaminergic neurotransmission is at the tuberoinfundibular neuron level or lies in the abnormal vascular transport of dopamine from the hypothalamus to the lactotrophs is uncertain. Moreover, the possibility of either the resistance of tumorous prolactin-secreting cells to central nervous system (CNS)-derived inhibitory inputs, or of a hyperprolactinaemia-induced central dopaminergic abnormality, has also been suggested. Even more uncertain is the hypothesis of a pathogenetic mechanism mediated by a prolactin-releasing factor. Recently, molecular studies on pituitary adenomas have more strongly supported the possibility of a primary pituitary origin. The monoclonality in origin of the majority of the pituitary tumours studied was clearly shown using the X-chromosomal inactivation suggesting the presence of genetic mutations in a progenitor cell with subsequent clonal expansion [9]. The genetic abnormalities so far studied,

Table 10.1 Incidence of micro- and macroprolactinoma in both sexes.

	Men	Women	Total
Microprolactinoma (≤10 mm)	1	86	87
Macroprolactinoma (>10 mm)	26	43	69
Total	27	129	156

including the loss of tumour suppressor genes or the activation of cellular proto-oncogenes, have been recently reviewed [10]. However, the finding of a known genetic mutation in prolactin-secreting tumour is exceptional, although this may change as our knowledge advances. Although oestrogens are known to stimulate the lactotroph, no association between the use of oral contraceptives or other therapeutic oestrogen preparations and the development of a pituitary tumour has been shown [11].

Natural history

Few data are available on the natural history of hyperprolactinaemic conditions, as most hyperprolactinaemic patients are now treated. While the precise risk of development of a large pituitary tumour is unknown, it must be presumed that only a minority of patients with microadenomas will show progressive increase in tumour size, and the development of the disease proceeds extremely slowly [12,13]. When serum prolactin levels are used as an indication of disease activity, either no change or a decrease in serum prolactin over time is seen in most patients in the absence of therapy; only in a few patients is there evidence of a significant increase in serum prolactin. On the other hand, the macroadenoma generally has a more rapid, invasive growth, and therefore needs more careful follow-up.

Pathophysiology

In chronic hyperprolactinaemia, 17-β-oestradiol and progesterone levels in women, and testosterone levels in men, are reduced. Indeed, the increase in prolactin concentration induces marked alterations in the mechanisms involved in reproductive function at hypothalamic and gonadal levels, while the release of gonadotrophins at the level of the pituitary does not seem to be inhibited [5,14,15]. In women, the ovulatory surge of gonadotrophins is abolished, and the frequency of secretory pulses of luteinising hormone (LH) is reduced. Moreover, the positive feedback of oestrogens on LH secretion is lost, and the rise of gonadotrophins in response to clomiphene is usually inhibited.

Induction of ovulation in women and of spermatogenesis in men (with an increase of gonadotrophins, 17-β-oestradiol, progesterone and testosterone) following the administration of pulsatile gonadotrophin-releasing hormone (GnRH) in hyperprolactinaemic patients demonstrates the presence of impaired GnRH secretion, and thus a fall in gonadotrophin secretion as a consequence. The mechanism by which hyperprolactinaemia alters hypothalamic GnRH hormone secretion is still unclear, but an inhibitory effect mediated by increased hypothalamic opiate and/or dopaminergic tone has been suggested [4].

Together with an abnormality at the level of the hypothalamus, hyperprolactinaemia also induces direct inhibition of progesterone and 17-β-oestradiol secretion and thus blockade of ovarian follicle maturation. The possibility of an inhibitory mechanism at the level of the testis is still debated, but there is some evidence that in men hyperprolactinaemia interferes with the peripheral conversion of testosterone to 5-dihydrotestosterone by inhibiting the activity of 5-α-reductase.

Clinical manifestations

The clinical manifestations of hyperprolactinaemia are related to gonadal dysfunction and to tumour mass. For such symptoms, prolactinoma patients may be initially referred to physicians of diverse specialities, such as neurologists, ophthalmologists, gynaecologists or urologists.

Hyperprolactinaemia-dependent symptoms

Chronic hyperprolactinaemia, independent of its cause, may induce in the woman various menstrual abnormalities: primary or secondary amenorrhoea, oligomenorrhoea, a short luteal phase, or infertility with regular cycles [2–5] (Table 10.2). Increased plasma prolactin levels have been demonstrated in nearly one-third of patients with secondary amenorrhoea. Galactorrhoea is found in 30–80% of patients, depending in part on the intensity with which it is sought. Galactorrhoea requires the presence of both oestrogen and prolactin and is thus less common than amenorrhoea alone, as chronic hypogonadism results in oestradiol deficiency. However, galactorrhoea has occasionally been found even in prepubertal children with hyperprolactinaemia.

Dyspareunia and osteoporosis are other findings correlated with chronic hyperprolactinaemia-induced hypo-oestrogenism. The bone density reduction has been attributed either to a direct effect of prolactin on bone or, more probably, is secondary to the oestrogen deficiency *per se*. Hyperprolactinaemic women have also been reported to have normoglycaemic hyperinsulinaemia and increases in adrenal androgen secretion. However, these abnormalities

Table 10.2 Symptoms, clinical signs and prolactin levels in 95 patients with surgically confirmed prolactinomas, 24 with pseudo-prolactinomas and 67 with idiopathic hyperprolactinaemias.

	Prolactinomas	Pseudo-prolactinomas	Idiopathic hyperprolactinaemias
Women			
No. of cases	75	15	63
Mean (range) age (years)	27 (16–57)	46 (23–68)	29 (16–47)
Primary amenorrhoea	7 (9%)	0	2 (3%)
Secondary amenorrhoea	59 (79%)	10 (67%)	15 (24%)
Oligomenorrhoea	5 (7%)	1 (7%)	22 (35%)
Short luteal phase	0	0	3 (5%)
Regular menses	3 (4%)	0	20 (32%)
Menopause	1 (1%)	4 (27%)	1 (2%)
Galactorrhoea	69 (92%)	6 (40%)	44 (70%)
Headache	37 (49%)	7 (47%)	11 (17%)
Visual field defects	5 (7%)	7 (47%)	0
Hypopituitarism	1 (1%)	1 (7%)	0
Mean (range) prolactin levels (ng/ml)	363 (28–4000)	38 (22–62)	55.9 (22–200)
Men			
No. of cases	20	9	4
Mean (range) age (years)	37 (15–61)	46 (19–63)	29 (20–27)
Impotence and reduction of libido	18/18 (100%)	9/9 (100%)	3 (75%)
Hypogonadism	3 (15%)	2 (22%)	0
Gynaecomastia	1 (5%)	1 (11%)	0
Galactorrhoea	3 (15%)	2 (22%)	0
Headache	10 (50%)	3 (33%)	0
Visual field defects	6 (30%)	5 (56%)	0
Hypopituitarism	5 (25%)	6 (67%)	0
Mean (range) prolactin levels (ng/ml)	473 (58–1800)	26.5 (13–50)	36 (20–69)

are usually mild and without obvious clinical relevance, although a polycystic ovary-type syndrome may sometimes be seen.

In men, loss of libido, impotence, reduction in seminal fluid and, more rarely, oligospermia, may occur. If the increase in prolactin levels occurs during puberty this may be arrested with a retardation of beard growth and body hair development. Gynaecomastia is rarely present, while galactorrhoea is found in 10–20% of patients, i.e. at a lower frequency when compared with women (Table 10.2).

Tumour mass-dependent symptoms

Together with hyperprolactinaemia-dependent symptoms, in patients with macroprolactinomas symptoms related to the compressive effects of the pituitary tumour also need to be considered. In these conditions, headache, visual field defects and paralysis of cranial nerves may occur. In addition, headache seems to occur more frequently in women with hyperprolactinaemia and presumed microadenomas [5]. The precise relationship between an elevated serum prolactin level in the setting of normal or near-normal radiological studies and headache is unclear. In patients with macroprolactinomas, a defect in the secretion of other hormones of the anterior pituitary (gonadotrophins, growth hormone, thyrotrophin, adrenocorticotrophic hormone) may also be present. The tumour mass-dependent symptoms appear to be more frequently present in men than in women (Table 10.2), at least in part because of later diagnosis in men.

Diagnosis

The principal diagnostic problem remains the differential diagnosis between hyperprolactinaemia due to a microprolactinoma in the absence of clear radiological evidence of abnormality in the sella turcica, and the so-called idiopathic or functional hyperprolactinaemia (see also Chapter 9). This latter may be defined as a condition in which modern radiological investigations reveal normal morphodensitometric pituitary structure, and any recognised cause of increased prolactin secretion (pregnancy, drugs, hypothyroidism, renal failure, etc.) has been excluded. Somewhat less difficult is the differential diagnosis between a prolactinoma and a non-prolactin-secreting tumour in patients with hyperprolactinaemia. These latter, which may also be referred to as 'pseudo-prolactinomas' [4], are usually either non-functioning pituitary tumours or other tumours of extrapituitary origin (craniopharyngiomas, meningiomas, ectopic pinealomas, third-ventricle tumours, etc.) which cause an increase in serum prolactin by interfering with the delivery of dopamine through pituitary-stalk compression. The diagnosis of these different causes of hyperprolactinaemia is of practical importance in view of the different therapeutic approaches.

The principal diagnostic investigations are radiological and hormonal. Formal visual field testing may also be performed, especially if there is any suggestion of a macroadenoma.

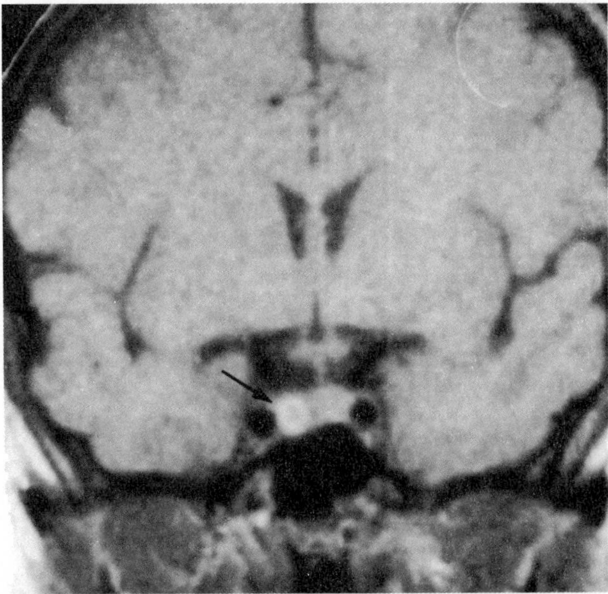

(a)

(b)

Fig. 10.1 (a) High-resolution magnetic resonance imaging (MRI) of microprolactinoma. (b) High-resolution MRI of macroprolactinoma, with suprasellar extension and involvement of optic chiasm.

Radiological investigations

Computed tomography (CT) and magnetic resonance imaging (MRI) are undoubtedly valuable techniques for the early diagnosis of pituitary adenoma (Fig. 10.1). The high-resolution CT technique has to be used either with direct coronal sections or reformatted sections in coronal and sagittal planes, preferably with contiguous images with 1.5-mm collimation through the pituitary gland. Intravenous contrast as a rapid bolus possibly followed by an infusion, should be administered to assess gland homogeneity and the presence or absence of focal lesions. The hallmark of a prolactinoma is a low-density area within the gland. The three-dimensional reconstruction of anatomical structures from CT data has been introduced with a better definition of normal anatomy of the sellar region and anatomical sites of pathology in the sella region, with particular regard to bone structures [16]. The improvement in the diagnosis especially occurs when calcification or erosions of bone structures are present.

MRI is characterised by a higher contrast resolution and a lack of ionising radiation: intravenous contrast enhancement is not always needed, but the use of gadolinium is able to increase the sensitivity of this technique. However, the superiority of MRI over high-resolution CT scanning has not been conclusively demonstrated. In one comparison of CT and MRI scans of patients with a pituitary adenoma, approximately 10% of investigations were judged superior by MRI, 10% superior by CT and 80% were equally effective in demonstrating the lesion [17]. MRI is less helpful than CT in visualising bone erosion, but is better for full definition of suprasellar masses and their proximity to the hypothalamus and optic chiasm (Fig. 10.1b).

High-resolution CT scanning (with contrast enhancement) and MRI are able to directly delineate sellar contents and para- and suprasellar structures, while conventional tomography is able only to evaluate sellar bone morphology. It is therefore possible to diagnose the presence of an adenoma even in patients with an apparently normal sella turcica (Fig. 10.2), and to identify other hypothalamo-pituitary abnormalities, especially a partial or totally empty fossa. Alternatively, CT and MRI may show the presence of a normal pituitary (Fig. 10.3), and therefore identify patients whose hyperprolactinaemia may be defined as idiopathic, although conclusive proof can only be obtained surgically. Therefore, all patients with significant hyperprolactinaemia (with the exclusion of drug-induced hyperprolactinaemia,

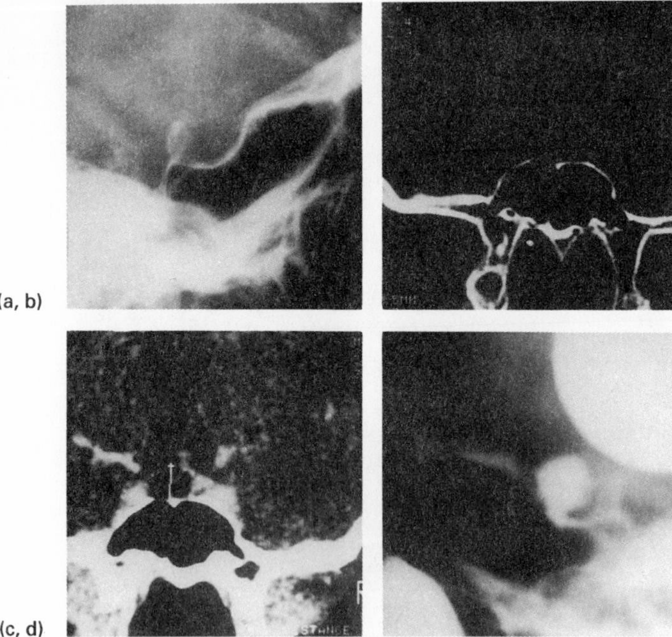

(a, b)

(c, d)

Fig. 10.2 Case of a 19-year-old woman with hyperprolactinaemia (64–70 ng/ml). (a) Normal sellar profile at standard radiography. (b) The normal sellar floor was also confirmed by computed tomography (CT). (c) However, CT showed a 12-mm adenoma. (d) After selective adenomectomy, injection of contrast showed the negative image of the adenoma, identical to that obtained by CT.

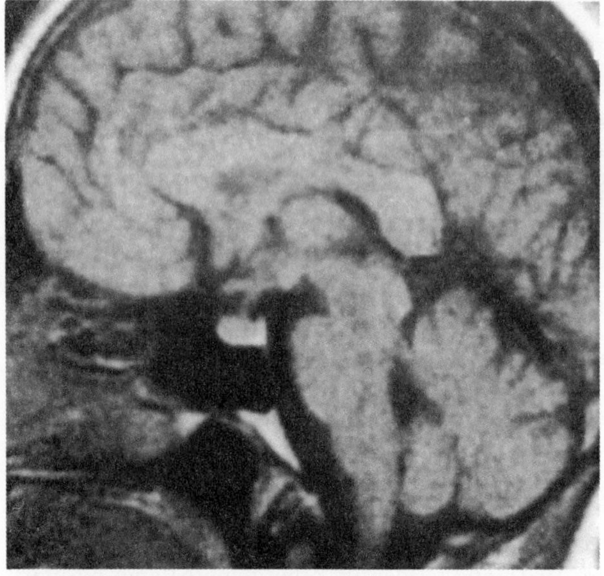

Fig. 10.3 High-resolution magnetic resonance imaging (MRI) (sagittal plane) of a normal pituitary in a 24-year-old woman with hyperprolactinaemia (68–74 ng/ml).

hypothyroidism, renal failure, etc.) need to be considered for such imaging after a standard radiograph (in lateral and frontal projection) and baseline hormonal investigation. Conventional tomography is no longer necessary or desirable. Indeed, some abnormalities of the sella, such as asymmetry of the floor or minor cortical changes, may be regarded as normal variations without pathological significance [18,19].

In a relatively high number of cases even the most sensitive CT or MRI are not conclusive. Moreover, focal defects may frequently be found in healthy subjects and may represent small cysts, areas of necrosis or artifacts [20]. These observations are important in terms of the diagnosis of a microadenoma. Furthermore, in an unselected autopsy series, a microadenoma was present in 27% of the pituitary glands examined without ante-mortem evidence of pituitary disease [19], suggesting that microadenomas may be common and insignificant. Thus, radiological findings must always be correlated with clinical and hormonal data.

Hormonal assessment

Prolactin is secreted in a pulsatile fashion and levels vary throughout a 24-hour period. For these reasons, the diagnosis of hyperprolactinaemia may be made on the basis of a single serum sample only if the level is sufficiently elevated. On the other hand, it is prudent to obtain several samples in the presence of a mildly elevated level which may reflect a random peak, or may be the result of stress. This can easily be achieved by obtaining a single sample on three separate days, or three sequential samples every 30 min when the patient is sufficiently relaxed (see also Chapter 9). Once the diagnosis of hyperprolactinaemia is established, the numerous secondary causes should be considered. After pregnancy, drugs, hypothyroidism and other pathological conditions have been excluded, a search for hypothalamic or pituitary disease is necessary. As already mentioned, despite the recent advances in technology, radiographic studies are not always conclusive. Patients diagnosed as having idiopathic hyperprolactinaemia may actually harbour small microadenomas not shown by CT or MRI scanning. It has generally been shown [2–5] that prolactin values of 100–200 ng/ml (2000–4000 mU/l) and above are almost always indicative of a prolactin-secreting tumour, but the presence of a prolactinoma cannot be excluded even if prolactin values are only minimally increased. Conversely, prolactin values higher than 100 ng/ml (2000 mU/l) have occasionally been found in patients with idiopathic hyperprolactinaemia or an empty sella (Fig. 10.4).

As has been discussed (see Chapter 9), dynamic function tests are useful for 'group' discrimination but cannot be used for individual patients, even when used in conjunction with high-resolution CT scanning [8] (Fig. 10.5). Further longitudinal studies are needed to ascertain whether the tumour-like neuroendocrine pattern in patients with idiopathic

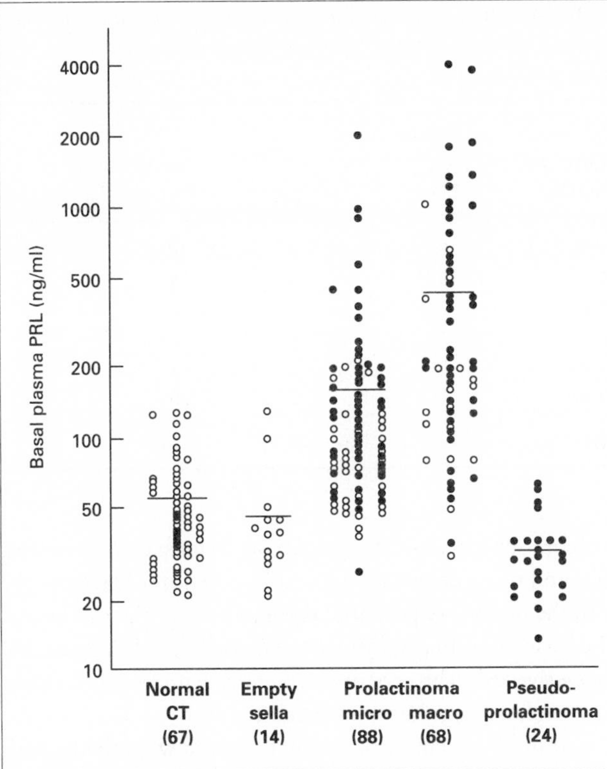

Fig. 10.4 Basal prolactin levels in 261 patients with hyperprolactinaemia. All patients were diagnosed based on computed tomographic scan (○) or histological evaluation (●). The number of patients is shown in parentheses. The horizontal lines indicate the mean prolactin levels for each group of patients.

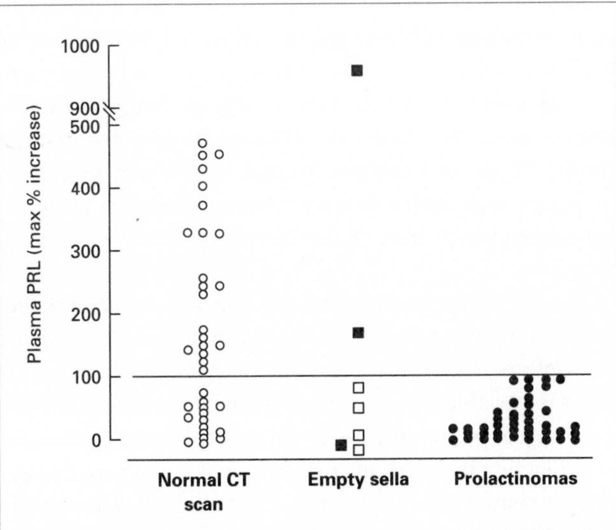

Fig. 10.5 Plasma prolactin changes after domperidone test (10 mg i.v.) in patients with normal computed tomograms, partial (■) or total (□) empty sella, and prolactinomas. The shaded line represents the lower normal limit.

hyperprolactinaemia does or does not represent a valid biological marker predicting the tumorous evolution of the disease.

Another diagnostic problem is the differential diagnosis between prolactinoma and 'pseudo-prolactinoma'. Identification of these forms of hyperprolactinaemia is an important issue as pseudo-prolactinomas are usually unresponsive to medical treatment with dopamine agonists. Prolactin levels that are only mildly elevated are usually found in non-prolactin-secreting tumours (Fig. 10.4; Table 10.2). Thus, the finding of mild hyperprolactinaemia in patients with macroadenomas may suggest the presence of a pseudo-prolactinoma, although, as already mentioned, this does not entirely exclude the existence of a prolactinoma. A normal or reduced thyrotrophin response to a dopamine-receptor antagonist is suggestive, but not diagnostic, of a pseudo-prolactinoma (Fig. 10.6). The administration of dopamine agonists may reduce plasma prolactin in both types of patients; however, only in patients with true prolactinomas is a drug-induced reduction in tumour size frequently observed; hence, a short course of dopaminergic drugs may be of some diagnostic value. The availability of α-subunit assay in specialised centres also may be of some help in detecting endocrine-inactive tumours.

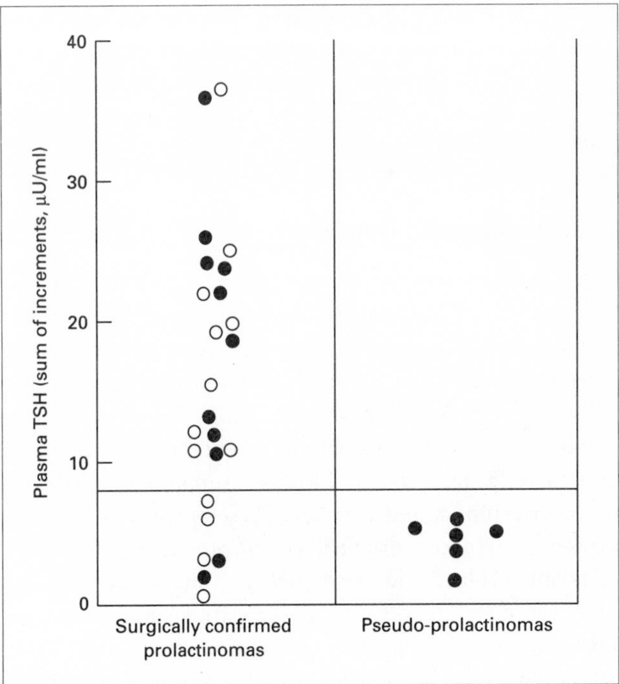

Fig. 10.6 Thyrotrophin (TSH) response to domperidone (10 mg i.v.) in 24 patients with surgically confirmed prolactinoma (left panel) or 'pseudo-prolactinoma' (right panel); ○, microadenomas; ●, macroadenomas. The horizontal line represents the upper normal limit.

It has been suggested that dynamic function tests may be helpful in evaluating the outcome of patients with prolactinoma who are successfully cured by adenomectomy, and in predicting which patients are at risk of relapse [21], but the evidence is far from conclusive.

Therapy

The treatment of prolactin-secreting tumours remains controversial although standardised treatment plans are becoming more frequently accepted. It may include pharmacological, surgical and radiotherapeutic procedures, either in isolation or in combination. Alternatively, in females with microadenomas or doubtful pituitary pathology and only mild hyperprolactinaemia, the possibility of careful follow-up in the absence of treatment may be considered, provided that clinical symptoms are absent or mild, and oestrogen levels are in the normal range.

In order to evaluate the efficacy of a form of treatment, the following goals need to be considered: (i) normalisation of prolactin levels and, subsequently, correction of the hypogonadism and the galactorrhoea; (ii) reduction of the tumour mass and the related pressure symptoms; (iii) preservation or restoration of other anterior pituitary function; and (iv) prevention of recurrence or progression of disease. Therefore, careful monitoring of prolactin levels and of the other pituitary hormones, of visual field and of pituitary morphology (using CT and/or MRI), need to be undertaken during therapy.

In patients likely to have a pseudo-prolactinoma, surgery is the treatment of choice, with or without subsequent radiotherapy (see Chapter 13).

Pharmacological treatment

The introduction of specific dopamine agonists into clinical medicine was a significant advance in the treatment of patients with hyperprolactinaemia and prolactinoma. Bromocriptine, a semisynthetic ergot alkaloid, is the prototype for other dopamine agonist preparations [2,4,5]. This drug directly stimulates specific neuronal and pituitary-cell membrane dopamine D_2 receptors and exerts a suppressive action on prolactin synthesis and secretion. Therefore, it is usually able markedly to reduce prolactin levels and produce normalisation of serum prolactin in most patients, independent of the presence of an adenoma. However, patients may vary considerably in their sensitivity to dopaminergic drugs (Table 10.3). This may be due either to the variable number of dopaminergic receptors present on the lactotrophs or to post-receptor events. Recently, bromocriptine-resistant prolactinomas that lack D_2 receptors were shown to express the receptors for nerve growth factor (NGF) [22]. After exposure to NGF human prolactinoma cells decreased their proliferation rate, lost their capability to form colonies in soft agar and re-expressed the typical D_2 receptor of lactotrophs with the inhibitory potential regulation of prolactin release. The possibility that treatment with NGF could restore the responsiveness to bromocriptine therapy in previously resistant patients has been therefore suggested.

Table 10.3 Dose of oral bromocriptine required to induce normal prolactin levels in 74 patients with tumorous or idiopathic hyperprolactinaemia.

Bromocriptine (mg/day)	Prolactinoma		Idiopathic hyperprolactinaemia
	Micro	Macro	
1.25–3.75	8	7	16
5	9	3	2
7.5	2	3	4
10	7	5	2
15–20	0	2	1
30–50	2	2	0
Total	28	22	25

It should be emphasised that in a few patients with macroadenomas, prolactin normalization may be achieved only with high doses of the drug and after many months of therapy (Fig. 10.7). This dose may not remain constant for long-term treatment, and continued suppression of serum prolactin may be maintained with progressively lower doses of the dopamine agonist. As the therapeutic effect usually disappears with drug discontinuation, treatment needs to be continuous.

Together with normalisation of prolactin levels, disappearance or reduction of the galactorrhoea and resumption of normal gonadal function in both sexes is usually apparent. Fertility may be restored early, and the patient may rapidly become pregnant even after many years of amenorrhoea. Amenorrhoea and changes in libido and potency respond to dopamine agonists unless there is associated gonadotrophin deficiency, which may occur in some patients with large tumours.

The dopaminergic agonist drugs may also induce a reduction in tumour mass (Fig. 10.8) with improvement of visual field defects and restoration of other pituitary functions. This effect is variable, may occur early or late, and seems to be unrelated to basal prolactin levels or the degree of reduction in prolactin. In addition, tumours will usually re-expand after discontinuation of treatment; prolactinomas are usually reversibly reduced in size and do not disappear. However, persistence of tumour regression after discontinuation of chronic therapy for many years has also been reported.

The mechanism of reduction of prolactin secretion and of prolactinoma volume occurs by interference with the

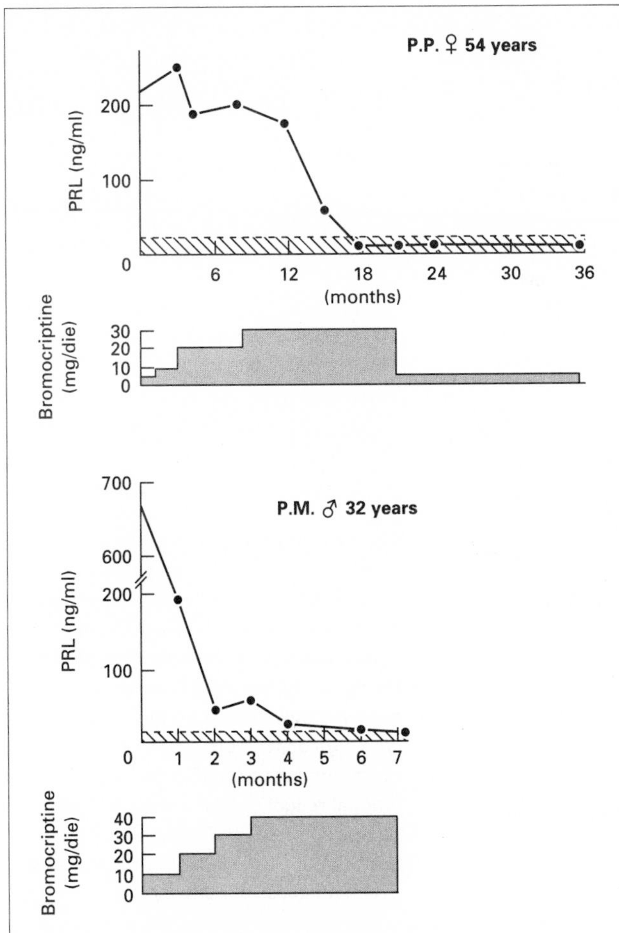

Fig. 10.7 Late normalization of prolactin levels in two bromocriptine-resistant macroprolactinomas. Prolactin levels normalised only after prolonged treatment with high doses of bromocriptine. The shaded area represents normal prolactin values.

transcriptional regulation of the prolactin gene and hence messenger RNA synthesis. The nucleolus of the prolactinoma cell shrinks by an average of 49%. The reduction in the cytoplasm is mainly caused by pronounced shrinkage of the rough endoplasmic reticulum and the Golgi cisterns [2].

While most patients show a satisfactory biochemical and clinical response to dopamine-agonist therapy, isolated reports of a few patients in whom progression of the disease has occurred during dopaminergic therapy have been described; this occurrence emphasises the need for close monitoring of all patients with prolactinomas.

Bromocriptine is usually administered orally in two or three daily doses; however, the efficacy of single evening dose administration has been clearly shown [23], and once-daily therapy is effective in most patients. The drug is usually well tolerated. Some side-effects (nausea, vomiting, postural hypotension) may be present initially, but they usually

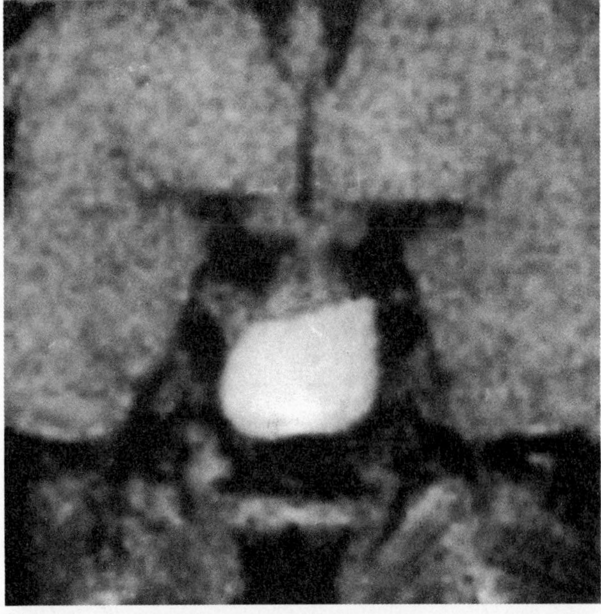
(a)

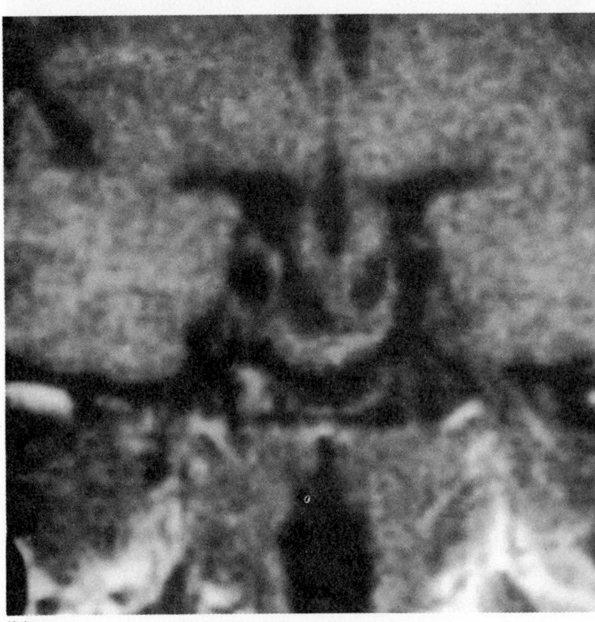
(b)

Fig. 10.8 Magnetic resonance imaging scan before (a) and 6 months after therapy (b) with bromocriptine in a patient with macroprolactinoma. The tumour completely disappeared on therapy.

disappear during therapy. To prevent or minimize such side-effects, it is usually advisable to start the treatment with a low dose, at bedtime, with a small meal. The dose is then gradually increased over days or weeks to that inducing a maximal therapeutic response, the drug always being taken during a bulk meal. Other less-commonly encountered side-effects include headache, fatigue, abdominal cramps, nasal congestion, constipation and hallucinations.

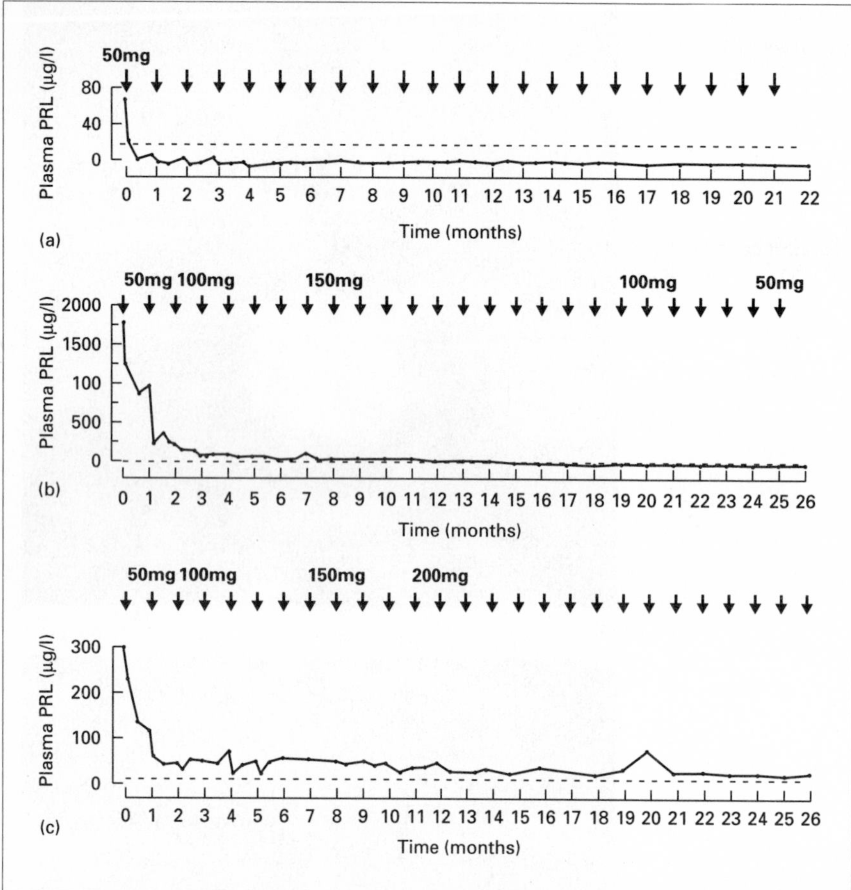

Fig. 10.9 Plasma prolactin (PRL) response to chronic treatment with Parlodel LAR. (a) The patient had normal PRL levels within 24 hours of the first injection, and this persisted throughout the study. (b) Normal PRL levels were achieved only after prolonged treatment with high doses. However, normoprolactinaemia persisted after gradual reduction of the drug. (c) The patient had a marked reduction of PRL, although this was never normalized, even with high doses of Parlodel LAR.

A new depot preparation of bromocriptine for parenteral use (Parlodel Long Acting Repeatable) has recently been developed. A single intramuscular injection of bromocriptine is usually able to induce a rapid decrease in prolactin levels and to maintain low hormonal levels for approximately 1 month [24]. The long-term administration of the drug, given once monthly in doses of 50–200 mg, is able rapidly to reduce and to maintain normal prolactin levels in most cases (Fig. 10.9a). In some cases, high doses are initially required to induce normalization of prolactin levels, which can subsequently be maintained with lower doses of the drug (Fig. 10.9b). Partial or complete resistance to high doses of bromocriptine is rarely found (Fig. 10.9c). Side-effects, if any, are usually initially present for only 1–2 days, and even they may be attenuated by coadministration of a glucocorticoid. Therefore, this parenteral preparation represents an important therapeutic approach as an alternative to oral bromocriptine.

Other dopaminergic drugs, all given by the oral route, have been introduced into medical practice. Lisuride seems to have a similar efficacy and duration of action to bromocriptine, although side-effects may be more marked. Terguride, the 9–10, dihydrogenated derivative of lisuride, has been shown to be better tolerated than bromocriptine. Metergoline and dihydroergokryptine seem to induce side-effects of lesser intensity; however, they also have a lower efficacy compared with bromocriptine. Pergolide and cabergoline are characterised by a very long-lasting prolactin-lowering activity. In particular cabergoline, which has been very recently introduced into clinical practice, can be given once or twice *weekly*. The therapeutic dose is 0.25–4 mg/week. Cabergoline has been shown to be as effective as bromocriptine but better tolerated [25]. Quinagolide is a non-ergot dopamine agonist which is effective once-daily, and has been reported to lower prolactin in bromocriptine-resistant patients. Occasionally, a patient who is intolerant of one drug may be more tolerant of another, so that a choice of agents is useful.

Oestrogens should never be given to a woman with undiagnosed menstrual irregularities unless she has been shown to have a normal serum prolactin level. However, in patients with microadenomas or idiopathic hyperprolactinaemia, if hyperprolactinaemia is controlled with dopamine agonists, combination with oral contraceptives may be prescribed as long as serum prolactin is monitored [4].

Surgical treatment (see Chapter 19)

Trans-sphenoidal adenomectomy is today the main surgical approach. Apart from individual preference, the availability of an expert neurosurgeon and other aspects such as the age or desire for pregnancy, the considerations for neurosurgical treatment include the diameter of the tumour and intolerance or resistance of the patient to medical therapy. Moreover, some patients request surgery in order to be independent of drug therapy, or because they are anxious regarding the presence of an intracranial tumour.

The efficacy of the surgical treatment depends on the diameter of the tumour and on the prolactin level [2,4,5] (Table 10.4). In general, patients with microprolactinomas show a normalisation of prolactin levels in 60–90% of cases. This frequency dramatically decreases (0–40%) in patients with macroprolactinomas or very high prolactin levels. In these latter, there is a high incidence of post-surgical hypopituitarism.

Preoperative short-term treatment with dopaminergic drugs may soften the macroprolactinoma and facilitate operation. However, there is some question as to whether prolonged pretreatment with bromocriptine makes the surgical approach more difficult and resection less successful due to the development of fibrosis [2]. Finally, 'cured' patients after adenomectomy have a significant risk of recurrence of hyperprolactinaemia, although the recurrence rate is highly variable in different surgical series.

Radiotherapy (see Chapter 20)

Pituitary irradiation is able to reduce plasma prolactin levels in most patients, but normalisation of hormonal levels may take some time to be achieved. Therefore, this treatment is usually followed by dopamine-agonist administration with intermittent withdrawal of medical treatment to determine the effectiveness of pituitary irradiation [4,5]. Due to the prolonged time required for the therapeutic effect to be manifest, and because of the possibility of pituitary insufficiency, radiotherapy is not usually the first-line treatment, but complements neurosurgery in patients with macroadenomas. Radiotherapy is also needed for aggressive, rapidly growing microadenomas, and may be useful in patients with non-surgically treated macroadenomas as definitive therapy after maximal shrinkage with dopaminergic drugs.

Table 10.4 Normalization of prolactin levels after selective trans-sphenoidal adenomectomy in 95 patients with prolactin secreting adenomas.

	No. of patients (%)	
Diameter of the adenoma		
≤10 mm	32/51	(63)
>10 mm	5/44	(11)
Preoperative prolactin level (ng/ml)		
<100	22/26	(85)
<200	34/56	(61)
>200	3/39	(8)

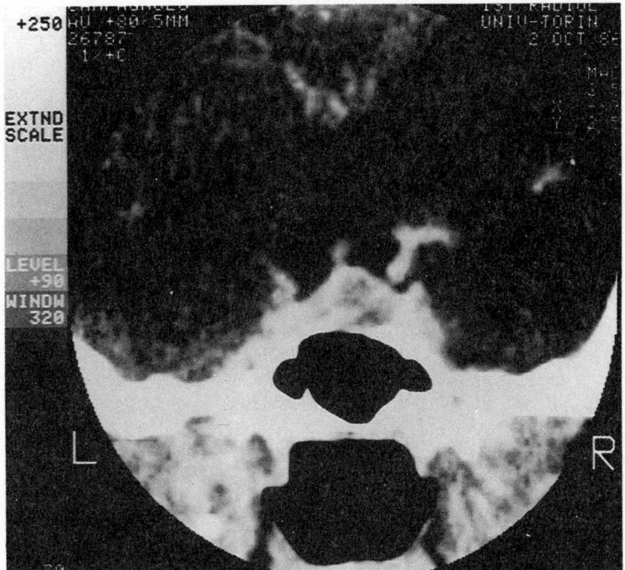

(a)

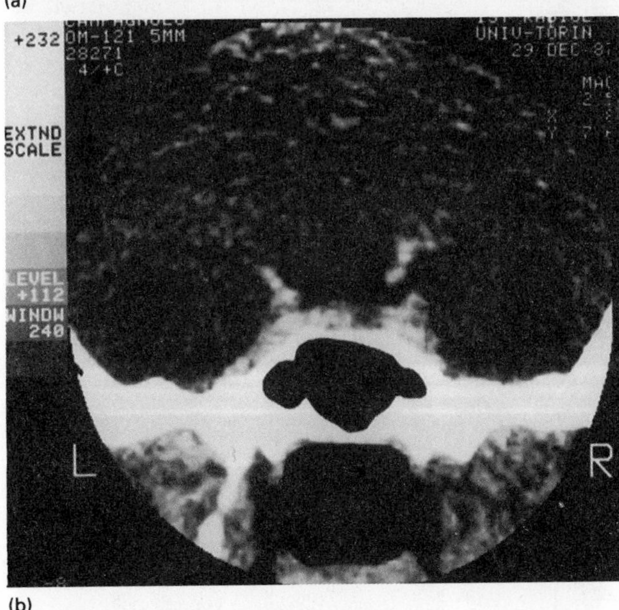

(b)

Fig. 10.10 (a) Computed tomography scan of a 28-year-old woman with a macroprolactinoma, maximal diameter 12 mm. She complained of oligomenorrhoea and galactorrhoea, with a mean prolactin level of 4800 mU/l. (b) Following a year's therapy with cabergoline 1 mg once weekly, shrinkage of the adenoma is clearly shown (diameter 6 mm).

General considerations relating to the choice of treatment

A proper therapeutic strategy for prolactin-secreting tumours may need one or more associated treatments in relation to the diameter of the adenoma, the desire for pregnancy, the age of the patient and the tolerability of dopaminergic drugs.

A macroprolactinoma should initially always be treated medically in order to reduce tumour mass, as neurosurgery is only rarely able to remove the tumour completely and to normalise prolactin levels. Moreover, in such cases the incidence of post-surgical hypopituitarism is high. Whenever medical treatment is able to decompress the optic chiasm and to reduce the tumour mass to within the pituitary fossa, chronic medical therapy, radiotherapy or neurosurgery should be considered. Surgery is advisable when, after some months of treatment with dopaminergic drugs, the tumour does not show any significant reduction with persistent extrasellar extension. If it is not possible to normalise prolactin levels by surgery and dopaminergic drugs, or drugs alone, radiotherapy may be necessary, particularly for invasive adenomas.

A microprolactinoma may be treated either medically or surgically. As medical therapy is usually well tolerated and effective, it should be considered the main therapeutic approach. On the other hand, transsphenoidal selective adenomectomy may be indicated in patients who do not tolerate or do not accept chronic medical therapy. Nevertheless, the finding of a relatively high

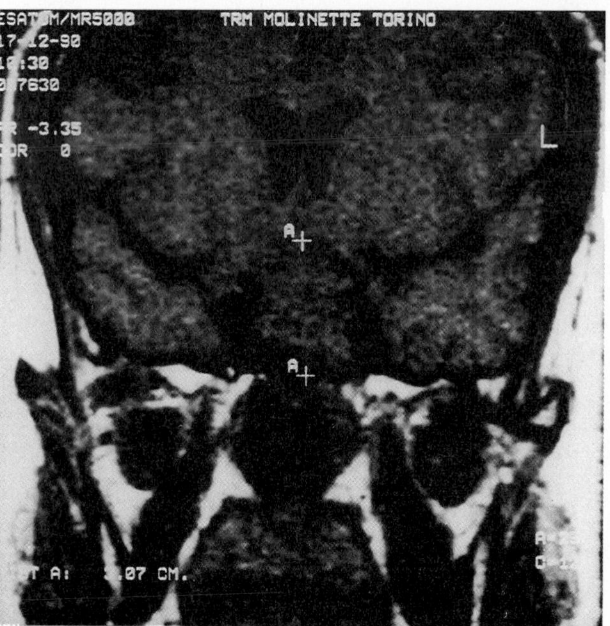

Fig. 10.11 Magnetic resonance image of a 42-year-old man with a macroprolactinoma and a large suprasellar extension invading the third ventricle; serum prolactin was 126 000 mU/l. This was an incidental discovery after loss of vision following a road traffic accident. On direct questioning, the patient admitted to headaches over the last 2 years with loss of libido and potency.

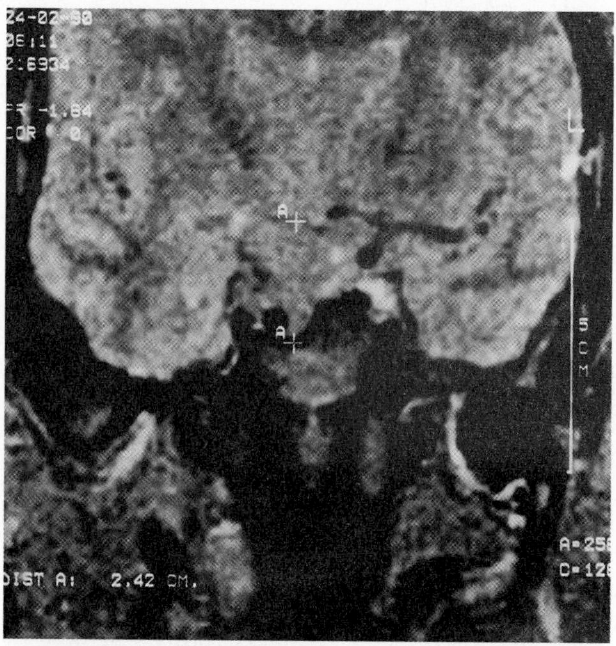

(a)

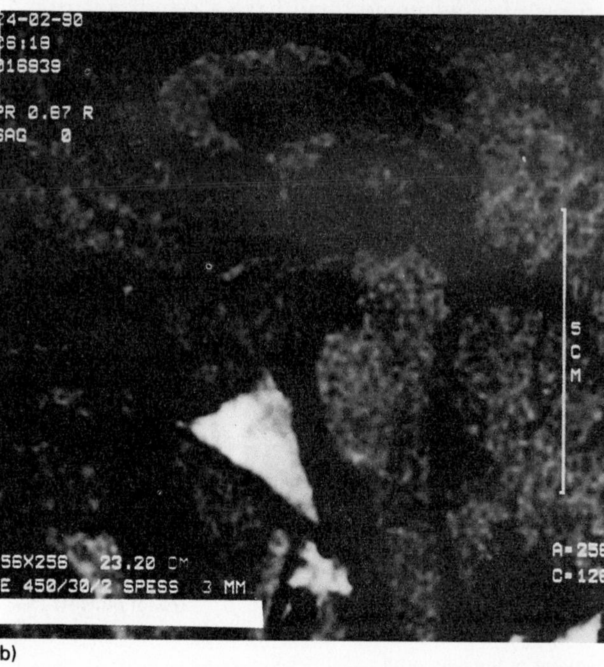

(b)

Fig. 10.12 Coronal (a) and sagittal (b) magnetic resonance images of a 33-year-old woman with a macroprolactinoma with suprasellar and lateral extension (diameter of the tumour 24×30 mm). Serum prolactin was 10 800 mU/l. She complained of secondary amenorrhoea, galactorrhoea, right quadrantinopia and headache. She had previously been operated upon transsphenoidally 4 years previously.

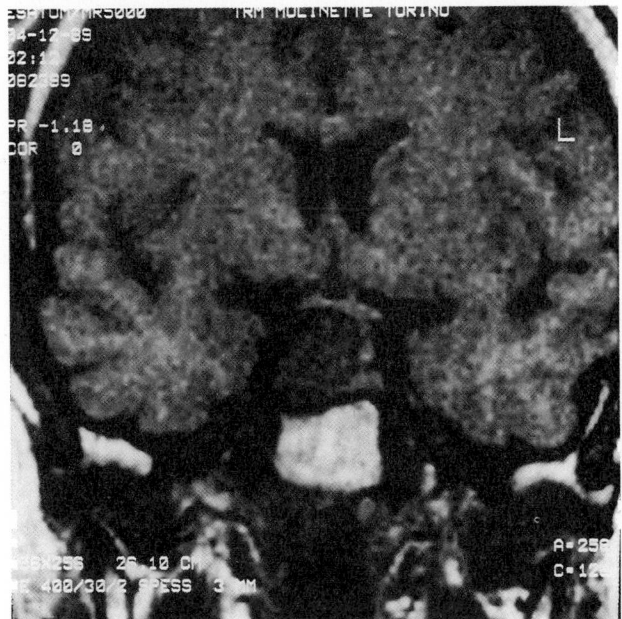

Fig. 10.13 Magnetic resonance image of a 19-year-old woman with a macroprolactinoma with suprasellar and lateral extension, reaching the chiasm (diameter of the tumour 19×20 mm); serum prolactin was 2400 mU/l. She complained of secondary amenorrhoea and galactorrhoea.

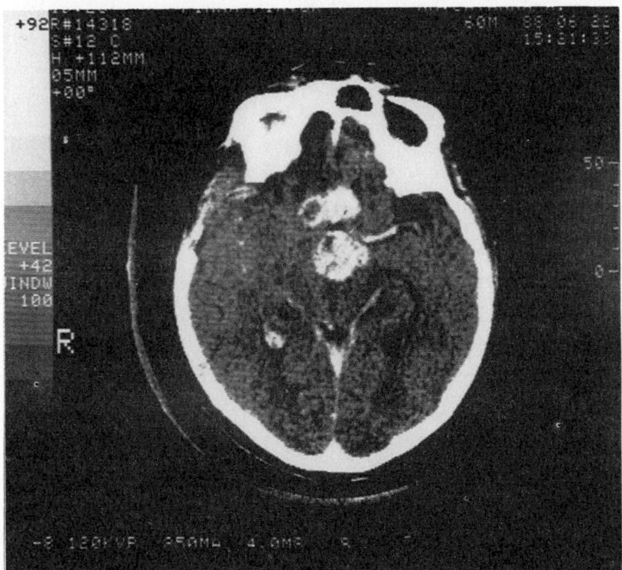

Fig. 10.14 Axial computed tomography scan of a 58-year-old man with a tumour showing suprasellar extension superiorly to the third ventricle and anteriorly to the frontal lobe; haemorrhage is shown inside the tumour; the prolactin level was 8800 mU/l. The tumour was an incidental discovery following a severe road traffic accident. The patient had had bitemporal hemianopia for 5 years, and was pan-hypopituitary. He underwent transcranial surgery 3 months after the accident, followed by radiotherapy.

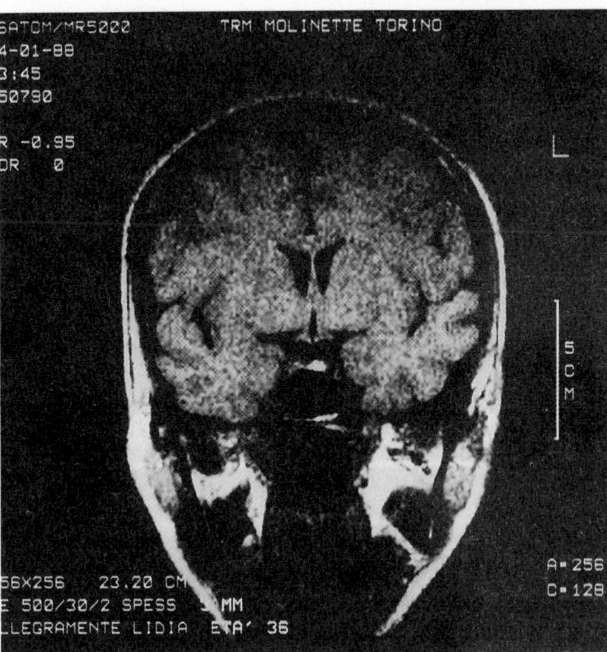

Fig. 10.15 Coronal magnetic resonance image of a 36-year-old female patient complaining of oligomenorrhoea and galactorrhoea; her serum prolactin level was 1300 mU/l. She was found to have a left-sided microprolactinoma at surgery (diameter 4 mm).

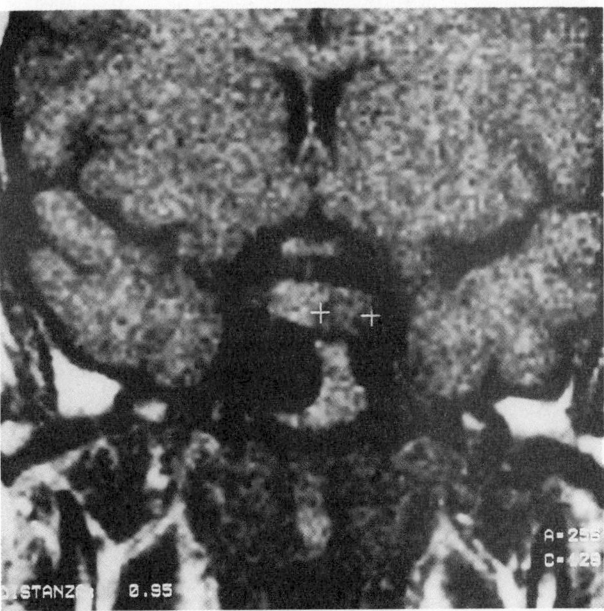

Fig. 10.16 Coronal magnetic resonance image of a 22-year-old female patient complaining of secondary amenorrhoea and galactorrhoea; her serum level was 1100 mU/l. A microprolactinoma (diameter 9.5 mm) was found at surgery.

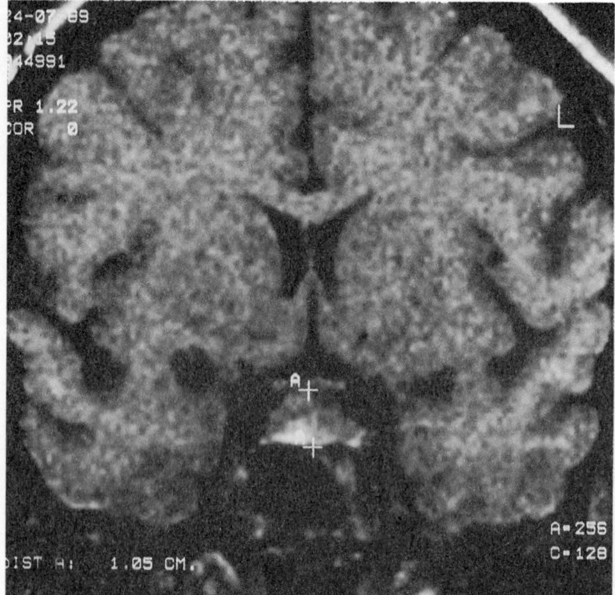

Fig. 10.17 Coronal magnetic resonance image of a 33-year-old female patient complaining of secondary amenorrhoea and galactorrhoea; her serum prolactin level was 2200 mU/l. The presence of a microprolactinoma with a diameter of 9×12 mm is shown.

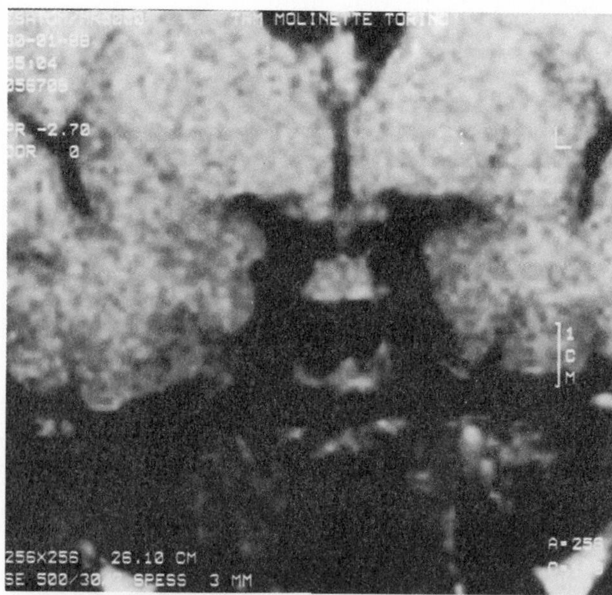

Fig. 10.19 Coronal magnetic resonance image of a normal pituitary in a 32-year-old female with normal endocrinology and regular ovulatory menses.

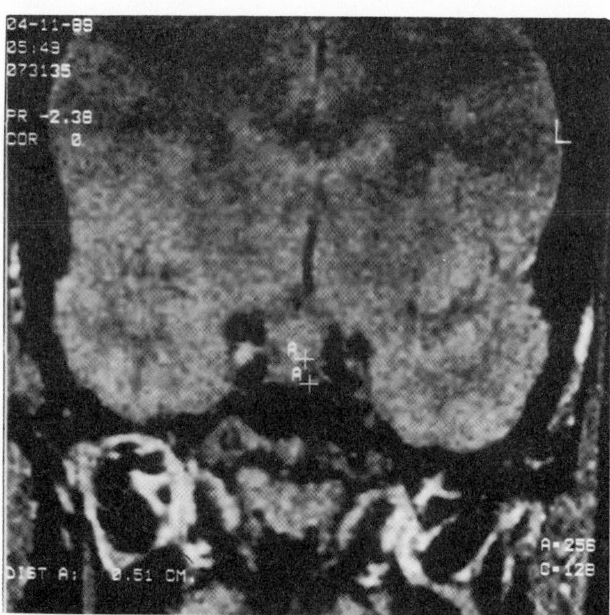

Fig. 10.18 Coronal magnetic resonance image of a 20-year-old female patient. She had regular menses with ovulation (she became spontaneously pregnant in 1990); her only complaint was of galactorrhoea. Her prolactin level was 1300 mU/l. The presence of a microprolactinoma (diameter 5 mm) is shown on magnetic resonance imaging.

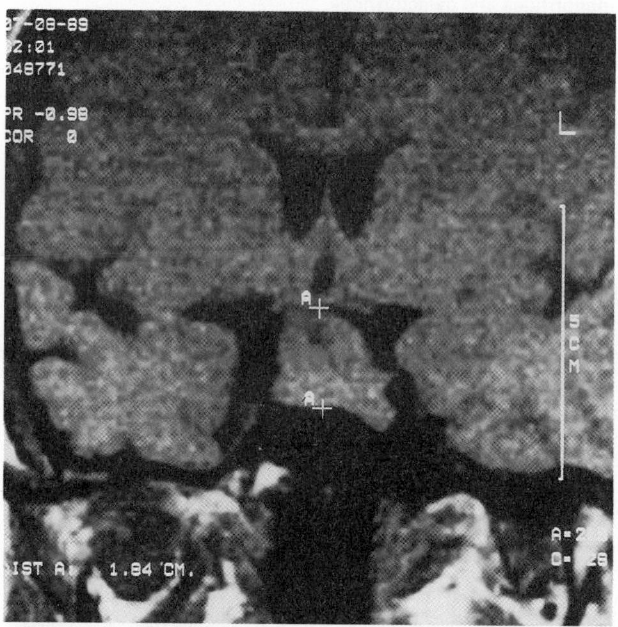

Fig. 10.20 Coronal magnetic resonance image of a 38-year-old female patient complaining of secondary amenorrhoea and galactorrhoea. Her prolactin level was 1500 mU/l. Magnetic resonance imaging shows the presence of a macroprolactinoma (diameter 18 mm). She was therefore treated with dopamine agonist drugs with normalisation of prolactin levels and of clinical symptoms, but with persistence of the large tumour. Following transsphenoidal surgery, a non-functioning tumour was found with negative immunostaining for prolactin ('pseudo-prolactinoma').

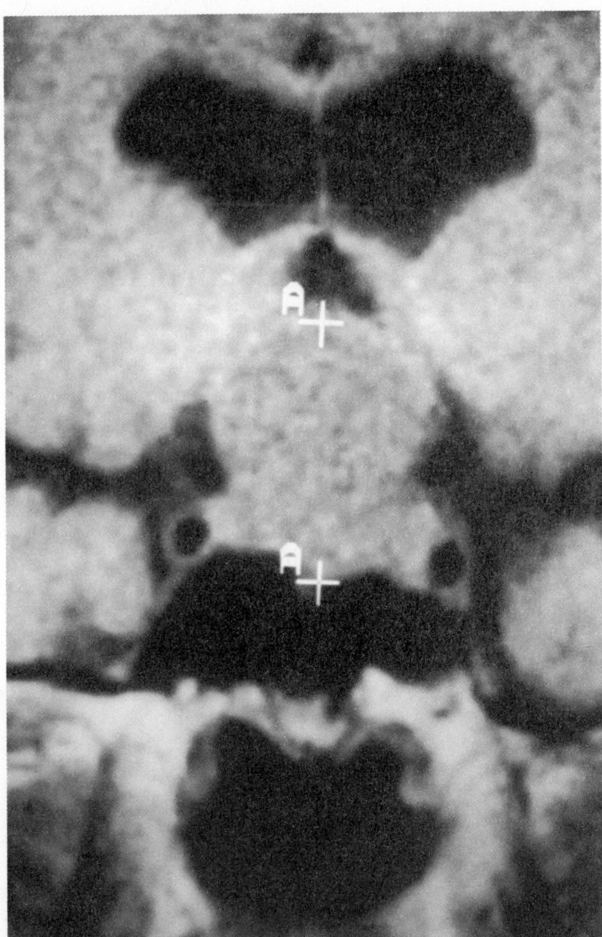

Fig. 10.21 Coronal magnetic resonance image of a 45-year-old female patient with a clinically non-functioning pituitary tumour, which was surgically confirmed. She complained of a visual field defect (bitemporal hemianopia) and 3 years of amenorrhoea without menopausal symptoms. She had a mildly elevated serum prolactin level of 800 mU/l. However, following dopamine agonist therapy the tumour enlarged and she was admitted to surgery.

incidence of late relapses after surgery appears to limit the place of surgical treatment. Finally, in some patients with mild hyperprolactinaemia without hypo-oestrogenism, the possibility of careful follow-up without treatment may be a possible option.

Pregnancy in patients with prolactinoma

Once a woman has received effective treatment for hyperprolactinaemia, fertility is usually restored. This may occur extremely rapidly, such that the patient needs to be informed about the possibility of becoming pregnant before the onset of menses.

As soon as pregnancy is confirmed, treatment with dopaminergic drugs is usually discontinued. However, bromocriptine has been uneventfully given throughout

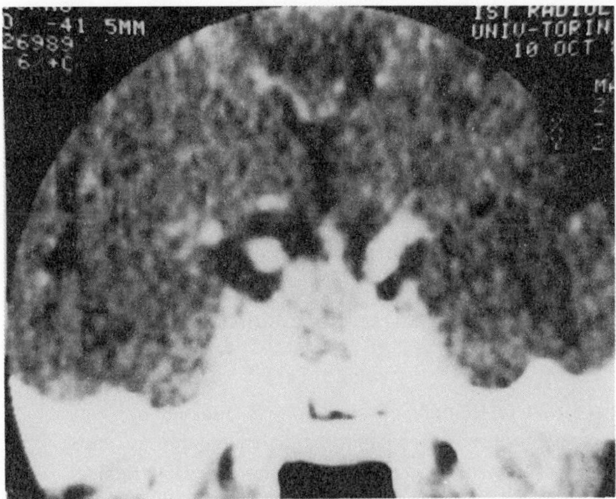

Fig. 10.22 Coronal computed tomography scan of a 72-year-old acromegalic woman with a macroadenoma and mild hyperprolactinaemia (GH 37 ng/ml; prolactin 480 mU/l).

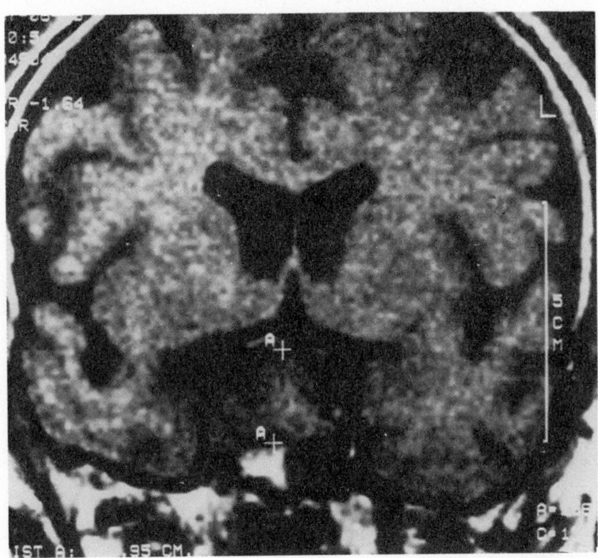

Fig. 10.23 Coronal magnetic resonance image of a 69-year-old man with a non-functioning pituitary macroadenoma and normal serum prolactin (260 mU/l).

pregnancy to prevent tumour expansion. Bromocriptine does not appear to interfere with pregnancy, and there is no increased risk of spontaneous abortion or congenital abnormality associated with exposure to the drug. Information regarding the newer dopamine agonists is much more limited. The management of women with prolactinoma during pregnancy remains controversial, although there is general agreement that these patients should be followed up closely for the development of symptoms of pituitary expansion, for example headache, visual field defects and ophthalmoplegia. Since the volume of the normal pituitary gland increases by approximately 70% during pregnancy, expansion in patients harbouring a prolactinoma is of particular concern. However, it appears that pregnant women with microadenomas have a very low risk for the development of complications related to pituitary expansion, perhaps of the order of 1% or slightly less. In women with macroadenomas, the risk is higher, but is probably less than 25% [4,5].

In the presence of a macroprolactinoma, before pregnancy either radiotherapy and/or neurosurgery is necessary; alternatively, bromocriptine may be administered throughout the pregnancy.

The development of significant pituitary expansion and of complications may be managed expectantly, medically with bromocriptine, or surgically. On the other hand, it is worth noting that a reduction or a normalisation of prolactin levels has been shown in some cases after pregnancy, probably due to spontaneous partial necrosis of the adenoma.

Neuroradiology of prolactinomas

Over the last decade, significant advances have been made in neuroradiological techniques which have influenced the diagnostic assessment of patients with pituitary tumours and, in particular, of prolactin-secreting tumours. Current neurodiagnostic procedures are less uncomfortable for patients and carry less risk, and the data provided are more easily interpreted than those afforded by older techniques such as pneumoencephalography. High-resolution CT scanning and MRI are the most important techniques used

Fig. 10.24 (a) Computed tomography (CT) scan of a macroadenoma showing lateral extension into the cavernous sinuses but without bony erosion (left, coronal scan; right, three-dimensional reconstruction). (b) CT scan of a macroadenoma showing inferior extension through the base of the sella and invasion and destruction of the bone (left, coronal scan; right, three-dimensional reconstruction).

(a)

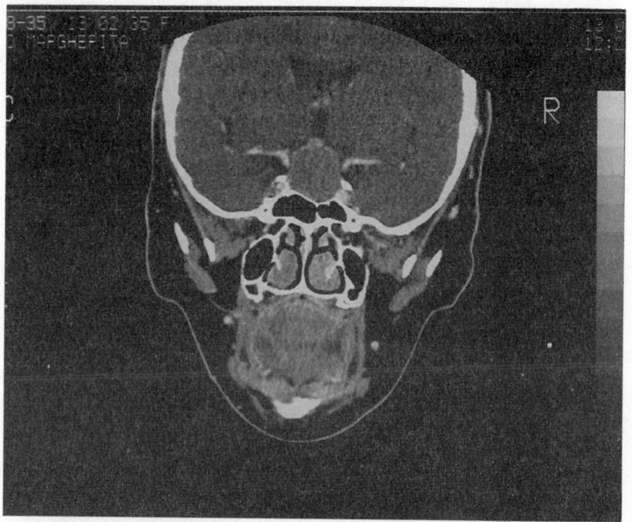

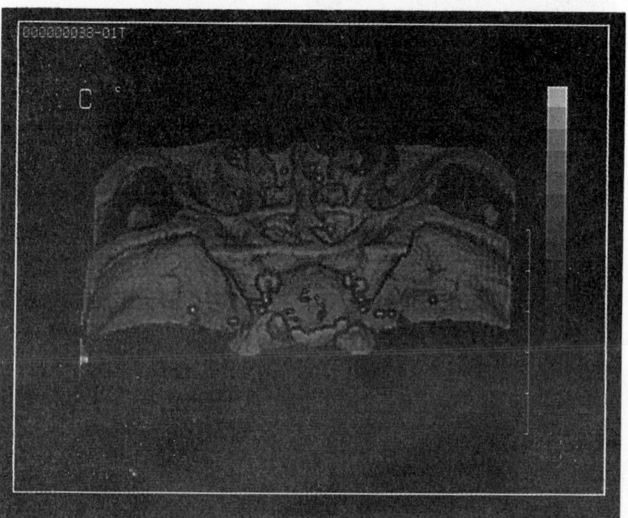

(b)

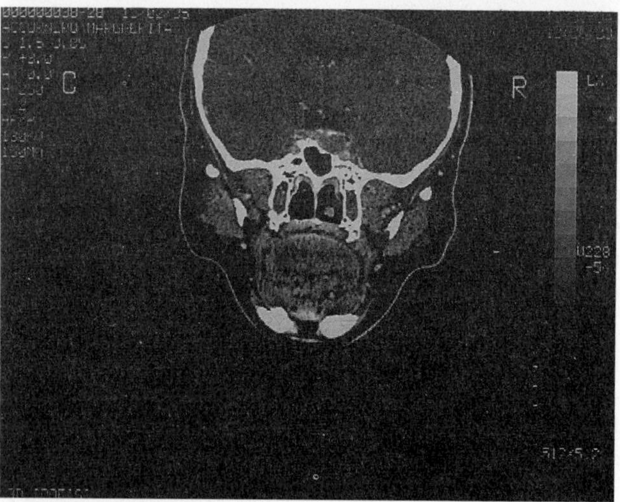

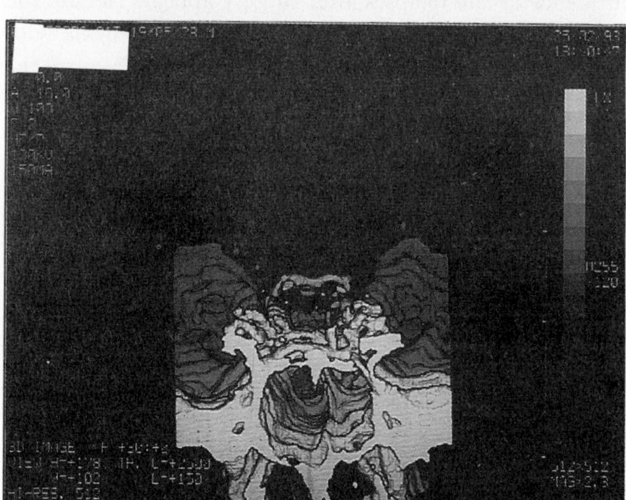

nowadays in the diagnosis of prolactinomas. In particular, MRI seems to be the ideal procedure for macroadenomas as it is best able to show the anatomy of hypothalamo-pituitary region, although details of bone structure are not clearly shown. In Figs. 10.10–10.24, some MRI or CT scans of patients with prolactinomas are shown. In addition, the normal pituitary, growth hormone-secreting tumours and 'pseudo-prolactinomas' are also shown for comparison. MRI scans were obtained using Esatom Esaote, 0.5 Tesla, 3-mm thickness, with a two signal acquisition 256×256 matrix and two-dimensional multislice data acquisition in coronal and sagittal planes. Each slice location was imaged with both a short repetition time (TR 500 ms) with a 30-ms echo delay (TE), and a long TR (1500 ms) with 100 ms TE. A gap of 2 mm was obtained between adjacent slices.

High-resolution CT was performed with a General Electric CT/T 8800 scanner, with direct coronal scans during contrast medium injection, or Tomoscan LX, Phyliphs, with three-dimensional reconstruction.

Radiological scans were kindly provided by T. Avataneo, MD, Institute of Radiology, University of Turin and by W. Liboni, Department of Neuroradiology, Ospedale Gradenigo, Turin.

References

1 Farid NR, Buehler S, Russel NA, Maroun FB, Allerdice P. Prolactinomas in familial multiple endocrine neoplasia syndrome type. *Am J Med* 1980; **69**: 874–80.

2 Labhart A, Proesch ER, Landolt AM, Prader A, Zachmann MJ, Zapf J. The adenohypophysis. In: Labhart A, ed. *Clinicial Endocrinology* (2nd ed.) Berlin: Springer Verlag, 1986: 124–6.

3 Schlechte J, Sherman B, Halmi N *et al.* Prolactin secreting pituitary tumors in amenorrheic women: a comprehensive study. *Endocr Rev* 1980; **1**: 295–308.

4 Grossman A, Besser GM. Prolactinoma. *Br Med J* 1985; **290**: 182.

5 Vance ML, Thorner MO. Prolactin: hyperprolactinemic syndromes and management. In: Degroot LY, ed. *Endocrinology*. WB Saunders, 1989: 408–18.

6 Asa SL, Kovacs K. Histological classification of pituitary disease. *Clin Endocrinol Metab* 1983; **12**: 567–96.

7 Landolt AM, Minder H. Immunohistochemical examination of the paraadenomatous 'normal' pituitary: an evaluation of prolactin cell hyperplasia. *Virchows Arch Pathol Anat* 1984; **403**: 181–93.

8 Camanni F, Ciccarelli E, Ghigo E, Muller EE. Hyperprolactinaemia neuroendocrine and diagnostic aspects. *J Endocrinol Invest* 1989; **12**: 653–68.

9 Herman V, Fagin J, Gonsky R, Kovacs K, Melmed S. Clonal origin of pituitary adenomas. *J Clin Endocrinol Metab* 1990; **71**: 1427–33.

10 Spada A, Vallar L, Faglia G. Cellular alterations in pituitary tumors. *Eur J Endocrinol* 1994; **130**: 43–52.

11 Franks S, Jacobs HS, Hull MGR. The oral contraceptive and hyperprolactinemia amenorrhea. In: Camanni F, Muller EE, eds. *Pituitary Hyperfunction, Physiopathology and Clinical Aspects*. New York: Raven Press, 1984: 175–8.

12 March CM, Kletzky OA, Davajan V *et al.* Longitudinal evaluation of patients with untreated prolactin secreting pituitary adenomas. *Am J Obstet Gynecol* 1981; **139**: 835–44.

13 Rjosk HK, Fahlbusch R, Van Werder K. Spontaneous development of hyperprolactinaemia. *Acta Endocrinol* 1982; **100**: 333–6.

14 Tolis G. Prolactin: physiology and pathology. In: Krieger DT, Hughes YC, eds. *Neuroendocrinology*. Sunderland: Sinauer Associates, 1980: 321–2.

15 Franks S. Hyperprolactinaemia and male reproductive function. In: Tolis G, Stefanis C, Mountokalakis T, Labrie F, eds. *Prolactin and Prolactinoma*. New York: Raven Press, 1983: 173–85.

16 Vannier MW, Marsh JI, Warren JO. Three dimensional CT reconstruction images for craniofacial surgical planning and evaluation. *Radiology* 1984, **150**: 179–84.

17 Baker HL, Berguist TH, Kispert DB *et al.* Magnetic resonance imaging in a routine clinical setting. *Mayo Clin Proc* 1985; **60**: 75–90.

18 Muhr C, Bergstrom K, Grimelis L. Larsson SG. A parallel study of the roentgen anatomy of the sella turica and the pathology of the pituitary gland in 205 autopsy specimens. *Neuroradiology* 1981; **25**: 55–61.

19 Burrow GN, Wortzman G, Rewcastle NB, Holgate RC, Kovacs K. Microadenomas of the pituitary and abnormal sellar tomograms in an unselected autopsy series. *N Engl J Med* 1981; **304**: 156–8.

20 Swartz YD, Russel KB, Basile BA, O'Donnel PC, Popky GL. High resolution computed tomographic appearance of the intrasellar contents in women of childbearing age. *Radiology* 1983; **147**: 115–17.

21 Ciccarelli E, Ghigo E, Miola C, Gandini G, Muller EE, Camanni F. Long-term follow-up of cured prolactinoma patients after successful adenomectomy. *Clin Endocrinol* 1990; **32**: 583–92.

22 Missale C, Boroni F, Losa M *et al.* Nerve growth factor suppresses the transforming phenotype of human prolactinomas. *Pharmacol* 1993; **90**: 7961–5.

23 Ciccarelli E, Mazza E, Ghigo E, Guidoni F, Barberis A, Massara F, Camanni F. Long term treatment with oral single administration of bromocriptine in patients with hyperprolactinaemia. *J Endocrinol Invest* 1987; **10**: 51–3.

24 Ciccarelli E, Miola C, Avataneo T, Camanni F, Grossman A, Besser GM. Long term treatment with a new repeatable injectable form of bromocriptine, Parlodel LAR, in patients with tumorous hyperprolactinaemia. *Fertil Steril* 1989; **52**: 930–5.

25 Rains CP, Bryson HM, Fitton A. Cabergoline: a review of its pharmacological properties and therapeutic potential in the treatment of hyperprolactinaemia and inhibition of lactation. *Drugs* 1995; **42**: 255–79.

CHAPTER 11

Galactorrhoea in women with normal basal prolactin concentrations

P.S. Sharp and D.G. Johnston

Physiological lactation

The female breast consists of alveoli surrounded by contractile myoepithelial cells, and is arranged in a lobular system [1]. The lobes and lobules are separated by connective tissue and by adipose tissue, and in the non-pregnant state fat and fibrous tissue are the major components. In pregnancy, the breasts are prepared for lactation by proliferation of the glandular tissue and an increase in blood flow. Expansion of the glandular components is hormone dependent: in animals it requires insulin, glucocorticoids and a lactogenic hormone such as prolactin or human placental lactogen.

The breast synthesizes colostrum in the second half of pregnancy, but true lactation begins only 2–3 days post-partum. Milk production (lactogenesis) requires the synthesis by the alveolar cells of unique components such as lactose, α-lactalbumin, casein and milk-fat triglyceride. The milk is released into the ductular system and 'let down' to the nipple. Once initiated, milk production is continued for a variable time post-partum (a process sometimes called galactopoiesis).

Lactogenesis is hormone dependent and requires prolactin, growth hormone, thyroid hormones, glucocorticoids, insulin and parathyroid hormone in different species [2]; in women, prolactin is paramount. It acts on alveolar epithelial cells via specific receptors which increase in number in pregnancy through an effect of prolactin to induce the synthesis of its own receptor [3]. Alveolar cells change from non-secretory to secretory with hyperplasia of the endoplasmic reticulum and dilatation of the Golgi. Prolactin is essential for these changes.

Although human growth hormone is lactogenic in lower species, women with growth-hormone deficiency breast feed normally [4]. Glucocorticoids have a permissive effect on prolactin-stimulated casein synthesis [5] but there is nothing to suggest that cortisol, thyroid hormones or insulin have effects which are other than permissive in women. Parathyroid hormone is necessary for the increased mobilization of Ca^{2+} from bone.

Removal of milk from the breast is essential for its production to continue, as increased alveolar luminal pressure inhibits further milk synthesis. Milk let-down is controlled by the milk-ejection reflex. Neural impulses generated during suckling release oxytocin which acts on the breast myoepithelial cells to stimulate contraction and milk expulsion. Suckling also stimulates myoepithelial cell contraction directly [6].

Continued milk production—galactopoiesis—also requires the secretion of prolactin. The importance of prolactin in galactopoiesis is illustrated by the efficacy of dopamine agonists in suppressing it. Basal prolactin levels are maximally elevated in the first 4 weeks post-partum and gradually fall to levels in the non-pregnant range [7]. Suckling releases prolactin in the first 5–10 min and this persists for 5–25 min. More frequent and prolonged suckling leads to more prolonged elevations in basal prolactin and in societies where suckling is on demand, basal prolactin may be elevated for 6–12 months [8]. Although prolactin levels do decrease with prolonged suckling, milk yields do not decrease in parallel, provided that suckling continues.

The primacy of prolactin in pathological lactation (galactorrhoea) in women

Although a variety of hormones play some role in preparing the breasts for milk production, in initiating lactogenesis and in maintaining it, prolactin plays a dominant role in women. Inappropriate milk production (galactorrhoea) occurs in the absence of pregnancy in women (and even in men) with prolactinomas or with hyperprolactinaemia for any other reason. Prolactin excess causes galactorrhoea even when other hormones (e.g. growth hormone, thyroid-stimulating hormone and adrenocorticotrophic hormone) are deficient, as may be observed in patients with macroprolactinomas [9]. Thus, despite abundant evidence for effects of other hormones *in vitro* and *in vivo* in different species, excess prolactin alone causes galactorrhoea in women.

Normoprolactinaemic galactorrhoea

Despite this prime role of prolactin, galactorrhoea occurs also in clinical situations in women in whom basal prolactin concentrations are normal. In several series of women with galactorrhoea, basal prolactin concentrations were normal in 28–55% [10,11]. The women affected are usually premenopausal, and galactorrhoea may have been present for many years. Unlike patients with hyperprolactinaemia and galactorrhoea, only one-third of the women have menstrual disturbances, usually oligomenorrhoea. In one series [12], galactorrhoea occurred either while taking an oral contraceptive or after stopping it in six of 20 women; the galactorrhoea represented continued milk production for more than 6 months after stopping breast feeding following a normal pregnancy in four of the 20 (formerly known as the Chiari–Frommel syndrome).

Several possibilities exist to explain the galactorrhoea in these patients. These include abnormalities in prolactin secretion or action, or the presence of alternative lactogenic substances in the circulation.

1 It has been suggested that true hyperprolactinaemia exists but is intermittent and is not recognized on basal blood samples. Circulating prolactin concentrations have been measured in frequent samples over 24 hours [12]. No difference was observed in circulating prolactin levels at any time of day, and the normal diurnal variation in prolactin concentrations was preserved (Fig. 11.1).

The possibility that hyperprolactinaemia occurs only at certain stages of the menstrual cycle has also been explored. Basal prolactin concentrations are similar in patients and controls when measured at intervals over a 5-week study period.

Follow-up of these patients for several years has demonstrated that basal prolactin levels remain normal in the majority (18 of 20 patients in one series).

2 Alternatively, the regulation of prolactin secretion may be abnormal, resulting in exaggerated responses to certain stimuli. Although basal prolactin concentrations are normal, the response to secretagogues may be exaggerated. Insulin-induced hypoglycaemia stimulates prolactin release through an action at the hypothalamic level, and is frequently used in clinical practice as a model of ‘stress’. Prolactin responses to hypoglycaemia are normal in these women with galactorrhoea [12]. Responses to thyrotrophin-releasing hormone are also normal [10,13]. The prolactin responses to dopamine antagonists have been reported as exaggerated, decreased and normal, with a normal response observed (to

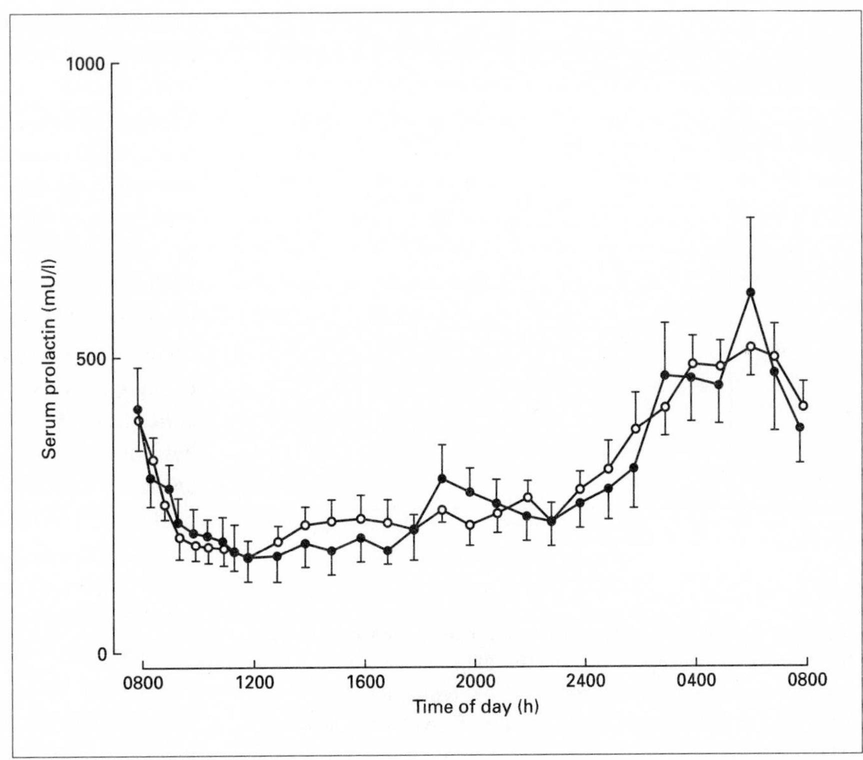

Fig. 11.1 Circulating prolactin levels over 24 hours in patients with galactorrhoea and in normal controls. Values shown are mean ± SEM for seven patients (●) and nine normal controls (○). Modified from [12].

domperidone) in the most detailed investigations [10,12,13]. An exaggerated prolactin response to a 5-hydroxytryptamine type 1A receptor agonist has been reported in normoprolactinaemic infertile women with galactorrhoea, in comparison with the prolactin responses in patients who did not have galactorrhoea [14]. The significance of this is uncertain currently.

3 Another possibility is that circulating prolactin is abnormal in that the antiserum employed in the immunoassay does not recognise it, although it is biologically active. This explanation is improbable in view of the observation in one series [12] that prolactin concentrations were normal using two different polyclonal antisera, and the prolactin values obtained with the different antisera correlated closely (Fig. 11.2). On gel electrophoresis, the proportion of prolactin variants (glycosylated and non-glycosylated) in the circulation in the basal state does not appear abnormal in patients with regular menstrual cycles and galactorrhoea [15].

4 Similarly, it has been suggested that the biological activity of circulating prolactin may be increased with normal immunoassayable levels. This hypothesis has been tested using an *in vitro* bioassay for lactogenic hormones, the Nb2 node rat lymphoma cell proliferation bioassay [16,17]. This assay recognises lactogenic hormones by their ability to stimulate proliferation of these cells in suspension culture. In normal human serum, prolactin and growth hormone account for the total lactogenic activity, as evidenced by disappearance of bioactivity when excess anti-growth hormone and anti-prolactin antisera are added to the assay system. Prolactin bioactivity assessed in the presence of excess anti-growth-hormone antiserum is normal from women with galactorrhoea and normal immunoassayable prolactin levels (Fig. 11.3). Basal prolactin levels by bioassay of 355 ± 43 mU/l have been described, compared with values of 348 ± 64 mU/l in serum from normal controls [12].

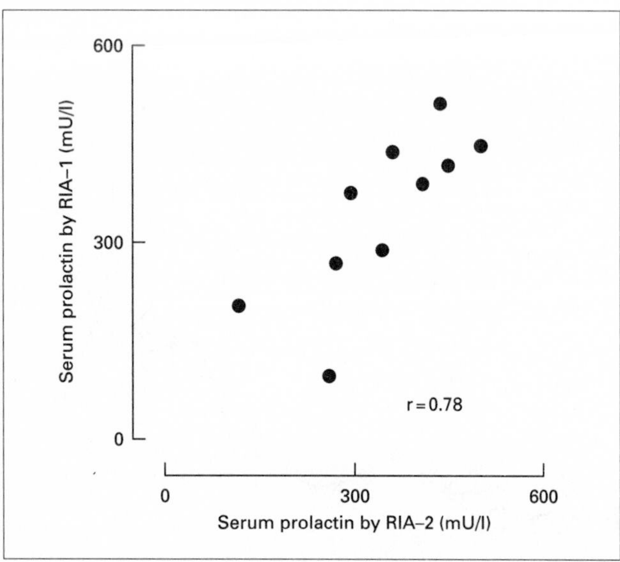

Fig. 11.2 Relationship between serum prolactin measured by two different immunoassays (RIA-1 and RIA-2) in women with normoprolactinaemic galactorrhoea. Linear regression was performed by the method of least squares. Experimental details are in [12].

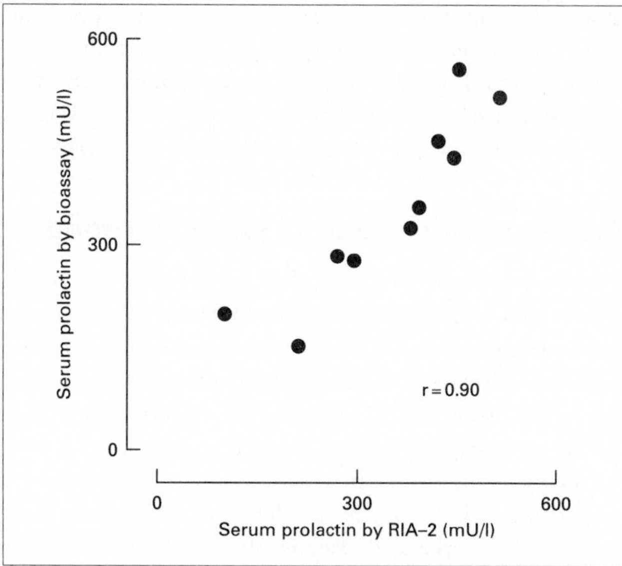

Fig. 11.3 Relationship between bioassayable and immunoassayable serum prolactin in women with normoprolactinaemic galactorrhoea. Experimental details are in [12].

5 There may be a lactogenic substance in serum other than prolactin. Human growth hormone is lactogenic in lower species, including primates [18]. Pituitary-derived growth hormone in large amounts increases breast milk in lactating women with deficient milk production [19]. Acromegalic patients may have galactorrhoea even when prolactin levels are normal [20]; this has been attributed to a spill-over effect with the excess growth hormone interacting with prolactin receptors [21]. Under physiological conditions in women the interaction of growth hormone with prolactin receptors is negligible, as growth hormone circulates in much lower concentrations than prolactin. In acromegaly, it has been hypothesised that the effects of the high growth-hormone levels, in combination with the normal concentrations of prolactin, are to increase the total lactogenic activity in serum. Growth hormone excess does not, however, appear to be important in women with galactorrhoea and normal basal prolactin concentrations, as immunoassayable growth-hormone levels are not elevated over a 24-hour period [12].

The data obtained from the Nb2 node bioassay also render very unlikely the possibility of another circulating lactogen, unless it is removed in the assay system by the growth-hormone antiserum. Human placental lactogen has not been measured. There is no information on oxytocin secretion in these women. Oestrogens have complex actions on milk production [2] and in high concentrations have an inhibitory effect in lactating women, but there is no information on oestrogen secretion or action in normoprolactinaemic galactorrhoea. A major sex-hormone abnormality is unlikely in view of the fact that most women continue to ovulate normally. A decline in circulating oestrogen and possibly progestogen, in association with oestrogen-stimulated prolactin release, contributes to the initiation of lactation in the post-partum period, and may be important in the galactorrhoea which develops in some women on stopping the oral contraceptive.

6 Finally, it may be that tissue sensitivity to prolactin is increased. This is the most likely explanation. The fact that in 50% of patients the galactorrhoea occurs during or after oral contraceptive use, or persists after pregnancy and breast feeding, suggests that the breasts may have become 'primed' in some way for milk production. The ability of prolactin to induce its own receptors may provide an explanation for this phenomenon, if the receptor number did not decline again as circulating prolactin levels fell after pregnancy or after stopping the oral contraceptive. Metabolic disturbances are observed in women with normoprolactinaemic galactorrhoea which are similar to those noted in hyperprolactinaemia [12,22]. These include mild hyperglycaemia with increased circulating levels of the gluconeogenic precursors, lactate, pyruvate and alanine. Circulating glycerol levels are decreased.

The clinical picture in normoprolactinaemic galactorrhoea is also similar to that observed in women with mild hyperprolactinaemia. The latter women have galactorrhoea but severe menstrual disturbance is not usually observed if the serum prolactin level is 2000 mU/l or less. These clinical and metabolic similarities suggest increased tissue sensitivity to the lactogenic and metabolic actions of prolactin in the normoprolactinaemic women. Further support for this hypothesis derives from the clinical observation that suppression of circulating prolactin levels to low normal or subnormal values with dopamine agonists frequently leads to improvement in, or abolition of, the galactorrhoea.

Finally, a laboratory normal range is derived from the values obtained in a normal population and the figures quoted are statistical estimates, such as the mean ± 2 standard deviations for this population. The normal range takes no account of biological activity. In an individual subject, prolactin levels within the statistical normal range may be elevated above the biological normal for that subject. Looked at in this way, tissue sensitivity is greater than average but prolactin hypersecretion also exists, although not to circulating levels outside the population normal range. Normal feedback mechanisms have not operated to decrease circulating prolactin levels to lower values, although the mechanism of this defect in feedback is unknown and no abnormality has been demonstrated in dynamic studies.

Clinical management of women with galactorrhoea

In assessing women with galactorrhoea, it is necessary first to take a careful history to ascertain if the onset was related to an event, such as pregnancy or breast feeding, or discontinuing the combined contraceptive pill. It is important to clarify whether the discharge is from one nipple or both, since a unilateral discharge may result from primary breast disease rather than an endocrine disorder. Features suggestive of acromegaly, Cushing's syndrome or hypothyroidism should be sought. In Cushing's syndrome, the galactorrhoea is usually associated with hyperprolactinaemia. Galactorrhoea occurs rarely in hypothyroidism in both children (in whom it may be associated with precocious puberty) and adults [23]. Serum prolactin levels in these patients may be in the normal adult range for women, or slightly elevated. A menstrual history is of paramount importance, since amenorrhoea suggests hyperprolactinaemia. Women with polycystic ovaries may have galactorrhoea and menstrual disturbance [24], and hyperprolactinaemia is sometimes intermittent in these patients. Other features of polycystic ovaries such as hirsutes or a positive family history should be sought. A history of visual disturbance indicates a pituitary macroadenoma. A detailed drug history is necessary, with particular reference to psychotrophic drugs and antiemetics which have dopamine antagonistic actions (see Chapter 9). Major surgery such as cholecystectomy or thoracotomy and conditions such as herpes zoster of the chest wall have been reported to be associated with galactorrhoea. It is usually assumed that the galactorrhoea results from hyperprolactinaemia, although circulating prolactin may be normal at the time the patient is investigated. Self-limited galactorrhoea occurs infrequently after augmentation mammaplasty [25].

Physical examination is directed towards finding the cause of the disorder, looking for features of acromegaly, Cushing's syndrome or hypothyroidism, examination of the optic discs for atrophy and assessment of the visual fields. It is important to confirm that the breast discharge is milky. Patients will generally feel most comfortable if asked to express the discharge themselves. True galactorrhoea is a milky or turbid white discharge; expression of clear fluid is suggestive of benign breast disease. Pustular discharges, black or grey-coloured secretions or blood-stained discharges suggest other pathology. Both breasts should be palpated, looking for evidence of primary breast disease. The breast conditions which most commonly lead to nipple discharge are duct ectasia, intraduct papillomatosis and sometimes fibroadenosis with cyst formation. Occasionally, in cases of duct ectasia, a single, solid cord will be felt, leading up to the nipple, and this finding is extremely valuable since not only the cause, but also the site, of the abnormality will have been demonstrated. Cysts associated with fibroadenosis are often palpable. Breast abscesses may discharge pus from the nipple. The discharge in women with breast carcinoma is frequently blood stained.

If doubt exists as to the nature of the discharge, further examination of the discharge itself is possible. This includes measurement of casein, α-lactalbumin or lactose, or, more usefully, microscopic examination for fat globules or pus cells. However, it is exceptional for these pathological examinations to be helpful in clinical practice, and if doubt exists as to the nature of a breast discharge, management in conjunction with a surgical breast specialist is advisable.

When it has been established that the discharge is true galactorrhoea, serum prolactin should be measured. In clinical practice, this is performed in working hours (morning or afternoon) despite some diurnal variation (see Fig. 11.1). If the value is marginally elevated, it is wise to repeat the estimation on samples taken in the morning 60–90 min following positioning of an intravenous cannula. If the level is unequivocally elevated, the clinical management as dealt with elsewhere in this book should be provided (see Chapter 10). If circulating prolactin levels are consistently mildly elevated (450–1500 mU/l), a prolactinoma or other disease of the hypothalamo-pituitary axis should be sought, but such values are compatible with disorders such as hypothyroidism or polycystic ovaries. With unequivocally normal prolactin concentrations (<450 mU/l in the authors' laboratory), careful clinical assessment and measurement of thyroid function are all that are usually required. Imaging of the pituitary is not necessary in these circumstances.

The treatment of true galactorrhoea is directed towards removal of the cause, such as cessation of psychotropic drug therapy if possible or treatment of hypothyroidism. Where no cause is known or if it cannot be removed, bromocriptine treatment is often effective. It is advisable to treat with low doses, for example 1.25 mg at night, as these patients are often unduly sensitive to the side-effects of dopamine agonists. More commonly, no specific therapy is required following reassurance as to the benign condition of the disorder.

References

1 Llewellyn-Jones D. Lactation and breast feeding. In: Shearman RP, ed. *Clinical Reproductive Endocrinology*. Edinburgh: Churchill Livingstone, 1985: 282–98.

2 Tucker HA. Lactation and its hormonal control. In: Knobil E, Neill J, eds. *The Physiology of Reproduction*. New York: Raven Press, 1988: 2235–63.

3 Djiane J, Durand P. Prolactin: progesterone antagonism in self regulation of prolactin receptors in the mammary gland. *Nature* 1977; **266**: 641–3.

4 Rimoin DL, Holzman GB, Merimee TJ *et al.* Lactation in the absence of growth hormone. *J Clin Endocrinol Metab* 1968; **28**: 1183–8.

5 Buttle HL, Forsyth IA. Placental lactogen in the cow. *J Endocrinol* 1976; **68**: 141–6.

6 Lucas A, Drewett RB, Mitchell MD. Breast feeding and plasma oxytocin concentrations. *Br Med J* 1980; **2**: 834–5.

7 Noel GL, Suh HK, Frantz AG. Prolactin release during nursing and breast stimulation in postpartum and non-postpartum subjects. *J Clin Endocrinol Metab* 1974; **38**: 413–23.

8 Howie RW, McNeilly AS, Houston MJ *et al.* Effect of supplementary food on suckling patterns and ovarian activity during lactation. *Br Med J* 1981; **2**: 757–9.

9 Johnston DG, Prescott RWG, Kendall-Taylor P *et al.* Hyperprolactinaemia—long-term effects of bromocriptine. *Am J Med* 1983; **75**: 868–74.

10 Kleinberg DL, Noel GL, Frantz AG. Galactorrhoea: a study of 235 cases, including 48 with pituitary tumors. *N Engl J Med* 1977; **296**: 589–600.

11 Tolis G, Somma M, van Campenhout J, Friesen H. Prolactin secretion in sixty-five patients with galactorrhea. *Am J Obstet Gynecol* 1974; **118**: 91–101.

12 Johnston DG, Haigh J, Prescott RWG *et al.* Prolactin secretion and biological activity in females with galactorrhoea and normal circulating prolactin concentrations at rest. *Clin Endocrinol* 1985; **22**: 661–78.

13 D'Agata RD, Aliffi A, Maugeri G, Mongiol A, Vicari E, Gulizia S. Dynamics of Prl release in galactorrhoeic normoprolactinaemic women. *Acta Endocrinol* 1982; **101**: 1–4.

14 Abdel-Gadir A, Khatim MS, Muharib NS, Shaw RW. The aetiology of galactorrhoea in women with regular menstruation and normal prolactin levels. *Human Reprod* 1992; **7**: 912–14.

15 Liu JH, Lee DW, Markoff E. Differential release of prolactin variants in postpartum and early follicular phase women. *J Clin Endocrinol Metab* 1990; **71**: 605–10.

16 Tanaka T, Shiu RPC, Gout RW, Beer CT, Noble RL, Friesen HG. A new sensitive and specific bioassay for lactogenic hormones: measurement of prolactin and growth hormone in human serum. *J Clin Endocrinol Metab* 1989; **51**: 1058–63.

17 Tanaka T, Shishiba Y, Gout PW, Beer CT, Noble RL, Friesen HG. Radioimmunoassay and bioassay of human growth hormone and human prolactin. *J Clin Endocrinol Metab* 1983; **56**: 18–20.

18 Kleinberg DL, Todd J. Evidence that human growth hormone is a potent lactogen in primates. *J Clin Endocrinol Metab* 1980; **51**: 1009–13.

19 Lyons WR, Li CH, Ahmad N, Rice-Wray E. Mammotrophic effects of human hypophyseal growth hormone preparations in animals and man. *Excerpta Medica International Congress Series* 1968; **158**: 349–63.

20 de Pablo F, Eastman RC, Roth J, Gorden P. Plasma prolactin in acreomegaly before and after treatment. *J Clin Endocrinol Metab* 1981; **53**: 344–52.

21 Fradkin JE, Eastman RC, Lesniak MA, Roth J. Specificity spill-over at the hormone receptor—exploring its role in human disease. *N Engl J Med* 1989; **320**: 640–5.

22 Johnston DG, Alberti KGMM, Nattrass M *et al.* Hyperinsulinaemia

in hyperprolactinaemic women. *Clin Endocrinol* 1980; **13**: 361–8.

23 Bigos ST, Ridgway EC, Kourides IA *et al.* Spectrum of pituitary alterations with mild and severe thyroid impairment. *J Clin Endocrinol Metab* 1978; **46**: 317–25.

24 Franks S. Polycystic ovary syndrome: a changing perspective. *Clin Endocrinol* 1989; **31**: 87–120.

25 Caputy GG, Flowers RS. Copious lactation following augmentation mammaplasty: an uncommon but not rare condition. *Aesthetic Plast Surg* 1994; **18**: 393–7.

CHAPTER 12

Acromegaly

S.W.J. Lamberts

Introduction

Acromegaly is a chronic, slowly developing, debilitating disease, which is characterised by progressive disfigurement and disability. Apart from the cosmetic changes, a multitude of complaints, mainly related to neuropathy and arthropathy, interfere with normal daily working life in most patients, while the secondary complications related to the cardiovascular system often cause premature death if no successful therapy is given.

In virtually all patients the clinical syndrome of acromegaly is caused by a growth hormone (GH)-secreting pituitary adenoma. Excessive GH production also results in increased production of GH-dependent tissue factors (insulin-like growth factor 1; IGF-1 = somatomedin C). An early diagnosis is difficult to make and the delay of many years in doing so results in the majority of patients in the development of irreversible complications in several organ systems.

Epidemiology

Acromegaly is encountered with equal frequency in both sexes. Most patients are diagnosed between the age of 40 and 60 years. A GH-secreting pituitary adenoma before puberty causes the clinical syndrome of gigantism. The familial presentation of acromegaly very seldom occurs, often as part of type 1 multiple endocrine adenomatosis.

Based on epidemiological studies, the annual incidence of acromegaly in western Europe was calculated to be approximately three to four cases per million, while the prevalence of diagnosed cases may be as high as 40–70 per million inhabitants.

Clinical signs and symptoms

The signs and symptoms of acromegaly can be the result of the long-standing overproduction of GH and/or IGF-1, but they can also be related to pressure effects of the pituitary adenoma causing loss of vision, visual field defects and/or a loss of anterior pituitary function (see Table 12.1; for review articles see [1–3]).

Acromegalic disfigurement of the face is in most patients very obvious (Fig. 12.1): however, a protruding chin, the rough facial features with deep nasolabial furrows, the thick lips and an enlarged nose become most evident if one examines a series of photographs of the patient taken over many years. Most patients have complaints of their teeth necessitating frequent visits to their dentist; widening of the spaces between teeth, as well as prominence of the lower jaw, cause malocclusion of the jaws and frequently pain of mastication, while non-fitting dentures can be an often recurring problem. The tongue is large and thick and the voice becomes rough and deep. Many patients snore loudly during their sleep. These changes are related to swelling in the larynx and upper airways. If extensive, sleep apnoea and intermittent drowsiness during the day occur.

Soft-tissue swelling of the cutis and subcutis, due to increased deposition of mucopolysaccharides, also causes many problems. The increased size of hands and feet gives them a plump appearance and there is a firm feeling on palpation (Fig. 12.2). The increased finger, hand and foot size often cause tightness of rings which cannot be removed and have to be cut off, as well as an increase in glove and shoe sizes. The subcutaneous swelling, especially in the hands, causes paraesthesiae of the fingers and eventually carpal tunnel syndrome due to compression of the median nerve at the wrist.

Hyperstimulation of the cutaneous appendages results in excessive sweating, stimulation of hair growth (which is especially evident in female patients) and an oily, seborrhoeic skin.

Table 12.1 Incidence and presentation of clinical signs and symptoms in 60 acromegalic patients. Adapted and extended from [2].

	Presentation which led to clinical diagnosis	Overall prevalence	
	n	*n*	%
Changes of appearance, acral enlargement and soft-tissue swelling	7	60	100
Excessive sweating	2	50	83
Hypertrichosis	1	43	72*
Acroparaesthesias/carpal tunnel syndrome	5	41	68
Headaches	8	32	53
Tiredness, weakness, decreased vitality and/or somnolence	1	32	53
Weight gain		29	48
Arthropathy	5	22	37
Ear, nose, throat or dental problems	5	19	32
Oligo- or amenorrhoea, infertility	8	33	55*
Impotence and/or loss of libido	1	25	42†
Galactorrhoea	1	24	40*
Goitre		21	35
Inguinal or umbilical hernia		15	25
Cardiac complications (tachyarrhythmias, congestive heart failure)	3	15	25
Hypertension	5	14	23
Impaired glucose tolerance		19	32
Manifest diabetes mellitus	1	3	5
Elevated serum phosphorus level		16	26
Evidence of pituitary adenoma at neuroradiological investigation		60	100
Loss of vision and/or visual field defect	4	10	17
Hyperprolactinaemia		25	42
Impaired gonadotrophin secretion		14	23
Impaired adrenal function		8	13
Lowered thyroxine level		5	8
Diagnosis by chance	3		

* Percentage of female patients.
† Percentage of male patients.

Headache is a frequent complaint both at presentation and during the course of the disease, and also after treatment. The cause of these headaches is not always apparent.

Hypersecretion of GH and IGF-1 before the end of puberty produces gigantism. In adult patients the musculoskeletal changes of acromegaly include localized increases in cartilage deposition in the ears, nose and joints, as well as slight periostal bone growth resulting in exostoses. Changes in the vertebral architecture cause kyphosis, compensatory scoliosis and backaches, while degenerative changes of the joints cause accelerated osteoarthrosis, especially of the hips, knees and hands.

Tiredness, weakness and a decreased vitality frequently occur in acromegalic patients. The cause of these complaints is not uniform. Long-standing acromegaly results in changes in body composition including an increase in the absolute amount of lean body mass (mainly muscle). Despite this, there may be myopathy, as well as symptoms such as chronic headaches, osteoarthrosis, cardiovascular symptoms, sexual and hypogonadal complaints, as well as other forms of hypopituitarism, which all contribute to ill-health to a variable extent in most patients.

Disorders of sexual function and hypogonadism frequently occur in acromegalic patients, and are also related to a variety of different pathogenetic mechanisms. First, the hyperprolactinaemia which is present in over one third of untreated patients causes galactorrhoea, loss of libido

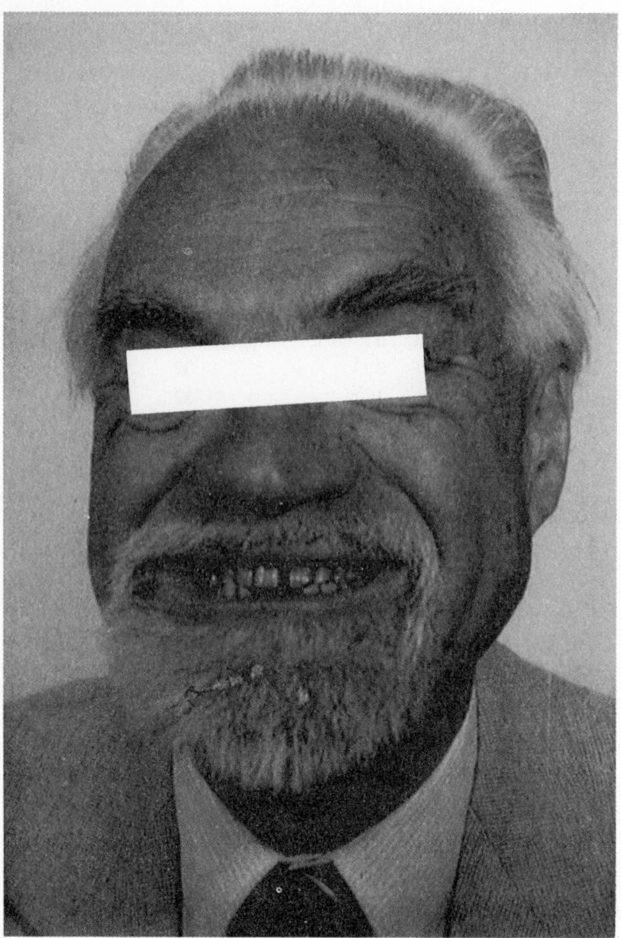

Fig. 12.1 The facial appearance of a 56-year-old patient with acromegaly. The enlargement of the nose, the thickening of the lips and a generalized coarsening of the features are evident. Widening of the spaces between teeth and a prominence of the lower jaw caused malocclusion of the jaws and pain of mastication. The diagnosis of acromegaly was made by the dentist.

and/or interruption of normal menstrual cycles (oligo- or amenorrhoea) as well as infertility in the females, and loss of libido and/or impotence in male patients. The origin of such hyperprolactinaemia is discussed below. In addition, hypogonadism caused by pressure effects of the pituitary adenoma on the normal anterior pituitary gonadotrophs often also contributes to this symptomatology.

Long-standing exposure of the human body to high GH and IGF-1 levels results in organomegaly. Nodular and sometimes diffuse goitres can be found in as many as one-third of untreated acromegalics. The liver and kidneys, as well as the gastrointestinal tract, increase in size without causing symptomatology. There is a high incidence of inguinal and umbilical hernias. In addition the heart increases in size. This is often not only part of the general organomegaly, but can also be secondary to hypertension and accelerated atherosclerosis. The pathogenesis of the increased blood pressure, as well as that of the varying degrees of cardiomyopathy and dilatation of the ventricles, is not well understood, but they may result in tachyarrhythmias and congestive heart failure, as well as premature death from cardiovascular complications in many patients.

Patients with acromegaly are at risk of developing adenomatous colonic polyps, which are considered to be preneoplastic lesions [4]. The prevalence of adenomatous colonic polyps was significantly increased in 103 acromegalic patients compared with 138 control subjects (22.3% versus 8.0%; $P < 0.003$) [5]. These studies indicate that colonoscopy should be part of the initial (and follow-up) examinations in acromegaly, especially in male patients above 50 years of age who have skin tags. A cohort of 1041 acromegalic men who were examined for subsequent cancer demonstrated after a mean follow-up of 8.3 years an increased rate of cancers of the digestive organs (oesophagus, stomach and colon), as well as melanomas [6].

Metabolic changes also contribute to the symptomatology of acromegalic patients. GH causes insulin resistance, and long-standing hypersecretion of GH causes a decrease in glucose tolerance which can result in clinically overt diabetes mellitus. Urinary calcium excretion and hydroxyproline excretion are often increased, while serum phosphate rises. Acromegalics have an increased incidence of renal stones.

The pituitary adenoma itself may contribute directly to the frequent complaint of headache. Slowly growing tumours cause an enlargement of the pituitary fossa and eventually pressure on the optic chiasm. Loss of vision and/or visual field defects may result from this. Parasellar extension of the tumour sometimes causes pressure on the cavernous sinus, resulting in external ophthalmoplegia and diplopia. Cosecretion of prolactin by the GH-secreting adenoma may result in hyperprolactinaemia and its associated features (see above), while the pressure effects of a slowly expanding pituitary tumour on the anterior pituitary gland can cause signs and symptoms of hypopituitarism.

Thus, the symptoms and signs in patients with acromegaly often progress relatively slowly. For this reason the diagnosis is often missed for many years. The mean delay between the onset of symptoms and the time of diagnosis in a group of 44 acromegalic patients was 6.5 years (4.1 years in the female and 8.6 years in the male patients) [2]. Changes in the appearance of acromegalic patients according to the evaluation of a series of photographs collected over many years is often of value. Change of appearance, acral enlargement, soft-tissue swelling, excessive sweating, hypertrichosis, acroparaesthesia, headaches, tiredness, arthropathy and hypogonadism are the main overall prevailing clinical signs and symptoms (Table 12.1). However, when we studied

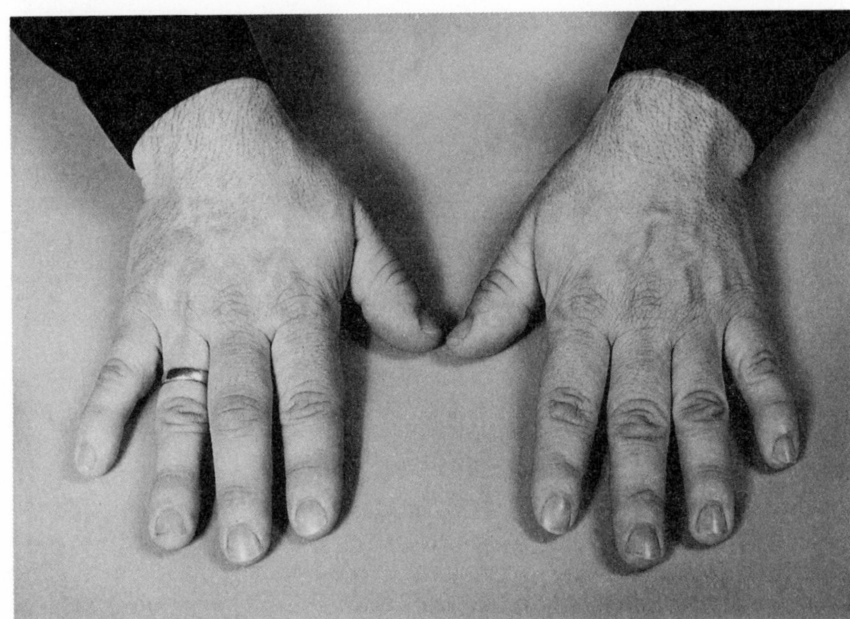

Fig. 12.2 The plump appearance of the fingers and hands of a 32-year-old acromegalic patient. The wedding ring had become too narrow and could not be removed.

the presenting symptoms which led to the clinical diagnosis in 60 of our patients, it became evident that the clinical alertness of specialists in different fields of medicine can contribute largely to an early diagnosis (Table 12.1). Apart from internists, rheumatologists, dentists, otorhinologists, ophthalmologists, neurologists, neurosurgeons and gynaecologists must all be aware of the clinical symptomatology of acromegaly. Finally, a new general practitioner, who doesn't know the patient, is often the first doctor to suggest the diagnosis.

Physiopathological and pathogenetic aspects

More than 99% of cases of acromegaly are the result of a GH-secreting pituitary adenoma. Very seldom acromegaly is the result of a gangliocytoma of the hypothalamus which secretes GH-releasing hormone (GHRH), while another very rare cause of acromegaly is a peripheral tumour which secretes GHRH. Around 25 of such endocrine pancreatic tumours, thymic tumours and bronchial, duodenal or jejunal carcinoids have been reported [7].

The group of pituitary adenomas causing the clinical syndrome of acromegaly is remarkably heterogeneous, both with regard to their size at presentation, their microscopic and electron-microscopic appearance, as well as to the cosecretion of hormones other than GH [8].

In our experience the majority of adenomas have a diameter of > 10 mm at the time of diagnosis. Extrasellar extension in supra- and/or parasellar directions is present in one-third of tumours; fewer than 35% are microadenomas. Between 30 and 40% of the tumours show localised or diffuse invasive growth in the surrounding structures, especially into the dura mater and bone. About 60% are eosinophilic pituitary adenomas, while the others are principally chromophobes. Electron microscopy demonstrates that the adenoma cells contain a variable number of secretory granules, reflecting the net balance between cellular hormone synthesis and hormone release. Both densely and sparsely granulated tumours can be recognised, but there is as yet no clinical significance attached to differentiating these groups of tumours [8]. In cases of (ectopic) GHRH-secreting tumours causing acromegaly, pituitary histology often reveals the presence of hyperplasia of GH-secreting cells [9], but adenoma formation has also been described [7].

Plurihormonal pituitary tumours are often found in acromegalic patients. Cosecretion of GH and prolactin by these adenomas occurs in as many as 40% of cases. Mammosomatotroph adenomas, in which both GH and prolactin are synthesised and released by the same tumour cells, occur in 5–10% of acromegalics, while in the other 30% of cases prolactin-containing cells are found at immunohistochemical examination scattered between the GH-containing tumour cells. Simultaneously synthesis of GH and prolactin often, but not always, results in hyperprolactinaemia; clinical symptomatology related to this includes the occurrence of galactorrhoea, menstrual disorders, infertility, a loss of libido and/or impotence, while the simultaneous presence of both hormones to a certain degree determines the sensitivity of hormone secretion to medical therapy (see below). However, not every case of hyperprolactinaemia in acromegalic patients is linked to cosecretion of GH and prolactin by the pituitary adenoma. Especially in very big tumours, disruption of the portal venous system by pressure on the pituitary stalk results in activation of prolactin release by normal lactotrophs which are no longer restrained by the tonic inhibition of hypothalamic dopamine (see Chapter 6).

More than 50% of GH-secreting pituitary adenomas cosecrete the α-subunit of the glycoprotein hormones; the pathophysiological significance of this is at present unknown. In a few cases of acromegaly, cosecretion of biologically active thyroid-stimulating hormone (TSH) results in hyperthyroidism, while cosecretion of GH and adrenocorticotrophic hormone (ACTH) has even more seldom been described.

GH is released by the anterior pituitary gland of adult humans in episodically occurring secretory bursts (see [5] for review). Fasting GH release is higher than after the ingestion of food, while GH release is also activated during (deep) sleep. Episodic GH secretion is thought to be regulated by dual stimulation of hypothalamic GHRH secretion, associated with a reduction in the tonic secretion of hypothalamic somatostatin. When the nutritional state is adequate, IGF-1 production in normal humans is dependent mainly on GH secretion, while both GH and IGF-1 also feed back at the pituitary and hypothalamic level to inhibit GH secretion.

The aetiology of GH-secreting pituitary adenomas is unknown. A primary hypothalamic disorder (increased release of GHRH and/or decreased release of somatostatin), which results in hyperplasia of GH-secreting pituitary cells and eventually in pituitary adenoma formation, has been hypothesised. In favour of such an assumption is the observation that the qualitative dynamics of GH secretion by cultured acromegalic pituitary tumour cells in response to GHRH and somatostatin (Fig. 12.3), as well as the reaction of GH secretion to these stimuli *in vivo*, are similar to those observed by normal pituitary cells as well as in normal individuals. Recent studies, however, suggest that most GH-secreting adenomas originate as a consequence of cellular alterations in the pituitary somatotrophs. Analyses of X-chromosomal inactivation have shown that these pituitary tumours are monoclonal in origin [10,11]. In addition, genetic mutations, which might be responsible for the selective expansion of a single cell clone, have been identified in subjects of GH-secreting pituitary adenomas [12,13]. The most frequently observed mutation involves the gene encoding the α-subunit of G_s, the protein that stimulates adenylyl cyclase. It was demonstrated that in these tumour cells the G_s α-subunit is converted to an oncogene designated *gsp* for G_s-protein. This results in a constitutive activation of G_s and these tumour cells are characterised by high levels of intracellular cyclic adenosine monophosphate (cAMP) and GH secretion. The clinical consequence of the presence of *gsp* mutations with regard to disease outcome and cure rate remain uncertain, but these tumours in general are very sensitive to somatostatin [14]. A second genetic alteration which frequently occurs in GH-secreting pituitary tumours is a loss of heterozygosity involving allelic deletions in chromosome 11, which are in agreement with the region which contains the multiple endocrine neoplasia 1 (MEN-1) gene (11q13) [15].

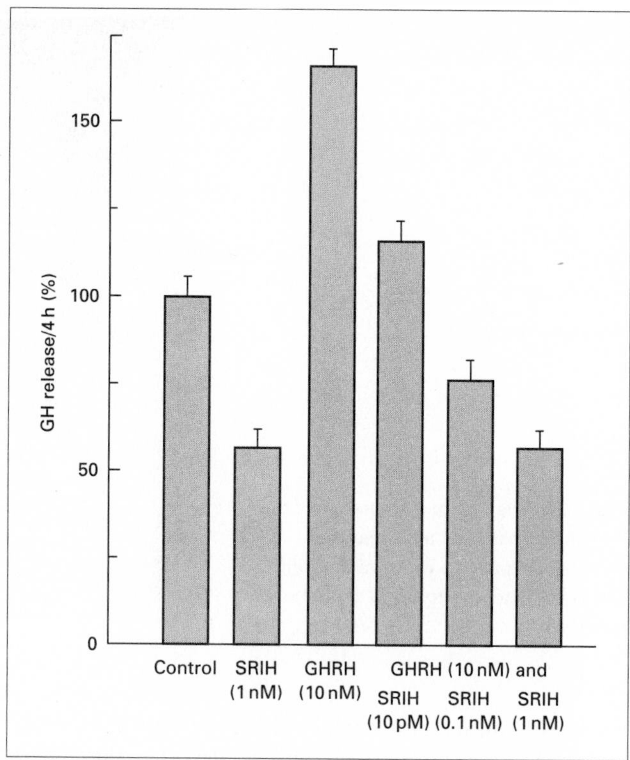

Fig. 12.3 The effect of growth hormone-releasing hormone (GHRH) and somatostatin (SRIH) on hormone release by cultured pituitary tumour cells obtained during transsphenoidal operation of an acromegalic patient. Note the qualitatively normal reaction of tumorous GH secretion to physiological hypothalamic regulators.

Laboratory and radiological diagnosis

Biochemical diagnosis

The laboratory diagnosis of acromegaly and the assessment of the clinical activity of the disease may be rapidly carried out by measuring the IGF-1 concentration in the serum. In normally fed individuals with normal liver and renal function, circulating IGF-1 levels reflect the integrated effect of GH at the tissue level, while they also correlate with mean 24-hour GH levels. Measurement of IGF-1 concentrations differentiates between active untreated acromegaly and normal individuals, while serum IGF-1 level also correlates well with the clinical activity of the disease [16]. The long half-life of IGF-1, which is mainly due to its binding to specific carrier protein(s), excludes the necessity for standardised or repeated sampling. In principle, the biochemical diagnosis of acromegaly can be made on the basis of the measurement of an elevated IGF-1 concentration of the serum. The measurement of the IGF-binding proteins 1 or 3 does not provide additional information [17].

While in some untreated acromegalic patients random serum GH concentrations are so high that they can be considered to be virtually diagnostic, multiple sampling is often necessary to exclude spontaneous fluctuations in normal values. In order to standardise this procedure, the suppressive reaction of GH secretion to glucose can be investigated by measuring GH levels after an oral glucose load (50–100 g). Normal GH secretion is suppressed by rising blood glucose levels; in the case of (untreated) acromegaly, the (often elevated) basal serum GH concentrations do not suppress within 30–120 min after glucose administration to undetectable levels (usually < 0.5 μg/l), and often even show a paradoxical increase. About 60% of acromegalics show a paradoxical increase (by more than 50% of basal values) of circulating GH levels in response to the intravenous administration of 100–200 μg TRH.

The availability of the measurement of serum IGF-1 concentrations has greatly facilitated the accurate diagnosis of active acromegaly on an out-patient base, precluding the (often in-hospital) collection of multiple serum samples for GH determinations in response to glucose and/or thyrotrophin-releasing hormone (TRH). As stated above, a significant association exists between the clinical symptomatology of acromegalic patients and the circulating IGF-1 levels [16], but there is also a correlation between fasting, post-prandial as well as mean 24-hour serum GH levels and IGF-1 concentrations [8]. However, circulating GH levels of 80–100 μg/l (1 μg/l = 2 mU/l) maximally activate IGF-1 generation in humans, and a further increase in GH secretion by pituitary adenomas will generally not result in a further increase in IGF-1 production [18]. In the assessment of the activity of acromegaly during and after different forms of therapy, a single IGF-1 determination is probably of equal value as the measurement of a 24-hour profile of GH secretion. In Fig. 12.4 the close relationship is shown between the course of the circulating IGF-1 and the mean 24-hour GH concentrations of 10 acromegalic patients during long-term medical therapy for more than 1 year [18].

A comparison between the value of measuring one single sample of GH and IGF-1 to define 'cure' in the follow-up of acromegalic patients remains unclear. The lowest GH during an oral glucose tolerance test correlates very well with IGF-1 [19], but random clinic GH levels are also well correlated with both the minimum GH and IGF-1 levels, suggesting that random GH measurements might also be valid parameters to be used in the follow-up of these patients after treatment [20].

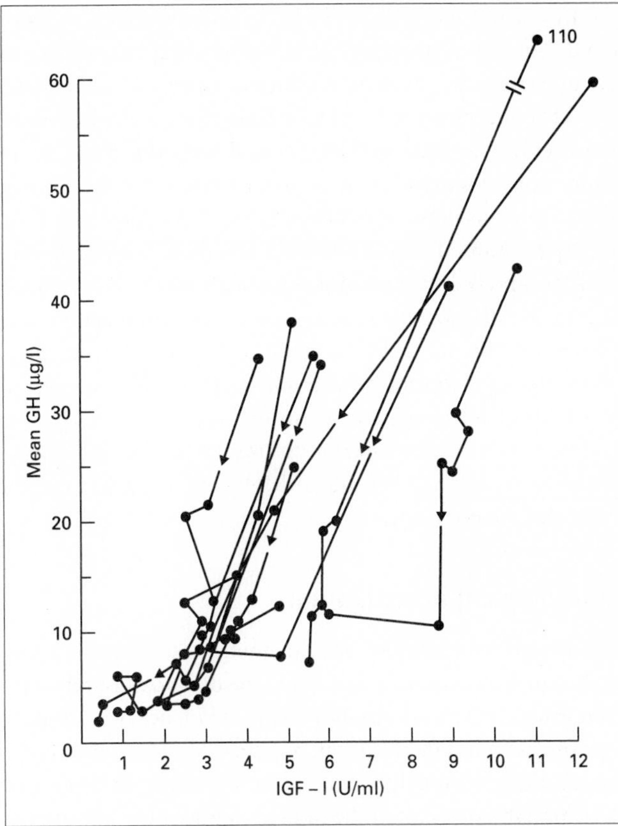

Fig. 12.4 The course of the mean 24-hour growth hormone (GH) concentrations (each point is the mean of 20 samples collected over a 24-hour period) and the circulating insulin-like growth factor 1 (IGF-1) levels in 10 acromegalic patients during treatment for more than 1 year with 300 μg octreotide daily (100 μg subcutaneously three times daily). Upper limit of normal of IGF-1 2.2 U/ml. Adapted from [18].

In the case of gigantism occurring during the pubertal growth spurt, the differential biochemical diagnosis between excessive but physiological growth and early gigantism is difficult if not impossible. Elevated IGF-1 and GH levels, which do decrease in response to glucose and often paradoxically increase in reaction to TRH, can be present in both conditions. Apart from a good physical examination (soft-tissue swelling), the radiological demonstration or exclusion of a pituitary tumour is essential in such cases.

Another biochemically difficult differential diagnosis is that between acromegaly caused by GH secretion from a pituitary adenoma and that from hyperplastic pituitary cells stimulated by GHRH secretion from a hypothalamic or peripheral endocrine tumour. Elevated IGF-1 and GH levels, which do not decrease in response to glucose and paradoxically increase to TRH, can be observed in both conditions [9]. Unnecessary transsphenoidal operation can be prevented by the routine measurement of circulating GHRH concentrations, and by the alertness of the physician in observing an enlarged liver containing metastases of an endocrine pancreatic tumour or a carcinoid or the finding of a suspicious mass on the chest X-ray (bronchial carcinoid or thymic tumour). Somatostatin receptor imaging is also valuable in visualising tumours throughout the body which secrete GHRH ectopically. However, as stated above this type of tumour occurs in less than 1% of cases of acromegaly, so the need for routine measurement of GHRH in the initial work-up of acromegaly is questionable.

The evaluation of anterior pituitary function in patients with acromegaly can best be carried by the standard function tests (see Chapter 83).

Radiological investigation

Computed tomography and magnetic resonance imaging techniques have greatly facilitated the diagnosis of pituitary abnormalities in acromegalic patients. Evidence of a pituitary tumour is found in almost all patients. Most adenomas are larger than 10 mm in diameter at the time of diagnosis. Extrasellar extension of the tumour is present in about one-third of cases. As mentioned above, tumours infiltrating the bone and other surrounding structures are frequent, and this can be recognized at neuroradiological examination in as many as 40% of cases. No firm radiological differentiation can be made between acromegaly caused by a pituitary adenoma and that caused by excessive GH secretion by a diffusely enlarged anterior pituitary, as occasionally found in cases of ectopic GHRH secretion.

Natural course of acromegaly

In a retrospective survey of 194 acromegalic patients it was found that the disease, if untreated, is associated with a reduced life expectancy [21]. Death rates amongst acromegalics were approximately twice those in the general population. This was largely due to cardiovascular, cerebrovascular and pulmonary (e.g. secondary to thoracic deformities) disorders. Clinical diabetes mellitus and hypertension were found to be important added risk factors. The data also suggest that patients given GH-lowering therapy had a lower mortality than those untreated (see below).

The terms 'inactive' or 'burnt-out' acromegaly refer to the occasional patient with a spontaneous cure of the clinical picture of acromegaly. In most cases this could be ascribed to the occurrence of apoplexy of the pituitary adenoma. Neuroradiological examination in such patients often shows the picture of a (partial) 'empty' sella turcica.

Therapy

General considerations and the definition of cure

Since acromegaly is a progressive disease which causes chronic and progressive disability and shortens life, therapy must be instituted in all patients with acromegaly, aimed at normalizing GH secretion. Optimally, however, a consistent normalization of GH secretion (and of circulating IGF-1 levels), should also be reached in parallel with a complete removal of the pituitary adenoma, or at least with a reduction in pituitary tumour size. This should ideally be accomplished without the production of secondary anterior pituitary insufficiency and with minimal side-effects and morbidity.

Three lines of therapeutic approach are currently used:
1 surgical therapy, in which the transsphenoidal approach has replaced transcranial surgery;
2 external pituitary irradiation with a linear accelerator; and
3 medical therapy with dopamine agonists and somatostatin analogues.

Many reports on single treatment modalities of acromegaly have been published, but there are few comparative studies of these different types of therapy.

The definition of 'cure' of acromegaly after surgical and/or radiotherapy and during medical therapy deserves some discussion. In the past, 'cure' after surgery was defined by many investigators as the lowering of serum GH concentrations to less than 10 or 5 μg/l. This unsatisfactory criterion was later amended by requiring a normalisation of circulating IGF-1 levels, a decrease of the mean 24-hour GH levels to 3 μg/l or less, and/or the disappearance of the paradoxical increase of GH to TRH [22]. The considerable variations in the criteria of 'cure' used by different investigators hamper objective interpretation of the results of the different forms of therapy which are currently used in the treatment of acromegaly.

Surgery

During transsphenoidal operation it is theoretically possible selectively to remove the adenoma and to preserve the normal surrounding pituitary gland. In a large series of patients postoperative serum GH levels of <5 μg/l were observed in 60–70% of acromegalic patients [23]. The size of the adenoma, the presence of invasive growth and the preoperative GH levels are all important factors which determine the outcome of transsphenoidal operation (Table 12.2). Only about 50% of patients with preoperative GH levels above 40 μg/l and/or who show signs of invasive growth of the tumour at neuroradiological examination can be expected

Table 12.2 Factors affecting the outcome of transsphenoidal surgery in 169 acromegalic patients. From [23].

	Outcome of surgery (%)	
Preoperative parameter	Normalized (GH <5μg/l; IGF-1 normal)	Not normalized (GH >5μg/l; IGF-1 elevated)
GH <40μg/l	81	19
GH >40μg/l	52	48
Non-invasive growth	84	16
Invasive growth	46	54

GH, growth hormone; IGF-1, insulin-like growth factor 1.

Table 12.3 Outcome of transsphenoidal surgery in 29 acromegalic patients in relation to different criteria of 'cure'. From [24].

Definition of 'cure'	Cases 'cured' (%)
Normal GH (<5μg/l)	66
Normal IGF-1	59
Normal IGF-1 + GH suppressed after glucose to <1μg/l	55
Normal IGF-1 + GH suppressed after glucose to <1μg/l + absent response to TRH/GnRH	45

GH, growth hormone; IGF-1, insulin-like growth factor 1; TRH, thyrotrophin-releasing hormone; GnRH, gonadotrophin-releasing hormone.

to be 'cured' after an operation by an experienced surgeon. In a very precise study [24] involving 29 consecutive acromegalic patients, a cure rate varying between 45 and 65% was observed, depending on the criteria used (Table 12.3). The availability of an experienced neurosurgeon is of crucial importance: Landolt, for example, observed a 63% cure rate in the first 87 acromegalics he operated upon between 1972 and 1981, and a 78% cure rate in the subsequent 82 patients he operated upon between 1982 and 1987 [23]. Postoperative hypopituitarism, diabetes insipidus, cerebrospinal fluid (CSF) rhinorrhoea (and sometimes subsequent meningitis) occur at varying frequency, but the mortality of the transsphenoidal operation is low.

Wrightson [25] studied the junctional area of 15 GH-secreting adenomas with the normal surrounding pituitary tissue: in three cases there was a sharp and well-defined boundary between adenoma cells and the normal gland for 1 or 2mm from the presumed junction. The other tumours showed an intermediate picture: invasion of tumour cells into the dura mater was present in 50% of the cases. These observations led some investigators to conclude that postoperative external pituitary irradiation is indicated in most patients in order to prevent regrowth of the tumour. However, recurrence of clinical acromegaly after an initially successful operation has not often been reported, although this may reflect the slow growth of this type of tumour.

Radiotherapy

Three different principles of radiotherapy have been used in the treatment of acromegaly: external pituitary irradiation, interstitial irradiation by the intrasellar implantation of yttrium (^{90}Y) and heavy particle irradiation with a proton beam. The results on the clinical course of acromegaly by all three treatment modalities are generally similar. The two last approaches of radiotherapy have been carried out only in a few highly specialised centres throughout the world and will not be further discussed here.

In modern radiotherapy virtually the whole dose of irradiation can be directed via a linear accelerator to the sella turcica without evoking damage to the surrounding structures; therefore, virtually no complications are encountered after external pituitary irradiation of GH-secreting tumors. However, radiotherapy will not only affect the pituitary adenoma, but eventually also diminishes anterior pituitary function in most individuals [26].

In general, an important reduction in circulating GH and consequently of the IGF-1 levels is accomplished by external pituitary irradiation, but 'normalisation' is not rapidly attained. The greatest disadvantage is the delay in response of tumorous hormone hypersecretion: a 50% decrease of pretreatment GH values can be expected within 2 years after an external irradiation with 4500cGy (rads), while the optimal effect is often even delayed for as long as 4–6 years or even longer. No mortality and only very low morbidity is seen, but as many as 50% of acromegalic patients will eventually develop secondary pituitary insufficiency in long-term follow-up 5–10 years after irradiation, necessitating life-long therapy with hydrocortisone, thyroxine and/or sex steroids [26].

In conclusion, external irradiation only slowly diminishes clinical signs and symptoms of acromegaly by decreasing GH and IGF-1 secretion. In spite of low morbidity rates, the frequent development of secondary pituitary insufficiency remains a major problem. Therefore, radiotherapy is only infrequently advised as a primary treatment for acromegaly, and it is mainly used as secondline treatment, for example, after an unsuccessful transsphenoidal operation.

Medical therapy

Two different lines of medical therapy have been proven to be effective in the majority of acromegalic patients: long-acting agonists of dopamine and of somatostatin.

Dopamine agonists

The discovery that drugs with long-acting dopamine agonistic activity such as bromocriptine acutely lower serum GH levels in many acromegalic patients raised high hopes with regard to their value as a chronic treatment in these patients. In an extensive study Wass *et al.* [27] reported definite and usually marked clinical and biochemical improvement (lowering of circulating GH and IGF-1 levels) in about 80% of acromegalic patients with daily doses of bromocriptine up to 60 mg. However, summarising a large number of studies carried out by numerous investigators, it emerges that about one-third of acromegalic patients do not significantly respond, even to high doses of bromocriptine. If a realistic parameter of the suppression of circulating GH levels during bromocriptine treatment to less than 5 μg/l is taken into account, only 20–30% of patients will achieve this goal during treatment with 20–40 mg of the drug daily. However, another 30–50% of patients react during such treatment with definite clinical improvement and/or lowering of GH levels. Reduction of pituitary tumour size during bromocriptine treatment is occasionally seen, but such shrinkage in acromegalic patients is less impressive than that observed in most patients with prolactinoma during therapy with the drug. Stopping bromocriptine therapy (even after several years) is in general accompanied within a few days by a rapid increase in serum GH concentrations to pre-treatment values. The relatively high dosages of bromocriptine required (20–40 mg daily) to maximally control the clinical signs and symptoms of acromegaly may cause side-effects, including nausea, vomiting, postural hypotension, dizziness, constipation and peripheral vasoconstriction, although if the drug is used carefully (see Chapter 10) these should not be dose limiting.

It has not been established with any certainty which factors determine whether dopamine receptors are present on GH-secreting pituitary adenomas, enabling successful treatment with bromocriptine. In several studies involving large groups of acromegalic patients, the presence of hyperprolactinaemia and/or the capacity of tumorous hormone secretion to react paradoxically to TRH have been found to be roughly predictive of a successful inhibitory effect of chronic bromocriptine treatment on GH secretion [28]. Investigating the relationship between the immunohistochemical presence of prolactin within the GH-secreting adenoma and the sensitivity of GH release *in vivo* to the acute administration of 2.5 mg bromocriptine, it was shown that hormone release by 'mixed' GH/prolactin containing pituitary adenomas is more sensitive to bromocriptine than that by 'pure' GH-containing adenomas (Fig. 12.5). However, hyperprolactinaemia, as an *in vivo* marker, was present in only 60% of these patients.

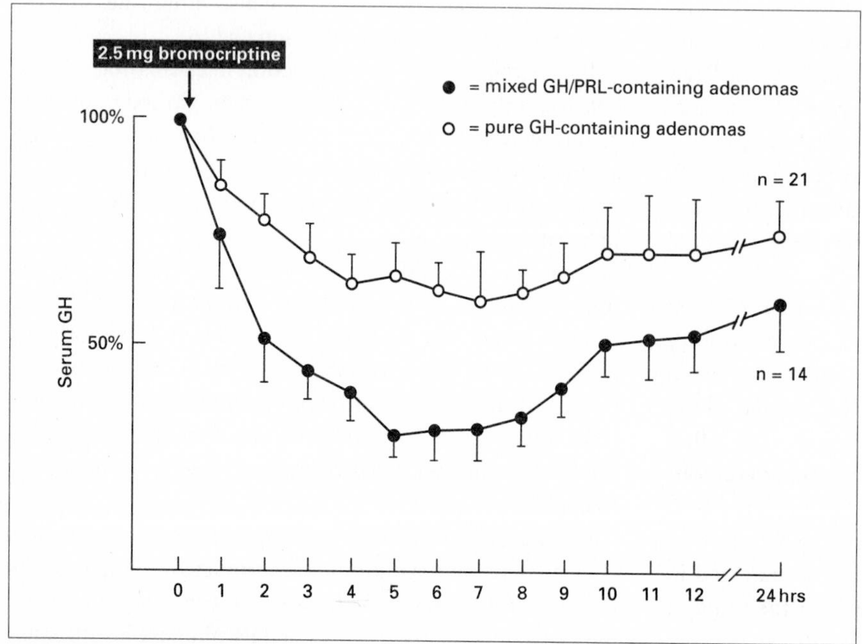

Fig. 12.5 The reaction of serum growth hormone (GH) levels to the oral administration of 2.5 mg bromocriptine at 0800 hours, followed for 24 hours in 35 untreated acromegalic patients. Immunohistochemical investigation of the subsequently transsphenoidally removed pituitary adenomas showed 21 'pure' GH-containing (open circles) and 14 'mixed' GH prolactin (PRL)-containing (closed circles) adenomas. GH secretion from 2 till 10 hours after bromocriptine administration was significantly more suppressed in the patients harbouring mixed GH/PRL-containing adenomas (mean ± SEM).

In conclusion, bromocriptine therapy is of value in the majority of acromegalic patients. However, clinical as well as biochemical 'cure' during chronic treatment with high dosages of the drug can be reached in only about 25% of patients, although about two-thirds of all acromegalics show clinical improvement during bromocriptine therapy. In view of the considerably greater sensitivity of hormone secretion by most acromegalic tumours to somatostatin analogues (see below), bromocriptine has in recent years become of less value in their treatment. However, the drug (or related dopamine agonist) still has a place in exceptional cases after unsuccessful surgery, and in the period before the full effect of radiotherapy appears, especially in young acromegalics of reproductive age who show signs and symptoms related to hyperprolactinaemia.

Somatostatin analogues

GH secretion by the pituitary tumour cells of acromegalic patients in most instances retains high sensitivity to the GH release-inhibitory effects of somatostatin (see Fig. 12.3). Most acromegalic tumours contain high numbers of high-affinity somatostatin receptors which are diffusely distributed over the adenoma. Intravenous administration of somatostatin to acromegalics markedly suppresses GH secretion in most cases, but rebound hypersecretion occurs after discontinuation of the infusion.

The availability of a long-acting analogue of somatostatin (octreotide; Sandostatin; SMS 201–995) has greatly changed the role of medical therapy in the overall treatment of acromegaly. Octreotide exerts a strong and prolonged inhibitory action on normal GH release, while its inhibitory effect on normal insulin release is only short-acting. The subcutaneous administration of a single dose of 50 μg octreotide to acromegalic patients usually suppresses GH secretion for several hours without rebound hypersecretion (Fig. 12.6). We have investigated the acute effect of 50 μg octreotide on GH levels in 46 consecutive acromegalics, in comparison with that of a placebo [28]. From 2 till 6 hours after drug administration the serum GH concentrations were suppressed to < 5 μg/l in 29 patients (63%), while a decrease by more than 50% was achieved in 39 (85%) of them. In later studies it was shown that the acute course of GH levels after a single subcutaneous dose of 50 μg octreotide closely predicts the ultimate success of chronic octreotide treatment in individual patients [12].

A growing number of reports has shown the high clinical and biochemical efficacy of chronic treatment of acromegalic patients with octreotide [28–30]. Clinical improvement occurs rapidly after the start of the injections: in virtually all patients excessive sweating, headache, paraesthesiae and tiredness decreased markedly within the first weeks of therapy, while these symptoms disappeared in most patients during longer treatment with octreotide (Fig. 12.7). A decrease in soft tissue swelling and remodelling, and improvement of the facial coarsening of most patients, was noted after longer periods of treatment. Additionally, cardiomyopathy and sleep apnoea are reduced or eliminated in most patients.

The optimal dose and dose scheme for the treatment of acromegalic patients with octreotide varies between individuals. Each subcutaneous administration of octreotide is followed by a rapid decline in circulating GH levels. However, after 5–7 hours the GH levels gradually increase again as the time for the next injection approaches (Fig. 12.8).

The usual initial dose of octreotide is thrice-daily subcutaneous injections of 100 μg each. Both the number of injections and the dose, however, can be increased to achieve the maximal benefit [28,29]. Among patients receiving 300–

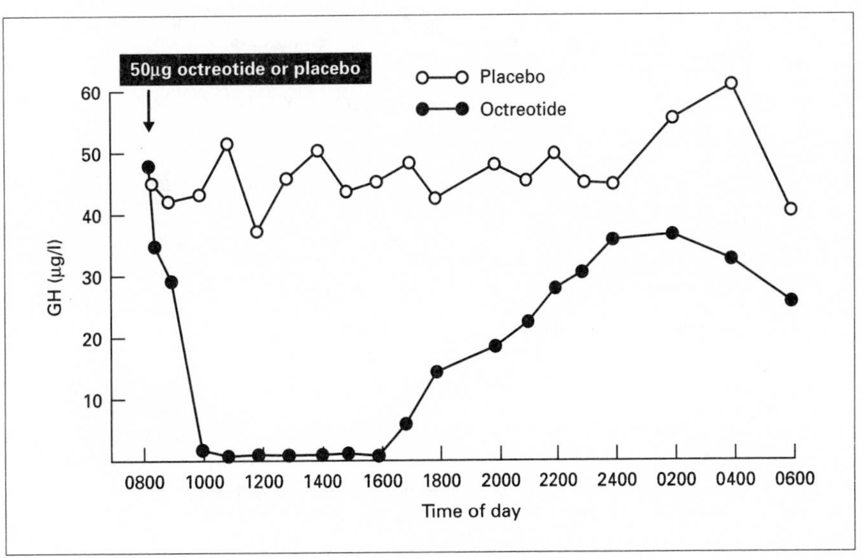

Fig. 12.6 The effect of the subcutaneous administration of 50 μg octreotide at 0815 hours on serum GH levels in comparison with the levels on a placebo day in an untreated acromegalic patient.

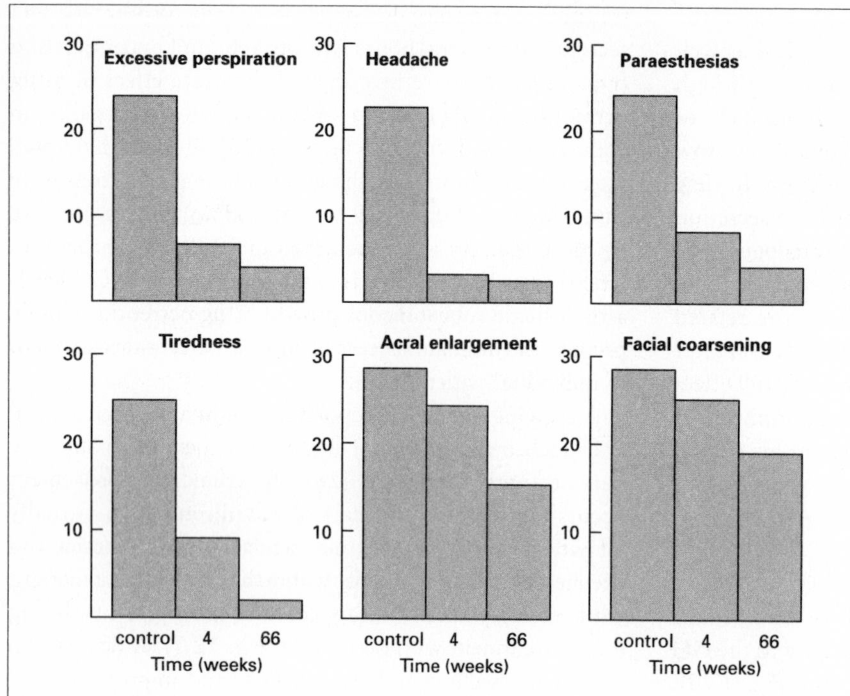

Fig. 12.7 Course of clinical features before (control) and after 4 and 66 weeks of treatment with octreotide (200–300 μg/day) of 10 acromegalic patients. Values indicate cumulative data according to an arbitrary scale between 0 (absent) and 3 (severe). In these 10 patients the presence of severe complaints in all cases would result in a maximal rating of 30.

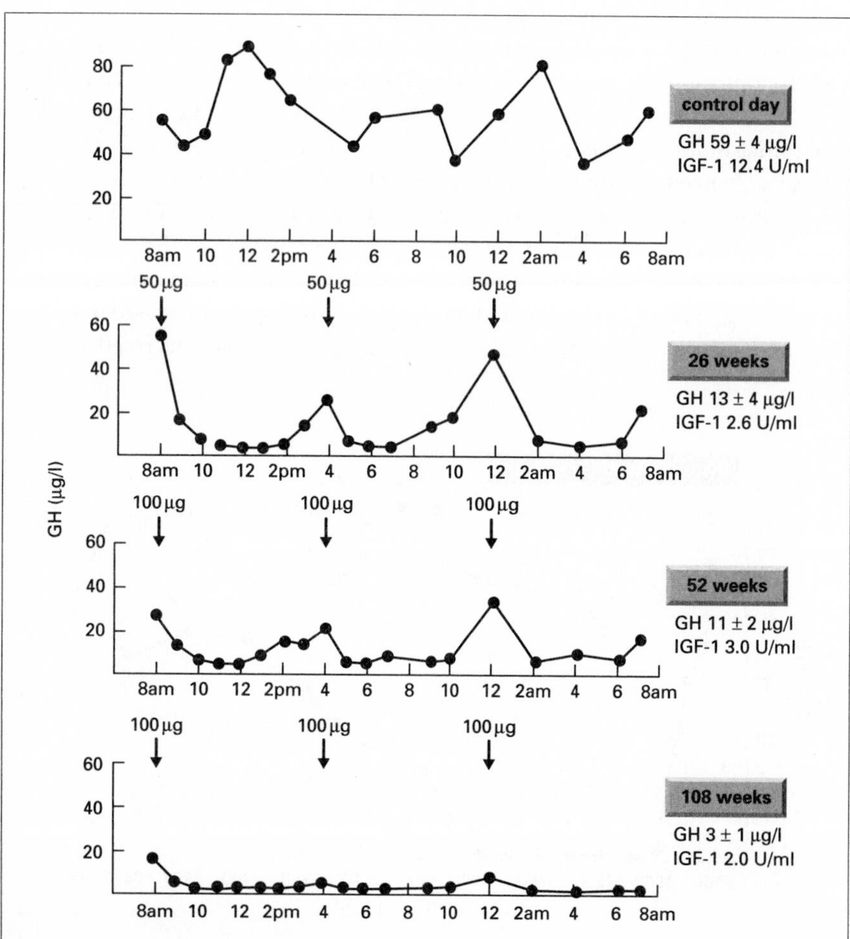

Fig. 12.8 The effect of long-term treatment with octreotide on circulating 24-hour growth hormone (GH) profiles and on mean 24-hour GH and the insulin-like growth factor 1 (IGF-1) levels in a previously untreated acromegalic patient. Data on different dosages of octreotide before and after 26, 52 and 108 weeks of treatment. Adapted from [30].

600 μg of octreotide daily, up to 90% have suppressed serum GH concentrations, over half have serum GH concentrations of <5 μg/l, and about 70% have normal serum IGF-1 concentrations [28,29,31]. Overall, in comparative studies in the same patients with acromegaly, octreotide is more effective than bromocriptine [28], while some patients show a better response to the combination of octreotide and bromocriptine than to either drug alone [28]. Increased serum prolactin concentrations, as well as galactorrhoea or secondary amenorrhoea, often resolve during treatment with octreotide in acromegalic patients who have pituitary adenomas secreting both GH and prolactin [28].

From a practical point of view, it is costly and troublesome to measure 24-hour GH profiles regularly in each individual patient in order to find the optimal dose and scheme of octreotide administration. The rapid clinical improvement which is observed in most patients during the first weeks of therapy does not help to optimise the dose scheme. A close correlation was found between the mean 24-hour GH levels and the serum IGF-1 concentrations before and during octreotide treatment in acromegalic patients (see Fig. 12.4). Therefore, regular IGF-1 measurements on an out-patient base enable optimisation of the daily dose and number of octreotide injections needed for each individual patient [9,14]. In many patients the subjective clinical benefits of octreotide therapy are greater than the decreases in serum GH and IGF-1 concentrations.

A slight decrease in pituitary tumour size during long-term octreotide treatment was observed in about 50% of acromegalic patients. The mechanism of tumour shrinkage evoked by octreotide might be a decrease in the size of individual tumour cells (caused by a decreased synthesis and content of GH within the tumour cells), rather than being the result of a cytotoxic or vascular effect of the drug. There is some evidence that pretreatment of acromegalic patients with octreotide might improve the efficacy of transsphenoidal surgery, especially in patients with macroadenomas.

Octreotide is well tolerated in most patients. Transient abdominal discomfort and/or steatorrhoea was observed in most patients. The injections are sometimes painful. Mean fasting serum glucose concentrations do not increase during chronic therapy in most patients, but post-prandial glucose levels tend to be slightly increased due to the (short-lasting) inhibitory effect of octreotide on normal insulin secretion. Gallstone formation was observed during long-term octreotide therapy in some patients [32], but this may increase in frequency over time.

Octreotide has to be administered subcutaneously twice or three times daily. A long-acting form that has recently been developed consists of 20 or 30 mg of octreotide mixed with microspheres of DL-lactide-co-glycolide polymer [33]. In most patients with acromegaly, an intramuscular injection of this preparation controls GH hypersecretion for 28–42 days as effectively as do multiple daily subcutaneous injections [34,35]. A long-acting intramuscular formulation of the somatostatin analogue lanreotide also controls GH secretion in patients with acromegaly, but its duration of action in 2 weeks at most [36,37].

In conclusion, the clinical introduction of the long-acting somatostatin analogue octreotide has added a new dimension to the medical therapy of acromegaly, especially in patients with large pituitary tumours which cannot be cured by surgery and/or radiotherapy [38]. In most patients, octreotide is more effective than bromocriptine. In all patients a marked clinical improvement with few side-effects is observed during the first weeks of therapy with the drug. During long-term octreotide therapy at a dose of 100 μg three times daily, normalization of circulating IGF-1 levels can be expected in about half of the patients. The effects of octreotide appear to be reversible, however, since both pretreatment GH and IGF-1 levels reappear within days to weeks after stopping treatment with octreotide.

Considerations on the choice of therapy

Acromegaly is a progressive disease which causes chronic disability and shortens life. In theory, the optimal therapeutic approach is the one which rapidly normalises circulating GH (and consequently IGF-1) levels, removing the pituitary tumour without the induction of secondary pituitary insufficiency and morbidity. Three lines of therapeutic approaches are currently used: surgical therapy, radiotherapy and medical therapy, but no single therapeutic approach is invariably curative [39,40].

Acromegaly is associated with an increased mortality rate due to excess deaths from cardiorespiratory and malignant diseases [21,41,42]. In recent years it has been demonstrated that the reduction of GH levels by surgical, radiotherapeutic and medical intervention is indeed associated with reduced mortality.

One study found that those patients in whom the post-treatment GH was <2.5 μg/l (5 mU/l, defined as the lowest mean GH of a series of day GH profiles) had a mortality which was not significantly different from the background population [41]. This was in contrast to those patients whose post-treatment GH was <5 μg/l (10 mU/l). In a further study it was observed that mortality in acromegalic subjects was more strongly associated with post-treatment GH values than with pretreatment GH levels [42].

These studies strongly suggest that a reduction of GH to <2.5 μg/l (5 mU/l) is essential to improve life expectancy in acromegalic patients after therapy. It also encourages those who advocate aggressive treatment of the disease in order to reach persistently lowered/normalised GH levels [20].

The conclusions of a consensus statement concerning the benefits versus risks of medical therapy for acromegaly include several options [43]. Medical management with octreotide is comparable in effectiveness to surgery and radiotherapy. In the case of radiotherapy, in which complete effectiveness may be delayed for years, octreotide can be used to suppress GH release until the radiation damage to the tumour reaches a significant level. The complications associated with octreotide are small relative to the benefits, but the inconvenience of thrice-daily subcutaneous injections and the cost are disadvantages. The documented higher incidence of gallstone formation necessitates the regular follow-up of these patients, but most of these gallstones will probably remain asymptomatic and require no treatment. The development of new, less invasive prophylactic or therapeutic approaches may further define management of these gallstones, making octreotide therapy a safer and more desirable option for the primary treatment of acromegalic patients. Surgical resection remains a mainstay of therapy for acromegaly, but improved delivery methods (e.g. long-acting formulations) and second-generation drugs would provide further advantages for pharmacotherapy in the future.

References

1 Nabarro JDN. Acromegaly. *Clin Endocrinol* 1987; **26**: 481–512.

2 Klijn JGM, Lamberts SWJ, de Jong FH, van Dongen KJ, Birkenhäger JC. Interrelationships between tumour size, age, plasma growth hormone and incidence of extrasellar extension in acromegalic patients. *Acta Endocrinol (Kbh)* 1980; **95**: 289–97.

3 Jadresic A, Banks LM, Child DF, Diamant L, Doyle FH, Fraser TR, Joplin GF. The acromegaly syndrome. *Quart J Med* 1982; **51**: 189–204.

4 Ezzat S, Strom C, Melmed S. Colon polyps in acromegaly. *Ann Intern Med* 1991; **114**: 754–5.

5 Delhougne B, Deneaux C, Abs R *et al.* The prevalence of colonic polyps in acromegaly: a colonoscopic and pathological study in 103 patients. *J Clin Endocrinol Metab* 1995; **50**: 3223–6.

6 Ron E, Gridley G, Hrubec Z, Page W, Arora S, Fraument JF, Jr. Acromegaly and gastrointestinal cancer. *Cancer* 1991; **68**: 1673–7.

7 Melmed S. Acromegaly. *N Engl J Med* 1990; **322**: 966–77.

8 Melmed S, Braunstein GD, Horvath E, Ezrin C, Kovacs K. Pathophysiology of acromegaly. *Endocr Rev* 1983; **4**: 271–89.

9 Thorner MO, Perryman RL, Cronin MJ *et al.* Somatotroph hyperplasia: successful treatment of acromegaly by removal of a pancreatic islet tumor secreting a growth hormone releasing factor. *J Clin Invest* 1982; **70**: 965–77.

10 Alexander JM, Biller BMK, Bikkal H, Zervas NT, Arnold A, Klibanski A. Clinically nonfunctioning pituitary tumors are monoclonal in origin. *J Clin Invest* 1990; **86**: 336–40.

11 Herman V, Fagin J, Gonsky R, Kovacs K, Melmed S. Clonal origin of pituitary adenomas. *J Clin Endocrinol Metab* 1990; **71**: 1427–33.

12 Landis C, Masters SB, Spada A, Pace AM, Bourne HR, Vallar L. GTPase inhibiting mutations activate the alpha chain of Gs and stimulate adenylyl cyclase in human pituitary tumours. *Nature* 1989; **340**: 692–6.

13 Vallar L, Spada A, Giannattasio G. Altered Gs and adenylate cyclase activity in human GH-secreting pituitary adenomas. *Nature* 1987; **330**: 566–7.

14 Spada A, Arosio M, Bochicchio D, Bazzoni N, Vallar L, Bassetti M, Falia G. Clinical, biochemical and morphological correlates in patients bearing growth hormone secreting tumors with or without constitutively active adenylyl cyclase. *J Clin Endocrinol Metab* 1987; **64**: 585–91.

15 Takker RV, Pook MA, Wooding C. Association of somatotropinomas with loss of alleles on chromosome 11 and with gsp mutations. *J Clin Invest* 1993; **91**: 2815–21.

16 Clemmons DR, van Wijk JJ, Ridgway EC, Kliman B, Kjellberg RN, Underwood LE. Evaluation of acromegaly by radioimmunoassay of somatomedin-C. *N Engl J Med* 1979; **301**: 1138–42.

17 de Herder WW, van der Lely AJ, Janssen JAMJL, Uitterlinden P, Hofland LJ, Lamberts SWJ. IGFBP-3 is a poor parameter for assessment of clinical activity in acromegaly. *Clin Endocrinol* 1995; **43**: 501–5.

18 Lamberts SWJ, Uitterlinden P, Verleun T. Relationship between growth hormone and somatomedin-C levels in untreated acromegaly, after surgery and radiotherapy and during medical therapy with Sandostatin (SMS 201–995). *Eur J Clin Invest* 1987; **27**: 354–9.

19 Dobrashian RD, O'Halloran DJ, Hunt A, Beardwell CG, Shalet SM. Relationship between insulin-like growth factor-I levels and growth hormone concentrations during diurnal profiles and following oral glucose in acromegaly. *Clin Endocrinol* 1993; **38**: 589–93.

20 Jenkins D, O'Brien I, Johnson A, Shakespear R, Sheppard MC, Stewart PM. The Birmingham pituitary database: auditing the outcome of the treatment of acromegaly. *Clin Endocrinol* 1995; **43**: 517–22.

21 Wright AD, Hill DM, Lowy C, Fraser TR. Mortality in acromegaly. *Quart J Med* 1970; **39**: 1–16.

22 Lamberts SWJ, Uitterlinden P, Schuijff PC, Klijn JGM. Therapy of acromegaly with sandostatin: the predictive value of an acute test, the value of serum somatomedin-C measurements in dose adjustment and the definition of a biochemical 'cure'. *Clin Endocrinol* 1988; **29**: 411–20.

23 Landolt AM, Illig R, Zapf J. Surgical treatment of acromegaly. In: Lamberts SWJ, ed. *Sandostatin in the Treatment of Acromegaly.* Berlin: Springer Verlag, 1988: 23–35.

24 Losa M, Oeckler B, Schopohl J, Muller OA, Alba-Lopez J, von Werder K. Evaluation of selective transsphenoidal adenomectomy by endocrinological testing and somatomedin-C measurement in acromegaly. *J Neurosurg* 1989; **70**: 561–7.

25 Wrightson P. Conservative removal of small pituitary tumours: is it justified by the pathological findings? *J Neurol Neurosurg Psych* 1978; **41**: 283–9.

26 Eastman RC, Gorden P, Roth J. Conventional supervoltage irradiation in an effective treatment for acromegaly. *Clin Endocrinol Metab* 1979; **48**: 931–40.

27 Wass JAH, Thorner MO, Morris DV *et al.* Long-term treatment of acromegaly with bromocriptine. *Br Med J* 1977; **I**: 875–9.

28 Lamberts SWJ. The role of somatostatin in the regulation of anterior pituitary hormone secretion and the use of its analogs in the treatment of human pituitary tumors. *Endocr Rev* 1988; **9**: 417–36.

29 Lamberts SWJ, Uitterlinden P, Verschoor L, van Dongen KJ,

Del Pozo E. Longterm treatment of acromegaly with somatostatin analogue SMS 201–995. *N Engl J Med* 1985; **313**: 1576–80.

30 Lamberts SWJ, Uitterlinden P, Del Pozo E. Sandostatin (SMS 201–995) induces a continuous further decline in circulating growth hormone and somatomedin-C levels during therapy of acromegalic patients for over two years. *J Clin Endocrinol Metab* 1987; **65**: 703–10.

31 Ezzar S, Snyder PJ, Young WF *et al*. Octreotide treatment of acromegaly. *Ann Intern Med* 1992; **117**: 711–18.

32 Lamberts SWJ, van der Lely AJ, de Herder WW, Hofland LJ. Octreotide. *N Engl J Med* 1996; in press.

33 Lancranjan I, Bruns C, Grass P *et al*. Sandostatin LAR: pharmacokinetics, pharmacodynamics, efficacy, and tolerability in acromegalic patients. *Metabolism* 1995; **44** (Suppl. 1): 18–26.

34 Stewart PM, Kane KF, Stewart SE, Lancranjan I, Sheppard MC. Depot long-acting somatostatin analog (Sandostatin-LAR) is an effective treatment for acromegaly. *J Clin Endocrinol Metab* 1995; **80**: 3267–72.

35 Kvistborg Fløgstad A, Halse J, Bakke S *et al*. Sandostatin LAR in acromegalic patients: long term treatment. *J Clin Endocrinol Metab* 1997; **82**: 23–8.

36 Heron I, Thomas F, Dero M. Pharmacokinetics and efficacy of a long-acting formulation of the new somatostatin analog BIM 23014 in patients with acromegaly. *J Clin Endocrinol Metab* 1993; **76**: 721–7.

37 Caron P, Morange-Ramos I, Cogne M, Jaquet P. Three year follow-up of acromegalic patients treated with intramuscular slow-release lanreotide. *J Clin Endocrinol Metab* 1997; **82**: 18–22

38 Robbins RJ. Editorial: Depot somatostatin analogs — A new first line therapy for acromegaly. *J Clin Endocrinol Metab* 1997; **82**: 15–17.

39 Jenkins D, O'Brien I, Johnson A, Shakespear R, Stewart PM. The Birmingham pituitary database: auditing the outcome of the treatment of acromegaly. *Clin Endocrinol* 1995; **43**: 517–22.

40 Sheaves R, Jenkins P, Blackburn P *et al*. Outcome of transsphenoidal surgery for acromegaly using strict criteria for surgical cure. *Clin Endocrinol* 1996; **45**: 407–13.

41 Rajasoorya C, Holdaway M, Wrightson P, Scott DJ, Ibbertson HK. Determinations of clinical outcome and survival in acromegaly. *Clin Endocrinol* 1994; **41**: 95–102.

42 Bates AS, Van't Hoff W, Jones JM, Clayton RN. An audit of outcome of treatment in acromegaly. *Quart J Med* 1993; **86**: 293–9.

43 Consensus Statement: benefits versus risks of medical therapy for acromegaly. Acromegaly therapy consensus development panel. *Am J Med* 1994; **97**: 468–73.

CHAPTER 13

Functionless pituitary tumours

G. Faglia and B. Ambrosi

Introduction

The term 'functionless pituitary adenoma' includes different types of tumours, which share the characteristic of not secreting any specific identified hormones in excess. As a consequence, they usually do not present with hypersecretory syndromes, but rather with pituitary insufficiency of variable degree, secondary to compression of either the normal pituitary tissue or the pituitary stalk and hypothalamus, thus preventing the hypophysiotrophic hormones from reaching the pituitary. The latter event may also induce a slight elevation in serum prolactin. In relation to the size and invasiveness of the adenoma, symptoms may be related to compression or invasion of adjacent structures. Indeed, the diagnosis is usually made when the size has become large enough to cause visual disturbances, headache and/or hypopituitarism, and thus it is relatively rare to identify small, non-functioning adenomas.

As far as their origin is concerned, the finding that many non-functioning adenomas are monoclonal [1], i.e. derived from a single precursor cell, has favoured the concept that the general model of tumorigenesis would also apply to these tumours [2]. This model implies that somatic mutations of proto-oncogenes and/or loss of oncosuppressor genes lead to neoplastic transformation (initiation) and then to the expansion of the mutated clone; stimulatory factors either of hypothalamic origin or locally produced by the tumor itself may also stimulate cell proliferation (promotion). The discovery of activating mutations in the gene coding for α-subunit of the G stimulatory protein (*gsp*) in about 40% of growth hormone (GH)-secreting pituitary adenomas has lent support to this expectation [3]. However, *gsp* mutations have been reported only in about 9% of non-functioning pituitary adenomas [4]. Interestingly, the presence of both *gsp* and *gip* mutations described in two tumours supports the concept of a multistep progression [5]. The role of oncosuppressor genes is still unclear. The accumulation of an oncosuppressor gene product, the P53 protein, not accompanied by the corresponding genetic mutation, reported in some non-functioning adenomas [6], suggests the existence of more complex and still unknown mechanisms. Furthermore, the loss of chromosome 11q13 sequences and deletions in chromosome 11 or other autosome (mainly chromosomes 10 and 22) described in some adenomas [7] reinforce the view that the inactivation of tumour-suppressor genes and the loss of heterozygosity at the retinoblastoma locus [8,9] may also be implicated.

Epidemiology

Functionless adenomas account for about 25% of all pituitary tumours. Their prevalence in the general population is estimated to be about 50 cases per million, and their incidence about 4.5 per million per year. Non-functioning adenomas most frequently present in middle age, mainly between 40 and 50 years (26%), while about 70% of all patients are in their fifth to eighth decades. There is no difference between sexes, the male to female ratio being approximately 1 [10].

Classification

The clinical classification of functionless pituitary tumors encounters several difficulties, and is still a matter of debate [33]. Efforts to correlate the absence of clinical evidence of secretory activity with common histopathological characteristics has been, for the most part, unsuccessful. In fact, the term 'chromophobe adenoma' is inappropriate, because the characteristic of not assuming any dye is shared with many prolactin- and thyrotrophin-secreting adenomas, while the term 'undifferentiated cell adenoma' has now been abandoned, since the tumours do not display anaplastic

Table 13.1 Classification of non-functioning pituitary adenomas.

Morphololologic characteristics	Immunoreactivity
Null-cell adenomas	Lacking distinctive fine-structural and/or immunocytochemical markers. Chromophobic, small polyhedral cells with irregular nuclei. Poorly developed RER, prominent Golgi. Clusters of ribosomes, small rod-shaped mitochondria. Sparse and small secretory granules, 100–250 nm
Oncocytomas	Extensively filled with mitochondria: 'dark mitochondria' (small, rod-shaped, eosinophilic) or 'light' mitochondria (large, ovoid or spherical, chromophobic)
Silent 'corticotroph' adenomas	Heterogeneous
Subtype 1	Indistinguishable from typical basophilic adenomas, but without ACTH or cortisol excess in patients
Subtype 2	Similar to ordinary corticotroph adenomas, but with smaller secretory granules and no type 1 microfilaments. Secretory granules up to 450 nm
Subtype 3	Not resembling ordinary corticotroph adenomas, but rather glycoprotein hormone-secreting adenomas. Chromophobe or slightly eosinophilic. Lightly PAS positive. Secretory granules up to 250 nm

RER, rough endoplasmic reticulum; ACTH, adrenocorticotrophic hormone; PAS, periodic acid–Schiff.

behaviour; the term 'null-cell adenoma' is now restricted to one particular histological type of non-functioning pituitary tumour. On the other hand, the purely clinical terms 'inactive', 'functionless', 'non-functioning' or 'non-secreting' are misleading, as it has been demonstrated by immunocytochemistry, *in situ* hybridization and *in vitro* studies that many of these tumours do indeed process secretory activity. For example, pure α-subunit-secreting adenomas are actively 'secreting', but clinically 'functionless'. Moreover, in some adenomas (e.g. subtype 1 silent corticotroph adenomas and gonadotrophinomas) there is no distinction between secreting and non-secreting forms. However, while, from a clinical point of view, a more appropriate term would possibly be 'clinically non-hypersecreting adenomas', the term 'functionless' is now generally accepted. A classification, based on comprehensive criteria is proposed in Table 13.1.

Pathology

Functionless pituitary tumours are usually approximately round and pink–yellow in colour, of variable size, from 0.5 mm to several centimetres, and occupy the pituitary fossa. The largest may present with suprasellar expansion up to Monro's foramina and/or extend laterally towards the cavernous sinuses or downward in the sphenoidal sinus. Some of them show considerable invasiveness, reaching the optic foramina and penetrating into the orbital cavity through the orbitosphenoidal fissure, or growing backward along the clivus sellae to the occipital foramen. They may include necrotic areas or degenerative cysts.

On light microscopy, neither acidic, basic or periodic acid–Schiff (PAS) dyes are positive. The immunoperoxidase technique does not show hormone production, although some tumours may contain granules positive for pituitary hormones or the α-subunit of glycoprotein hormones. A complete absence of immunoreactivity has been shown in about 36% of tumours, while positive immunostaining (for gonadotrophins, pro-opiomelanocortin (POMC), prolactin, etc.) in more than one-fifth of cells was present in about 25%, and sparse immunoreactivity in the remainder [11]. In some tumours, a small number of cells may show positive immunoreaction for cytokeratins and intermediate filaments composed of polypeptides [12].

On electron microscopy, most of the so-called 'null-cell' adenomas appear composed of small polyhedric cells with irregular nuclei. The rare cytoplasm contains a poor rough endoplasmic reticulum (RER) and organelles; the Golgi apparatus may be prominent, while mitochondria are small. Secretory granules are few, round, 100–125 nm in diameter, with a dense core. Some cells may undergo oncocytic transformation, characterized by an increased number and density of mitochondria, such that other cytoplasmic organelles are hidden [13]. The presence of many oncocytes produces the so-called 'oncocytomas'. These tumours may occasionally appear acidophilic in relation to the presence of cristae on mitochondria. Except for the abundance of mitochondria, oncocytomas are not distinguishable from null-cell adenomas; they also may present positive immunostaining for adenohypophysial hormones and α-subunit. This suggests that both types of tumours have a low secretory activity. Their origin is unclear, and oncocytomas have been suggested as originating from either normally existing oncocytes in the pituitary, neoplastic cells or intermediate lobe rests. It is of interest that oncocytes may be found also in all types of secreting adenoma [13].

Another heterogeneous group of clinically non-functioning pituitary tumours is constituted by the so-called 'silent corticotroph adenomas' [13]. These tumours contain POMC-derived peptide immunoreactivity, but are unassociated with clinical features of Cushing's disease. They are morphologically divided into three subtypes. *Subtype 1* adenomas are basophilic and their ultrastructural appearance resembles that of adrenocorticotrophic hormone (ACTH)-secreting pituitary tumours. *Subtype 2* adenomas are chromophobic, and may show sparse PAS-positive basophilic granulation. Ultrastructurally, the cells appear angular, with a well-developed RER and Golgi complex and secretory granules measuring 200–450 nm; no microfilaments are present. *Subtype 3* adenomas are chromophobic or slightly acidophilic. They are composed by large cells showing ultrastructural features similar to those of glycoprotein hormone-secreting tumours. They appear fast-growing and multidifferentiated: positive immunostaining for POMC derivatives, as well as for prolactin, growth hormone and glycoprotein hormones, may be present.

The study of chromosome number and cell phase by the flow cytometric technique has shown an aneuploid DNA pattern in about 50% of pituitary non-functioning adenomas [14]. Some tumours show a frequency of S-phase cells higher than 10%, indicating a certain degree of aggressiveness, although this does not correlate with their benign behaviour, clinical findings or follow-up observations.

Most non-functioning tumours are indeed able to produce hormones; in fact, the secretion of follicle-stimulating hormone (FSH), luteinizing hormone (LH), thyroid-stimulating hormone (TSH), α-subunit of glycoprotein hormones or POMC derivatives has been documented by *in vitro* hormone release from cultured adenomas under both basal conditions and after appropriate stimulation [15], while complementary DNA (cDNA) *in situ* hybridization shows the expression of messenger RNA (mRNA) of hormone genes [16].

Signs and symptoms

Due to the lack of hormone hypersecretion causing specific biological effects, there is no 'typical' presentation of patients. As the great majority of them have very large tumours, they usually present with ocular or neurological manifestations rather than endocrinological ones (Table 13.2). Compression of the optic nerve or the optic chiasm gives rise to visual field defects (quadrantanopia or hemianopia, mainly bitemporal). In other cases diplopia or ophthalmoplegia are the presenting symptoms. Overall, visual disturbances are the

Table 13.2 Comparison between the frequency of presenting symptoms and documented defects in a series of 164 patients with functionless pituitary tumours.

Presenting symptoms	Frequency (%)	Documented defects	Frequency (%)
Visual disturbances	56	Visual field defects (Goldman)	72
Gonadal function alterations	45	Low basal gonadotrophin levels	30
		Low basal sex hormone levels	64
		Impaired LH responses to GnRH	55
Galactorrhoea	10	Slightly elevated serum PRL	54
Symptoms suggestive on hypoadrenocorticism	18	Low basal cortisol levels	26
		Impaired cortisol responses to ITT	44
Symptoms suggestive of hypothyroidism	24	Low serum T_4 levels	34
		Altered TSH responses to TRH	46
Symptoms suggestive of GH deficiency	50	Impaired GH responses to ITT	70

LH, luteinising hormone; GnRH, gonadotrophin-releasing hormone; PRL, prolactin; ITT, insulin tolerance test; T_4, thyroxine; TSH, thyroid-stimulating hormone (thyrotrophin); TRH, thyrotrophin-releasing hormone; GH, growth hormone.

first presenting symptoms in 50–60% of cases. A deep, generally frontal, headache, due to the pressure over the dural structures, is common (35%). Much less frequent is the appearance of intracranial hypertension with headache, nausea, vomiting or of hypothalamic disturbances (as diabetes insipidus, hyperphagia, dysthermia, sleep–wake pattern and/or behavioural alterations). A sudden severe headache accompanied by rapid loss of sight, hypotension and mental confusion is typical of pituitary apoplexy due to haemorrhagic tumour infarction. The recognition of non-functioning pituitary tumours may occasionally occur in patients with unexplained headache, or with endocrine insufficiency undergoing computed tomography (CT) or magnetic resonance imaging (MRI) investigations. Sometimes, all symptoms go unobserved, and enlargement of the sella turcica is incidentally found on radiological examination.

Endocrine manifestations may not cause the patient concern, especially in the early stages of the disease. However, gonadal function defects are the most frequent features (40–45% of cases). About 40% of women in the fertile age range complain of menstrual disturbances (secondary amenorrhoea, hypo-oligomenorrhoea) which bring them to the physician; by contrast, men with loss of libido and sexual inadequacy (45% of patients) less frequently seek medical attention. Galactorrhoea may occur in 10–20% of affected women. Unfortunately, in many such patients skull radiology is not routinely performed. Less common is the presentation of signs of secondary hypothyroidism (apathy, hypothermia, dry skin, bradycardia, hypotension, etc.) or hypoadrenalism (weakness, tiredness, hypotension, etc.). These manifestations, which account for some 30% of cases, need to be carefully sought. Sometimes, external stress may precipitate latent hypoadrenocorticism into acute adrenal failure. Clinical features suggesting growth deficiency in adults are not clearly identifiable. Pan-hypopituitarism is clinically evident in about 10% of patients.

Diagnosis

Standard radiography of the skull with lateral and frontal projection is the first step in the evaluation of suspected non-functioning tumours. Owing to their large size, the existence of sellar alterations is almost invariably shown: 20% of patients show a completely destroyed sella turcica, 40% have diffuse alterations of the osseous walls, 35% have sellar enlargement without osseous deformity, while only 5% show a slight bulging, double floor or focal alterations. Axial and coronal CT scanning visualise tumours in the sellar and suprasellar region very well, and usually show homogeneous enhancement after contrast medium injection. The presence of necrotic or cystic areas is demonstrated by heterogeneous enhancement surrounded by a peripheral ring; calcification may also be present. MRI is at least as sensitive, and also gives precise three-dimensional information about surrounding structures and characteristics of tumour expansion. Sometimes, in the presence of very large adenomas, preoperative angiography may be required by the neurosurgeon to rule out vascular malformations such as a carotid aneurysm.

Ophthalmological study is also important in the clinical assessment of patients. Fundal examination may reveal the presence of optic pallor, atrophy or papilloedema. Although visual acuity may also be impaired, visual fields defects are the most common finding (70% of cases). They need to be carefully evaluated by the Goldmann perimeter or by computer-assisted perimetry.

Hormonal study is of great importance in order to detect the existence of overt or subtle alterations of the hypothalamo-pituitary function. In recent years, efforts have been made aimed at discovering other hormones or molecules secreted by 'functionless' adenomas to be used as tumour markers.

Preoperative testing includes the evaluation of pituitary function under basal conditions and in response to stimulating or inhibiting agents. Impairment of basal gonadal function is the most frequent finding in both sexes (> 50%). Absent or impaired responsivity of gonadotrophins to gonadotrophin-releasing hormone (GnRH) is found in about half the patients. LH or FSH hypersecretion may be occasionally observed [17]. However, it is worth noting that in many instances the high serum LH levels may result from the cross-reactivity of α-subunit in the LH radioimmunoassay. Indeed, in many of these patients LH determination with double monoclonal antibody immunometric methods and α-subunit measurement reveals normal or subnormal LH and high α-subunit levels, respectively [18]. Evaluation of the α-subunit of glycoprotein hormones may be useful in patients with functionless pituitary tumours, as its level has been found to be elevated in 12–18% of cases [18,19]. In this subset of patients, α-subunit constitutes a tumour marker, and its examination is of help in assessing the effects of therapy.

Elevations in serum prolactin levels are recorded in more than 50% of patients. Mild hyperprolactinaemia (usually lower than 100 ng/ml; 2000 mU/l) is the most common finding (two-thirds of cases), although levels up to 300–400 ng/ml (6000–8000 mU/l) have been reported.

Contrary to patients with prolactinomas, the majority (60–70%) of patients with non-functioning pituitary tumours show a rise in serum prolactin after thyrotrophin-releasing hormone (TRH) injection. On the other hand, only a minority of patients increase serum prolactin after administration of dopamine receptor blockers.

Under basal conditions, secondary hypoadrenocorticism is present in about one-third of cases. Impaired or absent responses to insulin-induced hypoglycaemia are shown in about 50% of patients, while the corticotrophin-releasing hormone (CRH) test elicits a normal response in most cases. Patients with silent corticotroph cell adenomas may show subtle alterations of ACTH secretion, such as plasma ACTH hyperresponsiveness to CRH or vasopressin and lack of suppression after the administration of opioid agonists [20].

Central hypothyroidism is a not uncommon finding (approximately 30%). Alterations of the TSH response to TRH are present in about 50% of cases: absent or impaired (40%) or sometimes delayed, exaggerated or prolonged responses (10%) may be found. There is a high frequency of absent GH responses (approximately 70% of cases in our experience) after insulin or GH-releasing hormone (GHRH) tests. The lack of a normal growth hormone rise after hypoglycaemia is a criterion for the diagnosis of GH deficiency in adult patients.

Clinical and endocrine features of pituitary non-functioning adenomas may be mimicked by other conditions, such as hypothalamic neoplasms and other intrasellar and parasellar lesions which will need to be differentiated. Craniopharyngiomas, metastatic cancers and histiocytosis X may present with diabetes insipidus, which occurs very seldom (if at all) in functionless pituitary tumours. MRI and CT scanning may be useful in distinguishing craniopharyngiomas (which frequently show a polycystic structure and calcification), intrasellar gliomas, empty sella, meningiomas, aneurysms and metastatic cancers. The presence of deposits from a widely disseminated primary neoplasm (in particular from lung, breast, kidney and gastrointestinal tract) generally suggests the diagnosis of pituitary metastasis. Lymphoid hypophysitis is not distinguishable on clinical and radiological grounds, but only with histopathological examination of surgical specimens.

Correlations and discrepancies between *in vivo* and *in vitro* findings and their clinical implications

High serum FSH, LH and α-subunit concentrations have been found in 4–23% of patients with functionless pituitary tumours [16,17,19]. This figure conflicts with many findings showing that a large number of non-functioning adenomas contain or release LH, FSH, α-subunit and LHβ, and express glycoprotein hormone genes [16,17]. Advances in immunocytochemical and molecular biology techniques and cell culture of non-functioning and gonadotroph pituitary adenomas indicate the existence of many similarities between the two entities, suggesting that they are part of a continuum [19]. In this respect, it is worth mentioning that tumour gonadotrophin secretion is more easily demonstrated in men than in women. Indeed, most female patients are postmenopausal and may have physiologically elevated serum gonadotrophin levels. In such patients, it may be difficult to ascertain whether high α-subunit or gonadotrophin levels are secreted by normal or tumoral gonadotrophs. The finding that, similar to patients with gonadotrophinomas, about one-third of patients with non-functioning pituitary adenomas show gonadotrophin or LHβ-subunit response to TRH administration, suggests the possible origin of non-functioning adenomas from gonadotroph cells [21].

Silent corticotroph adenomas have been demonstrated to release ACTH or POMC derivatives *in vitro* even in the absence of elevations in plasma ACTH and clinical features of hypercortisolism *in vivo*, a discrepancy that is probably due to the poor secretory activity of these tumours. A lack of inhibition of circulating ACTH and cortisol to opiates has been reported to occur in these rare cases given loperamide [20].

Nowadays, no value as specific markers of functionless tumours can be attributed to the occasional finding of high circulating gastrin, β-endorphin, calcitonin, β-chorionic gonadotrophin or chromogranin-A levels in occasional patients.

An interesting finding is the presence in the tumour of appreciable amounts of TRH, which is produced by the tumour itself and released in the culture medium [22], and of other releasing and inhibiting hypothalamic hormones (i.e. GnRH, GHRH, somatotrophin release-inhibiting hormone (SRIH), CRH, vasoactive intestinal peptide (VIP)). In addition, it has been demonstrated that non-functioning tumours are able to release in the culture media growth factors and interleukin-6, which might play a role in tumour progression [23].

Cell-membrane receptors for hypothalamic neurohormones including dopamine, somatostatin, TRH, GnRH, CRH, VIP, pituitaryadenylyl cyclase-activating peptide (PACAP) and vasopressin are present in the majority of non-functioning pituitary adenomas. Although their stimulation is not always followed by changes in hormone release, these receptors have been shown to be functional as the expected modifications in cytosolic Ca^{2+} or cyclic adenosine mono-phosphate (cAMP) occur [24]. However, defective inhibitory actions, or even paradoxical increases of intracellular Ca^{2+}, by somatostatin and dopamine have also been reported [24,25].

Therapy

The principal aims in the treatment of patients with non-functioning pituitary adenomas are: (i) to control tumour expansion and to remove mass effects; and (ii) to correct endocrine defects, if any.

The best way to attain the former is to resect the tumour surgically. However, as these adenomas are slow-growing, and no significant progression of the disease is observed in many asymptomatic patients during long-term follow-up, particularly in aged patients with intrasellar tumours and without neurological or visual problems, close follow-up alone might be indicated. On the contrary, a more aggressive approach is warranted in younger patients in whom a greater risk of tumour progression is expected.

While the transfrontal or the pterional routes are used only for very large and supra- or extrasellar extending tumours, the transsphenoidal route now constitutes the approach of choice. After transsphenoidal surgery serious complications and the mortality rate are rare, and even relatively large tumours with significant suprasellar extensions may be removed by this route.

Contrary to hypersecreting adenomas, there is at present no helpful hormonal criterion to assess the outcome of operation, although in some patients with high α-subunit circulating levels normalisation after successful surgery may be observed. Thus, the most valid criteria are clinical (regression of neurological and ocular symptoms) and radiological (disappearance of the tumour mass on CT or MRI).

In almost all cases, due to the incomplete resection of the adenoma, radiation therapy should follow. In many patients (60–80%), surgery is effective in normalizing or improving alterations in visual function, while radiotherapy augments the probability of long-term control.

The incidence of recurrences in patients in whom tumour remnants are not evident postoperatively ranges between 3 and 15%, while tumour regrowth is very common in patients with obvious remnants. In these last patients the risk of recurrence is reduced to 5–15% by subsequent radiation treatment (see Chapter 20).

As far as the hypothalamo-pituitary system is concerned, on the whole there is no substantial modification in endocrine function. Slight deterioration in pituitary secretion versus the preoperative situation is observed in 5–10% of patients, while a recovery of previously impaired endocrine function has also been reported [26]. However, after radiotherapy there may be a progressive loss of pituitary function in the long term.

Radiation therapy has also been used alone, mainly in untreated patients without important neurological or visual defects, in whom surgery was refused or contraindicated. In many centres, conventional radiation with ^{60}Co (3000–4500 cGy) or with a linear accelerator effectively completes the results of surgery in patients with macroadenomas. Similar to other types of pituitary adenomas, the efficacy of radiotherapy is slow and the regression of tumour growth requires several years. A poor response to irradiation is usually observed in patients bearing cystic tumours.

Stereotactic radiosurgery with the Leksell 'γ-knife' unit is becoming more widely available and constitutes an effective means of adjunctive therapy.

Contrary to hypersecreting adenomas, there is not as yet a well-defined place for medical therapy. Because most clinically non-functioning pituitary adenomas produce LH, FSH or α-subunit, the rationale for any medical treatment has been based on the possibility of reducing the secretion of these hormones. The observation that dopamine agonists are sometimes able to lower serum gonadotrophins and α-subunit levels has led to the evaluation of the possible role of bromocriptine in the treatment of non-functioning tumours. Currently, there is some evidence that 15–20% of patients show slight tumour shrinkage [27], but in most cases the size remains unchanged, while occasional growth has been reported [27]; thus, bromocriptine may constitute an alternative to other treatments in only a minority of patients.

The use of GnRH agonists has been suggested, as they can suppress gonadotrophin secretion from either normal pituitary gonadotroph or gonadotroph adenoma cells. However, only a few patients have been administered GnRH analogues, and their responsiveness has been highly variable and uncertain [28].

As already mentioned, in many tumours adenomatous cells have receptors for several other neuropeptides, particularly TRH, dopamine and somatostatin. As a proportion of surgically removed pituitary functionless tumours bear specific receptors for somatostatin, a potential therapeutic use of the drug has been suggested. The long-acting somatostatin analogue, octreotide, has been administered to a relatively small number of patients and it appeared to be effective in reducing tumour size in only a minority of cases [29], although a rapid but transitory amelioration in visual field defects may occur. Tumour expansion during octreotide therapy has also been reported. The recent availability of radiolabelled somatostatin analogues has allowed for the *in vivo* demonstration of somatostatin receptor-positive adenomas [30]. However, this procedure is unable to predict patients who will benefit from octreotide treatment [29].

On the whole, obvious shrinkage of adenomatous tissue has been documented in fewer than 20% of patients treated medically; however, the administration of either dopamine or somatostatin agonists may occasionally be advantageous in preventing further tumour growth in patients who have already received conventional therapies.

The second aim in the therapy of non-functioning pituitary adenomas is to correct hormonal deficiencies, if any. The endocrine management of patients with hypopituitarism mainly consists of peripheral gland hormone replacement: this is necessary in about 80% of cases (Fig. 13.1). In women of pre-menopausal age with secondary ovarian insufficiency, the administration of oestrogens and progestogens is advisable to restore menstrual bleeding and prevent osteoporosis. In hypogonadal men the administration of testosterone esters,

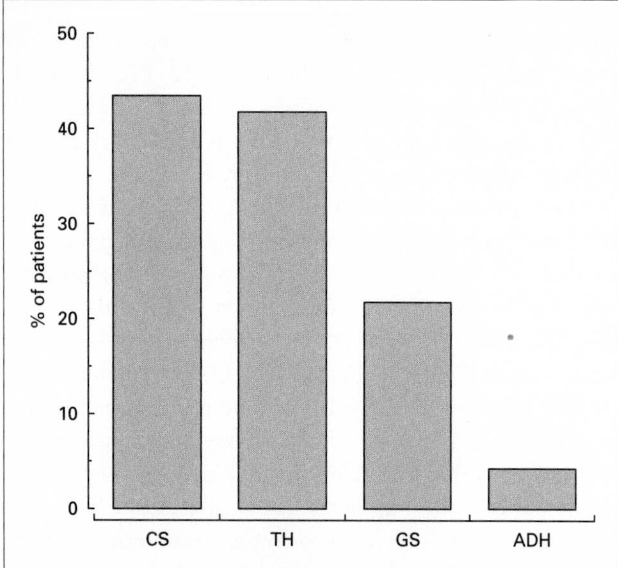

Fig. 13.1 Need for hormone replacement therapy in a series of 167 functionless pituitary tumours after the completion of antitumour treatment. Surgical treatment was done in 160 patients, of whom 16 and three required a second and a third operation, respectively. Radiant therapy was carried out in 61 patients after surgery and in four as unique treatment. Medical treatment (bromocriptine) was carried out in 13 patients after surgery and/or irradiation and in three as unique therapy. CS, corticosteroids; GS, gonadal steroids; TH, thyroid hormone; ADH, desmopressin.

either as injectable depot preparations (200–500 mg/month) or in an oral form (testosterone undecanoate, 120–160 mg/day) restores libido and sexual potency. In patients with central hypothyroidism, euthyroidism should be obtained by administering L-thyroxine (1.6–2 μg/kg bodyweight/day); the treatment should be instituted gradually and should follow cortisol replacement, as an increase in thyroid hormone supply can unmask latent secondary hypoadrenocorticism leading to acute adrenocortical insufficiency. In patients with secondary hypoadrenocorticism, 15–30 mg/day hydrocortisone in divided doses should be administered and adequately augmented during stress.

GH deficiency is very frequent and it worsens after surgery and/or radiotherapy [31]. In agreement with studies reporting beneficial effects of GH treatment together with the unlimited availability of human recombinant GH, the effectiveness of GH replacement therapy is currently under investigation in adult patients with impaired GH secretion. [32]. However, at the present time it cannot be routinely recommended.

Optimal treatment of hormonal defects permits normal activity and a good prognosis for life expectancy. On the whole, the available means of treatment, either alone or in combination, allow satisfactory control of the disease in more than 90% of patients.

References

1 Alexander JM, Biller BMK, Bikkai H, Zervas NT, Arnold A, Klibanski A. Clinically nonfunctioning pituitary tumors are monoclonal in origin. *J Clin Invest* 1990; **86**: 336–46.

2 Melmed S, Braustein GD, Horvath E, Ezrin C, Kovacs K. Pathophysiology of acromegaly. *Endocr Rev* 1983; **4**: 271–90.

3 Landis CA, Masters SB, Spada A, Pace AM, Bourne HR, Vallar L. GTPase inhibiting mutations activate the α chain of G_S and stimulate adenylyl cyclase in human pituitary tumours. *Nature* 1989; **340**: 692–6.

4 Tordjman K, Stern N, Ouaknine G, Yossiphov Y, Razon N, Nordenskjold M. Activating mutations of the Gs alpha gene in nonfunctioning pituitary tumors. *J Clin Endocrinol Metab* 1993; **77**: 765–9.

5 Williamson EA, Daniels M, Foster S, Kelly WF, Kendall-Taylor P, Harris PE. Gs alpha and Gi2 alpha mutations in clinically non-functioning pituitary tumours. *Clin Endocrinol* 1994; **41**: 815–20.

6 Buckley N, Bates AS, Broome JC, Strange RC, Perrett CW, Burke CW, Clayton RN. P53 protein accumulates in Cushings adenomas and invasive non-functional adenomas. *J Clin Endorinol Metab* 1994; **79**: 1513–16.

7 Boggild MD, Jenkinson S, Pistorello M *et al.* Molecular genetic studies of sporadic pituitary tumors. *J Clin Endocrinol Metab* 1994; **78**: 387–392.

8 Pei L, Melmed S, Scheithauer B, Kovacs K, Benedict WF, Prager D. Frequent loss of heterozygosity at the retinoblastoma susceptibility gene (RB) locus in aggressive pituitary tumors: evidence for a chromosome 13 tumor suppressor gene other than RB. *Cancer Res* 1995; **55**: 1613–16.

9 Woloschak M, Roberts JL, Post KD. Loss of heterozygosity at the retinoblastoma locus in human pituitary timors. *Exp Biol Med* 1994; **74**: 693–6.

10 Crichton M, Christy NP, Damon A. Host factors in 'Chromophobe' adenoma of the anterior pituitary: a retrospective study of 464 patients. *Metabolism* 1980; **30**: 248–67.

11 Kujas M, Pleau-Varet J, Peillon F, Derome P. Correlations between immunocytochemical and clinical data in 675 cases of pituitary adenomas. In: Landolt AM, Heitz PU, Zapf J, Girard J, Del Pozo E, eds. *Advances in the Biosciences*, Vol. 69. *Advances in Pituitary Adenoma Research*. Oxford: Pergamon Press, 1988: 21–2.

12 Heitz PhU, Oberholzer M, Zenklusen HR *et al.* Occurrence and pattern of cytokeratins in human pituitary adenomas. In: Landolt AM, Heitz PU, Zapf J, Girard J, Del Pozo E, eds. *Advances in the Biosciences*, Vol. 69. *Advances in Pituitary Adenoma Research* Oxford: Pergamon Press, 1988: 27–37.

13 Thapar K, Kovacs K, Muller PJ. Clinical–pathological correlations of pituitary tumours. In: Fagin JA, ed. *Pituitary Tumours. Baillière's Clinical Endocrinology and Metabolism*. Baillière Tindall, London, 1995; **9**: 225–42.

14 Anniko M, Wersall J. DNA studies for prediction of prognosis of pituitary adenomas. In: Landolt AM, Heitz PU, Zapf J, Girard J, Del Pozo E, eds. *Advances in the Biosciences*, Vol. 69. *Advances in Pituitary Adenoma Research* Oxford: Pergamon Press, 1988: 45–52.

15 Kwekkeboom DJ, de Jong FH, Lamberts SWJ. Gonadotropin release by clinically nonfunctioning pituitary adenomas *in vivo* and *in vitro*: relation to sex and effects of TRH, GnRH and bromocriptine. *J Clin Endocrinol Metab* 1989; **68**: 1111–18.

16 Jameson JL, Klibanski A, Black PMcL *et al.* Glycoprotein hormone

genes are expressed in clinically non-functioning pituitary tumors. *J Clin Invest* 1987; **80**: 1472–8.

17 Snyder PJ. Gonadotroph cell adenomas of the pituitary. *Endocr Rev* 1985; **6**: 552–63.

18 Beck-Peccoz P, Persani L, Medri G, Iglesias Guerrero M, Spada A, Faglia G. New aspects in 'non-functioning' pituitary tumors. In: Casanueva FF, Dieguez C, eds. *Recent Advances in Basic and Clinical Neuroendocrinology*. Amsterdam: Elsevier Science Publishers, 1989: 295–302.

19 Katznelson L, Alexander JM, Klibanski A. Clinically nonfunctioning pituitary adenomas. *J Clin Endocrinol Metab* 1993; **76**: 1089–94.

20 Ambrosi B, Colombo P, Bochicchio D, Bassetti M, Masini B, Faglia G. The silent corticotropinoma: is clinical diagnosis possible? *J Endocrinol Invest* 1992; **15**: 443–52.

21 Daneshdoost L, Gennarelli TA, Bashey HM *et al*. Recognition of gonadotroph adenomas in women. *N Engl J Med* 1991; **324**: 589–94.

22 Le Dafniet M, Blumberg-Tick J, Gozlan H, Barret A, Joubert (Bression) D, Peillon F. Altered balance between thyrotropin-releasing hormone and dopamine in prolactinomas and other pituitary tumors compared with normal pituitaries. *J Clin Endocrinol Metab* 1989; **69**: 267–71.

23 Levy A, Lightman SL. The pathogenesis of pituitary adenomas. *Clin Endocrinol* 1993; **38**: 559–70.

24 Spada A, Reza-Elahi F, Lania A, Gil-Del-Alamo P, Bassetti M, Faglia G. Hypothalamic peptides modulate cytosolic free Ca^{2+} levels and adenylyl cyclase activity in human nonfunctioning pituitary adenomas. *J Clin Endocrinol Metab* 1991; **73**: 913–18.

25 Lania A, Reza-Elahi F, Gil-del-Alamo P, Saccomanno K, Mantovani S, Spada A. Abnormal transduction of dopamine signal in human nonfunctioning pituitary adenomas. *J Endocrinol Invest* 1995; **18**: 265–70.

26 Arafah BM. Reversible hypopituitarism in patients with large nonfunctioning pituitary adenomas. *J Clin Endocrinol Metab* 1986; **62**: 1173–9.

27 Van Schaardenburg D, Roelfsema F, Van Seters AP, Vielvoye GJ. Bromocriptine therapy for non-functioning pituitary adenoma. *Clin Endocrinol* 1989; **30**: 475–84.

28 Klibanski A, Jameson JL, Biller BMK *et al*. Gonadotropin and α-subunit responses to chronic gonadotropin-releasing hormone analog administration in patients with glycoprotein hormone-secreting pituitary tumors. *J Clin Endocrinol Metab* 1989; **68**: 81–6.

29 Plockinger U, Reichel M, Fett U, Saeger W, Quabbe H-J. Preoperative octreotide treatment of growth hormone-secreting and clinically non-functioning pituitary macro-adenomas: effect on tumor volume and lack of correlation with immunohistochemistry and somatostatin receptor scintigraphy. *J Clin Endocrinol Metab* 1994; **79**: 1416–23.

30 de Herder WW, Lamberts SWJ. Imaging of pituitary tumours. In: Fagin JA, ed. *Pituitary Tumours. Baillière's Clinical Endocrinology and Metabolism*. Baillière Tindall, London, 1995; **9**: 367–89.

31 Hoeck, HC, Bang F, Laurberg P. Impaired growth hormone secretion in patients operated for pituitary adenomas. *Growth Reg* 1994; **4**: 63–7.

32 Bengtsson B-A, Eden S, Lonn L *et al*. Treatment of adults with growth hormone (GH) deficiency with recombinant human GH. *J Clin Endocrinol Metab* 1993; **76**: 309–17.

33 Kovacs K, Scheithauer BW, Horvathe G, Lloyd RV. The World Health Organization classification of adenohypophysial neoplasms. A proposed five-tier scheme. *Cancer* 1996; **78**: 502–10.

CHAPTER 14

Gonadotrophin-secreting pituitary adenomas

S.L. Atkin and M.C. White

Introduction

Gonadotrophin-secreting pituitary adenomas (gonadotrophinomas) are slow-growing, benign adenomas derived from the gonadotroph cells of the anterior pituitary gland. They comprise between 70 and 90% [1–9] of the clinically non-functioning (often called functionless, null-cell or non-secretory) pituitary adenoma subgroup. Although clinically non-functioning adenomas account for up to 50% of pituitary adenomas [10], only 3–4% of all patients with a gonadotrophinoma have inappropriately elevated serum gonadotrophins [2,5]. Gonadotrophinomas produce few clinical symptoms of hormonal excess, hence the relatively recent identification of this tumour group [11].

Pathogenesis

Monoclonality

There is increasing evidence that gonadotrophinomas are derived from the somatic mutation of a single cell which results in monoclonal cell growth [12], rather than due to hypothalamic stimulatory factors which may result in polyclonal cell growth. The monoclonal origin of gonadotrophinomas was shown for five non-functional adenomas secreting various combinations of the gonadotrophin α-subunits, follicle-stimulating hormone (FSH) or luteinising hormone (LH) β-subunits [12]. These elegant studies were based on the principle that during female embryogenesis one of the X chromosomes is randomly inactivated, which results in tissues whose X-chromosomal composition is 50% maternal and 50% paternal derived. The technique employed used X-linked restriction fragment length polymorphisms (silent mutations that alter where DNA can be cut by specific restriction enzymes) for the enzymes hypoxanthine phosphoribosyl transferase (HPRT) and phosphoglycerate kinase (PGK). These two enzymes are present only on the X chromosome. In normal polyclonal tissue, two products from the restriction-enzyme digest of the HPRT and PGK genes would be expected which correspond to the maternal and paternal alleles of HPRT and PGK, whilst if the tissue was monoclonal then only one product from *either* the maternal *or* paternal allele would be found. In the five patients studied both the maternal and paternal-derived alleles were found in peripheral leucocytes, whilst only a single allele was found in each of the adenomas, which indicated that the pituitary tumours were monoclonal [12]. However, this and other studies performed are limited because only a small proportion of tumours are suitable for analysis; all subjects have to be female, and each subject must be heterozygous for either the HPRT or PGK genes [13].

Factors implicated in gonadotrophinoma pathogenesis

The fundamental mutation(s) underlying the monoclonal growth of gonadotrophinomas and other factors that may contribute to their pathogenesis remain unknown. Research has focused on oncogenic mutations and other processes that may affect cell proliferation, the combination of which may allow the stepwise progression to tumour formation. Hypothalamic, oncogenic, autocrine and paracrine factors have been implicated.

Hypothalamic factors

Evidence suggests that trophic hypothalamic factors are important in hormonal secretion and may play a role in adenoma growth, whilst gonadal steroids may be involved in the inhibition of tumour development. Prolonged hypogonadism with unopposed hypothalamic stimulation may lead to pituitary enlargement [14,15], and anecdotal reports of long-standing hypogonadism associated with gonadotrophinomas have been described [16,17]. Experimentally, pituitary tumours can be induced in mice that have been orchidectomised [18]. Gonadotrophin-releasing hormone (GnRH)-receptor responses may be altered in these tumours, as demonstrated by the persistent elevation of gonadotrophin secretion following GnRH agonist-analogue treatment instead of the fall in FSH and LH normally expected [19]. However, treatment with a GnRH antagonist reduces elevated FSH levels to normal, as anticipated [20].

Oncogenic factors

It has been shown that chromosomal abnormalities are common in human pituitary adenomas [21], and recently allelic deletions on chromosome 11 were found in seven of 36 non-functional/gonadotrophinoma tumours [22], evidence for the multistep hypothesis of adenoma formation.

Specific mutations causing constitutive activation of adenoma intracellular metabolism and thereby facilitating cell proliferation may have role in tumorigenesis. Whilst 40% of human somatotrophinomas harbour mutant activating G_s regulatory proteins [23], this appears to be less important in gonadotrophinomas: mutations were only found in three of 22 adenomas in one study [24]. Another key intracellular factor, protein kinase Cα, has been found to be overexpressed in some non-functioning pituitary adenomas due to a point mutation [25]. Oncogenes which have been shown to be important in other tissue cancers have been investigated, but only the oncogene c-*myc* has been found to be overexpressed in a subset of tumours: six of 14 tumours overexpressed c-*myc* in one study, the importance of which is unclear [26].

Tumour-suppressor genes inhibit cell proliferation, and growth and inactivating mutations of the *p53* gene are found in 50% of human tumours [27]. However, whilst the p53 protein has been shown immunologically to be expressed in a few non-functioning tumours [28,29,106], no mutations of the *p53* gene have been found to date [29].

Autocrine and paracrine factors

Autocrine and paracrine mechanisms may be of importance in tumorigenesis, and the anterior pituitary is a rich source of many growth factors which have been shown to have potent proliferative actions in other tissue systems [30,31,107]. Whilst basic fibroblastic growth factor, epidermal growth factor, transforming growth factor-α, insulin-like growth factor 1, interleukin 1α and interleukin 6 have been found to be associated with gonadotrophinomas or effect gonadotrophin secretion [30,32–35], only insulin-like growth factor 1 has been shown to increase gonadotrophinoma cell proliferation indices to date [32].

Thus, somatic mutation coupled with hypothalamic, autocrine and paracrine factors may all play a role, either alone or in combination, in the pathogenesis of gonadotrophinomas.

Pathophysiology

Clinical secretory characteristics

Gonadotrophinomas have been shown to secrete every combination of intact FSH and LH together with the α-subunit FSH and LH β-subunits (Table 14.1). The majority of gonadotrophinomas secrete both FSH and LH (with or without subunits). The secretion of FSH alone (with or without α-subunit) is relatively uncommon and LH secretion (with α-subunit and/or LH β-subunit) is rare [36–38]: immunocytochemical and cell-culture studies show a similar pattern [2–4,7,8,39]. Anecdotal reports of FSH with thyroid-stimulating hormone (TSH) hypersecretion (without thyrotoxicosis) and LH with prolactin secretion (from different cells) have also been reported [40,41]. Clinically, FSH is the predominantly elevated serum hormone with LH levels usually being within the normal range or even subnormal. When intact tumorous LH is secreted the plasma testosterone may be either normal or elevated [42–46]. If the diagnosis of a gonadotrophinoma is made by immunohistochemistry or cell culture, fewer than 50% of cases are retrospectively identified as having inappropriate serum gonadotrophin levels [3,4,7,8].

Tumorous FSH has been shown to be biologically active [47]. Using gel electrophoresis tumorous FSH elutes to a similar location and appears to be identical to intact FSH [37,48,49]. However, tumorous FSH with a lower molecular weight than normal has been described [36]. Normal FSH bioactivity is associated with isoforms which have different oligosaccharide structures [50] and it is not known whether tumorous FSH may differ in the same fashion. Tumorous LH immunoreactivity may reflect the presence

Table 14.1 Characteristics of 22 gonadotrophin-secreting pituitary adenomas using *in vitro* cell culture.

Secretion characteristics	No.
FSH ± α-subunit	1
FSH + LH ± α-subunit ± LH β-subunit	17
FSH + LH + TSH ± α-subunit	3
LH ± α-subunit ± LH β-subunit	0
α-Subunit	1

FSH, follicle stimulating hormone; LH, luteinising hormone; TSH, thyroid-stimulating hormone.

of disassociated LH α- and β-subunits which cross-react in the assay for intact LH [49], leading to apparently normal or high serum LH values with low plasma testosterone levels. However, high inactive cross-reacting LH β-subunit levels are unlikely to be contributing significantly when the measured LH in men is associated with appropriate normal or high levels of testosterone. The structure of tumorous LH may also differ to that of normal; Northern blot analysis of LH β-subunit (from a single tumour) showed LH β-subunit messenger RNA (mRNA) of increased size [45]. These data suggest that, in addition to the heterogeneity of intact and gonadotrophin subunit secretion from gonadotrophinomas, there may also be specific defects of both pre- and post-translational tumorous gonadotrophin production.

Control of tumorous gonadotrophin secretion

Normal and tumorous gonadotrophin secretion occurs in pulses. In a series of 12 gonadotrophinomas all of the patients had pulsatile gonadotrophin secretion with pulses of normal frequency but varying amplitude [51]. In a smaller series, LH pulses were infrequent in three patients studied regardless of their circulating sex-steroid concentrations [8] and FSH pulses were random and asynchronous from the LH pulses, but the overall pulse frequency was equal to or greater than that anticipated for hypogonadal subjects without pituitary tumours. The role of hypothalamic GnRH in regulating the tumorous tissue is not clear, but evidence suggests that GnRH would appear to be important, although about 45% of subjects fail to show a rise in LH following intravenous GnRH [8]. Repetitive GnRH agonist-analogue treatment caused persistent gonadotrophin secretion in patients with gonadotrophinomas, rather than the normal expected fall in secretion [19]. However, GnRH antagonist treatment inhibits gonadotrophin secretion although tumour size may be unaffected [52].

A number of authors have administered testosterone in an attempt to suppress tumorous gonadotrophin secretion, but no effect has been demonstrated, at least in the short term [53–55]. Administration of oestrogen has been associated with both inhibition and stimulation of hormone release [44,48,53–57], both clinically and *in vitro*. However, clomiphene citrate (an anti-oestrogen) has not been found to alter tumorous gonadotrophin levels [54,56–58]. The gonadal peptide inhibin reduces FSH secretion and it is of interest that serum inhibin levels were shown to be significantly elevated when tumorous FSH levels were also increased [59]. All these data suggest that tumorous gonadotrophs may be insensitive to the normal negative feedback of gonadal steroids and peptides, a situation analogous to the reduced sensitivity to cortisol of tumorous corticotrophs seen in Cushing's disease.

Response to thyrotrophin-releasing hormone

Normal subjects do not show a gonadotrophin response to thyrotrophin-releasing hormone (TRH), but in gonadotrophinomas an abnormal LH response following intravenous TRH was first described in 1976 [60] and has subsequently been confirmed [8,49,61,62]. Approximately 50% of patients appear to show at least a twofold rise in LH and 30% a rise in FSH within 30 min of TRH administration. In some cases the LH rise can be accounted for by an increase in LH β-subunit rather than intact hormone [49]. In one series, 11 out of 16 women with a gonadotrophinoma showed an LH β-subunit response after TRH, but only three had an FSH response and only four an LH response, suggesting that measurement of the LH β-subunit after TRH may be a more specific diagnostic test [63].

Cell-culture studies

Cell-culture studies reveal that up to 100% of functionless tumours secrete gonadotrophins and/or their subunits into the culture medium [1,3,4,7,8,10]. In a series of 32 functionless tumours studied in culture by one of us (M.C.W.), 22 (69%) were associated with gonadotrophin secretion and one additional tumour with α-subunit alone; in many cases secretion rates were low, reflecting similar low serum gonadotrophin levels. Serum and cell-culture values may not correlate; individuals may hypersecrete only α-subunit in their serum, but both FSH and α-subunit in the culture medium [64]. The mechanism underlying this discrepancy is uncertain, but one possibility is that intact tumorous gonadotrophin secretion *in vivo* may be under inhibitory control.

In general, dynamic cell-culture studies have provided confirmation that the aberrant responses to hypothalamic factors seen *in vivo* are mediated by a direct effect on the tumorous gonadotrophs [65,66].

Pathology

Gonadotrophinomas compress surrounding structures by local growth and 88% of these tumours have evidence of suprasellar extension by the time of surgery [67] (Fig. 14.1). Gonadotrophinomas are benign tumours, although anecdotal reports have suggested possible malignant change [40,68]. Local invasion may be found in 21% of gonadotrophinomas, which is less than that found for other pituitary adenoma subtypes where the overall frequency of local invasion is 35%.

On light microscopy the cells are small to medium sized, often arranged in sheets and with pseudo-rosette formation

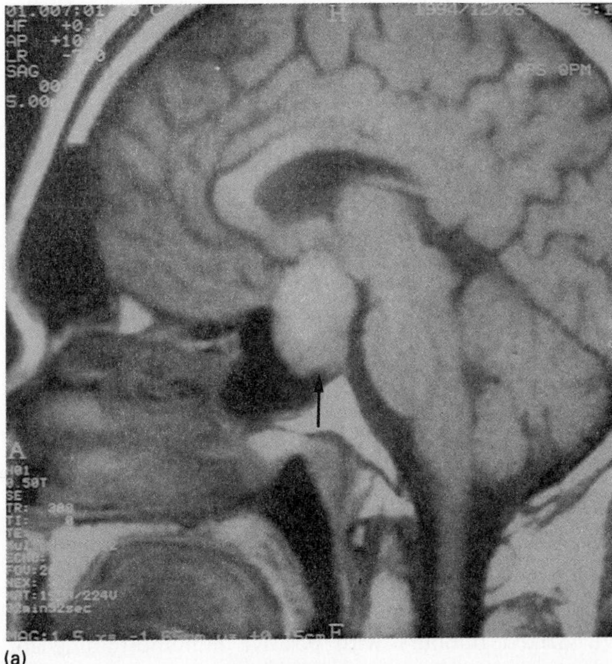

(a)

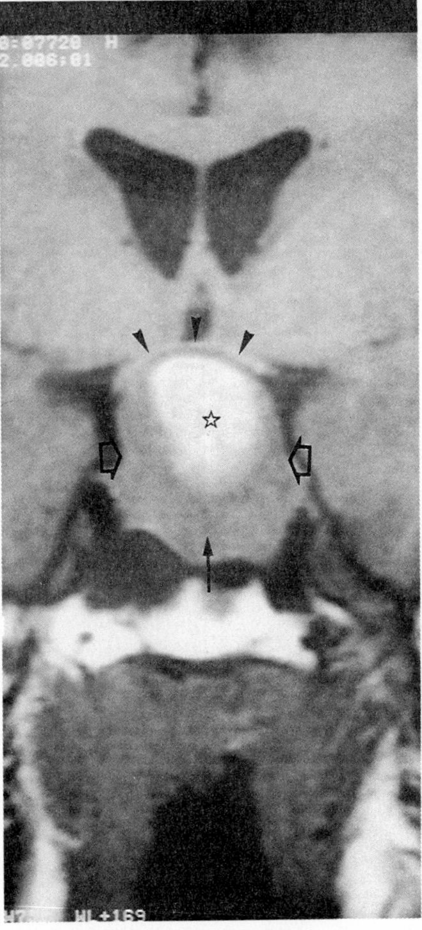

(b)

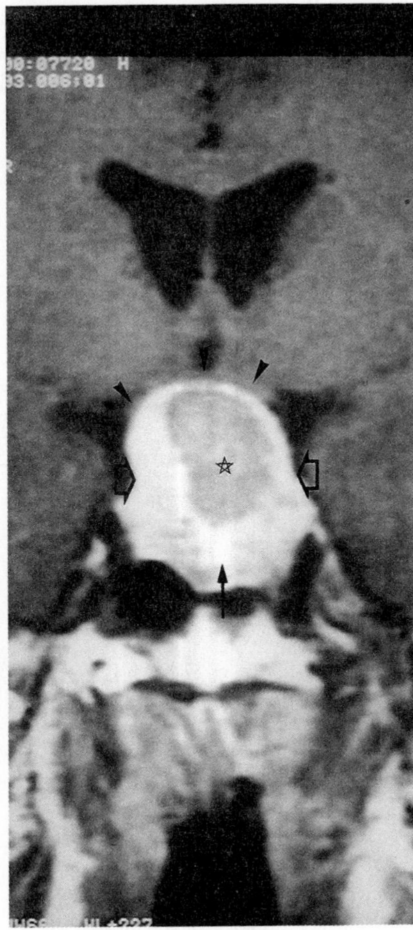

(c)

Fig. 14.1 (a) Sagittal T1-weighted magnetic resonance imaging showing a large gonadotrophinoma arising from the pituitary fossa with suprasellar extension (arrow). (b) Coronal image of the same patient before and (c) after gadolinium contrast injection showing the large gonadotrophinoma (arrow) compressing the optic chiasm (arrow head). The adenoma has a 'waist' due to its compression by the diaphragma sellae (open arrow). The value of magnetic resonance imaging in distinguishing lesions is shown by the large haemorrhagic cyst which is present within the adenoma (star).

occurring around blood vessels. Conventional histological stains generally show gonadotrophinoma cells to be chromophobic, although acidophilic staining may be seen [39] and periodic acid–Schiff (PAS)-positive cytoplasmic granules may be found. Immunohistochemical staining may demonstrate intact gonadotrophins or their β-subunits alone or in combination, in the same or in different cells; features which are in keeping with the colocalisation of FSH and LH in normal pituitary gonadotrophs [69,70]. It has been suggested that positive gonadotrophin immunostaining is more likely in tumours removed from male rather than female patients [39]. Immunopositive tumour cells may be scattered requiring serial tissue sections for diagnostic confirmation [71], which may explain the low incidence of gonadotrophinomas (1.4–4.7%) in some immunohistochemical studies [72–74] compared with those using cell culture or molecular biology methods [1,3,4,6–8]. However, a recent immunohistochemical study identified 80% of clinically non-functional adenomas as gonadotrophinomas [9]. Mixed tumours with positive immunostaining for gonadotrophins in combination with TSH, prolactin, GH or β-endorphin have also been described [70,71].

Gonadotrophinomas are the only pituitary adenomas where distinct sex differences have been observed on electron microscopy. In males, over 50% of adenomas are similar to null-cell adenomas having small cells with irregular nuclei, a poor-to-moderately developed cytoplasm with sparse rough endoplasmic reticulum (RER) and Golgi membranes and few secretory granules (≤250 nm): the remainder of adenomas have a well-developed RER. In women, by contrast, the cells are almost always clearly differentiated with a well-developed RER, and a characteristic honeycomb-like Golgi apparatus: secretory granules are also sparse [39].

Using markers of cell proliferation it is estimated that non-functional adenomas have a proliferation index of 0.1–2% [75–78], but evidence of mitoses are rare in tissue sections.

Clinical features

The majority of patients with gonadotrophinomas present between 30–70 years of age with a peak incidence occurring between 50 and 60 years and there is a slight male predominance (Fig. 14.2). The prevalence of gonadotrophinomas is unknown. Diagnostic difficulty arises in post-menopausal women in whom physiologically elevated serum FSH and LH levels may mask tumour-derived gonadotrophins. Consequently, most of the clinical descriptions have been

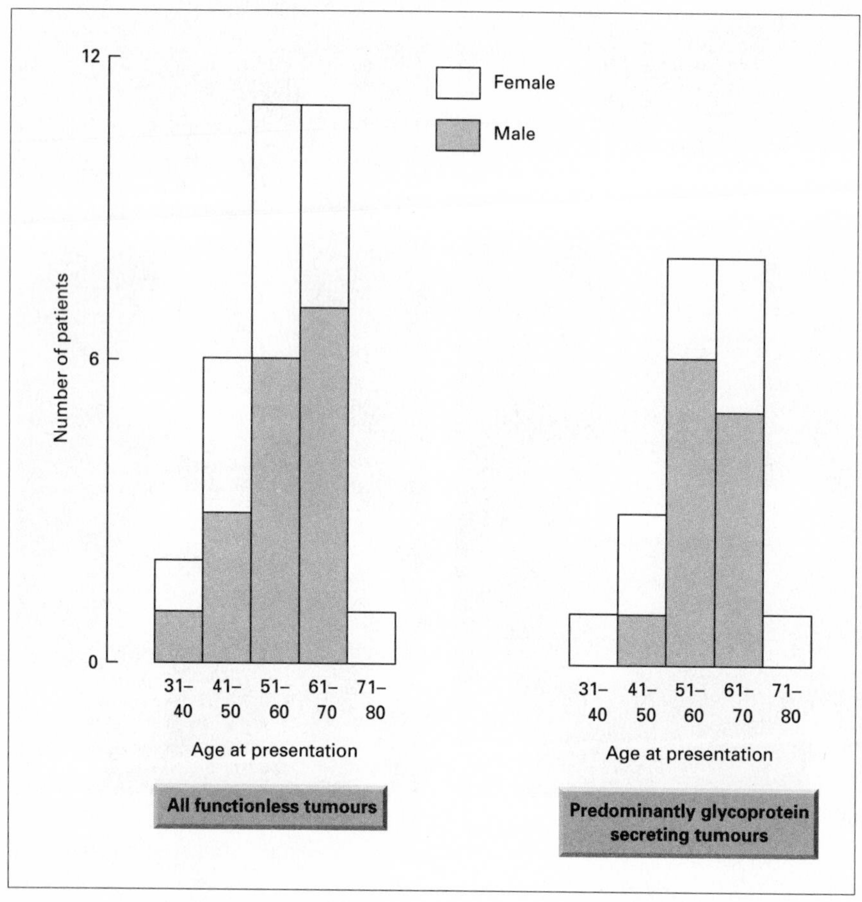

Fig. 14.2 Age of patients presenting with a functionless tumour. Glycoprotein-secreting adenomas confirmed by cell culture.

obtained from males. Gonadotrophinomas have rarely been described in children and adolescents [40,42,43].

The majority of patients present with large tumours causing neurological features and headaches, and over 80% are found to have a visual field defect at presentation [10]. The visual field defects are due to local pressure on the optic chiasm from suprasellar adenoma growth (see Fig. 14.1) which results in variable visual field loss. This may range from a mild asymmetrical bilateral upper temporal quadrantic hemianopia, classical bitemporal hemianopia through to complete loss of vision in extreme cases. Epileptiform seizures, diplopia from cavernous sinus invasion and other features from local invasion of surrounding structures are rare [10]. The length of history preceding diagnosis may be very variable, but usually ranges from 6 to 24 months. With the increased availability of computed tomography (CT) and magnetic resonance imaging (MRI) the second most common presentation of these tumours is that of an incidental finding [79]. The least common presentation results from hypopituitarism, although retrospective questioning may elicit such symptoms: in males loss of libido, impotence and infertility are seen in 50% of subjects, although increased libido may rarely be reported [44,45]. With excessive FSH hypersecretion testicular volume may be significantly increased [59] (Fig. 14.3). In premenopausal women gonadotrophinomas may present with oligomenorrhoea and be misdiagnosed as premature ovarian failure in the presence of elevated serum gonadotrophins [48].

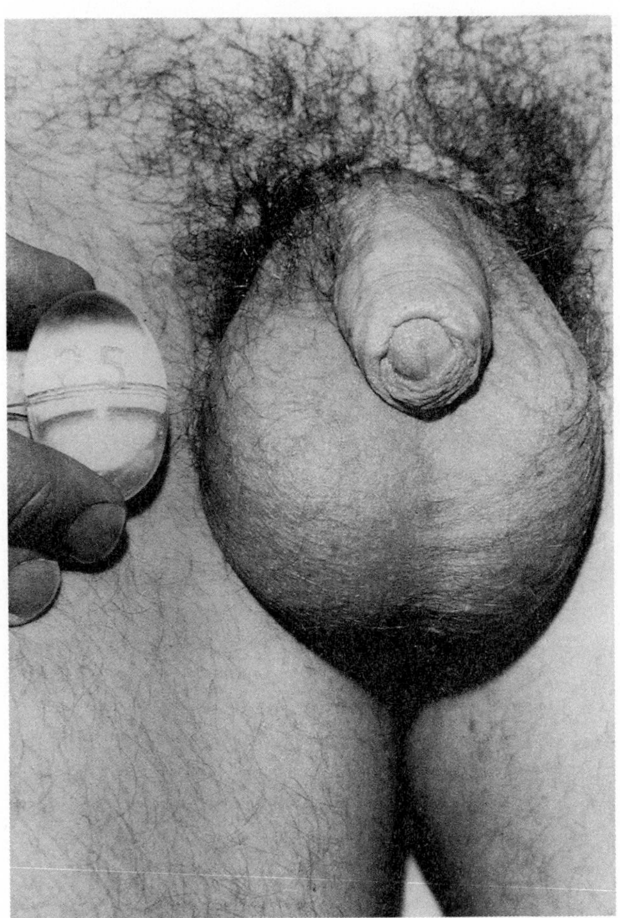

Fig. 14.3 Testes in a patient with gonadotrophin-secreting pituitary adenoma. From [59].

Testicular pathology

Testicular pathology has been described and the changes from normal would appear to relate in part to whether the serum level of LH and FSH is supraphysiological or subnormal (Table 14.2). In three of six cases with elevated serum LH levels, Leydig cell hypertrophy was recorded with an increased plasma testosterone in one. In contrast, Sertoli cell hyperplasia has been described in only one case of FSH hypersecretion. However, an interesting observation seen in a group of patients with elevated FSH levels was the dramatic increase in the total length of seminiferous tubules by up to 4–8 times the upper limits of normal, which may account for the increased testicular volumes which were seen in those cases [59].

In most subjects there was evidence of spermatogenesis, but with varying degrees of maturation arrest. This probably reflected the imbalance between the relative increase or decrease in secretion of either LH or FSH.

Diagnosis

The initial history and examination, including the careful examination of the visual fields, eliciting signs of hypopituitarism and testicular examination in males, will give the first suspicion of the diagnosis and will direct the urgency of the subsequent investigations. Formal assessment of the visual fields needs to be performed and radiological investigation of the pituitary fossa with MRI or CT scanning is required. MRI is the modality of choice for the initial evaluation of pituitary gland pathology because of the fine anatomical detail possible and the ability to distinguish blood vesells, haemorrhage and aneurysms [80] (see Fig. 14.1). CT scanning is now reserved for when MRI availability is limited [80] or where details of the surrounding bone anatomy are required. There is no role for the lateral skull radiograph in pituitary disease.

Many lesions may be found in the pituitary area and their management and treatment will depend on the diagnosis [79]. Initial endocrine investigation should include measurement of insulin-like growth factor 1, prolactin, a low-dose dexamethasone suppression test or a 24-hour urinary free cortisol to screen for 'silent' somatotrophinomas,

Table 14.2 Pathology of the testis in patients with gonadotrophin-secreting adenomas.

Reference	Serum luteinising hormone	Serum follicle-stimulating hormone	Plasma testosterone	Testicular biopsy findings
[16]	↑	↑	N	Slight Leydig-cell hyperplasia, spermatogenic arrest
[44]	↑↑	↓	↑	Leydig cell hyperplasia, decreased spermatocyte maturation
[53]	↑	↑↑	–	Leydig cells hypertrophy, active spermatogenesis
[55]	↓	↑	↓↓	Sparse Leydig cells, normal Sertoli cells, tubules well preserved, decreased spermatids, maturation rare
[59] Case 1	N	↑↑	N	Leydig cells normal, Sertoli cells normal
Case 2	↑	↑↑	↑	All stages of spermatogensis identified in 20% of tubules considered normal, but a reduction of germ cells in remainder
Case 3	↑	↑	↓	
[85]	N	↑↑	N	Sertoli-cell hyperplasia, tubules normal, reduced germ cells

↑, Elevated; ↓, reduced; N, in normal range.

prolactinomas and corticotrophinomas, respectively. However, the diagnosis of these tumours may only be made histologically [79].

Baseline FSH, LH and α-subunit estimation should be performed (FSH and LH β-subunit estimation is not routinely available as yet) and a marked difference between intact serum FSH and LH values may suggest the diagnosis of a gonadotrophinoma in post-menopausal women in whom gonadotrophin levels are physiologically elevated. When intact glycoprotein hormones are not increased the common α-subunit may be elevated and serve as a marker for the presence of a gonadotrophinoma [81]; even when the level of α-subunit is not elevated the ratio of α-subunit to LH or FSH may be raised, suggesting the diagnosis [7].

The TRH test may be diagnostic, as described above, with an elevation of intact FSH, LH or the LH β-subunit which may be particularly helpful in the difficult diagnosis of gonadotrophinomas in post-menopausal women.

The rise in gonadotrophin levels following GnRH administration provides no useful information as the gonadotrophin response may be from a gonadotrophinoma, the normal gonadotrophs or both. Indeed, there are reports documenting pituitary apoplexy of gonadotrophinomas following GnRH and GnRH-agonist administration, which argues against the use of GnRH in the evaluation of macroadenomas [82,83].

Plasma testosterone concentrations are normal in at least 50% of men, may be increased when LH levels are high [42–46] or low if LH levels are subnormal. When the testosterone level is low and the LH level is normal LH β-subunit assay cross-reactivity may be responsible, as discussed above [49].

In those patients with FSH hypersecretion, but reduced testosterone levels, gonadal testosterone production is increased following human chorionic gonadotrophin (hCG) administration [53,59,84,85] which indicates that the reduced gonadal function is secondary to pituitary pathology. The use of this test is valuable if there is any doubt as to the cause of elevated gonadotrophins in a male or a premenopausal female.

Various degrees of hypopituitarism are often found in patients with large macroadenomas [86,87]. In two series of patients with macroadenomas the majority of patients were growth-hormone deficient [86], 69–81% patients had thyroid insufficiency and 62–74% had adrenal insufficiency [86,87]. A degree of hyperprolactinaemia is found in 80% or more of these adenomas which is not of tumorous origin [86–88]. Diabetes insipidus is uncommon. The mechanism for the hypopituitarism and hyperprolactinaemia appears to be compression of the hypophysial portal vessels by the adenoma, with restoration of function and a reduction of prolactin levels within hours of transsphenoidal surgery [87]. Persistence of hypopituitarism has been suggested to be due to ischaemic necrosis of the anterior pituitary as a result of adenoma compression [87].

The hypogonadism that may occur in patients with gonadotrophinomas can be seen to be multifactorial and contributed to by insufficient intact gonadotrophin secretion, biologically inactive gonadotrophin-subunit secretion and mild hyperprolactinaemia.

Treatment

Surgery

Surgical decompression and removal of adenomatous tissue is the treatment of choice since the threat to sight is the major practical problem for most patients; visual field impairment may be dramatically alleviated in at least 50% and followed by some improvement in a further 20% of patients [89]. Cure is rare, but improvement in other clinical features such as secondary hypogonadism can be achieved and hypopituitarism may improve with the restoration of the hypophysial portal circulation [86,87]. Such change is usually associated with a reduction in serum gonadotrophin levels and the disappearance of the aberrant gonadotrophin responses to TRH. Postoperative recurrence is usually associated with an increase in serum gonadotrophin concentrations [89].

Transsphenoidal surgery is the procedure of choice for the operative removal of these tumours as the cranial fossa is not entered and it may be performed on elderly or ill patients [90]. The surgery-related mortality is less than 1%. Complications vary from 5–10% and include diabetes insipidus, syndrome of inappropriate antidiuretic hormone secretion, permanent hypopituitarism cerebrospinal fluid (CSF) rhinorrhoea, visual loss, oculomotor nerve palsy, hemiparesis, encephalopathy, meningitis and haemorrhage [90].

Endocrine assessment may be undertaken 6 weeks or more following surgery and should include basal hormone estimation, with gonadotrophin-subunit evaluation if available, and an assessment of the remaining pituitary function to determine hormonal replacement therapy. Radiological evaluation of the postoperative pituitary continues to be an area of particular difficulty in the search of residual or recurrent tumour [91]. It may be difficult to distinguish postoperative scarring and graft material from adenoma particularly in the first 6 months following surgery [91]. Routine postoperative radiological assessment may therefore be best performed at 6 months unless otherwise indicated.

External irradiation

External irradiation should be prescribed after surgery, unless there are specific contraindications, since the recurrence rate for large pituitary adenomas is reported to be as great as 80% at 10 years, but only 14% for those receiving adjuvant irradiation [92]. In a series of 100 macroadenomas, 12 of 50 patients who did not receive adjuvant irradiation and 18 of 50 patients who did receive irradiation had recurrence of their tumours [93]. However, comparison between studies is difficult because of patient-selection criteria. Approximately 50% of patients suffer partial or complete hypopituitarism at 10 years [94]. Because of progressive hypopituitarism following radiotherapy patients should be followed up 6-monthly for the first year and then yearly thereafter.

Radiotherapy is administered through multiple ports at a dose of 1.8–2 Gy daily up to a maximum of 45 Gy, at which dosage damage to the optic nerve is minimal [95].

Medical therapy

At present medical therapy is unsatisfactory for the treatment of gonadotrophinomas.

Dopamine agonist therapy with bromocriptine has been shown to suppress gonadotrophin release both acutely and chronically in just over half of the patients to whom the drug has been administered. In other patients little effect may be seen even when the drug has been administered chronically for up to 3 years; although tumour shrinkage is unpredictable [45,96–99], acute improvement of visual field defects may occur [97]. This contrasts with the dramatic effect the drug has on most prolactinomas. The newer dopamine agonists quinagolide (formerly known as CV 205–502) and cabergoline have also been shown to reduce tumorous hormonal secretion without affecting tumour size [100,101].

Most gonadotrophinomas express somatostatin receptors [102]. However, tumour shrinkage is uncommon with the somatostatin-analogue octreotide although visual field assessment may improve without a change in tumour size; the mechanism for this is unclear [43,103,104].

It would seem logical that GnRH-agonist treatment might be of value in the reduction of tumorous gonadotrophin levels, since these drugs can completely suppress gonadotrophin secretion in normal women. In practice, these agents are either without effect or cause a paradoxical persistent increase in gonadotrophin levels, whilst tumour size remains unchanged [19,105]. GnRH-antagonist therapy has been shown to suppress gonadotrophin and α-subunit secretion dramatically both acutely and over a period of 6 months, but tumour size was unaffected [20,52].

In a single case report, cyproterone acetate, an antiandrogen with antigonadotrophic properties, was found to have acutely suppressed LH in a young male patient with an LH- and prolactin-secreting adenoma [42].

With the increased availability of MRI and CT scanning the diagnosis of the pituitary incidentaloma may increase leading to the diagnosis of more gonadotrophinomas at an earlier stage. Currently, radiological studies on normal subjects have shown a 4–20% incidence of lesions <10 mm [79]. Further elucidation of the pathogenesis of gonadotrophinomas may facilitate the development of effective medical therapy to augment the surgical and adjuvant radiotherapy currently available.

References

1 Mashiter K, Adams EF, Van Noorden S. Secretion of LH, FSH and PRL shown by cell culture and immunocytochemistry of human functionless pituitary adenomas. *Clin Endocrinol* 1981; **15**: 103–12.

2 Beckers A, Stevenaert A, Mashiter K, Hennen G. Follicle stimulating hormone-secreting pituitary adenomas. *J Clin Endocrinol Metab* 1985; **61**: 525–8.

3 Asa SL, Gerrie BM, Singer W, Horvath E, Kovacs K, Smyth HS. Gonadotrophin secretion by human pituitary null cell adenomas and ancocytomas. *J Clin Endocrinol Metab* 1986; **62**: 1011–19.

4 Lawton NF, Evans AJ, Pickard JD, Perry S, Davies B. Secretion of neuron specific enolase, prolactin, growth hormone, lutinising hormone and follicle stimulating hormone by 'functionless' and endocrine-active pituitary tumours. *J Neurol Neurosurg Psychiatry* 1986; **49**: 574–80.

5 Black PM, Hsu DW, Klibanski A *et al.* Hormone production in clinically non functioning pituitary adenomas. *J Neurosurg* 1987; **66**: 244–50.

6 Jameson LJ, Klibanski A, Black P *et al.* Expression of gonadotrophin genes in non-functioning pituitary adenomas. *J Clin Invest* 1987; **80**: 1472–8.

7 Kwekkeboom DJ, De Jong FH, Lamberts SWJ. Gonadotrophin release by clinically nonfunctioning and gonadotrophin pituitary adenomas *in vivo* and *in vitro*: relation to sex and effects of thyrotrophin-releasing hormone gonadotrophin-releasing hormone and bromocriptine. *J Clin Endocrinol Metab* 1989; **68**: 1128–35.

8 White MC, Daniels M, Newland P *et al.* LH and FSH secretion and responses to GnRH and TRH in patients with clinically functionless pituitary adenomas. *Clin Endocrinol* 1990; **32**: 681–8.

9 Sano T, Yamada S. Histologic and immunohistochemical study of clinically nonfunctioning pituitary adenomas: special reference to gonadotropin positive adenomas. *Pathol Intl* 1994; **44**: 697–703.

10 Snyder PJ. Gonadotroph cell adenomas of the pituitary. *Endocr Rev* 1985; **6**: 552–63.

11 Woolf PD, Schenk EA. An FSH producing tumour in a patient with hypogonadism. *J Clin Endocrinol Metab* 1974; **38**: 561–8.

12 Alexander JM, Biller BMK, Bikkal H *et al.* Clinically nonfunctioning pituitary adenomas are monoclonal in origin. *J Clin Invest* 1990; **86**: 336–40.

13 Levy A, Lightman SL. The pathogenesis of pituitary adenomas. *Clin Endocrinol* 1993; **38**: 559–70.

14 Bower BF. Pituitary enlargement secondary to untreated primary hypogonadism. *Ann Intern Med* 1968; **69**: 107–9.

15 Samaan NA, Stephans AV, Danziger J, Trujillo J. Reactive pituitary abnormalities in patients with Klinefelter's and Turner's syndromes. *Arch Intern Med* 1979; **139**: 198–201.

16 Nicolis G, Shimshi M, Allen C, Halmi NS, Kourides IA. Gonadotropin-producing pituitary adenoma in a man with long-standing primary hypogonadism. *J Clin Endocrinol Metab* 1988; **66**: 237–41.

17 Kovacs K, Horvath, Rewcastle NB, Ezrin C. Gonadotroph cell adenoma of the pituitary in a woman with long standing hypogonadism. *Arch Gynaecol* 1980; **229**: 57–65.

18 Griesbach WE, Purves HD. Basophil adenomata in the rat hypophysis after gonadectomy. *Br J Cancer* 1960; **14**: 49–59.

19 Klibanski A, Jameson JL, Biller BM *et al.* Gonadotropin and alpha-subunit responses to chromic gonadotropin-releasing hormone analog administration in patients with glycoprotein hormone-secreting pituitary tumours. *J Clin Endocrinol Metab* 1989; **68**: 81–6.

20 Daneshdoost L, Pavlon SN, Molitch ME *et al.* Inhibition of follicle-stimulating hormone secretion from gonadotroph adenomas by repetitive administration of a gonadotropin-releasing hormone antagonist. *J Clin Endocrinol Metab* 1990; **71**: 92–7.

21 Mark J. Chromosomal characteristics of human pituitary adenomas. *Acta Neuropathol* 1971; **19**: 99–109.

22 Boggild MD, Jenkinson S, Pistorello M *et al.* Molecular genetic studies of sporadic pituitary tumours. *J Clin Endocrinol Metab* 1994; **78**: 387–92.

23 Landis CL, Masters SB, Spada A, Pace AM, Bourne HR, Valla L. GTPase inhibiting mutations activate the α chain of Gs and stimulate adenyl cyclase in human pituitary tumours. *Nature* 1989; **340**: 692–6.

24 Williamson EA, Daniels M, Foster S, Kelly WF, Kendall-Taylor P, Harris PE. Gsα and GI2α mutations in clinically non-functioning pituitary tumours. *Clin Endocrinol* 1994; **41**: 815–20.

25 Alvero V, Levy L, Dubray C *et al.* Invasive human pituitary tumours express a point-mutated α-protein kinase-C. *J Clin Endocrinol Metab* 1993; **77**: 1125–9.

26 Woloschak M, Roberts JL, Post K. c-Myc, c-fos and c-myb gene expression in human pituitary adenomas. *J Clin Endocrinol Metab* 1994; **79**: 253–7.

27 Hollstein M, Disransky D, Vogelstein B, Harris CC. p53 mutations in human cancers. *Science* 1991; **253**: 49–53.

28 Buckley N, Bates AS, Broome JC *et al.* p53 protein accumulates in Cushings adenomas and invasive non-functional adenomas. *J Clin Endocrinol Metab* 1995; **80**:4p following 692.

29 Levy A, Hall L, Yeudall A, Lightman SL. p53 gene mutations in pituitary adenomas: rare events. *Clin Endocrinol* 1994; **41**: 809–14.

30 Webster J, Scanlon MF. Growth factors and the anterior pituitary. *Growth Factors in Endocrinology. Baillière's Clin Endocrinol Metab* 1991; **5**: 699–726.

31 Halper J, Parnell PG, Carter BJ, Ren P, Scheithauer BW. Presence of growth factors in the pituitary. *Lab Invest* 1992; **66**: 639–45.

32 Atkin SL, Landolt AM, Jeffreys RV, Hipkin L, Radcliffe J, White MC. Insulin like growth factor-1 has differential effects on the hormonal product of glycoprotein secreting human pituitary adenomas. *J Clin Endocrinol Metab* 1993; **77**: 1059–66.

33 Chaidarun SS, Eggo MC, Sheppard MC, Stewart PM. Expression of epidermal growth factor (EGF), its receptor and related oncoprotein (ERB-2) in human pituitary tumours and response to EGF in vitro. *Endocrinology* 1994; **135**: 2012–21.

34 Atkin SL, Foy PM, Jeffreys RV, Hipkin L, Radcliffe J, White MC. Effects of basic fibroblastic growth factor on the function and proliferation of human clinically non-functional pituitary adenomas. *J Endocrinol* 1995; **144**: 173–8.

35 Ezzat S, Walpola IA, Ramyar L, Smyth HS, Asa SL. Membrane anchored expression of transforming growth factor-α in human pituitary adenoma cells. *J Clin Endocrinol Metab* 1995; **80**: 534–5.

36 Wide L, Lundberg PO. Hypersecretion of an abnormal form of follicle-stimulating hormone associated with suppressed luteinizing hormone secretion in a woman with a pituitary adenoma. *J Clin Endocrinol Metab* 1981; **53**: 923–30.

37 Chapman AJ, Macfarlane IA, Shalet SM, Beardwell GG,

Dutton J, Sutton ML. Discordant serum alpha subunit and FSH concentrations in a woman with a pituitary tumour. *Clin Endocrinol* 1984; **21**: 123–9.

38 Borges JL, Ridgway EC, Kovacs K, Rogol AD, Thorner MO. Follicle-stimulating hormone-secretng tumour with concomitant elevation of alpha subunit levels. *J Clin Endocrinol Metab* 1984; **58**: 937–41.

39 Horvath E, Kovacs K. Gonadotroph adenomas of the human pituitary: sex related fine structural dichotomy. *Am J Pathol* 1984; **117**: 429–40.

40 Spertini F, Dervaz J-P, Parentes E, Pelet B, Gomez F. Luteinizing hormone (LH) and prolactin releasing pituitary tumour: possible malignant transformation of the LH cell line. *J Clin Endocrinol Metab* 1986; **62**: 849–54.

41 Koide Y, Kugai N, Kimura S *et al.* A case of pituitary adenoma with possible simultaneous secretion of thyrotropin and follicle-stimulating hormone. *J Clin Endocrinol Metab* 1982; **54**: 397–403.

42 Faggiano M, Criscuolo T, Perrone L, Quarto C, Sinisi AA. Sexual precocity in a boy due to hypersecretion of LH and prolactin by a pituitary adenoma. *Acta Endocrinol* 1983; **102**: 167–72.

43 Vos P, Croughs RJM, Thijssen JHH, Vant Verlaat JW, Van Ginkel LA. Response of luteinizing hormone secreting pituitary adenoma to a long-acting somatostatin analogue. *Acta Endocrinol* 1988; **118**: 587–90.

44 Peterson RE, Kourides IA, Horwith M, Vaughn ED, Saxena BB, Fraser RAR. Luteinizing hormone and α-subunit secreting pituitary tumour: positive feedback of oestrogen. *J Clin Endocrinol Metab* 1981; **52**: 652–98.

45 Klibanski A, Deutsch PJ, Jameson JL *et al.* Luteinizing hormone-secreting pituitary tumour: biosynthetic characterization and clinical studies. *J Clin Endocrinol Metab* 1987; **64**: 536–42.

46 Zarate A, Fonseca ME, Mason M *et al.* Gonadotrophin-secreting pituitary adenoma with concomitant hypersecretion of testosterone and elevated sperm count treatment with LRH-agonist. *Acta Endocrinol* 1986; **113**: 29–34.

47 Galway AB, Hsueh AJW, Daneshdoost L, Zhou MH, Pavlov SN, Snyder PJ. Gonadotroph adenomas in men produce biologically active follicle stimulating hormone. *J Clin Endocrinol Metab* 1990; **71**: 907–12.

48 Cook DM, Watkins S, Snyder PJ. Gonadotrophin-secreting pituitary adenomas masquerading as primary ovarian failure. *Clin Endocrinol* 1986; **25**: 729–38.

49 Snyder PJ, Bashey HM, Kim Su, Chappel SC. Secretion of uncombined subunits of luteinizing hormone by gonadotroph cell adenomas. *J Clin Endocrinol Metab* 1984; **59**: 1169–75.

50 Creus S, Pellizzari E, Cigorraga SB, Campo S. FSH isoforms: bio and immuno-activities in post-menopausal and normal menstruating women. *Clin Endocrinol* 1996; **44**: 181–9.

51 Samuels MH, Henry P, Kleinschmidt-DeMasters BK, Lillehei K, Ridgeway EC. Pulsatile glycoprotein secretion in glycoprotein-producing pituitary tumours. *J Clin Endocrinol Metab* 1991; **73**: 1281–8.

52 McGrath GA, Gonclavez R, Udupa J *et al.* A new technique for quantitation of pituitary adenomas size: use in evaluating treatment of gonadotrophin adenomas with a GnRH antagonist. *J Clin Endocrinol Metab* 1993; **76**: 1363–8.

53 Demura R, Kubo O, Demura H, Shizume K. FSH and LH secreting pituitary adenoma. *J Clin Endocrinol Metab* 1977; **45**: 653–7.

54 Friend JN, Judge DM, Sherman BM, Santen RJ. FSH-secreting pituitary adenomas: stimulation and suppression studies in two patiens. *J Clin Endocrinol Metab* 1976; **43**: 650–7.

55 Cunningham GR, Huckins C. An FSH and prolactin-secreting pituitary tumour: pituitary dynamics and testicular histology. *J Clin Endocrinol Metab* 1977; **44**: 248–53.

56 Moses N, Goldberg V, Gutman R, Cacamo D. Combined LH and FSH secreting pituitary adenoma in a young fertile woman without primary gonadal failure. *Acta Endocrinol* 1986; **112**: 58–63.

57 Asa SL, Cheng Z, Ramyar L *et al.* Human pituitary null cell adenomas and oncocytomas *in vitro*: effects of adenohypophysiotropic hormones and gonadal steroids on hormone secreton and tumour morphology. *J Clin Endocrinol Metab* 1992; **74**: 1128–34.

58 Roman SH, Goldstein M, Kourites IA, Comite F, Bardin CW, Krieger DT. The luteinizing hormone-releasing hormone (LHRH) agonist (DTrp6-Pro9-NEt) LHRH increased rather than lowered LH and α-subunit levels in a patient with an LH-secreting pituitary tumour. *J Clin Endocrinol Metab* 1984; **58**: 313–19.

59 Heseltine D, White MC, Kendall-Taylor P, De Kretser DM, Kelly W. Testicular enlargement and elevated serum inhibin concentrations occur in patients with pituitary macroadenomas secreting follicle stimulating hormone. *Clin Endocrinol* 1989; **31**: 411–23.

60 Snyder PJ, Sterling FH. Hypersecretion of LH and FSH by a pituitary adenoma. *J Clin Endocrinol Metab* 1976; **42**: 544–50.

61 Snyder PJ, Muzyka R, Johnson J, Utiger RD. Thyrotrophin-releasing hormone provokes abnormal follicle stimulating hormone (FSH) and luteinizing hormone responses in men who have pituitary adenomas and FSH hypersecretion. *J Clin Endocrinol Metab* 1980; **51**: 746–8.

62 Lamberts SWJ, Verleum T, Oosterom R *et al.* The effects of bromocriptine, thyrotrophin-releasing hormone and gonadotrophin-releasing hormone or hormone secretion by gonadotropin-secreting pituitary adenomas *in vivo* and *in vitro*. *J Clin Endocrinol Metab* 1987; **64**: 524–30.

63 Daneshdoost L, Gennarelli TA, Bashey HM *et al.* Recognition of gonadotroph adenomas in women. *N Engl J Med* 1991; **324**: 589–94.

64 Snyder PJ, Bashey HM, Phillips JL, Gennarelli AT. Comparison of hormonal secretory behaviour of gonadotroph cell adenomas *in vivo* and in culture. *J Clin Endocrinol Metab* 1985; **61**: 1061–5.

65 Surmont DWA, Winslow CLJ, Loizon M, White MC, Adams EF, Mashiter K. Gonadotrophin and alpha-subunit secretion by human 'functionless' pituitary adenomas in cell culture: long term effects of luteinizing hormone releasing hormone and thyrotrophin releasing hormone. *Clin Endocrinol* 1983; **19**: 325–36.

66 Daniels M, Newland P, Dunn J, Kendall-Taylor P, White MC. Long term effects of a gonadotrophin-releasing hormone against (([D-Ser(Bu)6] GnRH(1–9) nonapeptide-ethylamide) on gonadotrophin secretion from human pituitary gonadotroph cell adenomas. *J Endocrinol* 1988; **118**: 491–6.

67 Scheithauer BW, Kovacs KT, Laws ER, Randall RV. Pathology of invasive pituitary tumours with special reference to functional classification. *J Neurosurg* 1986; **65**: 733–44.

68 O'Brien DP, Phillips JP, Rawluk DR, Farrel MA. Intracranial metastases from pituitary adenoma. *Br J Neurosurg* 1995; **9**: 211–18.

69 Childs GV, Hyde C, Naov Z, Catt K. Heterogeneous luteinizing

hormone and follicle stimulation hormone storage patterns in subtypes of gonadotrophs separated by centrifugal elutriation. *Endocrinology* 1983; **113**: 2120–8.

70 Giannattasio G, Bassetti M. Human pituitary adenomas. Recent advances in morphological studies. *J Endocrinol Invest* 1990; **13**: 435–54.

71 Trovillas J, Girod C, Sassolas G *et al.* Human pituitary gonadotropic adenoma: histological, immunocytochemical and ultrastructural and hormonal studies in eight cases. *J Pathol* 1981; **135**: 315–36.

72 Mukai K. Pituitary adenomas. Immunocytochemical study of 150 tumours with clinicopathologic correlation. *Cancer* 1983; **52**: 648–53.

73 Girod C, Mazzuca M, Trovillas J *et al.* Light microscopy, fine structure and immunocytochemistry studies of 278 pituitary adenomas. In: Derome PJ, Jedynak CP, Peillon F, eds. *Pituitary Adenomas, Biology, Physiopathology and Treatment*. France: Asclepios Publishers, 1980: 3–18.

74 Asa SL, Kovacs K. Histological classification of pituitary disease. *J Clin Endocrinol Metab* 1983; **12**: 576–96.

75 Nagashima T, Murovic JA, Hoshino T, Wilson CB, Dearmond SJ. The proliferative potential of human pituitary tumours *in situ*. *J Neurosurg* 1986; **64**: 588–93.

76 Landolt AM, Shibata T, Kleihues P. Growth rate of human pituitary adenomas. *J Neurosurg* 1987; **67**: 703–806.

77 Carboni P, Detta A, Hitchcock ER, Postans R. Pituitary adenoma proliferative indices and the risk of recurrence. *Br J Neurosurg* 1992; **6**: 33–40.

78 Tharpar K, Kovacs K, Scheithauer B *et al.* Proliferative activity and invasiveness among pituitary adenomas and carcinomas: an analysis using the MIB-1 antibody. *Neurosurgery* 1996; **38**: 99–107.

79 Molitch ME. Evaluation and treatment of the patient with a pituitary incidentaloma. *J Clin Endocrinol Metab* 1995; **80**: 3–6.

80 Elster AD. Modern imaging of the pituitary. *Radiology* 1993; **187**: 1–14.

81 Demura R, Jibiki K, Kubo O *et al.* The significance of α-subunit as a tumour marker for gonadotrophin-producing pituitary adenomas. *J Clin Endocrinol Metab* 1986; **63**: 564–9.

82 Masson EA, Atkin SL, Diver M, White MC. Pituitary apoplexy and sudden blindness following the administration of gonadotrophin-releasing hormone. *Clin Endocrinol* 1993; **38**: 109–10.

83 Chanson P, Schaison MD. Pituitary apoplexy caused by GnRH agonist treatment revealing gonadotroph adenoma (letter). *J Clin Endocrinol Metab* 1995; **80**: 2267–8.

84 Snyder PJ, Bigdeli H, Gardner DF *et al.* Gonadal function in fifty men with untreated pituitary adenomas. *J Clin Endocrinol Metab* 1979; **48**: 309–14.

85 Warnet A, Lubetzki J, Pestel M *et al.* Deux cas d'adenome hypophysaire a FSH. *Ann d' Endocrinol* 1980; **41**: 53–4.

86 Arafah BM. Reversible hypopituitarism in patients with large nonfunctioning pituitary adenomas. *J Clin Endocrinol Metab* 1986; **62**: 1173–9.

87 Arafah BM, Kailani SH, Neki KE, Gold RS, Selman WR. Immediate recovery of pituitary function after transsphenoidal resection of pituitary macroadenomas. *J Clin Endocrinol Metab* 1994; **79**: 348–54.

88 Randall RV, Scheithauer BW, Laws ER, Abboud CF, Ebersold MJ, Kao PC. Pituitary adenomas associated with hyperprolactinemia: a clinical and immunological study of 97 patients operated on transsphenoidally. *Mayo Clinic Proc* 1985; **60**: 753–62.

89 Harris RI, Schatz NJ, Gennarelli T *et al.* Follicle stimulating hormone-secreting pituitary adenomas: correlation of reduction of adenoma size with reduction of hormonal hypersecretion after transsphenoidal surgery. *J Clin Endocrinol Metab* 1983; **56**: 1288–93.

90 Wilson CB. Role of surgery in the management of pituitary tumours. *Neurosurg Clin North Amer* 1990; **1**: 139–59.

91 Kucharczyk W, Montanera W, Becker LE. The sella turcica and parasellar region. In: Scott WA, ed. *Magnetic Resonance Imaging of the Brain and Spine*, 2nd edn. Philadelphia: Lippincott–Raven, 1996: 871–928.

92 Sheline GE. Conventional radiation therapy in the treatment of pituitary tumours. In: Tindall GT, Collins WF, eds. *Clinical Management of Pituitary Disorders*. New York: Raven Press, 1979: 287–314.

93 Ebersold MJ, Quast LM, Laws ER. Scheithauer B, Randall RV. Long-term results in transsphenoidal removal of nonfunctioning pituitary adenomas. *J Neurosurg* 1986; **64**: 713–19.

94 Eastman RC, Gorden P, Roth J. Conventional supervoltage irradiation is an effective treatment for acromegaly. *J Clin Endocrinol Metab* 1979; **48**: 931.

95 Jones A. Review: radiation oncogenesis in relation to the treatment of pituitary tumours. *Clin Endocrinol* 1991; **35**: 379–97.

96 Bezerin M, Olchovsky D, Pines A, Tadmor R, Lunenfield B. Reduction of follicle-stimulating hormone (FSH) secretion in FSH-producing adenoma by bromocriptine. *J Clin Endocrinol Metab* 1984; **59**: 1220–3.

97 Vance ML, Ridgway EC, Thorner MO. Follicle stimulating hormone and α-subunit-secreting pituitary tumour treated with bromocriptine. *J Clin Endocrinol Metab* 1985; **61**: 580–4.

98 Grossman A, Ross R, Charlesworth M *et al.* The effect of dopamine against therapy on large functionless pituitary tumours. *Clin Endocrinol* 1985; **22**: 679–86.

99 Van Schaardenberg D, Roelfsema F, Van Seters AP, Vielvoye GJ. Bromocriptine therapy for non-functioning pituitary adenoma. *Clin Endocrinol* 1989; **30**: 475–84.

100 Kweckboom DJ, Lamberts SWJ. Long term treatment with the dopamine agonist CV 205 502 of patients with a clinically non-functioning gonadotroph, or α-subunit secreting pituitary tumour. *Clin Endocrinol* 1991; **36**: 171–6.

101 Paoletti AM, Depau GF, Mais V, Guerriero S, Ajossa S, Melis GB. Effectiveness of cabergoline in reducing follicle-stimulating hormone and prolactin hypersecretion from pituitary macroadenoma in an infertile woman. *Fertil Steril* 1994; **62**: 882–5.

102 de Buin TWA, Kwekkeboom DJ, Vsn't Verlaat JW *et al.* Clinically nonfunctioning pituitary adenomas and Octreotide response to long term high dose treatment, and studies *in vitro*. *J Clin Endocrinol Metab* 1987; **65**: 65–73.

103 Warnet A, Timsit J, Chanson P *et al.* The effect of somatostatin analogue on chiasmal dysfunction from pituitary macroadenomas. *J Neurosurg* 1989; **71**: 687–90.

104 Katznelson L, Oppenheim DS, Coughlin JF, Kliman B, Schoenfeld DA, Klibanski A. Chronic somatostatin analog administration in patients with α-subunit secreting pituitary tumours. *J Clin Endocrinol Metab* 1992; **72**: 1318–25.

105 Sassolas G, Le jeune H, Trouillas J *et al.* Gonadotropin-releasing hormone agonists are unsuccessful in reducing tumour

gonadotropin secretion in two patients with gonadotropin-secreting pituitary adenomas. *J Clin Endocrinol Metab* 1988; **67**: 180–5.
106 Thapar K, Scheithauer VW, Kovacs K, Pernicone PJ, Laws ER. p53 expression of pituitary adenomas and carcinomas: correlation with invasiveness and tumour growth. *Neurosurgery* 1996; **38**: 765–71.
107 Green VL, Atkin SL, Speirs V *et al*. Cytokine expression in human anterior pituitary adenomas. *Clin Endocrinol* 1996; **45**: 179–85.

CHAPTER 15

Thyrotrophin-secreting pituitary tumours

F.F. Casanueva, S.M. Webb and C. Dieguez

Introduction

When studying a patient with abnormally elevated serum thyrotrophin (TSH, thyroid-stimulating hormone), the differential diagnosis should include three distinct endocrinological entities:

1 TSH-secreting pituitary tumours leading to hyperthyroidism (TSH-oma);

2 elevated TSH levels due to peripheral resistance to thyroid hormone; and

3 TSH-secreting pituitary hyperplasia induced by primary hypothyroidism ('feedback adenoma').

All of these conditions are very rare and show unusual clinical presentations, but in the past few years they have been recognised with increasing frequency. The importance of these entities is based on the diagnostic and therapeutic challenges that they present. Indeed, due to both the small number of cases and to the variable clinical and biochemical presentation, erroneous initial diagnosis and management by the general practitioner or the less-aware specialist has been common (see reviews [1–7]).

Most authors still use the label of 'inappropriate secretion of TSH' to underline the paradoxical high levels of TSH concomitant with high levels of thyroid hormones (triiodothyronine (T_3), thyroxine (T_4)) presented in entities **1** and **2** [1,8]. However, this is only of historical interest, and should be changed. In fact, to call inappropriate the elevated levels of TSH in a TSH-secreting pituitary tumour is similar to labelling Cushing's disease as inappropriate secretion of adrenocorticotrophic hormone (ACTH); similarly, naming as inappropriate the secretion of TSH in the syndrome of peripheral resistance to thyroid hormone is similar to labelling Laron's syndrome as inappropriate secretion of GH; naming should be based on updated physiopathological knowledge.

The maintenance of normal thyroid function is dependent upon a complex of finely tuned interactions among different regulatory factors of the hypothalamo-pituitary–thyroid axis [3] (Fig. 15.1). The hypothalamus exerts dominant control over TSH release via thyrotrophin-releasing hormone (TRH) secretion. A classical feedback loop is operative between the TSH secretion by the pituitary, which stimulates the release of T_3/T_4, and those thyroid hormones in turn inhibit TSH release acting at the pituitary. There are other factors active on the regulation of TSH secretion, such as dopamine, corticosteroids and somatostatin, which are inhibitors, and oestrogens, which act as stimulants. However, the latter hormones have either a non-physiological or ancillary role, and for most, activity is only evident at pharmacological doses.

TSH is a glycoprotein of 30 000 Da molecular weight composed of two similar heavily glycosylated α- and β-chains. In addition to its role as a TSH secretagogue, TRH also increases the transcription of TSH β- and α-subunits. The TSH β- and α-subunits are encoded on different genes, and they are translated independently and glycosylated before they combine in the TSH molecule. It should be remembered that the rate-limiting step for the TSH molecule is the synthesis of the TSH β-subunit, because the α-subunit is produced in excess. T_3 inhibits TSH synthesis by binding to a nuclear thyroid hormone receptor/DNA thyroid hormone response element. Prior to being secreted, TSH undergoes further glycosylation, and, while the carbohydrate chains are not involved in hormone-receptor binding, the biological potency of TSH is dependent on the degree of glycosylation [9]. TRH, in addition to regulating the set point of the hypothalamo-pituitary–thyroid axis, determines the extent of TSH glycosylation, probably being responsible for the different TSH isoforms detected in plasma [9,10]. In humans, TSH is secreted in a dual fashion, with secretory bursts (pulses) superimposed upon tonic (non-pulsatile) secretion. In addition,

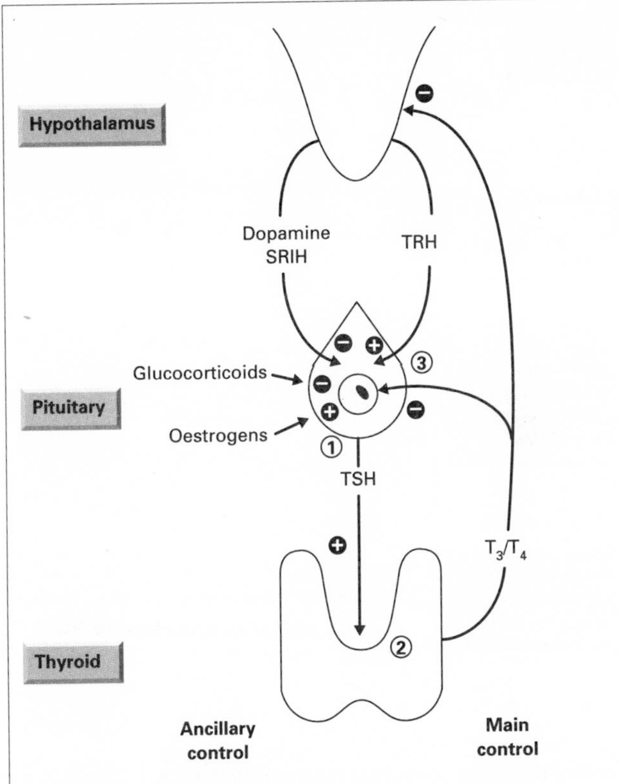

Fig. 15.1 General scheme of the hypothalamo-pituitary–thyroid axis. SRIH, somatostatin. Different levels of perturbation: (1) primary thyrotrophin (TSH)-secreting tumour inducing hyperthyroidism; (2) hypothyroidism-induced TSH adenoma; (3) resistance to thyroid hormone.

TSH is secreted in a circadian rhythm which leads to higher TSH levels between 2300 and 0500 hours. Thyroid hormones, dopamine and somatostatin decrease TSH secretion without affecting pulse frequency, while corticosteroids suppress both pulse frequency and the circadian rhythm [3].

TSH-secreting pituitary tumours leading to hyperthyroidism arise from a primary neoplastic transformation of the TSH-secreting pituitary cell [11] (Fig. 15.1, level 1). The resulting TSH increase leads to thyroid stimulation, with subsequent goitre and hyperthyroidism. Although it was originally proposed that these tumours might develop from abnormal thyrotroph stimulation by TRH, or from defective suppression by somatostatin or dopamine, there is no evidence to substantiate this theory. The small number of cases has impeded our discovery as to whether, similar to other pituitary adenomas, TSH-secreting tumours are monoclonal [12]. Similarly, the absence of suitable cell lines has hindered insight into the role of local growth factors or oncogene activation in their development. In addition, while only one case has been reported, it is important to consider the possibility of a tumour secreting an ectopic factor capable of releasing TSH and so leading to hyperthyroidism [13].

Primary hypothyroidism and prolonged thyroid hormone deficiency have been shown to lead to the development of pituitary TSH-secreting adenomas or to pituitary enlargement due to thyrotroph cell hyperplasia [14] (Fig. 15.1, level 2). The primary pathological event here is the lack of the negative feedback exerted by thyroid hormones, resulting in increased TSH synthesis and secretion. There is also increased responsiveness of the TSH cell to the stimulatory action of TRH, partly because the absence of thyroid hormones increases the number of TRH receptors as well as decreasing the activity of the membrane-bound TRH-degrading enzyme [3]. The ensuing TSH cell hyperplasia is accompanied by decreased sensitivity to the inhibitory actions of somatostatin. However, the transformation of such cells is completely different to the above-mentioned TSH tumours leading to hyperthyroidism, since replacement therapy with thyroid hormones reverses and indeed normalises the changes.

While not associated with pituitary tumours, it is relevant for the differential diagnosis to comment upon the syndrome of resistance to thyroid hormones [6,15] (Fig. 15.1, level 3). In that entity, abnormally high levels of TSH in the face of elevated levels of T_3 and T_4 are due to resistance to thyroid hormones caused by mutations in the T_3 receptor [16]. These patients will have elevated TSH, T_3 and T_4 while being clinically hyper-, eu- or hypothyroid.

These clinical entities are therefore diverse in aetiology and pathophysiology; however, all of them will present with elevated TSH levels (Fig. 15.2), and will challenge the diagnostic skills of the specialist.

TSH-secreting pituitary tumors

Clinical and biochemical hyperthyroidism caused by abnormally high TSH secretion due to neoplastic pituitary disease is a rare entity. As for most primary pituitary adenomas, the aetiology of TSH-secreting pituitary tumors is unknown. In the early stages of evolution, normal regulation by TRH and thyroid hormones is preserved, and the TSH tumour is able to grow, despite the negative feedback imposed by the elevated levels of thyroid hormones. At a later stage of development, the tumour becomes insensitive to both TRH and thyroid hormones.

Some 280 cases of TSH-secreting pituitary tumours have been reported to date [64] (Fig. 15.3); they account for 0.5–1% of all pituitary tumours and the prevalence in the general population may be 1–2 per million. It is slightly more frequent in women than in men (1.7 : 1) and more frequent in the middle age of life. A TSH-secreting pituitary carcinoma has also been described [60]. However, it is worth considering that as the data on prevalence and incidence have been

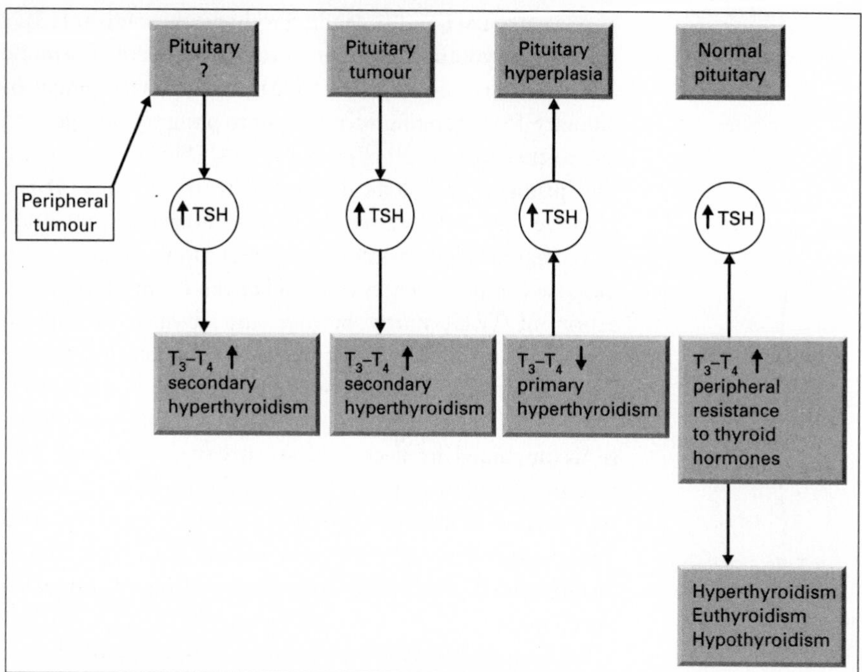

Fig. 15.2 General scheme of the clinical entities associated with elevated TSH levels.

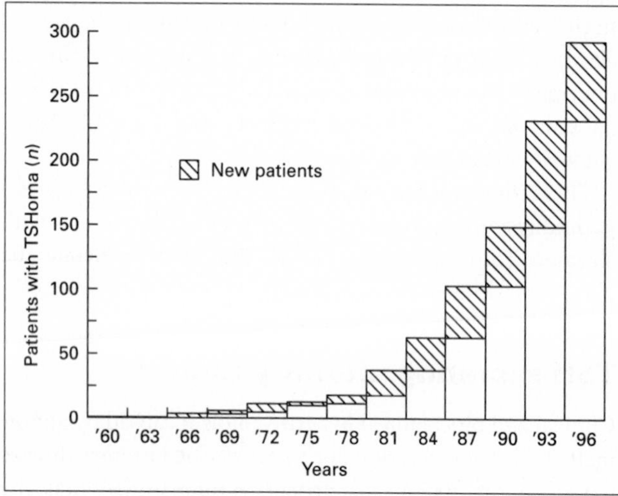

Fig. 15.3 Cumulative sum of patients with TSH-secreting pituitary tumours, showing the remarkable increase in recorded cases during the last 13 years. From [64] with permission.

calculated in the past few years, when (see Fig. 15.3) only a probable minority of such tumors were diagnosed and published, figures are likely to change in the near future. In fact, the number of reported cases has doubled in the last 6 years, and the disease is now observed at younger ages [17] and with unusual presentations [18]. The reasons for the increase in the reported cases of TSH-secreting pituitary tumors is probably twofold. First, the introduction and dissemination into clinical practice of ultrasensitive immunoradiometric assays for TSH measurement now allows a clear distinction of an individual hyperthyroid patient with abnormally elevated TSH levels from a patient with Graves' disease. Secondly, increased reporting of these tumours is making the general practitioner and even the specialist more aware.

The great majority of TSH-omas secrete TSH alone, although often accompanied by unbalanced secretion of α-subunit. The rest secrete in decreasing order of frequency: TSH-growth hormone (GH); TSH–prolactin (PRL); TSH–gonadotrophins and TSH–GH–PRL [5]. Practically all TSH-omas are macroadenomas and frequently highly invasive [2], with one carcinoma being reported [19]. The 'rule' until now was that patients harbouring a TSH-secreting tumour were initially misdiagnosed as having Graves' disease and treated with antithyroid drugs or by thyroid ablation. Invasive macroadenomas and tumours resistant to treatment are more common in patients initially treated as Graves' disease [20]. Histological analysis after surgery provides scarce information about the future behaviour of these tumours, and immunostaining shows the presence of TSH and its units in all adenomatous cells.

Neoplastic transformation of the thyrotrophs changes the normal expression of receptors. In fact, most TSH-secreting cells from such tumours lack TRH receptors [21], maintain somatostatin receptors [22], and show variable expression of dopaminergic receptors [23]. They demonstrate relative resistance to the inhibitory action of thyroid hormones [24], without detectable changes in the thyroid hormone receptor structure [5]. TSH-secreting pituitary tumours secrete

TSH molecules with different degrees of glycosylation and biological activity, a fact that may explain the discrepancy between TSH levels and the concomitant levels of thyroid hormones. To date no structural genetic abnormalities, such as mutations resulting in transcriptional activation, have been identified in TSH-omas [61].

Clinical presentation

The patient bearing a TSH-secreting pituitary tumour will usually seek medical attention with the signs and symptoms of either hyperthyroidism or the mass effect of an expanding intracranial tumour. Rarely, both kinds of symptoms are experienced during the early stages. Most patients have initially been misdiagnosed as having either Graves' disease or a non-functioning pituitary tumour.

Hyperthyroidism of a variable degree and diffuse enlargement of the thyroid gland is usually present, but without acropachy or pretibial myxoedema. Ophthalmopathy is rarely seen, and of the few reports of proptosis associated with such tumours, at least one was due to invasion of the orbit by the neoplasm [4]. Alternatively, a TSH-secreting tumour might first present with the classical symptoms of a mass effect produced by a pituitary adenoma, i.e. visual field defects and headache. Similarly, the initial manifestation may be endocrine, resulting from hormonal overproduction caused by cosecretion, or from hormonal underproduction due to tumour compression of the pituitary; thus, these tumours may occasionally present with acromegaly, hypogonadism or amenorrhoea. The mild hyperthyroidism found in the early stages of this entity contributes to delays in accurate diagnosis. The youngest case reported was 11 years old and the oldest 84 years old [4,17].

Laboratory studies

Elevated serum levels of T_3 and T_4 (preferably serum free T_3 and T_4 to exclude a protein-binding abnormality), and an enlarged thyroid gland with an enhanced radionuclide scan, are the hallmarks of this disease. Antithyroid antibodies are not detected in such patients. To differentiate this entity from conventional hyperthyroidism, in which the elevated thyroid hormone levels should lead to suppression of TSH, it is crucial to detect the abnormally high TSH values. However, diagnostic problems commonly arise in the evaluation of TSH, since in the past few years most commercially available radioimmunoassays (RIAs) have lacked sensitivity. These assays are not able to differentiate low from suppressed TSH levels, and they may be affected by the presence of circulating heterophilic or anti-TSH antibodies which cross-react with the α-subunit of the TSH molecule. With the introduction of highly sensitive immunoradiometric (IRMA) assays for TSH it is now possible to obviate such problems and to clearly discriminate between suppressed and non-suppressed TSH levels [25]. Therefore, the diagnosis of a TSH-secreting tumour combines elevated serum free thyroid hormones in association with non-suppressed or elevated levels of TSH as determined by a reliable assay, in the presence of clinical manifestations of hyperthyroidism. The clinical findings are of value when faced with the differential diagnosis of the syndrome of elevated TSH levels, as generalised resistance to thyroid hormone is generally associated with hypothyroidism, while selective pituitary resistance presents with clinical hyperthyroidism.

With regard to the elevation of TSH, the clinician should be aware of two important facts:

1 in the early stages of the TSH-secreting tumour, and at any stage in some patients, TSH levels measured by reliable assays may be within the normal range; and

2 a profound dissociation can exist between TSH values and both the tumour mass and the hyperthyroid status.

These facts are not well understood, and are probably caused by the different biological activities of the secreted TSH molecule(s). Case reports have been published of patients with TSH-secreting tumours who have hyperthyroidism in the face of low but detectable TSH levels, and also some cases of mild hyperthyroidism with extremely high levels of circulating TSH. For the same reasons, TSH macroadenomas with suprasellar extensions are not necessarily more frequently associated with higher TSH values than TSH microadenomas [2,26].

In addition to the determination of free T_3 and T_4, and TSH, the most useful biochemical measurement is that of the α-subunit of the TSH molecule [1], which is secreted by TSH tumors in large quantities but is not in other causes of TSH hypersecretion. α-Subunit values in plasma are always elevated in TSH-secreting tumours, while the α-subunit : TSH molar ratio is in most cases, but not always, greater than 1. This test remains reasonably specific, providing that the patient under study is neither hypogonadal nor a post-menopausal woman, since high levels of circulating gonadotrophins (which are also two-chain glycoproteins) may yield erroneously high results. Similarly, the α-subunit should be measured when in the hyperthyroid state because antithyroid drugs can affect the ratio.

Diagnostic studies

Despite previous expectations, dynamic tests of TSH function have not been particularly helpful in the diagnosis of these tumours. TRH-induced TSH secretion is absent or blunted in the majority, but not all, of such cases. The absence of a TSH response to TRH is quite useful in distinguishing tumour patients from other causes of elevated TSH secretion in which there is always hyperresponsiveness. Several of these tumours lack circadian rhythmicity in TSH secretion. Similarly, most of those tumours are unable to increase TSH secretion after dopamine antagonists such as domperidone, or to decrease TSH after dopamine agonists, for example bromocriptine [27]. However, such tests are associated with a large proportion of false negatives. Normal TSH suppression to T_3 has never been recorded in a patient with a TSH-secreting tumour, though the test needs further standardisation. It has been proposed that serum sex hormone-binding globulin (SHBG) may help differentiate TSH-secreting pituitary tumours, in which SHBG is elevated as in primary hyperthyroidism, from other causes of abnormally elevated TSH secretion [28]. Although none of these tests is of clear-cut diagnostic value, the combination of some of them may increase their usefulness.

Imaging studies and localisation

When considering the diagnosis of a TSH-secreting tumour, full imaging studies are necessary: the optimal procedure involves high-resolution magnetic resonance imaging (MRI) after gadolinium. However, it should be noted that some 10 patients with normal sella films or microadenomas have been reported. Most of the patients reported have been scanned late in the evolution of the tumour, such that macroadenomas with various degrees of suprasellar extension or sphenoidal sinus invasion have usually been found. Five tumours were reported invading the cavernous sinus, one the orbit and the base of the skull. One patient developed bony and peripheral metastases [19]. With the development of the octreoscan (radionuclide imaging after administration of radiolabelled Tyr-substituted octreotide), it has been possible to image the pituitary gland in patients with tumours endowed with somatostatin receptors. Some patients with TSH-secreting pituitary tumours were successfully imaged thus opening a new approach for diagnosis [29]. In a case with the biochemical diagnosis of TSH-secreting pituitary tumour and elevated α-subunit but no mass in the radiographic scans, a TSH-secreting tumour was successfully localised by bilateral petrosal sinus sampling of both basal and TRH-stimulated TSH secretion [30].

Complementary studies

After evaluating the degree of hyperthyroidism, the second step in the clinical investigation of a patient with a suspected TSH-secreting tumour involves evaluation of the secretory state of the other pituitary hormones, and the neurological effects of the tumour. Complete evaluation of the basal and stimulated secretion of GH, PRL, luteinising hormone (LH), follicle-stimulating hormone (FSH), and ACTH/cortisol by the pituitary should be undertaken. In this way one can obtain information regarding hormonal deficiencies induced by the expanding tumour, and about possible cosecretion of other hormones. Such information may even be useful as a guide to therapy; TSH-secreting pituitary tumours have a worse prognosis when they secrete multiple hormones [2], although when secreting TSH–GH they respond better to octreotide.

Visual field examination with Goldmann perimetry or computer-assisted methods should be undertaken in all patients with a large TSH-secreting tumour, and repeated at regular intervals to evaluate the evolution of the tumour and/or the effectiveness of treatment.

Differential diagnosis

Both TSH-secreting pituitary tumours and TSH adenomas due to primary hypothyroidism (feedback tumours) present with elevated TSH and a pituitary mass by imaging. However, the clinical and biochemical status is completely different, i.e. hyperthyroidism versus hypothyroidism, providing no challenges to diagnosis. More problematic is to differentiate a TSH-secreting tumour from the syndrome of resistance to thyroid hormone. While peripheral resistance to thyroid hormone shows elevated TSH levels and no pituitary mass, careful differential diagnosis from TSH-secreting pituitary tumours is mandatory because in a certain number of these latter tumours the pituitary is normal after imaging. Several cases of peripheral resistance to thyroid hormones show hypo- or euthyroidism, and in many there is a familial presentation of the disease, facts which will facilitate diagnosis. Contrary to TSH-secreting tumours, patients with resistance to thyroid hormone show marked TRH-mediated TSH secretion, and α-subunit levels are concordant with the TSH values. Finally, although there was no pituitary abnormality in the single case reported [13], a peripheral factor of tumoral origin, which activates TSH secretion, should be considered.

Treatment

Surgical resection is the recommended therapy for TSH-secreting pituitary tumours, with the aim of eliminating neoplastic tissue while normal pituitary–thyroid function is restored. Since these tumours are frequently invasive, surgical intervention should be undertaken as soon as possible. However, a therapeutic decision should involve consideration of the general health of the patient, previous treatment, and location and growth rate of the tumour, because these are crucial factors for determining prognosis after surgery. Prompt diagnosis while the tumour is still a microadenoma or a small macroadenoma normally allows for complete resection by either the transcranial or preferably the transsphenoidal route, with full recovery of the patient. By the same token, several intraoperative and perioperative deaths have been reported following surgical removal of TSH tumours, and in most of these cases previous misdiagnosis and inappropriate management had led to the development of invasive adenomas with serious injury to the hypothalamus. In any case, patients should undergo surgery when signs of visual compromise or neurological deterioration caused by the mass effect become evident. Partial or complete hypopituitarism may be the result of surgery; thus, a complete anterior pituitary evaluation should be undertaken with target hormone replacement therapy when needed. The success of surgery is demonstrated by normalisation of hyperthyroidism as well as of serum TSH and α-subunit levels. However, the most sensitive and specific tests to document the complete removal of a TSH-oma is the T_3 suppression test in which basal and TRH-stimulated TSH secretion are completely inhibited [62].

Few TSH tumours have been irradiated, such that the effectiveness of radiotherapy has not been clearly evaluated, nor has the radiosensitivity of the tumour been established [31]. Radiotherapy and conventional supervoltage radiation are generally available, and in experienced hands with modern equipment, adverse effects are minimal, the recommended dose being 4500 cGy [32]. However, it is our view that the most effective approach is to use radiation in combination with initial surgical debulking of the tumour. Regular follow-up thereafter should include estimation of circulating α-subunit levels in addition to TSH. Experience with proton-beam and heavy-particle radiotherapy in TSH-secreting tumours is lacking, though they have been successfully used in other pituitary tumours.

In terms of pharmacological therapy of neoplastic TSH-secreting tumours, one might be tempted to use antithyroid drugs to correct the hyperthyroid state of the patient. The administration of antithyroid drugs and the consequent reduction in the levels of circulating thyroid hormones would ameliorate the symptoms of the patient, but this could lead to a more rapid and unbridled growth of the tumour with invasion of the surrounding structures. Antithyroid drugs must not be used as definitive medical treatment of TSH-secreting tumours; we recommended employing them only as preparation of the patient for neurosurgery. For alleviating the symptoms of hyperthyroidism, β-adrenoceptor blockers such as propranolol can be employed. Glucocorticoids are usually effective in reducing TSH secretion in such patients, the effect being greater than the reduction in the levels of the α-subunit. Their striking ability to block TSH secretion is counterbalanced in the clinical setting by the deleterious side-effects they induce on long-term treatment. The fact that certain TSH tumours maintain some degree of responsiveness to thyroid hormones has led some authors to administer them in order to reduce TSH levels. However, the effectiveness of this treatment in reducing TSH levels is low, and in our opinion the adverse burden that thyroid hormones add to the already altered metabolic status of the patient precludes such treatment. Dopamine agonists in general, and bromocriptine in particular, have been employed in some TSH-secreting tumours, with variable results. In some cases a reduction in TSH with bromocriptine has been reported, but the positive effect diminished with time. In any case, it is not possible to know in advance if a particular patient will benefit from dopaminergic treatment, and a short-term trial is necessary.

Among the newer pharmacological treatments for tumoral TSH production, the use of somatostatin analogues is highly promising. It has been known for several years that somatostatin is able to decrease basal and stimulated TSH secretion from normal and tumorous pituitaries, but its short half-life precluded its use as a therapeutic agent. The development of octreotide, a somatostatin analogue which has a more prolonged half-life, led to its subcutaneous utilisation in TSH-secreting tumours with evident success. Octreotide therapy in these patients leads to a reduction in TSH and thyroid hormone levels and to a clear reduction in the effective tumour marker α-subunit, with an amelioration of the hyperthyroid symptoms [33] (Fig. 15.4). Patients with TSH tumours have been treated for years with daily injections of octreotide without any decrease in the beneficial effects, and in other cases octreotide has led to the improvement in visual field defects, suggesting an action on the tumour volume [34,35]. Only a single case of a TSH-secreting tumour has been described being both negative after octreoscan imaging and insensitive to octreotide therapy. Fortunately, the patient responded to dopamine agonists and to D-thyroxine, and was managed with those drugs [36]. A new slow-release formulation of a somatostatin analogue named lanreotide has been developed. In contrast to octreotide which must be administered t.i.d. in order to be effective, lanreotide is effective when given as one i.m. injection every 10–15 days. Lanreotide has been shown to be effective in TSH-secreting adenomas, opening a new avenue of treatment [37]. Lanreotide or any other long-acting somatostatin analogue seems to be the best pharmacological tool for restraining the growth or reducing the volume of TSH tumours, or as therapy in preparation for surgery. However, as surgery is commonly followed by relapse of tumour activity, it is likely that in the future some patients, at least with TSH-secreting tumours, will be treated exclusively with such long-acting somatostatin analogues.

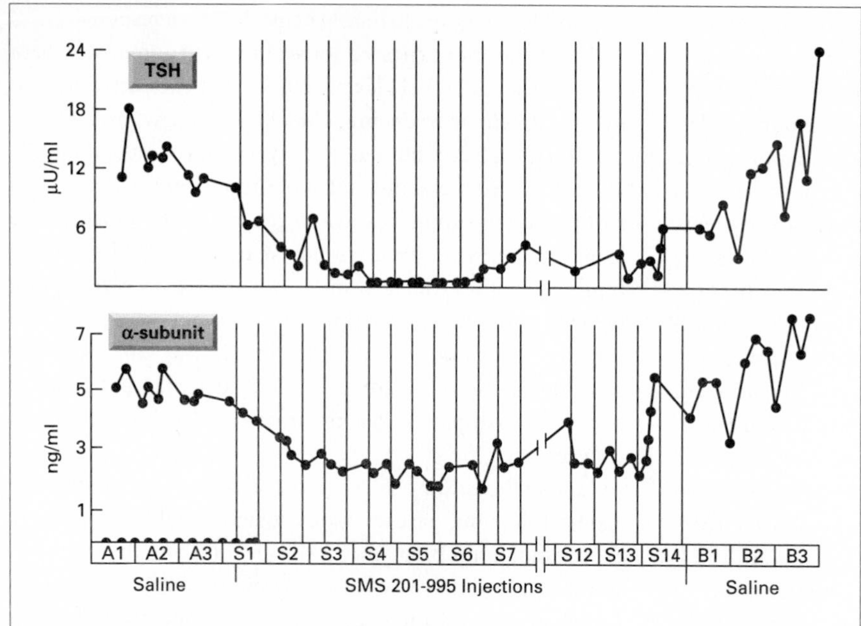

Fig. 15.4 Response to octreotide injection on serum thyrotrophin (TSH) and α-subunit in a patient with hyperthyroidism due to a TSH-secreting pituitary tumour. From [33].

Syndrome of resistance to thyroid hormone

The syndrome of resistance to thyroid hormone described in 1967 [38] is an inadequate response of the pituitary and/ or peripheral tissues to circulating free thyroid hormones, characterised by elevated serum free T_3 and T_4 in the presence of inappropriately elevated or normal TSH values [39,40]. This tissue resistance can be due to an isolated pituitary resistance or to generalised resistance in which the targets for thyroid hormone are affected to a varying degree, and is usually transmitted in an autosomal dominant form, though sporadic cases have also been described [6].

Thyroid hormone action is mediated through two types of nuclear receptors, α and β (TRα and TRβ) which have different organ distributions [41]. Resistance to thyroid hormone is due to mutations located in exon 9 and 10 which encode the T_3-binding domain of the TRβ gene [42,43]. Since most cases are heterozygotes and inherited as autosomal dominant traits, half of their TRβ receptors are abnormal and the other half normal. However, the abnormal receptor impairs T_3 binding as well as antagonising the function of normal receptors, either α or β (a dominant negative effect). The variable tissue distribution of TRβ explains the variable phenotype of this syndrome, which is traditionally defined as generalised resistance or selective pituitary resistance [1,44]. In generalised resistance, pituitary and peripheral tissues are not always affected to a similar degree, creating a variety of hypothyroid and hyperthyroid manifestations in the patient. If the degree of resistance is similar in pituitary and peripheral tissues, the feedback operates normally and the steady state is attained by maintaining a higher basal level of T_3; the clinical manifestation is then euthyroidism or hypothyroidism [45]. On the other hand, when the resistance is specific at the pituitary level, pituitary–thyroid feedback is reset through high levels of circulating T_3, but as the tissues are normally sensitive to thyroid hormones, hyperthyroidism is the clinical manifestation [45,46]. One case of isolated peripheral resistance without pituitary involvement has been published [47]. The prevalence of this syndrome is low but not precisely ascertained.

Clinical presentation

The phenotype is heterogeneous and ranges from highly symptomatic to subclinical manifestations [40,45]. Goitre, increased radionuclide uptake, enhanced thyroid hormone release and abnormally elevated or normal TSH are hallmarks of the disease (Table 15.1). There are two clinical forms of the disease which overlap, both clinically and biochemically, namely 'generalised resistance' characterised by absence of thyrotoxic symptoms, and a selective 'pituitary resistance' with characteristic thyrotoxic signs: both are clinical manifestations of the same single genetic entity. The disease is commonly mistaken for Graves' disease, which explains the fact that around 20% undergo thyroid ablation before reaching a correct diagnosis [6]. A clear association between resistance to thyroid hormone and attention-deficit hyperactivity disorder, as well as low IQ, has been frequently recorded [6]. Other manifestations are short stature and low body weight in children, tachycardia under non-basal conditions, enhanced frequency of ENT infections, and hearing loss [39,40].

Table 15.1 Elevated thyroid-stimulating hormone (TSH) secretion. From [32].

Parameter	TSH-tumours causing hyperthyroidism	Thyroid hormone resistance		Hypothyroidism-induced TSH adenomas
		Isolated pituitary	Generalized	
Occurrence	Sporadic	Sporadic–familial	Sporadic–familial	Sporadic
Metabolic status	Hyperthyroidism	Hyperthyroidism	Hypothyroidism or euthyroidism	Hypothyroidism
Goitre	Present	Present	Present	In 20%
Thyroid hormones	Increased	Increased	Increased	Decreased
Basal serum TSH	Increased or normal	Increased	Increased	Increased
TSH response to TRH injection	No increase or minimal	Increased	Increased	Increased
α-Subunit:TSH ratio	>1	Normal	Normal	Normal
Pituitary volume	Increased	Normal	Normal	Increased
TSH supression by:				
Thyroid hormones	Minimal or none	Minimal	Minimal	Yes
Dopamine agonists	Minimal	Yes	Yes	Yes
Glucocorticoids	Yes	Yes	Yes	Yes

Laboratory studies

The typical hormonal profile is elevated free and total thyroid hormone levels and normal or elevated TSH values; however, in mild pituitary resistance thyroid hormone levels are borderline. The TRH-induced TSH response is marked, reminiscent of that of hypothyroid patients; there is no hypersecretion of α-subunit. Indices of thyroid hormone action on the liver, such as thyroid hormone-binding globulin (TBG), ferritin or cholesterol, are in the normal range in persons with resistance, contrasting with the values that are expected for the high levels of thyroid hormones [6]. TSH values are resistant in the T_3 suppression test. When the syndrome of resistance to thyroid hormones is suspected, a genetic analysis of the patient and kindred is worthwhile. If the differential diagnosis from pituitary tumours secreting TSH is considered, MRI analysis of the pituitary will reveal a normal gland.

Treatment

Primary therapy in patients with resistance to thyroid hormones should be directed at suppression of TSH hypersecretion rather than at the reduction of thyroid hormone release [48]. Treatment directed at the ablation of the thyroid gland may induce a temporary improvement in the hyperthyroid state, but will further increase TSH release leading to a regrowth of the thyroid remnant. Thyroid hormone replacement is indicated in patients who suffered initial thyroid ablation due to misdiagnosis. A large variety of agents known to suppress the release of TSH have been used with variable results. In one family, T_3 therapy was able to suppress TSH oversecretion and the T_3-induced hyperthyroidism subdued after some months [49]; however, this treatment might have deleterious side-effects. A different approach is the use of thyroid hormone analogues or metabolites such as the sodium salt of 3,5,3′-triiodothyroacetic acid (TRIAC). At an appropriate dose, this natural metabolite of T_3 with less peripheral metabolic activity exerts a powerful inhibitory action on TSH at the pituitary level [50]. Recently, highly purified dextrothyroxine (D-thyroxine) has been shown to normalise both TSH and thyroid hormones in patients with resistance to thyroid hormone [51]. Octreotide has also been tested in these patients; however, when administered subcutaneously over a period of weeks, its suppressive effects on TSH secretion faded [52]. Similarly disappointing results were observed after treatment with dopamine agonists. The optimal therapeutic approach to patients with resistance to thyroid hormones is still a matter of debate.

TSH adenomas induced by hypothyroidism ('feedback adenomas')

It has been recognised for more than a century that longstanding primary hypothyroidism leads to pituitary enlargement. The first historical description in humans was that of Niepce in 1851, who observed an increase in pituitary volume in the autopsies of some cretins [53]. Other authors have confirmed these observations in hypothyroid patients [14,54], and in experimental animals prolonged deficiency of thyroid hormone has been shown to lead to the development of transplantable pituitary tumours. It is not known how long the hormonal deficiency needs to be maintained in order to induce pituitary hyperplasia, or if other factors are necessary as adjuvants of thyroid deficiency. In a large series of patients with long-standing hypothyroidism, pituitary alterations were common, ranging from hyperplasia to clear TSH-secreting adenomas [55], and a correlation can be observed in such situations between TSH levels and sella turcica volume [56]. A striking finding regarding these adenomas is the high prevalence in children and adults with untreated cretinism. One could argue that feedback adenomas reported in adults in some cases originated in infancy and only become unmasked during adulthood, suggesting an infancy-related growth stimulant in association with the thyroid deficiency.

Clinical presentation

Feedback TSH adenomas occur more commonly in females than in males, and the clinical presentation to the specialist is that of the symptoms of hypothyroidism. Alternatively, the patient may seek medical attention due to headache or visual field loss, which are manifestations of an intracranial mass effect; after taking skull radiographs an altered sella is found. In cases presenting with neurological findings, the symptoms of hypothyroidism can usually be elicited upon specific questioning. Nevertheless, some patients with large tumours generating neurological symptoms do not have any clinical hypothyroid manifestations. Goitre is present in 20% of cases [4].

Sometimes, children with hypothyroidism-induced TSH adenomas present with precocious puberty [57], i.e. menstrual bleeding, breast and uterine maturation, weight gain and growth acceleration. An alternative presentation in children is that of growth arrest, and the tumour is then suspected on radiography of the sella. In such cases, due to the mild clinical manifestations of hypothyroidism in infancy, the endocrinologist faces considerable diagnostic problems. In adults, TSH adenomas due to hypothyroidism have been reported in patients who presented hypogonadism, amenorrhoea–galactorrhoea with elevated PRL values, and loss of libido [58]. These protean endocrine presentations clearly indicate the difficulty in reaching a correct diagnosis, and the risk of mismanagement.

Laboratory studies

Low T_3 and T_4 and elevated TSH values are the biochemical hallmarks of this entity in patients with pituitary enlargement due to prolonged thyroid hypofunction. These results immediately permit the differential diagnosis from TSH-secreting tumours causing hyperthyroidism and from the situations of inappropriate secretion of TSH, both associated with high values of thyroid hormones. Antithyroid antibodies are positive in 80% of patients, and enhanced TSH discharge after TRH administration is a common finding. Skull radiographs should be obtained from all patients with suspected long-standing hypothyroidism and, if abnormal, MRI scans should follow. High-resolution MRI studies and formal visual field examination should be performed initially in all patients with neurological manifestations of an adenoma, and repeated at reasonable intervals to evaluate the effectiveness of treatment. One should bear in mind that, at diagnosis, TSH values can either be markedly high or only moderately elevated. Values for the α-subunit are elevated but always proportionately less than TSH, in contrast to TSH-secreting tumors leading to hyperthyroidism.

Treatment

Since these tumours are hyperplastic manifestations of long-term thyroid hormone deprivation, they may undergo involution after a few months of thyroid hormone replacement, and complete resolution is to be expected in most cases after 1 year of treatment [59] (Fig. 15.5). Alleviation of the clinical symptoms after T_4 administration is impressive, with cessation of the neurological signs and improvement in vision. In addition, endocrine manifestations such as hypogonadism or growth failure are rapidly corrected with treatment. Surgery should not be undertaken before at least 1 year of thyroid hormone replacement, and only if that treatment fails in reducing pituitary volume or if there is optic chiasm compression. In some cases an empty sella or pituitary enlargement has developed after thyroid hormone treatment. For these reasons, close follow-up of the patients is mandatory, at least in the first year of treatment.

Conclusions

TSH-secreting pituitary tumours causing hyperthyroidism, the syndrome of resistance to thyroid hormones, and 'feedback' TSH adenomas, were previously rare entities which have been reported with increasing frequency in the past few years. Unfortunately, the three entities are frequently misdiagnosed, and the ensuing mismanagement has led to a protracted deterioration in the clinical situation of the affected patients before initiation of the correct treatment.

We recommend that free T_3 and free T_4 assays, and highly sensitive assays of TSH, be introduced in the endocrine clinic as first-line diagnostic tools; availability of α-subunit determination is also extremely useful. In any case, the most sophisticated and up-to-date diagnostic armamentarium will be ineffective unless the endocrinologist is well aware and highly suspicious of these rare entities.

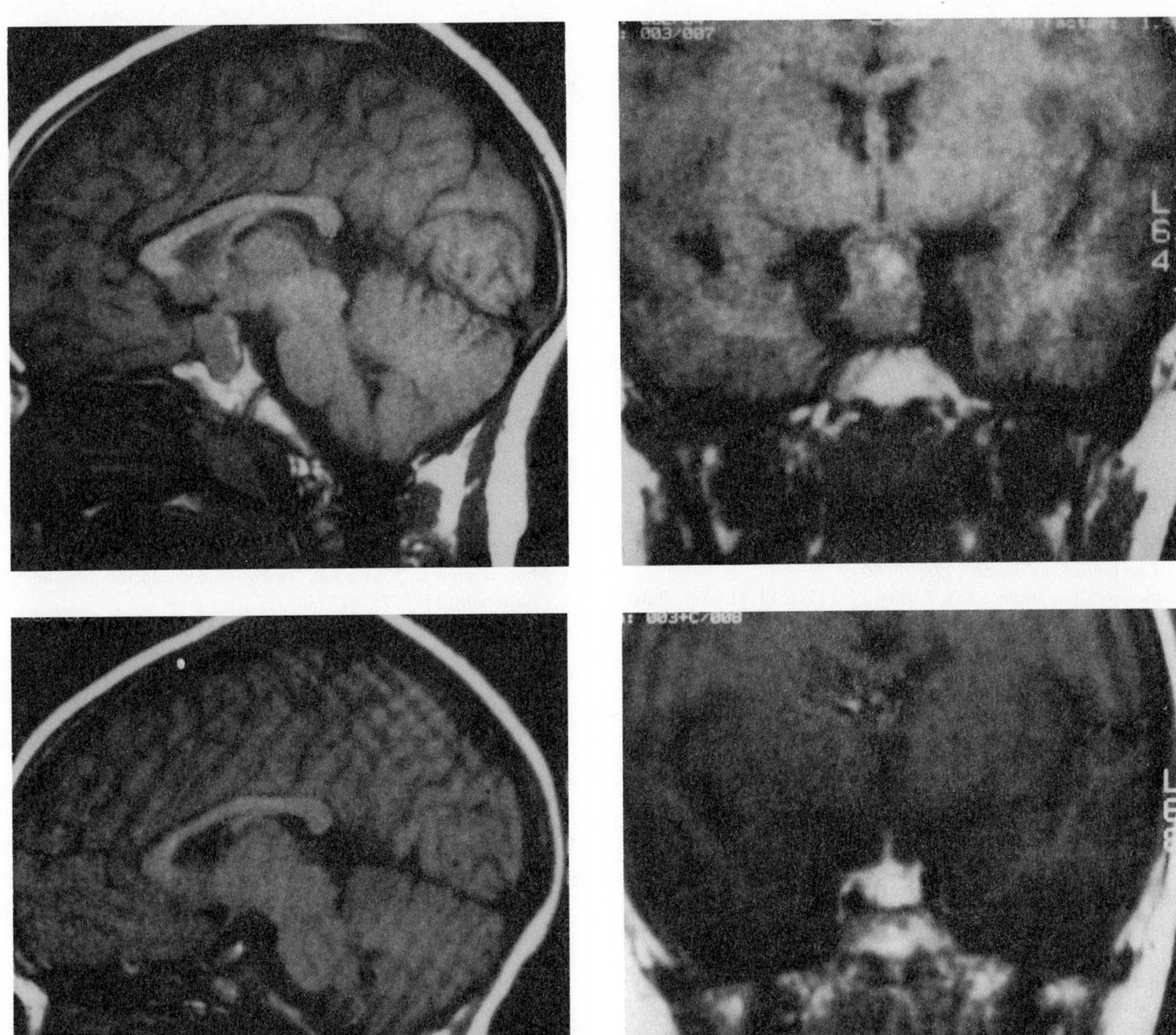

Fig. 15.5 Magnetic resonance image of a patient with a 'feedback adenoma' secreting TSH produced by long-term hypothyroidism before (a) and after (b) thyroid hormone replacement. From [59].

Acknowledgements

Supported by grants from Fundación Ramón Areces and Asociacion Española Contra el Cancer.

References

1 Weintraub BD, Gershengorn MC, Kourides IA, Fein H. Inappropriate secretion of thyroid-stimulating hormone. *Ann Intern Med* 1981; 95: 339–51.

2 Gesundheit N, Petrick PA, Nissim M *et al*. Thyrotropin-secreting pituitary adenomas: clinical and biochemical heterogeneity. *Ann Intern Med* 1989; **111**: 827–35.

3 Peters JR, Foord SM, Dieguez C, Scanlon MF. TSH neuroregulation and alterations in disease states. *Clin Endocrinol Metab* 1983; **12**: 669–94.

4 Smallridge RC Thyrotropin-secreting tumors. In: Mazaferri EL, Samaan NA, eds. *Endocrine Tumors*. Boston, MA: Blackwell Scientific Publications, 1993: 136–51.

5 Beck-Peccoz P, Persani L. TSH adenomas: clinical findings, endocrinology and treatment. In: Landolt AM, Vance M-L, Reilly PL, eds. *Pituitary Adenomas, Biology, Diagnosis and Treatment*. London: Churchill Livingstone, 1996: 139–55.

6 Brucker-Davis F, Skarulis MC, Grace MB *et al*. Genetic and clinical

features of 42 kindreds with resistance to thyroid hormones. *Ann Intern Med* 1995; **123**: 572–83.

7 Beckers A, Abs R, Mahler C *et al.* Thyrotropin-secreting pituitary adenomas: report of seven cases. *J Clin Endocrinol Metab* 1991; **72**: 477–83.

8 Smallridge RC, Wartofsky L, Dimond RC. Inappropriate secretion of thyrotropin: discordance between the suppressive effects of corticosteroids and thyroid hormone. *J Clin Endocrinol Metab* 1979; **48**: 700–5.

9 Amir SM, Kubota K, Tramontano D, Ingbar SH, Keutmann HT. The carbohydrate moiety of bovine thyrotropin is essential for full bioactivity but not for receptor recognition. *Endocrinology* 1987; **120**: 345–52.

10 Gesundheit N, Fink DL, Silverman LA, Weintraub BD. Effect of thyrotropin-releasing hormone on the carbohydrate structure of secreted mouse thyrotropin. *J Biol Chem* 1987; **262**: 197–203.

11 Saeger W, Lüdecke DK. Pituitary adenomas with hyperfunction of TSH. Frequency, histological classification immunocytochemistry and ultrastructure. *Virchows Arch* 1982; **394**: 255–67.

12 Herman V, Drazin NZ, Gonsky R, Melmed S. Molecular screening of pituitary adenomas for gene mutations and rearrangements. *J Clin Endocrinol Metab* 1993; **77**: 50–5.

13 Helzberg JH, McPhee MS, Zarling EJ, Lukert BP. Hepatocellular carcinoma: an unusual course with hyperthyroidism and inappropriate thyroid-stimulating hormone production. *Gastroenterology* 1985; **88**: 181–4.

14 Bergstrand CG. A case of hypothyroidism with signs of precocious sexual development. *Acta Endocrinol* 1995; **20**: 338–41.

15 Sakurai A, Takeda K, Ain K *et al.* Generalized resistance to thyroid hormones associated with a mutation in the ligand-binding domain of the human thyroid hormone receptor. *Proc Natl Acad Sci USA* 1989; **86**: 8977–81.

16 Sunthornthepvarakui T, Gottschalk ME, Hayashi Y, Refetoff S. Brief report: resistance to thyrotropin caused by mutations in the thyrotropin-receptor gene. *N Engl J Med* 1995; **332**: 155–60.

17 Avramides A, Karapiperis A, Triantafyllidou E, Vayas S, Moshidou A. TSH secreting pituitary macroadenoma in an 11-year-old girl. *Acta Paediatr* 1992; **81**: 1058–60.

18 Calle AL, Yuste E, Martin P *et al.* Association of a thyrotropin-secreting pituitary adenoma and a thyroid follicular carcinoma. *J Endocrinol Invest* 1991; **14**: 499–502.

19 Mixon AJ, Friedman TC, Katz DA *et al.* Thyrotropin-secreting pituitary carcinoma. *J Clin Endocrinol Metab* 1993; **76**: 529–33.

20 Weintraub BD, Petrick PA, Gesundheit N, Oldfield EH. TSH-secreting pituitary tumors. In: Medeiros-Neto G, Gaitan S, eds. *Frontiers in Thyroidology*. New York: Plenum Press, 1986: 71–7.

21 Chanson P, Li JY, LeDafniet M *et al.* Absence of receptors for thyrotropin (TSH)-releasing hormone in human TSH-secreting pituitary adenomas associated with hyperthyroidism. *J Clin Endocrinol Metab* 1988; **66**: 447–50.

22 Polak M, Bertherat J, Li JY *et al.* A human TSH-secreting adenoma: endocrine, biochemical and morphological studies. Evidence of somatostatin receptors by using quantitative autoradiography. Clinical and biochemical improvement by SMS 201–995 treatment. *Acta Endocrinol* 1991; **124**: 479–86.

23 Verhoeff NP, Bemelman FJ, Wiersinga WW, van Royen EA. Imaging of dopamine D2 and somatostatin receptors in vivo using single-photon emission tomography in a patient with a TSH/PRL-producing pituitary macroadenoma. *Eur J Nucl Med* 1993; **20**: 555–61.

24 LeDafniet M, Brandi AM, Kujas M, Chanson P, Peillon F. Thryotropin-releasing hormone (TRH) binding sites and thyrotropin response to TRH are regulated by thyroid hormones in human thyrotropic adenomas. *Eur J Endocrinol* 1994; **130**: 559–64.

25 Ross DS. New sensitive immunoradiometric assays for thyrotropin. *Ann Intern Med* 1986; **104**: 718–20.

26 Higuchi M, Mori S, Arita N *et al.* Two cases of TSH-secreting pituitary adenoma. *No Shinkey Geka* 1991; **19**: 883–9.

27 Caixas A, Infiesta F, Balsells M, Rodriguez J, Schwarzstein D, Webb SM. Secreción inadecuada de TSH. Rasgos clínicos, criterios diagnosticos y posibilidades terapeuticas. *Med Clin (Barc)* 1994; **102**: 776–80.

28 Beck-Peccoz P, Roncoroni R, Mariotti S *et al.* Sex hormone-binding globulin measurement in patients with inappropriate secretion of thyrotropin (IST): evidence against selective pituitary thyroid hormone resistance in nonneoplastic IST. *J Clin Endocrinol Metab* 1990; **71**: 19–25.

29 Lamberts SWJ, Van der Lely A-J, de Herder WW, Hofland LJ. Octreotide. *N Engl J Med* 1996; **334**: 246–54.

30 Frank SJ, Gesundheit N, Doppman JL *et al.* Preoperative lateralization of pituitary microadenomas by petrosal sinus sampling: utility in two patients with non-ACTH secreting tumours. *Am J Med* 1989; **87**: 679–82.

31 Mindermann T, Wilson CB. Thyrotropin-producing adenomas. *J Neurosurg* 1993; **79**: 521–7.

32 Kourides IA. Inappropriate secretion of thyroid stimulating hormone. Bardin CW, ed. *Current Therapy in Endocrinology and Metabolism*, 5th edn. St Louis: Mosby, 1994: 48–52.

33 Comi RJ, Gesundheit N, Murray L, Gorden P, Weintraub BD. Response of thyrotropin-secreting pituitary adenomas to a long-acting somatostatin analogue. *N Engl J Med* 1987; **317**: 12–17.

34 Sy RA, Bernstein R, Chynn KY, Kourides IA. Reduction in size of a thyrotropin- and gonadotropin-secreting pituitary adenoma treated with octreotide acetate (somatostatin analog). *J Clin Endocrinol Metab* 1992; **74**: 690–4.

35 Chanson P, Weintraub BD, Harris AG. Octreotide therapy for thyroid-stimulating hormone-secreting pituitary adenomas. A follow-up of 52 patients. *Ann Intern Med* 1993; **119**: 236–40.

36 Karlsson FA, Burman P, Kampe O, Westlin JE, Wide L. Large somatostatin-insensitive thyrotropin-secreting pituitary tumour responsive to D-thyroxine and dopamine agonists. *Acta Endocrinol* 1993; **129**: 291–5.

37 Gancel A, Vuillermet P, Legrand A, Catus F, Thomas F, Kuhn JM. Effects of a slow-release formulation of the new somatostatin analogue lanreotide in TSH-secreting pituitary adenomas. *Clin Endocrinol* 1994; **40**: 421–8.

38 Refetoff S, DeWind LT, DeGroot LJ. Familial syndrome of combining deaf–mutism, stippled epiphyses, goiter and abnormally high PBI: possible target organ refractoriness to thyroid hormone. *J Clin Endocrinol Metab* 1967; **27**: 279–94.

39 Refetoff S, Weiss RE, Usala SJ. The syndrome of resistance to thyroid hormone. *Endocr Rev* 1993; **14**: 348–99.

40 Refetoff S. Syndromes of thyroid hormone resistance. *Am J Physiol* 1982; **243**: E88–93.

41 Umesono K, Evans RM. Determinants of target gene specificity for steroid/thyroid hormone receptor. *Cell* 1989; **57**: 1139–46.

42 Usala SJ, Bale AE, Gesundheit N *et al.* Tight linkage between the syndrome of generalized resistance to thyroid hormone and the human c-erb A beta gene. *Mol Endocrinol* 1988; **74**: 49–55.

43 Beck-Peccoz P, Chatterjee VK, Chin WW *et al.* Nomenclature of thyroid hormone receptor beta gene mutations in resistance to thyroid hormone: consensus statement from the first workshop on thyroid hormone resistance. July 10–11 1993, Cambridge, UK.

J Clin Endocrinol Metab 1994; **78**: 990–3.

44 Salmeron J, Alonso C, Salazar A, Mutazzi E, Palacios Mateos JM. Syndrome of inappropriate secretion of thyroid-stimulating hormone by partial target organ resistance to thyroid hormones. *Acta Endocrinol* 1977; **97**: 361–8.

45 Beck-Peccoz P, Chatterjee VK. The variable clinical phenotype in thyroid hormone resistance syndrome. *Thyroid* 1994; **4**: 225–32.

46 Gershengorn MC, Weintraub BD. Thyrotropin-induced hyperthyroidism caused by selective pituitary resistance to thyroid hormone. A new syndrome of inappropriate secretion of TSH. *J Clin Invest* 1975; **56**: 633–42.

47 Kaplan MM, Swartz SL, Larsen PR. Partial peripheral resistance to thyroid hormone. *Am J Med* 1981; **70**: 1115–21.

48 Wynne AGA, Gharib H, Scheithauer BW, Davis DH, Freeman SL. Hyperthyroidism due to inappropriate secretion of thyrotropin in 10 patients. *Am J Med* 1992; **92**: 15–24.

49 Rosier A, Litvin Y, Hage C, Gross J, Cerasi E. Familial hyperthyroidism due to inappropriate thyrotropin secretion successfully treated with triiodothyronine. *J Clin Endocrinol Metab* 1982; **54**: 76–82.

50 Beck-Peccoz P, Piscitelli G, Cattaneo MG, Faglia G. Successful treatment of hyperthyroidism due to non-neoplastic pituitary TSH hypersecretion with 3,5,3′-triiodothyroacetic acid (TRIAC). *J Endocrinol Invest* 1983; **6**: 217–23.

51 Dorey F, Strauch G, Gayno JP. Thyrotoxicosis due to pituitary resistance to thyroid hormones. Successful control with D-thyroxine: a study in three patients. *Clin Endocrinol* 1990; **32**: 221–8.

52 Beck-Peccoz P, Mariotti S, Guillausseau PJ *et al.* Treatment of hyperthyroidism due to ectopic secretion of thyrotropin with the somatostatin analog SMS 201–995. *J Clin Endocrinol Metab* 1989; **68**: 201–14.

53 Niepce B. *Traite du Goitre et du Cretinisme*. Paris: Baillière, 1851.

54 Vagenakis AG, Dole K, Braverman LE. Pituitary enlargement, pituitary failure, and primary hypothyroidism. *Ann Intern Med* 1976; **85**: 195–8.

55 Scheithauer BW, Kovacs K, Randall RV. Pituitary gland in hypothyroidism. *Arch Pathol Lab Med* 1985; **109**: 499–505.

56 Yamada T, Tsukui T, Ikejiri K, Yukimura Y, Kotani M. Volume of the sella turcica in normal subjects and in patients with primary hypothyroidism and hyperthyroidism. *J Clin Endocrinol Metab* 1976; **42**: 817–22.

57 Bergstrand CG. A case of hypothyroidism with signs of precocious sexual development. *Acta Endocrinol* 1955; **20**: 338–41.

58 Groff TR, Shulkin BL, Utiger RD, Talbert LM. Amenorrhea-galactorrhea, hyperprolactinemia and suprasellar pituitary enlargement as presenting features of primary hypothyroidism. *Obstet Gynecol* 1984; **63**: 865–95.

59 Atchison JA, Lee PA, Albright AL. Reversible suprasellar pituitary mass secondary to hypothyroidism. *JAMA* 1989; **262**: 3175–7.

60 Mixson AJ, Freidman TL, Katz DA *et al.* Thyrotropin-secreting pituitary carcinoma. *J Clin Endocrinol Metab* 1993; **76**: 529–33.

61 Dong Q, Brucker-Davis F, Weintraub BD *et al.* Screening of candidate oncogenes in human thyrotroph tumours: absence of activation mutations in $G_{\alpha\gamma}$, G_{α}, G or thyrotrophin-releasing hormone receptor genes. *J Clin Endocrinol Metab* 1996; **81**: 1134–40.

62 Losa M, Giovanelli M, Persani J, Mortini P, Faglia G, Beck-Peccoz P. Criteria of cure and follow-up of central hyperthyroidism due to thyrotropin-secreting pituitary adenomas. *J Clin Endocrinol Metab* 1996; **81**: 3086–90.

63 Caron P, Gerbaud C, Pradayrol L, Simonetta C, Bayard F. Successful pregnancy in an infertile woman with a thyrotropin-secreting macroadenoma treated with a somatostatin analog (octreotide). *J Clin Endocrinol Metab* 1996; **81**: 1164–68.

64 Beck-Peccoz P, Brucker-Davis F, Persani L, Smallridge RC, Weintraub BD. Thyrotropin-secreting pituitary tumours. *Endocrine Rev* 1996; **17**: 610–38.

CHAPTER 16

Isolated adrenocorticotrophic hormone deficiency

S. Tsagarakis

Introduction

Isolated adrenocorticotrophic hormone (ACTH) deficiency is a rare cause of secondary adrenal insufficiency, characterised by a unitropic defect in the synthesis and/or release of ACTH, with preservation of function of all other pituitary trophic hormones [1]. The disease was first described by Steinberg *et al.* in 1954 [2], and since then an increasing number of well-documented cases have been reported in the world literature. The disease affects both sexes equally. It is primarily a disease of adult life with a peak incidence at around 40–50 years of age. Occasionally the disease has been diagnosed in childhood, when a history of birth trauma is often obtained. So far, only 13 cases have been reported under the age of 15 years, and only three presented in the neonatal period. Familial occurrence was described in two reports, suggesting an inherited defect [3].

Pathogenesis

Due to the rarity of the disorder, our understanding of the pathogenesis of isolated ACTH deficiency is currently limited. It is likely that a spectrum of different entities leading to varying degrees of corticortoph failure may exist. In theory, a lesion resulting in deficient ACTH secretion may be located at one of several sites including the pituitary, the hypothalamus, or even its central connections.

Pituitary origin

A pituitary defect is responsible for the majority of the described cases. Most convincing evidence favouring a pituitary defect has emerged following the application of the corticotrophin-releasing hormone (CRH) test in investigating hypothalamo-pituitary–adrenal axis dysfunction; this test is considered a good discriminatory tool between hypothalamic and pituitary causes of secondary adrenal insufficiency [4–6]. Hypothalamic defects are associated with a delayed and exaggerated response in ACTH secretion following bolus administration of CRH, but there is no response in ACTH release in the presence of pituitary defects. In the majority of patients with isolated ACTH deficiency tested so far, no ACTH responses to bolus CRH administration have been observed. Even consecutive injections of CRH in three patients reported by Koida *et al.* also failed to stimulate ACTH secretion [7]. Thus, it seems most likely that a pituitary defect, which involves the corticotrophs or their responsiveness to corticotrophin-releasing factors, is encountered in the majority of cases with adult-onset isolated ACTH deficiency. So far, in the world literature, there are only three reported patients demonstrating responsiveness of ACTH during the CRH test [8]; these patients may represent either a partial isolated ACTH deficiency or a hypothalamic CRH deficiency.

The nature of the process at the level of the pituitary leading to corticotroph failure is currently unclear. A few cases have been reported following post-partum haemorrhage, which imply that ischaemia may result in a partial form of Sheehan's syndrome, although isolated trophic hormone deficiencies have only rarely been described in this syndrome [9]. Histological studies of the pituitary have only rarely been performed in patients with isolated ACTH deficiency. In the limited existing studies [10–12], a marked decrease or complete loss of basophil cells of the anterior pituitary has been reported, with no bioassayable ACTH detected from the extracted gland. Lymphocytic infiltration was recorded in the majority of the reported cases. In fact, an autoimmune and/or lymphocytic involvement of the pituitary is probably responsible for the majority of cases, as suggested by the association of the disease with several other autoimmune conditions [13]. The strongest association of isolated ACTH deficiency is with cases of primary hypothyroidism with strongly positive antithyroid antibodies. This suggests that an autoimmune process might mutually involve both the pituitary and the thyroid [14]. Cases of the disease associated with polyglandular endocrinopathy have also been described [15]. Moreover, in patients with proven lymphocytic hypophysitis, ACTH deficiency represents the most common isolated type of anterior pituitary hormone deficiency encountered [16]. Lymphocytic hypophysitis commonly appears in the postpartum period, and this may well explain the frequent development of the disease in women during this period, even after uncomplicated labour (see also Chapter 17). Circulating pituitary autoantibodies have been detected in some but not all patients with the disease. The exact role, however, of these antibodies in the pathogenesis of corticotroph failure remains unclear. Recently, autoantibodies to corticotrophin antigens were detected in secretory granules that contained neither ACTH or other pro-opiomelanocortin (POMC)-derived peptide. It has been suggested that the antigen recognised by these antibodies may represent a cell-specific factor essential for the processing of POMC molecule [17], but more studies are required to clarify this issue.

It has been suggested that corticotroph gene defects lying in the CRH receptor or the POMC gene may be responsible for some rare cases, particularly of childhood or neonatal-onset isolated ACTH deficiency. In fact, evidence for a defect in the CRH receptor has emerged in some patients with dissociated ACTH responsiveness after lysine vasopressin and CRH [7]. In these patients, although there was no ACTH response following CRH administration, administration of lysine vasopressin, which is an alternative stimulatory test for the pituitary corticotrophs, resulted in ACTH secretion. Although such a selective corticotroph unresponsiveness to CRH may suggest a receptor or a post-receptor defect to its action, no abnormalities in the CRH receptor gene in isolated ACTH deficiency have yet been reported [3]. Defective POMC processing has been recently described by Nussey *et al.* [18] to result in isolated ACTH deficiency and secondary adrenocortical failure in a neonate, with elevated levels of ACTH precursors but no measurable ACTH. Since no abnormalities have been detected in the POMC precursor gene, it has been suggested that an enzymatic defect leading to abnormal processing of pituitary POMC products may be responsible. The frequency and clinical expression of abnormal POMC processing as a cause of isolated ACTH deficiency is currently unclear, but it may be relevant that an adult patient with high-molecular-weight ACTH immunoreactivity as the predominant circulating form, and a few patients with unexplained hyperpigmentation, have been described [1].

Hypothalamic origin

The possibility that a minority of cases of isolated ACTH deficiency may occur as a result of defective hypothalamic function has been suggested. Such a premise is indeed tenable, since hypothalamic deficiencies resulting in isolated pituitary hormone deficiencies of GH, gonadotrophins and thyroid-stimulating hormone (TSH) are well-recognised entities. As previously mentioned, so far, very few patients with adult-onset disease have been described to respond to exogenous administration of CRH. In contrast, it has been suggested that a hypothalamic defect may account for the majority of childhood-onset cases, particularly those developing as a result of complicated labour. However, since most of these cases were reported in the years preceding the use of CRH, evidence based only on lysine vasopressin responsiveness does not ascertain hypothalamic CRH deficiency. In fact, a case of childhood onset disease with unresponsive anterior pituitary corticotrophs to CRH administration has recently been described [19].

Hypothalamic defects leading to ACTH deficiency may in theory be due to decreased synthesis and/or release of CRH. CRH gene defects are probably incompatible with life and have not yet been reported in either animal models or humans. An intriguing hypothalamic mechanism has also been recently proposed by Redei *et al.* [20]: these investigators provided evidence that within the prepro-thyrotrophin-releasing hormone (TRH) gene there is a region responsible for the production of a prepro-TRH derived peptide with corticotrophin inhibiting activity. Thus, based on the observation that patients with isolated ACTH deficiency often demonstrate higher TSH levels, they speculated that overactivation of TRH-releasing neurons may be responsible. However, in view of the fact that in patients with primary hypothyroidism there is no gross evidence of impairment of ACTH secretion, involvement of such a mechanism in the pathogenesis of isolated ACTH deficiency seems unlikely.

Suprahypothalamic origin

Although defects in suprahypothalamic connections regulating hypothalamic CRH secretion may, in theory, result in impaired ACTH secretion, such a situation has not been convincingly confirmed in humans. It is of note, however, that an animal model, including Lewis and Fisher rats, showing a global impairment of hypothalamic CRH neuron function to several stimuli was recently described. In these animals, defective CRH secretion was associated with a predisposition to the development of several inflammatory processes [21], and it may be relevant that in humans a subgroup of patients with rheumatoid arthritis and hypothalamo-pituitary–adrenal axis hyporesponsiveness to the stress of surgery has been recently reported [22]. Thus, although there is no evidence that CRH hyporesponsiveness to suprahypothalamic stimuli may lead to gross impairment of ACTH secretion in humans, impaired activation of CRH neurons may be a significant predisposing factor in several human diseases, particularly those associated with autoimmune processes [23].

Clinical features

Manifestations of hypocortisolism due to ACTH deficiency are similar to those of Addison's disease. However, one should be alert to the non-specific nature and the great variability in the expression of the symptoms by which the disease is presented. It is, therefore, not unusual for unexplained fatigue, weakness and weight loss to occur for many years before a diagnosis is obtained. The major clinical findings of the disease, as reviewed by Stacpoole *et al.* [1], are given in Table 16.1. Hypoglycaemia is a frequent presenting symptom, encountered in more than 50% of the described cases. It is commoner in childhood and in the adult female, particularly during intervening pregnancies. Hypotension and orthostatic hypotension appear in approximately 25% of patients. In females, there is a sparsity of sexual hair, but this feature is less pronounced than in patients with Addison's disease. Electrolyte changes appear less commonly in isolated ACTH deficiency than in primary adrenal failure, due to preservation of aldosterone secretion. However, severe hyponatraemia can and does occur in some of the patients, and is aggravated by conditions leading to sodium depletion. This is probably due to some attenuation of the aldosterone secretory response in the presence of hypocortisolaemia, and is completely reversible with glucocorticoid treatment. In contrast to Addison's disease, acute adrenal crisis occurs less commonly in patients with isolated ACTH deficiency; precipitating factors are usually infections, anaesthesia and surgery. Classically, secondary adrenal failure is not associated with hyperpigmentation, and this is a reliable sign in differentiating this condition from primary adrenal disease. However, as previously mentioned, a few patients with isolated ACTH deficiency, including the original case of Steinberg *et al.*, have been described to express marked hyperpigmentation [2], which is probably due to high levels of circulating POMC precursor [18]. Finally, unusual presentations of the disease have been described, in the form of delayed puberty [8], secondary hypogonadism, the 'stiff-man' syndrome [24] or even the dramatic appearance of delirium in conjunction with neuromuscular symptoms [25]. These disturbances are readily reversible with glucocorticoid replacement treatment.

Table 16.1 Major clinical findings in isolated adrenocorticotrophic hormone deficiency. From [1].

Symptom/sign	%
Hypoglycaemia	56
Weight loss	32
Hypotension	26
Anaemia	26
Weakness/fatigue	26
Hair sparsity/loss	16
Nausea/vomiting	16
Inability to excrete water load	14
Hyponatraemia	9

Diagnosis

The diagnosis of isolated ACTH deficiency is based on the demonstration of adrenal failure in the presence of inappropriate low ACTH levels and preservation of the secretory responses of the other trophic pituitary hormones. A flow diagram of approaching the diagnosis of isolated ACTH deficiency is shown in Fig. 16.1.

The first step is to establish the diagnosis of adrenal failure by the presence of low basal cortisol levels and no cortisol response to ACTH administration (short Synacthen test). Evidence for secondary adrenal failure is then obtained by the finding of low or normal ACTH levels in the presence of hypocortisolaemia, and the resumption of adrenal cortisol responsiveness during prolonged ACTH administration (long Synacthen test). Insufficiency of the hypothalamo-pituitary unit is also confirmed by an insulin tolerance test. Lack of responsiveness in ACTH and in cortisol responsiveness (when adrenal atrophy has been reversed by prior ACTH administration) confirms the hypothalamo-pituitary dysfunction. At this stage it is important to exclude deficiencies of other pituitary hormones. This is best done with a combined test (insulin tolerance test (ITT), luteinising hormone-releasing hormone and TRH) and measurement of the responses of growth hormone, luteinising hormone, follicle-stimulating hormone, TSH and prolactin (see Chapter 83). It should, however, be mentioned that inadequate growth hormone responses should not be considered as evidence against isolated ACTH deficiency, as such responses can frequently be observed in the presence of low glucocorticoids, and they are completely reversed by glucocorticoid replacement. Of equal importance is also the exclusion of hypothalamo-pituitary destructive lesions by high-resolution computed tomography (CT) or magnetic resonance imaging (MRI) of the region. However, I would recommend a formal re-evaluation of the hypothalamo-pituitary region with the

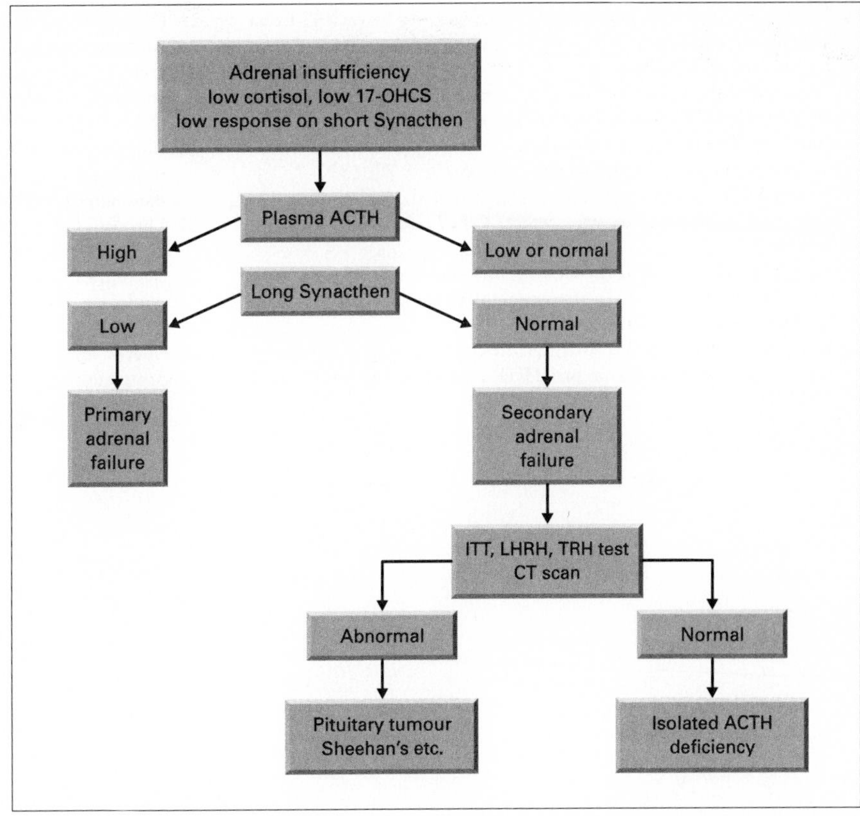

Fig. 16.1 Flow diagram for the diagnosis of isolated adrenocorticotrophic hormone (ACTH) deficiency.

combined test and MRI at least once following a year of glucocorticoid replacement. Finally, a CRH test should always be performed to confirm ACTH deficiency and to differentiate between hypothalamic and pituitary defects.

Treatment

The treatment of isolated ACTH deficiency consists of glucocorticoid replacement with hydrocortisone. The long-term prognosis is excellent.

References

1 Stacpoole PW, Interlandi JW, Nicholson WE, Rabin D. Isolated ACTH deficiency: a heterogeneous disorder. Critical review and report of four new cases. *Medicine* 1982; **63**: 13–24.

2 Steinberg A, Shetcher FR, Segal HI. True pituitary unitropic deficiency. *J Clin Endocrinol Metab* 1954; **14**: 1519–29.

3 Woods K, Weber A, Clark AJL. The molecular pathology of pituitary hormone deficiency and resistance. *Clin Endocrinol Metab* 1995; **9**: 453–87.

4 Schulte HM, Chrousos GP, Avgerinos P *et al.* The corticotropin releasing hormone stimulation test: a possible aid in the evaluation of patients with adrenal insufficiency. *J Clin Endocrinol Metab* 1984; **58**: 1064–7.

5 Tsukada T, Nakai Y, Koh T *et al.* Plasma adrenocorticotrophin and cortisol to ovine corticotropin-releasing factor in patients with adrenocortical insufficiency due to hypothalamic and pituitary disorders. *J Clin Endocrinol Metab* 1984; **58**: 758–60.

6 Lytras N, Grossman A, Perry L *et al.* Corticotrophin releasing factor: responses in normal subjects and patients with disorders of the hypothalamus and pituitary. *Clin Endocrinol* 1983; **20**: 71–84.

7 Koida Y, Kimura S, Inoue S *et al.* Responsiveness of hypophiseal-adrenocortical axis to repetitive administration of synthetic ovine corticotropin releasing hormone in patients with isolated ACTH deficiency. *J Clin Endocrinol Metab* 1986; **63**: 329–35.

8 Orme SM, Belchetz PE. Isolated ACTH deficiency. *Clin Endocrinol* 1991; 35: 213–17.

9 Kannan CR, Isolated ACTH deficiency. In: *The Pituitary Gland.* New York: Plenum Medical Book Company, 1987: 295–307.

10 Perkoff GT, Eik-nes K, Garnes WH, Tyler FH. Selective hypopituitarism with deficiency of anterior pituitary basophils: a case report. *J Clin Endocrinol* 1960; **20**: 1269.

11 Richsmeier AJ, Henry RA, Bloodworth JMB *et al.* Lymphoid hypophysitis with selective adrenocorticophin hormone deficiency. *Arch Intern Med* 1980; **140**: 1243–5.

12 Jensen MD, Handwerger BS, Scheitbauer BW, Carpenter PC, Mirakian R, Banks PM. Lymphocytic hypophysitis with isolated corticotropin deficiency. *Ann Intern Med* 1986; **105**: 200–3.

13 Yamamoto T, Fukuyana J, Hasegawa K, Sugiura M. Isolated corticotropin deficiency in adults: report of 10 cases and review of the literature. *Arch Intern Med* 1992; **152**: 1705–12.

14 Miller MJ, Horst TV. Isolated ACTH deficiency and primary hypothyroidism. *Acta Endocrinol* 1982; **99**: 573–6.

15 Kojima I, Nejima I, Ogata E. Isolated adrenocorticotropin deficiency associated with polyglandular failure. *J Clin Endocrinol Metab* 1982; **54**:182–6.

16 Thodou E, Asa SL, Kontogeorgos G, Kovacs K, Horvath E, Ezzat S. Lymphocytic hypophysitis: clinicopathological findings. *J Clin Endocrinol Metab* 1995; **80**: 2302–11.

17 Sauter NP, Toni R, McLaughlin CD, Dyess EM, Krizmann J, Lechan RM. Isolated ACTH deficiency associated with an autoantibody to corticotroph antigen that is not adrenocorticotropin or other POMC-derived peptides. *J Clin Endocrinol Metab* 1990; **70**: 1391–7.

18 Nussey SS, Shiu-Ching S, Gibson S *et al*. Isolated congenital ACTH deficiency: a cleavage enzyme defect? *Clin Endocrinol* 1993; **39**: 381–6.

19 Murch SH, Carter EP, Tsagarakis S *et al*. Isolated ACTH deficiency with absent response to corticotrophin-releasing factor-41. *Acta Paediatrica Scand* 1991; **80**: 259–61.

20 Redei E, Hilderbrand H, Aird F. Corticotropin release inhibiting factor is encoded within prepro-TRH. *Endocrinology* 1995; **136**: 1813–16.

21 Patchev VK, Kalogeras KT, Zelazowski P *et al*. Increased plasma concentrations, hypothalamic content, and *in vitro* release of arginine vasopressin in inflammatory disease prone, hypothalamic corticotropin releasing hormone deficient Lewis rats. *Endocrinology* 1992; **131**: 1453–7.

22 Chikanza IC, Petrou P, Kingsley G *et al*. Defective hypothalamic response to immune and inflammatory stimuli in patients with rheumatoid arthritis. *Arthritis Rheum* 1992; **35**: 1281–8.

23 Chrousos GP. The hypothalamo-pituitary-adrenal axis and immune-mediated inflammation. *N Engl J Med* 1995; **20**: 1351–62.

24 Gordon EE, Januszko DM, Kaufman L. A critical survey of stiffman syndrome. *Am J Med* 1967; **42**: 582.

25 Fang VS, Jaspan JB. Delirium and neuromuscular symptoms in an elderly man with isolated corticotroph-deficiency syndrome completely reversed with glucocorticoid replacement. *J Clin Endocrinol Metab* 1989; **69**: 1073–7.

CHAPTER 17

Lymphocytic hypophysitis

P.J. Jenkins

Introduction

Lymphocytic hypophysitis was first described by Goudi and Pinkerton in 1962, since when approximately 100 cases have been described worldwide [1]. The majority of early cases were diagnosed at autopsy, with death most likely resulting from secondary adrenal insufficiency. It was not until 1980 that the first ante-mortem diagnosis was made, but with increasing knowledge of the disorder it is becoming more readily diagnosed and earlier treatment instituted.

Clinical features

The vast majority of cases occur in women, usually but not invariably in relation to pregnancy when they tend to occur in the third trimester or puerperium. There is no correlation with parity, nor is there any racial predisposition. Outside of pregnancy, it may occur at any age with the oldest affected female patient being 67 years. Approximately 10% of cases are male, such patients tending to be older (median age 47 years; range 27–61 years) [2–7]. Overall, the clinical presentation is variable and similar to that of a pituitary adenoma; if occurring during pregnancy or the puerperium, it is often that of an enlarging pituitary mass lesion with increasing headaches and visual impairment, often bitemporal hemianopia, which may progress rapidly over a period of days [8–11]. In such cases, symptoms of endocrine deficiency secondary to pituitary failure may be non-existent or only become apparent on investigation. Outside of pregnancy, patients tend to present with symptoms of anterior and posterior pituitary deficiency, often insidious in onset. The extent of such hypopituitarism is variable, ranging from isolated deficiencies to severe pan-hypopituitarism, but is unrelated to the size of the pituitary mass. Unlike that associated with pituitary adenomas, it tends not to occur in the predictable sequence of growth hormone (GH), luteinising hormone (LH), follicle-stimulating hormone (FSH), adrenocorticotrophic hormone (ACTH) and thyroid-stimulating hormone (TSH); rather, ACTH and/or TSH are the commonest deficiencies, occurring in approximately 80% of patients, with LH and FSH tending to be preserved. In men, the disease appears to be more severe with four of the six cases described having pan-hypopituitarism [3,4,6,7]. Diabetes insipidus is present in approximately 10% of cases [2,4,5,12–14] which, if present, further differentiates the disorder from a pituitary adenoma. Associated autoimmune diseases occur in up to 30%, especially thyroiditis, adrenalitis and pernicious anaemia, giving rise to the suggestion that lymphocytic hypophysitis may be part of a pluriglandular syndrome. One case has also been reported in association with parathyroiditis and another with subsequent sarcoidosis [9]. Interestingly, many of the reported cases of thyroiditis have been sequential to ACTH deficiency, perhaps relating to perturbations in immunoendocrine homeostasis [4,9,15,16].

As alluded to above, the clinical course of this disease is unpredictable. Spontaneous resolution has been reported in a number of cases, almost invariably in pregnancy [2,4,8,12,17,18], although complete recovery from pan-hypopituitarism has been recorded in a 50-year-old woman [19]. Such recovery may be partial or complete and is independent of any changes in size of the pituitary mass. Alternatively, progressive hypopituitarism may occur over months to years. In males, the disease appears to be more severe; cavernous sinus extension and ophthalmoplegia has been reported in four patients, compared with only one female, together with a greater degree of hypopituitarism and less spontaneous recovery. To date, there have been no reports of recurrent disease after either prior resolution or surgical intervention.

Differential diagnosis

The major differential diagnosis of hypopituitarism in the post-partum period is Sheehan's syndrome, although the latter is extremely rare with modern obstetric care, requiring a clear history of a definite and significant haemorrhage causing hypotension. As such, it is likely that many cases previously attributed to this were actually lymphocytic hypophysitis, as has been suggested by other workers [20]. Prolactinomas are an alternative cause of an enlarging pituitary mass and visual impairment during pregnancy. Non-functioning adenomas may also present in a similar manner, but affect all age groups. Other possible diagnoses include Langerhans' cell histiocytosis and granulomatous hypophysitis secondary to diseases such as sarcoidosis, syphilis and tuberculosis.

Investigations

Full basal and dynamic pituitary investigations should be performed. As mentioned above, any degree of anterior pituitary hormone deficiency may occur. Serum prolactin levels may be low, normal or modestly elevated; in the latter case they tend to be lower than that seen in prolactinomas and most probably result from stalk compression. Diabetes insipidus occurs in approximately 10% of patients [4,12–14] and when present should alert the clinician to a diagnosis other than pituitary adenoma. Lymphocytic infundibulo-hypophysitis appears to be a different disease entity [21]. A chest X-ray should be performed, as well as measurement of erythrocyte sedimentation rate and serum angiotensin-converting enzyme, to aid in the differential diagnosis of alternative diseases such as sarcoidosis and tuberculosis. Formal visual field assessment with Goldmann perimetry is mandatory to document any chiasmal compression.

Radiology

Pituitary fossa X-rays may show an expanded fossa while the inflammatory nature of the disease may cause hyperostosis of the sella floor [22]. Computed tomography (CT) imaging has been the most common radiological investigation performed and typically shows a symmetrical enhancing mass, often with suprasellar extension, which is indistinguishable from a pituitary adenoma [23] (Fig. 17.1). An alternative appearance is that of an area of low attenuation with peripheral enhancement following contrast. As mentioned above, cavernous sinus involvement has been reported in several patients, males more often than females, and associated with ophthalmoplegia. With long-standing disease, the mass may become fibrotic with corresponding radiological shrinkage leading eventually to an empty fossa.

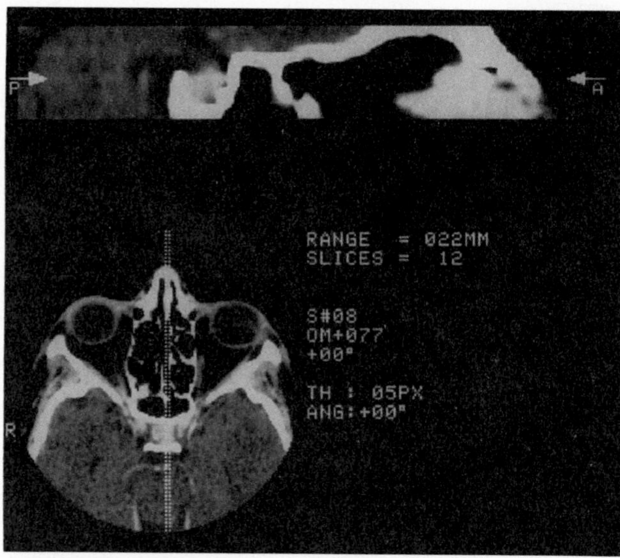

Fig. 17.1 Computed tomography scan (sagittal section) demonstrating a uniformly enhancing pituitary fossa mass with minimal suprasellar extension.

Although there has been less experience with magnetic resonance imaging (MRI), those that have been performed have shown a variable appearance, usually of a pituitary mass that is isointense with respect to brain parenchyma on T1- and T2-weighted images [2,23]. Alternatively, symmetrical enhancement following gadolinium contrast has been reported on T1- [3] and T2-weighted images [12], as has peripheral enhancement [2,13], a feature not seen in macroadenomas.

Pathogenesis

An autoimmune mechanism has been proposed in the pathogenesis of lymphocytic hypophysitis. Early work by Levine on mice suggested cellular-mediated mechanisms might play a role, with lymphocytic infiltration of the pituitary occurring after injection of pituitary extract and Freund's adjuvant into the foot pad [27]. A humoral mechanism has also been proposed with the discovery of anti-pituitary antibodies in the serum of some affected patients [28]. However, this does not occur in all patients [4] and such antibodies have also been reported in the serum of unaffected normal people [28]. Furthermore, the different methods of detection utilising rat, monkey, human fetal and human adult pituitary makes it difficult to draw any firm conclusions regarding their significance. Further circumstantial evidence in support of an autoimmune pathogenesis are the very similar histological appearances compared to those seen in other autoimmune diseases, such as Hashimoto's thyroiditis [11], and the frequent association with pregnancy, in which immunological function is known to be altered. The increasing pituitary size and blood flow that is a normal occurrence in pregnancy, secondary to prolactin-cell hyperplasia, may result in increased exposure to pituitary antigens, or alternatively, the exposure to fetal antigens and antibody may result in cross-reaction with maternal antigens. Putative loss of fetal suppressor substances in the post-partum period may also play a role, although, as yet, all these suggestions remain speculative and the precise pathogenesis of lymphocytic hypophysitis remains uncertain.

Histology

Histology of the pituitary mass typically shows a diffuse infiltrate of inflammatory cells, mostly comprising lymphocytes with a few plasma cells, often resulting in degeneration of normal anterior pituitary cells (Fig. 17.2). Lymphoid follicles may be present with occasional germinal centres (Fig. 17.3) and fibrous tissue is widespread. There are no granulomas or epithelial cells present, thus distinguishing from the similar condition, granulomatous hypophysitis. The histological findings are similar to those of other autoimmune diseases, particularly autoimmune thyroiditis but, as mentioned above, adjacent normal anterior pituitary tissue may be present and there have been two reports of coexisting growth hormone-secreting adenomas [4,5].

Treatment

The management of this rare condition remains controversial, with different authors recommending no treatment, medical therapy, pituitary biopsy or removal of the pituitary mass in its entireity. These opinions are based on experience with few numbers of patients with varied clinical manifestations.

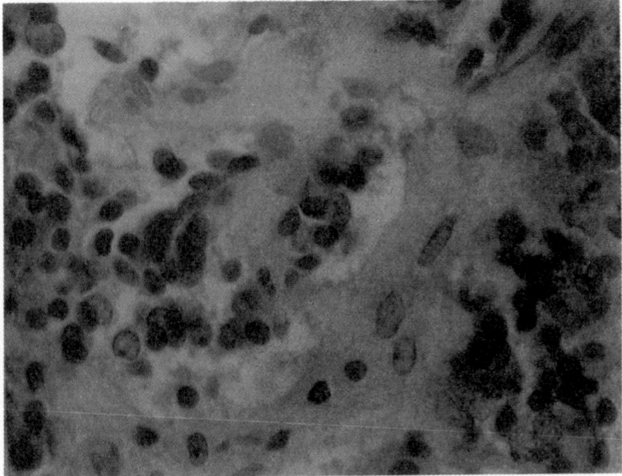

Fig. 17.2 Lymphocytes around degenerating anterior pituitary cells.

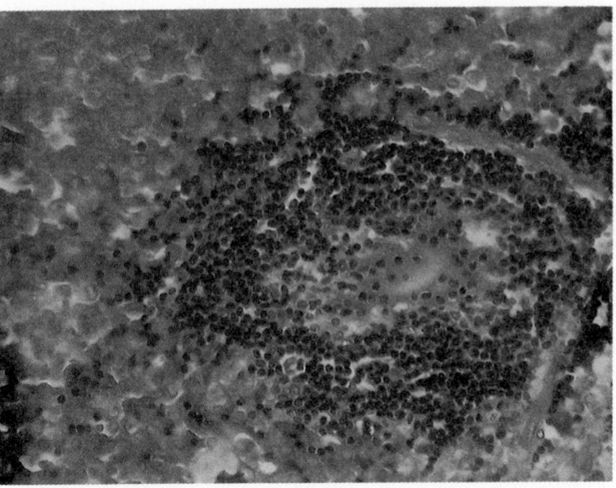

Fig. 17.3 Anterior pituitary with many lymphocytes comprising a lymphoid follicle.

A conservative approach has been associated with spontaneous resolution or, alternatively, the disease can progress to life-threatening pan-hypopituitarism. A trial of steroids has been reported to be beneficial [24], being associated with a rapid improvement in visual fields in one case [10], although other reports have shown no benefit [4,25]. Given the unpredictability of the disease process, it may be that any apparent benefit is coincidental. Furthermore, there is considerable morbidity associated with long-term high-dose glucocorticoid therapy. Taking these features into account, it is justifiable to adopt a conservative approach in a young woman with a pregnancy-related pituitary mass, although close monitoring is essential with frequent assessment of visual fields and pituitary function. With the major differential diagnosis in this group of patients being a prolactinoma, a trial of dopamine agonists should be performed if prolactin levels are elevated. Outside of pregnancy, the differential diagnosis widens considerably; as the definitive diagnosis can only be made on histological grounds, early surgery is indicated. It has been suggested that pituitary biopsy should be performed in preference to complete excision of the mass in order to minimise iatrogenic hypopituitarism [26]. However, such an approach is not without its draw-backs for a number of reasons. Firstly, due to the rarity of lymphocytic hypophysitis outside of pregnancy, a pituitary mass is more likely to be a pituitary adenoma, for which complete excision is the preferred treatment. Thus, if a biopsy only is performed as the initial manoeuvre, a second operation is likely to be subsequently required with its associated increased morbidity. Secondly, areas of lymphocytic infiltration have been reported to coexist with adjacent normal anterior pituitary [5] raising the possibility of an erroneous diagnosis if only normal pituitary is biopsied. Furthermore, areas of lymphocytic infiltration have also been reported to coexist with a functioning growth hormone-secreting adenoma [5] and may again be missed on biopsy findings. With these points in mind, it may be suggested that complete removal of the pituitary mass should be attempted, both for accurate diagnosis and as definitive therapy, although this aim is often difficult due to the dense and fibrotic nature of the mass and its frequent adhesion to surrounding structures. Needless to say, full hormone replacement should be instituted in all patients as required, and thorough reassessment performed at regular intervals.

Conclusions

Although lymphocytic hypophysitis is a rare disorder, it should be considered in the differential diagnosis of a pituitary mass, especially when occurring in relation to pregnancy. A conservative approach may be justified in such patients, but careful monitoring is required, particularly with regard to visual impairment, which may be rapidly progressive. As there are no reliable clinical or radiological diagnostic characteristics, surgery is indicated in other patients for definitive diagnosis and treatment. Although previously associated with a high mortality, earlier diagnosis and institution of hormone replacement should ensure a normal life expectancy.

References

1 Goudie RE, Pinkerton PH. Anterior hypophysitis and Hashimoto's disease in a young woman. *J Pathol Bacteriol* 1962; **83**: 584–5.

2 Lee J-H, Laws ER, Guthrie BL, Dina TS, Nochomovitz LE. Lymphocytic hypophysitis: occurrence in two men. *Neurosurgery* 1994; **34**: 159–63.

3 Supler ML, Mickle JP. Lymphocytic hypophysitis: report of a case in a man with cavernous sinus involvement. *Surg Neurol* 1992; **37**: 472–6.

4 Thodou E, Asa SL, Kontogeorgos G, Kovacs K, Horvath E, Ezzat S. Clinical Case Seminar: lymphocytic hypophysitis: clinicopathological findings. *J Clin Endocrinol Metab* 1995; **80**: 2302–11.

5 Jenkins PJ, Chew SL, Lowe DG, Afshar F, Charlesworth M, Besser GM, Wass JAH. Lymphocytic hypophysitis: unusual features of a rare disorder. *Clin Endocrinol* 1995; **42**: 529–34.

6 Pestell RG, Best JD, Alford FP. Lymphocytic hypophysitis. The clinical spectrum of the disorder and evidence for an autoimmune pathogenesis. *Clin Endocrinol* 1990; **33**: 457–66.

7 Guay AT, Agnello V, Tronic BC, Gresham DG, Freidberg SR. Lymphocytic hypophysitis in a man. *J Clin Endocrinol Metab* 1987; **64**: 631–4.

8 McGrail KM, Beyerl BD, Black PM, Klibanski A, Zervas NT. Lymphocytic adenohypophysitis of pregnancy with complete recovery. *Neurosurgery* 1987; **20**: 791–3.

9 Hayashi H, Yamada K, Kuroki T *et al*. Lymphocytic hypophysitis and pulmonary sarcoidosis. *Am J Clin Pathol* 1991; **95**: 506–11.

10 Stelmach M, O'Day J. Rapid change in visual fields associated with suprasellar lymphocytic hypophysitis. *J Clin Neuro-ophthalmology* 1991; **11**: 19–24.

11 Asa SL, Bilbao JM, Kovacs K, Josse RG, Kreines K. Lymphocytic hypophysitis of pregnancy resulting in hypopituitarism: a distinct clinicopathologic entity. *Ann Intern Med* 1981; **95**: 166–71.

12 Miura M, Ushio Y, Kuratsu J, Ikeda J, Kai Y, Yamashiro S. Lymphocytic adenohypophysitis: report of two cases. *Surg Neurol* 1989; **32**: 463–70.

13 Clinicopathologic conference. Headaches, diabetes insipidus and hyperprolactinaemia in a woman with an enlarged pituitary gland. *Am J Med* 1993; **95**: 332–9.

14 McDermott MW, Griesdale DE, Berry K, Wilkins GE. Lymphocytic adenohypophysitis. *Can J Neurol Sci* 1988; **15**: 38–43.

15 Jensen MD, Handwerger BS, Scheithauer BW, Carpenter PC, Mirakian R, Banks PM. Lymphocytic hypophysitis with isolated corticotropin deficiency. *Ann Intern Med* 1986; **105**: 200–3.

16 Richtsmeier AJ, Henry RA, Bloodworth JMB, Ehrlich EN. Lymphoid hypophysitis with selective adrenocorticotropic hormone deficiency. *Arch Intern Med* 1980; **140**: 1243–5.

17 Castle D, De Villiers JC, Melvill R. Lymphocytic adenohypophysitis. Report of a case with demonstration of spontaneous tumour regression and a review of the literature. *Br J Neurosurg* 1988; **2**: 401–6.

18 Bevan JS, Othman S, Lazarus JH, Parkes AB, Hall R. Reversible adrenocorticotropin deficiency due to probable autoimmune hypophysitis in a woman with postpartum thyroiditis. *J Clin Endocrinol Metab* 1992; **74**: 548–52.

19 Ozawa Y, Shishiba Y. Recovery from lymphocytic hypophysitis associated with painless thyroiditis: clinical implications of circulating antipituitary antibodies. *Acta Endocrinologica* 1993; **128**: 493–8.

20 Patel MC, Guneratne N, Haq N, West TET, Weetman AP, Clayton RN. Peripartum hypopituitarism and lymphocytic hypophysitis. *Quart J Med* 1995; **88**: 571–80.

21 Imura H, Nakao K, Shimatsu A, Ogawa Y, Sando T, Fujisawa I, Yamabe H. Lymphocytic infundibuloneurohypophysitis as a cause of central diabetes insipidus. *N Engl J Med* 1993; **329**: 683–9.

22 Clinicopathologic conference. Primary hypothyroidism and hypopituitarism in a young woman. *Am J Med* 1984; **77**: 319–28.

23 Levine SN, Benzel EC, Fowler MR, Shroyer III JV, Mirfakhraee M. Lymphocytic adenohypophysitis: clinical, radiological, and magnetic resonance imaging characterization. *Neurosurgery* 1988; **22**: 937–41.

24 Feigenbaum SL, Martin MC, Wilson CB, Jaffe RB. Lymphocytic adenohypophysitis: a pituitary mass lesion occurring in pregnancy. *Am J Obstet Gynecol* 1991; **164**: 1549–55.

25 Reusch JE, Kleinschmidt-DeMasters BK, Lillehei KO, Rappe D, Gutierrez-Hartmann A. Preoperative diagnosis of lymphocytic hypophysitis (adenohypophysitis) unresponsive to short course dexamethasone: case report. *Neurosurgery* 1992; **30**: 268–72.

26 Prasad A, Madan VS, Sethi PK, Prasad ML, Buxi TBS, Kanwar CK. Lymphocytic hypophysitis: can open exploration of the sella be avoided? *Br J Neurosurg* 1991; **5**: 639–42.

27 Levine S. Allergic adenohypophysitis: a new experimental disease of the pituitary gland *Science* 1967; **158**: 1190–1.

28 Crock P. Lymphocytic hypophysitis. *Curr Opin Endocrinol Diabetes* 1997 (in press).

CHAPTER 18

Craniopharyngiomas and other hypothalamic tumours

P.N. Plowman, J. Girard, C. Irwin and D. Sebag-Montefiore

Introduction

Central endocrine regulation may be disturbed by space-occupying lesions in the diencephalic and mid-brain areas.

Symptoms of anterior pituitary insufficiency and of disturbed body water homeostasis may be seen, as well as signs of autonomic dysfunction such as tachycardia, flushing and changes in body temperature. Anorexia or unexplained weight loss or weight gain, amenorrhoea and other menstrual disturbances may all be early signs. Behavioural and intellectual changes and focal motor weakness or seizures can also occur, and point directly to the central nervous system (CNS) localization of the possible lesion [1]. In children, the predominant symptom can be delay in growth and development, growth arrest or, less commonly, increased height velocity and precocious puberty. Larger or expanding lesions induce increased intracranial pressure with headache, vomiting and visual disturbance [2].

Evaluation of the hypothalamo-pituitary axis is part of the diagnostic investigation. It should be noted that not only the primary lesion itself, but the therapeutic modality such as surgery or irradiation, can eventually lead to involvement of the endocrine system [3–5].

The overall incidence of intracerebral tumours, as assessed from autopsy findings, is 2.7%; CNS tumours represent 9.8% of all malignant tumours. In children, of all malignancies only leukaemia is more frequent than intracranial neoplasm.

In adults and in children up to 4 years of age, a supratentorial location is most common. From 4 to 11 years 70% of all intracerebral tumours are infratentorial.

Forty to fifty per cent of all intracranial tumours are of brain parenchymal tissue origin: the great majority stem from neuroglial tissue, with only a minority being of neuronal origin.

Except for neurinomas and meningiomas there is a preponderance of males over females especially for medulloblastomas, craniopharyngiomas, dermoids and epidermoid cysts [6].

In children, pilocytic astrocytomas (spongioblastomas) and infratentorial medulloblastomas are the most frequent lesions. Ependymomas account for 12%, and ectodermal tumours account for 6% of all tumours. The location of these is the central neural axis (astrocytomas of the third ventricle, of the chiasmatic and pontine and mid-brain area). Malformation tumours such as teratomas, germinomas, dermoid and epidermoid cysts, hamartomas and craniopharyngiomas usually become symptomatic in the first or second decade of life.

Usually the growth of these tumours is slow and, as the skull of the child can expand, classical symptoms of increased intracranial pressure appear late. Obstruction to the flow of cerebrospinal fluid occurs more often in infratentorial tumours [7–9].

An absence of signs of increased intracranial pressure can be misleading, and suspicious symptoms suggestive of such tumours should be investigated even where evidence of raised intracranial pressure is absent.

In adults in the third and fourth decades, medulloblastomas and astrocytomas are more often found in the hemispheres. Glioblastomas and metastatic tumours usually appear at a later age.

Primary derangement of central endocrine regulation is to be expected with parasellar space-occupying lesions such as craniopharyngiomas, chondromas, chordomas, suprasellar meningiomas, astrocytomas of the optic nerve and primary tumours of the third ventricle. Signs and symptoms requiring further investigation to exclude or confirm the presence of an intracerebral lesion are summarized in Table 18.1; general investigations are listed in Table 18.2.

Table 18.1 Symptoms and signs compatible with an intracranial tumour (requiring diagnostic assessment for exclusion or confirmation).

Behavioural changes
Impaired motor and sensory activity
Increasing clumsiness/ataxia
Impaired growth (abnormal height velocity, delayed bone maturation)
Delayed or precocious puberty
Weight increase/weight loss
Other diencephalic symptoms
Anorexia/hypothermia/insomnia or hypersomnia, etc.
Hypoglycaemia
Symptoms of hormonal dysfunction, mostly deficiencies (diabetes insipidus)
Signs of increased intracranial pressure
Vomiting, headache, ocular symptoms such as visual impairment, double vision and abnormal positioning of the head (avoidance of double vision)

Table 18.2 General diagnostic procedures in suspected intracranial space-occupying lesions.

Personal history
Growth and development (related to family)
Intellectual changes
'Diencephalic symptoms'
Symptoms of increases intracranial pressure: headache, nausea, vomiting, visual impairment
General physical examination
Including height, height velocity, puberty rating, weight gain/loss, weight centile compared with height centile, and skinfold thicknesses, eventually psychological testing for psycho-organic syndromes
Neuro-ophthalmological examination
Visual fields, fundoscopy
Radiography
Bone age
Skull or computed tomography with enhancement
Magnetic resonance imaging

The hypothalamo-pituitary axis

Involvement of the hypothalamic centre regulating water homeostasis is easily diagnosed as overt diabetes insipidus if urine volumes and fluid requirements amount to more than 5 litres. Antidiuretic hormone insufficiency can, however, be partial and/or masked by a concomitant impairment of anterior pituitary function. Growth hormone, adrenocorticotrophic hormone (ACTH) (via cortisol) and thyroid-stimulating hormone (TSH) (via thyroxine) all enhance diuresis, either by a direct renal effect on glomerular filtration or by a permissive action on vasopressin (AVP) at the renal tubule. Acquired nocturia and/or fluid intake during sleeping hours are suspicious symptoms, particularly during childhood. Fluid requirements and 24-hour urine volume, together with measurement of osmolarity of the first early morning urine are the first steps in the diagnostic procedure. Comparing several paired plasma/urine osmolalities is an efficient screening procedure and can avoid the need for fluid restriction tests. A ratio of urine/plasma osmolality below 1 is characteristic of an impaired concentration capacity. Fluid deprivation followed by intranasal insufflation of the AVP derivative DDAVP (desaminoarginine vasopressin) usually leads to the diagnosis [10]. These tests are dealt with in more detail in Chapter 83.

Clinical symptoms of anterior pituitary dysfunction are usually mild. Biochemically, they are characterized by low concentrations of the hormones of the peripheral endocrine gland in the absence of an elevation of the trophic pituitary hormones seen in primary insufficiency. Pathologically, a low morning cortisol level without increased plasma ACTH, low T_4 and T_3 with 'normal' or diminished values for TSH (measured with an 'ultrasensitive' assay), and similarly abnormally low levels of sex steroids without the 'appropriate' increase in follicle-stimulating hormone (FSH) and luteinising hormone (LH) are characteristic, and may often render stimulation tests unnecessary. Urinary excretion of free cortisol, the gonadotrophins, sex steroids and of growth hormone may, where available, replace the more invasive and time-consuming dynamic tests, but are not in common use. With regard to the gonadotrophin–gonadal axis, the prepubertal and peri- or post-menopausal age groups have different biochemical profiles. In the latter, LH and more regularly FSH are normally grossly elevated, whereas the hormonal levels in the prepubertal age range are indistinguishable from secondary hypogonadism. The evaluation of growth hormone secretion is controversial; while it is considered that the growth hormone response to insulin-induced hypoglycaemia is the most reliable test, there is evidence from paediatric experience that false positives and false negatives may occur. There is no definition of the normal response for a specific age group for any of the various currently used stimulation tests [11–14]. Growth hormone-releasing hormone is of no diagnostic value in this situation [15]. Similarly, in childhood luteinising hormone-releasing hormone (LHRH) is of very little use.

Nevertheless, in order to corroborate the presence of an intracerebral lesion involving the hypothalamo-pituitary axis [16,17], dynamic tests may have their diagnostic value. They must be properly chosen with a specific indication, and interpreted with caution. This also applies to the post-operative or post-therapeutic assessment. When, however, modern imaging techniques such as enhanced computed tomography (CT) scans or magnetic resonance imaging (MRI) [18,19] have demonstrated the presence of a space-occupying lesion and surgical intervention is planned, the complete assessment of endocrine function can sometimes be postponed as steroid cover in the perioperative period is necessary anyway, and evaluation of pituitary function must be performed after operation.

It must also be remembered that irradiation as well as surgery, even to hemispheric or infratentorial tumours, can affect the hypothalamic centres.

For the paediatric age group it should be emphasised that growth and development are sensitive to any hypothalamic lesion. Auxological data must therefore be well documented at diagnosis, and followed closely for a prolonged period, i.e. over many years [20,21].

Perioperative care

It is essential to monitor water and electrolyte balance carefully, and to check that glucocorticoid reserve is sufficient for severe stress. Even if ACTH–adrenal function is unimpaired before operation, steroid cover in stress dosages is required the day before operation, on the day of surgery, and for the following 24–72 hours.

In Table 18.3 guidelines for perioperative care are summarised. The basal cortisol requirement of 15 mg/m²/day increases by a factor of 5–10 in stress situations. As a rule, cortisol supplementation should start on the evening before surgery and the'stress' dosage should be adjusted to oral substitution dosage around the fourth to sixth day after operation. Hydrocortisone can be replaced in one-fifth of the dosage by prednisone, or by dexamethasone in one-thirtieth of the dosage indicated for hydrocortisone.

Fluid balance must be closely watched. Perioperatively, transient diabetes insipidus within the first 12 hours after an operation near the hypothalamo-pituitary area is very frequently seen. During the first 24 hours fluid intake should not exceed urinary output; thereafter insensible losses must be replaced. DDAVP should be used if urinary volumes are large, urine osmolarity is low, and plasma osmolarity is above 300 mosmol/l. The duration of action of the drug varies to a great extent, and the dosage has to be adjusted individually. The end of the antidiuretic effect is indicated by an abrupt, dramatic increase in urine flow. There is no habituation to DDAVP; therefore, simple observation after withholding one dose of DDAVP will confirm or exclude the necessity for continuous treatment. It is obvious that through attention to water balance and control of bodyweight, overhydration must be avoided.

In some patients, hypothalamic damage may result in dysregulation of the sodium control centres with loss of thirst. High sodium levels without weight loss are signs that point to a chronic problem of hyperosmolarity, which is very difficult to handle in practice.

Long-term endocrine sequelae of space-occupying lesions and/or of surgical or irradiation therapy

Growth hormone appears to be most susceptible to damage of the hypothalamo-pituitary system. The diagnosis of partial growth hormone insufficiency is difficult; replacement is necessary in the growing child.

After irradiation, growth hormone deficiency may be suspected clinically because of impaired height velocity and 'confirmed' by a diminished response to stimulation tests. On treatment with appropriate amounts of growth hormone, only initial 'catch-up' growth may be observed, with little change in the final height. This is partly explained by a relatively early pubertal development. Thus, a concomitant deficiency of gonadotrophin secretion may improve the height prognosis.

If a complete lack of growth hormone is assumed, as after surgical intervention at the pituitary level, growth hormone replacement therapy is mandatory in the growing child. Whether replacement therapy is required in adults is currently a matter of debate. It should be kept in mind that

Table 18.3 Perioperative steroid cover: hydrocortisone sodium succinate is used for parenteral application, hydrocortisone for the oral medication. (During the perioperative period hydrocortisone can be replaced by prednisone in 20% or by dexamethasone in 3% of the hydrocortisone dose indicated.)

Day	Hydrocortisone (all doses per m² body surface per day)
−1 (24 hours before operation)	50 mg (i.m. evening, day before operation)
0 (operation)	50 mg i.m., 100 mg i.v. (drip)
1 (after operation)	50 mg i.m. (divided in three doses), 75 mg i.v. (drip)
2–3	50 mg i.m. (divided in three doses), 50 mg i.v. (drip)
4–5	50 mg i.m. (divided in three doses), 20 mg orally (divided in three doses)
Subsequently	20–15 mg orally (divided in three doses)

growth hormone has complex effects on carbohydrate, fat and protein metabolism, and is not only a 'growth' hormone [22–24].

The need for continuous treatment with DDAVP depends on water balance, i.e. urine volume and fluid intake. It is easily controlled by comparing paired urine and plasma osmolarity. Because growth hormone and cortisol positively affect water excretion, impaired adenohypophysial function can mask, and replacement therapy can unmask, the necessity for DDAVP therapy.

ACTH deficiency may in some instances not require cortisol replacement under normal conditions, whereas in stress situations replacement with 5–10 times the basic cortisol requirement of 15 mg/m^2/day is necessary. However, the patient, their relatives and, in children, their teachers, must be informed, and the patient should carry a 'medical alert' identification card. The decision for treatment must be taken individually. If, for safety reasons, replacement is required in children, hydrocortisone should be used and the daily dose should not exceed 15 mg/m^2/day. Higher dosages and the use of steroid derivatives are likely to interfere with growth.

Selected tumours frequently associated with endocrine disturbances

Of a total of 700 intracerebral tumours in childhood, 350, or 50%, were located in the posterior cranial fossa: 196 tumours were found in the cerebral hemispheres and the lateral ventricles; 154, or somewhat more than 40%, of the supratentorial tumours were found in the diencephalon–mid-brain area, where involvement of the hypothalamo-pituitary axis is most likely. Within this group, tumours were found mainly around the chiasm and the sella turcica. The mid-brain and pineal areas were less frequently involved, and in about 10–15% of cases the tumours were found around the third ventricle and in the hypothalamus. Malignant tumours included retinoblastomas and pinealoblastomas. Astrocytomas, ependymomas, oligodendrogliomas and pinealomas were classified as semimalignant. The benign tumours included craniopharyngiomas, spongioblastomas, epidermoids, osteomas and pituitary adenomas [2,3,7–9,25].

Craniopharyngiomas

Origin and location

The craniopharyngioma is the most common tumour of non-glial origin. It accounts for 8–13% of all intracranial tumours in patients below 14 years of age. Seventeen per cent of the supratentorial tumours, and more than half of all sellar–chiasmatic tumours, can be diagnosed as craniopharyngiomas. In childhood it is by far the most frequent tumour involving the hypothalamo-pituitary system. Like teratomas, dermoid and epidermoid cysts, the tumour is related to an embryonic maldevelopment; it stems from remnants of Rathke's pouch, and develops from squamous cells of the ectoderm of the buccal epithelium.

The pharynx contains a single ectodermal layer of epithelium which does not contribute to this tumour. The commonly used term craniopharyngioma is thus incorrect: Rathke's pouch cyst, suprasellar cyst, adamantinoma, cholesteatoma and hypophysial duct tumour are all synonyms. Craniopharygiomas grow very slowly. They can be solid but are usually cystic; the cysts are filled with cellular detritus, cholesterol crystals, etc. Fibrous reactions may compress the epithelial parts which form compact avascular masses with calcification. The tumour is non-functional (although there may be human chorionic gonadotrophin (hCG) in the cyst fluid) and varies in size from an olive to an orange.

Although the tumour is considered to have a benign pathology, its location, progressive nature and tendency to involve surrounding tissue of functional importance, as well as the high recurrence rate, make the craniopharyngioma a clinically malignant tumour.

The majority of craniopharyngiomas are suprasellar and may fill the cavity of the third ventricle or extend inferiorly and posteriorly along the dorsum sella and the clivus; 15% of the tumours are found within the sella [26–28].

Symptoms and diagnostic evaluation

Symptoms usually appear within the first or at the beginning of the second decade, and are present for from 0.1 to 9 years before the diagnosis is made [27]. In 85% of the patients, visual or neurological symptoms lead to the diagnosis. The hypothalamo-pituitary system is involved in more than 50% of the patients [26,28]. Visual complaints more frequently lead to the suspicion of the diagnosis than short stature, although growth is often obviously impaired. If impairment of endocrine function is suspected because of short stature, failure to grow (abnormally low height velocity), abnormalities in pubertal development (usually delayed puberty) or unexplained weight gain or weight loss, complete evaluation of the hypothalamo-pituitary–endocrine axis, examination of the visual fields and fundoscopy are required. Absence of neurological or visual abnormalities never excludes a sellar or suprasellar tumour. At the time of diagnosis, the following symptoms are usually present: headache, vomiting, polyuria/polydipsia, short stature and visual impairment; the latter includes visual field defects, often asymmetric or unilateral, central scotoma, signs of optic atrophy and/or papilloedema. If the tumour extends towards the frontal fossa, loss of memory, abnormal behaviour and neurological signs, such as hemiparesis, may occur. Radiological findings include a retarded bone age, an abnormal sellar configuration, intracranial calcifications and possibly separated skull sutures on plain radiology. Imaging by high resolution CT and/or MRI are always indicated (Figs 18.1 and 18.2).

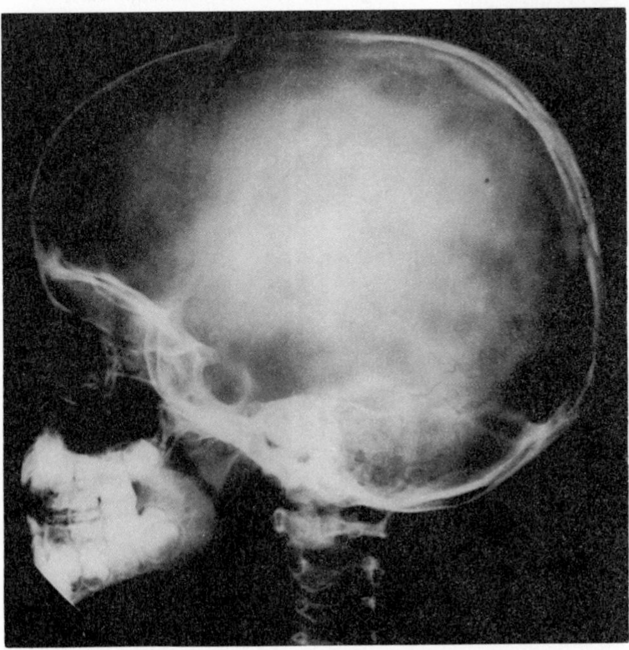

Fig. 18.1 Plain skull radiograph of a craniopharyngioma, demonstrating an enlarged pituitary fossa and suprasellar calcification. These features are not always present, while occasionally primary pituitary tumours, such as prolactinomas, may also calcify.

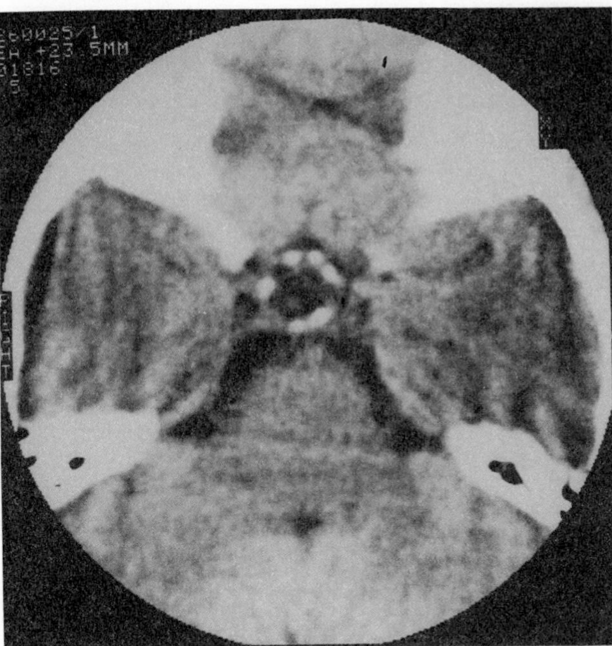

Fig. 18.2 Computed tomographic scan from a patient who presented with short stature in childhood, but no other endocrine abnormality. The characteristic calcification in a craniopharyngioma is clearly shown.

Therapy for craniopharyngiomas

The preferred treatment for craniopharyngiomas is complete excision of the tumour, if this is possible, without damaging the surrounding vital structures. Secondary operations are much more hazardous. In practice, attempts to do so may cause neurological, especially hypothalamic, damage. In most instances, therefore, subtotal excision followed by irradiation is the treatment of choice [26,27]. Radiotherapy greatly reduces the otherwise high recurrence rate of this congenital tumour. The total radiation dose should be approximately 5000 cGy in fractionated doses of less than 200 cGy/day. In children below 5 years of age a total dose of 4000–4500 cGy in 160 cGy fractions is delivered. In recurrent tumours, reoperation is more difficult; irradiation should be considered with decompression by cyst aspiration. Hypothalamic syndromes in this disorder are more likely to result from surgery and irradiation than to occur as primary symptoms. In purely intrasellar craniopharyngiomas (15%), long-term neuroradioloical surveillance without excision or radiotherapy has been suggested, since these tumours rarely spread beyond the sella [27]. Comprehensive perioperative endocrine management is absolutely essential. Cortisol cover is always necessary. During follow-up, re-evaluation of hypothalamo-pituitary function is necessary; total or partial hypopituitarism almost always occurs, whatever the strategy of treatment. While the mortality rate has been greatly reduced, the treatment of craniopharyngiomas is still not optimal. However, careful attention to water balance and steroid status has greatly reduced the mortality rate in recent years. ^{90}Y instillation into cystic recurrences can be very effective at reducing cyst size and refilling rates (Fig. 18.3).

Optic nerve glioma

Gliomas of the optic nerve account for 3% of intracranial tumours. Such gliomas are associated with the stigmata of von Recklinghausen's disease in 12–50% of cases.

Amblyopia, diplopia and exophthalmos (the tumour of the optic chiasm leads to unilateral exophthalmos as a late symptom) are clinical signs if the tumour grows intraorbitally. An extension above the chiasmatic area can lead

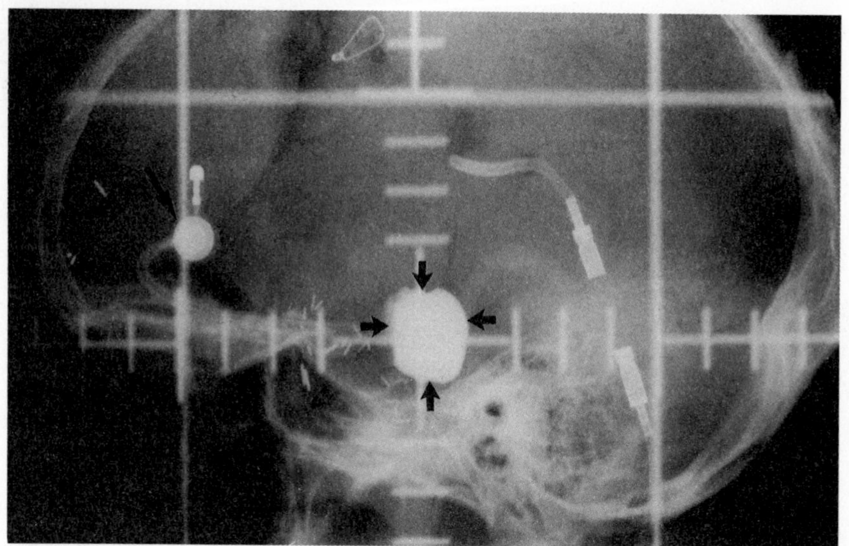

Fig. 18.3 Isohexal instillation via a Reckham reservoir positioned in the cystic part of a craniopharyngioma for volume estimation preparatory to β-emission isotope therapy. This 26-year-old woman had six craniotomies over a 13-year period, and external-beam radiotherapy. The 12–15 ml cyst required aspiration of 5–8 ml fortnightly before β-emission therapy.

to a compression of the third ventricle and can injure the pituitary stalk. Gliomas of the chiasm may therefore lead to bitemporal field defects and signs of pituitary dysfunction due to pituitary stalk section. The endocrine symptoms are very similar to those produced by an extrasellar craniopharyngioma: diabetes insipidus, obesity and retardation of growth and development in children.

The differential diagnosis between a tumour of the optic chiasm and a craniopharyngioma can be difficult. In the former, visual acuity is decreased in both eyes, whereas in the latter visual fields are usually more severely affected. The progress of tumours of the optic chiasm is more rapid than that of a craniopharyngioma, and there is no suprasellar calcification. Secondary pituitary insufficiency is not common in tumours of the optic chiasm, but very common in craniopharyngiomas. Cutaneous signs of von Recklinghausen's disease are confined to glioma of the optic chiasm. The assessment of endocrine function and the necessity for cortisol cover is the same as described for craniopharyngiomas.

Therapy for optic gliomas is controversial; surgery is the preferred therapy for lesions anterior to the chiasm and radiotherapy for lesions involving the chiasm. Chemotherapy has been used for infants.

Other tumours of the chiasmatic area

Three per cent of intracranial tumours in childhood occur in the thalamus and basal ganglia and may expand to the hypothalamus and third ventricle. This expansion can result in endocrine disturbances resembling those of craniopharyngiomas. The tumours lead to signs of increased intracranial pressure (headache, nausea, vomiting and papilloedema). Surgical attempts are only palliative and radiotherapy is indicated. Endocrine evaluation of hypothalamo-pituitary function is necessary.

Hypothalamic tumours and the diencephalic syndrome

Tumours in the hypothalamic area are usually gliomas, which grow more often in the anterior than in the posterior hypothalamus. They lead to symptoms from the newborn period to 4 years of age and have a peak incidence at 6 months. General symptoms include hyperkinesis, increased alertness, vomiting, inappropriate euphoria, pallor, nystagmus and extreme cachexia. Signs of occlusion of cerebrospinal fluid pathways may or may not be present. Tumour cells are often found in cerebrospinal fluid and the protein concentration is increased. The diencephalic syndrome can be associated with any endocrine defect following damage to the hypothalamo-pituitary regulatory centres [29].

The diagnosis is suspected from the clinical symptoms and supported by analysis of cerebrospinal fluid and CT. MRI is particularly valuable in imaging these tumours [30].

Tumours in the floor of the third ventricle, at the tuber cinereum, median eminence and of the pineal gland

Tumours in this area (hamartomas at the tuber cinereum, optic gliomas, teratomas, astrocytomas, ependymomas) are more frequently found in boys than in girls (5:1). If the tumour is small, precocious puberty may be the only

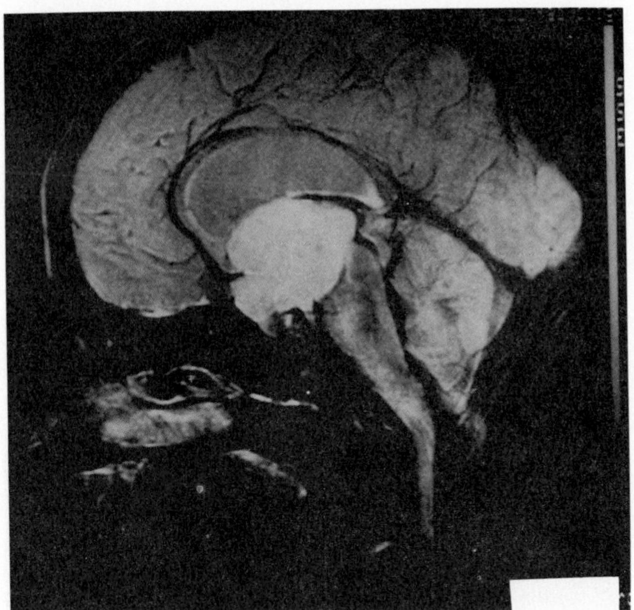

Fig. 18.4 Magnetic resonance image of a large hypothalmic astrocytoma. The patient was an adolescent female who was originally diagnosed as suffering from anorexia nervosa before the true diagnosis was ascertained.

manifestation. Larger tumours lead to increased intracranial pressure, visual loss, obesity, hypothalamic dysfunction such as changes in body temperature, diabetes insipidus and disturbance of growth and development (Fig. 18.4). The deep mid-line location of these tumours and their adherence to vital structures do not usually allow surgical treatment [31].

Craniocerebral trauma

Post-traumatic hypothalamo-pituitary dysfunction is a relatively rare disorder. Fractures, particularly of the temporal region, haemorrhagic contusions or subdural haematomas can induce lesions with the subsequent development of hormonal deficits. If diabetes insipidus develops, it is obvious that anterior pituitary function has to be assessed. More recently, however, attention has been focused on post-traumatic isolated anterior pituitary hormone deficiencies: the leading symptom in these patients is a decrease in growth in children, which can appear soon or only years after the head trauma. The difficulty in assessing growth hormone deficiency has been addressed above and in Chapters 61 and 62. Furthermore, precocious puberty has been observed following head trauma. These reports call for a strict follow-up of growth and development of children with head injuries in order to detect early and thus prevent developmental abnormalities. In adults, head trauma may lead to gonadotrophin deficiency which is usually reversible but may be prolonged.

Langerhans' cell histiocytosis

Previously called histiocytosis X, Langerhans' cell histiocytosis (LCH) encompasses a rare and diverse group of diseases, most commonly encountered in childhood. At one end of the spectrum comes a rather non-specific dermatitis in infants, whilst at the other is a rapidly progressive disease process destroying viscera (notably liver, lungs and bone marrow), again most commonly found in infants, previously called Letterer–Siwe disease. The common factor in all the clinical presentations of this spectrum is the underlying pathological process, which was formerly regarded as a malignant histiocytic infiltration of the organs affected. Recent research has narrowed the pathological cell type down to a particular subtype of histiocyte (reviewed in [32]). Two major histiocyte subsets are now recognized: the phagocytic or antigen-processing cells and the antigen-presenting or dendritic cells. One of the latter group of histiocytes is the Langerhans' cell—a tissue macrophage, particularly easily found histologically in normal skin but also physiologically present in other organs, and recognizable by unique surface antigen and other surface characteristics, as well as by the possession of the electron-microscopically unique Birbeck granule. It is an (apparently) uncontrolled proliferation of Langerhans' cells that is present in all LCH lesions, albeit with a secondary admixture or surrounding 'granuloma' of lymphocytes, neutrophils, eosinophils, other histiocytes and giant cells, and perhaps fatty change and fibrosis. The cause of the reactive or proliferation changes, and what determines its extent or pattern of tissue involvement in individual patients with LCH, is unclear, although disturbed immunoregulation is in some part involved [33]; there is no longer any evidence to support the historical viewpoint that this disease spectrum is a form of cancer. Indeed, the waxing and waning pattern of the disease, especially in less severely (particularly skin) affected childhood cases, never made this contention a satisfactory one.

In approximately 15% of cases of LCH in childhood diabetes insipidus occurs due to an LCH lesion/granuloma in the posterior pituitary/hypothalamus [34]; it is also well recognized in adults [35,36]. The occurrence of this lesion together with a lytic skull lesion and an orbital 'granuloma' produces the not uncommon triad of clinical features formerly called Hand–Schüller–Christian disease [37–39]. Other areas of the central nervous system are less commonly involved than the posterior pituitary and hypothalamus, but cerebellar [40,41], spinal cord [42,43] and more rarely cortical lesions are well documented.

The natural history of LCH is to wax and wane, to 'grumble chronically' (e.g. skin rash, mastoid or bone) for some years and then to 'burn out' or, rarely, to progress rapidly in multiple viscera to death. In childhood cases it is not uncommon to observe the patients off all therapy unless progressive visceral involvement is observed. When this occurs, steroids (prednisolone) are usually the first line of therapy with vinblastine as the traditional second-line drug. Recently, etoposide, an epipodophyllotoxin derivative, has been found to be a very effective and specific drug in LCH, and we have recently described a patient with adult multisystem LCH who achieved remission with etoposide as the first and only medication [36].

In patients with CNS disease, the diabetes insipidus observed may be partial or complete. Although in adult life some patients may no longer require their DDAVP, it is nevertheless difficult to show reversal of this aspect of CNS disease by either steroids or cytotoxic therapy, despite remission at other sites.

Local radiotherapy has been demonstrated to arrest and later to lead to reversal of LCH bone lesions: prescriptions of the order of 1000 cGy in six or seven fractions would be usual. Radiotherapy has also been described as reversing CNS disease, although patients with partial diabetes insipidus are more likely to benefit than those with complete diabetes insipidus [34,44]. Dose prescriptions of the order of 1200–1500 cGy in eight or 10 fractions are used. Radiotherapy has also been successfully used in low dosage in our unit for patients with LCH affecting the mastoid/middle ear, orbit and scalp. However, with the disease no longer carrying a malignant 'label', careful consideration for the use of a non-cytotoxic drug/radiation combination—notably steroids—should be given in all cases.

Neurosarcoidosis

'Sarcoidosis is a multisystem granulomatous disorder of unknown aetiology, most commonly affecting young adults and presenting most frequently with bilateral hilar lymphadenopathy, pulmonary infiltration and skin or eye lesions...' [45]. So begins the descriptive definition made at the Seventh International Conference on Sarcoidosis held in New York in 1976. However, sarcoidosis may involve the nervous system in 5–7% of cases [46]. The disease is commoner among Afro-Caribbeans, as are the neuroendocrine manifestations (Fig. 18.5).

Clinically, the diagnosis of neurosarcoid is easier if there are other features of a multisystem disease which may be confirmed by lung, skin or lymph node biopsy. However, when neurological dysfunction occurs in isolation or as the initial presenting complaint, diagnosis is more difficult [47]. Histological confirmation of non-caseating granulomas and exclusion of other conditions which can cause a granulomatous response, particularly tuberculosis, syphilis and fungal disease, is the most definitive means of establishing the diagnosis. A Kveim test complements other diagnostic procedures.

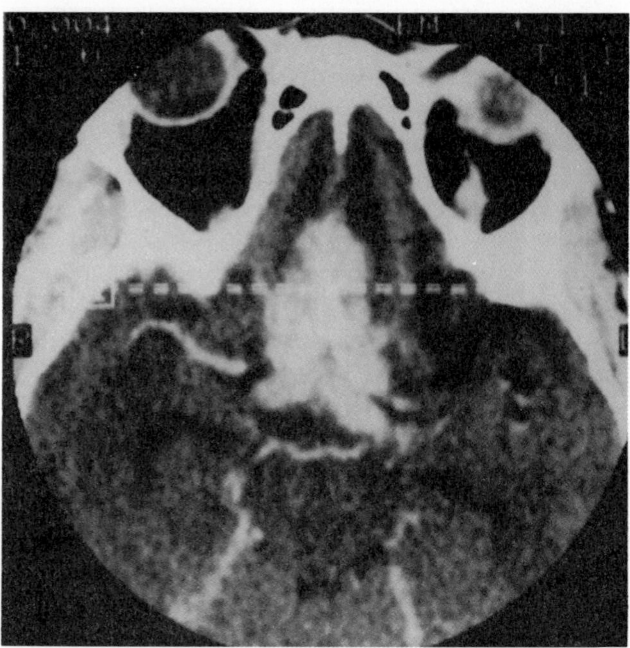

Fig. 18.5 Computed tomographic brain scan of 33-year-old West Indian woman showing an enhancing sarcoid lesion in the pituitary region.

The natural history of granulomas is variable. Spontaneous healing may occur with no scarring, or long-standing persistent lesions can hyalinize and fibrose with attendant scarring of normal tissues. This variable behaviour makes assessment of the efficacy of treatment modalities difficult [46,47].

Within the CNS, the cranial nerves, basal meninges, hypothalamus and pituitary gland are most likely to be affected. Of the cranial nerves, the facial nerve is the most frequently involved, and by itself is the commonest neurological manifestation in sarcoid. Onset is usually sudden and of lower motor neuron type, and may be bilateral in one-third of cases. Facial palsy may accompany parotitis but this is not universal. The next most likely affected is the optic nerve, giving rise to altered vision, field defects, pupillary abnormalities and even papilloedema. The visual pathway can be affected at any site along its course. The low incidence of oculomotor nerve dysfunction is noteworthy, but any cranial nerve can be involved. Although any part of the CNS may be affected by a localized granuloma, the major sites are the hypothalamus, pituitary and third ventricle. Because this region is not readily biopsied, a clinical diagnosis of sarcoid involvement is made on the basis of typical features elsewhere.

Diabetes insipidus occurs in up to 35% of all patients

with neurosarcoid, usually in association with disease outside the CNS; however, its overall prevalence in sarcoidosis is < 1%. Other features of hypothalamo-pituitary dysfunction may accompany diabetes insipidus—somnolence, weight gain, hypothermia, impotence, amenorrhoea, sleep disorder, hypothyroidism and hypogonadism.

Although it is the hypothalamus that is the principal site of functional damage in neurosarcoid, the anterior pituitary gland may be directly affected, with deficiency of one or more of the hormones secreted. Anterior hypopituitarism without diabetes insipidus is rare.

Space-occupying granulomas at the base of the brain may present with the more general features of a mass lesion and raised intracranial pressure—headache, seizures, lethargy, change in vision, papilloedema and optic atrophy if long standing. Raise intracranial pressure may also be due to obstructive hydrocephalus.

Seizures occur in up to 20% of patients with neurosarcoid and, if uncontrolled, carries a poor prognosis [48,49]. Meningitis in sarcoid is characterized by diffuse thickening of meninges as well as granulomatous nodules, and examination of the cerebrospinal fluid may show raised protein levels, a raised cell count, predominantly lymphocytes, and sometimes a low glucose concentration. It is important to note that cerebrospinal fluid may be biochemically normal with localized lesions.

Other manifestations of neurosarcoid include peripheral neuropathy in about 15% of cases, psychiatric disturbances and, more rarely, spinal cord involvement [49].

Management

Having established the diagnosis, Sharma suggests that the use of corticosteroids in neurosarcoid is standard therapy [47]. Whilst considering the range of features from facial palsy which may well be transient and self-limiting through to persistent and life-threatening intracranial sarcoid granuloma, Scadding and Mitchell [46] divide patients into two categories: those with 'labile' disease capable of resolution, and those with 'late-stage' disease with irreversible fibrotic changes.

Surgery may be performed to establish the diagnosis, or to relieve clamant symptoms of hydrocephalus or symptomatic tumour masses; a role for surgery is limited.

Corticosteroid treatment with prednisolone in high daily dosage of up to 80 mg/day in the acute phase is suppressive, not curative, and will help to control only active granulomas. However, neurosarcoid responds less well than the disease in other tissues. Those who do respond may require long-term maintenance therapy, the morbidity of which can be reduced by alternate-day scheduling. Immunosuppressive drugs have been used in a few patients who did not respond to steroids. Isolated case reports of sarcoid meningitis and seizures responding to low-dose external-beam radiotherapy to the whole brain have documented symptomatic as well as objective improvement [48,50–53]. Seizure activity is an adverse prognostic feature. Supportive treatment with anticonvulsants is important.

Chordomas

Chordomas arise from the remnants of the embryonic notochord: those at the skull base are rarer than their sacral counterparts [54–57]. They are slow growing, locally aggressive, malignant tumours. Despite their origin in primitive tissue, these tumours typically affect adults in middle age, and very rarely occur in children. Males are twice as likely to be affected.

The tumour is rarely controlled by either surgery or irradiation alone, nor by a combination of both modalities. Its tendency to local recurrence and invasion of neighbouring structures leads to the eventual death of the patient in most cases [54]. The average survival time in a group of 55 patients reported by Heffelfinger *et al.* in 1973 [58] was 7.4 years.

Metastases develop on average in 10% of cases, usually to the lung, lymph nodes and liver. When they do occur, metastases tend to occur late in the course of the disease.

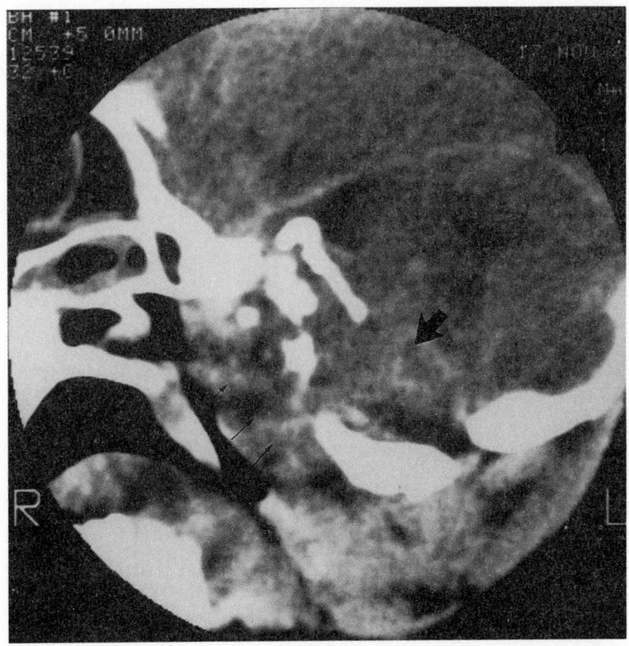

Fig. 18.6 Sagittally reconstructed computed tomographic scan through the skull showing destruction of the clivus by a chordoma (large arrow) with extension of the tumour into nasopharynx (small arrows).

Pathology

Chordomas appear grey and lobulated, and within soft tissue such as brain they appear soft and encapsulated with a 'pushing' margin. In bone, however, the tumour infiltrates along the line of least resistance and demarcation from normal tissue can be difficult. The tumour may expand and destroy bone [56,59].

Having arisen at the spheno-occipital synchondrosis, in the region of the clivus, the tumour may grow up and forwards towards, and into, the sellar and hypothalamic region. Other directions of spread may lead to involvement of the nasopharynx (Fig. 18.6), or more dangerously to pressure and invasion of the pons, medulla and upper cervical cord.

Tumours in the cranium tend to be smaller at diagnosis than those in the sacral area.

Microscopically, mitoses are usually infrequent, and mucin may be seen intracellularly, in the extracellular spaces and within cell nuclei. Dissolution of mucin in slide preparation causes a 'foamy' vacuolation and the commonly applied descriptive term 'physalliform'.

A significant chondroid component may cause problems in distinguishing chordoma from chondroma or chondrosarcoma. Heffelfinger *et al.* [58] suggested that a chondroid chordoma had a better outlook than the typical variant, with the average survival time being 15.8 years for the former and only 4.1 years for the latter group.

Clinical features

Symptoms are often present many months before diagnosis (range 4–24 months), and sometimes for even longer periods in chordomas of sacral origin [58].

Symptomatic headache of a generalized nature is a common complaint and may be associated with diplopia or deteriorating vision. The sixth cranial nerve is most often affected, causing a lateral rectus palsy.

Despite the tumour's mid-line origin, involved cranial nerves tend to be affected asymmetrically. Any nerve traversing the skull base may be compromised.

Unlike lesions arising within the pituitary gland, visual field defects tend to occur after the onset of headache. Marked superior extension may cause optic atrophy. Inferior extension of tumour into the nasopharynx may present as nasal obstruction or bleeding. Functional disturbances of the pituitary gland are uncommon.

Second to cranial nerve palsies, the next most common findings are due to compression of the pons, medulla and upper cervical spinal cord with attendant pyramidal tract signs and involvement of cranial nerve nuclei.

Radiology

Plain radiographic changes are characterised by osteolytic bony destruction without a periosteal reaction in the majority of intracranial chordomas. Bony sclerosis is uncommon. Soft-tissue swelling and distortion may be visible, as many calcium deposition within the tumour in a variety of patterns including a fine latticework or scattered flecks. Calcification has been reported in up to 50% of cases. The differential diagnosis includes tuberculosis, chondroma, chondrosarcoma, solitary plasmacytoma and lytic metastases, as well as craniopharyngioma and intracranial glioma [56,59]. CT scanning will provide more detailed information regarding the local extent of the tumour.

Management

Open surgical biopsy allows an adequate sample for definitive histological diagnosis. In view of their critical proximity to the brainstem, radical surgical removal is unlikely to be complete and should not be attempted in these locally aggressive tumours. Most groups now favour a combination of maximal but subtotal removal of tumour followed by external-beam radiotherapy to gain optimal palliation, yet appreciating the ultimate outcome in terms of survival is unlikely to be affected. Newer surgical approaches have been described which allow better access to the clivus: the Le Fort type I osteotomy approach to the clivus has been described by Uttley *et al.* [60]. By this technique, more extensive clival resections are possible, and it is likely that this will be the favoured first modality of therapy in future, followed by radiotherapy.

Radiotherapy delivered in high doses offers good palliation, the magnitude of dose required reflecting relative clinical radioresistance due to slow growth and low mitotic activity. No cures have been reported with radiotherapy alone. The proximity of critical normal structures, particularly brainstem and optic chiasm, limit the total dose that can be delivered by external-beam photon therapy, even with protracted fractionation. Tewfik *et al.* [57] suggested post-operative doses of 6000–6500 cGy in 6–7 weeks, increased to 7000–7500 cGy in unresectable lesions. Whilst this might be achieved in the sacral area, these doses could not be delivered safely to the region of the clivus by conventional external-beam photon technique. Recently, Rich *et al.* [61] have reported combined therapy with external-beam photons and 160 MeV protons to dose levels to the primary site in excess of 6500 cGy, with encouraging results both in the base of skull and cervical spine, albeit with limited length of follow-up. Further evidence that high radiation doses can be delivered by charged particle therapy with improved local control and an acceptable complication rate is provided by Castro *et al.* [62]. This group comments that irradiation after partial surgical excision is preferable, and this must now be advised as the best available therapy with several alternative focal radiotherapy methods competing for the ideal radiation boost to the clivus. No cytotoxic chemotherapy is known to be of benefit. With the historical 5-year disease-free survival rate being less than 10% [54], there are good reasons for exploring all these new approaches. Recently, improved survival in patients with skull base chordoma or chondrosarcoma has been reported using modern surgery and focused radiation [55].

Suprasellar germ-cell tumours

Despite their rarity, suprasellar germ-cell tumours attract considerable interest with their well-documented neuroendocrine presentation, their radiosensitivity and high cure rates. Primary intracranial germ-cell tumours comprise less than 1% of all intracranial neoplasms in the western world, with the highest incidence of 4–10% found in Japan [63,64].

The pathological appearance and classification of intracranial germ-cell tumours is identical to that applied to the more common gonadal primary, with the them 'germinoma' used intracranially for the analogous seminoma (Table 18.4). In common with other extragonadal germ-cell tumours, the primary intracranial sites are found in the mid-line, with the pineal the commonest followed by the suprasellar region. The latter were originally termed 'ectopic pinealomas' but this is, however, a misnomer, as no ectopic pineal cells have been found in the suprasellar region.

The natural history of suprasellar germ-cell tumours is enlargement with local infiltration producing characteristic neuroendocrine symptoms and signs. A coexisting pineal lesion may produce its own set of clinical signs. Germ-cell tumours may spread through the ventricular system and to the spinal canal via the cerebrospinal fluid.

Typically, suprasellar germ-cell tumour occurs in girls with a peak at the age of 10–12 years. Jennings *et al.* [65] reported, in a large retrospective review of the literature, that 75% of cases of primary intracranial germ-cell tumour in girls were suprasellar, whereas in boys the pineal region was involved in 67% of cases. They also found that 57% of all germinomas arose in the suprasellar region, whereas 68% of non-germinomatous germ-cell tumours occurred in the pineal site. The reason for the slightly higher incidence of germinomas in the suprasellar site and the relatively higher female incidence in this region is unknown.

Table 18.4 Pathological classification of intracranial germ-cell tumours.

Germinoma
Non-germinomatous germ-cell tumours
Embryonal carcinoma
Teratocarcinoma
Endodermal sinus tumour
Choriocarcinoma
Mixed
Differentiated teratoma

The typical clinical presentation of suprasellar germ-cell tumours includes the triad of diabetes insipidus, visual loss and hypopituitarism occurring in over 60% of patients [66–68]. Diabetes insipidus results from interruption of the hypothalamo-pituitary axis, and may precede the diagnosis of suprasellar germ-cell tumours by many months and sometimes years. Visual loss is slowly progressive, usually bitemporal, commencing in the inferior quadrants, and may be associated with a degree of optic atrophy. Hypopituitarism is usually clinically manifest as growth retardation, or delay or regression of sexual development; emaciation (the so-called 'diencephalic' syndrome), obesity, somnolence and precocious puberty may occur. Posterior hypothalamic lesions may present with part or all of Parinaud's triad—failure of upgaze, convergent nystagmus and Argyll Robertson pupils.

Skull radiography is usually normal but may show deformity of the pituitary fossa in the rare instance of intrasellar extension or pineal calcification if a coexistent lesion is present at this site. Unenhanced and enhanced CT scanning is the most useful investigation, and typically shows a mass of tissue homogeneity with strong uniform contrast enhancement (Fig. 18.7). Intracranial spread may be seen in the form of a second enhancing mass in the region of the pineal (Fig. 18.8), or involvement of the ventricular system with characteristic periventricular enhancement (Fig. 18.9), the latter being found more frequently in germinomas. Serum and cerebrospinal fluid estimations of β-hCG and α-fetoprotein (AFP) should be performed. While most germinomas are expected to be marker negative, an elevation of hCG in the cerebrospinal fluid may be found. The presence of elevated AFP in cerebrospinal fluid or serum is indicative of non-germinomatous germ-cell tumour [69]. Cerebrospinal fluid cytology may demonstrate the presence of the classical two-cell pattern of germinoma, although the incidence of this finding varies widely (0–55%) [70–72]. Unfortunately, this parameter alone is neither sensitive nor specific enough to correlate the incidence of spinal seeding accurately [68]. Myelography is the preferred investigation which reliably demonstrates synchronous spinal deposits and should be routinely performed; MRI is currently under evaluation, and the results of prospective correlation in conjunction with myelography are awaited before its role can be defined (Fig. 18.10).

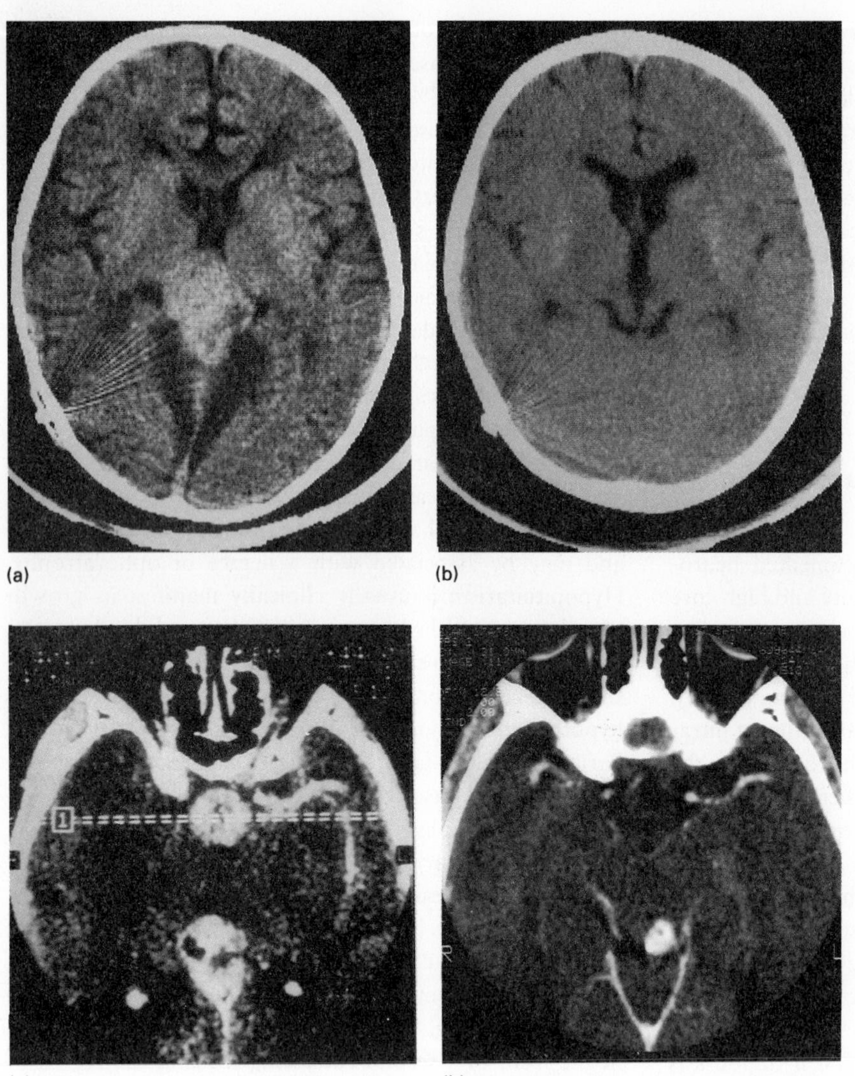

Fig. 18.7 Enhanced transaxial computed tomographic scans of a pineal germinoma before (a) and after (b) craniospinal irradiation. There is a burr hole artefact.

Fig. 18.8 Enhanced transaxial computed tomographic scans of a young girl with synchronous germ-cell tumours in both pineal and suprasellar sites before (a) and after (b) craniospinal irradiation.

Biopsy of the suprasellar region is now associated with a low morbidity rate when performed stereotactically. Histological diagnosis is required for diagnosis, and also to discriminate between germinoma and non-germinomatous germ-cell tumours, the latter requiring more aggressive therapy (see below). However, most authorities would accept elevated tumour markers and a mid-line mass in this region as diagnostic, certainly if the cerebrospinal fluid cytology was also positive.

Radical attempts at surgical resection no longer have a role in management.

Non-germinomatous germ-cell tumours are not as radiosensitive as germinoma and have poorer local control and survival rates. In the Royal Marsden Hospital series [73], Dearnley *et al.* reported an 18% actuarial 10-year survival rate for such tumours, compared with 69% for germinomas. Sano *et al.* [74] found that choriocarcinoma and yolk sac variants were particularly fatal.

In biopsy-confirmed suprasellar germ-cell tumours, irradiation is given to the entire craniospinal axis. Preradiotherapy staging by myelography and cerebrospinal fluid cytology is performed in the absence of raised intracranial pressure. Treatment is given with the patient prone, and the cranium is treated with parallel opposed megavoltage portals with a carefully matched posterior portal to the spine (two separate spinal fields may be required, depending on the total length). Meticulous attention to detail is essential at the sites of matching the radiation fields to avoid any unnecessary gap (underdosage) or overlap (the very real risk of overdosage of the spinal cord). Craniospinal irradiation delivers 30–35 Gy in 20–23 daily fractions to the whole brain and spine followed by a boost to the primary tumour, with a 2-cm margin giving a further 20 Gy in 12 daily fractions using a three-field technique. Any 'drop' spinal metastases would be boosted.

While craniospinal irradiation remains the 'gold standard',

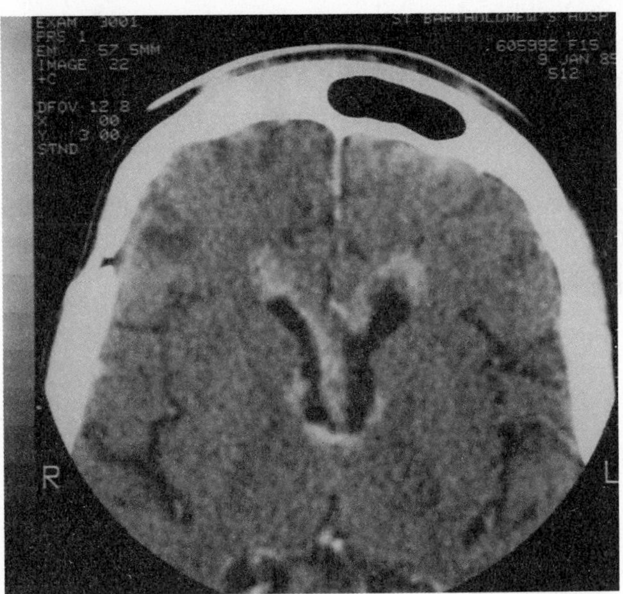

Fig. 18.9 Enhanced computed tomographic scan of a child with a suprasellar germ-cell tumour, demonstrating the characteristic periventricular enhancement.

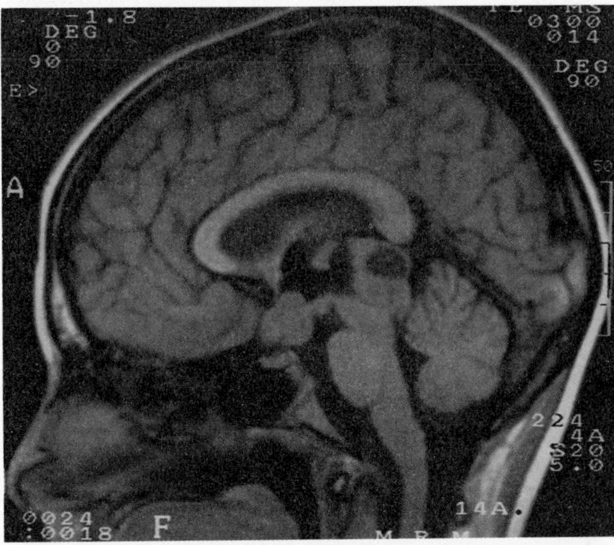

Fig. 18.10 Magnetic resonance image of a germinoma in a 14-year-old boy: tumour masses in the region of both the anterior hypothalamus and pineal region are shown. (Courtesy of Professor S. Webb, Hospital de la Santa Creu i Santa Pau, Barcelona, Spain.)

various authors have questioned the validity of routine spinal irradiation [70,75], particularly in young children where radiation will reduce spinal growth. The estimated incidence of spinal metastases varies widely (0–33%) [69,76–81], with an average of 12% for a total of 576 pooled patients [82]. A meaningful incidence applicable to germinoma alone is even less clear, as a significant number of patients were historically diagnosed on the basis of a 'radiosensitivity test' to the primary. However, the lack of successful salvage therapy for patients relapsing in the spine after local treatment [69,76,83] argues for very careful selection criteria to identify 'low-risk' patients for whom less than craniospinal irradiation may be contemplated; these would all be proven germinomas.

Unfortunately, the rarity of intracranial germ-cell tumours and the historical lack of histological verification in many patients means that the size of most published series of verified germinomas and non-germinomatous germ-cell tumours is small. Nevertheless, recent publications have demonstrated that 10-year survival rates of 70–100% are achievable (Table 18.5).

With excellent survival results for germinoma, attention has been directed at more accurately assessing and subsequently reducing the associated treatment morbidity, including significant intellectual retardation [84–88], neuroendocrine [89,90] and non-endocrine growth problems associated with craniospinal radiotherapy. Current novel approaches include the proposal that primary platinum-based combination chemotherapy, demonstrably very active in both systemic and brain germ-cell tumours [91], could allow a reduction in radiation doses for the subsequent cerebrospinal irradiation [92]. Thus, several groups, including our own, now employ two or more cycles of primary or neoadjuvant chemotherapy routinely before craniospinal irradiation in all of these patients [93]. There are good initial responses, and we believe that studies currently in progress will show that the dose to the craniospinal axis may be safely lowered in patients demonstrating good response.

Additionally, with the known radiosensitivity of seminoma and the prediction that disproportionate sparing of normal CNS tissues could be expected with a lower dose per fraction [95,96], we are currently studying a partial transmission block technique [97,98]. By such a technique, the total doses to all sites and the conventional dose per fraction to the primary site are maintained, but the dose per fraction to the rest of the cranium is reduced. The length of treatment is not prolonged. The advantage of this technique is perceived to be reduction in neuropsychological sequelae.

Table 18.5 Survival rates of patients with intracranial germinomas.

Series	No. of patients	Histological confirmation (%)	10-year survival rate (%)
Dearnley *et al.* [73]	34	26	69
Jenkin *et al.* [84]	21	76	90
Shibamoto *et al.* [71]	42	100	79

In conclusion, suprasellar germ-cell tumours usually present with the well-defined clinical triad of diabetes insipidus, visual field loss and hypopituitarism. Following histological verification, excellent cure results may be obtained with cerebrospinal irradiation, and systemic chemotherapy is establishing itself in primary treatment protocols. Further studies are on-going to minimize long-term, treatment-related morbidity without prejudicing the excellent long-term survival results.

Other conditions

Secondary deposits (metastases) show a preferential distribution in the posterior pituitary and present with diabetes insipidus. Primary carcinomas of the breast and bronchus are particularly noteworthy in this regard, although the overall incidence is low. It should also be pointed out that some cytotoxic drugs which might be used in the chemotherapy of these cancers, namely vincristine and cyclophosphamide, may temporarily stimulate antidiuretic hormone secretion. The treatment of such secondary deposits is radiotherapy (usually whole-brain radiotherapy in this context of brain metastases). We have seen at least one case of reversal of diabetes insipidus by such therapy.

Other mass lesions in this region are very rare. *Tuberculomas* in this region are well documented and other granuloma-like conditions must therefore be possible, namely fungal infections, cysticercosis, etc. The treatment is that of the underlying condition. *Meningiomas* of the sphenoid ridge or in the region of the clinoids may impinge upon the pituitary region, and we have seen several patients presenting with long-standing amenorrhoea and galactorrhoea. Surgical resection is the treatment of choice.

Giant-cell tumours are most commonly found near the epiphysial plates of long bones. Histologically, they comprise stromal cells and giant cells; the latter are now regarded as fusion products of the mesenchymal stromal cells, and are not now regarded as of osteoclast origin. Mitoses may be much in evidence and these tumours can be locally very aggressive.

Young adult women are most commonly affected. Surgical *en bloc* resection or curettage and, if incomplete, postoperative radiotherapy, are curative in the majority of cases [99,100]. There have been rare reports of sphenoid giant-cell tumours, and we have been referred two such cases (both young women) recently. Both patients have been successfully managed by surgery [60] and postoperative radiotherapy (45 Gy in 25 fractions). It may be noted that a young patient at Massachussetts General Hospital also did well following this approach [100]. The radiation dose is of the order that is prescribed for pituitary adenoma (see Chapter 20).

Lastly, there is the group of conditions that invade through the skull base from below—in the case of nasopharyngeal carcinoma, usually taking the line of least resistance through the foramen lacerum and causing oculomotor palsies before reaching the sella. In addition, malignant mid-line granuloma (of Wegener) and other conditions in this region may also invade in a similar manner.

References

1 Newman MM, Halmi KA. The endocrinology of anorexia nervosa and bulimia nervosa. *Endocrinol Metab Clin North Am* 1988; **17**: 195.

2 Cohen ME, Kressel-Duffner P. Diagnosis and management of common intracranial tumors of childhood. In: Cohen ME, Kressel-Duffner P, eds. *Brain Tumors in Children. Principles of Diagnosis and Treatment.* New York: Raven Press, 1984: 103–294.

3 Costin G. Endocrine disorders associated with tumors of the pituitary and hypothalamus. Symposium on Pediatric Endocrinology. *Pediatr Clin North Am* 1979; **26**: 15–31.

4 Cohen ME, Kressel-Duffner P. Long-term clinical effects of radiation and chemotherapy. In: Cohen ME, Kressel-Duffner P, eds. *Brain Tumors in Children, Principles of Diagnosis and Treatment.* New York: Raven Press, 1984: 308–27.

5 Oberfield SE, Allen JC, Pollack J, New MI, Levine LS. Long-term endocrine sequelae after treatment of medulloblastoma: prospective study of growth and thyroid function. *J Pediatr* 1986; **108**: 219–23.

6 Schröder JM. Zerebrale Raumfordernde Prozesse Allgemeine Pathologie, Klassifikation und biologische Wertigkeit der intrakraniellen raumfordernden Prozesse. In: Hopf HCh, Poeck K, Schliach H, eds. *Neurologie in Praxis und Klinik.* Stuttgart: G. Thieme, 1986: 6.1–6.13.

7 Voth D, Gutjahr P, Langmaid C, eds. *Tumours of the Central Nervous Systems in Infancy and Childhood.* Berlin: Springer-Verlag, 1982.

8 Schulte FJ. Intracranial tumors in childhood—concepts of treatment and prognosis. *Neuropediatrics* 1984; **15**: 3–12.

9 Leviton A. Principles of epidemiology. In: Cohen ME, Kressel-Duffner P, eds. *Brain Tumors in Children. Principles of Diagnosis and Treatment.* New York: Raven Press, 1984: 22–46.

10 Czernichow P, Robinson AG, eds. *Diabetes Insipidus in Man. Frontiers of Hormone Research*, Vol. 13. Basel: S. Karger, 1985.

11 Vanderscheueren-Lodeweckx M. Assessment of growth hormone secretion: what are we looking for practically? *Horm Res* 1990; 33 (Suppl. 4): 1–6.

12 Ho KY, Weiseberger AJ. Secretory patterns of growth hormone according to sex and age. *Horm Res* 1990; **33** (Suppl. 4): 7–11.

13 Girard J, Fischer Wasels T. Measurement of urinary growth hormone. *Horm Res* 1990; **33** (Suppl. 4): 12–18.

14 Reiter EO, Martha PM, Jr. Pharmacological testing of growth hormone secretion. *Horm Res* 1990; **33**: 121–7.

15 Frohman LA, Jansson JO. Growth hormone-releasing hormone. *Endocr Rev* 1986; **7**: 223–53.

16 Stalla GK, Stalla J, Schopohl J, von Werder K, Müller OA. Corticotropin-releasing factor in humans. I. CRF stimulation in normals and CRF radioimmunoassay. *Horm Res* 1986; **24**: 229–45.

17 Müller OA, Stalla GK, von Werder K. Corticotropin-releasing

factor in humans. II. CRF stimulation in patients with diseases of the hypothalamo-pituitary–adrenal-axis. *Horm Res* 1987; **25**: 185–98.

18 Chakeres DW, Curtin A, Ford G. Magnetic resonance imaging of pituitary and parasellar abnormalities. *Radiol Clin North Am* 1989; **27**: 265–81.

19 Kucharczyk W, Brant-Zawadzki M, Sobel D *et al.* Central nervous system tumors in children: detection by magnetic resonance imaging. *Radiology* 1985; **155**: 131–6.

20 Shalet SM, Clayton PE, Price DA. Growth and pituitary function in children treated for brain tumors or acute lymphoblastic leukaemia. *Horm Res* 1988; **30**: 53–61.

21 Packer RJ, Meadows AT, Rorke LB, Goldwein JL, Angio GD. Long term sequelae of cancer treatment on the central nervous system in childhood. *Med Pediatr Oncol* 1987; **15**: 241–53.

22 Job JC. Results of long term growth hormone replacement therapy in children: when and how to treat. *Horm Res* 1990; **33** (Suppl. 4): 69–76.

23 Sönksen PH. Replacement therapy in hypothalamo-pituitary insufficiency after childhood. Management in the adult. *Horm Res* 1990; **33**: 45–51.

24 Christiansen JS, Jorgensen JO, Pederson SA, Moller J, Jorgensen J, Skakkabaek N-E. Effects of growth hormone on body composition in adults. *Horm Res* 1990; **33** (Suppl. 4): 61–4.

25 Fahlbusch R, Marguth F. Raumfordernde Prozesse der Hypophyse und des sellanahen Bereiches. In: Hopf HCh, Poeck K, Schliach H, eds. *Neurologie in Praxis und Klinik*. Stuttgart: G. Thieme, 1986: 6.55–6.59.

26 Cohen ME, Kressel-Duffner P. Craniopharyngiomas. In: Cohen MC, Kressel-Duffner P, eds. *Brain Tumors in Children. Principles of Diagnosis and Treatment*. New York: Raven Press, 1984: 193–210.

27 Lalau Keraly J, Aubier F, Derome P, Kalifa Ch, Lemerle J, Canlorbe P, Chaussain JL, Job JC. Evolution à moyen terme des craniopharyngiomes de l'enfant en fonction des choix thérapeutiques initiaux. *Arch Fr Pediatr* 1986; **43**: 593–9.

28 Stahnke N, Grubel G, Lagenstein I, Willig RP. Long-term follow-up of children with craniopharyngioma. *Eur J Pediatr* 1984; **142**: 179–85.

29 Turpin G, Heshmati HM, Scherrer H, Metzger J, Bataini J, Philippon J, De Gennes JL. Tumeurs hypothalamiques primitives (en dehors des cranio-pharyngiomes). Etude endocrinienne et evolutive post-radiotherapique. A propos de 17 observations. *Ann Med Interne (Paris)* 1986; **137**: 395–400.

30 Barral V, Brunelle F, Brauner R, Rappaport R, Lallemand D. MRI of hypothalamic hamartomas in children. *Pediatr Radiol* 1988; **18**: 449–52.

31 Sharma RR. Hamartoma of the hypothalamus and tuber cinereum: a brief review of the literature. *J Postgrad Med* 1987; **33**: 1–13.

32 Ladisch S, Jaffe ES. The histiocytoses. In: Pizzo PA, Poplack DA, eds. *Principles and Practice of Pediatric Oncology*. Philadelphia: JB Lippincott, 1989; 491–504.

33 Osband ME, Lipton JM, Lavin O. Histiocytosis X: demonstration of abnormal immunity, T cell histamine H2 receptor deficiency and successful treatment with thymic extract. *N Engl J Med* 1981; **304**: 146–53.

34 Nesbit ME. Current concepts and treatment of histiocytosis X, (Langerhans cell histiocytosis X). In: Voute PA, Barrett A, Bloom HJG, Lemerle J, Neidhardt MK, eds. *Cancer in Children*. Berlin: Springer-Verlag, 1986: 176–84.

35 Smolik EA, Devecerski D, Nelson JS, Smith KR. Histiocytosis X in the optic chiasm of an adult with hypopituitarism. *J Neurosurg* 1968; **29**: 290–5.

36 Mayou S, Plowman PN, Munro D. Langerhans cell histiocytosis: excellent response to etoposide. *Clin Exp Dermatol* 1991; **16**: 292–4.

37 Hand A. Defects of membranous bones, exophthalmos and polyuria in childhood. Is it dyspituitarism? *Am J Med Sci* 1921; **162**: 509–15.

38 Schuller A. Uber eigenartige Schädeldefekte im Kindersalter. *Fortschr Rontgenstr* 1915; **23**: 12–18.

39 Christian HA. Defects in membranous bones, exophthalmos and diabetes insipidus: an unusual syndrome of dyspituitarism. *Med Clin North Am* 1920; **3**: 849–71.

40 Haslam RHA, Clark DBA. Progressive cerebellar ataxia associated with Hand–Schüller–Christian disease. *Dev Med Child Neurol* 1971; **13**: 174–9.

41 Iraci G, Chieco-Bianchi L, Giordano R, Gerosa M. Histiocytosis X of the central nervous system. Clinical and pathological report of a case with predominant cerebellar involvement. *Childs Brain* 1979; **5**: 116–30.

42 Salcman M, Quest DO, Mount LA. Histiocytosis X of the spinal cord. *J Neurosurg* 1974; **41**: 383–6.

43 Hewlett RH, Ganz JC. Histocytosis of the cauda equina. *Neurology (Minneapolis)* 1976; **26**: 472–6.

44 Greenberger JS, Cassady JR, Jaffe N, Vawter G, Crocker AC. Radiation therapy in patients with histiocytosis: management of diabetes insipidus and bone lesions. *Int J Radiat Oncol Biol Phys* 1979; **5**: 1749–55.

45 Subcommittee on Classification and Definition. Description of sarcoidosis. *Ann NY Acad Sci* 1976; **278**: 743.

46 Scadding J, Mitchell D. *Sarcoidosis*, 2nd edn. London: Chapman and Hall, 1985.

47 Sharma OP. *Sarcoidosis. Clinical Management*. London: Butterworths, 1984.

48 Grizzanti J, Knapp A, Schecter A, Williams MH. Treatment of sarcoid meningitis with radiotherapy. *Am J Med* 1982; **73**: 605–8.

49 Delaney P. Neurological manifestations in sarcoidosis. *Ann Intern Med* 1977; **87**: 336–45.

50 Bejar J, Kerby G, Ziegker D, Festoff B. Treatment of CNS sarcoidosis with radiotherapy. *Ann Neurol* 1985; **18**: 258–60.

51 Feibelman R, Harman E. Sarcoid meningoencephalitis treated with high dose steroids and radiation (letter). *Ann Intern Med* 1985; **102**: 136.

52 Scully R, Mark E, McNeely W, McNeely B. Case records of Massachusetts General Hospital. *N Engl J Med* 1991; **324**: 677–87.

53 Rubenstein I, Gray T, Moldofsky H, Hoffstein V. Neurosarcoid associated with hypersomnolence treated with corticosteroids and brain irradiation. *Chest* 1988; **94**: 205–6.

54 Perez C, Lindberg R, Montague E, Saxton J. Unusual non-epithelial tumours of the head and neck. In: Perez C, Brady L, eds. *Principles and Practice of Radiation Oncology*. Philadelphia: Lippincott Co., 1987; 619–35.

55 Gay E, Sekhar LN, Rubinstein E *et al.* Chordomas and chondrosarcomas of the skull base: Results and follow-up of sixty patients. *Neurosurgery* 1995; **36**: 887–95.

56 Phillips TL, Newman H. Chordomas. In: Deeley TJ, ed. *Modern Radiotherapy and Oncology: Central Nervous System Tumours*. London: Butterworths, 1974.

57 Tewfik H, McGinnis W, Nordstrom D, Latourette H. Chordoma. Evaluation of clinical behaviour and treatment modalities. *Int J Radiat Oncol Biol Phys* 1977; **2**: 959–62.

58 Heffelfinger M, Dahlin D, MacCarty C, Beaubout J. Chordoma and cartilaginous tumours at the skull base. *Cancer* 1973; **32**: 410–20.

59 Hankinson J, Banna M. *Pituitary and Parapituitary Tumours*. Philadelphia: WB Saunders, 1976.

60 Uttley D, Moore M, Archer D. Surgical management of midline skull base tumours: a new approach. *J Neurosurg* 1989; **71**: 705–10.

61 Rich T, Schiller A, Suit H, Mankin H. Clinical and pathological review of 48 cases of chordoma. *Cancer* 1985; **56**: 182–7.

62 Castro J, Collier J, Petti P *et al.* Charged particle radiotherapy for lesions encircling the brain stem or spinal cord. *Int J Radiat Oncol Biol Phys* 1989; **17**: 477–84.

63 Katsura S, Suzuki J, Wada TA. Statistical study of brain tumours in the neurosurgery clinics of Japan. *J Neurosurg* 1959; **16**: 570–88.

64 Koide O, Watanabe Y, Sata K. A pathological survey of intracranial germinoma and pinealoma in Japan. *Cancer* 1980; **45**: 2119–30.

65 Jennings MT, Geman R, Hochberg F. Intracranial germ cell tumours: natural history and pathogenesis. *J Neurosurg* 1985; **63**: 155–67.

66 Imura H, Kato Y, Nakai Y. Endocrine aspects of tumours arising from suprasellar, third ventricle regions. *Prog Exp Tumor Res* 1987; **30**: 313–24.

67 Kageyama N, Kobayashi T, Kida Y, Yoshida J, Kato K. Intracranial germinal tumours. *Prog Exp Tumor Res* 1987; **30**: 255–67.

68 Sung DI, Harisiadis L, Chang CH. Midline pineal tumours and suprasellar germinomas: highly curable by radiation. *Radiology* 1978; **128**: 745–51.

69 Arita N, Ustico Y, Hayakawa T *et al.* Role of tumour markers in the management of intracranial germ cell tumours. *Prog Exp Tumor Res* 1987; **30**: 289–95.

70 Linstadt D, Wara WM, Edwards MSB, Hudgins RJ, Sheline GE. Radiotherapy of primary intracranial germinomas: the case against routine craniospinal irradiation. *Int J Radiat Oncol Biol Phys* 1988; **15**: 291–7.

71 Shibamoto Y, Abe M, Yamashita J *et al.* Treatment results of intracranial germinoma as a function of irradiated volume. *Int J Radiat Oncol Biol Phys* 1988; **15**: 285–90.

72 Ueki K, Tanaka R. Treatments and prognosis of pineal tumours: experience of 110 cases. *Neurol Med Chir (Tokyo)* 1980; **20**: 1–26.

73 Dearnley DP, A'Hearn RP, Whittaker S, Bloom HJG. Pineal and CNS germ cell tumours: Royal Marsden Hospital Experience 1962–1987. *Int J Radiat Oncol Biol Phys* 1990; **18**: 773–81.

74 Sano K. So-called intracranial germ cell tumours: are they really of germ cell origin? *Br J Neurosurg* 1995; **9**: 391–401.

75 Amendola BE, McLatchey K, Amendola MA. Pineal region tumours: analysis of treatment results. *Int J Radiat Oncol Biol Phys* 1984; **10**: 991–7.

76 Abay EO, Laws ER, Grado GL *et al.* Pineal tumours in children and adolescents. Treatment by CSF shunting and radiotherapy. *J Neurosurg* 1981; **55**: 889–95.

77 Salazar OM, Castro-Vita H, Bakos RS, Feldstein ML, Keller B, Rubin P. Radiation therapy for tumours of the pineal region. *Int J Radiat Oncol Biol Phys* 1979; **5**: 491–9.

78 Waga S, Handa H, Yamashita J. Intracranial germinomas: treatment and results. *Surg Neurol* 1979; **11**: 167–72.

79 Maier JG, De Jong D. Pineal body tumour. *Am J Roentgenol* 1967; **99**: 826–32.

80 Wara WM, Jenkin DT, Evans A. Tumours of the pineal and suprasellar region: Children's Cancer Study Group treatment results 1960–75. *Cancer* 1979; **43**: 698–701.

81 Chapman PH, Lingood RM. The management of pineal area tumours. *Cancer* 1980; **46**: 1253–7.

82 Bloom HJG. Primary intracranial germ cell tumours. *Clin Oncol* 1983; **2**: 233–57 .

83 Griffin BR, Griffen TW, Tung DYK *et al.* Pineal region tumours: results of radiation therapy and indications for elective spinal radiation. *Int J Radiat Oncol Biol Phys* 1981; **7**: 605–8.

84 Jenkin D, Berry M, Chan H *et al.* Pineal region germinomas in childhood. Treatment considerations. *Int J Radiat Oncol Biol Phys* 1982; **8**: 1869–76.

85 Silverman C, Simpson J. Cerebellar medulloblastoma: the importance of posterior fossa dose to survival and patterns of failure. *Int J Radiat Oncol Biol Phys* 1982; **8**: 1869–76.

86 Cohen ME, Duffner PK. Ependymomas. In: Cohen ME, Duffner PK, eds. *Brain Tumours in Childhood. Principles of Diagnosis and Treatment*. New York: Raven Press, 1984; 136–55.

87 Janoun L, Bloom HJG. Long term psychological effects in children for intracranial tumours. *Int J Radiat Oncol Biol Phys* 1990; **18**: 747–53.

88 Walterhouse DO, Meadows AT. Late effects of childhood cancer therapy. In: Plowman PN, Meadows A, McElwain TI, eds. *The Complications of Cancer Management*. London: Butterworths, 1990: 95–113.

89 Blacklay A, Grossman A, Savage M. Cranial irradiation in children with cerebral tumours — evidence for a hypothalamic defect in growth hormone release. *J Endocrinol* 1986; **108**: 25–9.

90 Grossman A. Endocrine morbidity of cancer treatment. In: Plowman PN, Meadows A, McElwain TI, eds. *The Complications of Cancer Management*. London: Butterworths, 1990: 412–22.

91 Douek E, Kingston JE, Malpas JS, Plowman PN. Platinum-based chemotherapy for recurrent CNS tumours in young patients. *J Neurol Neurosurg Psych* 1991; **54**: 722–5.

92 Allen JC, Kim JH, Packer RJ. Neoadjuvant chemotherapy for newly diagnosed germ cell tumours of the central nervous system. *J Neurosurg* 1987; **67**: 65–70.

93 Sebag-Montefiore DJ, Douek E, Kingstion JE, Plowman PN. Intracranial germ cell tumours. I: Experience with platinum based chemotherapy and implications for the recommended craniospinal radiation dose. *Clin Oncol* 1992; **4**: 345–50.

94 Rustin GJS, Newlands ES, Bagshawe KD, Begent RHJ, Crawford SM. Successful management of metastatic and primary germ cell tumour in the brain. *Cancer* 1986; **57**: 2108–13.

95 Sheline GE. Irradiation injury of the human brain - a review of clinical experience. In: Gilbert HA, Kagan AR, eds. *Radiation Injury to the Central Nervous System*. New York: Raven Press, 39–58.

96 Thames HD, Hendry JH. *Fractionation in Radiotherapy*. London: Taylor and Francis.

97 Plowman PN, Doughty D. An innovative method for neuroaxis radiotherapy using partial transmission block technique—a recently adopted treatment regime for medulloblastoma/primitive neurectodermal CNS tumour/intracranial germ cell tumours/pineoblastoma/high risk ependymoma. *Br J Radiol* 1991; **63**: 745–51.

98 Sebag-Montefiore DJ, Doughty D, Plowman PN. Intracranial germ cell tumours. II: Craniospinal radiotherapy using the recently

adopted partial transmission block technique. *Clin Oncol* 1992; **4**: 351–4.

99 del Regato JA, Spjut HJ. In: del Regato, Spjut, eds *Cancer: Diagnosis, Treatment and Prognosis*. Chicago: CV Mosby Co., 1977: 877–916.

100 Schwartz LH, Okunieff PG, Rosenberg A, Suit HD. Radiation therapy in the treatment of difficult giant cell tumours. *Int J Radiat Oncol Biol Phys* 1989; **17**: 1085–8.

CHAPTER 19

The surgery of hypothalamo-pituitary tumours

C.B.T. Adams

Introduction

The surgery of pituitary tumours has changed considerably in the past 15 years. Formerly, it was directed to saving vision by removing the bulk of the tumour and so relieving chiasmal compression. Cairns [1,2] concluded in 1935: 'Pituitary tumour is a disease that destroys sight rather than life, and therefore the risks to life of operative treatment must be reduced to the lowest possible dimension.' However, in the past 15 years neurosurgical objectives have enlarged with the aim of eradicating secreting tumours and so producing biochemical cure while preserving pituitary function. Transsphenoidal surgery, using magnification and image intensification, is responsible for this improvement.

The history of transsphenoidal surgery extends back to Koenig in 1898, who is credited with having first approached the pituitary gland by this route. Halstead [3] in 1910 introduced the sublabial approach, which Cushing [4] adapted in 1912. Cushing later abandoned this approach in favour of transfrontal surgery, but his disciple, Norman Dott, continued its use. Guiot, who went to Edinburgh to learn the technique from Dott, in turn taught Hardy [5]. Hardy's use of the operating microscope and X-ray fluoroscopy ensured widespread acceptance, so the pendulum has swung back, and now the majority of pituitary tumours are approached transsphenoidally.

The treatment of pituitary tumours employs medical, surgical and radiotherapeutic methods. These differing therapies should not be thought to be in competition; the best results are obtained by the judicious use of all three methods, knowing the advantages, disadvantages and risks of each. Clearly, the aim of treatment is the eradication of the tumour, restoration of biochemical and visual abnormalities, and preservation of pituitary function without significant risk, complication or possibility of future recurrence. No one method of treatment can attain these ideals, but obviously which of the available treatments are used depends not only on the pathology of the tumour but also the availability of specialist skills and equipment. The best surgical results occur in centres where one surgeon has particular experience of this type of surgery; the occasional foray into the pituitary fossa should be discouraged, yet endocrinologists have to provide their chosen surgeon with a sufficient number of patients to establish and maintain his or her skills and interest.

Classification of pituitary tumours

While the histopathology of these tumours is dealt with in more detail in Chapter 5, for neurosurgical purposes the simpler the classification, the better [6]. There are two basic assessments necessary: the function (or non-function) of the tumour, and its size. Thus, although the term 'non-functioning' is a misnomer, for these tumours often secrete luteinising hormone (LH) and follicle-stimulating hormone (FSH), and perhaps other yet unidentified hormones, it is a convenient term used to denote a tumour that does not produce excess adrenocorticotrophic hormone (ACTH), growth hormone or prolactin. The diagnosis of prolactinoma may be difficult; a prolactinoma will secrete prolactin in tissue culture, and immunostaining will show prolactin-secreting cells. A non-functioning tumour may produce a stalk compression or disconnection phenomenon, interfering with tonic inhibition of prolactin secretion. Thus, hyperprolactinaemia is a blood test result and not a diagnosis.

Bevan [7] showed that a serum prolactin concentration of less than 3000 mU/l usually indicates a non-functioning tumour. A level over 8000 mU/l is always due to a prolactinoma, but between these limits either diagnosis may exist; cognizance of the size of the tumour in relation to the prolactin level will often clarify which type of tumour is present. It is interesting to classify the histological diagnosis in patients

Table 19.1 Non-adenomatous pathology found during transsphenoidal surgery (n = 14).

Pathology	*n*
Craniopharyngioma*†	4
Empty sella*	2
Sterile abscess	1
Arachnoid cyst*	1
Lymphocytic 'hypophysitis'*†	1
Carcinoid*	1
Chondrosarcoma	1
Meningioma*†	1
Dysgerminoma	1
Aspergilloma*	1

* Serum prolactin level elevated up to 5260 mU/l;
† Patients given bromocriptine elsewhere on the assumption that a prolactinoma was present, without 'tumour' shrinkage.

Table 19.2 Classification of pituitary tumours according to function and size.

Size	Determined by coronal MRI scanning
1 Microadenoma	< 10 mm. No suprasella extension
2 Mesoadenoma	10–20 mm, i.e. < 10-mm suprasella extension
3 Macroadenoma	> 20 mm, i.e. suprasella extension > 10 mm (a) No evidence of invasion (b) Invasive—radiological/CT evidence

referred to me, who were treated with bromocriptine on the assumption that they had a prolactinoma (Table 19.1).

I have found a simple classification of the size of pituitary tumours as determined by coronal magnetic resonance (MRI) scanning to be of considerable use (Table 19.2). It has always seemed to me incongruous that 1–2 mm may change a tumour classification from a microadenoma to macroadenoma. An intermediate size—a mesoadenoma—makes therapeutic as well as pathological sense. In our unit the management of prolactinomas very much depends on whether the adenoma is micro, meso or macro in size [6].

The advantages of transsphenoidal surgery

Transsphenoidal surgery has several advantages over transfrontal surgery. It is certainly less traumatic, and patients usually stay in hospital for only 4–5 days after surgery. The brain is undisturbed, obviating the mental confusion which not infrequently follows frontal lobe retraction, nor of course is there a risk of epilepsy, so that the patient can drive without delay. Visual recovery is quicker for two reasons: first, a

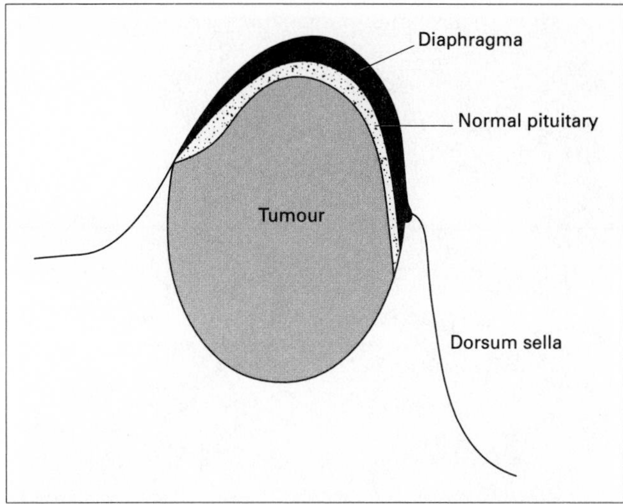

Fig. 19.1 Explanation of preservation of pituitary function following transsphenoidal surgery. Normal pituitary gland is displaced upwards to the subdiaphragmatic position. Thus, normal pituitary tissue is preserved following transsphenoidal surgery while it tends to be damaged following transfrontal surgery.

better decompression is obtained beneath the optic nerves; and, second, these nerves are not manipulated. I believe there is better preservation of pituitary function because the adenoma pushes the normal remnants of pituitary tissue against the diaphragma sella (Fig. 19.1), which is undisturbed when the tumour is removed transsphenoidally, whereas it is coagulated and incised by the transfrontal approach. Transsphenoidal surgery is most unlikely to cause hypopituitarism if pituitary function was normal before operation. Finally, I believe that the surgeon can obtain a much more complete removal of tumour transsphenoidally because this approach allows direct vision into the pituitary fossa (Fig. 19.2); transfrontal surgery must inevitably leave tumour in the fossa. When operating on a large pituitary tumour, I carry out a perioperative lateral cisternal puncture, which allows air to be injected intracranially, forcing the suprasellar tumour extension down into the evacuated pituitary fossa. This technique has the added advantage of allowing cerebrospinal fluid to be withdrawn in order to slacken the tense diaphragma, and so minimize the chance of cerebrospinal fluid leakage.

In my opinion, there are two absolute contraindications to the transsphenoidal approach. The first is when the tumour is highly unlikely to be a pituitary adenoma. In other words, if the history, signs and radiological findings suggest a meningioma, craniopharyngioma or particularly an aneurysm, then the approach should be transfrontal, unless the tumour is small and entirely intrasellar. The second absolute contraindication is if the surgeon finds at operation that the pituitary tumour is tough; no attempt should be

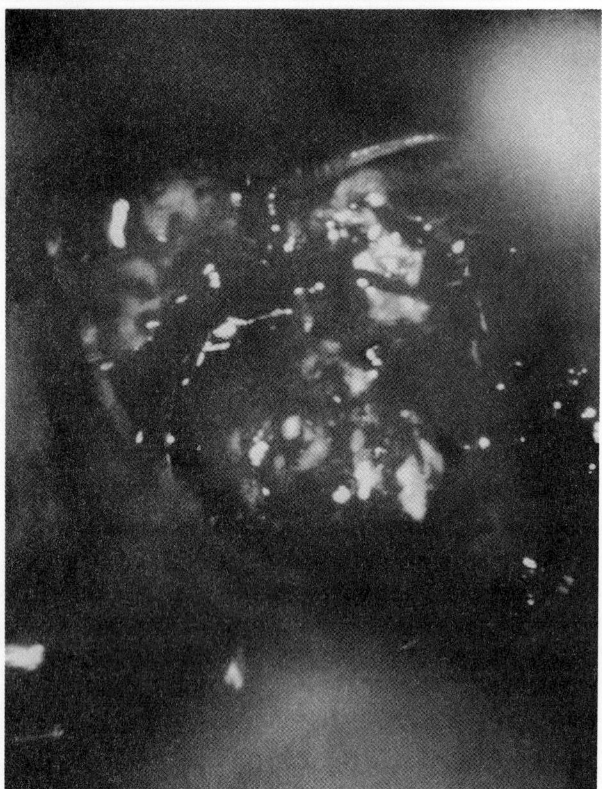

Fig. 19.2 A well-defined adenoma surrounded by normal anterior lobe of the pituitary gland. The transsphenoidal approach, unlike the transfrontal approach, allows not only selective removal of such microadenomas but also visualisation of the whole of the pituitary fossa and more complete removal of larger tumours.

made to remove such a tumour, but rather a small biopsy should be taken and the surgeon should abandon the operation, taking care to pack the sphenoid sinus with fat and fascia. Failure to do this will almost certainly lead to cerebrospinal fluid leakage after the subsequent transfrontal approach, and may also follow radiotherapy. However, it must be stressed that it is consistency, not size, that determines operability by the transsphenoidal approach. I have removed large tumours extending to the septum pellucidum via the transsphenoidal route. Fortunately, tough tumours are rare, < 1% in my personal series. Very occasionally a combined transfrontal/transsphenoidal approach is indicated when, for instance, there is tumour recurrence even after adequate surgery and radiotherapy. In these (rare) circumstances, I have used a transfrontal approach which allows one to drill through the tuberculum sella into the sphenoid sinus, and thus obtain the advantages of both approaches. This is a more major procedure, of course, but is useful to eradicate a biologically more active tumour which has not spread beyond surgical access, i.e. into the cavernous sinuses, middle or posterior fossae.

Preoperative assessment

It is necessary to classify the pituitary tumour by size and function. Pituitary function must be measured as well as, of course, the visual fields and acuity. Magnetic resonance imaging (MRI) and CT scanning are complementary, the former showing involvement of the cavernous sinuses particularly well, although the latter probably gives a better overall assessment of the size of the tumour. Which of the two methods is better for showing very small intrasellar adenomas is still debatable. The surgeon should be aware of the possibility of other pathologies; polydipsia or polyurea should raise the suspicion of a hypothalamic lesion (e.g. a craniopharyngioma) and question whether the transsphenoidal route is appropriate. Unilateral retro-orbital pain or a very asymmetrical field defect should also alert the surgeon to other pathology such as an aneurysm or meningioma. Most surgeons now avoid removing the nasal septum, merely displacing it to one side, as this approach has significantly reduced the rate of nasal morbidity. Patients can be told that there should be little postoperative discomfort; that they may feel thirsty, either temporarily or permanently; that they will have a pack in their nose for 24 hours; that fat or fascia may be taken (usually from the right thigh); and that they may experience a headache should it be necessary to carry out air encephalography. There is a risk—albeit small—of damage to pre-existing pituitary function, and if the tumour is large, a very small risk of postoperative visual deterioration; patients should be informed of these risks. I give patients a 5-day course of a broad-spectrum antibiotic, starting on the day of the operation, and this has reduced the incidence of sphenoid sinus infection and meningitis.

Non-functioning tumours

The difficulty diagnosing non-functioning tumours from prolactinomas has already been stressed. These tumours are usually large and present with visual failure, headache or hypopituitarism. Of our 64 patients with such tumours, 58 had macroadenomas. Transsphenoidal surgery improved vision in 29 of the 33 patients who presented in this way, with a return to normal vision in nine. Headache was relieved in all 10 patients in whom it was a major symptom. Figure 19.3 shows the pre- and postoperative pituitary function in this group; it is clear that no patient's pituitary function was made worse, and in some it was improved by tumour removal. What is the place of postoperative radiotherapy? This is discussed in detail in Chapter 20, and it is certainly indicated after transfrontal surgery, for some tumour is almost inevitably left in the sella, and there is indisputable evidence that radiotherapy reduces the recurrence rate. I advise radiotherapy after transsphenoidal surgery if either

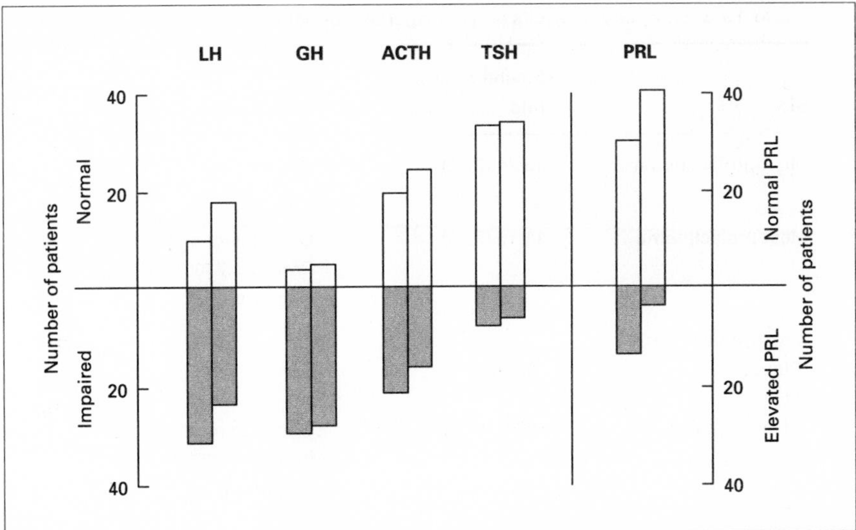

Fig. 19.3 Pre- and postoperative anterior pituitary function in patients operated on for non-functioning tumours. For each hormone the left-hand bar indicates the number of patients with normal and impaired function preoperatively and the right-hand bar shows the corresponding number postoperatively. Only patients with pre- and postoperative data are included.

the tumour excision is incomplete or if the patient already has hypopituitarism. There is good evidence in the literature [8,9] that radiotherapy does, in time, damage pituitary function, and I avoid its use if there is total tumour removal macroscopically and retained pituitary function. This policy seems particularly justified in young people of reproductive age, but this policy depends on vigorous follow-up.

Prolactinomas

The difficulties of diagnosis *vis-à-vis* other tumours causing disconnection hyperprolactinaemia have already been referred to. There are three factors that determine the management of these tumours. First, microprolactinomas seem to be biologically different to larger tumours, and usually do not enlarge to become meso- or macroadenomas; indeed, sometimes they spontaneously regress. Second, *invasive* macroprolactinomas are not cured by surgery (Table 19.3) and, third, radiotherapy is not without morbidity and so should not be used unless alternative therapy is unavailable or unsuccessful. The management depends on the size of the tumour. Thus, for patients with microprolactinomas who present usually with infertility or galactorrhoea, I advise bromocriptine in order to allow conception. Only if medical treatment is unsuccessful, poorly tolerated, unavailable, or there is doubt as to the diagnosis, do I then advise surgery. Our results show there is a small risk of pituitary damage following surgery for this group (Fig. 19.4, group 1), but we have had no recurrence so far with a median follow-up of 4.0 years. In my view undue prominence has been given to Hardy's results (see [10]); these are not representative of surgical results in general, and although I do not advocate surgery as the primary treatment for microprolactinomas, it is a good alternative option to advise, given the availability of a practised transsphenoidal surgeon.

I consider transsphenoidal surgery to be the best option for mesoprolactinomas (i.e. tumour size of 10–20 mm). This will cure 70% of patients without significant pituitary damage (see Fig. 19.4, group 2) and with a very low relapse rate (Table 19.3). If surgery is unsuccessful then bromocriptine and radiotherapy can be used, but by using surgery first approximately 70% of patients may avoid the need for radiotherapy with inevitable, delayed, pituitary damage.

Invasive tumours, in my experience, are large, i.e. macroprolactinomas. I have not seen a mesoadenoma behaving in an invasive fashion. My attempts to operate on invasive macroprolactinomas have not produced a cure (Table 19.3), and I would not advise surgery for this group. Bromocriptine and radiotherapy are indicated. Non-invasive macroprolactinomas can be operated on with a 40% chance of cure. Certainly, in theory, a 4–6-week preoperative course of bromocriptine to shrink the tumour would be advantageous, but whether this actually facilitates a cure that would not otherwise be possible is unclear. It is my experience that prolonged (over 3 months) bromocriptine therapy does make prolactinomas (but not other types of pituitary adenomas) tougher and more difficult to remove (see [11]). I would therefore urge endocrinologists to formulate a policy from the start, and fully discuss the options with the patient at that stage: whether to give bromocriptine for 4–6 weeks and proceed to surgery, or to rely on prolonged bromocriptine medication and radiotherapy. The alternative for non-invasive macroprolactinomas is bromocriptine and radiotherapy, but I consider surgery, particularly for the smaller macroprolactinoma, to be a worthwhile option, for it may well obviate the need for radiotherapy, and such surgery need not produce

Table 19.3 Summary of results and management of patients with prolactinomas at the Radcliffe Infirmary, Oxford.

Size	Biochemical cure rate	Relapse rate	Median (range) follow-up	Recommended management
Microprolactinoma	16/24 (67%)	0%	4.0 (0.3–8.9)	Bromocriptine, then surgery
Mesoprolactinoma	11/15 (73%)	One patient at 3.1 years Prolactin 2400 mU/l CT normal	0.9 (0.5–8.2)	Surgery, then bromocriptine and radiotherapy
Macroprolactinoma				
Invasive	0/8 (0%)			Bromocriptine and radiotherapy
Non-invasive	8/20 (40%)	One patient at 3 years Prolactin 1900 mU/l CT normal	1.1 (0.3–2.6)	Bromocriptine for 4 weeks then surgery or bromocriptine and radiotherapy

CT, computed tomography.

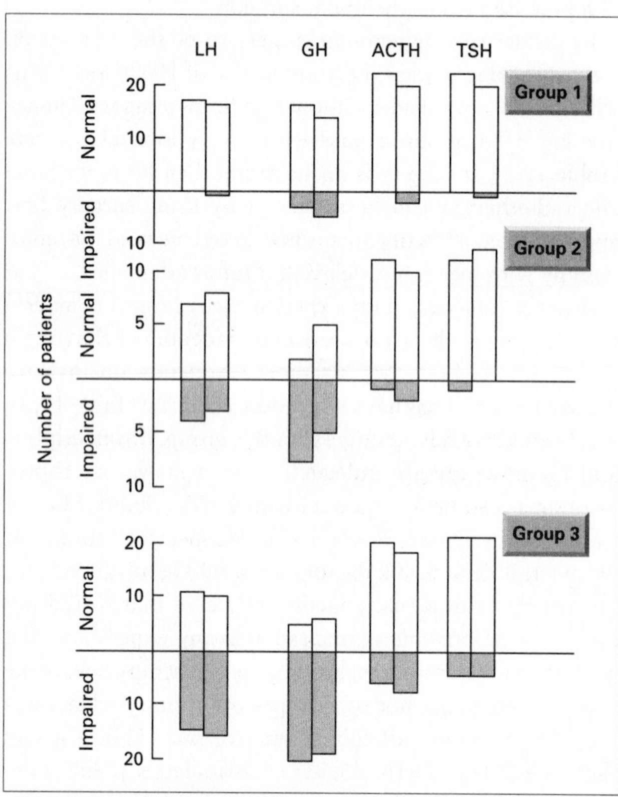

Fig. 19.4 Pre- and postoperative anterior pituitary function in the three groups of patients operated on for prolactinoma. Same format as for Fig. 19.3.

significant pituitary damage (Fig. 19.4, group 3) or relapse rate (Table 19.3). Unlike transfrontal surgery, transsphenoidal surgery for macroprolactinomas or (large) non-functioning tumours may occasionally be curative. Although one might expect more postoperative pituitary damage the larger the tumour, this is not so, although the *preoperative* pituitary function is more affected with large tumours. It seems that the preservation of remaining pituitary tissue depends on this being spread out as a thin rind over the summit of the pituitary tumour just beneath the diaphragma sella (see Fig. 19.2).

Growth hormone-secreting tumours

The results of transsphenoidal surgery for acromegaly are very similar to those of prolactinomas and are related to the size of the tumour. In our experience cure (defined as the attainment of a serum growth hormone level of less than 5 mU/l within 2.5 hours of 50 g oral glucose) was obtained in 82% of patients with a micro- or mesoadenoma, whereas 37% of patients with macroadenomas were 'cured' (median follow-up 4.3 years). One patient with an invasive adenoma later relapsed. As with prolactinomas, preoperative pituitary function is very little changed by transsphenoidal surgery.

Cushing's disease

The neurosurgeon relies heavily on the advice and assistance of the endocrinologist in deciding whether Cushing's syndrome is due to a pituitary adenoma (Cushing's disease), an ectopic tumour, or an adrenal tumour. Cushing's disease indeed challenges and tests both the endocrinologist and the surgeon. The surgeon is not only tested by the pathology, but also by the patient and the endocrinologist. The patients test the gentleness of the surgeon, for they are often ill, their tissues fragile and their blood vessels plentiful and easily ruptured. The endocrinologist can, as elsewhere with pituitary disease, critically analyse the surgeon's results in terms of cure, recurrence and preservation of pituitary function. The surgeon must be prepared to operate on a radiologically normal pituitary fossa, and to explore its contents carefully. Sometimes the endocrinologist cannot be certain of a pituitary source, even after determining ACTH gradients from both inferior petrosal sinuses; the reliability of this technique is still debatable. Ludecke [12] has recently advocated intraoperative assay of ACTH before and after corticotrophin-releasing factor 41 (CRF-41) stimulation in an effort to determine the lateralization of an adenoma in the pituitary fossa. The surgeon cannot expect help from frozen sections, for in 30% of my patients *cured* of Cushing's disease, the pathologist reported normal pituitary tissue; it is an extraordinary fact that the surgeon may recognize what appears to be abnormal tissue—pale, soft and diffluent (unlike the normal anterior lobe tissue which is yellow and firm)—yet the pathologist does not see abnormal cells. Possibly, examination of the non-cellular aspects of the tissue might be revealing; the blood vessels and fibrous tissue providing the 'scaffolding' of the pituitary cells may be different from the normal to produce such a characteristic and recognisable abnormality for the experienced pituitary surgeon.

Because of the seriousness of Cushing's disease (and more especially so in Nelson's syndrome with the adenoma's propensity for malignant change), the surgeon must adopt a more aggressive approach to these tumours. With prolactin- or growth hormone-secreting adenomas, the surgeon removes clearly abnormal tissue and leaves more doubtful tissue, especially in patients with microprolactinomas who wish to conceive. However, with Cushing's disease one leaves only unequivocally normal pituitary tissue, while in Nelson's syndrome one clears the fossa of all tissue, for such patients already require steroid replacement therapy anyway. There is debate as to what the surgeon should do if he or she fails to find abnormal tissue. In my view a 'blind' hypophysectomy should not be performed. The morbidity rate of trans-sphenoidal surgery is sufficiently low for the endocrinologist to ask an 'experienced' surgical colleague to explore the pituitary fossa if all other investigations still render the differential diagnosis between an ectopic source of ACTH (or CRF) and Cushing's disease uncertain. The results of the Oxford series are given in Table 19.4. One must be cautious reading the literature for there are some series with few patients, inadequate endocrine assessment and short follow-up, but the larger series show similar cure rates [13–20].

The results, and indeed postoperative pituitary function, do not depend on the size of the tumour and whether it is diffuse or localized. Fifty-nine per cent of the cured patients regain ACTH function (although this may take up to 3 years), often with the return of a normal cortisol diurnal rhythm. Gonadotrophin function was impaired in 48%, thyroid function in 25%, and the growth hormone response to hypoglycaemia was impaired in 21%. This impairment of pituitary function reflects the much more aggressive surgical approach employed, compared with other pituitary tumours. In the Oxford series, there is a greater incidence of permanent diabetes insipidus after transsphenoidal surgery for Cushing's disease than with other types of pituitary adenoma, which is surprising in view of the small size of these tumours. In summary, I advocate 'aggressively selective' adenomectomy for Cushing's disease; I do not think total

Table 19.4 Results of surgery for Cushing's syndrome from various centres in the world.

Centre	Cure rate	Recurrence rate	No tumour found
Selective surgery			
Hamburg	80/92 (87)	5/66 (8)	12/100 (12)
Nagoya	82/85 (96)	5/82 (6)	10/98 (10)
Mayo	77/98 (79)	4/77 (5)	10/98 (10)
Munich	71/96 (74)	5/75 (7)	5/101 (5)
Glasgow	17/19 (89)	1/19 (5)	0 (0)
San Francisco	67/85 (79)	3/67 (4)	15/100 (15)
Montreal	63/75 (84)	Not stated	15/75 (20)
Oxford*	42/50 (84)	2/50 (4)	1/58 (2)
Total hypophysectomy			
Cardiff	13/16 (81)	0 (0)	0 (0)
Birmingham	11/12 (92)	0 (0)	Not stated

Values in parentheses are percentages.
* The median follow-up for the Oxford series is 4.0 years.

hypophysectomy is required in the first instance unless the patient has Nelson's syndrome.

Rarer pituitary pathologies

Table 19.1 summarises some pathologies revealed by transsphenoidal surgery. Pituitary abscess may well be associated with an increased white cell count in the cerebrospinal fluid, but without organisms being found on Gram stain or culture. There is of course no difficulty in the surgeon recognizing such pathology. Lymphocytic hypophysitis appears to the surgeon as a tough white avascular mass that can be excised only with a scalpel blade: I have already stressed that toughness is an indication that the surgeon should take no more than a biopsy, and that is indeed all that is required for this condition [21]. There have been two thyrotrophin-secreting pituitary adenomas in the Oxford series, both treated by transsphenoidal surgery [22]. Metastatic tumours, especially from breast carcinoma, are not uncommon, but unlikely to be a diagnostic problem or an unexpected finding at operation. Non-neoplastic, simple pituitary cysts usually present with hypopituitarism, contain clear fluid, and are lined with fibrous tissue. Once evacuated they do not often recur. They should be distinguished from arachnoid cysts, which in fact communicate with the subarachnoid space, and small intrapituitary craniopharyngiomas.

Tumours rarely arise from the posterior pituitary gland; Bevan *et al.* [23] described an acromegalic patient with a gangliocytoma containing immunoreactive gastrin and growth hormone-releasing hormone in the neurons; the tumour, which was pale, tough and avascular, surrounded by soft tissue typical of a pituitary adenoma, was removed transsphenoidally with cure of the acromegaly. More frequently, gangliocytomas may be found in the hypothalamus.

Pituitary apoplexy

'Pituitary apoplexy' or haemorrhagic infarction of a pituitary adenoma may be used to describe either a sudden spontaneous cessation of pituitary function (which is not infrequent), or a sudden expansion of a pituitary tumour causing chiasmal compression. Should the haemorrhage rupture through the diaphragma sella, then subarachnoid haemorrhage occurs, producing signs of meningeal irritation. If blindness develops, or is threatened, emergency transsphenoidal surgery should be performed, and in my experience often produces very gratifying recovery of vision (and, in one patient of mine, cure of his acromegaly).

Surgical technique

Since the first edition of this book, the surgical technique has stayed the same. Most surgeons use the sublabial transnasal approach. The alternative—the transnasal (via the nostril) has its proponents who claim the shorter route to the pituitary fossa is advantageous although with the operating microscope this advantage seems less important than the under and more flexible approach allowed by the sublabial approach. Recently two papers [24,25] have highlighted the use of intraoperative ultrasound in the resection of pituitary adenomas, and this needs further evaluation.

Complications of surgery

The remarkable feature of transsphenoidal surgery is how little it upsets the patient, compared with transfrontal surgery. There have been no deaths in the Oxford series of over 400 patients, whose ages have ranged to 80 years and above. The patients usually leave hospital 4–5 days after operation.

Table 19.5 summarizes the complications of transsphenoidal surgery; postoperative pituitary damage has already been discussed for each type of adenoma and depends on the surgical aggressiveness used, which in turn depends on the type of pathology encountered, ranging from prolactinomas at one extreme to Nelson's syndrome at the other.

Why do we fail to cure some patients? MRI scanning suggests the most usual reason is tumour invaginating into the cavernous sinuses [26]. Of course, some benign-looking adenomas are biologically more active, and recur despite radiotherapy; it is this group of patients who may require radical combined transfrontal/transsphenoidal surgery. Frankly invasive tumours are not curable by surgery.

Thaper *et al.* [27] have shown that more aggressive tumours may (but not always) be identified by assessing the K1-67

Table 19.5 Complications of transsphenoidal surgery.

Complication	Prevention of treatment
CSF leak (5 patients, 1 required re-exploration)	Pack sphenoid sinus as well if CSF seen at operation
Nasal morbidity (2 patients)	Use paraseptal approach: avoid excising septum
Tough tumour—swelling after surgery (1 patient)	No more than a biopsy; pack sphenoid sinus
Visual deterioration (2 patients)	Immediate evacuation of haematoma
Diabetes insipidus (permanent in 2%)	Not known

CSF, cerebrospinal fluid.

cell cycle specific nuclear antigen growth functions using M1B-1 monoclonal antibody. The mean growth fraction was significantly higher for more active tumours. However, there were individual exceptions but this work is likely to be developed in future.

Cerebrospinal fluid leakage is more common early in a surgeon's experience. It may be difficult to diagnose. First, serum from an intranasal haematoma may be very similar to cerebrospinal fluid, but, more importantly, the patient may present not with an obvious rhinorrhoea, but with a low-grade meningitis partially treated by the routine postoperative antibiotics. This is the most dangerous and subtle postoperative complication; any patient who is generally 'unwell' postoperatively (given adequate steroid cover) should have brow-up lateral skull radiography or CT scan, looking for subarachnoid air. A lumbar puncture must also be done. Any patient complaining of a 'splashing' noise on sudden head movement is likely to have intracranial air denoting a fistula between the nasal and cranial cavities. Such a fistula must be closed immediately. These fistulae do not close spontaneously and, in my experience, lumbar drainage is not usually successful by itself. Reexploration of the pituitary fossa is indicated, with obliteration of the pituitary fossa and sphenoid sinus using fascia and fat. It is a straightforward procedure, but I emphasize the need for *immediate* and adequate closure of the fistula; prevarication is disastrous, leading to a patient gradually and subtly deteriorating from low-grade meningitis. It is essentially that both surgeon and endocrinologist are aware of the subtle nature of this complication so that early diagnosis and treatment can be instituted.

Postoperative visual deterioration

Table 19.6 summarises the possible causes of postoperative visual deterioration. Visual acuity should be checked routinely after any pituitary surgery, particularly if the tumour was large and there was preoperative chiasmal compression. If vision becomes worse then a scan must be performed; a haematoma in the tumour cavity must be immediately evacuated. This is an easy procedure transsphenoidally, with rapid improvement of vision if expeditiously performed. I have occasionally inserted a drain (brought out through the mucosa of the upper lip) into a particularly large tumour cavity to prevent such a haematoma developing; it is, in fact, surprisingly rare.

During transsphenoidal surgery for a large cystic or soft tumour, one sees the diaphragma sella rapidly herniating to the floor of the pituitary fossa as the tumour is removed. Presumably, the elongated optic nerves and chiasm must on many occasions acutely herniate into the sella as well. However, only one patient [28] has been described showing

Table 19.6 Causes of visual deterioration following pituitary surgery.

Time after operation	Cause
Immediately after operation	Haematoma Operative damage Acute empty sella syndrome
8 days after operation	Unilateral, probably ischaemic
Months after operation/irradiation	Recurrent tumour (gradual, progressive, symmetrical bitemporal hemianopia) Irradiation damage (suddent onset 10–18 months after irradiation, rapidly progressive, unilateral or asymmetrical field loss) Empty sella syndrome(?) (very doubtful) Scarring of chasm without displacement(?) (very doubtful)

acute postoperative visual deterioration for this reason, despite the many thousands of such operations performed since then. This also suggests that optic nerve or chiasmal damage due to 'chronic' herniation into an empty sella is, in fact, a very unusual event.

Morello and Frera [29] described a patient with unilateral loss of vision 8 days after surgery. I have had an identical occurrence, the explanation probably being ischaemic damage to the optic nerve.

Visual deterioration which occurs some months after operation may be due to recurrent tumour or radiation damage. I believe that the latter is underdiagnosed and has been frequently and mistakenly thought to be due to an 'empty sella'. The clinical features of post-irradiation damage are summarized in Table 19.6, and contrasted with those of tumour recurrence. The radiation dose is of great importance, and is discussed in greater detail in Chapter 20. The literature describing visual deterioration due to a 'secondary empty sella syndrome' is hopelessly muddled. Many patients so described have had radiotherapy in unspecified doses, the visual fields and acuity are often not recorded, and other ophthalmological causes have not been considered. McFadzean [30], an ophthalmologist, studied 14 such patients and could find no evidence to associate visual deterioration with the empty sella syndrome; in the majority he found an ocular cause. Furthermore, some authors have described the visual deterioration due to a secondary empty sella syndrome as occurring suddenly, a few months or several years after operation, the visual fields being characteristically asymmetrical, unilateral or bilateral, and concentric or eccentric [31,32]. These features are identical to the well-established chiasmal/optic nerve damage due to radiotherapy, which may cause damage to the vascular supply of these structures. There may be fairly rapid progress for 1–2 months with the eyes being asymmetrically affected [33–35]. It is my view that visual damage due to 'scarring' or the empty sella syndrome has been overdiagnosed and the operation of 'chiasmapexy' to replace the herniated chiasm should not be performed except after the greatest circumspection; if radiation damage is in fact the cause, such an operation is likely to make the patient's vision worse.

Craniopharyngiomas

Any patient presenting with diabetes insipidus is likely to have a hypothalamic tumour rather than a pituitary tumour. The commonest tumour affecting the hypothalamus is a craniopharyngioma. Sometimes the tumours may be sited entirely in the pituitary fossa (intrasellar craniopharyngioma), occasionally entirely in the third ventricle (presenting with slowly developing raised intracranial pressure and dementia) or, much more commonly, in the region of the hypothalamus and chiasm, causing diabetes insipidus, blindness and hypopituitarism. It is desirable to remove these lesions completely if possible, and the first operation is the best occasion to achieve this. However, the surgery of these lesions demands from the surgeon considerable judgement, not just from the neurological, but also from the endocrinological, point of view. Two factors mitigate against total removal: the size and the degree of surrounding fibrosis. Usually the areas most 'stuck' are those that are calcified, and so a small calcified lesion may be as irremovable as a large multiloculated cyst extending into both frontal and temporal lobes.

There are two particular considerations for the surgeon to be aware of. The first is that total removal of a craniopharyngioma, even without neurological deficit, may cause disastrous damage to the patient if the hypothalamic 'thirst' and 'appetite' centres are damaged. Permanent diabetes insipidus can of course be managed, but if thirst is no longer normally appreciated then control of fluid and electrolyte balance becomes an alarming problem, for which the surgeon will receive the thanks of neither the patient or endocrinologist.

Another difficult situation is the young, still growing, child with a small cystic craniopharyngioma which has not yet caused hypopituitarism. In these circumstances, simple aspiration of such a cyst (if causing optic chiasmal compression) may be preferable to total excision in order to preserve pituitary function for as long as possible during the growing phase. In adult patients, standard pituitary replacement therapy does not in my view confer pituitary normality to these patients, possibly due to the untreated growth hormone deficiency. Postoperative care requires not just steroid replacement therapy, but extremely careful management of fluid and electrolyte balance. Frequent weighing of the patient (a weigh-bed is invaluable) and 24-hour urinary fluid and electrolyte collections are needed. A low serum sodium can cause 'neurological' deterioration, confusion, drowsiness, coma and epilepsy. Indiscriminate use of mannitol or diuretics to 'shrink' the brain perioperatively can add to the endocrinologist's difficulties, and their use needs to be discussed by the team involved with caring for the patient.

Other hypothalamic tumours

Gliomas of the hypothalamus may present to the endocrinologist in other ways; hypothalamic 'wasting' is occasionally seen in children and the possibility of a lipolytic factor causing the extreme depletion of body fat in these children has been postulated. Precocious puberty is a well-known but rare manifestation of hypothalamic tumours. The pathology may be a glioma, and the place of surgery is confined to obtaining a histological diagnosis and, on occasions, to relieving optic chiasmal compression. Benign hamartomas should also be left alone.

Conclusions

The optimum treatment of pituitary and hypothalamic tumours demands close teamwork between endocrinologist, surgeon and radiotherapist. The differing therapeutic skills should not be considered to be in competition with each other; they all have an appropriate indication, and the judicious use of all three methods, appropriate to the individual patient, to the particular pathology and according to the skills available, combine to produce the best results. It is incumbent on the surgeon to have some understanding of the endocrine aspects of the tumours, for it is these that determine the aggressiveness or otherwise of the surgical approach. It has already been stressed that total removal of a craniopharyngioma even without neurological deficit may leave that patient an endocrine cripple.

Acknowledgements

I would like to thank the editor of *Acta Neurochirurgica* for his kind permission to produce figures and tables from the

Cairns Memorial Lecture published in that journal. It is a pleasure to acknowledge the debt I owe to my many colleagues in Oxford and elsewhere, many of whose ideas and data I have reproduced in this chapter.

References

1 Cairns H. The prognosis of pituitary tumours. I. *Lancet* 1935; ii: 1310–11.

2 Cairns H. The prognosis of pituitary tumours. II. *Lancet* 1935; ii: 1363–4.

3 Halstead AE. Remarks on the operative treatment of tumours of the hypophysis. *Surg Gynecol Obstet* 1910; **10**: 494–502.

4 Cushing H. *The Pituitary Body and its Disorders*. Philadelphia: JB Lippincott Co., 1912.

5 Hardy J, Wigger SM. Transsphenoidal surgery of pituitary fossa tumours with televised radio fluoroscopic control. *J Neurosurg* 1965; **23**: 612–19.

6 Adams CBT. The management of pituitary tumours and post-operative visual deterioration. *Acta Neurochir (Wien)* 1988; **94**: 103–16.

7 Bevan JS, Burke CW, Esiri MM, Adams CBT. Misinterpretation of prolactin levels leading to management errors in patients with sellar enlargement. *Am J Med* 1987; **82**: 29–32.

8 Eastman RC, Gorden P, Roth J. Conventional supervoltage irradiation is an effective treatment for acromegaly. *J Clin Endocrinol Metab* 1979; **48**: 931–40.

9 Sheline GE. Radiation therapy of pituitary tumours. In: Givens JR, ed. *Hormone Secreting Tumours*. Chicago: Year Book Publishers, 1982; 139.

10 Serri O, Rasio E, Beauregard H, Hardy J, Somma M. Recurrence of hyperprolactinaemia after selective transsphenoidal adenectomy in women with prolactinoma. *N Engl J Med* 1983; **209**: 280–3.

11 Esiri MM, Bevan JS, Burke CW, Adams CBT. Effect of bromocriptine treatment on the fibrous tissue content of prolactin secreting and non functioning macroadenomas of the pituitary gland. *J Clin Endocrinol Metab* 1986; **63**: 383–9.

12 Ludecke DK. Intraoperative measurement of adrenocorticotropic hormone in peripituitary blood in Cushing's Disease. *Neurosurgery* 1989; **24**: 201–5.

13 Boggan JE, Tyrell JB, Wilson CB. Transsphenoidal microsurgical management of Cushing's Disease: report of 100 cases. *J Neurosurg* 1983; **59**: 195–200.

14 Brand IR, Dalton GA, Fletcher RF. Long term follow-up of transsphenoidal hypophysectomy for Cushing's disease. *J Roy Soc Med* 1985; **78**: 291–3.

15 Fahlbusch R, Buchfelder M, Muller OA. Transsphenoidal surgery for Cushing's disease. *J Roy Soc Med* 1986; **79**: 262–9.

16 Kageyama N, Kuwayama A, Takahashi T, Khihara K, Kato T, Yokoe T. In: Lambers SWJ, Tilders FJH, van der Veen EA, Assies J, eds. *Trends in the Diagnosis and Treatment of Pituitary Adenomas*. Amsterdam: Free University Press, 1984: 325–38.

17 Ludecke DK. Present status of surgical treatment of ACTH secreting pituitary adenomas in Cushing's disease. In: Lamberts SWJ, Tilders FJH, van der Veen EA, Assies J, eds. *Trends in the Diagnosis and Treatment of Pituitary Adenomas*. Amsterdam: Free University Press, 1984: 315–23.

18 Salassa RM, Laws ER, Carpenter PC, Northcutt RC. Cushing's disease—50 years later. *Trans Am Clin Climatol Assoc* 1982; **94**: 122–9.

19 Semple CG, Thomson GA, Teasdale GM. Transsphenoidal microsurgery for Cushing's disease. *Clin Endocrinol* 1984; **21**: 621–9.

20 Thomas JP, Richards SH. Long term results of radical hypophysectomy for Cushing's disease. *Clin Endocrinol* 1983; **19**: 629–36.

21 McGrail KM, Beyerl BD, Black PMcL, Klibanski A, Zervas NT. Lymphocytic adenohypophysitis of pregnancy with complete recovery. *Neurosurgery* 1987; **20**: 791–3.

22 Bevan JS, Burke CW, Esiri MM, Adams CBT, Balabio M, Missim M, Falglia G. Studies of two thyrotrophine-secreting pituitary adenomas: evidence for dopamine receptor deficiency. *Clin Endocrinol* 1989; **3**: 59–70.

23 Bevan JS, Asa SL, Ross ML, Esiri MM, Adams CBT, Burke CW. Intrasellar gangliocytoma containing gastric and growth hormone-releasing hormone associated with a growth hormone-secreting pituitary adenoma. *Clin Endocrinol* 1989; **30**: 213–24.

24 Ram Z, Shawker TH, Bradford RDMS, Doppman JL, Oldfield EH. Intraoperative ultrasound-directed resection of pituitary tumours. *J Neurosurg* 1995; **83**: 225–30.

25 Yamasani T, Moritake K, Hatta J, Nagai H. Inoperative monitoring with pulse Doppler ultrasonography in transsphenoidal surgery: technique application. *Neurosurgery* 1996; **35**: 95–8.

26 Kaufman B, Kaufman BA, Arafah BM, Roessmann U, Selman WR. Large pituitary gland adenomas evaluated with magnetic resonance imaging. *Neurosurgery* 1987; **21**: 540–6.

27 Thaper K, Kovaks K, Scheithauer BW *et al.* Proliferative activity and invasiveness among pituitary adenomas and carcinomas: an analysis using the M1B-1 antibody. *Neurosurgery* 1996; **38**: 99–107.

28 Olson DR, Guiot G, Derome P. The symptomatic empty sella. Prevention and correction via the transsphenoidal approach. *J Neurosurg* 1972; **37**: 533–7.

29 Morello G, Frera C. Visual damage after removal of hypophyseal adenomas: possible importance of vascular disturbances of the optic nerve and chiasm. *Acta Neurochir (Wien)* 1966; **15**: 1–10.

30 McFadzean RM. The empty sella syndrome. A review of 14 cases. *Trans Ophthalmol Soc UK* 1983; **103**: 537–41.

31 Hodgson SF, Randall RV, Holman CB, Mccarthy CS. Empty sella syndrome. Report of 10 cases. *Med Clin North Am* 1972; **56**: 897–907.

32 Hodgson SF, Randall RV, Laws ER. Empty sella syndrome. In: Youmans J, ed. *Neurological Surgery*, Vol. 5, 2nd edn. Philadelphia: WB Saunders 1982: 3176.

33 Aristizabal S, Caldwell WL, Avila J. The relationship of time–dose fractionation factors to complications in the treatment. *Int J Radiat Oncol Biol Phys* 1977; **2**: 667–73.

34 Atkinson BA, Allen IV, Gordon DS, Hadden DR, Maguire CJF, Trimble ER, Lyons AR. Progressive visual failure in acromegaly following external pituitary irradiation. *Clin Endocrinol* 1979; **10**: 469–79.

35 Harris JR, Levene MB. Visual complications following irradiation for pituitary adenomas and craniopharyngiomas. *Radiology* 1976; **120**: 167–71.

CHAPTER 20

Radiotherapy for pituitary tumours

P.N. Plowman

Radiotherapy has an important place in the treatment of diseases of the hypothalamo-hypophysial region although this role, in conjunction with medical and surgical therapies, has considerably changed over the past 20 years [1].

Pituitary adenomas

Data from San Francisco provide us with a historical experience into relapse probabilities following transcranial surgery used alone in the treatment of pituitary adenomas. Sheline [1] found that the recurrence-free survival rate following radical transcranial surgery was 25% at 5 years and 9% at 10 years. However, with postoperative radiotherapy the recurrence-free survival rate was 79% at 10 years. In previous publications, Sheline *et al.* [2,3] had produced evidence from treating chromophobe adenomas that conventially fractionated radiotherapy with at least 4000 rad (cGy) was associated with a better control rate than lesser doses, and that small tumours were more easily controlled. More modern publications and using the transsphenoidal route, find lower rates of relapse after surgery alone. Bradley *et al.* [4] attempted to select a lower risk group of operated patients with non-functional tumours for whom they elected to 'watch and wait'. They followed a group of 73 unirradiated such patients, for whom they thought they had achieved a surgical cure. They demonstrated a 90% relapse-free survival rate in this selected population. These data are of interest but need to be confirmed in several respects: can they be reproduced in other surgical teams' hands? What is the recurrence rate in the second quinquennium? What selection criteria are to be used to select the low-risk group? The major difference between the latter data and the San Francisco data may relate to improvements in surgery as a whole but probably particularly to the improved surgical access to the pituitary fossa since the introduction of the transsphenoidal route.

The data on secretory adenomas are further discussed below, where a hormone may be used as a 'marker' for residual disease. Other series that demonstrate the high efficacy of modern surgery are often difficult to analyse fully because the authors have reported series of patients some (presumably the perceived higher-risk cases) of whom have received radiation therapy [5]—this is an aspect of surgical reporting that should be corrected in the future.

In an analysis of 411 patients presenting to the Royal Marsden Hospital over a 20-year period, all of whom received surgery and radiotherapy, Brada *et al.* [6] reported the actuarial progression-free survival rate to be 94% at 10 years and 88% at 20 years for all patients, and 97% at 10 years for patients with non-functioning adenomas. In their analysis of prognostic factors, only secretory state (which slightly negatively impacted on local control) was an independent prognostic factor for disease control. Presumably, if there was any selection bias by the referring neurosurgeons, it would have been in the direction of sending more perceived higher risk cases for radiotherapy. These data strongly support the concept that postoperative radiotherapy substantially reduces the local relapse risk. Indeed, single institution publications from the modern era would support this important function of radiotherapy. In a Parisian study, involving 57 non-secreting pituitary adenoma patients, 33 were treated by surgery alone and 24 by surgery and radiotherapy. With a mean follow-up of 7.1 years, there was a 27% relapse rate in the former group whereas there was only an 8% relapse rate in the irradiated group [7].

Acromegaly/gigantism

In 1909, Beclere [8] described a 16-year-old giant girl with visual disturbance whose vision and other symptoms improved after radiotherapy, while Gramegna [9] described a similar good result in a Parisian patient in that same year.

However, the important role of radiotherapy in the modern treatment of acromegaly has only recently been realised [10,11].

Owing to progress in diagnostic methods, the giant/acromegalic is frequently diagnosed earlier nowadays and consequently with a smaller tumour than the 'classically' large adenomas traditionally associated with this disease. This has allowed the group at St Bartholomew's Hospital to study the effects of radiotherapy on a large group of unoperated patients for a substantial period of follow-up [8] (Fig. 20.1). It may be seen in this series of 73 patients that mean growth hormone (GH) levels gradually but continuously decreased from a mean of 103 mU/ml to 12 mU/ml over the 10 years of follow-up. Furthermore, a significant further reduction of GH levels was observed in comparison with the results at 10 years in 18 patients in whom an assessment was carried out 11–15 years after radiotherapy, thereby showing the continuing beneficial effect of the radiotherapy [12]. Whilst we would probably not select radiotherapy alone for this patient group in this established transsphenoidal era, and whilst the hormone results over time may not reach the optimal cure criteria that we currently employ, nevertheless, they do demonstrate the durable and prolonged efficacy of this treatment modality. When used in the postoperative period with low bulk disease (and lower marker/hormone levels), this leads to the conclusion that radiotherapy is very effective at preventing relapse [11]. The dose prescription for radiotherapy is discussed below (usually *c.* 4500 cGy), but it is noteworthy that other data from the group in Manchester, UK, have suggested that lower total doses at irradiation may also be efficacious [13].

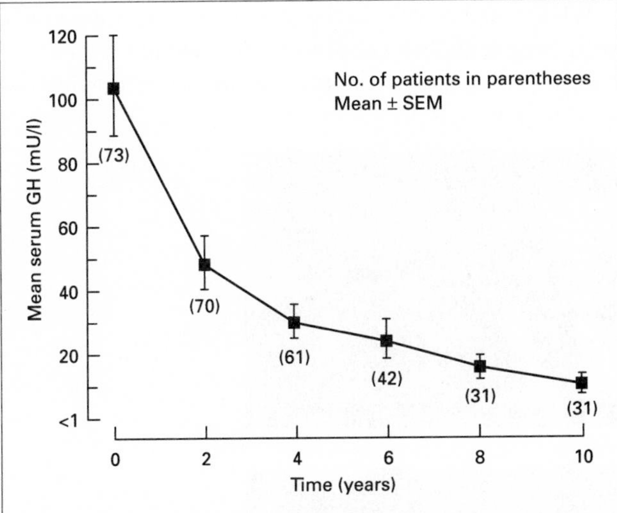

Fig. 20.1 Mean serum growth hormone levels before and with time after radiotherapy in a series of 73 unoperated acromegalic patients presenting to St Bartholomew's Hospital, London. All serum samples were taken with the patient off dopamine agonist therapy for a minimum of 4 weeks. Data from [12].

Dopamine agonists (e.g. bromocriptine) act directly on the somatotroph D_2 receptor and produce a symptomatic response in 70% of acromegalics, although only approximately one-third of treated patients show a fall in GH levels (and only rarely into the normal range). Dopamine agonist therapy is associated with relatively minor tumour shrinkage (except in mixed somatotroph/lactotroph tumours, see Chapter 12). Somatostatin analogues (e.g. octreotide) produce an excellent clinical and biochemical improvement in patients, with serum GH lowering in virtually all patients and normalisation of insulin-like growth factor 1 (IGF-1) values in approximately 60%. However, any effect on tumour size is far more modest and this shrinkage rebounds to pretreatment volume size on cessation of the drug, the same applying to any tumour shrinkage with dopamine-agonist therapy. Although octreotide rarely causes substantial tumour shrinkage, the combination of interim medical therapy and radiotherapy allows immediate hormonal control and long-term tumour control of small, intrasellar adenomas, when surgery may not be recommended. Large, suprasellar tumours, with or without visual field defects, demand (transsphenoidal) surgical resection. We no longer recommend postoperative radiotherapy *de rigueur*, but biochemically test for 'cure' (undetectable random serum GH levels and/or < 5 mU/l during a day profile or during a glucose tolerance test) before recommending radiotherapy for those (the majority) who have detectable GH postoperatively.

Thus, the modern recommendations for treatment of this condition are immediate medical therapy (dopamine agonist or somatostatin analogue) to control hormonal imbalance followed by definitive therapy. For large tumours this definitive therapy will be transsphenoidal resection with or without postoperative radiotherapy (depending on the postoperative GH levels). For small tumours, transsphenoidal resection with attempt at cure, and hopefully without immediate anterior pituitary dysfunction, is again followed by radiotherapy unless the stringent cure definition just outlined is met. The 'cost' of radiotherapy treatment is that, by 6 years after irradiation, approximately 25% of patients, who did not require replacement therapy beforehand, will require some form of replacement therapy. This figure may increase further with time.

Prolactinomas

Because assays for prolactin only became available relatively recently, the data on prolactinoma responses to radiotherapy are all relatively new, although the early data on chromophobe adenomas cited above would undoubtedly have included many of these tumours.

Macroprolactinomas

These are defined as tumours of > 10 mm in diameter, usually extrasellar. Since the observation in 1975 by Corenblum *et al.* [14] that bromocriptine therapy led to shrinkage of a prolactinoma, it is now quite clear that the great majority of prolactinomas will show significant tumour shrinkage with dopamine-agonist therapy, sometimes transforming a large tumour with extrasellar extension into a partially empty fossa (Fig. 20.2). The majority of such shrinkage will occur within the first 6 weeks of therapy, and the initial management of all but a few patients with macroprolactinomas is a 2–6-week course of bromocriptine or related drug. If the patient presents with visual field defects due to chiasmal compression, frequent (sometimes daily) visual field monitoring in the early weeks of bromocriptine therapy is necessary, with immediate neurosurgical back-up should the fields deteriorate. However, it is clear that initial bromocriptine/dopamine-agonist therapy is safe in the overwhelming majority of cases, and usually leads to rapid improvement in the visual fields. Following 6–8 weeks of medical therapy a decision is made on definitive therapy. Long-term bromocriptine is suppressive therapy, but in the majority of cases there is rapid re-expansion when treatment is stopped (Fig. 20.3). The patient is re-imaged after this time period, and if a large tumour persists then a (transsphenoidal) resection, probably followed by radiotherapy, is indicated. However, if the tumour has shrunk down into the fossa with dopamine agonist therapy, our definitive therapy is radiotherapy. An alternative approach is to recommend transsphenoidal surgery plus, probably, postoperative radiotherapy.

Fig. 20.2 Sagittal reconstruction computed tomographic scan of a male prolactinoma patient with a very large, apparently cystic, prolactinoma extending upwards and posteriorly out of the fossa (a). Following dopamine-agonist therapy, the tumour has shrunk back into the fossa (b).

Microprolactinomas

Patients with microprolactinomas are usually young women presenting with secondary amenorrhoea. Investigations will show subtle radiological changes in the pituitary fossa floor (a blister or double floor due to the downward compression by these predominantly anterolaterally situated pituitary adenomas), or more definite evidence of an abnormal pituitary on high-resolution computed tomography (CT) scan, in association with hyperprolactinaemia. Dopamine-agonist therapy quickly (often within days) restores normal menses and fertility, and it is the ensuing pregnancy (so often desired by this patient group) which induces a potential complication. Prolactinomas are oestrogen sensitive and pregnancy may produce rapid tumour expansion; although unusual (perhaps less than 5% of cases), such rapid expansion in pregnancy may, nevertheless, be dramatic and dangerous. Radiotherapy much reduces the risk of such pregnancy-related expansion, but we generally reserve its use for either large microadenomas or frank macroadenomas. Other authorities recommend transsphenoidal surgery, but risk immediate hypopituitarism with its problematic fertility consequences. Furthermore, the Montreal group reported a 40% 5-year recurrence rate after transsphenoidal surgery [15], although other reports are more sanguine. However, studies reporting a low rate of recurrence generally have short follow-up intervals.

Where patients with microprolactinomas are being treated with long-term bromocriptine, they should be imaged regularly (but not necessarily frequently) to monitor for

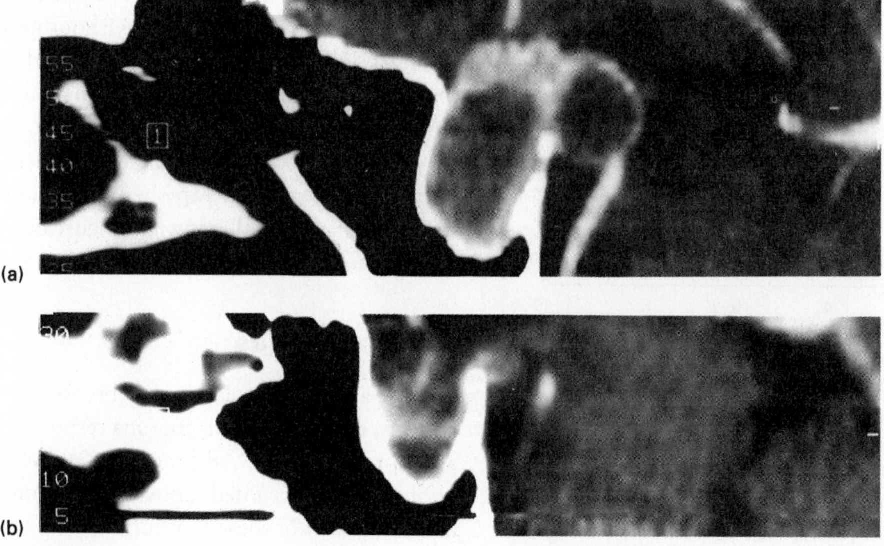

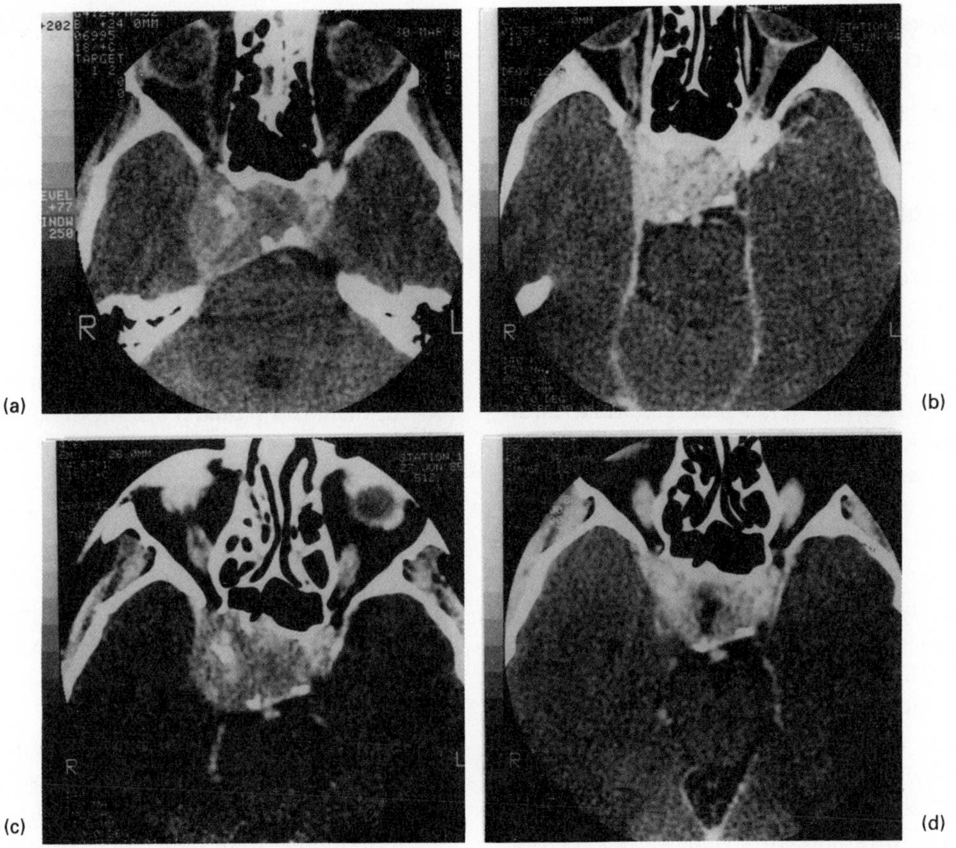

Fig. 20.3 High-resolution computed tomographic scans of a patient with a large prolactinoma: (a) at presentation (prolactin 20 600 mU/L) and (b) after 2 years on bromocriptine (prolactin 170 mU/L). The patient then stopped bromocriptine treatment for 5 weeks and his tumour enlarged rapidly as shown in (c), when his prolactin was 50 000 mU/l. He was restarted on bromocriptine and 3 months later his serum prolactin level had fallen to 400 mU/L and (d) the tumour had shrunk once more.

progression to a macroprolactinoma. If such a patient enters pregnancy without definitive treatment, assiduous monitoring of visual fields must be performed serially, as well as imaging should any complications arise.

With regard to radiotherapy in the management of prolactinomas, we may conclude that it is effective, causing a progressive decline in serum prolactin levels over the years following radiotherapy [16] (Fig. 20.4), in a manner analogous to that seen in acromegaly. In our institution, radiotherapy has an established definitive role in the management of macroprolactinoma and a selective role in the management of microprolactinoma. Radiotherapy has a particularly important therapeutic role in the management of the 15% of dopamine-agonist resistant cases, especially following transsphenoidal surgery when this appears not to be curative.

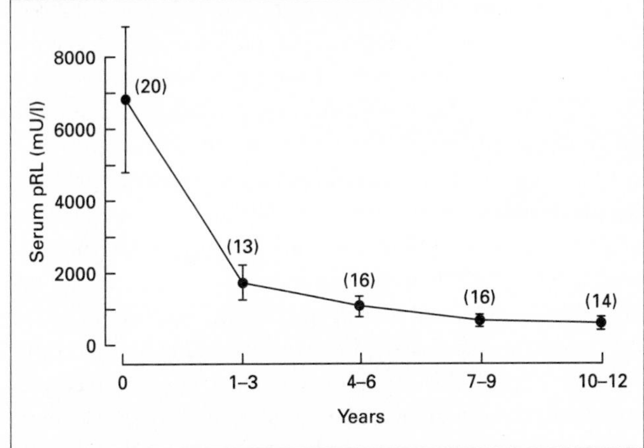

Fig. 20.4 Change in mean serum prolactin level (± SEM) in a group of patients treated with megavoltage radiotherapy for prolactinoma. The number of patients at each point is given in parentheses. We have individual data on the whole group of 36 patients, but this particular graph shows the prolactin levels in patients who had levels taken at every time-point. All samples taken off dopamine-agonist therapy for a minimum of 4 weeks. Data from [43].

Cushing's disease and Nelson's syndrome

Publications since the 1950s have described the efficacy of radiotherapy for Cushing's disease [17–20], but its role has until recently been placed very much in the shadow of transsphenoidal surgery, with only small series of patients with short follow-up intervals being published. However, Howlett *et al.* [21] recently analysed a series of 52 patients with Cushing's disease and Nelson's syndrome receiving radiotherapy at St Bartholomew's Hospital, London. Twenty-one of these patients had no preceding surgery; all were initially treated by metyrapone to induce normal mean plasma cortisol levels (all achieving clinical remission on this therapy), and then definitive pituitary radiotherapy. With a median follow-up of 9.5 years (range 5.8–15.5 years), 12 (57%) are off all therapy in clinical remission, and a further four patients require a steady reduction in medical therapy (accompanied by falling adrenocorticotrophic hormone (ACTH) levels), suggesting an overall final remission rate of approximately 76%. However, five of these 21 patients have not been controlled and have required alternative therapy with bilateral adrenalectomy or hypophysectomy.

Also noteworthy from Howlett *et al.*'s study is that although 12 of 21 showed clinical remission and were off all medical therapy with normal daytime serum cortisol, only two of these 12 had a normal midnight serum cortisol, suggesting incomplete cure. Howlett *et al.* [21] also analysed the results of radiotherapy in 15 patients with Nelson's syndrome, developing after bilateral adrenalectomy for Cushing's disease. The median follow-up of these 15 irradiated patients was 9.6 years. The results of the radiotherapy are extremely clear-cut: 14 of the 15 patients showed progressive depigmentation, shrinkage of the pituitary adenoma and falls in plasma ACTH to a mean 16% of preradiotherapy values. The 15th patient responded with falls in serum ACTH for 6 years and then progressed again to die 11 years after radiotherapy. Lastly, Howlett *et al.* [21] analysed the outcome of radiotherapy in nine patients who had received non-curative transsphenoidal surgery. Five of these nine patients (56%) were off all medical treatment and in clinical remission with a median of 3 years' follow-up. Of the three patients with large macroadenomas, however, two died from tumour regression and the third required bilateral adrenalectomy; this last patient is now well with a lower ACTH. In a more recent publication from the Barts group, Jenkins *et al.* examined the efficacy of post-adrenalectomy radiotherapy to the pituitary in the prevention of Nelson's syndrome. Of 56 patients available for long-term follow-up data, five of 20 who had received radiotherapy, and 18 of 36 who had not received the radiotherapy developed Nelson's syndrome ($P > 0.07$) [22]. It seems clear (and as predicted from the foregoing data) that radiotherapy is highly effective in this situation.

All these data support the inclusion of modern external-beam radiotherapy as part of the armamentarium in the management of Cushing's disease, either alone or postoperatively. The larger macroadenomas require the multimodality approach.

Craniopharyngioma

Craniopharyngiomas represent 2% of all intracranial tumours in adults, but are proportionately commoner in children. Indeed, there is a bimodal age incidence with one peak in the first decade of life and a second in the years from 50 to 70. The clinical presentation varies with age; very young children present with signs of hydrocephalus, whilst older children usually present with endocrinopathies such as growth failure or diabetes insipidus. Visual loss is also a relatively common presenting symptom in all age groups (see Chapter 18). Approximately half of all craniopharyngiomas are cystic, approximately 15% entirely solid and the rest equally cystic and solid.

Treatment approaches had, until the last decade, been largely influenced by the good results of radical surgery alone reported by Matson and Crigler [23], although subsequent long-term follow-up of these same patients showed a 27% relapse rate [24], and other workers have found radical attempts at resection difficult due to the tenacity with which the craniopharyngioma capsule adheres to adjacent normal and highly critical brain tissue. Although in recent years the advent of the operating microscope, dexamethasone and other advances in neurosurgery and neuroanaesthesia have increased technical standards in access and resection, it is clear from the literature that 'complete' resection is unusual, and that the neurosurgeon's assessment of completeness of resection is frequently incorrect. Amacher [25] amassed 111 cases of documented subtotally excised craniopharyngiomas from the literature and found an overall recurrence rate of 75%; thus, surgery alone is not a satisfactory form of treatment for craniopharyngioma.

There are now overwhelming data in support of the practice of postoperative radiotherapy, which is generally recommended for all patients [26–32]. These data confirm that following 'total' removal of a craniopharyngioma there is a recurrence rate of 20–25% that, following acknowledged subtotal removal, there is a 75% recurrence rate, but that subtotal surgery plus radiotherapy is attended by a recurrence rate of only 20–30%—a very substantial gain in control rate (and survival). Nevertheless, despite standard modern external-beam radiotherapy employed *de rigueur* in the postoperative setting, recurrences of craniopharyngiomas do occur, and occasionally recurrent fluid filling of cystic

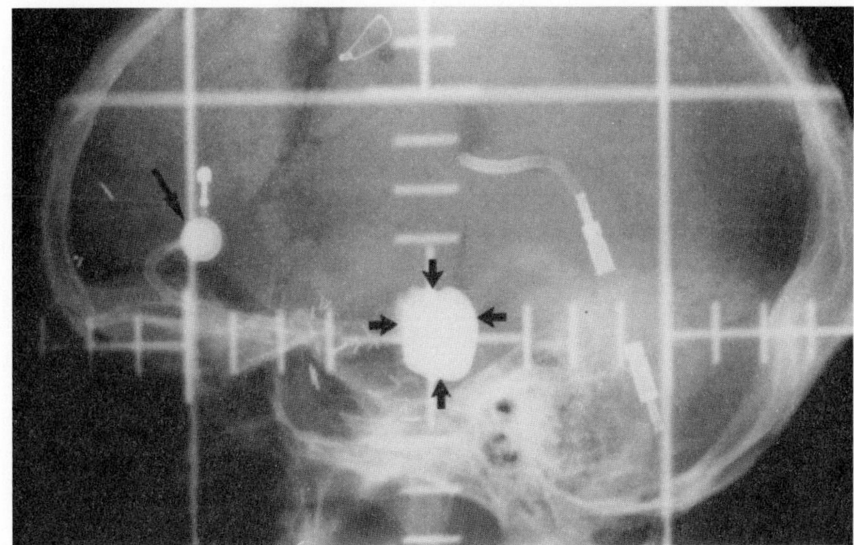

Fig. 20.5 Isohexal instillation via a Reckham reservoir positioned in the cystic part of a craniopharyngioma for volume estimation preparatory to remission isotope therapy. This 26-year-old woman had six craniotomies over a 13-year period and external-beam radiotherapy. The 12–15 ml cyst required aspiration of 5–8 ml fortnightly before β-emission therapy.

craniopharyngiomas repeatedly causes intracranial pressure problems. In these circumstances, intracystic instillation of β-emitting radioisotope provides an effective method of irradiating the secretory epithelium of the cyst wall to high dose (200–250 cGy) without (re-)irradiating adjacent brain tissue. There is a significant decrease in the 'refill rate' of the craniopharyngioma cyst after such therapy, and the procedure may be performed through an established reservoir into the cyst or by stereotactic puncture [33–40] (Fig. 20.5).

Thus, in the past 15 years the survival rate of patients with craniopharyngiomas has substantially improved due to the recognition of the importance of the routine use of external-beam therapy and the occasional use of intracystic isotope therapy. As Backlund [34] describes, it is possible to treat the cystic component with β-emitting isotope and adjacent solid portion with converging arc therapy.

Radiotherapy technique

The modern radiotherapeutic treatment of pituitary tumours is by multiple (almost always three) fixed, megavoltage (MV) X-ray portals. A head cast or shell is first made for the patient who lies in the supine position (the orbitomeatal line vertical) on the linear accelerator couch in this fixation device. The patient is next planned in a modern X-ray simulator, using modern imaging methods to determine the treatment volume. Noteworthy is the fact that our treatment volume is 5 mm around all imaged tumour boundaries, and also that we plan from the preoperative tumour size in postoperative cases but the post-bromocriptine tumour size in the primarily bromocriptine-shrunk prolactinomas. The simulator allows field centres and treatment volumes to be visualised on plain radiographs of the fossa, and the coaxial field centres are checked by lasers. Similar laser beams check the field centres on the linear accelerator couch, and a computed three-field isodosimetric plan is then actuated to deliver a dose of 4500 cGy in 25 fractions over 35 days, the final check being portal films on the first treatment day (Fig. 20.6).

The dose prescription just cited requires further comment. This dose was initiated by Professor Arthur Jones at St Bartholomew's Hospital some 25 years ago, and we have experience of some 400 pituitary adenoma patient follow-ups to testify to its safety and effectiveness. The daily dose (dose per fraction) is 180 cCy, and a daily dose below 200 cGy per day is felt to be important with regard to late optic chiasmal/hypothalamic/brainstem tolerance to radiation. It is accepted that the optic chiasm and hypothalamus, and probably the basilar artery, will be in the field. Other centres using yttrium implantation or proton-beam therapy also have good results, but nothing at present improves upon the results of carefully executed modern external beam X-ray therapy. The radiotherapy technique used for craniopharyngioma therapy is exactly the same as that used for pituitary radiotherapy, using the preoperative imaging for planning a three-field 6 or 8 MV X-ray plan at St Bartholomew's Hospital. However, our prescription takes the craniopharyngioma to 5000 cGy in 30 fractions over 42 days, a dose above which we would not deliver to the chiasm.

Recently, there has been considerable interest in focal radiotherapy techniques: proton beams, cobalt γ-knife and linear accelerator focal stereotactic radiotherapy/radiosurgery are all potentially applicable to pituitary adenomas. The conceptual beauty of using focal radiotherapy in this situation is that, being benign, a 'margin of safety' with regard to radiation volume around the adenoma is less necessary than with malignant tumours, and with so much critical adjacent nervous system it would seem highly appropriate

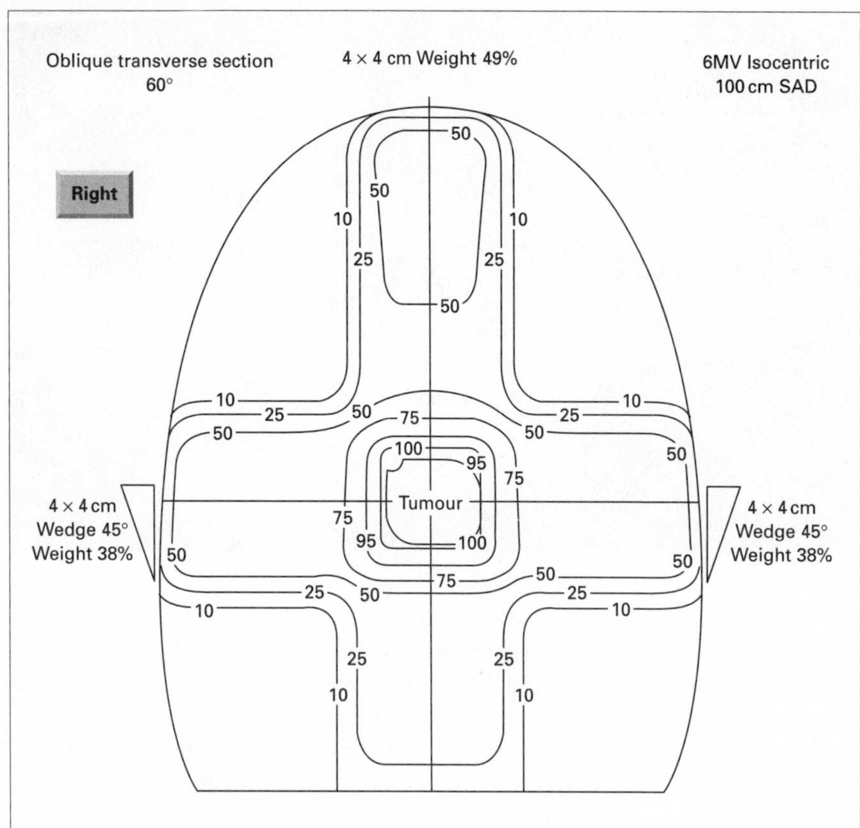

Fig. 20.6 Isodosimetric radiotherapy plan for pituitary adenoma treatment. Three fixed megavoltage X-ray fields.

to use a focal technique. However, the practicalities of focal radiotherapy make the situation not so clear-cut. Most of the focal radiotherapy techniques use one or 'a few' fractions of radiotherapy, necessarily of large size. This may not be of importance if the optic chiasm is outside the radiation volume but where the target volume abuts the chiasm, or other critically sensitive areas, not even the fast-falling radiation isodoses at the periphery of the radiation volume will spare these structures from high-dose fraction radiotherapy—a major factor in normal tissue morbidity. For these reasons, our own policy is to reserve these focal radiotherapy techniques for primary therapy of small adenomas lying low in the pituitary fossa or disease that is recurrent after conventional radiotherapy, especially recurrent disease extending laterally into the cavernous sinus regions. Having stated our own policy, I should state that the Pittsburgh group in the USA have used γ-knife technology to treat some 58 patients and report a low incidence of optic chiasmal damage.

Radiotherapy complications

The potential problems are those of hypopituitarism, chiasmal damage and late carcinogenesis. With increasing time after radiotherapy to pituitary adenomas, dynamic endocrine function tests will show worsening reserve in gonadotrophins, GH and later thyrotrophin/ACTH. Some patients who had normal pituitary reserve before radiotherapy will require anterior pituitary hormone replacement 10 years after therapy (we have never seen diabetes insipidus). The defect may well be mainly at the hypothalamic level [41] and such minor hypothalamic damage (probably to vasa nervorum) may also account for the late rise in serum prolactin concentration not infrequently encountered. These statements are even more relevant to patients irradiated for craniopharyngioma. Optic chiasmal damage should not be a problem if the dose prescription recommended above for pituitary adenoma is adhered to. However, optic chiasmal radiation tolerance is not much above this dose (and less far above the recommended craniopharyngioma dose prescription). The concern raised by Aristizabal and Boone [42] of increased radiosensitivity of the neurovascular connective tissue in this area in Cushing's disease is a theoretical increased risk, but the series reported by Howlett *et al.* [21] encountered no increased problems.

The risk of late malignancy following radiotherapy to pituitary adenomas is small, perhaps of the order of 10^{-3}. In our series of over 400 irradiated patients we have one patient who developed a temporal lobe glioma and a second patient who developed a malignant neuroendocrine tumour of the ethmoids. However, the difficulty in apportioning blame to radiotherapy is exemplified by the occurrence of a malignant glioma in another patient with pituitary adenoma at St Bartholomew's Hospital, who has never received radiotherapy.

References

1 Sheline G. Pituitary tumours: radiation therapy. In: Beardwell C, Robertson GL, eds. *Clinical Endocrinology 1. The Pituitary*. London: Butterworths, 1981: 106–39.

2 Sheline G, Boldrey EB, Philips TL. Chromophobe adenomas of the pituitary gland. *Am J Roentgenol Rad Ther Nucl Med* 1964; **92**: 160–73.

3 Sheline G. Treatment of chromophobe adenomas of the pituitary gland and acromegaly. In: Kohler PO, Ross G, eds. *Diagnosis and Treatment of Pituitary Tumours*. Amsterdam: Elsevier, 1973: 201–16.

4 Bradley KM, Adams CBT, Potter CPS *et al.* An audit of selected patients with non-functioning pituitary adenoma treated by transsphenoidal surgery without irradiation. *Clin Endocrinol* 1994; **41**: 655–9.

5 Laws ER. Surgical management of pituitary adenomas. In: *Pituitary Tumour's. Baillières Clin Endocrinol Metab* 1995; **9**: 391–405.

6 Brada M, Rajan B, Traish D *et al.* The long term efficacy of conservative surgery and radiotherapy in the control of pituitary adenomas. *Clin Endocrinol* 1993; **38**: 571–8.

7 Jaffrain-Rea ML, Derome P, Bataini JP, Thomopoulos P, Bertagna X, Luton JP. Influence of radiotherapy on long-term relapse in clinically non-secreting pituitary adenomas. *Eur J Med* 1993; **2**: 398–403.

8 Beclere J. The radiotherapeutic treatment of tumours of the hypophysis, gigantism and acromegaly. *Arch Roentgen Ray* 1909; **111**: 17–23.

9 Gramegna A. Un cas d'acromegalie traite par la radiotherapie. *Rev Neurol (Paris)* 1909; **17**: 15–20.

10 Sheline GE, Goldberg MB, Feldman R. Pituitary irradiation for acromegaly. *Radiology* 1961; **76**: 70–5.

11 Eastman RC, Gorden P, Roth J. Conventional supervoltage irradiation is an effective treatment for acromegaly. *J Clin Endocrinol Metab* 1979; **48**: 931–40.

12 Ciccarelli EC, Orsello SM, Plowman PN, Besser GM, Wass JAH. Prolonged lowering of growth hormone after radiotherapy in acromegalic patients followed over 15 years. *Biosci* 1988; **69**: 269–72.

13 Littley MD, Shalet SM, Swindell SR *et al.* Low dose pituitary irradiation for acromegaly. *Clin Endocrinol* 1990; **32**: 261–70.

14 Corenblum B, Webster BR, Mortimer CB, Ezrin C. Possible antitumor effect of 2-bromo-ergocryptine in two patients with large prolactin secreting pituitary adenomas. *Clin Res* 1975; **23**: 614A.

15 Serri O, Rasio E, Beanregard H *et al.* Recurrence of hyperprolactinemia after selective adenomectomy in women with prolactinoma. *N Engl J Med* 1983; **309**: 280–3.

16 Grossman A, Cohen BL, Charlesworth M *et al.* Treatment of prolactinomas with megavoltage radiotherapy. *Br Med J* 1984; **288**: 1105–9.

17 Dohan FC, Raventos A, Boucot N, Rose E. Roentgen therapy in Cushing's syndrome without adrenocortical tumor. *J Clin Endocrinol Metab* 1957; **17**: 8–32.

18 Soffer JL, Iannaconne A, Gabrilove JL. Cushing's syndrome. A study of fifty patients. *Am J Med* 1961; **30**: 129–46.

19 Henschele R, Lampe I. Pituitary irradiation for Cushing's syndrome. *Radiol Clin Biol* 1967; **36**: 27–31.

20 Orth DN, Liddle GW. Results of treatment in 108 patients with Cushing's syndrome. *N Engl J Med* 1971; **285**: 243–7.

21 Howlett TA, Plowman PN, Wass JAH, Rees LH, Jones AE, Besser GM. Megavoltage pituitary irradiation in the management of Cushing's disease and Nelson's syndrome: long term follow up. *Clin Endocrinol* 1989; **31**: 309–23.

22 Jenkins PJ, Trainer PJ, Plowman PN *et al.* The long term outcome after adrenalectomy and prophylactic pituitary radiotherapy in adrenocorticotrophin-dependent Cushing's syndrome *J Clin Endocrinol Metab* 1995; **79**: 165–71.

23 Matson DD, Crigler JF. Management of craniopharyngioma in childhood. *J Neurosurg* 1969; **30**: 377–90.

24 Katz EL. Late results of radical excision of craniopharyngiomas in children. *J Neurosurg* 1975; **42**: 86–96.

25 Amacher AL. Craniopharyngioma: the controversy regarding radiotherapy. *Childs Brain* 1980; **6**: 57–64.

26 Kramer S. Radiation therapy in the management of craniopharyngiomas. In: Deeley TJ, ed. *Modern Radiotherapy and Oncology, Central Nervous System Tumours*. London: Butterworths, 1974: 204–23.

27 McMurry FG, Hardy RW, Dohn DF, Sadar E, Gardner WJ. Long term results in the management of craniopharyngiomas. *Neurosurgery* 1977; **1**: 238–41.

28 Richmond IL, Wara WM, Wilson CB. Role of radiation therapy in the management of craniopharyngiomas in children. *Neurosurgery* 1980; **6**: 513–17.

29 Sung DI, Chang CH, Harisiadis L, Carmel PW. Treatment results of craniopharyngiomas. *Cancer* 1981; **47**: 847–52.

30 Stahnke N, Grubel G, Lagenstein I, Willig RP. Long term followup of children with craniopharyngioma. *Eur J Pediatr* 1984; **142**: 179–85.

31 Fischer EG, Welch K, Belli JA, Wallman J, Shillito JJ, Winston KR, Cassady R. Treatment of craniopharyngiomas in children 1972–1981. *J Neurosurg* 1985; **62**: 496–501.

32 Manaka S, Teramoto A, Takakura K. The efficacy of radiotherapy for craniopharyngioma. *J Neurosurg* 1985; **62**: 648–56.

33 Huk WJ, Mahlstedt J. Intracystic radiotherapy (^{90}Y) of craniopharyngiomas. CT-guided stereotaxic implantation of indwelling drainage system. *Nuc Roentgenol* 1983; **52**: 803–6.

34 Backlund EO. Stereotaxic treatment of craniopharyngiomas. *Acta Neurochir Suppl* 1974; **21**: 177–83.

35 Witt TC, Kondiolka D, Flickinger JC, Lansford LD. Stereotactic radiosurgery for pituitary tumours. In: Koudziolka D, ed. *Radiosurgery 1995*. Basel: Karger, 1996: 55–65.

36 Kobayashi T, Kageyama N, Ohara K. Internal irradiation for cystic craniopharyngioma. *J Neurosurg* 1981; **55**: 896–903.

37 Strauss L, Sturm V, Georgi P *et al.* Radioisotope therapy of cystic craniopharyngiomas. *Int J Radiat Oncol Biol Phys* 1982; **8**: 1581–5.

38 Huk WJ, Mahlstedt J. Intracystic radiotherapy (90Y) of craniopharyngiomas: CT guided stereotaxic implantation of indwelling drainage system. *Am J Neur Res* 1983; **4**: 803–6.

39 Julow J, Lanyi F, Hajda M *et al.* The radiotherapy of cystic craniopharyngioma with intracystic installation of 90Y silicate colloid. *Acta Neurochir* 1985; **74**: 94–9.

40 Pollack IF, Lunsford LD, Slamovits TL, Gumerman LW, Levine G, Robinson AG. Stereotaxic intracavitary irradiation for cystic craniopharyngiomas. *J Neurosurg* 1988; **68**: 227–33.

41 Blacklay A, Grossman A, Savage M, Plowman PN, Coy DH,

Besser GM. Cranial irradiation in children with cerebral tumours—evidence for a hypothalamic defect in growth hormone release. *J Endocrinol* 1986; **108**: 25–9.

42 Aristizabal S, Boone MLM. Radiation tolerance of nervous tissue: evidence of decreased tolerance in patients with Cushing's disease. *Int J Radiat Oncol Biol Phys* 1977; **2** (Suppl. 1): 56.

43 Tsagarakis S, Grossman A, Plowman PN *et al*. Megavoltage pituitary irradiation in the management of prolactinomas: long-term follow-up. *Clin Endocrinol* 1991; **34**: 399–406.

CHAPTER 21

Pituitary carcinoma and cytotoxic chemotherapy for aggressive pituitary tumours

P.A. Price

Classification and aetiology of malignant pituitary tumours

Pituitary tumours represent about 10% of all intracranial neoplasms, yet true pituitary carcinoma is extremely uncommon. The diagnosis of malignancy in pituitary tumours is based on the pattern of growth and spread rather than on histological criteria [1].

The malignancy of pituitary tumours cannot be defined histologically. In contrast to most human epithelial cancers, the generic histological criteria of malignancy (anaplasia, nuclear atypia and pleomorphism, mitotic activity and necrosis) are insufficient to secure a diagnosis of pituitary carcinoma, because these features may be seen in ordinary pituitary adenomas. The diagnosis is dependent on the tumour's biological behaviour and is relatively independent of histology [2].

Pituitary adenomas are benign and discrete, but not truly encapsulated, tumours. There is often a pseudo-capsule of compressed adjacent non-neoplastic gland. Microscopic cellular infiltration of the pseudo-capsule by adenoma cells is quite common [3]. In addition to suprasellar extension, infiltration and compression of neighbouring structures may occur: laterally into the cavernous sinus and downwards through the bony floor of the sella into the sphenoid air sinus. Adenomas have presented clinically as 'polyps' in the upper nasopharynx. In the past, many authors have regarded invasion of the cavernous sinuses with tumour cells and local infiltration of the adjacent nerves and adventitia of vessels as evidence of malignancy. These tumours were called 'malignant adenoma' or carcinoma. Jefferson [4] preferred to call these tumours 'invasive adenomas' to be distinguished from carcinomas by the absence of metastases. Jefferson surmised that probably 10% of all pituitary adenomas that come to surgery are invasive. True pituitary carcinomas according to this definition are much rarer, and there are less than 50 well documented cases in the literature [5]. Local invasion may be present, but in addition there is evidence of metastases within the central nervous system (CNS) or more rarely extracranial metastases. CNS dissemination appears to be the result of invasive extension into the subarachnoid space and subsequent dissemination by cerebrospinal fluid flow. Intracranial deposits involving brain substance probably develop as the result of tumour permeation of perivascular (Virchow–Robin) spaces or by venous sinus invasion. Extracranial spread of pituitary carcinomas involves both haematogenous and lymphatic routes. Invasion of the cavernous sinuses provides the necessary venous access for transport to the internal jugular vein via the petrosal system. The pituitary itself lacks lymphatic drainage; however, invasion of the tumour into the skull base provides access to a rich lymphatic network, which in turn mediates systemic dissemination [2].

The aetiology of pituitary carcinoma is unknown. In some cases a protracted course, often punctuated by multiple local recurrence, is then followed by metastatic dissemination. In many such cases clear escalation in histological aggressiveness from pituitary tumour to metastatic deposit is evident, suggesting that some pituitary carcinomas arise as a result of malignant transformation in a pre-existing benign tumour. In other cases the behaviour of a pituitary carcinoma suggests *de novo* malignancy, in that they do not appear to arise from malignant degeneration of a pre-existing benign adenoma. Instead, such tumours can be considered genuinely malignant cancers from the outset, beginning as locally invasive, cytologically atypical primary tumours which promptly give way to metastatic dissemination.

There is no evidence that pituitary carcinoma results from pituitary irradiation. Indeed, pituitary malignancy following pituitary irradiation is extremely rare, and reported cases are usually of fibrosarcoma or glioma [6].

Clinical features of pituitary carcinoma

The aggressive behaviour of pituitary carcinomas and indeed invasive adenomas cannot usually be predicted at the time of presentation. It is usually impossible to foresee whether any given pituitary tumour harbours metastatic potential, and in many patients the initial clinical course is indistinguishable from that of a benign adenoma [7]. Pituitary carcinomas are more likely to present preoperatively with diabetes insipidus because of hypothalamic invasion [7]; often, extracranial metastases are only identified years after the initial presentation of the tumour.

Metastases may be identified by histological, immunocytochemical or electron-microscopic features, and have been found in numerous sites including thoracic and cervical lymph nodes, liver, lung, bone, mediastinum, heart and kidney [2].

Extracranial metastases from five cases of malignant prolactinomas became evident between 4 and 14 years after the initial presentation of the tumour [8]. Indeed, metastases have been reported as late as 30 years after the initial diagnosis of the primary tumour [9].

Often, extracranial metastases are only identified at autopsy [10] and have not apparently contributed to the clinical course of the disease; death is usually the result of mass effect from extensive intracranial disease. The prevalence of micrometastatic extracranial pituitary carcinoma may therefore be underestimated. Intracranial metastases may occur many years following treatment, and apparent cure, of a pituitary adenoma without any evidence of recurrent local pituitary disease [11]. Pituitary carcinomas may be non-functioning or secrete growth hormone [12], prolactin [8] or adrenocorticotrophic hormone (ACTH) [13].

Treatment of pituitary carcinoma and invasive adenomas

The conventional treatment of large pituitary tumours consists of surgery, external radiotherapy and, where appropriate, non-cytotoxic chemotherapy, especially with a dopamine agonist such as bromocriptine. Pituitary carcinomas and often invasive adenomas recur repeatedly despite several attempts at radical surgery. The dose of radiotherapy which can be given is limited by the risk of radiation necrosis, although recent evidence suggests that stereotactic radiotherapy can be useful for well-circumscribed disease. Nevertheless, the outlook for invasive pituitary tumours and pituitary carcinomas is bleak, with visual loss, progressive neurological disability and death [4].

Cytotoxic chemotherapy

There have been a few promising reports of the value of combination cytotoxic chemotherapy in these recurrent aggressive tumours, leading to tumour shrinkage, improvement in vision and decrease in tumour or secretory status. Cytotoxic chemotherapy, whilst unlikely to be curative, may provide useful clinical remission where conventional therapeutic modalities have failed. Whilst there is very little published information in this difficult area, clinical details of the few reported cases where cytotoxic chemotherapy has been successfully used will be outlined to suggest the type of clinical settings in which cytotoxic chemotherapy might be used. Some broad recommendations on possible chemotherapeutic regimens will then be given.

Clinical characteristics of patients treated with cytotoxic chemotherapy

The three patients reported from the UK [14,15, P.E. Belchetz, personal communication] all presented with visual failure, and were found to have large pituitary tumours with massive extrasellar extensions at presentation. Histology at the first operation was of a chromophobe adenoma in each case. Table 21.1 details other relevant clinical information, and includes the chemotherapy regimen and the clinical response to this treatment. A fourth case from Poland [16] of a patient with a large pituitary adenoma causing acromegaly has also been described; tumour recurrence occurred following repetitive surgery, radiotherapy and bromocriptine. The tumour responded to combination chemotherapy with doxorubicin and lomustine (CCNU). Further surgery, however, may well have been possible before this chemotherapy was used: it seems that the benefits of conventional therapy had not been exhausted, although the response to cytotoxic chemotherapy is of some interest.

Cytotoxic chemotherapy regimens

The chemotherapy regimens chosen in the UK cases were based on the treatment of cerebral gliomas: the drugs used penetrate the blood–brain barrier and achieve demonstrable levels in the cerebrospinal fluid [17,18]. However, there is some evidence that, where an invasive tumour is present, the blood–brain barrier is less intact than in normal individuals, and thus such factors may be less important than previously considered.

The regimen successfully used in patients 1 and 3 is only moderately toxic in terms of side-effects, and can be given orally as out-patient therapy. This is particularly relevant, because treatment is likely to be palliative rather than curative. The detailed protocol is as follows:

Table 21.1 Results of combination chemotherapy in patients with aggressive pituitary tumours.

Patient no.	Age (years)	Sex	Tumour secretory status	Initial therapies: Mode	Date	Tumour status at time of chemotherapy	Chemotherapy	Response to chemotherapy
1 [2,3]	37	F	Non-functioning initially, adrenocorticotrophic hormone later	Surgery + R/T (36 Gy) Surgery + R/T (35 Gy) Surgery Surgery Adrenalectomy	1964 1973 1979 1982 1982	Parasellar tumour extending into temporal lobe and displacing brainstem	Procarbazine Etoposide Lomustine (CCNU)	Slight decrease in tumour size over 18 months with 2 years' remission; fall in adrenocorticotrophin levels
2 [2]	32	M	Growth hormone	Surgery + R/T (45 Gy) Surgery (twice)	1982 1983	Large tumour invading right cerebral hemisphere	Methotrexate Vincristine (+ folinic acid rescue then High-dose BCNU	No response 2 years' remission
3*	38	M	Prolactin	Surgery + R/T (45 Gy) Cyst drainage Bromocriptine Surgery	1979 1980 1981 1985	Huge tumour invading middle cranial fossa	Procarbazine Etoposide Lomustine (CCNU)	Marked tumour shrinkage with 15 months' remission

* P.E. Belchetz, personal communication. R/T, radiotherapy.

1 procarbazine, 50 mg three times daily for 7 days;
2 etoposide, 100 mg/m^2 for 3 days, followed by 2 days later by;
3 lomustine, 100 mg/m as a single dose.

This cytotoxic regimen may be repeated every 6–8 weeks. An alternative treatment plan, based on that used for carcinoid tumours and employing the relatively well-tolerated drugs 5-fluorouracil and lomustine [19], has also been shown to be of some value in the treatment of malignant prolactinomas; carboplatin has also been used, although its clinical efficacy was uncertain (A. Grossman, personal communication).

The exact scheme and doses used would be best designed in conjunction with a clinical oncologist, particularly in the light of current chemotherapeutic regimens for the treatment of other malignant cerebral tumours.

Conclusions

A proportion of pituitary tumours behave in an aggressive manner. Three categories of aggressive pituitary tumours may be defined:

1 invasive adenomas;
2 rare carcinomas with deposits restricted to the CNS;
3 even more rare carcinomas with extracranial systemic metastases.

Invasive adenomas and pituitary carcinomas may be non-functioning or secrete prolactin, growth hormone and/or ACTH.

Pituitary carcinomas and some invasive adenomas behave in an aggressive manner often recurring despite maximal therapy with surgery, radiotherapy, and in the case of prolactinomas, dopamine-agonist therapy. Cytotoxic chemotherapy is worthwhile in patients whose tumours cannot be controlled by these more conventional treatment modalities. Published experience is scant, but such treatment may provide a useful clinical remission in an otherwise fairly hopeless clinical setting. It is always worth considering other neurotransmitter manipulation for secretory tumours: octreotide for growth hormone-secreting tumours; cyproheptadine, bromocriptine and sodium valproate for those secreting ACTH. Bromocriptine-resistant prolactinomas have been reported to respond to other dopamine agonists such as pergolide and quinagolide [20,21] and to the combination of bromocriptine and the anti-oestrogen tamoxifen [22].

References

1 Doniach I. Histopathology of the pituitary. *Clin Endocrinol Metab* 1985; **14**: 765–89.

2 Thapar K, Kovacs K, Muller PJ. Clinico-pathological correlations of pituitary tumours. *Clin Endocrinol Metab* 1995; **9**: 243–70.

3 Doniach I. Pituitary carcinoma. *Clin Endocrinol* 1992; **37**: 194–5.

4 Jefferson G. The invasive adenomas of the pituitary. In: *The Sherrington Lectures* 1955; **III**: 3–63. Liverpool: University Press.

5 Pernicone J, Scheithauer BW. Invasive pituitary adenomas and pituitary carcinomas. In Lloyd RV, ed. *Surgical Pathology of the Pituitary Gland*. Philadelphia: WB Saunders, 1993: 121–36.

6 Plowman PN. Radiotherapy for pituitary tumours. *Clin Endocrinol Metab* 1995; **9**: 407–20.

7 Thapar K, Kovacs KT, Lawes ER, Muller PJ. Pituitary adenomas: current concepts in classification, histopathology and molecular biology. *The Endocrinologist* 1993; **3**: 39–57.

8 Walker JD, Grossman A, Anderson JV *et al.* Malignant prolactinoma with extracranial metastases: a report of three cases. *Clin Endocrinol* 1993; **38**: 411–19.

9 Scheithauer BW, Randall RV, Lawes ER *et al.* Prolactin cell carcinoma of the pituitary. Clinicopathological, immunohistochemical and ultrastructural study of a case with cranial and extracranial metastases. *Cancer* 1985; **55**: 598–604.

10 Mountcastle RB, Roof BS, Mayfield RK *et al.* Case report: pituitary adenocarcinoma in an acromegalic patient: response to bromocriptine and pituitary testing: a review of the literature in 36 cases of pituitary carcinoma. *Am J Med Sci* 1989; **298**: 109–18.

11 O'Brien DP, Phillips JP, Rawluk DR, Farrell MA. Intracranial metastases from pituitary adenoma. *Br J Neurosurg* 1995; **9**: 211–18.

12 Stewart PM, Carey MP, Graham CT, Wright AD, London DR. Growth hormone secreting pituitary carcinoma: a case report and literature review. *Clin Endocrinol* 1992; **37**: 189–95.

13 Nawata H, Higuchi K, Ikuyama S *et al.* Corticotrophin-releasing hormone and adrenocorticotrophin-producing pituitary carcinoma with metastases to the liver and lung in a patient with Cushing's disease. *J Clin Endocrinol Metab* 1990; **127**: 1068–73.

14 Price PA, Bloom HJG, McElwain TJ, Jenkins JS. Recurrent invasive pituitary tumours responsive to cytotoxic chemotherapy. *J Endocrinol* 1985; **104** (Suppl.): 54.

15 Vaughan NJA, Laroche CM, Goodman I, Davies MJ, Jenkins JS. Pituitary Cushing's disease arising from a previously non-functional corticotrophic chromophobe adenoma. *Clin Endocrinol* 1985; **22**: 147–53.

16 Kasperlik-Zaluska AA, Wislawski J, Kaniewska J, Zborzil J, Frankiewicz E, Zgliczynski S. Cytostatics for acromegaly—marked improvement in a patient with an invasive pituitary tumour. *Acta Endocrinol* 1987; **116**: 347–9.

17 Stewart DJ, Richard M, Hugenholtz H, Denney J. VP16 (VP) and VM26 (VM) penetration into human brain tumours (BT). *Proc Am Assoc Cancer Res* 1983; **24**: 133 (abstract).

18 O'Dwyer PJ, Leyland-Jones B, Alonso MJ, Parsoni S, Wittes RE. Etoposide—current status of an active anti-cancer drug. *N Engl J Med* 1985; **692**: 700.

19 Harris PE, Bouloux PMG, Wass JAH, Besser GM. Successful treatment by chemotherapy for acromegaly associated with ectopic growth hormone releasing hormone secretion from a carcinoid tumour. *Clin Endocrinol* 1990; **24**: 421–6.

20 Ahmad SR, Shalat SM. Discordant responses of a prolactinoma to two different dopamine agonists. *Clin Endocrinol* 1986; **24**: 421–6.

21 Duranteau L, Chanson P, Lavoinne A, Horlait S, Lubetzki J, Kuhn JM. Effect of the new dopaminergic agonist CV 205–502 on plasma levels and tumour size in bromocriptine-resistant prolactinomas. *Clin Endocrinol* 1991; **34**: 25–9.

22 Volker W, Gehring WG, Berming R *et al.* Impaired pituitary response to bromocriptine suppression: reversal after bromocriptine plus tamoxifen. *Acta Endocrinol (Copenh)* 1982; **101**: 491–500.

CHAPTER 22

Disorders of water balance

P.H. Baylis

Introduction

In recent years, our understanding of the mechanisms involved in the control of water balance and of the pathogenetic processes causing abnormalities of water homeostasis has increased substantially. With the development of radioimmunoassays capable of measuring the extremely low circulating concentrations of the antidiuretic hormone, vasopressin, and methods to assess thirst sensation, it is now possible to delineate more accurately the pathophysiology of disorders of water balance, investigate patients more appropriately and offer more rational treatment.

This chapter will describe briefly the basic physiology of osmoregulation and water homeostasis before dealing with the three major disturbances of water balance, polyuric, hypernatraemic and hyponatraemic states, with particular reference to the syndrome of inappropriate antidiuresis.

The physiology of water homeostasis

The maintenance of normal water balance is achieved principally by the interrelationship of three determinants, vasopressin, the kidney and thirst. There must be adequate secretion of osmotically stimulated vasopressin, which then acts upon the renal tubule to regulate solute-free water excretion. The kidney is capable of wide variations in urine output, ranging from 0.5–20 litres per 24 hours, without causing significant disturbance to the internal osmotic environment. The third determinant is osmoregulated thirst which stimulates the intake of fluid and is particularly important when the kidney is concentrating urine maximally but the body is still losing water. Under these circumstances it is the fluid input driven by thirst that maintains normal water homeostasis.

The importance of regulating water balance is to ensure that plasma osmolality, and therefore extracellular fluid osmolality, remains stable. The exquisite sensitivity of the function of the three major determinants allows plasma osmolality to be maintained within a narrow range, 285–295 mosmol/kg approximately.

In health, both vasopressin secretion and thirst are regulated mainly by plasma osmolality. Changes in plasma osmolality are detected by groups of specialised cells, the osmoreceptors. They are located in the anterior hypothalamus, the circumventricular organs, where fenestrations in the blood–brain barrier exist to allow circulating solutes (osmoles) to influence the brain osmoreceptors. Evidence from animal work has suggested at least two sites for osmoreceptors, the subfornical organ and the organum vasculosum laminae terminalis [1]. The osmoreceptor cells are believed to alter their volume by the transmembrane flux of water in response to changes in plasma osmolality, which initiates neuronal impulses that are transmitted to the supraoptic and paraventricular hypothalamic nuclei to release vasopressin and to the cerebral cortex to register thirst sensation.

Vasopressin, a nonapeptide, is derived from a large precursor molecule which comprises a signal peptide, vasopressin, its associated neurophysin and a glycoprotein moiety. Its gene is located on chromosome 20, close to the gene encoding for oxytocin (Fig. 22.1).

The functional characteristics of osmoregulated vasopressin secretion were defined originally in healthy adults by Robertson *et al.* [2], and have been confirmed by other groups [3]. Briefly, as plasma osmolality rises so there is a linear increase in plasma vasopressin concentration (Fig. 22.2). The relationship between the two variables, plasma vasopressin (p*Vp*) and plasma osmolality (p*Os*) can be expressed by the function, $pVp = 0.41\,(pOs–285)$. The abscissal intercept, 285 mosmol/kg, represents the osmotic threshold of vasopressin release, and the slope, 0.41 pmol *Vp*/1 per mosmol/kg, is a measure of the sensitivity of the vasopressin osmoreceptor and vasopressin-secreting unit. Thus, at plasma

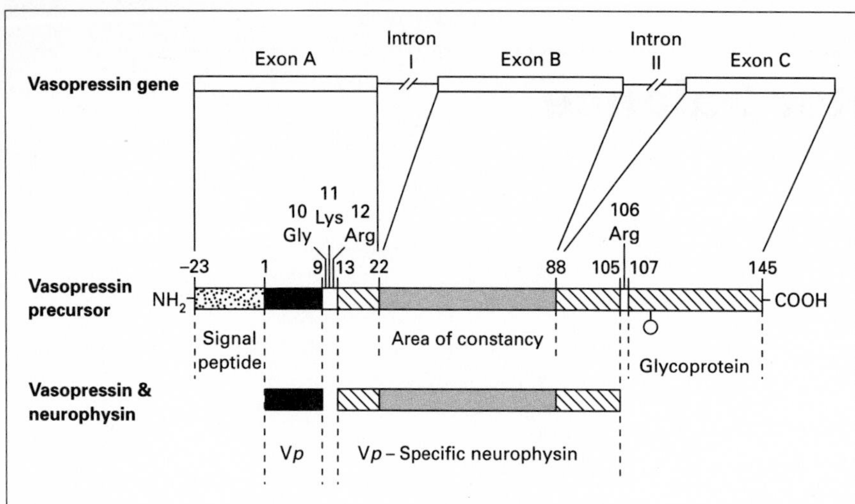

Fig. 22.1 Schematic representation of the vasopressin gene on chromosome 20, the precursor molecule, vasopressin and its specific neurophysin.

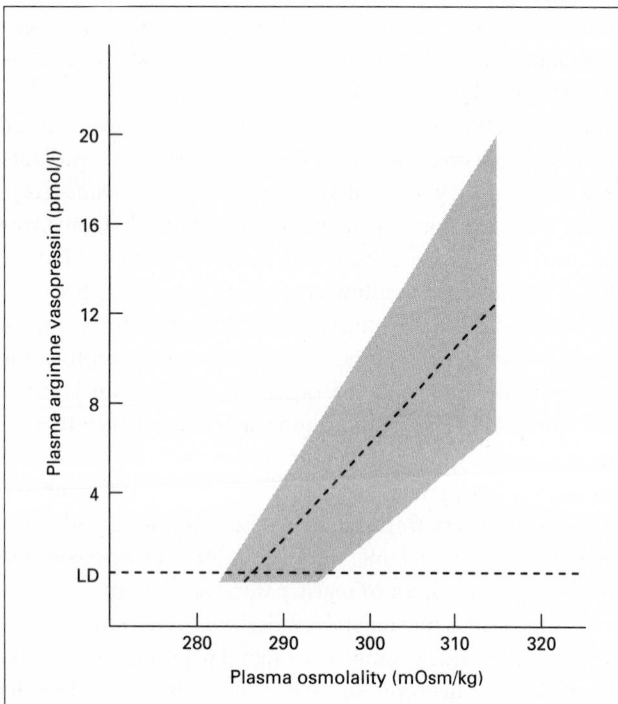

Fig. 22.2 The relationship between plasma arginine vasopressin and plasma osmolality. The stippled area represents the normal response of a group of healthy adults infused with hypertonic saline. The dashed line is the mean regression osmoregulatory line defining the function, p*Vp* = 0.41 (p*Os* – 285), *r* = +0.96, *P* < 0.001; p*Vp* being plasma vasopressin and p*Os*, plasma osmolality. LD is the limit of detection of the plasma vasopressin assay, 0.3 pmol/l. Adapted from [3], with permission.

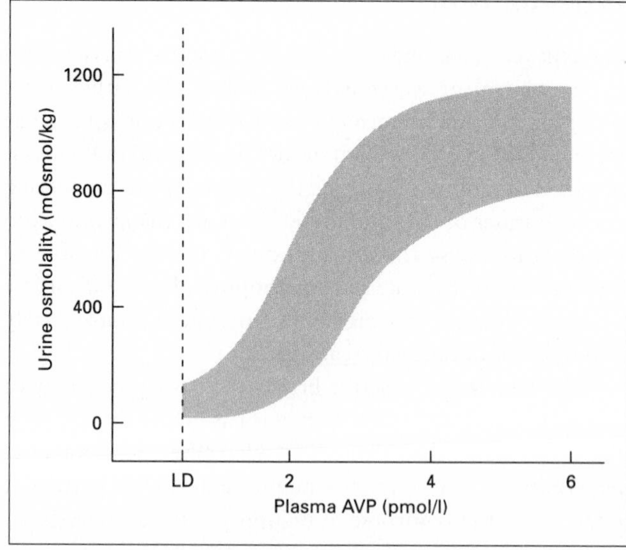

Fig. 22.3 The relationship between urine osmolality and plasma arginine vasopressin (AVP) from a group of healthy adults in various states of hydration. LD is the limit of detection of the plasma vasopressin assay, 0.3 pmol/l. From [33], with permission.

osmolality values of <285 mosmol/kg, on average, plasma vasopressin will be undetectable (< 0.3 pmol/l), maximum urine dilution occurs (urine osmolality 50–70 mosmol/kg) and the kidney excretes up to 15–20 litres of urine per 24 hours. As plasma osmolality increases to about 295 mosmol/kg, sufficient vasopressin is secreted to attain a maximum urinary concentration (Fig. 22.3). Alterations in the two indices describing osmoregulated vasopressin, the threshold and sensitivity, have been observed in some disorders of water balance.

A similar relationship exists between plasma osmolality and thirst assessed by a visual analogue scale [3] (Fig. 22.4). The sensation of thirst is minimal under basal resting conditions in healthy adults and increases progressively as plasma osmolality rises. The osmotic threshold for thirst onset, 281 mosmol/kg, is similar to the vasopressin threshold but the osmoreceptors serving thirst are probably anatomically distinct from those responsible for vasopressin secretion [4],

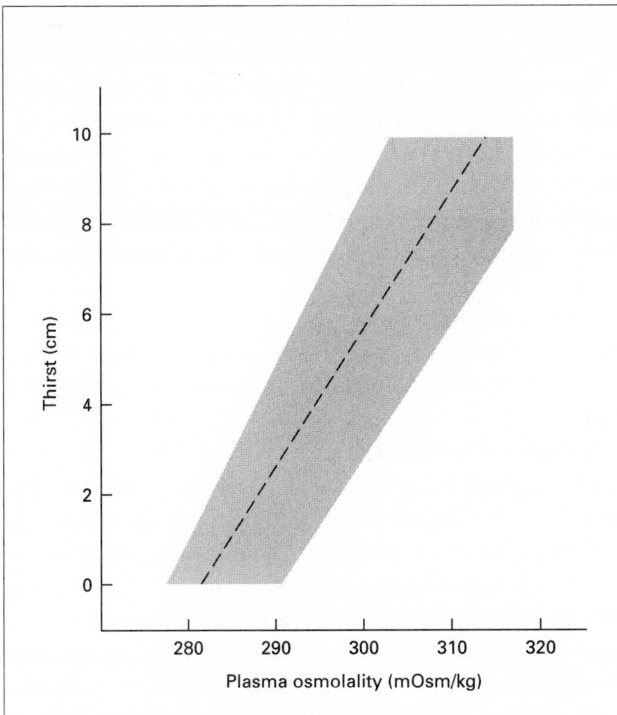

Fig. 22.4 The relationship between thirst and plasma osmolality. The shaded area represents the normal response of a group of healthy adults infused with hypertonic saline. The dashed line is the mean regression osmoregulatory line defining the function, $Th = 0.30\ (pOs - 281)$, $r = +0.91$, $P < 0.001$; *Th* being thirst and p*Os*, plasma osmolality. Adapted from [3], with permission.

although they too are situated in the circumventricular organs. Thus, at plasma osmolalities below the thirst threshold, there is no desire to drink at all, whereas increases in plasma osmolality above the threshold stimulate thirst.

It is recognised that each healthy individual has a unique threshold and sensitivity for both thirst and vasopressin secretion. These appear to change with age. Thirst is blunted in the elderly, but the sensitivity of the vasopressin osmostat (i.e. the slope of the regression line, Fig. 22.2) probably increases with age. This unusual physiological consequence of the ageing process, which results in more vasopressin secreted per unit rise in plasma osmolality, helps to compensate for the decline in renal concentrating ability.

Pregnancy is a 'physiological' condition associated with profound alterations in osmoregulation. Plasma osmolality falls by about 10 mosmol/kg, which is entirely due to a lowering of both thirst and vasopressin osmotic thresholds. The cause is not yet understood fully, but is probably due to the hormonal changes, particularly circulating human chorionic gonadotrophin, associated with pregnancy [5]. Similar but lesser changes in osmoregulation occur in the luteal phase of healthy cycling women [4].

It must be emphasised that the osmoregulatory system is not equally responsive to all plasma solutes. Plasma sodium and its anions elicit the greatest response whereas hyperglycaemia has minimal effects on thirst or vasopressin release [6]. Interestingly, the act of drinking causes precipitous falls in plasma vasopressin concentrations and thirst appreciation which are independent of plasma osmolality and are probably mediated by an oropharyngeal neuroendocrine reflex.

Thirst and vasopressin secretion can also be influenced by numerous non-osmotic factors, including changes in blood pressure and volume, nausea, hypoglycaemia and circulating substances (e.g. angiotensin II) [7]. None plays a significant role in the maintenance of water homeostasis in health, but each may assume major importance in some disorders of water balance.

Polyuric states

Polyuria may be defined as a state of excessive hypotonic urine secretion. Under conditions of *ad libitum* fluid intake, urine volumes > 2.5 litres/24 hours (40 ml/kg/24 hours) with persistent urine osmolalities < 300 mosmol/kg are regarded as abnormal. Only three pathogenetic mechanisms are responsible for polyuria. The first is a lack of osmoregulated vasopressin secretion which is termed as *cranial diabetes insipidus* but also known as central, neurogenic, hypothalamic or vasopressin-sensitive diabetes insipidus. The second mechanism is a reduction in the response of the renal tubule to adequate concentrations of circulating vasopressin, usually called *nephrogenic or vasopressin-resistant diabetes insipidus.* Thirdly, excessive persistent intake of fluid, referred to as *primary polydipsia* or dipsogenic diabetes insipidus will cause polyuria. Each will be discussed individually but their diagnostic differentiation will be described in a common section. The diabetes insipidus that occurs transiently in human pregnancy is rare and is probably caused by more than one mechanism (see below).

Cranial diabetes insipidus

This syndrome is defined as a disorder of urinary concentration resulting from deficient secretion of osmoregulated vasopressin. It has been estimated that at least 80% of vasopressin-synthesising neurons must be destroyed before overt clinical features become manifest. Cranial diabetes insipidus has been the subject of recent reviews [4,8–10] and a symposium [11].

Aetiology

The pathological causes of cranial diabetes insipidus are given in Table 22.1. In a recent survey of 104 cases [10], 27% were idiopathic, occurring between the ages of 1 and

Table 22.1 Causes of cranial diabetes insipidus.

Primary
Idiopathic
Familial (autosomal dominant)
DIDMOAD syndrome (autosomal recessive)
Secondary
Trauma (surgical, accidental)
Neoplasia (hypothalamic, pituitary, parapituitary)
Granulomas (histiocytosis, sarcoidosis)
Infections (encephalitis, meningitis)
Lymphocytic infiltration of neurohypophysis
Vascular incidents (Sheehan's syndrome, aneurysms)
Autoimmune (antibodies to vasopressin-producing neurons)

71 years, with a male preponderance of 70%. Rarely, the condition is familial (<5% of all cases). The mode of inheritance is usually autosomal dominant. Molecular studies in several kindreds have identified abnormalities unique to each family, and include single nucleotide substitutions or base-pair deletions, frequently involving the region encoding for vasopressin-associated neurophysin but rarely vasopressin itself or its signal peptide [12].

The DIDMOAD or Wolfram syndrome has generated interest out of proportion to its frequency of occurrence. The syndrome comprises DI (diabetes insipidus), DM (diabetes mellitus), OA (optic atrophy) and D (deafness). It has an autosomal recessive inheritance possibly due to a disorder of mitochondrial DNA, and patients may express some or all features of the syndrome. A few patients have, in addition, abnormalities of the renal tract with hydronephrosis and atonia of the bladder. The onset of polyuria in the familial causes of cranial diabetes insipidus is usually in early childhood but rarely in infancy. As a consequence of persistent polyuria in early life, patients develop enuresis, may not complain of the classical symptoms and regard their degree of thirst and polyuria as normal for their family. The pathological findings at autopsy of patients with idiopathic and familial cranial diabetes insipidus are neuronal degeneration of the supraoptic and paraventricular nuclei. Rarely, patients have an absent or small neurohypophysis [4].

The majority of patients with cranial diabetes insipidus develop the disorder secondary to an underlying abnormality (Table 22.1). Surgical injury to the posterior pituitary during hypophysectomy or selective adenomectomy often results in transient cranial diabetes insipidus, lasting a few hours to a few days with subsequent complete clinical recovery. Persistent cranial diabetes insipidus occurs more frequently after transfrontal than transsphenoidal approaches to the pituitary gland. In Moses' survey [10], at least 26% of all cases of cranial diabetes insipidus developed before or after surgery for pituitary or brain tumours. Head trauma, which may be a closed injury, accounted for about 18% of cases.

Primary pituitary tumours rarely cause cranial diabetes insipidus despite extending outside the pituitary fossa. Metastatic neoplasia involving the hypothalamic region, commonly from a primary bronchial or breast carcinoma, may be unusual but certainly can cause diabetes insipidus. Occasionally parapituitary tumours, for example meningioma, lymphoma and leukaemia, also result in cranial diabetes insipidus. The infectious causes include viral encephalitis, bacterial meningitis, syphilis and the Guillain–Barré syndrome. Some patients have lymphocytic infiltration of the pituitary stalk.

Peripartum haemorrhage with hypotension is the cause of Sheehan's syndrome and results in anterior pituitary dysfunction. Overt cranial diabetes insipidus is a rare association with this syndrome, but recent careful studies of posterior pituitary function have demonstrated minor abnormalities in osmoregulated vasopressin secretion in the majority of patients studied. Aneurysms of the anterior communicating artery can cause an interesting form of diabetes insipidus, particularly if the lesion bleeds or surgery to this area is attempted. Osmoreceptor function is lost in these patients leading to isolated defective osmoregulated vasopressin secretion with frequent loss of thirst sensation.

A few studies have suggested that circulating autoantibodies to the neurons that synthesise vasopressin in the hypothalamus in some patients are responsible for cranial diabetes insipidus. Interestingly, these patients tend to have a higher than normal prevalence of other autoimmune diseases. Circulating antibodies to vasopressin itself are present in some patients who have been treated with intramuscular injections of vasopressin or extract from the posterior pituitary gland (pitressin tannate in oil) but they do not cause cranial diabetes insipidus.

Clinical features

The major clinical manifestations of cranial diabetes insipidus are, of course, polyuria, nocturia, excessive thirst and increased drinking. Children may present with enuresis. There is a wide clinical spectrum to the disorder, ranging from mild degrees which fail to take patients to their medical practitioners and are diagnosed incidentally to severe polyuria of 15–20 l/24 hours. Each patient is able to maintain a stable plasma osmolality within the normal reference range provided thirst sensation remains intact and there is ready access to fluids to quench thirst. Ice-cold water appears to relieve thirst better than other fluids.

Glucocorticoid hormone deficiency caused by either pituitary or adrenal disease leads to impairment of water excretion due partly to persistent non-osmotic vasopressin secretion and partly to reduced water permeability of the distal nephron. In consequence, patients fail to normally excrete a water load. Thus, mild forms of cranial diabetes insipidus, associated with hypopituitarism for example, will be masked by glucocorticoid deficiency, and will only become apparent with correct steroid replacement therapy. Similar impairment of water excretion has been reported in severe thyroid hormone deficiency, due principally to enhanced non-osmotic vasopressin release.

Cranial diabetes insipidus secondary to head injury can follow various courses. Some patients may show the classical triple phase response to trauma which is characterised by an initial period of intense polyuria extending for a few hours or days, followed by a second phase of marked antidiuresis of variable duration which progresses finally to persistent diabetes insipidus. In practice, however, it is now recognised that these patients may make a clinical recovery after the first or second phase. The first and third phases are due to inadequate secretion of biologically active vasopressin, while the second is due probably to excessive release of vasopressin. Awareness of the possible clinical course is important to the clinician because continued treatment of the first phase with large quantities of fluid during the antidiuretic period will lead to acute profound hyponatraemia.

Pathophysiology

In cranial diabetes insipidus the primary defect is decreased or absent osmoregulated vasopressin secretion, which leads to excessive solute-free renal water exretion. Osmoregulated thirst remains intact. There is a consequent slight increase in plasma osmolality and serum sodium which stimulates thirst to enhance drinking and replenish body water. A high rate of water turnover therefore results with plasma osmolality stabilising at slightly higher values than normal and water balance is maintained.

Nephrogenic diabetes insipidus

In nephrogenic diabetes insipidus the renal tubules are totally, or more often partially, resistant to vasopressin.

Aetiology

Table 22.2 outlines the causes of nephrogenic diabetes insipidus. The hereditary sex-linked variety is uncommon. Patients present shortly after birth with profound polyuria, dehydration and failure to thrive. The antidiuretic (V_2) vasopressin receptor in the renal tubule has been characterised, its gene being located on Xq28. Recent molecular studies have identified a number of genetic mutations or deletions leading to vasopressin resistance of this transmembrane receptor [13]. With the discovery of aquaporin, the protein required for the formation of the apical membrane water channel and its gene, located on chromosome 12q13, other forms of nephrogenic diabetes insipidus may be elucidated in the next few years [14]; preliminary data suggest that aquaporin$_2$ mutations are associated with autosomal recessive nephrogenic diabetes insipidus.

Table 22.2 Causes of nephrogenic diabetes insipidus.

Primary
Idiopathic
Familial (X-linked recessive, autosomal recessive)
Secondary
Metabolic (hypercalcaemia, hypokalaemia)
Toxic (demeclocycline, lithium, methoxyflurane)
Vascular (sickle-cell disease)
Chronic renal disease (renal failure, pyelonephritis, amyloid, sarcoidosis)
Osmotic diuresis (glycosuria, post-obstructive nephropathy)

Metabolic causes of nephrogenic diabetes insipidus are well recognised. Hypercalcaemia not only impairs vasopressin function in the distal nephron but also enhances secretion of vasopressin. Renal concentrating ability after prolonged metabolic disturbance may take a few weeks to recover completely. Many drugs alter the renal effect of vasopressin. It is worthy of note that at least one-third of patients taking lithium will suffer from nephrogenic diabetes insipidus, occasionally severe, despite normal therapeutic serum lithium concentrations. In common with many drugs causing nephrogenic diabetes insipidus, lithium has numerous tubular effects. It inhibits cyclic adenosine monophosphate production, augments its metabolism by stimulating phosphodiesterase activity, and impairs its intracellular action.

Pathophysiology

This is similar to cranial diabetes insipidus. Renal resistance to circulating vasopressin leads to polyuria, increased thirst and a high turnover of water. Basal plasma osmolality is slightly increased. Osmoregulated vasopressin secretion is either normal or possibly enhanced.

Diabetes insipidus of pregnancy

In recent years a rare form of diabetes insipidus has been described in association with pregnancy [8]. Polyuria and thirst develops at mid-pregnancy and continues until shortly after delivery. One patient study has shown that in the non-pregnant state mild cranial diabetes insipidus exists but is not clinically troublesome (urine output 2–2.5 l/24 hours).

Polyuria becomes more severe with pregnancy, with urine output increasing to 5–6 l/24 hours. Since the metabolic clearance rate of vasopressin increases three- to fourfold in pregnancy, this may account for the worsening polyuria. Whether the enhanced clearance is entirely due to circulating vasopressinase, a cysteine-aminopeptidase enzyme of placental origin, is unknown. A characteristic observation in these patients is that they fail to respond to therapeutic arginine vasopressin, the natural hormone, but do respond to desmopressin, a long-acting synthetic analogue of vasopressin which partially resists degradation. A transient form of nephrogenic diabetes insipidus associated with pregnancy occurs very rarely.

Primary polydipsia

Primary polydipsia is a condition in which individuals drink large volumes of fluid greatly in excess of body requirements.

Aetiology

The causes of primary polydipsia are not as well understood as those of cranial and nephrogenic diabetes insipidus. Table 22.3 gives a classification. It is important to exclude drugs that cause dryness of the mouth as a cause of increased water intake. There is a group of individuals who appear psychologically normal but demonstrate a lowered osmotic threshold for thirst sensation but normal osmoregulated vasopressin secretion. This disturbance has been termed dipsogenic polydipsia [8]. It is most unusual to find an underlying structural abnormality leading to primary polydipsia.

Pathophysiology

Individuals with primary polydipsia increase fluid intake to lower plasma osmolality sufficiently to suppress vasopressin secretion. Urine osmolality falls and urine output increases. Again, there is a high turnover of water but in contrast to cranial and nephrogenic diabetes insipidus, plasma osmolality stabilises at a relatively low value.

Table 22.3 Causes of primary polydipsia.

Primary
Psychogenic (compulsive water drinking)
Psychotic (mania, schizophrenia)
Idiopathic
Secondary
Granulomas (sarcoid)
Vasculitis
Multiple sclerosis

Diagnostic evaluation of polyuric patients

Various investigations have been designed to differentiate between the three major causes of polyuria, cranial and nephrogenic diabetes insipidus and primary polydipsia. Before embarking on expensive, time-consuming tests, it is essential to document 24-hour urine volumes and basal plasma osmolality or serum sodium concentration. If the urine output is less than 2.5 l/24 hours and plasma osmolality or sodium is within the normal reference range, it is unlikely that there is a significant disturbance of water balance.

Routine biochemical investigations are of limited value. Although patients with cranial and nephrogenic diabetes insipidus tend to have higher plasma osmolalities than those with primary polydipsia, results of individual patients overlap considerably. Hypercalcaemia or hypokalaemia will suggest nephrogenic diabetes.

Dehydration tests

These tests are particularly useful in the diagnosis of severe cranial or nephrogenic diabetes insipidus. Although numerous tests have been described they all consist of two parts, the first a period of dehydration with measurements of plasma and urine osmolalities and possibly plasma vasopressin, the second an injection of a vasopressin to observe the renal concentrating response [15].

Prior to the test patients should be adequately hydrated overnight. Basal plasma and urine osmolalities are measured. The patient is weighed, and then deprived of fluid for up to 8 hours. Every 2 hours urine is collected to assess volume and osmolality, blood drawn to measure plasma osmolality and the patient weighed. If weight loss during dehydration exceeds 5% of the starting wieght the test is terminated. At the end of the dehydration period, urine and blood samples are collected to measure osmolalities. The patient is then given an intramuscular injection of desmopressin (DDAVP) 2 μg and urine collected at regular intervals for the next 16 hours to measure osmolality. Following the injection, patients can eat and drink. During the dehydration test, patients should be observed to avoid surreptitious drinking. Excessive drinking after desmopressin injection should be avoided to guard against profound hyponatraemia which can occur in primary polydipsic patients made antidiuretic.

A guide to the interpretation of results obtained from dehydration tests is given in Table 22.4. Plasma osmolality within the normal reference range (285–95 mosmol/kg) and maximum urine osmolality greater than 800 mosmol/kg excludes significant water imbalance. As discussed above, basal plasma osmolality tends to be higher in cranial and nephrogenic diabetes insipidus than primary polydipsia. Poor urinary concentration after adequate dehydration followed

Table 22.4 Interpretation of water deprivation test.

Urine osmolality (mosmol/kg)		
After dehydration	After desmopressin	Diagnosis
<300	>750	+CDI
<300	<300	NDI
300–800	<750	Partial CDI, partial NDI or PP

+CDI, cranial diabetes insipidus; NDI, nephrogenic diabetes insipidus; PP, primary polydipsia.

by a rise in urine osmolality to 750 mosmol/kg or more after desmopressin indicates cranial diabetes insipidus, while lack of response suggests nephrogenic diabetes. There is, however, a considerable area of overlapping results from which it is difficult to reach a firm diagnosis (Table 22.4).

Major difficulties in interpretation of dehydration tests arise occasionally. One reason for these difficulties is that prolonged polyuria, irrespective of the cause, leads to a reduction in maximum renal concentrating ability, probably due to loss of renal interstitial solute. Consequently the osmotic gradient across the tubular cell, so essential for the action of vasopressin on the kidney, decreases. The reduction in renal concentrating capacity is directly related to the severity of the polyuria; thus, the greater the urine output, the lower the maximum urine osmolality.

Measurement of plasma vasopressin after dehydration or osmotic stimulation

The measurement of plasma vasopressin at the end of the dehydration period may enhance the diagnostic accuracy of the test. An elevated plasma vasopressin in relation to urine osmolality will establish a diagnosis of nephrogenic diabetes insipidus (FIg. 22.5b). Cranial diabetes insipidus, either partial or complete, is diagnosed accurated by recording a subnormal response of vasopressin secretion to increasing plasma osmolality induced by infusion of hypertonic saline (Fig. 22.5a). The 2-hour infusion of 5% saline at a rate of 0.04 ml/kg/min with regular 30-min blood sampling for measurement of plasma vasopressin and osmolality is a convenient test [16], carrying little risk except in patients with cardiac failure.

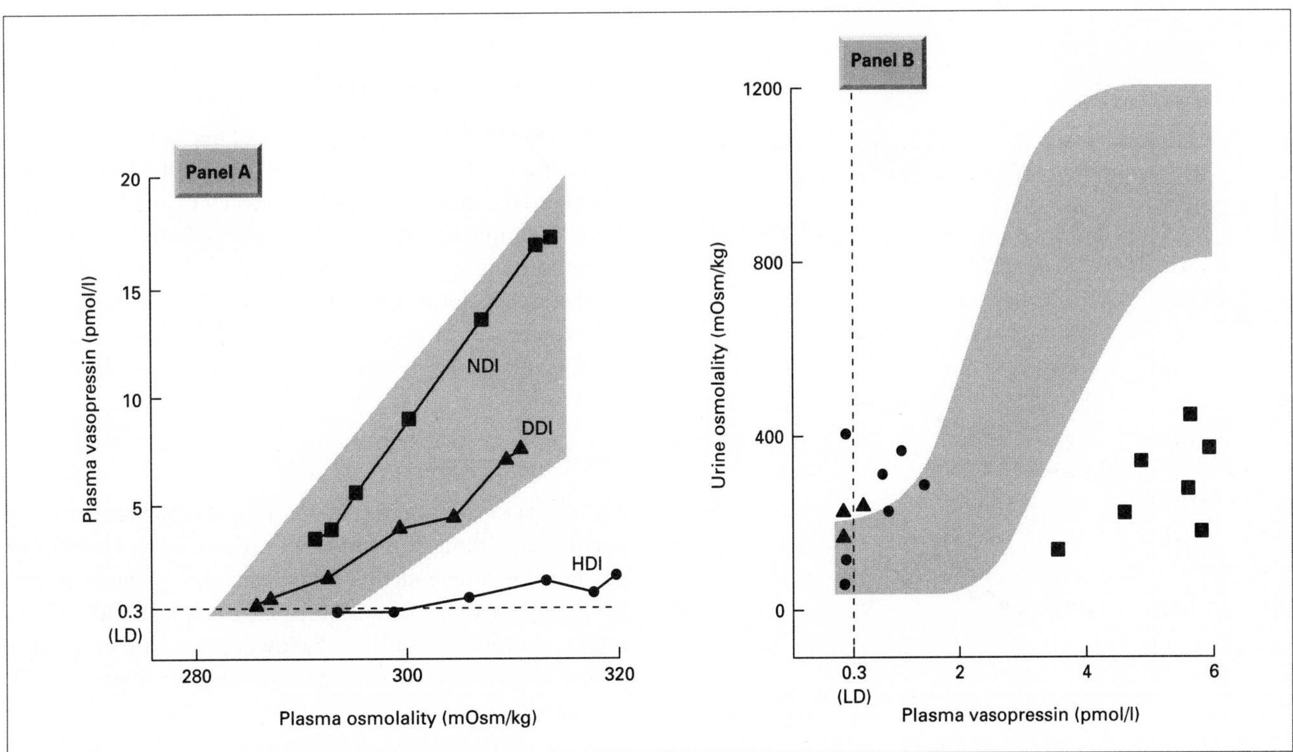

Fig. 22.5 Panel A.The relationship between plasma vasopressin and plasma osmolality during hypertonic saline infusion in typical patients with: (i) hypothalamic diabetes insipidus (HDI); (ii) nephrogenic diabetes insipidus (NDI); and (iii) dipsogenic diabetes insipidus (DDI). The shaded area represents the normal response. Panel B. The relationship between urine osmolality and plasma vasopressin in patients with HDI (●), NDI (■) and DDI (▲) after a period of dehydration. The shaded area is the normal relationship under various degrees of hydration. LD represents the limit of detection of the plasma vasopressin assay at 0.3 pmol/l.

Therapeutic trial of vasopressin analogue

If facilities to measure plasma vasopressin do not exist, and the cause of polyuria remains in doubt, then a therapeutic trial of desmopressin should be undertaken. Because of the potential hazard of water intoxication in primary polydipsic patients, the trial should be supervised closely, preferably in hospital. After a basal period of 3–4 days checking weight, and plasma and urine osmolalities, desmopressin is given intramuscularly, 1–2 μg daily, for at least 4 days. Patients with cranial diabetes insipidus will be identified by a reduction in thirst and polyuria and plasma osmolality will remain within the normal range. Nephrogenic diabetes insipidus is characterised by a lack of response with persistent thirst and polyuria. A subsequent 10-fold increase in the dose of desmopressin may result in a partial improvement. Primary polydipsic patients remain thirsty and develop progressive hyponatraemia (Fig. 22.6).

Having established the cause of the polyuria, it is important to search for the underlying aetiology (Tables 22.1–3). For example, appropriate investigation for cranial diabetes insipidus could include computed tomography (CT) and/or magnetic resonance imaging (MRI) scans of the hypothalamo-pituitary region, chest X-ray and possibly lumbar puncture. Interestingly, the hyperintense signal of the posterior pituitary and stalk seen on T1-weighted MRI scans is lost in many patients with cranial diabetes insipidus [17].

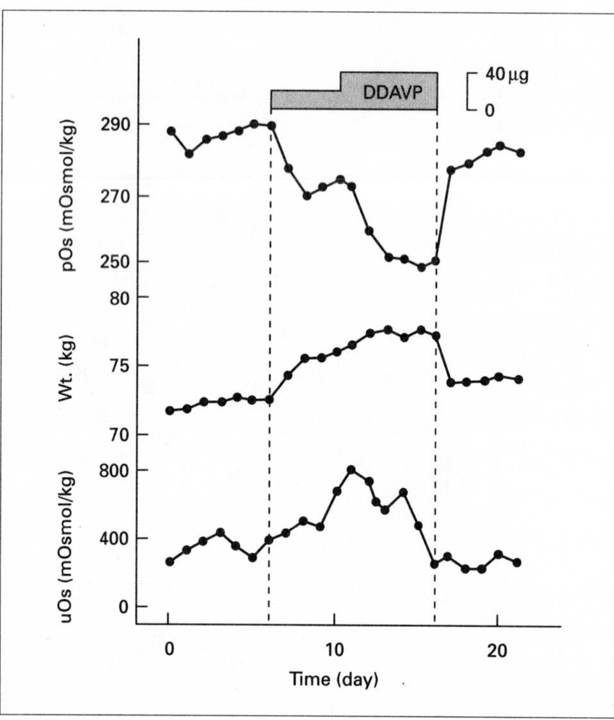

Fig. 22.6 The effect of desmopressin (DDAVP) given intranasally to a patient with primary polydipsia. Antidiuresis and persistent drinking leads to progressive hypotonicity and weight gain. From [34], with permission.

Treatment

Cranial diabetes insipidus

Mild forms of cranial diabetes insipidus (urine output <4 l/24 hours) may not require any specific therapy other than advice to ensure that thirst is quenched. In the more severe forms the drug of choice is desmopressin (DDAVP), a synthetic vasopressin analogue possessing little pressor activity and having a prolonged duration of action. There are wide individual variations in the intranasal dose required to control symptoms (5–80 μg daily). Oral desmopressin has become available recently, and patients require 100–1000 μg daily. In contrast to the aqueous form, oral desmopressin does not need to be stored at 4°C. It is particularly useful to treat children with oral desmopressin [18]. Dilutional hyponatraemia is a potential hazard if it is given in excess for a prolonged period. The shorter-acting drug, lysine vasopressin, is rarely used now because of its pressor activity.

Nephrogenic diabetes insipidus

Correction of the underlying cause of nephrogenic diabetes (e.g. hypercalcaemia or removal of drug) will allow recovery of maximal concentrating ability, which may take weeks to resolve completely. Specific therapies include thiazide and/or amiloride diuretics in combination with a prostaglandin synthetase inhibitor, e.g. indomethacin 100 mg daily.

The vasopressin-resistant diabetes of pregnancy is treated ideally with desmopressin in conventional doses (see above).

Primary polydipsia

No efficacious drug treatment is available for primary polydipsia, although propranolol in doses up to 120 mg/day has been recommended. Therapy directed towards underlying psychiatric problems may prove helpful. There is one report of reduction in thirst following steroid therapy in a patient whose polydipsia was attributed to hypothalamic sarcoidosis.

Hypernatraemic states

Hypernatraemia can be defined as a serum sodium concentration >150 mmol/l. It is uncommon, but is a subject of great interest [19,20].

Aetiology and pathophysiology

There are two broad categories of hypernatraemia based on extracellular volume status (Table 22.5). Hypervolaemic hypernatraemia is due to total body sodium excess, is usually transient, and often occurs as a result of accidental overdoses of sodium [9]. The disorder is usually self-limiting because the patient experiences severe thirst and quickly drinks sufficient fluid to lower plasma osmolality. Acute hypovolaemic hypernatraemia occurs in clinical situations where patients have large fluid losses which are not replenished.

Chronic hypovolaemic hypernatraemia is often due to deficient thirst, hypodipsia or adipsia, and is caused by lesions of the thirst osmoreceptor in the anterior hypothalamus (Table 22.5). Not infrequently the vasopressin osmoreceptor is also involved. Osmoregulatory studies on these patients have described four patterns of osmoregulatory dysfunction [4] (Fig. 22.7). The first (Fig. 22.7a) is a resetting of the osmostats for both thirst and vasopressin release such that the osmoregulatory lines are to the right of normal. Patients continue to dilute and concentrate urine normally but remain hypernatraemic. This has been called 'essential' hypernatraemia. The second type (Fig. 22.7b) is characterised by reduced sensitivity (slope of the osmoregulatory line) of both thirst appreciation and vasopressin secretion. The most serious type of chronic hypernatraemia, called adipsic hypernatraemia, is due to complete destruction of the osmoreceptors. Patients fail to sense thirst and never drink spontaneously (Fig. 22.7c). Interestingly, vasopressin secretion persists to give plasma concentrations about 1 pmol/l but fails to respond to osmotic changes. These patients can become hyponatraemic if forced to drink too much or hypernatraemic should fluid intake be inadequate. The fourth type (Fig. 22.7d) is a selective loss of thirst osmoregulation but normal osmoregulation of vasopressin secretion.

Table 22.5 Causes of hypernatraemia.

Hypervolaemic
Accidental (salt emetics, infant foods)
Iatrogenic (sodium bicarbonate infusion at cardiac resuscitation)
Hypovolaemic
Insufficient fluid intake
Hypodipsic
Tumours (primary and secondary neoplasia in hypothalamo-pituitary region)
Vascular (anterior communicating artery aneurysm)
Granulomas (sarcoidosis, histiocytosis)
Miscellaneous (trauma, hydrocephalus, ventricular cyst)
Decreased access
Desert travel
Limitation of movement (stroke)
Coma
Relative to excessive fluid loss
Gastrointestinal (vomiting, diarrhoea)
Burns

Clinical features

Severe hypernatraemia is characterised by neurological manifestations of irritability, hypotonia, seizures and coma. Clinical features of the hypovolaemic forms are related to dehydration. Since hypodipsia/adipsia is the fundamental abnormality in chronic hypovolaemic hypernatraemia it is essential to assess thirst. Simple enquiry may be all that is necessary, but semiquantitative measurement using a visual analogue scale is recommended.

Treatment

The principles of therapy of acute hypernatraemia have been reviewed [19]. Patients require water to lower serum sodium concentration. The safest mode of administration is oral, but unconscious individuals will need intravenous 5% dextrose. Care must be taken to avoid rapid falls in serum sodium concentration; the rate of correction should probably be no greater than 10 mmol/l per 24 hours.

The management of hypodipsic chronic hypernatraemia can be a challenge. 'Essential' hypernatraemia requires little specific therapy as patients are protected from extremes of hypo- and hypernatraemia. Patients with total osmoreceptor loss of both thirst and vasopressin (Fig. 22.7c) pose management difficulties. They should be instructed to drink a daily volume which is adjusted according to changes in bodyweight, usually about 1–2 l/24 hours. Regular checks of plasma osmolality or serum sodium are essential to reduce the wide fluctuations in plasma osmolality that can occur. If hypernatraemia does recur then extra oral fluid will be required, the volume of which can be calculated from information on the excess serum sodium concentration, the weight of the patient and the volume of distribution. Constant vigilance is necessary to maintain normal water balance in most chronic hypodipsic patients.

Hyponatraemic states

Hyponatraemia, defined as a serum sodium concentration < 130 mmol/1, is a common electrolyte disturbance. Up to 5% of hospital in-patients have hyponatraemia, but severe hyponatraemia (serum sodium < 115 mmol/l) affects only few patients (< 0.5%).

Clinical features

Many patients with mild chronic hyponatraemia do not

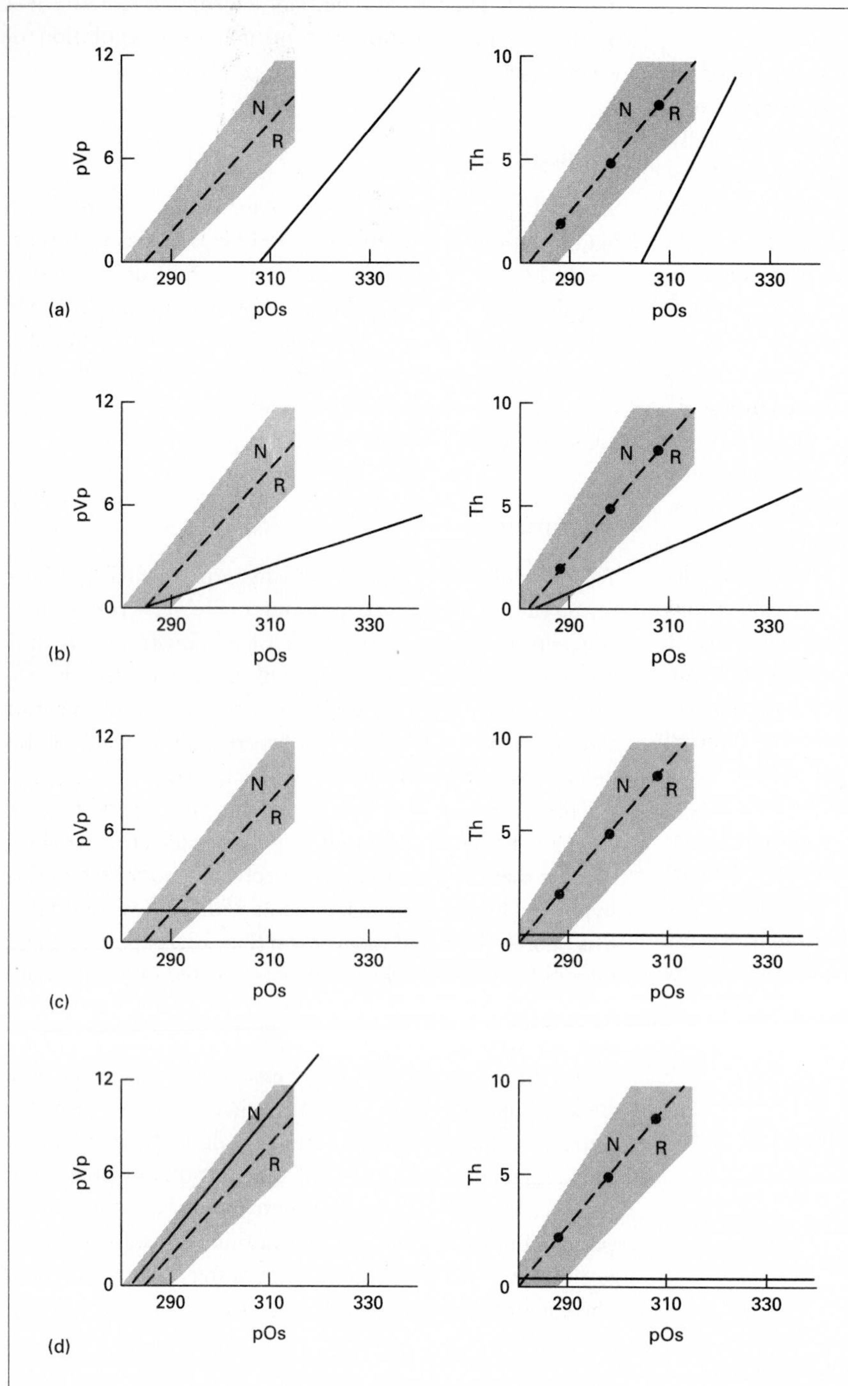

Fig. 22.7 Schematic representation of patterns of response of plasma vasopressin (pVp) and thirst (Th) to infusion of hypertonic saline in patients with chronic hypodipsic hypernatraemia. The shaded areas are the normal responses to increases in plasma osmolality (pOs). The line (●--●) represents the mean osmoregulatory lines for normal vasopressin release and thirst. (a) Reset osmostats for thirst and vasopressin release or 'essential' hypernatraemia; (b) decreased sensitivity of both thirst and vasopressin release; (c) complete destruction of both osmoreceptors; (d) normal osmoregulated vasopressin secretion but ablation of thirst osmoreceptor. From [4], with permission.

appear to have any symptoms related specifically to a low serum sodium concentration. Clinical features that have been attributed to hyponatraemia are described in Table 22.6 [21]. In general, the features worsen with the degree of hyponatraemia but the severity of symptoms depends on the rate of fall of serum sodium as well as the absolute value.

Some patients will have clinical evidence of extracellular volume disturbance (see below). One group with volume expansion will have characteristic signs of dependent oedema, raised jugular venous pressure and, possibly, ascites. In contrast, volume depletion will be recognised by tachycardia, orthostatic hypotension and reduced skin turgor.

Classification and aetiology

A pragmatic clinical approach to the classification of

Table 22.6 Clinical features of hyponatraemia.

Serum sodium < 120 mmol/l	Serum sodium < 110 mmol/l
Headache	Confusion
Anorexia	Drowsiness
Nausea	Diminished reflexes
Vomiting	Extensor plantar response
Irritability	Seizures
Depression	Coma
Personality change	Death
Cramps	
Muscle weakness	
Lethargy	

hyponatraemia is based on the extracellular fluid volume status of the patient [22]. Assessment of the patient at the bedside should allow the clinician to allocate the individual to one of three volaemic states, hypovolaemic, normovolaemic or hypervolaemic (Table 22.7). In hypovolaemic hyponatraemia there is a deficit of total body water but a greater deficit of total body sodium. Examples of causes of this type of hyponatraemia are given in Table 22.7. Pathogenetic mechanisms responsible for hypervolaemic hyponatraemia are an excess of total body sodium with a larger excess of water. Total body sodium is believed to be normal in normovolaemic hyponatraemia but total body water is in slight excess or there is abnormal distribution of water between intra- and extracellular compartments. The advantage of this approach to classification is that it leads immediately to groups of underlying causes of hyponatraemia and appropriate therapy.

Most of the examples of the causes by hyponatraemia assigned to the three volaemic groups are self-evident. The major cause of normovolaemic hyponatraemia which accounts for about 50% of all types of hyponatraemia is the syndrome of inappropriate antidiuresis (see below). Controversy still surrounds the 'sick cell' concept in which some believe that the primary abnormality is loss of intracellular solute due either to a catabolic state or cellular membrane dysfunction [23]. Hyponatraemia then develops secondary to intracellular hypotonicity to maintain osmotic equilibrium.

Diagnostic biochemical features

Factitious hyponatraemia or pseudo-hyponatraemia due to grossly elevated serum proteins or lipids must be excluded before proceeding to further investigations. Severe hyperglycaemia can also cause hyponatraemia due to a shift of water from the intracellular to exracellular compartments.

Routine biochemical tests may indicate prerenal azotaemia in the hypo- and hypervolaemic groups of hyponatraemia. Serum uric acid and urea are often low in the syndrome of inappropriate antidiuresis. Plasma osmolality is a useful measurement to confirm dilutional hyponatraemia. Measurements of plasma vasopressin are of no diagnostic benefit as over 95% of all hyponatraemic patients have detectable or elevated circulating vasopression concentrations [24]. Similarly, urine osmolality measurements are of little help because the majority of patients show values (> 450 mosmol/kg, on average) greater than plasma osmolality and they fail to distinguish between types of hyponatraemia [24]. In contrast, however, is the assessment of urinary sodium concentration which is a mandatory investigation in all

Table 22.7 Classification of hyponatraemia.

Clinical extracellular volume status	Hypovolaemia		Normovolaemia	Hypervolaemia	
Pathogenesis	Deficit of TBW Larger deficit of ExNa		Normal or slight excess of TBW	Excess of ExNa Larger excess of TBW	
	Renal loss	*Non-renal loss*	Syndrome of inappropriate antidiuresis	*Renal loss*	*Non-renal loss*
Aetiology (examples)	Mineralocorticoid deficiency Sodium-losing nephritis Diuretic excess	Vomiting Diarrhoea Burns Excessive sweating	Glucocorticoid deficiency Hypothyroidism Inappropriate IV therapy 'Sick-cell' concept	Acute and chronic renal failure	Cardiac failure Cirrhosis Nephrotic syndrome Inappropriate IV therapy
Urinary sodium concentration (mmol/l)	> 20	< 10	> 20	> 20	< 10

TBW, total body water; ExNa, extracellular sodium.

hyponatraemic patients. A guide to the interpretation of urinary sodium is given in Table 22.7. Finally, clinicians should not hesitate to assess adrenal function (by *Synacthen* test) or thyroid function as typical clinical features may be absent.

Management

Specific therapy for mild hyponatraemia is often not necessary; it is usually reserved for symptomatic patients. Treatment of the underlying cause of hyponatraemia is always essential and frequently corrects serum sodium concentration.

The principles of therapy are simple. For hypovolaemic hyponatraemia, volume replacement is necessary. Infusion of isotonic saline is normally sufficient but occasionally intravascular volume expanders are needed to maintain blood pressure in the acute situation. Water restriction is the treatment of choice for normovolaemic hyponatraemia, particularly the syndrome of inappropriate antidiuresis (see below). Hyponatraemia associated with hypervolaemic states responds to combined therapy with diuretic drugs and water restriction.

Although there is a high morbidity and mortality associated with severe hyponatraemia of any cause [21], rapid correction of the serum sodium can also lead to neurological sequelae and death, particularly central pontine myelinolysis or the osmotic demyelination syndrome [25]. It is recommended that serum sodium concentration should not be increased by more than 10 mmol/l per 24 hours.

Syndrome of inappropriate antidiuresis

This syndrome is the commonest cause of normovolaemic hyponatraemia. A number of criteria need to be fulfilled before a diagnosis can be made [26] (Table 22.8). Many clinicians rely only on the first two criteria to make the diagnosis, which is incorrect. As mentioned above, the measurement of plasma vasopressin is not helpful in differentiating this syndrome from other causes of hyponatraemia [24]. Persistent urinary sodium excretion with sodium concentrations of the order of 70 mmol/l is a characteristic feature.

Table 22.8 Criteria for the diagnosis of the syndrome of inappropriate antidiuresis.

Dilutional hyponatraemia
Urine osmolality generally greater than plasma osmolality
Persistent renal sodium excretion
Absence of hypotension, hypovolaemia and oedema-forming states
Normal renal and adrenal function

Table 22.9 Disorders associated with the syndrome of inappropriate antidiuresis (SIAD).

Malignant tumours	*Lung disease*
Ca lung, duodenum, pancreas, ureter, bladder, prostate	Pneumonia, TB, cavitation
Thymoma	Cystic fibrosis
Mesothelioma	Emphysema
Ewing's sarcoma	Pneumothorax
	Asthma
	Positive-pressure ventilation
Neurological disorders	*Drugs*
Meningitis, encephalitis, brain abscess	Vasopressin, oxytocin
	Vincristine, vinblastine, cisplatin
Brain tumour	Chlorpropamide
Guillain–Barré syndrome	Thiazide diuretics
Acute intermittent prophyria	Phenothiazines
Subarachnoid haemorrhage	Clofibrate
Cerebral and cerebellar atrophy	Carbamazepine
Shy–Drager syndrome	MAOI
Hydrocephalus	Nicotine
Cavernous sinus thrombosis	Tricyclic antidepressants
Miscellaneous	*Endocrine*
AIDS	Hypothyroidism
Idiopathic	Glucocorticoid insufficiency
Acute psychosis	
Porphyria	
Lupus erythematosus	
Burn injury	
Inappropriate IV therapy in the postoperative period	

AIDS, acquired immune deficiency syndrome; TB, tuberculosis; MAOI, monoamine oxidase inhibitor.

Aetiology

A large number of conditions have been associated with the syndrome of inappropriate antidiuresis (Table 22.9). The list of disorders continues to expand. The major groups of medical disorders include neoplasia, neurological disorders, non-malignant lung disease, a variety of drugs and acquired immune deficiency syndrome (AIDS). Excessive inappropriate intravenous therapy (5% dextrose or dextrose–saline) in the immediate postoperative period is a common, avoidable cause of the syndrome. Neurosurgery and intracranial haemorrhage can lead to hyponatraemia which appears to be due to cerebral salt wasting more frequently than the syndrome of inappropriate antidiuresis [27,28].

Pathophysiology

The combination of persistently detectable or frankly elevated concentrations of plasma vasopressin and continued intake of water is the fundamental basis of the syndrome of inappropriate antidiuresis. The syndrome can be easily reproduced experimentally by administration of vasopressin or desmopressin and water which leads to gradual accumulation of solute-free water, progressive expansion of body fluids and dilutional hyponatraemia [29]. When plasma volume expands by more than about 10% urinary sodium excretion increases, the exact mechanisms of which have yet to be elucidated fully. The natriuresis can be explained in part, however, by a decrease in proximal sodium reabsorption, a reduction in aldosterone secretion and, possibly, an increase in circulating atrial natriuretic factor or ouabain-like substances that inhibit renal sodium potassium adenosine triphosphatase activity.

Although measurement of plasma vasopressin plays no part in the diagnosis of the syndrome, subgroups based on osmoregulated vasopressin data have been described [30] (Fig. 22.8). Four patterns of secretion emerge. The first which shows erratic secretion of vasopressin (type A) accounts for about one-third of patients. A similar fraction has a reset in the vasopressin osmostat with a lowered vasopressin threshold (type B), while about 20% of patients demonstrate failure to suppress vasopressin secretion at low plasma osmolality but respond normally to osmotic stimulation at higher values (type C). A small proportion of patients appear to have normal osmoregulated vasopressin secretion (type D). Although interesting speculations can be made about the pathophysiology of these patterns of secretion [4,30], this approach is of little practical help since there is no correlation between the type of secretion pattern and the underlying cause of the syndrome. T1-weighted MR images of patients with the syndrome of inappropriate antidiuresis due to ectopic vasopressin secretion appear to lose the high-intensity signal from the neurohypophysis, suggesting that chronic hypo-osmolality stops vasopressin synthesis [31].

Treatment

The management of the syndrome of inappropriate antidiuresis is based on two principles. The first is the identification and then treatment of the underlying disorder (Table 22.9) and the second is removal of the excess body water. Again, it is worth emphasising that symptomatic or life-threatening hyponatraemia only requires specific therapy.

Fluid restriction to about 500 ml/24 hours to increase plasma sodium to approximately 130 mmol/l is the fundamental treatment. Should this approach be unsatisfactory then additional therapies are justified. A popular approach is the induction of mild nephrogenic diabetes insipidus with demeclocycline in divided doses up to 1200 mg daily. Maximal effect may take 2–3 weeks. This drug is preferable to lithium carbonate which also causes nephrogenic diabetes but is more toxic. An alternative approach is the administration of frusemide (40–80 mg daily) in combination with oral sodium chloride supplementation (3 g daily). A few drugs inhibit neurohypophysial vasopressin secretion; phenytoin is satisfactory in some patients whose vasopressin is secreted centrally.

The most logical therapy is the administration of a specific

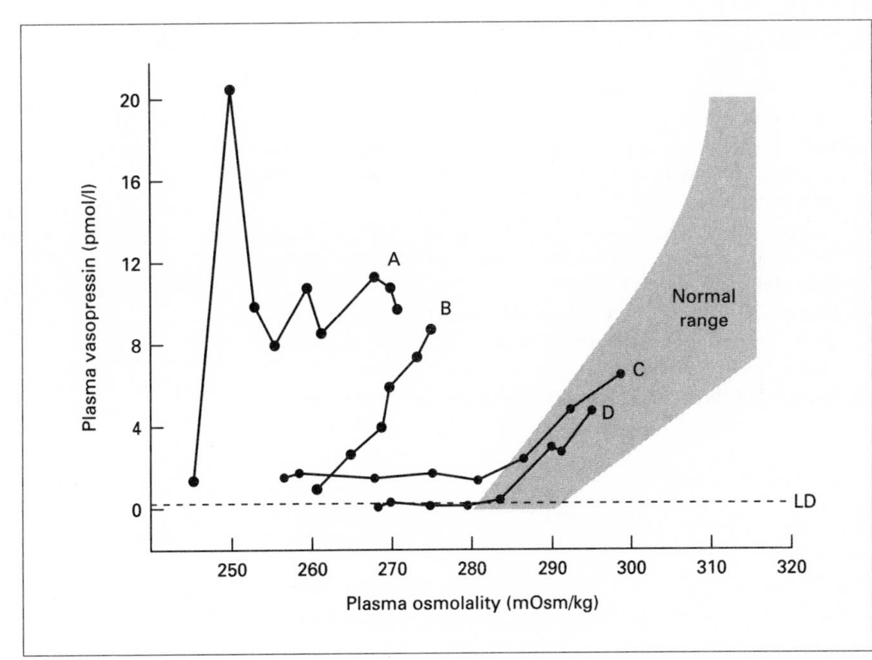

Fig. 22.8 The four patterns of plasma arginine vasopressin (AVP) response to osmotic stimulation by hypertonic saline infusion in patients with the syndrome of inappropriate antidiuresis. A, Erratic AVP secretion; B, reset AVP osmostat; C, failure of AVP suppression; D, normal. The shaded area represents the normal response and LD the limit of detection of the assay. From [30], with permission.

antagonist to the antiiduretic action of vasopressin. Peptide V-2 receptor antagonists have been uniformly unsuccessful in humans. The development of non-peptide antagonists which reverse the hyponatraemia of inappropriate antidiuresis in animals suggest an effective antagonist for humans will be available soon [32].

References

1 Thrasher TN, Keil LC, Ramsay DJ. Lesions of the organum vasculosum of the lamina terminalis (OVLT) attenuate osmotically induced drinking and vasopressin secretion in dogs. *Endocrinology* 1982; **110**: 1837–41.

2 Robertson GL, Shelton RL, Athar S. The osmoregulation of vasopressin. *Kidney Int* 1976; **10**: 25–37.

3 Thompson CJ, Bland J, Burd J, Baylis PH. The osmotic thresholds for thirst and vasopressin release are similar in healthy man. *Clin Sci* 1986; **71**: 651–6.

4 Baylis PH, Thompson CJ. Osmoregulation of vasopressin secretion and thirst in health and disease. *Clin Endocrinol* 1988; **29**: 549–76.

5 Lindheimer MD, Davison JM. Osmoregulation, the secretion of arginine vasopressin and its metabolism during pregnancy. *Eur J Endocrinol* 1995; **132**: 133–43.

6 Zerbe RL, Robertson GL. Osmoregulation of thirst and vasopressin secretion in human subjects: effect of various solutes. *Am J Physiol* 1983; **244**: E607–14.

7 Baylis PH. Posterior pituitary function in health and disease. *Clin Endocrinol Metab* 1983; **12**: 747–70.

8 Vokes TJ, Robertson GL. Disorders of antidiuretic hormone. *Endocrinol Metab Clin North Am* 1988; **17**: 281–99.

9 Wang LC, Cohen ME, Duffner PK. Etiologies of central diabetes in children. *Ped Neurol* 1994; **11**: 273–7.

10 Moses AM. Clinical and laboratory features of central and neurogenic diabetes insipidus and primary polydipsia. In: Reichlin S, ed. *The Neurohypophysis*. New York: Plenum Press, 1984; 115–38.

11 Czernichow P, Robinson AG. Diabetes insipidus in man. In: van Wimersma Greidanus TJ, ed. *Frontiers of Hormone Research*, Vol. 13. Basel: Karger, 1985: 1–314.

12 Miller WL. Molecular genetics of familial central diabetes insipidus. *J Clin Endocrinol Metab* 1993; **77**: 592–5.

13 Bichet DG, Birnbaumer M, Lonergan M *et al.* Nature and occurrence of AVPR2 mutations in X-linked nephrogenic diabetes insipidus. *Am J Hum Genet* 1994; **55**: 278–86.

14 Sasaki S, Fushimi K, Saito H *et al.* Cloning, characterisation, and chromosomal mapping of human aquaporin of the collecting duct. *J Clin Invest* 1994; **93**: 1250–6.

15 Dashe AM, Cramm RE, Crist CA, Habener JF, Solomon DH. A water deprivation test for the differential diagnosis of polyuria. *JAMA* 1963; **185**: 699–703.

16 Baylis PH, Robertson GL. Plasma vasopressin response to hypertonic saline to assess posterior pituitary function. *J Roy Soc Med* 1980; **73**: 255–60.

17 Sato N, Ishizaka H, Yagi H *et al.* Posterior lobe of the pituitary in diabetes insipidus: dynamic MR imaging. *Radiology* 1993; **186**: 357–60.

18 Fjellestad-Paulson A, Laborde K, Czernichow P. Water balance hormones during long-term follow-up of oral dDAVP treatment in diabetes insipidus. *Acta Paed* 1993; **82**: 752–7.

19 Ross EJ, Christie SBM. Hypernatraemia. *Medicine* 1969; **48**: 441–73.

20 Perez GO, Oster JR, Robertson GL. Severe hypernatraemia with impaired thirst. *Am J Nephrol* 1989; **9**: 421–34.

21 Arieff AI, Llach F, Massry SG. Neurological manifestations and morbidity of hyponatraemia: correlation with brain water and electrolytes. *Medicine* 1976; **55**: 121–9.

22 Berl T, Anderson RJ, McDonald KM, Schrier RW. Clinical disorders of water metabolism. *Kidney Int* 1976; **10**: 117–32.

23 Flear CTG, Gill CV, Burn J. Hyponatraemia: Mechanisms and management. *Lancet* 1981; **i**: 26–31.

24 Anderson RJ, Chung H-M, Kluge R, Schrier RW. Hyponatraemia: a prospective analysis of its epidemiology and the pathogenetic role of vasopressin. *Ann Intern Med* 1985; **102**: 164–8.

25 Sterns RH, Riggs J, Schochet SS. Osmotic demyelination syndrome following correction of hyponatraemia. *N Engl J Med* 1986; **314**: 1535–42.

26 Bartter FC, Schwartz WB. The syndrome of inappropriate secretion of antidiuretic hormone. *Am J Med* 1967; **42**: 790–806.

27 Kamoi K, Toyama M, Ishibashi M, Yamaji T. Hyponatraemia and osmoregulation of vasopressin secretion in patients with intracranial bleeding. *J Clin Endocrinol Metab* 1995; **80**: 2906–11.

28 Sivakumar V, Rajshekhar V, Chandy MJ. Management of neurosurgical patients with hyponatraemia and natriuresis. *Neurosurgery* 1994; **34**: 269–74.

29 Verbalis JG. Pathogenesis of hyponatraemia in an experimental model of the syndrome of inappropriate antidiuresis. *Am J Physiol* 1994; **267**: R1617–25.

30 Zerbe R, Stropes L, Robertson GL. Vasopressin function in the syndrome of inappropriate antidiuresis. *Ann Rev Med* 1980; **31**: 315–27.

31 Papapostolou C, Mantzoros CS, Evagelopoulou C, Moses AC, Kleefield J. Imaging of the sella in the syndrome of inappropriate secretion of antidiuretic hormone. *J Int Med* 1995; **237**: 181–5.

32 Okada K, Saito T. Therapeutic efficacy of non-peptide ADH antagonist OPC-31260 in SIADH rats. *Kidney Int* 1993; **44**: 19–23.

33 Baylis PH, Robertson GL. Physiological control of vasopressin secretion. In: Baylis PH, Padfield PL, eds. *The Posterior Pituitary*. New York: Marcel Dekker, 1985: 119–39.

34 Baylis PH. Polyuria and disorders of thirst. In: Baylis PH, Padfield PL, eds. *The Posterior Pituitary*. New York: Marcel Dekker, 1985: 195–225.

Part 4
The Thyroid

CHAPTER 23

The thyroid: development, structure and function

D.G. Lowe

Introduction

The thyroid gland is the largest discrete endocrine organ. It weighs 20–25 g in a normal adult, is usually heavier in women, and increases in size physiologically during menstruation and pregnancy. There is little difference in the size of the gland in boys and girls up to 14 years [1]. Clinically it has been shown that evaluation of the size of the thyroid by simple palpation is unreliable [2].

The thyroid was first described in the second century AD by Galen, who thought that its function was to lubricate the pharynx [3]. The name derives from the Greek *thyreos*, a shield. Some writers have considered that the thyroid was named from the likeness of its shape to a Greek shield [4] but the name (as 'thyroides') was in fact originally applied to what we now call the thyroid cartilage, which does resemble a shield. In 1656 Wharton named the gland after the cartilage on which it lies [5]. It is not really true, though, to say that the thyroid gland bears no resemblance to a shield [6]. While most Greek shields were round or oblong with a vertical keel reminiscent of the thyroid cartilage, the Dipylon shield of the Mycenaean Greeks certainly bears more than a passing likeness to the human thyroid gland (Fig. 23.1).

The shape of the gland varies among species but all vertebrates have the thyroid follicle as the basic unit. In fish such as teleosts there is no discrete organ: thyroid follicles are found diffusely in the pharyngeal tissues, and occasionally in the kidney, eye, brain, heart, oesophagus and spleen. The most primitive vertebrate, the larval lamprey, has a pharyngeal structure resembling the thyroglossal duct of a fetus of a higher vertebrate. This duct remains open for the first few years of life and drains a subpharyngeal gland that functions as a thyroid and secretes iodinated proteins into the alimentary system. The thyroid gland equivalent in primitive species, therefore, was exocrine rather than endocrine and depended on gut enzymes to release iodinated thyroid hormones from thyroglobulin [7,8]. The term thyroid hormones in this chapter will be used for the iodothyronine hormones and does not include calcitonin.

Embryology of the thyroid gland

The thyroid develops in the fourth week of intrauterine life as a thickening of the pharyngeal endoderm between the tuberculum impar and the copula. This collection of cells develops into the thyroglossal duct: a hollow cord of cells that becomes solid by the sixth week of life as the cells migrate caudally. The advancing end becomes bilobed and differentiation into thyroid parenchymal cells commences.

The developing thyroglossal duct and thyroid gland migrate anterior to, through, or sometimes posterior to, the mesenchyme that will become the hyoid bone. The final anatomical position of the gland anterior and inferior to the thyroid cartilage is reached in the seventh intrauterine week. The collections of cells that will mature into the lateral lobes of the thyroid are invaded by vascular mesenchyme and broken up into small clusters of cells by blood vessels. Intercellular clefts in the epithelial cell clusters begin to enlarge and form follicles at the 50-mm stage of development. By the 100-mm stage, recognisable follicular epithelial cells are present [9]. Colloid formation begins between the eighth and the 12th week. The thyroglossal duct degenerates and disappears around this time. Its most cranial aspect, in what will become the tongue, persists in many people as a shallow pit called the *foramen caecum*: its most distal part forms the isthmus of the thyroid gland [10]. The weight of the fetal thyroid increases proportional to the crown–rump length, the foot length and the fetal weight [11].

In some mammals and fish the ultimobranchial bodies, derived from the fifth branchial pouch, contribute cells to the thyroid anlage which become the C cells of the mature gland [12]. This probably occurs in human beings also.

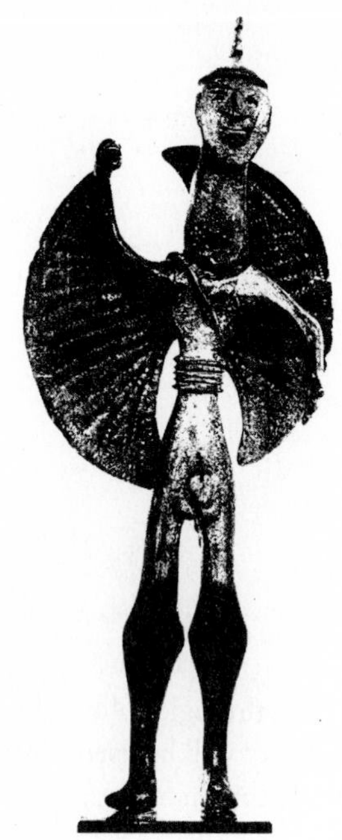

Fig. 23.1 Seventh century bronze figure in the heroic tradition of a warrior from the Karditsa region. He carries a Dipylon shield by a strap over his shoulder. He also appears to have a goitre. (Courtesy of Athens Museum.)

Serum thyroxine (T_4) and thyroxine-binding globulin concentrations begin to rise during the 12th gestational week and reach the concentrations found at term by the end of the second trimester. The fetal pituitary responds to maternal thyrotrophin-releasing hormone (TRH) [13]. Serum triiodothyronine (T_3) concentrations remain low until shortly after birth, probably because conversion of T_4 to T_3 is low in peripheral fetal tissues [14]. Thyroid-stimulating hormone (TSH) is detectable at about 10 weeks' gestation and rises to term concentrations by 16 weeks: levels are higher in the fetus and neonate than in later childhood and adulthood, probably because of the relatively low serum T_3 concentration. TSH is not necessary for the initiation of thyroid differentiation [15] though in rats, fetal thyroid development is delayed by maternal thyroidectomy [14]. When human fetal thyroid tissue is transplanted into nude mice, the number of follicle cells capable of proliferating without TSH stimulation decreases from about 58% soon after implantation to 1% after 60 days [15].

Factors influencing thyroid growth

Many hormones and other growth factors influence the development and function of the thyroid. Some have been found in animals but not in humans. Cervical sympathectomy in rats, for example, stimulates growth and inhibits hormone synthesis in the thyroid, and in chickens C cells are partly controlled by nerve stimuli [16]. It is not known whether these factors are applicable in humans.

TSH binds to membrane TSH receptors and activates the adenylyl cyclase and phosphoinositide/protein kinase C/Ca^{2+} systems [17,18]. These cellular responses to TSH are receptor specific rather than hormone specific: other ligands such as human chorionic gonadotrophin (hCG) and thyroid growth-stimulating antibodies can also activate the TSH receptor. Work with animal models suggests that there may be two or more types of receptor with different binding affinities [17]. The physiological significance of the different receptors is unknown. Alteration of the Ca^{2+} concentration within follicle cells by TSH has been suggested as one of the control mechanisms in the thyroid [19].

In experimental animals, TSH increases the mitotic rate of follicle cells and stimulates hypertrophy and eventually hyperplasia of the gland [20]. Raised concentrations of TSH induced by goitrogens or dietary iodine deficiency greatly augment the development of thyroid carcinoma in rats exposed experimentally to ionising radiation [21]. Clinically, TSH suppression by thyroid hormone replacement therapy in patients with papillary carcinoma of the thyroid has been found to decrease the rate of recurrence and improve survival [22] (see also Chapter 28).

There are factors that stimulate growth of the thyroid independently of TSH. Epidermal growth factor (EGF) is a 53-amino-acid polypeptide that has receptors principally on the basolateral plasma membrane of the thyroid follicle cell [23]. EGF stimulates proliferation of thyroid cells in many species including humans; thyroid carcinoma cells bind more EGF than normal cells [24]. EGF probably works in a paracrine or autocrine manner by activating the phosphoinositide/protein kinase C/Ca^{2+} system. In contrast to TSH, which promotes cell growth and differentiation, EGF promotes only growth and inhibits TSH-mediated thyroglobulin synthesis, iodine uptake and organification, and cytoplasmic structural development. Physiologically, TSH and EGF may work in concert [17].

hCG has the same α-subunit as TSH and probably acts via the TSH receptor to stimulate growth of thyroid cells [25]. High serum hCG levels in early pregnancy cause a rise in thyroid hormones and a slight decrease in circulating TSH, though the diurnal variation of TSH is preserved [26]. Thyroid growth in rats is affected by androgens in some species—male rats are twice as likely to develop experimental thyroid carcinomas as female rats, and the incidence in castrated rats is the same as in females [17]. Androgens seem less likely to be an important factor in humans.

Somatomedin and insulin have been found to stimulate thyroid cell growth *in vitro*. Other growth factors include interleukin 1 and vitamin C [17]. In human thyroid tissue culture, insulin-like growth factor 1 and transforming growth factor-α (TGF-α) stimulate growth. Their stimulatory effects are inhibited by TGF-β, which is produced by follicle cells, suggesting that TGF-β may be an autocrine growth inhibitor of thyroid follicle cells [27]. TGF-α has also been found to be a modulator of thyroid growth in pigs [28].

Anatomy and histology

The thyroid is a purple–brown gland consisting of two lateral lobes linked by an isthmus that lies anterior to the second and third tracheal rings. The lateral lobes lie on the thyroid and cricoid cartilages and extend caudally to the level of the sixth tracheal ring. A small pyramidal lobe is present at the isthmus, or the aspect of the lateral lobes adjacent to the isthmus, in about half of cases. The lateral lobes are usually about equal in size but one lobe (usually the right) can sometimes be considerably larger than the other in normal people [29].

The thyroid is composed of follicles ranging from 50 to 900 nm in diameter which consist of a central collection of hyaline colloid material enclosed by a single layer of cuboidal or columnar epithelial cells within a basement membrane. The follicles appear discrete and unitary on histological sections but in fact communicate, with a sheet of epithelial cells contributing to the lining of several follicles. There is no apparent difference in size or shape of follicles in the different parts of the human gland, unlike in the rat where peripheral follicles tend to be larger than central ones [21].

Two types of follicle can be demonstrated experimentally, with transition forms between them. Storage follicles have colloid with a low turnover of iodine and are lined by flattened follicular cells; active follicles are lined by cuboidal cells and have colloid with a rapid turnover. The number of active follicles is usually smaller than inactive ones, and it is the former that react to TSH first [21].

The intensity of staining of thyroid colloid with routine stains such as eosin depends on the glycoprotein content. Newly formed colloid is very pale pink, whilst colloid of some weeks' standing stains a deep orange–scarlet. This is in part due to the degree of polymerisation of the thyroglobulin subunits. The ovoid spaces commonly seen at the periphery of colloid on paraffin wax embedded sections are artifacts not seen in resin-embedded or frozen sections. They are thought to be the consequence of focally reduced viscosity of the colloid secondary to follicular cell activity. Needle-shaped and polygonal crystals of calcium oxalate dihydrate can often be demonstrated in colloid [30] (Fig. 23.2). These are present in greater numbers in deeply eosinophilic 'old' colloid and increase with the age of the patient [31].

During infancy and childhood, most thyroid follicles are spherical but after puberty larger follicles may show

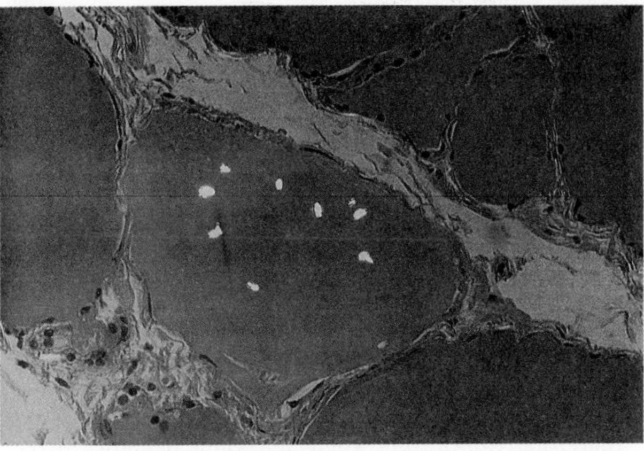

Fig. 23.2 Birefringent needle-shaped crystals of calcium oxalate dihydrate in thyroid colloid.

cushion-like infoldings with follicles in their cores ('Sanderson polsters'). Flattening of follicle lining cells may be seen in old age associated with a decrease in function of the gland [32].

On electron microscopy the organelles of the follicular epithelial cells are strikingly polarised. This reflects the functional differences, with thyroglobulin synthesis at the apex of the cell and exocytosis and thyroglobulin degradation with liberation of T_3 and T_4 at the base. The cytoplasm contains prominent cisternae of rough endoplasmic reticulum (RER). The nucleus is central or basal with a prominent nucleolus. At the apical side of the nucleus there are lysosomes containing acid phosphatase and other hydrolytic enzymes and a Golgi apparatus from which secretory vesicles migrate towards the lumen of the follicle.

The functions of follicle cells are site related. Maintenance of the intracellular architecture is important for iodine transport, though not essential [33]. The basal part of the cell actively transports from the plasma into the cell, and the apical plasma membrane has peroxidase and other enzymes for thyroid hormone synthesis. Thyroid peroxidase is also present in the perinuclear cisternae, RER, Golgi apparatus and apical vesicles [34], and is especially concentrated over the microvilli of the apical aspect. These microvilli are present even when the cell is in the resting state, and on TSH stimulation increase in length and become branched [35,36]. Within minutes of TSH administration, collections of resorbed thyroglobulin can be demonstrated in follicle cells [37].

Adult human thyroid glands also commonly have small areas in which the follicle cells have become large with large nuclei and deeply eosinophilic cytoplasm. These are called *oxyphil cells*, *Hürthle cells* or *Askanazy cells*. These cells have large numbers of mitochondria and scant RER; intermediate forms between oxyphil cells and typical follicle cells with smaller numbers of mitochondria can also be found. The cause of oxyphil cell change is unknown.

In addition to follicle cells the thyroid also contains C cells (also called parafollicular, light or clear cells). These epithelial cells lie between follicle cells and the basement membrane of the follicle and also form clusters in the parafollicular fibrous tissue [38] (Fig. 23.3). The proportion of C cells to follicle cells in human thyroids is relatively small compared with animals such as the dog [39]; C cells account for only about 1% of the total epithelial cell mass in human thyroids. C cells are found predominantly in the middle parts of the lateral lobes, and knowledge of the site of biopsy is therefore important when assessing whether C-cell hyperplasia is present. The number of C cells increases with age [40].

Ultrastructurally, C cells have numerous membrane-bound secretory granules in their cytoplasm which contain the storage form of calcitonin [41], probably in more than one form [42]. The calcium-lowering hormone katacalcin is also present in C-cell granules [43]. Helodermin, a vasoactive intestinal peptide (VIP)-like vasoactive peptide found in the salivary gland venom of the lizard *Heloderma suspectum*, is also present in C cells; this may be involved in local thyroid hormone regulation by stimulating basal T_4 secretion [44]. Chromogranin [45] and calcitonin gene-related peptide [46] are also found in C cells.

Follicle cells and C cells have low-molecular-weight keratins but high-molecular-weight keratins are not normally found. Follicular adenoma, follicular carcinoma and medullary carcinoma of thyroid immunostain strongly for low-molecular-weight keratins, and papillary carcinoma often has high-molecular-weight keratins in addition [47–49].

Another cell type demonstrable in about 60% of thyroids is the epidermoid cell. This forms so-called *solid cell nests*, in which plump epithelial cells form sheets, tubules and follicles [12,50]. The cells around lumens in these nests may contain mucin [50]. Epidermoid cells are considered to be derived from ultimobranchial remnants [51]. They immunostain for high- and low-molecular-weight keratins and for carcinoembryonic antigen. Some contain calcitonin in addition [12]. It is possible that the rare primary mucoepidermoid carcinoma of thyroid arises in these cells. Other epithelial cell types such as ciliated cells have been reported in rat but not human thyroids. Intrathyroid parathyroid glands are not uncommon, with the aberrant cells lying either below the thyroid capsule or deep within the gland [52].

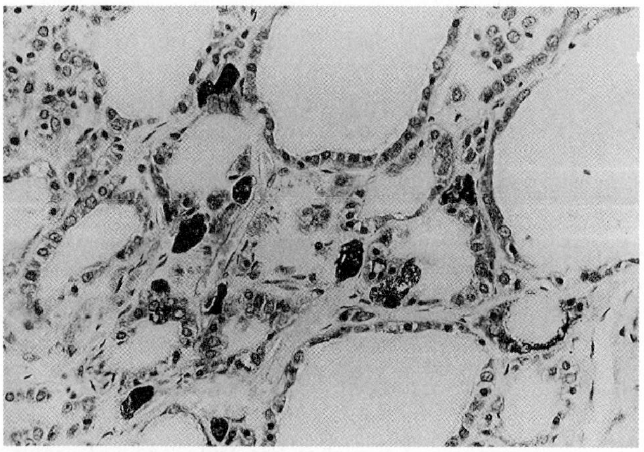

Fig. 23.3 C cells in the thyroid immunostained for calcitonin.

The innervation of the thyroid is mainly sympathetic from the three sympathetic cervical ganglia. The nerves form interstitial plexuses around arteries and follicles [53] and ganglia within the thyroid are occasionally found [54]. Adrenergic nerve terminals are associated with follicle cells and blood vessels. C cells in humans do not appear to have a direct nerve supply, though in chickens they have been found to be closely related anatomically to cholinergic axon terminals [16]. Thyroid growth may be determined to some extent by neural factors; axons containing VIP have been found in the thyroid, and VIP is known to increase adenyl cyclase levels and have an additive effect with TSH on thyroid tissue in culture [55].

Gastrin-releasing polypeptide (GRP), the mammalian homologue of bombesin, is expressed in normal C cells and in medullary carcinoma of the thyroid [55,56]. Calcitonin levels are 100 times higher than GRP levels in C cells and the two are closely related. Immunoreactivity for GRP in infants under 5 months old is 20 times that in adults; most C cells in fetuses and neonates contain GRP but only 5–18% of C cells in adult thyroids do so [57].

Thyroid biochemistry

The follicle cell traps, transports and oxidises iodide and makes thyroglobulin, which is needed in the synthesis and storage of iodotyrosines and iodothyronines and for storage of iodine. The requirement of dietary iodine is 100–200 μg/day.

The thyroid removes about 10 μg/hour from the plasma by actively transporting iodide into follicle cells—the intracellular concentration of iodine is over 30 times that in plasma [58]. This property of iodide trapping is not specific to the thyroid; cells in lactating mammary glands, salivary glands, gastric glands and hair follicles also concentrate iodine [21]. The inorganic iodide attaches to a specific thyroid peroxidase, a protoporphyrin haem-containing enzyme located at the apical (luminal) aspect of the follicle cell. At this location there are also binding sites for iodide and tyrosine residues on thyroglobulin. Both the iodide and the tyrosine are oxidised by peroxidase with hydrogen peroxide to form monoiodotyrosine (MIT) and diiodotyrosine (DIT). Neither of these is metabolically active.

Thyroglobulin is a large molecule (670 kDa, sedimentation coefficient 19S) composed of two identical subunits with sedimentation coefficients of 12S [59]. Oligosaccharides such as mannose that comprise about 10% of the molecule [60] are added in the Golgi apparatus of the follicle cell. There are about 120 tyrosine moieties per molecule, which in fact is not appreciably different from that in many other unrelated proteins. The steric arrangement of the tyrosine, however, probably facilitates iodination, as the number of DIT molecules formed is more than would be expected by chance iodination of MIT [21]. Thyroglobulin is stored in the follicle lumens as dimers, hexamers and other forms [61]. On the thyroglobulin molecule, coupling of one MIT and one DIT molecule by peroxidase and transaminase results in the formation of T_3, and of two DIT molecules in T_4 (Fig. 23.4). Coupling of two MIT molecules may occur to form 3,3′-diiodothyronine, but this has very little biological activity.

Thyroglobulin with its attached thyroid hormones is reabsorbed by endocytosis in the apical aspect of the follicle cells as colloid droplets. The thyroglobulin is hydrolysed by peptidases in secondary lysosomes and free T_3 and T_4 are allowed to diffuse through the basal part of the cell into the circulation. MIT and DIT, uncoupled from the hydrolysed thyroglobulin by lysosomal iodotyrosinase, are deiodinated and degraded to release iodine and tyrosine for recycling [62].

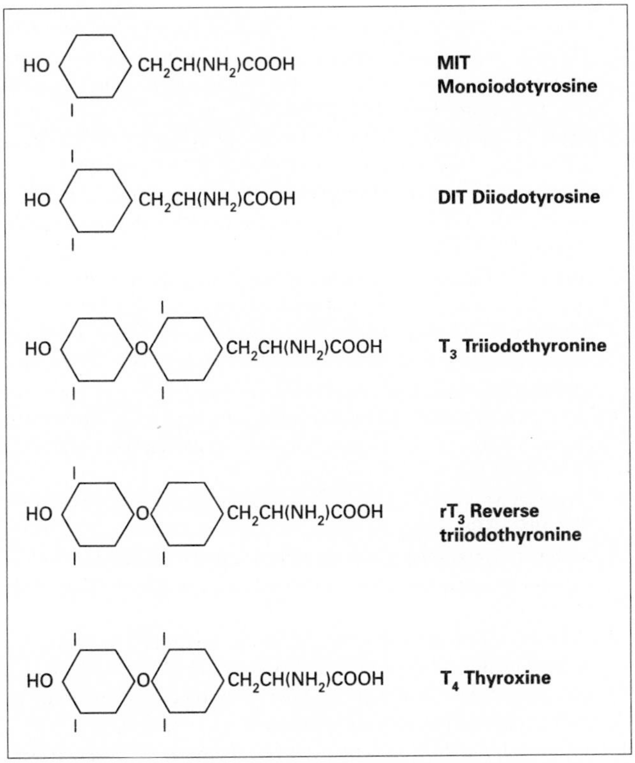

HO–(ring, I)–$CH_2CH(NH_2)COOH$ **MIT Monoiodotyrosine**

HO–(ring, I, I)–$CH_2CH(NH_2)COOH$ **DIT Diiodotyrosine**

HO–(ring, I, I)–O–(ring, I, I)–$CH_2CH(NH_2)COOH$ **T_3 Triiodothyronine**

HO–(ring, I, I)–O–(ring, I)–$CH_2CH(NH_2)COOH$ **rT_3 Reverse triiodothyronine**

HO–(ring, I, I)–O–(ring, I, I)–$CH_2CH(NH_2)COOH$ **T_4 Thyroxine**

Fig. 23.4 The biochemical structures of iodinated thyroid hormones and their precursors.

Minute amounts of thyroglobulin are detectable in serum, at a concentration of about 16 µg/l [63]. Patients with alcoholic cirrhosis have almost double this concentration, but patients with acute hepatitis have normal levels; it is not known whether the increase in cirrhotic patients is due to increased release from the thyroid or decreased clearance from the serum [63]. The thyroglobulin in serum is poorly iodinated, and so it seems likely that it represents newly synthesised protein rather than resorbed stored thyroglobulin [64,65].

Unlike T_4, which is produced solely by the thyroid, T_3 is produced mainly by conversion of T_4 by the cells of the kidney, heart, skeletal muscle, skin, liver, anterior pituitary and other tissues. Most of the T_3 in the body is intracellular. The conversion rate is reduced by starvation [66]; this also causes decreased TSH secretion and a reduction of the serum thyroglobulin concentration [66]. Growth hormone stimulates peripheral conversion of T_4 to T_3 [67].

Another form of T_3, reverse T_3 (rT3), is also produced in the thyroid (Fig. 23.4). Unlike T_3 (3′,3,5,-triiodothyronine), reverse T_3 (3,3′,5′-triiodothyronine) is metabolically inactive. In amniotic fluid and in umbilical cord blood in neonates, concentrations of rT_3 are much higher than in later life and are unrelated to the levels of T_3. Reverse T_3 concentrations do not decline to adult levels until the 10th neonatal day, whereas T_3 concentrations rise to adult levels within hours of birth [68]. In the adult, rT_3 may also be produced peripherally, especially in severely ill patients with a variety of diseases such as cirrhosis, chronic renal failure, pyrexia and starvation [68]. The mechanism controlling this is unknown, but does not appear to be related to the type of disease present (see Chapter 31).

Thyroid hormones in the circulation are largely bound to thyroxine-binding globulin, which has a high affinity for T_4 and a slightly lower affinity for T_3. Prealbumin binds small amounts of T_4 but T_3 is not bound to any significant extent. Small amounts of T_3 and T_4 bind to albumin, which has a low affinity but a high capacity for thyroid hormones. The concentration of free hormone dictates the patient's metabolic state. Free T_3 and free T_4 serum concentrations are normal in patients with congenital deficiency of thyroxine-binding globulin [69] (see Chapter 24).

The rate of production of T_4 is about 90 µg/day, and of T_3 30 µg/day. There are circadian variations in serum TSH concentrations but not of T_4, which stays remarkably constant; the daily variation in T_4 concentration stems principally from the effects of haemoconcentration from standing. Less than 1% of the intrathyroid pool of iodinated thyroglobulin is needed to achieve the normal daily output of thyroid hormones [70]. Ten per cent of the serum T_4 and 75% of T_3 are metabolised each day; the total-body T_4 and T_3 are therefore 900 μg and 40 μg, respectively. Only free T_3 has been found to decrease as a specific effect of the menopause; both T_3 and T_4 decrease with age and this is unrelated to TSH secretion [71].

Calcitonin secretion is considerably lower in women than in men and has been reported to decrease with age, though this is disputed [72]; in rats, calcitonin secretion increases with age [73]. In cell culture, somatostatin significantly inhibits calcitonin secretion and serotonin increases it [74].

Action of T_3 and T_4

Most hormones modify the activity of the target tissues so that the exigencies of life, such as stress, reproduction and nutrition, can be met. To do so they are secreted in varying amounts according to need. Control of thyroid secretion, paradoxically, seems to have evolved in the human to maintain thyroid hormone at a constant level in most circumstances.

Thyroid hormones have been known for many years to increase oxygen consumption by tissues; deficiency greatly decreases consumption. This in fact applies only to certain tissues—lymph nodes, spleen, thymus, lung, dermis and gonads do not change their rate of oxygen consumption as a response to thyroid hormone synthesis, but all other tissues do [75]. Maintenance of sodium and potassium gradients across cytoplasmic membranes may consume up to half of the total energy generated by a cell. Thyroid hormones increase sodium pump activity and increase concentrations of intracellular adenosine triphosphatase [76].

Nuclei have binding sites for T_3 and T_4; thyroid hormones act on specific messenger RNA synthesis to increase the production of proteins, particularly enzymes but also albumin and haemoglobin [77]. Three types of thyroid hormone receptor have been described [78]. Tissues unresponsive to thyroid hormone such as the testis and spleen have a much lower number of nuclear binding sites than tissues that respond with an increase in oxygen consumption [79]. Binding sites for thyroid hormones are also demonstrable on the inner membranes of mitochondria, cytoplasmic membranes, and microsomes [78].

The mitochondrion is the organelle most affected by changes in thyroid hormone concentration. Thyroxine has been shown experimentally to increase the number of mitochondrial cristae and adenosine diphosphate uptake by mitochondria is also increased [80]. T_3 does not appear to influence mitochondrial function directly, though both T_3 and T_4 increase the concentration of mitochondrial α-glycerophosphate dehydrogenase 20-fold. Other cellular enzymes that increase as a result of the action of thyroid hormones include glucose-6-phosphate dehydrogenase, pyruvate carboxylase and phosphoenolpyruvate carboxykinase [81].

Thyroid hormones have been shown to stimulate the biochemical and morphological differentiation of human fetal lung cells in organ culture [82], to modulate the synthesis of γ- and δ-globin chains in the fetus [77] and to stimulate the release of growth factors such as EGF in some tissues [83]. T_4 acts with adrenocorticotrophic hormone (ACTH) to stimulate 3-β-hydroxysteroid dehydrogenase production in cell cultures of fetal adrenal cortex [84].

Calcitonin is secreted in response to a high serum ionised calcium concentration and has been shown to stimulate growth and maturation of embryonic chick pelvic cartilage *in vitro* [85]. Watery diarrhoea is a feature in patients with medullary carcinoma of the thyroid and high calcitonin levels, but it is thought unlikely that fluid secretion in the small intestine is increased by a direct effect of calcitonin [86].

References

1 Langer P, Tajtakova M, Podoba J, Jr, Kostalova L, Gutekunst R. Thyroid volume and urinary iodine in school children and adolescents in Slovakia after 40 years of iodine prophylaxis. *Exp Clin Endocrinol* 1994; **102**: 394–8.

2 Jarlov AE, Hegedus L, Gjorup T, Hansen JE. Accuracy of the clinical assessment of thyroid size. *Danish Med Bull* 1991; **38**: 87–9.

3 Goodman HM, van Middlesworth L. The thyroid gland. In: Mountcastle VB, ed. *Medical Physiology*, 14th edn. London: CV Mosby, 1980: 1495.

4 Hoyes AD, Kershaw DR. Anatomy and development of the thyroid gland. *Ear Nose Throat J* 1985; **64**: 11–42.

5 Wharton T. *Adenographia: Sive, Glandularum Totius Corporis Descriptio. De Glandularis Thyreoidis*. London: Typ. JG impens, Authoris (printed privately), 1656.

6 Halmi NS. Anatomy and histochemistry. In: Ingbar SH, Braverman LE, eds. *Werner's The Thyroid*, 5th edn. Philadelphia: Lippincott, 1986: 24–42.

7 Clements M, Gorbman A. Protease in ammocoete endostyle. *Biol Bull* 1955; **108**: 258–63.

8 Gorbman A. Some aspects of the comparative biochemistry of iodine utilization and the evolution of thyroid function. *Physiol Rev* 1955; **35**: 336–46.

9 Chan AS. Ultrastructural observations on the formation of follicles in the human fetal thyroid. *Cell Tissue Res* 1983; **233**: 693–8.

10 Mansberger AR, Jr, Wel JP. Surgical embryology and anatomy of the thyroid and parathyroid glands 1993; **73**: 727–46.

11 Bocian-Sobkowska J, Malendowicz LK, Wozniak W. Morphometric studies on the development of human thyroid gland in early fetal life. *Histol Histopathol* 1992; **7**: 415–20.

12 Harach HR. Solid cell nests of the thyroid. *J Pathol* 1988; **155**: 191–200.
13 Thorpe-Beeston JG, Nicholaides KH, McGregor AM. Fetal thyroid function. *Thyroid* 1992; **2**: 207–17.
14 Morreale de Escobar G, Obregon MJ, Escobar del Rey F. Fetal and maternal thyroid hormones. *Horm Res* 1987; **26**: 12–27.
15 Peter HJ, Studer H, Groscurth P. Autonomous growth, but not autonomous function in embryonic human thyroids: a clue to understanding autonomous goiter growth? *J Clin Endocrinol Metab* 1988; **66**: 698–73.
16 Kameda Y, Okamoto K, Ito M, Tagawa T. Innervation of the C cells of chicken ultimobranchial glands studies by immunohistochemistry, fluorescence microscopy and electron microscopy. *Am J Anat* 1988; **182**: 353–68.
17 Duh Q-Y, Clark OH. Factors influencing the growth of normal and neoplastic thyroid tissue. *Surg Clin North Am* 1987; **67**: 281–99.
18 Dumont JE. The action of thyrotropin on thyroid metabolism. *Vitam Horm* 1971; **29**: 287–412.
19 D'Arcangelo D, Silleta MG, Di Francesco AL *et al.* Physiological concentrations of thyrotropin increase cytosolic calcium levels in primary cultures of human thyroid cells. *J Clin Endocrinol Metab* 1995; **80**: 1136–43.
20 Dumont JE, Roger P, van Heuverswyn B, Erneux C, Vassart G. Control of growth and differentiation by known intracellular signal molecules in endocrine tissues: the example of the thyroid gland. *Adv Cyclic Nucleotide and Protein Phosphorylation Res* 1984; **17**: 337–42.
21 Doniach I, Gray AB. The thyroid. In: Beck F, Lloyd JB, eds. *The Cells in Medical Science*, Vol. 3. London: Academic Press, 1975: 107–53.
22 Clark OH. TSH suppression on the management of thyroid nodules and thyroid cancer. *World J Surg* 1981; **5**: 39–47.
23 Carpenter G, Cohen S. Epidermal growth factor. *Ann Rev Biochem* 1979; **48**: 193–216.
24 Errick JE, Ing KA, Eggo MC *et al.* Growth and differentiation in cultured human thyroid cells: effects of epidermal growth factor and thyrotropin. *In Vitro* 1986; **22**: 28–36.
25 Hershman JM, Lee HY, Sugawara M *et al.* Human chorionic gonadotropin stimulates iodide uptake, adenylate cyclase, and deoxyribonucleic acid synthesis in cultured rat thyroid cells. *J Clin Endocrinol Metab* 1988; **67**: 74–9.
26 Pekonen F, Alfthan H, Stenman UH, Ylikorkala O. Human chorionic gonadotropin (hCG) and thyroid function in early human pregnancy: circadian variation and evidence for intrinsic thyrotropic activity of hCG. *J Clin Endocrinol Metab* 1988; **66**: 853–6.
27 Grubeck-Loebenstein G, Buchan R, Sadeghi M *et al.* Transforming growth factor beta regulates thyroid growth. Role in the pathogenesis of nontoxic goiter. *J Clin Invest* 1989; **83**: 764–70.
28 Arai M, Tsushima T, Isozaki O *et al.* Effects of transforming growth factor alpha (TGF-alpha) on DNA synthesis and thyrotropin-induced iodine metabolism in cultured porcine thyroid cells. *Eur J Endocrinol* 1995; **132**: 242–8.
29 Meissner WA. Pathology. In: Werner SC, Ingbar SH, eds. *The Thyroid*, 4th edn. New York: Harper and Row, 1978: 444–79.
30 Reid JD, Chang-Hyun C, Oldroyd NO. Calcium oxalate crystals in the thyroid. *Am J Clin Pathol* 1987; **87**: 443–54.
31 Wahl R, Fuchs R, Kallee E. Oxalate in the human thyroid gland. *Eur J Clin Chem Clin Biochem* 1993; **31**: 559–65.
32 Charepper HA, Pearlstein A, Bourne GH, ed. *Structural Aspects of Ageing*. London: Pittman, 1961: 265–76.
33 Tong W, Kerkof P, Chaikoff IL. Iodine metabolism of dispersed thyroid cells obtained by trypsinisation of sheep thyroid glands. *Biochem Biophys Acta* 1962; **60**: 1–19.
34 Mizukami Y, Nonomura A, Michigishi T *et al.* Immunohistochemical demonstration of thyroid peroxidase (TPO) in human thyroid tissues from various thyroid diseases. *Anticancer Res* 1994; **14**: 1329–34.
35 Wetzel BK, Spicer SS, Wollman SH. Changes in fine structure and acid phosphatase localization in rat thyroid cells following thyrotropin administration. *J Cell Biol* 1965; **255**: 593–618.
36 Hayakawa N, Hirakawa S, Nakai H, Suzuki S, Ota Z. The effects of thyroid-stimulating hormone and thyroid microsomal antibody on thyroid peroxidase activity in human follicular cells: a mini organ culture study. *Endocrine J* 1993; **40**: 149–61.
37 Nadler NJ, Sarkar SK, Leblond CP. Origin of intracellular colloid droplets in the rat thyroid. *Endocrinology* 1962; **71**: 120–9.
38 Scopsi L, Arias J, Houen G, Racchetti G, Fossati GL, Galante YM. Monoclonal antibodies against calcitonin. Characterization and application in light and electron microscopy immunocytochemistry. *Histochemistry* 1988; **88**: 113–25.
39 Kameda Y. Fine structural and endocrinological aspects of thyroid follicular cells. In: Coupland RE, Fujita T, eds. *Chromaffin, Enterochromaffin and Related Cells*. Amsterdam: Elsevier, 1976: 155–70.
40 Lietz H. C cells: source of calcitonin. A morphological review. *Curr Top Pathol* 1971; **55**: 109–46.
41 Wolfe HJ, Melvin KEW, Cervi-Skinner SJ *et al.* C cell hyperplasia preceding medullary thyroid carcinoma. *N Engl J Med* 1973; **289**: 437–41.
42 Cohen R, Delehaye MC, Minvielle S *et al.* CCP II: a novel calcitonin carboxy terminal peptide is expressed in normal thyroid tissue. *Biochem Biophys Res Commun* 1992; **185**: 330–4.
43 Ali Rachedi A, Varndell IM, Facer P *et al.* Immunocytochemical localisation of katacalcin, a calcium-lowering hormone cleaved from the human calcitonin precursor. *J Clin Endocrin Metab* 1983; **57**: 680–2.
44 Grunditz T, Persson P, Hakanson R. Helodermin-like peptides in thyroid C cells: stimulation of thyroid hormone secretion and suppression of calcium incorporation into bone. *Proc Natl Acad Sci USA* 1989; **86**: 1357–61.
45 Murray SS, Burton W, Deftos J. The effects of forskolin and calcium ionophore A23187 on secretion and cytoplasmic RNA levels of chromogranin-A and calcitonin. *J Bone Miner Res* 1988; **3**: 447–52.
46 Haller-Brem S, Muff R, Fischer JA. Calcitonin gene related peptide and calcitonin secretion from a human medullary thyroid carcinoma cell line: effects of ionomycin, phorbol ester and forskolin. *J Endocrinol* 1988; **119**: 147–52.
47 Miettinen M, Franssila K, Lehto VP, Paasivuo R, Virtanen I. Expression of intermediate filament proteins in thyroid gland and thyroid gland tumours. *Lab Invest* 1984; **50**: 262–70.
48 Pemanetter W, Nathrath WBJ, Löhrs U. Immunohistochemical analysis of thyroglobulin and keratin in benign and malignant thyroid tumours. *Virchows Arch (A)* 1982; **398**: 221–8.
49 Yagi Y, Yagi S, Saku T. The localization of cytoskeletal proteins and thyroglobulin in thyroid microcarcinoma in comparison with clinically manifested thyroid carcinoma. *Cancer* 1985; **56**: 1967–71.
50 Harach HR. A study on the relationship between solid cell nests and mucoepidermoid carcinoma of the thyroid. *Histopathology* 1985; **9**: 195–207.

51 Harach HR, Vujanic GM, Jasani B. Ultimobranchial body nests in human fetal thyroid: an autopsy, histological and immunohistochemical study in relation to solid cell nests and mucoepidermoid carcinoma of the thyroid. *J Pathol* 1993; **169**: 465–9.
52 Harach HR, Vujanic GM. Intrathyroidal parathyroid. *Ped Pathol* 1993; **13**: 71–4.
53 Nilsson OR, Karlberg BE. Thyroid hormones and the adrenergic nervous system. *Acta Med Scand Suppl* 1983; **672**: 27–32.
54 Sarrat R, Torres A, Whyte J, Lostale F. Peculiarities of the thyroid gland structure (with special reference to the presence of ganglion cells). *Histol Histopathol* 1994; **9**: 95–103.
55 Siperstein AE, Miller RA, Clark OH. Stimulatory effect of vasoactive intestinal polypeptide on human normal and neoplastic thyroid tissue. *Surgery* 1988; **104**: 985–91.
56 Spindel ER, Zilberberg MD, Chin WW. Analysis of the gene and multiple messenger ribonucleic acids (mRNAs) encoding human gastrin-releasing peptide: alternate RNA splicing occurs in neural and endocrine tissue. *Mol Endocrinol* 1987; **1**: 224–32.
57 Sunday ME, Wolfe HJ, Roos BA, Chin WW, Spindel ER. Gastrin-releasing peptide gene expression in developing, hyperplastic and neoplastic human thyroid C-cells. *Endocrinology* 1988; **122**: 1551–8.
58 Taurog A. Hormone synthesis: thyroid iodine metabolism. In: Ingbar SH, Braverman LE, eds. *Werner's The Thyroid*, 5th edn. Philadelphia: Lippincott, 1986: 53–97.
59 Lissitzky S. Thyroglobulin entering into molecular biology. *J Endocrinol Invest* 1984; **7**: 65–76.
60 Spiro MJ. Presence of a glucuronic acid-containing carbohydrate unit in human thyroglobulin. *J Biol Chem* 1977; **252**: 5424–30.
61 Saboori AM, Rose NR, Kuppers RC, Butscher WG, Bresler HS, Burek CL. Immunoreactivity of multiple molecular forms of human thyroglobulin. *Clin Immunol Immunopathol* 1994; **72**: 121–8.
62 Ishii H, Inada M, Tanaka K. Induction of outer and inner ring monodeiodinases in human thyroid gland by thyrotropin. *J Clin Endocrinol Metab* 1983; **57**: 500–5.
63 Hegedus L, Kastrup J, Feldt-Rasmussen U, Petersen PH. Serum thyroglobulin in acute and chronic liver disease. *Clin Endocrinol (Oxf)* 1983; **19**: 231–7.
64 Schneider AB, Ikekubo K, Kuma K. Iodine content of serum thyroglobulin in normal individuals and patients with thyroid tumours. *J Clin Endocrinol Metab* 1983; **57**: 1251–6.
65 Metcalfe RA, Davies R, Weetman AP. Analysis of fibroblast-stimulating activity in IgG from patients with Graves' dermopathy. *Thyroid* 1993; **3**: 207–12.
66 Unger J. Fasting induces a decrease in serum thyroglobulin in normal subjects. *J Clin Endocrinol Metab* 1988; **67**: 1309–11.
67 Jorgensen JO, Moller J, Laursen T, Orskov H, Christiansen JS, Weeke J. Growth hormone administration stimulates energy expenditure and extrathyroidal conversion of thyroxine to triiodothyronine in a dose-dependent manner and suppresses circadian thyrotrophin levels: studies in GH-deficient adults. *Clin Endocrinol* 1994; **41**: 609–14.
68 Chopra IJ, Sack J, Fisher DA. Circulating 3,3′,5′-triiodothyronine (reverse T3) in the human newborn. *J Clin Invest* 1975; **55**: 1137–41.
69 Byfield PG, Lalloz MR, Pearce CJ, Himsworth RL. Free thyroid hormone concentrations in subjects with various abnormalities of binding proteins: experience with amerlex free-T4 and free T3 assays. *Clin Endocrinol (Oxf)* 1983; **19**: 277–83.
70 De Costre P, Buhler U, DeGroot LJ, Refetoff S. Diurnal rhythm in total serum thyroxine levels. *Metabolism* 1971; **20**: 782–91.
71 Bottiglioni F, de Aloysio D, Nicoletti G, Mauloni M, Mantuano R, Capelli M. A study of thyroid function in the pre- and post-menopause. *Maturitas* 1983; **5**: 105–14.
72 Tiegs RD, Body JJ, Barta JM, Heath H III. Secretion and metabolism of monomeric human calcitonin: effects of age, sex and thyroid damage. *J Bone Miner Res* 1986; **1**: 339–49.
73 Kurosawa M, Sato A, Shiraki M, Takahashi Y. Secretion of calcitonin from the thyroid gland increases in aged rats. *Arch Gerontol Geriatr* 1988; **7**: 229–238.
74 Endo T, Saito T, Uchida T, Onaya T. Effects of somatostatin and serotonin on calcitonin secretion from cultured rat parafollicular cells. *Acta Endocrinol (Copenh)* 1988; **117**: 214–18.
75 Barker SB, Klitgaard HM. Metabolism of tissues excised from thyroxine-injected rats. *Am J Physiol* 1952; **170**: 81–6.
76 Oppenheimer JH, Surks MI. The peripheral action of the thyroid hormones. *Med Clin North Am* 1975; **59**: 1055–61.
77 Kuhn JM, Rieu M, Rochette J *et al.* Influence of thyroid status on hemoglobin A2 expression. *J Clin Endocrinol Metab* 1983; **57**: 344–8.
78 Nakai A, Sakurai A, Bell GI, DeGroot LJ. Characterization of a third human thyroid hormone receptor coexpressed with other thyroid hormone receptors in several tissues. *Mol Endocrinol* 1988; **2**: 1087–92.
79 Murad S, Freedland RA. The *in vivo* effects of thyroxine on citrate cleavage enzyme and NADP linked dehydrogenase activities. *Life Sci* 1965; **4**: 527–31.
80 Reith A, Brdiczka D, Nolte J, Staudte HW. The inner membrane of mitochondria under influence of triiodothyronine and riboflavin deficiency in rat heart muscle and liver: a quantitative electron-microscopical and biochemical study. *Exp Cell Res* 1973; **77**: 1–14.
81 Rall JE. Mechanism of action of T4. In: Werner SC, Ingbar SH, eds. *The Thyroid*. New York: Harper and Row, 1978: 138–50.
82 Gonzales LW, Ballard PL, Ertsey R, Williams MC. Glucocorticoids and thyroid hormones stimulate biochemical and morphological differentiation of human fetal lung in organ culture. *J Clin Endocrinol Metab* 1986; **62**: 678–91.
83 Westermark K, Alm J, Skottner A, Karlsson A. Growth factors and the thyroid: effects of treatment for hyper- and hypothyroidism on serum IGF-I and urinary epidermal growth factor concentrations. *Acta Endocrinol (Copenh)* 1988; **118**: 415–21.
84 Simonian MH. ACTH and thyroid hormone regulation of 3 beta hydroxysteroid dehydrogenase activity in human fetal adrenocortical cells. *J Steroid Biochem* 1986; **25**: 1001–6.
85 Burch WM. Calcitonin stimulates growth and maturation of embryonic chick pelvic cartilage *in vitro*. *Endocrinology* 1984; **114**: 1196–202.
86 Rambaud JC, Jian R, Flourie B. Pathophysiological study of diarrhoea in a patient with medullary thyroid carcinoma. Evidence against a secretory mechanism and for the role of shortened colonic transit time. *Gut* 1988; **29**: 537–43.

CHAPTER 24

Assessment of thyroid function

J.P. Monson

Introduction

The high prevalence of thyroid disease and its protean manifestations have stimulated progressive developments in the laboratory assessment of thyroid function. As a consequence the clinician is in a position to document subtle degrees of thyroid dysfunction with relatively high precision. However, the technical improvements in hormone assay techniques, and the attempt to define thyroid dysfunction at the earliest possible stage in its natural history, may result in problems of interpretation. There is no single test of thyroid function which provides maximum diagnostic precision for all manifestations of thyroid dysfunction; measurements of the individual thyroid hormones and thyroid-stimulating hormone (TSH) each have complementary roles in defining thyrotoxicosis, hypopituitary hypothyroidism and thyroid failure. Furthermore, artifactual results due to intercurrent illness or extraneous factors, such as drug interference or alteration in thyroid hormone metabolism, are frequently encountered. An awareness of all these factors is an essential prerequisite for the successful management of thyroid disease.

The earliest attempts to quantify thyroid function precisely depended on measurement of basal metabolic rate. Whilst this had the theoretical advantage of measuring whole-body energy expenditure, the technique was cumbersome and not widely available. Furthermore, perturbations of basal metabolic rate by intercurrent illness created problems in interpretation in those patients in whom the clinical assessment of disease activity was most difficult. The subsequent development of radioiodine-uptake studies was particularly useful in the assessment of hyperthyroidism and dyshormonogenetic states. The era of thyroid hormone measurement commenced with the development of protein-bound iodine assays. This was followed by the successive development of radioimmunoassays for total thyroxine (T_4), triiodothyronine (T_3) and TSH, indirect assessment of thyroid hormone binding capacity in plasma, equilibrium dialysis and monoclonal antibody methods for determination of free thyroid hormone concentrations in serum and the development of high-precision assays for TSH.

This chapter reviews the basic physiology of pituitary–thyroid function, describes the available isotopic and chemical methods for assessing thyroid function, discusses their utility in the various manifestations of thyroid disease and reviews those intercurrent medical conditions and pharmacological therapies which may either disturb thyroid function or, alternatively, perturb thyroid hormone assays.

Basic physiology of the hypothalamo-pituitary–thyroid axis and peripheral thyroid hormone action

Normal thyroid function depends on a precisely controlled relationship between synthesis of hypothalamic thyrotrophin-releasing hormone (TRH), its secretion into the hypophysial portal system, stimulation of production and release of TSH by anterior pituitary thyrotroph cells and the subsequent endocrine action of TSH on thyroid follicular cells. TSH secretion is also modulated by hypothalamic somatostatin which reduces the thyrotroph response to TRH. Negative-feedback control of TSH secretion is achieved by the inhibitory action of T_4 on hypothalamic TRH and pituitary TSH production. TSH interacts with its specific receptor on thyroid follicular cell plasma membranes leading to activation of adenylate cyclase, generation of cyclic adenosine monophosphate (cAMP), stimulation of iodide transport, organification of iodine, coupling of iodine to tyrosines, and ultimately synthesis and secretion of thyroid hormones, predominantly T_4 with a minor quantity of T_3. TSH is also a major determinant of thyroid growth and all of these processes are energy dependent. Serum concentrations of free thyroid hormones are held within a narrow range by the negative-feedback effect of thyroxine, predominantly on TSH production. In addition, thyroid stores of thyroxine are autoregulated by alterations in the rate of iodide transport into the thyroid under the influence of the quantity of available iodide. Iodine depletion leads to an increase in iodide transport whereas increased exogenous iodine results in partial blockade of iodine transport and trapping, the Wolff–Chaikoff effect [1], and a consequent reduction in thyroid hormone secretion [2]. The mechanism of the inhibitory effect of iodine on iodide incorporation and thyroid hormone secretion is poorly understood and furthermore the effect is temporary; after approximately 3 weeks of iodine therapy, thyroid function may be enhanced, particularly when there is an underlying predisposition to thyroid dysfunction.

TRH and TSH

TRH is a modified tripeptide (pyroglutamyl-histidyl-prolineamide) which is synthesised in the supraoptic and paraventricular nuclei of the hypothalamus and stored in the median eminence prior to secretion into the hypophysial portal system. Stimulation of TSH secretion by TRH depends on activation of Ca^{2+} influx into thyrotrophs and also activation of phospholipase C; this process is exquisitely sensitive to prevailing levels of thyroid hormone such that marginal reductions of serum T_4 will result in substantial augmentation of TSH secretion [3], while increments in serum T_4 will have the opposite effect. TRH is also a secretagogue for prolactin, secretion of the latter being largely determined by dopamine inhibition. In addition, TRH may have a more generalised neurotransmitter role and is located in the neural plexus of the gastrointestinal system, the brain and spinal cord.

The rapid stimulatory effect of TRH on TSH secretion may be utilised diagnostically in the *intravenous TRH test* in which the serum TSH response is measured at 20 and 60 min after an intravenous injection of 200 μg synthetic TRH. Prior to the availability of high-precision assays for TSH, this test was used to document mild degrees of thyroid overactivity which are associated with blunting of TSH response to TRH [4]; borderline hypothyroidism results in an exaggerated response [5]. The test may also be used to investigate the hypothalamo-pituitary axis in suspected hypopituitarism, and attempts have been made to distinguish hypothalamic from pituitary failure on the basis of the relative values of serum TSH at 20 and 60 min. However this is rarely useful in clinical practice and may, in fact, be misleading [6]. Furthermore, intravenous TRH may result in acute haemorrhagic infarction of a pituitary macroadenoma and is therefore relatively contraindicated in patients with hypothalamo-pituitary space-occupying lesions. Intravenous TRH may be utilised to augment TSH secretion prior to radioiodine scanning for thyroid carcinoma [7].

TSH is a glycoprotein consisting of two subunits, α and β (each approximately 14 kDa); the latter is specific to TSH whereas the α-subunit is ubiquitous to the glycoprotein hormones follicle-stimulating hormone (FSH), luteinising hormone (LH) and human chorionic gonadotrophin (hCG). It interacts with a specific receptor on the thyroid follicular cell membrane with resulting trophic effects and stimulation of thyroid hormone synthesis and release. TSH secretion demonstrates a minor degree of circadian rhythmicity. The earliest assays for TSH in serum lacked precision at the lower end of the range and had their major utility in the diagnosis of primary thyroid failure. Currently available assays are useful in the diagnosis of both hypothyroidism and thyrotoxicosis (see below) and may also aid in the definition of the rare instances of TSH hypersecretion from pituitary tumours and of syndromes of thyroid hormone resistance [8].

Circulating thyroid hormones

T_4, formed by the combination of two molecules of diiodotyrosine, is the major secretory product of the thyroid. Thyroglobulin and T_3 are also released but the direct contribution of the thyroid to circulating T_3 is relatively minor. T_4 enters cells by means of a specific, stereoselective, energy-dependent carrier mechanism [9] and undergoes intracellular monodeiodination to yield approximately equal quantities of T_3 and reverse T_3 (5′ and 5 monodeiodination, respectively), the latter having no recognised biological activity. T_3 thus formed in the periphery constitutes >80% of the circulating hormone and is largely responsible for the physiological effects of thyroid hormone. Small quantities of diiodothyronines are also produced by deiodination of T_4 and T_3 but do not appear to have any demonstrable physiological action.

Thyroid hormones in the circulation are virtually completely bound to three binding proteins, namely T_4-binding globulin (TBG), albumin and T_4-binding prealbumin (TBPA). The relative contributions of the individual binding proteins to the total concentration of thyroid hormones in plasma is dependent on their concentration and binding affinity; the approximate distribution of binding is depicted in Fig. 24.1. Although T_4 demonstrates greater affinity for binding than T_3, the latter is >99.5% bound, almost exclusively to thyroxine (thyronine)-binding globulin.

Precise control of TSH secretion (and therefore, indirectly, of T_4 production) depends on the intracellular 5′ deiodination of T_4 to T_3 by type II deiodinase in pituitary thyrotroph

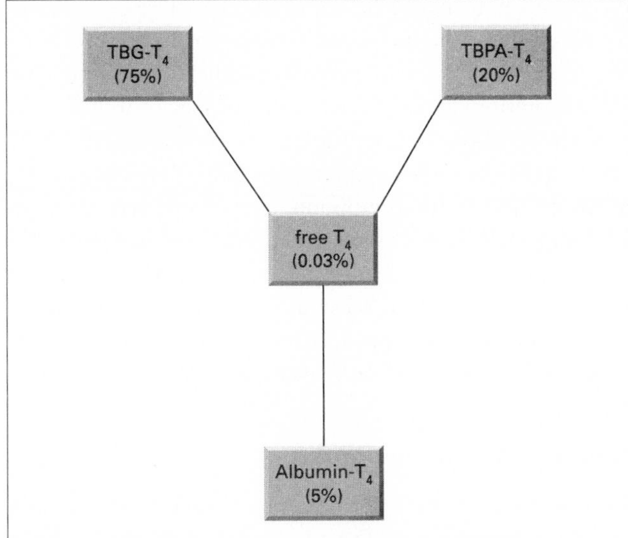

Fig. 24.1 Total serum thyroxine (T_4): percentage free T_4 and distribution of binding between T_4-binding globulin (TBG), T_4-binding prealbumin (TBPA) and albumin. Relative binding is dependent on individual binding-protein concentration and binding affinity.

cells [10]. Because thyrotroph exposure to T_4 is proportional to the free concentration of hormone, it follows that the negative-feedback mechanism will maintain a stable concentration of free thyroid hormone. It will be appreciated, however, that the total concentration of thyroid hormone will remain substantially dependent on the concentration of thyroid binding proteins. Alterations in the latter, either genetic or resulting from intercurrent conditions, will produce alterations in total thyroid hormone measurements without altering free thyroid hormone concentrations (see below); the changes are therefore not of physiological significance. None the less, a knowledge of these artifactual changes is essential for the interpretation of total thyroid hormone assays.

Thyronine-binding proteins

T_4-binding globulin

TBG is a glycoprotein of 54 kDa molecular weight, encoded by a gene on chromosome Xq and synthesised in the liver [11]. It is composed of approximately 20% carbohydrate moieties and sialic acid residues. The rate of hepatic clearance of the compound is determined by the degree of sialylation and the latter depends on, amongst other things, prevailing concentrations of oestrogen; this phenomenon underlies the increased concentration of TBG evident during pregnancy or during exogenous oestrogen therapy [12]. Although present at a lower circulating concentration than the other thyroid binding proteins (Table 24.1), its high affinity renders it quantitatively the most important thyronine-binding protein. TBG provides a high-capacity system for thyroid hormone binding, accounting for >70% of T_4 carriage in plasma, with each molecule of TBG potentially binding one molecule of T_4 or T_3, the latter with somewhat lower affinity. TBG concentrations will be elevated under conditions of reduced hepatic clearance including pregnancy, combined oral contraceptive use, acute and chronic liver disease and hypothyroidism. With the obvious exception of hypothyroidism, these conditions therefore give rise to elevations in serum total thyroid hormone levels. Decrease in serum TBG concentration, with consequent reduction in serum total thyroid hormone concentration, may occur in protein-losing states, for example nephrotic syndrome or protein-losing enteropathy. Total serum thyroid hormone concentrations may also decrease as a result of displacement of T_4 or T_3 from high-affinity binding sites on TBG by certain drugs, including salicylates, phenytoin and barbiturates.

Congenital deficiency of TBG is well described as an X-linked recessive characteristic, possibly due to point mutations, abnormal gene transcription or translation since the TBG gene is grossly intact [13]. A spectrum of TBG deficiency is found in heterozygotes [14] and the overall prevalence of the condition is 1:5000 live births. X-linked TBG excess and abnormalities of TBG binding are also recognised, the

Table 24.1 Thyroid hormone binding proteins in serum: concentration ranges, approximate binding affinities and production rates.

	Concentration (μg/l)	Affinity constant K_a (mole^{-1}) T_4	T_3	Production rate (mg/day)
T_4-binding globulin	6–16	1×10^{10}	1×10^9	15
T_4-binding prealbumin	150–350	1×10^8	1×10^7	650
Albumin	$35–50 \times 10^3$	2×10^6	2×10^5	17000

T_4, thyroxine; T_3, triiodothyronine.

latter being described in Australian aborigines [15] and black Americans [16] and being associated with alteration in heat lability of TBG. Suspected abnormalities in circulating TBG may be investigated by specific radioimmunoassays.

T_4-binding prealbumin

TBPA is present in substantially higher concentration than TBG but has a lower affinity for T_4 binding and does not contribute significantly to T_3 binding. It is synthesised in the liver and consists of four identical polypeptide subunits forming a tetramer [17] which has the capacity to bind two molecules of T_4, but only one with high affinity. TBPA is partly complexed to retinol-binding protein in the circulation but this does not alter T_4-binding characteristics. A dominantly inherited trait associated with increased binding of T_4 and reverse T_3 by TBPA has been described [18]; this may not alter circulating total T_4 concentrations and, predictably, does not affect free thyroid hormone levels. Familial increments in circulating TBPA and total T_4 levels have also been described [19]. The condition of familial amyloidotic polyneuropathy is due to the deposition of mutant variations of the TBPA subunit in peripheral nerves [20]; it is not associated with alterations in conventional thyroid function tests.

Serum albumin

Serum albumin provides high-capacity, low-affinity binding sites for T_4 and T_3 which are quantitatively less important than TBG and TBPA. However, artifactually elevated serum total T_4 concentrations may be found in certain individuals in whom albumin has an increased binding affinity for T_4. This is inherited as an autosomal dominant trait and is termed familial dysalbuminaemic hyperthyroxinaemia [21]. Its major importance from a clinical point of view is to avoid an incorrect diagnosis of thyrotoxicosis. Importantly, the analogue employed in 'analogue free T_4 assays' demonstrates high affinity for the mutant albumin therefore producing spuriously high free-T_4 levels by this method.

Other thyronine-binding proteins

Minor contributions to serum thyroid hormone binding may be made by high-density lipoproteins [22]. In addition, some binding of circulating antibodies to thyroglobulin may occur in patients with autoimmune thyroid disease.

Measurement of thyroid function *in vivo*

Isotopic uptake studies of the thyroid may be carried out to define total thyroid function, to characterise particular forms of dyshormonogenesis and to document the functional characteristics of thyroid nodules. Three isotopes are conventionally employed. The isotopes of iodine (^{131}I, half-life 8.1 days; ^{123}I, half-life 0.55 days) are predictably taken up by the iodide trapping mechanism and eventually incorporated into thyroglobulin; in contrast, pertechnetate ($^{99m}TcO_4$, half-life 0.25 days) enters via the iodide pump but is not retained. Pertechnetate and ^{123}I are used for scanning imaging of the thyroid whereas ^{131}I has utility in studies of thyroid hormone production and the assessment of functional uptake of iodine by metastatic thyroid carcinoma.

Radioactive iodine uptake

Measurements of radioactive iodine uptake by the thyroid provide information on the uptake of iodide by the gland, subsequent organification and coupling to tyrosine residues in thyroglobulin and the eventual rate of thyroid hormone formation. The results, expressed as a percentage of administered labelled iodine, depend not only on the prevailing level of thyroid function but also on iodine content of the diet and pharmacological exposure, including topical preparations such as povidone iodine. Measurements are made at 4–6, 24 and 48 hours after administration of tracer. Thyrotoxicosis is associated with increased initial uptake and reduced retention at 48 hours reflecting increased throughput. Uptake is typically reduced in hypothyroidism and absent in subacute thyroiditis and following exposure to excess iodine. The development of reliable serum thyroid hormone assays has largely eliminated the use of iodine uptake studies for the diagnosis of thyroid dysfunction. None the less, iodine or pertechnetate scanning has a role in establishing a diagnosis of subacute thyroiditis and in the distinction between Graves' disease and autonomous thyroid adenoma, particularly when extrathyroidal manifestations of the former are absent.

Iodine uptake studies performed after administration of T_3 have previously been used to determine whether thyroid function is suppressible and therefore mediated by TSH rather than thyroid-stimulating immunoglobulins (*T_3 suppression test*). A modification of this principle, using pertechnetate scanning after T_3 administration, has been employed in an attempt to predict remission of Graves' thyrotoxicosis in patients on medical therapy [23], but probably adds relatively little to the demonstration of a measurable serum TSH on a high-precision assay (see below).

Prior to the development of serum TSH assays, measurement of iodine uptake after intramuscular TSH administration was utilised as a means of distinguishing hypopituitary hypothyroidism from primary thyroid failure (*TSH stimulation test*). The test may also be used to confirm a diagnosis of thyroid hemiagenesis and to establish the presence of functioning thyroid parenchyma in patients on long-standing thyroid hormone therapy. However, the investigation requires the administration of bovine TSH which may be associated with allergic reactions and is difficult to obtain; recombinant human TSH is not currently available for clinical use.

The administration of perchlorate during radioiodine uptake study may be used to confirm a diagnosis of a peroxidase defect as the cause of dyshormonogenetic, goitrous hypothyroidism. The test depends on the principle that in patients with organification defects (e.g. Pendred's syndrome—a thyroid peroxidase type of defect with nerve deafness) the perchlorate inhibition of iodine uptake by the thyroid combined with failure of oxidation of iodide and incorporation into thyroglobulin results in release of labelled iodine from the gland (*positive perchlorate discharge test*).

Measurement of serum thyroid hormone concentrations

The initial investigation of suspected thyroid dysfunction depends on measurement of thyroid hormone concentrations in serum. Predictably, thyrotoxicosis is characterised by elevation of serum T_4 and T_3 and hypothyroidism the reverse (Table 24.2). However, there are a variety of clinical situations in which results may be difficult to interpret because

Table 24.2 Typical changes in serum thyroxine (T_4), free T_4, triiodothyronine (T_3) and thyroid-stimulating hormone (TSH) in thyrotoxicosis, primary hypothyroidism, hypopituitary hypothyroidism, thyroid hormone resistance and autonomous TSH secretion.

	Total T_4	Free T_4	Total T_3	TSH
Thyrotoxicosis	↑	↑	↑	↓
Borderline thyrotoxicosis	↑ or N	↑ or N	↑	↓
Thyroid failure	↓	↓	↓ or N	↑
Borderline thyroid failure	↓ or N	↓ or N	↓ or N	↑
Hypopituitarism	↓	↓	↓ or N	↓ or N
Thyroid hormone resistance	↑	↑	↑	↑ or N
Thyrotroph adenoma	↑	↑	↑	↑ or N

N, within reference range.

Table 24.3 Causes and direction of change in serum total thyroxine (T_4) in the euthyroid subject.

	Serum T_4
Pregnancy	+
Oestrogen therapy	+
Non-thyroidal illness	−
Nephrotic syndrome	−
Chronic liver disease	+
Anticonvulsant therapy	−
Amiodarone therapy	+

of artifactual increments or decrements in total thyroid hormone levels (Table 24.3). Anomalies arising as a result of changes in thyroid hormone-binding proteins may be partially circumvented by the use of 'free' thyroid hormone assays, although the original analogue free-T_4 methods produced spuriously high results in a small number of subjects who exhibited increased binding of the labelled analogue by albumin (dysalbuminaemic hyperthyroxinaemia) [21]. The development of high-precision assays for serum TSH which were capable of distinguishing completely suppressed levels on the one hand from low and normal levels on the other raised the possibility that a single TSH measurement might be used for the initial definition of thyroid function in an individual with some precision [24]. The major problem with this approach is that it may fail to diagnose hypopituitary hypothyroidism, in which the serum TSH concentration is usually within the reference range.

There are significant differences in reference ranges for both total and free thyroid hormone concentrations depending on laboratory and methodology. For this reason, reference data will not be provided in this chapter. It is clearly essential that clinicians should maintain a close working relationship with their laboratory colleagues in the interpretation of the investigations described.

Total thyroid hormone assays

Measurements of total T_4 and T_3 were amongst the first radioimmunoassays (RIA) used in general clinical practice. The basic methodology depended on the displacement of bound thyroid hormone from binding proteins by chemical means followed by conventional immunoassay utilising radioiodine-labelled ligand and antibodies relatively specific to either T_4 or T_3. Separation of bound from free ligand was achieved by either precipitation or solid phase techniques. Subsequent developments in total thyroid hormone assays have included the use of enzyme-linked immunosorbent assays (ELISA) and fluorescence excitation techniques.

As indicated above, these assays will produce spurious results in any situation in which binding-protein concentrations are altered or competition for binding sites occurs (Table 24.3). In addition, artifactual results may occur in the presence of circulating antibodies directed against either the hormogenic sequence of thyroglobulin or against thyroid hormones.

Indirect assays of thyroid hormone binding capacity

These assays are based on the principle that T_3 has a lower affinity for the major thyroid binding proteins than T_4; labelled T_3 is added to serum followed by separation of bound from free T_3 using, for example, sephadex resin binding. The indirect measurement of thyroid hormone capacity thus achieved is known as a *T_3 resin uptake test* or *thyroid hormone uptake test (THUT)*. The numerical value of the assay will depend on whether results are expressed in terms of T_3 taken up by the serum binding proteins or subsequently bound by the resin, a high value of resin uptake indicating a lower availability of serum thyroid hormone binding sites.

These measurements, or direct assays of TBG, may be combined with total thyroid hormone assays to give a so-called *free thyroxine index*. The values obtained have a reasonable correlation with measurements of free thyroid hormone measured by equilibrium dialysis methods and consequently they relate more precisely to the patient's clinical state of thyroid function.

Free thyroid hormone assays

Direct measurement of circulating 'free' thyroid hormones represents the ideal in biochemical assessment of thyroid function, but this is difficult to achieve for at least three important reasons. Firstly, the quantity of free hormone is very small (0.03% of total T_4; 0.3% of total T_3) and thus an extremely high degree of assay sensitivity is required; secondly, any assay method must avoid perturbing the equilibrium between bound and free hormone; and thirdly, the patient's serum may contain factors which interfere with the *in vitro* assay method.

Serum free T_4 and T_3 may be measured directly by *equilibrium dialysis* or ultracentrifugation followed by immunoassay [25]. Isotopic equilibrium dialysis methods provide an indirect method of assessing free hormone concentration and although this constitutes a reference method, there are substantial variations evident between laboratories. Furthermore, dialysis methods are labour intensive and not applicable to the routine laboratory. Alternative methods for the indirect measurement of free thyroid hormones include the following.

1 *Two-step immunoassays*—free hormone is immuno-extracted from serum by an antibody bound to a solid support followed by washing and the addition of labelled tracer which binds to the remaining unoccupied antibody binding sites.

2 *Analogue methods*—the tracer used is a radioiodine-labelled T_4 or T_3 analogue which binds to the relevant antithyroid antibody but not to serum thyroid hormone binding proteins. This latter requirement in the assay may not be borne out in practice; in particular, there may be significant binding of the analogue to albumin with consequent spurious results which are most evident (for free T_4) in the condition of familial dysalbuminaemic hyperthyroxinaemia (FDH). These assays may also be variously perturbed by drug interactions, do not perform well in dilution and may produce artifactual results under conditions of non-thyroidal illness. The latter, sometimes referred to as the *sick euthyroid syndrome* is associated with increased conversion of T_4 to reverse T_3, reduction in thyroid hormone binding proteins and a consequent decrease in total T_4 concentration; free T_4 concentrations by dialysis methods are normal or slightly increased but analogue methods tend to give reduced results.

3 *Enhanced radiolabelled or chemiluminescence labelled-antibody methods*—these one-step assays employ a monoclonal antibody to T_4 which competes for binding with free T_4 or with an immobilised conjugate of a protein and T_3. In the case of the chemiluminescence assay, the signal is generated by an antibody–peroxidase conjugate with luminol as substrate [26]. They compare favourably with analogue methods, are more robust in dilution, are relatively unaffected by changes in serum binding proteins and fulfil the recently proposed minimum requirements for free thyroid hormone assays [27].

Measurement of free T_3, in contrast to free T_4, has little diagnostic advantage over measurement of total T_3.

Measurement of serum TSH

The initial RIA methods for serum TSH measurement were used to diagnose primary hypothyroidism, in which the concentration is almost invariably raised. The subsequent development of second- and third-generation immunometric assays have resulted in dramatic improvements in precision, thus making it possible to distinguish between normal and suppressed levels of TSH [28]. These assays depend on a 'sandwich' principle in which two or more antibodies are directed against different portions of the TSH molecule. One solid-phase antibody serves to extract TSH from serum and the second antibody has an attached signalling system for quantification of antibody-bound TSH. Different assays are referred to as immunoradiometric, immunoenzymometric or immunochemoluminometric, depending on whether the signalling system is radioactive, enzymatic (e.g. peroxidase) or chemiluminescent (e.g. luminol or dioxetanes), respectively. 'Third-generation' assays can achieve a reliable functional sensitivity of 0.01–0.02 mU/l [29].

High-precision TSH assays are particularly valuable in the following circumstances.

1 The diagnosis of early (compensated) primary hypothyroidism in which serum TSH is elevated despite thyroid hormone levels remaining within the reference range. However, it should be remembered that untreated primary adrenal failure may produce an identical profile.

2 The diagnosis of mild thyrotoxicosis due to Graves' disease, autonomous thyroid adenoma or multinodular goitre.

3 The documentation of measurable serum TSH in the presence of raised thyroid hormone concentrations. In the absence of thyroid hormone binding assay anomalies, this finding raises the possibility of either primary TSH hypersecretion from a thyrotroph adenoma or, alternatively, central (and peripheral) thyroid hormone resistance [8]. These possibilities may be further distinguished by measurement of peripheral markers of thyroid hormone action (serum sex hormone binding globulin, SHBG), serum TSH response to intravenous TRH (increased in thyroid hormone resistance), serum α-subunit (may be increased with thyrotroph tumours) and pituitary imaging.

4 The distinction between the hypothyroxinaemia of non-thyroidal illness and primary hypothyroidism. However, the exclusion of hypopituitary hypothyroidism may be problematic.

5 Determining optimum T_4 replacement dose in hypothyroidism [30].

Adjunctive tests in the investigation of thyroid function

The measurement of tissue exposure to thyroid hormone is difficult. However, further assessment of the peripheral action of thyroid hormone may be made by measurement of serum SHBG, which is increased in thyrotoxicosis and provides a sensitive indicator of tissue exposure to thyroid hormone. Cardiac systolic time intervals have also been used to indicate subtle degrees of thyroid hormone excess [31]. Measurement of basic metabolic rate and reflex relaxation times are useful research techniques in the investigation of the hypothyroid patient.

Thyroid antiperoxidase (antimicrosomal) antibodies are a useful marker of the presence of autoimmune thyroid disease; they are frequently present in titres of 1:400–6400 in Graves' disease and in higher titre in autoimmune thyroiditis. Measurements of TSH receptor antibodies are rarely carried out in routine clinical practice but may be of some value in determining the potential risk of neonatal thyrotoxicosis in the antenatal assessment of patients with Graves' disease, particularly when the patient has previously undergone surgery or radioiodine therapy and therefore no longer provides a bioassay of thyroid-stimulating activity (see Chapter 27).

Measurements of serum thyroglobulin do not have a role in the investigation of thyroid dysfunction but are particularly useful in the follow-up of patients with differentiated thyroid carcinoma.

The influence of intercurrent illness and drug therapy on thyroid function tests

Artifactual alterations in thyroid function tests or overt thyroid dysfunction may occur in various clinical situations and pharmacological interventions (Table 24.3). The most commonly encountered examples are outlined below.

Severe systemic illness or starvation

Serum total T_4 and T_3 levels are reduced in the presence of a normal serum TSH concentration (sick euthyroid syndrome). There is evidence for preferential conversion of T_4 to reverse T_3. Free T_4 measured by analogue methods may be normal or reduced (see Chapter 31).

Protein-losing states

Nephrotic syndrome and severe protein-losing enteropathy may result in decreased TBG concentrations and consequent low serum total T_4. Free T_4 concentrations are normal.

Chronic liver disease

Serum TBG may be decreased or increased giving spurious concentrations of serum total T_4. Serum SHBG is also increased and therefore can not be used as a marker of peripheral thyroid hormone action. Free T_4 concentrations may decrease (see Chapter 77).

Pregnancy and oestrogen therapy

Reversible increments in thyroid hormone binding proteins and SHBG. Free T_4 concentrations are slightly reduced and TSH concentrations are normal.

Glucocorticoid excess and deficiency

Exogenous or endogenous glucocorticoid excess is associated

with a modest reduction in TSH secretion, decreased concentration of serum TBG and reduced peripheral conversion of T_4 to T_3. The net result is a decrease in serum total-T_4 concentration but little change in free T_4 and no clinically discernible change in thyroid function. Glucocorticoid deficiency may be associated with a transient decrease in serum total and free T_4 and modest increment in TSH.

Anticonvulsants

Phenytoin may compete with T_4 for binding to TBG and thus reduce serum total-T_4 concentration. A similar effect is produced by salicylates and sulphonylurea drugs. Free thyroid hormone concentrations are unchanged.

Amiodarone

Effects of the antiarrhythmic drug, amiodarone, on thyroid function are complex [32]. In the majority of patients studied, the initial effect is one of inhibition of peripheral conversion of T_4 to T_3 and enhanced conversion to reverse T_3; minor changes in TBPA and albumin are also noted. The net effect is an increment in serum total and free T_4 and a slight rise in TSH which is evident within a week or two of commencing treatment. Clinically normal thyroid function is maintained. However, after prolonged therapy, both hypothyroidism and hyperthyroidism may occur and are manifest by characteristic changes in thyroid function. This phenomenon is related to the high iodine content of the drug and is seen in approximately 2% of subjects treated in the UK but to a greater extent in iodine-deficient areas worldwide. Patients with pre-existing nodular thyroid disease and evidence of thyroid autoimmunity are particularly susceptible. Amiodarone-induced thyrotoxicosis should only be diagnosed on the basis of elevated thyroid hormone concentrations in the presence of TSH suppression.

Propranolol

By virtue of intrinsic membrane-stabilising activity, propranolol may decrease peripheral conversion of T_4 to T_3. This may have some therapeutic benefit in the treatment of thyrotoxicosis but is not associated with significant alteration of serum thyroid function tests during routine clinical use.

Lithium

Lithium may induce hypo- or hyperthyroidism in susceptible individuals, more commonly the former. Serum thyroid hormone and TSH concentrations are characteristic.

References

1 Wolff J. Physiological aspects of iodide excess in relation to radiation protection. *J Mol Med* 1980; **4**: 151–65.
2 Buhler UK, De Groot LJ. Effect of stable iodine on thyroid iodine release. *J Clin Endocrinol* 1969; **29**: 1546–52.
3 Saberi M, Utiger RD. Augmentation of thyrotrophin responses to thyrotrophin releasing hormone following small decreases in serum thyroid hormone concentration. *J Clin Endocrinol Metab* 1975; **40**: 435–41.
4 Morgans ME, Thompson BD, Whitehouse SA. Sporadic non-toxic goitre: an investigation of the hypothalamic-pituitary-thyroid axis. *Clin Endocrinol* 1978; **8**: 101–8.
5 Ridgway EC, Kourides IA, Chin WW, Cooper DS, Maloof F. Augmentation of pituitary thyrotrophin response to thyrotrophin releasing hormone during subphysiological triiodothyronine therapy in hypothyroidism. *Clin Endocrinol* 1979; **10**: 343–53.
6 Snyder PJ, Jacobs LS, Rabello MM *et al.* Diagnostic value of thyrotrophin-releasing hormone in pituitary and hypothalamic disease. *Ann Intern Med* 1974; **81**: 751–7.
7 Fairclough PD, Cryer RJ, McAllister J *et al.* Serum TSH responses to intravenously and orally administered TRH in man after thyroidectomy for carcinoma of the thyroid. *Clin Endocrinol* 1973; **2**: 351–9.
8 Refetoff S, Weiss RE, Usala SJ. The syndromes of resistance to thyroid hormone. *Endocr Rev* 1993; **14**: 348–99.
9 Blondeau JP, Osty J, Francon J. Characterization of the thyroid hormone transport system of isolated hepatocytes. *J Biol Chem* 1988; **263**: 2685–92.
10 Silva JE, Larsen PR. Pituitary nuclear 3,5,3′-triiodothyronine and thyrotrophin secretion: an explanation for the effect of thyroxine. *Science* 1977; **198**: 617–19.
11 Hocman G. Human thyroxine binding globulin (TBG). *Rev Physiol Biochem Pharmacol* 1981; **91**: 45–89.
12 Ain KB, Mori Y, Refetoff S. Reduced clearance rate of thyroxine-binding globulin (TBG) with increased sialylation: a mechanism for estrogen-induced elevation of serum TBG concentration. *J Clin Endocrinol Metab* 1987; **65**: 689–96.
13 Mori Y, Refetoff S, Flink IL *et al.* Detection of the thyroxine-binding-globulin (TBG) gene in six unrelated families with complete TBG deficiency. *J Clin Endocrinol Metab* 1988; **67**: 727–33.
14 Burr WA, Ramsden DB, Hoffenberg R. Hereditary abnormalities of thyroxine binding globulin concentration. *Q J Med* 1980; **49**: 295–313.
15 Murata Y, Refetoff S, Sarne DH, Dick M, Watson F. Variant thyroxine-binding globulin in serum of Australian aborigines. *J Endocrinol Invest* 1985; **8**: 225–32.
16 Murata Y, Takamatsu J, Refetoff S. Inherited abnormality of thyroxine-binding globulin with no demonstrable thyroxine-binding activity and high serum levels of denatured thyroxine-binding globulin. *N Engl J Med* 1986; **314**: 694–9.
17 Cody V. Thyroid hormone interactions: molecular conformation, protein binding and hormone action. *Endocr Rev* 1980; **1**: 140–66.
18 Lalloz MRA, Byfield PGH, Goel KM, Loudon MM, Thomson JA, Himsworth RL. Hyperthyroxinaemia due to co-existence of two raised affinity thyroxine binding proteins (albumin and prealbumin) in one family. *J Clin Endocrinol Metab* 1987; **64**: 346–52.
19 Skiest D, Braverman LE, Emerson CH. Concentration of free thyroxin in serum of a patient with euthyroid hyperthyroxinaemia secondary to increased thyroxin-binding prealbumin: results by various methods compared. *Clin Chem* 1986; **32**: 687–9.

20 Refetoff S, Dwulet FE, Benson MD. Reduced affinity for thyroxine in two of three structural thyroxine-binding prealbumin variants associated with familial amyloidotic polyneuropathy. *J Clin Endocrinol Metab* 1986; **63**: 1432–7.

21 Ruiz M, Rajatanavin R, Young RA *et al.* Familial dysalbuminemic hyperthyroxinemia, a syndrome that can be confused with thyrotoxicosis. *N Engl J Med* 1982; **306**: 635–9.

22 Benvenga S. The 27-kilodalton thyroxine (T4)-binding protein is human apolipoprotein A-1: identification of a 68-kilodalton high density lipoprotein that binds T4. *Endocrinology* 1989; **124**: 1265–9.

23 Shimmins J, Alexander WD, McLarty DG, Robertson JWK, Sloane DJP. ^{99m}Tc pertechnetate for measuring thyroid suppressibility. *J Nucl Med* 1971; **12**: 51–4.

24 Caldwell G, Gow SM, Sweeting VM, Kellett HA, Beckett GJ, Seth J, Toft AD. A new strategy for thyroid function testing. *Lancet* 1985; **i**: 1117–19.

25 Ekins R. Measurement of free hormones in blood. *Endocr Rev* 1990; **11**: 5–46.

26 Christofides ND, Sheehan CP. Enhanced chemiluminescence labeled-antibody immunoassay (Amerlite-MAB^{TM}) for free thyroxine: design, development, and technical validation. *Clin Chem* 1995; **41**: 17–23.

27 Hay ID, Bayer MF, Kaplan MM, Klee GJ, Larsen PR, Spencer CA. American thyroid association assessment of current free thyroid hormone and thyrotrophin measurements and guidelines for future clinical assays. *Clin Chem* 1991; **37**: 2002–8.

28 Squire CR, Fraser WD. Thyroid stimulating hormone measurement using a third generation immunometric assay. *Ann Clin Biochem* 1995; **32**: 307–13.

29 Spencer CA, Takeuchi M, Kazarosyan M, MacKenzie F, Beckett GJ, Wilkinson E. Interlaboratory/intermethod differences in functional sensitivity of immunometric assays of thyrotrophin (TSH) and impact on reliability of measurement of subnormal concentrations of TSH. *Clin Chem* 1995; **41**: 367–74.

30 Bearcroft C, Toms GC, Williams SJ, Noonan K, Monson JP. Thyroxine replacement in post-radioiodine hypothyroidism. *Clin Endocrinol* 1991; **34**: 115–18.

31 Price DE, O'Malley BP, Northover B, Rosenthal FD. Changes in circulating thyroid hormone levels and systolic time intervals in treated hypothyroidism. *Clin Endocrinol* 1991; **35**: 67–9.

32 Gammage MD, Franklyn JA. Amiodarone and the thyroid. *Q J Med* 1987; **238**: 83–6.

CHAPTER 25

Thyroid imaging

M.N. Maisey

Introduction

The effective management of thyroid diseases depends on an accurate diagnosis followed by appropriate treatment and follow-up. Since being introduced nearly half a century ago, imaging techniques, particularly those using radionuclides, have always played a leading part in the diagnosis and management of thyroid diseases: radioimmunoassay (RIA) revolutionised the investigation of thyroid dysfunction, while radionuclide scanning has long been the main method of investigating the thyroid *in vivo*. During the last decade the role of thyroid imaging in clinical practice has been expanded by the introduction of new radiopharmaceuticals (Table 25.1); the development of other imaging techniques has altered the role of radionuclide scanning in the management of some thyroid disorders. For example, the use of ultrasound scanning of the thyroid and the widespread use of fine-needle aspiration (FNA) cytology have both changed the way the thyroid nodule is investigated. The increasing use of diagnostic imaging techniques other than radionuclide scans, such as radiography, computed tomography (CT) and magnetic resonance imaging (MRI), have also had an impact on the use of radionuclides for investigating thyroid disease, but have not significantly decreased their use. Radioactive iodine (^{131}I) has become established as a simple, cheap and effective method of treating thyrotoxicosis, and in most instances represents the treatment of choice. Fear that its use might result in an increased risk of cancer and other genetic complications has not been substantiated after worldwide experience for more than four decades. Radioactive iodine is also important in the treatment and follow-up of differentiated thyroid cancer (see Chapter 28).

Thyroid imaging is currently used for the investigation and management of thyrotoxicosis, thyroid nodules, goitre, ectopic thyroid and thyroid cancer.

Hyperthyroidism

The diagnosis of hyperthyroidism is incomplete unless its cause is also established, because the choice of management and prognosis depend on the underlying cause.

In practice, Graves' disease and single or multiple autonomous toxic nodules (uninodular or multinodular Plummer's disease) account for the majority of cases of thyrotoxicosis. Nevertheless, the remaining causes are clinically important and should always be borne in mind because their management and clinical course follow entirely different lines. A summary of the causes of hyperthyroidism is shown in Table 25.2.

Role of thyroid scanning in the diagnosis of hyperthyroidism

The appropriate management of patients with hyperthyroidism depends on an accurate initial diagnosis; the value of the thyroid scan in thyrotoxicosis has been reviewed by us [1]. The radionuclide scan has three main uses in managing hyperthyroidism: (i) establishing the cause of thyrotoxicosis; (ii) the measurement of tracer uptake and gland size for the selection of appropriate ^{131}I therapy regimens; and (iii) for the follow-up of patients after treatment. There are a number of patients in whom the type of hyperthyroidism cannot be confirmed clinically or biochemically and, without the thyroid scan, an incorrect diagnosis may be assumed. This may result in inappropriate treatment; in a review [2] we found that 22% of patients with toxic nodules (Plummer's disease) had received long-term antithyroid medication without a correct diagnosis being established and more appropriate treatment instituted.

Table 25.1 Radiopharmaceuticals used in the investigation of thyroid diseases.

Radiopharmaceutical	Applications
Technetium-99m (^{99m}Tc) pertechnetate	Routine thyroid scanning
Iodine-123	Thyroid scanning when a radioisotope of iodine is required
Iodine-131	The investigation of thyroid cancer
Gallium-67 citrate	Investigation of thyroid lymphoma, silent thyroiditis, thyroid infection and amyloid
Thallium-201	Investigation of thyroid cancer, thyroid nodules, demonstration of suppressed thyroid tissue
^{99m}Tc pentavalent DMSA	Investigation of medullary thyroid carcinoma
$^{131}I/^{123}I$ MIBG	Investigation of medullary thyroid carcinoma
^{18}F-FDG	Thyroid cancer

DMSA, dimercaptosuccinic acid; MIBG, meta-iodobenzylguanidine; FDG, fluorodeoxy-glucose.

Table 25.2 Causes of hyperthyroidism.

Graves' disease (diffuse or nodular variants)
Solitary or multiple toxic autonomous nodules (toxic adenoma, Plummer's disease)
Thyroid hormone 'leakage'
Subacute (De Quervain's) thyroiditis
Painless (silent) thyroiditis
Hashimoto' thyroiditis
Post-partum thyroiditis
Iodide induced hyperthyroidism (Jod–Basedow's phenomenon)
Excess thyroid hormone ingestion
Rare causes including:
Pituitary TSH-dependent hyperthyroidism
Ectopic TSH-secreting tumour
Extensive functioning differentiated thyroid cancer
Trophoblastic tumour
Struma ovarii

TSH, thyroid-stimulating hormone.

The solitary thyroid nodule and thyrotoxicosis

When a patient with thyrotoxicosis is found to have a solitary thyroid nodule on clinical examination, this is usually an autonomous toxic nodule. However, clinical examination is unreliable; 32% of cases were incorrectly diagnosed in one series [3]. Other causes which may be identified by scanning include a solitary non-functioning nodule in a patient with Graves' disease, a very asymmetric goitre, or diffuse enlargement of a single lobe with agenesis of the other lobe all of which simulate a toxic nodule. It is usually possible to differentiate between these on the initial scan, but further investigations may be required, for example repeating the scan after stimulation with exogenous thyroid-stimulating hormone (TSH) (Fig. 25.1) will demonstrate suppressed tissue [4]; scanning with thallium-201 [5] will often show uptake in tissue which is not accumulating $^{99m}TcO_4$ or $^{123}I/^{131}I$; ultrasonography will demonstrate a lobe which is present but not taking up tracer, or a hypoplastic or aplastic lobe; and the use of X-ray fluorescent measurements or scans [6] will establish the presence of ^{127}I-containing tissue on the contralateral side. The simple method of shielding the active nodule with lead on routine thyroid scintigraphy may be sufficient to show the presence of the contralateral lobe.

The importance of making a correct diagnosis lies in the choice of treatment and subsequent follow-up. Patients with toxic nodules respond well to radioiodine treatment, and the nodule usually decreases in size to approximately 60% of the volume [7] with complete cure being the normal outcome and hypothyroidism a rare sequel [3]. In contrast, a single lobe with Graves' disease will be treated in a conventional manner, usually with antithyroid drugs, followed by ablative therapy only when a relapse occurs. A patient with Graves' disease who has an incidental non-functioning nodule on the radionuclide scan is usually treated by subtotal thyroidectomy in order to detect possible malignancy, the incidence of which has been reported to be as high as 21% [8]. Our own experience would, however, suggest that

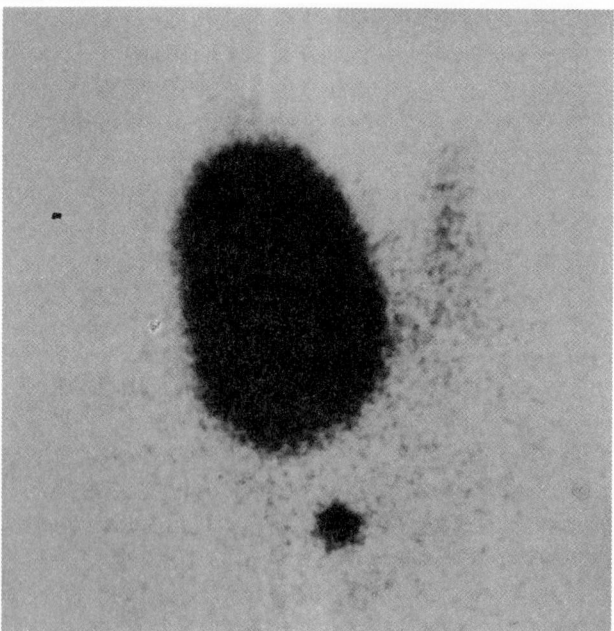

(a)

(b)

Fig. 25.1 ^{99m}Tc thyroid scan from a patient with thyrotoxicosis. The first scan (a) could be a toxic nodule or Graves' disease associated with agenesis of the left lobe. A repeat scan after thyroid-stimulating hormone (b) shows a normal left lobe together with visualisation of the upper pole of the right lobe confirming a toxic nodule.

the true incidence of malignancy is very much lower. An alternative approach is FNA cytology examination of the nodule followed by radioiodine treatment of the toxic diffuse goitre, after which some non-functioning TSH-dependent nodules which are present will function after resolution of disease (Marine–Lenhart syndrome) [9,10]. These nodules probably do not require surgical treatment, but a definitive study has not been carried out.

Nodular goitre associated with thyrotoxicosis

When a thyrotoxic patient presents with a multinodular goitre they are frequently diagnosed as having a 'toxic nodular goitre'. There are, however, three possible clinical diagnoses:

1 multiple toxic nodules developing in a long-standing multinodular goitre (Plummer's disease);

2 Graves' disease occurring in a patient with a previous multinodular goitre; and

3 a patient with long-standing Graves' disease in whom the enlarged gland has become nodular.

The latter two can be differentiated only by the presence or absence of a previous history of nodular goitre. The scan appearances of Plummer's disease in a nodular goitre may vary from that of a single toxic nodule to multiple, clearly defined nodules throughout the gland. Occasionally it may be difficult to differentiate from Graves' disease in a multinodular gland when the nodules appear almost confluent on the scan (Fig. 25.2).

The diagnosis can usually be made from the scan, although appearances do overlap and further investigations may be necessary. These include the measurement of serum thyroid-stimulating antibody and a repeat scan after TSH to demonstrate stimulation of suppressed tissue. This effect may also be achieved when the serum TSH rises if antithyroid drugs are given [4]; alternatively, a diagnosis may be established retrospectively when patients are rescanned after radioiodine treatment. As mentioned previously for the single nodule, ^{201}thallium can also be used to demonstrate tissue in which the uptake function, but not the metabolic activity, is suppressed, and may demonstrate the suppressed perinodular thyroid tissue of Plummer's disease.

The impalpable gland and thyrotoxicosis

If the thyroid is small it may be difficult to palpate; when it is not obviously enlarged a thyroid scan should generally be performed. The scan may demonstrate any of the recognised patterns associated with thyrotoxicosis, i.e. diffuse uptake of Graves' disease, low uptake or functioning nodules of Plummer's disease. This is particularly important in elderly patients with atrial fibrillation, who should have a scan to detect toxic nodules which may not be producing obvious clinical disease as these can be easily treated with radioiodine. In a recent series of patients with toxic nodules, 10% were impalpable and some of these nodules could not be palpated even after identification on the scan [2].

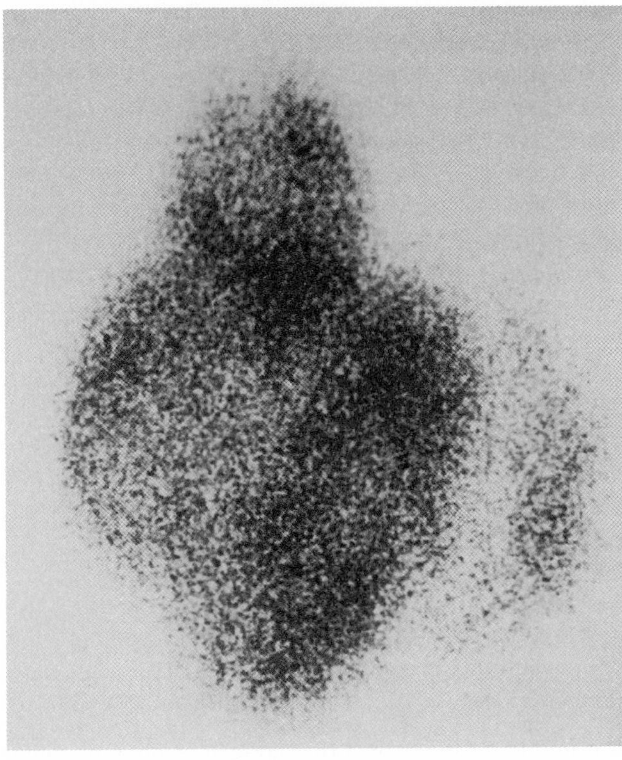

(a)

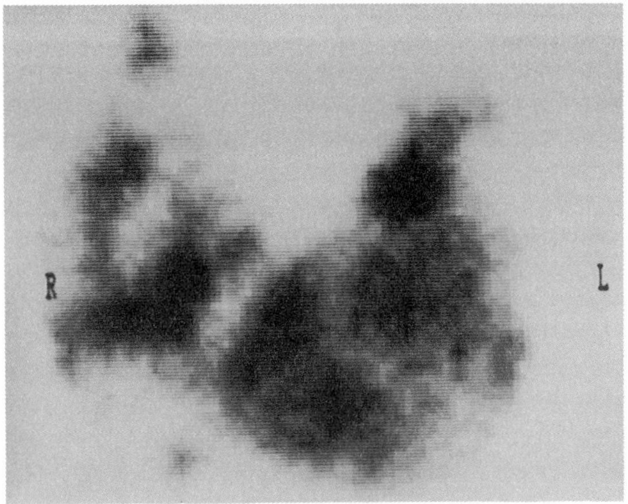

(b)

UPTAKE=4.0 %

R

L

(c)

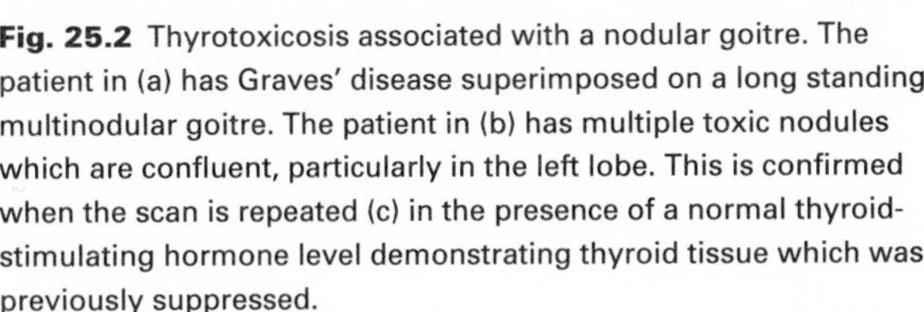

Fig. 25.2 Thyrotoxicosis associated with a nodular goitre. The patient in (a) has Graves' disease superimposed on a long standing multinodular goitre. The patient in (b) has multiple toxic nodules which are confluent, particularly in the left lobe. This is confirmed when the scan is repeated (c) in the presence of a normal thyroid-stimulating hormone level demonstrating thyroid tissue which was previously suppressed.

Low tracer uptake and thyrotoxicosis

The thyroid scan in patients with thyrotoxicosis may show a low uptake of tracer. This often indicates a cause for thyrotoxicosis which may be self-limiting and thus the administration of radioiodine or long-term antithyroid drugs may be avoided. These conditions are shown in Table 25.3.

Table 25.3 Causes of low tracer uptake in hyperthyroidism.

Subacute thyroiditis
Iodine-induced thyrotoxicosis (Jod–Basedow)
Amiodarone-induced thyrotoxicosis
Ectopic thyroid tissue
Thyrotoxicosis factitia (excess thyroid hormone administration)
Recent high iodine load (due to dilutional effects)

Ectopic tissue may rarely cause hyperthyroidism and suppress the 'normal' thyroid on routine scanning. Ober *et al.* [11] describe a case of thyrotoxicosis due to metastatic follicular cancer which was resistant to conventional treatment; in addition to drawing attention to the rarity of this case, it again emphasises the potential importance of a thyroid scan before therapy is undertaken. A retrosternal goitre may contain a toxic nodule. Tang Fui *et al.* [12] and Fogelfield *et al.* [13] have described patients with ectopic intrathoracic goitre causing thyrotoxicosis. In both cases the cervical uptake was low either due to suppression or absence of tissue. In females the scan in such cases should include the pelvis to identify a very rare struma ovarii. Post-partum thyroiditis is now recognised [14], and may be associated with both hypo- and hyperthyroidism (or occasionally both), and is usually transient. The scan reveals low tracer uptake in both (see Chapter 30).

Subacute thyroiditis continues to be a regular cause of transient hyperthyroidism. This is usually diagnosed clinically in a patient with a painful thyroid and a low ^{99m}Tc or iodine uptake on the scan. Occasionally the diagnosis may be more difficult and White *et al.* [15] described two cases of subacute thyroiditis being investigated for pyrexia in whom intense gallium-67 uptake in the thyroid identified the origin of the pyrexia and hyperthyroidism.

Treatment of hyperthyroidism

The thyroid scan before ^{131}I treatment

One of the factors involved in calculating the radiation dose from a therapeutic dose of ^{131}I is the thyroid mass. There have been a number of formulae proposed for calculating the thyroid mass, derived from the thyroid scan, which make assumptions about the geometry of the lobe [16]. Thyroid volume is best calculated using a combined radionuclide and ultrasound method. However, for calculating the dose of ^{131}I for therapy, the functional tissue volume as opposed to the total tissue volume is more important. Positron emission tomography using ^{124}I may be the optimal technique [17,18], although SPECT (single photon emission computed tomography) studies which will be more widely available may eventually be able to achieve this.

A second important factor in dose calculation is the peak uptake of ^{131}I. At the present time, no careful studies have been performed comparing the early ^{99m}Tc uptake, which can be routinely obtained, with the 24 hour ^{131}I uptake, although the diagnostic accuracy is equal [19]. ^{123}I uptake measured at 4–5 hours using a γ camera can replace the ^{131}I uptake [20].

It has been suggested that the thyroid scan together with an uptake measurement may be used to assess the activity of the thyroid during anithyroid drug treatment to provide an indication as to the likelihood of a relapse when the patient discontinues treatment [21]; this has been found to be valuable in children [22]. However, others found that the ^{99m}Tc uptake was a poor predictor of relapse in 49 patients with Graves' disease compared with the TSH-receptor antibody, which was superior. Turner *et al.* [23], in a study of 76 patients with Graves' disease using 21 clinical, biochemical, scan and tracer-kinetic parameters, concluded that no single or combination of treatment variables was able to predict outcome of ^{131}I treatment.

Treatment of toxic autonomous nodules (Plummer's disease)

It is important to obtain a thyroid scan before radioiodine is used to treat autonomous toxic nodules (Plummer's disease), particularly for patients who have received antithyroid drug therapy. This is to be sure that the normal thyroid tissue is fully suppressed at the time of ^{131}I administration to prevent subsequent hypothyroidism. When patients with

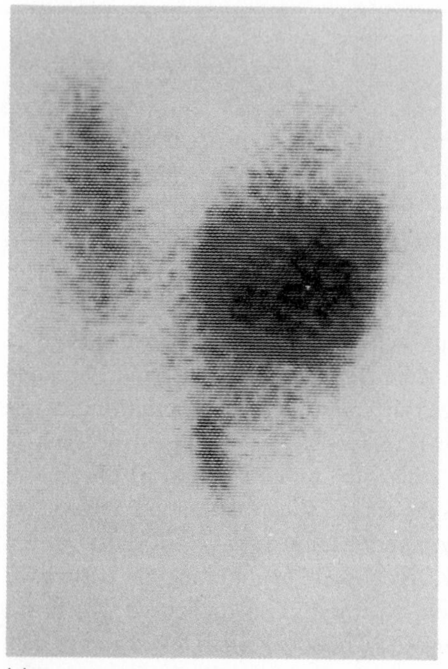

(a)

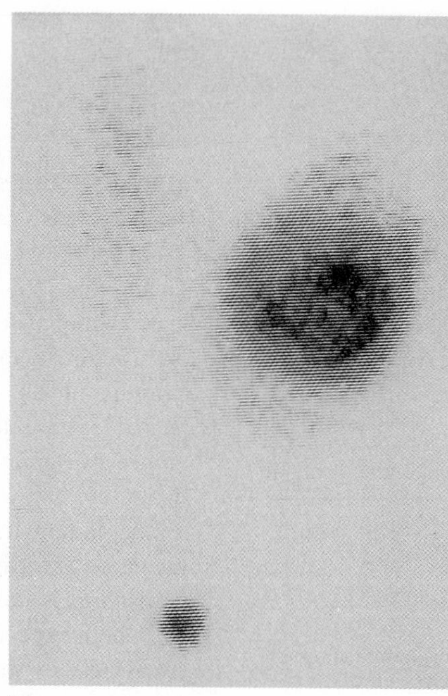

(b)

Fig. 25.3 This patient has thyrotoxicosis due to a toxic nodule treated with antithyroid drug therapy. The treatment has resulted in a rise in thyroid-stimulating hormone which in turn has stimulated the suppressed normal tissue (a). The scan was repeated (b) after triiodothyronine (T_3) administration before ^{131}I was given.

toxic nodules are treated in this way, the likelihood of hypothyroidism is very low. In a series of 48 patients treated with 500 MBq of ^{131}I, no patient became hypothyroid in the follow-up period (mean 37 months) [5]. The only patients who become hypothyroid are those who have received antithyroid drugs before ^{131}I treatment and without first establishing that the normal thyroid tissue was suppressed and the TSH was not elevated at the time of ^{131}I administration. If normal thyroid tissue is not fully suppressed because the TSH has risen during treatment then a further period of time off antithyroid drugs is required; alternatively the administration of thyroid hormone may be used, if clinically acceptable, and the thyroid scan repeated before ^{131}I (Fig. 25.3).

Follow-up

After radioiodine treatment, patients are usually reviewed at 1, 3, 6, 9 and 12 months. A repeat thyroid scan in cases of Plummer's disease is carried out at 6 months, at which time most patients will be clinically and biochemically euthyroid and have a normal TSH response to thyrotrophin-releasing hormone (TRH). The thyroid scan can be used to establish that radioiodine therapy has successfully destroyed an autonomous nodule or nodules (Fig. 25.4). Successfully treated nodules will be non-functional on the scan by 6 months after treatment, whereas those liable to relapse retain some functional activity. The scan at 6 months can thus be valuable as an indicator of long-term outcome. Those patients who are not cured at 6 months may be given a second dose of ^{131}I and followed up as before. Once the patient is cured, annual examination is sufficient, although post-radiation hypothyroidism is very rare.

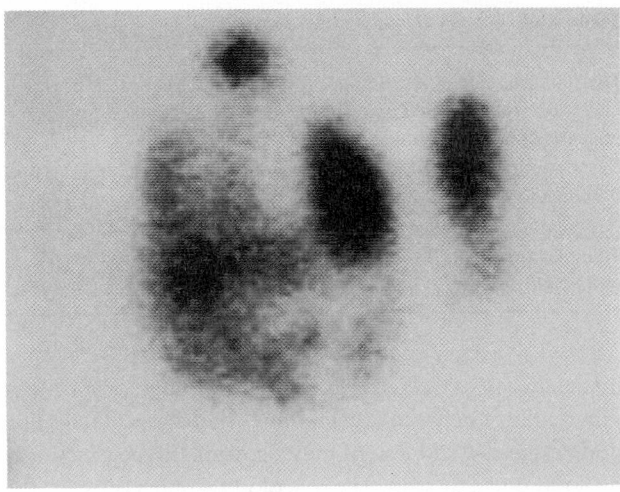

(a)

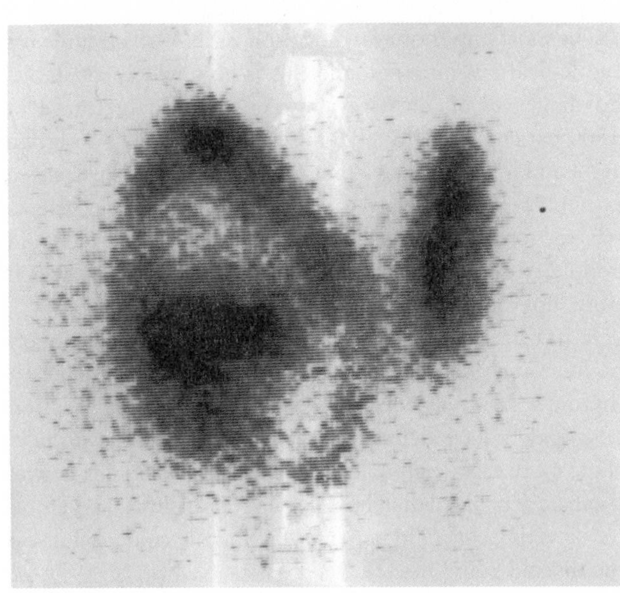

(b)

Fig. 25.4 This patient has toxic nodules (a) as a cause of thyrotoxicosis. Six months after ^{131}I therapy a repeat scan (b) shows resolution of the nodules with returning function of suppressed tissue and persistent cold nodules due to non-functional cysts and colloid nodules.

Solitary thyroid nodules

Solitary thyroid nodules are a common clinical problem: as many as 15.5% of the population may have palpable nodules [24], with 3.2% solitary in women and 0.8% solitary in men in England. In the USA, 4–7% of the population has been reported to have thyroid nodules [25]. The causes of a thyroid nodule are shown in Table 25.4.

The clinical problem is how to detect the 5–10% of solitary thyroid nodules with cancer without the need to perform unnecessary operations on the other 90%. It has been this goal, i.e. to identify benign disease with a high degree of accuracy without loss of sensitivity for detecting cancer, that has driven the diagnostic developments in this area.

The thyroid scan (with ^{99m}Tc or ^{123}I) has been the most widely used method for investigating a thyroid nodule on the premise that finding a solitary cold nodule increases the probability of malignancy, whereas finding a functioning nodule or a simple multinodular goitre without a dominant nodule reduces the chance of malignancy to low levels. Occasionally, a repeat scan after triiodothyronine (T_3) suppression may be necessary to clearly demonstrate an autonomously functioning solitary thyroid nodule (Fig. 25.5).

Ultrasonography provides a valuable method for demonstrating thyroid abnormalities, and in particular to discriminate between solid and cystic lesions [26]. It can be used to measure thyroid volumes and to detect nodules. Most

Table 25.4 Causes of solitary thyroid nodules.

Thyroid cyst
Local subacute thyroiditis
Local Hashimoto's disease
Functioning adenoma (hot nodule)
Benign adenoma
Colloid nodule
Thyroid cancer
Metastatic deposit

malignancies are echogenic, but ultrasonography cannot differentiate between functioning and non-functioning nodules, and cystic lesions may occasionally be functional on a radionuclide scan. The role of ultrasonography for the evaluation of thyroid disease has been reveiwed by Leisner [27].

The most important investigation is FNA of a nodule for cytological examination, and this is now widely available. Lowhagen *et al.*, in a review of the world literature of 3500 patients [28], found a false-negative rate of less than 10% and a false-positive rate of less than 2%. Christensen *et al.* [29] in a prospective study of 100 consecutive patients selected for surgical treatment of a clinically solitary thyroid nodule who had FNA, confirmed that all 12 cases which were 'hot' on the scan were benign.

It has been suggested that all patients with a solitary nodule should have FNA as their initial investigation and a thyroid scan is not required. However, clinical examination frequently fails to detect that the 'clinically solitary nodule' is the more easily palpable nodule of a multinodular goitre. It can be concluded that FNA cytology is an efficient method for detecting cancer in patients who have a 'cold' nodule on the thyroid scan [30–32].

The thyroid scan may also be used for the follow-up of patients who have had thyroid cysts aspirated.

Other methods are used in attempts to reduce the surgical rate for thyroid nodules. X-ray fluorescence, which measures stable ^{127}I, is accurate for the identification of benign disease [6] with a sensitivity of 63% and specificity of 99%, but the technique is not widely available. More controversial is the use of thallium-201 for evaluating the thyroid nodule. It is well known that thallium-201 is taken up into the thyroid and may show thyroid tissue not identified by ^{99m}Tc or iodine isotopes, and also that malignant thyroid lesions take up thallium-201 preferentially. An early evaluation [33] obtained good results, differentiating between benign and malignant nodules with a 94% sensitivity rate and 90% specificity; when there was no fading of activity on a delayed image as a criterion of malignancy the specificity reached 100%. However, in further studies [34–36] with semi-quantitative assessments of thallium uptake in cold nodules

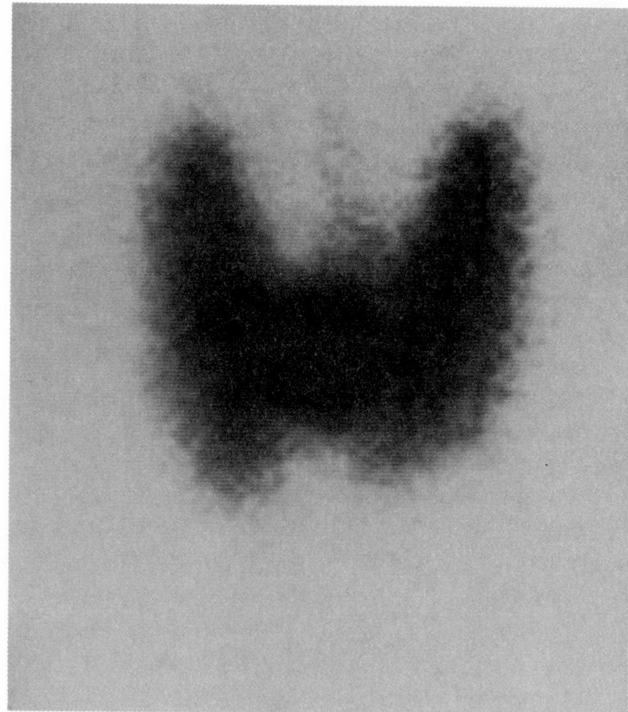

(a)

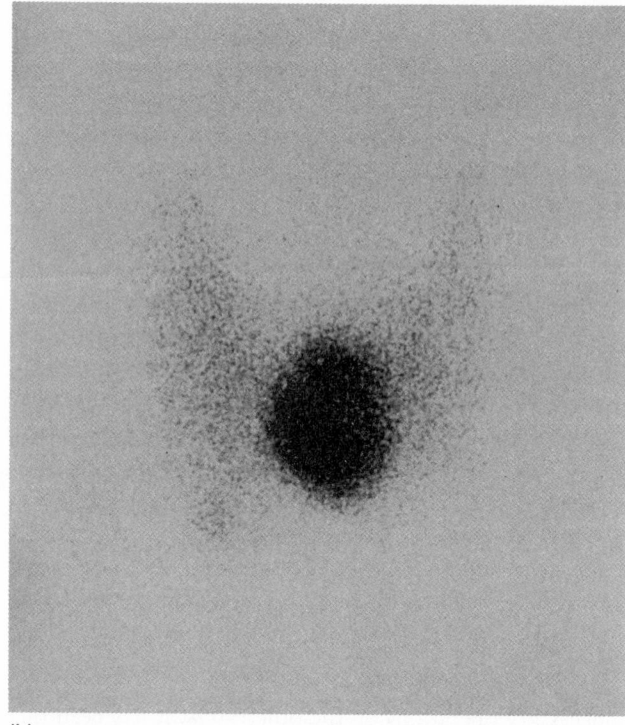

(b)

Fig. 25.5 This patient has a solitary nodule in the isthmus which is not clearly visualised on the ^{99m}Tc scan (a). After triiodothyronine (T_3) suppression it appears clearly against the low suppressed background of normal tissue (b).

on ^{99m}Tc scans, all 37 patients with malignant lesions had equal or more tracer uptake than perinodular tissue, whereas benign lesions ranged from no uptake to uptakes well in excess of the perinodular tissue. No uptake or uptake less than perinodular tissue confirmed benign disease and would allow a reduction in surgical rate. While there may be a role for thallium in the evaluation of the thyroid nodule, the definitive study has not yet been performed and its routine use cannot be recommended.

If the thyroid scan shows the solitary nodule to be functioning ('hot'), the probability of malignancy is very low since most hot nodules are benign, autonomously functioning adenomas; however, there have been occasional reports of malignancy. Ashcroft and Van Herle [37] in a review of the literature reported a 9% malignancy in warm and hot nodules. Nagai *et al.* [38] reported three cases of malignancy in hot nodules on ^{123}I scans, and Evans [39] found that 44% of patients with thyroid malignancy presented with warm nodules. Three problems can be identified in these reports.

1 Some malignancies, while not organifying the isotopes, do trap ^{99m}Tc and iodine, and appear as hot or warm nodules on ^{99m}Tc scans or early ^{123}I scans but cold on delayed ^{123}I scans (Fig. 25.6). If we call 'functioning' only those nodules that suppress TSH, cause a flat TRH test response, or remain hot on a ^{123}I scan after a perchlorate discharge test or delayed imaging, then the likelihood of malignancy is very low.

2 Nodules often occur in multinodular glands and the 'hot nodule' may be close to an 'incidentally' found malignancy and may behave differently to those cancers that present clinically.

3 Many adenomas and carcinomas have a good blood supply and it is the blood volume that creates the 'warm' nodule on a ^{99m}Tc scan and not true metabolic uptake of tracer (Fig. 25.7).

Walfish *et al.* [40] reviewed their experience of 12 FNA cases of functioning nodules to evaluate the consequences of not obtaining a radionuclide scan first. They concluded that not performing a scan to diagnose a functioning nodule could expose some unprepared patients with thyrotoxicosis to surgical morbidity, and could induce hyperthyroidism in patients with functioning nodules if they were treated with suppression therapy. FNA cytology was not able to differentiate a functioning from a non-functioning adenoma. There is as yet, therefore, no absolute consensus on the optimal investigations for this common clinical problem. Routine removal of all clinically apparent thyroid nodules no longer seems justified, and results in a great deal of unnecessary surgery. A reasonable policy would be a ^{99m}Tc or ^{123}I scan in the first instance; this is a cheap, accurate and widely available test. Functioning nodules will be identified, and these patients should have a TSH measurement to confirm true biological function with subsequent follow-up and

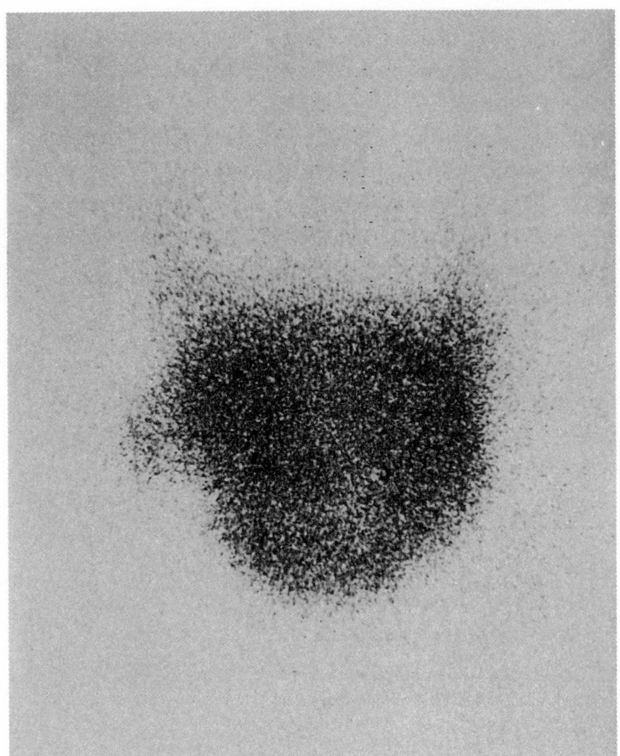

(a)

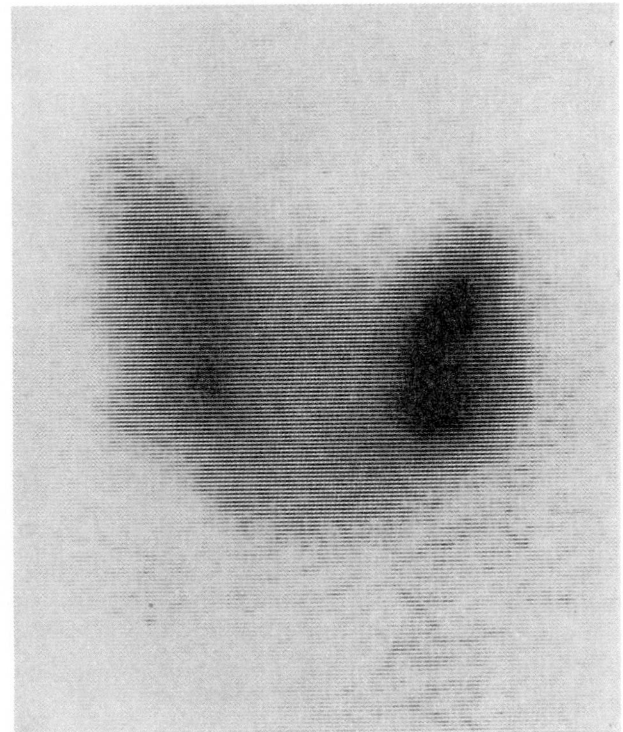

(b)

Fig. 25.6 This scan shows an apparent functioning nodule with ^{99m}Tc (a) but on a delayed ^{123}I scan it is clearly non-functional (b).

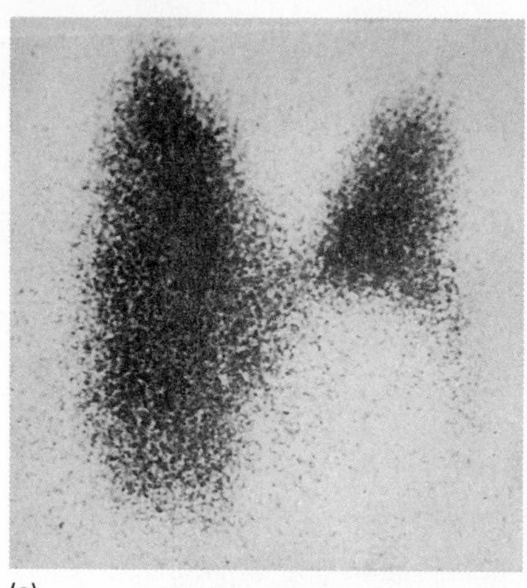
(a)

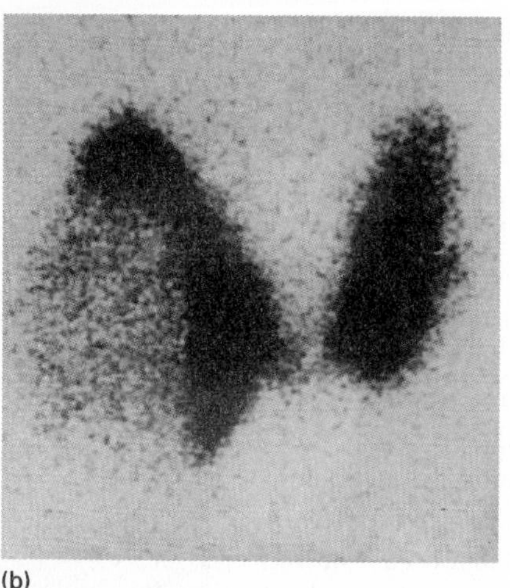
(b)

Fig. 25.7 These two scans compare a typical cold nodule (a) with a 'warm' nodule (b) which is non-functional but has a relatively good blood supply giving a tissue background of radioactivity in the nodule.

treatment for thyrotoxicosis as necessary. The evidence for any significant likelihood of malignancy in this group is not convincing. If reliable cytology is available, then all non-functioning solitary nodules should have FNA cytology which will result in a reduction in unnecessary surgery. Ultrasonography is necessary as an adjunct to the scan when FNA cytology is not available. Simple cysts can be aspirated and recurrences may be considered for injection with sclerosants. Thallium-201 can be used when there is a relative contra-indication to surgery; a negative or positive scan will help in making a decision, but it is probably not justified otherwise.

A proportion of patients who are thought to have a solitary nodule on palpation are shown to have a multinodular goitre on scanning. The frequency with which this is noted depends on the experience of the clinician in palpating the thyroid, the ease with which the patient's thyroid can be palpated, and the technique of the scan. Alderson *et al.* [41] reported that approximately 36% of clinically diagnosed solitary nodules were multiple on scan; an even higher percentage was found at operation or autopsy [42]. It is often possible to palpate previously unsuspected nodules in the light of the scan findings.

Finding a simple multinodular goitre when a solitary nodule was suspected clinically reduces the probability of thyroid cancer in the absence of any clinically suspicious features of malignancy; a 'solitary nodule' which is found to be part of a multinodular goitre on scanning does not need surgical excision.

The presence of a dominant cold nodule in a gland with otherwise generally irregular uptake on scanning does not reduce the probability of malignancy to that of a typical multinodular goitre [41]. Such dominant cold nodules should therefore be investigated with ultrasonography and aspiration cytology as for a solitary nodule, and excised if indicated.

Goitre (see also Chapter 26)

A goitre may be diffuse or multinodular on examination, although occasionally it may be difficult describe it clearly as one type or the other. Outside endemic areas of iodine deficiency, the main causes of a non-toxic goitre are shown in Table 25.5 with the associated appearances on a thyroid scan.

Investigations of a non-toxic goitre include thyroid function tests, estimation of serum thyroid microsomal or thyroglobulin antibodies, and a thyroid scan. Further investigations which may be necessary include a perchlorate discharge test, studies of iodine kinetics *in vivo*, and a thyroid biopsy.

Simple colloid goitre and simple multinodular goitre

These are the commonest causes of a sporadic diffuse or nodular non-toxic goitre. Thyroid function tests, including TSH, are usually normal, and thyroid antibodies are usually absent or in low titre. Uptake of ^{99m}Tc or radioiodine is normal. The distribution of uptake on the scan is diffuse in a simple colloid goitre, but markedly irregular, often with discrete areas of diminished uptake, in a multinodular goitre. Oblique scan views may be helpful. Occasionally the goitre may contain one or more areas of increased uptake which indicate developing functioning nodules. If nodules are autonomous, TSH level will be suppressed in spite of normal serum T_3 and thyroxine (T_4) concentrations.

The appearance of symmetrical nodules in both lobes of

Table 25.5 Role of the thyroid scan in the assessment of goitre.

Scan findings	Cause	Comment
Diffuse, normal uptake of tracer	Diffuse non-toxic of tracer (simple) goitre	
Diffuse, with high uptake of tracer	Diffuse toxic goitre (Graves' disease)	May be first indication of hyperthyroidism
	Lymphocytic thyroiditis (Hashimoto's disease)	Occurs in early disease
	Iodine deficiency Organification defects (inherited or goitrogens)	May be difficult to distinguish from each other
Diffuse, low uptake	Subacute thyroiditis (De Quervain's) Iodine-induced goitre Hashimoto's disease Lymphoma	} May be indistinguishable on the scan
Multifocal irregularity, normal uptake of tracer	Simple multinodular goitre	Detection of autonomous nodule is important
	Hashimoto's disease	Diagnosis by antibodies
Irregular replacement of thyroid tissue	Diffuse cancer	Usually clinically apparent, but may be confused with mutlinodular goitre

a goitre should raise the suspicion of a medullary thyroid cancer, and will increase the likelihood of it being the familial type which has arisen from symmetrically distributed C-cell hyperplasia. A calcitonin measurement in addition to FNA cytology may be helpful in making a preoperative diagnosis, as may a scan using ^{99m}Tc (V) DMSA or ^{123}I/^{131}I MIBG [43,44]. This will be of particular value in cases of multiple endocrine neoplasia, and phaeochromocytoma must be excluded before surgery (see Chapter 47).

A thyroid lymphoma may develop spontaneously, with the patient usually presenting with a rapidly enlarging diffuse goitre, or may occur in a patient with Hashimoto's disease as there is recognised to be an increased risk of lymphoma in this condition. A radionuclide thyroid scan is not helpful because in this condition the patient will be hypothyroid and receiving T_4 treatment; in the absence of Hashimoto's disease the scan will usually show diffuse enlargement with an overall low uptake due to the diffuse infiltration. In these instances it is best to proceed directly to surgical biopsy, but there may be clinical circumstances when this is not advised and a gallium scan, which shows avid accumulation in lymphoma, may provide valuable information.

Familial dyshormonogenesis should be considered in the differential diagnosis of goitre in the younger patient with a family history of goitre, absent thyroid antibodies and subclinical or frank hypothyroidism. The thyroid scan normally shows a high diffuse uptake and the perchlorate test may be positive.

Hashimoto's thyroiditis

The diagnosis of this condition depends on three main features:

1 the presence of a goitre which is typically bosselated and firm on palpation;

2 subclinical or frank hypothyroidism, i.e. a raised TSH with borderline-low or low serum T_4; and

3 serum thyroid antibodies which are usually strongly positive although they have been reported to be negative in a small proportion of cases of biopsy-proven Hashimoto's thyroiditis.

The thyroid scan is of limited diagnostic value; for example, it may show high, normal or low uptake of radionuclide with varying distribution which may be uniform, irregular or nodular, according to the degree of fibrosis. We have reviewed 32 cases, and shown that a wide variety of scan patterns can be obtained [45]. The most common scan appearances were either of an enlarged gland with diffusely increased tracer uptake similar to Graves' disease, or those of a multinodular gland. However, other scans appeared normal, showed a focal defect or reduced tracer uptake throughout one lobe or generally low uptake by the whole gland. The perchlorate discharge test shows excess discharge of radioiodine in many of the cases.

Painful goitre

Pain originating from the thyroid associated with palpable

enlargement may be due to one of the following conditions:

1 subacute (De Quervain's) thyroiditis;
2 acute onset of Hashimoto's thyroiditis;
3 Haemorrhage into a thyroid nodule or cyst;
4 thyroid cancer, particularly anaplastic carcinoma;
5 acute suppurative thyroiditis.

A careful history and clinical examination will often suggest the diagnosis, but should always be supplemented with appropriate investigations for confirmation. The most useful investigations include a full blood count and erythrocyte sedimentation rate (ESR), thyroid function tests, a radionuclide thyroid scan with ^{99m}Tc or ^{123}I, a perchlorate discharge test and serum thyroid antibodies. Rarely a biopsy may be necessary. Sudden onset of pain in the thyroid is most often caused by haemorrhage in a thyroid nodule or cyst which may either be solitary or part of a multinodular goitre. Thyroid function tests in these cases are usually normal; a thyroid scan shows a solitary cold nodule or a multinodular goitre with one or more cold nodules. Pain due to haemorrhage into a thyroid nodule usually lasts only a few days and the nodule appears very rapidly, usually over a few hours. The nodule gets smaller and may disappear completely after a few weeks. The patient should therefore be reviewed after 2–3 months and the thyroid scan repeated to confirm resolution or reduction of the nodule. If symptoms persist, and the nodule enlarges, excision is advisable.

Subacute onset of pain over the neck, associated with a recent upper respiratory infection, fever, malaise, anorexia and a tender, diffuse goitre, are characteristic of subacute thyroiditis (see Chapter 29). However, similar features may sometimes be caused by acute onset of Hashimoto's thyroiditis. A mild leucocytosis and moderately elevated ESR may occur in both conditions, but subacute thyroiditis is characterised by mild biochemical hyperthyroidism in the early stages, a diffusely low uptake on ^{99m}Tc scan and absence of thyroid antibodies or only a transient rise in low titre. In Hashimoto's thyroiditis, thyroid function tests usually show frank or compensated hypothyroidism; a thyroid scan characteristically shows a high ^{99m}Tc uptake, but a low radioiodine uptake indicating trapping of iodine without organic binding. This can also be shown by a perchlorate discharge test which may show increased discharge of radioiodine.

Confusion may be caused when subacute thyroiditis involves only one lobe with the characteristic low uptake in that lobe only on the scan. This may then resolve and the other lobe may be affected; this may occur in as many as 20% of cases. Difficulty may arise if it simulates a thyroid cancer [46].

Ectopic thyroid

Thyroid tissue may occur in anatomical positions other than the normal position, when it may constitute a diagnostic or therapeutic problem. The commonest sites are at the back of the tongue (lingual thyroid), in the mid-line position of the upper neck (sublingual or subhyoid thyroid), inside the thoracic cavity (anterior or posterior mediastinal goitre) and in ovarian tumours (struma ovarii).

For investigating ectopic thyroid cases the ^{123}I thyroid scan is better because the higher uptake avoids confusion with vascular structures, saliva and salivary glands on a ^{99m}Tc scan. The radiation dose with either radionuclide is small compared to ^{131}I, and the scan can therefore be used in infants, children or adolescents. The whole area from the mouth to the sternal notch should be imaged and reference markers are placed on any palpable nodule and appropriate anatomical landmarks, for example the sternal notch. In the case of a lingual thyroid, a lateral view is important for accurate three-dimensional localisation. Radionuclide uptake in the nodule confirms the presence of ectopic thyroid, whereas other types of nodule, for example a thyroglossal cyst, are non-functional. The presence or absence of a normal thyroid is also established at the same time. Rarely, if the normal thyroid is not visualised the scan should be repeated after TSH stimulation to exclude the possibility that its function may be suppressed by autonomous function of ectopic tissue.

Patients who have undergone previous thyroid surgery may have congenital remnants of thyroid tissue along the thyroglossal tract which hypertrophy to produce a mid-line swelling in the upper neck, particularly with recurrence of Graves' disease. This can be confirmed by a thyroid scan.

A normally situated thyroid gland may enlarge downward into the anterior mediastinum to produce a retrosternal goitre, or less commonly it may extend behind the trachea and oesophagus downwards as a posterior mediastinal goitre.

To confirm intrathoracic goitre and assess extent, a radiograph of the thoracic inlet and a thyroid scan with ^{123}I should be performed. Although the presence of radioiodine uptake below the sternal notch confirms the diagnosis of intrathoracic goitre, its absence does not exclude a non-functioning intrathoracic goitre. In such cases, mediastinoscopy and tissue biopsy or thoracotomy may be necessary. Mediastinal CT or MRI may be necessary to assess the extent and to evaluate tracheal compression.

The thyroid scan will delineate the anatomy of infants with congenital hypothyroidism, but in addition provides functional information. A scan should be obtained if possible before commencing treatment with thyroxine. Anatomical findings may be broadly characterised to four groups based on scan findings [47]:

1 a normal gland;
2 ectopic location;
3 no dectectable thyroid activity; and

4 normal location with increased size of gland or increased tracer uptake.

An ectopic thyroid gland is found in approximately 45% of cases and athyreosis in 35%; 10% will have a normal gland and 10% will have other abnormalities [48]. In the latter cases, it is presumed that there is a disorder of thyroid hormonogenesis and a number will have defects of thyroid hormone synthesis. A perchlorate discharge test will identify those cases with an organification defect. Two cases of a congenital defect in iodide trapping have been reported where the scan showed absence of not only thyroid but gastric uptake [49]. Further, the scan findings in isolation are misleading in terms of prognosis as there is no tracer uptake by the thyroid and this will erroneously suggest athyreosis.

Thyroid cancer

Treatment and follow-up of thyroid cancer

Differentiated thyroid cancers (see Chapter 28) account for at least 80% of all thyroid malignancies. Follicular carcinomas consist entirely of neoplastic thyroid follicles whereas papillary carcinomas contain cells in a papillary arrangement with a varying proportion of follicular structures. Both types of tumours may have functioning endocrine properties which are similar to, but less efficient than, normal thyroid cells. Thus, under certain conditions which include total ablation of all normal thyroid tissue and TSH stimulation, these tumours may concentrate and organify small but significant amounts of iodine, an important property which can be exploited for their detection and treatment with radioiodine.

Most thyroid cancers are diagnosed when a hemithyroidectomy is performed for a solitary non-functioning thyroid nodule or after removal of a cervical lymph node. Usually a total thyroidectomy will have been performed at the time of the first operation or as a second procedure. Total thyroidectomy enables subsequent effective follow-up of patients to be performed with thyroglobulin estimations and whole-body ^{131}I scans.

After the total thyroidectomy a period of 4 weeks should elapse to allow the TSH level to rise before a scan is performed. If only a subtotal operation has been performed, the scan and ^{131}I ablation therapy can be started immediately. Postoperatively the scan at 4 weeks will usually demonstrate some residual tissue in the neck which may be tumour or normal tissue, there being no reliable way to distinguish these two. Doses of ^{131}I postoperatively should be kept low to avoid 'stunning' with consequent decreased uptake of ablative doses [50].

Subsequent ^{131}I scans are usually performed at 6 monthly or annual intervals with repeated ^{131}I therapy until tumour ablation is complete. These scans are performed after discontinuing thyroid hormone for at least 4 weeks (T_4) or 2 weeks (T_3), and establishing that the TSH is > 30 mU/l. Scans will identify most functioning metastases which most usually occur locally in the neck, in the lung or in bone. Lung metastases are well shown on the ^{131}I scan which is more sensitive than other imaging modalities. Piekarski *et al.* [51] reviewed their experience with ^{131}I scans, CT scanning and chest X-ray in 27 patients with micronodular metastases and showed that 19 out of 27 had normal chest X-rays while CT scanning demonstrated micronodules in 14 of these 19 cases. CT scanning also demonstrated micronodules in seven out of 13 patients with known, previously treated metastases with no ^{131}I uptake, some of whom had detectable thyroglobulin levels. It was suggested that these nodules may be a result of fibrosis. They concluded that the ^{131}I scan was the most sensitive investigation, but CT scanning was a valuable complementary procedure. There is no doubt about the clinical importance of pulmonary metastases. Samaan *et al.* [52] reviewed 101 patients with lung metastases; of these 67 died from the disease, with the majority being over 40 years of age (16% survival). The prognosis was better when the ^{131}I scan was positive and radiography was negative, and it was found that pulmonary metastases occurred more frequently in patients who had not initially had a total thyroidectomy. De Groot and Reilly [53] looked at the detectability of thyroid metastases in 108 patients using ^{131}I scan, chest X-ray, skeletal survey and bone scan. They found that physical examinations, chest X-ray, and ^{131}I scans detected all metastases, while skeletal surveys and bone scans did not contribute significantly. Occasionally metastases occur in the brain, and it is important to identify them on the ^{131}I scan as cerebral oedema may occur following ^{131}I therapy.

While uncommon, false positives on the ^{131}I scan may occur. We have recently seen a patient with accumulation of trapped ^{131}I within a plaque of psoriasis which was thought to be a metastasis in a lumbar vertebra. Wu *et al.* [54] reported striking radioiodine and ^{99m}Tc localisation in a disseminated gastric adenocarcinoma. Ziessman *et al.* [55] looked at the frequency of hepatic uptake of ^{131}I, which may represent a possible false positive and found hepatic visualisation in 44% of cases which was related to the ^{131}I dose and functional activity of metastatic disease. Kim *et al.* [56] reported ^{131}I uptake in a benign serous cystadenoma of the ovary, while Hoschl *et al.* [57] reported uptake in inflammatory lung disease as a potential pitfall.

The definition of ablation of tumour or thyroid tissue to some extent depends on the dose of ^{131}I used for scanning the patient. Some patients will show positive uptake at 400 MBq, but negative at lower dose levels. It is recognised that a scan performed after a therapeutic dose of ^{131}I may detect additional lesions. Doses used for scanning in different centres vary from 8 to 500 MBq. However, some potentially treatable lesions will still be missed even at the higher dose level. Therefore, the choice of dose is a balance between detecting treatable lesions and radiation dose to the patient. In practice, we now use 400 MBq which is the highest dose that can be given such that the patient can return home using public transport if necessary. The optimal scanning time is at 72 hours. Lithium has been used as an adjunct to increase ^{131}I uptake by preventing its release from the thyroid [58]. Positron emission tomography (PET) scanning may provide more reliable dosimetry but is not widely available [17].

Thyroglobulin is an adjunct to the ^{131}I scan in the follow-up of thyroid cancer, and there is no doubt that most well-differentiated tumours both take up ^{131}I and produce thyroglobulin, but in a few cases these aspects of cellular function appear to be separated [59]. Ericsson *et al.* [60] reviewed 262 patients with differentiated cancer, and concluded that thyroglobulin can replace ^{131}I scans, while Ronga *et al.* [61] reviewed 233 patients and found 43 thyroglobulin-positive cases without ^{131}I uptake and three with a positive scan and negative thyroglobulin, thus urging caution in replacing the ^{131}I scan, and stressing the complementary role of the two tests. Girelli *et al.* [62] reviewed 429 patients and found high thyroglobulin levels in 76% of patients with metastases detected by other diagnostic procedures which were unable to take up ^{131}I. Moser *et al.* [63] reviewed 158 patients following thyroidectomy, and found a positive ^{131}I scan with negative thyroglobulin in 21% of patients, confirming that thyroglobulin could not replace the scan at this stage in the management. The incidence of positive scans with negative thyroglobulin is low (<4%), but may be very important as illustrated by a report of three cases with lung and bone metastases shown with ^{131}I, but with negative thyroglobulin levels [64].

For management decisions it is probably wise to treat all patients with an elevated thyroglobulin and a negative scan with ^{131}I and scan following the treatment dose. Pacini *et al.* [65] found 17 such patients of whom 16 showed a positive scan using the therapeutic dose of ^{131}I for imaging. An alternative when PET scanning is available is to use ^{18}F-fluorodeoxyglucose (FDG) to identify sites of malignancy undetected by ^{131}I scanning [66].

Thyroglobulin probably cannot be relied on exclusively for follow-up on T_4 suppression, but a reasonable compromise is annual physical examination, chest X-ray and thyroglobulin estimation after two whole-body ^{131}I and thyroglobulin levels have been negative 1 year apart, and some centres would add a whole-body ^{131}I scan at 5-yearly intervals.

Khammash *et al.* [67] evaluated the use of ^{99m}Tc pertechnetate when compared with ^{131}I in 66 patients with thyroid carcinoma, and found five false-negative ^{99m}Tc studies and one false-negative ^{131}I study, confirming that ^{99m}Tc is less reliable than ^{131}I in the detection of thyroid cancer.

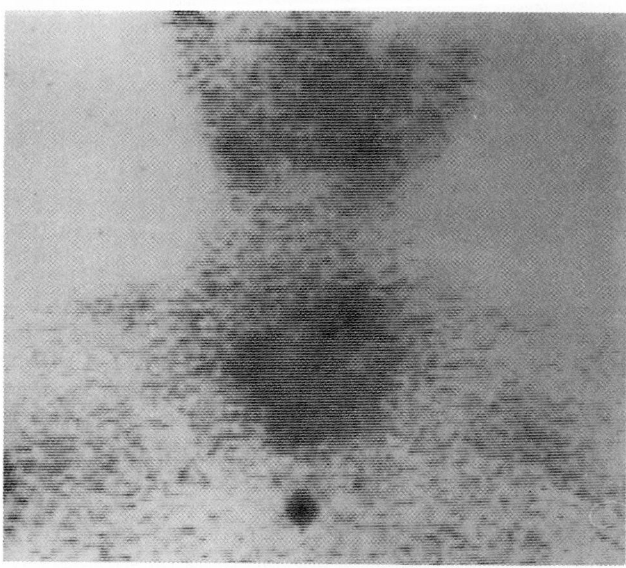

Fig. 25.8 A thallium-201 scan of a patient under follow-up for follicular thyroid cancer. The ^{131}I scan was negative and thyroglobulin elevated. The thallium-201 demonstrates the active thyroid cancer tissue.

Other agents have been used to investigate and follow up patients with thyroid carcinoma, usually in an attempt to avoid having to discontinue thyroid hormone replacement treatment and the associated clinical hypothyroidism. The most widely used radiopharmaceutical is thallium-201 chloride. Hoefnagel *et al.* [68] compared thallium-201 with ^{131}I in 620 scans in 303 patients, and found positive thallium in 39 with negative ^{131}I (but eight medullary cases were included) and three negative thallium with positive ^{131}I and concluded that thallium was superior. On the other hand Varma and Reba [69] concluded that thallium was only of use in widespread disease and could not replace ^{131}I for routine use. While there were differences in administered doses, it was recommended that thallium should not be used for follow-up of patients with differentiated thyroid carcinoma. It was suggested that thallium may be helpful in localising metastases in patients with a negative ^{131}I scan and abnormal levels of serum thyroglobulin (Fig. 25.8).

Medullary carcinoma (see Chapter 47)

The management of a patient who is suspected to have a medullary carcinoma of the thyroid should include a radionuclide thyroid scan to localise the tumour. Magnified and oblique views should be performed if a thyroid nodule is not palpable. The tumour may not be detectable by palpation or scanning even when plasma calcitonin is raised, as the latter is a more sensitive investigation. Radiography, CT and ultrasonography may all be used to localise the tumour if the radionuclide scan is negative.

The specific treatment for medullary thyroid carcinoma is a total thyroidectomy, as the tumour may be multicentric, or may recur in the remaining thyroid tissue. Postoperatively, plasma calcitonin should be measured as a marker for residual, metastatic or recurrent tumour. If significant levels are present, investigations such as chest radiography, liver and bone scans or CT scanning will help localise the lesions. Until recently there were no specific imaging techniques for this tumour but there are now several possibilities. Ochi *et al.* [70] showed uptake of pentavalent ^{99m}Tc dimercaptosuccinic acid (DMSA) and this has been confirmed by others [71]; its role is particularly valuable in relation to repeated surgical exploration (Fig. 25.9). Thallium-201 was evaluated by Hoefnagel *et al.* [68], who reported eight positive uptakes. Uptake of ^{131}I meta-iodobenzylguanidine (MIBG) in these tumours has also been reported, but in general the frequency of uptake has been lower and less predictable than with ^{99m}Tc pentavalent DMSA [43]. In animal studies (nude mice with medullary thyroid cancers), Guilloteau *et al.* [72] showed good uptake of ^{131}I MIBG but failed to find uptake using ^{131}I anticalcitonin antibody. Reiners *et al.* [73] evaluated the use of anticarcinoembryonic monoclonal antibody in nine patients, but only showed uptake when there were very large secondaries. High-resolution ultrasonography or CT scanning with iodine enhancement may also be useful. Rarely, venous sampling along the jugular veins or inferior vena cava for measurement of plasma calcitonin may be necessary to localise persistent tumour. Recently ^{18}FDG and ^{111}In octreotide scans have proved useful in this group of patients [74].

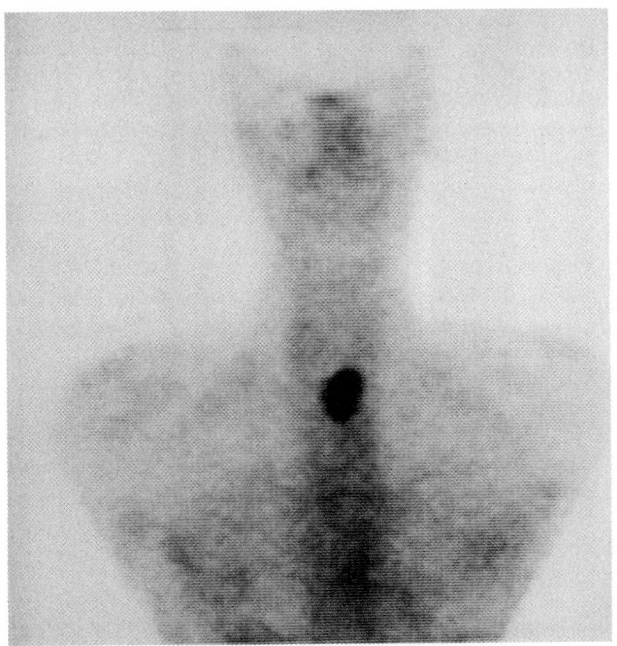

Fig. 25.9 An example of recurrent medullary thyroid cancer. The ^{99m}Tc pentavalent dimercaptosuccinic acid (DMSA) clearly localised the site of recurrence associated with elevation of the serum calcitonin.

Given the risk of malignancy in the relatives of patients with medullary carcinoma, the most sensitive screening method is the measurement of plasma calcitonin. When this is positive a thyroid scan with magnified views should also be carried out, but often the tumour is too small to be identified on the scan. The ^{99m}Tc pentavalent DMSA scan may be helpful, as is an iodine-enhanced CT scan of the neck. Some clinicians prefer to recommend a total thyroidectomy after the basal calcitonin level has been raised on two occasions, particularly if the level is rising.

Radionuclide thyroid scan

The thyroid scan is now most commonly performed with ^{99m}Tc and to a lesser extent with ^{123}I. ^{99m}Tc pertechnetate is concentrated but not organified by the thyroid follicle, so that imaging with ^{99m}Tc is a reflection of the trapping property of the thyroid whereas the radioiodine scan reflects both the trapping and organification properties of the gland. Rarely, there may be a disparity between these two functions of the thyroid, which results in dissimilar appearances of the image obtained with ^{99m}Tc and radioiodine.

In view of the emission of high-energy γ-rays and short-range β-particles and its long half-life (hence high radiation dose to the patient), ^{131}I has now been largely replaced by ^{99m}Tc or ^{123}I for routine thyroid scanning. ^{123}I is the ideal scanning agent for physiological and physical reasons, but unlike ^{99m}Tc it cannot be produced in the laboratory from 'generators', and at present its high cost and limited availability restrict its widespread clinical use. ^{123}I is especially useful to confirm true organification of nodules, for mediastinal goitres, for low uptake, and when a perchlorate discharge test is performed with the scan.

The following technical points are important when performing a ^{99m}Tc thyroid scan.

1 Inject 40–200 MBq ^{99m}Tc pertechnetate intravenously.

2 Image after 20–30 min when the thyroid/background count rate ratio is maximum.

3 Give the patient a drink of water immediately before imaging to flush away any secreted radionuclide in saliva which may pool in the pharynx or upper oesophagus.

4 Image with a γ-camera fitted with a pinhole or special parallel-holed collimator.

5 The patient should lie down comfortably with the head

slightly extended and the collimator about 10 cm above the neck.

6 Image for a fixed count of 100 K with the γ-camera.

7 Whenever indicated, locate the position of anatomical landmarks such as the sternal notch, and any relevant palpable nodules with appropriate radionuclide markers for reference on the image.

8 Repeat images with oblique or magnified views are sometimes necessary.

9 Whenever possible, the percentage uptake by the thyroid should be measured by comparing the count rate over the thyroid against the total amount of radionuclide injected, allowance being made for background and decay.

^{123}I scan

The technique is similar, but instead of giving intravenous ^{99m}Tc pertechnetate, 8–20 MBq ^{123}I sodium iodide is administered orally and imaging is carried out after 4–24 hours.

Whole-body radiodine scan

This is the most sensitive investigation for detecting and localising persistent or recurrent differentiated thyroid cancer after initial thyroid ablation.

1 A high serum TSH (30 mU/l) is essential for tumour uptake of radioiodine to take place. T_4 or T_3 therapy should therefore be discontinued for at least 4 weeks and 2 weeks, respectively, prior to scanning, and the serum TSH checked.

2 A low iodine diet reduces the stable iodide pool of the body and improves radioactive iodine uptake and tumour visualisation.

3 An adequate dose, for example 200–600 MBq ^{131}I, is given orally because small scanning doses of ^{131}I may fail to produce sufficient uptake in some lesions which become apparent only after bigger doses.

4 The optimal time for imaging is 72 hours after the dose of ^{131}I has been administered when the target/background activity is maximal.

5 Imaging is carried out with a γ-camera with multiple static views or one that can image in a whole-body scanning mode. A high-energy collimator for ^{131}I is essential.

Perchlorate discharge test

This test is used to assess what proportion of the radioiodine uptake into the thyroid is organified, and it is therefore useful in the diagnosis of organification defects in the thyroid. Its principle is based on the ability of perchlorate to block further thyroidal uptake of a previously administered dose of radioiodine, allowing free radioiodine but not organified iodine to be discharged from the gland. In normal subjects $< 10\%$ of radioiodine activity is discharged from the thyroid after perchlorate.

A tracer dose of ^{131}I or ^{123}I is given orally, and the count rate over the thyroid region at a standard distance from the detector is measured at intervals for 2 hours. One gram of potassium perchlorate (10 mg/kg in children) is then given orally and measurement of the count rate is continued at 15-min intervals for 1 hour. A fall in count rate of 10% or more 1 hour after perchlorate administration (allowing for decay) indicates an organification defect. A quicker variant of the test has also been described. The tracer dose of ^{131}I or ^{123}I is given intravenously and the count rate is measured regularly for 10 min. Sodium perchlorate (200 mg) is then given intravenously and counting is continued for further 10 min. The test may also be peformed using a γ-camera. The test is considered abnormal if the count rate 10 min after perchlorate administration has fallen by more than 0.5% of its value beforehand.

The sensitivity of either test may be improved by giving 0.5–1 mg stable iodide at the time the radioiodide tracer is given.

An abnormal perchlorate discharge test is seen in patients with congenital organification defect (e.g. Pendred's syndrome), in Hashimoto's thyroiditis, in patients on antithyroid drugs which block organification, for example carbimazole, or after treatment with radioiodine.

References

1 Fogelman I, Cooke SG, Maisey MN. The role of thyroid scanning hyperthyroidism. *Eur J Nucl Med* 1986; **11**: 397–400.

2 Cooke SG, Ratcliffe GE, Fogelman I, Maisey MN. Prevalence of inappropriate drug treatment in patients with hyperthyroidism. *Br Med J* 1986; **291**: 1491–2.

3 Hegedus L, Veiergang D, Karstrup S, Hansen JM. Compensated 131I-therapy of solitary autonomous thyroid nodules: effect on thyroid size and early hypothyroidism. *Acta Endocrinol (Copenh)* 1986; **113**: 226–32.

4 Reschini CC, Peracchi M. Thyroid scintigraphy during antithyroid treatment for autonomous nodules as a means of imaging extranodular tissue. *Clin Nucl Med* 1993; **18**: 597–600.

5 Ratcliffe GE, Cooke S, Fogelman I, Maisey MN. Radioiodine treatment of solitary functioning thyroid nodules. *Br J Radiol* 1986; **59**: 385–7.

6 Fragu P, Briancon C. Macroscopic and microscopic imaging of stable iodine (127I) in the thyroid (review). *Thyroidology* 1992; **4**: 57–67.

7 Jonckheer MN. Clinical usefulness of thyroid imaging by means of X-ray fluorescence. *Horm Res* 1987; **26**: 42–7.

8 Livadas D, Psarvas A, Koutras DA. Malignant cold nodules in hyperthyroidism. *Br J Surg* **63**: 726–8.

9 Marine D, Lenhart CH. Pathological anatomy of exophthalmic goiter. *Arch Intern Med (Chicago)* 1911; **8**: 265–316.

10 Charkes, ND. Graves' disease with functioning nodules (Marine–Lenhart Syndrome). *J Nucl Med* 1982; **13**: 885–92.

11 Ober KP, Cowan RJ, Sevier RE, Poole GJ. Thyrotoxicosis caused

by functioning metastatic thyroid carcinoma. A rare and elusive cause of hyperthyroidism with low radioactive iodine uptake. *Clin Nucl Med* 1987; **12**: 345–8.

12 Tang Fui S, Prior J, Saunders AJ, Maisey MN. Posterior intrathoracic goitre as a cause of thyrotoxicosis. *Br J Radiol* 1979; **52**: 995–7.

13 Fogelfeld L, Rubinstein U, Bar On J, Feigl D. Severe thyrotoxicosis caused by an ectopic intrathoracic goiter. *Clin Nucl Med* 1986; **11**: 20–2.

14 Lazarus JH, Othman S. Thyroid disease in relation to pregnancy (review). *Clin Endocrinol* 1991; **34**: 91–8.

15 White WB, Spencer RP, Sziklas JJ, Rosenberg RJ. Incidental finding of intense thyroid radiogallium activity during febrile illness. *Clin Nucl Med* 1985; **10**: 71–4.

16 Becker DV, Hurley JR. Current status of radioiodine treatment of hyperthyroidism. Freeman LM, Weissman HS, eds. *Nucleic Medicine Annual*. New York: Raven Press, 1982: 265–90.

17 O'Connell ME, Flower MA, Hinton PJ, Harmer CL, McCready VR. Radiation dose assessment in radioiodine therapy. Dose-response relationships in differentiated thyroid carcinoma using quantitative scanning and PET. *Radiother Oncol* 1993; **28**: 16–26.

18 Flower MA, al-Saadi A, Harmer CL, McCready VR, Ott RJ. Dose–response study on thyrotoxic patients undergoing positron emission tomography and radioiodine therapy. *Eur J Nucl Med* 1994; **21**: 531–6.

19 Maisey MN, Natorajam TK, Harley PJ, Wagner HN. Validation of a rapid computerised method of measuring ^{99m} pertechnetate uptake for routine assessment of thyroid structure and function. *J Clin Endocrinol Metab* 1973; **36**: 317–22.

20 Floyd JL, Rosen PR, Borchert RD, Jackson DE, Weiland FL. Thyroid uptake and imaging with iodine-123 at 4–5 hours: replacement of the 24-hour iodine-131 standard. *J Nucl Med* 1985; **26**: 884–7.

21 Wilson R, McKillop JH, Pearson DWM, Cuthbert GF, Thomson JA. Relapse of Graves' disease after medical therapy: predictive value of thyroidal technetium-99m uptake and serum thyroid stimulating hormone receptor antibody levels. *J Nucl Med* 1985; **26**: 1024–8.

22 Duck SC, Sty J. Technetium thyroid uptake ratios in paediatric Grave's disease. *J Paediatr* 1985; **107**: 905–9.

23 Turner J, Sadler W, Brownlie B, Rogers T. Radioiodine therapy for Graves' disease: multivariate analysis of pre-treatment parameters and early outcome. *Eur J Nucl Med* 1985; **11**: 191–3.

24 Tunbridge WMG, Evered DC, Hall R *et al.* The spectrum of thyroid disease in a community: the Wickham survey. *Clin Endocrinol* 1977; **7**: 481–93.

25 Rojeski MT, Gharib H. Nodular thyroid disease evaluation and management. *N Engl J Med* 1985; **313**: 428–36.

26 Simeone JF, Daniels GH, Mueller RP *et al.* High resolution real time sonography of the thyroid. *Radiology* 1982; **145**: 431–5.

27 Leisner B. Ultrasound evaluation of thyroid disease. *Horm Res* 1987; **26**: 33–41.

28 Lowhagen T, Willems JS, Lundell G *et al.* Aspiration biopsy cytology in the diagnosis of thyroid cancer. *World J Surg* 1981; **5**: 61–73.

29 Christensen SB, Bondeson L, Ericsson UB, Lindholm K. Prediction of malignancy in the solitary thyroid nodule by physical examination, thyroid scan, fine-needle biopsy and serum thyroglobulin. A prospective study of 100 surgically treated patients. *Acta Chir Scand* 1984; **150**: 433–9.

30 Dworkin HJ, Meier DA, Kaplan M. Advances in the management of patients with thyroid disease (review). *Sem Nucl Med* 1995; **25**: 205–20.

31 Wool MS. Thyroid nodules. The place of fine-needle aspiration biopsy in management (review). *Postgrad Med* 1911; **94**: 111–12.

32 Woeber KA. Cost-effective evaluation of the patient with a thyroid nodule. (review). *Surg Clin North Amer* 1995; **75**: 357–63.

33 Ochi H, Sawa H, Fakuda T. *et al.* ^{201}Thallium chloride thyroid scinigraphy to evaluate benign and malignant thyroid nodules. *Cancer* 1982; **50**: 236–40.

34 Henze E, Roth J, Boerer H, Adam WE. Diagnostic value of early and delayed 201Tl thyroid scintigraphy in the evaluation of cold nodules for malignancy. *Eur J Nucl Med* 1986; **11**: 413–16.

35 Hoschl R, Murray PC, McClean RG. Radio thallium scintigraphy in solitary non functioning thyroid nodules. *World J Surg* 1984; **8**: 956–62.

36 Bleichrodt RP, Vermey A, Piers DA, Langen ZJ. Early and delayed thallium 201 imaging: diagnosis of patients with cold nodules. *Cancer* 1987; **60**: 2621–3.

37 Ashcroft MW, Van Herle AJ. Management of thyroid nodules 11: scanning techniques, 64 thyroid suppressive therapy and fine needle aspiration. *Head Neck Surg* 1981; **3**: 297–322.

38 Nagai GR, Pitts WC, Basso L, Cisco JA, McDoungall IR. Scintigraphic hot nodules and thyroid carcinoma. *Clin Nucl Med* 1987; **12**: 123–7.

39 Evans DM. Diagnostic discriminants of thyroid cancer. *Am Surg* 1987; **153**: 569–70.

40 Walfish PG, Strawbridge HT, Rosen IB. Management implications from routine needle biopsy of hyperfunctioning thyroid nodules. *Surgery* 1985; **98**: 1179–88.

41 Alderson PO, Summer HW, Siegel BA. The single palpable thyroid nodule. *Cancer* 1976; **37**: 258–65.

42 Maisey MN, Moses DC, Hurley PJ, Wagner NH, Jr. Improved methods for thyroid scanning. *JAMA* 1963; **223**: 761–3.

43 Clarke SEM, Lazarus CR, Wraight P, Sampson C, Maisey MN. Pentavalent (^{99m}Tc)DMSA, (^{131}I)MIBG, and (^{99m}Tc)MDP—an evaluation of three imaging techniques in patients with medullary carcinoma of the thyroid. *J Nucl Med* 1988; **29**: 33–8.

44 Udelsman R, Ball D, Baylin SB, Wong CY, Osterman FA, Jr, Sostre, S. Preoperative localization of occult medullary carcinoma of the thyroid gland with single-photon emission tomography dimer-captosuccinic acid. *Surgery* 1993; **114**: 1083–9.

45 Ramtoola S, Maisey MN, Clarke SEM, Fogelman I. The thyroid scan in Hashimoto's thyroiditis: the great mimic. *Nucl Med Commun* 1988; **9**: 639–45.

46 Ramtoola S, Maisey MN. Subacute (De Quervains) thyroiditis. *Br J Radiol* 1988; **61**: 515–16.

47 Wells RG, Sty JR, Duck SC. Technetium 99m pertechnetate thyroid scintigraphy: congential hypothyroid screening. *Pediatr Radiol* 1986; **16**: 368–73.

48 Brooks PT, Archard ND, Carty HML. Thyroid screening in congenital hypothyroidism: a review of 41 cases. *Nucl Med Comm* 1988; **9**: 613–17.

49 Leger FA, Doumith R, Courpotin C *et al.* Complete iodine trapping defect in two cases with congenital hypothyroidism: adaptation of thyroid to huge iodine supplementation. *Eur Clin Invest* 1987; **17**: 249–55.

50 Park HM. Stunned thyroid after high-dose I-131 imaging. *Clin Nucl Med* 1992; **17**: 501–2.

51 Piekarski JD, Schlumberger M, Leclere J, Couanet D, Masselot J, Parmentier C. Chest computed tomography (CT) in patients with micronodular lung metastases of differentiated thyroid carcinoma. *Int J Radiat Oncol Biol Phys* 1985; **11**: 1023–7.

52 Samaan NA, Schultz PN, Naynie TP, Ordonez NG. Pulmonary metastases of differentiated thyroid carcinoma treatment results in 101 patients. *J Clin Endocrinol Metab* 1985; **65**: 376–80.

53 De Groot LJ, Reilly M. Use of isotope bone scans and skeletal survey X-rays in the follow-up of patients with thyroid carcinoma. *J Endocrinol Invest* 1984; **7**: 175–9.

54 Wu SY, Kollin J, Coodley E *et al.* I-131 total body scan: Localization of disseminated gastric adenocarcinoma. Case report and survey of the literature. *J Nucl Med* 1984; **25**: 1204–9.

55 Ziessman HA, Bahar H, Fahey FH, Dubiansky V. Hepatic visualization on iodine-131 whole-body thyroid cancer scans. *J Nucl Med* 1987; **28**: 1408–11.

56 Kim EE, Pjura G, Gobuty A, Verani R. 131-I uptake in a benign serous cystadenoma of the ovary. *Eur J Nucl Med* 1984; **9**: 433–5.

57 Hoschl R, Choy DHL, Gandevia B. Iodine-131 uptake in inflammatory lung disease: a potential pitfall in treatment of thyroid carcinoma. *J Nucl Med* 1988; **29**: 701–6.

58 Pons F, Carrio I, Estorch M, Ginjaume M, Pons J, Milian R. Lithium as an adjuvant of iodine-131 uptake when treating patients with well differentiated thyroid carcinoma. *Clin Nucl Med* 1987; **12**: 644–7.

59 Sheppard MC. Serum thyroglobulin and thyroid cancer. *Q J Med* 1986; **59**: 429–33.

60 Ericsson UB, Tegler L, Lennquist S, Christensen SB, Stahl E, Thorell JI. Serum thyroglobulin in differentiated thyroid carcinoma. *Acta Chir Scand* 1984; **150**: 367–75.

61 Ronga G, Fiorentino A, Fragasso G, Fringuelli FM, Todino V. Complementary role of whole body scan and serum thyroglobulin determination in the follow-up of differentiated thyroid carcinoma. *Ital J Surg Sci* 1986; **16**: 11–15.

62 Girelli ME, Busnardo B, Amerio R *et al.* Serum thyroglobulin levels in patients with well-differentiated thyroid cancer during suppression therapy: study on 429 patients. *Eur J Nucl Med* 1985; **10**: 252–4.

63 Moser E, Fritsch S, Braun S. Thyroglobulin and I-131 uptake of remaining tissue in patients with differentiated carcinoma of thyroidectomy. *Nucl Med Commun* 1988; **9**: 262–6.

64 Arning G, Ehrenheim C, Schober O, Hundeshagen H. 131I-accumulating pulmonary and bone metastases of differentiated thyroid cancer with low serum thyroglobulin levels—an exception in tumor follow-up? *Nuklearmedizin*1987; **26**: 139–42.

65 Pacini F, Lippi F, Formica N, Elisei R, Anelli S, Ceccarelli C, Pinchera A. Therapeutic doses of iodine-131 reveal undiagnosed metastases in thyroid cancer patients with detectable serum thyroglobulin levels. *J Nucl Med* 1987; **28**: 1888–91.

66 Sisson JC, Ackermann RJ, Meyer MA Wahl RL. Uptake of 18-fluoro-2-deoxy-D-glucose by thyroid cancer: implications for diagnosis and therapy. *J Clin Endocrinol Metab* 1993; **77**: 1090–4.

67 Khammash NF, Halkar RK, Dayen-Abdel HM. The use of technetium-99m pertechnetate in post operative thyroid carcinoma: comparative study with iodine-131. *Clin Nucl Med* 1988; **13**: 17–22.

68 Hoefnagel CA, Delprat CC, Marcuse HR, Vijlder JMM. Role of thallium-201 total-body scintigraphy in follow-up of thyroid carcinoma. *J Nucl Med* 1986; **27**: 1854–7.

69 Varma V, Reba R. Comparative study of Tl-201 and I-131 scintigraphy in post operative metastatic thyroid carcinoma. In: Raynaud C, ed. *Nucleic Medicine and Biology*. Oxford: Pergamon Press, 1982: 103–4.

70 Ochi H, Yamamoto K, Endo K *et al.* A new imaging agent for medullary carcinoma of the thyroid. *J Nucl Med* 1984; **25**: 323–5.

71 Clarke SEM, Lazarus CR, Fogelman I, Maisey MN. Technetium-99m(V)-DMSA in the imaging of medullary thyroid carcinoma. *J Nucl Med* 1987; **25**: 252–3.

72 Guilloteau D, Baulieu JL, Besnard JC. Medullary-thyroid carcinoma imaging in an animal model: use of radiolabelled anticalcitonin F(ab′)2 and meta-iodobenzylguanidine. *Eur J Nucl Med* 1985; **11**: 198–200.

73 Reiners C, Eilles C, Spiegel W, Becker W, Borner W. Immuno-scintigraphy in medullary thyroid cancer using an 123-I or 111In-labelled monoclonal anti-CEA antibody fragment. *Nuklearmedizin* 1986; **25**: 227–31.

74 Krausz Y, Ish-Shalom S, Dejong RB *et al.* Somatostatin-receptor imaging of medullary thyroid carcinoma. *Clin Nucl Med* 1994; **19**: 416–21.

CHAPTER 26

Goitre and hypothyroidism

A.P. Weetman

Goitre

The term goitre indicates enlargement of the thyroid but cannot be defined precisely as the distribution of thyroid size in the population forms a continuous, positively distributed curve with variations due to age, sex and geographical location. Single nodules are generally considered as separate entities, in view of their malignant potential, although often an apparently solitary nodule turns out to be part of a nodular goitre on close examination.

The common causes of goitre are shown in Table 26.1. From a practical standpoint there are two broad groups, endemic and non-endemic goitre. Endemic goitre is defined arbitrarily as >10% prevalence of goitre in children aged 6–12 years in a particular geographical region and is usually due to iodine deficiency. Although endemic goitre is common in the Himalayas, Andes and parts of Africa, areas of Europe are still iodine deficient [1] and of course endemic goitre may present in immigrants to non-endemic areas. Non-endemic goitre affects around 5% of the UK population, and is four times more frequent in women.

Aetiology

Endemic goitre

Endemic goitre frequency increases with the severity of iodine deficiency; the prevalence of goitre exceeds 30% in populations whose median urinary iodide concentration is below 15 μg/l [1]. The pathogenesis of endemic goitre is not simply related to excessive thyroid-stimulating hormone (TSH) stimulation. Endemic goitres are often large and filled with colloid; such glands may be incapable of adequate iodine organification and, therefore, leak iodide, aggravating the iodine deficiency. While modest goitre formation is an adaption to iodine deficiency, large goitre is probably a maladaptation, with disordered and useless thyroid overgrowth [2].

Goitrogens in the environment or diet also contribute to endemic goitre. Natural goitrogens are found in vegetables of the *Brassica* family, which contain thiocyanates, and these compounds are also formed by metabolism of cyanoglucosides found in cassava and other vegetables. Iodine excess plus goitrogens found in seaweed contribute to the endemic coast goitre of Japan and China, whereas bacterial and chemical pollution of water are goitrogenic in parts of the USA [3]. Conversely, when selenium deficiency is combined with iodine deficiency, there is thyroid cell destruction and fibrosis, and a consequent reduction in the frequency and size of endemic goitre.

Sporadic non-toxic goitre

The aetiology of goitre resulting in hypothyroidism is considered in detail in the second half of this chapter. Sporadic non-toxic goitre is a benign thyroid enlargement which evolves over years, usually with a change from a diffuse to a multinodular character. A distinction must be drawn between adenoma and nodule formation in sporadic goitres. Adenomas are often found as single lesions, have a fibrous capsule and arise from a heritable alteration in growth control in a single thyroid cell, whereas nodules are usually multiple, consist of unencapsulated colloid-rich follicles and are polyclonal in origin [4]. Thyroid nodules are very heterogeneous in size, colloid content and iodine metabolism, both within and between individuals, resulting from heterogeneity of single thyroid cells. A few predestined cells give rise to daughter follicles which amplify the heterogeneity [5]. This accounts for the characteristic 'hot' and 'cold' areas on scintiscans of these glands, reflecting areas of different functional capacity. Ultimately, nodules undergo degenerative changes with haemorrhage, fibrosis, necrosis and cyst formation.

Table 26.1 Causes of goitre.

Endemic goitre
Iodine deficiency
Environmental and dietary goitrogens
Sporadic goitre
Non-toxic diffuse or nodular goitre (aetiology obscure)
Autoimmune thyroid disease (Hashimoto's thyroiditis, Graves' disease)
Thyroiditis (post-partum, subacute, Riedel's)
Dyshormonogenesis
Thyroid hormone resistance syndrome
Goitrogens, especially drugs
Genetic disorders (McCune–Albright syndrome, TSH-receptor mutations)
Infiltration (amyloidosis, sarcoidosis)
Secondary hyperthyroidism (due to a TSH-secreting tumour or acromegaly)

TSH, thyroid-stimulating hormone.

Table 26.2 World Health Organization classification of goitre size.

Grade	
0	No palpable or visible goitre
1a	Goitre detected by palpation only
1b	Goitre palpable and visible with neck extended
2	Goitre visible with neck in normal position
3	Large goitre visible from a distance

The basis for these changes is not clear. Mild iodine deficiency during childhood may initiate changes which progress in adult life to goitre formation even when iodine intake is normalised; in other patients there may be modest enzymatic defects or goitrogen intake, insufficient to cause hypothyroidism. Smoking is mildly goitrogenic, possibly due to thiocyanate intake. Other factors may also be involved. It is now clear that TSH is the major element controlling thyroid growth, but a large number of endocrine, paracrine and autocrine factors modulate thyroid cell growth [6], and their disordered regulation in some individuals may result in goitre. Certain growth factors, such as insulin-like growth factor 1 (IGF-1), are derived from the stroma, and disordered growth could therefore be due to a defect in the thyroid epithelial cell, the stromal fibroblast, or the interaction between these. A role for thyroid growth-stimulating antibodies, operating independently of the TSH receptor, has been proposed, but there is no agreement yet over the nature and importance of these antibodies in endemic or sporadic goitre [7].

Clinical presentation

Endemic goitre

It is usually obvious from the geographical situation that a patient has endemic goitre. Before puberty boys are less affected than girls; prevalence declines in adult men but persists or increases during the childbearing period in women. The goitre is initially diffuse but becomes more nodular with age and increasing iodine deficiency. Goitre size may be graded according to the World Health Organization system (Table 26.2). However, ultrasound is far more precise and is the recommended method for surveys of goitre prevalence [1].

The main complications are mechanical effects of the goitre (although these are in fact surprisingly rare), late diagnosis of coincidental thyroid cancer in the presence of an already nodular goitre and, most importantly, the irreversible mental and physical changes termed endemic cretinism. Two distinctive syndromes occur, although there may be considerable overlap between these in some areas: (i) a predominantly neurological disorder, with speech and hearing defects, mental deficiency and gait abnormalities; and (ii) hypothyroidism and stunted growth. In China and Indonesia particularly it seems likely that maternal hypothyroidism impairs the small but significant transplacental transfer of thyroxine (T_4) during the first and second trimesters of pregnancy, resulting in brain damage at a critical stage of fetal development and the predominantly neurological syndrome, whereas congenital hypothyroidism after birth produces the hypothyroid features [8]. However, in other regions, severe maternal hypothyroidism may be associated with a predominantly hypothyroid picture, so other factors besides the timing of hypothyroidism must be involved.

As indicated previously, endemic goitre is not simply related to iodine deficiency and this accounts for the appearance of endemic cretinism, in the absence of goitre, in parts of Zaire and China. In mild iodine deficiency, for instance in many parts of Europe, goitre trends to appear during puberty when iodine metabolism is increased, or after pregnancy, following the fall in T_4 and rise in TSH with borderline iodine intake during pregnancy. Transient neonatal hypothyroidism is also more common when there is mild iodine deficiency.

Sporadic non-toxic goitre

The presenting features usually are confined to the neck swelling, sometimes noticed by relatives or incidentally during a medical consultation. Key points to elicit in the

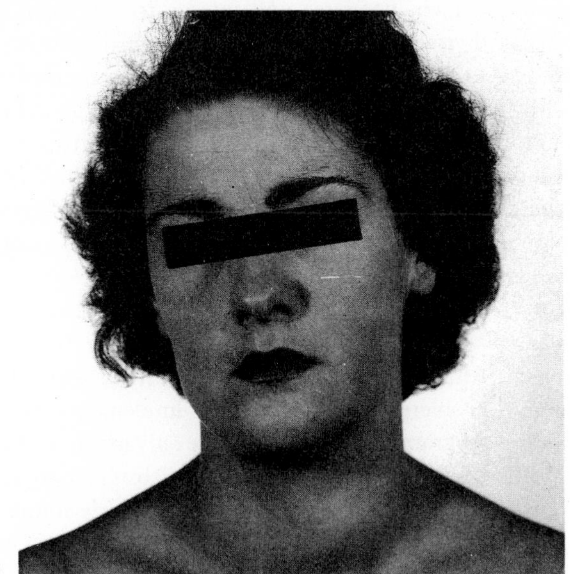

(a)

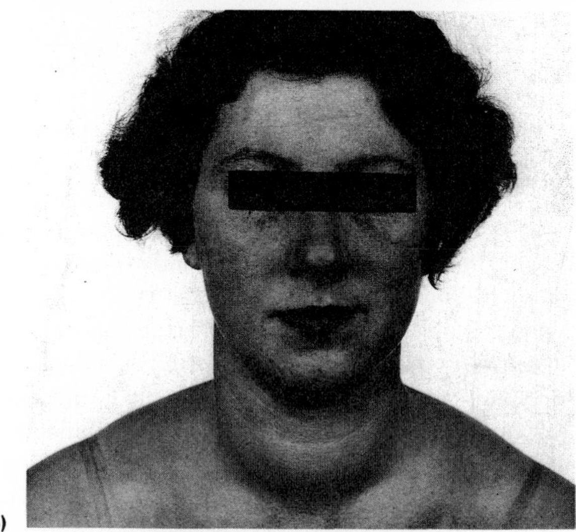

(b)

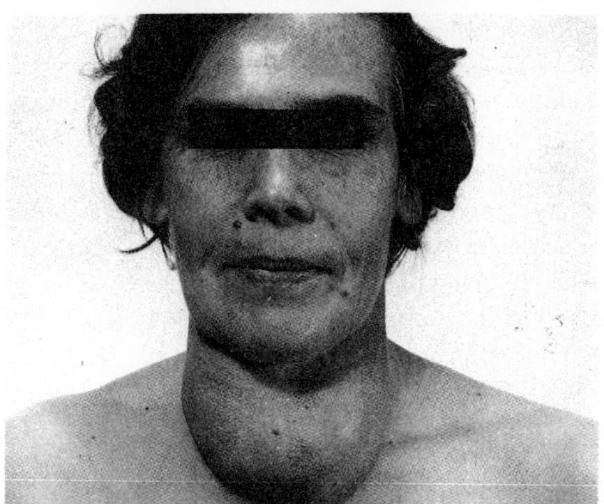

(c)

Fig. 26.1 Three examples of goitre: (a) grade 1b; (b) grade 2; (c) grade 3. (Courtesy of Professor D.S. Munro.)

history include the duration of swelling and symptoms of pain or tightness, dysphagia, hoarseness, dyspnoea or wheeze. Pain and tenderness usually imply subacute thyroiditis or haemorrhage into a cyst, although these features may also occur in anaplastic carcinoma or lymphoma. Evidence of hypothyroidism or thyrotoxicosis should also be sought. A family and drug history, including ingestion of iodine (e.g. as kelp tablets), can provide important clues in the diagnosis.

Examination of the thyroid begins with inspection; if visible, the thyroid is enlarged (Fig. 26.1). Mobility on swallowing indicates that the swelling is indeed in the thyroid, although in Riedel's thyroiditis or anaplastic carcinoma, this feature may be lost. As well as determining size (Table 26.2), palpation should identify whether the goitre is nodular or diffuse, soft, firm or hard, tender or painless, mobile or fixed, and whether there is an associated lymphadenopathy. A retrosternal goitre may cause dyspnoea and facial congestion when the arms are raised.

Investigations

Field survey investigation of endemic goitre is detailed elsewhere [1]. In sporadic goitre the first step is to determine whether the patient is euthyroid. This is most simply done by estimating the level of serum TSH as modern assays can readily detect suppressed as well as elevated TSH levels. If the TSH is abnormal, free triiodothyronine (T_3) and free T_4 levels help to confirm thyroid dysfunction. In many centres, the free T_4 alone is requested, free T_3 being reserved for those patients in whom the TSH is suppressed but the free T_4 is normal, raising the possibility of T_3 toxicosis. T_3 levels are normal in around 25% of hypothyroid patients with an elevated TSH and low free T_4, making T_3 a poor discriminator of hypothyroidism [9].

A frequently encountered problem is the elderly patient with a suppressed TSH but normal free T_3 and T_4. These patients usually have a multinodular goitre and their subclinical hyperthyroidism presumably results from an increase in the autonomous function of 'hot' nodules within the gland. Dietary iodine has increased in many western countries and may account for this change because patients with nodular goitre are particularly susceptible to hyperthyroidism after excess iodine intake. It remains unclear whether it is worthwhile treating subclinical hyperthyroidism or awaiting its further evolution [10]. New fourth-generation assays for TSH may help to discriminate between low and undetectable levels of TSH, the latter indicating the need for treatment. If untreated, such patients should be offered regular follow-up (at least annually).

At the same time as checking TSH, thyroid antibodies should be sought, as their presence (particularly at a high concentration) suggests an autoimmune basis for the goitre. However, these antibodies do not necessarily confirm that a goitre is due to Hashimoto's thyroiditis, as some patients with non-toxic multinodular goitre also have antibodies, reflecting the presence of a usually mild focal lymphocytic thyroiditis. Even if the TSH is normal, the presence of thyroid antibodies is associated with an increased risk of future hypothyroidism [11] and such patients should be offered follow-up. Although it is usual to check both thyroglobulin (TG) and thyroid peroxidase (TPO; previously called microsomal) antibodies, TG antibodies alone are infrequent and screening for TPO antibodies may be sufficient in many patients.

The value of imaging is debated and depends to some extent on the clinical experience of the clinician, the frequency of goitre in the local population and the availability of the patient for follow-up. Certainly ultrasound can determine the size and number of nodules accurately and allows discrimination between solid and cystic lesions. Thyroid scintiscanning provides unique information on the functional activity of nodules, characteristically showing multiple 'hot' and 'cold' areas [12]. How much this information influences the cost-effective management of patients is unclear (and to my mind doubtful). The main questions in patients with non-toxic sporadic goitre are: (i) is there a malignancy within the gland, (ii) is there tracheal compression; and (iii) are the signs and symptoms sufficient to warrant treatment? Fine-needle aspiration of a clinically apparent dominant nodule and regular follow-up is the optimal initial approach to the first of these questions, whereas neither ultrasound nor scintiscanning can exclude a malignancy. Clinical suspicion of tracheal compression, particularly by a retrosternal goitre, is best confirmed by airway flow loop studies, followed by computed tomography (CT) scanning or magnetic resonance imaging (MRI) of the neck and thoracic inlet; neck and chest X-rays are much less satisfactory. Finally, a decision on the need for treatment is largely based on the patient's attitude to the goitre; sometimes reassurance is provided by repeated imaging studies for patients who are experiencing neck discomfort or difficulty swallowing. The value of radio-nucleotide studies in confirming subacute or post-partum thyroiditis, in which there is suppression or absence of tracer isotope uptake, is undisputed.

Management

Endemic goitre

Most affected populations live in underdeveloped countries, but 50–100 million people are at risk of mild to moderate iodine deficiency in Europe [1]. Iodine supplementation is the obvious answer to endemic goitre, particularly targeting pregnant women, neonates and infants to minimise the effects of thyroid failure on the neurological system. In developed countries the most successful strategy for meeting the daily recommended adult requirement of 100 μg iodine/day (150 μg/day for pregnant and lactating women) has been the supplementation of food, particularly salt and bread.

Where access and expense prevent this approach in developing countries, an alternative has been to use a single intramuscular or oral dose of iodised oil which acts as a depot for the sustained release of iodine. Iodine must be administered before pregnancy to avoid neurological cretinism. Although highly effective, political, social and economic problems have limited the implementation of iodisation programmes worldwide. The only major medical complication is the occurrence of thyrotoxicosis in a variable proportion of individuals [13]. This is particularly common in older subjects and is attributed to the increased iodine available to autonomous nodules for thyroid hormone synthesis.

Sporadic non-toxic goitre

In many patients with either a diffuse or nodular non-toxic goitre, no treatment is needed. However, if the patient has discomfort or is worried about the appearance, treatment aimed at goitre shrinkage is indicated. Of course airways obstruction or a suspicion of a coincidental malignancy are further indications for active intervention.

T_4 is the simplest therapy, given with the aim of suppressing TSH levels. Prior to the widespread use of sensitive TSH assays, unselected patients treated with T_4 showed a variable response, related in part to underlying mild iodine deficiency in a proportion, and the inclusion of patients with hypothyroidism (who may respond favourably) or with subclinical hyperthyroidism (who would be unlikely to respond). Even so, the results of uncontrolled studies, as well as placebo-controlled trials, indicate that around 60% of sporadic non-toxic goitres may shrink on T_4 therapy [14,15]. The optimum results occur when the TSH is suppressed and a good response is more likely with diffuse rather than nodular goitres, although at least one-third of the latter may improve. Size reduction is usually evident by 3 months and there is little further benefit after this. Continuous treatment is needed to maintain benefit in the short term. It is unclear whether the long-term outcome is altered by T_4.

A simple strategy is to check the TSH and give T_4 100 μg/day if the TSH is above the lower end of the normal reference range. This dose is increased by 25 μg increments every 2 months until TSH levels fall below 0.1 mU/l. If there is no change 6–12 months after achieving TSH suppression, T_4 should be discontinued. In those patients who respond, it may be worth seeing if shrinkage can be sustained with a modest reduction in T_4 dosage, sufficient to keep the TSH within the lower end of the normal range. This is particularly important in the elderly who may have underlying cardiovascular disease or osteoporosis; indeed, these complications may even prevent successful T_4 treatment in some due to the appearance of frank thyrotoxicosis.

Radioiodine has also been used to treat large non-toxic multinodular goitres, particularly when these recur after surgery. In one study, the doses used ranged from 750–3400 MBq and were based on the size of the goitre and tracer uptake studies [16]. Even with such large doses, hypothyroidism was uncommon and the treatment was effective in relieving obstructive symptoms, despite the theoretical risk of radiation-induced acute thyroid swelling. High-dose steroids may prevent this latter complication and all patients with threatened obstruction at the thoracic inlet or in the neck should be monitored carefully.

Surgery is the treatment of choice for non-toxic goitre when there is a suspicion of malignancy in one part of the gland. The presence of a substernal goitre is also an indication for surgical removal in all but the highest risk patients, even in the absence of symptoms, because malignancy cannot be excluded reliably and serious pressure effects may occur unexpectedly [17]. Most retrosternal goitres arise from the thyroid in the neck and can be removed using the standard collar incision. True ectopic or aberrant goitres are rare, and are defined by the absence of a cervical blood supply or any connection with the normal thyroid. They can occur anywhere within the thorax.

Tracheal compression, dysphagia and rarely Horner's syndrome are other complications from a non-toxic goitre which require surgery (generally a subtotal thyroidectomy). Concern about the appearance of a large goitre is a relative indication for surgery, although many patients prefer at least a trial of T_4 suppression before considering this option. A major problem with subtotal thyroidectomy is the risk of recurrence. There are few convincing trials showing that T_4 therapy after surgery prevents regrowth of non-toxic goitre, partly due to the inclusion of many patients who have already had a failure of medical treatment prior to their surgery [14]. Needless to say, avoidance of post-surgical hypothyroidism, demonstrated by an elevation of TSH, with appropriate T_4 treatment is still necessary.

Hypothyroidism

The previous section has dealt with the general causes of goitre, many of which are associated with hypothyroidism. The commonest cause worldwide of thyroid underactivity is iodine deficiency. In this section the other causes of hypothyroidism will be detailed; these are summarised in Table 26.3. In non-iodine-deficient regions, autoimmune thyroiditis and destruction of thyroid tissue in the course of treatment for hyperthyroidism are by far the major mechanisms for thyroid failure. These will be discussed before the other rarer causes. Secondary hypothyroidism due to TSH deficiency is frequently associated with pituitary disease and loss of other pituitary-dependent hormones; it is considered in detail in Chapter 8. Isolated TSH deficiency is very rare [18].

Table 26.3 Aetiology of hypothyroidism, with common causes in parentheses.

Primary
Iodine deficiency and excess
Autoimmune hypothyroidism (Hashimoto's thyroiditis, primary myxoedema)
Iatrogenic (following thyroid surgery, ^{131}I treatment or external-beam radiotherapy)
Congenital hypothyroidism due to structural thyroid abnormalities
Dyshormonogenesis
Infiltration (amyloidosis, sarcoidosis)
Drugs (antithyroid drugs, lithium)
Transient
Subacute thyroiditis
Post-partum thyroiditis
Silent thyroiditis
Secondary
Pituitary disease
Hypothalamic disease
Generalised thyroid hormone resistance

Natural history of autoimmune hypothyroidism

Several different variants of autoimmune hypothyroidism have been identified whose interrelationship is unclear. Broadly, patients can be classified as having primary myxoedema (atrophic thyroiditis), in which there is hypothyroidism but no goitre, or Hashimoto's thyroiditis (goitrous thyroiditis), in which a goitre or hypothyroidism may be the presenting feature. There is considerable fibrosis, atrophy of the thyroid follicles and a mild to moderate lymphocytic infiltrate in primary myxoedema, but these features are also found in the fibrous variant of Hashimoto's thyroiditis. The majority of patients with Hashimoto's thyroiditis, however, have a marked lymphocytic infiltrate with germinal centre formation, atrophic follicles with oxyphil metaplasia of thyroid cells, absent colloid and variable fibrosis. In juvenile lymphocytic thyroiditis, follicular atrophy and oxyphil metaplasia are focal or absent. These variants appear to have a distinct but overlapping pathogenesis. Whilst it is possible that these features represent a spectrum of the same disease, with some patients progressing from goitre to atrophy, the histological features in Hashimoto's thyroiditis are largely unaltered over

10–20 years [19] and there is no clear evidence that patients with primary myxoedema have a preceding goitre.

A recent follow-up to a large-scale epidemiological survey of hypothyroidism in the UK [11] has shown that the annual incidence rate of spontaneous (autoimmune) hypothyroidism over a 20-year period was 3.5/1000 women and 0.8/1000 men. A further 0.6/1000 women/year developed hypothyroidism secondary to destructive therapy for hyperthyroidism. The mean age at diagnosis was around 60 years. Over this period, 21% of the women aged 35–45 years at the start of the survey developed thyroid antibodies. The annual risk of developing hypothyroidism in women was 4.3% when thyroid antibodies were present in association with an elevated TSH level, with lesser but none the less significant risks of future hypothyroidism if either abnormality was present. Indeed, independent of age or antibodies, the higher the TSH level was above 2 mU/l, the greater was the risk of hypothyroidism.

These observations confirm the clinical impression that autoimmune hypothyroidism evolves slowly from a high background prevalence of autoimmune thyroiditis, predominantly in women. Circulating thyroid antibodies reflect the presence of an underlying thyroiditis, which is usually focal but may be sufficient to cause a goitre during an initial euthyroid phase. As thyroid destruction continues, the TSH rises and this is sufficient to keep circulating T_4 levels normal and the patient euthyroid. Finally, however, thyroid cell insufficiency despite high levels of TSH leads to overt hypothyroidism.

Aetiology of autoimmune hypothyroidism

Autoimmune thyroiditis is the result of a complex and poorly understood interplay between genetic and environmental factors. The frequent occurrence of autoimmune hypothyroidism and Graves' disease in different members of the same family suggests that there is a shared genetic susceptibility in these two diseases, which may, for instance, determine the formation of thyroid antibodies in both conditions. However, in many patients there is no clear family history of thyroid or other endocrine autoimmunity and in them environmental factors play a more substantial role.

The genetic loci determining susceptibility are largely unknown. Human leucocyte antigen (HLA)-DR3, -DR4 and -DR5 are weakly associated with both Hashimoto's thyroiditis and primary myxoedema in Caucasians, whereas the supertypic specificity HLA-DRw53 is associated (again weakly) with Hashimoto's thyroiditis in Japanese patients [7]. Animal models of autoimmune thyroiditis suggest that genes involved in controlling self-reactive T cells and thyroid cell function may be crucial [20] but in humans there are no clearly analogous data.

The excess of women with autoimmune thyroiditis is probably related to sex hormones. The clearest evidence for this comes from experimental animal models in which testosterone inhibits the development of thyroiditis whereas oestrogens exacerbate it [20]. Pregnancy is another endogenous factor influencing autoimmune thyroiditis; thyroid antibody levels decline during pregnancy and rise 3–6 months post-partum at which time thyroid dysfunction may appear in previously euthyroid women. This is termed post-partum thyroiditis and is discussed further in Chapter 30. Although usually transient, it is now clear that an episode of post-partum thyroiditis is an important marker of future autoimmune hypothyroidism; in one UK survey, 23% of women who had had post-partum thyroiditis were hypothyroid 2–4 years later [21]. Since the peak age of onset of autoimmune hypothyroidism is around 60, these results suggest that pregnancy alters the natural history of the underlying thyroiditis.

There is no clear proof that infection precipitates autoimmune thyroiditis, except for a high prevalence of autoimmune hypothyroidism in the congenital rubella syndrome [22]. Dietary iodine may be important, with epidemiological and experimental evidence that excessive iodine stimulates thyroid antibody production and exacerbates thyroiditis [7]. Other dietary components and environmental toxins may also be involved. One clearly established iatrogenic cause is the administration of recombinant cytokines, such as α-interferon, interleukin 2 and granulocyte/macrophage colony-stimulating factor, which exacerbate pre-existing autoimmune thyroiditis [7].

The appropriate combination of genetic and environmental factors causes autoimmune thyroid disease by altering the regulation of thyroid-specific, autoreactive T cells [7,23]. Normally, such T cells are either deleted during early life or rendered non-responsive (or tolerant) to thyroid antigens by one of a number of mechanisms, including peripheral tolerance and active suppression [7]. Certain genetic factors may alter the developing T-cell repertoire, permitting survival of more autoreactive T cells, whilst both genetic and environmental factors may interfere with T-cell tolerance.

Although the mechanisms involved remain unclear, there is now little doubt that one of the primary events in autoimmune thyroiditis is the activation and expansion of thyroid-specific $CD4^+$ T-helper cells. Via release of cytokines, the $CD4^+$ cells promote the development of cytotoxic T cells and the production of autoantibodies by B cells. These then contribute to the various pathogenic mechanisms, summarised in Fig. 26.2, leading to thyroid failure in autoimmune hypothyroidism. Patients will differ in the relative importance of each mechanism, and this contributes to the clinical and pathological heterogeneity of autoimmune hypothyroidism.

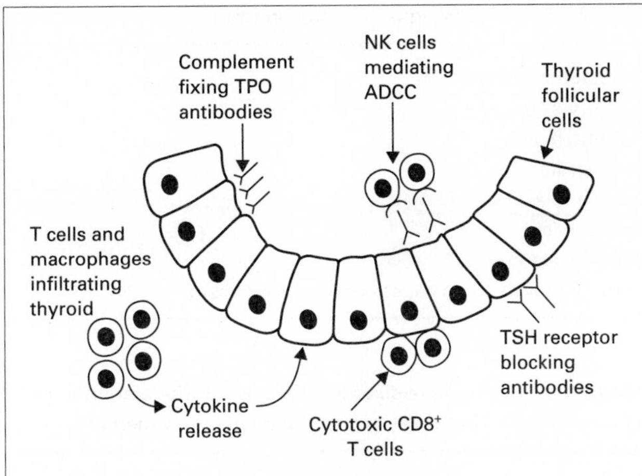

Fig. 26.2 The pathogenetic mechanisms thought to mediate autoimmune hypothyroidism. Cytokines may modulate thyroid cell function and induce the expression of immunologically important molecules such as human leucocyte antigen (HLA)-DR and adhesion molecules. Cytotoxic $CD8^+$ T cells destroy thyroid cells specifically; natural killer (NK) cells may destroy thyroid cells with TPO antibodies bound to their surface via antibody-dependent cell-mediated cytotoxicity (ADCC).

Most, if not all, of these immunological phenomena occur in Graves' disease, although this is distinguished from autoimmune hypothyroidism by the presence of TSH-receptor-stimulating antibodies. Destructive mechanisms may supervene in around 15% of patients with Graves' disease several years after successful treatment with antithyroid drugs, leading to autoimmune hypothyroidism [24], and there is some evidence that autoimmune mechanisms may even have an impact on the iatrogenic hypothyroidism seen after subtotal thyroidectomy or radioiodine treatment for Graves' disease. This close association between Graves' disease and autoimmune hypothyroidism also accounts for the occasional patient who shows rapid, spontaneous fluctuations between hyper- and hypothyroidism but the mechanisms modulating the immunological changes involved are unknown.

Clinical presentation

The main presenting symptoms are shown in Table 26.4. As already indicated, autoimmune hypothyroidism is an insidious disease and often patients have few complaints at presentation, although they become aware of their ill health when euthyroidism is restored. Many symptoms such as fatigue and weight gain are vague and non-specific, but the ready availability of simple thyroid function tests makes exclusion of primary thyroid failure as a cause straightforward. This, combined with the frequency of autoimmune

Table 26.4 The main symptoms of hypothyroidism.

Fatigue and lethargy
Cold intolerance
Dry skin and lifeless hair
Impaired memory
Hoarse voice
Increased weight with decreased appetite
Constipation
Paraesthesiae, especially carpal tunnel syndrome
Menorrhagia; later oligomenorrhoea
Arthralgia
In childhood: delayed development
In adolescence: delayed or rarely precocious puberty

thyroiditis, has resulted in calls for screening certain populations such as the elderly. It is not yet clear whether this would be cost effective, particularly as non-thyroidal illness may interfere with the interpretation of biochemical tests [25]. However, there should be a low threshold for pursuing the diagnosis in at-risk groups such as patients who have had previous treatment for thyrotoxicosis or radiotherapy to the head or neck, or who have a goitre or family history of autoimmune thyroid disease.

Examination may not reveal any specific abnormalities if there is mild to moderate hypothyroidism, the characteristic features tending to occur with long-standing severe disease (Fig. 26.3 and Table 26.5). The goitre in Hashimoto's thyroiditis can be small or large, but is characteristically firm to hard in consistency and often rather irregular (or 'bosselated'). These features may be accompanied by considerable asymmetry, giving rise to the suspicion of malignancy. Although the frequency of cancer of the thyroid epithelium is not increased in Hashimoto's thyroiditis, it is not reduced either. Primary lymphoma of the thyroid occurs almost exclusively in the presence of Hashimoto's thyroiditis and may present as an enlarging thyroid mass with or without pain [26]. For these reasons, fine-needle aspiration biopsy may be needed to rule out malignancy in a Hashimoto goitre. Rarely, there may be a painful goitre with uncomplicated Hashimoto's thyroiditis, sometimes accompanied by transient thyrotoxicosis [27]. Management of these patients can be difficult. After excluding lymphoma and anaplastic carcinoma, some patients respond to corticosteroids with or without azathioprine, while others may require thyroidectomy. In primary myxoedema, no goitre is apparent and the thyroid can be shown to be atrophic by ultrasound, but there are no clinical grounds for performing this investigation.

A number of disorders may be associated with autoimmune hypothyroidism, either in an individual patient or in his or her family (Table 26.6). The prevalence of autoimmune hypothyroidism plus Graves' disease is 30–

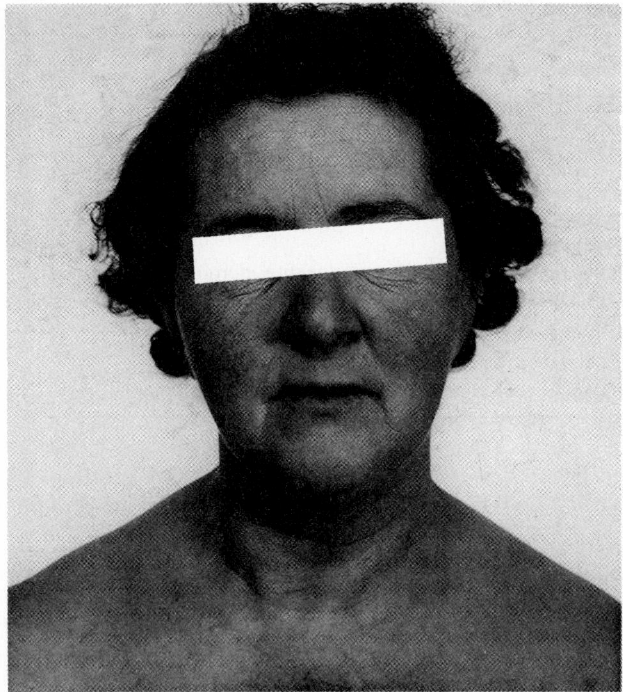

(a)

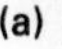

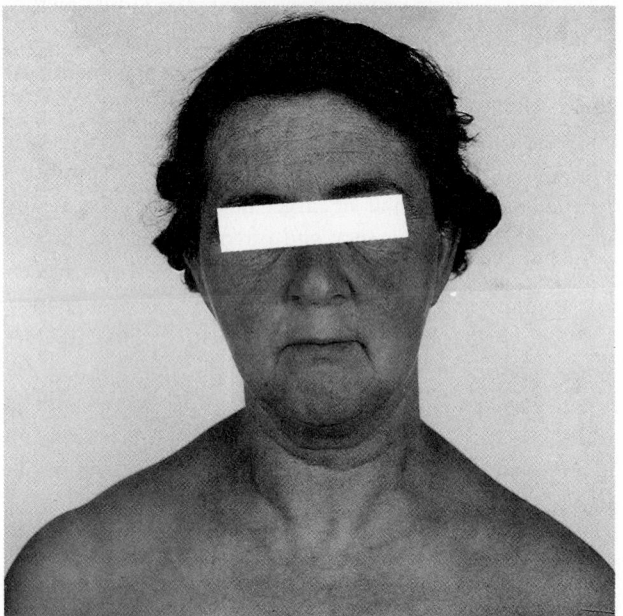

(b)

Fig. 26.3 Typical facial appearance in hypothyroidism (a) and improvement after thyroxine (b). (Courtesy of Professor D.S. Munro.)

50% in autoimmune Addison's disease and annual screening for thyroid dysfunction is clearly warranted in these patients. Around 5% of patients with type I diabetes mellitus also have thyroid disease; if screening is not performed, a low threshold for thyroid function testing should be maintained.

Table 26.5 The main signs of hypothyroidism.

Characteristic facies
Cool, dry skin
Thinning hair
Bradycardia
Delayed relaxation of reflexes
Hoarse voice
Bradykinesia
Goitre only with some causes of hypothyroidism

Table 26.6 Autoimmune disorders associated with autoimmune hypothyroidism. These may also be found in family members.

Common
Vitiligo
Alopecia
Type I diabetes mellitus
Addison's disease
Pernicious anaemia
Thyroid-associated ophthalmopathy
Less common
Chronic active hepatitis
Coeliac disease, dermatitis herpetiformis
Systemic lupus erythematosus
Rheumatoid arthritis
Sjögren's syndrome

Autoimmune hypothyroidism is also increased in Turner's syndrome and Down's syndrome.

Effects of hypothyroidism

The most important features which contribute to the clinical picture are outlined below.

Skin

The characteristic dry skin is the result of thinning of the epidermis and hyperkeratosis of the stratum corneum. The dermal content of glycosaminoglycans, predominantly hyaluronate and chondroitin sulphate, increases and the elastic fibres decrease. The skin acquires a yellowish tinge due to hypercarotenaemia. Hair growth is impaired and there is reduced function of the sweat glands with eventual atrophy.

Cardiovascular system

There is no specific cardiomyopathy due to hypothyroidism. Myocardial contractility is impaired, leading to a decreased stroke volume, and there is increased peripheral vascular resistance. A redistribution of blood flow occurs with diversion away from the skin. Diminished adrenergic sensitivity may contribute to the bradycardia. A pericardial effusion occurs in up to 30% of hypothyroid patients but rarely causes tamponade. Patients with moderate hypothyroidism are at increased risk of hypertension, despite low renin levels, probably due to increased peripheral vascular resistance. The development of atherosclerosis is accelerated in hypothyroidism, in part related to hypercholesterolaemia.

Respiratory system

Resting pulmonary function is normal in hypothyroidism but ventilatory drive may be impaired in some patients. Pleural effusions, a myopathy affecting the respiratory muscles and upper airways obstruction due to goitre can all contribute to the symptom of dyspnoea in individual patients. Sleep apnoea may also occur.

Neurological system

Hypothyroid myopathy affects patients of all ages but is most severe in childhood. The muscles increase in volume, with slow contraction and relaxation (pseudo-myotonia). The aetiology is unclear. Entrapment neuropathies, especially at the carpal tunnel, are common. Reversible cerebellar ataxia is an unusual complication in some adults but does not occur in hypothyroid children. Deafness may result from an effusion in the middle ear. Dementia and psychosis are rare, serious manifestations of severe hypothyroidism.

Haematological changes

Erythropoiesis is diminished, with a low red-cell mass and hypocellular marrow. This is mediated by a decrease in erythropoietin (as a result of decreased oxygen requirements) and by a direct effect of hypothyroidism on erythrocyte precursors. The result is a nomochromic, normocytic anaemia. In many patients macrocytosis occurs, related in some but not all patients to vitamin B_{12} or folate deficiency. A microcytic hypochromic anaemia in hypothyroidism can be due to iron deficiency, secondary to menorrhagia, or decreased iron absorption, but may have no obvious cause. White cells and platelets are generally normal.

Investigations

As indicated in the section on goitre, a normal serum TSH essentially rules out primary hypothyroidism, although this test does not exclude secondary hypothyroidism. If the TSH is elevated (or pituitary dysfunction is suspected) a free T_4 should be requested to confirm the presence of hypothyroidism. The combination of an elevated TSH but normal free T_4 is termed subclinical hypothyroidism. Free T_4 is inferior to TSH as a screening test because subclinical hypothyroidism is not diagnosed and even current free T_4 assay may be affected by T_4 antibodies, non-esterified fatty acids or drugs such as phenytoin. There is no place for T_3 or free T_3 measurement in the diagnosis of hypothyroidism. Serum enzymes, including creatine phosphokinase; and cholesterol are usually elevated in overt hypothyroidism, and although they have no diagnostic role such changes may cause confusion.

Thyroid antibodies, particularly against TPO, are generally present in autoimmune hypothyroidism and help to confirm the aetiology [28]. TSH-receptor-blocking antibodies can be found in 10–20% of patients but their assay is not required for routine management. Some patients have anaemia, hypergammaglobulinaemia or an elevated erythrocyte sedimentation rate (ESR); in the absence of any obvious cause, the effects of T_4 treatment should be awaited before pursuing extensive investigation of these abnormalities.

Management

In patients with overt hypothyroidism, treatment is simple [29–32]. Unless there are cardiovascular problems or the patient is elderly, 50–100 μg T_4 daily can be given at the time of diagnosis; in the remainder it is wise to start with 25 μg daily and increase the dose cautiously (see below). Patients should be reviewed at 3-month intervals and the dose adjusted by 25 μg increments or decrements with the aim of normalising the TSH. There is generally no urgent need to correct hypothyroidism and biochemical testing at more frequent intervals can be misleading as the TSH levels may still not have stabilised after the last change in T_4 dose. Most patients require 100–150 μg T_4 daily depending on weight and the initial TSH value [29]. Requirements of greater than 200 μg should raise the question of poor compliance, particularly if the free T_4 is normal despite a high TSH level. Once the TSH level is normal the patient should be offered regular follow-up, usually by means of a computerised register. Recall intervals range from 1–3 years. In patients with secondary hypothyroidism the TSH cannot be used for monitoring treatment, and reliance must be placed on clinical assessment and free T_4 levels.

There are several situations in which therapy may need to be adjusted (Table 26.7). A mildly elevated TSH in a newly diagnosed Addison's patient should simply be followed as steroid replacement often normalises the TSH; if needed, T_4 should always be started after glucocorticoids. During pregnancy TSH should be measured each trimester as the level can rise despite maintenance of the pre-pregnancy dose of T_4. Some women require an increment of 25–50 μg T_4

Table 26.7 Conditions which may require an increase in thyroxine (T_4) replacement.

Malabsorption
 Gastrointestinal disease—short bowel syndrome, coeliac disease
 Cirrhosis
Pregnancy
Drugs
 Impaired absorption—cholestyramine, aluminium hydroxide, ferrous sulphate, sucralfate, lovastatin
 Increased clearance—rifampicin, carbamazepine, phenytoin
 Impaired T_4 to T_3 conversion—amiodarone
Ongoing thyroiditis
 If treatment is begun before there is total thyroid failure, T_4 requirements will tend to increase as destruction continues

during pregnancy [8]. Patients with ischaemic heart disease may experience worsening of angina with a full replacement dose of T_4, even with a slow and gradual introduction of treatment, and sudden death and myocardial infarction are also rare but well-recognised complications. Hypothyroidism is not a contraindication to coronary artery bypass grafting, or any other major surgery, although under ideal circumstances T_4 replacement should precede an operation. Unless the patient's adrenal function is known to be satisfactory, glucocorticoid cover should be provided for emergency surgery on a hypothyroid patient. There may be a need for a small reduction in T_4 dosage with age, T_4 requirements being about 10% less in the elderly; monitoring TSH levels will prevent overtreatment.

The need for T_4 treatment in subclinical hypothyroidism is largely a matter of clinical judgement. Epidemiological evidence indicates the high risk of progression to overt thyroid failure if an elevated TSH is accompanied by positive thyroid antibodies, although either abnormality alone is associated with a significant (but reduced) risk [11]. If the TSH alone is mildly elevated, this should be rechecked after 2–3 months, in case the original value was the result of non-thyroidal illness. If the patient has symptoms and the TSH is still raised, a trial of T_4 is worthwhile. If this is not instituted, the patient requires regular follow-up as do those individuals with thyroid antibodies alone. For patients with an elevated TSH plus thyroid antibodies, T_4 treatment is probably indicated to prevent the emergence of overt hypothyroidism, irrespective of the presence or absence of hypothyroid symptoms. Subclinical hypothyroidism is common immediately after thyroid surgery and, unless symptomatic, patients should simply be followed until 6 months after their operation, as in many the TSH will become normal without T_4.

The goitre in Hashimoto's thyroiditis usually shrinks with T_4 treatment and thyroid antibody levels also tend to decrease. Remission has been reported in a small proportion (around 10%) of patients in whom T_4 could be discontinued several years after starting treatment, and was associated with a fall in TSH-receptor-blocking antibodies in one study [33]. As yet it is unclear whether such remissions are permanent. This fact, and the low frequency of remission, means that at present there is little justification for trials of withdrawing T_4 routinely.

Considerable attention has been paid recently to the potential adverse effects of excessive T_4. With the introduction of sensitive TSH assays, it should be possible to adjust replacement to avoid this problem, but there are patients who have taken T_4 over many years in doses sufficient to suppress their TSH and who feel unwell if the dose is reduced. Osteoporosis has been the main concern. Although bone density is reduced by excessive T_4, there is no increase in fracture rate and, therefore, the risks must be extremely small [34]. Particularly in the elderly, suppression of TSH by excessive T_4 may cause cardiovascular side-effects, including atrial fibrillation [35,36]. The risk are lower than with overt hyperthyroidism, but this remains the best reason to maintain TSH levels within normal limits.

Myxoedema coma

A number of events may precipitate decompensation of unsuspected or poorly treated hypothyroidism, particularly in the elderly, leading to the rare, life-threatening complication of myxoedema coma (Table 26.8). The three key features are altered mental state, defective thermoregulation and a precipitating cause [37]. True coma is not necessary for the diagnosis, as patients may present with confusion or psychosis. Temperature must be judged in the clinical context, for instance being inappropriately normal during an infection.

Prompt action based on clinical suspicion alone is needed to minimise mortality which is around 50%; awaiting biochemical confirmation of hypothyroidism is mistaken. Emergency investigations usually reveal non-specific changes, including hyponatraemia, hypoglycaemia, hypoxia, hypercapnia, an elevated creatine phosphokinase and a

Table 26.8 Factors that may precipitate myxoedema coma.

Infection
Trauma
Congestive heart failure
Myocardial infarction or stroke
Respiratory failure—CO_2 retention
Hypothermia
Hypoglycaemia
Drugs—diuretics, sedatives, anaesthetics, antidepressants

low-voltage electrocardiogram. Supportive measures include intravenous fluids, glucose and gradual warming. External warming is only indicated with profound hypothermia (30°C or less) because there is a risk of cardiovascular collapse. Broad-spectrum antibiotics pending urine and blood cultures should be given, as infection is a common precipitant, and other underlying causes should be sought and treated. Parenteral hydrocortisone is also given empirically. Ventilatory support may be needed.

The best method of starting thyroid hormone replacement is unclear [29]. A single 500 μg dose of T_4 by nasogastric tube or as an intravenous bolus will be sufficient to cover the patient's needs for several days, although maintenance T_4 is generally given at 50–100 μg/day. A large bolus of T_4 has few adverse consequences because T_4 is protein bound and requires conversion to T_3 for its activity. As this conversion is impaired in severe illness, T_3 is advocated by some clinicians. An appropriate dose is 10 μg by nasogastric tube or intravenously every 4–6 hours.

Congenital disorders of the thyroid

Transient or permanent hypothyroidism in the neonatal period is relatively common, with a prevalence of around one in 4000 [38]. The main causes of congenital hypothyroidism are shown in Table 26.9. Highly effective neonatal screening programmes have been established, based on the need to begin T_4 treatment as soon as possible after birth to avoid neurological damage. Reliance cannot be placed on clinical signs of hypothyroidism in the newborn, although if unidentified by screening, a hypothyroid baby may have prolonged jaundice, feeding problems, hypotonia, delayed bone maturation and an umbilical hernia, as well as the predictable features of constipation, dry skin and inactivity. Screening relies on estimation of TSH and free T_4 in heel-prick blood specimens collected by drying on filter paper. Estimation of TSH alone may miss central hypothyroidism and thyroid hormone resistance.

Table 26.9 Causes of neonatal hypothyroidism.

Permanent hypothyroidism
Iodine deficiency
Abnormal thyroid development—agenesis, hypoplasia, ectopic thyroid
Insensitivity to TSH—abnormal TSH or its receptor
Dyshormonogenesis—see text for details
Thyroid hormone resistance
Secondary hypothyroidism—pituitary or hypothalamic disease
Transient hypothyroidism
Fetal immaturity
Transplacental passage of TSH-receptor-blocking antibodies
Transplacental transfer of drugs—antithyroid drugs, iodine

TSH, thyroid-stimulating hormone.

It is important to exclude drugs and the transplacental passage of TSH-receptor-blocking antibodies which can cause transient hypothyroidism by taking a careful history and testing maternal serum for thyroid hormone levels and thyroid antibodies [39]. If the diagnosis of neonatal hypothyroidism is made, however, T_4 treatment is required; treatment can safely be withdrawn for 4 weeks when the child is 3 years old to reassess the diagnosis [31], but the developing brain has a critical need for T_4 in the period immediately after birth. Relatively large doses of T_4 (8–10 μg/kg/day) are needed to treat congenital hypothyroidism, with adjustment depending on TSH levels checked every 2 months. TSH levels may remain modestly elevated despite normal free T_3 and T_4 levels, suggesting impaired pituitary responsiveness. If suspected before birth, because of polyhydramnios or a fetal goitre, the diagnosis can be confirmed by cordocentesis and intrauterine T_4 treatment commenced [40].

Between 80 and 90% of permanent neonatal hypothyroidism is due to thyroid dysgenesis. Girls are two to three times more commonly affected than boys. Thyroid scans may reveal an absent thyroid, a hypoplastic remnant in the normal position or ectopic thyroid tissue located between the tongue and the anterior mediastinum. The pathogenesis is unknown but genetic factors may operate in some cases. A number of genetic disorders resulting in dyshormonogenesis are responsible for about 10% of all cases of neonatal hypothyroidism. Patients usually have a significant family history and a goitre [38]. These conditions are generally inherited as autosomal recessive disorders: defects in TPO activity and TG expression are the commonest [41,42].

Impaired iodide transport

The nature of this defect is unclear but probably involves the iodide transporter which actively concentrates iodide in the thyroid cell and in other tissues such as salivary glands, gastric mucosa and choroid plexus. In these patients, radioiodine is not accumulated by the thyroid or salivary glands.

Defective TPO

A spectrum of abnormalities has been described giving rise to a quantitative or qualitative impairment of TPO and resulting in varying degrees of thyroid dysfunction [41]. In some patients, TPO has apparently normal activity *in vitro* but iodine organification is impaired and this variant is associated with unexplained deafness in Pendred's syndrome

[43]. The diagnosis of this group of disorders depends on demonstrating a rapid discharge of a tracer dose of radioiodine from the thyroid after administration of perchlorate.

Defective iodotyrosyl coupling

These are rare, poorly understood disorders in which iodotyrosines do not couple to form T_3 and T_4. Diagnosis tends to be by exclusion of other causes, demonstration of an iodine leak in kinetic studies and, where possible, estimation of iodotyrosine, T_3 and T_4 content in a thyroid biopsy.

Defective TG synthesis and secretion

Several mutations have been described which result in abnormal TG synthesis [42]. Tissue studies reveal low TG levels, but TG can also be measured in serum and the levels fail to rise after TSH stimulation in these disorders. Iodoalbumin and other iodinated proteins are detectable in the blood. In some patients there are qualitative defects in TG structure, glycosylation or transport.

Defective iodotyrosine deiodination

Thyroid hormone secretion depends on endocytosis of TG in colloid and lysosomal hydrolysis, releasing T_3, T_4 and iodotyrosines. Iodine is rapidly removed from these free iodotyrosines for re-use in thyroid hormone synthesis but, when intrathyroidal deiodination is impaired, there is a leak of iodotyrosines into the urine, leading essentially to iodine deficiency. Such patients have a rapid uptake and turnover of radioiodine in the thyroid and a negative perchlorate discharge test. Treatment with iodine may reverse the condition.

Other causes of goitre or hypothyroidism

Transient hypothyroidism occurs in subacute thyroiditis, silent thyroiditis and post-partum thyroiditis, considered in detail in Chapters 29 and 30. A few patients with generalised thyroid hormone resistance, due to mutations in the thyroid hormone receptor, have features of hypothyroidism including cretinism, but the majority of patients are euthyroid. A diffuse goitre is found in 85% of patients. This condition is readily distinguished from primary hypothyroidism by the raised free T_4 and normal or elevated levels of TSH: further tests are required to rule out a TSH-secreting pituitary tumour.

Rarely, infiltration of the thyroid by amyloid, sarcoidosis, haemochromatosis and other unusual disorders may cause hypothyroidism and/or goitre. Drugs may also be implicated, particularly iodide-containing medications and lithium. Riedel's thyroiditis is a rare inflammatory condition of unknown aetiology, leading to thyroid fibrosis and presenting as a painless, hard, fixed goitre [44]. This frequently produces dysphagia or airways obstruction; hypothyroidism may occur in advanced disease and the condition is associated with fibrosis elsewhere (e.g. retroperitoneal fibrosis, orbital pseudo-tumour or sclerosing cholangitis). Treatment to relieve compression is surgical, but is frequently unsatisfactory.

References

1 Delange F. The disorders induced by iodine deficiency. *Thyroid* 1994; **4**: 107–27.

2 Dumont JE, Ermans AM, Maenhaut C, Coppée F, Stanbury JB. Large goitre as a maladaptation to iodine deficiency. *Clin Endocrinol* 1995; **43**: 1–10.

3 Gaitan E. *Environmental Goitrogenesis*. Boca Raton: CRC Press, 1989.

4 Thomas GA, Williams ED. Aetiology of simple goitre. *Baillière's Clin Endocrinol Metab* 1988; **2**: 703–18.

5 Studer H, Peter HJ, Gerber H. Natural heterogeneity of thyroid cells: the basis for understanding thyroid function and nodular goiter growth. *Endocr Rev* 1989; **10**: 125–35.

6 Dumont JE, Maenhaut C, Pirson I, Baptist M, Roger PP. Growth factors controlling the thyroid gland. *Baillière's Clin Endocrinol Metab* 1991; **5**: 727–45.

7 Weetman AP, McGregor AM. Autoimmune thyroid disease—further developments in our understanding. *Endocr Rev* 1994; **15**: 788–830.

8 Burrow GN, Fisher DA, Larsen PR. Maternal and fetal thyroid function. *N Engl J Med* 1994; **331**: 1072–8.

9 Stockigt JR. Serum thyrotropin and thyroid hormone measurements and assessment of thyroid hormone transport. In: Braverman LE, Utiger RD, eds. *Werner and Ingbar's The Thyroid*, 6th edn. Philadelphia: JB Lippincott Co., 1991: 463–85.

10 Jayme JJ, Ladenson PW. Subclinical thyroid dysfunction in the elderly. *Trends Endocrinol Metab* 1994; **5**: 79–86.

11 Vanderpump MPJ, Tunbridge WMG, French JM *et al.* The incidence of thyroid disorders in the community: a twenty-year follow-up of the Whickham survey. *Clin Endocrinol* 1995; **43**: 55–68.

12 Sandler MP, Patton JA, McCook BM. Multimodality imaging of the thyroid gland. *Baillière's Clin Endocrinol Metab* 1989; **3**: 89–119.

13 Dremier S, Coppée F, Delange F, Vassart G, Dumont JE, Van Sande J. Thyroid autonomy: mechanism and clinical effects. *J Clin Endocrinol Metab* 1996; **81**: 4187–93.

14 Ross DS. Thyroid hormone suppressive therapy of sporadic non-toxic goiter. *Thyroid* 1992; **2**: 263–9.

15 Cooper DS. Thyroxine suppression therapy for benign nodular disease. *J Clin Endocrinol Metab* 1995; **80**: 331–4.

16 Kay TWH, d'Emden MC, Andrews JT, Martin FIR. Treatment of non-toxic multinodular goiter with radioactive iodine. *Am J Med* 1988; **84**: 19–22.

17 Mack E. Management of patients with substernal goiters. *Surg Clin North Am* 1995; **75**: 377–93.

18 Peacey SR. Price A, Giles M, Weetman AP. Isolated TSH deficiency with a partially empty sella. *J Endocrinol Invest* 1995; **18**: 792–33.

19 Hayashi Y, Tamai H, Fukata S *et al.* A long term clinical, immunological, and histological follow-up study of patients with goitrous chronic lymphocytic thyroiditis. *J Clin Endocrinol Metab*

1985; **61**: 1172–7.

20 Charreire J. Immune mechanisms in autoimmune thyroiditis. *Adv Immunol* 1989; **46**: 263–334.

21 Othman S, Phillips DIW, Parkes AB *et al.* A long-term follow-up of postpartum thyroiditis. *Clin Endocrinol* 1990; **32**: 559–64.

22 Tomer Y, Davies TF. Infection, thyroid disease and autoimmunity. *Endocr Rev* 1993; **14**: 107–20.

23 Eguchi K, Matsuoka N, Nagataki S. Cellular immunity in autoimmune thyroid disease. *Baillière's Clin Endocrinol Metab* 1995; **9**: 71–94.

24 Tamai H, Kasagi K, Takaichi Y *et al.* Development of spontaneous hypothyroidism in patients with Graves' disease treated with antithyroid drugs: clinical, immunological and histological findings in 26 patients. *J Clin Endocrinol Metab* 1989; **69**: 49–53.

25 Danese MD, Powe NR, Sawin CT, Ladenson PW. Screening for mild thyroid failure at the periodic health examination: a decision and cost-effectiveness analysis. *JAMA* 1996; **276**: 285–92.

26 Matsuzuka F, Miyauchi A, Katayama S *et al.* Clinical aspects of primary thyroid lymphoma: diagnosis and treatment based on our experience of 119 cases. *Thyroid* 1993; **3**: 93–9.

27 Shigemasa C, Ueta Y, Mitani Y *et al.* Chronic thyroiditis with painful tender thyroid enlargement and transient thyrotoxicosis. *J Clin Endocrinol Metab* 1990; **70**: 385–90.

28 Mariotti S, Anelli S, Ruf J *et al.* Comparison of serum thyroid microsomal and thyroid peroxidase autoantibodies in thyroid diseases. *J Clin Endocrinol Metab* 1987; **65**: 987–93.

29 Roti E, Minelli R, Gardini E, Braverman LE. The use and misuse of thyroid hormone. *Endocr Rev* 1993; **14**: 401–23.

30 Mandel SJ, Brent GA, Larsen PR. Levothyroxine therapy in patients with thyroid disease. *Ann Intern Med* 1993; **119**: 492–502.

31 Toft AD. Thyroxine therapy. *N Engl J Med* 1994; **331**: 174–80.

32 Vanderpump MPJ, Ahlquist JAO, Franklyn JA, Clayton RN. Consensus statement for good practice and audit measures in the management of hypothyroidism and hyperthyroidism. *BMJ* 1996; **313**: 539–44.

33 Takasu N, Yamada T, Takasu *et al.* Disappearance of thyrotropin-blocking antibodies and spontaneous recovery from hypothyroidism in autoimmune thyroiditis. *N Engl J Med* 1992; **326**: 513–18.

34 Faber J, Galloe AM. Changes in bone mass during prolonged subclinical hyperthyroidism due to L-thyroxine treatment: a meta-analysis. *Eur J Endocrinol* 1994; **130**: 350–6.

35 Sawin CT, Geller AN, Wolf PA *et al.* Low serum thyrotropin concentrations as a risk factor for atrial fibrillation in older persons. *N Engl J Med* 1994; **331**: 1249–52.

36 Biondi B, Fazio S, Cuocolo A *et al.* Impaired cardiac reserve and exercise capacity in patients receiving long-term thyrotropin suppressive therapy with levothyroxine. *J Clin Endocrinol Metab* 1996; **81**: 4224–8.

37 Nicoloff JT, LoPresti JS. Myxedema coma: a form of decompensated hypothyroidism. *Endocrinol Metab Clin North Am* 1993; **22**: 279–290.

38 Beck Peccoz P, Medri G. Congenital thyroid disease. *Baillière's Clin Endocrinol Metab* 1988; **2**: 737–59.

39 McKenzie JM, Zakarija M. Fetal and neonatal hyperthyroidism and hypothyroidism due to maternal TSH receptor antibodies. *Thyroid* 1992; **2**: 155–63.

40 Perelman AH, Johnson RL, Clemons RD, Finberg HJ, Clewell WH, Trujillo L. Intrauterine diagnosis and treatment of fetal goitrous hypothyroidism. *J Clin Endocrinol Metab* 1990; **71**: 618–21.

41 Medeiros-Neto GA, Billerbeck AEC, Wajchenberg BL, Targovnik HM. Defective organification of iodide causing hereditary goitrous hypothyroidism. *Thyroid* 1993; **3**: 143–59.

42 Medeiros-Neto G, Targovnik HM, Vassart G. Defective thyroglobulin synthesis and secretion causing goiter and hypothyroidism. *Endocr Rev* 1993; **14**: 165–81.

43 Forrest D. Editorial: Deafness and goiter: molecular genetic considerations. *J Clin Endocrinol Metab* 1996; **81**: 2764–7.

44 de Lange WE, Freling NJM, Molenaar WM, Doorenbos H. Invasive fibrous thyroiditis (Riedel's struma): a manifestation of multifocal fibrosclerosis? A case report with review of the literature. *Q J Med* 1989; **72**: 709–17.

CHAPTER 27

Thyrotoxicosis

P. Kendall-Taylor

Introduction

Thyrotoxicosis is the condition that results when there is an elevation of circulating thyroid hormone (thyroxine (T_4) and/or triiodothyronine (T_3)) resulting in increased thyroid hormone action in peripheral tissues. This excess usually results from increased production of thyroid hormone, in which case the term hyperthyroidism is used, but it can also result from excess intake of thyroxine, or from release into the circulation of stored thyroid hormone, as occurs in thyroiditis. The causes of thyrotoxicosis are given in Table 27.1. The commonest of these is Graves' disease, which is discussed in detail later in this chapter.

Clinical features of thyrotoxicosis

The clinical features resulting from excess thyroid hormone in the circulation are common to the various types of thyrotoxicosis regardless of the cause. Additional clinical features are associated with specific types of thyrotoxicosis and these are discussed under the appropriate headings. Similarly, many of the biochemical changes are a direct effect of thyroid hormone on peripheral tissues and may be found in any case of thyrotoxicosis. However, the symptoms, clinical signs and biochemical abnormalities discussed in this section will not all be found in every patient, but will depend upon such factors as severity of the disease, the length of the history, the age of the patient and perhaps the presence of additional pre-existing disease. Clinical features and laboratory tests, associated with specific diseases in which thyrotoxicosis occurs, are discussed in the appropriate sections.

Metabolic effects

The increase in metabolic rate resulting from excess thyroid hormone reaching the peripheral tissues leads to loss of weight, which is typically associated with an increased appetite. In about 10% of patients the increase in appetite is of such degree as to outweigh the increased metabolism and then weight may be gained rather than lost. In occasional patients, usually the middle-aged or elderly, the appetite is not increased and then weight loss may be profound. There is a general feeling of warmth, the extremities are warm and moist from excess sweating, and there is intolerance of hot weather. Hyperactivity is common and there is sometimes a feeling of excessive energy, but this is associated with easy fatiguability and a general feeling of tiredness.

Cardiovascular features

Palpitations are common and may be associated with sinus tachycardia, supraventricular tachycardia or atrial fibrillation. The pulse rate is increased during sleep as well as in waking hours. The pulse pressure tends to be wide and the character of the pulse may be collapsing. A pulse rate of <80 beats/min is unusual in thyrotoxicosis, but it should be remembered that some patients when first seen in a hospital clinic will already be taking β-adrenoceptor blocking drugs and this should obviously be noted in the interpretation of the physical findings. The hyperdynamic circulation may be evidenced by a systolic flow murmur and patients may complain of flushing. The cardiovascular effects may be complicated by high-output congestive cardiac failure. Angina is not directly associated with thyrotoxicosis, but where there is pre-existing ischaemic heart disease this may become worse with the development of thyrotoxicosis.

Catecholamine-like effects

The features of thyrotoxicosis are suggestive of increased catecholamine activity, and it has long been considered that

Table 27.1 Causes of thyrotoxicosis.

Autoimmune
Graves' disease
Hashimoto's thyroiditis
Autonomous
Toxic multinodular goitre
Solitary toxic adenoma
Transient
Post-partum thyroiditis
Subacute thyroiditis
Painless thyroiditis
Drug-induced
Iodine-induced (Jod–Basedow)
T_4 or T_3 (factitious)
Secondary
TSH-secreting tumour
Syndromes of inappropriate TSH secretion
Trophoblastic tumours
Ectopic
Struma ovarii
Metastatic follicular carcinoma

T_4, thyroxine; T_3, triiodothyronine; TSH, thyroid-stimulating hormone.

thyrotoxic patients have increased sensitivity to catecholamines [1]. Moreover, some of these effects can be blocked by the use of β-adrenergic blocking drugs. The circulating levels of catecholamines are not increased, but there appears to be an increase in tissue β-adrenoceptors. The features which respond to β-adrenergic blocking agents include a fine tremor of the outstretched hands, excess sweating, tachycardia, nervousness and a staring appearance of the eyes due to retraction of the eye lids.

Neuropsychiatric features [2]

Nervousness and irritability are very common symptoms. Insomnia and inability to relax despite fatigue are also encountered frequently. Patients are hyperkinetic and this is most readily apparent by their inability to sit still during a consultation, giving a general impression of constant fidgeting, with rapid jerky movements. Hyperreflexia is common and in patients with severe thyrotoxicosis there may also be evidence of mild spasticity. Occasionally, apathy may be the predominant feature, usually in the elderly, and can be misdiagnosed as depression or dementia. Chorea is another rare manifestation of hyperthyroidism.

Muscle function [3]

Proximal myopathy is common and, if carefully looked for, evidence for this will be found in most patients [4]. It is characterised by atrophy and weakness, but there is no fasciculation; these abnormalities are non-specific and can be detected by electromyography in almost all patients. The changes are thought to be a direct result of thyroid hormone excess, acting at the level of myosin heavy-chain genes, causing a switch from slow to fast fibres. Weakness of respiratory muscles also occurs and may account for the complaint of dyspnoea. The ophthalmopathy associated with Graves' disease is not due to myopathy of extraocular muscles (see section on thyroid-associated ophthalmopathy). In Oriental populations thyrotoxicosis is sometimes associated with periodic paralysis [5].

Gastrointestinal system

Transit time through the gastrointestinal tract is shortened and results in increased stool frequency, although not diarrhoea. This perhaps contributes to the weight loss.

Reproductive system

Menstrual blood flow is reduced, leading progressively to oligomenorrhoea and sometimes to amenorrhoea. Ovulation is usually preserved, but in some women it is lost and then infertility may result. Some male patients develop gynaecomastia.

Cutaneous manifestations

The extremities are usually warm and moist and there may be palmar erythema. Patients may complain of generalised itching, but without any visible skin change. Alterations in the quality of hair may be noticed and sometimes the hair has a tendency to fall out (as of course it also does in hypothyroidism). Changes in the nails are also noted and onycholysis is sometimes present.

Eyes

A staring appearance with lid lag and lid retraction are features of excess circulating thyroid hormone from any cause, and do not indicate the presence of thyroid-associated ophthalmopathy.

Other features

Increased thirst and polyuria are sometimes present. Mild hepatomegaly, splenomegaly and also lymphadenopathy are occasionally found, but their presence is more likely to reflect active autoimmune disease than the thyrotoxicosis itself. Osteoporosis and loss of bone mineral occurs in thyrotoxicosis and may occasionally be symptomatic, particularly in patients who have an additional reason for bone disease. In children with thyrotoxicosis, skeletal growth tends to be accelerated.

Laboratory tests in thyrotoxicosis

In most cases of thyrotoxicosis both the serum T_4 and T_3 are elevated. However, in some patients only the T_4 is increased; reasons for this may relate to a high iodine intake, severe intercurrent illness or starvation leading to preferential conversion of T_4 to reverse T_3, or inhibition of deiodination by drugs such as β-adrenergic blockers or dexamethasone. Conversely, in some cases the T_3 is elevated with a normal T_4 (termed 'T_3 toxicosis'); this may occur in any type of patient but is more likely to be associated with toxic nodular goitre or with relative iodine deficiency. It follows from this that the finding of a normal level of either T_4 or T_3 does not exclude a diagnosis of thyrotoxicosis. However, regardless of whether it is the T_4 or T_3 or both which are elevated, the serum thyroid-stimulating hormone (TSH) level is suppressed in patients with thyrotoxicosis; TSH is therefore the first-line test for diagnosis, but a highly sensitive TSH assay is necessary in order to achieve clear-cut differentiation between euthyroid and hyperthyroid TSH levels. Where a reduced level of TSH is found (< 0.1 mU/l) the serum thyroid hormone levels should be checked. Some knowledge of the factors influencing the levels of total T_4 and T_3 is required (see Chapter 24), but most laboratories now also offer direct measurements of free T_4. Since the introduction of highly sensitive TSH assays the TRH test for the diagnosis of thyrotoxicosis has been superseded.

The effects of thyroid hormones on peripheral tissues and the metabolic effects have been reviewed in detail elsewhere [6]; from them some of the effects of excess thyroid hormone levels can be deduced. Basal metabolic rate is increased and there is negative nitrogen balance. Glycogenolysis, lipolysis and calorigenesis are increased; impaired glucose tolerance may develop in predisposed individuals. Calcium turnover is increased and mild hypercalcaemia is common. There is also an increase in some liver enzymes. Some of the resulting abnormalities may come to light during the routine investigation of patients, and are therefore listed in Table 27.2, but these tests are not used for the diagnosis of thyrotoxicosis.

Table 27.2 Abnormal tests in thyrotoxicosis due to peripheral effects of thyroid hormones.

Test	Increased	Decreased
Sex hormone-binding globulin	+	
Glucose tolerance test		
Glucose	+ (delayed peak)	
Insulin	+	
NEFA and glycerol	+	
Cholesterol		+
Liver enzymes (transaminases, alkaline phosphatase and γ-glutamyl transferase)	+	
Serum Ca^{2+}	+	
Urine Ca^{2+} and phosphate	+	
Urine OH-proline	+	
Vital capacity		+
Electromyogram	abnormal	

NEFA, non-esterified fatty acid.

Graves' disease

Definition

Graves' disease is an autoimmune disorder which is characterised by hyperthyroidism, goitre and in some cases ophthalmopathy and less often dermopathy. The hyperthyroidism is the direct effect of the stimulating action of an autoantibody directed to the TSH receptor. Although not an inherited disease as such, it occurs in those who have a genetically determined susceptibility.

Prevalence

The prevalence of hyperthyroidism in the population of the UK is about 2.2%, with an estimated annual incidence of three per 1000. These figures were derived from a population survey which was conducted in the north of England [7]. The disease is rare in juveniles but the frequency increases up to a peak in the fourth decade, thereafter declining (Fig. 27.1). There is a female preponderance of between 7 : 1 and 10 : 1.

Pathology [8,9]

The thyroid is enlarged to a variable degree; the enlargement is diffuse not nodular, involving both lobes symmetrically and sometimes the isthmus. Vascularity is increased. Histologically, the follicles are small and lined by hyperplastic columnar epithelium. Colloid within the follicular lumen is scanty or absent and gives the appearance of scalloping (Plate 27.1a, opposite p. 332). Epithelial projections into the lumen are seen; the nuclei may show occasional mitoses. In addition to these changes in the thyroid follicles, the other striking change is the infiltration of the gland with lymphocytes and plasma cells. These are seen to be infiltrating throughout the gland (Plate 27.1a) although their distribution is uneven,

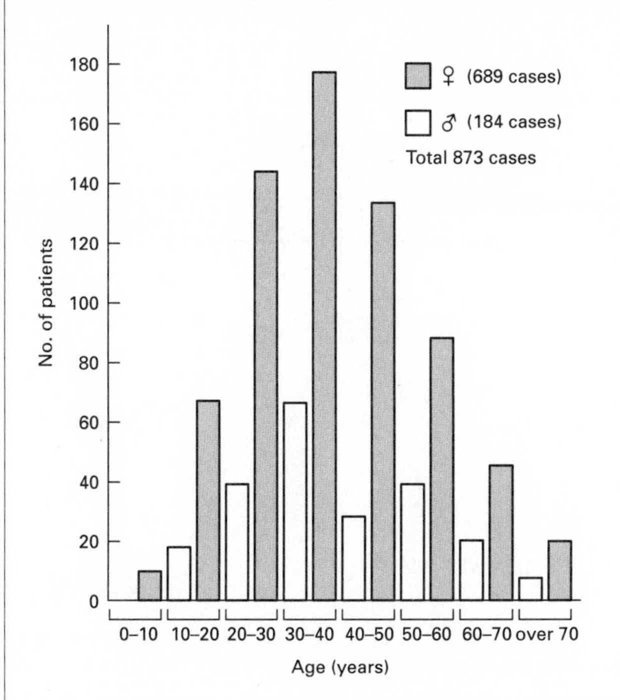

Fig. 27.1 Age and sex incidence of Graves' disease.

and aggregations may form into lymphoid follicles (Plate 27.1b). After treatment with antithyroid drugs (Plate 27.1b) some of these changes regress; the follicles become larger and the lining epithelium flatter. Patients who have been treated with antithyroid drugs for several months have diminished thyroidal lymphocytic infiltration compared with untreated patients.

In Graves' disease, as in other autoimmune endocrine diseases, the target cells display aberrant expression of major histocompatibility complex (MHC) class II antigens; the significance of this is discussed below. Expression of the DR antigen by thyroid follicular cells is shown by immunoperoxidase staining, with a monoclonal antibody directed to the non-polymorphic region of the DR antigen (Plate 27.1c). Activated lymphocytes within the thyroid also express MHC Class II antigens on their surface and this is shown in Plate 27.1d.

Pathogenesis

Several pathogenic factors have been implicated in Graves' disease.

Age and gender

The age-specific incidence has already been referred to (see Fig. 27.1). The explanation for the female sex preponderance, which also occurs in some other organ-specific autoimmune diseases, is not clear; there is a known effect of oestrogen on immune responsiveness and it is also possible that immunomodulatory genes may be located on the sex chromosomes [10].

Genetic factors

A family history of autoimmune endocrine disease can be obtained in approximately 50% of patients with Graves' disease and the frequency of hyperthyroidism in first-degree relatives is increased, for example the frequency in children of the proband in one study was 6% and for siblings of the proband 21%. In another study the concordance rate for monozygotic twins was found to be 30% and for dizygotic twins 5%, from which can be inferred the existence of both genetic and environmental factors in the aetiology. Family studies have also shown that there is a nearly equal incidence of Graves' disease and Hashimoto's disease in relatives of probands, suggesting that what is inherited is a predisposition to thyroid autoimmunity rather than to hyperthyroidism. There is also an association with other organ-specific autoimmune diseases, such as Addison's disease, insulin-dependent diabetes mellitus and premature ovarian failure, as well as with pernicious anaemia and myasthenia gravis.

There is an association with expression of certain genes encoded for by loci of the MHC [11], which are involved in regulation of immune responses. Those most closely associated with Graves' disease are B8, DR3, in Caucasian populations, but the relative risk is rather weak (<5 in many different studies), and this haplotype is also common in other organ-specific autoimmune diseases. Other candidate genes have been postulated, for example genes encoding the T-cell receptor, immunoglobulin heavy-chain allotypes and the lambda light-chain constant region, but no clear association has yet been identified.

It is clear that genetic factors are involved in the aetiology of Graves' disease, but it is equally clear that this is not a simple pattern of inheritance, nor is a single gene likely to be involved; current understanding indicates that the disease results from interaction of environmental factors with MHC genes (or possibly disease-susceptibility genes in linkage disequilibrium with the MHC), and perhaps other minor immunomodulatory genes, to induce the autoimmune response. Thus, what is inherited is a genetic susceptibility rather than the disease itself, and no genotype reliably predicts the development of Graves' disease.

Autoimmunity

The clinical features of Graves' disease appear to result from the effects of autoantibodies to thyroid tissues, and thus the hyperthyroidism of Graves' disease results from the action of TSH-receptor antibodies (TSH-RAb); these antibodies are directed against the TSH receptor and when they bind to it they activate the receptor, mimicking the effects of TSH and leading to the stimulation of thyroid hormone biosynthesis and secretion. Antibody production requires the processing of antigen by accessory cells and the subsequent presentation of antigen, in conjunction with the MHC molecules, to T cells. The defect in immune surveillance which permits the development of antibodies to self antigen is not fully understood and the initiating event triggering the autoimmune process is not known. For more detailed explanation see [12] and [13].

Thyroid autoantibodies

IgG autoantibodies (Ab) develop in autoimmune thyroid disease against several thyroid antigens, the most important of which have now been cloned and characterised.

Thyroglobulin

Thyroglobulin is a large glycoprotein dimer of 660 kDa, which is secreted by the thyroid cell across the apical cell membrane, where it is iodinated by thyroid peroxidase (TPO) and stored in the follicular colloid. Thyroglobulin antibody (TgAb) is a marker for autoimmune thyroid disease, but appears to have no biological activity. Occasionally TgAb will bind thyroid hormones and interfere with their measurement by radioimmunoassay (RIA). Immune complex-mediated nephritis involving TgAb has been reported but is extremely rare.

Thyroid peroxidase

TPO is a 107-kDa protein, essential for thyroid hormone biosynthesis, and is the antigen to which thyroid microsomal antibodies are directed. These antibodies occur in several types of autoimmune thyroid disease including Graves' disease; in thyroiditis TPO Ab are involved in complement-mediated cell lysis and antibody-dependent cell cytotoxicity.

Thyroid-stimulating hormone receptor

TSH-R has also been cloned and sequenced [14,15]. Two transcripts of 4.6 and 4.4 kb were identified in the human thyroid. The receptor protein has seven transmembrane domains and an extracellular domain of 418 amino acids. It has been transfected and expressed in mammalian (CHO and COS7) cells, with resulting binding and stimulation of adenylate cyclase by TSH. There are approximately 1000 receptor-binding sites for TSH on the surface of a human thyroid cell. Like the luteinising hormone (LH)/human chorionic gonadotrophin (hCG) receptor, with which it shares some sequence homology, the receptor is linked to a G-protein and its effects are mediated by cyclic adenosine monophosphate (cAMP) (Fig. 27.2).

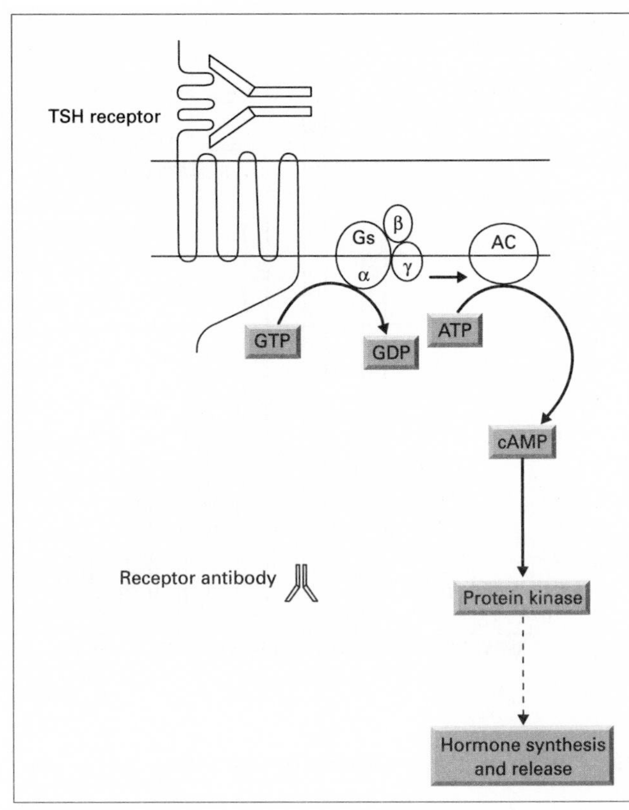

Fig. 27.2 The actions of thyroid-stimulating hormone receptor antibodies (TSH-RAb). AC, adenylate cyclase.

Antibodies to TSH-R in Graves' disease may have several effects, of which the major one is the stimulation of thyroid hormone biosynthesis; receptor antibodies may also stimulate cell proliferation leading to goitre, or they may block thyroid hormone synthesis and possibly inhibit thyroid cell growth. These antibodies are usually referred to as thyroid-stimulating antibodies (TSAb), thyroid growth-stimulating immunoglobulins (TGSI), or TSH-blocking antibodies (TBAb). Antibodies to the TSH-R are measured by their capacity to bind to the receptor in the thyrotrophin-binding inhibiting immunoglobulin (TBII) assay, but this does not define their biological activity. The differing biological effects of TSH-RAb are assumed to be mediated via binding to different epitopes of the TSH-R, but as yet there are no data to support this.

TSH-RAb is produced to a large extent in the thyroid itself and in most, though not all, patients, removal of the

(a)
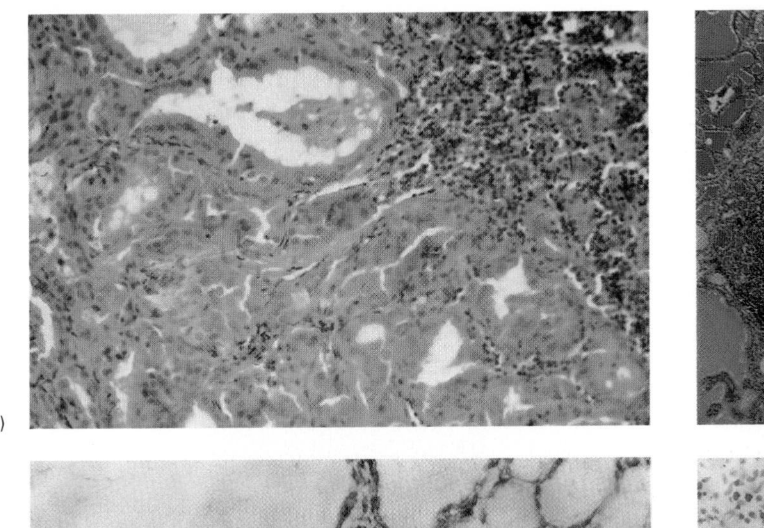

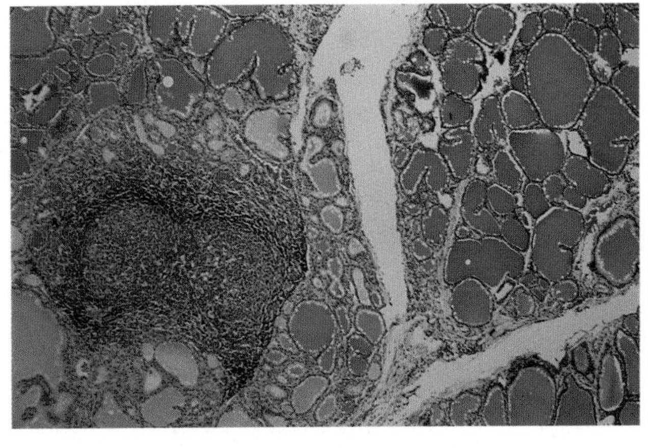
(b)

(c)
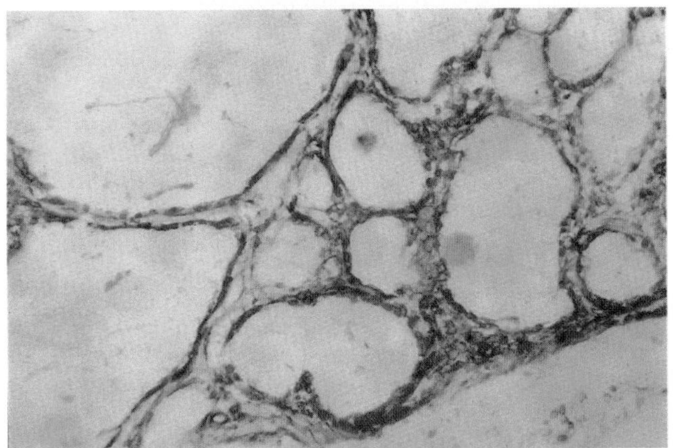

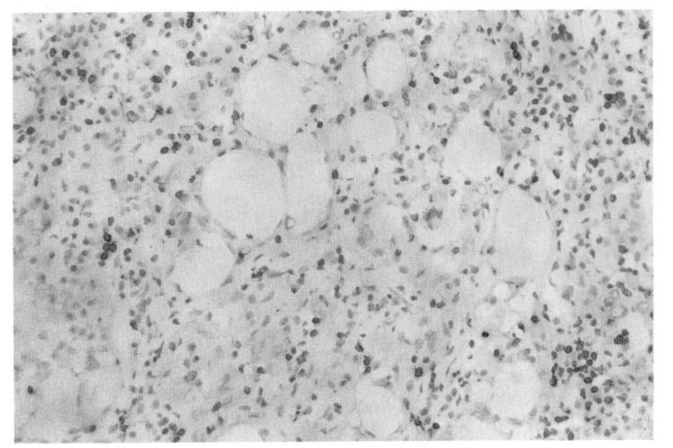
(d)

Plate 27.1 Histological changes in thyroid in Graves' disease. (a) Untreated (preoperative propranolol only); changes in thyroid follicular cells, as described in text, and lymphocytic infiltration. (b) After treatment with carbimazole; note the differences in thyroid follicular cells; formation of lymphoid follicles is also seen. (c) Immunoperoxidase stain, with antiserum to the DR antigen, showing expression on thyroid follicular cells. (d) DR staining of lymphocytes but not of follicular cells.

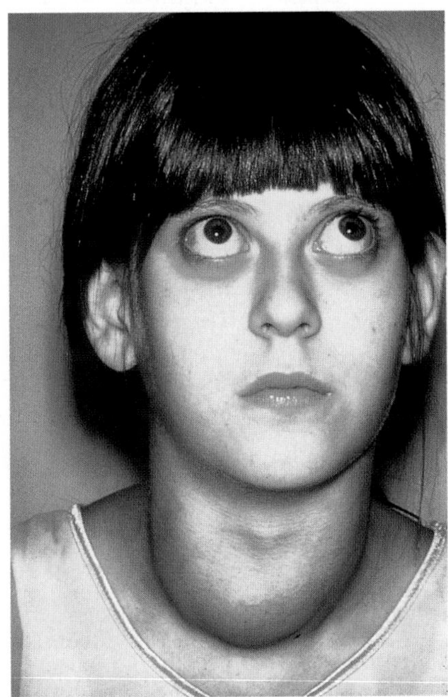

Plate 27.2 Patient with florid hyperthyroidism and clearly visible diffuse symmetrical enlargement of the thyroid.

Plate 27.3 Histological appearance of eye muscle in thyroid-associated ophthalmopathy, showing lymphocytic infiltration, proliferation of fibroblasts, deposition of collagen (stained green) and some destruction of muscle fibres. (Masson trichrome stain. Courtesy of Professor W. Lees.)

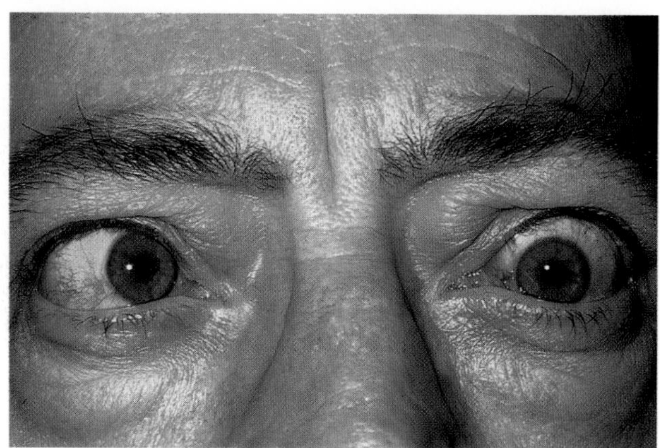

(a)

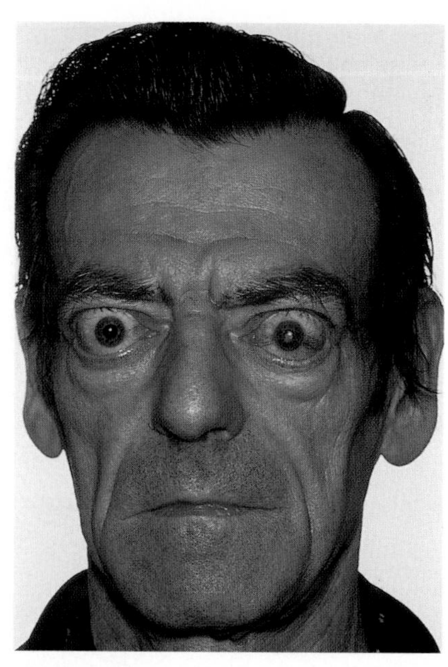

(b)

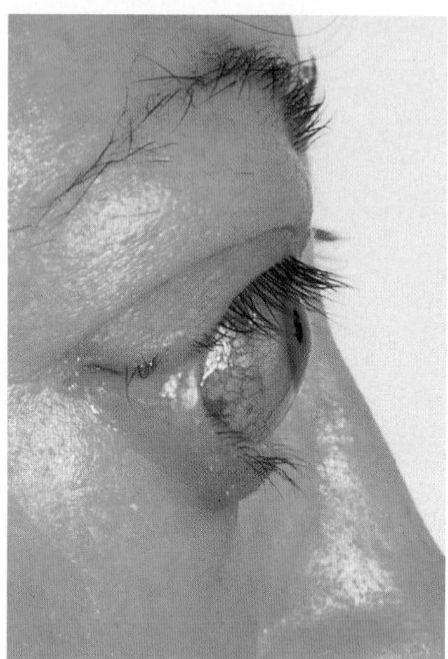

(c)

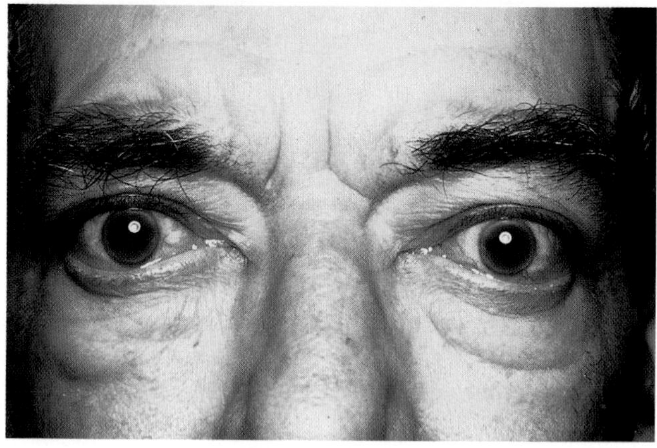

(d)

Plate 27.4 Clinical features of thyroid-associated ophthalmopathy. (a) Inflammation, oedema and diplopia. (b) Proptosis and inflammation over the insertion of lateral rectus; note the previous tarsorrhaphy. (c) The proptosis has resulted in corneal scarring on the left. (d) Low-grade inflammatory change in a patient with severe congestive ophthalmopathy (poor visual acuity and bilateral disc oedema).

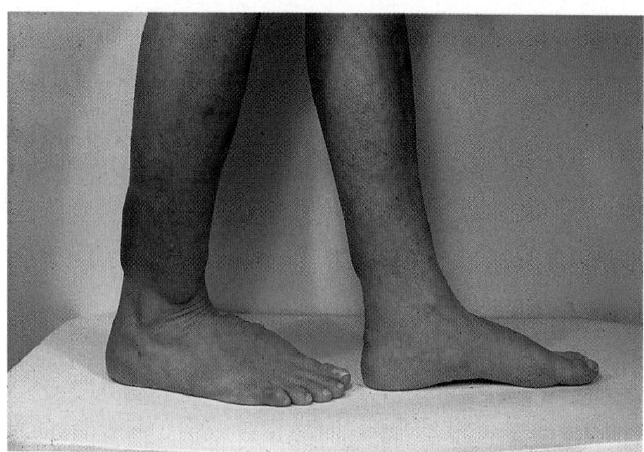

Plate 27.5 Thyroid-associated dermopathy.

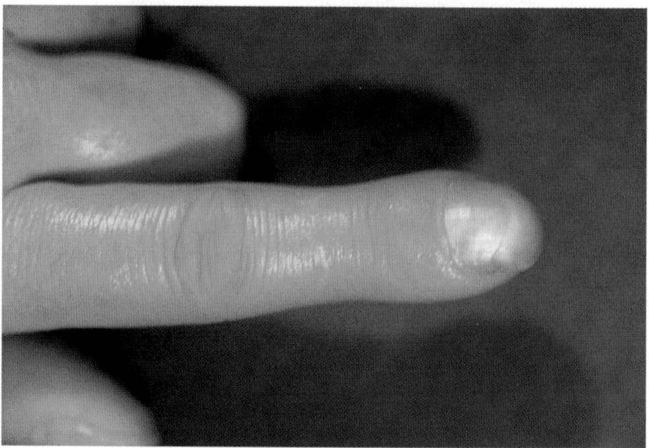

Plate 27.6 Thyroid acropachy, same patient as Plate 27.5.

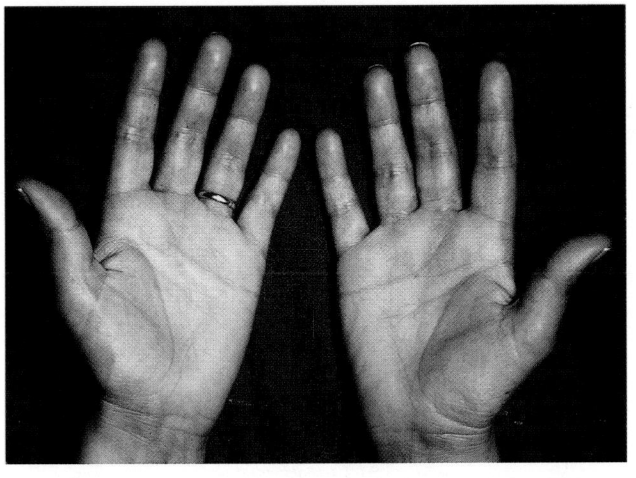

(a)

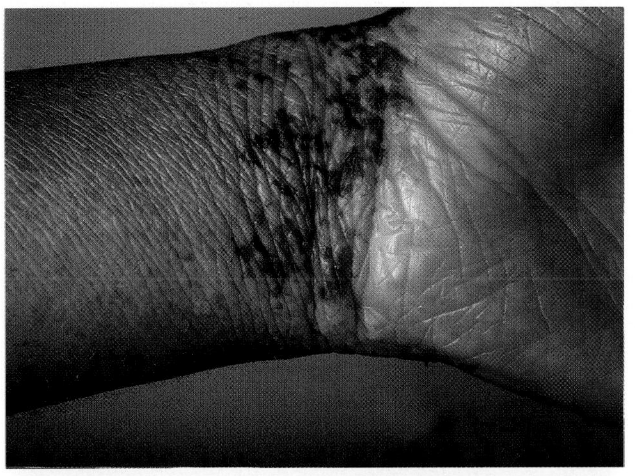

(b)

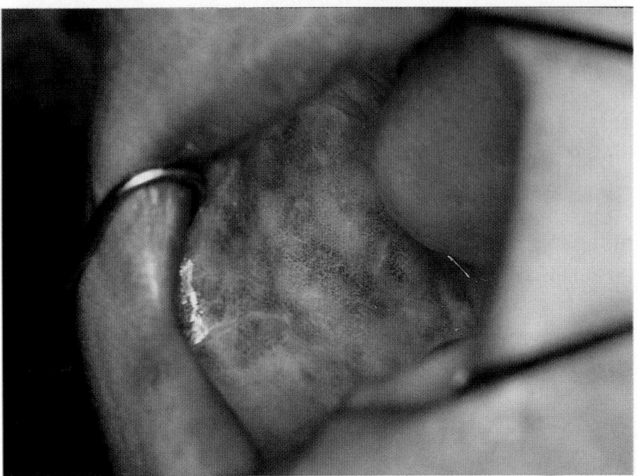

(c)

Plate 36.1 ACTH-dependent pigmentation is present in 90% of patients with primary adrenal failure at diagnosis. It is seen in light exposed areas, skin creases (a), flexures (b) and mucosal membranes (c).

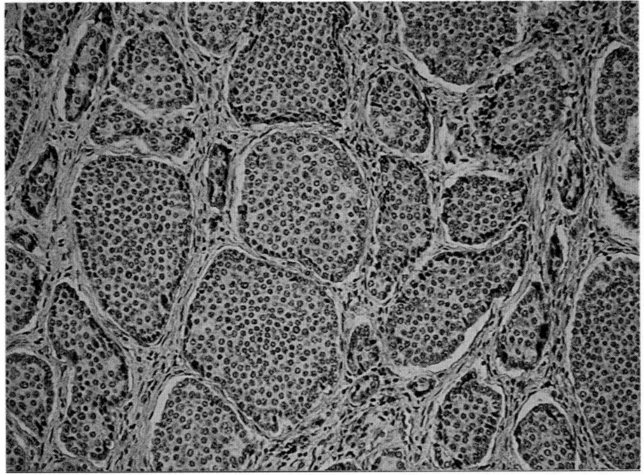

Plate 45.1 Eosin staining of a midgut carcinoid tumour. Note the regular 'insular' growth pattern.

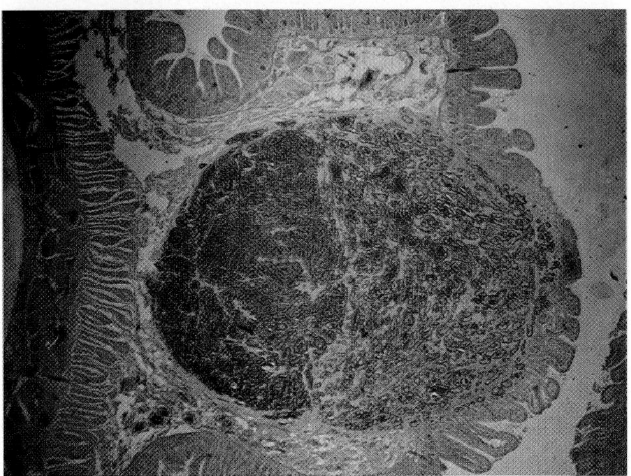

Plate 45.2 Grimelius silver staining of a midgut carcinoid localised in the small bowel wall. Note the intact mucosal layer.

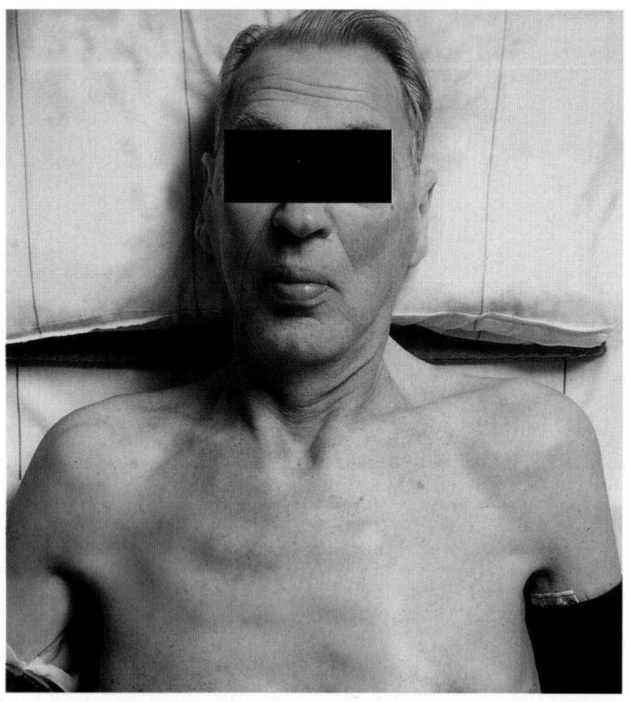

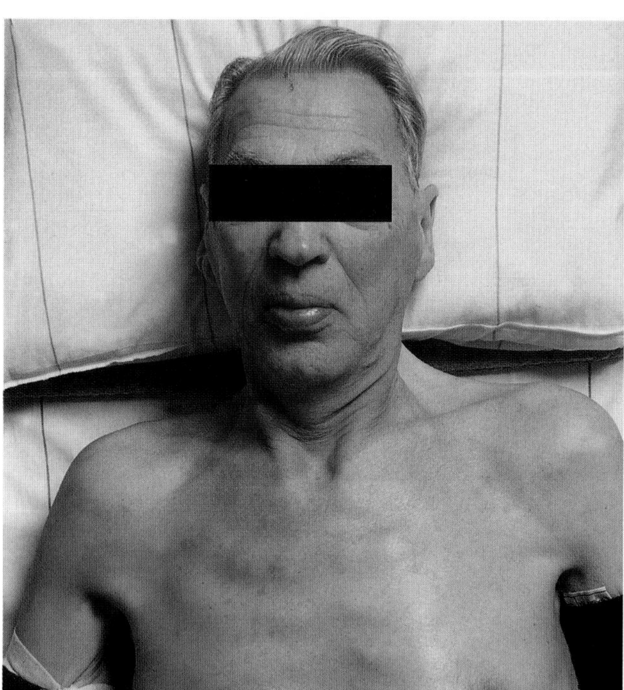

Plate 45.3 Patient with midgut carcinoid and carcinoid syndrome. (a) Before, (b) after pentagastrin-induced flush.

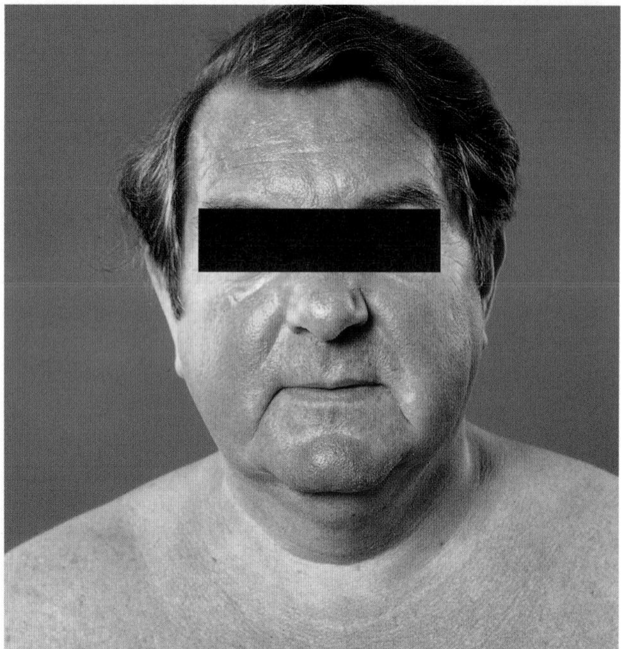

Plate 45.4 Flush reaction in a patient with a long-standing carcinoid tumour. Notice the bluish-red colour and telangiectasia.

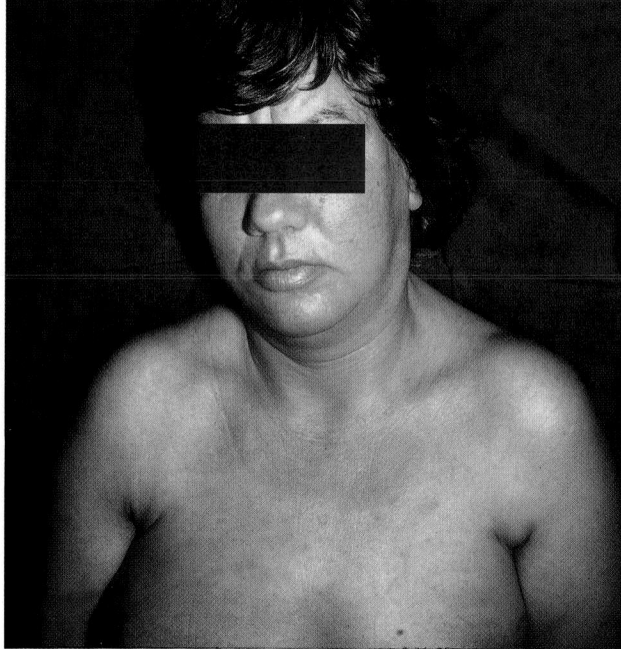

Plate 45.5 Patient with a bronchial carcinoid. Notice the dark red flush, swelling and lacrimation.

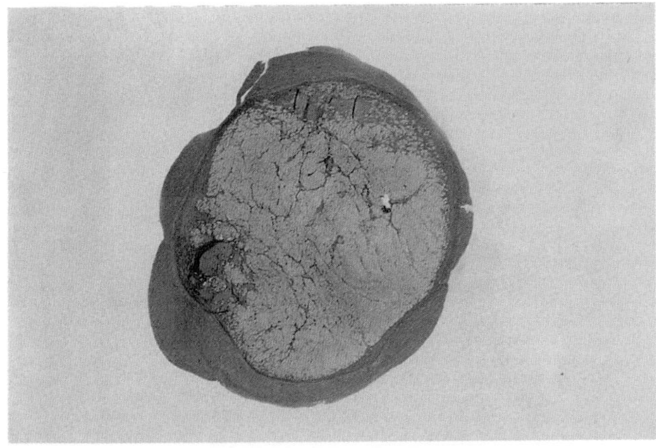

Plate 45.6 Photomicrograph of a cross-sectioned tricuspid papillary muscle from a patient with carcinoid heart disease. The carcinoid lesion completely encircles the central muscle. H&E staining.

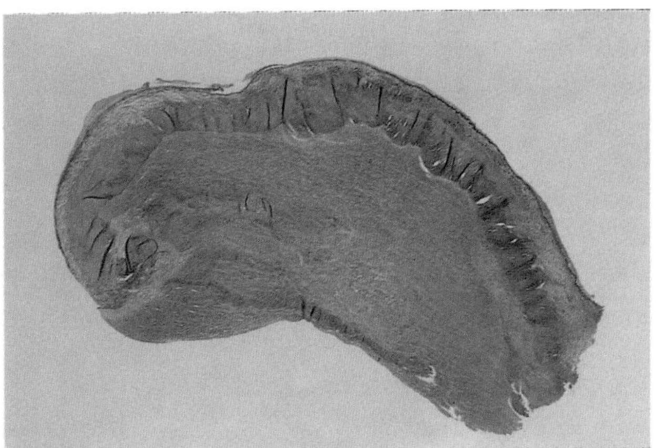

Plate 45.7 Pulmonary cusp with a typically curly thickened edge embedded in a thick carcinoid lesion. H&E staining.

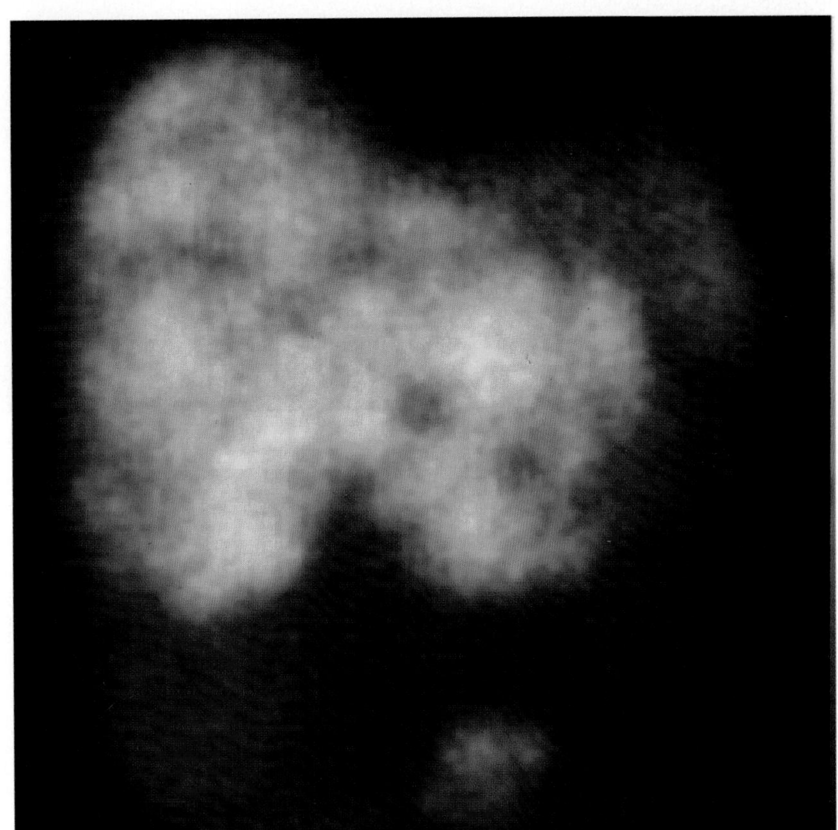

Plate 45.8 ^{111}In-DTPA-D-Phe^{1}-octreotide scintigraphy of a patient with a midgut carcinoid tumour and multiple liver metastases. (The picture is a kind gift from Assoc. Prof. J-E Westlin, Dept of Oncology, University Hospital, Uppsala, Sweden.)

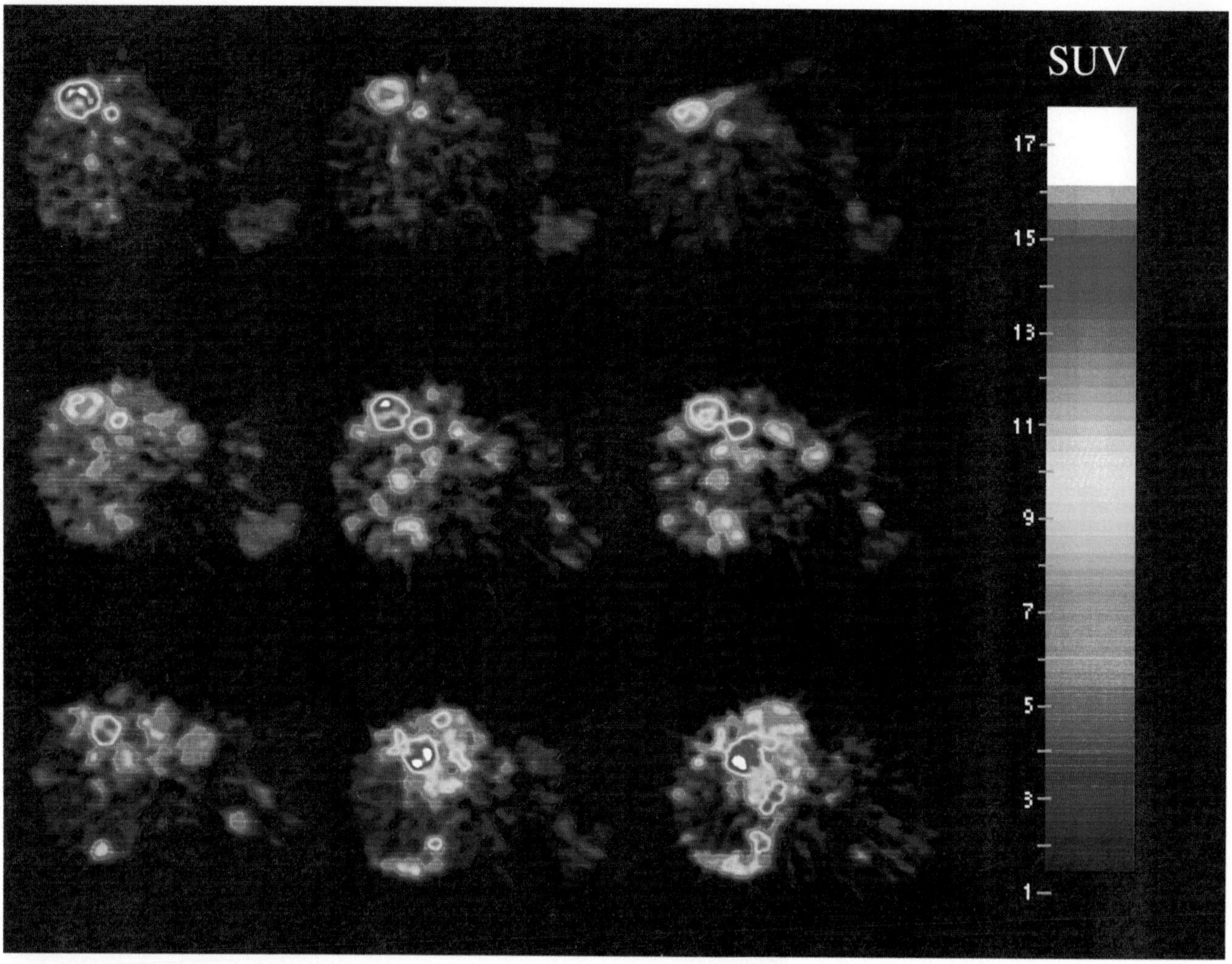

Plate 45.9 ^{11}C-5-hydroxytryptamin (5-HTP) positron emission tomography of a patient with midgut carcinoid and liver metastases. Sections through the liver during 36 months of follow-up. Notice the initial response to biotherapy which however only lasts for 9 months. Significant tumour progression is seen in the last two scans. (The picture is a kind gift from Assoc. Prof. Anders Sundin, PET-center, Uppsala, Sweden.)

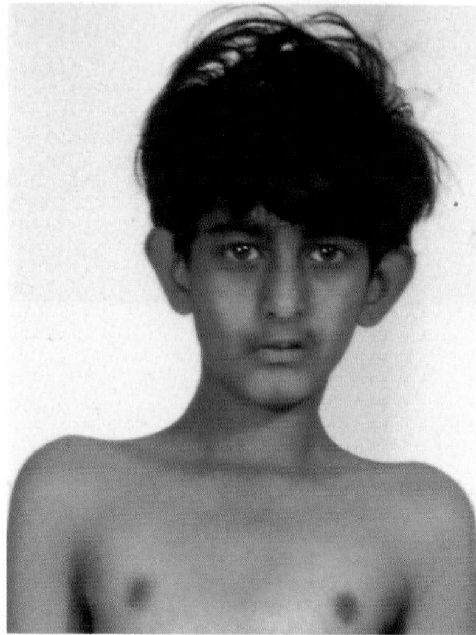

Plate 62.1 Boy with Russell–Silver syndrome showing the triangular shaped facies and body asymmetry.

Plate 63.1 Typical skin pigmentation in McCune–Albright syndrome.

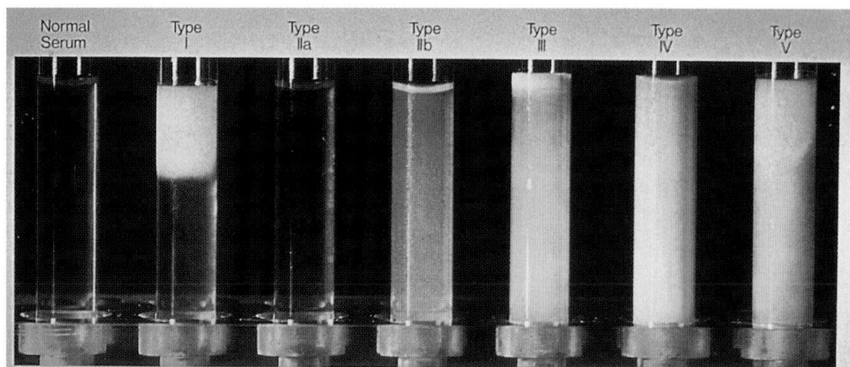

Plate 72.1 The Fredrickson classification of the hyperlipidaemias according to the appearance of the plasma.

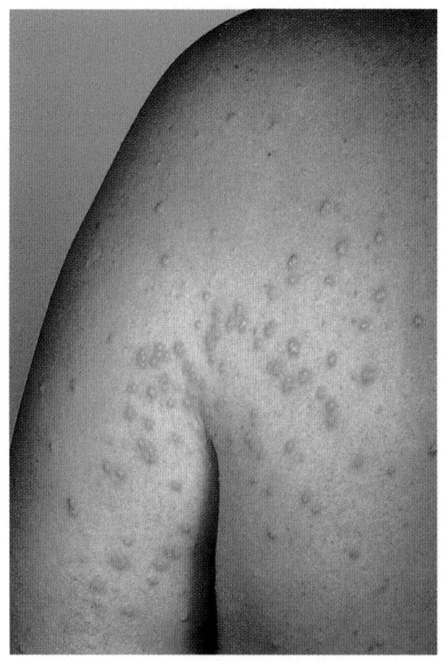

Plate 72.2 Crops of eruptive xanthomata over the skin of a patient with familial hypertriglycerideaemia.

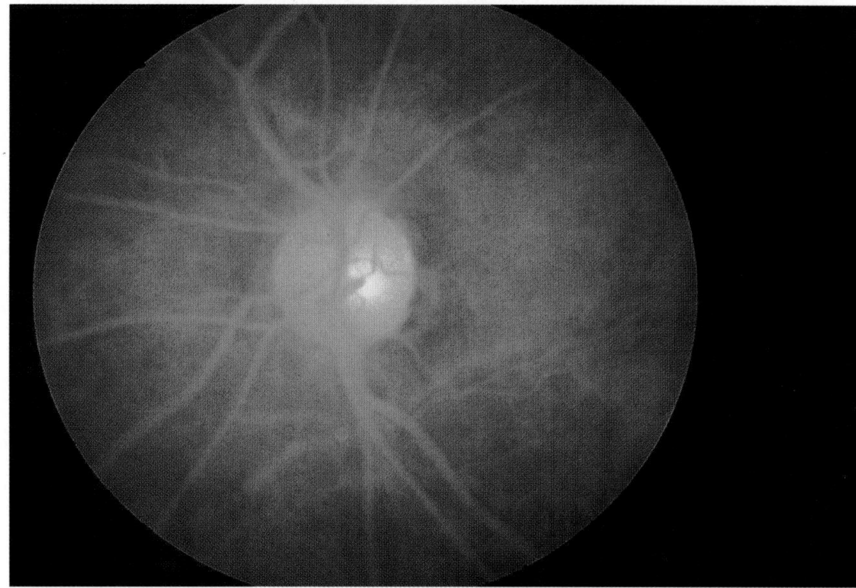

Plate 72.3 Lipaemia retinalis in a patient with familial hypertriglyceridaemia.

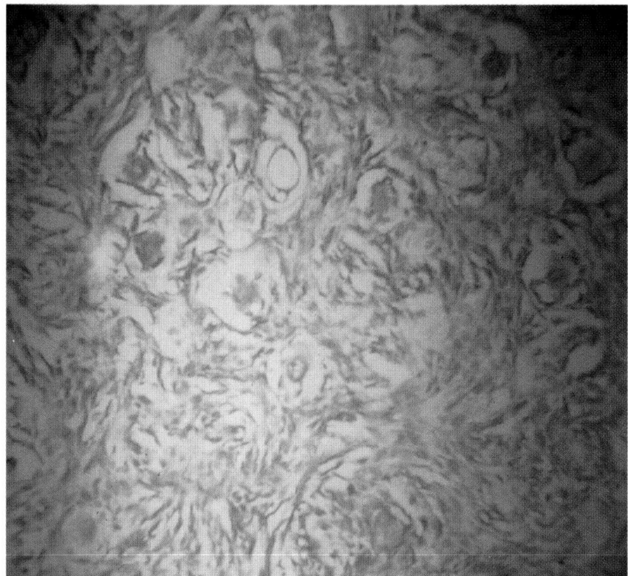

Plate 81.1 Reduction of primordial follicles in the ovary without siderosis in a thalassaemic patient with hypogonadism.

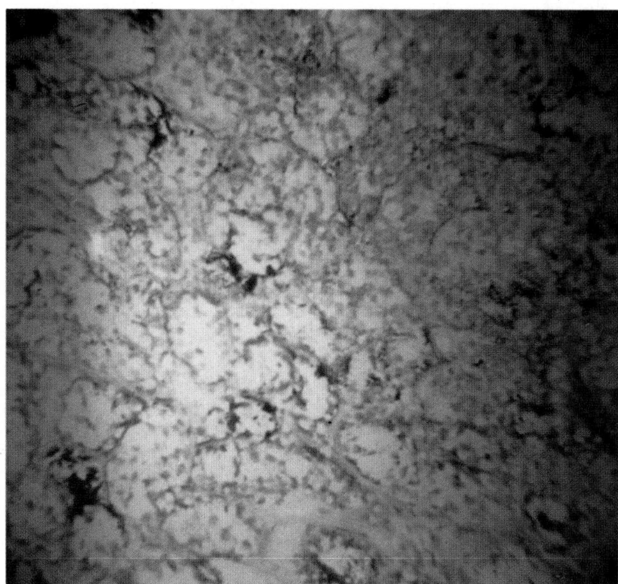

Plate 81.2 Heavy iron deposition in the seminiferous tubules and interstitial tissue in a thalassaemic male patient with hypogonadism.

thyroid results in the disappearance of TSH-RAb from the circulation. Other antibodies have also been described in relation to Graves' disease and may be of importance in thyroid-associated ophthalmopathy and thyroid-associated dermopathy (see relevant sections).

Antigen recognition and antibody production (Fig. 27.3) [12,16]

Antigen processing and presentation

Antibodies are produced by B-cells in response to antigen and to activated helper T cells. For this to occur, antigen must be 'presented' to the T lymphocytes in a form which they are able to recognise. Antigen is processed (broken down) in 'accessory cells' or 'antigen-presenting cells' (APC), such as macrophages, dendritic cells and B cells; the fragmented antigen combines in the APC with a protein molecule of the MHC, which is peculiar to the individual, and the complex of MHC molecule plus processed antigen is displayed on the cell surface.

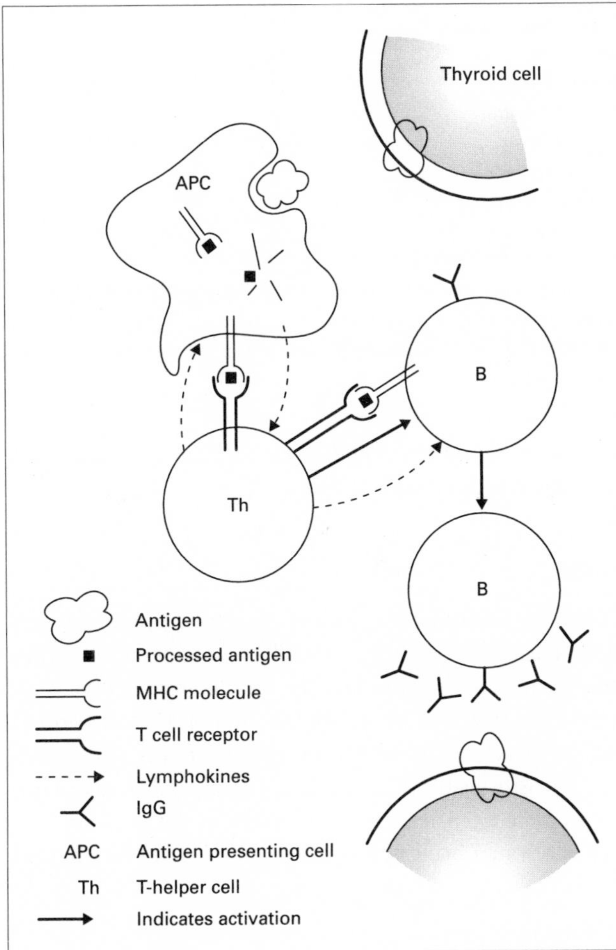

Fig. 27.3 Antigen recognition and T-cell activation, leading to antibody production.

T-cell activation

T cells are identified by their surface antigens, some of which are common to all T cells and others specific for certain classes of T cells. Cells which express the CD8 antigen are known as cytotoxic T cells and those which express CD4 are helper T cells. $CD8^+$ T cells recognise antigen combined with MHC class I molecules, which are present on most somatic cells. In contrast, $CD4^+$ helper T cells recognise antigen in conjunction with class II molecules, which are normally present only on APCs. T cells respond, through the T-cell antigen receptor (TCR), to processed antigen (a sequence of amino acids in the antigen protein chain, not the complete protein) only when it is complexed to the MHC molecule. When this occurs the T cells are activated to produce lymphokines (e.g. interleukin 2) which stimulate further T-cell proliferation, and also induce B-cell maturation and immunoglobulin production.

Importance of the MHC [17]

The MHC molecules are highly polymorphic and susceptibility to Graves' disease is at least in part a genetic trait consequent upon the MHC. Not all peptide fragments of a protein are able to bind to a given MHC molecule, and not all antigen–MHC complexes are able to induce a T-cell response. Thus, the MHC molecules confer selectivity on the immune response. This would be in keeping with the observation that Graves' disease occurs more commonly in individuals expressing B8 and DR3 molecules; but the binding of TSH-R peptides to DR3 β-chains, and the activation of helper T cells by these complexes, will require further detailed study before this can be explained on a molecular basis. Also, the correlation of B8 DR3 with Graves' disease is not particularly close and many individuals with this haplotype do not develop the disease.

Aberrant MHC class II expression

Class II MHC molecules are normally expressed on the surface of the APC. However, in Graves' disease, thyroid follicular cells also express MHC class II (DR and DP). This class II expression is not the primary event in the development of Graves' disease, but the mechanism by which it is induced is not known; however, *in vitro* interferon-γ is a potent stimulator of class II expression by thyroid follicular cells and this action is enhanced by TSH. Thyroid follicular cells may thus be themselves able, by virtue of this aberrant class II expression, to present antigen to T cells.

Antibody production by B cells

B cells carry immunoglobulin molecules on their surface which enable them to recognise a specific antigen. This elicits T-cell help and the lymphokines produced by activated helper T cells induce B-cell maturation and also the secretion of immunoglobulin molecules. In Graves' disease much of the RAb is produced by B cells actually within the thyroid tissue.

Strict conditions must therefore be met before auto-antibody production can take place: (i) antigen must be processed, and presented in association with MHC class II antigens by APC; (ii) the processed antigen–MHC Class II complex must be recognised by specific $CD4^{+}$ cells via the TCR, leading to T-cell activation; and (iii) specific B-cell clones, in turn, must be activated by T cells, in order to produce antibody.

Initiating events

The key question in the pathogenesis of Graves' disease is what triggers the development of the autoimmune process. Given the genetic susceptibility, Graves' disease does not in general have the characteristics of an inherited condition. The trigger factor in susceptible individuals may be infection with a microorganism [18] (*Yersinia enterocolitica* is one candidate) but convincing evidence for this does not exist. Other factors such as stress, sex hormones and thyroidal iodide levels may have a modulatory role in the induction of the immune response.

Stress or emotional trauma

Starting with Parry's original description, published in 1825, of what we now call Graves' disease, many have held that the initiating event may be stress related. Attempts to confirm this using scientific methods have suffered from the difficulty of comparing the effects of stress or trauma in two similar, genetically predisposed populations. However, it is known that psychosocial factors influence susceptibility to other conditions, such as infections and cancer; furthermore, stress leads to detectable changes in lymphocyte function. The effect of stress in the induction of the autoimmune response leading to Graves' disease is therefore still an open question but one which deserves an answer.

Clinical features (Table 27.3)

Hyperthyroidism

The characteristics of Graves' disease are hyperthyroidism, goitre, ophthalmopathy and dermopathy. The clinical features of hyperthyroidism are common to any condition in which there is an excess of circulating thyroid hormone, and have been described in detail above.

Table 27.3 Incidence of physical features in Waynes index in toxic and euthyroid groups. From [63].

Feature	Incidence (%)	
	Toxics	Euthyroids
Preference for cold	64*	34
Preference for heat	2	10
Increased sweating	73	62
Loss of appetite	23	28
Increased appetite	32†	8
Loss of weight	71*	49
Increased weight	5	16
Palpitations	61	60
Tiredness	84	80
Dyspnoea	64	54
Palpable thyroid	91†	58
Thyroid bruit	61†	3
Exophthalmos	43†	4
Lid retraction	32†	3
Lid lag	30†	3
Hyperkinesis	46†	11
Fine finger tremor	82†	41
Coarse finger temor	11	5
Hot hands	73*	41
Moist hands	57	40
Atrial fibrillation	2	1
Tachycardia		
>90/min	77	13
80–90 per min	21	58
<80/min	2	29

* Significantly more common in toxic group at 0.50 level (χ^2 with Yates' correction).
† Significantly more common in toxic group at 0.001 level (χ^2 with Yates' correction).

Goitre

Goitre or thyroid enlargement is almost always present in Graves' disease. It is typically a symmetrical, diffuse enlargement, without nodularity. Most commonly the gland is enlarged to about 30 or 40 g (about 3 or 4 times normal), but on occasion is greatly in excess of this. The gland may be easily visible (Plate 27.2, opposite p. 332), vascularity is apparent from increased pulsation in the neck and, on auscultation, a bruit is very often audible over the thyroid.

Ophthalmopathy

This is described in detail later in this Chapter. It is found in moderate severity in about 10% of patients with Graves' disease, severe in about 3%, and mild in approximately 60% of patients.

Dermopathy

Dermopathy is a rare accompaniment of the above features, occurring in around 3% of patients. It is closely associated with ophthalmopathy, with a high titre of TSH-RAb and often with recurrent hyperthyroidism.

Additional features

Features also found in thyrotoxicosis, when it is due to Graves' disease, include thyroid acropachy (see below), lymphadenopathy and splenomegaly. There may be additional evidence of autoimmunity, such as vitiligo or association with myasthenia gravis or with other autoimmune endocrine disorders.

Clinical history

At the time of presentation, symptoms will usually have been apparent for a few months, but the length of history varies from weeks to several years; the former usually indicates rather severe illness and the latter, chronic low-grade hyperthyroidism. Patients may present with any of the clinical features noted, of which the most common include weight loss, palpitations, heat intolerance, flushing and sweating, goitre, muscle weakness and menstrual change. In younger patients, the presenting symptoms are more likely to be those of weight loss with large appetite, or heat intolerance. In the older age group, cardiovascular symptoms predominate and patients may present with signs of cardiac failure or, more likely, complaining of palpitations, often associated with tachyarrhythmias. Enquiries should be made as to the presence of other autoimmune conditions. In addition a detailed family history should be taken with respect to thyroid disorders or other autoimmune diseases, such as type I diabetes mellitus, pernicious anaemia, Addison's disease, etc.

Clinical examination (Plate 27.2)

Typically, the patient sitting in the surgery will appear thin, nervous, hyperactive and unable to sit still without fidgeting. He or she may appear flushed, with a wide-eyed expression. The extremities will be warm and moist in contrast to the merely nervous patient whose hands will be cold and clammy. Palmar erythema should be noted and there may be changes in the nails of onycholysis or acropachy. The presence of a fine tremor can best be assessed by asking the patient to extend the arms and hands, spreading the fingers out, and then placing a sheet of paper on the fingers. The pulse rate will be increased, the volume full and its nature often bounding with a wide pulse pressure. Atrial fibrillation is a fairly common complication, particularly in older patients. On inspection of the neck symmetrical thyroid enlargement may be apparent and will be seen to move on swallowing; when palpated, this is found to be a soft smooth enlargement of both lobes. A bruit can usually be heard over the thyroid in these patients and this is a very useful diagnostic sign in Graves' disease, but must be carefully distinguished from a venous hum or carotid bruit. There is a hyperdynamic circulation, which may be suggested by obvious precordial pulsation and a systolic flow murmur in addition to the increased pulse rate. Lymphadenopathy, splenomegaly or hepatomegaly should be noted, but are unusual findings in Graves' disease. Proximal myopathy can usually be demonstrated even in those patients who have not themselves noticed muscle weakness, and is particularly found in the upper limbs. The lower limbs should be carefully checked, by palpation as well as inspection, for dermopathy, the favoured sites being the pretibial area, the back of the lower leg above the Achilles tendon, the dorsum of the foot and the dorsum of the great toe. Examination of the eyes will take note of widening of the palpebral aperture with lid retraction and lid lag, which are features simply of the hyperthyroid state and do not indicate ophthalmopathy; signs of ophthalmopathy itself must be carefully sought. Occasionally vision-threatening, congestive ophthalmopathy is present in the virtual absence of obvious inflammatory change and for this reason it is important always to examine the fundi for evidence of disc oedema and to assess the visual acuity. Hyperreflexia is commonly present and is on occasion associated with an increase in tone.

Cardiovascular complications [19]: these take the form of sinus tachycardia, supraventricular paroxysmal tachycardia, atrial fibrillation, and high-output congestive cardiac failure. With the exception of the first two, these are found much more commonly in older patients in whom the other features of hyperthyroidism may be inapparent. Therefore, in any patient with atrial fibrillation or cardiac failure of undetermined origin, hyperthyroidism should be excluded.

Diagnosis

Laboratory confirmation of the diagnosis of thyroid overactivity is made as described above (p. 330). However, before commencing treatment a definitive diagnosis of Graves' disease must be made, and other causes of thyrotoxicosis, listed in Table 27.1, excluded. Useful points should be noted in the history and physical examination. Nodular thyroid enlargement suggests that the thyrotoxicosis may be autonomous or secondary to Hashimoto's thyroiditis.

Table 27.4 Differentiation of different causes of thyrotoxicosis by laboratory tests.

	Antibodies to TPO or thyroglobulin	TSH-RAb	Isotope scan: Uptake	Isotope scan: Scan
Graves' disease	+	+	↑	Diffuse, symmetrical
'Hashitoxicosis'	+++	±	↑	Irregular
Post-partum thyroiditis	+	0	↓	Diffuse
Subacute or painless thyroiditis	0	0	↓	
Toxic multinodular goitre	0	0	Normal or ↑	Irregular with 'hot' or 'cold' nodules
Toxic adenoma	0	0		Single 'hot' nodule, reduced elsewhere
Iodine or T_4 ingestion	±	0	↓	

These results give a general guideline but exceptions will be seen from time to time.
TPO, thyroid peroxidase; TSH-RAb, thyroid-stimulating hormone receptor antibodies; T_4, thyroxine.
+, positive; +++, strongly positive; ↑, increased; ↓, decreased; 0, negative; ±, positive or negative.

Transient post-partum thyroid dysfunction, with a hyperthyroid phase, is remarkably common [20,21], complicating 10% or more of normal pregnancies; thus, an important question to ask is the length of time since the last pregnancy and, if less than 6 months, this possibility should be seriously considered. Subacute thyroiditis may readily be confused with Graves' disease, and here the clue is recent onset of a goitre associated with some local discomfort and tenderness. Painless thyroiditis on the other hand can only be differentiated from autoimmune hyperthyroidism by laboratory investigations. Hyperthyroidism may be precipitated by the recent ingestion of iodine or the use of iodine-containing contrast media, so this should be enquired after; it should be noted also that iodine-containing vitamin preparations are available over the counter in the UK. Secondary causes of thyrotoxicosis, though very rare, would be suggested by a history of previous trophoblastic tumour or of pituitary adenoma.

Laboratory tests (Table 27.4) will also be required to substantiate the diagnosis of Graves' disease (in addition to the tests used to confirm the diagnosis of hyperthyroidism).

Autoantibody tests

Autoantibodies to TPO, previously termed thyroid microsomal antigen, can be detected in about 90% of patients with autoimmune hyperthyroidism. As far as is known they are not pathogenic in Graves' disease, and they are not specific for Graves' disease, in that they are found in other types of autoimmune thyroid disease also. However, measurement of TPO antibodies in a patient with thyrotoxicosis is useful in that it points to the probability of an autoimmune cause. Thyroglobulin antibodies may also be detected, though rather less commonly; where these are present in high titre, the possibility of thyrotoxicosis due to Hashimoto's disease is suggested. The antibodies directed to the TSH receptor, which have thyroid stimulating activity, can be measured by their capacity to compete with TSH for binding to the receptor (TBII). For the routine diagnosis of Graves' hyperthyroidism the measurement of TBII does not offer any great advantage over that of anti-TPO antibodies, which with currently available technology is both simpler and cheaper. Measurement of TBII is useful in certain circumstances, such as pregnancy.

Radioisotope thyroid scan

Unless the diagnosis is obvious from the history and examination, for example a typical goitre together with ophthalmopathy, then a scan should generally be arranged in order to exclude other causes of thyrotoxicosis (see Table 27.1). Although radioiodine can be used for this purpose, ^{99m}Tc is usually to be preferred; it is cheap, quick and convenient, and gives good imaging with a low radiation

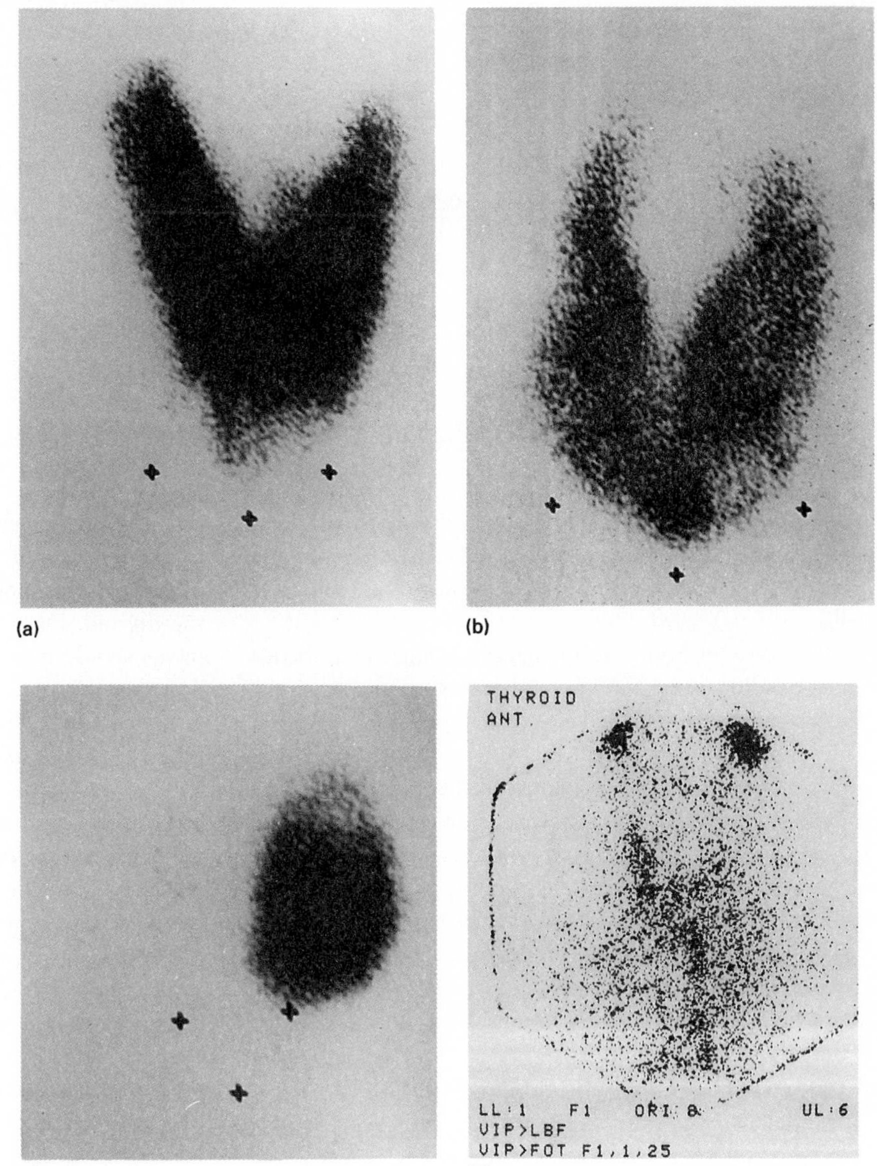

Fig. 27.4 Thyroid isotope scans. (a) Graves' disease; (b) toxic multinodular goitre; (c) solitary toxic nodule; (d) subacute thyroiditis.

dose to the patient as well as to the thyroid. Fig. 27.4a shows the typical thyroid enlargement with uniformly increased uptake, which is found in Graves' disease. This can be compared with the appearance found in toxic multinodular goitre (Fig. 27.4b) where the gland is also enlarged and uptake increased, but the distribution patchy and irregular; and with the appearance of a solitary toxic adenoma (Fig. 27.4c), where the increased uptake is confined to the area of the nodule, with the uptake over the remainder of the thyroid suppressed. Not infrequently, the radioisotope scan will demonstrate unexpectedly decreased thyroid uptake (Fig. 27.4d), when the most likely diagnosis is thyroiditis, but the other possibilities which should be carefully considered are iodine or thyroxine ingestion.

Cardiac tests

Where there is evidence of cardiac dysfunction, such as dysrhythmia, heart murmur or cardiac failure, electrocardiography, chest X-ray and sometimes echocardiography will be required.

Management of Graves' hyperthyroidism

The objectives of treatment of Graves' disease at the present time are to render the patient euthyroid as soon as possible and without the need for long-term drug treatment, to avoid the complications of treatment, and in particular to prevent the development or deterioration of ophthalmopathy. The

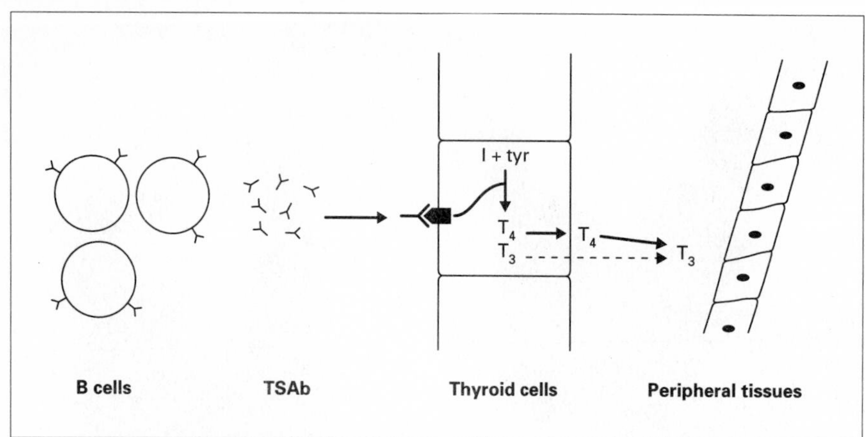

Fig. 27.5 The mechanisms which result in thyrotoxicosis. T_4, thyroxine; T_3, triiodothyronine; TSAb, thyroid-stimulating antibody.

management of the ophthalmopathy itself is dealt with in a later section. Current treatment is directed to correcting the hypersecretion of thyroid hormones by the thyroid follicular cells.

Objectives for future treatment, which must await better understanding of the autoimmune pathogenic mechanisms, must include prevention and the possibility of clonal deletion. The possible sites at which the disease process might be attacked are shown in Fig. 27.5. A further possibility is the inhibition of thyroid hormone action on peripheral tissues (e.g. with propranolol); this approach is sometimes useful as an adjunct to other treatment, but is unsatisfactory by itself in that it does not affect the hyperthyroidism.

The alternatives available for treatment of the hyperthyroidism are:

1 antithyroid drugs;
2 surgery; and
3 radioiodine.

Antithyroid drugs

The agents in use are carbimazole, methimazole and propylthiouracil, comprising the thionamide group of drugs. Their major action is to block thyroid hormone biosynthesis, which they do by inhibition of iodide oxidation and organification and by blocking the coupling of iodotyrosines to form T_4 and T_3.

Administration

In the UK carbimazole is the antithyroid drug of first choice and therefore the details of administration will be discussed with regard to carbimazole, but the principles apply to the other two drugs also. The usual starting dose is 40 or 45 mg daily given in divided doses, although in patients with very severe hyperthyroidism or with excessively large goitres a dose of 60 mg daily may be advisable. This should be continued until a euthyroid state is achieved, which usually takes 4–6 weeks, the delay presumably reflecting the amount of thyroid hormone already synthesised and stored within the thyroid. Once the patient becomes euthyroid, adjustments should be made to the dose schedule, which can be done in one of two ways.

1 Reducing the dose of carbimazole to a maintenance level of around 10 mg daily. If this is done the patient will need to be seen frequently for clinical and biochemical assessment and further adjustments to dosage made as appropriate. This method of using antithyroid drugs tends to cause fluctuations in thyroid status which are undesirable and it also necessitates frequent visits of the patient to the doctor.

2 The alternative is to continue with a high dose (e.g. 40 mg carbimazole daily), producing complete blockade of thyroid hormone biosynthesis, but to it add a replacement dose of T_4, which is usually 125 μg daily. This is the simpler procedure, demanding fewer visits of the patient to the doctor, leading to fewer fluctuations in thyroid status, and, according to recent evidence, the larger total dose of the drug resulting in an improved remission rate after discontinuation.

The length of time for which the drug is given varies from 6 months to 2 years or more. The remission rate can be improved to a small degree by prolonging the course of treatment [22]. Thus, in patients with mild disease where the expectation of remission is high, a 6-month course of treatment may be adequate, whereas in those with more severe disease 2 years is probably to be recommended.

The outcome of antithyroid drug treatment

When carbimazole administration is discontinued, approximately 60% of patients will continue to be in remission (Fig. 27.6). Those who relapse are most likely to do so early after discontinuation and the relapse rate later than 1 year after finishing a course of treatment is small. Bad prognostic factors [23] for relapse include large goitre or severe

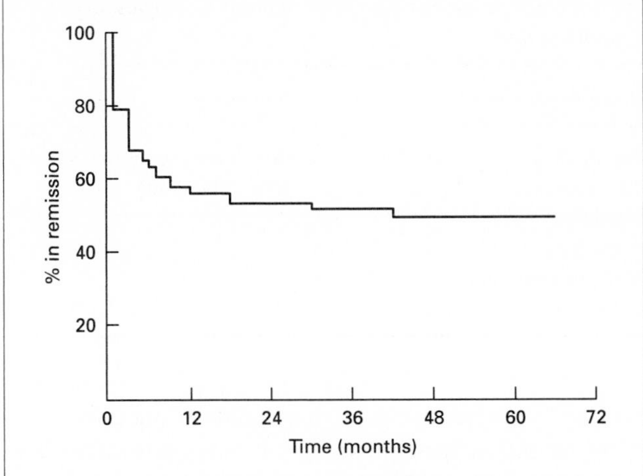

Fig. 27.6 The outcome of treatment with carbimazole in Graves' disease. Relapse of all patients. From [23].

hyperthyroidism at the time of diagnosis (Fig. 27.7a,b) and a very high level of TSH-RAb. In patients having these characteristics, it is sensible either to prescribe a long course of carbimazole or to recommend alternative treatment for the hyperthyroidism. It would be helpful if it were possible to determine precisely when drug treatment could safely be discontinued without fear of relapse; this has been investigated in some detail but there is no reliable way of determining this point.

During the course of drug treatment, measurement of thyroid hormones and clinical assessment should be undertaken periodically to ensure continued euthyroidism; after discontinuation of treatment, patients are seen at intervals (e.g. 2-monthly) during the first year, so that relapse can be detected early.

Why do antithyroid drugs induce remission? [24]

Since the action of the drug is to block thyroid hormone synthesis, and since the development of hyperthyroidism is due to the action of TSH-RAb, it would be expected that when the drug is discontinued hyperthyroidism would recur. That this is not usually the case is probably accounted for by the decrease in levels of TSH-RAb that occurs during treatment (Fig. 27.8). These drugs appear to have a local immunosuppressive effect within the thyroid, where most of the TSH-RAb is produced; whether this is a direct effect of the drug or mediated by some effect on the hormone biosynthetic pathway is not clear.

Indications

Indications for the use of antithyroid drugs are listed in Table 27.5.

Adverse effects

The commonest are pruritis and a rash, which is usually urticarial. These tend to occur early in the course of treatment and do not usually necessitate drug withdrawal. Other adverse effects which are less common include nausea, vomiting and arthralgia. The most important of the adverse effects are neutropenia and agranulocytosis. This is reversible if the drug is discontinued; therefore, it is mandatory to warn patients of the possibility and advise them that should a severe sore throat and/or febrile illness develop the drug should be discontinued and the white blood cell count checked. Other adverse effects result from overtreatment, causing symptoms of hypothyroidism, and, by virtue of increased serum TSH, an increase in goitre size. Carbimazole can be given with apparent safety during pregnancy (see below).

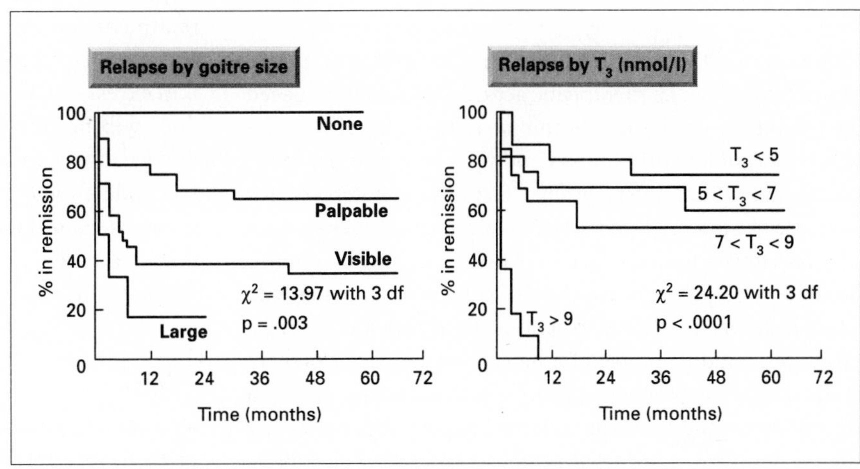

Fig. 27.7 Factors associated with the outcome of treatment with carbimazole. The graph on the left shows relapse by goitre size; the graph on the right shows serum triiodothyronine (T_3) at the time of diagnosis. From [23].

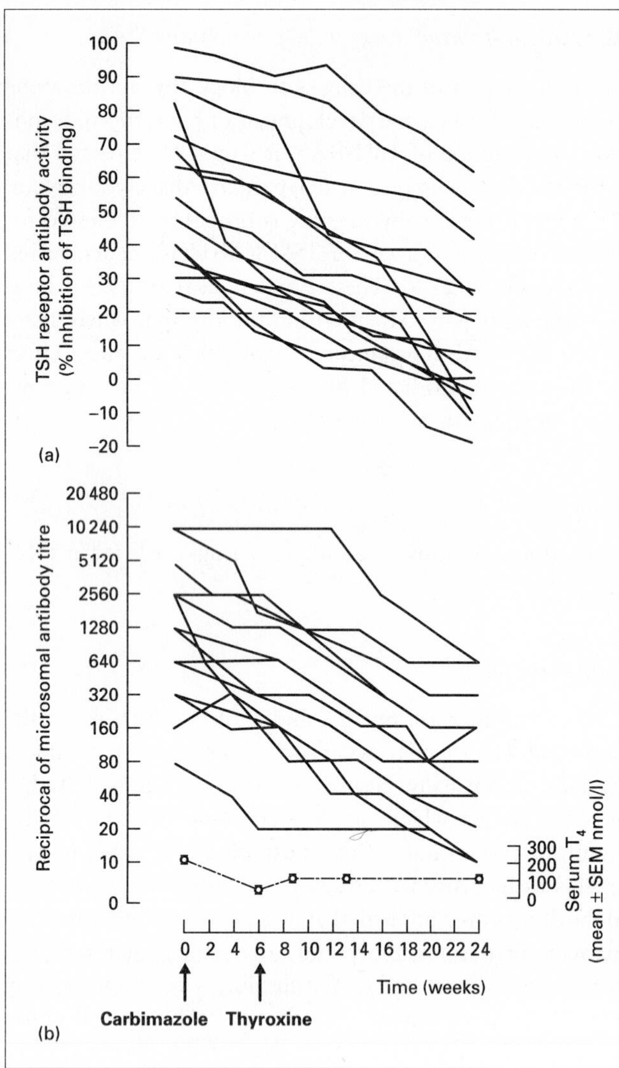

Fig. 27.8 Changes in antibody levels during treatment with carbimazole. From [61].

Iodine

Iodine is used only rarely now in the management of hyperthyroidism. Its therapeutic action is probably achieved by inhibition of thyroid hormone release. Its effects are achieved rapidly within hours and thus its major use is for patients in whom a very prompt response is necessary, for example treatment of thyrotoxic crisis, or emergency surgery in a previously undiagnosed thyrotoxic patient; it can also be used in preparation for thyroid surgery in patients who have developed adverse reactions to thionamide drugs. However, if iodide is given for more than a few weeks there is the danger of an escape phenomenon occurring in which thyroid hormone release is no longer suppressed, but rather there is increase in hormone synthesis and secretion. Iodine is given in the form of potassium iodide 15 mg three times daily, or the iodine-containing contrast material sodium ipodate can be used [25]. Lithium carbonate can be given in place of iodide in patients with allergy to iodine.

Table 27.5 Indications for antithyroid drugs for Graves' hyperthyroidism.

Definitive treatment	Adjunctive
Young adults	Preparatory to thyroid surgery
Juveniles	After ^{131}I therapy
Neonates	
Pregnancy	
Mild hyperthyroidism	
Severe ophthalmopathy	

β-Adrenoceptor-blocking drugs [26]

Propranolol is the β-blocker most commonly used for symptomatic treatment in thyrotoxicosis and it has some advantages over more selective agents. It acts at the level of the β-adrenoceptors on peripheral tissue cells and also blocks the conversion of T_4 to T_3, as well as having a direct effect on myocardium. Propranolol is used only as an adjunct to other forms of treatment which are directed more specifically at the thyroid itself; for example, in a newly diagnosed patient while awaiting a decision concerning definitive treatment, or to suppress symptoms pending a response to carbimazole or to radioiodine. It is particularly useful in patients with supraventricular arrhythmias due to thyrotoxicosis. It can also be used in an emergency situation, for example to prepare patients for urgent surgery or, together with other agents, in the treatment of thyroid crisis. It should not be used in patients with asthma or in pregnant patients; it is normally contraindicated in patients with heart failure but in those with thyrotoxicosis-induced high-output failure it may have a place, but only in conjunction with diuretic treatment and careful monitoring.

The dose of propranolol necessary to induce β-blockade is in excess of that required in euthyroid patients. The initial dose will usually be 160–240 mg per day, given either in divided doses or as a depot preparation; adequacy of β-blockade should be checked by measurement of exercise pulse rate and the dose increased as necessary. The average dose required in one series of hyperthyroid patients was 480 mg daily.

Surgery

Subtotal thyroidectomy is one of the most effective methods of treatment for hyperthyroidism due to Graves' disease.

A small remnant of thyroid tissue (approximately 8g of tissue) is left; postoperatively the majority of patients go into permanent remission and within the course of a few months the thyroid remnant becomes normal both functionally and histologically. Careful preparation of the thyrotoxic patient for surgery is mandatory, such that the patient is euthyroid and stable at the time of operation; if this is not done and the patient is hyperthyroid at operation there is then a risk of thyrotoxic crisis, which may be fatal. Carbimazole and thyroxine are given together until the day of operation and then discontinued; this procedure gives smooth perioperative control. Alternatives are the use of propranolol, in dosage adequate to produce demonstrable β-blockade (short-term treatment only), or iodine; neither of these agents given alone is satisfactory for routine preoperative treatment.

Postoperative complications are shown in Table 27.6. Hypoparathyroidism due to trauma to, or removal of, the parathyroid glands gives rise 1–2 days after surgery to tingling and numbness in the extremities or around the mouth, tetany and occasionally fitting; Chvostek's sign and Trousseau's sign should be sought and the serum calcium checked. Early postoperative hypoparathyroidism is treated with intravenous calcium gluconate, given by continuous infusion if severe. The problem usually resolves within a few days or weeks, but if prolonged maintenance treatment is necessary, a vitamin D analogue should be given. Laryngeal nerve damage causes vocal cord paralysis and it is wise to check the vocal cords before and after surgery. Haemorrhage into the operative site can be a serious complication causing respiratory embarassment and may necessitate surgical drainage and ligation of the bleeding site. Thyrotoxic crisis should be a thing of the past and will not occur when the patient has been adequately prepared and is euthyroid.

The results of surgery for Graves' hypethyroidism are excellent. Between 70 and 80% of patients can be expected to become euthyroid and remain in permanent remission. In the majority of these patients TSH-RAb have disappeared from the circulation by 4 weeks after surgery, which is in keeping with the contention that most of the TSH-RAb is produced by thyroidal lymphocytes. The incidence of recurrent hyperthyroidism is small, being about 1% per annum. The incidence of postoperative hypothyroidism is between 20 and 30% in most series; this relates partly to the amount of thyroid tissue removed, but probably depends to some extent also on the nature of the autoimmune condition. An early fall in T_4 level is of course to be expected but this is usually followed by a compensatory increase in TSH and ultimately return to normality of both serum T_4 and TSH (Fig. 27.9); T_4 treatment is only required if the patient is symptomatic.

Table 27.6 Complications of thyroidectomy.

Hypoparathyroidism
Haemorrhage
Laryngeal nerve damage
Thyroid crisis
Recurrent hyperthyroidism
Hypothyroidism

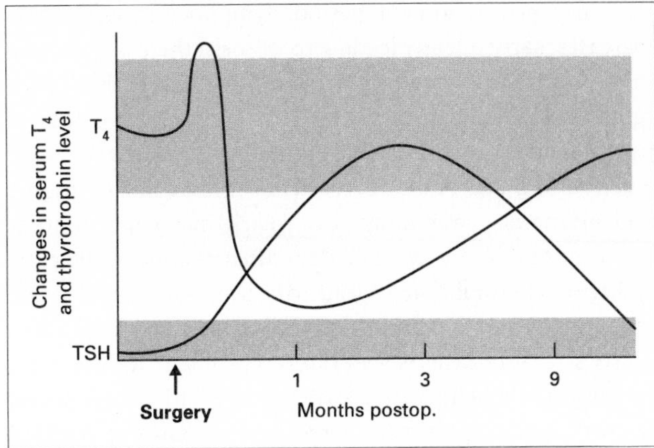

Fig. 27.9 The changes in serum thyroxine (T_4) and thyroid-stimulating hormone (TSH) which occur after subtotal thyroidectomy for Graves' disease. Shaded areas indicate normal ranges.

Indications for surgery

When it appears likely that a patient will not go into remission after a course of antithyroid drugs, surgery should probably be recommended early in the course of the disease, for example in those patients with a very large goitre or with very severe hyperthyroidism. Patients who have relapsed after an adequate course of antithyroid drugs may be offered surgery, although radioiodine therapy is an alternative. Thyroidectomy for Graves' disease should only be contemplated when an experienced thyroid surgeon is available, but where this is the case the results are so good in terms of long-term euthyroidism without the need for medication that patients should be given the option of surgical treatment.

Radioiodine therapy

Radioiodine is conveniently and effectively used to produce thyroid ablation by medical means; ^{131}I is the isotope used and, although others have been tried, there is no evidence that they offer any advantage over ^{131}I. ^{131}I has a destructive effect on thyroid epithelial cells which is progressive. In the early post-treatment period, lymphocytic infiltration increases, subsequently leading to fibrosis; there is reduction in the blood supply to the thyroid and also inhibition of cell replication. These features lead to a progressive loss of function and death of thyroid epithelial cells, such that over a period of weeks or months patients become first euthyroid and ultimately, over months or years, many will become hypothyroid. In the first 5–7 days after treatment, the early radiation thyroiditis may lead to a transient exacerbation of hyperthyroid symptoms, as well as to some increase in goitre size. While this is very rarely a problem, it should not be forgotten when treating patients with either very severe hyperthyroidism, or very large goitres causing tracheal compression. During the first few weeks after radioiodine treatment the titre of TSH-RAb increases reaching a peak at around 12 weeks, and subsequently declining, becoming undetectable by 1 or 2 years after treatment.

The two most important undesirable effects of radioiodine are the late development of hypothyroidism, or continued inadequately controlled hyperthyroidism; these result from the problems of dosimetry. Giving a large dose of ^{131}I leads to earlier and more profound destructive effects, with early hypothyroidism, whereas a smaller dose may result in inadequately controlled hyperthyroidism. Many studies have attempted to define an optimum dose which would result in early control of hyperthyroidism, and prolonged euthyroidism without the ultimate risk of hypothyroidism [27]. Unfortunately this has not proved to be possible, and it must be accepted that all patients treated in this way are at risk of developing hypothyroidism at some stage, the incidence increasing in a linear fashion with time (Fig. 27.10a). The physician thus has to choose whether to administer a dose of say 200 MBq, when patients may need to be monitored for years for delayed development of hypothyroidism, or whether to administer a dose of say 500 MBq, when the majority of patients will become hypothyroid within 6 months (Fig. 27.10b) and can then be established on T_4 replacement treatment.

Patients with very severe hyperthyroidism, in whom there is a small risk of thyroid crisis developing early after treatment, or patients with congestive cardiac failure due to the hyperthyroidism, should receive prior treatment with antithyroid drugs for 2 or 3 months to control the hyperthyroidism before the administration of radioiodine; this is because of the transient worsening of clinical features which may occur due to radiation thyroiditis, mentioned above.

Other adverse effects seen occasionally after radioiodine treatment are radiation thyroiditis, exacerbation of hyperthyroidism 3–10 days after therapy, mild hypoparathyroidism, presumably due to radiation destruction of parathyroid glands or interference with their vascular supply; also very occasionally, late recurrence of hyperthyroidism may occur in patients who have previously been rendered euthyroid.

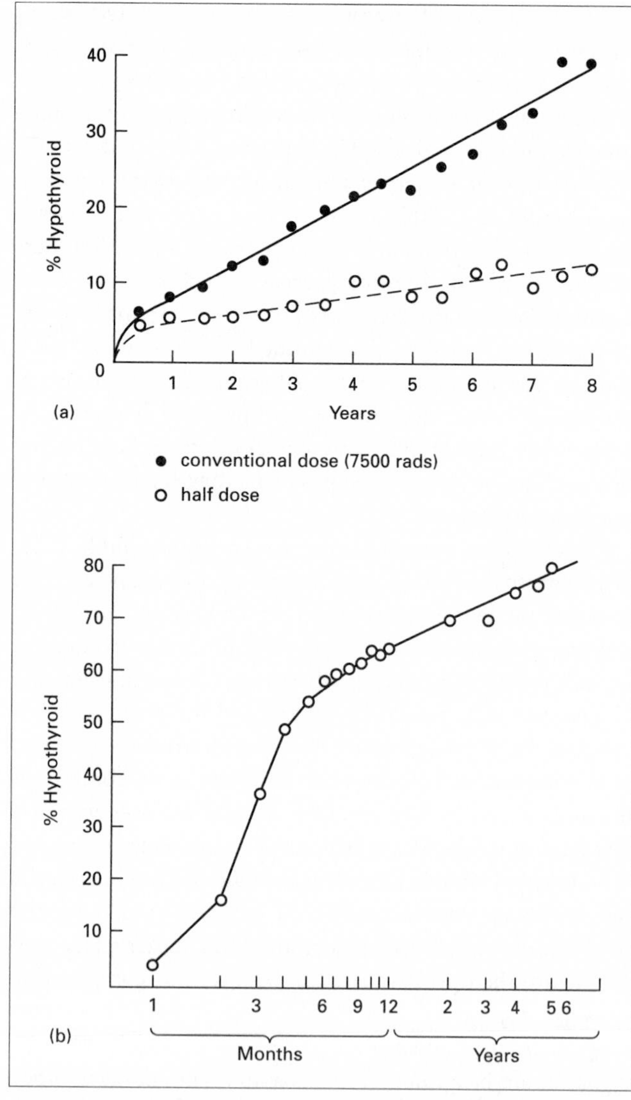

Fig. 27.10 The development of hypothyroidism after ^{131}I therapy in Graves' disease, (a) using a calculated dose to the thyroid of 7500 or 3250 cGy [27]; (b) with a dose of 15 mCi (550 MBq). From [62].

Radioiodine therapy should not be given to patients who are pregnant or lactating and it is wise for conception to be deferred for at least 6 months after treatment. This advice applies to men as well as women. However, there is no evidence for either a teratogenic or a carcinogenic effect of this treatment [28–30]. Despite this, stringent regulations were introduced in 1990 in the UK governing the use of radioiodine treatment. These have the effect of limiting the size of a single dose of ^{131}I which can be given to an out-patient. Contact with small children after treatment is restricted, which limits the usefulness of this form of treatment for patients in close contact with small children.

A further important point to be considered before administering ^{131}I is the presence of thyroid-associated ophthalmopathy (TAO). Several reports have commented on the deterioration in TAO which may occur within a few months of ^{131}I treatment, and in some cases ophthalmopathy develops *de novo* after treatment. There are still many unanswered questions surrounding this observation, but it occurs with sufficient frequency to recommend that ^{131}I therapy requires special care if TAO is recognised as a potential problem. Preventive measures which can be taken are either to reduce the dose administered at any one time, or to pretreat for a few months with carbimazole. In patients with established TAO, in whom there are good reasons for administering radioiodine, the risk of deterioration can be reduced by the use of steroids (in moderate dosage) to start a few days after the therapy dose, or administration of thyroxine 100 µg daily starting 2 weeks after therapy.

Indications for radioiodine therapy

Since this treatment is cheap, effective, convenient and relatively free of serious adverse effects, its use can be considered for the majority of patients with proven Graves' disease, excluding those who are:

1 pregnant or lactating;
2 have TAO;
3 very young.
4 It should be remembered that in a number of patients attending a thyroid clinic with hyperthyroidism and a small diffuse goitre, the diagnosis is in fact thyroiditis and not Graves' disease; in these patients destructive therapy for the thyroid is not appropriate. It is therefore to be recommended that a definitive diagnosis of Graves' disease be made before destructive therapy is prescribed, and this will in most cases require that an isotope thyroid scan be done.
5 Patients with mild Graves' hyperthyroidism are probably better treated with antithyroid drugs, since the likelihood of permanent remission is then high.
6 Patients with exceptionally large goitres in association with Graves' disease may be better treated by thyroidectomy, although the goitre size does eventually reduce after radioiodine treatment.

After noting these various points, the decision whether or not to administer radioiodine therapy to a patient with newly diagnosed hyperthyroidism becomes a matter of personal preference, which will be influenced by the local situation; for example, it will be recommended more frequently where there is no specialist thyroid surgeon available. In addition, radioiodine treatment is indicated for patients who have relapsed after thyroidectomy or antithyroid drugs and for patients in whom there is a contraindication to either antithyroid drug treatment or to surgery.

If it is considered advisable to control the symptoms of hyperthyroidism pending the outcome of radioiodine treatment, propranolol is effective, providing it is given in adequate dosage. If the patient has very severe hyperthyroidism, ophthalmopathy or cardiac failure, then carbimazole should be administered for at least 2 months before radioiodine treatment. Where an antithyroid drug is being taken by the patient, this will need to be discontinued prior to radioiodine administration (3–4 weeks if high dose, 1 week if low dose) to allow effective uptake of ^{131}I into the thyroid gland. Patients should be warned in advance of the requirement to restrict interpersonal contact and detailed written instructions will need to be given at the time of treatment. Further details regarding use of ^{131}I therapy in the UK can be found in [31].

Juvenile thyrotoxicosis

Graves' hyperthyroidism is infrequently seen during childhood and adolescence but deserves a special mention because of the different pattern of response to treatment. The clinical features are those of the adult, but in addition there may be an increased growth velocity, behavioural disturbance and declining academic performance.

Patients respond well to the administration of carbimazole, providing it is given in a manner with which the child is able to comply, but discontinuing the carbimazole after a course of treatment is most unlikely to result in remission. For this reason the recommendation to use carbimazole for a 1- or 2-year course is inappropriate for juvenile thyrotoxicosis, when carbimazole is best given continuously until the age of about 18 years. Attempts to titrate the dose of carbimazole against the clinical response are unlikely to be successful and it is preferable to give a fully suppressive dose of carbimazole together with a replacement dose of T_4. Furthermore, children are usually unable to comply with a thrice-daily dose schedule. The recommendation would therefore be to commence with a dose of carbimazole of 40 mg or 60 mg daily (the bigger dose to be given only to patients with very large goitres), to be given as a 20-mg capsule twice daily. Once the patient is shown to be euthyroid, which may take 4–12 weeks, T_4 is added in a once-daily dose of 100–150 µg.

Thyroidectomy is generally to be avoided for juvenile thyrotoxics because of the high frequency of relapse; if surgery is indicated, total thyroidectomy is preferable. Radioiodine therapy is also to be avoided in this age group because of the possible risk of carcinogenesis (theoretical rather than proven).

Thyrotoxicosis in pregnancy (see also Chapter 30)

Hyperthyroid women who are pregnant will quite frequently be encountered in a thyroid clinic; most of these patients will have been diagnosed previously and will already be taking carbimazole. A number of changes occur during pregnancy which have a bearing on thyroid disease.

1 Vascular changes—the blood volume is increased and there is also increased blood flow and vascular supply to the thyroid, which may become enlarged with an audible bruit.

2 The concentration of T_4-binding globulin (TBG) increases, so that the normal levels of total T_4 and T_3 are above that in the normal non-pregnant subject.

3 Iodine status—the thyroid iodine uptake and iodide clearance rate are increased and there is also an increase in renal iodide clearance, which results in some degree of iodine deficiency. These changes, which occur in the normal pregnant woman, give rise to clinical changes which can be mistaken for hyperthyroidism and in addition, because of the increase in circulating thyroid hormone levels, confuse the laboratory assessment of hyperthyroidism. Thus, in a pregnant woman not previously known to be hyperthyroid this diagnosis may be missed, or in a patient known to be hyperthyroid and receiving carbimazole it may be difficult to accurately assess her thyroid status.

4 A further feature of pregnancy relevant to Graves' disease is the immunosuppression which occurs naturally and has the effect of preventing rejection of the fetal allograft; this also leads to some suppression of autoimmunity, such that in Graves' disease there is a decline in titre of antibodies including TSH-RAb during pregnancy (Fig. 27.11) and a general tendency to amelioration of the hyperthyroidism, with a consequent diminution in the requirement for antithyroid drug.

5 Hyperemesis gravidarum in early pregnancy is sometimes associated with hyperthyroidism.

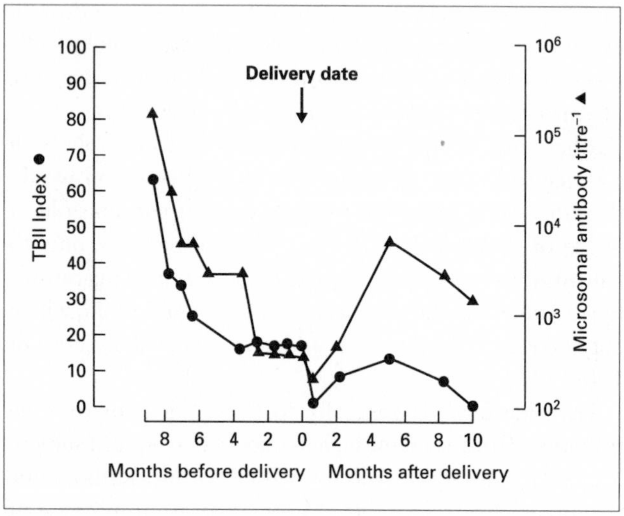

Fig. 27.11 Changing titres of thyroid microsomal antibody and thyrotrophin-binding inhibiting immunoglobulins (TBII), occurring during pregnancy and after delivery.

Treatment of hyperthyroidism in pregnancy

The role of the placenta in permitting access of drugs, antibodies or hormones to the fetal circulation (Fig. 27.12) must be remembered. Carbimazole readily crosses the placenta, so that after the fetal thyroid becomes functional at around 20 weeks of gestation, too high a dose of carbimazole can have adverse effects on fetal thyroid function leading eventually to goitre, and secondarily on fetal development. The amount of T_4 and T_3 crossing the placenta is very small and inadequate to counteract the carbimazole effect, although in early pregnancy maternal thyroid hormone does reach the fetus.

Treatment is best achieved with antithyroid drugs, but given in the appropriate dose and without the addition of thyroxine. Patients will need to be seen more frequently during pregnancy and, because of the difficulty in evaluating thyroid status, require clinical asesssment, measurement of thyroid hormones and TSH; the latter is probably the most useful of the tests to evaluate thyroid function in pregnancy. The dose of carbimazole is kept to the minimum required, avoiding hypothyroidism. When the third trimester of pregnancy is reached, by which time the fetal thyroid is

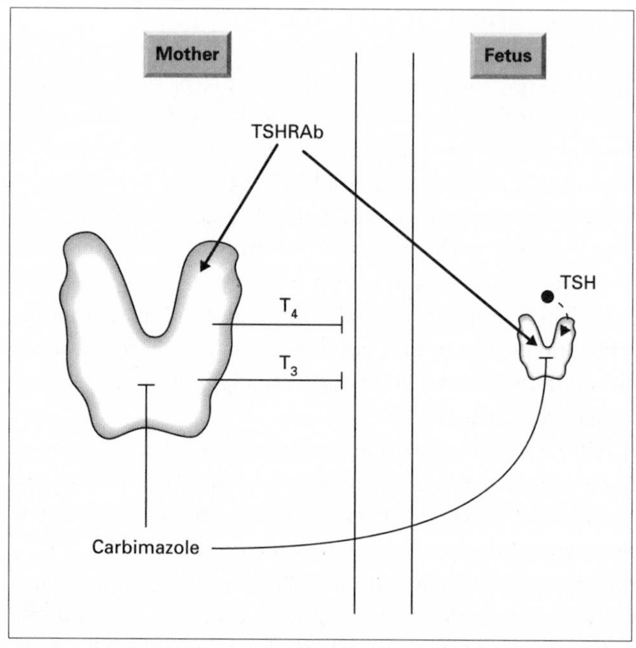

Fig. 27.12 The role of the placenta in relation to Graves' disease.

fully responsive to carbimazole, the dose should be further reduced and discontinued when possible to avoid the risk of neonatal goitre. Since there is often a tendency to remit during pregnancy, reduction or discontinuation of carbimazole dosage is rarely a problem. After delivery the naturally occurring non-specific immunosuppressive factors associated with pregnancy disappear within a few weeks and, probably associated with this, there is a tendency to relapse of hyperthyroidism within days or weeks post-partum, which is likely to be associated with recrudescence of specific antibodies. Patients should therefore be seen within a few days after delivery and regularly thereafter so that early relapse can be treated promptly.

Intrauterine thyrotoxicosis and neonatal thyrotoxicosis

Aetiology and prediction

In a woman with Graves' disease, present or previous, in whom there is a high titre of TSH-RAb, intrauterine fetal hyperthyroidism, and/or neonatal hyperthyroidism may develop. This results from the transplacental passage of the TSH-RAb stimulating the fetal thyroid (Fig. 27.12). The fetal pituitary and thyroid glands [32] are well formed by about 12 weeks' gestation but are relatively inactive; pituitary TSH secretion increases between 18 and 24 weeks, when the thyroid starts to respond, with a progressive increase in fetal thyroid hormone secretion occurring during the last trimester of pregnancy. Thus, from about 24 weeks on, it can be assumed that the fetal thyroid is potentially responsive to the action of thyroid-stimulating antibody reaching it from the maternal circulation. Whether or not a hyperthyroid state develops depends directly upon the titre of maternal antibody. Thus, the risk to the fetus, and hence the neonate, can be predicted by measurement of TSH-RAb in the maternal circulation, which should be done at the time of antenatal booking if the mother is known to have, or to have been treated for, Graves' disease. The measurement of TBII, which is routinely available, is adequate for prediction, but if combined with a measure of thyroid stimulation the predictive capacity is further increased [33].

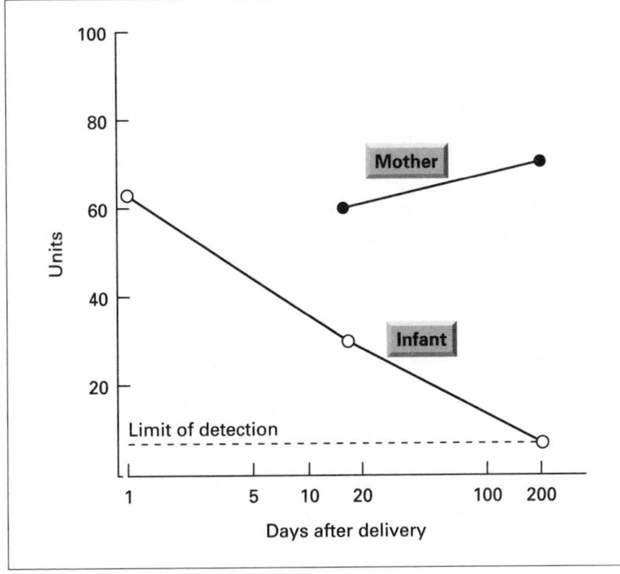

Fig. 27.13 Changes in TSH receptor antibodies (TSH-RAb) after delivery, in mother and infant.

Neonatal thyrotoxicosis is fortunately rather rare, occurring in about one in 70 of thyrotoxic pregnancies. It is unrelated to the maternal thyroid status; thus, one cannot assume that because a woman has been successfully treated for hyperthyroidism, her baby is therefore not at risk. The reverse may be the case; indeed, some of the babies most severely affected are born to women who have undergone successful thyroidectomy, becoming either euthyroid, or hypothyroid stabilised on T_4, but in whom the level of TSH-RAb continues to be high. This is particularly likely to be the case where ophthalmopathy and or dermopathy persist.

Clinical features

Intrauterine thyrotoxicosis

The possibility that the fetal thyroid may be affected should be considered from around the 28th week on. If the mother is receiving adequate doses of antithyroid drugs this is unlikely, but becomes more of a risk when the mother has previously been treated successfully for hyperthyroidism and may perhaps be taking T_4 replacement therapy. The main feature to watch for is fetal tachycardia and the fetal heart rate should be checked regularly. If the rate reaches or exceeds 160 beats/min it should be assumed that intrauterine thyrotoxicosis has occurred and appropriate treatment should be instituted. Other features which will probably be apparent are hyperactivity of the fetus and perhaps a small-for-dates baby.

Neonatal thyrotoxicosis

The features most likely to be encountered are tachycardia, hyperirritability and feeding problems. The birthweight may be a little lower than expected and there will probably be poor weight gain. Other features which may occur are tachypnoea, arrhythmia and cardiac failure. Stillbirth may occur in undiagnosed pregnancies and there is also a significant mortality in the early neonatal period.

If the mother has been receiving antithyroid drugs, the thyrotoxicosis in the neonate will probably not become apparent till 5–10 days post-partum. This obviously constitutes a danger since most post-natal patients will have been discharged home with their infants by this time. The reason for the delay can be construed from Fig. 27.12, illustrating the fact that carbimazole, like TSH-RAb, readily crosses the placenta; thus, hyperthyroidism in the infant only becomes apparent when the thyroid has recovered from the suppressive effects of the carbimazole. The TSH-RAb level in cord blood approximates to that in the maternal circulation; the half-life of maternal IgG in the neonatal circulation is of the order of 12–20 days; therefore, whereas the maternal TSH-RAb tends to rise in the post-partum period, in the neonate the level of TSH-RAb progressively falls and disappears usually by about 3 months (Fig. 27.13).

Some babies with neonatal thyrotoxicosis appear to have exophthalmos, but it is not known whether this represents a true increase in the bulk of orbital tissues, or whether it is simply due to lid retraction, secondary to the increased serum thyroid hormone. Clearly if the former, it would strongly suggest that thyroid-associated ophthalmopathy is an antibody-mediated condition. Enlargement of the thyroid gland is also found in neonatal thyrotoxicosis, indicating that maternal IgG can stimulate thyroid growth as well as thyroid hormone biosynthesis.

Laboratory diagnosis

Cord blood should be collected from affected pregnancies for measurement of TSH-RAb, T_4, T_3 and TSH. Some normal ranges are given in Table 27.7 and it should be remembered that TSH secretion increases dramatically within 30 min of delivery, gradually falling through the first week of life. Consequently, the secretion of T_4 and T_3 increases during the first week. In premature babies the levels of thyroid hormones are significantly lower than those shown here for full-term babies. It should again be remembered that if the mother has been treated with carbimazole until the time of delivery, then the cord blood levels of T_4 and T_3 may be low, but may rise into the thyrotoxic range during the following 4 or 5 days.

Table 27.7 Levels of thyroid hormones in the newborn. From [32].

	T_4* (nmol/l)	T_3* (nmol/l)	TSH (mU/l)
Cord blood	140 (85–225)	0.8 (0.2–1.3)	2.1–25
30 min			70–100
5–10 days			1–14
1–4 weeks	160 (105–210)	2.7 (1.5–4.8)	<20

T_4, thyroxine; T_3, triiodothyronine; TSH, thyroid-stimulating hormone.

* levels quoted are mean ± 2SD.

Prevention and treatment

In women at risk for the development of intrauterine thyrotoxicosis, antithyroid drugs may be administered from around the 28th week, even though the woman herself may not be thyrotoxic. The mother can be maintained in a euthyroid state by the simultaneous administration of thyroid hormone, only a negligible amount of which is able to cross the placenta. When antithyroid drugs are used in this way there is also a risk of hypothyroidism at birth; therefore it is probably best to reserve such treatment for cases where there is evidence, from the fetal heart rate, that intrauterine thyrotoxicosis is indeed developing. In the mother with active hyperthyroidism requiring treatment, in whom there is an unusually high titre of TSH-RAb, it may be wise to continue antithyroid drug treatment until parturition, rather than discontinuing it in the final month as would often be recommended. Following delivery the baby will need to be carefully observed during the first 2 weeks for the onset of hyperthyroidism and if treatment is required, carbimazole can be given in a dose of 1 mg 8-hourly (or 0.5 mg/kg/day). This can be withdrawn after a few weeks of treatment, the precise time depending on the severity of the hyperthyroidism and the level of TSH-RAb. If the baby is severely affected iodine can be given in the form of Lugol's iodine 1 drop 8-hourly. Propranolol can be used for tachyarrhythmias (1 mg/kg/day); digoxin and a diuretic may be necessary for heart failure. Sedation may also be indicated.

Providing the baby survives the initial thyrotoxic phase, the prognosis is excellent with spontaneous resolution occurring. These babies do not have an increased likelihood of developing Graves' disease in later life, compared with their unaffected siblings. However, it has been noted that they tend to be hyperactive during childhood (and possibly beyond) and short stature may also result.

Thyrotoxic crisis

This severe, potentially fatal disorder associated with hyperthyroidism has now become exceedingly rare in developed countries. It occurs in patients with untreated or inadequately treated hyperthyroidism, in response to stress factors such as infection, trauma or surgery. The clinical features which characterise it are: fever or hyperpyrexia, profuse sweating, tachycardia or tachyarrythmia, congestive cardiac failure, extreme nervousness, behavioural disorder or even psychosis on occasion, nausea and vomiting; later, the development of hypotension, coma and death occurs within a few hours or days. The onset is acute and the progress rapidly downhill so that the condition calls for immediate treatment.

Management is directed at counteracting the excess thyroid hormones and increased catecholaminergic activity, treatment of the precipitating condition and general supportive measures. *Iodide* produces the most prompt reduction in thyroid hormone secretion; it can be given as potassium iodide 15 mg every 4 or 6 hours by mouth, or specially prepared as an intravenous preparation; alternatively, ipodate (an iodine-containing contrast medium) can be given intravenously. *Carbimazole* is started at the same time to block further thyroid hormone synthesis (60 or 80 mg daily in divided dosage). *Propranolol* is given to block the conversion of T_4 to T_3, to counteract the peripheral effects of thyroid hormone and to block adrenoceptors and reduce cardiac effects; 80 mg 6-hourly by mouth may be adequate but more may be required. *Dexamethasone* is traditionally recommended but may not be necessary; it blocks conversion of T_4 or T_3 and may help to counteract the onset of shock. *Intravenous saline* may be required to correct salt and water loss, maintain adequate hydration and blood pressure. In patients with congestive cardiac failure, the use of propranolol and infusion of intravenous saline may not be appropriate, though this will depend on the aetiology of the congestion. Additional treatment with a diuretic and an antiarrhythmic may be required. In addition, steps should be taken to reduce the fever with aspirin, fans or wet packs.

Thyrotoxicosis from causes other than Graves' disease

Hashimoto's thyroiditis

Hyperthyroidism may occur during the course of Hashimoto's disease, characteristically in an early phase, and has been termed 'Hashitoxicosis'. This condition may be difficult to differentiate from Graves' hyperthyroidism, but, as it is self-limiting, it is of some importance to do so since ablative treatment is not required.

Clinically the hyperthyroidism will be indistinguishable from that of Graves' disease but the thyroid is more likely to be nodular, as determined by both palpation and isotope scanning. Ophthalmopathy is less likely to be present, but is not unknown in Hashimoto's disease. A family history is likely to be found, as it is in Graves' disease. Thyroid antibodies will be positive, but a high titre of thyroglobulin antibodies points to the greater likelihood of Hashimoto's thyroiditis rather than Graves' hyperthyroidism. TSH-RAb, as determined by TBII, may be present so do not distinguish this condition from Graves' disease.

Treatment

The hyperthyroidism of Hashimoto's thyroiditis is self-limiting; thus, the appropriate treatment is with the short-term use of carbimazole, or if the hyperthyroidism is very mild, propranolol alone may be adequate. Thyroid surgery is usually only considered in Hashimoto's thyroiditis if there is any suspicion of malignancy in a thyroid nodule. Radioiodine therapy is inappropriate.

Toxic multinodular goitre

Here the hyperthyroidism results from thyroid autonomy and not from stimulation by antibodies, nor by TSH. The aetiology is unknown but useful discussions of the subject can be found in [34] and [35]. A multinodular non-toxic goitre will often have been present for many years before the development of hyperthyroidism, which will probably have been of insidious onset. Patients tend to be older than those with Graves' disease. The symptoms of hyperthyroidism may be mild and fluctuating, but the condition frequently presents as a result of cardiovascular complications such as tachyarrhythmias or cardiac failure. The thyroid gland (Fig. 27.4b) will be irregularly and often asymmetrically enlarged with palpable nodules, sometimes with retrosternal extension and with tracheal compression. Thyroid autoantibodies are occasionally positive, probably coincidentally, but TSH-RAb are not found.

Treatment

Whereas carbimazole will suppress thyroid hormone synthesis and secretion, it cannot be expected to induce remission as it frequently does in Graves' disease, since the pathogenesis of the hyperthyroidism here is different. Therefore, carbimazole is useful only as a prelude to definitive treatment. Probably the most appropriate and effective form of therapy for patients with toxic multinodular goitre is with radioiodine, not forgetting that there may be an initial brief phase of increased gland size and increased thyroid hormone secretion. If the gland is very large then a dose of ^{131}I considerably in excess of 400 MBq may be required, and for convenience this may be better given as two separate doses. The ^{131}I will suppress hyperactive nodules but will have little or no effect on thyroid tissue which does not concentrate the isotope; therefore, as the treatment becomes effective, the previously non-functioning areas of thyroid will resume normal function, so that the expected response to therapy is euthyroidism rather than the hypothyroidism which is commonly seen with Graves' disease. However, this cannot be guaranteed and there is no alternative to long-term follow-up of such patients to ascertain that they continue to be euthyroid. After ^{131}I therapy the gland itself gradually regresses, although may remain palpably enlarged.

Solitary toxic adenoma

Again, the hyperthyroidism is autonomous and in some ways the picture in this condition resembles that of toxic multinodular goitre. In these patients the thyroid as a whole is not enlarged and the single adenoma may or may not be palpably enlarged. The underlying lesion is a follicular adenoma and patients not infrequently present with the complaint of a swelling in the thyroid, and are subsequently found to be mildly hyperthyroid. Alternatively, they may present with features of mild hyperthyroidism, which may be long-standing, and subsequently shown by isotope thyroid scanning to be due to a solitary adenoma.

Investigations show the changes associated with hyperthyroidism but with a tendency to 'T_3 toxicosis', i.e. an elevated serum T_3 with normal serum T_4. The TSH will be reduced, autoantibodies are usually negative and there is no association with TSH-RAb. The isotope scan shows an increased uptake in the nodule with suppressed uptake elsewhere in the thyroid (Fig. 27.4c).

Treatment

As with toxic multinodular goitre, carbimazole is not effective as definitive treatment, but is used in preparation for thyroid surgery. Definitive treatment can be achieved with either thyroid surgery (lobectomy) or with radioiodine. In the latter case the unaffected and suppressed part of the thyroid will eventually be restored to normal thyroid function as the nodule undergoes atrophy, so that the development of hypothyroidism and the need for T_4 replacement is unlikely.

A condition seen not infrequently is that of the 'warm nodule' in which the clinical features of hyperthyroidism are equivocal, the biochemical tests euthyroid but the scan shows a hyperfunctioning nodule with suppression of the remainder of the thyroid. The need for therapy is less apparent, but since the autonomous nodule will not remit spontaneously, once a clear diagnosis has been made, radioiodine treatment or surgery should probably be recommended.

Transient thyroiditis

As shown in Table 27.1 thyroiditis may have different aetiologies, but in each case may be associated with hyperthyroidism and in each case the hyperthyroidism will be transient.

Transient post-partum thyroid dysfunction [20,21,36]

Transient post-partum thyroid dysfunction occurs between 1 and 6 months after delivery. The patient may have a short-lived (a few weeks) hyperthyroid phase followed by hypothyroidism, followed by spontaneous resumption of euthyroidism; alternatively, but less commonly, transient hyperthyroidism may follow a hypothyroid phase, or the initial hyperthyroidism may resolve back to euthyroidism. The clinical features are misleading since the patient may have symptoms more suggestive of hyperthyroidism at a time when the tests indicate hypothyroidism. A family history of thyroid autoimmune disease is common. Thyroid antibodies are usually present, as also is a small goitre, but TSH-RAb are not present. The hyperthyroid phase is usually so short-lived that antithyroid treatment is not required. The condition is discussed in detail elsewhere.

A diagnosis of Graves' disease developing in the post-partum period has to be differentiated from transient thyroid dysfunction; this is done by isotope scanning (Table 27.4), which should of course be avoided if the patient is breast feeding. In Graves' disease, the isotope uptake will be increased (Fig. 27.4a), whereas in post-partum hyperthyroidism due to thyroiditis the isotope uptake is decreased as in Fig. 27.4d at the time when the serum T_4 and T_3 are elevated; in an ensuing hypothyroid phase isotope uptake is likely to be increased when serum TSH increases.

Subacute thyroiditis (De Quervain's thyroiditis)

Subacute thyroiditis is believed to be viral in origin. As with post-partum thyroiditis, there is frequently an initial hyperthyroid phase which is transient; this results from the inflammation causing release of preformed stored thyroid hormone into the circulation. Features of thyrotoxicosis may be present and are often relatively severe but of very recent onset. However, this is not true hyperthyroidism in that the thyroid function is in fact suppressed not increased, as can be shown by much reduced isotope uptake. The characteristic clinical feature of the condition is the pain and tenderness in the thyroid tissue. Apart from the symptoms that this disease causes, which may be considerable, its significance lies in the possible confusion with Graves' disease. Thus, all thyrotoxic patients should be asked about discomfort in the gland and subacute thyroiditis excluded for example by isotope scan, before arranging antithyroid treatment.

Painless thyroiditis

Painless thyroiditis is a very uncommon condition, at least in the UK. The features are identical to those of subacute thyroiditis, except that the thyroid is neither painful nor tender to palpation; thus, the potential for confusion with Graves' disease is greater. Again, the possibility can be excluded by an isotope scan. Antithyroid treatment is not required.

Iodine-induced thyrotoxicosis

The ingestion of iodine in excess of that required for normal thyroid function, or the administration of iodine-containing intravenous contrast media, can induce thyrotoxicosis [37]. This has been noted particularly in areas of iodine deficiency following the introduction of iodide supplements, but occurs also in areas of iodine sufficiency. Frequently these patients have had an underlying goitre, either nodular or autoimmune. In the former case, it would seem that a non-toxic multinodular goitre or solitary functioning adenoma is converted to the thyrotoxic state by the iodine, or, in the case of autoimmune disease, the iodine appears to unmask hyperthyroidism in a susceptible individual. On laboratory investigation thyroid hormone levels will be elevated, antibodies detectable if there is underlying autoimmune disease, and TSH suppressed, but the isotope scan will demonstrate reduced uptake of ^{99m}Tc or radioiodine. The diagnosis can be confirmed by measurement of urinary iodine excretion. Obviously a detailed history is required. In addition to the agents already mentioned, medicines containing iodine are used in some countries for treatment of chronic chest disease; in two recent cases of iodine-induced thyrotoxicosis seen by the author one followed angiography and the other was associated with an 'over-the-counter' vitamin preparation containing iodine.

Amiodarone

Amiodarone presents special problems [38,39]. This drug, which is widely used for treatment of cardiac arrhythmias, contains 37.2% iodine (75 mg of iodine per 200 mg tablet). It is fat soluble and accumulates in many tissues, having a very long half-life (40–100 days), so that its effect on thyroid function continues for weeks after it has been discontinued.

Diagnosis

Amiodarone has complex effects on thyroid function, making it difficult to assess thyroid status: it enhances TSH synthesis by a direct effect on TSH-α- and β-subunit gene expression; it competes with thyroid hormone for the thyroid receptor; it inhibits deiodination of T_4 to T_3; and it has β-adrenergic blocking action. Therefore thyroid tests are frequently abnormal in a euthyroid patient. More serious is the development of iodine-induced hyperthyroidism, which occurred in 20% of patients in one series. The clinical features in these patients are likely to be non-diagnostic. Serum T_3 is likely to be elevated and TSH reduced, but this is not invariable; T_4 is often increased in euthyroid patients so is unhelpful. Isotope uptake is suppressed by amiodarone, so this test is not indicated. Measurement of serum thyroglobulin may be useful to discriminate thyrotoxic from euthyroid individuals on this drug, but it has not been properly evaluated as yet.

Because of these difficulties, patients about to commence amiodarone should have their thyroid status assessed first, by examination for goitre, with measurement of T_4, T_3, TSH, thyroglobulin and thyroid antibodies. Those with goitre or thyroid autoimmunity are more likely than others to develop iodine-induced hyperthyroidism and in these patients amiodarone should be avoided if possible.

Treatment

There is no easy solution to this problem. If possible the amiodarone should be discontinued and alternative therapy given for the cardiac arrhythmia; even when this is done it is weeks or months before the hyperthyroidism resolves. Radioiodine therapy cannot be used because thyroidal uptake is suppressed. Thyroidectomy is generally contraindicated by the patient's cardiac condition and in any case cannot be undertaken while the patient is thyrotoxic. Thionamide drugs (propylthiouracil (PTU) may have advantages over carbimazole) are used but with less effect than in other thyrotoxic patients; they should not be given in combination with T_4 because amiodarone blocks conversion to T_3. Perchlorate might be the logical choice despite the risk of agranulocytosis: it has been used with variable response [40]. β-Adrenergic blocking agents in high dose can be considered. Corticosteroids may also be useful. The response to treatment can be monitored by measurement of T_3, TSH and thyroglobulin.

Thyrotoxicosis due to excess thyroid hormone ingestion [41]

This condition is most commonly encountered in the thyroid clinic as a result of overtreatment of hypothyroidism. The patient will have clinical signs of overtreatment, the serum T_4 and T_3 concentrations will be increased and serum TSH suppressed into the undetectable range. Occasionally thyroid hormone ingestion may come from unexpected sources, as in the recent epidemic of thyrotoxicosis which was attributed to hamburgers made from beef contaminated with thyroid tissue [42]. This was at first confused with painless thyroiditis, in which the clinical and biochemical features are indistinguishable, but clustering of cases has led to the true diagnosis.

Thyrotoxicosis secondary to stimulation by TSH

The finding of an elevated serum TSH in a patient with clinical features of hyperthyroidism and raised serum T_4 and

T_3 is always interesting. If an artifact of the TSH assay can be excluded then the possibilities of a TSH-secreting pituitary tumour or the syndrome of inappropriate hypersecretion of TSH should be considered.

TSH-secreting pituitary tumour

A TSH-secreting pituitary tumour is one of the rarest of the pituitary tumours. It may be associated with modest hyperprolactinaemia, amenorrhoea and galactorrhoea, and is usually a rather large tumour with often some intrasellar calcification. Investigations should include skull X-ray, measurements of prolactin and of other pituitary hormones including α-subunit, since this is secreted in excess giving a raised α-subunit : TSH ratio. TSH-secreting pituitary tumours are discussed in Chapter 15.

The syndrome of inappropriate TSH hypersecretion

This is a condition characterised by biochemical, but not usually clinical, thyrotoxicosis, with inappropriately normal or elevated serum TSH. It is due to thyroid hormone receptor resistance to stimulation by TSH, and is a familial disorder which usually follows an autosomal dominant pattern of the inheritance. In the original description somatic abnormalities were also present, but in subsequent families these have not featured. The degree of tissue refractoriness to thyroid hormone action is variable among different kindreds and in some a selective pituitary resistance has been noted.

In patients with generalised tissue resistance, clinical thyroid status will be either normal or hypothyroid, despite the elevated thyroid hormone levels. The elevated TSH results in the development of goitre. In the occasional patient with selective pituitary resistance hyperthyroidism results, again in association with a goitre. Generalised thyroid hormone resistance has recently been shown to be linked to the thyroid hormone receptor gene, TR-β; different mutations involving the T_3-binding domain may account for the variable phenotypes of thyroid hormone resistance [43].

Confusion may arise regarding the diagnosis and frequently patients will have undergone numerous attempts at normalising their thyroid function tests which makes interpretation of tests more difficult. It emphasises the importance of a good clinical assessment in the evaluation of laboratory results, and this is particularly so where raised thyroid hormone levels are associated with elevation of serum TSH. This condition has to be differentiated from TSH hypersecretion from a thyrotroph–pituitary tumour; thus skull X-ray and computed tomography (CT) scan of the pituitary are indicated. In thyroid hormone resistance the TRH test will result in exaggerated TSH secretion, whereas in a pituitary thyrotroph tumour the TSH response to TRH is usually, though not always, flat. The measurement of α-subunit is also helpful since TSH producing tumours result in an increase in the α-subunit : TSH ratio.

Reduction of secretion of thyroid hormone with antithyroid drugs or radioiodine is not appropriate for these patients, but surgery may be indicated for a large goitre. The TSH hypersecretion can be reduced by the use of corticosteroids, dopamine agonists or somatostatin analogues. A thyroid hormone analogue, 3,5,3′-triiodothyroacetic acid (TRIAC), which does not have thyroid hormone action on peripheral tissues, may effectively reduce TSH secretion. In the occasional patient who is hypothyroid, supraphysiological doses of T_3 may be appropriate. The response to treatment must be assessed by clinical examination and by tests of peripheral thyroid hormone action.

Trophoblastic tumours

Trophoblastic tumours such as choriocarcinoma or hydatidiform mole may be associated with secretion of a thyroid-stimulating factor, which is identical or very similar to human chorionic gonadotrophin (hCG) [44]. The clinical signs are those of mild hyperthyroidism with little or no thyroid enlargement and no evidence of thyroid autoimmunity. Laboratory tests show, in addition to raised T_4 and T_3, a marked elevation of hCG; TSH may be detectable but is unresponsive to thyrotrophin-releasing hormone (TRH). Treatment is directed to the causative condition.

Thyrotoxicosis from ectopic thyroid tissue

Gonadal teratomas may contain thyroid tissue. This should be remembered as a possible though very rare site of thyroid hyperfunction, for example struma ovarii.

Thyroid follicular carcinoma may accumulate iodine, and when metastatic deposits are present and functional, these may secrete sufficient thyroid hormone to produce thyrotoxicosis. These patients have also been observed on occasion to have associated ophthalmopathy. Treatment is with an ablative dose of radioiodine.

Thyroid-associated ophthalmopathy

TAO [45–47] is probably an autoimmune condition of the orbit which has been variously termed dysthyroid eye disease, Graves' ophthalmopathy or orbitopathy. It is closely associated with Graves' hyperthyroidism, though either condition may exist without the other. It may ante-date, coincide with or follow hyperthyroidism. Assessment of the frequency of the association depends on the method used for detecting ophthalmopathy; with sensitive methods subclinical ophthalmopathy can be demonstrated in 60–70% of patients with hyperthyroidism, whereas it is clinically apparent and moderately severe in about 10%. The clinical features of the disorder vary from a mild grittiness of the eyes to severe diplopia, loss of vision and disfiguring proptosis. The pathogenesis is poorly understood. Available methods for prevention and treatment are far from ideal.

Pathology (Plate 27.3, opposite p. 332) [47,48]

The most obvious pathological change within the orbit is the enlargement of extraocular muscles. In most cases microscopy reveals that the muscle fibres are preserved and the increase in muscle bulk probably reflects changes in the connective tissue: fibroblasts are very numerous and there is excessive deposition of collagen and of glycosaminoglycans, which lead to interstitial oedema. There is also some lymphocytic infiltration.

The muscles most frequently affected are the medial rectus and inferior rectus. Functionally the effect is of tightness (rather than weakness) or contraction of the muscles, and thus the patient may experience difficulty with upward or lateral gaze. The increased bulk of the muscles and of orbital connective tissue leads to an increase in pressure within the orbit, which results in some cases in proptosis, and in other cases, where the tissues at the apex of the orbit are involved, in optic neuropathy and disc oedema.

Pathogenesis

At the present time a clear account of the pathogenesis of TAO cannot be given [47]; much research is currently being directed to its elucidation, from which it seems likely to be multifactorial.

Gender

By comparison with hyperthyroidism, the moderate to severe form of the condition occurs rather more frequently in males, the sex ratio female/male, being 2 : 1, and in hyperthyroidism 7 : 1.

Age

By comparison with hyperthyroidism the age of onset is older, peaking in the 5th or 6th decade.

Genetic

As with hyperthyroidism there is a linkage with human leucocyte antigen (HLA)-B8 and -DR3. Linkage with the P1 blood group has also been found.

Cigarettes

There is a greater incidence of cigarette smoking among patients with TAO compared with either normal subjects or hyperthyroid patients without ophthalmopathy. The significance of this observation is not known.

Autoimmunity

The evidence that TAO is an autoimmune condition is based firstly on the pathological findings (characterised by lymphocytic infiltration), and on its close association with autoimmune thyroid disease; in addition, autoimmune responses to orbital tissues have been described. As yet induction of the condition by transfer of antibody or immune response cells has not been demonstrated and the responsible autoantigen(s) have not yet been characterised. The target tissues for autoimmunity may be the orbital connective tissue or the extraocular muscle fibres or both. Autoantibodies have been described which bind specifically to orbital fibroblasts or to antigen prepared from eye muscle. When IgG, purified from serum of patients with TAO, is incubated with either orbital fibroblasts or orbital myoblasts in culture, functional changes can be observed. This suggests that these autoantibodies have biological activity and thus may be pathogenic, but conclusive proof is not yet available. Lymphocyte-mediated cytotoxicity or antibody-dependent cellular cytotoxicity (ADCC) have also been proposed as mechanisms for induction of muscle damage, but there is no clear evidence of a cytotoxic effect on eye muscle *in vivo*. A role for cytokines in TAO seems likely: fibroblasts, muscle and lymphocytes all produce cytokines; it may be that the autoimmune response evokes the local production within the orbit of cytokines which cause fibroblast stimulation and hence the production of collagen and glycosaminoglycans.

Association with autoimmune thyroid disease

Although TAO is most commonly associated with active hyperthyroidism this is not necessarily the case. It may present many years before the development of hyperthyroidism; alternatively, TAO may develop some years after the treatment of hyperthyroidism when the patient is euthyroid and stable. There is thus no clear association with hyper- or hypothyroidism although either of these conditions may exacerbate the ophthalmopathy. Early studies suggested an association of TAO with antithyroglobulin antibodies, but this has not been confirmed. Ophthalmopathy is not a direct result of TSH-RAb activity; however, it seems likely that the autoantigens on orbital tissues would share common epitopes with TSH-R or other thyroidal antigens. This is an attractive hypothesis, which would explain the association with autoimmune thyroid disease, and for which there is some experimental evidence. More detailed discussion of autoimmunity and the pathogenesis of TAO may be found elsewhere [46,47,49].

Clinical features

In Plate 27.4a–d (opposite p. 332) are shown some of the clinical features of thyroid associated ophthalmopathy. Plate 27.4a illustrates the inflammatory nature of the disorder showing the periorbital oedema, conjunctival inflammation and oedema, as well as the muscle dysfunction resulting from involvement of medial and lateral recti. Plate 27.4b shows severe proptosis with inflammation localised over the insertion of the lateral rectus muscle, which is a characteristic feature; in addition, note that a lateral tarsorrhaphy has been performed to reduce the effects of the proptosis. Plate 27.4c shows a patient with long-standing, now quiescent TAO in which the major feature is the proptosis, which has been complicated by the development of corneal scarring with blindness in the left eye. Plate 27.4d represents the most dangerous form of the disease: inflammation is apparent though not severe, but proptosis is not obvious; this patient had marked loss of visual acuity in both eyes (optic neuropathy) with bilateral papilloedema, due to congestive or malignant ophthalmopathy.

The symptoms which patients may have noticed include: grittiness, soreness, or excessive watering of the eye, periorbital puffiness or conjunctival inflammation, double vision particularly on upward or lateral gaze, a staring appearance or protruberance of the orbit, discomfort on extreme lateral or upward gaze, and visual disturbance. Involvement of the eyes is often asymmetrical.

Clinical assessment

When examining a patient for possible TAO, the physical findings should be assessed in detail and graded, as shown in Tables 27.8 and 27.9. This will enable an accurate diagnosis to be made and, more important, will facilitate an accurate assessment of progress of the disease or response to therapy. Traditionally the NO SPECS classification has been used (Table 27.8), its main value being as a memory aid. In class 1, upper lid retraction and lid lag are not deemed to be features of ophthalmopathy, but occur simply as a result of excess circulating thyroid hormones. Features listed in classes 2–6 are associated with TAO; detailed measurements should be made in relation to each of these features where ever possible (Table 27.9). The proptosis is measured with an exophthalmometer, and the palpebral aperture can also be measured. Muscle dysfunction is assessed by: simple clinical examination, Hess chart, the field of binocular single vision and by applanation tonometry to measure intraocular pressure on forward gaze and upgaze (the differential between these two reflects the degree of muscle involvement). Visual loss (due to optic nerve involvement) is assessed by: fundoscopy, measurement of visual acuity (corrected), colour vision and visual evoked responses. Visual failure may also result from corneal opacity so exposure keratitis or corneal ulceration must be noted. A clinical activity score may be useful, and is based on the presence of retrobulbar pain, pain on eye movement, eyelid erythema, conjunctival injection, chemosis, swelling of the caruncle, and eyelid

Table 27.8 The NO SPECS classification of features of thyroid-associated ophthalmopathy.

Class	Definition
0	**N**o physical signs or symptoms
1	**O**nly signs, no symptoms (e.g. upper lid retraction, stare, and eyelid lag)
2	**S**oft tissue involvement (symptoms and signs)
3	**P**roptosis
4	**E**xtraocular muscle involvement
5	**C**orneal involvement
6	**S**ight loss (optic nerve involvement)

Table 27.9 Evaluation of features of thyroid-associated ophthalmopathy.

Class	Feature
2	Periorbital oedema
	Conjunctival oedema
	Conjunctival injection
	Injection of lateral rectus insertion
	Swelling of caruncle
	Eyelid erythema and oedema
3	Exophthalmometry
	Width of palpebral aperture
4	Intraocular pressure
	Primary position
	Upgaze
	Hess chart
	Field of binocular single vision
5	Corneal examination
6	Visual acuity (corrected)
	Distance
	Near
	Fundoscopy
	Colour vision
	Visual evoked potentials

oedema. It should be emphasised that visual loss due to optic neuropathy (congestive ophthalmopathy) can occur in the absence of severe superficial features of the disease, as shown in Plate 27.4d; thus, fundoscopy and measurement of visual acuity should not be omitted.

Diagnostic investigations

In most cases the diagnosis can be readily made by careful clinical assessment, done in conjunction with an ophthalmologist and noting the above-mentioned features. Additional investigations will be useful in the following circumstances.

1 In a patient with hyperthyroidism to determine if ophthalmopathy is present, or to assess its severity prior to treatment.

2 In a patient presenting with ophthalmopathy to determine thyroid status. In some 10 or 15% of patients presenting with features of TAO there is no evidence of thyroid dysfunction nor of thyroid autoimmunity. In these patients alternative diagnoses must be considered (Table 27.10). If none can be found or if the patient is euthyroid but with positive thyroid antibodies, then the diagnosis is deemed to be that of euthyroid Graves' ophthalmopathy.

3 To exclude other orbital pathology. This is important where there is no evidence of associated thyroid disease, and becomes even more essential where the orbital disease is unilateral.

Thyroid function tests

In the untreated patient the serum TSH will usually be suppressed into the hyperthyroid range. The introduction of highly sensitive TSH assays has superseded the need for TRH testing to detect subclinical degrees of hyperthyroidism. Serum T_4 and/or T_3 may be elevated before hyperthyroidism has become clinically apparent.

Table 27.10 The differential diagnosis of orbital disease with features similar to thyroid-associated ophthalmopathy.

Orbital pseudo-tumour
Orbital myositis
Vascular malformations
Granulomatous disease, e.g. sarcoidosis, Wegener's
Vasculitic diseases
Amyloidosis
Infection with microorganisms
Neoplastic disease
Lymphoma
Leukaemia
Primary carcinoma (e.g. ethmoidal)
Metastatic carcinoma

Detection of autoantibodies

The finding of autoantibodies to thyroid peroxidase or thyroglobulin is useful in the euthyroid patient, denoting the probability of autoimmune thyroid disease. TSH-RAb (usually measured as TBII) point to Graves' disease, although they have no particular significance with regard to TAO. Antibodies to orbital connective tissue or eye muscle have been studied, but their clinical significance is unknown.

Imaging techniques

Where available, orbital ultrasound may be useful diagnostically and also to evaluate the severity of eye muscle involvement. The more generally available techniques are orbital CT scan (Figs 27.14a,b) or orbital magnetic resonance imaging (MRI) scan (Fig. 27.15). These are particularly useful for diagnostic purposes where other orbital pathology, for example tumour, may need to be excluded; they also usefully demonstrate optic nerve compression at the apex of the orbit. The CT scan delivers a significant radiation dose to the lens, which if repeated constitutes a risk for cataract development. For this reason MRI is preferable, particularly if repeat scans are required to assess response to treatment.

Management of thyroid-associated ophthalmopathy

The aims of treatment of ophthalmopathy are to relieve the symptoms, to suppress the disease process, to decrease the bulk of the eye muscles and restore muscle contractility, and lastly but not least to improve the cosmetic appearance. There is as yet no treatment available which will reliably achieve these aims. Indeed, the condition can be difficult to treat, for several reasons:

1 the mechanisms involved in the development of the disease are not fully understood, so it is difficult to formulate a rational approach to therapy, apart from the general one of immunosuppression;

2 knowledge of the natural history of the condition, and of the factors which determine the outcome, is incomplete; and

3 there have been few properly conducted controlled trials of different treatment regimens, and where such studies have been performed the population studied is generally very small, making interpretation difficult.

Fortunately, in most cases the ophthalmopathy is mild and remits either spontaneously or during the course of antithyroid treatment, without the need for any specific treatment for the ophthalmopathy. Patients with severe disease should be seen in a centre with a major interest in this condition and with the collaboration of an ophthalmologist. The features of the disease should be documented carefully, as indicated

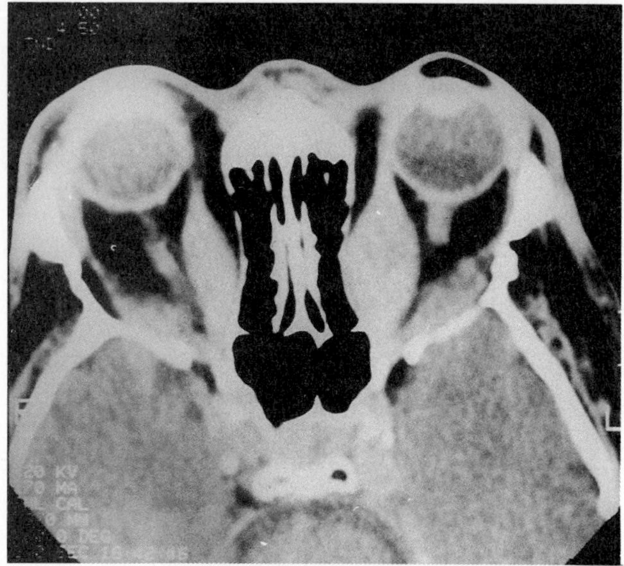

(a)

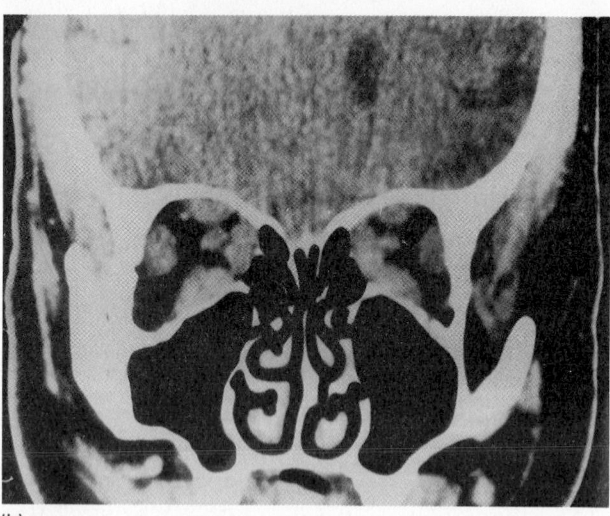

(b)

Fig. 27.14 Computed tomography scans of the orbit in thyroid-associated ophthalmopathy. (a) Axial plane scan: note the gross enlargement of medial rectus, also with enlargement of lateral rectus. Constriction at the apex of the orbit is seen, which resulted in severe optic neuropathy. (b) Coronal plane scan of a different patient, showing enlarged rectus muscles in cross-section.

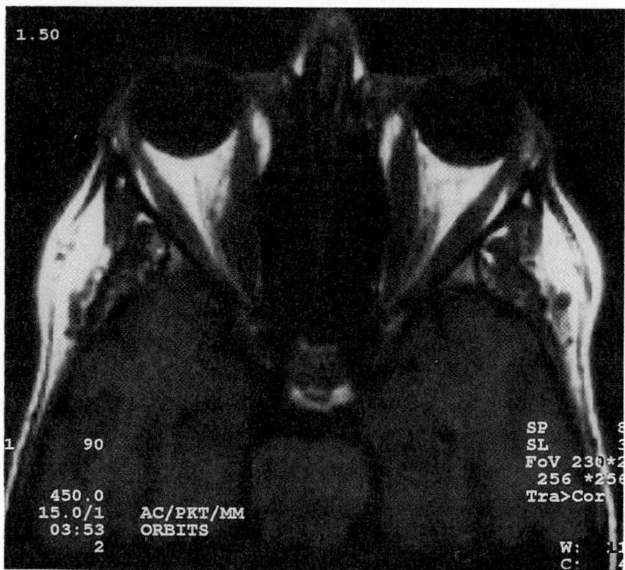

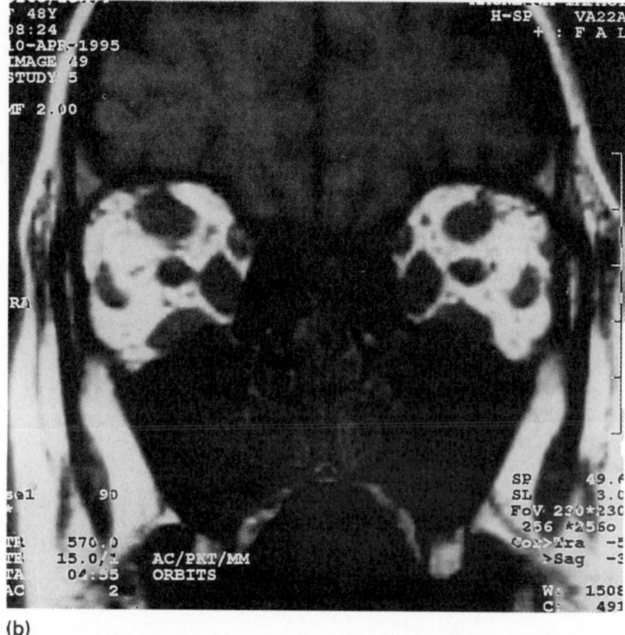

(b)

Fig. 27.15 Magnetic resonance imaging of orbits. (a) Axial plane; (b) coronal plane (same patient). Note enlargement of superior, inferior and medial rectus. There is crowding of the optic nerve at the orbital apex, mainly by the medial rectus muscle enlargement.

in Table 27.9, so that an accurate assessment can be made of response to treatment or deterioration.

The different aspects of the management of ophthalmopathy are summarised in Table 27.11.

Treatment of the associated thyroid disease

The patient should be rendered euthyroid as quickly as possible and fluctuations in thyroid status should be avoided. Some patients presenting with TAO are already hypothyroid, either occurring spontaneously, or as a result of previous treatment for hyperthyroidism; if this is the case then treatment with T_4 is simple, but overtreatment is best avoided. Most patients with TAO are hyperthyroid and the question then arises as to which method of treating the hyperthyroidism is most likely to prove beneficial to the ophthalmopathy. Treatment with *antithyroid* drugs, in patients with mild

Table 27.11 Management of ophthalmopathy.

Local
Methylcellulose eye drops
Prism lenses
Orbital irradiation
Thyroid
Antithyroid drugs
Surgical ablation
Immunomodulation
Corticosteroids (± azathioprine)
Cyclosporin A
Plasma exchange
Surgical
Tarsorrhaphy
Squint surgery
Eyelid surgery
Orbital decompression

orbital disease, is usually associated with some improvement in the eye signs. Although most physicians would agree with this general observation, it has not been studied in detail and it is not clear whether the carbimazole has a direct effect in suppressing the disease process, or whether the effect is mediated by the reduction in excessive levels of thyroid hormone. However, it is known that antithyroid drugs can at least partially suppress the immune response in the thyroid, and that the production of TSH-RAb within the thyroid is reduced. Thus, if the orbital disease results, as it may well do, from cross-reactivity with thyroidal antigens, this would represent one mechanism of action for carbimazole in improving ophthalmopathy. The place of total or subtotal *thyroidectomy* for treatment of TAO is controversial, but should probably be considered in patients with severe disease and large goitre, in whom other methods of treatment have not proved beneficial. *Radioiodine* may have a deleterious effect on ophthalmopathy [50] and therefore is better not used as first-line treatment for hyperthyroidism complicated by ophthalmopathy. Where it is considered essential, patients should receive a prior course of carbimazole. Prophylactic treatment with steroids, commencing 1–2 days after radioiodine therapy, may help to prevent the development or deterioration of ophthalmopathy [51]. The early use of T_4 (100 μg starting 2 weeks after therapy) is also beneficial [52].

Local treatment applied to the orbit

Methyl cellulose eye drops can be used to relieve the sensation of soreness and grittiness. Local steroid applied by the subconjunctival or retrobulbar route is occasionally used but there is no evidence for its efficacy. Orbital radiotherapy is effective treatment for patients with severe ophthalmopathy if given in conjunction with systemic corticosteroids. A dose of 2000 cGy is administered by linear accelerator or by a cobalt unit. Prism lenses are valuable for the management of diplopia, although once the condition has stabilised surgical correction would usually be undertaken.

Immunomodulatory treatment [53,54]

Corticosteroid drugs are the most effective for immunosuppression in TAO; a high dose (in excess of 60 mg daily of prednisolone) is required for immunosuppression and adverse effects are a disadvantage. Steroids are the first-line treatment for patients with severe ophthalmopathy, particularly where there is a threat to vision. They are most effective when given early in the course of the disease. After an initial dose of 80–120 mg per day of oral prednisolone, the dose can be reduced stepwise over the ensuing few weeks depending on the response, which needs to be monitored frequently by ophthalmometric assessment. Prophylactic potassium supplements and ranitidine may be given, and additional monitoring made of blood pressure, blood glucose and body weight. A maintenance dose of 10 or 15 mg per day may be required for several months.

An alternative approach, which may be particularly useful in patients with congestive ophthalmopathy, is the use of intravenous methyl prednisolone, given as 500 mg in 200 ml normal saline over 30–60 min, repeated on 3 consecutive days, and followed with oral prednisolone in reducing doses. High-dose steroids, whether oral or intravenous, should probably be commenced in hospital where the patient can be closely observed; patients with cardiovascular disease are excluded from the use of intravenous methyl prednisolone. One advantage of the intravenous regimen is the rapidity of the response in responsive patients; thus, if no response occurs within the first 3–4 days of treatment and if visual acuity is reduced, then referral for orbital decompression should be considered. Because of the risk of adverse effects, high-dose steroids should not be recommended for patients with mild ophthalmopathy.

Cyclosporin A may be a useful immunosuppressive drug in patients with severe disease who have a poor response to corticosteroids. This drug should probably not be regarded as a first-line treatment in that it has a wide spectrum of adverse effects, it is expensive, and it is probably less effective than prednisolone. However, it does have a place in resistant cases and may be useful in combination with prednisolone.

Plasma exchange has been tried but in general the results are disappointing and it is not without risk.

Each of the above methods is more likely to be effective if used early in the course of the disease. Other drugs which have been directed at the immune response include cyclophosphamide, azathioprine and ciamexone are not generally recommended, although azathioprine may have a place as a steroid-sparing agent. Optic neuropathy requires urgent treatment. Corticosteroids may be used first, but if there is no prompt improvement surgical decompression should not be delayed.

Surgical management

Orbital decompression [55–57] is usually carried out via the transantral transethmoidal route with removal of the ethmoidal sinuses and the orbital floor, which allows the orbital contents to herniate medially and downwards. There is a high incidence of complications after this procedure, the commonest being diplopia, which occurs in more than 50% of patients; others include numbness of the lip, nasolacrimal duct obstruction, cerebrospinal fluid rhinorrhoea, oroantral fistula and, rarely, blindness. The procedure is therefore reserved for cases of severe ophthalmopathy; indications include optic neuropathy with decreased visual acuity, and/or optic disc oedema, particularly if there is failure of response to steroids; it may also be indicated where there is severe proptosis associated with orbital pain or exposure keratitis. Orbital decompression is not usually performed for cosmetic reasons, but if the appearance of the proptosis and chemosis are exceptionally distressing it can be considered, though in the absence of diplopia it is probably best avoided.

Lateral tarsorrhaphy is a simple out-patient procedure aimed at reducing the degree of corneal exposure and improving the cosmetic appearance. Diplopia can be corrected by muscle surgery, but this should be deferred until the condition of the eye muscles has been unchanged for several months and the patient is euthyroid. Also, when the active phase of the disease has resolved, the possibility of cosmetic surgery may be considered: correction of upper or lower lid retraction, or of ptosis, or removal of herniated orbital fat may be beneficial.

In summary, whereas mild ophthalmopathy usually remits during treatment of the hyperthyroidism, moderate or severe ophthalmopathy may be difficult to treat. The following recommendations should be noted.

1 Patients should be evaluated fully by an endocrinologist working with an ophthalmologist, both of whom have special experience of managing this disease.

2 Patients with severe disease should be treated as early as possible in the course of the disease. Sometimes it is not clear whether the disease is severe enough to warrant treatment and in these cases a useful guide can be obtained by repeated ophthalmometric assessments, from which deterioration will be apparent and taken as an indication for treatment.

3 Patients undergoing treatment should be assessed accurately and frequently by objective criteria.

More detailed discussions of the treatment of TAO can be found in [47,57].

Thyroid-associated dermopathy and acropachy [58]

Dermopathy occurs in a minority of patients with Graves' disease, probably <5%, and is accompanied by ophthalmopathy in almost all cases and by thyroid acropachy in some. The dermopathic lesions are slightly raised, indurated and discoloured areas (Plate 27.5, opposite p. 332) occurring usually either on the lower legs (front or back), or on the dorsum of the foot or great toe. The lesions can often be detected more readily by palpation than by inspection, and they may also on palpation be tender. The term pretibial myxoedema refers to these lesions when they occur in the pretibial area, but since they occur with equal frequency in the other areas mentioned, the term thyroid-associated dermopathy is preferable. The term thyroid acropachy refers to finger clubbing associated with periosteal new bone formation occurring in patients with Graves' disease [59] (Plate 27.6 opposite p. 332).

Where dermopathy is present there is invariably a high titre of TSH-RAb. The nature of this association is not known, and the pathogenesis of the dermopathy is not known. Specific dermopathy-associated antibodies have also been described [60].

Treatment is indicated where the lesions are painful or tender, and is also appropriate where the swelling makes the wearing of shoes impossible. Local steroids are effective, given either by intradermal injection or by a topical steroid preparation together with an occlusive dressing.

References

1 Levey GS. The heart and hyperthyroidism. Use of beta-adrenergic blocking drugs. *Med Clin North Am* 1976; **59**: 1193–9.
2 Swanson JW, Kelly JJ, McConahey WM. Neurologic aspects of thyroid dysfunction. *Mayo Clin Proc* 1981; **56**: 505–12.
3 Kendall-Taylor P, & Turnbull DM. Endocrine myopathies. *Br Med J* 1983; **287**: 705–708.
4 Ramsay I. *Thyroid Disease and Muscle Dysfunction.* London: Heinemann, 1974.
5 McFadzean AJS, Yeung R. Periodic paralysis complicating thyrotoxicosis in Chinese. *Br Med J* 1967; **1**: 451–5.
6 Franklyn JA. The molecular mechanisms of thyroid hormone action. *Baillière's Clin Endocrinol Metab* 1988; **2**: 891–909.
7 Tunbridge WMG, Evered DC, Hall R *et al.* The spectrum of thyroid disease in a community: the Whickham Survey. *Clin Endocrinol* 1977; **7**: 481–93.
8 Doniach I. The thyroid gland. In: Symmers WStC, ed. *Systematic Pathology*. Edinburgh: Churchill Livingstone, 1978: 1975–2037.

9 Heimann P. Ultrastructure of human thyroid in thyrotoxicosis. In: *Thyrotoxicosis*. In: Irvine WJ, ed. *Thyrotoxicosis*. Edinburgh: Livingstone, 1967: 155–63.

10 Talal N. Autoimmunity and sex revisited. *Clin Immunol Immunopathol* 1989; **53**: 355–7.

11 Tiwari JL, Terasaki PI. *HLA and Disease Associations*. Heidelberg: Springer-Verlag, 1986: 214–20.

12 Jones DEJ, Diamond AG. The basis of autoimmunity: an overview. *Baillière's Clin Endocrinol Metab* 1995; **9**: 1–24.

13 Fisfalen ME, DeGroot LJ. Graves' disease and autoimmune thyroiditis. In: Weintraub BD, ed. *Molecular Endocrinology: Basic Concepts and Clinical Correlations*. New York: Raven Press, 1995: 319–70.

14 Parmentier M, Libert F, Maenhaut G *et al.* Molecular cloning of the thyrotropin receptor. *Science* 1989; **246**: 1620–2.

15 Vassart G, Dumont JE. The thyrotropin receptor and the regulation of thyrocyte function and growth. *Endocr Rev* 1992; **13**: 596–611.

16 Grey HM, Sette A, Buus S. How T cells see antigen. *Sci Am* 1989; **261**: 38–46.

17 Todd JA, Acha-orbea H, Bell JI *et al.* A molecular basis for MHC class II-associated autoimmunity. *Science* 1988; **240**: 1003–9.

18 Tomer Y, Davies TF. Infections and autoimmune endocrine disease. *Baillière's Clin Endocrinol Metab* 1995; **9**: 47–70.

19 Woeber KA. Thyrotoxcicosis and the heart. *N Engl J Med* 1992; **327**: 94–8.

20 Amino N, Miyai K. Postpartum autoimmune endocrine syndrome. In: Davies TF, ed. *Autoimmune Endocrine Disease*. New York: John Wiley & Sons, 1983: 247–72.

21 Fung HY, Kologlu M, Collison K *et al.* Postpartum thyroid dysfunction in mid Glamorgan. *Br Med J* 1988; **296**: 241–4.

22 Romaldini JH, Bromberg N, Werner RS *et al.* Comparison of effects of high and low dosage regimens of antithyroid drugs in the management of Graves' hyperthyroidism. *J Clin Endocrinol Metab* 1983; **57**: 563–70.

23 Young ET, Steel NR, Taylor JJ *et al.* Prediction of remission after antithyroid drug treatment in Graves' disease. *Q J Med* 1988; **66**: 175–89.

24 Ratanachaiyavong S, McGregor AM. Immunosuppressive effects of antithyroid drugs. *J Clin Endocrinol Metab* 1985; **14**: 449–66.

25 Shen DC, Wu SY, Chopra JJ *et al.* Long-term treatment of Graves' hyperthyroidism with sodium ipodate. *J Clin Endocrinol Metab* 1985; **61**: 723–7.

26 Utiger RD. Beta-adrenergic antagonist therapy for hyperthyroid Graves' disease. *N Engl J Med* 1984; **310**: 1597–8.

27 Smith RN, Wilson GM. Clinical trial of different doses of 131-I in treatment of thyrotoxicosis. *Br Med J* 1967; **1**: 129–31.

28 Dobyns BM, Sheline GE, Workman JB *et al.* Malignant and benign neoplasms of the thyroid in patients treated for hyperthyroidism. *J Clin Endocrinol Metab* 1974; **38**: 976–98.

29 Holm LE, Dahlqvist I, Israelsson A, Lundell G. Malignant thyroid tumours after iodine-131 therapy. A retrospective cohort study. *N Engl J Med* 1980; **303**: 188–91.

30 Saenger EL, Thomas GE, Tompkins EA. Incidence of leukaemia following treatment of hyperthyroidism. *JAMA* 1968; **205**: 855–62.

31 Royal College of Physicians. Guidelines for the use of radioiodine in the management of hyperthyroidism: a summary. *J Roy Coll Phys Lond* 1995; **29**: 464–9.

32 Fisher DA. The thyroid gland. In: Brook GD, ed. *Paediatric Endocrinology*. Oxford: Blackwell Scientific Publications, 1988: 309–337.

33 Tamaki H, Amino N, Aozasa M *et al.* Universal predictive criteria for neonatal overt thyrotoxicosis requiring treatment. *Am J Perinatol* 1988; **5**: 152–8.

34 Studer H, Peter HJ, Gerber H. Toxic nodular goitre. *J Clin Endocrinol Metab* 1985; **14**: 351–72.

35 Studer H, Peter HJ, Gerber H. Natural heterogeneity of thyroid cells: the basis for understanding thyroid function and nodular goitre growth. *Endocr Rev* 1989; **10**: 125–35.

36 Walfish PG, Chan JYL. Postpartum hyperthyroidism. *J Clin Endocrinol Metab* 1985; **14**: 417–47.

37 Vagenakis AG, Wang C, Burger A *et al.* Iodide induced thyrotoxicosis in Boston. *N Engl J Med* 1972; **287**: 523–7.

38 Franklyn JA, Davis JR, Gammage MD *et al.* Amiodarone and thyroid hormone action. *Clin Endocrinol* 1985; **22**: 257–64.

39 Himsworth RL. Hyperthyroidism with a low iodine uptake. *J Clin Endocrinol Metab* 1985; **14**: 397–415.

40 Newnham HH, Topliss DJ, Legrand BA, Chosich N, Harpir RW, Stockigt JR. Amiodarone-induced hyperthyroidism: assessment of the predictive value of biochemical testing and response to combined therapy using prophylthiouracil and potassium perchlorate. *Aust NZ J Med* 1987; **18**: 37–44.

41 Cohen JH, Ingbar SH, Braverman LE. Thyrotoxicosis due to ingestion of excess thyroid hormone. *Endocr Rev* 1989; **10**: 113–24.

42 Hedberg CW, Fishbein DB, Janssen RS *et al.* An outbreak of thyrotoxicosis caused by the consumption of bovine thyroid in ground beef. *N Engl J Med* 1987; **316**: 993–8.

43 Refetoff S, Weiss RE, Usala SJ. The syndromes of resistance to thyroid hormones. *Endocr Rev* 1993; **14**: 348–99.

44 Kenimer JG, Hershman JM, Higgins HP. The thyrotropin in hydatidiform moles is human chorionic gonadotropin. *J Clin Endocrinol Metab* 1975; **40**: 482–91.

45 Jacobson DH, Gorman CA. Endocrine ophthalmopathy: current ideas concerning aetiology, pathogenesis and treatment. *Endocr Rev* 1984; **5**: 200–20.

46 Burch HB, Wartofsky L. Graves' ophthalmopathy: current concepts regarding pathogenesis and management. *Endocr Rev* 1993; **14**: 747–93.

47 Perros P, Kendall-Taylor P. Thyroid-associated ophthalmopathy: pathogenesis and clinical management. *Baillière's Clin Endocrinol Metab* 1995; **9**: 115–35.

48 Hufnagel TJ, Hickey WF, Cobbs WH *et al.* Immunohistochemical and ultrastructural studies on the exenterated orbital tissues of a patient with Graves' disease. *Ophthalmologica* 1984; **91**: 1411–19.

49 Lamberg BA, Välimäki M. (eds) Advances in endocrine ophthalmopathy of Graves' disease. *Acta Endocrinol* 1989; **121**(Suppl. 2).

50 Tallstedt L, Lundell G, Törring O *et al.* Occurrence of ophthalmopathy after treatment for Graves' hyperthyroidism. *N Engl J Med* 1992; **326**: 1733–8.

51 Bartalena L, Marcocci C, Chiovato M *et al.* Orbital cobalt irradiation combined with systemic corticosteroids for Graves' ophthalmopathy: comparison with systemic corticosteroids alone. *J Clin Endocrinol Metab* 1983; **56**: 1139–44.

52 Tallstedt L, Lundell G, Blomgren H, Bring J. Does early administration of thyroxine reduce the development of Graves' ophthalmopathy after radioiodine treatment. *Eur J Endocrinol* 1994; **130**: 494–7.

53 Prummel MF, Mourits MP, Berghout A *et al.* Prednisone and cyclosporine in the treatment of severe Graves' ophthalmopathy. *N Engl J Med* 1989; **321**: 1353–9.

54 Wiersinga WM. Immunosuppressive treatment of Graves'

ophthalmopathy. *Thyroid* 1992; **2**: 229–33.

55 Grahne B, Lamberg BA, Rinne J *et al*. Transantral orbital decompression in the treatment of Graves' disease. *J Laryngol Otol* 1985; **99**: 865–70.

56 Garrity JA, Fatourechi V, Bergstrach EJ *et al*. Results of transantral orbital decompression in 428 patients with severe Graves' ophthalmopathy. *Am J Med* 1993; **116**: 533–47.

57 Gorman CA, Waller RR, Dyer JA. *The Eye and Orbit in Thyroid Disease*. New York: Raven Press, 1984.

58 Smith TJ, Bahn RS, Gorman CA. Connective tissue, glycosaminoglycans and diseases of the thyroid. *Endocr Rev* 1989; **10**: 366–91.

59 Gimlette TMD. Thyroid acropachy. *Lancet* 1960; **i**: 22–4.

60 Tao TW, Leu SL, Kriss JP. Biological activity of autoantibodies associated with Graves' dermopathy. *J Clin Endocrinol Metab* 1989; **69**: 90–9.

61 McGregor AM, Petersen MM, McLachlan SM, Rooke P, Rees Smith B, Hall R. Carbimazole and the autoimmune response in Graves' disease. *N Engl J Med* 1980; **303**: 302–7.

62 Kendall-Taylor P, Keir M, Ross WM. Longterm follow up of treatment of hyperthyroidism with an ablative dose of radioiodine. *Br Med J* 1984; **289**: 361–3.

63 Gurney C, Hall R, Harper M, Owen SG, Roth M, Smart GA. Newcastle thyrotoxicosis index. *Lancet* 1970; **ii**: 1275–8.

CHAPTER 28

Thyroid carcinoma

F. Pacini and L.J. De Groot

Introduction

Thyroid carcinoma, although representing no more than 1% of all cancers, is the most common malignancy of the endocrine glands. Cancers of the follicular thyroid epithelium include papillary and follicular histotypes, usually referred to as 'differentiated thyroid carcinomas', and undifferentiated (or anaplastic) carcinoma. Those of the parafollicular epithelium (the C cells) are represented by medullary thyroid carcinoma, in its sporadic or hereditary form. Much less frequent malignancies of the thyroid are sarcomas, lymphomas and metastases from other cancers. Because of the peculiar biological, pathogenetic and clinical features associated with the tumours of the follicular and parafollicular epithelium, these two entities will be reviewed separately.

Thyroid carcinoma of the follicular epithelium

Incidence

The estimated incidence of thyroid nodules is of about one per 1000 persons per year, and that of thyroid carcinoma is of approximately three to four per 100 000 persons per year. Thus, 3–4% of patients with thyroid nodules have thyroid cancer. Although this figure seems to reflect well the incidence of clinically important thyroid carcinomas, several geographical and environmental factors contribute to generating confusion over the true incidence of thyroid carcinoma. First of all, the continuous improvement of diagnostic methods, mainly ultrasound and fine-needle aspiration cytology, increase the discovery of minimal thyroid carcinomas, which might have been biologically unimportant, as demonstrated in autopsy studies. Similarly, accurate pathological examination of resected multinodular goitres, frequent in areas of iodine deficiency, is able to detect many occult tumours which, again, might be of no relevance from the clinical point of view. The presence of these tumours makes it difficult to define the true incidence of thyroid carcinoma. Thyroid cancer accounts for about 1% of all malignant neoplasms, and it is among the five most frequent cancers in the second, third and fourth decades of life. With regard to other malignancies it is probably the most curable cancer, with very high long-term survival rates, at least in the well-differentiated histotypes. Geographic variations in thyroid cancer incidence have been reported, but they are of minor magnitude. A significant predilection of the differentiated cancers for females is reported in all series. However, the female predominance decreases in prepubertal and post-menopausal ages, suggesting that sex hormones might play some role in the pathogenesis.

Aetiology

Oncogenes

With the advent of molecular biology, significant achievements have been made in our understanding the pathogenesis of thyroid carcinoma over the last 10 years. Gene rearrangements, involving the *ret* and *trk* proto-oncogenes, have been demonstrated as causative events specific for the papillary histotype. The oncogenic activation of these genes is accomplished by the fusion of their tyrosine kinase domain with unlinked amino-terminal sequences following intrachromosomal rearrangements involving chromosomes 10 and 1 in the case of *ret* and *trk*, respectively. The *trk* oncogenes are created by a specific rearrangement of *ntk*-1 gene, encoding a receptor for nerve growth factor, linking it to at least three different activating genes. In the case of *ret* rearrangements, the resulting chimaeric oncogenes have been called *ptc* as acronyms for papillary thyroid cancer

[1,2]. Three chimaeric forms have been identified up to now (*ret/ptc*-1, -2, and -3). All of them have shown transforming activity when transfected in cell cultures. Although *ptc* oncogenes are strictly associated with papillary thyroid carcinoma, they are found in no more than one-third of cases, with geographical differences ranging from as low as 2.5% in Saudi Arabia to 33% in Italy [2–5]. Whether these differences are due to ethnic and/or environmental reasons or to different mutagenic events, remains to be established. Indeed, it is also worth mentioning the high rates of *ret/ptc* activation (nearly 55%) reported in papillary thyroid carcinomas diagnosed in children in Belarus, heavily exposed to radiation after the Chernobyl nuclear disaster in 1986 [6–8]. The oncogenes involved in these radiation-induced tumours are mainly *ret/ptc*-2, -3, and, recently, -4 [90] while in spontaneous tumours, not exposed to radiation, the *ret/ptc*-1 is the predominant rearrangement. Based on this finding, one can speculate that *ret/ptc*-2 and -3 are specifically linked to radiation as a mutagenic event. The other possibility is that *ret/ptc* activation is a distinctive character of papillary tumours arising in young patients (most Belarus cancers were diagnosed in children), with or without the cooperation of radiation. This second hypothesis is supported by recent data showing a significant correlation between high rates of *ret/ptc* activation and a lower age at diagnosis in Italian patients not exposed to radiation [9].

Mutated forms of the H-*ras*, K-*ras* and N-*ras* oncogenes are found in differentiated thyroid cancer, but in this case the mutations are not specifically restricted to malignant lesions, since the same mutations have also been found in benign thyroid nodules. Based on this finding it is conceivable that mutations of the *ras* gene family may represent early events in thyroid tumorigenesis. In an attempt to define a new prognostic indicator, *ras* overexpression, detected by immunohistochemistry, has been associated with poor outcome [10].

Anaplastic carcinomas, whether arising as a primary event or as a progression from pre-existing follicular or papillary carcinomas, have a very high prevalence of point mutations of the *p53* gene [11–13], a tumour-suppressor gene implicated in several human cancers; *p53* mutations could be the transitional step necessary for the progression from differentiated to undifferentiated thyroid carcinoma.

Recently, point mutations of the thyroid-stimulating hormone (TSH) receptor gene have been described in a few cases of differentiated thyroid cancer, mainly follicular, selected on the basis of a high level of cyclic adenosine monophosphate (cAMP) activation [14]. This finding, which is reminiscent of the mutations found in toxic adenomas, deserves further studies in order to investigate whether it is a relevant event in the malignant transformation of thyroid cells.

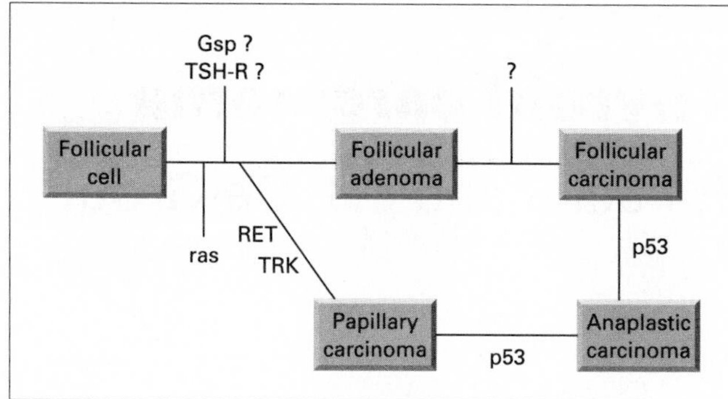

Fig. 28.1 Schematic representation of the proposed genetic lesions involved in the malignant transformation of follicular thyroid cells.

Based on the gene defects discovered in the different types of thyroid carcinomas, a hypothetical model for the sequential changes involved in tumorigenesis of the follicular thyroid cell is suggested in Fig. 28.1.

Ionising radiation

The carcinogenic effects of radiation exposure in the development of thyroid carcinoma are very well recognised. Several studies have demonstrated that external radiation on the head and neck, used in the past for the treatment of a number of benign diseases in children, carries a high risk of inducing thyroid carcinoma, mostly papillary, in the subsequent years [15–17]. The latency period between exposure and diagnosis of thyroid cancer ranges between 10 and 30 years, with a peak at about 20 years. There is a linear dose–response relationship between external radiation and thyroid cancer, starting from radiation doses as low as 50 cGy up to 1500 cGy. Beyond this point the risk of thyroid cancer decreases, probably due to complete destruction of thyroid cells. This finding might explain why there is no relative increase in the risk of thyroid cancer in patients treated with large doses of radioiodine for benign conditions such as Graves' disease and toxic adenoma.

Administration of radioactive iodine (^{131}I) does not seem to be associated with an increased risk for thyroid cancer. Analysis of large series of patients treated with therapeutic doses of ^{131}I for hyperthyroidism or exposed to diagnostic doses for thyroid scanning failed to show an excess risk of thyroid cancer [18]. However, the recent epidemic of papillary thyroid cancer observed in Belarus and Ukraine, as a consequence of the Chernobyl nuclear reactor accident [19,20], has strongly pointed towards a direct carcinogenetic effect of radioactive isotopes of iodine, both ^{131}I and/or short-lived isotopes. At variance with the cancers observed after external irradiation, the post-Chernobyl cancers developed in children and young adults after a very short mean latency period (6.5 ± 1.7 years) between exposure and diagnosis. Whether these discrepancies are due to different radiation doses to the thyroid, or to the very young age of the patients (when the growing thyroid is particularly sensitive to radiation) or to a combination of these and other environmental (iodine deficiency) factors is still a matter of discussion.

Other factors

Other epidemiological factors associated with thyroid carcinoma include iodine deficiency and familial predisposition. Iodine deficiency, exposing the thyroid to mild and chronic hyperstimulation by TSH, has been considered a potential risk factor. Although there is no definite demonstration of an increased number of thyroid cancers in iodine-deficient countries, it is well recognised that there is in such areas a relative increase of follicular cancers with respect to papillary tumors as a general rule.

Cases of familial thyroid cancer have been reported both with the follicular [21] and the papillary histotype (associated with familial adenomatous polyposis coli) [22]. A higher frequency of thyroid tumours has also been reported in association with several inherited syndromes, such as multiple endocrine neoplasia type 1, Cowden's disease and Gardner's syndrome, implying that genetic factors may also be involved.

Pathology

Papillary thyroid carcinoma

Papillary thyroid carcinoma represents nearly 80% of all thyroid carcinomas in iodine-sufficient areas of the world; a lower incidence, 60–70%, is found in areas of severe or moderate iodine deficiency, due to a relative increase in the frequency of the follicular histotype. Females are more affected (ratio of about 4 : 1).

The typical appearance of papillary thyroid carcinoma is that of an invasive neoplasm with papillary and follicular structures and characteristic nuclear changes. The papillae have a fibrovascular core covered by a single layer of neoplastic cells. The typical nuclear features include large size, clear nuclei and nuclear grooves. Cytoplasmic invaginations into the nuclei, termed pseudo-inclusions, are also typical. Another distinctive feature of papillary carcinoma is the presence, in 40–50% of the cases, of psammoma bodies, degenerative calcified changes within the papillae, which, when present, are almost pathognomonic of papillary thyroid carcinoma both in a primary tumour as well as in node metastases. The tumour spreads through lymphatics to the regional lymph nodes and, less frequently, to the lung.

Table 28.1 Histological variants and their relative proportions in papillary thyroid carcinoma.

Variant	Relative (%)
Classical type	70
Encapsulated	10
Follicular	10
Tall cell	4
Diffuse sclerosing	3
Clear cell	2
Others	1

The typical histological appearance described above accounts for nearly 70% of papillary carcinomas. As reviewed in a recent publication [23], the remaining cases are composed of several variants, including encapsulated, follicular, tall-cell, diffuse sclerosing and clear-cell variants. The relative proportion of these variants is listed in Table 28.1.

Follicular thyroid carcinoma

Depending on the degree of iodine intake this histotype accounts for 10–30% of all thyroid carcinomas. As in papillary carcinoma, females are more frequently affected. Histologically, this tumour is characterised by a follicular structure resembling the normal thyroid, with follicles filled with colloid. The neoplasia is limited by a capsule which is invaded by tumour cells. Vascular invasion is also found. The last two findings, invasion of the capsule and vessels, are the key features distinguishing between benign and malignant follicular proliferation, and must be carefully searched for to avoid diagnostic failure. The pattern of invasion may vary between a minimally invasive and a widely invasive form. The growth pattern may also vary, ranging from diffuse solid growth with high degree of atypia to a macrofollicular structure resembling that of the normal thyroid. Lymph-node involvement is rare, while distant metastases, mainly to the lung and bone, are relatively frequent due to hematogenous spread.

Hürthle-cell (oncocytic) and insular variants are the two more frequent subtypes of follicular carcinoma; they are characterised by a more aggressive behaviour. From a biological point of view, these variants are much less well differentiated and show a more aggressive growth potential. The clinical behaviour is also more aggressive; the ability to take up radioiodine and to produce thyroglobulin is frequently lost and the clinical outcome is poor. For these reasons, several authors now consider these two variants as separate categories.

Undifferentiated (anaplastic) thyroid carcinoma

Undifferentiated thyroid cancer, large cell type, comprises about 10% of all thyroid carcinomas. It is typical of older patients, frequently with a history of simple or multinodular goitre present for many years. It is supposed that the tumour represents the transition from a benign or well-differentiated lesion to an undifferentiated one, possibly due to the loss of function of the *p53* tumour-suppressor gene by somatic point mutation, as reported in several series [11–13]. The appearance is that of a large mass with many necrotic areas, and extremely aggressive invasion both locally and at distance. By local spread it invades the soft tissues of the neck, particularly the trachea and oesophagus, making radical surgery impossible. Metastases to the lung are quite common and occur early in the course of the disease. Death is usually within the first 12 months, usually from local complications, despite any therapeutic intervention.

The rare small-cell histotype, previously considered a variant of undifferentiated thyroid carcinoma, has been shown by immunohistochemical studies to represent medullary and follicular carcinomas or small cell lymphomas, erroneously diagnosed as undifferentiated carcinomas.

Diagnosis

The clinical picture of most thyroid tumours is largely dependent on the histology. The presenting feature of differentiated (papillary and follicular) thyroid carcinomas is often the discovery, sometimes fortuitous, of an asymptomatic thyroid nodule. Sometimes, particularly in children, one or more metastatic lymph nodes may be the first sign of disease. More rarely, distant metastases in the lung or bone from follicular carcinoma may be the presenting symptom. Hoarseness, dysphagia and/or dyspnoea may seldom be the first indication of the tumour; this presentation is suggestive of advanced stages of the disease. On physical examination the nodule, usually single, is firm, freely moveable during swelling and poorly distinguishable from a benign lesion. The malignant nature of a thyroid nodule should be suspected when it is found in children or adolescents, in males, in an otherwise normal thyroid, and particularly when a history of previous exposure to external radiation is present. Whatever the presentation, the final diagnosis of malignancy must rely upon the results of fine-needle aspiration cytology, which should be perfomed in any palpable nodule. Other diagnostic procedures are seldom useful in the diagnostic work-up of thyroid nodules. Measurement of thyroid hormones and TSH may help in revealing the small proportion of 'hot', almost invariably benign, nodules to be further assessed by radioiodine thyroid scan. Positive thyroid autoantibodies suggest the presence of an underlying autoimmune disease which reduces (but does not abolish) the possibility of an association with thyroid malignancy. Thyroid ultrasonography, although unable to differentiate benign and malignant lesions, is useful for assessing the number and the size of nodule(s), the structure of the extranodular thyroid, and for guiding the cytology of poorly palpable nodules.

Quite different findings are found in undifferentiated carcinomas. In such cases the patient presents with a rapidly enlarging thyroid mass. The tumour is hard in consistency and fixed to the soft tissues of the neck. Local symptoms, such as dysphagia and dysphonia, are frequent, due to infiltration of the oesophagus and the recurrent laryngeal nerves, respectively. Involvement of the skin with ulceration is also possible. The picture of an undifferentiated thyroid cancer is so impressive that the diagnosis is usually readily made on physical examination.

Management of differentiated thyroid carcinoma

Treatment of primary tumour

The initial treatment for differentiated thyroid cancer is surgery. Although controversy still exists as to the extent of thyroid surgery to be performed, we are in favour of the so called 'near-total thyroidectomy', a procedure intended to leave only a small amount of thyroid tissue near the recurrent nerve and parathyroid glands. There are two main arguments in favour of this approach. First, even when the lesion is apparently single, multicentric tumours, particularly papillary carcinoma, are found in 30–60% of cases according to different series. Secondly, removal of all the thyroid gland is the prerequisite for the subsequent discovery of occult local or distant metastases by means of diagnostic radioiodine whole-body scanning and serum thyroglobulin measurement, and for their treatment by administration of therapeutic doses of radioiodine. The argument against a radical surgical procedure is the increased risk of surgical complications such as recurrent laryngeal nerve injuries and hypoparathyroidism. However, both these complications are almost absent in the hands of an experienced surgeon, and should not be advocated as reasons against near-total thyroidectomy.

In the context of papillary thyroid carcinoma, some authors guide their surgical decision on the basis of prognostic factors identifying 'low-risk' patients, to be treated with limited surgery, and 'high-risk' patients, to be treated with more radical surgery. Prognostic factors defining low-risk patients are papillary tumours, age <40 years, a single nodule <20 mm in size, no clinical evidence of local or distant metastases, and no history of previous exposure to external radiation.

The influence of initial treatment on the outcome of differentiated thyroid cancer has been the object of several publications from centres with large series of patients and long-term follow-up. In general, there is considerable evidence that recurrence rates and death rates tend to be higher when subtotal thyroidectomies are performed [24–26]. In the series of papillary thyroid carcinomas treated at the Mayo Clinic [24], the extent of surgery significantly affected the risk of local recurrence. In the series of the Ohio State University [25], both the 30-year cancer-recurrence rate and the 30-year cancer-specific mortality were higher after subtotal thyroidectomy than after total or near-total thyroidectomy. Similarly, in the series of papillary thyroid cancer patients treated at the University of Chicago [26], performance of less extensive initial surgery (lobectomy or bilateral subtotal thyroidectomy) was associated with a non-significant trend to increased risk of death and a significantly increased risk of recurrence when compared to more extensive surgery (lobectomy plus contralateral subtotal lobectomy or near-total or total thyroidectomy). Furthermore, both a significant increase in risk of death and of recurrence was associated with less extensive surgery if tumour size was > 10 mm.

Another controversial issue is whether a post-surgical thyroid remnant should be ablated by therapeutic doses of radioiodine. Again, ablation of any thyroid residue should be performed whenever the subsequent strategy is based on serum thyroglobulin measurement and radioiodine whole-body scan (WBS). We are convinced that this should be the basic treatment program to be offered to all cases of differentiated thyroid carcinoma, especially in view of a growing number of studies demonstrating that completion of surgery by radioiodine ablation is associated with decreased tumour recurrence and fewer cancer-related deaths, at least in patients with tumours larger than 10 mm [26]. In addition to thyroidectomy, clinically evident lymph-node metastases must be treated by ipsilateral neck dissection. More extensive surgery may be required in individual cases with invasive tumours. By general agreement, follicular carcinomas should always be treated by near-total thyroidectomy followed by radioiodine thyroid ablation: with this treatment a better prognosis has been reported in patients with follicular carcinoma [27].

Diagnosis and treatment of distant metastases

According to several large series the frequency of distant metastases in differentiated thyroid carcinoma ranges between 10 and 18% of cases [28–34]. Sometimes, distant metastases, particularly in bone, may be the presenting symptom of the disease but usually (two-thirds of cases) they are discovered at the time of the primary diagnosis or soon after thyroidectomy when performing the first WBS with ^{131}I [28]. However, distant metastases may develop later in the course of follow-up, even as late as 20 years after initial treatment [28], suggesting that follow-up of differentiated thyroid cancer should continue throughout the patient's life.

Lung metastases are the most common site of distant metastases, followed by bone metastases. The combination of lung and bone disease is found in about one-third of patients with distant metastases. Other less common sites are in the brain, the liver, and the skin; all are more likely to occur in association with lung and/or bone metastases.

The pattern of metastatic lung involvement may vary from one or more macronodular (> 10 mm in diameter) nodules to a diffuse micronodular spread [28,29,31]. The latter are usually not detected by chest X-ray, and sometimes not even by computed tomography (CT) scanning, but can be easily diagnosed with ^{131}I WBS. Not infrequently, especially in papillary tumours, enlarged lymph nodes in the mediastinum may also be identified [33,35].

Bone metastases are mainly associated with the follicular histotype and tend to occur in older patients (Fig. 28.2). The vertebrae, pelvis and ribs are the sites more frequently affected, but occasionally any skeletal segment may be affected. Single lesions are present in one-third of patients. Most metastases are detectable both by WBS and plain X-rays, but a minority (about 25%) are visible only by WBS [28,36]: this latter group is more likely to respond to ^{131}I therapy.

Diagnostic procedures

After thyroidectomy and ablation of thyroid residues, two powerful tools are used to identify and localise distant metastases, serum thyroglobulin (Tg) measurement and ^{131}I WBS.

Serum Tg measurement. As a rule, distant metastases are associated with elevated serum Tg concentrations when measured after withdrawal of thyroxine (T_4) therapy. During T_4 treatment serum Tg concentrations are reduced, but still detectable, with respect to off-therapy values [29,37] (Fig. 28.3). The comparison between the results of serum Tg measurement and those of ^{131}I WBS shows that there is close agreement between the two techniques [38,39]. As shown in Fig. 28.4, detectable serum Tg levels are usually associated with positive WBS, indicating the presence of residual or metastatic disease. Undetectable serum Tg levels are found in patients with negative scans, indicating that the patient is in complete remission. However, serum Tg is superior to WBS in predicting the presence of metastases in a significant proportion of patients who have increased serum Tg levels but a false-negative WBS [40].

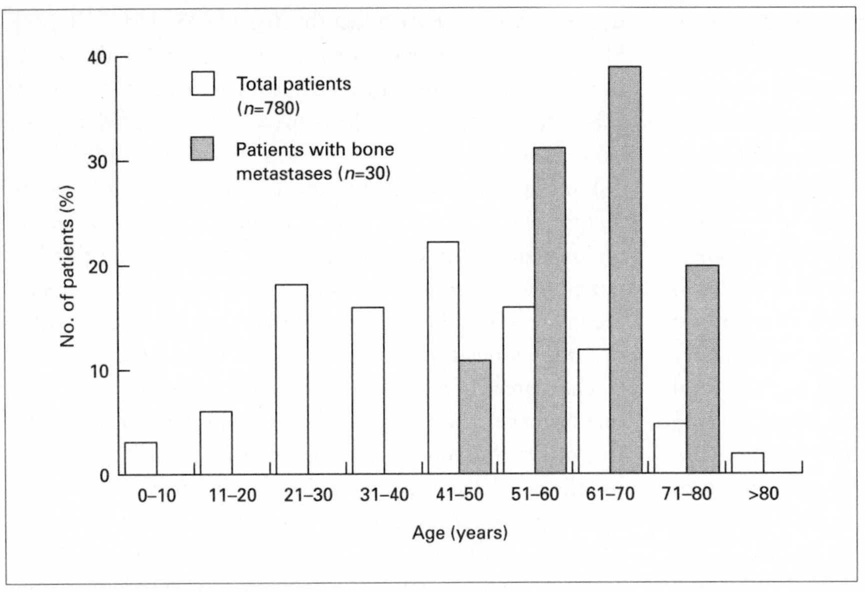

Fig. 28.2 Age distribution of patients with bone metastases at diagnosis.

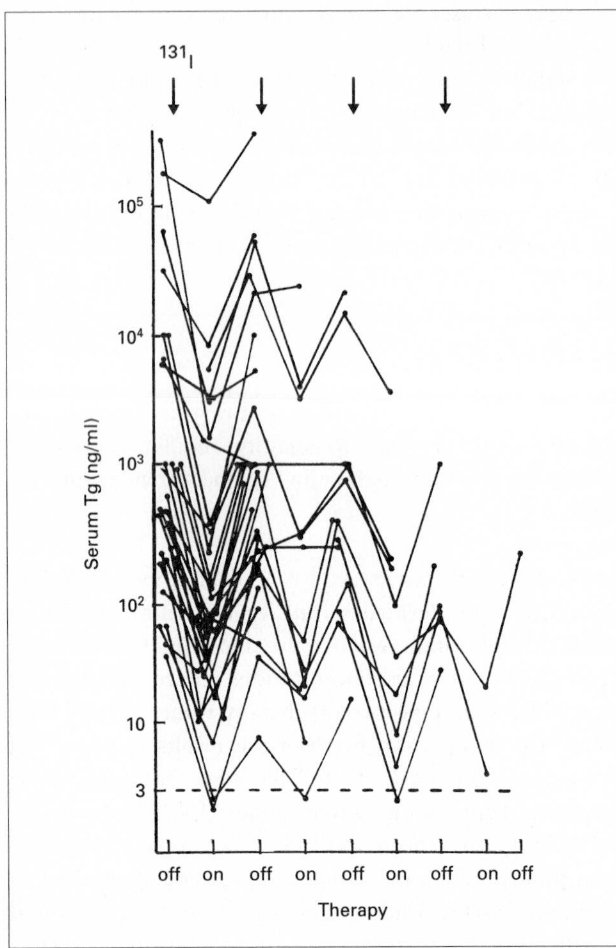

Fig. 28.3 Behaviour of serum thyroglobulin (Tg) levels in patients with distant metastases (bone and/or lung) studied on and off thyroxine (T_4) therapy. When off T_4, all patients have elevated serum Tg levels; on T_4 serum Tg levels usually drop, but are still detectable.

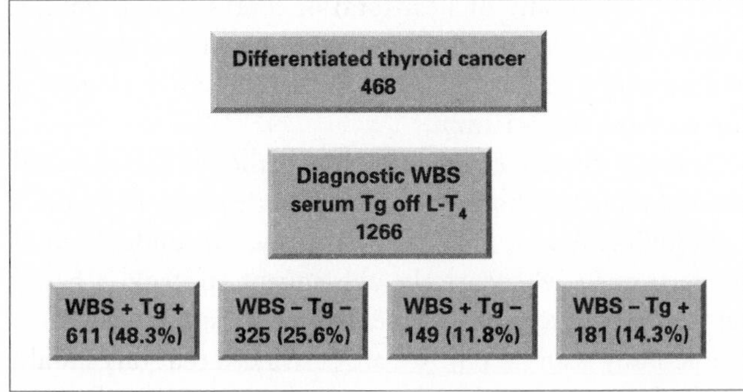

Fig. 28.4 Comparison between the results of ^{131}I whole-body scan (WBS) and serum thyroglobulin (Tg) assay off thyroxine (T_4) therapy in patients with differentiated thyroid cancer.

^{131}I WBS. Metastatic well-differentiated thyroid cancer retains the ability to concentrate iodine, as do normal follicular cells. This notion is the rationale for the traditional diagnostic and therapeutic use of ^{131}I in metastatic thyroid cancer. Radioiodine uptake by metastatic tissue is dependent on TSH stimulation, thus requiring a state of hypothyroidism. For this reason, thyroidectomy and ablation of post-surgical thyroid residues is the fundamental prerequisite for radioactive imaging. The other important point is the withdrawal of T_4 therapy for a period of time long enough to induce high serum levels of endogenous TSH [41,42]. The minimum level of serum TSH required for adequate incorporation of ^{131}I in neoplastic tissues is around 30 μU/ml, a level which is traditionally achieved after 30–45 days off T_4, and 2 weeks off triiodothyronine (T_3). We now prepare most patients for scanning by having them take half their usual T_4 dose, which raises TSH to an adequate

level in 5–6 weeks, and induces only mild hypothyroidism. Another requirement for effective ^{131}I uptake is that the patient is not contaminated by the recent consumption of stable iodine which would prevent the uptake of radioactive iodine by metastases. Serum TSH concentrations should be checked before performing ^{131}I WBS and ^{131}I therapy.

WBS is performed 48–72 hours after the administration of ^{131}I, using either a rectilinear scan or γ-camera. ^{131}I doses of 2–5mCi (74–185MBq) are usually employed as tracer; higher doses are not indicated due to the possibility that they will produce a sublethal radiation effect in the metastatic cells (stunning effect), thus preventing the uptake of the therapeutic dose of ^{131}I to be administered after a few days [43].

If no abnormal ^{131}I uptake is found, despite the elevation of serum Tg off T_4, the search for metastases should include chest X-ray, CT scanning, bone scintigraphy and liver echography. If no localisation is found, a WBS performed 5–7 days after the administration of 100mCi of ^{131}I will often allow the localisation of small neoplastic foci not seen in the conventional WBS, and will have a therapeutic effect in most patients in lowering Tg [44–46]. However, the long-term benefit of this treatment is not yet known.

Whenever a metastasis has been localised by WBS, a complete radiological assessment should also be obtained. In bone metastases the aim is to assess whether the localisation is accessible to radical surgical therapy, which, in the case of a single localisation, may be curative [36,47]. In the case of lung metastases it is extremely important to establish whether there are one or more macronodular lesions or multiple micronodules, not visible on the plain chest X-ray but only on the CT scan. This is of relevant prognostic utility, since diffuse lung metastases, not detectable by X-ray but able to take up radioiodine, such as those frequently encountered in children, are highly responsive to treatment with ^{131}I [45,48,49].

Treatment

Surgery. The decision to treat distant metastases with surgery depends on their nature, localisation, diffusion, ability to concentrate radioiodine and radiological pattern.

Lung metastases are frequently cured by radioiodine therapy, leaving the choice of surgical therapy for the treatment of a minority of selected cases. Patients eligible for surgery are those with a single macronodular lesion, or more than one in the same lobe, with or without mediastinal lymph node involvement, particularly when they are devoid of radioiodine uptake. Too few patients have been operated on for lung metastases to draw statistical conclusions as to the outcome; however, the feeling is that some may achieve long-term remission, and, in less advanced cases (a single pulmonary nodule), even definitive cure [50].

In cases of bone metastases, the surgical approach is gaining interest due to their relative insensitivity to radioiodine therapy [36,47,50,51]. The purpose of bone surgery may be palliative or curative. Palliation is required in the case of pathological fractures or to ameliorate neurological symptoms due to spinal cord compression by vertebral metastases; curative surgery is possible in the case of single, localised metastases. In the case of large metastases, not radically resectable, surgery may be of help in reducing tumour mass, thus allowing a more effective action of radioiodine therapy.

Brain metastases are extremely rare, ranging from 0.15 to 1.3% in different series [52–55] and, when present, carry a very poor prognosis. Although they are usually associated with ^{131}I uptake, whenever feasible surgery is indicated because of severe neurological symptoms.

Radioiodine. The role and the indications of ^{131}I therapy in the management of distant metastases from differentiated thyroid carcinoma are well established. Its results are reproducible in large series of patients and indicate a percentage of complete responses ranging between 35 and 45% [28,29,31,32,49]. Lung metastases show a better response than bone metastases. In the adult patient, the treatment dose is usually 100–150 mCi, repeated every 8–12 months. Lower doses (empirically 1 mCi/kg bodyweight) should be employed in children with lung metastases, particularly of the diffuse type, to avoid the risk of radiation-induced pulmonary fibrosis [48,56]. Less than 65 mCi ^{131}I should be deposited in the lungs.

In a review of 118 patients with distant metastases treated with ^{131}I therapy at the Institute of Endocrinology in Pisa [28] (Table 28.2), 43 patients (36.4%) were cured (defined as negative WBS and undetectable serum Tg off T_4), 28 (23.7%) died of their disease, while the remainder have persistent disease. Of those who died, 10 had lung metastases, eight had bone metastases, and nine had both. Better results were obtained in patients with metastases limited to lymph nodes. Metastases from papillary tumours showed a better response than follicular tumours. The risk of dying was higher if lung metastases were macronodular and detectable by chest X-ray, if bone metastases were multiple, and if both lung and bone metastases were present. The mean cumulative dose of ^{131}I employed in cured patients was 233 mCi, delivered in 2.2 treatment courses, over 3.4 years. Loss of radioiodine uptake was seen in four (5.2%) patients after a mean cumulative dose of 161 mCi, 2.7 years from the beginning of treatment. Six patients with single bone metastases and one with a macronodular lung metastasis were treated surgically. In these cases histology revealed that the metastatic tumour was less well differentiated than the corresponding primary tumour.

Table 28.2 Effect of ^{131}I therapy in differentiated thyroid cancer with metastases to lymph nodes (n = 191) and to distant sites (n = 118).

	Cured (%)	Continued disease (%)	Dead (%)
Lymph nodes	73.0	23.4	3.6
Distant	36.4	39.9	23.7

As previously mentioned, there is a group of patients who have elevated serum Tg levels and no uptake in the diagnostic WBS [38,39]. This situation, which accounts for 15–20% of the cases, has important diagnostic and therapeutic implications. From the diagnostic point of view, it has been well demonstrated [44–46] that the site of metastatic involvement in such patients is usually the lung or mediastinal lymph nodes, which may be detected by WBS performed 5–7 days after the administration of high doses of ^{131}I (100 mCi). From the therapeutic point of view, the open question is whether the administration of such high doses of ^{131}I have a therapeutic effect in metastatic foci with low radioiodine uptake. Indirect evidence that this procedure is of therapeutic value comes from the finding that a few days after the administration of ^{131}I therapy there is a transient increase in serum Tg concentrations, which may be explained as the massive release into the circulation of stored Tg from radiation-damaged tumour cells (Fig. 28.5). Furthermore, progressive normalisation of WBS and serum Tg levels over the years [44,45], and the normalisation of chest CT scans in patients with radiographic evidence of micronodular lung metastases [46], have been observed in patients periodically treated with this modality.

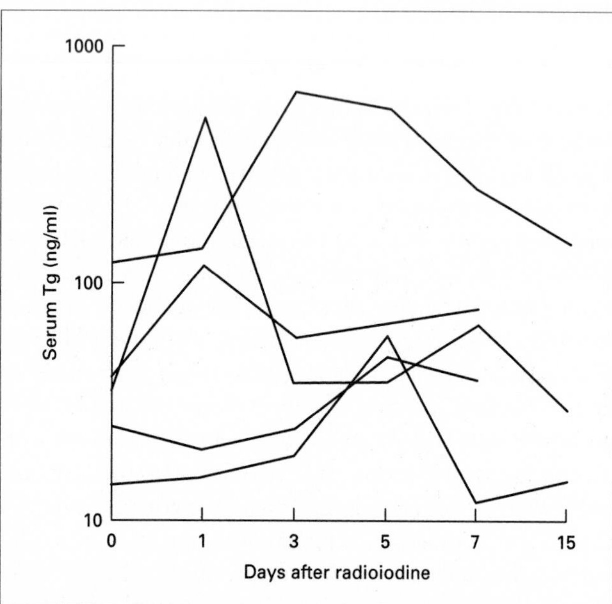

Fig. 28.5 Release of serum thyroglobulin (Tg) after the administration of a therapeutic dose of ^{131}I in patients with detectable serum Tg and negative diagnostic whole-body scan (WBS).

Side-effects after the administration of therapeutic ^{131}I doses are frequent, but usually very mild and reversible in a few days. They consist mainly of gastrointestinal symptoms, nausea and occasionally vomiting, and acute sialoadenitis. More serious complications are those related to blood and bone marrow. An increased risk of leukaemia of the order of five cases per 1000 treated patients has been found in several published series [49]. The risk increases with increasing cumulative doses, reducing the intervals between each treatment, and giving total blood doses per treatment >2 [57]. Pan-cytopenia has been reported in 4.4% of patients treated with mean ^{131}I doses of 536 mCi by Schober *et al.* [58]. In the same study, anaemia was found in about 25% of the patients and thrombocytopaenia in one-third.

Another complication of radioiodine therapy is radiation-induced pulmonary fibrosis, which may develop in patients repeatedly treated for lung metastases, particularly of the diffuse type. Children seem to be particularly prone to this complication. We observed a 22-year-old woman, who was treated at another institution with high doses of ^{131}I from the age of 10 for lung metastases, who died, apparently free of disease, with pulmonary fibrosis [48].

The occurrence of a second solid cancer following radioiodine treatment has been addressed in a few studies [59], reporting three excess cases of bladder and three of breast carcinomas out of 258 patients treated for differentiated thyroid cancer. All of them had been treated with more than 900 mCi of ^{131}I. The issue of a second malignancy is still controversial.

Equally controversial is whether radioiodine treatment can promote the anaplastic transformation of well-differentiated thyroid cancer. Although varying degrees of 'dedifferentiation' are observed in almost all series of thyroid cancer, the question is whether this is due to radioiodine or whether it is an independent biological event concluding the natural history of papillary and follicular thyroid carcinoma. Recent studies in molecular biology [12,60] have shown that anaplastic thyroid carcinoma is associated with the loss of expression or function of the tumour-suppressor gene *p53*. It is possible, but not proven, that differentiated thyroid cancers, through a (radiation-induced?) second mutation in the *p53* gene, shift toward the poorly differentiated or totally undifferentiated histotype.

Finally, the occurrence of both transient and permanent testicular damage has been reported, limited to the germinal epithelium, in men treated with high levels of administered activity of ^{131}I, particularly when treated for bone metastases close to the testis [61].

Prognostic factors

The effective treatment of distant metastases depends largely on the size, location, number of metastatic lesions, and their ability to take up radioiodine. Micronodular diffuse lung metastases and, to a lesser extent, small metastatic bone foci revealed by WBS in the absence of radiographic changes, have the greatest chance of cure. This is particularly true in children, who often have this pattern of metastatic pulmonary spread, and do exceptionally well with radioiodine therapy [48,62]. Macronodules in the lung and large bone metastases have a poor prognosis. Loss of radioiodine uptake is also a prognostic indicator of poor outcome. Together, these findings emphasise the concept that early recognition and early treatment of distant metastases is of paramount importance to the final outcome.

The importance of T_4 suppressive therapy

Both the function and the growth of metastatic thyroid cells are under TSH control. It is a common observation that bone or lung metastases increase in size and take up radioiodine during periods of T_4 withdrawal, while a reduction in size and no uptake is observed on T_4. Serum Tg, a marker of cell function, increases dramatically during hypothyroidism, while it returns to low levels during hormone therapy. In the classical paper by Mazzaferri [52], thyroid hormone therapy significantly influenced both recurrence rate and survival, as an independent variable. In this regard, suppression of endogenous TSH to undetectable levels is to be regarded as a true antineoplastic therapy and should never be omitted in patients with active disease.

The drug of choice is T_4, and the effective dosage is between 2.2 and 2.8 μg/kg bodyweight. A relatively higher dosage is usually required in children. In any patient, attempts should be made to use the smallest dose necessary to suppress TSH secretion [63]. The adequacy of therapy is monitored by measurement of serum TSH. In patients with known or possible active disease, TSH should be suppressed as far as possible towards 0.1 μU/ml. The therapeutic value of suppression below the normal range has in fact not been proven in patients believed to be free of disease; who can probably safely be maintaned with TSH in the 0.3–1.0 μU/ml range.

Therapy of undifferentiated thyroid carcinoma

Undifferentiated thyroid carcinoma is among the most aggressive malignant tumours in the human. Its frequency is approximately 5–15% of all thyroid carcinomas. The management of this type of cancer is a cause of major concern since no effective treatment, other than palliative, is available. Patients usually die within 12 months from diagnosis [64,65]. As soon as a diagnosis of undifferentiated thyroid cancer has been made, total thyroidectomy should be attempted. Unfortunately, the infiltration of soft tissues of the neck, almost invariably present at operation, makes radical surgery impossible. In an attempt to control local disease external radiotherapy is used after surgery, but this treatment is usually unsatisfactory [66]. Several chemotherapeutic protocols, including single (doxorubicin) and combination (doxorubicin plus cisplatin) drugs, have been uniformly disappointing [67,68]. The combination of radiotherapy and chemotherapy has been employed with very modest advantages [60]. With any form of treatment, mean survival ranges between 3 and 6 months from diagnosis [66–68], although individual survivals exceeding 2–3 years have been reported. Since radical surgery, as mentioned above, is rarely feasible, it has been proposed to use hyperfractionated radiotherapy in combination with chemotherapy as initial treatment, leaving surgery as the second step. The idea is to control and to reduce the primary tumour with medical therapy, thus giving the surgeon a better chance to perform a radical thyroidectomy. Further radiotherapy and chemotherapy may be added after surgery to stabilise the results of treatment. Using this integrated therapeutic approach, relatively longer survivals have been reported, and several patients have achieved long-term remission, at least of local disease [70–73].

In the future, the recent discovery of point mutations of the *p53* tumour-suppressor gene specifically associated with undifferentiated thyroid carcinoma [11–13] may lead to the development of more effective treatment strategies at the molecular level.

Medullary thyroid carcinoma (see also Chapter 47)

Medullary thyroid carcinoma (MTC) is a tumour of the parafollicular thyroid cells (C cells). These cells are physiologically directed to the synthesis and release of calcitonin (CT). MTC is a rare tumour, accounting for about 10% of all thyroid carcinomas. Most MTCs (nearly 80%) occur as sporadic tumours with a peak of incidence in the fourth and fifth decades, the rest (20%) occurs as inherited tumours usually earlier in life, associated with other endocrine neoplasms as part of familial syndromes known as multiple endocrine neoplasia type 2 (MEN-2). Germline point mutations of the *ret* proto-oncogene, a gene coding for a tyrosine kinase membrane receptor, have been demonstrated as causative of MEN-2 [74–76], with a specificity of almost 100%. As

Table 28.3 *ret* proto-oncogene mutations in sporadic medullary thyroid carcinoma.

Ref	Mutated/all (%)	Exon			
		10	11	15	16
Zedenius *et al.* [88]	6/9 (66.6)				6
Marsh *et al.* [78]	22/32 (68.7)			1	21
Romei *et al.* [77]	10/20 (50.0)	1*	3		6

* In this case the mutation was a 48-bp deletion; in all the other cases it was a point mutation.

reported in Table 28.3, somatic mutations of the same gene have been also found in nearly 50% of sporadic MTC [77,78].

In the normal human thyroid, a few C cells are found around thyroid follicles, mixed with the follicular cells. Their embryological origin is from the neural crest, from which they migrate during fetal life to reach their final destination. Within the thyroid, C cells are preferentially located at the junction between the upper one-third and the lower two-thirds of both thyroid lobes. This is the region where most MTCs will develop. Despite close contact between para-follicular and follicular cells, no paracrine interaction seems to exist between these two types of cells.

The product of the C cells is a 32-amino-acid hormone, CT, whose gene acts with an alternative RNA splicing coding for CT in the normal C cells and for an other peptide, calcitonin gene-related peptide (CGRP), in several cells of the central nervous system [79]. Unlike normal C cells, neoplastic C cells are able to produce both CT and CGRP [80]. The action of CT, once released into the bloodstream, is to bind to specific receptors on osteoclasts, thus inhibiting bone resorption. Specific receptors for CT have been demonstrated in the kidney and brain. CT release is regulated by the extracellular concentration of calcium. Other substances, mainly pentagastrin, may stimulate CT secretion. On this basis, both calcium infusion and pentagastrin injection are commonly used as stimulating agents in the diagnosis and follow-up of MTC [81].

Pathology

Sporadic MTC presents as a white–red, hard lesion. Microscopically it presents as sheets of spindle or rounded cells, typical of endocrine tumours. Nuclei are usually uniform with rare mitoses. Secretory granules are found in the cytoplasm. Deposits of amyloid, a product of the CT gene, are frequently found and are a distinctive feature of MTC. This pattern is not always the case, and sometimes MTC can mimic other thyroid tumours, mainly Hürthle cell, anaplastic or even papillary carcinoma. In these cases, immunohistochemistry with anti-CT antibodies will help in establishing the diagnosis [82]. Accompanying C-cell hyperplasia, a distinctive feature of familial MTC, is seldom found in sporadic cases.

Metastatic spread of MTC to regional lymph nodes is very frequent, even in the earliest phase of the disease. Metastatic nodes, not clinically evident, are frequently found by the surgeon when careful exploration of the central neck compartment and lateral chains is performed. Distant metastases, usually slow-growing, are also frequent both at diagnosis or during follow-up. The sites most frequently affected are the liver, the lungs and the bone.

Clinical manifestation

The mode of presentation of MTC is usually the discovery of a 'cold' thyroid nodule indistinguishable from thyroid nodules of any other nature. Cervical lymph node involvement is very frequent. The diagnosis may be suspected only if there is a familial history of MTC, or in the presence of secretory diarrhoea, typically, but not frequently, associated with MTC [83]. Most of the time the diagnosis is made on histology. Cytology is an excellent diagnostic procedure for thyroid carcinoma in general; however, the specific diagnosis of MTC may be missed with routine staining, especially if the pathologist is not alerted by suspicion of MTC. In a recent prospective study [84] performed in more than 1000 unselected thyroid nodules undergoing diagnostic evaluation, routine measurement of serum CT allowed the preoperative diagnosis of unsuspected MTC in a surprisingly high number of patients (0.57% of all nodules), with a diagnostic accuracy superior to fine-needle aspiration cytology. Based on this finding, recently confirmed in another study [85], we believe that serum CT measurement should be considered in the diagnostic evaluation of thyroid nodules.

Therapy

A number of studies have shown that the outcome of sporadic MTC is largely, if not entirely, dependent upon the effectiveness of the first surgical procedure. Minimal therapy for MTC is total thyroidectomy with dissection of the central node compartment, which is the first site of lymphatic spread [86]. Dissection of other lymph-node chains will depend upon the clinical presentation.

After surgery, one should allow for the clearance of CT from the circulation before measuring the serum CT concentration. Thirty to forty days are usually sufficient, since the half-life of serum CT has a rapid component of about 3 hours and a longer component of 30 hours [87]. If at that time basal and pentagastrin-stimulated serum

CT concentrations are undetectable, the patient has a high probability of having achieved definitive cure. Unfortunately, even after careful surgery, no more than 40–50% of the patients will appear cured (including normalization of serum CT concentrations) in the subsequent follow-up. Many will have a sustained increase in serum CT which is evidence of persistent disease. The localisation of suspected metastases is based on diagnostic imaging techniques, including neck and liver ultrasound, CT scanning of the mediastinum and lung, and bone scintigraphy. Several other scanning techniques, such as MIBG and ^{99m}Tc DMSA scanning, have been successfully employed in the detection of macroscopic lesions, but their usefulness in detecting microscopic disease is questionable. Recently, WBS with radiolabelled somatostatin analogues has been proposed, but its level of diagnostic accuracy does not seem to be superior to other traditional methods. In selected cases venous catheterisation for measurement of serum CT has been successfully employed.

From a practical point of view, if local disease has been detected in the neck a second operation is indicated. Patients with continued CT elevation but without identifiable disease may have careful dissection of the supraclavicular nodes on the side ipsilateral to the tumor. This intensive approach may remove nodal tissue and return CT to normal in 15–30% of patients. If no disease is found, despite elevation of serum CT, it is probably better to wait and to re-evaluate the patient after 6–12 months, and then consider other treatment modalities. External radiotherapy is useful, but chemotherapy has been disappointing in the treatment of MTC. Considering all stages of MTC, the usual 10-year survival in several series is around 50–60%. Survival may be prolonged and the quality of life acceptable even in the presence of diffuse metastatic involvement.

References

1 Fusco A, Grieco M, Santoro M *et al.* A new oncogene in human thyroid papillary carcinomas and their lymph-nodal metastases. *Nature* 1987; **328**: 170–2.

2 Santoro M, Carlomagno F, Hay ID *et al.* *Ret* oncogene activation in human thyroid neoplasms is restricted to the papillary cancer subtype. *J Clin Invest* 1992; **89**: 1517–22.

3 Zou M, Shi Y, Farid NR. Low rate of ret proto-oncogene activation (PTC/ret TPC) in papillary thyroid carcinomas from Saudi Arabia. *Cancer* 1994; **73**: 176–80.

4 Wajjwalku W, Nakamura S, Hasegawa Y *et al.* Low frequency of rearrangements of the *ret* and *trk* proto-oncogenes in Japanese thyroid papillary carcinomas. *Jpn J Cancer Res* 1992; **83**: 671–5.

5 Namba H, Yamashita S, Pei HC *et al.* Lack of PTC gene (*ret* proto-oncogene rearrangement) in human thyroid tumors. *Endocrinol Jpn* 1991; **38**: 627–32.

6 Ito T, Seyama T, Iwamoto KS *et al.* Activated RET oncogene in thyroid cancers of children from areas contaminated by Chernobyl accident. *Lancet* 1994; **344**: 259.

7 Fugazzola L, Pilotti S, Pinchera A *et al.* Oncogenic rearrangements of the RET proto-oncogene in papillary thyroid carcinomas from children exposed to the Chernobyl nuclear accident. *Cancer Res* 1995; **55**: 5617–20.

8 Klugbauer S, Lengfelder E, Demidchik EP, Rabes HM. High prevalence of RET rearrangement in thyroid tumors of children from Belarus after the Chernobyl reactor accident. *Oncogene* 1995; **11**: 2459–67.

9 Bongarzone I, Fugazzola L, Vigneri P *et al.* Age-related activation of the tyrosine kinase receptor protooncogenes RET and NTRK1 in papillary thyroid carcinoma. *J Clin Endocrinol Metab* 1996; **81**: 5.

10 Basolo F, Pinchera A, Fugazzola L *et al.* Expression of p21 *ras* protein as a prognostic factor in papillary thyroid cancer. *Eur J Cancer* 1994; **30A**: 171–4.

11 Ito T, Seyama T, Mizuno T. Unique association of p53 mutation with undifferentiated but not differentiated carcinomas of the thyroid gland. *Cancer Res* 1992; **52**: 1369–71.

12 Fagin JA, Matsuo K, Karmar A, Chen DL, Tang SH, Koeffler HP. High prevalence of mutation of p53 gene in poorly differentiated human thyroid carcinomas. *J Clin Invest* 1993; **91**: 179–84.

13 Pollina L, Pacini F, Fontanini G, Vignati S, Bevilacqua G, Basolo F. bcl-2, p53 and proliferating cell nuclear antigen expression is related to the degree of differentiation in thyroid carcinoma. *Br J Cancer* 1996; **73**: 139–42.

14 Russo D, Arturi F, Schlumberger M *et al.* Activating mutations of the TSH receptor in differentiated thyroid carcinomas. *Oncogene* 1995; **11**: 1907–11.

15 Favus MJ, Schneider AB, Stachyra ME. Thyroid cancer occurring as a late consequence of head-and-neck irradiation. *N Engl J Med* 1976; **294**: 1019–24.

16 Refetoff S, Harrison J, Karanfilski BT. Continuing occurrence of thyroid carcinoma after irradiation to the neck in infancy and childhood. *N Engl J Med* 1975; **292**: 171–5.

17 DeGroot L, Paloyan E. Thyroid carcinoma and radiation: a Chicago endemic. *JAMA* 1973; **255**: 487–91.

18 Franceschi S, Boyle P, Maissonneuve P. The epidemiology of thyroid carcinoma. *Crit Rev Oncogenesis* 1993; **4**: 25–9.

19 Pacini F, Vorontsova T, Demidchik EP *et al.* Diagnosis, surgical treatment and follow-up of thyroid cancers. In: Karaoglou A, Desmet G, Kelly GN, Menzel HG, ed. *The Radiological Consequences of the Chernobyl Accident*. Luxembourg: *EUR* 16544 EN, 1996; 755–63.

20 Tronko N, Bogdanova T, Kommisarenko I *et al.* Thyroid cancer in children and adolescents in Ukraine after the Chernobyl accident (1986–1995). In: Karaoglou A, Desmet G, Kelly GN, Menzel HG, eds. *The Radiological Consequences of the Chernobyl Accident*. Luxembourg: EUR 16544 EN, 1996; 683.

21 Cooper DS, Axelrod L, DeGroot LJ *et al.* Congenital goitre and the development of metastatic follicular carcinoma with evidence for a leak of non-hormonal iodide: Clinical, pathological, kinetic and biochemical studies and a review of the literature. *J Clin Endocrinol Metab* 1981; **52**: 294–7.

22 Bell B, Mazzaferri EL. Familial adenomatous polyposis (Gardner's syndrome) and thyroid carcinoma: a case report and review of the literature. *Dig Dis Sci* 1993; **38**: 185–7.

23 Ain KB. Papillary thyroid carcinoma. *Endocrinol Metab Clin North Am* 1995; **24**: 711.

24 McConahey WM, Hay ID, Woolner LB, van Heerden JA, Taylor WF. Papillary thyroid cancer treated at the Mayo Clinic, 1946

through 1970: initial manifestations, pathologic findings, therapy and outcome. *Mayo Clin Proc* 1986; **61**: 978–88.

25 Mazzaferri EL, Jhiang SM. Long term impact of initial surgical and medical therapy on papillary and follicular thyroid cancer. *Am J Med* 1994; **97**: 418–23.

26 DeGroot LJ, Kaplan EL, McCornick M, Straus FH. Natural history, treatment, and course of papillary thyroid carcinoma. *J Clin Endocrinol Metab* 1990; **71**: 414–19.

27 DeGroot LJ, Kaplan EL, Shukla MS, Salti G, Straus FH. Morbidity and mortality in follicular thyroid cancer. *J Clin Endocrinol Metab* 1995; **80**: 2946–50.

28 Pacini F, Cetani F, Miccoli P *et al.* Outcome of 309 patients with metastatic differentiated thyroid carcinoma treated with radioiodine. *World J Surg* 1994; **18**: 600–4.

29 Schlumberger M, Tubiana M, De Vathaire F *et al.* Long-term results of treatment of 238 patients with lung and bone metastases from differentiated thyroid carcinoma. *J Clin Endocrinol Metab* 1986; **63**: 960–7.

30 Hoie J, Stenwig AE, Kullmann G, Lindegaard M. Distant metastases in papillary thyroid cancer. A review of 91 patients. *Cancer* 1988; **61**: 1–4.

31 Brown AP, Greening WP, McCready VR, Shaw HJ, Harmer CL. Radioiodine treatment of metastatic thyroid carcinoma: the Royal Marsden Hospital Experience. *Br J Radiol* 1984; **57**: 323–7.

32 Samaan NA, Schultz PN, Haynie TP, Ordonez NG. Pulmonary metastasis of differentiated thyroid carcinoma: treatment results in 101 patients. *J Clin Endocrinol Metab* 1985; **60**: 376–81.

33 Massin JP, Savoie JC, Garnier H, Guiraudon G, Leger FA, Bacourt F. Pulmonary metastases in differentiated thyroid carcinoma. Study of 58 cases with implications for the primary tumor treatment. *Cancer* 1984; **53**: 982–5.

34 Ruegemer JJ, Hay ID, Bergstralh EJ, Ryan JJ, Offord KP, Gorman CA. Distant metastases in differentiated thyroid carcinoma: a multivariate analysis of prognostic variables. *J Clin Endocrinol Metab* 1988; **67**: 501–5.

35 Beierwaltes WH, Nishiyama RH, Thompson NW *et al.* Survival time and 'cure' in papillary and follicular thyroid carcinoma with distant metastases: Statistics following University of Michigan therapy. *J Nucl Med* 1982; **23**: 561–5.

36 Marcocci C, Pacini F, Elisei R *et al.* Clinical and biological behaviour of bone metastases from differentiated thyroid carcinoma. *Surgery* 1989; **106**: 960–6.

37 Pacini F, Lari R, Mazzeo S *et al.* Diagnostic value of a single serum thyroglobulin determination on and off thyroid suppressive therapy in the follow-up of patients with differentiated thyroid cancer. *Clin Endocrinol* 1985; **23**: 405–9.

38 Pacini F, Pinchera A, Giani C *et al.* Serum thyroglobulin concentrations and 131-I whole body scans in the diagnosis of metastases from differentiated thyroid carcinoma (after thyroidectomy). *Clin Endocrinol* 1980; **13**: 107–10.

39 Ashcraft MW, Van Herle AJ. The comparative value of serum thyroglobulin measurements and iodine-131 total body scans in the follow-up study of patients with treated differentiated thyroid cancer. *Am J Med* 1981; **71**: 806–10.

40 Pacini F, Ceccarelli C, Elisei R, Grasso L, Pinchera A. Serum thyroglobulin determination in thyroid cancer: a ten year experience. In: Nagataki S & Torizuka K, eds *The Thyroid*. Amsterdam: Elsevier Science Publishers, 1988: 685–8.

41 Schlumberger M, Charbord P, Fragu P, Lumbroso J, Parmentier C, Tubiana M. Circulating thyroglobulin and thyroid hormones in patients with metastases of differentiated thyroid carcinoma: relationship to serum thyrotropin levels. *J Clin Endocrinol Metab* 1980; **51**: 513–17.

42 Schneider AB, Line BR, Goldman JM, Robbins J. Sequential serum thyroglobulin determination 131-I scan and 131-I uptakes after triiodothyronine withdrawal in patients with thyroid cancer. *J Clin Endocrinol Metab* 1981; **53**: 1199–204.

43 Jeevanram RK, Shah DH, Sharma SM *et al.* Influence of initial large dose on subsequent uptake of therapeutic radioiodine in thyroid cancer patients. *Nucl Med Biol* 1986; **13**: 277–9.

44 Pacini F, Lippi F, Formica N *et al.* Therapeutic doses of iodine-131 reveal undiagnosed metastases in thyroid cancer patients with detectable serum thyroglobulin levels. *J Nucl Med* 1987; **28**: 1888–91.

45 Pineda JD, Ain LK, Reynolds JC, Robbins J. Iodine-131 therapy for thyroid cancer patients with elevated thyroglobulin and negative diagnostic scan. *J Clin Endocrinol Metab* 1995; **80**: 1488–92.

46 Schlumberger M, Arcangioli O, Piekarski JD *et al.* Detection and treatment of lung metastases of differentiated thyroid carcinoma in patients with normal chest x-ray. *J Nucl Med* 1988; **29**: 1790–4.

47 Roy-Camille R, Leger FA, Merland JJ, Saillant G, Savoie JC, Riche MC. Perspectives actuelles dans le traitement des metastases osseuses des cancers thyroidiens. *Chirurgie* 1980; **106**: 32–5.

48 Ceccarelli C, Pacini F, Lippi F *et al.* Thyroid cancer in children and adolescents. *Surgery* 1988; **104**: 1143–7.

49 Maxon HR, Smith HS. Radioiodine-131 in the diagnosis and treatment of metastatic well differentiated thyroid cancer. *Endocrinol Metab Clin North Am* 1990; **19**: 685–96.

50 Niederle B, Roka R, Schemper M, Fritsch A, Weissel M, Ramach W. Surgical treatment of distant metastases in differentiated thyroid cancer: Indication and results. *Surgery* 1986; **100**: 1088–95.

51 Proye CAG, Dromer DHR, Carnaille BM *et al.* Is it still worthwhile to treat bone metastases from differentiated thyroid carcinoma with radioactive iodine? *World J Surg* 1992; **16**: 640–6.

52 Mazzaferri EL. Papillary and follicular thyroid cancer: a selective approach to diagnosis and treatment. *Ann Rev Med* 1981; **32**: 73–91.

53 Parker LN, Wu SY, Kim DD *et al.* Recurrence of papillary thyroid carcinoma presenting as a focal neurological deficit. *Arch Intern Med* 1986; **146**: 1985–7.

54 Hay ID. Brain metastases from papillary thyroid carcinoma. *Arch Intern Med* 1987; **147**: 607–10.

55 Venkatesh A, Leavens ME, Samaan NA. Brain metastases in patients with well-differentiated thyroid carcinoma: study of 11 cases. *Eur J Surg Oncol* 1990; **16**: 448–52.

56 Rall JE, Alpers JB, Lewallen CG, Sonemberg M, Berman M, Rawson RW. Radiation pneumonitis and fibrosis: a complication of radioiodine treatment of pulmonary metastases from cancer of the thyroid. *J Clin Endocrinol Metab* 1957; **17**: 1263–5.

57 Leeper R. Controversies in the treatment of thyroid cancer: The New York Memorial Hospital approach. *Thyroid Today* 1982; **V**: 1.

58 Schober O, Gunter HH, Schwarzrock R *et al.* Hämatologische Langzeitveranderungen bei der Schilddrüsenkarzinoms. *Strahlenther Onkol* 1987; **163**: 464–7.

59 Edmonds CJ, Smith T. The long-term hazard of the treatment of thyroid cancer with radioiodine. *Br J Radiol* 1986; **59**: 45–50.

60 Pacini F, Pinchera A, Mancusi F *et al.* Anaplastic thyroid carcinoma: a retrospective clinical and immunohistochemical study. *Oncol Rep* 1994; **1**: 921–5.

61 Pacini F, Gasperi M, Fugazzola L *et al.* Testicular function in patients

with differentiated thyroid carcinoma treated with radioiodine. *J Nucl Med* 1994; **35**: 1418–22.

62 Schlumberger M, De Vathaire F, Travagli JP *et al.* Differentiated thyroid carcinoma in childhood: long term follow-up of 72 patients. *J Clin Endocrinol Metab* 1987; **65**: 1088–93.

63 Marcocci C, Golia F, Bruno-Bossio G, Vignali E, Pinchera A. Carefully monitored levothyroxine suppressive therapy is not associated with bone loss in premonopausal women. *J Clin Endocrinol Metab* 1994; **78**: 818–23.

64 Nel CJ, van Heerden JA, Goellner JR. Anaplastic carcinoma of the thyroid: a clinicopathological study of eighty-two cases. *Mayo Clin Proc* 1985; **60**: 51–4.

65 Venkatesh YSS, Ordonez NG, Schultz PN, Hickey RC, Goepfert H, Samaan NA. Anaplastic carcinoma of the thyroid: a clinicopathological study of 121 cases. *Cancer* 1990; **66**: 321–4.

66 Smedal MI, Messner WA. The results of x-ray treatment in undifferentiated carcinoma of the thyroid. *Radiology* 1961; **76**: 927–30.

67 Shimaoka K, Schoenfeld DA, DeWys WD. A randomized trial of doxorubicin versus doxorubicin plus cisplatin in patients with advanced thyroid carcinoma. *Cancer* 1985; **56**: 2155–9.

68 Sokal M, Harmer GI. Chemotherapy for anaplastic carcinoma of the thyroid. *Clin Oncol* 1978; **4**: 3–7.

69 Pacini F, Pinchera A, Mancusi F *et al.* Anaplastic thyroid carcinoma: a retrospective clinical and immunohistochemical study. *Oncol Rep* 1994; **1**: 921.

70 Tallroth E, Wallin G, Lundell G, Lowhagen T, Einhorn P. Multimodality treatment in anaplastic giant cell thyroid carcinoma. *Cancer* 1987; **60**: 1428–33.

71 Kim JH, Leeper RD. Treatment of anaplastic giant and spindle cell carcinoma of the thyroid gland with combination adriamycin and radiation therapy: a new approach. *Cancer* 1983; **52**: 954–8.

72 Werner B, Abele J, Alveryd A *et al.* Multimodal therapy in anaplastic giant cell thyroid carcinoma. *J World Surg* 1984; **8**: 64–9.

73 Tenval J, Tallroth E, El Hassan A *et al.* Anaplastic thyroid carcinoma. Doxorubicin, hyperfractionated radiotherapy and surgery. *Acta Oncol* 1990; **29**: 1025–8.

74 Mulligan LM, Kwok JBJ, Healey CS *et al.* Germ-line mutations of the RET proto-oncogene in multiple endocrine neoplasia type 2A. *Nature* 1993; **363**: 458–60.

75 Donis-Keller H, Dou S, Chi D *et al.* Mutations of the RET proto-oncogene are associated with MEN 2A and FMTC. *Hum Molec Genet* 1993; **2**: 851–6.

76 Hofstra RMW, Landsvater RM, Ceccherini I *et al.* A mutation in the RET proto-oncogene associated with multiple endocrine neoplasia type 2B and sporadic medullary thyroid carcinoma. *Nature* 1994; **367**: 375–6.

77 Romei C, Elisei R, Pinchera A *et al.* Somatic mutation of the ret protooncogene in sporadic medullary thyroid carcinoma are not restricted to exon 16 and are associated with tumor recurrence. *J Clin Endocrinol Metab* 1996; **81**: 1619–22.

78 Marsh DJ, Learoyd DL, Andrew SD *et al.* Somatic mutations in the RET proto-oncogene in sporadic medullary thyroid carcinoma. *Clin Endocrinol (Oxf)* 1996; **44**: 249–57.

79 Rosenfeld MG, Mermod JJ, Amara SG *et al.* Production of a novel neuropeptide encoded by the calcitonin gene via tissue specific RNA processing. *Nature* 1983; **304**: 129–32.

80 Pacini F, Fugazzola L, Basolo F, Elisei R, Pinchera A. Expression of calcitonin gene-related peptide in medullary thyroid cancer. *J Endocrinol Invest* 1992; **15**: 539–42.

81 Wells SA, Jr, Baylin SB, Linehan WM *et al.* Provocative agents and the diagnosis of medullary carcinoma of the thyroid gland. *Ann Surg* 1978; **188**: 139–43.

82 Pacini F, Basolo F, Elisei R, Fugazzola L, Cola A, Pinchera A. Medullary thyroid cancer. An immunohistochemical and humoral study using six separate antigens. *Am J Clin Pathol* 1991; **95**: 300–308.

83 Bernier JJ, Rambaud JC, Cattan D *et al.* Diarrhoea associated with medullary carcinoma of the thyroid. *Gut* 1970; **10**: 980–2.

84 Pacini F, Fontanelli M, Fugazzola L *et al.* Routine measurement of serum calcitonin in nodular thyroid diseases allows the preoperative diagnosis of unsuspected sporadic medullary thyroid carcinoma. *J Clin Endocrinol Metab* 1994; **78**: 826–9.

85 Rieu M, Lame MC, Richard A *et al.* Prevalence of sporadic medullary thyroid carcinoma: the importance of routine measurement of serum calcitonin in the diagnostic evaluation of thyroid nodules. *Clin Endocrinol (Oxf)* 1995; **42**: 453–7.

86 Grauer A, Raue F, Gagel RF. Changing concept in the management of hereditary and sporadic medullary thyroid carcinoma. *Endocrinol Metab Clin North Am* 1990; **19**: 613–21.

87 Fugazzola L, Pinchera A, Luchetti F *et al.* Disappearance rate of serum calcitonin after total thyroidectomy for medullary thyroid carcinoma. *Int J Biol Markers* 1994; **9**: 21–4.

88 Zedenius J, Walliw G, Hamberger B, Nordenskjold H, Weber G, Larsson C. Somatic and MEN2A *de novo* mutations identified in the RET proto-oncogene by screening of sporadic MTCs. *Hum Mol Genet* 1994; **3**: 1259–62.

89 Bongarzone I, Pierotti AM, Monzini N, *et al.* High frequency of activation of tyrosine kinase oncogenes in human papillary thyroid carcinoma. *Oncogene* 1989; **4**: 1457–62.

90 Fugazzola L, Pierotti MA, Vigano E, Pacini F, Vorontsova TV, Bongarzone I. Molecular and biochemical, analysis of RET/PTC4, a novel oncogenic rearrangement between RET and ELE1 genes, in a post-Chernobyl papillary thyroid cancer. *Oncogene* 1996; **13**: 1093–97.

CHAPTER 29

Subacute thyroiditis

A.D. Toft and P. Perros

Introduction

Subacute or de Quervain's thyroiditis is an inflammatory disorder, usually affecting women aged 30–60 years, in which there is pain arising in the thyroid gland characteristically associated with systemic upset, tender thyroid enlargement and mild hyperthyroidism. It is a rare cause of hyperthyroidism, however, accounting for only 3% of all new cases referred to the authors' clinic. The true incidence of subacute thyroiditis is difficult to assess as patients with mild forms of the disorder either do not seek medical attention or are considered by their primary care physicians to be suffering from pharyngitis. As the pain and hyperthyroidism resolve there is usually a transient period of hypothyroidism followed by eventual recovery by the sixth month (Fig. 29.1).

Subacute thyroiditis is probably the result of infection with one of a variety of viruses, although conclusive proof, which depends upon the demonstration of virus inclusion bodies in the thyroid follicular cells of affected patients, is lacking. There is often a history of recent upper respiratory tract infection or of symptoms suggestive of viraemia such as headache, malaise and myalgia. Furthermore, there have been frequent reports of an association between subacute thyroiditis and viral infections such as mumps, measles, influenza, common cold, adenovirus, infectious mononucleosis, myocarditis, Coxsackie, catscratch fever [1], and an epidemic affecting 23 individuals has been described [2]. In almost 50% of patients without clinical evidence of viral infection, antibodies can be detected against common viruses, most often Coxsackie B [3], but it is possible that the antibody response is an anamnestic reaction. A seasonal distribution of subacute thyroiditis is recognised. For example, the majority of cases present in Italy between June and September when enteroviral infections are most common [4]. Recently, subacute thyroiditis has been reported following interferon-α therapy [5].

There is no evidence, however, that subacute thyroiditis is an organ-specific autoimmune disease like Hashimoto's thyroiditis or Graves' disease [6]. The transient appearance in the serum of autoantibodies to thyroglobulin, to thyroid microsomes and to the thyroid-stimulating hormone (TSH) receptor in a minority of cases [7–9] represents a normal and appropriate response to antigen released by the damaged follicles, although thyroid-blocking antibodies may be implicated in the hypothyroid phase of some patients with subacute thyroiditis [10]. In addition, the histological appearance of subacute thyroiditis is quite distinct from that of autoimmune thyroid disease and is characterised by the presence of multinucleated giant cells (Fig. 29.2) derived from mononuclear histiocyte cells [11]. There is also a strong association between subacute thyroiditis in Caucasian patients and the histocompatibility antigen B35 but not with human leucocyte antigen (HLA)-B8, -DR3 or -DR5, which are over-represented in patients with autoimmune thyroid disease [12,13].

Clinical features

These depend upon the stage at which the patient presents. In the early weeks of the illness there is pain, which may be excruciating, in the region of the thyroid which may radiate to the jaws and ears, and is made worse by swallowing, coughing and movement of the neck. There may be associated lassitude, myalgia, feverishness and symptoms of mild hyperthyroidism such as tremor, irritability and weight loss of 3–4 kg. On examination the thyroid gland is usually slightly but diffusely enlarged and tender. Discomfort may be localised initially to one lobe. Cervical lymphadenopathy is rare. Pyrexia which may reach 40°C is present in less than half of all patients. Lid retraction may be evident during the hyperthyroid phase but exophthalmos, pretibial myxoedema, thyroid acropachy, and a bruit over the thyroid are *never* present.

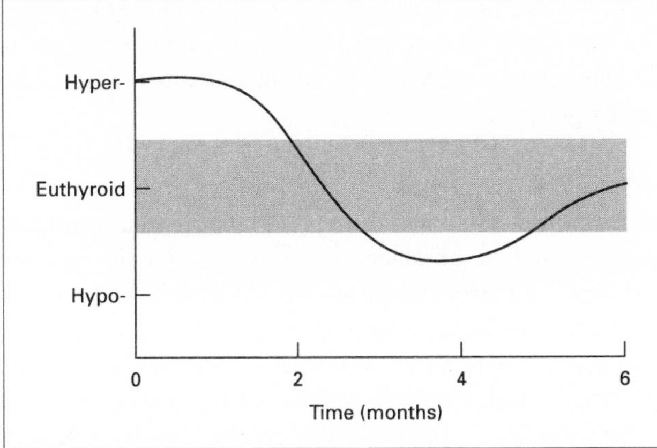

Fig. 29.1 Pattern of changes in thyroid function in patients with subacute thyroiditis. The degree of hyper- and hypothyroidism varies from patient to patient, is rarely severe, and depends upon the timing of blood sampling. Permanent hypothyroidism is rare and probably only occurs in patients with underlying autoimmune thyroid disease.

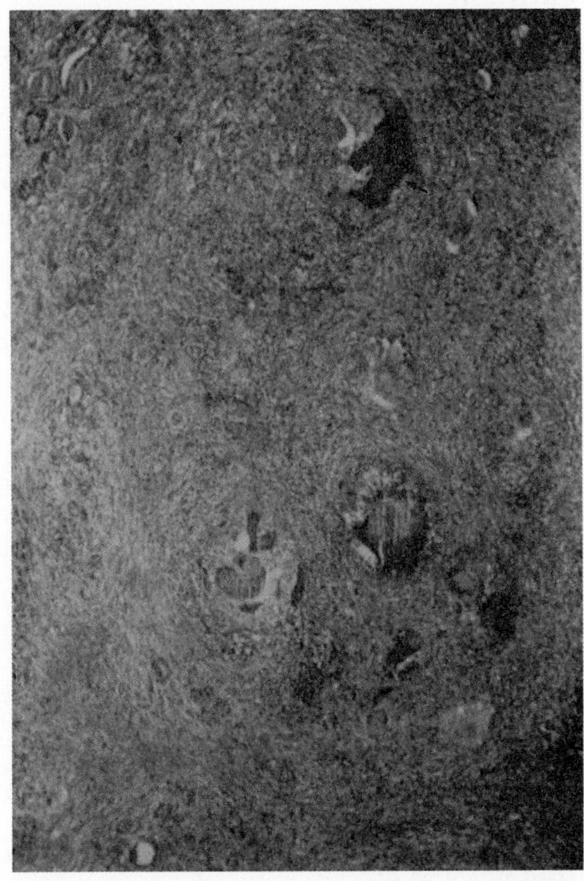

Fig. 29.2 Early phase of subacute thyroiditis. The normal thyroid architecture is destroyed with the appearance of giant cells (arrowed). It is remarkable that such an appearance is compatible with restoration to normal structure and function, (H&E, ×40).

Eight weeks after the onset of illness thyroid tenderness has usually resolved and by 12–16 weeks there may be clinical evidence of mild hypothyroidism. Rarely, subacute thyroiditis may recur several years after the first episode [14].

Investigations (Table 29.1)

In the initial stages the inflammatory reaction within the gland disrupts the follicles and causes release of colloid and its constituents into the peripheral circulation. Serum concentrations of thyroxine (T_4) and triiodothyronine (T_3) are raised, usually slightly, and account for the early mild hyperthyroidism which lasts for a few weeks until the preformed colloid is depleted. Uptake of isotope (^{99m}Tc, ^{123}I or ^{131}I) by the thyroid during the phase of hyperthyroidism is negligible for two reasons. First, the damaged follicular cell is unable to trap iodine and, secondly, there is suppression of endogenous TSH by the elevated serum thyroid hormone concentrations.

The erythrocyte sedimentation rate (ESR) is high and often exceeds 80 mm in the first hour. The white blood cell count is usually normal. Serum thyroglobulin concentrations may be increased and antibodies appear transiently in the serum in weak titre to thyroglobulin, thyroid peroxidase and the TSH receptor in some patients.

Table 29.1 Features of 21 patients presenting to the Endocrine Clinic, Royal Infirmary NHS Trust, Edinburgh, with hyperthyroidism due to subacute thyroiditis during a 3-year period. Results expressed as mean and (range).

Female/male	18 : 3
Age	49 years (31–73)
June–September presentation	14/21
Initial investigations	
Free T_4	33.8 pmol/l (25–47)
Total T_3	3.1 nmol/l (28–4.1)
TSH	Undetectable in all cases
4-hour ^{131}Iuptake	Negligible in all cases
ESR	72 (51–107)
Autoantibodies to peroxidase, thyroglobulin or TSH receptor	3/21
Follow-up investigations	
TSH at 4 months	18.3 mU/l (3.0–98.2)
Normal TSH at 4 months	5/21
Permanent hypothyroidism	0/21

Normal ranges: free T_4 9–21 pmol/l; total T_3 1.1–2.6 nmol/l; TSH 0.15–3.5 mU/l. T_4, thyroxine; T_3, triiodothyronine; TSH, thyroid-stimulating hormone; ESR, erythrocyte sedimentation rate.

The acute phase of the disease is accompanied by high concentrations of interleukin 6 in the serum of patients, released from damaged thyrocytes [15,16], and this measurement may prove to be a useful marker of destructive thyroiditis.

Not all patients enter a phase of hypothyroidism at 3–4 months. In those who do the degree of thyroid failure varies from a minor elevation of serum TSH with normal thyroid hormone concentrations (subclinical hypothyroidism) to overt hypothyroidism. If measured, radioiodine uptake by the thyroid at this stage will be normal or even high under the influence of TSH as the follicular cells recover normal function. Although serum T_3, T_4 and TSH concentrations have usually returned to normal by 6 months, subtle thyroid defects remain. Thyroidal iodine stores measured by X-ray fluorescence are still depleted 12 months after clinical remission [17] and ultrasonographic [18] and magnetic resonance imaging (MRI) [19] abnormalities and antibodies directed against thyroid antigens other than thyroglobulin, peroxidase or the TSH receptor persist for 3–4 years [20].

Permanent hypothyroidism develops in approximately 5% of patients and in these there is thought to be a background of autoimmune thyroid disease [21].

Differential diagnosis

Subacute thyroiditis is one of a number of causes of hyperthyroidism associated with a negligible radioiodine uptake by the thyroid, some of which may be associated with thyroid tenderness (Table 29.2). In the great majority of cases of pyogenic thyroiditis the patient is euthyroid. The swelling is usually confined to one lobe, is fluctuant, and is extremely tender and associated with a high white blood cell count. Fine-needle aspiration will yield pus. Infiltration of the thyroid by amyloid [22], carcinoma [23] or lymphoma [24] causing a subacute thyroiditis-like syndrome is rare and cytological examination of a thyroid aspirate should resolve any diagnostic dilemma. Other causes of a painful thyroid gland include Hashimoto's thyroiditis [25], albeit rarely, haemorrhage into a nodular goitre, secondary deposits and very rarely Graves' disease [26], but in none of these is the combination of hyperthyroidism and a low radioiodine uptake present.

Table 29.2 Causes of hyperthyroidism with a negligible radioiodine uptake.

Subacute (de Quervain's) thyroiditis*
Acute bacterial thyroiditis*
Silent thyroiditis especially post-partum
Iodide-induced
Factitious
Struma ovarii
Functioning metastatic thyroid carcinoma
Infiltration of thyroid by malignancy or amyloid†

* Always associated with discomfort in the neck.
† May be associated with discomfort in the neck.

Due to the delay between onset of subacute thyroiditis and medical consultation, particularly if neck discomfort has been mild and constitutional upset absent, a history of pain may not be obtained, and if isotope studies are not performed, an erroneous diagnosis of Graves' disease made and inappropriate treatment given.

In recent years there has been confusion between de Quervain's and silent thyroiditis which was considered to be a painless variant of subacute thyroiditis. Although the pattern of thyroid function tests may be similar, silent thyroiditis is an immunologically mediated destructive form of hyperthyroidism with low radioiodine uptake, commonly presenting in the post-partum period [27]. Pain is not a feature and the histological and cytological appearances of the gland are those of a lymphocytic thyroiditis.

Treatment

In the majority of cases the neck discomfort and associated systemic symptoms such as pyrexia and myalgia respond to simple analgesics such as aspirin 600 mg every 4–6 hours orally. Occasionally it is necessary to administer oral prednisolone in a total daily dose of 30–40 mg for 3–4 weeks. Corticosteroids produce relief of symptoms within 24 hours but do not modify the natural history of the disease.

Symptoms of mild hyperthyroidism should be controlled by a non-selective β-adrenoceptor antagonist, such as propranolol 160 mg daily. Antithyroid drugs are of no benefit since the hyperthyroidism is due to the release of preformed thyroid hormones by the damaged follicles and not due to increased synthesis of new hormones as in Graves' disease.

It is not necessary to treat the phase of transient hypothyroidism but thyroid failure persisting beyond the sixth month should be regarded as permanent and T_4 prescribed.

References

1 Volpe R, Row VV, Ezrin C. Circulating viral and thyroid antibodies in subacute thyroiditis. *J Clin Endocrinol Metab* 1967; **27**: 1275–84.

2 deBruin TW, Riekhoff FP, deBoer JJ. An outbreak of thyrotoxicosis due to atypical subacute thyroiditis. *J Clin Endocrinol Metab* 1990; 70: 396–402.

3 Volpe R. Subacute (de Quervain's) thyroiditis. *Clin Endocrinol Metab* 1979; **8**: 81–95.

4 Martino E, Buratti L, Bartalena L *et al.* High prevalence of subacute thyroiditis during summer season in Italy. *J Endocrinol Invest* 1987; **10**: 321–3.

5 Gonzalez-Fernandez B, Arrenz A, Penarrubia MJ, Marazuela M.

Subacute thyroiditis associated with interferon-alpha 2a therapy. *Horm Metab Res* 1995; **27**: 45–6.

6 Tomer Y, Davies TF. Infections and autoimmune endocrine disease. *Baillière's Clin Endocrinol Metab* 1995; **9**: 47–70.

7 Strakosch CR, Joyner D, Wall JR. Thyroid-stimulating antibodies in patients with subacute thyroiditis. *J Clin Endocrinol Metab* 1978; **46**: 345–8.

8 Mitani Y, Shigemasa C, Kouchi T, Tanigushi S, Ueta Y, Yoshida, Mashiba H. Detection of thyroid-stimulating antibody in patients with inflammatory thyrotoxicosis. *Horm Res* 1992; **37**: 196–201.

9 Yoshikawa N, Arreaza G, Morita T, Resetkova E, Miller N, Volpe R. Studies of human peripheral blood mononuclear calls (PBMC) from patients with subacute thyroiditis in severe combined immunodeficient (SCID) mice: less production of human interferon gamma than that seen for Graves' disease. *Horm Metab Res* 1994; **26**: 419–23.

10 Tamai H, Nozaki T, Mukuta T *et al.* The incidence of thyroid stimulating blocking antibodies during the hypothyroid phase in patients with subacute thyroiditis. *J Clin Endocrinol Metab* 1991; **73**: 245–50.

11 Mizukami Y, Michigishi T, Kawato M, Matsubara F. Immunohistochemical and ultrastructural study of subacute thyroiditis with special reference to multinucleated giant cells. *Hum Pathol* 1987; **18**: 929–35.

12 Bech K, Nerup J, Thomsen M *et al.* Subacute thyroiditis de Quervain: a disease associated with a HLA-B antigen. *Acta Endocrinol* 1977; **86**: 504–9.

13 Rubin RA, Guay AT. Susceptibility to subacute thyroiditis is genetically influenced: familial occurrence in identical twins. *Thyroid* 1991; **1**: 157–61.

14 Iitaka M, Momotani N, Ishi J, Ito K. Incidence of subacute thyroiditis recurrences after a prolonged latency: 24-year survey. *J Clin Endocrinol Metab* 1996; **81**: 466–9.

15 Bartalena L, Brogioni S, Grasso L, Martino E. Increased serum interleukin-6 concentration in patients with subacute thyroiditis: relationship with concomitant changes in serum T4-binding globulin concentration. *J Endocrinol Invest* 1993; **16**: 213–18.

16 Bartalena L, Brogioni S, Grasso L, Rago T, Vitti P, Pinchera A, Martino E. Interleukin-6: a marker of thyroid-destructive processes? *J Clin Endocrinol Metab* 1994; **79**: 1424–7.

17 Fragu P, Rougier P, Schlumberger M, Tubiana M. Evolution of thyroid 127-I stores measured by X-ray fluorescence in subacute thyroiditis. *J Clin Endocrinol Metab* 1982; **54**: 162–6.

18 Benker G, Olbricht T, Windeck R *et al.* The sonographical and functional sequelae of de Quervain's subacute thyroiditis: long-term follow-up. *Acta Endocrinol* 1988; **117**: 45–41.

19 Otsuka N, Nagai K, Morita K *et al.* Magnetic resonance imaging of subacute thyroiditis. *Radiat Med* 1994; **12**: 273–6.

20 Weetman AP, Smallridge RC, Nutman TB, Burman KD. Persistent thyroid autoimmunity after subacute thyroiditis. *J Clin Lab Immunol* 1987; **23**: 1–6.

21 Tikkanen MJ, Lamberg BA. Hypothyroidism following subacute thyroiditis. *Acta Endocrinol* 1982; **101**: 348–53.

22 Ikenoue H, Okamura K, Kuroda T, Sato T, Yoshinari M, Fujishima M. Thyroid amyloidosis with recurrent subacute thyroiditis-like syndrome. *J Clin Endocrinol Metab* 1988; **67**: 41–5.

23 Watts NB, Sewell CW. Carcinomatous involvement of the thyroid presenting as subacute thyroiditis. *Am J Med Sci* 1988; **296**: 126–8.

24 Gochu J, Piper B, Montana J, Park HS, Poretsky L. Lymphoma of the thyroid mimicking thyroiditis in a patient with the acquired immune deficiency syndrome. *J Endocrinol Invest* 1994; **17**: 279–82.

25 Anonymous. The painful thyroid. *Lancet* 1986; i: 1308–9.

26 Stanley JM, Najjar SS. Painful thyroid gland: an atypical presentation of Graves' disease. *Clin Endocrinol* 1992; 37: 468–9.

27 Anonymous. Post-partum thyroiditis. *Lancet* 1987; i: 962.

CHAPTER 30

Thyroid disease and pregnancy

J.H. Lazarus

During pregnancy there are complex hormonal and metabolic changes in the mother and the fetus. Diseases of the thyroid may affect the pregnant woman (Table 30.1), and the fetus and neonate may also be at risk. The subject has been recently reviewed [1–3, 39].

Effect of pregnancy on thyroid function

Maternal thyroid function

The rise in oestrogen concentration associated with pregnancy stimulates the hepatic synthesis of thyroxine (T_4) binding globulin (TBG) to double its normal concentration, thus producing elevations in serum total T_4 and, to a lesser extent, total triiodothyronine (T_3). Measurement of 'free' thyroid hormones together with the availability of the 'sensitive' thyroid-stimulating hormone (TSH) assay gives a reasonable guide to maternal thyroid status, but it must be remembered that there is a drop in free T_4 and free T_3 in the third trimester, although they remain within the normal range. Serum thyroglobulin also rises during pregnancy despite the lack of TSH elevation. This implies that other 'TSH-like' stimulators, such as human chorionic gonadotrophin (hCG), which shares a common α-subunit with TSH, may be responsible for the increase in thyroglobulin. Thyroid volume, as measured by ultrasonography, increases in early pregnancy and remains elevated. During pregnancy urinary iodine excretion increases due to increased glomerular filtration rate and decreased tubular reabsorption [4]. In areas of mild iodine deficiency there will be a compensatory increase in thyroid volume and a significant decrease of T_4 and T_3 into the hypothyroid range in up to 50%, depending on the severity of the iodine deficiency [5]. These changes may persist for up to a year post-partum and in some cases may never be reversed. TSH levels, measured with 'sensitive' assays, are found to be within normal limits during pregnancy, as is the TSH response to thyrotrophin-releasing hormone (TRH). A schematic picture of the changes in maternal and fetal thyroid function is shown Fig. 30.1.

Fetal thyroid function

The fetal thyroid starts hormone production at 12 weeks' gestation. At about this time fetal TSH is detectable, but remains low until about 20 weeks. Thus, a functional fetal pituitary–thyroid axis exists at 12 weeks' gestation. Contrary to older views, it has been recently shown that placental transfer of T_4 and T_3 occurs near to term [7] and also earlier in pregnancy (11–25 weeks of gestation). Recent data obtained from sampling of embryonic cavities during the first trimester of pregnancy clearly show that maternal T_4 reaches the embryonic cavity at 3–8 weeks after conception [8]. The implication is that the increase in maternal T_4 occurring during the first trimester may be functionally important for the developing embryo when its thyroid is not yet functioning. There is no doubt that low maternal T_4 concentration during early pregnancy results in impairment of fetal brain development. It should be noted that transplacental passage of iodide, thionamide drugs, thyroid-stimulating antibodies and TRH readily occurs, whereas there is no transfer of TSH. The placenta contains deiodinase enzymes which presumably regulate the quantity of iodothyronines that can cross to the fetus [9].

Hyperthyroidism in pregnancy [10]

Hyperthyroidism is rare (prevalence 0.05–0.2%) in pregnancy, and its presence is associated with a significant increase in neonatal mortality. Congenital abnormalities may be more common in infants of mothers with untreated Graves', as are low-birthweight infants and premature labour. The

Table 30.1 Diseases of the thyroid occurring during and after pregnancy.

Graves' hyperthyroidism
Autoimmune hypothyroidism
Post-ablation hypothyroidism
Non-toxic goitre
Thyroid cancer
Post-partum thyroid disease
Exacerbation of previous Graves' hyperthyroidism
De novo Graves' hyperthyroidism
Post-partum thyroiditis
Thyrotoxicosis
Hypothyroidism
Autoimmune hypothyroidism

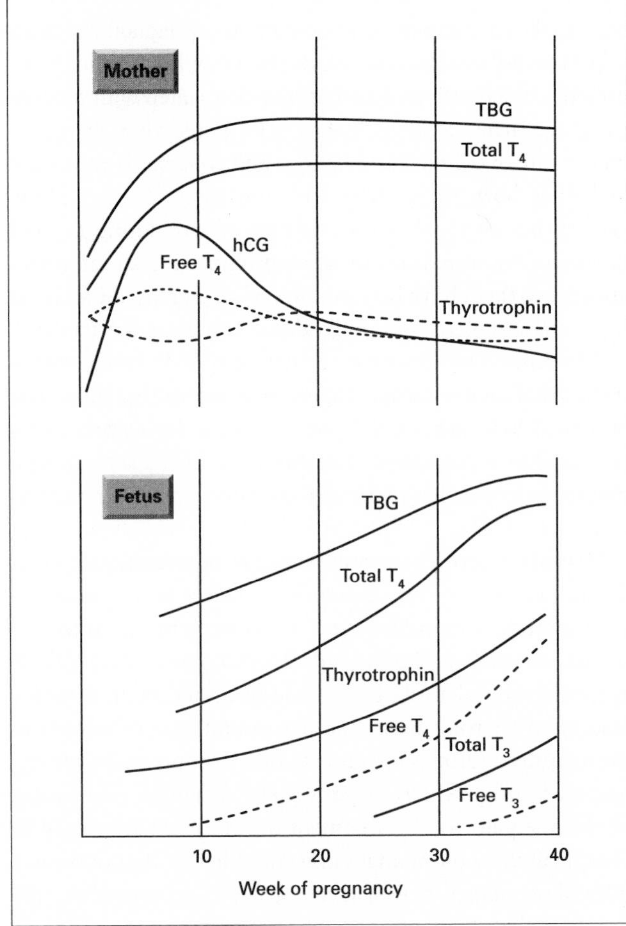

Fig. 30.1 Changes in maternal and fetal thyroid function during gestation. TBG, thyroxine-binding globulin. hCG, human chorionic gonadotrophin. From [6], with permission.

commonest cause of hyperthyroidism in pregnancy is Graves' disease. The condition may remit spontaneously during pregnancy due to the changes in maternal immunological activity at this time; in particular, this is likely to be due to a fall in circulating thyroid-stimulating immunoglobulins (TSH receptor antibodies). The reason for this is complex, but may involve changes in the reactivity of both T and B lymphocytes as well as the secretion of placental factors which may modulate the immune response [11]. The role of the placenta is crucial in maternal/fetal immune interaction. The influence of class II human leucocyte antigens (HLA) on relapse of another autoimmune disease (rheumatoid arthritis) [12] and even abortion [13] has been discussed. In some patients the hyperthyroidism is mild and may even go unnoticed, only to relapse in the post-partum period. Other causes of hyperthyroidism include toxic multinodular goitre, toxic uninodular goitre and trophoblastic tumours. The latter are characterised by the presence of large amounts of hCG, leading to very high circulating thyroid hormone concentrations, but with few clinical findings of hyperthyroidism.

Hyperemesis gravidarum, characterised by severe vomiting in the first trimester, is also associated with modestly raised thyroid hormone values due to hCG normally produced at this stage of pregnancy. The condition is relatively rare ($<0.5\%$ of all pregnancies), but may be difficult to diagnose clinically because of the frequency of nausea and vomiting of early pregnancy. Hyperthyroidism due to other causes may also present with vomiting. About one-third of patients with hyperemesis gravidarum are found to have high total and free T_4 concentrations, with a lesser number having high free T_3 [14]. There are molecular variants of hCG with altered glycosylation and enhanced thyrotrophic activity which are responsible for the increased level of thyroid hormones in some cases of hyperemesis [15]. The hCG level has been found to correlate with the degree of thyroid stimulation together with the severity of the clinical symptomatology [16], and patients with gestational thyrotoxicosis have circulating hCG with high biological activity [17]. This condition, although potentially serious due to the persistent vomiting, is likely to resolve by the second trimester. Occasionally it is necessary to treat such patients with propylthiouracil. The clinical diagnosis of hyperthyroidism in pregnancy is difficult because many of the clinical symptoms and signs (e.g. heat intolerance, tachycardia, nervousness and goitre) may occur in normal pregnancy. Peripheral manifestations of Graves' disease, such as eye signs and pretibial myxoedema, will alert the clinician to the presence of thyroid disease but do not help in establishing thyroid status.

Maternal thyroid function should be assessed by measuring free T_4, free T_3 and TSH. Careful attention should be paid to the 'normal' ranges of these hormones in pregnancy when interpreting the results. Thyroid-stimulating immunoglobulins, which can cross the placenta, are present in Graves' disease, and their detection at 36 weeks' gestation is a good (but not invariable), guide to the likelihood of transient neonatal hyperthyroidism [18]. However, the usual assays for thyroid-stimulating antibodies do not differentiate between stimulating and blocking antibodies thus causing doubt about the interpretation of results in some cases. It is important to remember that women previously treated for Graves' hyperthyroidism who are euthyroid during gestation may have significantly raised circulating concentrations of thyroid-stimulating antibodies.

Management of hyperthyroidism in pregnancy [19]

The risks of hyperthyroidism in pregnancy are twofold: first, on the mother, and secondly, on the fetus. There is an increased risk of abortion in untreated pregnant thyrotoxic women. Treatment of hyperthyroidism during pregnancy is best done using antithyroid drugs. The aim should be to maintain the dose at the lowest level compatible with euthyroidism. The dose is important because thionamide antithyroid drugs cross the placenta, and if given in too large a quantity may induce fetal goitre, thus potentially causing difficulties in labour. A suitable regimen is to render the patient rapidly euthyroid with a moderate dose of propylthiouracil (e.g. 100 mg three times a day) and then reduce to say 50–100 mg a day if possible. A blocking/replacement therapy regimen of propylthiouracil and T_4 should *not* be used because T_4 will not cross the placenta in sufficient quantities and the dose of antithyroid drug will be too high (thereby resulting in fetal goitre and hypothyroidism). Although carbimazole is the commonest antithyroid drug used in the UK, a fetal scalp lesion (aplasia cutis) associated with this drug has been described [20] and it is generally thought that propylthiouracil should be the antithyroid drug of choice in hyperthyroidism occurring in early pregnancy. This drug also blocks peripheral conversion of T_4 to T_3 (unlike carbimazole). It is usual to continue the antithyroid drugs right up to and during labour. Adjunctive administration of propranolol to reduce peripheral manifestations of hyperthyroidism may be carried out cautiously during the pregnancy, but should not be given during labour in view of its potentially deleterious effect on the fetus. A pregnant patient with hyperthyroidism should be monitored regularly through the pregnancy as well as post-partum in case of relapse. Hashizume *et al.* [21] from Japan have reported that T_4 administration to pregnant women with Graves' hyperthyroidism during pregnancy and after delivery, together with methimazole, was effective in reducing the incidence of post-partum recurrence of hyperthyroidism, but these results have not been confirmed in other countries. Treatment of the hyperthyroidism by bilateral subtotal thyroidectomy may be undertaken most conveniently in the second trimester. Operation in other stages of pregnancy carries an increased risk of fetal loss. Patients should be carefully prepared with antithyroid drug administration before surgery. It may be necessary to give postoperative T_4 therapy to maintain euthyroidism during the remainder of the pregnancy. Radioiodine therapy for hyperthyroidism in pregnancy is completely contraindicated. Thyrotoxic patients who have had radioiodine and who are later found to be in the very early stages of pregnancy have grounds for requesting a termination because of the increased sensitivity of fetal tissue. Women of reproductive age who receive radioiodine treatment should be sure that they are not pregnant at the time and should not conceive for 4 months after the therapy.

Hypothyroidism

Maternal hypothyroidism is uncommon in pregnancy because hypothyroid females are relatively infertile. Although the presence of hypothyroidism has been associated with successful pregnancies to term, it has been noted that there is a higher rate of stillbirths, abortions and congenital anomalies in babies born to mothers with untreated disease. However, although there is no evidence of circulating thyroid hormone abnormalities in women who have spontaneous abortions, there have been reports of an increased incidence of antithyroid peroxidase antibodies in recurrent aborters [40].

The aim of treatment is to maintain TSH levels within the normal range. Recent studies have shown that there may be a 50–100% increase in T_4 requirements during pregnancy [22] and it is suggested that the dose of T_4 replacement therapy should be increased as soon as pregnancy is confirmed [23].

Hypothyroidism may present either before pregnancy or during gestation. The commonest cause is Hashimoto's autoimmune thyroiditis, and measurement of autoantibodies to thyroglobulin and thyroid peroxidase (TPO) (antimicrosomal antibody) should be undertaken. A family history of thyroid disease is often obtained. Treatment of the hypothyroidism is the same as for a non-pregnant patient, namely oral T_4, usually in a dose of 0.15 mg/day. Assessment of the adequacy of T_4 treatment during pregnancy may be complicated by the changes in metabolic rate that occur in a normal pregnancy, as well as the variations in normal thyroid function already mentioned. The best guides as to adequate replacement therapy are the patient's weight and sense of well-being, together with the maintenance of the serum T_4 concentration at the upper limit of normal as for a non-pregnant person [24]. As transplacental passage of thyroid autoantibodies can occur, neonatal hypothyroidism may be detected and should be routinely looked for. In a few of these infants, TSH-receptor-blocking antibodies may be found [25].

Goitre in pregnancy

The thyroid gland may enlarge during pregnancy due to iodine deficiency, and is clinically manifest as a diffuse soft enlargement; it requires no further evaluation. Any other thyroid enlargement occurring in pregnancy where the patient has been shown to be euthyroid should be investigated along the usual lines. Fine-needle aspiration cytology is a safe procedure in pregnancy. A diagnosis of papillary cancer may be made, but follicular cancer cannot readily be diagnosed using fine-needle aspiration. Thyroid cancer in pregnancy is rare and the treatment is by surgery, preferably during the second trimester.

Effect of maternal thyroid disease in pregnancy on fetal and neonatal thyroid function

Fetal thyroid function

The development of normal fetal thyroid function has been described. The fetal thyroid may be affected by maternal thyroid disease due to substances, including drugs, which cross the placental barrier. Thyroid-stimulating immunoglobulins can produce fetal hyperthyroidism in patients with Graves' disease, and TSH-receptor-blocking antibodies or growth-blocking antibodies, seen in some patients with autoimmune thyroiditis, may result in fetal hypothyroidism (Table 30.2). Congenital hyperthyroidism may also be due to a mutation in the TSH-receptor gene which causes constitutive activation of thyroid hormone synthesis [26]. Diagnosis of the fetal thyroid state may be difficult, but sustained fetal tachycardia or bradycardia in the absence of other causes in a woman with thyroid disease is suggestive. The mother need not necessarily be thyrotoxic or hypothyroid. Fetal thyroid state may also be diagnosed by measurement of thyroid hormones in amniotic fluid samples obtained at amniocentesis for other diagnostic purposes. Treatment of fetal hyperthyroidism can be performed by administration of thionamide drugs to the mother as they cross the placenta. Treatment of fetal hypothyroidism is difficult, because thyroid hormones do not cross the placenta in large quantities, but an artificial thyroid hormone analogue, such as dimethylisopropyl thyronine (DIMIT), which crosses the placenta more efficiently than T_4 or T_3, may be beneficial.

Neonatal thyroid function

The maternal diseases associated with neonatal thyroid dysfunction and the specific causes are shown in Table 30.2 and have been reviewed [27].

Neonatal thyrotoxicosis is due to thyroid-stimulating antibodies derived from the mother, and the disease is self-limiting consistent with the short half-life of IgG. Neonatal hypothyroidism occurs independently of maternal thyroid disease and in many countries is routinely screened for by TSH estimations carried 5–7 days post-partum. Transient

Table 30.2 Fetal and neonatal transplacental disease.

Disease	Maternal disease	Cause
Fetal hyperthyroidism	Graves'	TsAb
Fetal hypothyroidism	Hashimoto	TBAb, TGBAb, excess iodides or antithyroid drugs
Fetal goitre	Goitre or Hashimoto	Iodides, antithyroid drugs, TGAb
Neonatal hyperthyroidism		TsAb
Neonatal hypothyroidism	Endemic goitre	Severe iodine deficiency (associated with subnormal maternal T_4), TBAb
	Hashimoto	TPOAb, TGBAb
	Maternal drug ingestion	Iodides, antithyroid drugs
Neonatal pseudohypothyroidism		'High' TSH due to circulating TSH antibody

TsAb, thyrotrophin-receptor-stimulating antibodies; TBAb, thyrotrophin-receptor-blocking antibodies, TGBAb, thyroid growth-blocking antibodies; TGAb, thyroid growth-stimulating antibodies; TPOAb, thyroid peroxidase antibodies; TSH, thyroid-stimulating hormone (thyrotrophin); T_4, thyroxine.

neonatal hypothyroidism may occur in iodine-deficient areas and also in babies born to mothers with autoimmune thyroid disease who have TSH-receptor-blocking antibodies. Some infants have transient congenital hypothyroidism associated with the presence of anti-thyroid peroxidase (TPO) (microsomal) antibodies normally seen in Hashimoto's disease. There is controversy relating to the percentage of babies with congenital hypothyroidism who have TSH-receptor-blocking antibodies and thyroid growth-blocking antibodies because of apparent differences in assay methodology and sensitivity. Figures for positive antibodies in neonates with congenital hypothyroidism range from 10 to 70%. Transient hyperthyrotrophinaemia may occur in the neonate due to the transplacental passage of antibodies to TSH which are not pathogenetic for hypothyroidism. The baby is euthyroid; if such a condition is suspected, the mother should be checked for thyroid disease and a falsely raised TSH level.

Fetal and neonatal goitre may be due to maternal ingestion of iodides or antithyroid drugs. If the goitre is large it may cause obstruction during labour.

Post-partum thyroid dysfunction

The immune suppression associated with pregnancy is not seen in the post-partum period, with the result that there may be an exacerbation of autoimmune diseases such as systemic lupus erythematosus, rheumatoid arthritis and myasthenia gravis. Circulating levels of thyroid antibodies, for example thyroid-stimulating antibodies and anti-TPO, fall during pregnancy in patients with autoimmune thyroid disease, though the mechanism underlying these changes is not understood. The immunological rebound phenomenon, the details of which are not clear, is also relevant to the syndromes of post-partum thyroiditis.

As early as 1948, Roberton [28] documented the occurrence of symptoms of hypothyroidism occurring up to 6 months' post-partum and he instituted treatment with T_4. The prevalence of post-partum thyroid dysfunction (PPT) has been reported to vary widely depending on the method of ascertainment, frequency of blood sampling and hormone measurement methodology. Reports of large series show a prevalence of 5–9% of thyroid dysfunction occurring within 6 months of delivery. Patients with insulin-dependent diabetes mellitus during gestation have a threefold risk of developing PPT [29] and this group should therefore be screened for anti-TPO antibodies during pregnancy. Clinically, the patient may develop transient hyperthyroidism (at about 13 weeks post-partum) followed by transient hypothyroidism (at about 18 weeks post-partum); some patients develop only transient hyperthyroidism while others only show a hypothyroid phase. However, of those patients who develop hypothyroidism 25–30% develop permanent hypothyroidism [30]. The course of thyroid function in susceptible women is shown in Fig. 30.2. Of the 10% of women who are anti-TPO antibody positive at 12–16 weeks' gestation approximately 50% will develop thyroid dysfunction post-partum. The different clinical presentations (see above) account for about 33% of patients in each group (i.e. hyperthyroid only, hyper–hypo and hypothyroid only). Thyrotoxicosis in the post-partum period may thus be due to exacerbation of previous Graves' disease, a new presentation of Graves' disease, or transient post-partum thyrotoxicosis. Differentiation is aided by radioiodine uptake measurements and thyroid-stimulating antibody concentrations. The diagnosis of post-partum thyrotoxicosis may easily be missed

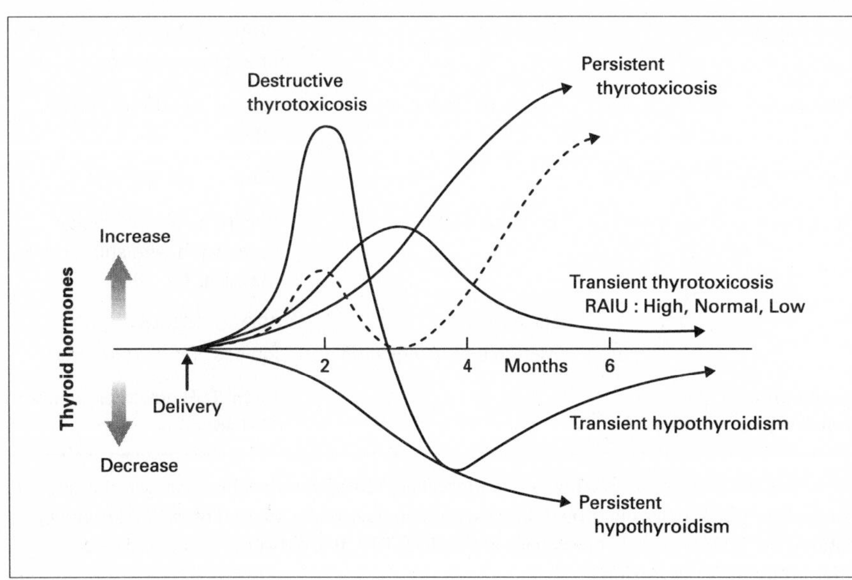

Fig. 30.2 Diagram showing possible development of post-partum thyroid dysfunction in susceptible women. RAIU, radioactive iodine uptake. From [31], with permission.

because of the transient nature of the disease. Patients may present with classic symptoms of hyperthyroidism associated with goitre: radioiodine uptake is low, antibodies to thyroglobulin and thyroid peroxidase are usually present, but thyroid-stimulating antibodies are absent. In the more severe cases the symptoms may be treated with propranolol. Subsequently, many patients go on to develop an episode of hypothyroidism which also may be transient. Again, the diagnosis may be overlooked by the medical attendant because of the non-specific nature of many of the symptoms, perhaps attributed to difficulty in caring for the infant. Psychiatric symptomatology is common. Clinically the patient may appear hypothyroid with weight increase, and a goitre may be noted. A family history of thyroid disease may be obtained and the goitre may be painful. Investigations show a low T_4 with a high TSH level. Fine-needle aspiration cytology of the thyroid shows evidence of infiltration, somewhat similar to that seen in Hashimoto's autoimmune thyroiditis. The thyroid condition is similar to Hashimoto's thyroiditis with lymphocytic infiltration [32] but there is evidence of a destructive thyroiditis with resulting low thyroidal radioiodine uptake, increase in urinary iodine and serum thyroglobulin. Further immunological and genetic studies have shown that while T cell changes accompany normal pregnancy, distinct phenotypic differences can be identified in women who develop PPT [33]. In addition, a role for complement in the genesis of thyroid damage in PPT has been suggested by the finding of an increase in that part of the total TPO antibody activity able to interact with the complement system [34]. It is unlikely that iodine status plays an important role in the pathogenesis of PPT. There is disagreement about the HLA association with this condition, but it has been reported to be associated with DR3, DR4 and DR5 [3,35]. Symptoms of hypothyroidism may be severe enough to warrant therapy with T_4, and it is usual to treat patients for up to a year. Although post-partum hypothyroidism is transient, in many cases there is evidence that at least some of the psychiatric symptomatology of the post-partum period is associated with thyroid dysfunction. Post-partum depression occurs in about 15–20% of normal women. Evidence has accrued that women with anti-TPO antibodies have an increased incidence of post-partum depression (up to 30%) independent of their post-natal thyroid function [36,37].

In view of the numbers of women with positive anti-TPO antibodies who are then likely to develop PPT and/or depressive symptomatology, there is a case to be made for routine screening for TPO antibodies in early gestation in all women.

Breast feeding

Although the thionamide drugs, carbimazole, methimazole and propylthiouracil appear in breast milk, breast feeding is not contraindicated provided the dosage of these agents is low. The amount of propylthiouracil that crosses into the breast is less than the other thionamide drugs and its safety has been documented [38].

References

1 Burrow GN. Thyroid diseases in pregnancy. In: Burrow GN, Oppenheimer JH, Volpe R, eds. *Thyroid Function and Disease.* Philadelphia: WB Saunders, 1989: 292–323.

2 Kendall-Taylor P. Pregnancy and the thyroid. *Fetal Maternal Med* 1993; 5: 89–103.

3 Hall R. Pregnancy and autoimmune endocrine disease. *Baillière's Clin Endocrinol Metab* 1995: 137–55.

4 Glinoer D, De Nayer P, Bourdoux P. Regulation of maternal thyroid during pregnancy. *J Clin Endocrinol Metab* 1990; **71**: 276–87.

5 Glinoer D, Delange F, Laboureur I *et al.* Maternal and neonatal thyroid function at birth in an area of marginally low iodine intake. *J Clin Encrinol Metab* 1992; 75: 800–5.

6 Burrow GN, Fisher DA, Larsen PR. Mechanisms of disease: maternal and fetal thyroid function. *N Engl J Med* 1994; **331**: 1072–8.

7 Vulsma T, Gons MH, de Vijlder Jan JM. Maternal–fetal transfer of thyroxine in congenital hypothyroidism due to a total organification defect or thyroid agenesis. *N Engl J Med* 1989; **321**: 13–16.

8 Contempre B, Jauniaux E, Calvo R *et al.* Detection of thyroid hormones in human embryonic cavities during the first trimester of pregnancy. *J Clin Endocrinol Metab* 1993; **77**: 1719–22.

9 Roti E, Gnudi A, Braverman LE. The placental transport, synthesis and metabolism of hormones and drugs which affect thyroid function. *Endocr Rev* 1983; **4**: 131–49.

10 Emerson CH. Thyroid disease during and after pregnancy. In: Braverman LE, Utiger R, eds. *Werner and Ingbar's The Thyroid*, 7th edn. Philadelphia: JB Lippincott, 1996: 1021–31.

11 Froelich CJ, Goodwin JS, Bankhurst AD, Williams RC, Jr. Pregnancy, a temporary fetal graft of suppressor cells in autoimmune disease? *Am J Med* 1980; **69**: 329–31.

12 Nelson JL, Hughes KA, Smith AG *et al.* Maternal–fetal disparity in Class II alloantigens and the pregnancy-induced amelioriation of rheumatoid arthritis. *N Engl J Med* 1993; **329**: 466–71.

13 Ober C, Simpson JL, Ward M *et al.* Prenatal effects of maternal–fetal HLA compatibility. *Obstet Gynecol* 1987; **15**: 354.

14 Swaminathan R, Chin RK, Lao TTH, Mak YT, Panesar NS, Cockram CS. Thyroid function in hyperemesis gravidarum. *Acta Endocrinol (Copenh)* 1989; **120**: 155–60.

15 Cole LA, Kardana A, Park S-Y, Braunstein GD. The deactivation of hCG by nicking and dissociation. *J Clin Endocrinol Metab* 1993; **76**: 704–10.

16 Goodwin TM, Montoro M, Mestman JH *et al.* The role of chorionic gonodotropin in transient hyperthyroidism of hyperemesis gravidarum. *J Clin Endocrinol Metab* 1992; **75**: 1333–7.

17 Kimura M, Amino N, Tamaki H *et al.* Gestational thyrotoxicosis and hyperemesis gravidarum; possible role of hCG with higher stimulating activity. *Clin Endocrinol* 1993; **38**: 345–50.

18 Munro DS, Dirmikis SM, Humphries H, Smith T, Broadhead DG. The role of thyroid stimulating immunoglobulins in Graves' disease in neonatal thyrotoxicosis. *Br J Obstet Gynaecol* 1978; **85**: 837–43.

19 Lazarus JH. Treatment of hyper- and hypothyroidism in pregnancy. *J Endocrinol Invest* 1993; **16**: 391–6.

20 Van Duke CP, Heyendael RJ, Dekleine MJ. Methimazole,

carbimazole and congenital skin defects. *Ann Intern Med* 1987; **106**: 60.

21 Hashizume K, Ichikawa K, Nishii Y *et al.* Effect of administration of thyroxine on the risk of postpartum recurrence of hyperthyroid Graves' disease. *J Clin Endocrinol Metab* 1992; **75**: 6–10.

22 Mandel SJ, Larsen PR, Seely EW, Brent GA. Increased need for thyroxine during pregnancy in women with primary hypothyroidism. *N Engl J Med* 1990; **323**: 91–5.

23 Hall R, Richards CJ, Lazarus JH. Review: the thyroid and pregnancy. *Br J Obstet Gynaecol* 1993; **100**: 512–15.

24 Toft AD. Drug therapy—thyroxine therapy. *N Engl J Med* 1994; **331**: 174–80.

25 Matsuura N, Yamanda Y, Nohara J *et al.* Familial neonatal transient hypothyroidism due to maternal TSH-binding inhibitor immunoglobulins. *N Engl J Med* 1980; **303**: 738–41.

26 Kopp P, Vansande J, Parma J *et al.* Brief report—congenital hyperthyroidism caused by a mutation in the thyrotropin-receptor gene. *N Engl J Med* 1995; **332**: 150–4.

27 Foley TP, Jr. Maternally transferred thyroid disease in the infant: recognition and treatment. In: Bercu BB, Shulman DI, eds. *Advances in Perinatal Thyroidology*, Vol. 299. New York: Plenum Press, 1991: 209–26.

28 Roberton HEW. Lassitude, coldness, and hair changes following pregnancy, and their response to treatment with thyroid extract. *Br Med J* 1948; **2**: 93–4.

29 Gerstein HC. Incidence of postpartum thyroid dysfunction in patients with Type 1 diabetes mellitus. *Ann Intern Med* 1993; **118**: 419–23.

30 Othman S, Phillips DIW, Parkes AB *et al.* Long term follow up of post-partum thyroiditis. *Clin Endocrinol* 1990; **32**: 559–64.

31 Amino N, Postpartum thyroid disease. In: Bercu BB, Shulman, eds. *Advances in Perinatal Thyroidology*. New York: Plenum Press, 1991; **299**: 167–80.

32 Mizukami Y, Michigishi T, Nonomura A *et al.* Postpartum thyroiditis. A clinical, histologic, and immunopathologic study of 15 cases. *Am J Clin Pathol* 1993; **100**: 200–5.

33 Stagnaro-Green A. Postpartum thyroiditis: prevalence, etiology, and clinical implications. *Thyroid Today* 1993; **XVI**: 1–11.

34 Parkes AB, Othman S, Hall R, John R, Lazarus JH. The role of complement in the pathogenesis of postpartum thyroiditis: relationship between complement activation and disease presentation and progression. *Eur J Endocrinol* 1995; **133**: 210–15.

35 Parkes AB, Darke C, Othman S *et al.* MHC Class II and complement polymorphism in postpartum thyroiditis. *Eur J Endocrinol* 1996; **134**: 449–53.

36 Pop VJ, De Rooy HAM, Vader HL *et al.* Postpartum thyroid dysfunction and depression in an unselected population. *N Engl J Med* 1991; **324**: 1815–16.

37 Harris B, Othman S, Davies JA *et al.* Association between postpartum thyroid dysfunction and thyroid antibodies and depression. *Br Med J* 1992; **305**: 152–6.

38 Momotani N, Yamashita R, Yoshimoto M, Noh J, Ishikawa N, Ito K. Recovery from foetal hypothyroidism: evidence for the safety of breast-feeding while taking propylthiouracil. *Clin Endocrinol* 1989; **31**: 591–5.

39 Mestman JH, Goodwin TM, Montoro MM. Thyroid disorders of pregnancy. *Endocrinol Metab Clin North Am* 1995; **24**: 41–71.

40 Singh A, Dantas ZN, Stone SC, Asch RH. Presence of thyroid antibodies in early reproductive failure: biochemical versus clinical pregnancies. *Fertil Steril* 1995; **63**: 277–81.

41 Lazarus JH, Hall R, Othman S *et al.* The clinical spectrum of post partum thyroid disease. *Quart J Med* 1996; 89: 429–35.

CHAPTER 31

Alterations of thyroid function in non-thyroidal illness: the 'euthyroid sick' syndrome

A.G. Vagenakis

Introduction

It has generally been accepted that the quantity of thyroid hormones secreted by the thyroid determines the metabolic status of the individual in health and disease. However, over the past two decades it has become evident that the thyroid gland is no longer the only organ responsible for metabolic control; intracellular events in various tissues modulate by self-regulating mechanisms the production of an active hormone such as triiodothyronine (T_3) or a calorigenically inactive reverse T_3 (rT_3) through local deiodinating pathways of thyroxine (T_4). Under normal circumstances, about 100 μg of T_4 are produced daily, all of thyroidal origin, and approximately 30 μg of T_3, 20% of which is secreted by the thyroid and 80% is produced in extrathyroidal tissues from 5′-deiodination of T_4, a process called T_3 neogenesis. The rest of the T_4 is converted either to rT_3 generating 25 μg daily, or to a conjugated form in the liver which is secreted via the bile into the intestine.

It was initially thought that the deiodination of T_4 to T_3 or rT_3 was an unregulated and random process. However, it soon became apparent that because T_4 and T_3 secretion from the thyroid is regulated by thyroid-stimulating hormone (TSH), deiodination of T_4 to its active or 'inactive' metabolites is regulated by the activity of type I and type II 5′-deiodinases and type III 5-deiodinase. It has been subsequently found that various disease states have different effects on the local production of T_3 or rT_3. For example, hypothyroidism greatly enhances the type II 5′-deiodinase activity in the brain and pituitary whereas it decreases the activity of type I in liver and kidneys as well as the type III deiodinase activity in the central nervous system. Thus, in this example tissue activity of 5′- or 5-deiodinases determines the local tissue concentration of T_3 by enhancing T_4 to T_3 conversion (5′-deiodinases) and inhibiting the waste of T_4 substrate by decreasing the 5-deiodinase activity (For a recent review see [1]).

In 1963, Oppenheimer *et al.* [2] reported the first detailed analysis of alterations in thyroid function in hospitalised patients with non-thyroidal illness. A decrease in plasma protein binding of T_4, a decrease in serum T_4-binding prealbumin (now called transthyretin) and a normal or decreased level of protein-bound iodine was found in the majority of the patients. These initial observations have been amplified and extended by many investigators over the past two decades by employing sensitive and accurate methods of measurement of the thyroid hormones and their deiodinative products.

Ten years later, Reichlin *et al.* [3], and Portnay *et al.* [4] made two original and important observations. Patients with terminal, non-thyroid originated illness, displayed a profound decrease of T_3 in serum and tissue [3]. Acute starvation also resulted in a dramatic decrease in T_3 production, and increase in serum rT_3 concentration without changes in T_4 production [4]. Subsequently, it was found that many abnormalities in pituitary–thyroid function, serum thyroid hormone binding, and extrathyroidal thyroid hormone metabolism occur in patients with non-thyroidal illness, including those with voluntary or forced food deprivation. These abnormalities result in a decreased serum T_3 concentration, less often in decreased serum T_4 concentration, and occasionally in decreased free T_4 and/or TSH concentration. In general, the degree of the abnormality in thyroid hormone metabolism correlates with the severity of the underlying disease [5–8].

In general, these findings mimic those of hypothyroidism either primary or secondary. They are often referred to as the 'euthyroid sick syndrome' [5] but this term is inappropriate for several reasons. First, although there is no conclusive evidence that these patients are hypothyroid, thyroid hormone action at least in some tissues may be decreased. Secondly, these findings are transient in nature since successful treatment of the underlying disease quickly normalises pituitary–thyroid function. It is possible, therefore, that a transient hypothyroid state exists, which represents an 'adaptation' to the disease, serving to reduce the availability of T_3, the active form of thyroid hormone to the tissue, and thus lessening the deleterious impact of the illness to various tissues such as the muscle and liver. In other words, there may be transient tissue hypothyroidism which may be a beneficial adaptation to illness or starvation.

The derangements that contribute to the so-called 'euthyroid sick syndrome' are summarised in Table 31.1; a relatively detailed analysis is given below, the pathophysiology of

Table 31.1 Alterations in pituitary–thyroid function in non-thyroidal illness.

	Disease state				
Parameter	Mild	Moderate	Severe	Site	Cause
Serum T_3	Decreased	Decreased	Greatly decreased	Extrathyroidal tissue (liver, kidney)	Decreased 5′-deiodinase (type I)
Production rate of T_3	Decreased	Decreased	Greatly decreased		Increased formation of T_3 sulphate and TRIAC
Serum T_4	Usually normal Occasionally increased	Normal Occasionally increased or decreased	Decreased Normal	Thyroid	Decreased serum binding protein(s) Inhibitors of T_4 binding to serum proteins Increased T_4 clearance
Production rate of T_4	Normal	Usually normal	Moderately decreased	Thyroid	
Serum TSH	Normal	Normal or slightly decreased	Decreased	Pituitary, hypothalamus (?)	Decreased TRH secretion Cortisol excess Increased cytokine production Decreased biological activity of TSH
Diurnal variation of TSH	Absent	Absent	Absent	Pituitary	
TSH response to TRH	Normal, decreased	Blunted	Severely blunted	Pituitary	
T_3 action	Decreased (in some tissues)	Decreased (in some tissues)	Decreased (in some tissues)		Decreased cellular uptake of T_3 and T_4 Decreased T_3 receptors or post-receptor effects
Serum rT_3	Increased	Increased	Increased Occasionally normal or decreased	Extrathyroidal tissue (liver)	Decreased 5′-deiodinase (type I)

T_3, triiodothyronine; T_4, thyroxine; TRIAC, triiodothyroacetic acid; TSH, thyroid-stimulating hormone; TRH, thyrotrophin-releasing hormone; rT_3, reverse T_3.

each parameter is discussed and an approach to exclude underlying primary thyroid disease is proposed.

Low serum T_3 and decreased T_3 production

A decreased serum T_3 concentration occurs in almost all patients with acute or chronic non-thyroidal diseases. Many investigators have measured, among other parameters, serum T_3 levels in patients who were hospitalised for a variety of different disorders [5–8]. Serum T_3 concentration was invariably decreased in all patients when compared with healthy individuals, and approximately 70% had serum T_3 values in the hypothyroid range. Almost invariably, low serum T_3 levels have been found in a very wide spectrum of non-thyroidal illness such as diabetes mellitus, chronic liver disease, acute and chronic infections, renal, cardiac and pulmonary disease, neoplastic disease, and following surgery and trauma [8]. A decreased serum T_3 level as well as decreased production of T_3 is also seen in acute and chronic starvation, protein-calorie malnutrition, in normal fetuses and in newborns at birth and for a few hours therafter [9–11].

The cause of the decreased serum T_3 concentration in these conditions is decreased extrathyroid deiodination of T_4 to T_3, a process regulated mainly by type I 5′-deiodinase.

As discussed elsewhere, type I 5′-deiodinase is responsible for approximately 90% of the circulating T_3 since type I 5′-deiodinase is found mainly in tissues outside the brain, particularly in liver and kidney [8]. It may be expected, therefore, that T_3 production will fall due to a decrease in action of type I and not type II 5′-deiodinase which is found mainly in the brain and pituitary. In fact, under certain conditions, such as starvation, hypothyroidism, and during fetal and neonatal life, the activity of *type II* 5′-deiodinase is *increased* and thus (provided the T_4 substrate is adequate) T_3 neogenesis in the brain and pituitary under these circumstances may be increased [1,11,12]. Simultaneously, measured type I 5′-deiodinase activity in these conditions is much decreased and the overall T_3 production rate is therefore also decreased. It thus appears that different organs, under certain circumstances, sense the need for T_3 neogenesis in an opposite way. Non-brain tissues in some respect may be hypothyroid while others, such as brain and pituitary, are not.

Thus, in non-thyroidal disease the decreased local production of T_3 in some organs such as liver, kidney and muscles, may be beneficial and may counteract the sequelae inflicted upon them by the disease, while in other organs such as the pituitary and brain the maintenance of normal T_3 neogenesis may be essential for their function.

The mechanism(s) whereby the T_3 production in liver and other tissues is altered remains elusive (Table 31.2). The systemic diseases decreasing the T_3 production are diverse, including a variety of acute and chronic systemic illness as well as calorie deprivation and drugs. In the majority of these conditions the decrease in serum T_3 may result by the action of a 'tissue inhibitor' upon the type I 5′-deiodinase activity which is triggered by cytokines released from macrophages and monocytes as part of the immune response [13]. Recent studies indicate that infusion of cytokines (interleukin 2, (IL-2), tumour-necrosis factor-α (TNF-α) and IL-6) in healthy volunteers induces characteristic changes in serum thyroid hormone concentration observed in the low T_3 state [14,15, 53]. Circulating soluble cytokine receptors and cytokine-receptor antagonists have a strong negative relation with the serum T_3 levels in patients with systemic illness [16,17]. The hypothetical 'tissue inhibitor' also may be triggered by fasting, diabetes, glucocorticoids, ketogenic diets, whereas drugs such as propranolol, propylthiouracil (PTU) and cholecystographic agents, decrease serum T_3 by direct inhibition of type I 5′-deiodinase activity.

Table 31.2 Proposed mechanisms involved in the pathogenesis of the euthyroid sick syndrome.

Increased production of cytokines (TNF-α, IL-2, IL-6)
Inhibition of 5′-deiodinase by a 'tissue factor' of unknown nature
Decreased delivery ot T_4 to intracellular deiodinases
T_4-binding 'inhibitor' to serum proteins and to intracellular cytosolic proteins
Acceleration of T_3 conjugation to T_3 sulphate
Increased TRIAC production
Decreased T_3 nuclear receptor number

TNF-α, tumour-necrosis factor-α; IL, interleukin; T_4, thyroxine; T_3, triiodothyronine; TRIAC, triiodothyroacetic acid.

Other mechanisms proposed to explain the low T_3 state include alterations in substrate entry into the cell [8], diminished type I 5′-deiodinase activity due to decreased enzyme mass, deficiency of cofactor(s), and extracellular and an intra-cellular T_4-binding defect. Recently, the formation of T_3 sulphate (T3S) at the apparent expense of circulating T_3 by activating liver sulphotransferase enzyme system has been proposed as a possible mechanism [18]. The recent developments of molecular and biochemical tools for studying the action of deiodinases, and the recognition of the role that selenium plays in the catalytic reaction involving the type I and III deiodinases, provides a new insight into the mechanism of T_4 deiodination. There is evidence that selenium deficiency in animals results in a marked decrease in type I deiodinase activity (for recent review see [1]). However, in patients with euthyroid sick syndrome there was no significant independent relationship between plasma selenium concentration and thyroid function indices [19].

Serum total and free T_4 concentrations are usually normal in patients with impaired extrathyroidal T_3 production. Serum rT_3 concentration is usually high but in severe illness it may be decreased or normal. However, the production rate of rT_3 is usually normal or only slightly increased [20,21]. This is due to decreased extrathyroidal 5′-deiodination of rT_3, a process catalysed by the type I 5′-deiodinase in the liver, which is the same enzyme which converts T_4 to T_3. The activity of type III 5′-deiodinase is believed to remain unaltered [10]. Thus, not only is T_4 to T_3 conversion impaired, but so is rT_3 to diiodothyronine (T_2) conversion.

Decreased serum T_4 concentration

In the majority of patients with mild or moderately severe non-thyroidal disease, the serum T_4 concentration remains normal, accompanied invariably by a decreased serum T_3 concentration. A low serum T_4 level in addition to a low serum T_3 concentration is found in critically ill patients with various infections, cardiac diseases, malignant tumours, burns [22] and severe trauma [8].

Usually, only total serum T_4 level is decreased while serum T_3 resin uptake values are normal or increased, and free T_4 levels and the free thyroid index are usually normal. Despite the profound reduction in total serum T_4 concentrations, kinetic data obtained in a few patients have shown that the T_4 production rate is usually within the normal range or, at most, is only modestly reduced [23,24].

It is not easy to explain these alterations in serum T_4 concentration. It is generally accepted that in the majority of patients serum concentration of T_4-binding globulin (TBG), transthyretin and albumin are decreased, resulting in an accelerated turnover rate of T_4. Recently, inhibitor(s) of T_4 binding to proteins have been described but the nature and the importance of the inhibitor(s) are uncertain. There is evidence both supporting and refuting the motion that the inhibitor(s) are either fatty acids or protein. In some patients the administration of drugs such as salicylates, frusemide and heparin, which are competitive inhibitors of T_4 and T_3 binding to TBG, may be partially or totally responsible for decreased serum T_4 concentrations (for extensive review see [8]).

It should be emphasised that misinterpretation of the thyroid status of the patient may occur when tests involving serum free thyroid hormone measurements are applied in patients with severe non-thyroidal illness. The results obtained from commercially available kits which measure free T_4 and free T_3 'directly' are very frequently misleading. The best method currently available for measurement of free T_4 in such patients is equilibrium dialysis [25], but this technique is too cumbersome and slow to be applied in everyday practice. New reliable methods for measuring free T_4 concentrations such as the two-step free T_4 assays are now available, but 2–10% of patients still present with falsely high or low free T_4 values [26].

Serum TSH concentration

Serum TSH concentration is usually normal in patients with non-thyroidal illness. In normal individuals, a diurnal variation of TSH is observed with the nadir at 1100 hours and a zenith at 2300 hours. In patients with mild to moderate non-thyroidal illness there is an absence of diurnal variation and a loss of the usual nocturnal increase of TSH pulse amplitude [27–29].

A puzzling finding concerning TSH secretion in patients with non-thyroidal illness and starvation is the inappropriately low TSH concentration despite low T_3 production. In some patients, especially in those with severe illness, serum TSH may be very low or undetectable, the serum TSH response to TRH may be subnormal or absent, and T_4 production may be low to normal or decreased, providing further evidence that TSH secretion is indeed decreased. It has been found that approximately 3% of patients display TSH values < 0.1 mU/l and 1% above 15 mU/l. Furthermore non-thyroidal illness-induced TSH alterations are transient, usually normalising within a few days [30].

The mechanism(s) responsible for impaired TSH secretion are unknown. It may include increased somatostatin secretion or the effects the increased production of cortisol or dopamine on the pituitary. The latter is rendered improbable by the fact that dopamine antagonists do not increase the sensitivity of the pituitary thyrotroph to TRH in patients with non-thyroidal illness (personal observations). A possible role of cytokines on the suppression of hypothalamo-hypophysial–thyroid axis is emerging. Acute recombinant IL-6 administration in patients with metastatic renal cell carcinoma decreased serum TSH concentration although chronic IL-6 administration had no effect [31]. Hypophysial TSH-β messenger RNA (mRNA) and hypothalamic pro-TRH mRNA were decreased in rats after infusion of IL-1β but not by IL-6 [14,32].

There is no doubt that quantitative changes in TSH secretion occur in patients with non-thyroidal illness. However, qualitative changes of the molecule of TSH *per se* may occur. We have observed (unpublished observations) that the thyroidal T_3 response to endogenous TSH secretion following TRH administration is reduced in patients with non-thyroidal illness, suggesting decreased biological action of TSH. This finding is strengthened by the finding that circulating TSH in patients with non-thyroidal illness is biologically less active due to altered glycosylation of its molecule [33]. Altered glycosylation of TSH molecule *in vivo* occurs in patients with hypothalamic hypothyroidism [34]. These findings are in agreement with the suggestion that patients with severe non-thyroidal illness may have central hypothyroidism, possibly due to decreased TRH secretion which results in altered glycosylation of TSH.

Variants of euthyroid sick syndrome

(Table 31.3)

Non-thyroidal illness usually produces very consistent and predictable responses in serum TSH and thyroid hormone concentrations. However, various diseases may affect several parameters of thyroid hormone metabolism in a pattern entirely different from that described so far. The clinician therefore should be aware to avoid misinterpretation of the thyroid status of the patients [13]. Liver disease, acute and chronic, usually presents with increased serum T_4 concentration whereas serum free T_4 and T_3 remain normal. The cause of increased serum T_4 is secondary to elevation of serum TBG probably due to increased production in the liver (see also Chapter 77). It has been proposed that the inflammatory process, acting on the hepatocyte, increases TBG synthesis [35]. Serum rT_3 show a tendency to decrease. Acute and chronic viral hepatitis, alcoholic cirrhosis, acute intermittent porphyria are the most common liver diseases in which these alterations are observed. For reasons not well understood serum TSH may be mildly elevated.

Chronic renal disease usually presents with normal rT_3 and mildly elevated serum TSH levels. The clearance of rT_3 is normal whereas in fasting and in other low T_3 states it is usually decreased [36]. The increased serum parathyroid hormone (PTH) usually observed in chronic renal failure may be responsible for the decrease in rT_3 clearance [37].

Table 31.3 Systemic diseases with thyroid indices diverging from those observed in the euthyroid sick syndrome.

Disease	T_4	Free T_4	T_3	rT_3	TSH
Hepatic disease	I	N	N	D	I
Chronic renal failure	N	N	D	N	I
AIDS	I	N	N	D	N
Pregnancy with intercurrent illness	I	N	N	N	N
Acute psychosis	I	I	N	–	N or D
Aged population	N	N	N or D	–	I, N OR D

T_4, thyroxine; T_3, triiodothyronine; rT_3, reverse triiodothyronine; TSh, thyroid-stimulating hormone; N, normal; I, increased; D, decreased.

Patients infected with human immunodeficiency virus (HIV) usually display elevated serum T_4, normal T_3 and decreased rT_3 while maintaining normal serum TSH. A progressive elevation of serum TBG accompanying the decline of CD4 lymphocyte count and associated with a concomitant increase in the serum T_4 values has been reported (for review see [38]). Even in the most severely ill HIV-infected patient, the low T_4 state is rarely observed.

Pregnant women with intervening illness display a remarkable 'resistance to adjust' the thyroid hormone indices to those observed in the euthyroid sick syndrome. Except the well-known increased serum T_4 due to oestrogen-induced increase in serum TBG, all the other thyroid hormone indices show little changes during illness.

An intriguing but poorly understood pattern of thyroid hormone indices is occasionally encountered in acute psychosis. Both T_4 and free T_4 may be elevated, serum T_3 remains normal and TSH may be normal or slightly decreased, and in some cases slightly increased. These abnormalities rapidly resolve in a few days after hospitalisation and appropriate therapy. No specific treatment is required for the apparent thyroid dysfunction, which might possibly relate to changes in pituitary–adrenal function (see also Chapter 82) [38].

The most prevalent cause of low T_3 state is advanced age [39]. It is not clear whether ageing or concurrent unrecognised illness is responsible for such a low T_3 state. However, in a highly selected, physically active, healthy elderly population, values of serum T_3 are similar to those observed in normal young adults [40]. In a small number of the elderly (over 65 years of age), a persistent low serum TSH concentration has been observed in the face of both normal T_4 and free T_4 values. A resetting of the pituitary 'thyrotrophinostat' has been proposed as an explanation of these findings [41]. Incipient hyperthyroidism due to micronodular thyroid diseases which is very common in the elderly may impose difficulties in the distinction between these two conditions.

Metabolic consequences

An experimental model designed to permit study of the alterations described in patients with non-thyroidal illness is calorie deprivation. However, it must be kept in mind that the low T_3 state produced by fasting or calorie deprivation is not fully analogous with a low T_3 state of the euthyroid sick syndrome. This model was developed several years ago when we observed that a young female patient of Greek origin admitted to hospital in Boston for evaluation of hypoglycaemia exhibited a profound decrease in serum T_3 concentration during 72-hour fast. Serum T_3 concentration returned to normal shortly after refeeding [9]. In normal subjects who ingest 600 calories or less each day, serum T_3 concentrations decrease by 50% while rT_3 increases by

100% in 72 hours following calorie deprivation. Serum T_4 and free T_4 concentrations change very little if at all, while the serum TSH concentration as well as the TSH response to thyrotrophin-releasing hormone (TRH) may decline slightly. The pituitary thyrotroph displays exquisite sensitivity to increased amounts of T_3: administration of T_3 in quantities sufficient to restore serum T_3 values to prefasting levels decreases serum TSH and abolishes the TSH response to TRH. Similarly, when serum T_4 and T_3 levels are further decreased in fasting individuals by administration of inorganic iodine, the sensitivity of the thyrotroph is evidenced by an increase in serum TSH level and an increased TSH response to TRH [42]. The cause of this apparent increased sensitivity of the pituitary thyrotroph to circulating thyroid hormones is unknown.

During fasting, urinary nitrogen and 3-methylhistidine excretion are decreased in parallel with decreased T_3 production. This is believed to be an adaptation to prevent protein breakdown in fasting as well as in patients with non-thyroidal illness. When the serum T_3 concentration is brought back to prefasting levels by exogenous T_3 administration, urinary nitrogen and 3-methylhistidine excretion increase, suggesting that the decrease in protein catabolism is an adaptive phenomenon rather than a 'side-effect' of fasting [43].

After refeeding with protein, carbohydrates or both, all metabolic derangements observed during fasting gradually attenuate and disappear in a few days or weeks. This depends upon the weight loss inflicted upon the individual during fasting. Refeeding with fat does not restore the metabolic effects or fasting to normal [9].

Some manifestations of hypothyroidism occur when T_3 neogenesis is reduced. The basal metabolic rate (BMR) is decreased, cardiac contractility and rate may be reduced, and the Na^+/K^+ adenosine triphosphatase (ATPase) activity in skeletal muscle is decreased and restored to normal after T_3 replacement [44,45]. In animals bearing transplantable carcinoma, reduced T_3 neogenesis is accompanied by changes in the hepatic production of certain enzymes, suggesting that post-receptor factors may result in augmentation of some and depression of other biologic responses to thyroid hormones. Also, in starved animals a reduction of myosin isoenzymes, Ca^{2+} myosin ATPase activity, and cardiac β-adrenergic receptors is observed. There is also evidence that a greater than expected quantity of T_3 is required to restore these changes to normal, suggesting resistance to the action of thyroid hormones [46].

It appears, therefore, that reduction in T_3 neogenesis is accompanied by responses in some tissues, suggesting diminished biological effects similar to those observed in hypothyroidism. These responses should act to conserve fuel substrate and maintain tissue integrity. It is accomplished by a reduction in T_3 neogenesis and decreased T_3 action at the nuclear level, at least in some tissues. This is accompanied by adaptation in hypothalamo-pituitary function to prevent increases in TSH secretion in response to decreased T_3 production. These findings indicate that decreased T_3 neogenesis reflects an adaptation to stress and is probably beneficial to the sick or starved individual.

Differential diagnosis (Fig. 31.1)

Clinical manifestations of hypothyroidism are not usually apparent in seriously ill patients who display alterations in thyroid hormone metabolism. However, when true hypothyroidism is present in these patients, the diagnosis is not difficult. The serum TSH concentration is invariably elevated in patients with primary hypothyroidism who become ill from a non-thyroidal illness, although the serum TSH level may be somewhat decreased compared with values obtained before the onset of the extrathyroidal disease. More difficulties arise when hypothalamic or pituitary disease is suspected, since decreased serum T_3, serum T_4 and TSH levels are seen in patients with central hypothyroidism. In such cases, however, other hormones such as serum cortisol are usually depressed, whereas in patients with non-thyroidal illness cortisol is invariably increased and the diurnal variation of cortisol is not observed, resulting in high serum cortisol values in the afternoon and evening. Also, in women after the menopause, measurements of serum follicle-stimulating hormone (FSH) and luteinising hormone (LH) are helpful since they are usually elevated, suggesting a normal hypothalamo-pituitary axis. Thus, low serum T_3, T_4, and TSH levels in the presence of increased serum cortisol and normal pituitary function as judged from other pituitary hormones suggest adaption of hypothalamo-pituitary–thyroid axis towards central hypothyroidism and thus no treatment is warranted.

Difficulties in the differential diagnosis of hyperthyroidism may be encountered when serum T_4 and free T_4 levels are elevated. Clinical manifestations of hyperthyroidism are absent in these patients and the serum T_3 level is invariably decreased, but may be normal in patients with acute psychiatric illness. Most importantly, the serum TSH level is usually normal and, in some cases, may be slightly increased. When true thyrotoxicosis coexists with concurrent non-thyroidal illness serum TSH concentration measured by the so-called 'third-generation assays' is invariably undetectable. Currently, therefore, the only reliable test to diagnose primary thyroid disease in these patients is the measurement of serum TSH level by an ultrasensitive assay and interpretation of these results in relation to the clinical picture and serum thyroid hormone values.

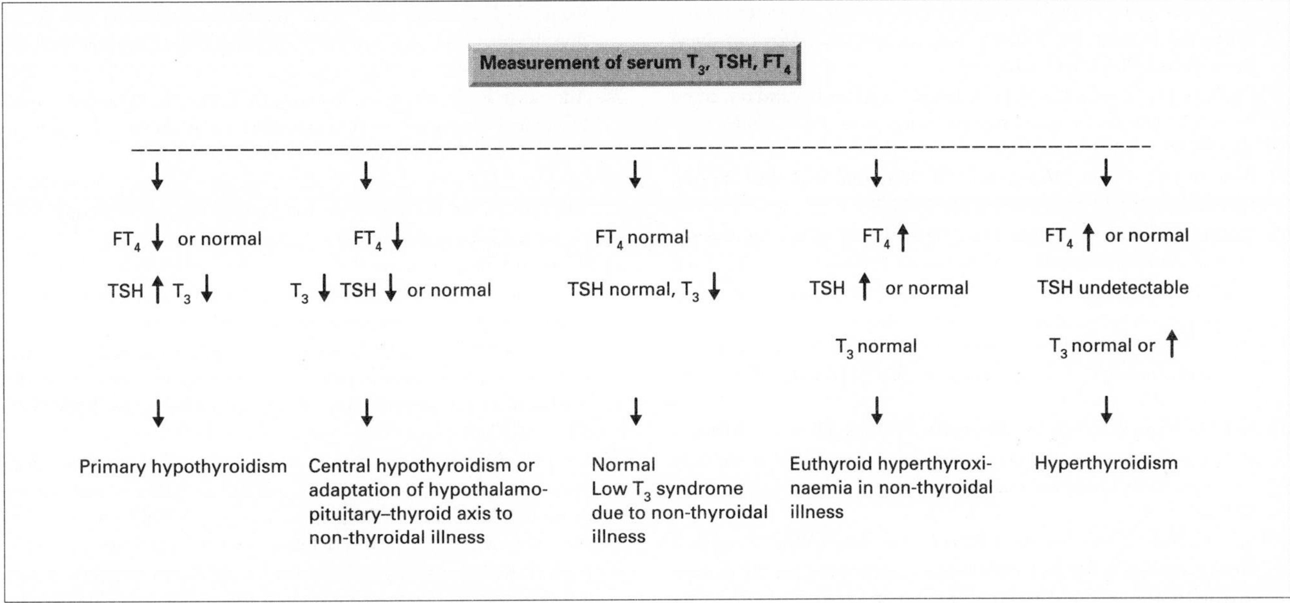

Fig. 31.1 Laboratory diagnosis of thyroid dysfunction in patients with non-thyroid illness. T_3, triiodothyronine; TSH, thyroid stimulating hormone; FT_4, free thyroxine.

Treatment and prognosis

It is obvious that our knowledge concerning the role of thyroid hormone alterations in patients with non-thyroidal illness is limited. However, a few generalisations concerning the use of T_3 administration in these patients should be made. From the outset it appears that thyroid hormone replacement therapy is not required in patients with non-thyroidal illness. Thyroid hormone therapy has been given to heterogeneous groups of seriously ill patients but the outcome of the underlying disease was not altered [47].

There is evidence that low serum T_3, T_4 and TSH concentrations in patients with non-thyroidal illness indicate a grave prognosis: in two studies more than 60% of patients with low serum free T_4 index values died [48,49]. Among patients with congestive heart failure, low serum T_3 values are associated with poor outcome [50] and short-term T_3 administration does not improve survival, despite the increase in cardiac output [54]. This reflects the severity of the underlying disease and is not due to altered thyroid hormone metabolism, since T_4 therapy [48,49] did not improve survival. Recently, it has been proposed that thyroid hormone treatment in patients undergoing coronary artery bypass surgery results in a better outcome [51]. However, in a large group of these patients [45] the decreased level of serum T_3 was raised to supraphysiological levels by intravenous T_3 administration. A slight increase in cardiac indices and lower systemic vascular resistance was observed in the T_3-treated patients but there was no difference in the mortality and morbidity between the T_3 and placebo groups. It appears, therefore, that at present, based on current knowledge on the effects of thyroid hormone in the patients with non-thyroidal illness, thyroid hormone replacement therapy is not recommended [52].

Patients with elevated serum T_4 concentrations due to non-thyroidal illness are not usually severely ill. As in patients with low serum T_4 levels, specific treatment addressed to the thyroid is not required.

References

1 St Germain DL. Thyroid hormone deiodination. *Curr Opin Endocrinol Diabetes* 1995; **2**: 421–8.

2 Oppenheimer JH, Squef R, Surks MI, Hauer H. Binding of thyroxine by serum proteins evaluated by equilibrium dialysis and electrophoretic techniques: alterations in nonthyroidal disease. *J Clin Invest* 1963; **42**: 1769–82.

3 Reichlin S, Bollinger J, Nejad I, Sullivan P. Tissue thyroid hormone concentration of rat and man determined by radioimmunoassay: biologic significance. *Mt Sinai J Med* 1987; **40**: 502–10.

4 Portnay GI, O'Brian JT, Vagenakis AG *et al.* The effect of starvation on the concentration and binding of thyroxine and triiodothyronine in serum and on the response to TRH. *J Clin Endocrinol Metab* 1974; **39**: 199–202.

5 Wartofsky L, Burman KD. Alterations in thyroid function in patients with thyroid illness: the euthyroid sick syndrome. *Endocr Rev* 1982; **3**: 164–217.

6 Kaptein EM. Thyroid hormone metabolism in illness. In: Henneman G, ed. *Thyroid Hormone Metabolism*. New York: Marcel Dekker, 1986: 297–333.

7 Vagenakis AG. Non-thyroid diseases affecting thyroid hormone metabolism in the low T_3 syndrome. In: Hesch R-D, ed. *Serono Symposium 40*. New York: Academic Press, 1981: 128–39.

8 Docter R, Krenning EP, deJong M, Henneman G. The sick euthyroid syndrome: changes in thyroid hormone serum parameters and hormone metabolism. *Clin Endocrinol* 1993; **39**: 499–518.

9 Vagenakis AG. Thyroid hormone metabolism in experimental starvation in man. In: Vigersky RA, ed. *Anorexia Nervosa*. New York: Raven Press, 1977: 127–39.

10 Lo Presti JS, Gray D, Nicoloff JT. Influence of fasting and refeeding on 3, 3′ 5′ triiodothyronine metabolism in man. *J Clin Endocrinol Metab* 1991; **72**: 130–36.

11 Burrow GD, Fisher DA, Larsen PR. Maternal and fetal thyroid function. *N Engl J Med* 1994; **331**: 1072–8.

12 Balsam A, Sexton F, Ingbar SH. The influence of fasting and the thyroid state on the activity of thyroxine 5′ deiodinase in rat liver. A kinetic analysis of microsomal formation of triiodothyronine from thyroxine. *Endocrinology* 1981; **108**: 472–7.

13 Nicoloff JN, Lo Presti J. Nonthyroidal illness. In: De Groot L, ed. *Endocrinology*, 3rd edn. London: WB Saunders, 1995: 665–75.

14 Van Haastern GA, Van der Meer MJ, Hermus AR *et al.* Different effects of continuous infusion of interleukin-1 and interleukin-6 on the hypothalamic-hypophysial thyroid axis. *Endocrinology* 1994; **135**: 1336–45.

15 Van der Poll T, Van Zee KJ, Endert E *et al.* Interleukin-1 receptor blockade does not affect endotoxin induced changes in plasma thyroid hormone and thyrotropin concentrations in man. *J Clin Endocrinol Metab* 1995; **80**: 1341–6.

16 Boelen A, Platvoet Ter Schiphorst MC, Wiersinga WM. Soluble cytokine receptors and the low T_3 syndrome in patients with non thyroidal diseases. *J Clin Endocrinol Metab* 1995; **80**: 971–6.

17 Bartalena L, Brogioni S, Grasso L, Martino E. Interleukin-6 and the thyroid *Eur J Endocrinol* 1995; **132**: 386–93.

18 Lo Presti JS, Nicoloff JT. 3, 5, 3′ Triiodothyronine sulfate: a major metabolite in T_3 metabolism in man. *J Clin Endocrinol Metab* 1994; **78**: 688–92.

19 Van Lente F, Daher R. Plasma selenium concentrations in patients with euthyroid sick syndrome. *Clin Chem* 1992; **38**: 1885–8.

20 Eisenstein Z, Haag S, Vagenakis AG *et al.* Effect of starvation on the production of peripheral metabolism of 3, 3′, 5′ triiodothyronine in euthyroid obese subjects. *J Clin Endocrinol Metab* 1978; **47**: 889–93.

21 Lo Presti JC, Eigen A, Kaptein E *et al.* Alterations in 3, 3′, 5′ triiodothyronine metabolism in response to propylthiouracil, dexamethasone and thyroxine administration in man. *J Clin Invest* 1989; **84**: 1650–6.

22 Becker RA, Vaugham GM, Ziegler MG *et al.* Hypermetabolic low T_3 syndrome of burn injury. *Crit Care Med* 1982; **10**: 870–5.

23 Kaptein EM, Grieb DA, Spencer CA *et al.* Thyroxine metabolism in the low thyroxine state of critical non-thyroidal illness. *J Clin Endocrinol Metab* 1981; **53**: 764–71.

24 Kaptein EM, Robinson WJ, Grieb DA, Nicoloff JI. Peripheral serum thyroxine, triiodothyronine and reverse triiodothyronine kinetics in low thyroxine state of acute non thyroidal illness. *J Clin Invest* 1982; **69**: 526–35.

25 Nelson JC, Tomei RI. Direct determination of free thyroxine in undiluted serum by equilibrium dialysis/radioimmunoassay. *Clin Chem* 1988; **34**: 1737–44.

26 Konno N, Hirokawa J, Tsuji M *et al.* Concentrations of free thyroxine in serum during nonthyroidal illness. Calculation or measurements? *Clin Chem* 1989; **35**: 159–63.

27 Lampropoulou C, Makri M, Vagenakis A. Absence of nyctohemeral variation of TSH and thyroid hormone secretion in humans with non thyroidal illness. *62nd Annual Meeting of the American Thyroid Association* 1987; Abstr. No. 16.

28 Romijin JA, Wiersinga WM. Decreased nocturnal surge of thyrotropin (TSH) in non thyroidal illness. *J Clin Endocrinol Metab* 1990; **70**: 35–42.

29 Adriaanse R, Romijin JA, Brabant G, Endert E, Wiersinga WM. Pulsatile thyrotroph secretion in nonthyroidal illness. *J Clin Endocr Metab* 1993; **77**: 1313–17.

30 Spencer CA, Eigen A, Shen D *et al.* Sensitive TSH tests—specificity and limitations for screening for thyroid disease in hospitalized patients. *Clin Chem* 1987; **33**: 1391–6.

31 Stouthard JML, Van der Poll, Endert E *et al.* Effects of acute and chronic interleukin-6 administration on thyroid hormone metabolism in humans. *J Clin Endocrinol Metab* 1994; **79**: 1342–6.

32 Kakucska I, Romero LI, Clark BD *et al.* Suppression of thyrotropin-releasing hormone gene expression by interleukin-1-beta in the rat: implications for nonthyroidal illness. *Neuroendocrinology* 1994; **59**: 129–37.

33 Lee HY, Suhl J, Pekary AE *et al.* Secretion of thyrotropin with reduced concanavalin-A-binding activity in patients with severe nonthyroidal illness. *J Clin Endocrinol Metab* 1987; **65**: 942–5.

34 Horimoto M, Niskikawa M, Ishihara T *et al.* Bioactivity of TSH in patients with central hypothyroidism: comparison between in vivo T3 response to TSH and in vitro bioactivity of TSH. *J Clin Endocrinol Metab* 1995; **80**: 1124–8.

35 Yamanaka T, Ido K, Kumura K, Saito T. Serum levels of thyroid hormone in liver disease. *Clin Chim Acta* 1980; **101**: 45–55.

36 Kaptein EM, Feinstein EI, Nikoloff JT, Massary SG. Serum reverse triiodothyronine and thyroxine kinetics in patients with chronic renal failure. *J Clin Endocrinol Metab* 1983; **57**: 181–9.

37 Kaptein EM, Massry SG, Quion-Verde H *et al.* Serum thyroid hormone indexes in patients with primary hyperparathyroidism. *Arch Intern Med* 1984; **1448**: 313–15.

38 Lambert M. Thyroid dysfunction in HIV infection. *Baillière's Clin Endocrinol Metab* 1994; **8**: 825–35.

39 Lipson A, Nicoloff EL, Hsu TH *et al.* A study of age-dependent changes in thyroid changes in thyroid function tests in adults. *J Nucl Med* 1979; **20**: 1124–30.

40 Kabadi UM, Rosman PM. Thyroid hormone indices in adult healthy subjects: no influence of aging. *J Am Geriat Soc* 1988; **36**: 312–16.

41 Lewis GF, Alessi GA, Imperial JG, Reffetoff S. Low serum free thyroxine index in ambulatory elderly is due to resetting of the threshold of thyrotropin feed back suppression. *J Clin Endocrinol Metab* 1991; **73**: 843–9.

42 Gardner DF, Kaplan MM, Stanley CA, Utiger RD. Effect of triiodothyronine replacement on the metabolic and pituitary responses to starvation. *N Engl J Med* 1979; **300**: 579–84.

43 Burman KD, Wartofsky L, Dinterman RE, Kesler P, Wannemacher RW. The effect of T3 and reverse T3 administration on muscle protein catabolism during fasting as measured by 3-methylhistidine excretion. *Metabolism* 1979; **28**: 805–13.

44 Matsumura M, Kuzuya N, Kawakami Y, Yamashita K. Effects of fasting, refeeding and fasting with T3 administration on Na-K ATPase in rat skeletal muscle. *Metabolism* 1992; **41**: 995–99.

45 Klemperer JD, Klein I, Comez M *et al.* Thyroid hormone treatment after coronary-artery bypass surgery. *N Engl J Med* 1995; **333**: 1522–7.

46 Tibaldi JM, Surks MI. Animal models of nonthyroidal disease. *Endocr Rev* 1985; **6**: 87–102.

47 Brent GA, Hershman JM. Thyroxine therapy in patients with severe nonthyroidal illnesses and low serum thyroxine concentration. *J Clin Endocrinol Metab* 1986; **63**: 1–8.

48 Slag MF, Morley JE, Elson MK *et al.* Hypothyroxinaemia in critically ill patients as a predictor of high morality. *JAMA* 1981; **245**: 43–5.
49 Kaptein EM, Weiner JM, Robinson WJ, Wheeler WS, Nicoloff JT. Relationship of altered thyroid hormone indices to survival in nonthyroidal illness. *Clinical Endocrinol* 1982; **16**: 565–74.
50 Hamilton MA, Stevenson LW, Luu M, Walden JA. Altered thyroid hormone metabolism in advanced heart failure. *Am J Coll Cardiol* 1990; **16**: 91–5.
51 Novitzky D, Cooper DK, Barton CI *et al.* Triiodothyronine as an inotropic agent after open heart surgery. *J Thorac Cardiovasc Surg* 1989; **98**: 972–8.
52 Utiger RD. Altered thyroid function in nonthyroidal illness and surgery: to treat or ot to treat? *N Engl J Med* 1995; **333**: 1562–3.
53 Wiersinga WM, Boelen A. Thyroid hormone metabolism in non-thyroidal illness. *Curr Opin Endocrinol Diabetes* 1996; **3**: 422–7.
54 Hamilton MA, Stevenson LW. Thyroid hormone abnormalities in heart failure: possibilities for therapy. *Thyroid* 1996; **6**: 527–9.

Part 5
The Adrenal Cortex

CHAPTER 32

Structure and function of the adrenal cortex

G.P. Vinson, B.J. Whitehouse and J.P. Hinson

Structure of the adrenal cortex

In the mammal the adrenals are paired glands lying anterior to the kidneys. In humans they are situated close to the kidney's cephalic pole (hence also the older term suprarenal capsules). Their combined wet weight is about 0.01–0.02% of the total bodyweight, and thus they weigh about 8 g in the adult. In the human, and in some other species, such as dog, sheep and cattle, the glands are similar in males and females, although in many rodent species there is a degree of sexual dimorphism; frequently, as in the rat, the female gland is bigger. The gland receives arterial blood through a number of small arteries which originate directly from the dorsal aorta, and the blood is dispersed from these through a network of arterioles in the connective tissue capsule of the gland. The drainage is through a single vein which discharges directly into the vena cava (Fig. 32.1).

Morphology

Histologically, the cells of the mammalian adrenal cortex entirely surround those of the medulla, and are arranged as three major layers, or zones, organised as concentric shells. The cells of the different zones are generally distinguished by their shape and size, and by their ultrastructure, as well as by their arrangement and position within the gland. The three zones are called *zona glomerulosa*, *zona fasciculata* and *zona reticularis*. In general, the zona glomerulosa lies just below the connective tissue capsule, and consists of an arrangement of cells described variously as loops, whorls or baskets. Cells of the zona fasciculata are invariably arranged as a series of centripetally oriented cords, which abut on to the less clearly organised network of cells which form the zona reticularis.

Other zones are recognised, although these are usually smaller and may be transient. In the human the most prominent of these is the fetal cortex (see below). In general, the cells of the cortex are now thought to arise from a region just below the glomerulosa; this may be the role of the cells of the zona intermedia, which has been described as a small band of cells in some species. In the classical literature, this was described as a sudanophobe zone (i.e. containing relatively little lipid). Recently it has been shown that, in the rat at least, it contains neither aldosterone synthase nor 11-β-hydroxylase, and has been renamed 'white zone' (i.e. unstained by antibodies for either of these two enzymes), perhaps supporting the view that this is a pluripotential layer of cells. Certainly, mitoses are more frequent in this region, and the cells may presumably be recruited by the zona glomerulosa, as demand arises, or move centripetally through the cortex, undergoing sequential transformation into first zona fasciculata then zona reticularis cells. Cell death is more frequent in the zona reticularis than in the other zones.

In humans, the zona glomerulosa is smaller than in many other species, and seldom occupies more than 5% of the total cortical volume. This is because it does not form a continuous shell in the outer part of the gland, but its cells occur in the form of more or less isolated islets. The cells are relatively small and round, with a high nuclear/cytoplasmic ratio. In common with those other species, the mitochondria of zona glomerulosa cells are characterised by their lamelliform or shelf-like cristae. The smooth endoplasmic reticulum is sparse; ribosomes and polysomes are visible throughout the cytoplasm.

The zona fasciculata cells are larger, with abundant cytoplasm, and the mitochondria contain tubulovesicular cristae, although these may vary between the outer and inner parts of the zone. In conventional stains, these cells are lighter in appearance than zona reticularis cells, and hence have been termed 'clear cells' as opposed to the 'compact cells' of the zona reticularis, which stain more deeply.

The zona reticularis occupies one-third of the cortex, and

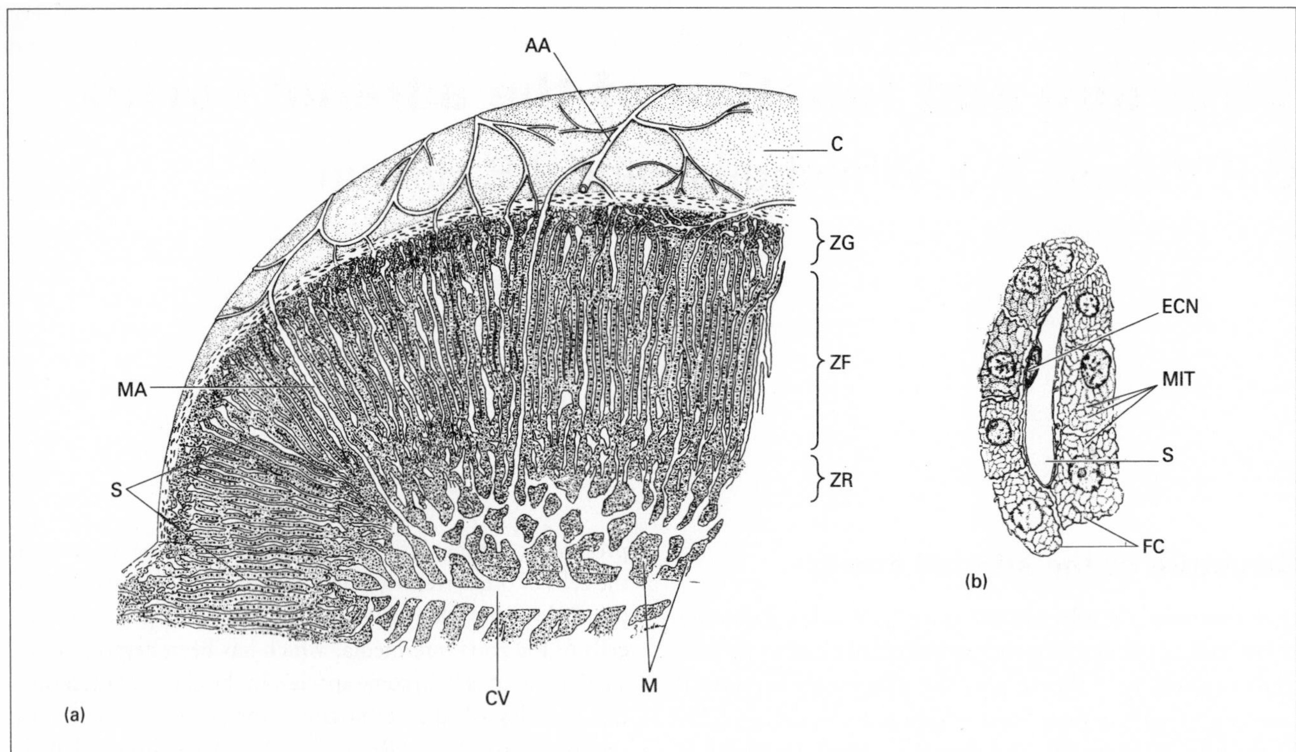

Fig. 32.1 (a) General morphology of the mammalian adrenal gland. ZG, zona glomerulosa; ZR, zona reticularis; ZF, zona fasciculata; M, medullary tissue; CV, central vein; S, sinusoids; MA, medullary artery; AA, afferent arterioles; C, capsule. (b) Transverse section of a sinusoid in the zona fasciculata. ECN, endothelial cell nucleus; MIT, mitochondria. From [1].

its cells are intermediate in size between those of the zona glumerulosa and zona fasciculata. The mitochondria of zona reticularis cells are elongated with tubulovesicular cristae; microbodies (lipofuchsin granules) and lipid droplets also occur (Fig. 32.2).

In the human the adrenal is important in fetal life, when it reaches a maximum of about 0.3% of bodyweight. This declines slightly in the third trimester, and precipitously in the neonate. The large size of the gland is attributable to the presence of an additional zone—the fetal zone—which lies between the definitive cortex and the medulla (Fig. 32.3). In contrast to the small basophilic cells of the outer definitive zones, the larger cells (20–50 μm) of the fetal zone are eosinophilic. In the fetus, the cells of the definitive cortex contain lamelliform cristae (like the zona glomerulosa of the adult gland), whereas the mitochondria of the fetal zone cells are tubulovesicular. Studies on the origin and ultimate fate of the cells of the fetal zone are inconclusive. The cells of the cortex arise from a proliferation of cortical *anlagen* between the dorsal mesentery and the germinal ridge, and some have held that the fetal zone cells arise from a second discrete proliferation, although this has been contested, and they may arise, like the reticularis, from the outer zones. Similarly, some have held that the zone involutes after birth, while others find that it is transformed into elements of the definitive cortex.

Circulation and innervation

The intraglandular circulatory system deserves some attention, particularly because of its responses during stimulation. The adrenal is one of the most highly vascularised organs within the body, and detailed studies have shown that virtually every cell borders on to the thin and attenuated endothelial cells which line the vascular space. Although different descriptions have been given at various times, it is reasonable to summarise the arrangement in mammals as follows: a variable number of arteries supply the gland, which divide in the capsular or subcapsular region to form an arteriolar plexus. Two types of vessels arise from this plexus; first, there are the thinly walled capillaries, frequently called sinuses, which run centripetally in all regions of the cortex. These are the most abundant of the cortical vessels and may be assumed to supply all of the cortical cells. Second, there are the much more sparsely distributed medullary arteries, with thicker walls, which run through the cortex to supply the medulla direct. It is likely that blood from the cortical sinuses and the medullary arteries is mixed in the medulla, and, on the basis of the relative abundance of the vessels, it is reasonable to assume that the medulla receives most of its supply from

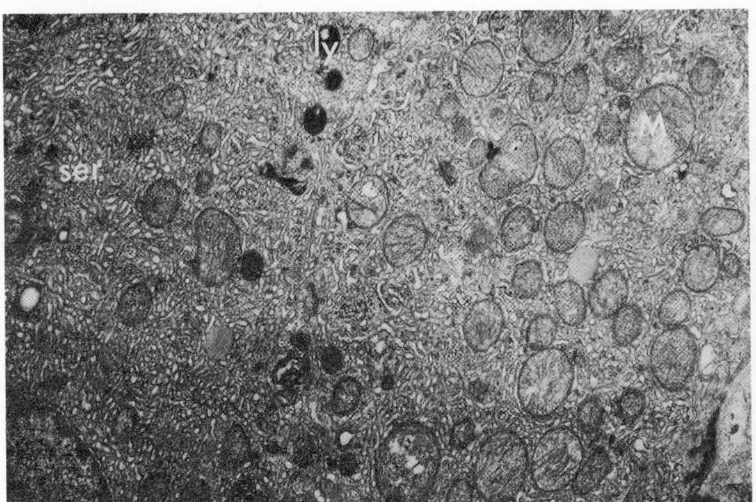

(a)

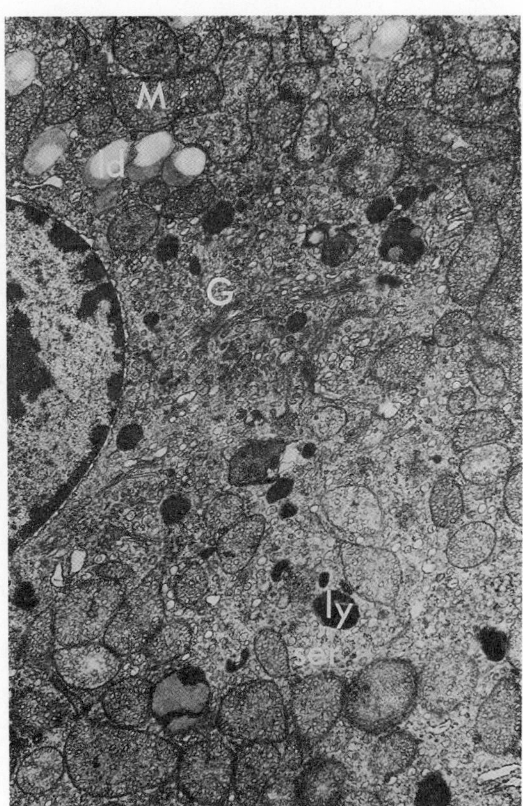

(b)

Fig. 32.2 Ultrastructure of adrenocortical cells. (a) Transmission electron micrograph of human zona glomerulosa cells, showing mitochondria (M) with tubulolaminar cristae, abundant smooth endoplasmic reticulum (ser) and lysosomes (ly) (×9000). (b) Transmission electron micrograph of human adrenal zona fasciculata cells. Mitochondria showing vesicular cristae, rather abundant smooth endoplasmic reticulum and a well-developed Golgi apparatus (G) (×11 000). From [2], with permission.

the sinuses. It is in the medulla that the sinuses are drained into the single common vein for the whole gland (Fig. 32.1).

Two main ways in which the vasculature of the human gland varies from this generalised mammalian picture are: (i) in the human gland there also exist arteriovenous loops in which blood is apparently carried from the subcapsular arterioles in vessels which sweep down through the zona glomerulosa and the zona fasciculata, then loop back to the exterior of the gland to sites close to their origins; (ii) as the vein leaves the gland, a portion of the cortex is introverted from the exterior to surround the vessel as the 'cortical cuff' (Fig. 32.4).

Most early studies reported that nerve fibres which entered the gland passed straight to the medulla without branching, and with no evidence of nerve endings. Although the picture is not clear for the human gland, certainly evidence exists from animal studies that nerve fibres occur, arising partly from the medulla, but also partly through direct innervation. In general, neural arborisation is most dense in the capsular and subcapsular region and nerves may contact both adrenocortical cells and blood vessels. Both catecholaminergic and peptidergic fibres have been identified.

Hormones of the adrenal cortex

The hormones of the adrenal cortex are steroids: compounds that contain the perhydrocyclopentanophenanthrene structure consisting of four linked rings, three of six carbon atoms, and one of five. There are four major groups of these compounds, classified according to the number of carbon atoms they contain (Fig. 32.5).

C_{27} compounds. These are related to cholestane, and include cholesterol.

C_{21} steroids. These include progesterone, the hormone of pregnancy and of female cyclic reproductive function, as well as the compounds produced more or less exclusively by the adrenal cortex. The adrenal C_{21} steroids, collectively termed corticosteroids, are of two major types according to their activities, the *mineralocorticoids* and the *glucocorticoids*. The activity of the mineralocorticoids is primarily concerned with the regulation of electrolyte metabolism, mainly sodium and potassium. The most potent mineralocorticoid in all mammals is aldosterone, although other corticosteroids possess some mineralocorticoid activity. In most tests, deoxycorticosterone is the next most potent mineralocorticoid, although its secretion is not known to be closely linked to physiological demand for mineralocorticoid function. The glucocorticoids were originally defined on the basis of their actions on gluconeogenesis, but are known to have a wide variety of functions (see below). In humans and many other

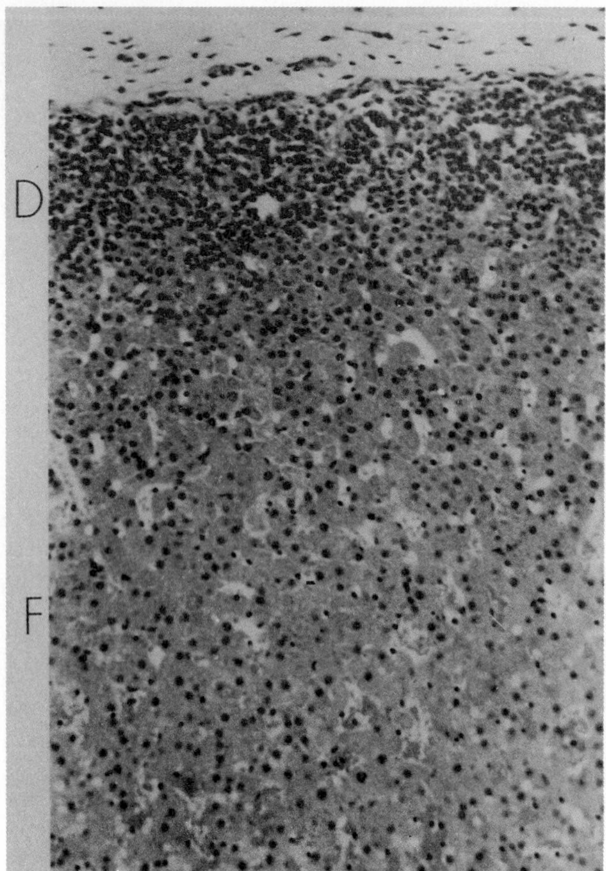

Fig. 32.3 Light micrograph illustrating the structure of the fetal adrenal (18 weeks). The relatively small cells of the definitive cortex (D) surround the larger cells of fetal zone (F). (Courtesy of I. Doniach, Royal Hospitals Trust).

species (including dog, sheep, bovine) cortisol (hydrocortisone) is the most prominent secreted glucocorticoid, and smaller amounts of cortisone and corticosterone are also produced. In the rat and some other rodents (and in many non-mammalian vertebrates), adrenal 17α-hydroxylase activity (see below) is weak, and corticosterone is the major secreted adrenocortical product.

C_{19} steroids. These are related to androstane, and include the androgens, which support male structure and reproductive function. Of these, testosterone is the most potent, but is normally produced in only small amounts by the adrenal. However, androstenedione is a prominent adrenal secretory product, which may be converted to testosterone peripherally. In humans, and some of the primates, other major C_{19} secretory products are dehydroepiandrosterone (DHEA) and its sulphate (DHEAS).

C_{18} steroids. These are related to oestrane, and are the oestrogens, female sex hormones, which are not usually secreted by the adrenal. However, androstenedione from the adrenal may be converted peripherally to oestrogens, and this is the major source of circulating oestrogen in post-menopausal women. In the fetus, DHEAS from the fetal adrenal is converted first to 16α-hydroxy-DHEAS and then to oestriol sulphate by placental enzymes.

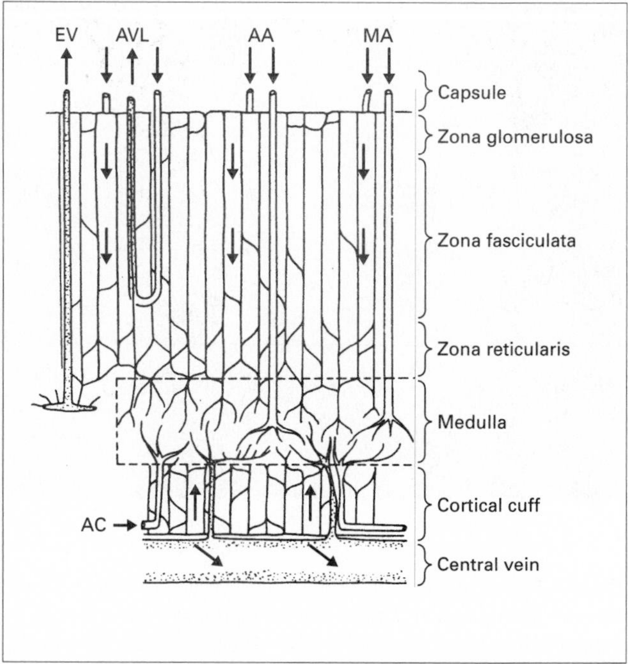

Fig. 32.4 Vascular arrangement of the adrenal gland showing the presence of the cortical cuff and vascular loops. MA, medullary artery; AA, afferent arteriole; AVL, arteriovenous loop; AC, arteriae comitantes; EV, emissary vein. From [3], with permission.

The circulating concentrations of the major adrenal steroids are shown in Table 32.1.

Biosynthesis of the corticosteroids

Steroid hormones are formed from cholesterol. Cholesterol may be formed *de novo* from acetate in the adrenal, or it may be imported into the gland from circulating low-density lipoprotein (LDL) through a process of receptor-mediated endocytosis, as is known to occur in the hepatocyte. These two sources of cholesterol have varying importance in different species, but it is likely that both occur in the human adrenal. Cholesterol is stored as esters in the lipid droplets within the adrenocortical cell.

Several groups of enzymes are concerned with the biosynthesis of adrenal steroids.

1 Enzymes concerned with cholesterol synthesis from acetate. Of these, hydroxymethylglutaryl coenzyme A (HMG CoA) reductase has an important role as a regulatory site for cholesterol synthesis.

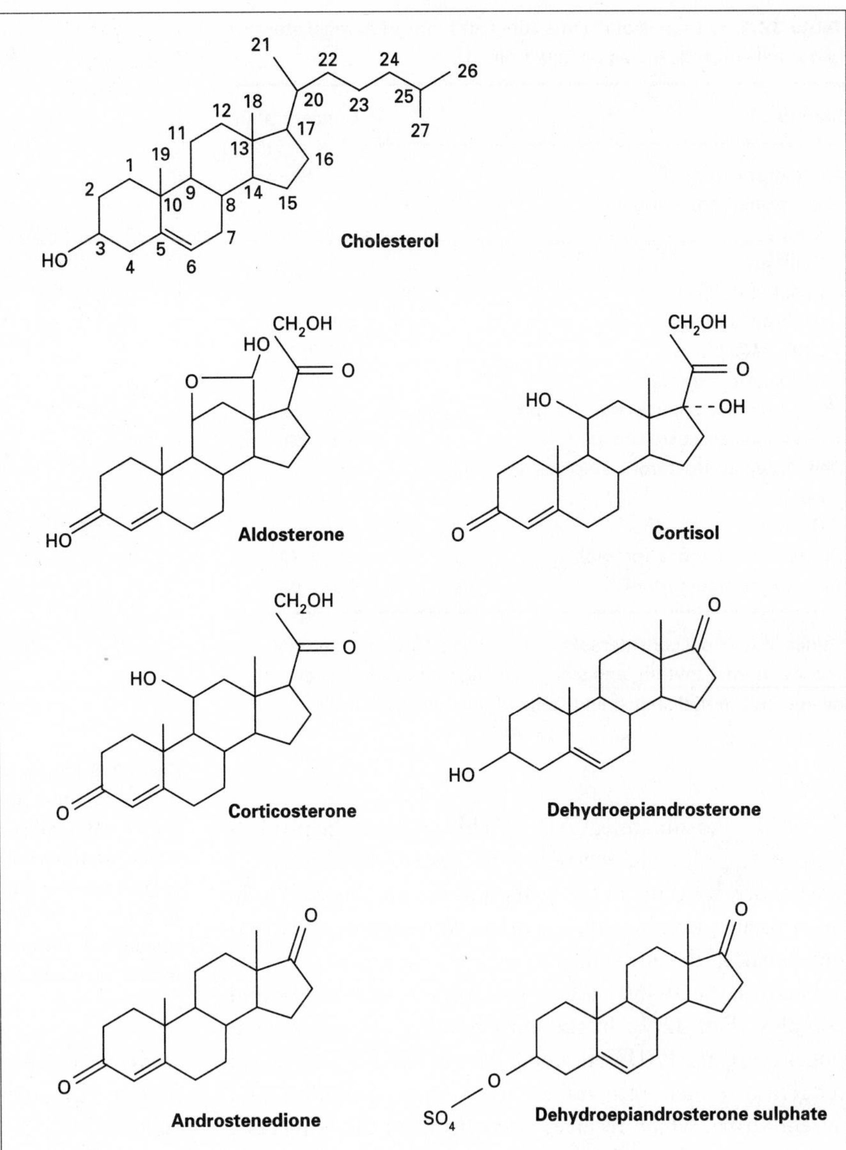

Fig. 32.5 Structures of the major hormones secreted by the adrenal cortex, showing the conventional steroid numbering system.

2 Enzymes concerned with esterification and hydrolysis of cholesterol esters within the lipid droplets. Principally these are acyl CoA: cholesterol acyl transferase (ACAT) and cholesterol ester hydrolase (CEH).

3 Hydroxylases. These are nicotinamide adenine dinucleotide phosphate (NADPH)-linked enzymes of the cytochrome P-450 family. They occur both in mitochondrial and in microsomal compartments.

4 Dehydrogenases. These NAD^+-linked enzymes are microsomal. These include Δ^5,3β-dehydroxysteroid dehydrogenase, and 11β-dehydrogenase. The 17β-dehydrogenase is relatively weak in the adrenal.

Much is known about the function of the P-450 hydroxylases. Five types may be involved in steroid biosynthesis, and four of these occur in the adrenal. The five types are as follows.

1 P-450_{scc} (CYP11A). This catalyses cholesterol hydroxylation at C-22 and C-20, and side-chain cleavage (hence 'scc'). It occurs on the inner mitochondrial membrane.

2 P-$450_{11\beta/18}$ (11β-hydroxylase, CYP11B1). This also occurs on the inner mitochondrial membrane in the cells of the zona fasciculata and zona reticularis. It catalyses 11β- and 18-hydroxylation. Aldosterone synthesis, involving production of the 18-aldehyde function which precedes formation of the hemiacetal form of aldosterone, is catalysed by the zona glomerulosa-specific isoenzyme, aldosterone synthase (P-450_{aldo}, CYP11B2).

3 P-450_{21} (21-hydroxylase, CYP21). This special microsomal enzyme catalyses 21-hydroxylation.

4 P-$450_{17\alpha}$ (17α-hydroxylase/lyase, CYP17). This microsomal enzyme catalyses 17α-hydroxylation, and also the lyase reaction which generates C_{19} steroids from 17α-hydroxy C_{21} precursors.

Table 32.1 Examples of plasma concentrations of adrenal steroids in normal subjects. Based on data from [1].

Steroid	Concentration
Aldosterone (pmol/l)	100–400
Androstenedione (nmol/l)	
Adults	2–13
Children	<2
Cortisol (nmol/l)	
0700–0900 hours	280–720
2100–2400 hours	60–340
Corticosterone (nmol/l)	2.3–23
18-Hydroxydeoxycorticosterone (pmol/l)	156 ± 20
18-Hydroxycorticosterone (pmol/l)	635 ± 60
Dehydroepiandrosterone sulphate (μmol/l)	
Adults	2–11
Children	<2
Deoxycorticosterone (pmol/l)	202 ± 70
11-Deoxycortisol (nmol/l)	1.51 ± 0.83

Values may show considerable variation as all adrenal steroids show a diurnal rhythm, and steroid secretion may also be affected by age, nutritional status, and stage of the menstrual cycle.

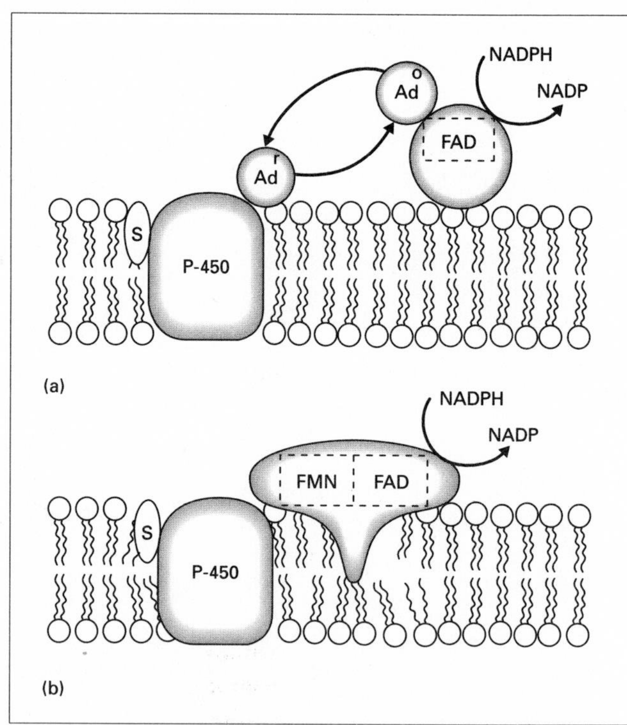

Fig. 32.6 Membrane arrangement of adrenocortical cytochrome P-450s: (a) mitochondrial; (b) microsomal. Each obtains electrons from nicotinamide adenine dinucleotide phosphate (NADPH), which are transmitted to the P-450 via adrenodoxin (Ad) and the FAD-containing adrenodoxin reductase (mitochondrial P-450s), and by a single FMN/FAD-containing reductase in the microsomal systems. S, steroid; FAD, flavin adenine dinucleotide; FMN, flavin mononucleotide. From [4].

5 P-450_{arom} (aromatase, CYP19). This catalyses the production of C_{18} phenolic steroids—the oestrogens—from C_{19} precursors. It occurs in the ovary and placenta as well as in other tissues, notably adipose tissue, although its activity is only weak in the adrenal.

Each of the P-450s forms part of a membrane-bound complex (Fig. 32.6). In the mitochondria the other components are: the FAD-containing flavoprotein, adrenodoxin reductase, which receives electrons from NADPH, and adrenodoxin, which receives electrons from the reductase, and in turn reduces P-450, as part of the P-450 catalytic cycle. In the microsomal P-450s, a single reductase transfers electrons from NADPH to P-450. The NADPH required for steroid hydroxylation may be generated by the glucose-6-phosphate dehydrogenase reaction in the cytosol, and by the $NADP^+$-linked isocitrate dehydrogenase in the mitochondrion. Other sources may be the malic enzyme reaction, and from succinate, by reversed electron transport from ubiquinone to NAD^+, and thence to $NADP^+$ by the energy-linked transhydrogenase reaction.

A general account of corticosteroid biosynthesis can therefore be drawn from this knowledge of the individual components of the scheme (Fig. 32.7).

Cholesterol, derived from either *de novo* biosynthesis or from circulating cholesterol, is stored in esterified form within the adrenal cell. When required for steroid synthesis, stored cholesterol esters are hydrolysed and transferred to the mitochondrion. Mitochondrial cholesterol is the intermediate substrate for steroid biosynthesis. It is hydroxylated first at C-22, then at C-20, and the side-chain is cleaved to yield the C_{21} steroid pregnenolone, with isocaproic acid. Pregnenolone leaves the mitochondrion and passes to the smooth endoplasmic reticulum where it is either hydroxylated at 17α, to give 17α-hydroxypregnenolone, or converted by the Δ^5,3β-hydroxysteroid dehydrogenase/isomerase system to yield progesterone. 17α-Hydroxypregnenolone is converted by the same enzyme to 17α-hydroxyprogesterone. Progesterone and 17α-hydroxyprogesterone are both then sequentially hydroxylated at C-21, and returned to the mitochondrion, where they may be 11β-hydroxylated. At this stage the final products in the inner zones, which are secreted, are cortisol and corticosterone, respectively. In the glomerulosa cell, deoxycorticosterone can be directly converted to aldosterone by aldosterone synthase. However, other substrates such as 18-hydroxydeoxycorticosterone or corticosterone may also be converted. Since these can only be provided by other cell types, primarily the fasciculata, such a mechanism would depend on their close functional contact. Aldosterone is formed after hydroxylation at C-18, and the aldehyde

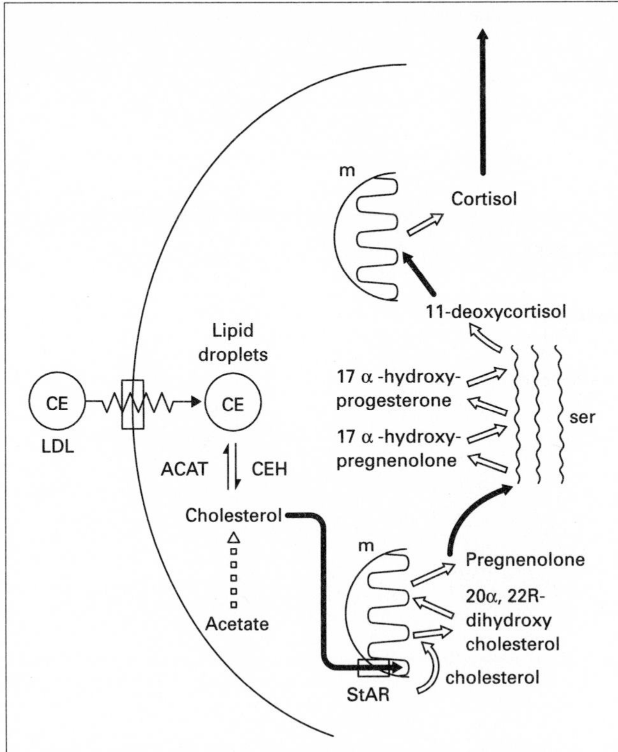

Fig. 32.7 Steroid biosynthetic pathway shown in relation to adrenal cell morphology. LDL, low-density lipoprotein; CE, cholesterol esters; ACAT, acyl CoA : cholesterol acyl transferase; CEH, cholesterol ester hydrolase; StAR, steroidogenic acute regulatory protein; SER, smooth endoplasmic reticulum; m, mitochondrion; ➔ = transport; ⇒ = conversions.

function at C-18 is generated, not by a dehydrogenase as originally thought, but by a second hydroxylation at the same site, which generates the aldehyde through spontaneous loss of water molecule.

The rate-limiting steps in these sequences are thought to be as follows.

1 The delivery of cholesterol to the inner mitochondrial membrane, and $P450_{scc}$. Current evidence suggests that this is primarily facilitated by a specific protein, designated the steroidogenic acute regulatory (StAR) protein.

2 Much evidence suggests that a second 'late-pathway' rate-limiting step lies between 18-hydroxydeoxycorticosterone or corticosterone and aldosterone. However, since aldosterone synthase can catalyse all of the steps between deoxycorticosterone and aldosterone, this could only be achieved by the regulation of supply of the alternative precursors.

Knowledge of the mechanisms for corticosteroid biosynthesis has led to the development of numerous more-or-less specific inhibitors of adrenal steroidogenesis. Some of these, with their sites of action, are illustrated in Fig. 32.8.

Transport and metabolism of corticosteroids

Under normal conditions around 90% of the circulating cortisol is bound to a specific plasma binding protein, corticosteroid-binding globulin (CBG). This protein is present in the plasma at a concentration of approximately 550 nmol/l, and has a single binding site for corticosteroids with a dissociation constant of between 100 and 10 nmol/l. There is no comparable binding protein for aldosterone, and thus aldosterone in plasma is largely unbound, although there is low affinity binding to plasma albumin.

It is generally considered that only the unbound steroid fraction is biologically active, and thus salivary steroid measurements may be used to assess adrenal function, particularly in children, because this test is believed to reflect the concentration of unbound steroid in plasma. This view has, however been questioned, but the conditions required for bioactivity of the bound fraction remain unclear.

The liver is the major site for corticosteroid metabolism, and in humans metabolites are generally excreted in the urine rather than by the biliary/faecal route which predominates in some other species. The main reactions involved are reduction of ring A, hydroxylation and conjugation as sulphates or glucuronides.

A summary of the kinetics of adrenal steroids in plasma is shown in Table 32.2.

Control of adrenocortical secretion

Control of cortisol secretion

Cortisol (together with cortisone and corticosterone) is produced virtually exclusively by the zona fasciculata and zona reticularis of the adrenal cortex. Its secretion is almost entirely related to the degree of stimulation by adrenocorticotrophic hormone (ACTH). Following hypophysectomy, glucocorticoid levels in the blood fall to about 5% of normal values within 2 hours and this fall may be reversed by administration of ACTH. The action of administered ACTH is shown in Fig. 32.9. Under normal conditions cortisol secretion has a clear diurnal rhythm, paralleling the pattern of ACTH secretion, with an early morning peak and an evening nadir (Fig. 32.10).

Physiologically, the acute actions of ACTH are:

1 to increase secretion of corticosteroids;

2 to increase blood flow through the gland;

3 to cause a massive depletion of ascorbic acid from the gland.

The role of ascorbic acid is still not clarified, but it may act as an antioxidant in the unstimulated gland, preventing the action of cytochrome P-450 on non-specific substrates with potentially harmful products. Alternatively, it may

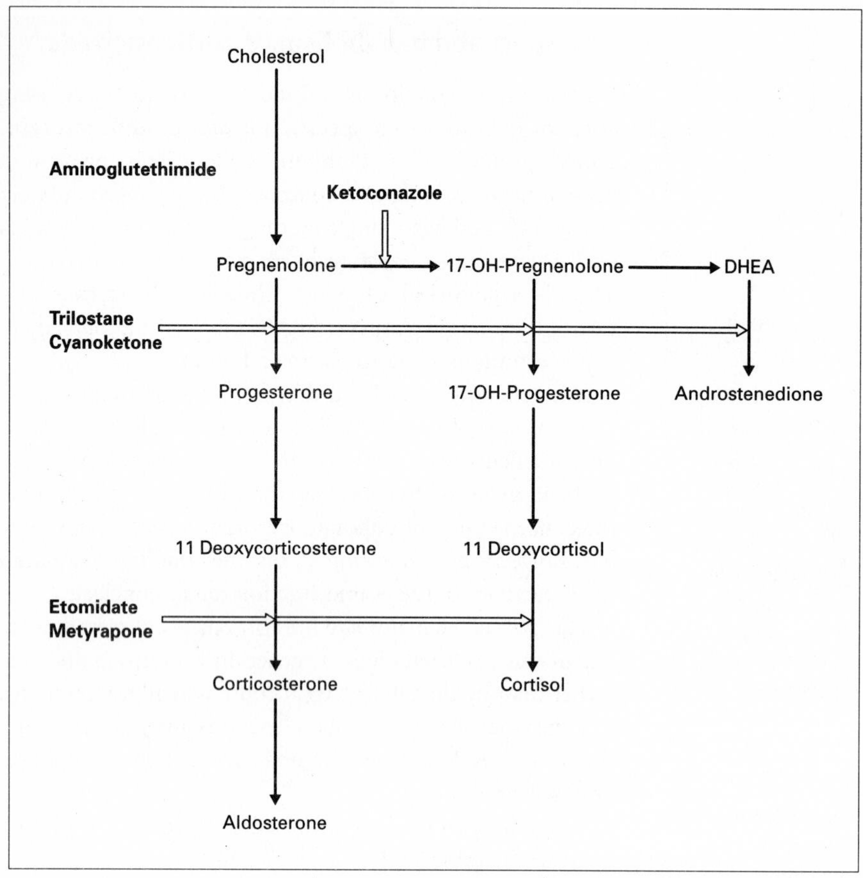

Fig. 32.8 Sites of action of some of the inhibitors of steroid biosynthesis.

Table 32.2 Kinetics of adrenal steroids in plasma. Data from [5].

	Cortisol	Corticosterone	Aldosterone
Mean extra-adrenal pool (nmol)	6215	290	20
Turnover time (time constant) (min)	130	43	43
Virtual volume of distribution (at plasma conc) (litres)	15	9	47
Metabolic clearance rate (l/min)	0.1	0.2	1.1
24-hour secretion rate (μmol/day)	60	10	0.7

function as part of an auxiliary electron transport system, providing electrons for P-450-catalysed hydroxylation. Clearly, the stimulated increases in steroid secretion and blood flow are functionally related, and serve to maximise the efficiency of the secretory process and the distribution of secretory products to the body. Increased steroid secretion is seen 2–5min after ACTH administration in intact gland pre-parations, although maximal responses may take longer to be achieved.

Chronically, as well as maintaining elevated glucocorticoid levels, ACTH also brings about increased gland weight, which is attributable both to increases in adrenocortical cell number and size, and to increased blood content. ACTH is also required to maintain steroid synthetic enzymes, including the P-450s, which decline after a few days in the hypophysectomised animal.

Morphologically, the effects of hypophysectomy on adrenal weight are attributable to the degeneration of the zona fasciculata and zona reticularis, while the zona glomerulosa is comparatively unaffected at the light microscopic level, although transitory decreases in nuclear and mitochondrial volumes can be detected. In the inner zones, cell numbers decline markedly (through the mechanism of apoptosis), and the remaining cells are shrunken because of major decreases in mitochondrial volume and smooth endoplasmic reticulum.

Stimulation with ACTH also produces morphological changes. Acutely, inner-zone cells ‘round up’ and generate filopodia (microvilli) on the plasma membrane. Internally,

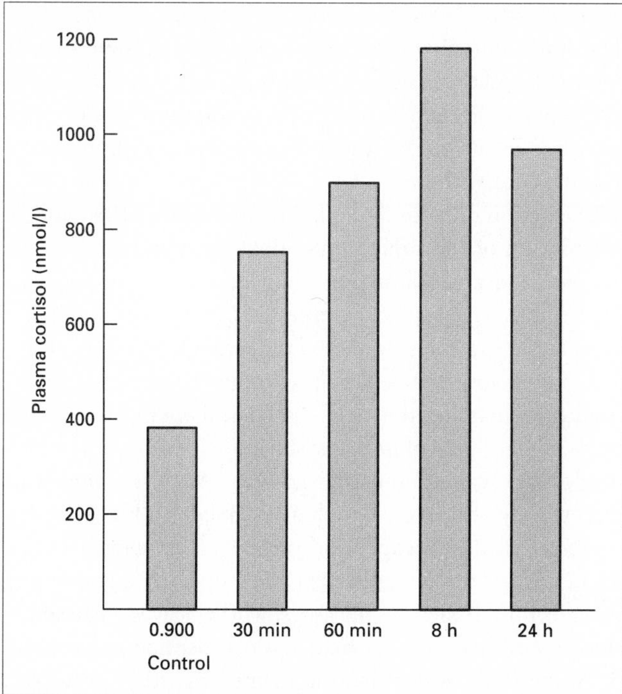

Fig. 32.9 Effects of adrenocorticotrophic hormone (ACTH) on plasma cortisol levels. One milligram of depot Synacthen ($ACTH_{1-24}$) was given intramuscularly at 0900 hours. Blood samples were taken at the time intervals shown and assayed for cortisol. This protocol forms the basis of the Synacthen tests of adrenocortical function (see Chapter 83).

Fig. 32.10 Diurnal rhythm of adrenocorticotrophic hormone (ACTH) and cortisol secretion. There is a characteristic peak of ACTH and cortisol in the morning, with an evening nadir.

there are increases in endosomes and Golgi apparatus which may be related to the internalisation of LDL, or with the hydrolysis of cholesterol esters. Dilatation of the sinusoids, consistent with the increased blood flow noted above, is also visible in suitably preserved material. Chronically, the effects can be partly interpreted as continuations of these acute effects. Thus, the gland may become massively hyperaemic, and the cells increase in number, and also in size, as a result of increased mitochondria and smooth endoplasmic reticulum. In addition, however, the cells of the zona glomerulosa may lose their characteristic morphology, and become indistinguishable from inner-zone cells, or intermediate between the zona glomerulosa and zona fasciculata cell types. In particular, the characteristic shelf-like cristae of the normal zona glomerulosa cell mitochondria are transformed into the tubulovesicular type of the inner zone cells, and cell volume is increased, with the increase of the cytoplasmic compartment. The changes in zona glomerulosa morphology are broadly correlated with changes in cellular function, as the transformed cells lose their capacity to synthesise aldosterone or to respond to the specific zona glomerulosa stimulants, such as angiotensin II or potassium (see below). These changes are clinically important as they may be seen in patients in chronic illness, or other conditions, where levels of ACTH may be mildly but chronically elevated.

Control of glomerulosa function and aldosterone secretion

Physiologically, the most important stimuli for aldosterone

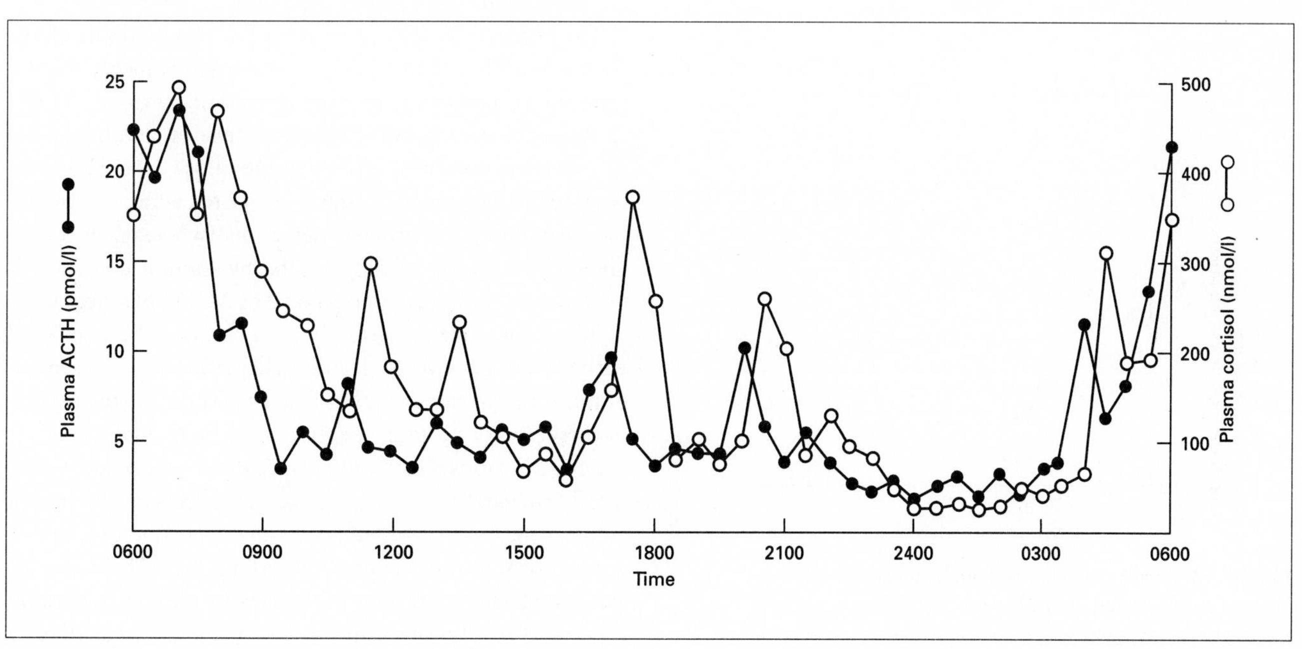

secretion are altered electrolyte and fluid status (particularly sodium loss) or extracellular fluid volume reduction, for example by haemorrhage, the use of diuretics, and postural changes; aldosterone levels are increased by upright posture. Restriction of dietary sodium intake in experimental animals causes hypertrophy of the zona glomerulosa, and elevation of secreted aldosterone and circulating aldosterone concentrations, with no concomitant effect on glucocorticoids (Fig. 32.11). The hypertrophy of the zona glomerulosa arises from increased mitochondrial and smooth endoplasmic reticulum volumes, and zona glomerulosa cell number also increases. The inner mitochondrial membrane may become greatly enlarged, and the cristae may consequently take the form of stacks of parallel lamelli, unlike the normal appearance. Such increases in surface area may be associated with increased aldosterone synthase.

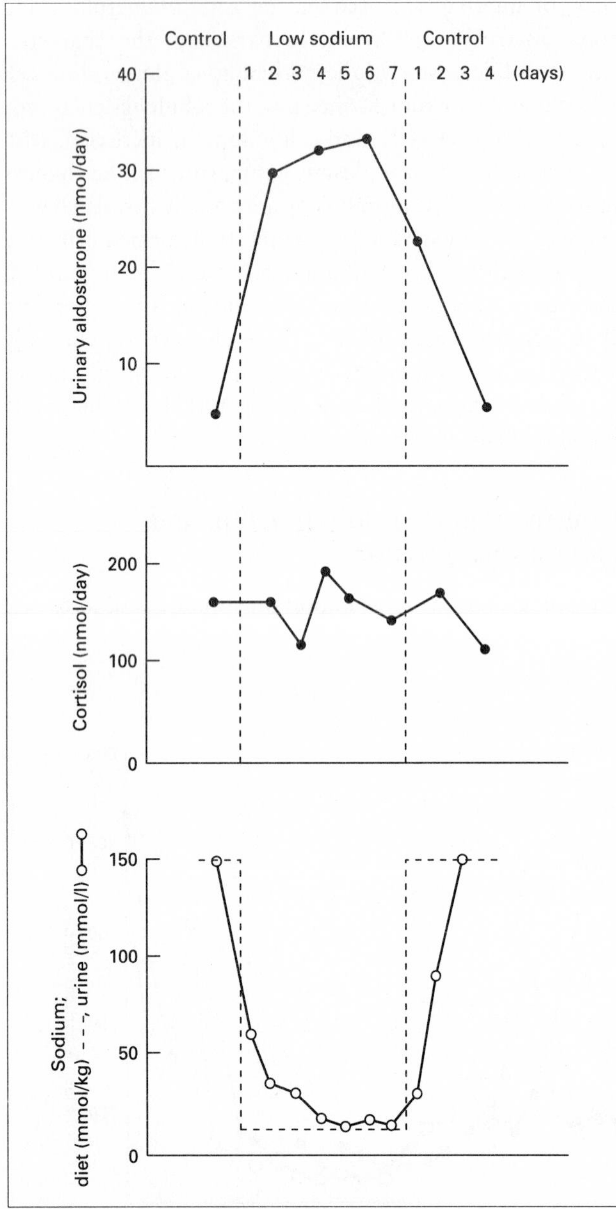

Fig. 32.11 Effects of dietary sodium restriction on daily aldosterone excretion. A low sodium diet causes a dramatic increase in aldosterone output, while cortisol is unaffected.

The action of sodium depletion, and other physiological stimulation of the zona glomerulosa, is attributable to the actions of several stimulants which may act in concert. The renin–angiotensin system is especially important. Renin is a proteolytic enzyme secreted by the juxtaglomerular cells of the kidney, and the secretion of renin is increased under conditions of reduced sodium intake, sodium loss or reduced extracellular fluid volume. The substrate for renin is a plasma α_2-globulin called angiotensinogen. Angiotensinogen is secreted by the liver, which is cleaved by blood-borne renin to yield a decapeptide product, angiotensin I (Fig. 32.12). Angiotensin I is in turn acted upon by a converting enzyme, found chiefly in the lungs, which cleaves the terminal leucine and histidine to yield the octapeptide angiotensin II. Angiotensin II can also be formed by other proteases, although the physiological significance of these reactions is unclear. Angiotensin II has a short half-life in plasma of only 2 min. It is cleaved by various aminopeptidases, one of which removes the terminal aspartate to form the heptapeptide, angiotensin III. Intra-adrenal sources of renin and angiotensin-converting enzyme also exist, and their physiological contribution appears to be to reinforce the actions of the systemic system. Angiotensin II acts on zona glomerulosa cells to stimulate the synthesis and secretion of aldosterone. Administered chronically, it can also reproduce the morphological changes in the zona glomerulosa which are associated with sodium depletion.

The pituitary is also involved in the regulation of aldosterone secretion, and hypophysectomised subjects show a reduced response to sodium depletion. Infused ACTH causes a rise in circulating aldosterone level, and this is due to a direct action of ACTH on glomerulosa cells. However, because this increase is invariably associated with concomitant increases in glucocorticoid secretion (whereas, as noted above, stimulation of aldosterone by sodium depletion is not), the physiological importance of ACTH in aldosterone regulation is unclear. Certainly, ACTH cannot be associated with the chronic effects of sodium depletion on enlargement of the zona glomerulosa, because its actions are the reverse of these. Other pituitary peptides may be involved.

Potassium ions also stimulate aldosterone secretion. Chronically, increased potassium intake has effects on circulating aldosterone, and on zona glomerulosa morphology, which are identical to those caused by sodium loss. These may be associated with only minor changes in plasma potassium concentrations, however, and although potassium can directly

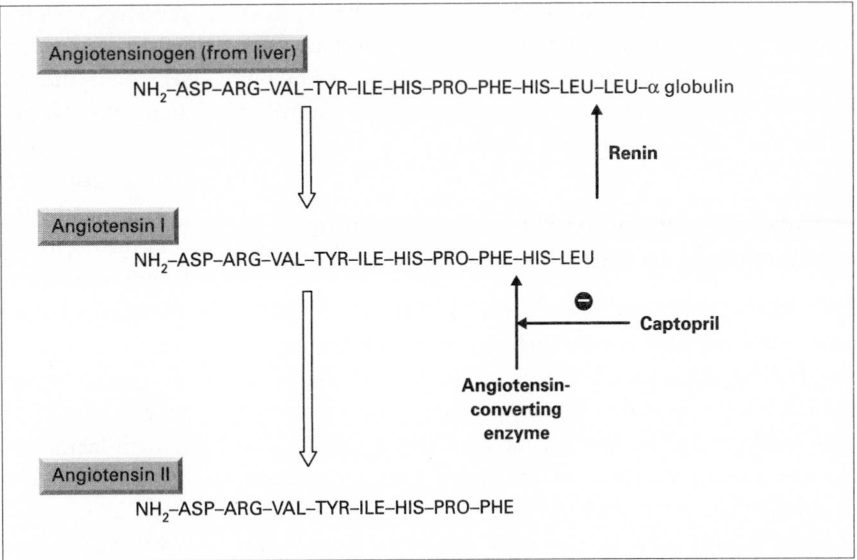

Fig. 32.12 The renin–angiotensin system. Renin secretion from the juxtaglomerular cells of the kidney is provoked by a decrease in renal perfusion pressure or by a decreased plasma sodium concentration. Renin circulates in the blood and cleaves the decapeptide angiotensin I from the circulating α-globulin, angiotensinogen. Angiotensin I is cleaved to form angiotensin II by the actions of a 'converting enzyme' located mainly in the lung. The actions of this enzyme, and the formation of angiotensin II, are inhibited by captopril. Angiotensin II acts to elevate blood pressure and also to stimulate aldosterone secretion.

stimulate steroidogenesis in glomerulosa cells, this is seen only as relatively high concentrations of potassium, which are not usually achieved in plasma. It is probable that physiologically the most important effect of potassium is to increase the sensitivity of the zona glomerulosa response to angiotensin II, and this effect is seen when potassium ion concentrations are increased only marginally.

The discovery of the atrial natriuretic peptides (ANP) illuminated the possibility that they might also play a part in the regulation of aldosterone secretion. Infusion of ANP in humans and in experimental animals causes a decrease in circulating aldosterone concentrations. In part this may be due to decreased renin activity, but a direct effect on the cells of the zona glomerulosa is also involved. ANP inhibits the response of aldosterone secretion to angiotensin II stimulation in zona glomerulosa cells, while there is no effect on glucocorticoid secretion, or on the zona fasciculata or zona reticularis.

These are numerous other factors that stimulate aldosterone secretion and zona glomerulosa function under experimental conditions, although the physiological importance of their actions remains to be clarified. These include serotonin, catecholamines, acetylcholine, vasoactive intestinal peptide, vasopressin, oxytocin, α-melanocyte-stimulating hormone other neuropeptides and prostaglandin E. Other inhibitors include somatostatin and dopamine.

Control of adrenal androgen secretion

Adrenal androgen secretion (androstenedione and DHEA) rises throughout childhood, paralleling the increase in adrenal size, and peaks in puberty, a period that has been termed adrenarche (Fig. 32.13). Secretion of these hormones

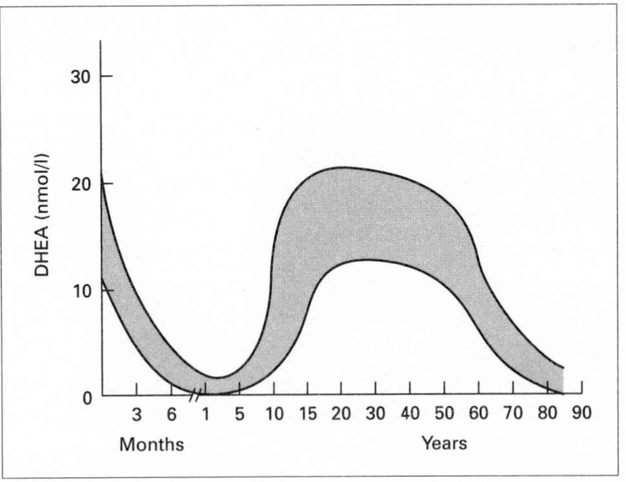

Fig. 32.13 Pattern of dehydroepiandrosterone (DHEA, the most abundant adrenal androgen) secretion throughout life in women. There is a rise in adrenal androgen secretion at puberty, and levels of DHEA remain elevated until around the time of menopause, when there is a gradual decline in plasma levels of these steroids. These phenomena are termed adrenarche and adrenopause, respectively. A similar pattern is seen in men.

remains high until 40–50 years of age, then they begin to decline (the 'andrenopause'). The mechanism for regulation of adrenal androgen secretion is not completely clear, and although ACTH is a potent stimulant, the secretion of cortisol and the adrenal androgens may be dissociated under some conditions. During adrenarche, for example, adrenal androgen secretion rises while cortisol is unchanged. This has led to a search for a specific adrenal androgen-stimulating peptide. Candidates for this role have included prolactin, a novel peptide isolated from bovine pituitaries, and the 'joining peptide' in the ACTH precursor, but the evidence is weak. Alternatively, intra-adrenal mechanisms have been suggested in which the accumulation of cortisol may favour transformation of steroid precursors along the androgen rather than the glucocorticoid pathway.

Intracellular mechanisms for the control of corticosteroid secretion

Peptides and other stimulants of the adrenal cortex (except potassium) act, like many other hormones, by binding to specific receptors located in the cell membrane. This binding is of high affinity, with dissociation constants in the region of 10^{-11} mol/l for ACTH, and 10^{-9} mol/l for angiotensin II. The number and affinity of the receptors, and hence the response to stimulation, may vary according to physiological status.

Both ACTH and angiotensin receptors have been cloned. At least five subtypes of the ACTH/melanotrophin receptor are known, and all are members of the seven transmembrane domain, G-protein-linked receptor family. Their primary mode of intracellular transduction is through adenylyl cyclase activation (see below). Depending on their inhibition by subtype specific antagonists, angiotensin receptors are subdivided into two primary subtypes, AT_1 and AT_2. Most known actions of angiotensin II, including those on the adrenal cortex, are thought to be modulated through the AT_1 receptor, which is also a classical G-protein-linked receptor, but which acts primarily through the inositol triphosphate (IP_3)/diacylglycerol/Ca^{2+} signalling pathway. Two minor variants exist, which seem to be similarly active, and are similarly regulated. These are designated AT_{1a} and AT_{a1b}. The functional significance and mode of action of the AT_2 receptor is not entirely clear, and although it is a seven transmembrane receptor, with low homology to the AT_1 receptor, there appear to be two subtypes, of which AT_{2a} is sensitive to guanine nucleotides and pertussis toxin, while AT_{2b} is not.

The act of hormone binding to receptors triggers a sequence of events related to the production and actions of one or more of a series of intracellular modulators, sometimes termed 'second messengers' (the hormone being the 'first messenger'). The principal second messengers identified to date in the adrenal cortex are cyclic adenosine monophosphate (cAMP), IP_3, diacylglycerol and Ca^{2+} (see also Chapter 4). From a combination of experimental approaches it is possible to conclude that any or all of these modes of intracellular signal modulation may be involved in the stimulation of adrenal steroidogenesis (Fig. 32.14). Thus, ACTH produces increases in adenylyl cyclase activity, and increased cAMP generation precedes the steroidogenic response to ACTH. Activation of cAMP-dependent protein kinase results in the phosphorylation of many cellular proteins, possibly including StAR protein. Other agents also increase adenylate cyclase activity in the adrenal, including serotonin and potassium ions in glomerulosa cells, while angiotensin II may inhibit cAMP production. Cyclic AMP also reproduces most, if not all, of the effects of ACTH on steroidogenesis, enzyme induction, RNA transcription and protein synthesis.

However, the trophic actions of ACTH, or angiotensin II, are almost certainly modulated through the effects of intraglandular paracrine mechanisms, which will include members of the growth-factor family, including especially the insulin-like growth factors (IGFs) and basic fibroblast growth factor (bFGF). Either directly, or indirectly through growth-factor activity, the trophic effects of the systemic hormones are characterised by the initial induction of the early intermediate genes, for example c-*fos* and c-*jun*. Growth-factor receptors are generally of the insulin-receptor family, which are trans-membrane proteins incorporating a tyrosine kinase domain at an intracellular site. Like other actions of this group of receptors, the intracellular signalling pathways that are involved in regulation of adrenal growth and modelling therefore involve a cascade of protein kinases, including mitogen-activated protein kinase (MAP-kinase) and others. These may ultimately act through the induction of c-*fos* and c-*jun* and the formation of the the heterodimer of their gene products, the transcription factor AP-1.

Angiotensin II clearly does not act through stimulation of cAMP, on which its effects are inhibitory. Instead, angiotensin II operates through the classical IP_3–Ca^{2+} signalling system. It increases phospholipase-C activity and IP_3 generation, and, in consequence, cytosolic free Ca^{2+} is also increased. As in other systems, this increase may be oscillatory. The magnitude of the Ca^{2+} response correlates with, but precedes, the steroidogenic response.

The actions of potassium ions on steroidogenesis also depend on increases in intracellular Ca^{2+}. However, in this case, the small increases in extracellular potassium which can produce increased steroid output are sufficient to bring about depolarisation of the plasma membrane, which results in the opening of voltage-dependent Ca^{2+} channels. The system is complex, and potassium is also observed to stimulate cAMP production in some preparations.

Inhibition of aldosterone production by ANP may depend on enhanced cyclic guanosine monophosphate (cGMP), which is thought to be the second messenger that modulates the actions of this peptide in several systems.

Arachidonic acid metabolites, including prostaglandins and leucotrienes, have also been implicated by some authors as second messengers in the adrenal, but the evidence is weak.

The mode of action of the second-messenger systems, and of the specific protein kinases which they activate, on the steroidogenic process is only partly understood.

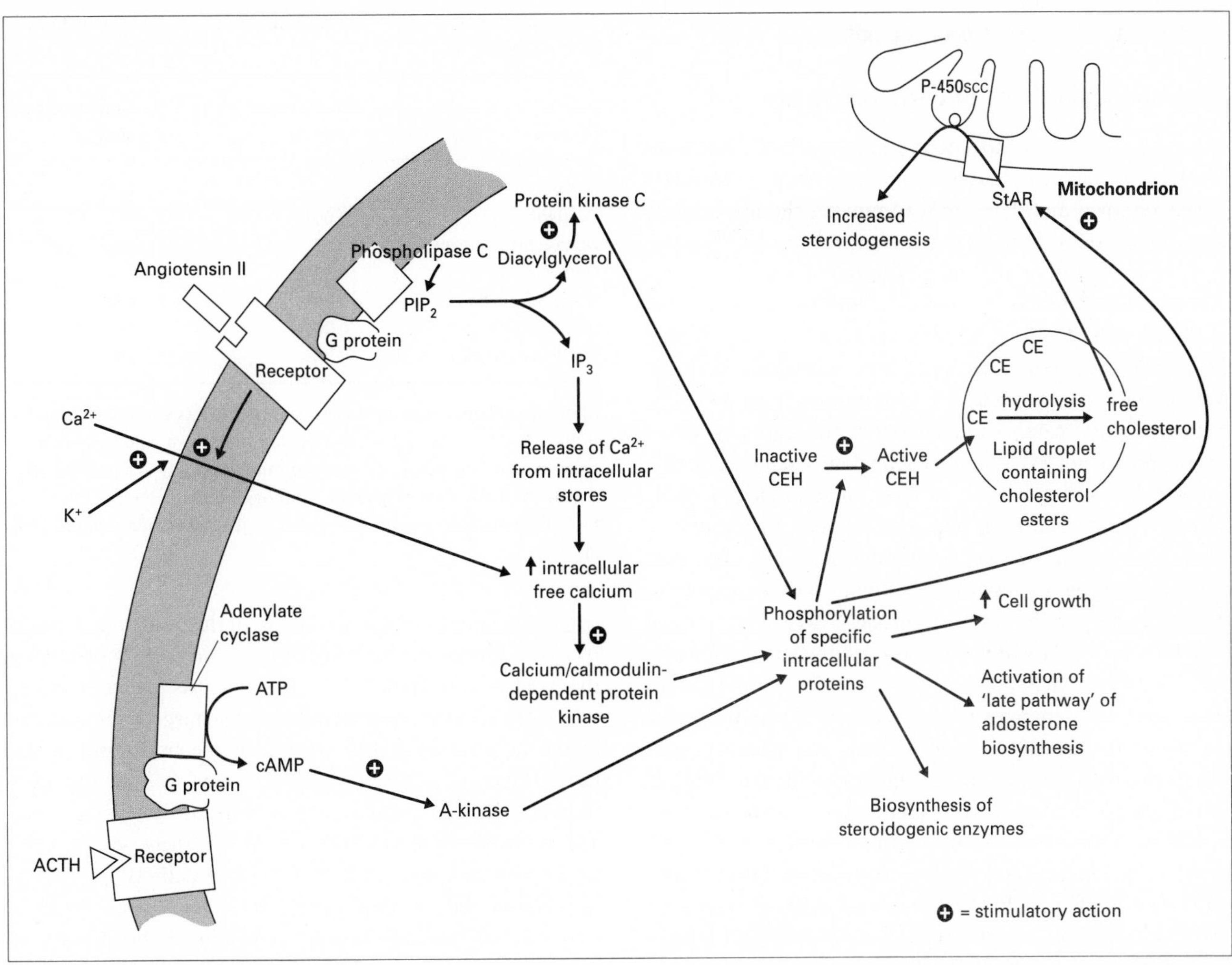

Fig. 32.14 The role of second messengers in the response to the major stimulants of adrenocortical hormone secretion. IP_3, inositol trisphosphate; PIP_2, phosphatidyl inositol bisphosphate; CE, cholesterol esters; CEH, cholesterol ester hydrolase. A-kinase, cyclic AMP-dependent protein kinase.

There are five sites at which steroidogenesis is enhanced by stimulation:

1 LDL internalisation;
2 activation of HMG CoA reductase;
3 activation of CEH;
4 activation of processes leading to cholesterol side-chain cleavage;
5 the conversion of 'late pathway precursors' to aldosterone.

With the exception of CEH activation, the role of protein phosphorylation in any of these processes is unclear. However, it is known that increased specific peptide or protein synthesis, through increased translation of pre-existing messenger RNA (mRNA) species, is required for ACTH action. From the evidence available it seems probable that this agent increases the rate of cholesterol side-chain cleavage by increasing the availability of cholesterol to the inner mitochondrial membrane and to cytochrome $P\text{-}450_{scc}$.

Although several candidates for this role have been proposed in the past, the most convincing evidence is now that this is the function of the StAR protein. This 30-kDa protein is a member of a family of mitochondrial proteins and phosphoproteins present in adrenocorticol cells (and other steroid-producing cells) that rapidly appear in response to ACTH. Transfected transiently into steroid-secreting cell lines, StAR induces increased steroid output in the absence of other stimulation. It is likely that transcription is not required in the initial stages of stimulation; instead, the protein is from pre-existing mRNA. The congenital loss of this protein leads to the condition of lipoid congenital adrenal hyperplasia, characterised by the failure to form corticosteroids, and the presence of large adrenals that contain very high concentrations of cholesterol and its esters. Without steroid replacement therapy, the condition in newborn children results in death within a few weeks.

Actions of corticosteroids

Physiological effects of corticosteroids

The classical approach to determining the role of a hormone is to remove the organ that produces it, to observe the effects of this removal and, later, to readminister the hormone to see whether the effects of organ removal can be reversed. Early in the study of adrenal physiology it was discovered that the gland's function is essential for life, and that most of the numerous effects of adrenalectomy are attributable to loss of the adrenocortical and not the medullary products. Among these effects are loss of sodium ions from the body, decreased blood volume and onset of hypotension, increased plasma potassium levels, muscular weakness, reduced cardiac contractility and depletion of liver and muscle glycogen, together with a generally impaired capacity to respond to physical stress. From these beginnings it became clear that two distinct types of activity were involved in the actions of the hormones of the adrenal cortex. These were termed mineralocorticoid (actions associated with changes in water and electrolyte metabolism) and glucocorticoid (actions associated with changes in intermediary metabolism and resistance to stress). As noted above, the primary mineralocorticoid is aldosterone, and in humans the predominant glucocorticoid is cortisol although in rats it is corticosterone.

Although the hormones were first classified on the basis of their physiological actions, they may also be differentiated on the basis of their binding affinity for tissue receptors. Two main types of receptor were described in early studies in animals: type I, originally detected in the kidney, was considered to be the mineralocorticoid receptor, and bound aldosterone and deoxycorticosterone with higher affinity than cortisol or corticosterone; type II, considered to be the glucocorticoid receptor, bound the synthetic glucocorticoid, dexamethasone, with greatest affinity and cortisol with somewhat lower affinity. More recently, with the cloning and characterisation of the receptors an unexpected finding has been that the recombinant mineralocorticoid (type I) receptor binds both aldosterone and the glucocorticoids, cortisol and corticosterone, with equal affinity *in vitro*. This raises the problem of how a specific mineralocorticoid effect can be exerted in the intact animal where the free plasma levels of the glucocorticoids may be up to 100 times higher than those of aldosterone. A suggestion which helps to explain this conundrum is that glucocorticoids are prevented from exerting their effects at mineralocorticoid target tissues by being converted to their 11-keto derivatives (cortisone and 11-dehydrocorticosterone) which do not bind effectively to the receptor. This transformation is achieved by the type 2 isozyme of 11β-hydroxysteroid dehydrogenase present in the kidney and other tissues, and which

Table 32.3 Relative glucocorticoid and mineralocorticoid activity of corticosteroids.

Steroid	Mineralocorticoid activity	Glucocorticoid activity
Aldosterone	1	0.15
Cortisol	0.001	1
Deoxycorticosterone	0.03	0.02
Corticosterone	0.004	0.4
11-Deoxycortisol	0.002	0.06
Dexametasone	0.001	20
9α-Fluorocortisol	0.15	10

Mineralocorticoid activity is assessed on the basis of the change in urinary Na^+/K^+ in the adrenalectomised rat, where aldosterone is given a standard value of 1. Glucocorticoid activity is assessed on the basis of the level of glycogen deposition in the liver of the fasted adrenalectomised rat. Cortisol is given a standard value of 1 [1].

can be thought of as the 'guardian' of the mineralocorticoid receptor. There are also 'unprotected' binding sites showing the biochemical characteristics of type I receptors in tissues which are not obvious mineralocorticoid targets, for example in the hippocampus and septum in the brain and in the heart. Here, the type I receptor seems to function as a 'non-classical' glucocorticoid receptor; low levels of cortisol and corticosterone are able to interact freely with it since no 11β-hydroxysteroid dehydrogenase activity is present. In addition, the possibility of a further mechanism of aldosterone action has been raised recently, involving interaction with membrane (rather than cytosolic) receptors that trigger rapid, non-genomic, changes in electrolyte transport (see below).

Table 32.3 shows the relative glucocorticoid and mineralocorticoid activity *in vivo* of some common steroids, and it can be seen that, in practice, few corticosteroids are completely specific in their effects. Thus, cortisol, which normally shows about one-thousandth of the mineralocorticoid activity of aldosterone *in vivo*, may have appreciable effects on electrolyte metabolism when plasma levels are elevated as in Cushing's syndrome.

Mineralocorticoid actions

The main actions of hormones which bind to type I (mineralocorticoid) receptors are to increase the reabsorption of sodium in the kidney and at other secretory epithelial sites, thus reducing the sodium content of urine, sweat, saliva etc. Effectively, sodium ions are exchanged for hydrogen and potassium ions, leading to decreased sodium and increased potassium excretion, and increased urine acidity. With prolonged mineralocorticoid treatment, extracellular

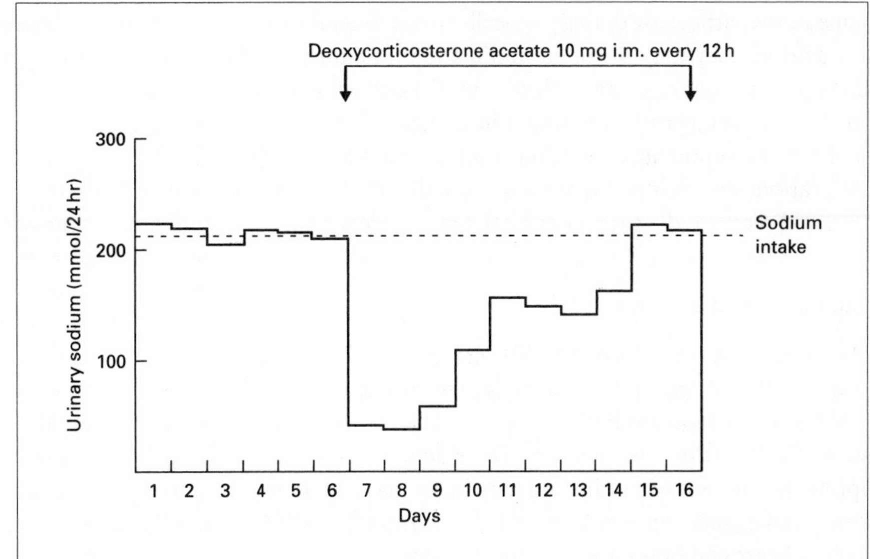

Fig. 32.15 Effects of mineralocorticoid administration on urinary sodium excretion. Mineralocorticoid 'escape' is the gradual resumption of control levels of sodium excretion, despite continued treatment. Adapted from [6], with permission.

fluid volume expansion occurs and renin production is reduced in response. After a few days, however, the kidney escapes from the mineralocorticoid effect on sodium retention but not potassium excretion (Fig. 32.15), and thus a major effect of prolonged mineralocorticoid exposure is that serum and total body potassium levels are reduced. Hypertension is a well-known consequence of excess corticosteroid secretion, and is seen in conditions with elevated aldosterone secretion such as Conn's syndrome as well as in conditions of elevated cortisol secretion such as Cushing's syndrome. The mechanism of the hypertensinogenic effect of steroids is not fully understood, but it is thought to be due in part to their sodium-retaining effect leading to expansion of extracellular fluid volume (Fig. 32.16). Other mechanisms which have been postulated recently include direct actions of mineralocorticoids in the central nervous system.

Glucocorticoid actions

The effects of glucocorticoid receptor activation are varied and complex. Almost all tissues of the body have been found to contain type II receptors and a large number of systems and processes are affected by these steroids. They are essential for the maintenance of cardiovascular and metabolic

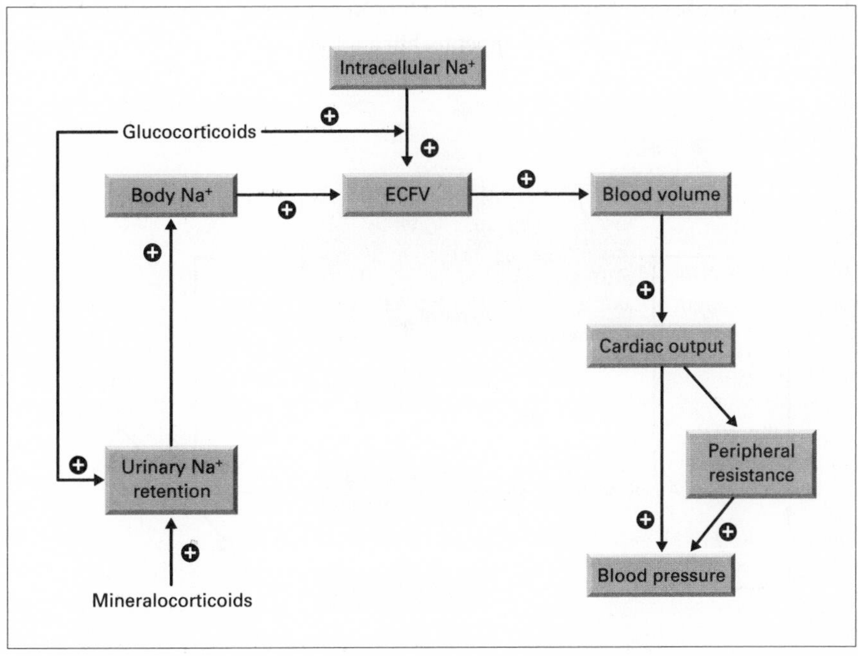

Fig. 32.16 Possible mechanisms for glucocorticoid- and mineralocorticoid-induced increases in blood pressure. ECFV, extracellular fluid volume

homeostasis particularly during physically stressful conditions. In addition, they play a role in modulating inflammatory and immune responses and affect central nervous system function. In the perinatal period, glucocorticoids are particularly important in controlling lung development and maturation, and transgenic mice with a disrupted glucocorticoid receptor die soon after birth from asphyxia.

Intermediary metabolism

The major effects of glucocorticoids are the stimulation of protein catabolism, and hepatic glycogenesis and gluconeogenesis; in most body tissues the results are catabolic but in the liver they are anabolic. These actions essentially oppose the actions of insulin and may be seen as providing protection against long-term glucose deprivation for tissues such as heart and brain; they are most evident in the unfed state. Thus, glucose uptake in many tissues is reduced and amino acids and glycerol are released as a result of the catabolic (and antianabolic) actions of the glucocorticoids. These contribute to increased gluconeogenesis in the liver where glucose output is increased (Fig. 32.17). The hepatic actions arise through a combination of two effects: (i) the freeing of glycogen synthesis from the normally tight control exerted by glucose (thus, glycogen, synthesis occurs even when plasma glucose levels are low); and (ii) stimulation of transamination and other steps in the gluconeogenic process which further enhance the production of glycogen.

The effects of glucocorticoids on fat metabolism are complex. In some situations increased lipolysis is seen, partly through direct stimulation of lipase, but also through enhancement of the actions of other hormones, including glucagon. The obesity characteristic of Cushing's syndrome is partly attributable to increased appetite, but a differential sensitivity of different fat depots to glucocorticoids may be involved in the typical redistribution of body fat.

Growth

A conspicuous effect of corticosteroid administration is inhibition of growth in young subjects. This is in part explained by general inhibition of protein synthesis but further possibilities are that glucocorticoids inhibit tissue growth factor production and interfere with the processes that regulate growth hormone release. Glucocorticoids may also bring about a negative calcium balance, through inhibition of calcium uptake in the gut and increased urinary calcium excretion. In excess, glucocorticoids can interfere with the second, remodelling, stage of wound healing (in addition to inhibiting the first, inflammatory, stage; see below). This may also be associated with effects on the local production and actions of growth factors.

Effects on water and electrolyte metabolism and the cardiovascular system

One of the classical signs of adrenocortical insufficiency is the inability to excrete a water load; this is related to glucocorticoid, not mineralocorticoid, deficiency. In part this is explained by elevated plasma vasopressin levels, but glucocorticoids are also known to affect kidney function directly through an action on glomerular filtration rate.

Hypotension is also one of the characteristics of adrenocortical insufficiency, and can be corrected very rapidly by administration of cortisol. The speed of this effect suggests that cortisol has actions on the cardiovascular system which are independent of its relatively slow action on redistribution of sodium from the intracellular into the extracellular

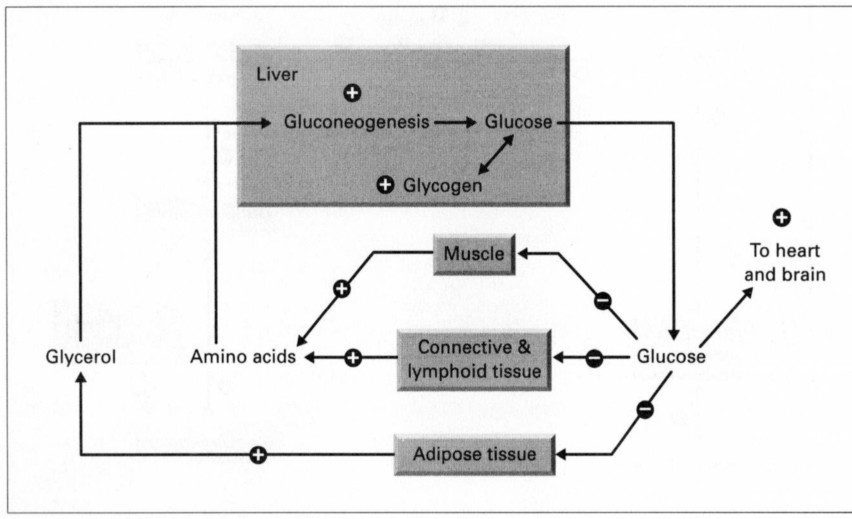

Fig. 32.17 Effects of glucocorticoids on intermediary metabolism. ⊕ Stimulatory action; ⊖ Inhibitory action on glucose uptake.

compartment as well as those mediated through mineralocorticoid receptors (Fig. 32.16). In the absence of glucocorticoids there is reduced myocardial efficiency and a loss of arteriolar tone, as vascular smooth muscle becomes unresponsive to catecholamines. Glucocorticoids are beneficial in the treatment of endotoxin shock; this action appears to be mediated in part by preventing the induction of nitric oxide synthase. Inhibition of prostacyclin synthesis may also contribute to the effects on blood pressure.

Inflammation

The inflammatory response to a wound, infection, or other foreign protein invasion consists of a number of components, including vasodilatation, increased capillary permeability, and accumulation of platelets and leucocytes at the site of damage. A large number of mediators of these effects have been identified, including cytokines, eicosanoids, histamine, kinins and components of the complement system. Glucocorticoids reduce inflammation by inhibiting the production of many of the mediators of the vascular response and thus reducing tissue fluid accumulation and the severity of the granulation response. One mode of action of the glucocorticoids is through the inhibition of phospholipase A2 activity and reduced production of lipid mediators of inflammation such as leukotrienes, prostaglandins and platelet-activating factor. In part, this action seems to be achieved through the induction of a peptide mediator, lipocortin 1, a member of the annexin family of Ca^{2+}-binding proteins. However, direct effects of steroids on the transcription of enzymes have also been found. Glucocorticoids also reduce cytokine-mediated inflammation, both by inhibiting their production and counteracting their effects.

Immunosuppression

One sensitive response to glucocorticoids is the cytotoxic response in cells of the immune system. This is particularly visible in young animals, in which relatively low doses can cause massive involution of the thymus. However, there are considerable species differences, and the response is much less marked in humans. The major cell targets are lymphocytes, monocytes and macrophages, in which many cell functions are disrupted; in addition, antibody production and B-cell proliferation are suppressed by high doses of glucocorticoids. One of the major routes to their overall immunosuppressive effect is the inhibition of the production of cytokines, including that of interferon-γ and interleukins 2, 3 and 6 by T cells. Lipocortin 1 may also mediate some of these effects of glucocorticoids.

Effects on the central nervous system

Corticosteroids can freely cross the blood–brain barrier, and both type I and type II receptors are found in brain tissue. The effects of glucocorticoid excess on behaviour are complex and variable, and some of the reported changes may not be due to direct actions of the hormones themselves. The psychological consequences of adrenocortical malfunction are well known; approximately 70% of patients with Cushing's syndrome are reported to be depressed. In contrast, acute treatment with exogenous glucocorticoid is more commonly associated with improved mental state. There is also evidence of hypersecretion of cortisol in patients suffering from severe depression, and a causal role for alterations in the activity of the hypothalamo-pituitary–adrenal axis in the illness appears possible (see also Chapter 82).

Glucocorticoids exert powerful inhibitory feedback effects on the secretion of ACTH and corticotrophin-releasing hormone (CRH); these actions are mediated by three distinct mechanisms which operate over different time spans. Rapid feedback effects which occur over a very short period (< 10 min) are exerted primarily at the level of the hypothalamus and may involve rapid, non-genomic action of the steroids at the cell membrane. The early and late phases of delayed feedback involve mainly glucocorticoid (type II) receptors in the pituitary, hypothalamus and hippocampus. In the early phase of delayed feedback both the release and synthesis of CRH and ACTH are affected, probably as the results of impairment of processing at the level of translation. These actions may be mediated by lipocortin 1. The late phase of steroid feedback requires that plasma levels of glucocorticoid are elevated for at least 24 hours; in the case of long-term treatment the inhibition of the hypothalamo-pituitary–adrenal axis can persist when the steroid is withdrawn, with potentially catastrophic consequences. This phase of inhibition is associated with suppression of gene expression and reduced synthesis of pituitary and hypothalamic products.

Stress

Although ACTH secretion and consequently corticosteroid secretion have long been known to be increased in response to stresses of many different types, the exact way in which glucocorticoids confer resistance to stress is still debated. There is general agreement that the many actions of glucocorticoids in the cardiovascular system which improve vascular reactivity and cardiac performance are beneficial under stressful conditions. Another possibility is that glucocorticoids, by virtue of their ability to suppress the production of many mediators of the response to infection and injury, may protect against the over-reaction of these systems and the risk of excessive vasodilatation, oedema and other damaging effects. It may seem paradoxical that in some cases glucocorticoids appear to regulate defence mechanisms in two opposing ways, being both necessary for proper expression of a response and also capable of suppressing it. This may be rationalised by the suggestion that in their 'permissive' mode (at levels found in the normal diurnal cycle) the hormones act to prime the body's defences for normal activity, whereas the suppressive actions (at levels found during severe stress) prevent the reactions from overshooting.

Cellular mode of action of corticosteroids

As with all other hormones, the primary event in corticosteroid action is to bind to a specific receptor. In the case of the steroid hormones, which can freely penetrate cells, the receptors are intracellular, and are mostly located in the nucleus. In the case of glucocorticoid receptors, unoccupied receptors are also found in the cytoplasm. The corticosteroid receptors, like those of other steroids, are members of a large family of related proteins which also includes receptors for 1,25-dihydroxycholecalciferol, thyroid hormones, retinoic acid and the ecdysteroids (hormones that control moulting in insects). The structures of the major types are known, and each consists of relatively highly conserved functional domains separated by more poorly conserved regions. The DNA-binding domain, of about 70 amino-acid residues, is the most highly conserved region, while the hormone-binding domain also shows considerable homology (Fig. 32.18). The glucocorticoid receptor is a monomer of molecular weight of about 94 000 present in target organs at concentrations of 25 000 molecules per cell, and its K_D is in the nanomolar range. The mineralocorticoid receptor has a molecular weight of 107 000.

The intracellular sequence of events of hormonal stimulation is similar for all the steroids, although variations in detail occur (Fig. 32.19). In essence, the binding of hormone to its receptor results in receptor activation. The unactivated receptor probably exists as a dimer in association with two 90-kDa heat-shock protein molecules. Ligand binding brings about a tranformational change that results in the dissociation of the heat-shock proteins, and higher-affinity binding of the receptor dimer to DNA hormone response elements (HRE) in the promoter region of target genes. Generally, corticosteroid receptors bind to HREs as homodimers, though in the case of other nuclear receptors, heterodimers frequently occur. By analogy, it may eventually emerge that glucocorticoid/mineralocorticoid receptor heterodimers have particular physiological roles. By comparison with the ligand-binding domains of the retinoic acid receptors, the unliganded RXR-α and the liganded RAR-γ for which three-dimensional structures have been derived, it has been possible to generate a general alignment of the ligand-binding domain (LBDs) of all of the nuclear receptors. A 20-amino-acid region constitutes a nuclear receptor-specific signature and contains most of the conserved residues that stabilise the core of the canonical fold of their ligand binding domains.

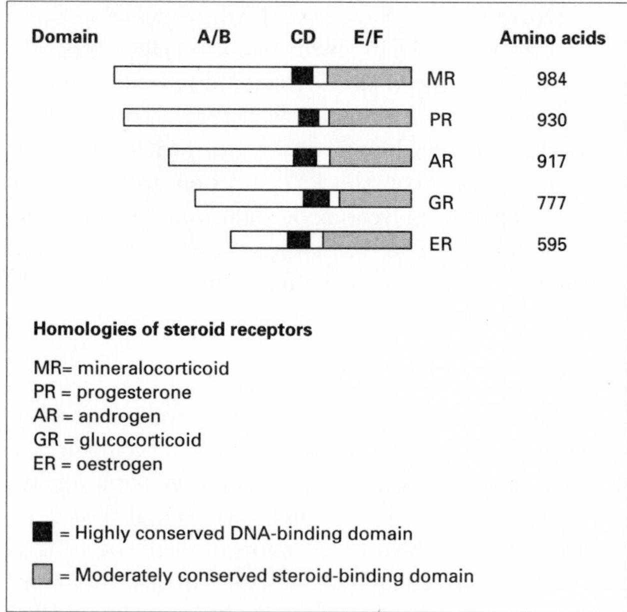

Fig. 32.18 Homologies of steroid hormone receptors.

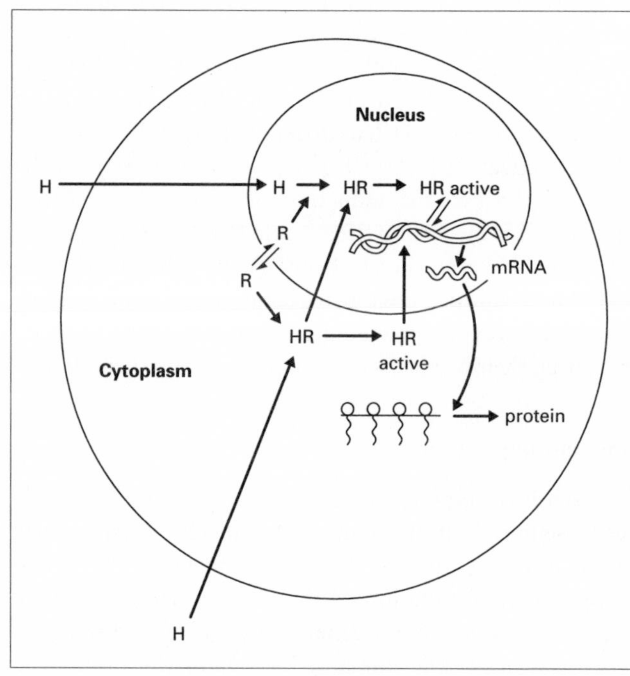

Fig. 32.19 Nuclear action of glucocorticoids. H, hormone; R, receptor; HR, hormone–receptor complex.

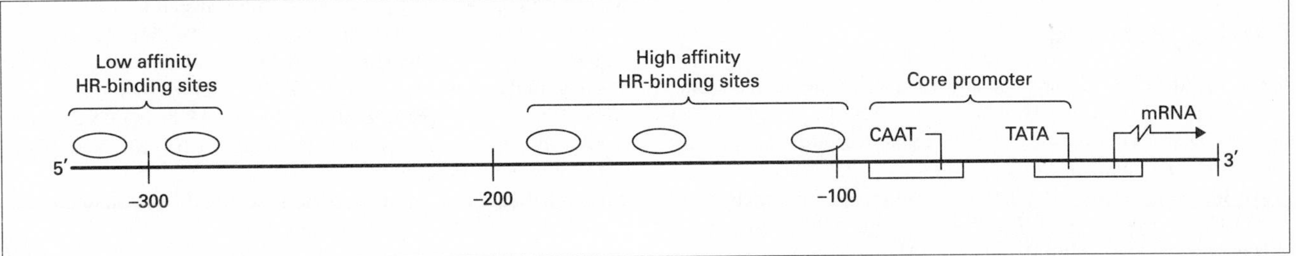

Fig. 32.20 Gene activation by corticosteroids. From [1].

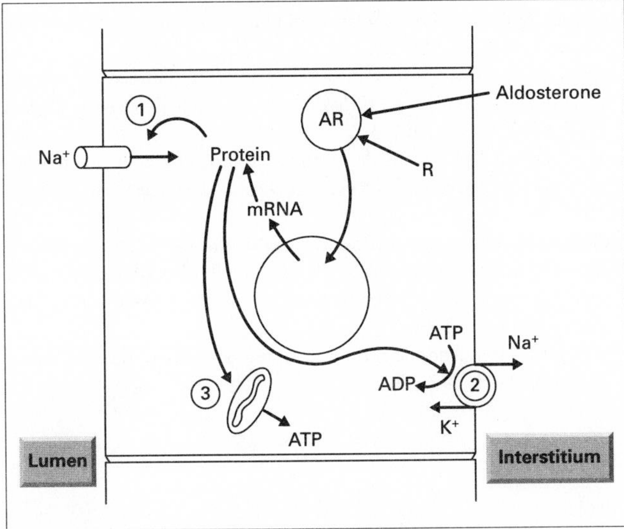

Fig. 32.21 Possible mode of action of aldosterone on an epithelial cell. R, receptor; AR, aldosterone–receptor complex. Possible sites of action of aldosterone-induced proteins are: (1) recruitment of amiloride-sensitive sodium channels; (2) activation of Na^+/K^+ adenosine triphosphatase (ATPase); and (3) stimulation of mitochondrial enzymes involved in ATP production.

A common ligand-binding pocket, involving predominantly hydrophobic residues, has been inferred by homology modelling of the human RXR-α and glucocorticoid receptor ligand-binding sites according to the RAR-γ holo-LBD structure. Hormonal responses to the steroids are then generated by the finding of the activated hormone–receptor complex to HREs in DNA, which bring about the activation of specific genes (Fig. 32.20). This results in the increased production of specific mRNAs and protein synthesis. It is probable, however, that the presence of one or more additional transcription factors is also necessary before gene activation occurs. According to this model, then, it is axiomatic that, like all steroids, the actions of the glucocorticoids are modulated by production of specific cellular protein mediators of the response (but see below). Some of these, like lipocortin-1, are known. However, it is possible that there are a variety of other mediators both stimulatory and inhibitory. Possible intracellular mechanisms for aldosterone action are shown in Fig. 32.21.

Non-genomic effects of steroids

Although the primary attention of research has been directed towards elucidation of the nuclear actions of steroids, substantial evidence now supports the view that non-genomic actions may be extremely important. There are various mechanisms that may be involved. One example is the action of 5α-reduced metabolites of deoxycorticosterone and of progesterone which act on the central nervous system to produce sedation and anaesthesia, apparently through binding to the γ-amino butyric acid A (GABA-A) receptor/chloride channel complex. Like the barbiturate anaesthetics, these steroids may therefore act by potentiating the action of the inhibitory neurotransmitter GABA. In addition, some effects of aldosterone on human leucocytes, vascular smooth muscle or kidney cells, including changes in intracellular electrolyte concentration and cell volume, IP_3 generation, and Na^+-proton exchanger activity are incompatible with an action via the classical nuclear pathway. Instead it is thought that a membrane aldosterone receptor is responsible for these effects. Functional characterisation of these receptors reveals a distinct receptor class, with 10-fold higher affinity for aldosterone than the classical nuclear receptor, and 10 000-fold greater specificity for aldosterone than for cortisol.

References

1 Vinson GP, Whitehouse BJ, Hinson JP. *The Adrenal Cortex*. Englewood Cliffs, NJ: Prentice Hall Endocrinology Series, 1992.
2 Belloni AS, Mazzochi G, Mantero F, Nussdorfer G. The human adrenal cortex – ultrastructure and base-line morphometric data. *J Submicrosp Cytol* 1987; **19**: 657–8.
3 Neville AM, O'Hare MJ. *The Human Adrenal Cortex*. Berlin: Springer-Verlag, 1982.
4 Takemori S, Kominami S. The role of cytochrome P-450 in adrenal steroidogenesis. *TIBS* 1984; **9**: 393–6.
5 Yates FE, Marsh DJ, Maran JW. The adrenal cortex. In: Mountcastle VB, ed. *Medical Physiology*. St Louis: CV Mosby, 1980: 1558–60.
6 Ganong WF. *Review of Medical Physiology*, 15th edn East Norwalk, CT: Appleton and Lange, 1991.

Further reading

Barnes PJ, Adcock I. Anti-inflammatory actions of steroid: molecular mechanisms. *TIPS* 1993; **14**: 438–41.

Beato M, Herrlich P, Schütz G. Steroid hormone receptors: many actors in search of a plot. *Cell* 1995; **83**: 851–7.

Bravo EL. Aldosterone and other adrenal steroids. In: Zanchetti A, Tarzi RC, eds. *Handbook of Hypertension, vol 8. Pathophysiology of Hypertension-regulatory Mechanisms*. Amsterdam: Elsevier 1986: 603–25.

Clark BJ, Stocco DM. StAR – a tissue specific acute mediator of steroidogenesis. *Trends Endocr Metab* 1996; 7: 277–33.

Cone RD, Mountjoy KG. Molecular genetics of the ACTH and MSH receptors. *Trends Endocr Metab* 1993; **4**: 243–7.

Flower RJ, Rothwell NJ. Lipocortin-1: cellular mechanisms and clinical relevance. *TIPS* 1994; **15**: 71–6.

Funder J. Target tissue specificity of mineralocorticoids. *Trends Endocrinol Metab* 1990; **1**: 145–8.

Gaillard RC, Al-Damluji S. Stress and the pituitary-adrenal axis. *Baillère's Clin Endocrinol Metab* 1987; **1** (2): 319–54.

Gomez Sanchez EP. Mineralocorticoid modulation of central control of blood pressure. *Steroids* 1995; **60**: 69–72.

Goulding NJ, Guyre PM. Glucocorticoids, lipocortins and the immune response. *Curr Opinion Immunol* 1993; **5**: 108–13.

Hornsby PJ. The mechanism of action of ACTH in the adrenal cortex. In: Cooke BA, King R, van der Molen HJ eds. *Hormones and their Actions* Part 2. Amsterdam: Elsevier, 1988: 193–210.

James VHT ed. *The Adrenal Gland*. New York: Raven Press 1992.

McEvan BS, De Kloet ER, Rostene W. Adrenal steroid receptors and actions in the nervous system. *Physiol Rev* 1986; **66**: 1121–88.

Mangelsdorf DJ, Thummel C, Beato M *et al.* The nuclear receptor superfamily: the second decade. *Cell* 1995; **83**: 835–9.

Miller WL, Tyrell JB. The adrenal cortex. In: Felig P, Baxter JD, Frohman LA, eds. *Endocrinology and Metabolism*. 3rd ed. New York: McGraw-Hill, 1994: 555–711.

Muller J. Regulation of aldosterone biosynthesis: physiological and clinical aspects. *Monogr Endocrinol* 1988.

Munck A, Guyre AP, Holbrook NJ. Physiological functions of glucocorticoids in stress and their relation to pharmacological actions. *Endocr Rev* 1984; **5**: 24–44.

Munck A, Naray-Fejes-Toth A. The ups and downs of glucocorticoid physiology. Permissive and suppressive effects revisisted. *Mol Cell Endocrinol* 1992; **90**: C1–C4.

Quinn SJ, Williams GH.Regulation of aldosterone secretion. *Ann Rev Physiol* 1988; **50**: 409–26.

Stewart PM, Edwards CRW. Specificity of the mineralocorticoid receptor. Crucial role of 11β-hydroxysteroid dehydrogenase. *Trends Endocrinol Metab* 1990; **1**: 225–30.

Stocco, DM, Clark, BJ. Role of the steroidogenic acute regulatory protein (StAR) in steroidogenesis. *Biochem Pharmacol* 1996; **51**: 197–205.

Vallotton M. The renin-angiotensin system. *TIPS* 1987; **8**: 64–74.

Vinson GP, Ho MM, Puddefoot JR. The distribution of angiotensin II type 1 receptors, and the tissue renin-angiotensin systems. *Mol Med Today* 1995; **1**: 35–9.

Wehling M. Non-genomic action of steroid hormones. *Trends Endocr Metab* 1994; **5**: 347–53.

CHAPTER 33

Cushing's syndrome

K. von Werder and O.A. Müller

Introduction

Although Cushing's syndrome was first described almost 60 years ago [1], diagnosis and management of this clinical entity remains one of the most difficult problems in clinical endocrinology [2]. The syndrome is represented by the combination of distinctive clinical features, which were already described in Harvey Cushing's detailed case reports, and associated biochemical changes resulting from persisting hypercortisolism. Inappropriately elevated corticosteroid levels may be caused by adrenal autonomous hypersecretion due to an adrenal adenoma, carcinoma or bilateral nodular hyperplasia, pituitary adrenocorticotrophic hormone (ACTH)-dependent adrenal hyperplasia, ectopic ACTH or corticotropin-releasing hormone (CRH) production, and exogenous corticosteroid or ACTH administration in supraphysiological doses. The latter is the most common cause of Cushing's syndrome. Furthermore, hypercortisolism and its clinical consequences may also be due to excessive alcohol intake, so-called alcoholic pseudo-Cushing, or due to endogenous depressive disorders [3].

Pathophysiology of ACTH and cortisol secretion

The pathophysiological disturbance responsible for spontaneously occurring Cushing's syndrome is excessive cortisol secretion by the adrenal cortex. This cortisol excess can be autonomous or ACTH dependent. A rare cause of hypercortisolism is present in food-induced Cushing's syndrome: adrenal cortical cells of hyperplastic adrenals express abnormally receptors of gastric inhibitory polypeptide (GIP) which are stimulated by food-induced rises of GIP blood levels [4,5].

Adrenal autonomous hypercortisolism

Autonomous cortisol-producing adenomas or carcinomas of the adrenal cortex are found in about 10% of adult patients with endogenous Cushing's syndrome. In contrast, adrenal cortisol-producing tumours are more common in childhood, more than 50% being malignant [3,6], though the most common cause of Cushing's syndrome in adolescence is also bilateral adrenal hyperplasia driven by pituitary ACTH [6].

Malignant adrenal tumours often produce, in addition to cortisol, substantial amounts of androgens and androgen precursors, which cause hirsutism and often virilisation in women, who are affected 2.5 times more frequently than men.

Due to the autonomous cortisol hypersecretion from the adrenal tumour, pituitary ACTH secretion is suppressed (Fig. 33.1a,b). Due to suppressed ACTH secretion, the para-adenomatous tissue of the adrenal cortex and the contralateral adrenal are atrophic. A rare exception is the primary bilateral nodular hyperplasia of the adrenal gland which is also ACTH independent, leading to suppression of ACTH levels (Fig. 33.1c). This condition has been described to occur as a familial form of Cushing's syndrome in which primary pigmented nodular adrenocortical hyperplasia is combined with other endocrine and neuronal tumours and pathological skin pigmentation [7]. It has been speculated that the underlying pathophysiology of this rare syndrome may be the presence of adrenal cortex-stimulating immunoglobulins comparable to the pathophysiology of thyroid-stimulating antibodies in Graves' disease [7]. However, the autoimmune pathogenesis has never been proven unequivocally. Equally rare is bilateral macronodular hyperplasia, which is not familial and occurs in an older age group.

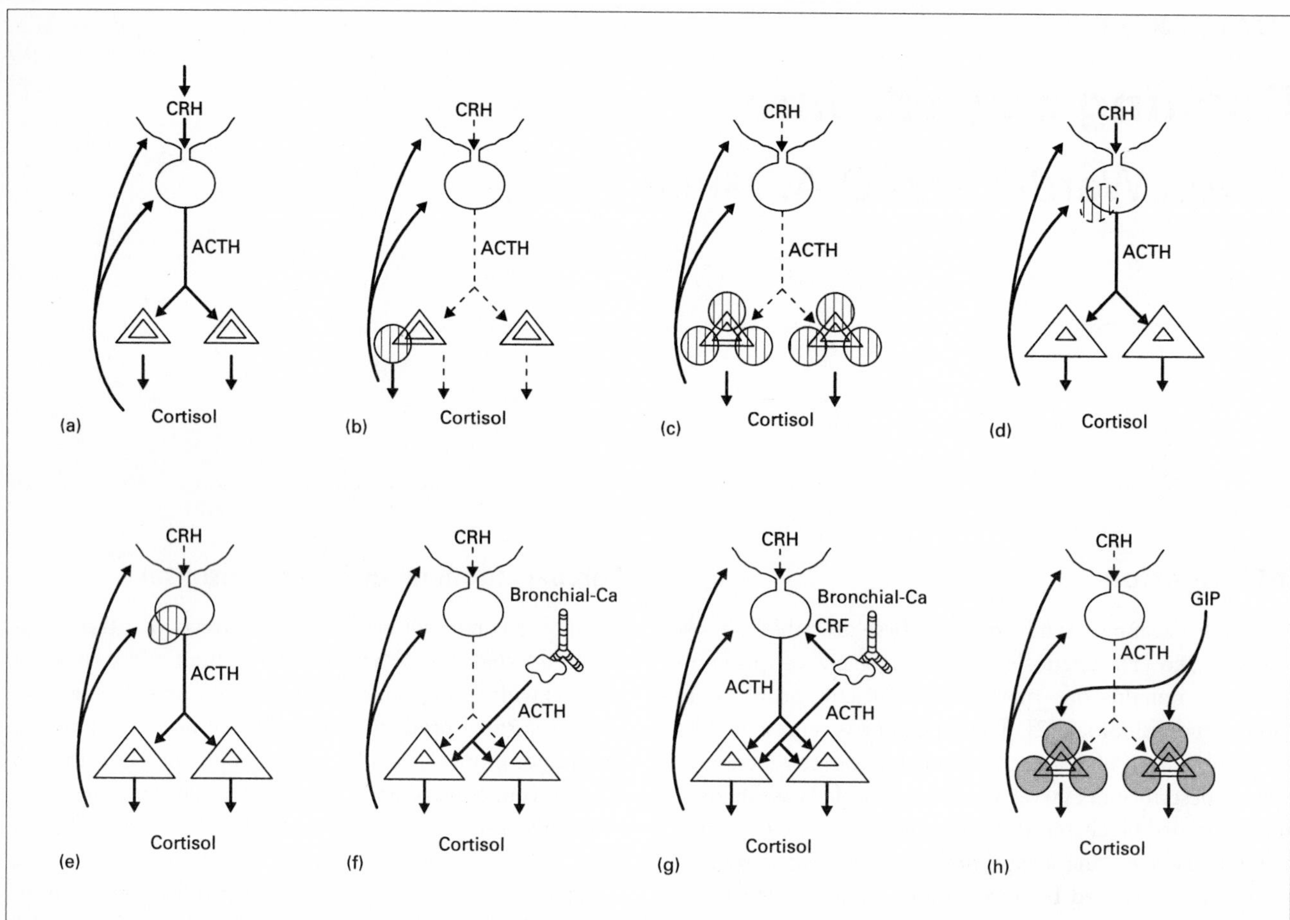

Fig. 33.1 Hypothalamo-pituitary–adrenal axis in different states of endogenous hypercortisolism: (a) normal; (b) adrenal Cushing's syndrome due to an adrenal adenoma or carcinoma; (c) adrenal Cushing's syndrome due to bilateral nodular hyperplasia; (d) hypothalamic Cushing's disease; (e) pituitary Cushing's disease; (f) ectopic adrenocorticotrophic hormone (ACTH) syndrome; (g) ectopic corticotrophin-releasing hormone (CRH) syndrome (often associated with ectopic coproduction of ACTH); (h) illicit expression of the gastrointestinal polypeptide (GIP) receptor in the adrenal which leads to nodular adrenocortical hyperplasia and food-induced Cushing's syndrome.

ACTH independence is also shown in the bilateral nodular hyperplasia with illicit expression of GIP receptors leading to food-dependent hypercortisolism [4,5].

ACTH-dependent Cushing's syndrome

ACTH hypersecretion, regardless of its origin, leads to bilateral adrenal hyperplasia with hypersecretion of cortisol from the zona fasciculata and adrenal androgens from the zona reticularis.

Pituitary-dependent Cushing's syndrome (Cushing's disease)

Pituitary ACTH hypersecretion is the most common cause of endogenous Cushing's syndrome in adulthood. Thus, 70–80% of all adult patients with endogenous Cushing's syndrome have bilateral adrenal hyperplasia with eutopic pituitary ACTH hypersecretion. Theoretically, two forms of pituitary ACTH excess may be discerned. First, an ACTH-producing adenoma may arise from hyperplasia caused by hypothalamic derangement leading to hypersecretion of CRH or other ACTH-stimulating neurohormones into the portal circulation (Fig. 33.1d). There is no absolute biochemical proof that this situation exists, although the outcome of endocrinological function tests as well as clinical and therapeutic data support this hypothetical pathophysiology of ACTH hypersecretion. Thus, ACTH levels can usually be suppressed with higher doses of dexamethasone and can be stimulated with exogenous CRH [8]. Furthermore, drugs which may act centrally at the hypothalamic level, such as cyproheptadine, can alter ACTH levels in patients with Cushing's disease [9]. In addition, other anterior pituitary hormones such as growth hormone and prolactin are often affected, which may point to a more general hypothalamic derangement [9]. Furthermore, ACTH hypersecretion in Cushing's syndrome may persist after histologically documented removal of an ACTH-producing adenoma [10]. Finally, true recurrence of pituitary ACTH hypersecretion after complete normalisation of ACTH and cortisol secretion dynamics may indicate an underlying hypothalamic defect [10,11].

However, against this concept is the fact that at transsphenoidal exploration of the pituitary, microadenomas can be visualised in 80–96% of patients. The experience that persisting normalisation of ACTH and cortisol secretion dynamics occur in 74–96% of these patients after selective adenomectomy (after initial postoperative adrenal failure of varying duration) also suggests that the majority of patients do in fact have an autonomous corticotrophinoma of the pituitary [10,11]. This is also supported by the recent evidence that most corticotrophinomas are monoclonal [12]. Autonomous pituitary ACTH secretion followed by bilateral adrenal hypersecretion of cortisol leads to long-lasting suppression of hypothalamic CRH release, with consecutive para-adenomatous atrophy of the corticotrophic cells of the pituitary (Fig. 33.1e).

That corticotrophinomas may be autonomous is also supported by the observation that some patients harbour large tumours leading to ballooning or even destruction of the sella turcica; this is particularly seen in 10–20% of patients in whom therapy was not directed against the underlying pituitary disease but against the ACTH target organ, the adrenal gland [9,13]. Thus, adrenalectomised patients with Cushing's disease may develop large, invasively growing tumours with extremely high ACTH levels causing pronounced pigmentation of the skin—Nelson's syndrome. Whether the aggressiveness of tumour growth is stimulated by the diminished negative-feedback activity of circulating cortisol levels is still unclear, and it may be that 10% or so of all patients with Cushing's disease harbour aggressive tumours regardless of the modality of therapy.

There is only one situation in which the CRH dependency of pituitary ACTH hypersecretion leading to Cushing's syndrome is unequivocally demonstrable: this is the case when paraneoplastic production of CRH [14] or substances facilitating CRH bioactivity are the cause of ACTH hypersecretion from the pituitary (see below). In all other cases, most authorities now consider that all other neuroendocrine changes which are observed in patients with corticotroph adenomas are a consequence of the pituitary adenoma, rather than indicating a primary hypothalamic defect.

Alcohol-induced (Pseudo-) Cushing's syndrome

Occasionally, patients with the history of heavy alcohol consumption (varying from 4 litres of gin per week to 6–12 pints of beer daily) may develop the clinical picture of Cushing's syndrome with elevated basal cortisol levels, abnormal circadian variation, increased cortisol production rate and increased urinary free cortisol excretion. These patients do not suppress adequately with dexamethasone. Similarly, patients with depression often have abnormally elevated cortisol levels as in Cushing's syndrome. These patients also have increased free urinary cortisol excretion and impaired dexamethasone suppression (see also Chapter 83). After remission of the depressive disorder or discontinuance of alcohol ingestion, clinical and laboratory abnormalities disappear, usually within weeks [9].

Paraneoplastic Cushing's syndrome

Ectopic ACTH secretion (see also Chapter 73)

Ectopic ACTH production is the most common paraneoplastic hormone syndrome that leads to a well-defined clinical picture [14,15]. About 10% of all cases with endogenous Cushing's syndrome are due to ectopic ACTH hypersecretion (Fig. 33.1f). The most common cause of paraneoplastic ACTH secretion is the small-cell carcinoma of the lung, but additionally pancreatic carcinomas, thymomas and other mediastinal tumours, ovarian and prostatic cancers, phaeochromocytomas and C-cell carcinomas of the thyroid and neoplastic blood cells can produce ACTH ectopically.

Typically, ACTH levels are excessively elevated and can neither be stimulated with CRH nor suppressed with dexamethasone [3,8,15]. Frequently, the underlying tumours are particularly malignant leading to a rapid clinical course which does not allow development of the full picture of Cushing's syndrome. However, these patients usually develop hyperpigmentation, extreme muscle wasting, hypertension and hypokalaemic alkalosis.

It has been recently speculated that the latter two signs, which are evidence for a mineralocorticoid excess, are due to defective 11β-hydroxysteroid-dehydrogenase (11β-HSD) activity in patients with ectopic ACTH syndrome. Reduced activity of 11β-HSD would allow the elevated cortisol level access to the mineralocorticoid receptor leading to hypertension and hypokalaemia [16]. Occasionally, benign or semibenign tumours can produce ACTH ectopically leading to only slightly elevated ACTH levels; this situation is easily confused with pituitary ACTH hypersecretion and represents one of the most difficult diagnostic dilemmas of Cushing's syndrome (see below).

Ectopic CRH secretion

The ectopic production of CRH [15], leading to systematically elevated CRH levels and thus causing corticotroph pituitary hyperplasia (Fig. 33.1g), is a very rare cause of paraneoplastic Cushing's syndrome. This is in contrast to paraneoplastic acromegaly, which is almost always due to ectopic production of growth hormone-releasing hormone and is only very rarely caused by the ectopic secretion of growth hormone itself [17]. Unfortunately, the few cases of ectopic CRH syndrome that have been reported in the literature have been incompletely investigated. Thus, we know very little about the regulation of ACTH secretion in this situation, for example does exogenous CRH stimulation lead to a further rise of ACTH levels, and can the ACTH levels be suppressed with dexamethasone? The pathophysiology of this syndrome is further confused by the fact that almost always tumours which produce and secrete CRH are also able to produce and secrete pro-opiomelanocortin-derived products, including ACTH [14,15]. A unique cause of Cushing's syndrome due to an extrapituitary tumour has been described in a single patient with a medullary thyroid tumour. This tumour did not secrete either ACTH or CRH, but a bombesin-like peptide, which was demonstrated to enhance the biological activity of CRH at the pituitary level leading to eutopic ACTH hypersecretion [18].

Table 33.1 Frequency of clinical manifestation of Cushing's syndrome according to Labhart [21].

Symptom	Frequency (%)
Moon face (red face with 'plethora')	90
Truncal obesity	85
Impaired glucose tolerance	85
Hypertension	80
Hypogonadism (menstrual irregularity in women, loss of libido and potency in men)	75
Osteoporosis	65
Purple striae, haemorrhagic diathesis	60
Muscular weakness	65
Hirsutism (in women)	70
Ankle oedema	55
Buffalo hump	55
Acne	55
Backache and other skeletal pains	50
Mental changes	45
Impaired wound healing, crural ulcers	35
Polyuria and polydipsia	30
Kyphosis	25
Renal calculi	20
Minor polycythaemia	20

Clinical features

Endogenous Cushing's syndrome is observed in all races at all ages, although it occurs more frequently between 20 and 60 years of age. The overall incidence in the general population is estimated to be between 0.7 and 2.4 cases/million inhabitants per year [19,20]. Cushing's syndrome occurs in both sexes, though there is a clear preponderance of female patients in whom the disease occurs three times more frequently than in males [11].

The main clinical findings of Cushing's syndrome and their frequency are summarised in Table 33.1. While weight gain and truncal obesity are the most common presenting features, the vast majority of patients with severe obesity do not have Cushing's syndrome. Fat distribution in Cushing's syndrome is predominantly centripetal, involving the trunk and abdomen. Characteristic features are the plethoric 'moon face', the 'buffalo hump', and relatively thin extremities with muscle atrophy as a result of protein wasting leading occasionally to extreme muscle weakness. Typically these patients, when sitting, cannot stand up without help from their arms; also characteristic are the skin changes with thin skin and easy bruising (particularly useful clinical features), which are also due to protein catabolism, and abdominal striae which are bright red or purple in colour. The striae rubrae are due to small haemorrhages in the stretched skin: these haemorrhages also occur spontaneously and after mild trauma. Hirsutism and acne occur in women due to the hypersecretion of adrenal androgens. Overt virilisation is usually seen only in women with adrenal cancer. The skin can also be pigmented, particularly in patients with the ectopic ACTH syndrome and very elevated ACTH levels. Osteoporosis can be very severe, leading to back pain and vertebral collapse with loss of height, kyphosis, and rib fractures. Patients have gonadal dysfunction with oligo- or amenorrhoea in females and loss of libido and sexual impotence in males. Hypertension is usually present, as may be impaired carbohydrate tolerance, thus being associated with a high incidence of cardiovascular complications. Furthermore, patients complain of polyuria and polydipsia, and also nocturia, which may be caused by overt diabetes mellitus or direct effects of steroids on vasopressin activity. Particularly common are psychiatric symptoms, which range from severe depression to other forms of agitated psychoses, and may be present to some degree in 60–70% of patients. On the other hand, depressed patients without Cushing's syndrome may have deranged ACTH and cortisol secretion, i.e. abnormal dexamethasone suppressibility, which has to be differentiated from true Cushing's syndrome with appropriate biochemical tests (see below).

Prognosis

Cushing's syndrome is a very severe illness which almost never remits spontaneously, although cyclic forms of the syndrome with intermittent spontaneous remissions and recurrences have been described [3,9]. In general, 50% of patients affected are dead within 5 years of the onset of symptoms in the absence of treatment [9,21], mostly due to infections, cardiovascular disease, metastatic disease in those who have adrenal cancer or the ectopic ACTH syndrome, and suicide due to severe depressive illness. Furthermore, osteoporosis and arteriosclerosis lead to severe disability in patients with Cushing's syndrome. However, advances in diagnostic and therapeutic measures have improved the prognosis for all patients, and most can now be cured or at least improved with the exception of those harbouring adrenal cancers or small-cell carcinomas of the lung, in whom complete cure of disease cannot usually be accomplished.

Table 33.2 Wrong initial diagnosis in 33 patients with later established Cushing's syndrome (see Fig. 33.2).

Diagnosis	*n*
Hypertension	11
Obesity	20
Menstrual irregularity	10
Impaired glucose tolerance	9
Oedema	4
Renal calculi	4
Hirsutism	3
Growth retardation	2
Muscular weakness	2
Hypokalaemia	1
Purple striae	1

Diagnostic procedures

Cushing's syndrome should now be diagnosed at an early stage before the obvious Cushingoid features become apparent, but even today there is a considerable lag time between the first subtle symptoms and the final diagnosis (Fig. 33.2). Thus, patients may be treated for many years for hypertension, obesity, gonadal problems, diabetes mellitus, psychiatric disturbances and other symptoms before the combination of symptoms suggests the correct diagnosis (Table 33.2). In a recent European survey in which data of 668 patients with Cushing's disease were collected, the estimated mean interval between onset and diagnosis of Cushing's disease was 4 years [11].

Special clinical symptoms, which are helpful for the *differential diagnosis* of obvious Cushing's syndrome, are rarely present. Thus, extreme hyperpigmentation may indicate very elevated ACTH levels which are highly suggestive of the ectopic ACTH syndrome. Furthermore, hypokalaemic alkalosis and pronounced muscle wasting may be taken as evidence for the very pronounced ACTH stimulation of the adrenal cortex typical of this syndrome. Normally, however, only special endocrine function tests allow the differential diagnosis of the various causes of Cushing's syndrome [2,3,6,8,15]. There are three important phases in the endocrine evaluation of patients with Cushing's syndrome:

1 the primary evaluation or exclusion of the syndrome in patients who present with uncertain clinical features;

2 the definitive establishment of the diagnosis of Cushing's syndrome;

3 identification of the cause of the disease, i.e. differential diagnosis (Table 33.3).

These three steps are performed with endocrine function tests. Imaging studies should be performed only after the cause of the disease has been identified biochemically (Table 33.3).

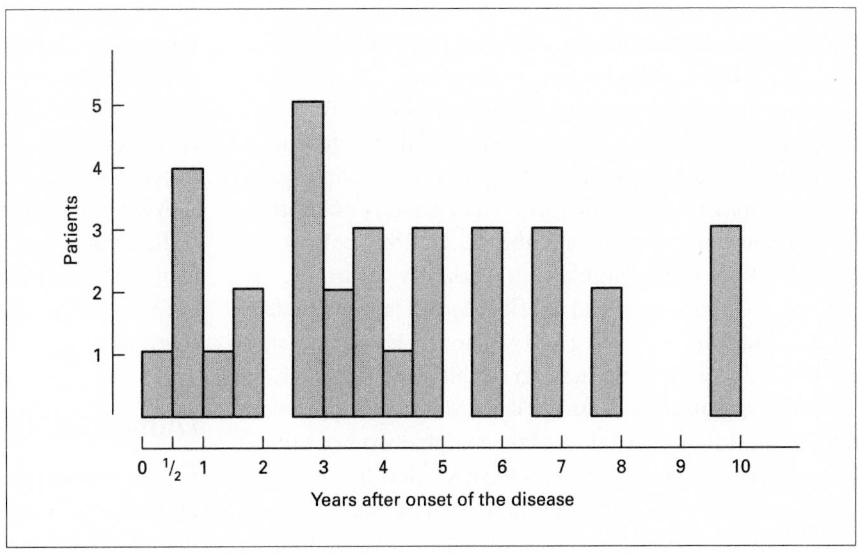

Fig. 33.2 Lag time in 33 patients with different forms of Cushing's syndrome between the first symptom and the final diagnosis. The initial diagnoses of these patients are listed in Table 33.2.

Table 33.3 Diagnostic procedures for establishment of diagnosis, differential diagnosis and tumour localisation of Cushing's syndrome.

Primary evaluation
Overnight dexamethasone suppression (1 or 2 mg)
Establishment of diagnosis
Free urinary cortisol
Diurnal variation
Insulin hypoglycaemia
Dexamethasone suppression (Liddle test)
Differential diagnosis
ACTH RIA
CRH test
High-dose dexamethasone suppression (8 mg overnight)
ACTH RIA after catheterisation
Tumour localisation
ACTH RIA after catheterisation
MRI, CT, ultrasonography, scintigraphy

ACTH RIA, adrenocorticotrophic hormone radioimmunoassay; CT, computed tomography; MRI, magnetic resonance imaging; CRH, corticotrophin-releasing hormone.

Primary evaluation

There are laboratory findings other than the clinical picture and specific endocrine studies which are not diagnostic, but represent additional data that are compatible with the disease, such as an elevated haemoglobin level and diminished percentage of lymphocytes and eosinophils in the white cell differential. Furthermore, fasting hyperglycaemia or impaired glucose tolerance occurs two or three times more frequently in Cushing's syndrome than it does in the general population. Hypokalaemia in patients not treated with diuretics is typical of adrenocortical carcinoma or ectopic ACTH production. Furthermore, hypercalciuria with renal stones (see Tables 33.1 and 33.2) is not infrequently observed.

For many endocrinologists, the first step of the endocrine diagnostic investigation of patients suspected of endogenous Cushing's syndrome is the 1–2 mg dexamethasone overnight suppression test, which serves as a primary evaluation test for Cushing's syndrome (Table 33.3). Only patients in whom this test is compatible with Cushing's syndrome, i.e. cortisol levels not suppressed to below 2 μg/dl (approximately 50 nmol/l) the next morning at 0900 hours should be tested further with confirmatory tests to establish the diagnosis. In the interpretation of the overnight dexamethasone suppression test, account should be taken of the fact that women taking oestrogens (oral contraceptives) have an elevated cortisol-binding globulin (CBG) and may therefore have higher cortisol levels the next morning after dexamethasone. Furthermore, it should not be forgotten that patients with agitated depression may not suppress their cortisol levels overnight into the normal range in the absence of Cushing's syndrome. It should therefore be noted that a number of endocrinologists believe that the specificity of the overnight test is so low that it is of little use. However, the single dose dexamethasone suppression test is the easiest out-patient procedure and therefore still frequently employed as a screening test [3,6,8,21]. Isolated plasma ACTH and cortisol determinations are of limited value, since both hormones are secreted episodically and in a circadian fashion, and their secretion is influenced by physical and emotional stress. Patients with Cushing's disease very often have single ACTH and cortisol levels within the normal range [3].

It is important that all laboratories establish their own normal range for the single dexamethasone suppression test as well as the others described below.

Confirmation of the diagnosis

The diagnosis of Cushing's syndrome is confirmed by measuring free cortisol in the urine, examining the circadian variation of cortisol secretion or the cortisol response to insulin hypoglycaemia, and by using the dexamethasone suppression test according to Liddle, which measures cortisol and cortisol metabolites in the urine or blood [3,9,21]. In patients with Cushing's syndrome, excretion of urinary free cortisol usually exceeds 100 μg/day; furthermore, in contrast to normal subjects there is no circadian variation of serum cortisol levels which remain elevated at midnight (or at least within the same range as the morning cortisol levels). Regardless of the cause of cortisol hypersecretion, there is no rise of cortisol levels during insulin hypoglycaemia in 80% of patients, and the growth hormone response is also usually blunted during this test (as it may also be in simple obesity). Giving dexamethasone in a dosage of 0.5 mg every 6 hours for 2 days does not lead to suppression of cortisol metabolites in the urine (17-hydroxy-corticosteroids) on the second day of dexamethasone administration, or of serum cortisol in most patients. However, as noted above, normal ranges for each test vary according to laboratory and assay.

After establishment of the diagnosis, the next and most difficult part is that of differential diagnosis of the various causes of Cushing's syndrome. The latter must be performed in order to provide patients with the most appropriate treatment.

Differential diagnosis

For the differential diagnosis between ACTH-dependent and autonomous cortisol hypersecretion, ACTH radioimmunoassay (RIA), particularly after CRH stimulation, is most important [8]. However, since this test may occasionally be misleading, other tests such as the high-dose dexamethasone suppression test (with 8 mg) and catheterisation studies, as well as sophisticated radiological or nuclear medicine-based evaluation, may finally become necessary. The dexamethasone suppression test in combination with the CRH stimulation test is the most reliable biochemical test procedure for the differential diagnosis of the various causes of Cushing's syndrome [22,23].

The basal level of ACTH can provide significant information for the differential diagnosis of Cushing's syndrome, if the RIA for this hormone is satisfactory. RIA for ACTH is more difficult than those for other anterior pituitary hormones because of the low basal hormone level, the possible dissociation of immunoactivity and bioactivity, and interfering factors in the plasma which often necessitate extraction procedures before assay. However, when the ACTH RIA is accurate, reproducible and of high sensitivity, normal or non-suppressed ACTH levels which occur in pituitary ACTH-dependent Cushing's disease are clearly separated from suppressed levels in patients with adrenal autonomous hypercortisolism (Fig. 33.3). However, there is always an overlap between pituitary and ectopically derived ACTH levels (Fig. 33.3). More information is obtained if the ACTH levels are measured before and after stimulation with 100 μg (1 μg/kg) human (h) or ovine (o) CRH given intravenously. Whereas 80% of patients with pituitary ACTH-dependent Cushing's disease show an exaggerated response of ACTH to CRH, ACTH secretion remains suppressed in patients with adrenal autonomous hypercortisolism (Fig. 33.4). In patients with ectopic ACTH secretion the elevated basal ACTH levels usually remain unchanged, although very occasionally a further rise of the ACTH after CRH may be observed without subsequent changes in cortisol levels. There is often no cortisol rise after an increase of ACTH levels because cortisol levels are usually already maximally stimulated in the basal state in this situation (Fig. 33.5). The high-dose dexamethasone suppression test (with 8 mg) usually leads to partial suppression (> 50% fall in 80–90% of patients) of cortisol level in eutopic pituitary ACTH-dependent hypercortisolism, in contrast to autonomous adrenal hypercortisolism and ectopic ACTH-dependent hypercortisolism in which cortisol levels remain unchanged. If the results of the CRH test and/or high-dose dexamethasone suppression test are equivocal, i.e. do not allow the confident differential diagnosis between eutopic or ectopic ACTH secretion, catheterisation

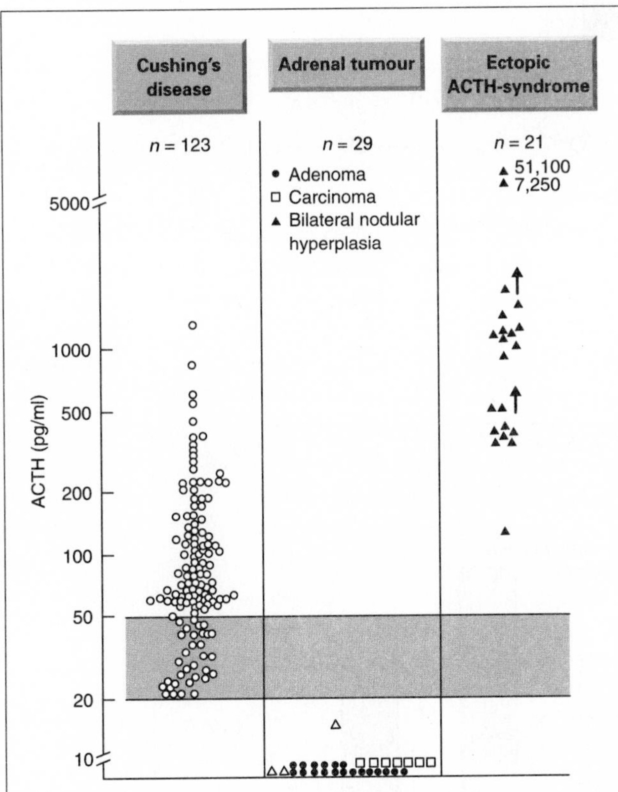

Fig. 33.3 Adrenocorticotrophic hormone (ACTH) levels in 173 patients with Cushing's syndrome.

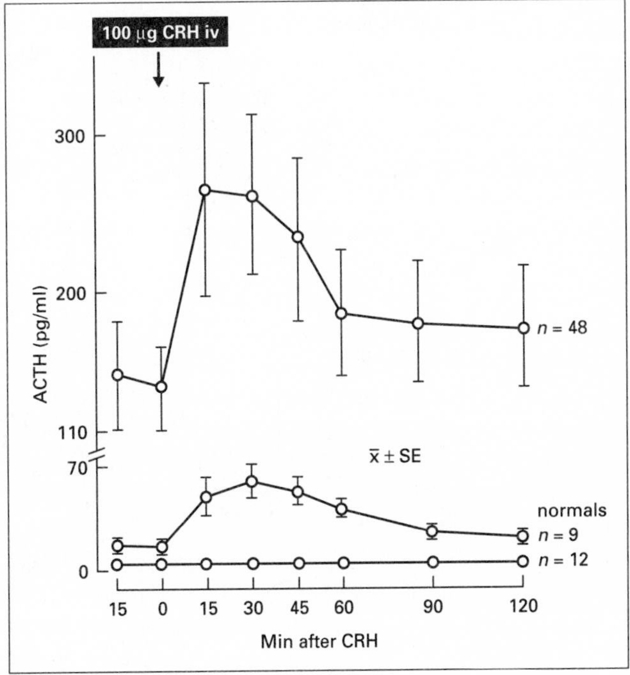

Fig. 33.4 Corticotrophin-releasing hormone (hCRH)-stimulation test in patients with Cushing's syndrome; mean values of the adrenocorticotrophic hormone (ACTH) levels before and after stimulation with CRH are shown in normal controls, in patients with untreated pituitary ACTH-dependent Cushing's disease (n = 48) and in patients with autonomous cortisol secretion (n = 12).

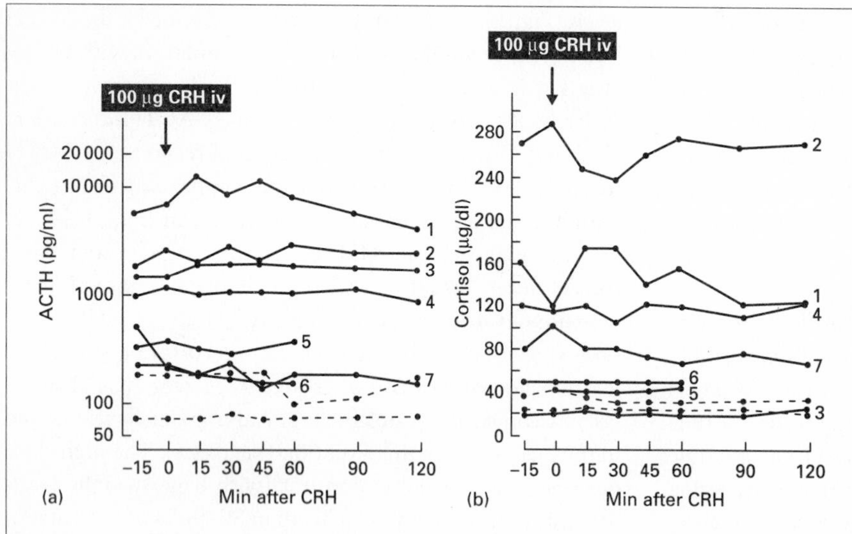

Fig. 33.5 Corticotrophin-releasing hormone (hCRH)-stimulation test in patients with Cushing's syndrome: adrenocorticotrophic hormone (ACTH) (a) and cortisol (b) levels before and after CRH stimulation in seven patients with ectopic ACTH production due to bronchocarcinomas. The dotted lines show the CRH-stimulation test in two female patients with ectopic ACTH production due to small carcinoid tumours of the lung.

studies of the cerebral sinuses which drain the pituitary gland may be necessary [24]. Lack of a gradient between the ACTH level in the inferior petrosal sinus and the periphery suggest that the source of the ACTH hypersecretion is not localized to the pituitary but is elsewhere (Fig. 33.6).

Fig. 33.6 Test results in a female patient with ectopic adrenocorticotrophic hormone (ACTH) production as a cause of her Cushing's syndrome. From [2].

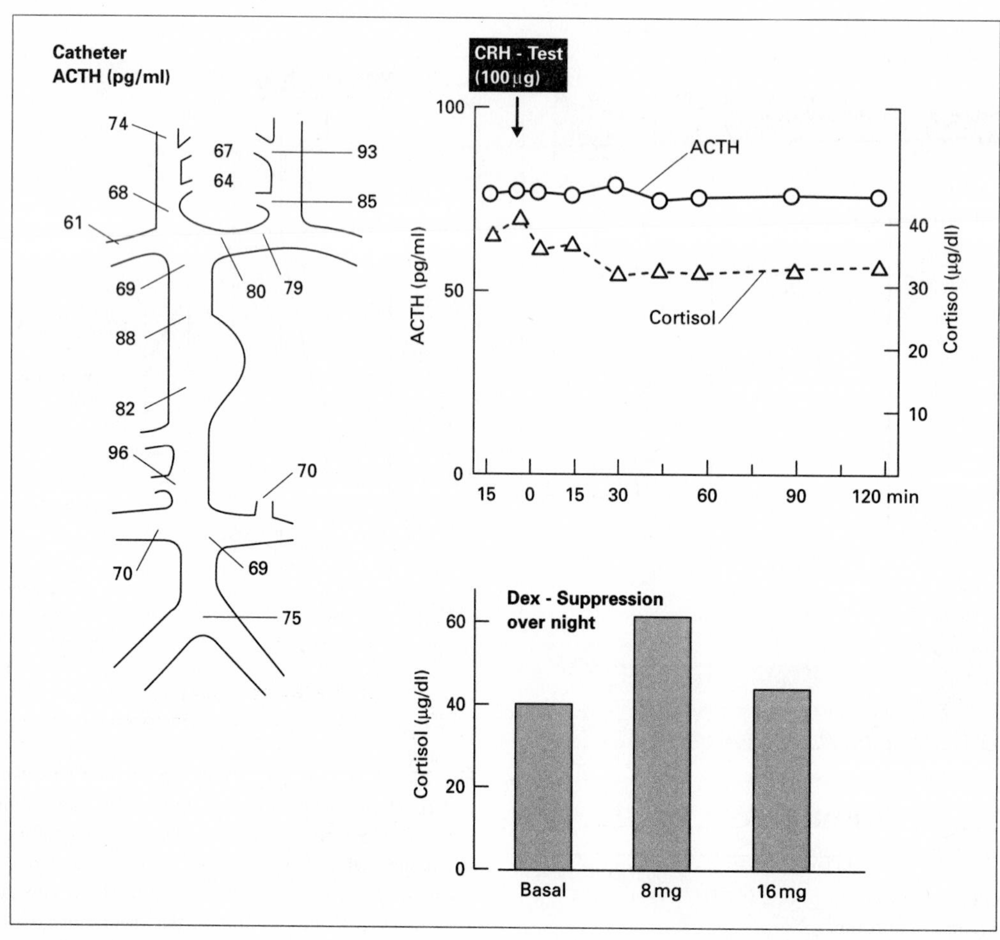

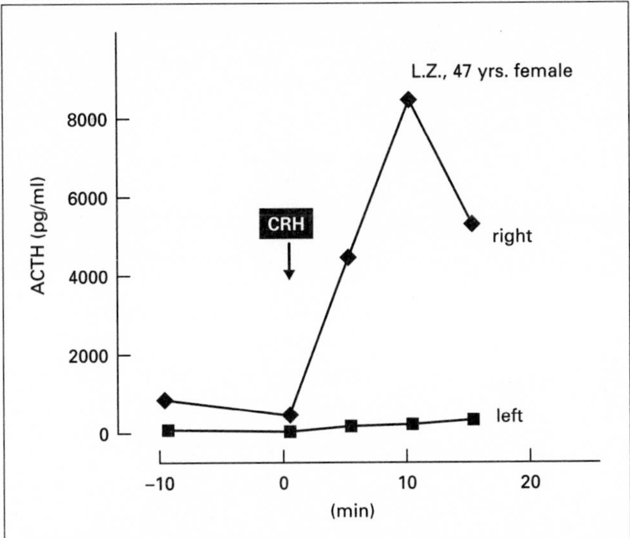

Fig. 33.7 Corticotrophin-releasing hormone (CRH) test in a female patient with Cushing's disease after bilateral catheterisation of the inferior petrosal sinus. Most of the CRH-stimulated adrenocorticotrophic hormone (ACTH) is drained in the right petrosal sinus. In this case the pituitary microadenoma was found at surgery in the right side.

However, while a significant gradient between the petrosal sinus and peripheral venous blood (particularly after CRH stimulation, Fig. 33.7) virtually always points to pituitary ACTH-dependent hypersecretion, localisation of the ectopic source by selective peripheral catheterisation—lung, pancreas, etc.—can often not be demonstrated (Fig. 33.6). However, in the study from the National Institute of Health in Bethesda measurement of inferior petrosal ACTH and CRH had a 100% accuracy in differentiating pituitary from ectopic sources of Cushing's syndrome, and its use in all patients lacking an obvious adrenal tumour is recommended [24].

Localisation studies

Pituitary Cushing's disease

When the pituitary gland has been demonstrated to be the source of ACTH hypersecretion by endocrine function tests, imaging studies can sometimes be helpful in depicting the pituitary corticotrophinoma. The method of choice is magnetic resonance imaging (MRI); alternatively, cranial computed tomography (CT) can be performed. According to the European Cushing's Disease Survey, the adenoma could be visualised using these imaging studies in 48% of 589 patients [11]. However, these tumours often cannot be visualised despite high-resolution MRI techniques. The reason for the failure to demonstrate the corticotrophinoma is the small size of the microadenomas, which are usually around 4–6 mm in diameter, and often centrally localised in the pituitary gland (Fig. 33.8). However, these microadenomas can frequently be localised indirectly by bilateral catheterisation of the petrosal sinus with simultaneous ACTH measurements: this procedure allows localisation of the microadenoma within the pituitary in those cases in which lateralisation of the ACTH excess can be demonstrated. CRH stimulation exaggerates the ACTH response and is therefore helpful in this procedure (Fig. 33.7), a recent analysis showing correct lateralisation in 71% of 105 patients [23].

Is Cushing's disease due to a primary pituitary or hypothalamic defect?

There is no endocrine function test to differentiate the two possible forms of pituitary ACTH excess, primary pituitary ACTH excess and hypothalamic CRH hypersecretion (Fig. 33.1d,e). Lamberts *et al.* have postulated that ACTH hypersecretion may originate from a persisting intermediate lobe of the pituitary [25], but there is little histological evidence to support this hypothesis. That the ACTH excess may originate from the intermediate lobe was originally suggested on account of the observation that some patients with pituitary ACTH-dependent Cushing's disease respond to dopamine agonists with a lowering of the ACTH and cortisol levels; it is well established that the secretion of pro-opiomelanocortin-derived peptides from the intermediate lobe is under inhibitory dopaminergic control in rodents. However, in contrast to what one would anticipate in patients with intermediate-lobe Cushing's syndrome, the ACTH response to dopamine agonists in these patients with pituitary ACTH-dependent Cushing's disease does not correlate with the findings during transsphenoidal exploration of the sella turcica or with the outcome of pituitary microsurgery [2]. CRH measurements in peripheral blood and blood obtained from the cavernous sinus during transsphenoidal microsurgery are also unable to differentiate between primary pituitary and hypothalamic CRH-dependent ACTH hypersecretion [26]. There are patients with either high or unmeasurable CRH levels in the groups with and without clinical remission following transsphenoidal microsurgery.

Van Cauter and Refetoff have postulated that the evaluation of the episodic secretion of cortisol may help in differentiating between primary pituitary and hypothalamic CRH-induced ACTH hypersecretion [27]. They postulated that a cortisol secretory pattern with minor and few secretory pulses points to autonomous pituitary ACTH secretion, whereas hyperpulsatility of cortisol secretion reflects exaggerated CRH pulses and therefore points to a hypothalamic origin of the disease. However, our experience shows that there is no clear correlation between the preoperative pulsatile secretion pattern of ACTH and cortisol and the therapeutic

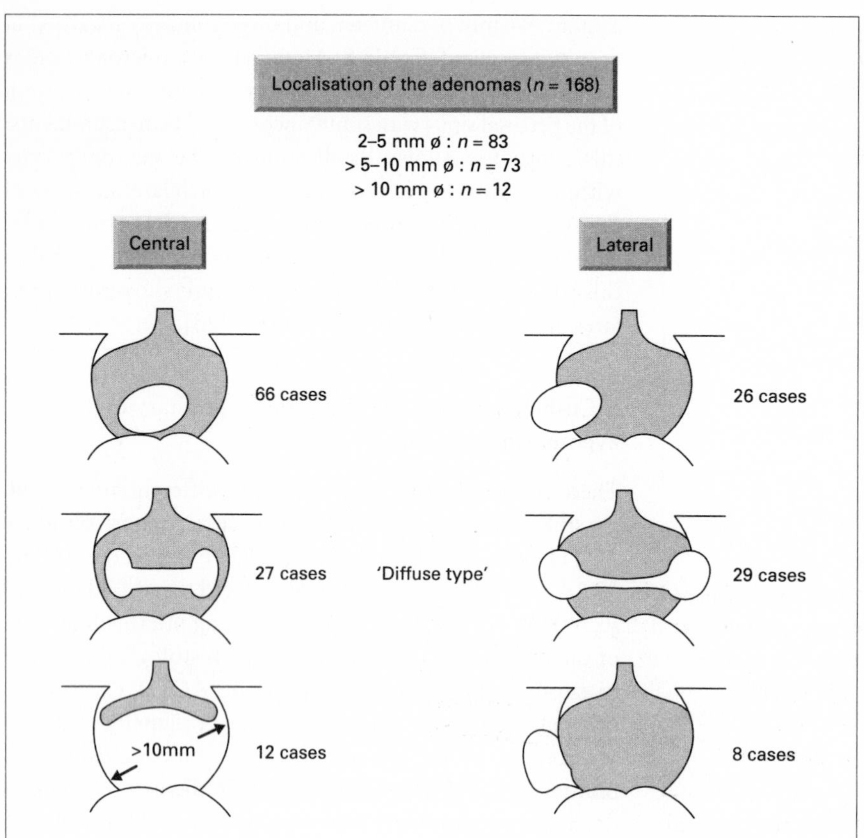

Fig. 33.8 Localisation of adenomas in 168 patients with adrenocorticotrophic hormone (ACTH)-dependent Cushing's disease who were operated on. (Unpublished results of M. Buchfelder and R. Fahlbusch.)

outcome following transsphenoidal microsurgery, although we did find a higher remission rate in the group of patients who had a hypopulsatile type of cortisol secretion compared with the hyperpulsatile group. In the individual situation, evaluation of the cortisol secretion pattern did not allow prediction as to whether transsphenoidal surgery would be successful or not. In contrast, in patients in whom imaging studies demonstrated a distinct corticotrophinoma the surgical results were significantly better to those which were obtained in patients in whom no adenoma could be demonstrated by preoperative imaging studies [11].

Ectopic ACTH syndrome

In most cases with paraneoplastic ACTH secretion, the localisation of the tumour producing and secreting ACTH is obvious at the time of the diagnosis of Cushing's syndrome. However, there are occasional benign or semibenign small carcinoid tumours which may be detected and localised using only CT or MRI studies (Fig. 33.9), and even then only with difficulty. When imaging studies do not allow localisation of the source of exaggerated ACTH secretion, catheterisation studies with ACTH measurements can be performed [14,17,24]. However, though catheterisation

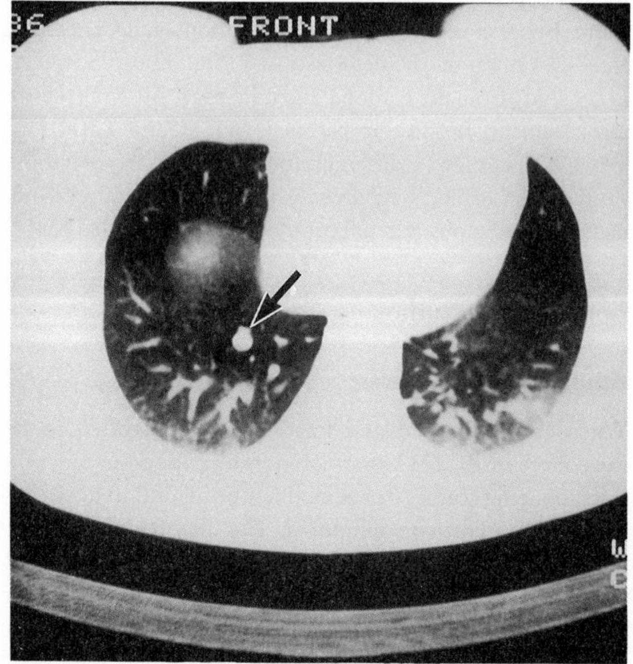

Fig. 33.9 Computed tomography of the chest in a 23-year-old female patient with ectopic ACTH syndrome (see also Fig. 33.13). In this patient conventional chest X-ray did not depict the lesion shown in the right half of the thorax.

studies with measurement of ACTH particularly after stimulation with CRH will allow to make the differential diagnosis between eutopic and ectopic ACTH syndrome with confidence [24], it will not always lead to detection of the tumour responsible for paraneoplastic ACTH hypersecretion (Fig. 33.6). These patients may harbour very small carcinoid tumours with the diameter < 10 mm which evade detection by imaging studies with CT or MRI. However, these tumours usually express somatostatin receptors at the cell surface which are functionally active (see below), and may be visualised by somatostatin-receptor scintigraphy [28]. Thus, occult ACTH-secreting bronchocarcinoid tumours with a diameter of 6 mm have been localised by using receptor scintigraphy (octreoscan) with labelled octreotide [29].

Autonomous adrenal hypercortisolism

In patients with ACTH-independent autonomous adrenal cortisol hypersecretion, abdominal ultrasonography or CT scanning is usually sufficient to localise the adrenal adenoma or carcinoma, or to depict bilateral nodular hyperplasia in the rare cases where both adrenals are affected (Figs 33.10 and 33.11). The latter may have different aetiologies (unknown, hereditary or food-induced, see above). Recently, it has been speculated that autonomous nodular hyperplasia may present tertiary hypercortisolism on account of the observation of pituitary tumours in this syndrome [30]; the fact that pituitary enlargement may occur in bilateral nodular hyperplasia demonstrates the need for ACTH measurements in the documentation of autonomous adrenal hypercortisolism.

In contrast to primary hyperaldosteronism, catheterisation studies with cortisol measurements in adrenal venous blood, or scintigraphy with ^{131}I-labelled cholesterol, are rarely needed [9,21].

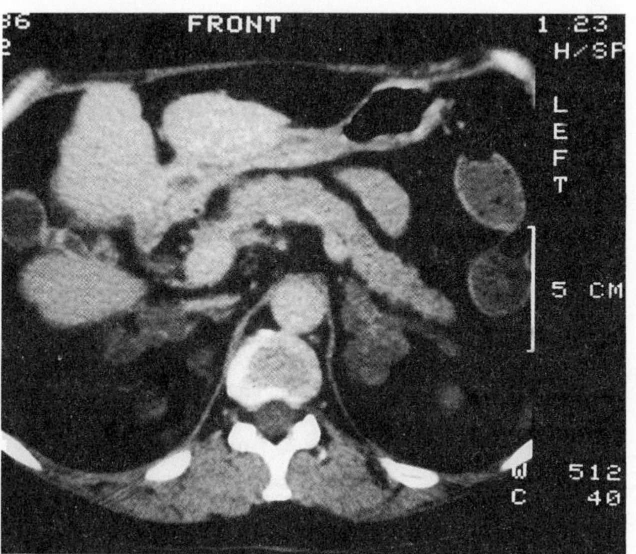

Fig. 33.10 Computed abdominal tomography in a patient with ACTH-independent Cushing's syndrome due to nodular bilateral hyperplasia. The scan clearly shows the enlarged adrenals on both sides (see Fig. 33.11).

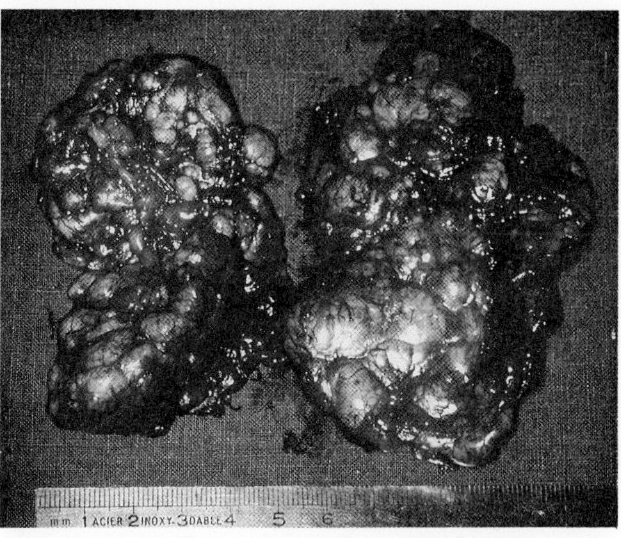

Fig. 33.11 Nodular adrenal hyperplasia in a patient with ACTH-independent Cushing's syndrome. After demonstrating autonomous adrenal hypercortisolism and demonstrating bilateral hyperplasia (Fig. 33.10) by abdominal computed tomography, the patient was cured by bilateral adrenalectomy.

Therapy for Cushing's syndrome

The primary aim of treatment is the abolition of cortisol hypersecretion and the preservation of normal anterior pituitary function. In patients with space-occupying lesions or even malignancy, treatment must also be specifically directed against the underlying tumour.

Surgery

Surgery or neurosurgery is the treatment of choice in spontaneously occurring Cushing's syndrome. Thus, surgical extirpation of an adrenal adenoma or carcinoma is always attempted as first-line therapy. In the rare cases of bilateral ACTH-independent nodular adrenal hyperplasia, bilateral adrenalectomy is indicated. Surgery is also attempted to eliminate the tumour that is the source of ectopic ACTH or CRH secretion. In patients with eutopic pituitary ACTH hypersecretion, transsphenoidal pituitary microsurgery has become the initial treatment of choice; according to the recently published European Cushing's Disease Survey Group, clinical and biochemical remission occured in 510

Reference	Date	Success rate: number of cases cured (%)	Recurrence rate (percentage recurred)	Duration of follow-up (years)
Nakane *et al.* [32]	1987	86/100 (86.0)	8/86 (9.3)	3
Guilhaume *et al.* [33]	1988	42/61 (68.9)	6/42 (14.3)	2
Mampalam *et al.* [34]	1988	171/216 (79.2)	9/71 (5.3)	4
Burke *et al.* [35]	1990	44/54 (81.5)	2/44 (4.5)	5
Tindall *et al.* [36]	1990	46/53 (86.8)	1/46 (2.1)	5
Robert and Hardy [37]	1991	60/78 (76.9)	5/60 (8.3)	$6^1/_2$
Tahir and Sheeler [38]	1992	34/45 (75.6)	7/34 (20.6)	$5^1/_2$
Trainer *et al.* [31]	1993	39/48 (81.2)	3/39 (7.7)	Not stated
Ram *et al.* [39]	1994	205/222 (92.3)	Not stated	Not stated
European Cushing's disease survey group [11]	1995	510/668 (76.3)	65/510 (12.7)	4

Table 33.4 Results of transsphenoidal surgery for Cushing's disease in the last decade. Only series with more than 30 reported cases are listed. Modified from [11].

out of 668 (76.3% of the patients). The success rates and the number of recurrences of those series which have been published in the last 10 years are summarised in Table 33.4. Pre- or intraoperative identification of the tumour by neuroradiological imaging with histopathological corroboration is highly associated with postoperative remission of hypercortisolism. Recurrence of the disease after initial remission occurred in the European Cushing's Disease Survey in 65 out of 510 patients (12.7%). Low postoperative steroid levels and absence of cortisol or ACTH respond to CRH, and the need for long-term substitutional therapy with glucocorticosteroids, is highly correlated with a high probability of long-term remission (Fig. 33.12). For this reason, the CRH-stimulation test in the first days after transsphenoidal surgery is a good predictive test for prognosis of long-lasting outcome after microadenomectomy, although some groups would use the basal cortisol alone.

Patients who do not develop postoperative secondary adrenal failure after microsurgery, but have normal cortisol levels in the immediately postoperative period, may also show clinical remission after operation: it has been suggested that these patients need early reoperation or radiotherapy [31]. However, in the European Cushing's Disease Survey Group only 33 out of 135 patients (24%) with normal postoperative circulating cortisol had a relapse of the disease [11]. Thus, normal steroid levels after surgery are not necessarily followed by recurrence of the disease; the aggressive policy of early reoperation and radiotherapy is therefore not

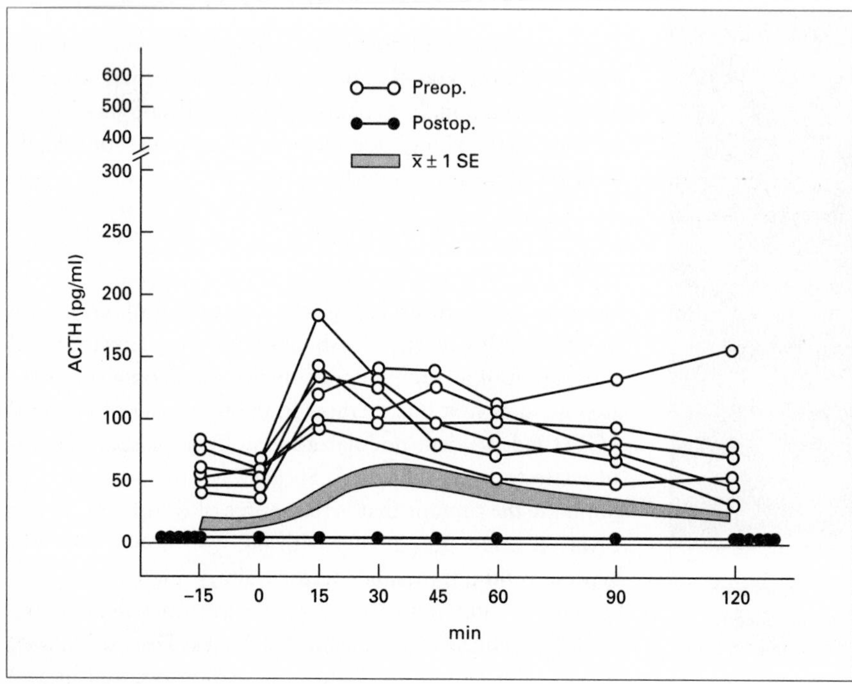

Fig. 33.12 Preoperative and postoperative corticotrophin-releasing hormone (100 μg hCRH)-stimulation test in six patients with adrenocorticotrophic hormone (ACTH)-dependent Cushing's disease. Whereas preoperatively a high ACTH level could be stimulated in an exaggerated manner, the unmeasureable, low ACTH levels found postoperatively could not be stimulated by CRH. This observation only days after operation corresponded to persisting remission of the disease during long-term follow up.

universally accepted, particularly since they often result in hypopituitarism or persisting diabetes insipidus [31].

If transsphenoidal surgery is not successful, pituitary irradiation or bilateral adrenalectomy are further therapeutic options [9,21].

Bilateral adrenalectomy usually leads to definitive cure in patients with failed transsphenoidal pituitary exploration. It is therefore indicated, especially in patients with the severe form of the disease, preferably after a course of adrenolytic therapy [10]. However, others advise postoperative radiotherapy in these patients, particularly when the disease is milder and interim control with medical therapy is possible [46].

Radiotherapy

When patients have a relatively mild form of Cushing's syndrome, pituitary irradiation with 4500 cGy from a high voltage source can be instituted as primary or secondary therapy [3,9,21,46]. While conventional teaching suggests that cure is rare, except in very young patients, Howlett *et al.* [41] demonstrated that 12 out of 21 patients without preceding surgery but only metyrapone treatment (see below) were in remission after radiotherapy, with a follow-up ranging from 5.8 to 15.5 years. In four further patients medical therapy could be reduced after radiotherapy, whereas five of the 21 patients required alternative therapy such as bilateral adrenalectomy or pituitary surgery [41]. In this respect, it is important to note that those 12 of the 21 patients who showed clinical remission and did not need further medical therapy were not biochemically cured when strict criteria for the assessment of cure in Cushing's disease were applied [42].

Medical therapy

Another alternative for the treatment of patients with Cushing's syndrome is medical treatment, although it is rarely used as primary long-term therapy. Only in a few selected cases, such as patients with inoperable adrenal carcinoma or paraneoplastic Cushing's syndrome, may drug treatment be the only palliative form of treatment. Furthermore, those patients in whom the adrenal carcinoma cannot be totally removed, or in whom metastases are already present, or in whom ectopic ACTH secretion persists after tumour removal, may also benefit from such a therapeutic regimen.

One important indication for medical therapy of hypercortisolism is severe catabolism in a patient who is otherwise a perfect candidate for pituitary microsurgery or removal of a unilateral adrenal tumour. Such pretreatment prevents postoperative complications such as disturbances of wound healing and infections. Finally, medical therapy has a place in the temporary management of patients in whom the precise source of ACTH has yet to be located, or those following pituitary irradiation in whom tumour ACTH secretion is still present.

The drugs that are used for suppressing hypercortisolism in endogenous Cushing's syndrome can be divided into substances that act at the adrenal gland as adrenolytic agents, at the pituitary level inhibiting ACTH secretion, and on the central nervous system influencing putative neurotransmitters involved in the release of CRH (Table 33.5).

Metyrapone is the most frequently used drug, which acts by blocking the final step in cortisol biosynthesis. It is generally well tolerated, but may lead to marked virilisation as the precursors will be shifted towards androgen synthesis [43].

For the adrenolytic agent o,p'DDD (mitotane), an additional cytotoxic effect on adrenocortical tissue has been documented. It has therefore become the drug of choice in patients with metastasising adrenal carcinoma [44]. Impure preparations contain DDT and may cause nausea and ataxia at low doses, but this is much less of a problem with purified formulations. Unfortunately, recent studies have shown that the drug causes significant hypercholesterolaemia which will diminish its long-term usefulness.

It has also been shown that the imidazole derivatives, for example ketoconazole or etomidate, do not only interfere with steroidogenesis in the adrenal gland but have also an ACTH-suppressive effect at the pituitary level [45]. Patients with pituitary ACTH-dependent hypercortisolism who have been subjected to long-term therapy with ketoconazole do not have elevated ACTH levels following normalisation of peripheral cortisol levels, as is observed in patients with the same disease who have been subjected to bilateral adrenalectomy receiving substitution therapy with hydrocortisone. However, ketoconazole use is limited by hepatotoxicity.

Whereas adrenolytic agents are usually quite effective, at least as short-term therapy, centrally acting drugs lead to remission of the disease only in individual cases. Bromocriptine, cyproheptadine and sodium valproate may all occasionally be temporarily useful in such cases.

Somatostatin usually does not affect pituitary ACTH hypersecretion in Cushing's disease. Elevated cortisol levels suppress the expression of somatostatin receptors at the cell membranes of the tumorous corticotroph [47]. Accordingly, octreotide is of limited use in patients with Cushing's disease in whom the suppression of ACTH and cortisol levels into the normal range is the exception.

In contrast, patients with ectopic ACTH syndrome, in whom the ACTH-secreting tumour can be visualised by octreoscan due to its somatostatin receptors [28,48], octreotide is often also effective in controlling Cushing's

Table 33.5 Adrenolytic drugs and other substances that inhibit corticotrophin releasing hormone, adrenocorticotrophic hormone or cortisol secretion.

Drug	Main site of action	Mechanism of action	Daily dosage	Main side-effects
Cyproheptadine	Central	Serotonin antagonist	8–24 mg	Sedation, increase of appetite, dry mouth, disturbance of urination
Sodium valproate	Central	γ-Aminobutyric acid amino transferase inhibitor	0.6–2 g	Loss of hair, clotting disturbances, liver and pancreatic damage
Bromocriptine	AP	Dopamine agonist	5–30 mg	Nausea, vomiting, hypotension
Octreotide	Ectopic ACTH	Somatostatin analogue	300 μg (s.c.)	Hyperglycaemia, diarrhoea, nausea
o,p'DDD (mitotane)	AC	3β-Hydroxydehydrogenase blocker induces necrosis of the zona reticularis and fasciculata	2–12 g	Nausea, vomiting, diarrhoea, exanthema, cerebral symptoms, hypercholesterolaemia
Aminoglutethimide	AC	3β-Hydroxydehydrogenase and 11β-hydroxylase blocker	1–2 g	Nausea, sleepiness, exanthema, myalgia
WIN 24,540 (Trilostane)	AC	3β-Hydroxydehydrogenase blocker	0.2–1 g	Increased saliva, gastrointestinal symptoms
Metyrapone	AC	11β-Hydroxylase blocker	2–4.2 g	Gastrointestinal disturbances, vertigo, headaches, exanthema, hypotension
Ketoconazole	AC (AP)	Blocker of cytochrome P-450-dependent enzymes, mainly 11β-hydroxylase	0.6–1 g	Nausea, diarrhoea, itching, headaches, transaminase increase, hypogonadism
Etomidate	AC (AP)	Blocker of cytochrome P-450-dependent enzymes, mainly 11β-hydroxylase	2.5–30 mg (i.v.)	Myoclonia, painful veins, sleepiness, hypotension

AP, Anterior pituitary; AC, adrenal cortex; RR, hypotension.

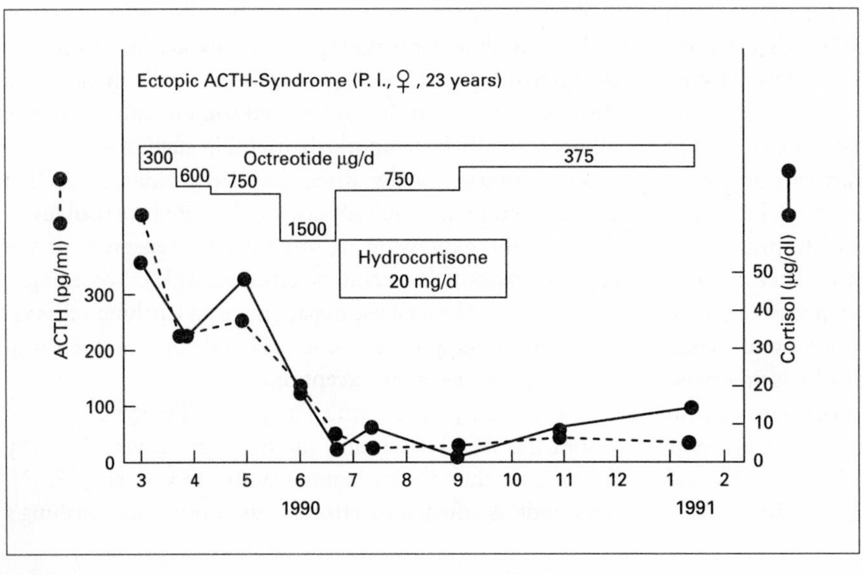

Fig. 33.13 Treatment of recurrent ectopic ACTH syndrome with octreotide. This patient was brought into complete remission after thoracotomy and removal of the carcinoid tumour in her right lung (see also Fig. 33.9). After recurrence of hypercortisolism, the source of ectopic ACTH syndrome could not be detected though octreoscan was not available at that time. She was treated with octreotide which lowered her ACTH and cortisol levels into the hypoadrenal state necessitating hydrocortisone replacement [48].

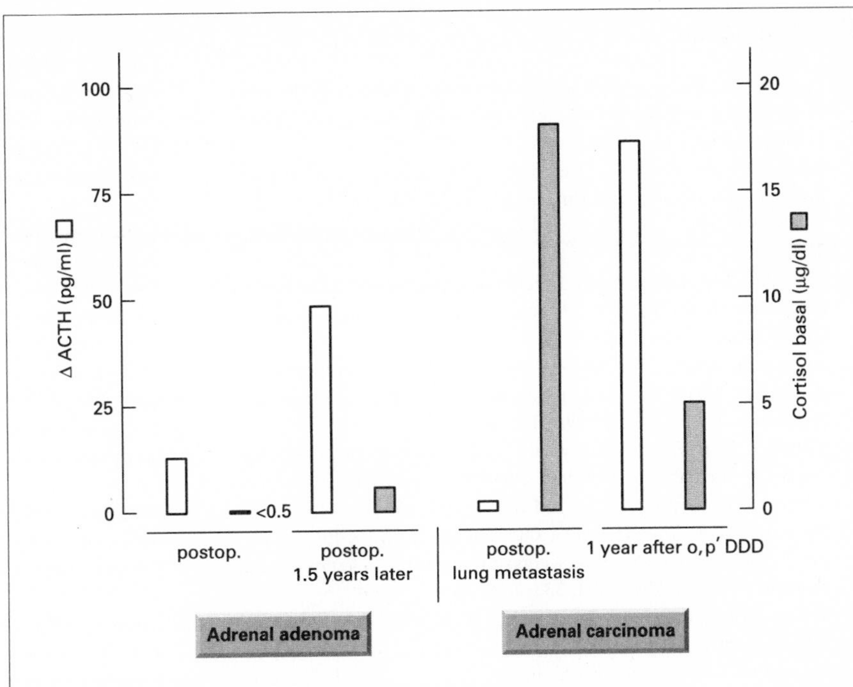

Fig. 33.14 Corticotrophin-releasing hormone (CRH)-stimulation tests in two patients with autonomous cortisol-producing adrenal adenoma or carcinoma at different times after therapy.

syndrome by suppressing ACTH and cortisol levels to such an extent necessitating hydrocortisone replacement therapy (Fig. 33.13). This documents that somatostatin receptors which can be demonstrated by receptor scintigraphy may be functional in respect of regulating tumorous ACTH secretion [15,29,47].

The success of drug therapy in patients with autonomous cortisol-secreting carcinomas can be documented in the same fashion as the success of unilateral adrenalectomy by a CRH-stimulation test (Fig. 33.14). The secondary adrenal insufficiency after successful removal of an autonomous cortisol-secreting adrenal tumour may last occasionally for several years, and therefore needs long-term substitution therapy with hydrocortisone followed by periodic withdrawal and reassessment.

Therapeutic strategy in Cushing's syndrome

The therapeutic recommendations in patients with Cushing's syndrome are summarised in Fig. 33.15.

In ACTH-dependent Cushing's disease transsphenoidal surgery is the therapy of first choice; this holds for adults as well as for children. In cases with contraindications to pituitary surgery, radiotherapy is the principal second-line treatment. In cases in whom transsphenoidal surgery did not lead to clinical remission, pituitary irradiation is the most likely next step of therapy with medical treatment until the effects of radiotherapy become manifest. In severe cases, bilateral adrenalectomy should be seriously considered, since only removal of the adrenals leads to rapid definitive abolition of the cortisol excess.

Only selected cases, particularly those with inoperable ectopic ACTH syndrome, are candidates for primary long-term octreotide or adrenolytic therapy. However, this form of treatment may be used for a limited period of time preoperatively in patients with severe catabolic states before transsphenoidal or retroperitoneal surgery is performed.

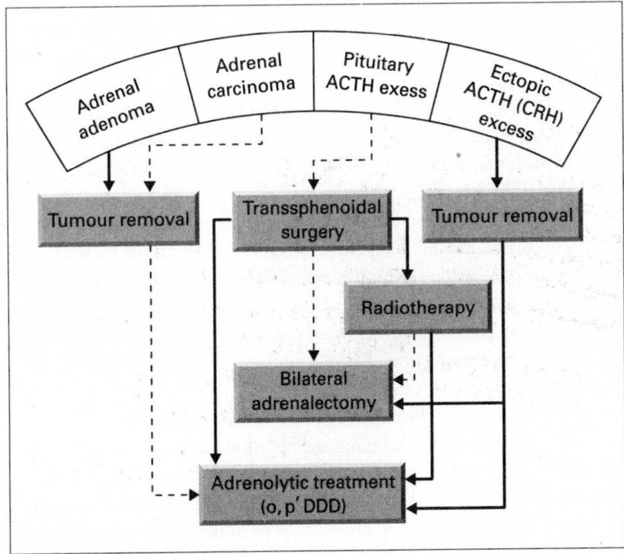

Fig. 33.15 Therapeutic steps in the different forms of Cushing's syndrome.

References

1 Cushing H. The basophil adenomas of the pituitary body and their clinical manifestations (pituitary basophilism). *Bull Johns Hopkins Hosp* 1932; **50**: 137–95.

2 Müller OA, von Werder K. Diagnostic dilemmas in hypercortisolism: investigation and management. In: Müller EE, MacLeod RM, eds. *Neuroendocrine Perspectives*, Vol. 6. Berlin: Springer-Verlag, 1989: 293.

3 Magiakou MA, Chrouros GP. Diagnosis and treatment of Cushing's disease: In: Imura H, ed. *The Pituitary Gland*, 2nd edn. New York: Raven Press, 1994: 491–508.

4 Lacroix A, Bolté E, Tremblay J. Gastric inhibitory polypeptide-dependent cortisol hypersecretion—a new cause of Cushing's syndrome. *N Engl J Med* 1992; **327**: 974–80.

5 Reznik Y, Allali-Zerah V, Chayvialle JA. Food-dependent Cushing's syndrome mediated by aberrant adrenal sensitivity to gastric inhibitory polypeptide. *N Engl J Med* 1992; **327**: 981–6.

6 Magiakou MA, Mastorakos G, Oldfield EH *et al.* Cushing's syndrome in children and adolescents: presentation, diagnosis, and therapy. *N Engl J Med* 1994; **331**: 629–36.

7 Young WF, Carney JA, Byron UM, Wulffraat NM, Lens JW, Drexhage HA. Familial Cushing's syndrome due to primary pigmented nodular adrenocortical disease. *N Engl J Med* 1989; **321**: 1659–64.

8 von Werder K, Müller OA. The role of corticotropin releasing factor in the investigation of endocrine diseases. In: *Corticotropin Releasing Factor*, Ciba Foundation Symposium 172. Chichester: John Wiley and Sons, 1993: 317–33.

9 Krieger DT. *Cushing's Syndrome*. Berlin: Springer-Verlag, 1982.

10 Fahlbusch R, Buchfelder M, Müller OA. Transsphenoidal surgery for Cushing's disease. *J Roy Soc Med* 1986; **79**: 262–9.

11 Bochicchio D, Losa M, Buchfelder M and the European Cushing's Disease Study Group. Factors influencing the immediate and late outcome of Cushing's disease treated by transsphenoidal surgery: a retrospective study by the European Cushing's Disease Survey Group. *J Clin Endocrinol Metab* 1995; **80**: 3114–120.

12 Herman V, Fagin J, Gonsky R, Kovacs K, Melmed S. Clonal origin of pituitary adenomas. *J Clin Endocrinol Metab* 1990; **71**: 1427–33.

13 Moore TJ, Dluhy RG, Williams GH, Cain JP. Nelson's syndrome: frequency, prognosis and effect of prior pituitary irradiation. *Ann Intern Med* 1976; **85**: 731–4.

14 Müller OA, von Werder K. Ectopic CRH and ACTH secretion. In: Clifford Rose F, ed. *The Control of the Hypothalamo-Pituitary–Adrenocortical Axis*. Madison, CT: International Universities Press, 1989: 371–80.

15 Wajchenberg BL, Mendonca BB, Liberman B. *et al.* Ectopic adrenocorticotropic hormone syndrome. *Endocr Rev* 1994; **15**: 752–87.

16 Stewart PM, Walker BR, Holder G, O'Halloran D, Shackleton CHL. 11-β-hydroxysteroid dehydrogenase activity in Cushing's syndrome: explaining the mineralocorticoid excess state of the ectopic adrenocorticotropin syndrome. *J Clin Endocrinol Metab* 1995; **80**: 3617–20.

17 von Werder K, Schopohl J, Wolfram G. Ectopic production of pituitary hormones and releasing hormones. *Adv Biosci* 1988; **69**: 87–95.

18 Howlett TA, Price J, Hale AC. Pituitary ACTH-dependent Cushing's syndrome due to ectopic production of bombesin-like peptide by a medullary carcinoma of the thyroid. *Clin Endocrinol* 1985; **22**: 91–107.

19 Ambrosi B, Faglia G and the Multicenter Pituitary Tumor Study Group, Lombardia Region. Epidemiology of pituitary tumors. In: Faglia G, Beck-Peccoz P, Ambrosi B, Travaglini P, Spada A, eds. *Pituitary Adenomas: New Trends in Basic and Clinical Research*. Amsterdam: Excerpta Medica, 1991: 159–68.

20 Extabe J, Vazquez JA. Morbidity and mortality in Cushing's disease: an epidemiological approach. *Clin Endocrinol (Oxf)* 1994; **40**: 479–84.

21 Labhart A. *Clinical Endocrinology—Theory and Practice*, 2nd end. Berlin: Springer-Verlag, 1986.

22 Hermus ARMM, Pieters GFFM, Pesman GJ, Smals AGH, Benraad TJ, Kloppenborg PWC. The corticotropin-releasing-hormone test versus the high-dose dexamethasone test in the differential diagnosis of Cushing's syndrome. *Lancet* 1986; **ii**: 540–4.

23 Grossman A, Howlett TA, Savage MO. CRF in the differential diagnosis of patients with Cushing's syndrome: a comparison with the dexamethasone suppression test. *Clin Endocrinol* 1988; **29**: 167–78.

24 Oldfield EH, Doppman JL, Nieman LK *et al.* Petrosal sinus sampling with and without corticotropin-releasing hormone for the differential diagnosis of Cushing's syndrome. *N Engl J Med* 1991; **325**: 897–905.

25 Lamberts SWJ, de Lange SA, Stefanko SZ. Adrenocorticotropin-secreting pituitary adenomas originate from the anterior or intermediate lobe in Cushing's disease: difference in the regulation of hormone secretion. *J Clin Endocrinol Metab* 1982; **54**: 286.

26 Müller OA, Stalla GK, von Werder K. CRH in Cushing's syndrome. *Horm Metabol Res Suppl* 1987; **16**: 51.

27 Van Cauter E, Refetoff S. Evidence for two subtypes of Cushing's disease based on the analysis of episodic cortisol secretion. *N Engl J Med* 1985; **312**: 1343.

28 De Herder WW, Krenning EP, Malchoff CD. Somatostatin receptor scintigraphy: its value in tumour localization in patients with Cushing's syndrome caused by ectopic corticotropin or corticotropin-releasing hormone secretion. *Am J Med* 1994; **96**: 305–12.

29 Philipponneau M, Nocaudie M, Epelbaum J. *et al.* Somatostatin analogs for the localization and preoperative treatment of an adrenocorticotropin-secreting bronchial carcinoid tumour. *J Clin Endocrinol Metab* 1994; **78**: 20–24.

30 Sturrok NDC, Morgan C, Jeffcoate WJ. Autonomous nodular hyperplasia of the adrenal cortex: tertiary hypercortisolism? *Clin Endocrinol* 1995; **43**: 753–8.

31 Trainer PJ, Lawrie HS, Verhelst J *et al.* Transspenoidal resection in Cushing's disease: undetectable serum cortisol as the definition of successful treatment. *Clin Endocrinol (Oxf)* 1993; **39**: 73–8.

32 Nakane T, Kuwayama A, Watanabe M *et al.* Longterm results of transsphenoidal adenomectomy in patients with Cushing's disease. *Neurosurgery* 1987; **21**: 218–22.

33 Guilhaume B, Bertagna X, Thomsen M *et al.* Transsphenoidal pituitary surgery for the treatment of Cushing's disease: results in 64 patients and longterm followup studies. *J Clin Endocrinol Metab* 1988; **66**: 1056–64.

34 Mampalam TJ, Tyrrell JB, Wilson CB. Transspenoidal microsurgery for Cushing's disease: a report of 216 cases. *Ann Intern Med* 1988; **109**: 487–93.

35 Burke CW, Adams CBT, Esiri MM, Morris C, Bevan JS. Transsphenoidal surgery for Cushing's disease: does what is removed determine the endocrine outcome? *Clin Endocrinol (Oxf)* 1990; **33**: 525–37.

36 Tindall GT, Herring CJ, Clark RV, Adams DA, Watts NB. Cushing's disease: results of transsphenoidal microsurgery with emphasis on surgical failures. *J Neurosurg* 1990; **72**: 363–9.

37 Robert F, Hardy J. Cushing's disease: a correlation of radiological, surgical and pathological findings with therapeutic results. *Pathol Res Pract* 1991; **187**: 617–21.

38 Tahir AH, Sheeler LR. Recurrent Cushing's disease after transsphenoidal surgery. *Arch Intern Med* 1992; **152**: 977–81.

39 Ram Z, Nieman LK, Cutler, GB, Jr, Chrousos GP, Doppman JL, Oldfield EH. Early repeat surgery for persistent Cushing's disease. *J Neurosurg* 1994; **80**: 37–45.

40 Schrell U, Fahlbusch R, Buchfelder M, Riedl S, Stalla GK, Müller OA. Corticotropin-releasing hormone stimulation test before and after transsphenoidal selective microadenomectoma in 30 patients with Cushing's disease. *J Clin Endocrinol Metab* 1987; **64**: 1150–9.

41 Howlett TA, Plowman PN, Wass JAH, Rees LH, Jones AE, Besser M. Megavoltage pituitary irradiation in the management of Cushing's disease and Nelson's syndrome: long-term followup. *Clin Endocrinol* 1989; **31**: 309–23.

42 McCance DR, Besser M, Brew Atkinson A. Assessment of cure after transsphenoidal surgery for Cushing's disease. *Clin Endocrinol* 1996; **44**: 1–6.

43 Verhelst JA, Trainer PJ, Howlett TA *et al.* Short- and longterm responses to metyrapone in the medical management of 91 patients with Cushing's syndrome. *Clin Endocrinol* 1991; **35**: 169–78.

44 Luton J-P, Cerdas S, Billaud L. *et al.* Clinical features of adrenocortical carcinoma, prognostic factors, and the effect of Mitotane therapy. *N Engl J Med* 1990; **322**: 1195–201.

45 Stalla GK, Stalla J, Huber M. Ketoconazole inhibits corticotropic cell function *in vitro*. *Endocrinology* 1988; **122**: 618–23.

46 Estrada J, Boronat M, Mielgo M *et al.* The long-term outcome of pituitary irradiation after unsuccessful transspheniodal surgery in Cushing's disease. *New Engl J Med* 1997; **336**: 172–7.

47 Von Werder K, Müller OM, Stalla GK. Somatostatin analogs in ectopic corticotrophin production. *Metabolism* 1996; **45** (Suppl.1): 129–31.

48 Stalla GK, Brockmeier SJ, Renner U *et al.* Octreotide exerts different effects *in vivo* and *in vitro* in Cushing's disease. *Europ J Endocrinol* 1994; **130**: 125–31.

CHAPTER 34

Disorders of mineralocorticoid hormone secretion

C.R.W. Edwards

Introduction

Aldosterone, the most important mineralocorticoid steroid produced by the zona glomerulosa, plays a key role in sodium homeostasis. Excess production leads to sodium retention with concomitant loss of potassium, whilst aldosterone deficiency results in the reverse. The resultant changes in body electrolyte composition and cardiovascular control have important effects on blood pressure, renal function, and both cardiac and skeletal muscle. Disorders of mineralocorticoid hormone secretion are common in routine clinical practice (Fig. 34.1), and thus need to be understood by all practising physicians and surgeons.

Mineralocorticoids are defined as steroid hormones which promote the unidirectional transport of sodium across epithelia. In humans, the epithelia involved are in the distal nephron (principally the cortical collecting tubule), salivary and sweat glands, and the distal part of the large bowel. The steroids act via specific cytoplasmic receptors, so-called type 1 mineralocorticoid receptors, which are structurally similar to the type 2 glucocorticoid receptors (Fig. 34.2). The structure of the mineralocorticoid receptor is not sufficiently different to the glucocorticoid receptor to prevent the major glucocorticoid cortisol from binding to, and activating, the type 1 receptor; protection is essential because the circulating free levels of cortisol are 100 times those of aldosterone. To overcome this lack of receptor specificity, the aldosterone-selective tissues have high levels of a particular isoform of the enzyme 11β-hydroxysteroid dehydrogenase (11β-HSD); this isoform converts cortisol to inactive cortisone but does not metabolise aldosterone which is protected by its 11–18 hemiketal bridge (Fig. 34.3). Thus, the non-specific aldosterone receptor does not 'see' cortisol. In certain circumstances this protective mechanism may be either congenitally absent or inhibited, thus leading to mineralocorticoid excess mediated not by aldosterone but by cortisol (see below).

The control of aldosterone secretion is complex, and multiple factors appear to be involved. This is perhaps not surprising given the importance of sodium homeostasis in relation to survival. The dominant control mechanism is the renin–angiotensin system (Fig. 34.4). Adrenocorticotrophic hormone (ACTH) and elevated plasma potassium are both stimuli to aldosterone secretion, but are usually less important than angiotensin II (AII). Low sodium intake can stimulate aldosterone by two different mechanisms. The first involves activation of the renin–angiotensin system resulting in the release of AII and the direct effect of this on the zona glomerulosa. The second is due to the indirect effect of sodium deprivation on enhancing the action of AII on the adrenal. It would also appear that the stimulant effect of hyperkalaemia requires the presence of AII. This would explain why the hyperkalaemia found in patients with hyporeninaemic hypoaldosteronism does not result in an increase in aldosterone secretion.

Hypokalaemia is an important pointer to the possibility of mineralocorticoid excess and is usually associated with a metabolic alkalosis. However, this clue is commonly either overlooked, obscured or absent. Factors that may obscure hypokalaemia include red-cell haemolysis, long delay in the separation of red cells from plasma, and use of a tourniquet with muscular effort involving the forearm muscles when the blood sample is being taken. If the patient is taking a low-salt diet this may have a significant effect on the plasma potassium, as the low filtered load of sodium results in less sodium being available for sodium–potassium exchange in the distal nephron and hence a rise in plasma potassium concentration.

Hyperkalaemia may indicate mineralocorticoid deficiency. The lack of aldosterone results not only in a failure of renal sodium–potassium exchange but also in a shift of potassium out of cells. The latter occurs in other causes of acidosis and in insulin deficiency.

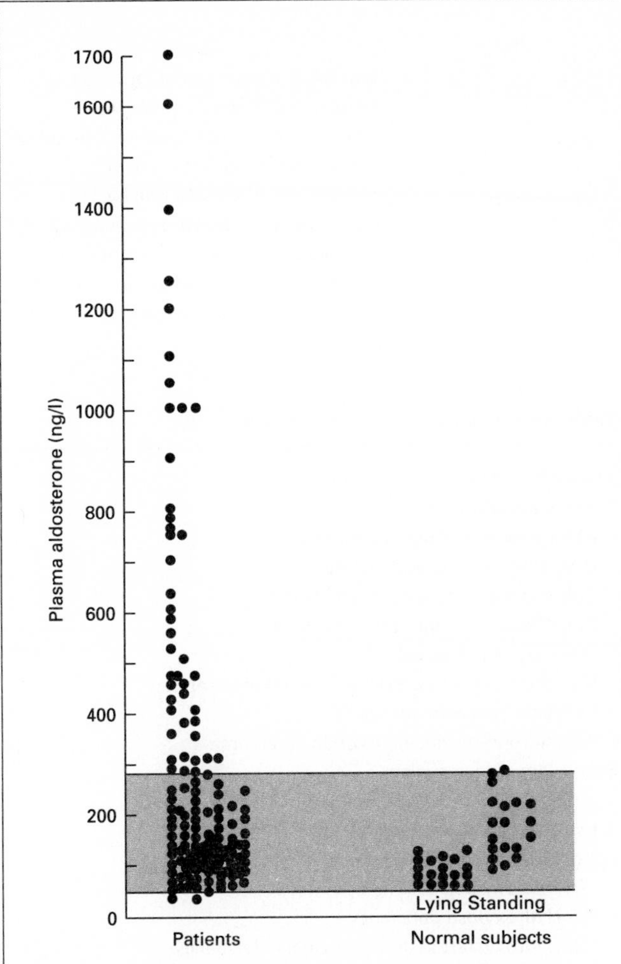

Fig. 34.1 Results of plasma aldosterone screening on 160 consecutive routine electrolyte samples. Because blood samples were taken without the patients being in a fixed posture the reference ranges for lying and standing normal subjects are included.

Impaired excretion of potassium is an important problem in acute renal failure and in severe chronic renal failure. In the clinical context of Addison's disease, hyperkalaemia should present no major diagnostic problems. More commonly, hyperkalaemia is due to the patient taking a potassium-sparing diuretic, often with inappropriate potassium supplements. With primary renin deficiency (hyporeninaemic hypoaldosteronism), where the patient is usually elderly, presents with an arrhythmia, has moderate renal impairment and is on multiple drugs other than potassium-sparing diuretics or supplements, the diagnosis is often missed. In rare patients, hyperkalaemia results from a defect in the red cell which results in rapid leakage of potassium into plasma when the blood sample has been taken. This is thus described as pseudo-hyperkalaemia.

Mineralocorticoid excess syndromes

A list of the causes of mineralocorticoid excess is given in Table 34.1. They are most conveniently divided into a major group in which there is overproduction of aldosterone, and a minor one in which there is excess of mineralocorticoids other than aldosterone.

Primary aldosteronism

This diagnosis should be suspected in any patient with hypertension and hypokalaemia, either spontaneous or provoked by diuretic therapy. Conn *et al.* originally suggested that 20% of patients with essential hypertension had aldosterone-producing adenomas [1] but this proved to be a gross overestimate. Others have suggested that about 1–2% of unselected patients with essential hypertension have primary aldosteronism [2,3]. In the context of a hypertension clinic one might expect to find a higher prevalence, as patients with this syndrome respond poorly to many commonly used antihypertensive agents and may thus be referred to hospital. We looked at this in a study of 254 consecutive patients in a London hypertension clinic. The patients were initially screened by measurement of plasma potassium concentration. If this was < 3.5 mmol/l, then full evaluation of the renin–angiotensin–aldosterone axis was carried out

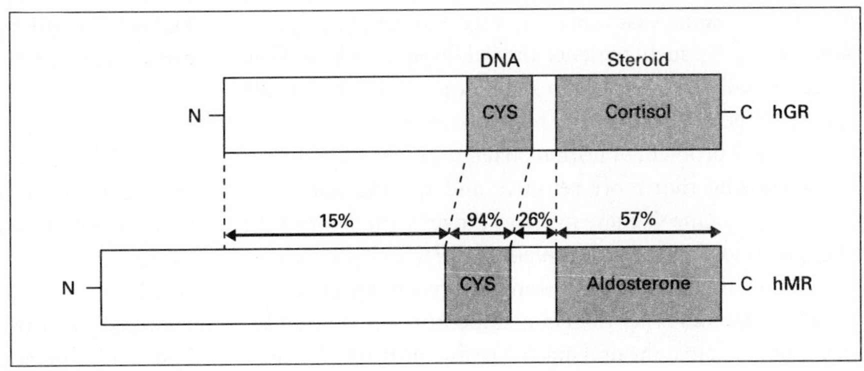

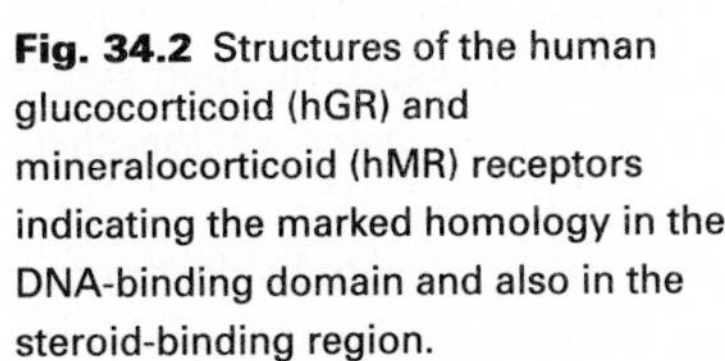
Fig. 34.2 Structures of the human glucocorticoid (hGR) and mineralocorticoid (hMR) receptors indicating the marked homology in the DNA-binding domain and also in the steroid-binding region.

Fig. 34.3 Conventional formulae of aldosterone. Recent studies using magnetic resonance spectroscopy taken in conjunction with the lack of metabolism of aldosterone by 11β-hydroxysteroid dehydrogenase indicate that aldosterone is not present in the form having a free hydroxyl group in the 11 position but usually exists as the 11–18 bridge structure.

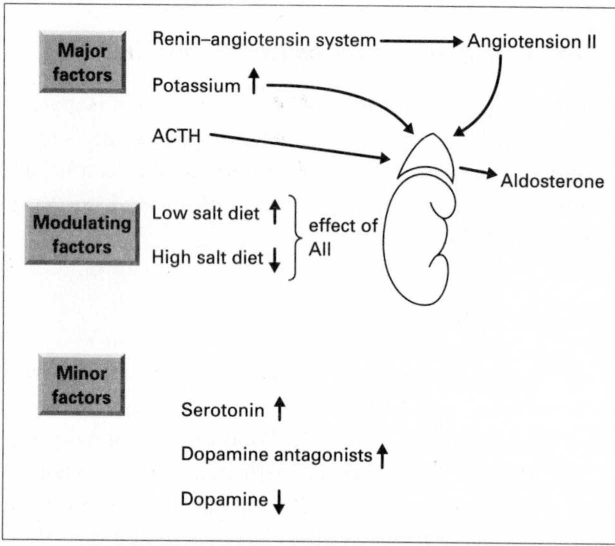

Fig. 34.4 Control mechanisms for aldosterone secretion.

(Table 34.2). A surprisingly high prevalence of primary aldosteronism was found (5.2%). Of the 13 patients identified, four were diagnosed as having aldosterone-producing adenomas and the rest as having idiopathic hyperplasia. When diuretic therapy was stopped, 62% of the patients became normokalaemic. These patients would therefore *not* have been identified if they had not been on thiazide therapy. Many other groups have also described normokalaemic primary aldosteronism [4], but as already discussed in some cases this may relate to a relatively low salt intake. In such patients the addition of 6 g sodium chloride daily for a week to their normal intake usually results in the development of hypokalaemia.

Given the problem of normokalaemic aldosteronism, it is not surprising that more sensitive and specific tests have been sought. One of these involves the measurement of the effect of aldosterone on the potential difference (PD) across the wall of the rectum. Unfortunately, this is affected by a variety of factors other than mineralocorticoids. To obviate these the PD across the oral mucosa is also measured, because this is influenced by the non-steroidal factors but not by aldosterone. The resultant subtraction PD (rectal PD–oral PD) relates directly to the plasma aldosterone level. A value greater than 25 mV indicates mineralocorticoid excess [5].

Table 34.1 Causes of mineralocorticoid excess.

Elevated aldosterone
Primary aldosteronism
Aldosterone-producing adenoma
Idiopathic hyperaldosteronism
Aldosterone-producing carcinoma
Angiotensin II-responsive adenoma
Unilateral hyperplasia
Glucocorticoid-suppressible hyperaldosteronism
Familial hyperaldosteronism
Aldosterone-producing ovarian carcinoma
Secondary aldosteronism
Suppressed or normal aldosterone
Congenital enzyme defects
17α-Hydroxylase deficiency
11β-Hydroxylase deficiency
11β-Hydroxysteroid dehydrogenase deficiency
Pseudo-hyperaldosteronism (includes acquired enzyme defects)
Liddle's syndrome
Liquorice
Carbenoxolone
Exogenous mineralocorticoid
Cushing's syndrome
Primary cortisol resistance
Isolated deoxycorticosterone excess
Isolated corticosterone excess

Diagnosis of primary aldosteronism

The conventional approach is that if the screening tests suggest that there may be mineralocorticoid excess, the next step is to measure renin and aldosterone to determine whether there is either:

1 primary aldosteronism (low renin, elevated aldosterone);
2 secondary aldosteronism (high renin and aldosterone);

Table 34.2 Screening hypertension clinic for prevalence of primary aldosteronism.

254 consecutive hypertensive patients
83 plasma potassium <3.5 mmol/l
47 high plasma aldosterone
26 low plasma renin activity
13 high aldosterone, low PRA (i.e. elevated aldosterone/PRA ratio) (see text)

13 patients identified as having primary aldosteronism
(a) Trial of spironolactone
One patient unable to tolerate drug
6/12 blood pressure < 140/95 mmHg
Other six patients mean systolic blood pressure drop of 42 mmHg (range 25–64) and mean diastolic pressure fall of 19 mmHg (range 14–27)

(b) Computed tomography scanning: 3/13 patients' scans indicated adenomas

(c) 4/13 had fall of plasma aldosterone on standing compatible with adenoma

PRA, plasma renin activity.

3 other forms of mineralocorticoid excess (low renin and low aldosterone).

However, some authors feel that this approach will miss a very significant number of patients with primary aldosteronism and that all patients with moderate or severe hypertension should have plasma aldosterone and plasma renin activity measured.

Even though direct renin assays are now becoming more readily available, their sensitivity is a problem in this context, and thus plasma renin activity is usually the assay of choice. Plasma aldosterone concentration is now more frequently measured than urinary aldosterone. In the past our usual practice was to measure 0800 hours plasma renin activity and plasma aldosterone concentration with the patient recumbent and on *ad libitum* sodium intake. (In occasional patients with severe hypokalaemia, the plasma aldosterone level may be in the normal reference range; such patients should have the test repeated after potassium supplementation.) However, this has the disadvantage that the patient's posture has to be controlled. This has been largely overcome by looking at the ratio of plasma aldosterone to plasma renin activity in random blood samples with no control of posture or sodium intake.

Aldosterone–renin profiling

Because of the problems of making the diagnosis, several groups have looked at the value of using the aldosterone/renin ratio as a screening test. This approach has revealed a surprisingly large number of patients with primary aldosteronism. As indicated above, in our own series of 254 consecutive hypertensives (Table 34.2), 13 (5.1%) had an aldosterone/renin ratio suggestive of primary aldosteronism with four probably having aldosterone-producing adenomas (APA) (1.6%). In the series of 348 patients with hypertension studied by Hiramatsu *et al.* [6], nine patients had APA (2.6%) as confirmed by scintigraphy, venography and surgical excision. Hiramatsu found that in patients with APA the aldosterone/PRA ratio (aldosterone pg/ml: PRA ng/ml/hour) was always more than 400 whereas in 323 patients with essential hypertension the aldosterone/PRA ratio was less than 200. Six of these nine were normokalaemic (67%). In our series 62% of the patients with primary aldosteronism were normokalaemic off diuretic treatment but all had plasma potassium < 3.5 mmd/l on thiazide therapy.

McKenna *et al.* [7] found that a single elevated aldosterone/renin ratio associated with an elevated or normal plasma aldosterone correctly diagnosed primary aldosteronism in 10 patients, five with hyperplasia and five with APA. The only problem they had with false positives was in patients with chronic renal failure. Secondary aldosteronism was characterised by elevated plasma aldosterone values together with a normal ratio.

Gordon's group have recently reviewed their experience of this screening test [8]. They diagnosed 48 patients as having primary aldosteronism in the previous 12 months. This compared with 90 patients with primary aldosteronism diagnosed in the period 1970–90. Of the 48 patients, 34 (71%) were normokalaemic on presentation (14 out of 24 with APA; 58%). The results of the aldosterone/renin ratio studies suggest that the conventional approach of using plasma potassium as the sole guide to the need for further investigation is probably inappropriate.

Effect of drug therapy on renin–angiotensin–aldosterone system in suspected primary aldosteronism

One of the common problems facing a physician is investigation of possible secondary causes of hypertension in a patient on medication likely to interfere either with the tests or their interpretation. Some drugs such as spironolactone and β-adrenoceptor-blocking drugs have long-lasting effects on the renin–angiotensin–aldosterone axis and thus should be stopped several weeks before testing; others, such as thiazide and loop-acting diuretics and Ca^{2+}-channel-blocking agents, have shorter effects, and some do not interfere at all. This latter group can thus be used if the patient develops severe hypertension off their drug therapy; it includes prazosin and bethanidine. We normally use bethanidine at a starting dose of 10 mg three times daily. As with other adrenergic neuron-blocking agents, postural hypotension may be a problem. However, it is usually possible to control severe high blood pressure satisfactorily for a period of a few weeks off other drug therapy.

Differential diagnosis of primary aldosteronism

The various causes of primary aldosteronism and their approximate prevalence are listed in Table 34.3. With the exception of glucocorticoid-suppressible hyperaldosteronism (GSH) (alternatively called dexamethasone-suppressible hyperaldosteronism, DSH or glucocorticoid-remediable hyperaldosteronism, GRH), the precise molecular aetiology has not been determined. GSH is an autosomal dominant disorder with hypertension, variable hypokalaemia, aldosterone excess with suppression of plasma renin activity and excess production of 18-hydroxycortisol and 18-oxocortisol (see below). The key difference from other forms of aldosteronism is that aldosterone secretion is under ACTH control and can be suppressed by glucocorticoid therapy. Lifton *et al.* have shown this results from ectopic expression of aldosterone synthase in the zona fasciculata, an enzyme normally only found in the zona glomerulosa [9]. The genes encoding aldosterone synthase and 11β-hydroxylase (which is expressed in both the glomerulosa and the fasciculata) are 95% homologous and both lie on chromosome 8. Lifton *et al.* have shown linkage of GSH to a gene duplication arising from unequal crossing over which has fused the 5′ regulatory region of 11β-hydroxylase (under ACTH control) to the coding sequence of aldosterone synthase (Fig. 34.5). Subsequent studies with other pedigrees have shown similar mutations but with at least five independent breakpoints. *In vitro* work has indicated that all breakpoints should be within or to the left of exon 4. Hybrids which contained exons 1, 2, 3 and up to mid-exon 4 coded for an enzyme which synthesised aldosterone. Hybrids containing exons 5, 6 and 7 did not result in aldosterone production. The reason why most kindreds are normokalaemic despite clear aldosterone excess remains obscure. Family screening using Southern blotting to identify the chimaeric gene, a test with absolute sensitivity and specificity, has shown that there is a poor correlation between phenotype and genotype. Some patients with the chimaeric gene and aldosterone excess are normotensive. Such screening suggests that the condition is much more common than previously thought.

No abnormality of aldosterone synthase has been found in either APAs or idiopathic aldosteronism. Indeed, there is very little known about the aetiology of zona glomerulosa hyperplasia, but in contrast to the generally beneficial effects

Table 34.3 Causes of primary aldosteronism.

Cause	Approximate percentage
Aldosterone-producing adenoma	60
(Probably 10% of adenomas are angiotensin-II responsive)	
Idiopathic zona glomerulosa hyperplasia	
Bilateral, symmetrical	20
Bilateral, multinodular	17
Unilateral, nodular	1
Glucocorticoid-remediable	?1 (see text)
Aldosterone-producing carcinoma	<1
Aldosterone-producing ovarian carcinoma	Very rare

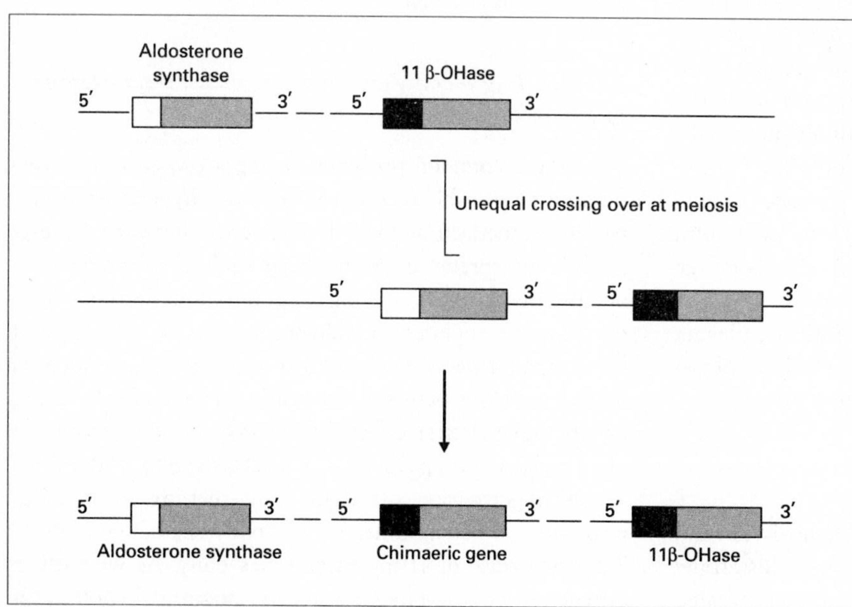

Fig. 34.5 Mechanism for the production of the chimaeric gene responsible for glucocorticoid remediable aldosteronism.

Table 34.4 Tests used in differential diagnosis of primary aldosteronism.

Aldosterone response to time and posture
Measurement of 18-hydroxycortisol
Dexamethasone suppression
Southern blotting or equivalent to detect chimaeric gene
Angiotensin converting enzyme inhibition
Adrenal vein catheterisation
Adrenal scanning
Computed tomography or magnetic resonance imaging
Labelled cholesterol scanning

of surgical removal of APAs, bilateral adrenalectomy in patients with hyperplasia is much less satisfactory. The tests used in making the differential diagnosis are detailed in Table 34.4.

Effect of time and posture

The patient has blood taken when lying down at 0800 hours for aldosterone, cortisol and plasma renin activity. The same assays are then repeated at 1200 hours after 4 hours in the upright posture. In patients with aldosterone-producing adenomas, the plasma aldosterone level will usually fall during the morning, in keeping with the circadian rhythm of cortisol as the adenoma is ACTH responsive (Fig. 34.6). If, however, the patient is stressed by the test, aldosterone levels will rise and hence there is a need to measure plasma cortisol as well as aldosterone levels. In glucocorticoid-remediable aldosteronism the plasma aldosterone levels will also fall. In contrast, the levels rise in most patients with idiopathic zona glomerulosa hyperplasia because the adrenal in this condition is very sensitive to angiotensin II (AII), and the positive response parallels that resulting from AII infusion. It is important to recognise that possibly 10% of adenomas are responsive to AII [10], and that patients with unilateral hyperplasia may also show a rise in aldosterone concentration on standing. Both these conditions are amenable to surgery.

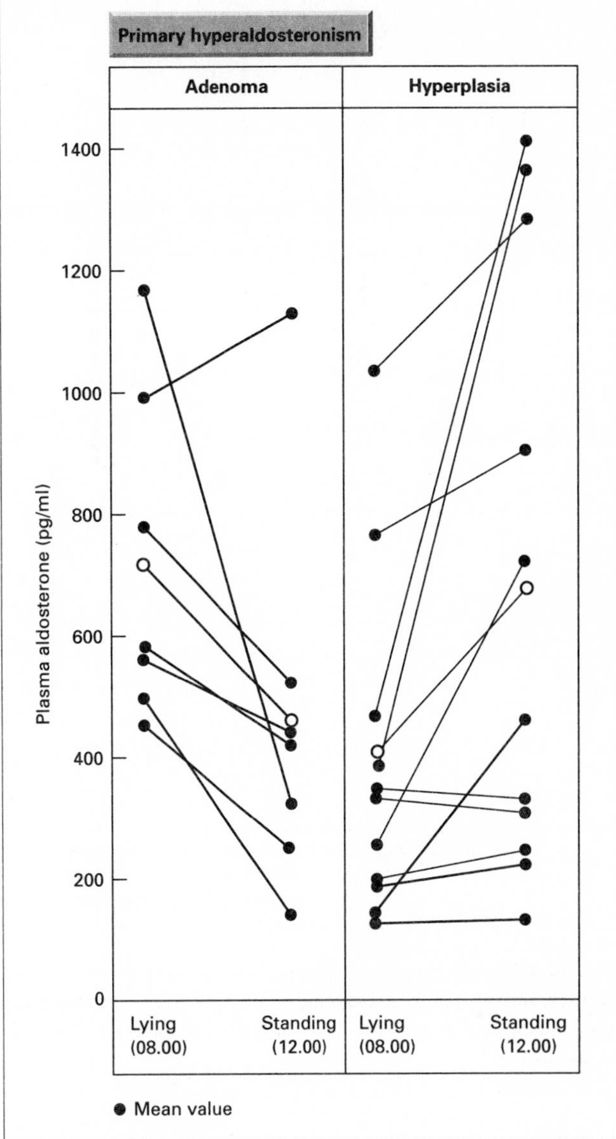

Fig. 34.6 Effects of time and posture on plasma aldosterone levels in patients with aldosterone secreting adenomas as compared with idiopathic zona glomerulosa hyperplasia. One patient with an adenoma had a rise in plasma aldosterone between 0800 and 1200 hours. In this patient the plasma cortisol also rose indicating that the individual had been stressed. When this test was repeated both plasma aldosterone and plasma cortisol levels fell during the course of the morning.

Measurement of 18-hydroxycortisol

This steroid, first identified by Ulick and Chu [11], has been shown to be the most abundant urinary free steroid in patients with primary aldosteronism. The levels in both plasma and urine are significantly higher in patients with aldosterone-producing adenomas in comparison to idiopathic adrenal hyperplasia [12,13], and patients with glucocorticoid-remediable aldosteronism have even higher levels (Figs 34.7 and 34.8) [14]. We have found that measurement of this steroid is an extremely useful screening test in hypertensive patients with suspected mineralocorticoid excess. However, it is essential to demonstrate that there is primary mineralocorticoid excess (i.e. that plasma renin activity is low) because elevated 18-hydroxycortisol may be found in some patients with secondary aldosteronism. If the level is in the adenoma range or above, then full investigation is indicated. 18-Oxocortisol has also been shown to be of similar value

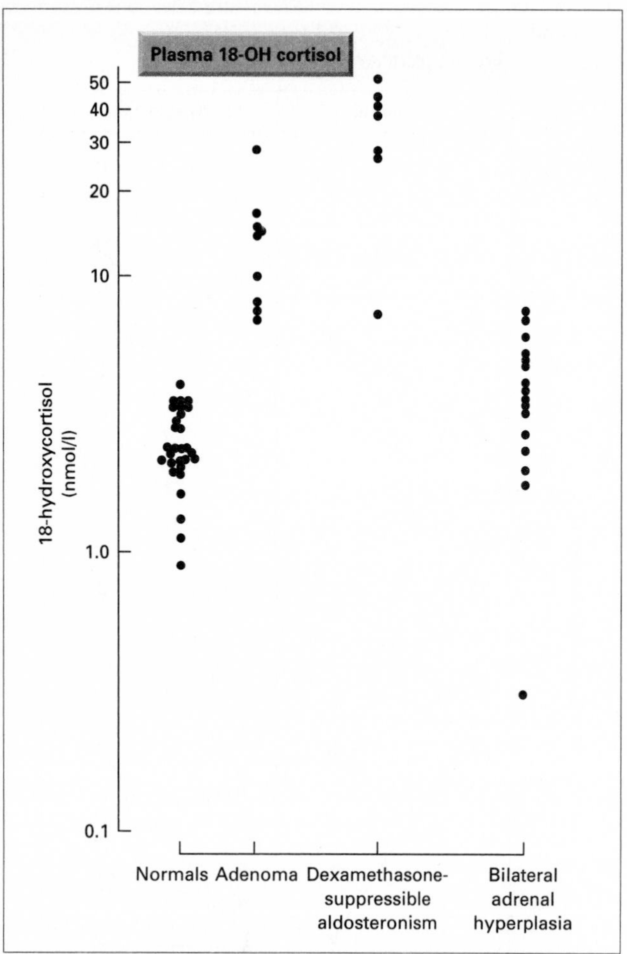

Fig. 34.7 Plasma 18-hydroxycortisol levels in normal subjects, in patients with aldosterone-secreting adenomas, in dexamethasone-suppressible aldosteronism and in idiopathic bilateral adrenal hyperplasia.

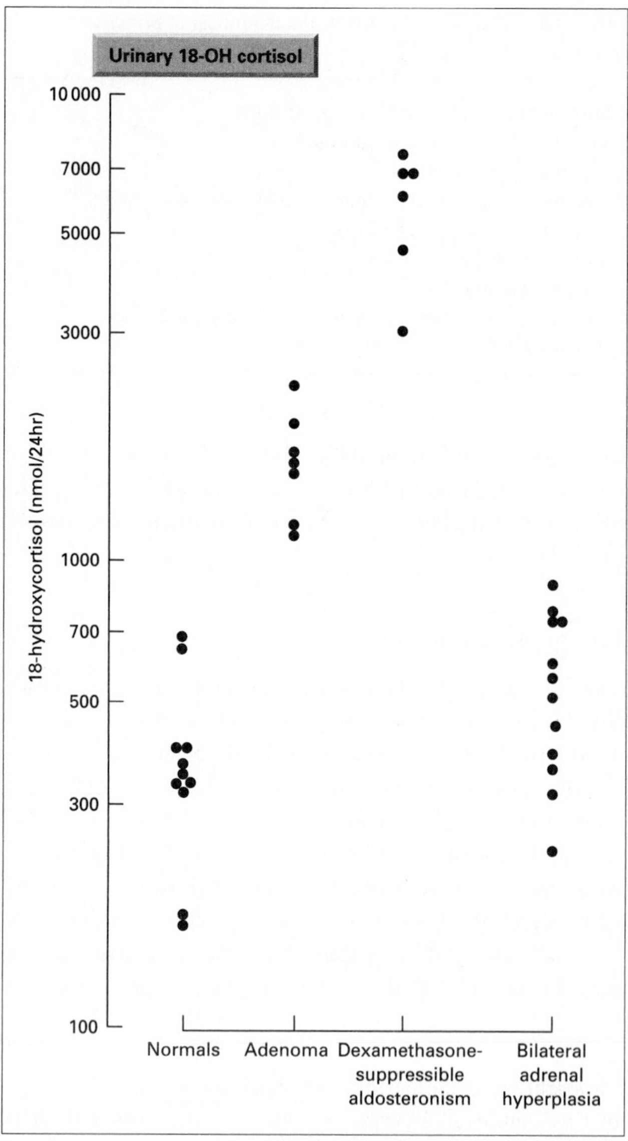

Fig. 34.8 Urinary 18-hydroxycortisol levels in normal subjects, in patients with aldosterone-secreting adenomas, in dexamethasone-suppressible aldosteronism and in idiopathic bilateral adrenal hyperplasia.

[15]. In our experience, measurement of 18- hydroxycortisol is more valuable than 18-hydroxycorticosterone in making the differential diagnosis of primary aldosteronism. Plasma levels of 18-hydroxycorticosterone tend to be higher in adenoma than hyperplasia, but there is often overlap (Fig. 34.9). Plasma 18-hydroxydeoxycorticosterone levels are frequently elevated in primary aldosteronism but are of little value in distinguishing adenoma from hyperplasia.

Dexamethasone suppression

Suppression of ACTH with dexamethasone (0.5 mg 6-hourly) will transiently suppress plasma aldosterone in patients with APA, but only in glucocorticoid-remediable aldosteronism will aldosterone remain suppressed when dexamethasone is given for more than 5 days [16]. Dexamethasone will also lower the blood pressure in this condition and result in recovery of the renin–angiotensin system.

Detection of chimaeric gene

As indicated above, the molecular pathology of glucocorticoid-remediable aldosteronism is now known. This has resulted in a specific test with 100% sensitivity and specificity; the chimaeric gene is detected by either Southern blotting or a version of the polymerase chain reaction.

Angiotensin-converting enzyme inhibition

In patients with bilateral hyperplasia of the zona glomerulosa, administration of captopril results in a fall in plasma aldosterone concentration [17]. This reflects the AII re-

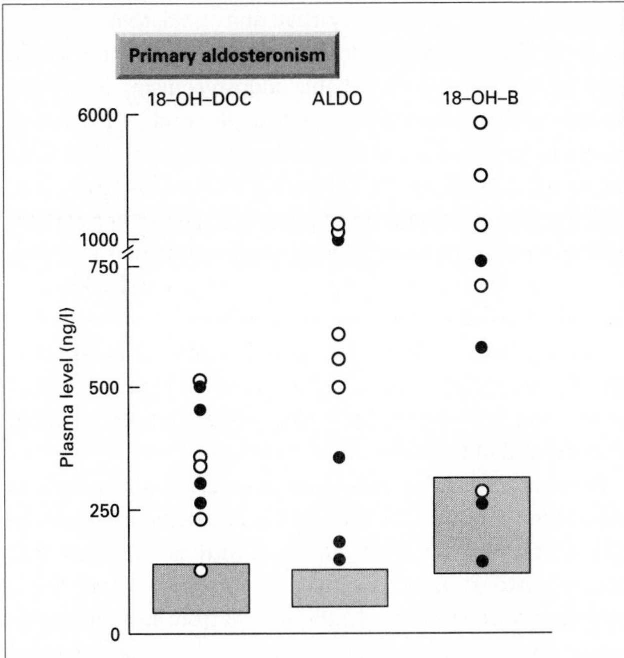

Fig. 34.9 Plasma levels of 18-hydroxydeoxycorticosterone, aldosterone and 18-hydroxycorticosterone in patients with aldosterone-producing adenomas (○) and in idiopathic zona glomerulosa hyperplasia (●). Box shows normal reference range.

sponsiveness of the adrenal. In most patients with APA the aldosterone levels are not AII responsive. It is important to compare the test with a control day because the plasma aldosterone level in patients with APA will fall during the test, as ACTH levels fall if the test is done in the morning.

Adrenal vein catheterisation

This is obviously an invasive procedure and is normally necessary only when there is doubt about the diagnosis. It is important to measure both aldosterone and cortisol (and/or adrenaline) levels so as to be certain about the position of the catheter, and it is useful to take blood simultaneously from a peripheral vein to compare the plasma cortisol and aldosterone values with those in the adrenal vein. The left adrenal vein which drains into the left renal vein is relatively easy to catheterise but the right, which enters directly into the inferior vena cava, is much more difficult. In APA, the side of the adenoma will have elevated aldosterone values in contrast with the suppressed contralateral gland, where the adrenal vein level will be similar to the periphery. In hyperplasia, the levels in both adrenal veins will be elevated in comparison to the peripheral samples (Fig. 34.10).

Adrenal scanning

Either computed tomography (CT) or magnetic resonance imaging (MRI) is useful in demonstrating the presence of an adrenal tumour, even if this is <10mm in diameter (Fig. 34.11). However, it is important to recognise that many adrenal tumours are non-functioning 'incidentalomas', and thus simple demonstration of an adrenal lesion augments but does not replace the tests detailed above (see also Chapters 37 and 65).

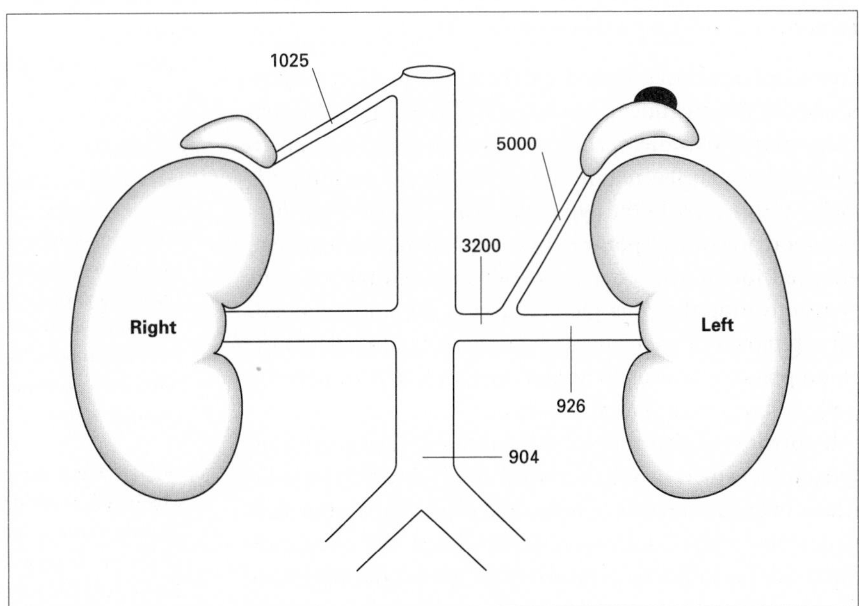

Fig. 34.10 Plasma aldosterone levels in samples taken during differential venous catheterisation indicating a left-sided aldosterone-secreting tumour.

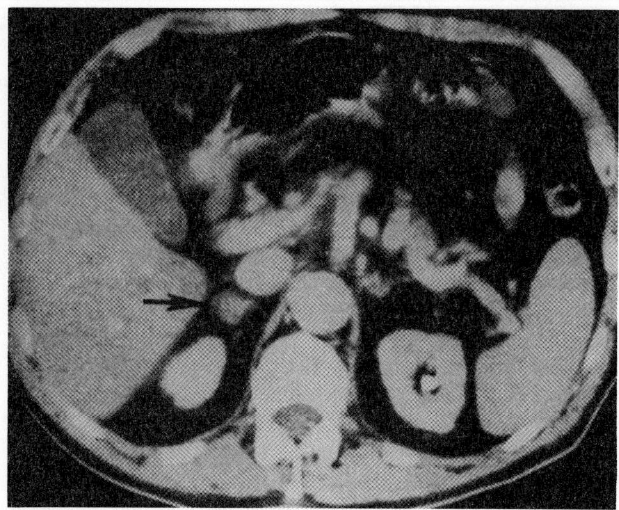

Fig. 34.11 Computed tomography scan of the abdomen showing adrenal adenoma (arrowed) in a patient with Conn's syndrome.

Labelled cholesterol scanning

This scanning technique, using either iodine or selenium labelling of cholesterol, has been useful in demonstrating unilateral uptake in an adenoma. However, its value, even when the label is given after dexamethasone suppression of uptake by zona fasciculata, has been less than in Cushing's syndrome. It is important to realize that long-term treatment with spironolactone in a patient with APA will reactivate the renin–angiotensin system and thus the contralateral zona glomerulosa. Scanning these patients will then often give bilateral rather than mainly unilateral uptake of the isotope.

Treatment of primary aldosteronism

Treatment obviously depends on the cause. In APA, surgery is usually the treatment of choice unless contraindicated. Preoperative treatment with spironolactone (doses up to 400 mg/day may be required) for 6–8 weeks or longer is useful as this corrects the hypokalaemia and usually predicts the blood pressure response to operation. It may also obviate the need for postoperative mineralocorticoid replacement by reactivating the zona glomerulosa in the normal gland. After removal of an adenoma by unilateral adrenalectomy, blood pressure returns to normal in about 70% of patients [18], but may take several months.

If surgery is contraindicated or refused, then long-term spironolactone is usually satisfactory. However, the side-effects of gynaecomastia in males and menstrual dysfunction in females often mean that other drugs are necessary. Amiloride (an inhibitor of renal tubular ionic transport rather than an aldosterone-receptor-blocking drug) is frequently used, but is less satisfactory than spironolactone in many patients, even when high doses (up to 40 mg/day) are given.

In glucocorticoid-remediable aldosteronism, long-term therapy with dexamethasone will usually produce resolution of the hypertension and hypokalaemia. The smallest dose necessary to suppress ACTH secretion should be given (e.g. 0.75 mg dexamethasone on going to bed and 0.25 mg at 0800 hours). In some patients, blood pressure control is lost with long-term therapy and other treatment is required (e.g. a thiazide diuretic with potassium supplements, or amiloride or spironolactone). Relatives should be screened (using the specific genetic test as indicated above or 18-hydroxycortisol in addition to blood pressure, electrolytes and plasma renin activity, and aldosterone concentration).

Patients with idiopathic zona glomerulosa hyperplasia require long-term medical treatment. Some will respond to spironolactone, but often blood pressure is not controlled despite restoration of normal plasma electrolytes. These patients may receive considerable benefit from an angiotensin-converting enzyme (ACE) inhibitor [19] or a Ca^{2+}-channel blocking agent [20].

Secondary aldosteronism

The conditions associated with this are listed in Table 34.5. The term 'secondary' indicates that the aldosterone excess results from stimulation of the zona glomerulosa by an external factor (almost invariably AII). The normal physiological response to standing, salt depletion, haemorrhage or severe sweating involves activation of the renin–

Table 34.5 Aetiology of secondary aldosteronism.

Physiological
Sodium deprivation/volume depletion
Pregnancy
Pathological
Associated with normal or low blood pressure
Congestive heart failure
Nephrotic syndrome
Reduction of 'effective' intravascular volume
Cirrhosis with ascites
Bartter's syndrome
Salt-losing renal or bowel disease
Idiopathic oedema
Diuretic abuse
Associated with hypertension
Malignant or accelerated phase hypertension
Diuretic therapy in hypertensive patient
Renin-secreting tumours
Some cases of renal artery stenosis or ischaemia

angiotensin–aldosterone system in an attempt to restore the effective intravascular volume. In pregnancy, elevated progesterone levels block the effect of aldosterone and hence produce a natriuresis which stimulates a compensatory increase in renin and aldosterone. This antagonistic; effect of progesterone may explain why the hypertension in patients with aldosterone-producing adenomas may resolve in pregnancy and return post-partum [21].

Various hypotheses have been put forward to explain the stimuli to salt and water retention found in normotensive causes of secondary aldosteronism associated with oedema. It has been suggested that in one group renal sodium and water retention is initiated by a fall in cardiac output (low-output cardiac failure, hypovolaemic nephrotic syndrome), and in the other by peripheral arterial vasodilatation (high-output cardiac failure, cirrhosis, vasodilator therapy). Both result in a fall in effective arterial blood volume which then provokes the release of renin and vasopressin, and activation of the sympathetic nervous system. These in turn act to restore the effective volume by retention of salt and water (see also Chapter 79). For a full review of the conditions associated with secondary aldosteronism, see [22].

Excess production of mineralocorticoids other than aldosterone

Congenital adrenal hyperplasia

Two forms of congenital adrenal hyperplasia are associated with mineralocorticoid excess, 17α-hydroxylase and 11β-hydroxylase deficiency. These are very rare in comparison with 21-hydroxylase deficiency (see Chapter 35).

17α-Hydroxylase deficiency

In 17α-hydroxylase deficiency the defective production of cortisol activates ACTH negative-feedback control, which then stimulates production of corticosterone and deoxy-corticosterone (DOC). Aldosterone secretion is usually low [23] but gradually returns towards normal with glucocorticoid replacement therapy, indicating that there is not a separate block in the aldosterone biosynthetic pathway. The enzyme defect is also present in the gonads. Thus, females present with primary amenorrhoea and males with pseudo-hermaphroditism in addition to hypertension and hypokalaemia.

It would seem very likely that the DOC and corticosterone originate from the zona fasciculata. Other steroids produced in excess are 18-OH-DOC and 18-OH-corticosterone. Both the basal and ACTH stimulated levels of DOC, corticos-terone, 18-OH-DOC and 18-OH-corticosterone are elevated in heterozygotes [24].

Two sisters with 17α-hydroxylase deficiency and hyper-aldosteronism have been reported [25]. In the untreated state, ACTH regulated the plasma aldosterone levels, but during glucocorticoid replacement therapy control was by the renin–angiotensin system.

11β-Hydroxylase deficiency

In this condition there is impaired conversion of DOC to corticosterone and of 11-deoxycortisol to cortisol. The increased secretion of ACTH results in elevation of DOC with sodium retention and hypertension. In addition, there is increased androgen production with clitoromegaly in the female and precocious puberty in the male. However, there may be no correlation between the degree of virilisation and the mineralocorticoid excess [26], and even in those who are hypertensive hypokalaemia may not be present. Several cases have now been described where the defect has been partial and the condition has presented in adults with menstrual dysfunction, acne and hypertension [27].

Both forms of congenital adrenal hyperplasia should be treated with glucocorticoid replacement therapy, as discussed in Chapter 35. As indicated above, patients with 17α-hydroxylase deficiency will usually have a gradual recovery of zona glomerulosa function. In 11β-hydroxylase deficiency glucocorticoid therapy alone should be given initially, but the plasma renin activity should be monitored and, if this is elevated, mineralocorticoid replacement with fludrocortisone should be added.

11β-Hydroxysteroid dehydrogenase deficiency

11β-Hydroxysteroid dehydrogenase (11β-HSD) is the enzyme complex responsible for the interconversion of the active glucocorticoid cortisol and inactive cortisone (Fig. 34.12). The complex is now known to consist of two isoforms, 11β-HSD1 which is found principally in the liver and converts cortisone to cortisol, and 11β-HSD2 which is located in all aldosterone-selective target tissues such as the distal nephron, colon and salivary glands, and which metabolises cortisol to cortisone. Even though this metabolic pathway has been known for many years, it is only relatively recently that its full biological importance has been appreciated [28]. This understanding has stemmed from the study of congenital and acquired 11β-HSD deficiency. In congenital 11β-HSD deficiency there is severe hypertension and hypokalaemia with suppression of the renin–angiotensin–aldosterone axis. The diagnosis has usually been made by measuring the urinary cortisol metabolites (Fig. 34.12). In normal subjects the ratio of tetrahydrocortisol plus allotetrahydrocortisol/ tetrahydrocortisone is usually about 1.3. In 11β-HSD deficiency it is markedly increased. The condition has been called

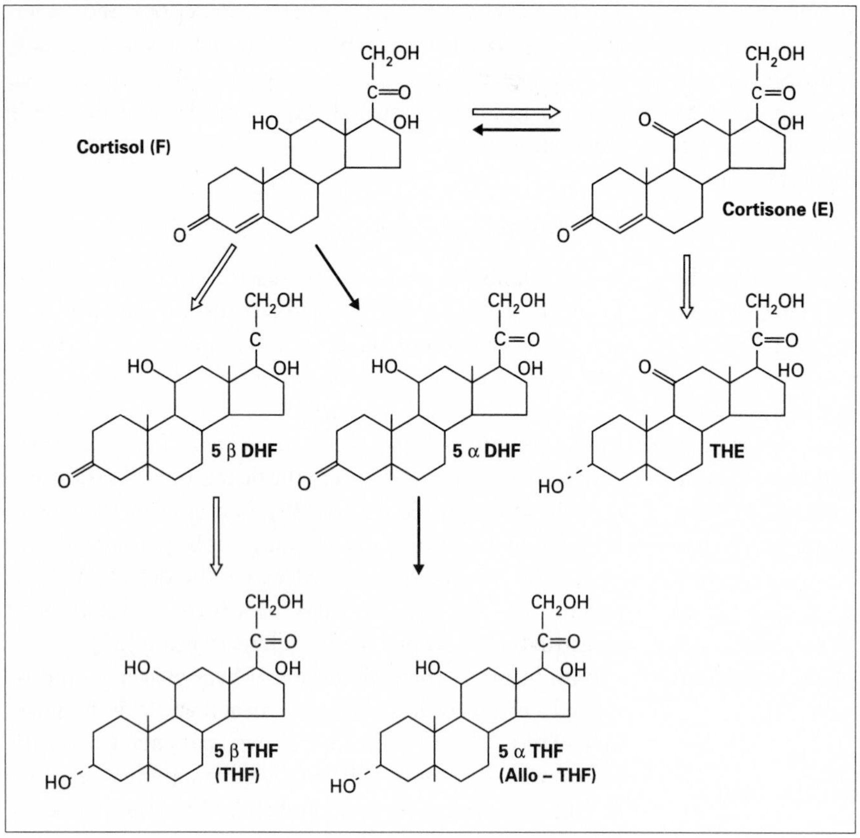

Fig. 34.12 Pathways of cortisol metabolism indicating key role played by 11β-hydroxysteroid dehydrogenase in the interconversion of cortisol and cortisone.

'the syndrome of apparent mineralocorticoid excess' because, despite the clinical and biochemical picture, no excess mineralocorticoid production can be demonstrated [29]. Our own studies have shown that in these patients cortisol in physiological amounts acts as a very potent mineralocorticoid [30]. We suggested that in the normal kidney the non-specific renal mineralocorticoid receptor was protected from cortisol by the metabolism of cortisol to inactive cortisone [31], but this mechanism was absent in patients with 11β-HSD deficiency. Our further work demonstrated that liquorice produced sodium retention and hypertension by inhibition of 11β-HSD (see below).

Congenital 11β-HSD deficiency is a rare condition of which about 30 cases have been reported in children and one in an adult. Several of the children have died, usually from cardiovascular complications secondary to poor control of hypertension. In several cases, administration of dexamethasone in a dose adequate to suppress cortisol production has lowered blood pressure and restored plasma potassium concentration to normal. The explanation for this is that dexamethasone binds type 2 glucocorticoid receptors more selectively than type 1 mineralocorticoid receptors, in contrast to cortisol which in the absence of 11β-HSD has a high affinity for the mineralocorticoid receptor. It has recently been shown that this condition is due to a mutation in the gene coding for the 11β-HSD2 enzyme [32].

Pseudo-hyperaldosteronism

Several conditions have been described in which there is mineralocorticoid excess mimicking Conn's syndrome but in which aldosterone levels are not elevated. The term 'pseudo-hyperaldosteronism' has been applied to these. However, recent advances have shown that this is a very heterogeneous group.

Liddle's syndrome

In this condition there is abnormal renal tubular ionic transport which results in excessive sodium reabsorption and potassium loss. The sodium excess leads to suppression of the renin–angiotensin–aldosterone system. The patients present with hypertension and have a biochemical picture indicative of mineralocorticoid excess. The condition is inherited as an autosomal dominant. The molecular pathology of this syndrome has recently been described. It relates to dysfunction of the amiloride-sensitive sodium channel which is responsible for sodium reabsorption in the distal nephron,

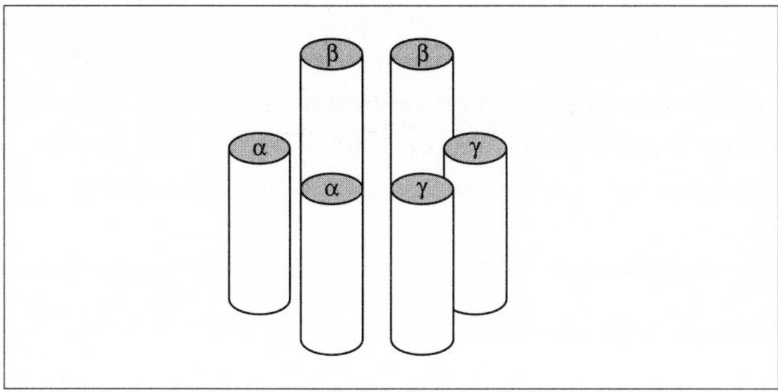

Fig. 34.13 Hexameric arrangement of subunits in epithelial sodium channel.

salivary glands, colon and lung. This channel consists of three homologous subunits called α, β and γ ENaC. These are arranged in pairs to form a hexamer (Fig. 34.13). Liddle's syndrome has been shown to be due to mutations in the C-terminal intracellular domain of the β-subunit (or in some cases of the γ-subunit) (Fig. 34.14) [33]. The mutations result in constitutive activation of the channel; this could be due to a failure of the normal process by which the channel is recycled.

The patients present with hypertension and have a biochemical picture indicative of mineralocorticoid excess (i.e. suppressed plasma renin activity and hypokalaemia but with low plasma aldosterone levels). The condition responds to inhibitors of renal tubular ionic transport such as amiloride (which bind to the sodium channel) but not to mineralocorticoid-receptor antagonists such as spironolactone.

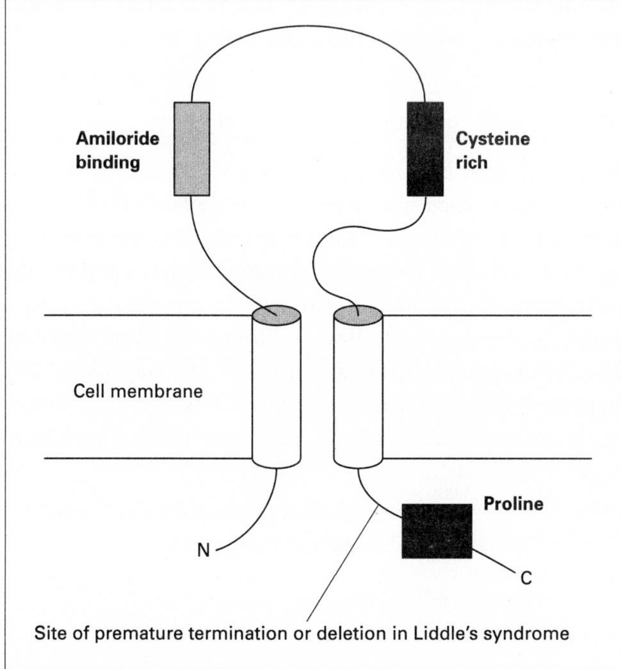

Fig. 34.14 Molecular pathogenesis of Liddle's syndrome showing site of mutations in the intracellular domain of the β-subunit of the epithelial sodium channel.

Liquorice ingestion

Liquorice abuse has long been known to be associated with hypertension and hypokalaemia. This was thought to be due to a direct effect of the active components of liquorice, glycyrrhetinic acid and glycyrrhizic acid. At high doses these were shown to displace aldosterone from the mineralocorticoid receptor. However, previous studies had shown that liquorice did not produce sodium retention when given to adrenalectomised animals or humans, indicating that this could not be a direct effect. Our own studies have shown that liquorice administration has marked effects on cortisol metabolism [34], and that glycyrrhetinic acid is a potent inhibitor of 11β-hydroxysteroid dehydrogenase [35]. These results explain why dexamethasone blocks the mineralocorticoid effect of liquorice.

Carbenoxolone

This is the hemisuccinate derivative of glycyrrhetinic acid which has been used in the treatment of peptic ulcer and reflux oesophagitis. Its administration produces sodium retention and hypokalaemia. However, unlike liquorice the hypokalaemia is not associated with a kaliuresis. Interestingly, carbenoxolone is a potent inhibitor of 11β-HSD1 and 2, unlike liquorice which only blocks the oxidation of cortisol to cortisone (i.e. 11β-HSD2) [36]. It is unclear why this might allow renal sodium retention but not potassium loss.

Exogenous mineralocorticoids

The administration of excess mineralocorticoids such as fludrocortisone will produce hypertension and hypokalaemia. This is not usually a diagnostic problem because the patient is known to be on mineralocorticoid replacement therapy. However, there can be diagnostic difficulty if the physician fails to appreciate that some drugs thought to be glucocorticoids can have profound mineralocorticoid effects. Thus, several patients have developed severe hypertension and hypokalaemia with suppressed plasma renin activity and aldosterone following the chronic use of a nasal spray containing 9α-fluoroprednisolone for chronic rhinitis [37]. A 2-month-old breast-fed infant was also found to be severely hypertensive and hypokalaemic secondary to the mother using 9α-fluoroprednisolone on her bruised nipples. In a further case, the same features stemmed from this steroid being used in the chronic treatment of eczema.

Cushing's syndrome

Patients with the ectopic ACTH syndrome almost invariably have a hypokalaemic alkalosis, whereas this is uncommon in those with pituitary-dependent Cushing's disease. Recent studies have demonstrated that in the ectopic ACTH syndrome there is an elevated cortisol/cortisone ratio in comparison to other forms of Cushing's syndrome [38]. This suggests that there is inhibition of 11β-hydroxysteroid dehydrogenase and that the hypokalaemia may relate to the same aetiology as in the apparent mineralocorticoid excess syndrome with cortisol gaining access to the non-specific, unprotected mineralocorticoid receptor. Patients with the ectopic ACTH syndrome also tend to have higher ACTH and cortisol levels; in addition, plasma DOC and corticosterone levels are elevated. However, with chronic ACTH excess, aldosterone levels are either normal or low.

Cushing's syndrome in pregnancy, whether pituitary dependent or due to an adrenal adenoma, is commonly associated with severe hypokalaemia (Table 34.6). It is interesting to speculate whether the profound changes in renal function during pregnancy might also result in the normal mineralocorticoid receptor protection by 11β-hydroxysteroid dehydrogenase being less effective.

Some patients with Cushing's syndrome have activation of the renin–angiotensin system, presumably reflecting effects of glucocorticoid on plasma renin substrate among other actions. Some authors have reported elevated AII and a positive correlation with the serum cortisol [43]. Others have found that there may be a significant response of blood pressure to captopril in Cushing's syndrome and this, as in other forms of hypertension, relates to the pretreatment level of plasma renin activity [44].

As in essential hypertension, several researchers have looked for mineralocorticoids other than aldosterone which might explain hypertension in Cushing's syndrome. Elevated levels of 19-nor-deoxycorticosterone (a steroid which lacks the 19-methyl group) have been found in both pituitary-dependent Cushing's syndrome and in patients with adrenal tumours producing Cushing's syndrome [45]. The relationship of this steroid to the blood pressure elevation is unknown.

Adrenal carcinomas producing aldosterone are a rare cause of primary aldosteronism. These tumours may produce a wide variety of steroids in addition to aldosterone, including cortisol and androgens. The clinical picture may thus be a mixture of mineralocorticoid, glucocorticoid and androgen excess.

Primary cortisol resistance

A small number of patients with primary cortisol resistance have been described [46–48]. This is a familial condition in which there may be mineralocorticoid excess with hypertension, hypokalaemia and metabolic alkalosis. The patients have elevated cortisol secretion rates and high plasma and urinary free cortisol levels, but do not develop the features of Cushing's syndrome. The plasma ACTH levels are high and do not suppress with conventional low-dose dexamethasone. The mineralocorticoid excess has been thought to be due to the elevated levels of corticosterone and DOC, but the role played by cortisol acting on mineralocorticoid receptors is unclear. Studies on the glucocorticoid receptor have shown that it is abnormal with a low affinity for dexamethasone, and in some cases mutations in the gene encoding the receptor protein have been found. The condition can be treated by giving a dose of dexamethasone which is sufficient to suppress ACTH (usually about 3 mg/day). The clinical presentation of this condition is not invariably with hypertension; in women, severe hirsutism may be the presenting problem, with high levels of adrenal androgens secondary to the increased ACTH drive.

Isolated DOC or corticosterone excess

Rarely, adrenal tumours may produce either DOC or corticosterone as their major product. In isolated DOC excess a clinical picture similar to primary aldosteronism may be seen [49]. In such patients aldosterone levels have usually been normal and not suppressed as one might expect. Some of these patients have subsequently been found to have primary aldosteronism with intermittent aldosterone hypersecretion. Corticosterone-producing adrenal tumours are usually carcinomas, and again may present with min-

Table 34.6 Hypokalaemia in Cushing's syndrome in pregnancy.

Reference	Year	Cause of Cushing's syndrome	Plasma [K^+] (mmol/l)
Kreines *et al.* [39]	1964	Adrenal adenoma	2.3
Parra and Cruz-Krohn [40]	1966	Adrenal adenoma	3.1
Wieland *et al.* [41]	1971	Pituitary dependent	2.2
Semple *et al.* [42]	1985	Pituitary dependent	2.2

Table 34.7 Causes of mineralocorticoid deficiency.

Adrenal hypoplasia
Congenital adrenal hyperplasia
Pseudo-hypoaldosteronism
Hyporeninaemic hypoaldosteronism
Aldosterone biosynthetic defects (CMO types I and II)
Addison's disease
Adrenoleucodystrophy
Drug induced

CMO, corticosterone methyl oxidase.

eralocorticoid hypersecretion [50]. The prognosis in such patients is very poor.

Mineralocorticoid deficiency syndromes

The causes of mineralocorticoid deficiency are given in Table 34.7. They can be subdivided into a congenital and an acquired group.

Adrenal hypoplasia

This is a rare X-linked condition which presents in infancy with features of salt-losing adrenocortical insufficiency and is frequently associated with hypogonadotrophic hypogonadism. Mutations in the X-chromosome gene DAX-1 (dosage-sensitive sex critical region in the X gene 1) have recently been identified and shown to be responsible for this disorder. In contrast to 21-hydroxylase deficiency, the patients do not have ambiguous external genitalia and the urinary 17-oxosteroids and pregnanetriol and the plasma 17-hydroxyprogesterone are not elevated. CT scanning of the adrenals confirms the adrenal hypoplasia (see also Chapter 36).

Adrenoleucodystrophy

This is an X-linked recessive disorder characterised by adrenal insufficiency, demyelinating lesions in the central nervous system and elevated circulating levels of very long chain fatty acids. The adrenal insufficiency can range from the patient being asymptomatic with elevated ACTH levels to complete adrenal insufficiency.

Congenital adrenal hyperplasia

This subject is covered in detail in Chapter 35. The commonest enzyme defect is that of 21-hydroxylase. In about three-quarters of cases of so-called classical (i.e. presenting at birth) 21-hydroxylase deficiency, there is salt wasting with deficient aldosterone synthesis. This is a higher percentage than originally thought, and reflects a variety of factors including more sensitive methods of ascertainment including measurement of plasma renin activity and aldosterone. Usually within a family there is a consistent pattern with regard to the presence or absence of salt wasting [51]. Even though the salt wasting may improve with age, it is common to find that adults who are not thought to be salt losers have elevated plasma renin activity.

In the simple virilising form of 21-hydroxylase deficiency, plasma aldosterone levels may actually be elevated. This is thought to be a compensatory response to the elevated levels of natriuretic steroids such as progesterone. In addition to aldosterone, plasma levels of DOC and 18-hydroxycorticosterone are also elevated in these patients, thus providing further evidence that the 21-hydroxylase in the zona glomerulosa differs from that in the zona fasciculata [52].

Maintaining sodium balance is critical in optimal control of patients with 21-hydroxylase deficiency and hence in height prognosis. In children with this condition, the addition of mineralocorticoid replacement therapy to the glucocorticoid regimen produces a very significant improvement in control as judged by further reduction of 17-hydroxyprogesterone and androgens together with increased linear growth [53,54]. This is true not only in severe salt losers, but also in those who do not require mineralocorticoids yet have elevated plasma renin activity. The reason for this is not clear. It was initially thought to relate to a stimulatory effect of AII on ACTH release. However, studies in which AII levels have been altered by either manipulation of sodium status or by AII infusion have not shown changes in plasma ACTH levels but have demonstrated that high levels of AII stimulate 17-hydroxyprogesterone (17-OHP), whereas 17-OHP falls when AII is low [55].

As with 21-hydroxylase deficiency, patients with 3β-HSD deficiency may or may not have salt wasting (see [56] for review).

The condition of lipoid adrenal hyperplasia is an autosomal recessive disorder with associated profound deficits of all adrenal and gonadal steroids. This is a very rare defect with only 32 cases in the literature. Only rarely has a child survived beyond infancy. The molecular defect in this condition has now been discovered. There is a defect in the function of the so-called StAR protein (*St*eroidogenic *A*cute *R*egulatory protein) which is responsible for translocating cholesterol into the mitochondrial membrane. Several mutations have now been reported in the StAR gene in patients with the disease.

Pseudo-hypoaldosteronism

This condition usually presents in infancy with severe salt wasting and failure to thrive. The child has hyponatraemia, hyperkalaemia, high urinary sodium excretion and very high levels of plasma renin activity and aldosterone. Mineralocorticoid-receptor studies have been carried out using monocytes which, in normal subjects, bind labelled aldosterone with high affinity. In affected children either no binding or a very reduced level has been found [57]. The abnormality appears to be transmitted in an autosomal recessive manner. Despite extensive studies no mutations have been found in the mineralocorticoid-receptor gene. The heterozygotes have been shown to have a reduced number of monocyte aldosterone-binding sites.

Some interesting patients with so-called type II pseudo-hypoaldosteronism have been described. These have mineralocorticoid-resistant hyperkalaemia but do not have the salt wasting found in the type I condition. It has been suggested that the primary abnormality in these patients is excessive reabsorption of chloride by the distal nephron which reduces the sodium and mineralocorticoid-dependent driving force for potassium and hydrogen ion secretion (thus producing hyperkalaemia and acidosis), and increases sodium chloride reabsorption which produces hyperchloraemia, volume expansion, hyporeninaemia and hypertension [58]. A similar hyperkalaemic distal renal tubular acidosis may be associated with obstructive uropathy.

Hyporeninaemic hypoaldosteronism

Patients with this condition are often elderly and may present with recurrent arrhythmias. Investigation reveals hyperkalaemia, acidosis and mild to moderate impairment of renal function. Further study shows isolated aldosterone deficiency with otherwise intact adrenal function and low levels of plasma renin activity. A wide variety of renal diseases have been thought to lead to damage to the juxtaglomerular apparatus. Of these, diabetic nephropathy is the commonest. Dynamic function testing with salt depletion, erect posture and frusemide administration demonstrates subnormal responses of plasma renin activity and aldosterone. Some patients, but not all, show an aldosterone response to AII infusion.

Fludrocortisone is the obvious first-line treatment to replace aldosterone, together with dietary potassium restriction. However, this often leads to problems because of expansion of the extracellular fluid volume with resultant hypertension. In these patients the addition of frusemide is of value. This drug alone increases acid excretion and thus improves the metabolic acidosis. However, the acid response is limited by aldosterone deficiency and the addition of fludrocortisone increases acid excretion [59].

Patients with suspected hyporeninaemic hypoaldosteronism often present a complex problem in which several factors may contribute to the hyperkalaemia. These include drugs inhibiting renin release such as prostaglandin synthetase inhibitors and β-adrenoceptor blockers, insulin deficiency, inappropriate potassium supplementation and the use of inhibitors of renal tubular ionic transport or aldosterone antagonists. Withdrawal of the appropriate drug or improved control of diabetes is then necessary to determine whether the problem is entirely drug related or due to the drug exacerbating an underlying defect in renin secretion.

Aldosterone biosynthetic defects

Isolated aldosterone deficiency has been postulated to result from defective conversion of corticosterone to 18-hydroxycorticosterone by corticosterone methyl oxidase type I (CMO-I; 18-hydroxylase), or of 18-hydroxycorticosterone to aldosterone by corticosterone methyl oxidase type II (CMO-II; 18-dehydrogenase). Congenital deficiency of these enzymes was then suggested to result in hyponatraemia and hyperkalaemia. Recently it has been shown that the two steps in the synthesis of aldosterone are catalysed not by two different enzymes but by a single multifunctional one called steroid 18-hydroxylase (P-450C18) or aldosterone synthase (P-450_{aldo}). The CMO-deficient patients have null mutations of the gene encoding the enzyme (CYP11B2) with a complete lack of aldosterone synthase activity. The CMO-II-deficient patients have leaky mutations with altered aldosterone synthase activity. The specific defect can be identified by measuring plasma corticosterone, 18-hydroxycorticosterone and aldosterone levels or the urinary metabolites. These conditions are inherited as autosomal recessive disorders.

Rosler has studied the natural history of salt wasting in the type II defect and has compared this with pseudo-hypoaldosteronism [60]. In both conditions there was progressive normalisation of sodium balance with increasing age. In the type II defect the plasma 18-hydroxycorticosterone/aldosterone ratio ranged between 160 and 760, whereas it was normal in pseudo-hypoaldosteronism (6.9 ± 5.1 (SD)). In addition to elevated 18-hydroxycorticosterone, patients with both conditions had increased deoxycorticosterone levels.

In some patients defective aldosterone secretion has been due to an acquired biosynthetic defect. For a full review of this area see [61].

Addison's disease

This is an important cause of mineralocorticoid deficiency and is covered in detail in Chapter 36. Unfortunately, investigation of mineralocorticoid production in these patients is often neglected, and there are thus few data comparing zona glomerulosa with zona fasciculata function either before or during glucocorticoid replacement therapy. The latter is relevant as chronic ACTH excess will stimulate zona glomerulosa DOC secretion. Measurement of plasma renin activity is an important part of the assessment of the adequacy of glucocorticoid replacement. Many patients appear to require only hydrocortisone replacement as judged by plasma electrolytes and yet have elevated plasma renin activity. As with 21-hydroxylase deficiency, the addition of fludrocortisone may improve glucocorticoid control as judged by a fall in plasma ACTH before the morning dose of hydrocortisone.

Drug-induced mineralocorticoid deficiency

Several of the drugs which affect mineralocorticoid secretion either directly (e.g. aldosterone antagonists) or indirectly (e.g. ACE inhibitors) have been mentioned in the section on hyporeninaemic hypoaldosteronism. In addition to these, heparin has been shown to inhibit aldosterone production as indicated by a fall in plasma aldosterone levels during heparin therapy coupled with a rise in plasma renin activity [62]. The authors suggest that in normal subjects with an intact renin–angiotensin–aldosterone axis the effect is not clinically relevant. However, in patients with defective aldosterone production, such as in some diabetics, mineralocorticoid deficiency could be produced.

Another significant drug interaction is that of phenytoin with fludrocortisone. Patients with adrenal insufficiency who are on fludrocortisone may require a large increase in fludrocortisone dose if given phenytoin [63]. Even though phenytoin also enhances the metabolic clearance of hydrocortisone with increased 6β-hydroxycortisol production, this is less marked. Lithium has been found to block the action of fludrocortisone on the kidney.

Summary

Disorders of mineralocorticoid secretion are common in clinical practice and may be life-threatening if not correctly diagnosed and appropriately treated. In the majority of cases there is secondary hyperaldosteronism with activation of the renin–angiotensin system. Primary mineralocorticoid excess is relatively rare but should be considered in all patients with hypertension and hypokalaemia, and in those with drug-resistant hypertension. Recent advances in our understanding of the role played by 11β-hydroxysteroid dehydrogenase in the protection of the mineralocorticoid receptor from cortisol have led to an appreciation of how, when this enzyme is inhibited (e.g. by liquorice), cortisol can produce mineralocorticoid excess.

Salt wasting with hyperkalaemia is the commonest presentation of aldosterone biosynthetic or receptor defects. Even though the salt wasting found in children improves with age, mineralocorticoid replacement is usually required to achieve normal growth velocity. In adults with 21-hydroxylase deficiency the addition of mineralocorticoid to glucocorticoid therapy will also facilitate control. In the elderly patient with hyperkalaemia, hyporeninaemic hypoaldosteronism should be considered and needs to be distinguished from a variety of drug-induced and other conditions.

References

1 Conn JW, Morita R, Cohen EL, Beierwaltes WH, McDonald WJ, Herwig KR. Normokalemic primary aldosteronism: its masquerade as 'essential hypertension'. *JAMA* 1972; **195**: 21–6.

2 Fishman LM, Kuchel O, Liddle GW, Michelakis AM, Gordon RD, Chick WT. Incidence of primary aldosteronism in uncomplicated 'essential' hypertension. *JAMA* 1968; **205**: 497–502.

3 Laragh JH, Sealey JE, Sommers SC. Patterns of adrenal secretion and urinary excretion of aldosterone and plasma renin activity in normal and hypertensive subjects. *Circ Res* 1966; **19** (Suppl. I): 158–74.

4 Bravo EL, Tarazi RC, Fouad FM, Textor SC. A reappraisal of the diagnostic criteria for primary aldosteronism. *Clin Sci* 1982; **63**: 975.

5 Skrabal F, Aubock J, Edwards CRW, Braunsteiner H. Subtraction potential difference: *in vivo* assay for mineralocorticoid activity. *Lancet* 1978; i: 298–302.

6 Hiramatsu K, Yamada T, Yukimura Y *et al.* A screening test to identify aldosterone-producing adenoma by measuring plasma renin activity. Results in hypertensive patients. *Arch Intern Med* 1981; **141**: 1589–93.

7 McKenna TJ, Sequeira SJ, Heffernan A, Chambers J, Cunningham S. Diagnosis under random conditions of all disorders of the renin–angiotensin–aldosterone axis, including primary hyperaldosteronism. *J Clin Endocrinol Metab* 1991; **73**: 952–7.

8 Gordon RD, Stowasser M, Tunny TJ, Klemm SA, Rutherford JC. High incidence of primary aldosteronism in 199 patients referred with hypertension. *Clin Exp Pharmacol Physiol* 1994; **21**: 315–8.

9 Lifton RP, Dluhy RG, Powers M *et al.* A chimaeric 11β-hydroxylase/aldosterone synthase gene causes glucocorticoid-remediable aldosteronism and human hypertension. *Nature* 1992; **355**: 262–5.

10 Gordon RD, Hamlet SM, Tunny TJ, Klemm SA. Aldosterone-producing adenomas responsive to angiotensin pose problems in diagnosis. *Clin Exp Pharmacol Physiol* 1987; **14**: 175–8.

11 Ulick S, Chu MD. Hypersecretion of a new corticosteroid, 18-hydroxycortisol in two types of adrenocortical hypertension. *Clin Exp Hypertens* 1982; **4**: 1771–7.

12 Corrie JET, Edwards CRW, Budd PS. A radioimmunoassay for 18-hydroxycortisol in plasma and urine. *Clin Chem* 1985; **31**: 849–52.

13 Corrie JET, Edwards CRW, Jones DB, Padfield PL, Budd PS. Factors

affecting the secretion of 18-hydroxycortisol, a novel steroid of relevance to Conn's syndrome. *Clin Endocrinol* 1985; **23**: 579–86.

14 Davis JRE, Burt D, Corrie JET, Edwards CRW, Sheppard MC. Dexamethasone-suppressible hyperaldosteronism: studies on over-production of 18-hydroxycortisol in three affected family members. *Endocrinol* 1988; **29**: 297–308.

15 Gomez-Sanchez CE, Montgomery M, Ganguly A *et al.* Elevated urinary excretion of 18-oxocortisol in glucocorticoid-suppressible aldosteronism. *J Clin Endocrinol Metab* 1984; **59**: 1022–4.

16 Woodland E, Tunny TJ, Hamlet SM, Gordon RD. Hypertension corrected and aldosterone responsiveness to renin–angiotensin restored by long-term dexamethasone in glucocorticoid suppressible hyperaldosteronism. *Clin Exp Pharmacol Physiol* 1985; **12**: 245–8.

17 Lyons DF, Kem DC, Brown RD, Hanson CS, Corollo ML. Single dose captopril as a diagnostic test for primary aldosteronism. *J Clin Endocrinol Metab* 1983; **57**: 892–6.

18 Young WF, Klee GG. Primary aldosteronism. Diagnostic evaluation. *Endocrinol Metab Clin North Am* 1988; **17**: 367–95.

19 Griffing GT, Melby JC. The therapeutic effect of a new converting enzyme inhibitor, enalaprilat maleate in idiopathic hyperaldosteronism. *J Clin Hypertens* 1985; **3**: 265–76.

20 Nadler JL, Hsueh W, Horton R. Therapeutic effect of calcium channel blockade in primary aldosteronism. *J Clin Endocrinol Metab* 1985; **60**: 896–9.

21 Gordon RD, Tunny TJ, Aldosterone-producing adenoma: effect of pregnancy. *Clin Exp Hypertens* 1982; **4**: 1685–93.

22 Schrier RW. Symposium on hormonal control of blood pressure and hydro-electrolytic metabolism. 33 EMES journees internationale Henri-Pierre Klotz. *D'endocrinologie Clinique* 1990: 8–19.

23 New MI, Wight PC, Speiser PW, Crawford C, DuPont B. Congenital adrenal hyperplasia. In: Edwards CRW, Lincoln DW, eds. *Recent Advances in Endocrinology and Metabolism*, Vol. 3. Edinburgh: Churchill Livingstone, 1989: 29–76.

24 D'Armiento M, Reda G, Kater C, Shackleton CH, Biglieri EG. 17α-hydroxylase defidency: mineralocorticoid hormone profiles in an affected family. *J Clin Endocrinol Metab* 1983; **56**: 697–701.

25 Monno S, Takasu N. A new variant of 17α-hydroxylase defidency with hyperaldosteronism in two Japanese sisters. *Endocrinol Jpn* 1989; **36**: 315–23.

26 Rosler A, Leiberman E, Sack J *et al.* Clinical variability of congenital adrenal hyperplasia due to 11β-hydroxylase defidency. *Horm Res* 1982; **16**: 133–41.

27 Cathelineau G, Breurault JL, Fiet J, Julien R, Arux C, Canivet J. Adrenocortical 11β-hydroxylation defect in adult women with post-menarchial onset of symptoms. *J Clin Endocrinol Metab* 1980; **51**: 287–91.

28 Stewart PM, Edwards CRW. Specificity of the mineralocorticoid receptor: crutial role of 11β-hydroxysteroid dehydrogenase. *Trends Endocrinol Metab* 1990; **1**: 225–30.

29 Ulick S, Levine LS, Gunczler P *et al.* A syndrome of apparent mineralocorticoid excess associated with defects in the peripheral metabolism of cortisol. *J Clin Endocrinol Metab* 1979; **49**: 757–64.

30 Stewart PM, Corrie JET, Shackleton CHL, Edwards CRW. Syndrome of apparent mineralocorticoid excess: a defect in the cortisol–cortisone shuttle. *J Clin Invest* 1988; **82**: 340–9.

31 Edwards CRW, Stewart PM, Burt D *et al.* Localisation of 11β-hydroxysteroid dehydrogenase: tissue specific protector of the mineralocorticoid receptor. *Lancet* 1988; **ii**: 986–8.

32 Mune T, Rogerson FM, Nikkila H, Agarwal AK, White PC. Human hypertension caused by mutations in the kidney isozyme of 11β-hydroxysteroid dehydrogenase. *Nature Genet* 1995; **10**: 394–9.

33 Shimkets RA, Warnock DG, Bositis CM *et al.* Liddle's syndrome: heritable human hypertension caused by mutations in the β-subunit of the epithelial sodium channel. *Cell* 1994; **79**: 407–14.

34 Stewart PM, Valentino R, Wallace AM, Burt D, Shackleton CHL, Edwards CRW. Mineralocorticoid activity of liquorice: 11β-hydroxysteroid dehydrogenase deficiency comes of age. *Lancet* 1987; **ii**: 821–4.

35 Monder C, Stewart PM, Lakshmi V, Valentino R, Burt D, Edwards CRW. Liquorice inhibits corticosteroid 11β-dehydrogenase of rat kidney and liver: *in vivo* and *in vitro* studies. *Endocrinology* 1989; **125**: 1046–53.

36 Stewart PM, Wallace AM, Atherden SM, Shearing CH, Edwards CRW. Mineralocorticoid activity of carbenoxolone: contrasting effects of carbenoxolone and liquorice on 11β-hydroxysteroid dehydrogenase activity in man. *Clin Sci* 1990; **78**: 49–54.

37 Mantero F, Armanini D, Opocher G *et al.* Mineralocorticoid hypertension due to a nasal spray containing Gα-flurprednisolone. *Am J Med* 1981; **71**: 352–7.

38 Walker BR, Campbell JC, Fraser R, Stewart PM, Edwards CRW. Mineralocorticoid excess and inhibition of 11β-hydroxysteroid dehydrogenase in patients with ectopic ACTH syndrome. *Clin Endocrinol* 1992; **27**: 483–92.

39 Kreines K, Perin E, Salzer R. Pregnancy in Cushing's syndrome. *J Clin Endocrinol* 1964; **24**: 75–9.

40 Parra A, Cruz-Krohn J. Intercurrent Cushing's syndrome and pregnancy. *Am J Med* 1966; **40**: 961–6.

41 Wieland O, Siess E, Schulze-Wethmar FH *et al.* Active and inactive forms of pyruvate dehydrogenase in rat heart and kidney: effect of diabetes fasting, and re-feeding on pyruvate. *Arch Biochem Biophys* 1971; **143**: 593–601.

42 Semple CG, McEwan H, Teasdale GM, McNicol AM, Thomson JA. Recurrence of Cushing's disease in pregnancy. Case report. *Br J Obstet Gynaecol* 1985; **92**: 295–8.

43 Luton JP, Vidal-Trecan G, Mouveroux F, Bricaire H. Hypertension and Cushing's disease. *Ann Med Interne (Paris)* 1983; **134**: 203–8.

44 Greminger P, Vetter W, Groth H, Luscher T, Tenschert W, Siegenthaler W, Vetter H. Captopril in Cushing's syndrome. *Klin Wochenschr* 1984; **62**: 855–8.

45 Ehlers ME, Griffing GT, Wilson TE, Melby JC. Elevated urinary nordeoxycorticosterone glucuronide in Cushing's syndrome. *J Clin Endocrinol Metab* 1987; **64**: 926–30.

46 Vingerhoeds ACM, Thijssen JHH, Schwartz F. Spontaneous hypercortisolism without Cushing's syndrome. *J Clin Endocrinol Metab* 1976; **43**: 1128–30.

47 Chrousos GP, Vingerhoeds A, Brandon D *et al.* Primary cortisol resistance in man. A glucocorticoid receptor-mediated disease. *J Clin Invest* 1982; **69**: 1261–9.

48 Chrousos GP, Loriaux DL, Brandon D *et al.* Primary cortisol resistance: a familial syndrome and an animal model. *J Steroid Biochem* 1983; **19**: 567–75.

49 Brown JJ, Ferriss JB, Fraser R *et al.* Apparently isolated excess deoxycorticosterone in hypertension. A variant of the mineralocorticoid excess syndrome. *Lancet* 1972; **ii**: 243–7.

50 Fraser R, James VHT, Landon J *et al.* Clinical and biochemical studies of a patient with a corticosterone-secreting adrenocortical tumour. *Lancet* 1968; **ii**: 1116.

51 New MI, Wight BC, Speiser PW, Crawford C, Dupont B. Congenital adrenal hyperplasia. In: Edwards CRW, Lincoln DW, eds. *Recent Advances in Endocrinology and Metabolism*, Vol. 3. Edinburgh:

Churchill Livingstone, 1989: 29–76.

52 Biglieri EG, Wajchenberg BL, Malerbi DA, Okada H, Leme CE, Kater CE. The zonal origins of the mineralocorticoid hormones in the 21-hydroxylation deficiency of congenital adrenal hyperplasia. *J Clin Endocrinol Metab* 1981; **53**: 964–9.

53 Kuhnie U, Rosler A, Pareira JA, Gunzcler P, Levine LS, News MI. The effects of long-term normalisation of sodium balance on linear growth in disorders with aldosterone deficiency. *Acta Endocrinol (Copenh)* 1983; **102**: 577–82.

54 Jansen M, Wit JM, van den Brande JL. Reinstitution of mineralocorticoid therapy in congenital adrenal hyperplasia. Effects of control and growth. *Acta Paediatr Scand* 1981; 70: 229–33.

55 Schaison G, Couzinet B, Gourmelen M, Elkik F, Bougneres P. Angiotensin and adrenal steroidogenesis: study of 21-hydroxylase defident congenital adrenal hyperplasia. *J Clin Endocrinol Metab* 1980; **51**: 1390–4.

56 Pang S, Levine LS, Stoner E *et al.* Non salt-losing congenital adrenal hyperplasia due to 3β-hydroxysteroid dehydrogenase deficiency with normal glumerulosa function. *J Clin Endocrinol Metab* 1983; **56**: 808–18.

57 Armanini D, Kuhnle U, Strasser T *et al.* Aldosterone-receptor deficiency in pseudo-hyperaldosteronism. *N Engl J Med* 1985; **313**: 1178–81.

58 Schambelan M, Sebastian A, Rector FC, Jr. Mineralocorticoid resistant renal hyperkalaemia without salt-wasting (type 11 pseudo hypoaldosteronism): role of increased renal chloride reabsorption. *Kidney Int* 1981; **19**: 716–27.

59 Sebastian A, Schambelan M, Sutton JM. Amelioration of hyperchloraemic acidosis with frusemide therapy in patients with chronic renal insufficiency and type IV renal tubular addosis. *Am J Nephrol* 1984; **4**: 287–300.

60 Rosler A. The natural history of salt-wasting disorders of adrenal and renal origin. *J Clin Endocrinol Metab* 1984; **59**: 689–700.

61 Veldhuis JD, Melby JC. Isolated aldosterone defidency in man: acquired and inborn errors in the biosynthesis or action of aldosterone. *Endocr Rev* 1981; **2**: 495–517.

62 O'Kelly R, Magee F, McKenna TJ. Routine heparine therapy inhibits adrenal aldosterone production. *J Clin Endocrinol Metab* 1983; **56**: 108–12.

63 Keilholz U, Guthrie GP, Jr. Adverse effect of phenytoin on mineralocorticoid replacement with fludrocortisone in adrenal insufficiency. *Am J Med Sci* 1986; **291**: 280–3.

CHAPTER 35

Congenital adrenal hyperplasia

M.C. Young and I.A. Hughes

Introduction

The management of congenital adrenal hyperplasia (CAH) has traditionally fallen to the paediatrician, reflecting the propensity for this disorder to present in childhood. Recently however, there has been increasing recognition of less severe forms of CAH which present atypically to diverse medical specialties. That these 'non-classical' versions may be remarkably common, in conjunction with recent investigations into the molecular genetics of CAH, has led to a resurgence of interest in the condition. This review emphasises the clinical aspects of CAH—when to suspect CAH, how to diagnose it, and what to do about it. Biochemical and physiological principles are touched upon where necessary, but for details the reader is referred elsewhere [1–3].

Definitions and classification

The taxonomy of CAH has developed historically and can be confusing. Therefore, we have attempted to adopt a consistent and clinically pertinent classification and terminology throughout. 'Congenital adrenal hyperplasia' is the name given to inborn errors of cortisol biosynthesis. It is not a single disease entity, but comprises five disorders which share similar pathophysiology and symptomatology (Table 35.1). Disorders affecting exclusively aldosterone synthesis, often included for convenience, will not be discussed.

'Congenital' originally described the presentation of CAH during early infancy, but now denotes the inherited nature (autosomal recessive) of the disorder.

'Adrenal hyperplasia' refers to the characteristic finding of grossly enlarged adrenals in neonatal deaths due to this condition, occasionally demonstrable in living subjects.

'Classical' refers to the traditional, severe forms of CAH predominately occurring in the neonate and young infant. Its counterpart, 'non-classical', describes milder variants presenting in later childhood or thereafter.

The term 'adrenogenital syndrome' is not synonymous with CAH and has no place in current practice.

Pathophysiology

The biosynthesis of adrenal corticosteroids is complex [4]; a simplified version is shown in Fig. 35.1. Table 35.2 shows abbreviations used for steroids and related substances throughout this review.

Three major classes of steroids are produced: mineralocorticoids (principally aldosterone), glucocorticoids (principally cortisol) and androgens (principally androstenedione and dehydroepiandrosterone).

The synthesis of cortisol from cholesterol involves at least five steps, each enzymatically controlled. CAH represents a deficiency in one of these steps. This may involve a reduction in the amount of enzyme present or impaired functional activity, depending on the genetic basis for the disorder in each individual [3]. In 21-hydroxylase deficiency (21-OHD), complete deletion of the gene encoding this enzyme—and hence a probable absolute deficiency—is present in some cases, whilst in others mutational changes in the gene probably result in a less active version of the enzyme [5–8]. This genotypic variability undoubtedly accounts for some of the remarkable phenotypic variability of CAH. Some individuals can produce normal amounts of cortisol under basal conditions, and may remain totally undetected ('cryptic') unless deliberately, sought, or may present with mild symptoms at a later age ('late onset'). Others have a profound deficiency and manifest early with severe disease. Phenotypic variability has been most well documented for 21-OHD [9], but less severe (non-classical) forms of 11β-hydroxylase deficiency (11β-OHD) and 3β-hydroxysteroid dehydrogenase (3β-HSDD) have been described [1,2,10,11].

Table 35.1 Classification and types of congenital adrenal hyperplasia.

Type	Subtype	Abbreviation	Synonyms
21-Hydroxylase deficiency		21-OHD	
	Classical	C	
	Simple virilising	SV	
	Salt-wasting	SW	Salt-losing
	Non-classical	NC	Acquired adrenal hyperplasia
	Late onset		
	Cryptic		Asymptomatic, biochemical
11β-Hydroxylase deficiency		11β-OHD	CYPIIBI deficiency, Steroid 11-hydroxylase deficiency
	Classical	C	
	Non-classical	NC	
3β-Hydroxysteroid dehydrogenase deficiency		3β-HSDD	3β*ol*-dehydrogenase deficiency $\Delta^5 \rightarrow \Delta^4$ isomerase deficiency
	Classical	C	
	Non-classical	NC	
17α-Hydroxylase deficiency		17α-OHD	17,20-lyase deficiency, P-450c17 deficiency
20,22-Desmolase deficiency		20,22-DD	Cholesterol desmolase deficiency Congenital lipoid adrenal hyperplasia Prader syndrome, P-450scc deficiency

The pathophysiology of CAH resembles other inborn errors of metabolism (Fig. 35.2). Normally 'A' is principally converted to 'B' and little to 'C'. If conversion is blocked, the precursor 'A' accumulates and spills over to increase production of 'C'. Production of 'B' becomes deficient. The principle is applicable to any of the five steps in cortisol synthesis, so that Fig. 35.1 can be used to predict which steroids will be present in deficiency or excess. This is usually reflected by alterations in either the absolute concentrations or relative ratios of these steroids in the plasma under basal or stimulated conditions. The general pattern of changes for each type of CAH is listed in Table 35.3, whilst more detailed information is given in Table 35.4. The clinical manifestations of CAH can be explained in terms of these changes, as discussed below.

Glucocorticoids

Diminished secretion of cortisol results in reduced feedback inhibition of pituitary so that plasma adrenocorticotrophic hormone (ACTH) levels rise. This causes an increase in size and functional activity of the adrenal cortex. If the enzymatic deficiency is mild, the increased ACTH drive may overcome the block, so that plasma cortisol levels are restored, but at the expense of increased precursors and 'spill-over' products. Despite the physiological importance of cortisol, its deficiency is well tolerated and symptoms are few. Two important corollaries are that CAH rarely presents as 'hypocortisolism', and measurements of plasma cortisol are unhelpful in diagnosis, as they may be normal.

Mineralocorticoids

Depending upon the site of the enzyme deficiency, mineralocorticoids may be present in deficiency or excess. In the latter case, salt and water retention occur, often accompanied by hypertension, possibly due to raised levels of 11-deoxycorticosterone (DOC). In deficiency states, a situation analogous to that for glucocorticoids may be seen. Decreased aldosterone synthesis leads to salt and water loss and a raised plasma renin level (PRA). This, acting through the renin–angiotensin–aldosterone pathway, may restore aldosterone secretion if the enzyme block is mild. However, for many the situation is precarious and any adverse shift in homeostasis will result in acute dehydration, hypovolaemia and hypotension—typically described as a 'salt-wasting (losing) crisis'.

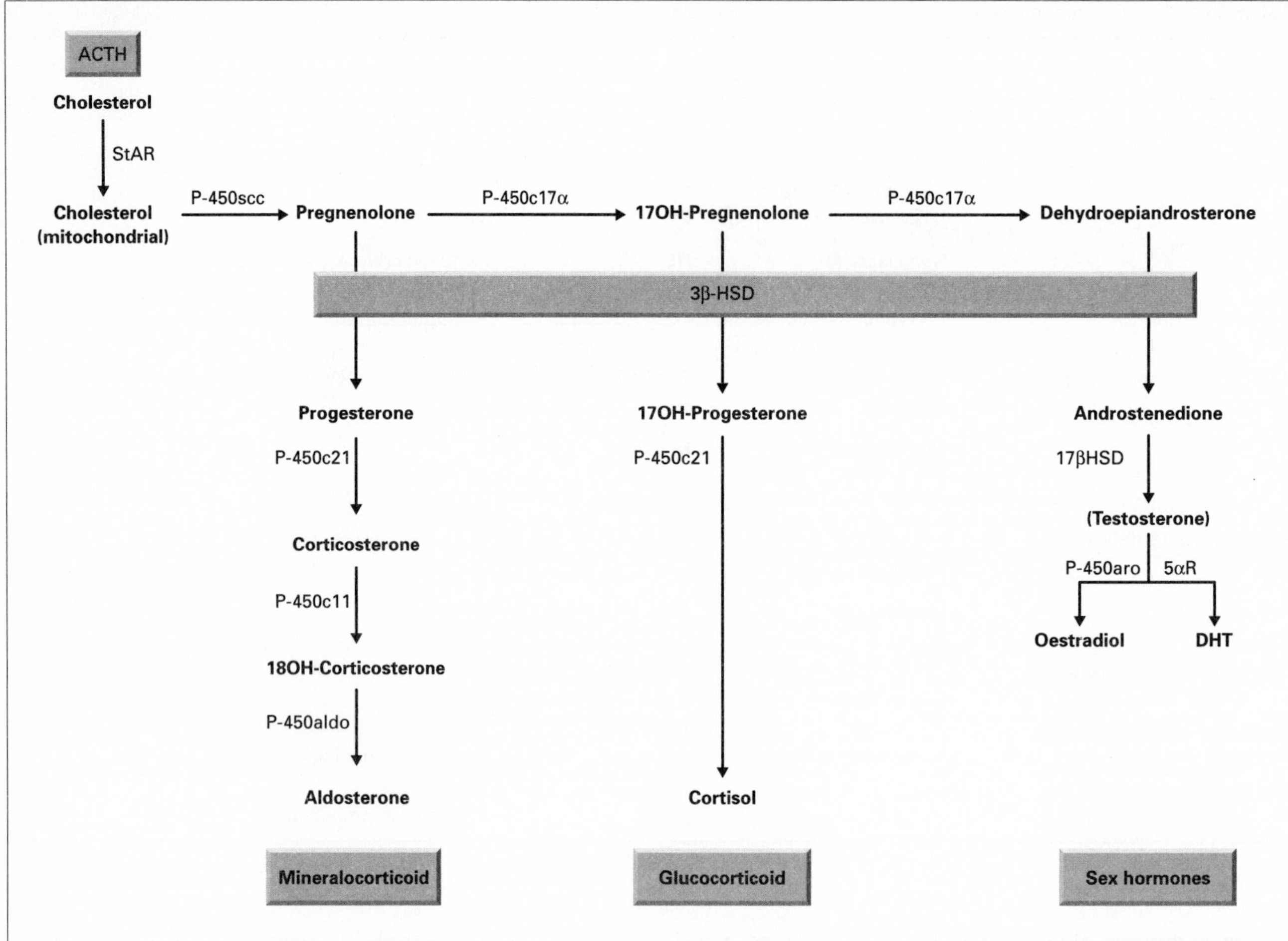

Fig. 35.1 Pathway of adrenal steroidogenesis including the enzymes involved (the production of testosterone and its metabolites is mainly extra-adrenal). StAR, steroid acute regulatory protein.

Table 35.2 Abbreviations for adrenal corticosteroids and related substances used in the text.

Δ^5-Pregnenolone	Preg
17α-Hydroxypregnenolone	17-OHPreg
Progesterone	P
17α-Hydroxyprogesterone	17-OHP
11-Deoxycorticosterone	DOC
11-Deoxycortisol	S
Corticosterone	B
Aldosterone	ALD
Cortisol	F
Dehydroepiandrosterone	DHEA
Δ^4-Androstenedione	D_4
Testosterone	T
Urinary 17-ketosteroids	U_{17}-KS
Urinary pregnanetriol	UPtriol
Plasma renin activity	PRA
Dehydroepiandrosterone sulphate	DS

Sex steroids

CAH may result in increased or decreased secretion of sex steroids (Table 35.5). In the commoner forms (21-OHD, 11β-OHD) androgen production is increased; androstenedione (D_4) is the chief product but the more androgenic testosterone (T), formed through peripheral conversion, is responsible for the clinical manifestations.

Fetal life

For the genetic female (XX), inappropriate androgen secretion during fetal life will result in virilisation, constituting a 'female pseudo-hermaphrodite'. Changes vary from mild clitoromegaly through ambiguous genitalia, severe perineal hypospadias in an apparent 'male', to a complete male phenotype (with phallic urethra) marked only by undescended (really absent) testes [12,13].

In those forms of CAH where androgen production is reduced, the genetic male (XY) may fail to masculinize adequately, becoming a 'male pseudohermaphrodite'. Severity

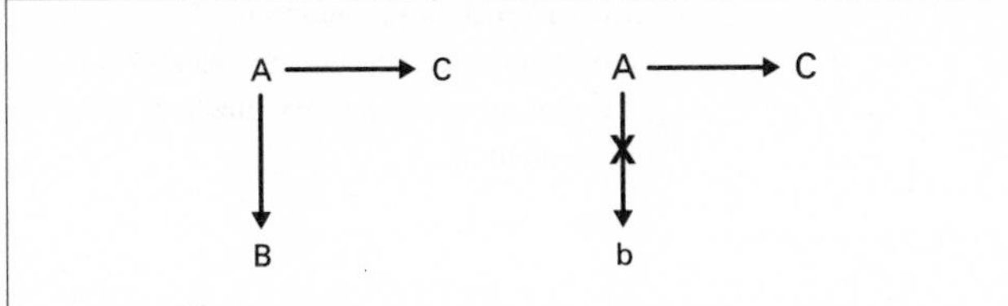

Fig. 35.2 Pathophysiology of inborn errors of metabolism. Left diagram shows normal condition of conversion of 'A' principally to 'B'. Right diagram shows accumulation of 'A' and 'C' in inborn error of 'A' → 'B' conversion.

Table 35.3 Patterns of secretion of adrenal corticosteroids in the various types of congenital adrenal hyperplasia.

CAH type	Mineralocorticoids	Glucocorticoids	Sex steroids
21-OHD			
SW	↓↓	↓↓	↑↑
SV	N/↓	↓	↑↑
NC	N	N/↓	N/↑
11β-OHD	↑†	↓↓	↑↑↑
3β-HSDD	↓↓	↓↓	↓↓*
17α-OHD	↑†	↓↓	↓↓
20,22-DD	↓↓↓	↓↓↓	↓↓↓

N, normal; ↑, increased; ↓, decreased.
* DHEA (weak androgen) increased.
† DOC (potent mineralocorticoid) increased.

is variable up to apparent complete female phenotype. In such cases the disorder may not be suspected at all until later, the child passing for female.

Infancy and early childhood

Hyperandrogenaemia arising at this age will result in virilisation of both genetic male and female. In the former, the appearance of rapid growth with penile enlargement, rugated scrotum and pubic hair, but normal-sized (< 4 ml in volume) testes, denotes 'pseudo-precocious puberty'. In the latter, clitoromegaly, pubic hair and rapid growth may be termed 'heterosexual precocity'.

Late childhood and adolescence

Some cases of premature pubarche previously labelled as idiopathic may in fact represent mild versions of 21-OHD, 11β-OHD or even 3β-HSDD [9,14,15].

Very rarely, phenotypic females (both genetic females and complete male pseudo-hermaphrodites) with classic 3β-HSDD or 17α-hydroxylase (17α-OHD) deficiency (or inadequate) have inadequate secondary sexual characteristics, due to deficient sex steroid synthesis.

Adult life

Increased secretion of androgens in adult females ('female

Table 35.4 Changes in plasma and urine concentrations of adrenal corticosteroids, their metabolites, and related compounds in the various forms of congenital adrenal hyperplasia. (Abbreviations as in Table 33.2.)

	20,22-DD	17α-OHD	3β-HSDD	11β-OHD	21-OHDSW	21-OHDSV	21-OHDNC
Preg			↑				
P							
DOC		↑		↑			
B		↑					
ALD	↓	↓		↓			
17-OHPreg			↑				
17-OHP	↓	↓	N/↑	N/↑	↑↑	↑↑	↑
S				↑			
F					N/↓	N/↓	N
DHEA	↓	↓	↑	↑	N/↑	N/↑	
D_4	↓	↓	N/↑	↑	↑↑	↑↑	
T	↓	↓		↑	↑	↑	
PRA	↑	↓	↑	↓	N/↑	N/↑	N
ACTH	↑	↑	↑	↑	↑	↑	N
U17-KS	↓↓	↓↓	↑	↑↑	↑↑	↑↑	N/↑

N, normal; ↑, increased; ↓, decreased.

Table 35.5 Consequences of inappropriate secretion of sex steroids in congenital adrenal hyperplasia at different periods of life.

Life period	Sex steroid secretion: Increased	Sex steroid secretion: Decreased
Fetal life	Female pseudo-hermaphrodite	Male pseudo-hermaphrodite
Infancy and early childhood	Female virilisation Male pseudo-precocious puberty	
Late childhood and adolescence	Premature pubarche True precocious puberty	Delayed puberty
Adult life	Female hyperandrogenaemia Infertility	

hyperandrogenaemia') may manifest as any combination of the following: hirsutism, menstrual disturbance, severe acne, infertility, and male pattern hair loss [9,11].

Excessive adrenal androgen production in males can lead to subfertility through suppression of the hypothalamo-pituitary–testicular axis.

Pathophysiology of individual disorders

A detailed discussion of the pathophysiology of the individual adrenal hyperplasias is inappropriate for a clinically orientated text, and the interested reader is referred elsewhere [1–3]. However, some important specific aspects are covered below.

21-Hydroxylase deficiency CAH

21-OHD is the commonest CAH, comprising 96% of all 'classic' cases, with an incidence of about one in 12 000. It is the archetypical CAH and the most extensively studied [5–8].

There is decreased synthesis of cortisol and aldosterone, and increased production of androgens via 17-hydroxyprogesterone (17-OHP) (see Fig. 35.1, Tables 35.3 and 35.4). As already mentioned, the degree of enzyme deficiency is variable. This variability has led to a rather awkward classification of 21-OHD into classic salt-wasting (C21-OHDSW), classic simple virilising (C21-OHDSV), and non-classical (NC21-OHD) late-onset and cryptic (Table 35.1). Although useful, it is more helpful to think of 21-OHD as comprising a spectrum of deficiency, as depicted in Fig. 35.3.

C21-OHDSW constitutes approximately 75% of C21-OHD cases and exhibits the severest enzyme deficiency of the group. Activity is diminished in both the zona fasciculata and glomerulosa, such that production rates of both cortisol and aldosterone are absolutely low. Androgen secretion rates are high. Presentation is as ambiguous genitalia (females) or salt-losing crisis during the first few weeks of life (males) [13].

In C21-OHDSV the deficit is only moderate. Indeed, cortisol secretion is typically well maintained and

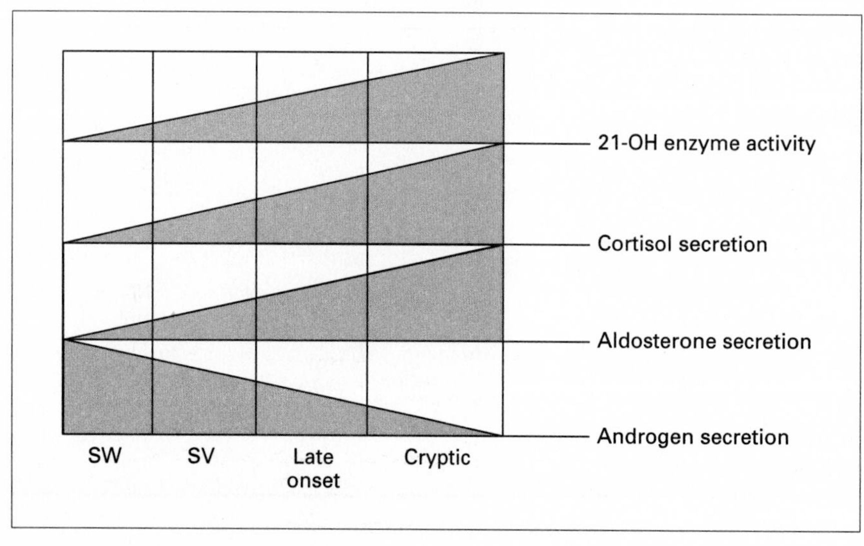

Fig. 35.3 Stylised diagram of 21-hydroxylase enzyme activity and adrenal steroid secretion rates in the various subtypes of 21-hydroxylase deficiency. SW, salt-wasting; SV, simple virilising.

aldosterone secretion may be normal or even increased. Various hypotheses have been proposed to explain the relative sparing of the zona glomerulosa in this type [16], but it should be understood that the distinction between the SW and SV types is to some extent artificial. A defect in mineralocorticoid metabolism clearly exists in the latter [17]; PRA is increased consequent upon either deficient production or action of aldosterone, the latter perhaps arising through competitive inhibition by increased levels of circulating progesterone and 17-OHP at the renal tubular receptor. Recognition of this has important consequences for treatment.

Cortisol and aldosterone production in NC21-OHD are adequate in almost all circumstances. Problems arise from the overproduction of androgens which may be so mild as to go unnoticed (cryptic/asymptomatic/biochemical cases—discernible only on biochemical testing), or which may produce clinical features of fluctuating severity in later life (late-onset cases) [9,14,15,18,19].

11β-Hydroxylase deficiency

11β-OHD results from an abnormality of the CYP11B1 gene and accounts for about 5% of classical CAH cases. With an incidence of one in 100 000 it is rare [20–22]. Although the block in the conversion of 11-deoxycortisol (S) to cortisol is usually incomplete, synthesis of the latter is absolutely reduced. Accumulation of DOC leads to a paradoxical increase in mineralocorticoid activity despite diminished aldosterone secretion, so that PRA is low. Androgen production may exceed that seen in C21-OHD.

3β-Hydroxysteroid dehydrogenase deficiency

This is a proximal block in steroid synthesis and in its classical form (comprising 1% of classical CAH cases) affects both adrenal and gonad [3]. All three classes of steroids are diminished. However, the weak androgen dehydroepiandrosterone (DHEA) accumulates in excess, causing mild virilisation (typically clitoromegaly alone) in female neonates with the classical version. Non-classical forms presenting as hyperandrogenaemia in later life are being reported with increasing frequency and may exceed the classic type in incidence [1,10,18]. The hallmark of 3β-HSDD is a rise in the plasma levels of Δ^5 steroids (especially 17-OHPreg and DHEA) compared to the Δ^4 steroids (principally 17-OHP and D_4). In classic cases absolute values may be raised and lowered, respectively; in non-classic cases absolute values may be normal, but ratios (17-OHPreg/17-OHP; DHEA/D_4) become elevated, especially with ACTH stimulation.

17α-Hydroxylase deficiency

This very rare form of CAH affects both adrenals and gonads, reducing synthesis of both glucocorticoids and sex steroids. Increased levels of DOC, which is the second most potent mineralocorticoid after aldosterone, may produce mild hypertension and hypokalaemia (despite inhibiting aldosterone secretion through depressing PRA). The glucocorticoid properties of DOC and another steroid precursor that accumulates in excess—corticosterone (B)—partially compensate for the deficiency of cortisol. As a result the presentation is often delayed until adolescence when the deficient production of ovarian oestrogens and adrenal androgens becomes evident [23,24].

20,22-Desmolase deficiency

Deficiency of this enzyme in this extremely rare form of CAH is devastating for the fetal adrenal and gonad. Cholesterol cannot be converted to pregnenolone (Preg) and simply accumulates in the cortical cells as lipid globules. Synthesis of all three steroid classes is seriously impaired, so that death is usual in early infancy [1], though survival has been reported.

Clinical features of CAH

Rather than presenting as distinct clinical entities, CAH enters into the differential diagnosis of a wide variety of symptoms and signs, indicated in Table 35.6. The diagnostic approach to many of these presenting syndromes is more properly detailed elsewhere in this book, but consideration from the view of CAH will be given below, following the order of the table.

Abnormal genitalia

Abnormalities of the genitalia present at birth may be seen in all five types of CAH. Genital ambiguity is the commonest; indeed, C21-OHD is the most frequent cause of this state and should be strongly suspected where gonads are impalpable (suggesting a female pseudo-hermaphrodite). Males with C21-OHD typically escape notice at birth as the genitalia are usually normal. The classic description of 'macrogenitosomia praecox', with large pigmented penis and rugated scrotum, is rarely seen.

Most male hypospadias is idiopathic, but severe cases should be regarded with suspicion. Impalpable testes suggest C21-OHD, palpable 3β-HSSD. The extremely virilised female ('complete female pseudo-hermaphrodite') may escape notice altogether as a case of 'undescended testes, [12]. Similarly, males (XY) with deficient androgen production due to 3β-HSSD, 17α-OHD or 20,22-DD may pass for normal females ('complete male pseudo-hermaphrodite'), but fortunately this is rare.

Salt-wasting crisis

Only 11β-OHD and 17α-OHD are spared this phenomenon, although its occasional surprising absence in 3β-HSDD has been reported, as has its equally surprising presence in rare cases of 11β-OHD [22]. C21-OHDSW is its principal cause. As most females with genital abnormalities will have been detected at birth, the presentation is typically confined to males. Frequently there is poor weight gain, followed by an acute illness usually at 2–3 weeks of age, involving vomiting, diarrhoea and circulatory collapse [13]. A clue to the aetiology is provided by the plasma electrolyte concentrations; a metabolic acidosis accompanied by hyperkalaemia, hyponatraemia and mild uraemia suggests CAH. The hyperkalaemia may precede the crisis by as much as 2 weeks. Levels may peak above 10 mmol/l and cause cardiac arrest.

Virilisation in early childhood

Both C21-OHDSV and C11β-OHD may present for the first time in infancy and early childhood due to hyperandrogenaemia. Rapid growth with an advance in bone age may be the first manifestation: eventually virilization appears. Girls will show clitoromegaly and boys show penile enlargement, but testes remain small.

Delayed puberty

Individuals with poorly controlled or undiagnosed C21-OHD may suffer from either delayed puberty (due to suppression of gonadotrophins by adrenal androgens) or true precocity (consequent upon premature activation of the gonadal axis secondary to rapid maturation). The latter typically predominates. Diagnosis at an early age and appropriate treatment leads to normal pubertal timing.

Patients with the very rare 17α-OHD may present as delayed puberty. Both genetic (XY) males and females (XX) with this type have a female phenotype; if the condition goes undetected, the first presentation may be as failure of sexual maturation at puberty due to sex steroid deficiency [23,24].

Primary amenorrhoea

Those with slightly milder variants of 17α-OHD, especially in genetic males, may succeed in attaining poorly developed secondary sexual characteristics and instead present as primary amenorrhoea, as may the occasional male (XY) with C3β-HSDD and female phenotype.

Initial presentation may be as delayed puberty (both gonadarche and adrenarche) due to deficient production of ovarian oestrogen (but not progesterone, which is produced in excess) and adrenal androgens. The typical appearance is a rather tall eunuchoid appearing phenotypic female with absent breast development (thelarche) and absent sexual hair (pubic and axillary) (pubarche). Plasma oestrogen and DHEA levels are low, but P and gonadotrophins are elevated. Definitive diagnosis depends upon measurement of appropriate corticosteroids and metabolites (Table 35.4). Of course, the hyperandrogenic forms of CAH (21-OHD and 11β-OHD) can produce amenorrhoea (typically secondary) or other menstrual irregularities (usually oligomenorrhoea), but are distinguished by other signs of hyperandrogenism, for example hirsutism and virilisation.

Non-classical presentations

Although certain classical forms of CAH may not be *diagnosed* until later life, 'non-classical' variants produce clinical features *for the first time* only in later childhood or beyond. Non-classical forms of 21-OHD, 11β-OHD and 3β-HSSD have been documented and are probably much commoner than their classical counterparts [9,11]. The exact incidence of these forms is racially dependent; for example, NC21-OHD has an overall incidence of 1:100 in Caucasians, but as many as one in 27 Ashkenazi Jews may be affected. The incidence is also high in Italians, Hispanics and Slavic people [2,3].

Non-classic CAH shows broad phenotypic diversity, although salt loss is never a feature. Presenting syndromes are shown in Table 35.6 and are discussed below.

Precocious pubarche

Early onset of sexual hair with a slight increase in growth velocity and/or bone age is most often due to 'idiopathic precocious adrenarche' [25], but there is increasing realisation that many cases may represent NC21-OHD, NC11β-OHD or even NC3β-HSSD. The exact incidence of NCCAH in such circumstances is debatable but may be substantial (e.g. up to 30%) [14,15,26,27]. NCCAH should particularly be suspected where precocious pubarche shows 'atypical' features, for example considerable increase in growth velocity or bone age, marked acne or clitoromegaly [25]. Correct diagnosis is important as stature may be reduced if not treated, and progression to polycystic ovarian (PCO) disease may occur in later adolescence.

Hypertension

Endocrine causes of hypertension are uncommon at any age.

Table 35.6 Presenting syndromes of the various types of congenital adrenal hyperplasia listed according to age. The presentations, divided roughly into 'classical' and 'non-classical', are discussed in the text.

	11β-OHD	3β-HSDD	17α-OHD	20,22-DD	21-OHDSW	21-OHDSV	21-OHDNC
CLASSICAL							
Neonatal period							
Abnormal genitalia							
Ambiguity							
M		+	+	+			
F	+	+			+	+	
Complete pseudo-hermaphrodite							
M		+	+	+			
F	+				+	+	
Perineal hypospadias		+			+	+	
Infancy and early childhood							
Salt-losing crisis		+		+	+		
Virilisation							
M	+					+	
F	+					+	
Rapid growth alone	+					+	
Late childhood and adolescence							
Delayed puberty							
M			+				
F			+				
Primary amenorrhoea		+	+				
NON-CLASSICAL							
Precocious pubarche	+	+					+
Adult							
Hypertension	+		+				
Female hyperandrogenaemia	+	+					+
Infertility							
M		+					+
F	+	+					+
Cryptic	+	?					+

The purpose of the table is to allow physicians rapidly to identify which type of CAH is a possible cause in that clinical context, not to describe comprehensively features of the CAH types. Thus, for example, although 21-OHDSW may subsequently cause virilisation in infancy/early childhood, it invariably presents as a salt-losing crisis in the neonatal period and is therefore listed under the latter but not the former.
M, male; F, female.

However, both NC11β-OHD and C17α-OHD can present as mild to moderate hypertension in later life. The presence of hypokalaemia and/or difficulty in achieving control with conventional therapy provide clues. An elevated plasma concentration of DOC with depressed PRA indicates the need for further investigation.

Although the mineralcorticoid action of DOC is usually blamed for the hypertension, this does not provide a full explanation for its aetiology in 11β-OHD. Approximately two-thirds of cases of C11β-OHD exhibit hypertension, though presentation is usually as androgen excess in this more severe form. Blood pressure falls with adequate glucocorticoid therapy.

Female hyperandrogenaemia

The clinical features of androgen excess in women are as varied as the possible causes. NCCAH can produce signs and symptoms indistinguishable from other adrenal or ovarian androgen-producing disorders, although frank virilisation is unusual. Both NC21-OHD and NC3β-HSDD can mimic PCO [9,10,28,29]. Aetiological distinction is important, as NCCAH is responsive to steroid treatment, and rests upon hormonal studies described later. Again the incidence of the various NCCAH types is unsure.

NC21-OHD and NC3β-HSSD probably each account for 1% of hirsute women and NC11β-OHD 2% [9,10,15,18, 19,30]. In the latter, androgens are produced by the adrenals and the ovaries, and through peripheral conversion of Δ5 to Δ4 steroids in the skin.

Infertility

NC21-OHD causes increased fetal wastage, and infertility in both sexes. A diagnosis of C21-OHD is not incompatible with fertility provided good therapeutic control is achieved.

Cryptic CAH

By strict definition the person with 'cryptic' CAH has no clinical features, but is only revealed (often in the course of investigating the family pedigree of a patient with classical CAH) by biochemical studies. This has been most well documented for 21-OHD but also occurs in 11β-OHD. Although such individuals are deemed to carry the mildest allelles there is overlap with 'symptomatic' forms in NC21-OHD; the two forms are indistinguishable in their response to ACTH challenge, and many individuals transfer between the categories as symptoms and signs wax and wane during life.

Diagnosis of CAH

The first step in diagnosis is to consider CAH in any of the circumstances in Table 35.6. Tests specific for CAH will form only part of those involved but are crucial, as CAH is always a biochemical diagnosis. Close liaison with the laboratory performing steroid assays, regarding choice and interpretation of tests, is essential. Normal ranges quoted here can serve only as a rough guide. Diagnosis invariably rests upon the pattern of concentrations of the various adrenal steroids in plasma viewed in conjunction with the clinical findings.

Ambiguous genitalia

Table 35.7 shows the tests that should be performed initially. Blood should be drawn for 17-OHP, S, T and D_4, preferably on more than one occasion. The first sample should be taken at least 24 hours after birth to allow for elimination of 17-OHP of placental origin (Fig. 35.4). Although a single sample *may* suffice, our experience has shown that levels of adrenal steroids fluctuate unpredictably in the newborn; in C21-OHD, 17-OHP levels may drop spontaneously, temporarily achieving values seen in sick term, preterm or sick preterm infants (Fig. 35.5), or even in 11β-OHD. T levels may also dip to within the normal range. In those destined to become salt losers, PRA may not show a rise for 2–3 days.

In C21-OHD, 17-OHP levels are grossly elevated. Somewhat misleadingly, S levels may also be raised substantially above the normal range due to peripheral conversion of 17-OHP to S, although the ratio of the increase leaves no doubt as to the diagnosis. In the rare case of C11β-OHD the situation is reversed; S is highly elevated in comparison with a modest rise in 17-OHP. A confusing elevation of 17-OHP is also sometimes seen in C3β-HSDD (Table 35.4); low levels would be expected from the pathophysiology (Fig. 35.1), but extra-adrenal 3β-HSD activity (largely occurring in the liver through the activity of an entirely separate enzyme) can result in increased synthesis [1]. Abdominal ultrasonography should confirm the presence of uterus and ovaries and may help support the diagnosis by demonstrating an increase (four-to-sevenfold) in adrenal size [31]. The choice of radiological contrast procedures is best made in conjunction with radiological and surgical colleagues. Should plasma 17-OHP and S levels prove normal, C3β-HSDD may be suspected from a raised DHEA level or increased DHEA/D_4 ratio; otherwise, non-CAH causes should be sought.

In cases of doubt, analysis of urine steroid secretion patterns (Table 35.8) can be helpful, but requires sophisticated chromatography [32]. Twenty-four-hour urinary excretions of 17-ketosteroids (U17-KS) and pregnanetriol (UPtriol) are *not* reliable for the diagnosis of C21-OHD during the neonatal period.

Salt-wasting crisis

Blood samples (multiple samples are again prudent) should be drawn before commencing steroid therapy, although general resuscitative procedures should not be delayed. Raised 17-OHP, T, D_4 and PRA, as in Table 35.7, confirm the diagnosis of C21-OHDSW. A raised PRA with normal or only midly elevated 17-OHP, T, D_4, or even low values, should raise the suspicion of C3β-OHD or 20,22-DD, respectively (see Table 35.4).

Important differential diagnoses include renal disease with associated renal failure and salt-losing nephropathy, and obstructive uropathy with severe coexisting acute urinary tract infection.

Diagnosis in early childhood

The diagnosis of C21-OHD and C11β-OHD can be made

Table 35.7 Diagnostic investigations pertinent to congenital adrenal hyperplasia in the differential diagnosis of ambiguous genitalia in the newborn.

Test	Normal	21-OHD	11β-OHD	Comments
Karyotype	46XX or 46XY	46XX	46XX	Venous blood sample
Plasma 17-OHP	Term healthy <15 (495)	>200 (6600)	Slightly raised	Multiple venous samples taken over a 24-hour period not within 24 hours of birth
	Term sick <30 (990) Preterm healthy <40 (1320) Preterm sick <100 (3300)			
Plasma T	<2 (58) approx.*	>20 (500) typically	>20 (500) typically	As above
Plasma D_4	<4.3 (150) approx.*	Raised	Raised	As above
Plasma S	<5.5 (160)	Normal or slightly raised	Extremely raised	As above
PRA	Term <35 Preterm <167	Normal or raised	Normal or low	Single venous sample drawn after 3–4 days
Abdominal ultrasonograph		Normal female internal genitalia, adrenals may be enlarged (typically 3–4 times normal)		Standard scan with specific assessment of adrenal size
Vaginogram		Normal female internal genitalia, but variable external genital anatomy		Discuss choice of test with radiologist

Plasma steroid values are given in nmol/l (ng/dl), plasma renin activity in ng/ml/hour.
These values should be treated with caution as levels change rapidly in the normal newborn in the first week of life.

using a single blood sample provided the time of sampling is well chosen. Levels of androgens and precursor steroids are typically raised to well above the normal range (Table 35.9). In C21-OHD, 17-OHP levels will be > 100 nmol/l and usually in excess of 1000 nmol/l. Compound S will be well above 60 nmol/l in 11β-OHD. However, because of the circadian rhythm of secretion of these steroids, samples drawn late in the day may fall close to the normal range. It is often prudent to admit the patient for sampling of relevant plasma steroids and androgens, and U17-KS, over a 24-hour period (Fig. 35.6), followed by a short ACTH test the next morning; 250 μg synthetic ACTH (no allowance for weight is necessary) is given i.v. or i.m. and sampling is performed at 0 and 60 min. The additional stimulation this provides further unmasks the enzymatic 'block'. The 60-min sample shows an excessive increase in precursors over post-block products. Thus, in 21-OHD there is an exaggerated rise in 17-OHP levels from (normal or elevated) baseline. These changes permit diagnosis by reference to the nomogram of responses produced by New *et al.* [33] (Fig. 35.7). A typical C21-OHD patient will show a post-stimulation value of between 490 and 1525 nmol/l. For C11β-OHD, a rise in S from (normal or elevated) baseline to well in excess of 11.5 nmol/l (more typically > 35) is diagnostic. Such an approach allows a confident diagnosis to be made and fully defines the degree of androgen production in the individual patient.

The diagnosis of C11β-OHD can be complicated by the finding of mildly elevated 17-OHP levels (since this is a

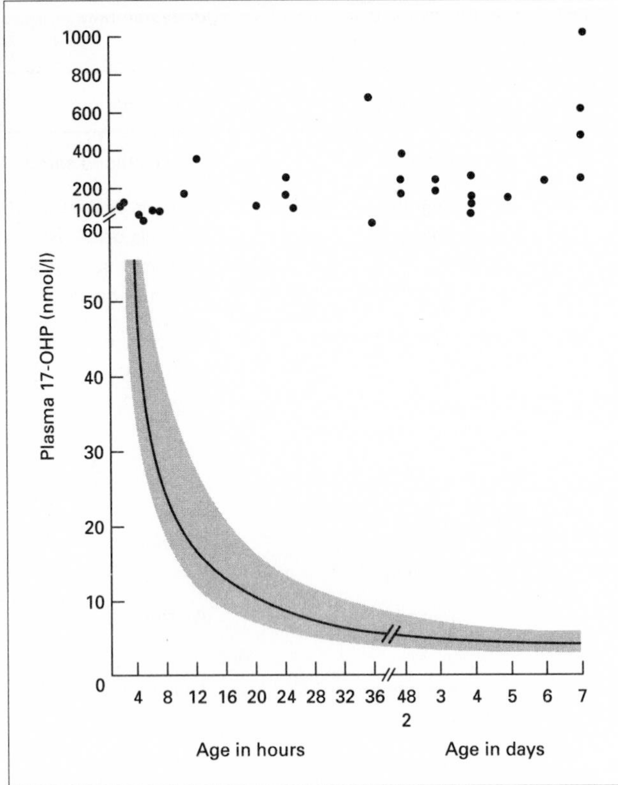

Fig. 35.4 Plasma 17-hydroxyprogesterone concentrations in normal term and infants with congenital adrenal hyperplasia (•) during the first 7 days of life. The line represents the mean and the shaded area encompasses the range in normal infants. (Reproduced with permission of *Archives of Disease in Childhood* [70].)

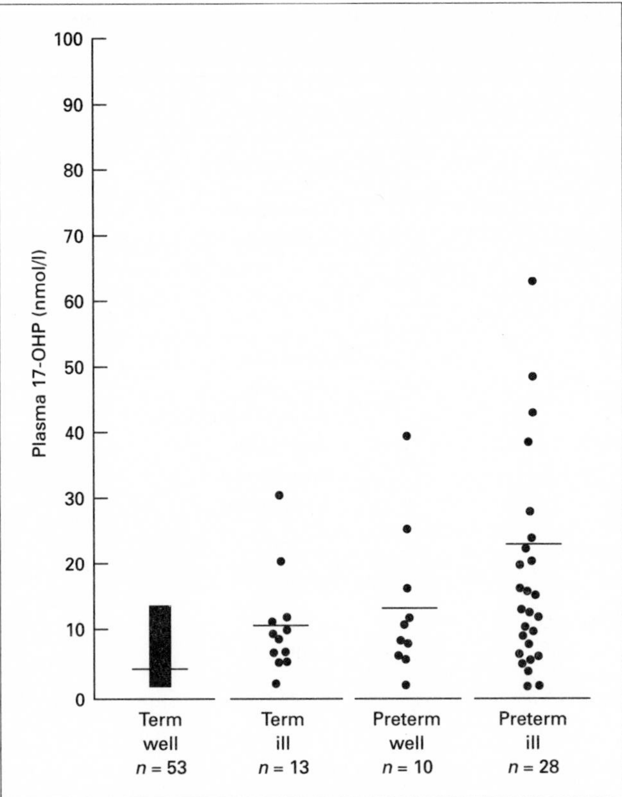

Fig. 35.5 Plasma 17-hydroxyprogesterone (17-OHP) concentrations in term and preterm infants in relation to illness. The data represent the mean and range of values in each group of infants. Repeat blood samples were collected from some infants; '*n*' refers to the number of 17-OHP measurements in each group. (Reproduced with permission of *Archives of Disease in Childhood* [71].)

precursor steroid). However, levels are not as high as in C21-OHD, and the finding of a depressed PRA and ALD with a raised DOC helps confirm the diagnosis. In cases of doubt urine chromatography is useful (Table 35.8). Unlike C21-OHD, heterozygotes for C11β-OHD are not diagnoseable on ACTH testing.

Differentiation of CAH from other causes of virilisation at this age, including adrenal tumour, testicular Leydig cell tumour and true precocious puberty, is vital. Adrenal tumour is suggested by disproportionately raised DS levels, ultrasonographic findings and failure of androgen suppression with steroid treatment (dexamethasone 1.25 mg/m^2/day for 7 days). True precocity is indicated by testicular enlargement and elevated follicle-stimulating hormone (FSH) and luteinising hormone (LH) levels, or a typical response to gonadotrophin-releasing hormone (GnRH) administration.

Table 35.8 Urine steroid excretion profiles in the various types of congenital adrenal hyperplasia.

CAH type	Characteristic metabolites	17-Oxosteroid excretion
20,22-DD	Absent 17-Oxogenic steroids Pregnanediol Pregnanetriol	None
3β-HSDD	Pregnenediol	Low or normal
17α-OHD	Pregnenediol Pregnanediol	Low or normal
11β-OHD	Tetrahydro-11-deoxycortisol	High
21-OHD	Pregnanetriol	High

Diagnosis of non-classical CAH

Distinction of NCCAH from other causes of hyperandrogenism cannot be made on the basis of clinical findings or plasma androgen levels alone. As for classical CAH, diagnosis is made by demonstrating raised concentrations, or abnormal ratios, of plasma steroids. However, as elevation tends to be less, the timing of the sample is more critical. Afternoon

Table 35.9 Upper limits of normal ranges for certain plasma steroids, urinary metabolites and plasma renin activity, used as measures of therapeutic control in congenital adrenal hyperplasia, expressed according to age and/or stage of pubertal development [40].

Age	17P	T		D_4	S	PRA	U17-KS		UPtriol
		M	F				M	F	
Prepuberty	<3 (99)			<1.8 (50)	<5.5 (160)				
0–7 days			<1 (29)						
7 days to 1 month		<13 (380)	<1 (29)			<35	<2	<2	
1 month to 1 year			<0.5 (15)			<37	<0.5	<0.5	<0.1
1–4 years						<11			<0.2
5–7 years		<0.5 (15)					<2	<2	<0.4
Puberty	<8 (264)				<5.5 (160)				
P2		<5.0 (150)	<1.0 (29)	<5.3 (150)			<3.5	<4.4	
P3		<11.0 (330)				<6	<6.1	<9.1	<1.0
P4		<21 (620)	<1.2 (35)	<8.0 (225)			<18.8		
P5		<33* (970)				<3	<20	<15	

The values have been drawn from several sources and are given in nmol/l (ng/dl) for 17P, T, D_4 and S, ng/ml/hour for PRA, and mg/24 hour for U17-KS and UPtriol. The values given should be taken as a rough guide only and wherever possible local laboratory normal ranges should be substituted.

* Even in poorly controlled 21-OHD or 11β-OHD, T levels will rarely exceed this value which represents predominantly testicular production.

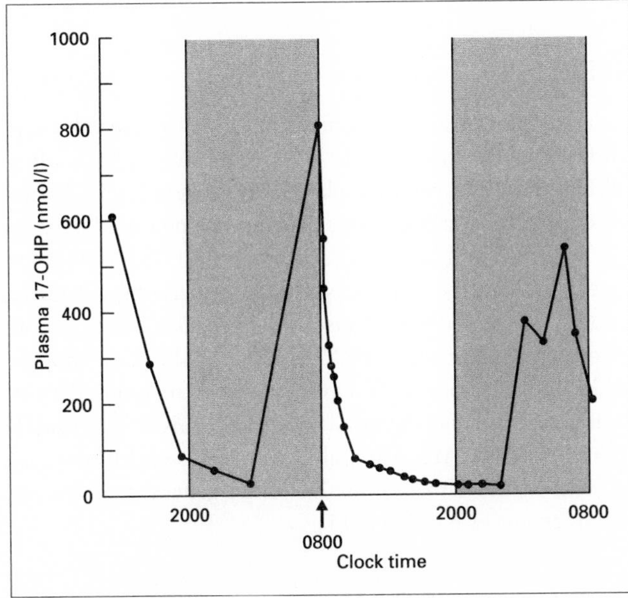

Fig. 35.6 Plasma 17-hydroxyprogesterone (17-OHP) levels in a girl with 21-hydroxylase deficiency. Values before the arrow represent those in the untreated state, showing the natural circadian rhythm. Dexamethasone 0.5 mg administered at the arrow produced a precipitous fall but the nocturnal circadian rise is still evident. (Reproduced with permission of *Hormone Research* [40].)

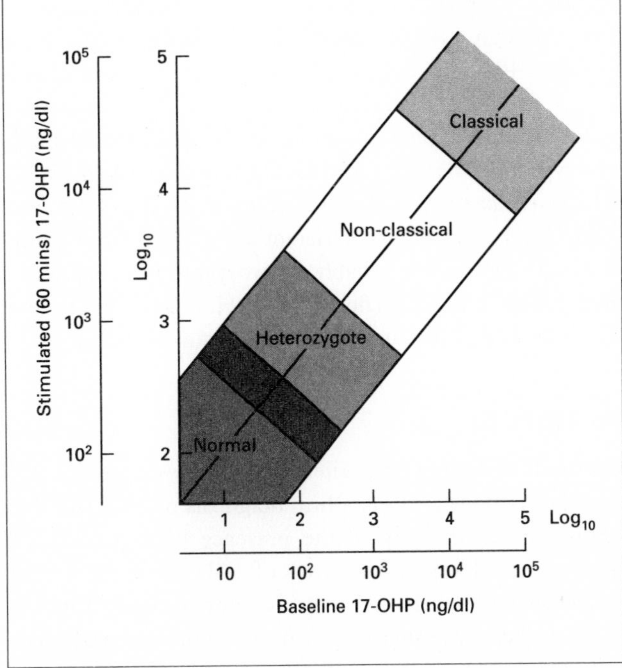

Fig. 35.7 Nomogram for genotyping 21-hydroxylase deficiency (21-OHD) based on plasma 17-hydroxyprogesterone (17-OHP) concentrations before (baseline) and after (stimulated) intravenous injection of an adrenocorticotrophic hormone analogue (Synacthen). Note the considerable area of overlap between heterozygote and unaffected regions; differentiation of these two categories on hormonal data alone is therefore unreliable. (33 ng/dl = 1 nmol/l). Modified from [33].

values may fall misleadingly to within the normal range. Collection at 0700–0900 hours is most sensitive but levels may still be borderline. In such cases an ACTH-stimulation test as described above should be used. Where ACTH-induced responses clearly exceed the normal range, the diagnosis is easily made. However, in many NC individuals, the response may be less marked. This, plus lack of clear normative data on post-stimulation plasma steroid ranges (a variety of such ranges are to be found in the literature and between various laboratories) can make the diagnosis less certain. Careful analysis of the data by an experienced endocrinologist can be valuable. An excellent overview of the problem is provided by Azziz *et al.* [11]. In situations of extreme difficulty, the diagnosis of NCCAH is strongly supported by the ability of steroid therapy (see above) to suppress mildly elevated levels and/or restore equivocal ratios into the normal range.

NC21-OHD

Baseline levels of relevant steroids (17-OHP, T, D_4 DHEA, F and ACTH) may be normal or just outside the normal range, depending on collection time. Plasma 17-OHP concentration in samples drawn between 0700 and 0900 hours >6 nmol/l are suspicious [11], >10 nmol/l are highly likely to be due to, and >50 nmol/l virtually diagnostic of, NC21-OHD. Saliva 17-OHP can also be used for screening; a concentration >300 pmol/l at these same times is highly suggestive [34], though affected individuals typically have values between 400 and 7000 pmol/l [35]. The ACTH-stimulation test is definitively diagnostic (Fig. 35.7). Post-stimulation values should exceed 10 nmol/l, are invariably >30 nmol/l and typically fall in the range 45–500 nmol/l [9,10,14,19,36]. The response to ACTH will distinguish NC21-OHD from C21-OHD, but cannot differentiate cryptic from symptomatic varieties, nor (reliably) heterozygous from unaffected individuals. Like all forms of NCCAH, NC21-OHD can at times be difficult to diagnose with certainty [19,36].

NC11β-OHD

Methods of testing and criteria for diagnosis are not well standardised. Therefore, a firm diagnosis of NC11β-OHD should be made only in the presence of a post-ACTH compound S level well in excess of 2 SD above the normal response for age-matched controls (approximately 10nmol/l [15]). Others have suggested 3 SD as a more acceptable cut-off [11] in conjunction with other supportative clinical or biochemical evidence (e.g. raised 24-hour urinary S or tetrahydro-S excretion). Values typically seen are 10–30 nmol/l [10].

NC3β-HSDD

Contrary to expectation plasma levels of D_4 and T are occasionally elevated, possibly due to hepatic conversion of excess circulating precursors. Baseline levels of these (Δ5 steroids—17-hydroxypregnenolone (17-OHPreg), DHEA and its sulphate) may be normal or elevated, whilst 17-OHP and cortisol levels are normal. Diagnosis is difficult and controversial and chiefly rests upon the presence of an abnormal ratio of Δ5/Δ4 steroids. This may be present on a random plasma sample if timed carefully, but may require ACTH stimulation; both 17-Preg and DHEA will show a greater than normal rise, although these absolute increases are insufficient for diagnosis alone, due to overlap with the response shown by NC21-OHD patients. The diagnosis is made when a significant rise in 17-OHPreg (>3 SD above the normal mean has been suggested [11], i.e. above approximately 45 nmol/l) occurs in conjunction with a 17-OHPreg/17-OHP ratio elevated well in excess of 5 (prepubertal) and 10 (pubertal and adult) [10,15]. In NC21-OHD this ratio is typically <0.5 after stimulation. The DHEA/D_4 ratio may or may not become elevated, but is significant if >6 (prepubertal) and >8 (pubertal and adult). A 17-Preg/F ratio >50 is further supportive evidence. These ratios should be treated with caution as normal values are based on studies of limited numbers of subjects. In cases of doubt, suppression of both Δ5 and Δ4 plasma steroid levels by dexamethasone (see above) is confirmatory.

Differential diagnosis of NCCAH

Adrenal tumour, idiopathic hirsutism and PCO are important differential diagnoses. PCO can be particularly difficult to differentiate, as random plasma androgen levels do not discriminate, and polycystic ovaries may be found in up to 30% of cases of NCCAH [11]. Only the ACTH stimulation test will identify those cases with underlying NCCAH, though as usual dexamethasone suppression will help confirm the difficult ones. NCCAH is probably best thought of as one aetiology of PCO rather than a separate identity. Adrenal tumor is suggested by grossly raised DS, usually normal in NCCAH. Adrenal ultrasound is useful, showing a focal lesion with tumour but often generalised bilateral enlargement in NCCAH [11].

Treatment of CAH

C21-OHD is sufficiently common that many paediatricians care for one or more such patients, and often do so remarkably well. However, management can be difficult and a successful outcome is most likely with an experienced practitioner.

Classical 21-OHD

The aims of treatment are listed in Table 35.10. Glucocorticoid therapy, introduced by Wilkins *et al.* [37] and

Table 35.10 Long-term goals in the treatment of classical 21-OHD congenital adrenal hyperplasia.

Correction of cortisol deficiency
Correction of mineralocorticoid deficiency
Suppression of virilisation
Permission of normal growth and ultimately normal final height
Normal gonadal maturation
Normal fertility in adult life

Bartter *et al.* [38] in the 1950s, remains the mainstay of treatment in all forms of CAH today. General aspects will be discussed before addressing more specific details.

Glucocorticoid therapy

The actions of glucocorticoids in C21-OHD are complex (Table 35.11) [1]. The principal effect is often described as 'cortisol replacement', but this is misleading. As already seen, many patients secrete normal amounts of cortisol under basal conditions. For these, 'replacement' is strictly necessary only during times of stress when increased demands cannot be met by endogenous production. Therapeutically, the most important action is suppression of excessive adrenal androgen production, through inhibition of ACTH release, generally interpreted as achieving plasma androgen levels and/or U17-KS excretion within the normal range for age/sex (see Table 35.9).

Glucocorticoid therapy may produce unwanted effects, even at the small doses used in CAH. Growth suppression is a particular problem and may be seen without other signs of hypercortisolism. The difficulty in treating CAH is to select a glucocorticoid preparation, total daily dose and dose schedule that satisfy these three interrelated actions: we wish to provide physiological replacement whilst at the same time suppressing androgen production, yet avoiding growth inhibition. For most this is possible, but for a substantial number it is difficult. Considerable research has been devoted to finding an optimal regimen for C21-OHD, but this has not been completely successful. Once the efficacy of glucocorticoids had been established, attempts were made to define a 'safe' total daily dose. However, this was

Table 35.11 Therapeutic actions of glucocorticoids in the treatment of congenital adrenal hyperplasia.

Action	Classification
Cortisol replacement	Physiological
Adrenal androgen suppression	Pharmacological
Growth suppression	Toxic

Table 35.12 Relative potencies of various glucocorticoids when used in the treatment of congenital adrenal hyperplasia.

Compound	Relative potency
Hydrocortisone	1
Cortisone	0.8
Prednisolone	5
Prednisolone	4
Dexamethasone	80

hampered by a lack of appreciation that total daily dose is not the only determining factor in therapeutic efficacy, and that the measures used to monitor efficacy were inadequate. Nevertheless, it was established that a total daily dose close to the normal adrenal cortisol production rate (12 mg/m^2/day; more recently established as 7 mg/m^2/day) provided a satisfactory starting point. The questions of optimal preparation, dose division and timing of administration remain unresolved. Theoretical considerations can lead to opposing conclusions, and experimental evidence is undecided. Heavy nocturnal dosing might theoretically cause suppression of nocturnal growth hormone release. Conversely, as maximal androgen secretion occurs in the morning coincident with circadian ACTH release, a proportionately larger dose at bedtime might achieve superior suppression. Some studies suggest little effect of dose division and timing on overall adrenal steroid production whilst others have demonstrated marked changes with even slight alterations. One important factor is the choice of glucocorticoid. Cortisone acetate was originally employed but other compounds are now available. The question of relative potencies is difficult to address but Table 35.12 provides a rough guide. Those with a longer half-life are generally more potent. Long-acting depot preparations have been tried but, although extremely effective in providing adrenal suppression, are devastating in terms of steroidal side-effects. A final source of variability is the patients themselves. There is tremendous idiosyncracy in therapeutic requirements between individuals, and these may change over time. The source of this variability is not entirely clear but may relate to differences in the pharmacokinetics [39], pharmacodynamics [40], and drug interaction [41]. Although variability represents a problem, it can be turned to advantage. Careful manipulation of the choice of preparation, total daily dose, dose division and timing can be used in conjunction with appropriate measures of therapeutic control to tailor a regimen for each patient that maximizes the chances for a successful outcome.

Mineralocorticoid treatment

Traditionally, less importance is placed upon mineralocorticoid replacement therapy, as aldosterone secretion stays relatively constant throughout childhood. Thus, the typical C21-OHDSW patient often receives a fixed daily dose of oral mineralocorticoid such as 9α-fludrocortisone (9α-FC) with little change. This provides protection against salt wasting but overlooks an important aspect of therapeutic control. Many patients with C21-OHDSV also show a tendency to salt loss (see Fig. 35.3), as evidenced by an increased PRA. In such patients mineralocorticoid therapy, while not strictly necessary from the 'replacement' aspect, will not only suppress PRA but also reduce ACTH levels and hence androgen secretion [1,42], leading to a reduction in glucocorticoid dose and an improvement in growth pattern.

Treatment during infancy

In the case of C21-OHD or 11β-OHD presenting at birth with ambiguous genitalia, the diagnosis should be firmly established before proceeding to steroid therapy. A full discussion of surgical aspects is not appropriate here, but in most a reduction in the size of the clitoris and division of the fused labial folds to exteriorise the vaginal opening are the minimum requirements. The timing of surgery is variable, but the former is usually performed in infancy, the latter near puberty. The choice of sex of rearing in these circumstances is virtually always female, as female internal genitalia and ovaries are present, and full female reproductive ability in adult life is possible. For 17α-OHD and C3β-HSDD male pseudo-hermaphrodites, the sex of rearing is also usually female, although reproductive potential will be lacking.

The precise therapy for the infant with a salt-losing crisis is given in standard paediatric texts, and will not usually come to the attention of the 'adult' endocrinologist. However, children with CAH may be seen by both paediatricians and non-paediatric endocrinologists.

Following confirmed diagnosis, the infant with C21-OHD should commence steroid treatment. Glucocorticoids are indicated for all and mineralocorticoids for overt salt losers and those with an elevated PRA. Traditionally, an initial period of high dose (often parenteral) glucocorticoid therapy was given in order to suppress androgen secretion rapidly. This is of no proven benefit, and may be detrimental through contribution to glucocorticoid overdosage often seen in infancy [43]. A starting dose of hydrocortisone at 10–30 mg/m^2/day will result in a fall in plasma adrenal steroid concentrations to acceptable levels by 3 months [44]. Doses in excess of 30 mg/m^2 day inevitably produce growth failure and >40 mg/m^2/day produces overt hypercortisolism. An initial dose as low as 15–20 mg/m^2/day may be prudent as many previous studies have demonstrated significant and irreversible loss of height by 1–2 years of age with more standard doses. Most infants can therefore be commenced on 1.5 mg hydrocortisone given 8-hourly. After the age of 6 months, the doses are probably best confined to the earlier part of the day (e.g. 0800, 1200, 1600 hours) so as to mimic the natural circadian rhythm of endogenous cortisol secretion that establishes itself at about this age, or a little earlier. We prefer hydrocortisone because it is the natural hormone and has a short half-life and low potency, making dose adjustment easier. To achieve such small doses, hydrocortisone may need to be specially prepared by the pharmacy in solution. When slightly older the child can be given hydrocortisone lozenges (Corlan pellets) containing 2.5 mg hydrocortisone.

Where indicated 9α-fludrocortisone should be started at 0.1 mg/day as a single oral daily dose. Overt salt wasters should also receive oral sodium supplements (2–3 g sodium chloride = approx. $^1/_2$ tsp) until taking solid foods which can be salted.

During the first 6 months of life the child should be seen monthly both to ensure compliance and to adjust treatment. Two-monthly visits thereafter are probably adequate for the first 2 years. The aim is to ensure normal growth, permit a normal advance in bone age (1 year per year of chronological age) and avoid virilisation. The dose of hydrocortisone should be adjusted according to growth velocity and plasma steroid levels; optimum levels of the latter are difficult to set but 17-OHP should probably be <70 nmol/l and D_4 <1.8 nmol/l. Plasma T is useful in girls (<0.5 nmol/l) but cannot be used in boys aged <9 months because of testicular T production during this period. In many the dose may be allowed to fall naturally with growth to 10 mg/m^2/day with safety. In making dose adjustments close attention should be paid to the pattern of growth and bone age, although judgement is rendered difficult by the tendency for infants to cross the centiles during the first 6–9 months of life.

The dose of fludrocortisone should be adjusted to keep PRA in the normal range (Table 35.9); a dose >0.3 mg/day is rarely required.

Treatment during childhood

Although 9α-fludrocortisone dosage usually requires little adjustment to maintain PRA within the normal range, glucocorticoid requirements are often idiosyncratic and there may be difficulty in avoiding growth suppression or even overt hypercortisolism at times. Hydrocortisone 10–25 mg/m^2/day is given orally in three divided doses with approximately half of the total daily dose given in the morning [45]. More potent steroids such as prednisolone (dose approximately 5 mg/m^2/day) should be employed with caution. The latter can be helpful in certain circumstances when given last thing at night to suppress the early morning steroid surge. Because the dose and schedule require constant

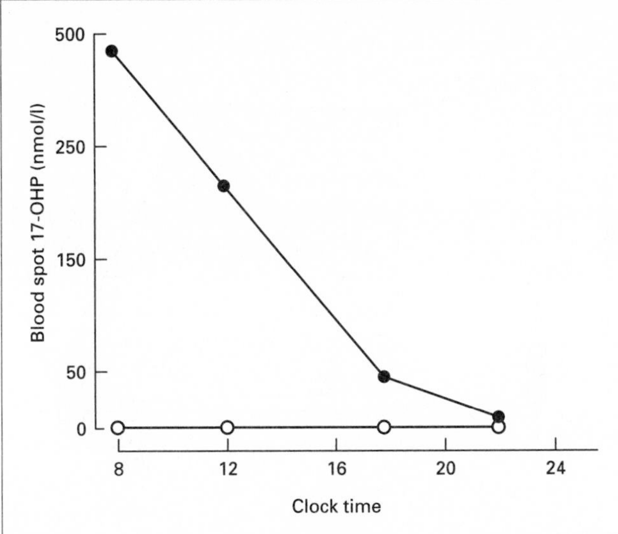

Fig. 35.8 Blood-spot 17-hydroxyprogesterone (17-OHP) concentrations measured over a 24-hour period on two separate occasions 1 month apart in a single patient. On the first occasion, the patient was undertreated and exhibited the typical large diurnal swing associated with this state (•). On the second occasion (o), the patient had become inadvertently overdosed due to drug interaction and 17-OHP levels were suppressed throughout the day. A second month later the patient had developed a Cushingoid appearance.

revision, patients should be seen at least 6 monthly. Changes should be made according to the various measures of therapeutic control listed in Table 35.13. Growth velocity and bone age are useful but suffer from being retrospective and, in addition to U17-KS excretion, are prone to measurement error. However, some authorities use them as the best criteria of adequate therapy [46]. Measurements of plasma steroid levels on single occasions are more useful but have drawbacks; both plasma 17-OHP and D_4 show a circadian rhythm so that untimed sampling is useless and afternoon collection may be misleading. They (and plasma T) also lack a lower limit of normal by which overtreatment can be detected. These parameters are therefore useful in setting a lower limit for total daily dose of glucocorticoid but may not prevent inadvertent overdosage. Fine tuning is now possible using steroid *profiling*.

Several studies [47–49] have shown that the characteristics of the circadian rhythm of 17-OHP in C21-OHD correlate with both androgen secretion and growth velocity. The poorly treated CAH patient shows high 17-OHP levels throughout a 24-hour period but with particularly high values in the morning, resulting in a very exaggerated diurnal swing. Over-treatment typically produces low values (often within the normal range for healthy unaffected individuals and thus often misinterpreted as constituting good control), and a suppressed rhythm (Fig. 35.8). The diurnal pattern under these circumstances is remarkably consistent from day to day.

We have defined an 'optimal' profile, for both 17-OHP, measured in either blood or saliva, and D_4 in saliva, associated with normal androgen secretion and growth. Patients are instructed to collect blood (obtained by finger pricking using an 'autolet' type device and spotted on to filter paper) and saliva (obtained by spitting into a sterile bottle after first rinsing the mouth 5 min before) at home at 0800, 1200, 1800 and 2200 hours on the two consecutive days of a weekend half-way between routine clinic visits,

Table 35.13 Measures of therapeutic control in the prepubertal child with classical 21-OHD congenital adrenal hyperplasia. Measurement category refers to the value of the parameters in terms of adjusting the therapeutic regimen.

Measurement category	Parameter	Desired range	
Coarse	Growth velocity	25th-75th centile for age	
	Bone age	ΔBA/ΔCA = 1	
	Urine 17-KS	Within normal range for age/sex	
Moderate	Plasma testosterone (nmol/l)	<0.5 (male and female)	
	Plasma androstenedione (nmol/l)	<2.0	
	Plasma 17-hydroxyprogesterone (nmol/l)	5–70 (measured at 0800 hours)	
Fine	17-Hydroxyprogesterone profiling	0800 hours	Thereafter
	Blood spot (nmol/l)	30–70	<10
	Saliva (pmol/l)	260–1000	<150
	Saliva androstenedione profiling (pmol/l)	0800 hours <1500	Thereafter See nomogram

Δ, change in parameter; BA, bone age; CA, chronological age.

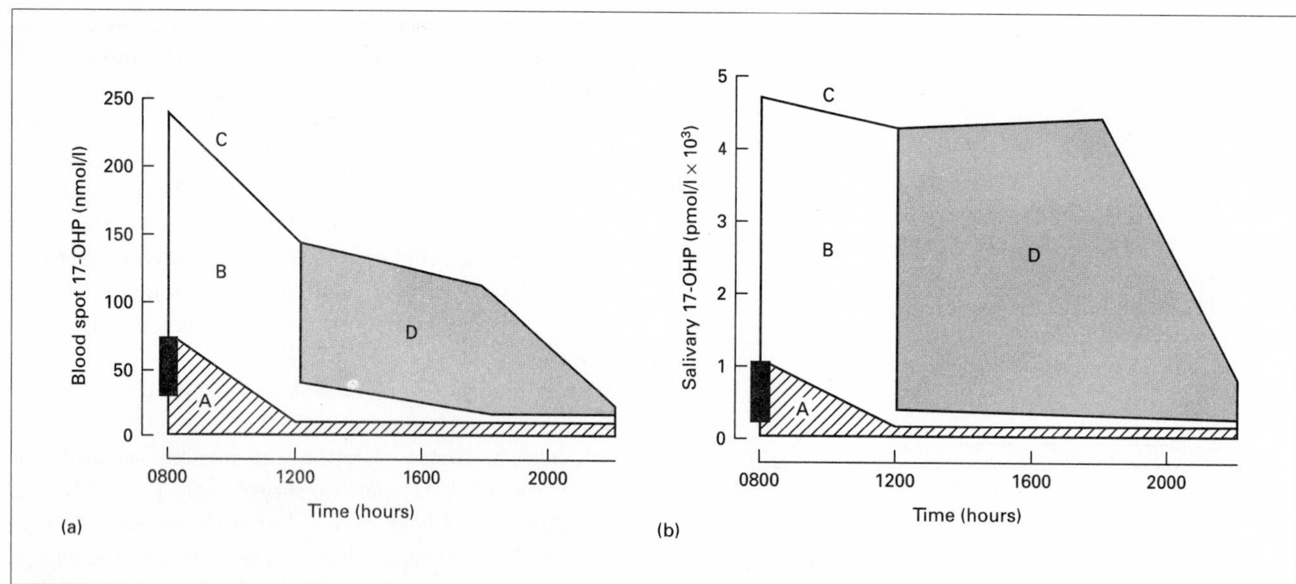

Fig. 35.9 (a) Nomogram to monitor control in congenital adrenal hyperplasia using blood-spot 17-hydroxyprogesterone (17-OHP) profiles. The shaded bar denotes a 17-hydroxyprogesterone range of 30–70 nmol/l at 0800 hours which avoids overtreatment. (b) Nomogram to monitor control in congenital adrenal hyperplasia using salivary 17-hydroxyprogesterone profiles. The shaded bar denotes a 17-hydroxyprogesterone range of 260–1000 pmol/l at 0800 hours. A, good control; B, poor control; C, extremely poor control; D, area where values from B and C overlap. (Reproduced with permission of *Archives of Disease in Childhood* [48].)

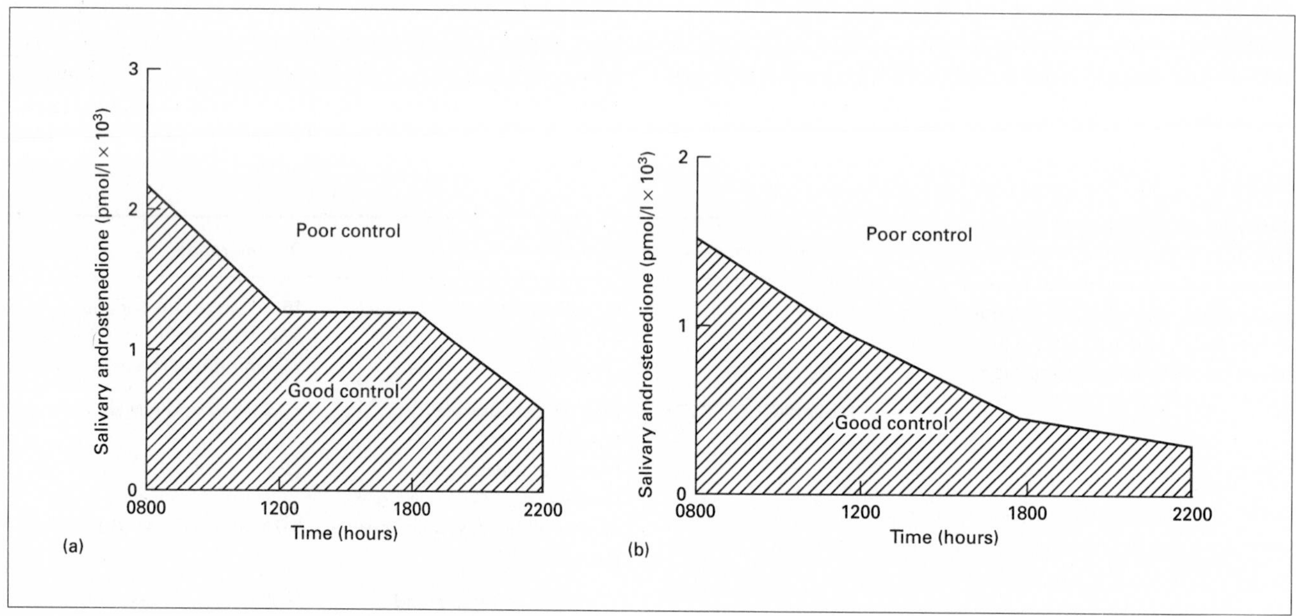

Fig. 35.10 (a) Nomogram to monitor control in pubertal female patients with congenital adrenal hyperplasia using androstenedione profiles in saliva. Area labelled 'good control' is associated with plasma testosterone concentrations within normal range. (b) Nomogram to monitor control in prepubertal children with congenital adrenal hyperplasia using androstenedione profiles in saliva. Area labelled 'good control' is associated with plasma testosterone concentrations of <0.5 nmol/l. (Reproduced with permission of *Archives of Disease in Childhood* [49].)

whilst continuing to take their usual medication. These are then mailed to the laboratory so that the values of 17-OHP and D_4, plotted on specially constructed nomograms of therapeutic control (Figs 35.9 and 35.10), are available at the next clinic visit. Choice of glucocorticoid, total daily dose, dose schedule and loading can then be adjusted in a very accurate manner to achieve a profile pattern within the desired range. Experience has shown this to be of particular value in reducing the incidence of subtle overtreatment in patients apparently well treated according to other, less sensitive, measures.

Treatment during puberty

The wide variation of the onset of puberty means that bone age and growth velocity are less useful as measures of therapeutic control. Plasma D_4 levels should probably be kept at < 18 nmol/l. Plasma T should be kept < 1.5 nmol/l in girls but cannot be used in boys. However, these levels should not be adhered to slavishly. Steroid profiling is again valuable. Changes in compliance can make control extremely difficult; once statural growth is near completion, conversion from hydrocortisone to dexamethasone can offer advantages. Once-daily dosage is adequate for most, and women show improved regulation of menses; dexamethasone should be introduced judiciously at 5 μg/kg/day, taken in the morning. Cautious increases in combination with steroid profiling will avoid side-effects, although increased appetite is commonly reported.

Treatment in adult life

Once growth is complete therapeutic control becomes less critical. Dexamethasone given once or twice daily in doses between 0.25 and 0.75 mg/day is usually adequate [50]. The need for glucocorticoid treatment in adult males has been questioned, but probably ensures optimal health and fertility. If stopped, stress events should still be covered. As the tendency to salt loss appears to wane with age, many patients can safely discontinue 9α-fludrocortisone therapy in adult life.

Females are reported to have low fertility rates [72,73]. However, there is the potential for improved fertility after treatment is monitored more closely and the external genitalia have been adequately reconstructed [74].

Treatment during stress

Minor infections unaccompanied by fever and/or significant systemic upset require no increase in glucocorticoid dose. This is particularly important in infancy when frequent dose increases can lead to stunting. For most other illness, a doubling of the total daily dose is adequate. For major stresses, such as severe illness, trauma or labour, treble the dose. Surgical procedures require maximum coverage with 5–10 times the daily dose [1,45].

The difficult patient

Many individuals with CAH run a smooth therapeutic course, but some seem doomed to difficulty. Brittle patients undergo frequent transformation between good and bad control for no immediately apparent reason. Compliance is always the chief suspect but such changes can also be due to stressful life events, or unreported self-initiated changes in dose scheduling. Patients should be instructed to take their medication at the same time each day and under the same circumstances (e.g. food). Brittleness can also be an artifact due to changes in sampling time, for example through a change from morning to afternoon clinic.

Occasional prepubertal patients show a pattern of rapidly advancing bone age and growth velocity despite normal plasma androgen levels. In some, intermittent random sampling may fail to detect significant periods of hyperandrogenaemia, for example, at night. In others there appears to be a genuine oversensitivity to androgens at the tissue level.

Some patients appear to be resistant to glucocorticoid therapy in that androgen levels do not suppress and growth velocity and bone age advance, despite large doses. Compliance is nearly always the problem, although there are those who are apparently genuinely resistant. A distressing subgroup show high androgen levels with poor growth and/or Cushingoid features; doses of glucocorticoid seem inadequate to control androgen production but sufficient to produce side-effects. Ensuring that PRA is within the normal range by commencing or adjusting the dose of fludrocortisone is the first step. Strenuous efforts to adjust the schedule in conjunction with steroid profiling may help; this should be done in hospital where compliance can be ensured.

Uncontrollable hyperandrogenism may be helped by the use of specific anti-androgens. The US National Institutes of Health are currently evaluating the value of flutamide (an androgen blocker) and testolactone (an aromatase inhibitor) as an adjunct to glucocorticoid therapy in CAH [75].

Other forms of classical CAH

Due to their rarity, there is much less therapeutic experience with the other forms of classical CAH. Treatment is generally along the lines of C21-OHD with replacement of glucocorticoid and mineralocorticoids; doses of the former may be less in those forms uncomplicated by androgen overproduction. Dose adjustment is more difficult due to lack of satisfactory markers of control.

In C11β-OHD, glucocorticoid dose is usually adjusted to keep plasma S and T and/or urinary tetrahydro-S within the normal range and PRA unsuppressed. The measurement of blood pressure, plasma DOC and D_4 can also be useful. Hydrocortisone doses of 10–20mg/m²/day are usually adequate [21]. In some cases hypertension persists despite adequate glucocorticoid therapy and specific antihypertensive drugs may be necessary. Overtreatment appears to be a particular problem and the prognosis for height is less good [51].

In those forms marked by sex steroid deficiency appropriate supplementation will be required at the time of puberty.

Non-classical CAH

Lower doses of glucocorticoid (usually hydrocortisone or dexamethasone) are required to suppress androgen levels. The dexamethasone dose is typically 0.25–0.5 mg/day often given as a single bedtime dose. Mineralocorticoids are hardly ever necessary. Antiandrogens such as spironolactone or cyproterone acetate can help [11]. Care should be taken when making a decision to treat precocious pubarche due to NCCAH. Pros and cons should be carefully weighed; although glucocorticoid treatment can reduce troublesome androgenic symptoms and prevent adult short stature, and may even prevent ultimate progression to PCO, it can produce growth stunting and rapid weight gain [25].

Molecular genetics of CAH

The genes encoding each of the enzymes required for adrenal steroid biosynthesis have now been cloned and their chromosomal location identified. Figure 35.11 depicts these genes superimposed on the pathway of steroidogenesis illustrated in Fig. 35.1; chromosomal loci and some details about the genes are summarised in Table 35.14.

Deleterious mutations have been identified in each of the cognate genes to account for the corresponding enzyme deficiencies except in the case of P-450_{scc} deficiency [52]. This rare enzyme deficiency has recently been shown to arise on account of a defect in cholesterol transport across the mitochondrial membrane. Several proteins are involved in cholesterol transport but notably mutations in StAR (*st*eroidogenic *a*cute *r*egulatory protein) have been identified in patients with P-450_{scc} deficiency [53]. Closely homologous genes on chromosome 1 encode two isoenzymes of 3β*ol*-dehydrogenase; type 1 is expressed primarily in placenta and skin whereas the type II isoenzyme is expressed in the adrenal,

Fig. 35.11 Pathway of adrenal steroidogenesis indicating the genes encoding the enzymes involved.

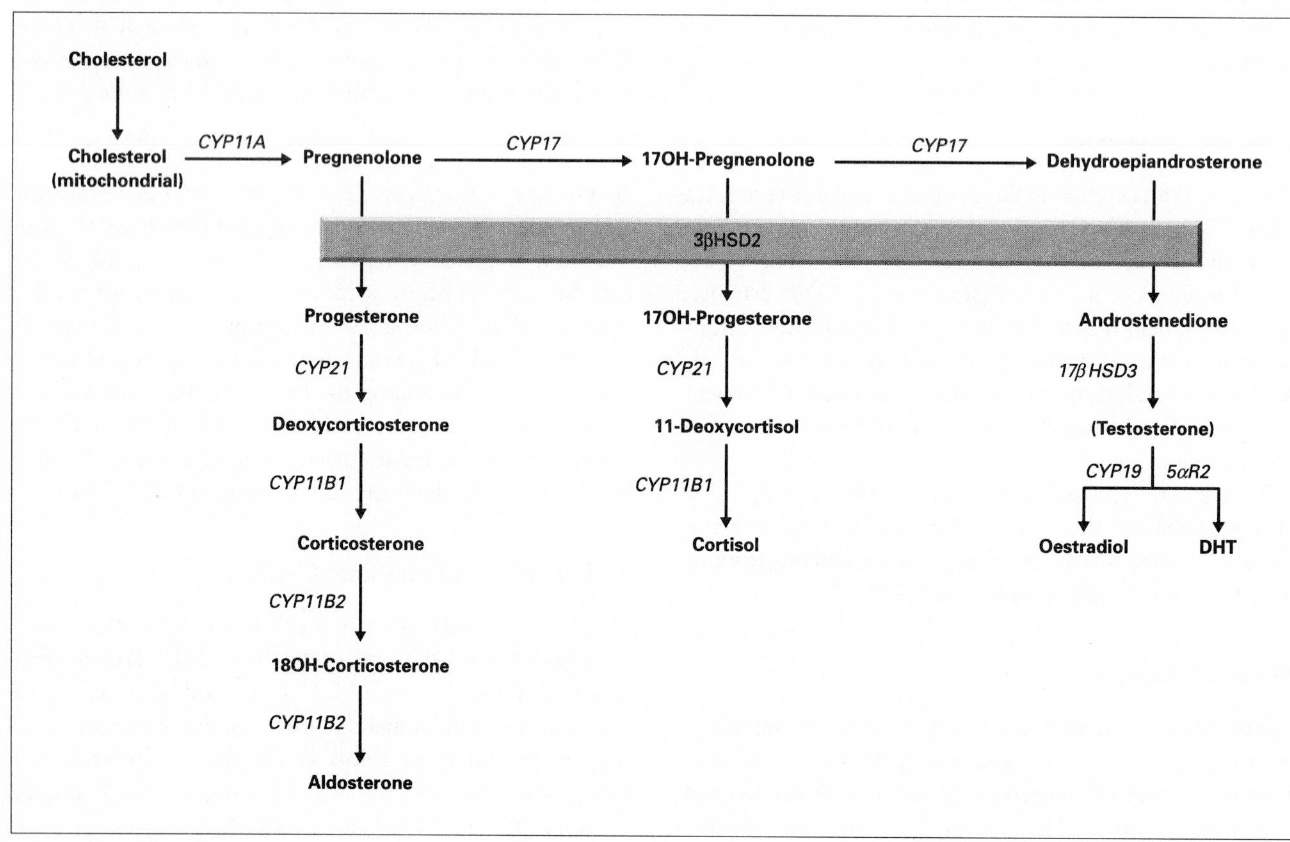

Table 35.14 Genes and enzymes involved in adrenal steroidogenesis.

Enzyme activity	Gene label	Chromosome
20,22-desmolase (P-450scc)	CYP11A	15
3β-hydroxysteroid dehydrogenase	3βHSD2	1p13
17α-hydroxylase (P-450c17α)	CYP17	10
21-hydroxylase (P-450c21)	CYP21	6p23
11β-hydroxylase (P-450c11)	CYP11B1	8q21-q22
18-hydroxylase (P-450c18; P-450aldo)	CYP11B2	8q21-q22

testis and ovary. In classical 3β*ol*-dehydrogenase deficiency, all mutations identified are exclusive to the type II gene [54]. The increased levels of Δ^4 steroids such as 17OH-progesterone observed in some patients are presumably due to substrate use of the intact type I isoenzyme. The late-onset or non-classical form of 3β*ol*-dehydrogenase deficiency is not associated with any identifiable mutation in either the type I or type II gene.

Both 17α-hydroxylase and 17,20-lyase enzyme activities are mediated by a single cytochrome P-450c17 enzyme encoded by the CYP17 gene on chromosome 10. The clinical phenotype associated with mutations of the CYP17 gene depends on which enzyme deficiency is predominant. Ambiguous genitalia is the result in an affected male with 17,20-lyase deficiency whereas hypertension can be profound in either affected sex when 17α-hydroxylase deficiency is severe. This second enzyme deficiency may only arise with increasing age [55]. Mutational analysis of the CYP17 gene demonstrates a heterogeneous nature to the defects with some correlation between mutation type and degree of enzyme deficiency as based on studies of mutant enzymes expressed *in vitro*. CYP11B1 and CYP11B2, two closely related genes about 4.5 kb apart on chromosome 8, encode enzymes responsible for cortisol and aldosterone synthesis, respectively. Both possess 11β-hydroxylase activity while CYP11B2 encodes an enzyme which also has 18-hydroxylation and 18-oxidation activities. The latter enzyme function is also referred as P-450aldo or aldosterone synthase. Isolated congenital aldosterone deficiency is rare and molecular studies have demonstrated substitution of a highly conserved arginine by proline at amino-acid position 384 which is involved in haeme binding [56]. An arginine substitution in a similar position of the CYP11B1 gene causes classical 11β-hydroxylase deficiency. The disorder is relatively frequent (one in 5000–7000 births) in Moroccan Jews where the genetic abnormality is a missense arginine to histidine mutation at amino-acid position 448 which completely abolishes enzyme activity [57].

The molecular genetics of CAH is best characterised for 21-OHD in which the disorder was known for some time to be closely linked with the genes encoding the major histocompatibility complex on the short arm of chromosome 6. Thus, the C21-OHDSW form is closely correlated with the uncommon HLA-BW-47 antigen. An active (CYP21) and an inactive pseudo-gene (CYP21P) are in tandem duplication with two C4 genes as depicted in Fig. 35.12. Approximately 20–25% of classical 21-OHD cases are the result of a

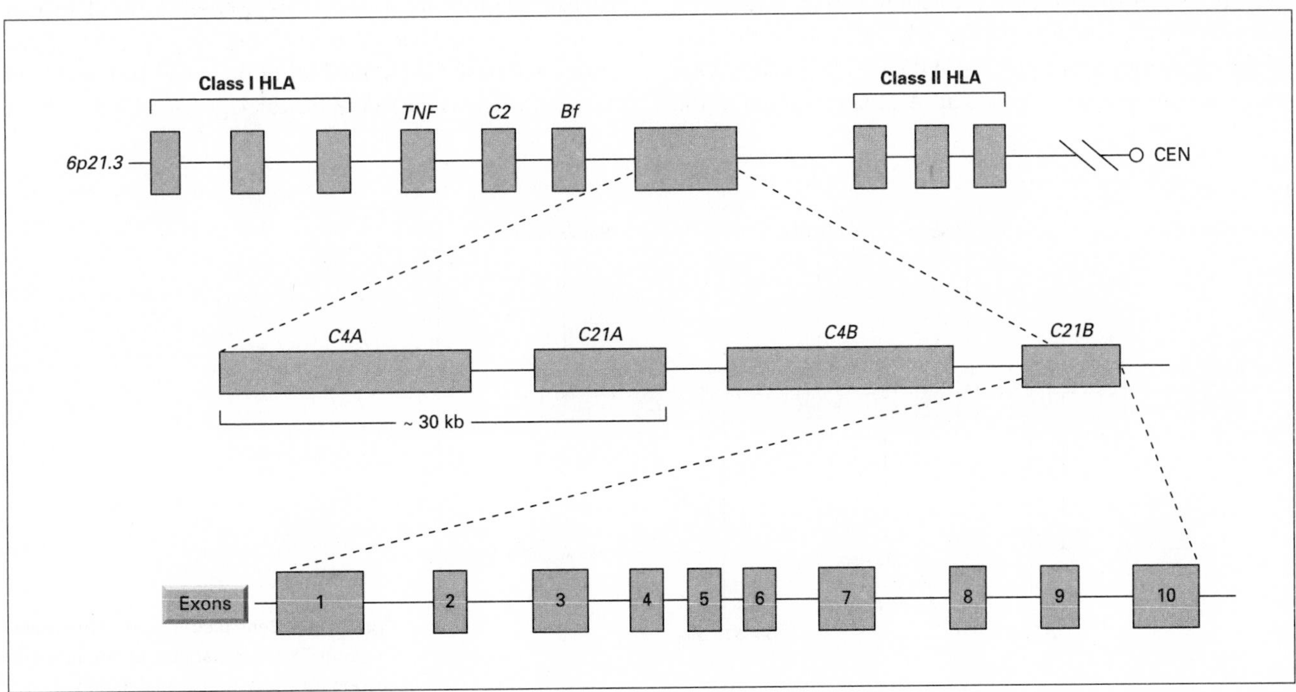

Fig. 35.12 Organisation of the CYP21 gene on chromosome 6p.

Table 35.15 Clinical phenotypes and types of CYP21 mutations.

Phenotype	Mutation
Salt wasting	Deletion (15–30%) Intron 2(20–50%) Arg 356 Trp Δ 8bp, exon 3 Cluster of mutations, exon 6 Glu 318 STOP Insertion, exon 7
Simple virilising	Ile 172 Asu (10–20%) Arg 356 Trp
Non-classical	Val 281 Leu (5–15%) Pro 30 Leu Pro 453 Ser
No mutation detected in 10–12% patients	

Percentages in brackets refer to range of frequencies reported.

recombination event with unequal crossing over during meiosis resulting in deletion of the active CYP 21 gene. The CYP21P pseudo-gene has become inactivated as a result of a series of deleterious mutations and the active CYP21 gene can acquire such mutations as a result of a gene conversion event [6]. Table 35.15 lists the more frequent types of mutations which lead to the three forms of 21-OHD recognised clinically and their distribution throughout the exon organisation of the gene is illustrated in Fig. 35.13. The concordance between the type of mutation and clinical manifestation is generally close, although there are always exceptions reported [58,59]. Predictions can be made from prenatal testing which is particularly valuable in the case of the salt-wasting form of 21-OHD affecting males. One of the commonest mutations is an A to G transition in the second intron which results in abnormal splicing of exons 2 and 3 and the synthesis of a truncated protein with no enzymatic activity. The mutation is universally found in those Yupick Eskimos of Alaska who have CAH suggesting a founder effect in this inbred population. Occasionally, the splicing mutation can result in a salt-wasting syndrome which is delayed beyond the neonatal period, perhaps the result of variable splicing producing some normal enzyme [60]. Another example to highlight is a valine to leucine substitution at amino-acid position 281 which invariably is associated with the non-classical or late-onset form of 21-OHD.

Prenatal diagnosis and treatment

Prenatal diagnosis of CAH is obviously only applicable where there is already an affected child in the family. The ultimate purpose of diagnosis is to offer either *in utero* treatment or, more rarely, termination of an affected pregnancy [61–63].

Early diagnosis using chorionic villus biopsy (CVB) performed between 7 and 12 weeks of gestational age is now possible. Villus tissue so obtained is first cultured, then used to ascertain the sex and HLA status of the fetus. This can be done either with conventional genetic techniques (HLA microcytotoxicity testing and standard karyotyping) or, where available, newer molecular genetic techniques such as HLA-specific probes and PCR sex determination. A variety of techniques are now also available to evaluate the CYP21B gene directly, including Southern blotting and specific probes that will permit detection of the commoner mutations. The adjacent C4 genes can be similarly probed [64,65]. The risk/benefit ratios must be carefully weighed; the chance of a fetus requiring therapy is only 1:8 (one-quarter of the fetuses will have CAH, one-half of these will be female, on average), whereas the risk of miscarriage from CVB is about

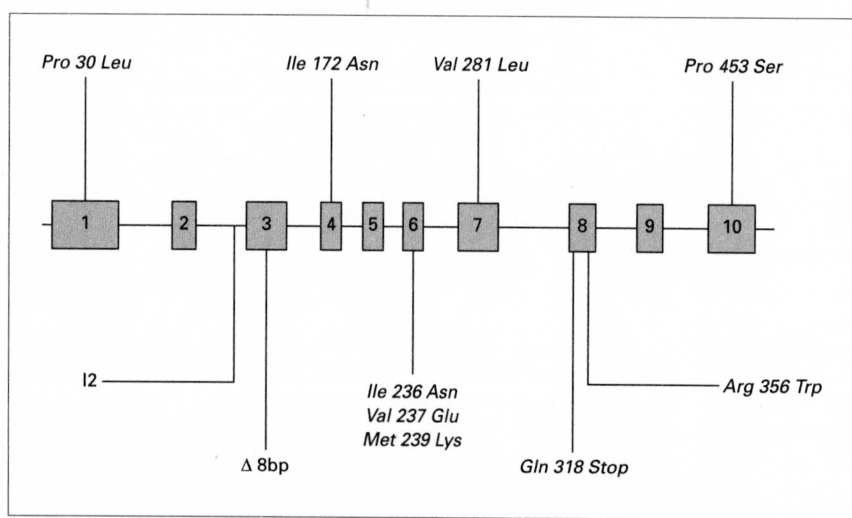

Fig. 35.13 Gene distribution of the most frequent CYP21 mutations. I2: mutation in second intron. Δ: indicates deletion.

1%. Furthermore, prenatal treatment cannot guarantee an unaffected fetus.

Amniocentesis is usually performed during the second trimester (15–18 weeks). Over 80% of cases can be reliably diagnosed; prediction is most accurate where measurement of amniotic fluid 17-OHP (normally < 30 nmol/l) is used in conjunction with full HLA typing of cultured amniotic cells [62,66].

Measurement of Δ^4 steroid concentrations may also be useful if the affected sibling has C21-OHDSV, as 17-OHP levels are occasionally falsely normal in the similarly affected fetus, whereas Δ^4 steroids will be raised. If dexamethasone was com-menced in the first trimester and amniocentesis is now being performed in order to establish that the fetus is indeed an affected female, it should be discontinued at least 5 days previously, otherwise a falsely low level may result.

Prenatal treatment is indicated only for affected female fetuses, but for maximum effect needs to be commenced before the sex of the fetus is known, i.e. at 5–7 weeks' gestational age. The aim is to suppress fetal adrenal androgen production and prevent virilisation. Dexamethasone in doses of 0.5–1.5 mg/day or 20 μg/kg/day (range 10–45) in two or three divided doses has been used with variable success. Treatment is continued until the fetal status is ascertained at CVB or amniocentesis and then continued if the fetus is female and HLA type is identical with the index case [67,68]. The dose of dexamethasone may be adjusted by reference to maternal serum/urine oestriol levels, and the amniotic fluid 17-OHP concentration in the second trimester. Dose increase for increasing maternal weight during the pregnancy is not necessary, and indeed a reduction after mid-pregnancy may be possible. Severe maternal side-effects are rare, though about 10% experience excessive weight gain, hypertension, glucose intolerance, mild oedema, hypertrichosis and abdominal pain. There appear to be no adverse fetal effects and teratogenicity has not been reported. The success of therapy in preventing virilisation increases with earlier onset (< 7 weeks), adequate dosage (both total daily dose and division into twice or thrice daily) and uninterrupted therapy. Virilisation is usually reduced to the degree where corrective surgery is not necessary. Further studies are needed to determine any long-term adverse effects of this treatment, both to the mother and to the fetus [69].

Prenatal diagnosis of C11β-OHD is possible by estimating S concentration in amniotic fluid. Prenatal treatment is also theoretically possible, but there is much less experience with this rarer type of CAH.

References

1 Miller WL. Congenital adrenal hyperplasias. *Endocrinol Metab Clin North Am* 1991; **20**: 721–49.

2 New MI. Genetic disorders of adrenal hormone synthesis. *Horm Res* 1992; **37** (Suppl. 3): 22–33.

3 Kalaitzoglou G, New MI. Congenital adrenal hyperplasia. Molecular insights learned from patients. *Receptor* 1993; **3**: 211–22.

4 Waterman MR, Lund J, Ahlgren R, Win D, Simpson ER. Regulation of steroid hydroxylase gene expression and steroid hormone biosynthesis. *Biochem Soc Transac* 1990; **18**: 26–8.

5 New MI. Steroid 21-hydroxylase deficiency (congenital adrenal hyperplasia). *Am J Med* 1995: **98** (Suppl. 1A); 2S–8S.

6 White DC, Tusie-Luna MT, New MI, Spenser PW. Mutations in steroid 21-hydroxylase (CYP21). *Human Mutation* 1994; **3**: 373–8.

7 White PC, New MI. Genetic basis of endocrine disease 2: congenital adrenal hyperplasia due to 21-hydroxylase deficiency. *J Clin Endocrinol Metab* 1992; **74**: 6–11.

8 Migeon CJ, Donohoue PA. Congenital adrenal hyperplasia caused by 21-hydroxylase deficiency. Its molecular basis and its remaining therapeutic problems. *Endocrinol Metab Clin North Am* 1991; **20**: 277–96.

9 Azziz R. 21-hydroxylase-deficient nonclassic adrenal hyperplasia. *Endocrinologist* 1995; **5**: 297–303.

10 Eldar-Geva T, Hurwitz A, Vecsei P, Palti Z, Milwidsky A, Rosler A. Secondary biosynthetic defects in women with late-onset congenital adrenal hyperplasia. *N Engl J Med* 1990; **323**: 855–63.

11 Azziz R, Dewailly D, Owerbach D. Clinical review 56: nonclassic adrenal hyperplasia: current concepts. *J Clin Endocrinol Metab* 1994; **78**: 810–15.

12 Harinarayan CV, Ammini AC, Karmarkar MG *et al.* Congenital adrenal hyperplasia and complete masculinization masquerading as sexual precocity and cryptorchidism. *Ind Ped* 1992; **29**: 103–06.

13 Donaldson MDC, Thomas PH, Love JG, Murray GP, McNinch AW, Savage DCL. Presentation, acute illness and learning difficulties in salt-wasting 21-hydroxylase deficiency. *Arch Dis Child* 1994; **70**: 214–18.

14 Vasconcelos M, Mendonca BB, Arnold IJP *et al.* Identification of non-classical 21-hydroxylase deficiency in girls with precocious pubarche. *J Endocrinol Invest* 1991; **14**: 11–15.

15 Hawkins LA, Chasalow FI, Blethen SL. The role of adrenocorticotrophin testing in evaluating girls with premature adrenarche and hirsutism/oligomenorrhea. *J Clin Endocrinol Metab* 1992; **74**: 248–53.

16 Speiser PW, Agdere L, Ueshiba H. White PC, New MI. Aldosterone synthesis in salt-wasting congenital adrenal hyperplasia with complete absence of adrenal 21-hydroxylase. *N Engl J Med* 1991; **324**: 145–9.

17 Rosler A, Levine IS, Schneider B, Novogroder M, New MI. The interrelationship of sodium balance, plasma renin activity and ACTH in congenital adrenal hyperplasia. *J Clin Endocrinol Metab* 1977; **45**: 500–12.

18 Siegel SF, Finegold DN, Lanes R, Lee PA. ACTH stimulation tests and plasma dehydroepiandrosterone sulfate levels in women with hirsutism. *N Engl J Med* 1990; **323**: 849–54.

19 Rouach M, Blumenfeld Z. Diagnosis of late onset congenital adrenal hyperplasia. *Harefuah* 1993; **124**: 249–53.

20 Menon PSN, Harinarayan CV, Forest MG. Congenital adrenal hyperplasia due to 11-beta-hydroxylase deficiency. *Ind Ped* 1992; **29**: 98–103.

21 White PC, Speiser PW. Steroid 11-beta-hydroxylase deficiency and related disorders. *Endocrinol Metab Clin North Am* 1994; **23**: 325–39.

22 White PC, Curnow KM, Pascoe L. Disorders of steroid 11-beta-hydroxylase isozymes. *Endocr Rev* 1994; **15**: 421–38.

23 Kater CE, Biglieri EG. Disorders of steroid 17α-hydroxylase deficiency. *Endocrinol Metab Clinic North Am* 1994; **23**: 341–57.

24 Yanase T, Simpson ER, Waterman MR. 17-α-hydroxylase/17,20-lyase deficiency: from clinical investigation to molcecular definition. *Endocr Rev* 1991; **12**: 91–108.

25 Editorial. Premature adrenarche: a normal variant of puberty? *J Clin Endocrinol Metab* 1992; **74**: 236–8.

26 Cathro DM, Golombek SG. Non-classical 3-beta-hydroxysteroid dehydrogenase deficiency in children in central Iowa. Difficulties in differentiating this entity from cases of precocious adrenarche without an adrenal enzyme defect. *J Ped Endocrinol* 1994; **7**: 19–32.

27 Siegel SF, Finegold DN, Urban M, McVie R, Lee PA. Premature pubarche: etiological herterogeneity. *J Clin Endocrinol Metab* 1992; **74**: 239–47.

28 Winter JS. Hyperandrogenism in female adolescents. *Curr Opin Ped* 1993; **5**: 488–93.

29 Rosenfield R. Hyperandrogenism in peripubertal girls. *Ped Clin North Amer* 1990; **37**: 1333–59.

30 Bailey-Pridham DD, Sanfilippo JS. Hirsutism in the adolescent female. *Ped Clin North Amer* 1989; **36**: 581–99.

31 Bryan PJ, Caldamone AA, Morrison SC, Yulish BS, Owens RO. Ultrasound findings in the adreno-genital syndrome (congenital adrenal hyperplasia). *J Ultrasound Med* 1988; **7**: 675–9.

32 Honour JW, Rumsby G. Problems in diagnosis and management of congenital adrenal hyperplasia due to 21-hydroxylase deficiency. *J Steroid Biochem Mol Biol* 1993; **45**: 69–74.

33 New MI, Lorenzen F, Lerner AJ *et al.* Genotyping steroid 21-hydroxylase deficiency; hormonal reference data. *J Clin Endocrinol Metab* 1983; **57**: 320.

34 Zerah M, Pang S, New MI. Morning salivary 17-alpha-hydroxyprogesterone is a useful screening test for non-classical 21-hydroxylase deficiency. *J Clin Endocrinol Metab* 1987; **65**: 227–32.

35 Zerah M, Ueshiba H, Wood E *et al.* Prevalence of non-classical steroid 21-hydroxylase deficiency based on a morning salivary 17-hydroxyprogesterone screening test: a small sample study. *J Clin Endocrinol Metab* 1990; **70**: 1662–7.

36 Innanen VI, Vale JM. Assessment of the one hour adrenocorticotrophic hormone test in the diagnosis of attenuated 21-hydroxylase deficiency. *J Clin Pathol* 1990; **43**: 493–5.

37 Wilkins L, Lewis RA, Klein R, Rosemberg E. The suppression of androgen secretion by cortisone in a case of congenital adrenal hyperplasia. *Bull Johns Hopkins Hosp* 1950; **86**: 249–52.

38 Bartter FC, Albright F, Forbes AP, Leaf A, Dempsey E, Carroll E. The effects of adrenocorticotrophic hormone and cortisone in the adrenogenital syndrome associated with congenital adrenal hyperplasia: an attempt to explain and correct this disordered hormonal pattern. *J Clin Invest* 1951; **30**: 237–51.

39 Young MC, Cook N, Read CF, Hughes IA. The pharmacokinetics of low-dose dexamethasone in congenital adrenal hyperplasia. *Eur J Clin Pharmacol* 1989; **37**: 75–77.

40 Shen SX, Young MC, Hinohosa-Sandoval M, Hughes IA. The 17OH-progesterone response to acute dexamethasone administration in congenital adrenal hyperplasia. *Horm Res* 1989; **32**: 136–41.

41 Young MC, Hughes IA. Loss of therapeutic control in congenital adrenal hyperplasia due to interaction between dexamethasone and primidone. *Acta Paediatr Scand* 1991; **80**: 120–24.

42 Tilul'pakov AN, Kasatkina EP, Ibragimova GV. Mineralocorticoids (MC) in the treatment of congenital adrenal hyperplasia due to 21-hydroxylase deficiency (21-OHD). *Ped Res* 1993; **33** (Suppl): S25 (abstract 128).

43 Rappaport R, Cornu G, Royer P. Statural growth in congenital adrenal hyperplasia treated with hydrocortisone. *J Pediatr* 1968; **75**: 760–6.

44 Young MC, Hughes IA. The response to treatment of congenital adrenal hyperplasia in infancy. *Arch Dis Child* 1990; **65**: 441–4.

45 Anonymous. Corticosteroid replacement: getting it right. *Drug Ther Bull* 1990; **28**: 71–2.

46 Appan S, Hindmarsh PC, Brook CGD. Monitoring treatment in congenital adrenal hyperplasia. *Arch Dis Child* 1989; **64**: 1235–9.

47 Hughes IA, Read G. Control in congenital adrenal hyperplasia monitored by frequent saliva 17OH-progesterone measurements. *Horm Res* 1984; **19**: 77–85.

48 Young MC, Robinson JA, Read CF, Riad-Fahmy D, Hughes IA. 17OH-progesterone rhythms in congenital adrenal hyperplasia. *Arch Dis Child* 1988; **63**: 617–23.

49 Young MC, Walker RF, Riad-Fahmy D, Hughes IA. Androstenedione rhythms in congenital adrenal hyperplasia. *Arch Dis Child* 1988; **63**: 624–8.

50 Horrocks PM, London DR. Effects of long term dexamethasone treatment in adult patients with congenital adrenal hyperplasia. *Clin Endocrinol* 1987; **27**: 635–41.

51 Hochberg Z, Schechter J, Benderly A, Liebman E, Rosler A. Growth and pubertal development in patients with congenital adrenal hyperplasia due to 11β-hydroxylase deficiency. *Am J Dis Child* 1985; **139**: 771–6.

52 Fukami M, Sato S, Ogata T, Matsuo N. Lack of mutations in P450scc gene (CYP11A) in six Japanese patients with congenital adrenal hyperplasia. *Clin Ped Endocrinol* 1995; **4**: 39–46.

53 Lin D, Sugawara T, Straus III JF *et al.* Role of steroidogenic acute regulatory protein in adrenal and gonadal steroidogenesis. *Science* 1995; **267**: 1828–31.

54 Simard J, Rhéaume E, Sanchez R *et al.* Molecular basis of congenital adrenal hyperplasia due to 3β-hydroxysteroid dehydrogenase deficiency. *Mol Endocrinol* 1993; **7**: 716–28.

55 Zachmann M. Prismatic cases: 17,20 Desmolase (17,20-lyase) deficiency. *J Clin Endocrinol Metab* 1996; **81**: 457–9.

56 Geley S, Jöhrer K, Peter M *et al.* Amino acid substitution R384P in aldosterone synthase causes corticosterone methyl-oxidase Type I deficiency. *J Clin Endocrinol Metab* 1995; **80**: 424–9.

57 Rösler A, White PC. Mutations in human 11β-hydroxylase genes: 11β-hydroxylase deficiency in Jews of Morocco and corticosterone methyl-oxidase II deficiency in Jews of Iran. *J Steroid Biochem Mol Biol* 1993; **45**: 99–106.

58 Wedell A, Thilén A, Ritzén EM, Stengler B, Luthman H. Mutational spectrum of the steroid 21-hydroxylase gene in Sweden: implications for genetic diagnosis and association with disease manifestation. *J Clin Endocrinol Metab* 1994; **78**: 1145–52.

59 Wilson RC, Mercado AB, Cheng KC, New MI. Steroid 21-hydroxylase deficiency: genotype may not predict phenotype. *J Clin Endocrinol Metab* 1995; **80**: 2322–9.

60 Kohn B, Day D, Alemzadeh R *et al.* Splicing mutation in CYP21 associated with delayed presentation of salt-wasting congenital adrenal hyperplasia. *Am J Med Genet* 1995; **57**: 450–4.

61 Forest MG, David M, Morel Y. Prenatal diagnosis and treatment of 21-hydroxylase deficiency. *J Steroid Biochem Mol Biol* 1993; **45**: 75–82.

62 Speiser PW, New MI. Prenatal diagnosis and treatment of congenital adrenal hyperplasia. *J Ped Endocrinol* 1994; **7**: 183–91.

63 Levine LS, Pang S. Prenatal diagnosis and treatment of congenital

adrenal hyperplasia. *J Ped Endocrinol* 1994; **7**: 193–200.

64 Speiser PW, LaForgia N, Kato K *et al.* First trimester prenatal treatment and molecular genetic diagnosis of congenital adrenal hyperplasia (21-hydroxylase deficiency). *J Clin Endocrinol Metab* 1990; **70**: 838–48.

65 Y Morel, Murena M, Forrest MG, Cerel JC, Leger J, Nivelon JL, David M. Prenatal diagnosis of congenital adrenal hyperplasia due to 21-hydroxylase deficiency. *Ped Res* 1993; **33** (Suppl.): S3 (abstract).

66 Hughes IA, Dyas J, Riad-Fahmy D, Laurence KM. Prenatal diagnosis of congenital adrenal hyperplasia; reliability of amniotic fluid steroid analysis. *J Med Genet* 1987; **24**: 344–7.

67 Forest MG, Door HG. Prenatal treatment of congenital adrenal hyperplasia (CAH) due to 21-hydroxylase deficiency: european experience in 223 pregnancies at risk. *Ped Res* 1993; **33** (Suppl): S3 (abstract). (Also *Clinical Courier* 1993; **11**: 2–8.)

68 Speiser PW. Prenatal treatment of congenital adrenal hyperplasia. *Clinical Courier* 1993; **11**: 3.

69 Kelnar CJ. Congenital adrenal hyperplasia (CAH)—the place for prenatal treatment and neonatal screening. *Early Human Dev* 1993; **35**: 81–90.

70 Hughes IA, Fahmy DR, Griffiths K. Plasma 17-OH-progesterone concentrations in newborn infants. *Arch Dis Child* 1979; **54**: 347–9.

71 Murphy JF, Joyce BG, Dyas J, Hughes IA. Plasma 17-hydroxyprogesterone concentrations in ill newborn infants. *Arch Dis Child* 1983; **58**: 532–4.

72 Mulaikal RM, Migeon CJ, Rock JA. Fertility rates in female patients with congenital adrenal hyperplasia due to 21-hydroxylase deficiency. *N Engl J Med* 1987; **316**: 178–82.

73 Holmes-Walker DJ, Conway GS, Honour JW, Rumbsy G, Jacobs HS. Menstrual disturbance and hypersecretion of progesterone in women with congenital adrenal hyperplasia due to 21-hydroxylase deficiency. *Clin Endocrinol* 1995; **43**: 291–6.

74 Premawardhana LDKE, Hughes IA, Read GF, Scanlon MF. Longer-term outcome in females with congenital adrenal hyperplasia (CAH): the Cardiff experience. *Clin Endocrinol* 1997; **46**: 327–32.

75 Lane L, Rennet OM. Congenital adrenal hyperplasia: molecular genetics and alternative approaches to treatment. In: *Advances in Pediatrics*, vol. 42; St Louis: Mosby Year Book Inc 1995; 113–43.

CHAPTER 36

Primary adrenocortical failure

P.J. Trainer and G.M. Besser

Introduction

The adrenal glands weigh approximately 5 g each and can be subdivided anatomically into the cortex and medulla, the former being responsible for steroid synthesis and secretion and the latter catecholamines [1]. The cortex accounts for 90% of the gland and consists of three histologically and functionally distinct components: the zona fasciculata and zona reticularis of the inner cortex are responsible for the synthesis and the secretion of glucocorticoids under the regulation of adrenocorticotrophic hormone (ACTH), and the zona glomerulosa for release of aldosterone, the main mineralocorticoid, under the regulation of the renin–angiotensin system. In primates, the dog and rabbits, cortisol is the principal glucocorticoid whereas corticosterone is the main glucocorticoid in rodents. In humans, cortisol is secreted at a rate of 9.9 mg per day under basal conditions [2]. The medulla secretes three principal catecholamines: adrenaline, noradrenaline and dopamine, under the modulation of preganglionic cholinergic neurons. The clinical manifestations of primary adrenal failure are a consequence of combined cortisol and aldosterone deficiency and occur only when there is destruction of at least 90% of adrenocortical tissue; adrenomedullary catecholamine deficiency is of no clinical importance since adequate levels are achieved from noradrenergic neurons [3,4].

Disease affecting the hypothalamo-pituitary unit results in ACTH hyposecretion leading to secondary adrenal insufficiency and is manifest as isolated cortisol deficiency either alone (see Chapter 16) or in combination with other pituitary hormone deficiencies. Isolated ACTH deficiency is also imitated by mutations of the ACTH receptor, with consequent resistance to ACTH actions on the adrenal cortex, and the related Allgrove's syndrome [5–7]. Aldosterone secretion is usually adequately sustained by renin in the absence of ACTH. Isolated aldosterone deficiency is extremely rare and is characterised by hyperkalaemia with cardiac dysrhythmias, acidosis and muscle weakness.

In 1855, Thomas Addison described, with remarkable perception and clarity, the clinical consequences of destruction of the adrenal glands [8]. Nearly 150 years later and with the advantages of hormone measurement, hypoadrenalism is still overlooked and the diagnosis delayed, but once considered can usually be rapidly confirmed. Lethargy, fatigue and weakness are uniform among patients but are of low specificity to this syndrome, and possibly because of their insidious onset and apparently nebulous nature diagnosis is all too often delayed. Gastrointestinal symptoms such as weight loss, anorexia, nausea, abdominal pain and diarrhoea are common, as are muscle and joint pains. Postural hypotension of 20 mmHg can be found in the majority of patients even with subclinical compensated hypoadrenalism; it is uniform in patients acutely unwell, and is a useful diagnostic aid. Increased skin pigmentation, particularly of the palmar creases, scars, buccal mucosa and pressure points such as knuckles, knees and under the belt, is specific for primary hypoadrenalism and a consequence of elevated plasma ACTH which has melanocyte-stimulating activity (Plate 36.1; opposite p. 332). ACTH shares a peptide sequence contained within melanocyte-stimulating hormones (MSH) of subhuman species, for example α-MSH and β-MSH, but there is no MSH peptide hormone secreted in normal humans post-partum. Recent work suggests that this is due to interaction of ACTH with a specific MSH receptor in the skin.

Gradual destruction of the adrenal glands can result in a prolonged period during which basal plasma cortisol levels are maintained but ACTH levels are high (compensated hypoadrenalism). Symptoms are minimal but Addisonian pigmentation is present; the lack of adrenal reserve and consequent inability to mount a 'stress' response can result in decompensation during 'trivial' illness and delayed recovery. In women, reduced adrenal androgen secretion may result in loss of body hair. Vitiligo and other associated autoimmune endocrine disease such as diabetes mellitus or thyroid dysfunction may accompany autoimmune adrenal failure (see below). The first presentation may be in a crisis with dehydration, hypotension, vomiting and diarrhoea with hyponatremia, hyperkalaemia, hypoglycaemia and hypercalcaemia as the main clues to the correct diagnosis (see below).

Aetiology (Table 36.1)

Worldwide, tuberculosis is still the most common cause of adrenal insufficiency. Mycobacterial infection of the adrenal gland initially causes enlargement followed by fibrosis, shrinkage and calcification with the characteristic caseating granulomas on histology in both the cortex and medulla [9]. In the developed world autoimmune adrenal insufficiency accounts for over 80% of cases and often occurs as a part of the autoimmune polyglandular syndromes (APGS) [10]. Pernicious anaemia, hypothyroidism, vitiligo, alopecia and gonadal failure are common to both type I and II APGS [11]. Type II APGS typically presents in early adult life and, in addition to the above, may be associated with hyperthyroidism, insulin-dependent diabetes mellitus and myasthenia gravis; it is of autosomal dominant inheritance and is linked to human leucocyte antigen (HLA) DR3 and 4 [12]. Type I APGS is a rare autosomal recessive condition with no recognised HLA haplotype and presents in childhood with mucocutaneous candidiasis and hypoparathyroidism; hypoadrenalism often develops later [13,14]. Humoral and cell-mediated autoimmune mechanisms are involved in the destruction of all layers of the adrenal cortex in autoimmune adrenalitis, with much work having been devoted to the identification of serological markers of disease activity. Complement-fixing anticytoplasmic adrenal antibodies, mainly of the IgG class, are present in the serum of at least 80% of patients with 'idiopathic' hypoadrenalism at diagnosis, but may disappear with time; antibodies are present in only between 0.1 and 0.2% of the general population [15]. Anti-'steroid-producing cell' antibodies have been identified that react with adrenal cytoplasmic antigens, Leydig cells, placental trophoblasts and theca cells, and are associated with hypoadrenalism and premature primary gonadal failure [16]. Autoantibodies to the ACTH receptor and steroid synthetic enzymes have been identified in the plasma of patients with autoimmune adrenal failure but are unlikely to play an aetiological role in causing the adrenal failure [17].

All types of fungi, with exception of *Candida*, are being recognised with increasing frequency as the causative agents in primary adrenal insufficiency, particularly where fungal infection is endemic and in immune-compromised individuals. Histoplasmosis is endemic in regions of the mid-western and southern states of the USA, while in South America blastomycosis and paracoccidioidomycosis are the common fungal infections and important causes of adrenal failure [18,19]. Cryptococcosis and coccidioidomycosis are rare

Table 36.1 Causes of primary adrenal failure.

Autoimmune
Infection
Tuberculosis
Fungal infection
Histoplasmosis
Blastomycosis
Coccidiomycosis
Cryptococcosis
Paracoccidoidomycosis
Acquired immune deficiency syndrome (AIDS)
Cytomegalovirus
Congenital or hereditary
Adrenal hyperplasia (see Chapter 35)
Lipoid adrenal hyperplasia (cholesterol 20, 22 desmolase defect)
Adrenal hypoplasia
Adrenal cysts
ACTH receptor gene mutations
Allgrove's syndrome (triple A syndrome)
Adrenoleucodystrophy
Adrenomyeloneuropathy
Drugs inhibiting cortisol synthesis
Aminoglutethamide
Metyrapone
*o,p'*DDD
Ketoconazole
Suramin
Drugs increasing cortisol clearance
Barbiturates
Phenytoin
Rifampicin
Other
Haemorrhage
Infection (Waterhouse–Friderichsen Syndrome)
Neisseria meningitides
Haemophilus influenzae
Pseudomonas aeruginosa
Escherichia coli
Pneumococcus
Anticoagulant therapy
Metastatic tumour (commonly lung)
Amyloidosis
Haemochromatosis
Sarcoidosis
Bilateral adrenalectomy

ACTH, adrenocorticotrophic hormone.

causes of adrenal destruction but have increased in incidence with the advent of acquired immune deficiency syndrome (AIDS). The pathological process is comparable with tuberculosis of the adrenals with formation of caseating granulomas and subsequent shrinkage and calcification. Cytomegalovirus adrenalitis is an occasional cause of hypoadrenalism in patients with AIDS, as is infection with atypical microbacteria such as *Mycobacterium avium-intracellulare* [20–23].

X-linked adrenoleucodystrophy (ALD, Addison–Schilder's disease) is a rare inherited disorder of very-long-chain fatty acid (VLCFA) metabolism that results in progressive demyelination of the central nervous system and hypoadrenalism affecting glucocorticoid secretion preferentially. The ALD gene has been identified and is responsible for defective peroxisomal β-oxidation of VLCFA, particularly C24 : 0 and C26 : 0 [24]. The clinical phenotype varies greatly, even in the same family, from at one extreme rapidly progressive spastic tetraparesis, dementia, epilepsy, coma and death, through to adrenomyeloneuropathy (AMN) in which the gene defect is the same but cerebral cortical function is spared [25]. Adrenal insufficiency is also very variable, often omitting glomerulosa-aldosterone deficiency and is only seen in males; females may show mild spasticity.

Congenital adrenal hyperplasia (see Chapter 35) or hypoplasia can result in neonatal hypoadrenalism with either a salt-losing crisis or present more insidiously with lethargy and hyperpigmentation in the first month of life or virilism later. Congenital adrenal hypoplasia is present in one in 12 500 births and is the common end-point of several pathological processes. The affected adrenals have a combined weight < 1 g and the medulla is spared [26]. Three distinct histological types have been described; cytomegalic or primary (abnormal architecture, giant cells), anencephalic (commonest form, fetal zone absent, adult cortical zone well differentiated) and miniature (normal architecture, just very small, may be a subclassification of anencephalic type) [26–28]. Familial X-linked and autosomal recessive inheritance as well as sporadic forms are recognised [29,30]. Primary or cytomegalic congenital adrenal hypoplasia is an X-linked condition that can occur in association with delayed puberty (hypogonadotrophic hypogonadism); the genetic mutation is known and probably relates to mutations of a recently identified nuclear hormone receptor gene (DAX-1) [31,75,76]. As noted above, isolated glucocorticoid deficiency may occur as an autosomal recessive abnormality due to ACTH-receptor mutations, and also in association with alacrima and achalasia and a variety of neurological problems; this latter is termed Allgrove's or the 'triple A' syndrome [7].

In the last decade it has been recognised that end-organ insensitivity to glucocorticoids, including cortisol, can mimic mild adrenal failure. Familial glucocorticoid resistance is a rare disorder of variable severity in which patients have elevated plasma cortisol and ACTH levels and adrenal hyperplasia but no signs of Cushing's syndrome; indeed, they may show symptoms and signs of hypoadrenalism. The high ACTH levels result in excess adrenal androgen secretion. Hence, women present with hirsutism, acne and menstrual irregularities, while in men, because androgen excess may not be clinically apparent, the phenotype is more difficult to recognise with mild hypertension and hypokalaemia, due to excess mineralocorticoid activity of cortisol precursors, being the main features [32,33]. The variable severity of the signs and symptoms reflects the differing degrees of glucocorticoid resistance consequent upon the diverse point mutations and microdeletions of the glucocorticoid-receptor gene described in these families [34]. Presumably, severe mutations are incompatible with life.

Acquired glucocorticoid resistance can occur as an adjunct to non-endocrine illness. Norbiato *et al.* [35] described a cohort of patients with advanced AIDS and clinical stigmata of hypoadrenalism (postural hypotension, hyperpigmentation, hyponatremia) but elevated plasma cortisol and ACTH levels which did not suppress in response to dexamethasone. Glucocorticoid-receptor ligand-binding studies on peripheral lymphocytes demonstrated reduced affinity for ligand, and reduced bioactivity measured by thymidine incorporation. The clinical significance of these changes and their therapeutic implications are the subject of intense study.

Biochemical features

Urea and electrolytes

The electrolyte abnormalities of primary hypoadrenalism are the result of a combination of aldosterone deficiency, causing a failure to reabsorb sodium and excrete potassium in the distal tubules and collecting ducts of the kidney and the distal colon, and glucocorticoid deficiency, causing loss of vascular tone and hypovolaemia, which in turn causes an *appropriate* vasopressin response, water retention and haemodilution. In decompensated primary adrenal failure the plasma urea is elevated, hyponatremia is uniform and is often accompanied by hyperkalaemia. Potassium loss due to vomiting or diarrhoea can normalise the serum potassium. Hyponatraemia is the result of a combination of chronic renal sodium loss and an appropriate vasopressin response to hypovolemia. Aldosterone is unaffected by ACTH deficiency and hence in secondary adrenal failure aldosterone secretion is usually maintained; the serum potassium is usually normal and hyponatraemia, secondary to vasopressin secretion, is mild.

Hypercalcaemia is seen in a variable proportion of patients with hypoadrenalism, and rapidly reverses with glucocorticoid therapy [36].

Hypoglycaemia

The initial presentation of hypoadrenalism in childhood may be a hypoglycaemic fit, and hypoglycaemia, due to impaired gluconeogenesis, is present in 90% of children and neonates with hypoadrenalism and approximately one-third of adults [3,4]. Hypoadrenalism is part of the differential diagnosis of any child or adult with hypoglycaemia. Symptoms of hypoglycaemia such as weakness, anxiety and sweating may precede convulsions and require prompt intervention as untreated hypoglycaemia can be fatal. Adrenal failure causing hypoglycaemia may complicate bacterial septicaemia, as in fulminating meningococcal infection. Hypoglycaemia is glucocorticoid responsive but initially treatment should be combined with glucose administration.

Haematology

A normocytic, normochromic anaemia and neutropenia with eosinophilia commonly accompany cortisol deficiency and reverse with treatment. In autoimmune adrenal failure, a peripheral blood macrocytosis may indicate the coexistence of pernicious anaemia.

Thyroid function tests

Interpretation of thyroid function tests in a hypoadrenal patient may be difficult. As in any seriously ill patient, the sick-euthyroid syndrome (normal thyroid-stimulating hormone (TSH), low thyroxine (T_4) and triiodothyronine (T_3)) may accompany hypoadrenalism (see Chapter 31). Difficulty arises in patients with hypoadrenalism and an elevated serum TSH in combination with low T_4 and T_3. The coexistence of autoimmune hypoadrenalism and primary hypothyroidism is one explanation, but cortisol deficiency itself may cause the same biochemical picture which resolves with glucocorticoid therapy alone [37–39]. In this context, if primary hypothyroidism is thought to coexist and to require treatment, T_3 should be used in preference to T_4 for replacement therapy once cortisol treatment is established, as the shorter half-life allows treatment to be discontinued conveniently and thyroid function tests followed weekly to see if the TSH rises again. Conversely but very rarely, hypothyroidism with an elevated TSH is the first presentation of hypoadrenalism, under which circumstances T_4 therapy will worsen the situation by exacerbating the glucocorticoid deficiency. It is prudent to measure serum cortisol in all patients prior to commencing T_4 replacement therapy. Another pitfall for the unwary is the coexistence of TSH and ACTH deficiency in secondary hypoadrenalism.

Diagnosis

Emergency diagnosis

No patient ever died of an extra dose of hydrocortisone, but alas many have perished for want of glucocorticoid; the commonest reason for delay in treatment is failure to consider the diagnosis of hypoadrenalism. In any unwell patient with the signs and symptoms and the electrolyte abnormalities outlined, particularly hyponatraemia and hypoglycaemia, blood should be drawn for measurement of serum cortisol, and hopefully also plasma ACTH, and thereafter treatment commenced immediately and continued until the result of the acute serum cortisol measurement is available.

A plasma cortisol of < 200 nmol/l in combination with a ACTH of > 80 ng/l is diagnostic of primary adrenal failure, while a serum cortisol > 550 nmol/l excludes the diagnosis. Usually, plasma ACTH is > 200 ng/l. Other combinations of results require elective investigation once the patient has recovered.

Elective diagnosis

The investigation of patients with suspected adrenal insufficiency involves three steps: confirmation of hypoadrenalism, differentiation between pituitary and adrenal aetiology, and establishing the underlying pathology.

In suspected hypoadrenalism, differentiation between adrenal and pituitary aetiology is rarely difficult. A history of pituitary disease, head or neck radiotherapy, headaches and visual field disturbance, associated signs of hypogonadism and pallor are suggestive of secondary adrenal failure, while the presence of hyperpigmentation, hyponatraemia and hyperkalaemia suggests primary adrenal failure. An ACTH-stimulation test should be undertaken for suspected primary adrenal failure and an insulin tolerance test for secondary hypoadrenalism.

ACTH testing (see also Chapter 83)

The plasma cortisol response to 250 μg of soluble synthetic ACTH (N-terminal 1–24 amino acids) (tetracosactrin, Synacthen, Cortrosyn) is the 'gold standard' for the diagnosis of primary hypoadrenalism with plasma cortisol and ACTH being measured in the early morning at baseline with additional measurement of cortisol at 30 and 60 min. There is a lack of consensus in the definition of the cortisol response required to exclude hypoadrenalism, although the diagnosis of primary hypoadrenalism is usually clear-cut; greater difficulty arises in the diagnosis of secondary hypoadrenalism (see below). In our hands, a plasma cortisol response of

550 nmol/l or above excludes hypoadrenalism [40,41]. In untreated primary adrenal failure the baseline ACTH is elevated and the cortisol is low, although possibly within the normal range. There appears to be little difference in response whether the ACTH is given intramuscularly or intravenously, but some authorities maintain that only the 30-min post-stimulation level has been validated.

Exogenous glucocorticoid therapy, typically in the form of skin cream or inhaler, can suppress spontaneous and ACTH-induced cortisol secretion, and such patients are at risk of hypoadrenalism on discontinuing therapy. False negatives occur in patients with pituitary disease and impaired ACTH secretion, as the pharmacological dose of ACTH used in the short Synacthen test can result in a peak cortisol response of > 550 nmol/l.

Moreira *et al.* [42] performed short tetracosactrin tests on patients with paracoccidioidomycosis, but without clinical evidence of hypoadrenalism, and noted greater impairment of androgen and mineralocorticoid pathways than that of cortisol secretion, suggesting the failing adrenal diverts synthetic capacity from androgen and mineralocorticoid to the essential cortisol pathway. By implication, measurement of adrenal androgens and mineralocorticoids following ACTH stimulation might allow early identification of insidious adrenal failure, but this is not currently used in clinical practice.

The failure to respond to depot Synacthen (1 mg i.m. of depot Synacthen, measurement of plasma cortisol at 0, 30, 60, 90 and 120 min 4, 6, 8, 12, 24 hours; see Chapter 83) can be used to confirm primary adrenal failure as patients with secondary adrenal atrophy will mount a cortisol response with such prolonged stimulation. If serum cortisol levels are low but rise at 12 hours or later after a depot injection of ACTH (e.g. 1 mg i.m. depot Synacthen or Cortrosyn), then prolonged ACTH deficiency must have been present producing adrenocortical atrophy [43,44].

Secondary hypoadrenalism

The combination of a low 0900-hour plasma ACTH and serum cortisol (< 100 nmol/l) is diagnostic of secondary adrenal failure, and no dynamic provocation test is necessary. Exogenous glucocorticoid therapy must be excluded. If cortisol levels exceed 100 nmol/l at 0900 hours a dynamic test of ACTH reserve is needed in the absence of elevated plasma ACTH levels; the insulin tolerance test (see Chapter 83) is the investigation of choice [45–47]. A suboptimal response indicates an inadequate ACTH reserve but not necessarily the need for replacement therapy (see below). Basal serum cortisol levels of 500 nmol/l or above are almost always a predictor of a normal response to hypoglycaemia and the test may be avoided [48]. Insulin-induced hypoglycaemia is contraindicated in individuals with a history of cardiac disease, epilepsy or black-outs, in which case the glucagon test should be used.

The short Synacthen test is being increasingly advocated as a test for secondary hypoadrenalism as it is simpler to perform and free of the risks and contraindications of the insulin tolerance test. Several studies have demonstrated high concordance between the plasma cortisol responses to insulin-induced hypoglycaemia and Synacthen stimulation, but the diagnostic criteria used to exclude secondary hypoadrenalism have varied between plasma cortisol responses of > 500 and > 600 nmol/l, but usually > 550 nmol/l [49–53]. The concern with the 250-μg short Synacthen test is that the 'wrong' component of the hypothalamo-pituitary–adrenal axis is stimulated by a pharmacological dose of ACTH and that the test will fail to detect minor degrees of ACTH insufficiency as illustrated by the case report of Soule *et al.* [54]. Preliminary studies of small numbers of patients suggest that an intravenous bolus of a more physiological dose of ACTH, either 250 ng or 1 μg, may be superior to 250 μg of ACTH, but much more data are required before such a test can be routinely used [55–59].

Investigation of the aetiology of hypoadrenalism

Primary adrenal failure (Table 36.1)

Autoimmune adrenalitis is a diagnosis of exclusion, with adrenal autoantibodies being present in 80% of patients (see above) who often have evidence of other autoimmune diseases. The adrenal glands are small on computed tomography (CT) or magnetic resonance imaging (MRI), in contrast to most other processes such as tuberculosis and fungal infection, which result in enlarged glands. Evidence of tuberculosis on chest radiographs or elsewhere, or a strongly positive tuberculin skin test, are indications for a course of antituberculosis chemotherapy.

Many systemic processes can affect the adrenal glands but there are usually other manifestations to guide investigation. The adrenal blood flow is disproportionately great for their mass, receiving 11% of cardiac output and as a consequence are a frequent site of metastatic deposits, most commonly from lung carcinoma, occasionally bilaterally, resulting in hypoadrenalism [60]. Bilateral adrenal haemorrhage either due to septicaemia (Waterhouse–Friderichsen syndrome) or anticoagulant therapy, particularly in the elderly, may be signalled by loin pain and symptoms of hypoadrenalism [61]. Other clinical manifestations of systemic amyloidosis are usually apparent prior to the development of hypoadrenalism, although disturbance of adrenal function may be detected much earlier [62–64].

Secondary adrenal failure (Table 36.2)

Pituitary and hypothalamic imaging by either CT or MRI scanning will identify structural abnormalities, and pituitary function (see Chapter 83) must be fully assessed as ACTH secretion is usually among the last hormones to be affected by any insult to the pituitary or hypothalamus. In cases where the aetiology remains obscure, a meticulous history of ACTH and glucocorticoid therapy must be taken, particularly including treatments such as a steroid creams or inhalers.

Treatment

Emergency treatment

Parenteral hydrocortisone should commence as soon as blood samples have been obtained for serum cortisol and ACTH assay. An intravenous infusion of hydrocortisone at a rate of 4 mg/hour or 100 mg i.m. every 6 hours will ensure adequate serum cortisol levels, with conversion to oral hydrocortisone (20 mg three times per day) once the patient is better and able to tolerate oral fluids. Mineralocorticoid therapy is unnecessary during high-dose parenteral hydrocortisone administration.

In hypoadrenalism, hypovolaemia is rarely as severe as might at first seem, and improved vascular tone following hydrocortisone may correct many of the features of apparent hypovolaemia. In most circumstances, 1 litre of normal saline intravenously over 4 hours followed by additional fluids as appropriate is adequate.

Long-term treatment

Cortisol, marketed under the generic name of hydrocortisone, is the glucocorticoid of choice in the treatment of adrenal failure as therapy can be monitored by measurement of serum cortisol and its relatively short half-life allows individualised dose adjustment. In an attempt to reproduce the circadian rhythm of cortisol, the first dose should be taken on waking on an empty stomach before rising and the final dose with an early evening meal. The total daily dose of hydrocortisone can vary greatly, the range usually being 10–30 mg/day. The daily dose is traditionally divided into two-thirds in the morning and one-third in the evening, although it is often necessary to administer the daily dose divided three ways, because of inappropriately low blood levels in the middle of the day; we would suggest giving half the total daily dose in the morning and a quarter before lunch and a quarter before the evening meal [65,66]. Many factors alter cortisol metabolism, most notably hepatic enzyme inducers such as rifampicin, phenytoin and carbamazepine, which result in rapid clearance of corticosteroids as well as gonadal steroids, and it is important to adjust the dose for the individual and monitor treatment (67–69).

Alternative glucocorticoids are available but their use is rarely indicated. Cortisone acetate was the first glucocorticoid available but is itself inactive and requires hepatic 11β-hydroxysteroid dehydrogenase to convert it to cortisol. Absorption and conver-sion of cortisone is variable and often idiosyncratic and should now not be used [70]. Potent synthetic glucocorticoids such as dexamethasone and prednisolone cannot be satisfactorily monitored in blood as a routine and precise dose adjustment is difficult, frequently resulting in overtreatment.

Patients with secondary adrenal failure and a suboptimal response to hypoglycaemia but a normal baseline plasma cortisol, for example following pituitary radiotherapy, do not automatically require replacement therapy, but should carry a 'steroid card'and be aware of the need for glucocorticoid therapy at times of illness.

Education is pivotal to successful long-term treatment. Patients should be given a steroid card to carry at all times and be encouraged to register with a reference agency such as the MedicAlert Foundation (9 Hanover Street, London W1R 9HF, UK) and wear a bracelet or necklace indicating their therapy. Patients need to be taught what to do at times of intercurrent illness and in emergencies and preferably given written explanations and instructions [66]. The importance of doubling glucocorticoid therapy at times of intercurrent illness must be stressed, and patients should keep an ampoule of hydrocortisone in the refrigerator contained within an 'emergency pack' containing a syringe, needles and swabs for use in an emergency, for example when vomiting. If possible, a relative should be taught how to administer an intramuscular dose of hydrocortisone, or alternatively it can be handed to the primary-care physician on arrival.

The necessity of and optimal means for assessment of glucocorticoid therapy is controversial. Measurement of serum cortisol profiles allows dose adjustment in an attempt to approximate to the normal circadian rhythm of cortisol in blood while avoiding overtreatment. At least 90% of circulating cortisol is bound to cortisol-binding globulin (CBG), and changes in plasma CBG levels can cause difficulty in interpretation as routine assays measure total rather than free plasma cortisol [71]. To circumvent CBG-related problems, salivary and urinary free cortisol measurement have been advocated but both have major limitations [72]. Plasma CBG, and hence cortisol, are increased by exogenous oestrogen and pregnancy, making it difficult to assess the adequacy of replacement therapy; if in doubt, oestrogen therapy should be discontinued for 6 weeks and a plasma cortisol profile performed. It should be noted that the increased plasma capacity for transport of cortisol caused by high CBG levels

Table 36.2 Causes of secondary adrenal failure.

Pituitary

1 Compression of pituitary stalk vasculature and the gland
- Functionless tumour
- Prolactinoma
- Growth hormone-secreting tumour
- Metastatic (commonly breast or lung)
- Infiltrative (commonly sphenoid ridge meningioma)
- Craniopharyngioma
- Rathke's pouch cyst
- Pituitary abscess
- Lymphocytic hypophysitis

2 Vascular
- Infarction of tumour (pituitary apoplexy)
- Post-partum haemorrhage (Sheehan's syndrome)
- Surgical trauma
- Head injury

3 Other
- Sarcoidosis
- Langerhans' cell histiocytosis (histocytosis X)
- Acute intermittent porphyria
- Haemochromatosis
- Irradiation
- Hypophysectomy
- Exogenous glucocorticoid therapy (including skin creams and inhaled steroids)
- ACTH therapy
- Idiopathic
- Isolated ACTH deficiency
- Tuberculosis

Suprapituitary

1 Tumours
- Craniopharyngioma
- Pinealoma
- Chordoma
- Third ventricle
- Meningioma of the sphenoidal ridge
- Optic chiasm (commonly glioma)
- Metastatic

2 Vascular
- Aneurysms
- Arteriovenous malformations
- Acute epidural and subdural haematoma (post-traumatic)
- Subarachnoid haemorrhage

3 Other
- Tuberculosis
- Norcardosis
- Actinomycosis
- Sarcoidosis
- Langerhans' cell histiocytosis (histocytosis X)
- Anencephaly
- Irradiation
- Exogenous glucocorticoid therapy (including skin creams and inhaled steroids)
- ACTH therapy
- Anorexia nervosa
- Isolated CRH deficiency
- Idiopathic

ACTH, adrenocorticotrophic hormone.

is not an indication to increase the dose of replacement therapy as changes in plasma CBG levels are gradual and free cortisol levels are maintained [73].

Although not routinely necessary, in primary adrenal failure plasma ACTH, measured at predose and 2 hours post-dose, can be used as a measure of the overall adequacy of glucocorticoid replacement therapy. Persistent elevation of the 120-min sample suggests poor compliance or inadequate hydrocortisone dosage.

In patients with primary adrenal failure, mineralocorticoid therapy is administered in the form of fludrocortisone and monitored by measurement of the plasma electrolytes and plasma renin activity measured after lying down for 30 min (120 min after the oral dose) and plasma electrolytes [74]. The daily requirement of fludrocortisone is usually 0.2–0.4 mg, divided into a morning and evening dose; it is now realised that higher doses than have been used in the past are often needed.

In conclusion, nearly 150 years after the definitive description of the consequences of adrenal destruction the greatest challenge for the clinician is recognition of the many guises under which hypoadrenalism can present. Once considered, the diagnosis can usually be rapidly substantiated and treatment instigated. Treatment is effective and should result in restoration of health, a normal lifestyle and life expectancy; the most important determinant of long-term well-being is the underlying process that resulted in adrenal failure. With patient education and close monitoring of treatment, the long-term adverse effects of glucocorticoids should be minimal.

References

1 Symington T. *Functional Pathology of the Adrenal Gland.* Edinburgh: Churchill Livingstone, 1969.
2 Esteban NV, Loughlin T, Yergey, AL *et al.* Daily cortisol production rate in man determined by stable isotope dilution/mass spectrometry. *J Clin Endocrinol Metab* 1991; **72**: 39–45.
3 Aynsley-Green A, Moncrieff MW, Ratter S, Benedict CR, Storrs CN. Isolated ACTH deficiency. Metabolic and endocrine studies in a 7-year-old boy. *Arch Dis Child* 1978; **53**: 499–502.
4 Stacpoole PW, Interlandi JW, Nicholson WE, Rabin D 1982. Isolated ACTH deficiency: a heterogeneous disorder. Critical Review and Report of four new cases. *Medicine* **61**: 13–24.
5 Clark AJL, Mcloughlin L, Grossman A. Familial glucocorticoid deficiency associated with point mutation in the adrenocorticotropin receptor. *Lancet* 1993; **341**, 461–2.
6 Weber A, Toppari J, Harvey RD *et al.* Adrenocorticotropin receptor gene mutations in familial glucocorticoid deficiency: relationships with clinical features in four families. *J Clin Endocrinol Metab* 1995; **80**: 65–71.
7 Allgrove J, Clayden GS, Grant DB, Macaulay JC. Familial glucocorticoid deficiency with achalasia of the cardia and deficient tear production. *Lancet* 1978; **1**: 1284–6.
8 Addison T. On the constitutional and local effects of disease of the suprarenal capsules. In a collection of the published writings of the late Thomas Addison MD physician to Guy's Hospital 1868. *Metab Classics* 1937; **2**: 244–93.
9 Guttman PH. Addison's disease, a statistical analysis of 566 cases and a study of the pathology. *Arch Pathol Lab Med* 1930; **10**: 742–85.
10 Nerup J. Addison's disease—serological studies. *Acta Endocrinolog* 1974; **76**: 142–58.
11 Neufeld M, Maclaren NK, Blizzard RM. Two types of autoimmune Addison's disease associated with different polyglandular autoimmune (PGA) syndromes (Review). *Medicine* 1981; **60**: 355–62.
12 Neufeld M, Maclaren N, Blizzard R. Autoimmune polyglandular syndromes (Review). *Ped Ann* 1980; **9**: 154–62.
13 Weetman AP, Zhang L, Tandon N, Edwards OM. HLA associations with autoimmune Addison's disease. *Tiss Ant* 1991; **38**: 31–3.
14 Ahonen P, Koskimies S, Lokki ML, Tiilikainen A, Perheentrupa J. The expression of autoimmune polyglandular disease type I appears associated with several HLA-A antigens but not with HLA-DR. *J Clin Endocrinol Metab* 1988; **66**: 1152–7.
15 Betterle C, Caretto A, Pedini B, Rigon F, Bertoli P, Peserico A. Complement-fixing activity to melanin-producing cells preceding the onset of vitiligo in a patient with type 1 polyglandular failure (Letter). *Arch Dermatol* 1992; **128**: 123–4.
16 Anderson JR, Goudie RB, Gray K, Stuart-Smith DA. Immunological features of idiopathic Addison's disease: an antibody to cells producing steroid hormones. *Clin Exp Immunol* 1968; **3**: 107–17.
17 Wardle CA, Weetman AP, Mitchell R, Peers N, Robertson WR. Adrenocorticotropic hormone receptor-blocking immunoglobulins in serum from patients with Addison's disease: a reexamination. *J Clin Endocrinol Metab* 1993; **77**: 750–3.
18 Abernathy RS, Melby JC. Addison's disease in North American blastomycosis. *NEJM* 1962; **266**: 552–4.
19 Osa SR, Peterson RE, Roberts RB. Recovery of adrenal reserve following treatment of disseminated South American blastomycosis. *Am J Med* 1981; **71**: 298–301.
20 Glasgow BJ, Steinsapir KD, Anders K, Layfield LJ. Adrenal pathology in the acquired immune deficiency syndrome. *Am J Clin Pathol* 1985; **84**: 594–7.
21 Glasgow BJ, Layfield LJ, Anders KH. Mycobacterium avium-intracellulare and adrenal insufficiency in AIDS (Letter). *Human Pathol* 1988; **19**: 245–6.
22 Guarda LA, Luna MA, Smith JL, Jr, Mansell PW, Gyorkey F, Roca AN. Acquired immune deficiency syndrome: postmortem findings. *Am J Clin Pathol* 1984; **81**: 549–57.
23 Reichert CM, O'Leary TJ, Levens DL, Simrell CR, Macher AM. Autopsy pathology in the acquired immune deficiency syndrome (Review). *Am J Pathol* 1983; **112**: 357–82.
24 Mosser J, Douar AM, Sarde CO *et al.* Putative X-linked adrenoleukodystrophy gene shares unexpected homology with ABC transporters [see comments]. *Nature* 1993; **361**: 726–30.
25 Moser HW, Naidu S, Kumar AJ, Rosenbaum AE. The adrenoleukodystrophies (Review). *Crit Rev Neurobiol* 1987; **3**: 29–88.
26 Favara BE, Franciosi RA, Miles V. Idiopathic adrenal hypoplasia in children. *Am J Clin Pathol* 1972; **57**: 287–96.
27 Mamelle JC, David M, Riou D, Gilly J, Trouillas J, Dutruge J, Gilly R. Hypoplasie surrenalienne congenitale de type cytomegalic. Forme recessive liée au sexe. A propos de trois observations. *Arch Franc Pediat* 1975; **32**: 139–59.
28 Winquist PG. Adrenal hypoplasia. *Arch Pathol Lab Med* 1961; **71**: 324–9.

29 Hay ID, Smail PJ, Forsyth CC. Familial cytomegalic adrenocortical hypoplasia: an X-linked syndrome of pubertal failure. *Arch Dis Child* 1981; **56**: 715–21.

30 Ohlbaum P, Hehunstre PP, Bouchet JL, Deminiere C. Insuffisance surrénale chronique et hyalinose segmentaire et focale familiale. Une nouvelle association. *Pediatrie* 1986; **41**: 86 (abstract).

31 Yanase T, Takayanagi R, Oba K, Nishi Y, Ohe K, Nawata H. New mutations of DAX-1 genes in two Japanese patients with X-linked congenital adrenal hypoplasia and hypogonadotropic hypogonadism. *J Clin Endocrinol Metab* 1996; **81**: 530–5.

32 Malchoff CD, Reardon G, Javier EC, Rogol AD, McDermott P, Loriaux DL. Dexamethasone therapy for isosexual precocious pseudopuberty caused by generalised glucocorticoid resistance. *J Clin Endocrinol Metab* 1994; **79**: 1632–6.

33 Chrousos GP. Syndromes of glucocorticoid resistance. *Ann Intern Med* 1993; **119**: 1113–24.

34 Karl M, Arai K, Stratakis CA, Accili D, Chrousos GP. *Molecular Studies of the Glucocorticoid Receptor Patients with Generalised Glucocorticoid Resistance and Steroid Resistant Asthma*. Washington, DC: The Endocrine Society, 1995: 3–55 (abstract).

35 Norbiato G, Bevilacqua M, Vago T *et al.* Cortisol resistance in acquired immunodeficiency syndrome. *J Clin Endocrinol Metab* 1992; **74**: 608–13.

36 Nerup J. Addison's disease—clinical studies. A report 108 cases. *Acta Endocrinolog* 1974; **76**: 127–41.

37 Gharib H, Hodgson SF, Gastineau CF, Scholz DA, Smith LA. Reversible hypothyroidism in Addison's disease. *Lancet* 1972; **ii**: 734–6.

38 Topliss DJ, White EL, Stockigt JR. Signifiance of thyrotropin excess in untreated primary adrenal insufficiency. *J Clin Endocrinol Metab* 1980; **50**: 52–6.

39 De Nayer P, Dozin B, Vandeput Y, Bottazzo FC, Crabbe J. Altered interaction between triiodothyronine and its nuclear receptors in absence of cortisol: a proposed mechanism for increased thyrotrophin secretion in corticosteroid deficiency. *Eur J Clin Invest* 1987; **17**: 106–10.

40 Wang TWM, Wong SM, Falconer-Smith J, Howlett TA. The use of the short tetracosactrin test for the investigation of suspected pituitary hypofunction. *Ann Clin Biochem* 1996; **33**: 112–18.

41 Price A, Ross RJM. Interpretation of cortisol response to synacthen. *Ann Clin Biochem* 1996; **33**: 175–6.

42 Moreira AC, Martinez R, Castro M, Elias LLK. Adrenocortical dysfunction in paracoccidioimycosis: comparison between plasma beta-lipoprotrophin/adrenocorticotropin levels and adrenocortical tests. *Clin Endocrinol* 1992; **36**: 545–52.

43 Besser GM, Butler PW, Plumpton FS. Adrenocorticotrophic action of long-acting tetracosactrin compared with corticotrophin-gel. *Br Med J* 1967; **4**: 391–4.

44 Galvao-Telves A, Burke CW, Fraser TR. Adrenal function tested with tetracosactrin depot. *Lancet* 1971; **i**: 557–60.

45 Landon J, Greenwood FC, Stamp TCB, Wynn V. The plasma sugar, free fatty acid, cortisol, and growth hormone response to insulin, and the comparison of this procedure with other tests of pituitary and adrenal function. II. In patients with hypothalamic of pituitary dysfunction or anorexia nervosa. *J Clin Invest* 1966; **45**: 437–49.

46 Greenwood FC, Landon J, Stamp TCB. The plasma sugar, free fatty acid, growth hormone and cortisol response to insulin in normal control subjects. *J Clin Invest* 1966; **45**: 429–36.

47 Plumpton FS, Besser GM. The adrenocortical response to surgery and insulin-induced hypoglycaemia in corticosteroid-treated and normal subjects. *Br J Surg* 1969; **56**: 216–19.

48 Jones SL, Trainer PJ, Perry L, Wass JAH, Besser GM, Grossman A. An audit of the insulin tolerance test in adult subjects in an acute investigation unit over one year. *Clin Endocrinol* 1994; **41**: 123–8.

49 Lindholm J, Kehlet H, Blichert-Toft M, Dinesen B, Riishede J. Reliability of the 30-minute ACTH test in assessing hypothalamic-pituitary–adrenal function. *J Clin Endocrinol Metab* 1978; **47**: 272–4.

50 Lindholm J, Kehlet H. Re-evaluation of the clinical value of the 30 min ACTH test in assessing the hypothalamic-pituitary–adrenocortical function. *Clin Endocrinol* 1987; **26**: 53–9.

51 Stewart PM, Corrie J, Seckl JR, Edwards CRW, Padfield P. A rational approach for assessing the hypothalamo-pituitary–adrenal axis. *Lancet* 1988; **i**: 1208–10.

52 Hurel SJ, Thompson CJ, Watson MJ, Harris MM, Baylis PH, Kendall-Taylor P. The short Synacthen and insulin stress tests in the assessment of the hypothalamic-pituitary–adrenal axis. *Clin Endocrinol* 1996; **44**: 141–6.

53 Clayton RN. Short synacthen test versus insulin stress test for assessment of the hypothalamo-pituitary–adrenal axis: controversy revisited. *Clin Endocrinol* 1996; **44**: 147–9.

54 Soule SG, Fahie-Wilson M, Tomlinson S. Failure of the short ACTH test to unequivocally diagnose long-standing symptomatic secondary hypoadrenalism. *Clin Endocrinol* 1996; **44**: 137–40.

55 Crowley S, Hindmarsh PC, Honour JW, Brook CGD. Reproducibility of the cortisol response to stimulation with a low dose of ACTH (1–24)—the effect of basal cortisol levels and comparison of low-dose with high-dose secretory dynamics. *J Endocrinol* 1993; **136**: 167–72.

56 Crowley S, Hindmarsh PC, Holownia P, Honour JW, Brook CG. The use of low doses of ACTH in the investigation of adrenal function in man. *J Endocrinol* 1991; **130**: 475–9.

57 Daidoh H, Morita H, Mune T *et al.* Responses of plasma adrenocortical steroids to low dose ACTH in normal subjects. *Clin Endocrinol* 1995; **43**: 311–15.

58 Tordjman K, Jaffe A, Grazas N, Apter C, Stern N. The role of the low dose (1 microgram) adrenocorticotropin test in the evaluation of patients with pituitary diseases. *J Clin Endocrinol Metab* 1995; **80**: 1301–5.

59 Broide J, Soferman R, Kivity S *et al.* Low-dose adrenocorticotropin test reveals impaired adrenal function in patients taking inhaled corticosteroids. *J Clin Endocrinol Metab* 1995; **80**: 1243–6.

60 Hasan RI, Yonan NA, Lawson RA. Adrenal insufficiency due to bilateral metastases from oat cell carcinoma of the oesophagus. *Eur J Cardio-Thorac Surg* 1991; **5**: 336–7.

61 Siu SC, Kitzman DW, Sheedy PF, Northcutt RC. Adrenal insufficiency from bilateral adrenal hemorrhage (Review). *Mayo Clin Proc* 1990; **65**: 664–70.

62 Arik N, Tasdemir I, Karaaslan Y, Yasavul U, Turgan C, Caglar S. Subclinical adrenocortical insufficiency in renal amyloidosis. *Nephron* 1990; **56**: 246–8.

63 Erdkamp FL, Gans RO, Hoorntje SJ. Endocrine organ failure due to systemic AA-amyloidosis. *Neth J Med* 1991; **38**: 24–8.

64 Harvey CJ, Gower PE, Hawkins PN, Pepys MB, Phillips ME. Occult adrenal insufficiency secondary to amyloidosis in the context of chronic renal failure. *Nephrol Dial Transplant* 1995; **10**: 1237–9.

65 Groves RW, Toms GC, Houghton BJ, Monson JP. Adrenal steroid replacement—twice or thrice daily. *J Roy Soc Med* 1988; **81**: 514–16.

66 Trainer PJ, Besser GM. *The Bart's Endocrine Protocols*. Edinburgh: Churchill Livingstone, 1995.

67 Kyriazopolou V, Paparousis O, Vagenakis AG. Rifampicin-induced adrenal crisis in Addisonian patients receiving corticosteroid replace-

ment therapy. *J Clin Endocrinol Metab* 1984; **59**: 1204–6.

68 Ediger SK, Isley WL. Rifampicin-induced adrenal insufficiency in the acquired immunodeficiency syndrome: difficulties in diagnosis and treatment. *Postgrad Med J* 1988; **64**: 405–6.

69 Hey AA, Conaglen JV, Espiner EA, Thornley PE. Rifampicin-induced adrenal crisis (Letter). *NZ Med J* 1983; **96**: 988–9.

70 Fariss J, Hane S, Shinsako H. Comparison of absorption of cortisone acetate and hydrocortisone hemisuccinate. *J Clin Endocrinol Metab* 1978; **47**: 1137–40.

71 Rosner W. Plasma steroid-binding proteins (Review). *Endocrinol Metab Clin North Am* 1991; **20**: 697–720.

72 Laudat MH, Cerdas S, Fournier C, Guiban D, Guilhaume B, Luton JP. Salivary cortisol measurement: a practical approach to assess pituitary-adrenal function. *J Clin Endocrinol Metab* 1988; **66**: 343–8.

73 Burke CW, Roulet F. Increased exposure of tissues to cortisol in late pregnancy. *BMJ* 1970; i: 657–9.

74 Stockigt JR, Hewitt M, Topliss DJ. Renin and renin substrate in adrenal insufficiency: contrasting effects of glucocorticoid and mineralocorticoid deficiency. *Am J Med* 1979; **66**: 915–22.

75 Mc Cabe ERB. Sex and the single DAX-1: too little is bad, but can we have too much? *J Clin Invest* 1996; **96**: 881–2.

76 Mc Cabe ERB. Adrenal hypoplasia congenita with hypogonadotropic hypogonadism: evidence that DAX-1 mutations lead to combined hypothalamic and pituitary defects in gonadotropin production. *J Clin Invest* 1996; **96**: 1055–62.

CHAPTER 37

The management of adrenal incidentalomas

S. Tsagarakis

Introduction

Adrenal incidentalomas are defined as adrenal masses discovered during abdominal imaging in patients with no gross evidence of adrenal disease. Over the last two decades, due to the introduction of high-resolution imaging techniques (computed tomography (CT), magnetic resonance imaging (MRI) and ultrasound), adrenal incidentalomas have become recognised as a common clinical problem [1]. As a result, endocrinologists worldwide are currently facing a new 'epidemic' to which the acronym AIDS (adrenal incidentalomas discovered serendipitously) has been applied [2]. While the vast majority of incidentally discovered adrenal masses are benign and non-hypersecreting, there is always some concern about the twin possibilities of hormonal hypersecretion or malignancy. It is therefore important to define cost-effective strategies to understand the exact nature of the underlying adrenal nodule and proceed to appropriate decision making to minimise patients' morbidity or mortality.

Prevalence and aetiology of adrenal nodules

The current frequency of adrenal incidentalomas in different series ranges from 0.35 to 4.5% of patients undergoing abdominal imaging [3,4,5]. When the adrenals are examined at autopsy, however, nodules are much more frequent. This is due to the fact that smaller nodules detected at autopsy escape detection with the current imaging techniques. Thus, it is possible that a further increase in the prevalence of incidentally discovered adrenal masses will occur by applying higher-resolution imaging.

Consideration of the aetiology of adrenal masses covers a wide range of pathology (Table 37.1) [6]. Benign or malignant neoplasms from all zones of the adrenals, and metastases to the adrenals, constitute the most frequently seen pathologies. Rarely, the adrenals may be affected by various infiltrative diseases. Occasionally, lesions arising from adjacent structures may be misdiagnosed as primary adrenal tumours (adrenal pseudo-tumours). These latter lesions, and certain other masses, by virtue of pathognomonic imaging characteristics, are diagnosed by CT findings alone. Histologically, the vast majority of the remaining adrenal nodules (70–94%) are benign adrenocortical adenomas, and in clinical practice the major diagnostic challenge for the physician is to differentiate these commonly seen benign tumours from the less frequently occurring hypersecretory or malignant adrenal masses.

Adrenal masses with specific CT features

These include myelolipomas, haemorrhage, cysts and adrenal pseudo-tumours. Recognition of these masses with a great degree of confidence by an experienced radiologist makes further work-up unnecessary.

Myelolipomas (Fig. 37.1)

Myelolipomas are benign neoplasms composed of mature fat and myeloid tissue similar to that found in the bone marrow. Unenhanced CT scans are usually sufficient in establishing the diagnosis. The proportion of fat within an adrenal myelolipoma detectable by CT is variable, but even minute amounts in an otherwise water-density mass establish the diagnosis, and further investigation is not indicated [7].

Adrenal haemorrhage (Fig. 37.2)

Adrenal haemorrhage can be unilateral or bilateral. When bilateral it is commonly associated with symptoms and signs of acute adrenal failure, and death can result if not properly treated. Sepsis, anticoagulant therapy, collagen vascular

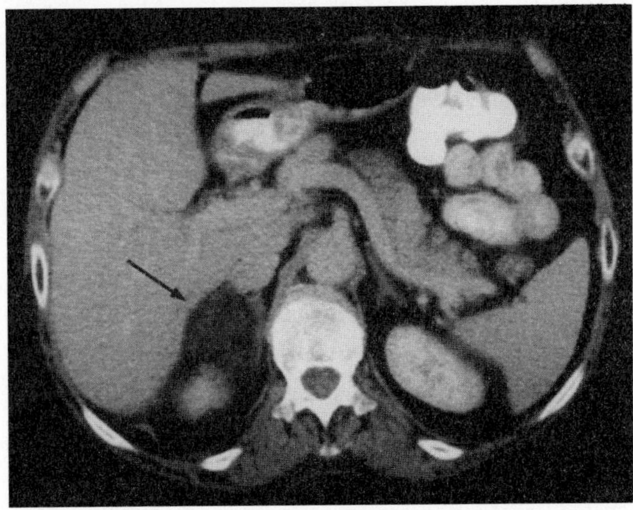

Fig. 37.1 Myelolipoma (arrowed). Macroscopic fat is clearly detected on computed tomography scan. (Courtesy of Dr C. Malagari Evangelismos Hospital, Athens.)

Table 37.1 Incidentally discovered adrenal masses.

Adrenal cortex
Adenoma
Nodular hyperplasia
Carcinoma
Adrenal medulla
Phaeochromocytoma
Ganglioneuroma
Ganglioneuroblastoma
Other adrenal masses
Myelolipoma
Neurofibroma
Hamartoma
Teratoma
Xanthomatosis
Amyloidosis
Cyst
Haematoma
Granulomatosis
Metastases
Breast carcinoma
Lung cancer
Lymphoma
Leukaemia
Other
Pseudo-adrenal masses (e.g. arising from kidney, pancreas, spleen, lymph nodes, and vessels)
Technical artefacts

disease and the post-partum state are the most common associated conditions. The CT appearance of bilateral adrenal haemorrhage is that of bilateral asymmetric masses of high density [8].

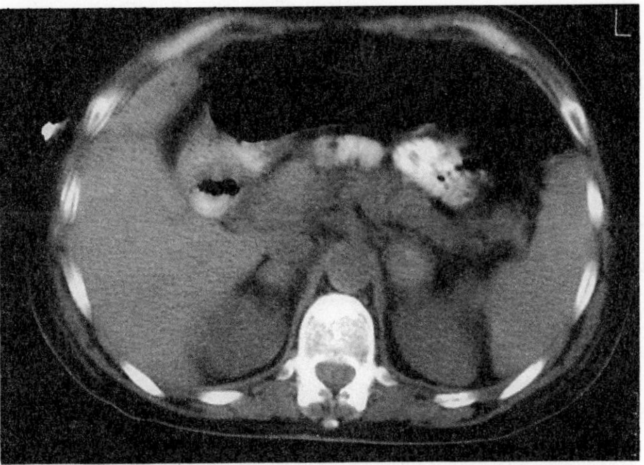

Fig. 37.2 Adrenal haemorrhage. Computed tomography scan shows bilateral high-density adrenal masses in a patient with acute onset abdominal pain and collapse. (Courtesy of Dr C. Malagari.)

Adrenal cysts

Cysts of variable size may be detected as oval or round sharply demarcated masses with homogeneous water density on CT and walls of varying thickness. The presence of soft-tissue component in the cyst requires further investigation.

Adrenal pseudo-tumours

Adrenal pseudo-tumours are most common on the left; the superior tip of the spleen, a tortuous splenic artery or a posterior gastric diverticulum of the fundus may resemble a left adrenal mass. Fewer pseudo-tumours occur on the right; most commonly, a right renal vein ascending adjacent to adrenal medial or lateral limbs. Intravenous or oral contrast is required to make the distinction from a true adrenal tumour [9].

Benign adrenocortical adenomas

Benign adrenocortical adenomas occur equally in males and females and their frequency increases linearly with age. There is some evidence of a higher prevalence in patients with diabetes mellitus, obesity and hypertension [10,11]. This association, however, remains controversial, and at present there is much uncertainty regarding any possible cause-and-effect relationship. Histologically, benign adrenocortical adenomas consist of clear lipid-laden cells similar in size and appearance to those of the normal zona fasciculata (Fig. 37.3). The cells are arranged in cords and clusters separated by prominent fibrovascular trabeculae. They are commonly located in the periphery of the cortex or in cortical tissue surrounding the central vein. Large nodules may compress the adjacent adrenal cortex. Macroscopically, they appear

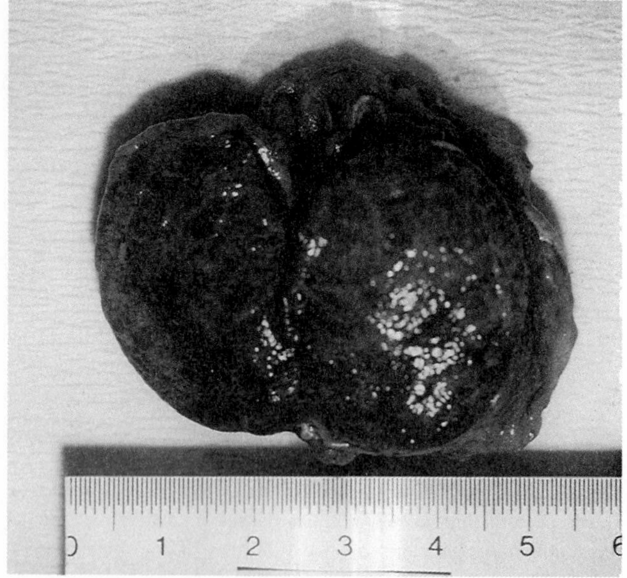

(a)

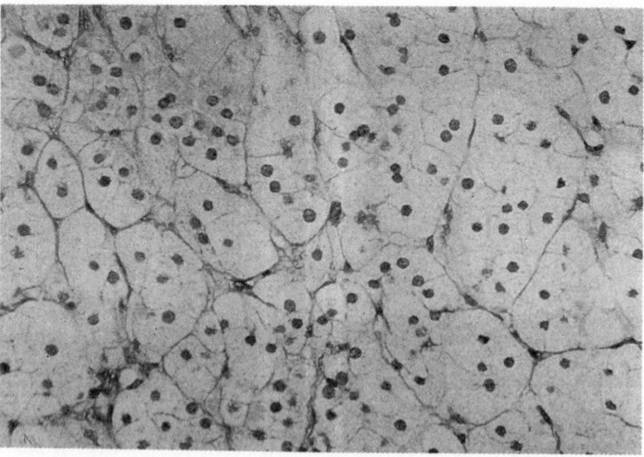

(b)

Fig. 37.3 Benign adrenocortical adenoma: (a) macroscopic appearance; (b) clear lipid-laden cells of the zona fasciculata type. (Courtesy of Dr G. Kontogeorgos, Athens General Hospital.)

as yellow nodules. Rarely they appear black; these latter nodules contain compact cells with increased amounts of lipofuscin [12].

The pathogenesis of benign adrenocortical adenomas is currently obscure. It has long been suggested that they may develop from vascular damage leading to cortical ischaemic atrophy and compensatory nodular hyperplasia in the less ischaemic areas of the adrenal cortex [12]. This may well account for the high frequency with which such nodules are related to the central vein, which is less frequently affected by vascular damage. Alternatively, as in the thyroid, adrenal nodule formation may represent a variant of neoplastic cell transformation due to preferential replication of constitutively predisposed cells. However, so far, oncogenetic abnormalities in adrenal adenoma cells have not been extensively investigated [13].

Functional activity of benign adrenocortical adenomas

For many years benign adrenocortical adenomas had been considered as non-functioning and thus non-secreting tumours. In fact, while in most cases these tumours are not accompanied by, at least, overt clinical evidence of hormone production, recent studies have shown that benign adenomas may retain some functional activity. Almost all such tumours demonstrate the ability to accumulate radiocholesterol on scintigraphy [14]. Moreover, the messenger RNA (mRNA) for all steroidogenic enzymes is well expressed in cells from such adrenal adenomas, and variable concentrations of all active adrenal steroids are present in extracts of such tumours [15]. Thus, most authors prefer to define such adenomas as non-hypersecreting to underline their finite functional steroidogenic activity [16,17]. It is of note, as shown by *in vitro* and *in vivo* studies, that in a substantial number of such adenomas a partial deficiency of 21-hydroxylase had been detected. This finding may well explain the absence of overt hypersecretion of active steroids by these tumours [18].

Subclinical Cushing's syndrome

Glucocorticoid secretion from benign adrenocortical adenomas has been more extensively investigated. Several studies have now indicated a wide range of biochemical abnormalities on elaborate testing of the hypothalamo-pituitary–adrenal (HPA) axis in variable proportions of patients harbouring such tumours. Biochemical findings in patients with benign adrenal adenomas are heterogeneous. Thus, blunting of the diurnal variation of cortisol, incomplete suppression by dexamethasone, decreased adrenocorticotrophic hormone (ACTH) responsiveness to corticotrophin-releasing hormone (CRH) and excessive urinary cortisol excretion have been detected with a decreasing order of frequency, due to varying degrees of autonomous cortisol production by such tumours [16,17,18]. Many authors have drawn parallels with functioning ('warm') thyroid nodules, where a spectrum of thyroid hormone excess also exists with symptomatic thyroid hormone hypersecretion eventually occurring in approximately 20% of these patients, the rest being asymptomatic. Accordingly, glucocorticoid excess, responsible for manifestations of Cushing's syndrome, may eventually evolve in a subpopulation of patients with benign adrenocortical adenomas. Since such glucocorticoid excess is not sufficient to produce overt Cushing's syndrome on clinical grounds, many authors have used terms such as 'preclinical or pre-Cushing's syndrome' to define this subclinical situation

[1,16]. However, the definition of such a clinical situation is not clear-cut and several questions remain to be answered. First, there are no widely accepted biochemical criteria for the definition of preclinical Cushing's syndrome; most authors have used the dexamethasone-suppression test as the most sensitive index of autonomous cortisol production, but different 'cut-offs' of post-dexamethasone cortisol values have been used. Secondly, there is still much uncertainty about the clinical implications of the condition; it has been suggested but not proven that depending on the amount and the duration of cortisol excess clinical problems such as obesity, insulin resistance, excess bone loss, and hypertension may develop. Thirdly, controversy still exists about the risk of progression from preclinical to full-blown hypercortisolism. Finally, the need for tumour removal remains still questionable; so far there are only few reports in the literature indicating improvement of existing hypertension and biochemical alterations of bone remodelling after tumour removal. To summarise, although there is good evidence suggesting that at least a subpopulation of patients with significant hypercortisolism exists for which surgical intervention may be beneficial, future studies correlating biochemical, clinical and epidemiological data are urgently required, in order to develop widely agreed guidelines for decision making. The term subclinical Cushing's syndrome might more accurately describe the situation as this makes no assumptions as to the clinical progression.

Hypersecretory adrenal nodules

Secretory products from a hypersecreting adrenal mass are: glucocorticoids, androgens or oestrogens, aldosterone, and catecholamines. Overt clinical signs of glucocorticoid excess are not, by definition, compatible with the characterisation of an adrenal mass as incidentally discovered. As previously mentioned, glucocorticoid excess commonly appears in the form of subtle hypercortisolism and is of uncertain clinical significance. Androgen- or oestrogen-secreting adrenal tumours are extremely rare, and in the absence of virilisation in females or feminisation in males detailed hormonal testing is not indicated. Although some evidence for hormonal hypersecretion of aldosterone or catecholamines may often be provided by careful history and physical examination, clinically unsuspected cases are well represented in the literature.

Aldosterone-producing tumours

The prevalence of aldosterone-producing adenomas may be as high as 7% in patients with adrenal incidentalomas [19]. Aldosterone hypersecretion invariably produces hypertension. Thus, the absence of hypertension precludes the need for routine biochemical exclusion of an aldosterone-secreting adrenal mass. However, biochemical exclusion hypertension is a common disease, and the incidence of hypertension may be even higher in patients with adrenal incidentalomas. Therefore, exclusion of aldosterone hypersecretion will be eventually required in a significant proportion of patients with an adrenal mass. Although the absence of hypokalaemia is strongly against the diagnosis of hyperaldosteronism, it should be remembered that sodium restriction may mask the hypokalaemia.

Catecholamine-producing tumours

Although catecholamine-producing tumours are characteristically associated with paroxysmal hypertension, silent phaeochromocytomas may be more common than previously thought. In one series, 76% of 54 autopsy-proven cases were clinically unsuspected before death and many of these patients died of causes possibly related to the phaeochromocytoma [20]. According to Ross and Aron [19], the expected prevalence of phaeochromocytomas among patients with an incidental adrenal mass may be as high as 6.5%. For these reasons, screening for catecholamine hypersecretion is strongly recommended in all patients with an adrenal mass. This is of primary importance for those patients who are candidates for surgery or biopsy, since a lethal hypertensive crisis may be provoked by these procedures. Most recent studies suggest that 24-hour urinary catecholamines are the optimal screening test [21].

Malignant adrenal masses

Adrenocortical carcinoma

Primary adrenocortical carcinoma is fortunately an uncommon malignancy with a frequency of approximately one to five cases per million people [22]. The majority of these tumours are >50 mm in diameter at presentation. In up to 10% of cases they may be bilateral. Approximately one-half of these tumours are functional and manifestations of excess cortisol, androgen or oestrogen, and/or mineralocorticoids, may be detected. Some of these patients may only have elevated urinary excretion rates of steroid metabolites, without obvious clinical manifestations of hormonal excess, due to inefficient hormone biosynthesis. Adrenal carcinomas may frequently lack histological features of malignancy; nuclear pleomorphism, mitotic figures and in particular vascular or lymphatic invasion when present suggest the diagnosis.

Metastases to the adrenals

The adrenal gland is a common site of metastatic disease;

8–38% of patients with known extra-adrenal malignancies have adrenal metastases at autopsy [23,24]. The most common primary malignancies metastasising to the adrenals are of breast, lung, kidney, melanoma and lymphoma. In view of the fact that in patients with known malignancies abdominal imaging is commonly performed for staging, the presence of an adrenal mass requires a distinction to be made between a metastasis and the commonly seen benign adrenocortical adenomas.

Diagnostic evaluation and management of incidentally discovered adrenal masses

Since most adrenal nodule morbidity is related to either hormonal hypersecretion or malignancy, clinical evaluation focuses on the identification of these possibilities. The first step in the evaluation of any adrenal mass is to determine if the mass is functional. The next step is to exclude malignancy. Thus, the major role of a physician dealing with incidentally detected adrenal masses is:

1 the exclusion of unsuspected overt hormonal hypersecretion;

2 the identification of patients with clinically significant subtle hormonal hypersecretion;

3 the exclusion of adrenal primary malignancy or the exclusion of adrenal secondaries in patients with known primary malignancy.

Exclusion of unsuspected overt hormonal hypersecretion

The primary aim is to exclude the possibility of a hyperfunctioning aldosterone or catecholamine-producing adrenal tumour. Aldosterone-producing adenomas appear as small (< 30 mm) rounded homogeneous masses with well-defined margins, and a substantially lower than water density on CT scan [25] (Fig. 37.4). Phaeochromocytomas are depicted on CT as variable in size, inhomogeneous masses with significant enhancement after intravenous contrast. On MRI they often demonstrate high signal intensity on T2-weighted images [26] (Fig. 37.5). Screening tests for catecholamine and aldosterone overproduction are best illustrated in the relevant chapters. Briefly, at least two 24-hour urinary collections for catecholamines and a paired sample for the measurement of plasma potassium, renin and aldosterone are generally required as the initial screening to exclude these entities [21,27].

Identification of patients with clinically significant subtle hormonal hypersecretion

In view of the most recent reports indicating subclinical glucocorticoid hypersecretion in a substantial number of patients with benign adrenocortical adenomas, it has been suggested that the cortisol secretory status should be screened in all patients with incidentally discovered adrenal masses, even in the absence of clinical stigmata of Cushing's syndrome. The primary aim by testing the HPA axis is to define a subpopulation of patients with glucocorticoid excess responsible for less pronounced manifestations of Cushing's syndrome. However, the selection of the best screening test for the biochemical assessment of glucocorticoid secretion of these patients, and the biochemical criteria of what constitutes significant hypercortisolism, has not yet been accurately defined.

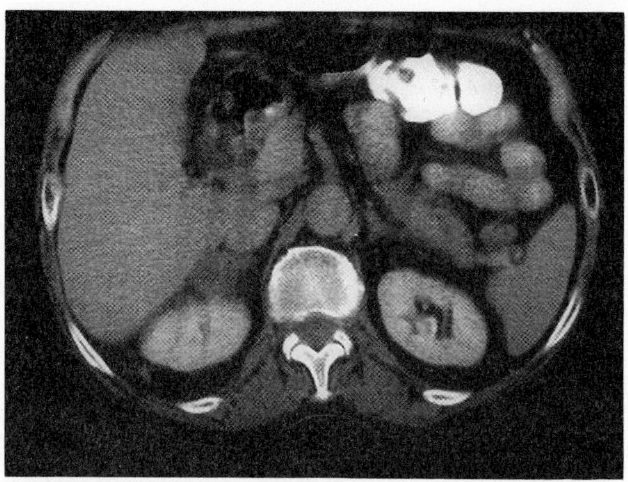

Fig. 37.4 Aldosterone-producing adenoma. Computed tomography scan showing a 2-cm well-defined low-density right adrenal mass. (Courtesy of Dr C. Malagari.)

Problems in the biochemical definition of subclinical Cushing's syndrome

Current tests in clinical practice rely upon the demonstration of an excess integrated cortisol secretion and/or abnormal feedback regulation of the hypothalamo-pituitary–adrenal (HPA) axis. The most commonly used tests include: 24-hour urinary free-cortisol (UFC) measurements, and the overnight and low-dose dexamethasone-suppression tests [28].

UFC excretion provides an integrated measure of cortisol secretion. In different series 5–10% of patients with adrenal adenomas have elevated UFC excretion. This, however, may well be an underestimate of significant hypercortisolism, since UFC excretion is an insensitive test, with false negative rates ranging from 5 to 11% even in patients with overt Cushing's syndrome [28].

Dexamethasone-suppression tests have been considered more sensitive, but assessment of deranged feedback by either the overnight or the low-dose dexamethasone-suppression

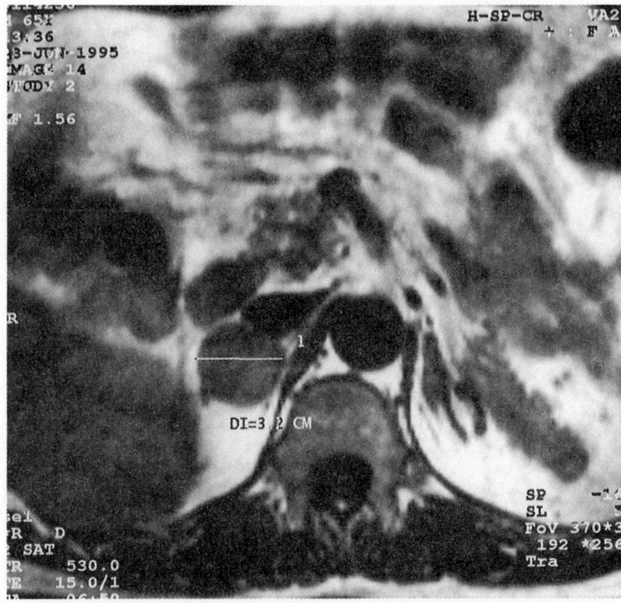

(a)

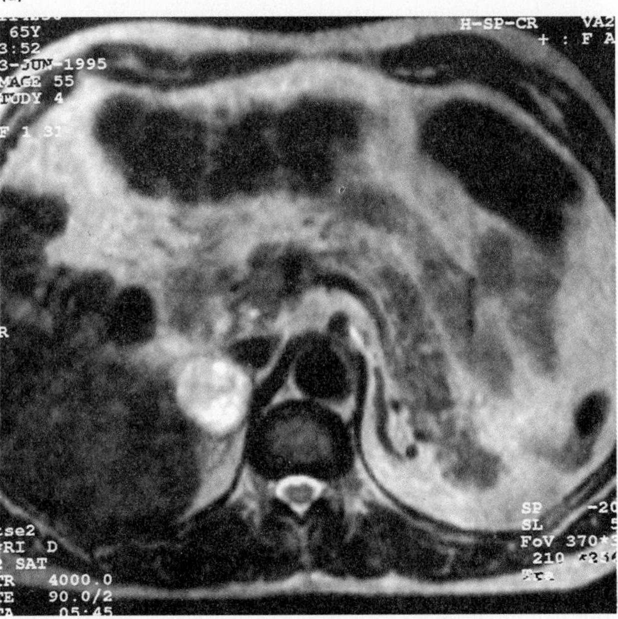

(b)

Fig. 37.5 Phaeochromocytoma. (a) Magnetic resonance imaging appearance of a right-sided adrenal phaeochromocytoma on T1-weighted image; (b) note the high signal intensity on T2-weighted image, in an asymptomatic patient with normal metanephrine and VMA excretion but high catecholamine 24-hour urinary excretion. A chromaffin-cell tumour was confirmed on histology.

tests may be difficult to interpret. The criteria of what constitutes an abnormal post-dexamethasone cortisol response have been largely anecdotal. Most authors have suggested a post-dexamethasone level of >140 nmol/l (5 µg/dl) as indicating inadequate suppression [29]. However, following a 2-day dexamethasone-suppression test cortisol levels

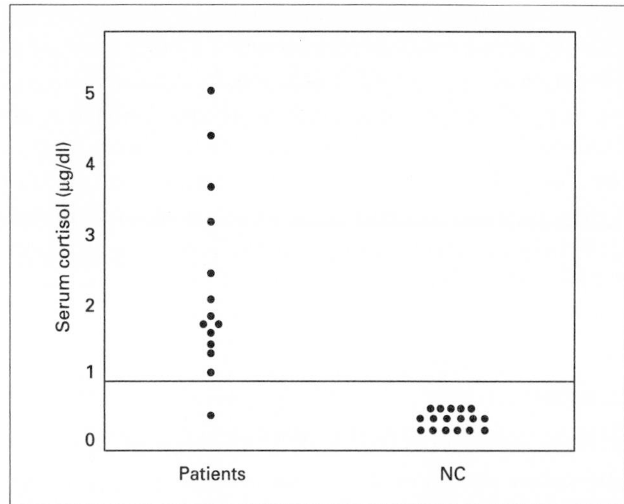

Fig. 37.6 Cortisol levels following a low-dose dexamethasone-suppression test in 14 consecutive patients with adrenal incidentalomas. NC, normal controls. (S. Tsagarakis and N. Thalassinos, unpublished.)

usually become undetectable in normal subjects. In patients with the pituitary-dependent form of Cushing's syndrome, in which inadequate suppression provides an indication of dexamethasone-resistant and therefore abnormal corticotrophs, even barely detectable cortisol levels following dexamethasone suppression may provide good confirmatory evidence in diagnosing Cushing's syndrome. This led most investigators to define post-dexamethasone cortisol levels much lower than 140 nmol/l (5 µg/dl) as indicating inadequate suppression [30,31,32]. However, the introduction of lower cut-off post-dexamethasone cortisol levels in patients with adrenal adenomas will lead to a dramatic increase in the number of non-suppressors [33] (Fig. 37.6). In such patients, 'incomplete suppression' by dexamethasone is probably due to ACTH-independent secretion of even minute amounts of cortisol by the adrenal mass. Therefore, inadequate suppression with dexamethasone in these patients is a sensitive index even of a very low-grade and therefore clinically insignificant autonomous glucocorticoid secretion. It could be suggested that post-dexamethasone cortisol levels may in fact provide a measure of the degree of autonomous (i.e. non ACTH-dependent) glucocorticoid secretion, but cut-off levels corresponding to clinically significant autonomous production remain to be defined.

Exclusion of adrenal primary malignancy or adrenal secondaries in patients with known primary malignancy

Primary malignancies of the adrenal are fortunately rare. Metastases to the adrenals, however, are common, and in the setting of a known primary malignancy exclusion of adrenal secondaries may be of primary importance. The distinction is most critical for those patients with no other evidence of metastatic disease, as they may benefit from curative surgery of their primary malignancy if the adrenal lesion is not a metastasis. In contrast, the presence of an adrenal mass in a patient with obvious evidence of metastatic disease is of little importance to the patient, since staging is not altered. Judicious use of laboratory tests, imaging techniques, scintigraphy and fine-needle aspiration biopsy, constitute the current tools for diagnostic evaluation of these patients.

CT scan

It is generally agreed that the CT appearance of an adrenal mass does not allow for confident separation of benign from malignant lesions. However, certain morphological characteristics may be suggestive of a malignant rather than a benign lesion [34]. Metastases and adrenocortical carcinomas appear as inhomogeneous soft tissue density masses of variable size with irregular margins, and marked contrast enhancement (Fig. 37.7). Adrenocortical carcinomas most commonly are larger than 60 mm in diameter and signs of local invasion may be prsent [35]. Metastases are often bilateral. In contrast, benign adrenocortical adenomas appear as small (< 30 mm) rounded homogeneous masses with well-defined margins, and a substantially lower than water density on CT scan.

The single most specific discriminating feature between benign and malignant adrenal masses is the measurement of attenuation values on non-contrast-enhanced CT scans.

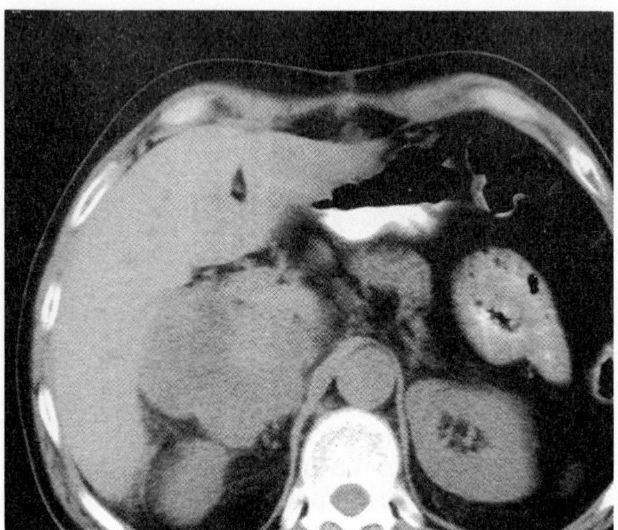

Fig. 37.7 Adrenal carcinoma. Computed tomography scan appearance of a large adrenal inhomogeneous mass with irregular margins infiltrating the liver and the inferior vena cava. (Courtesy of Dr C. Malagari.)

Low-attenuation values reflect lipid content which is specific for benign adrenocortical tissue. Thus, with a threshold of 0 Hounsfield units, Lee *et al.* reported a 100% specificity in distinguishing benign from malignant masses [36]. Even with a threshold between 0 and 10 Hounsfield units specificity is also high (96%). With CT attenuation values > 10 Hounsfield units, however, cortical adenomas, phaeochromocytomas and malignant adrenal masses cannot be distinguished [36].

MRI scan

The MRI features of benign versus malignant adrenal lesions have been investigated extensively. It has been suggested that on T2-weighted images, adrenal adenomas have a lower signal than malignant masses and phaeochromocytomas [37] (Fig. 37.8). However, several studies have now shown a 20–30% overlap between these groups of patients [38]. Recently, chemical-shift MRI has been introduced as a promising tool in differentiating benign adenomas from malignant masses [39]. The technique is based on the difference in resonance frequency between protons in water and triglyceride molecules. Signal intensity loss on chemical shift is suggestive of a high lipid content, and thus of a benign adrenocortical adenoma. So far, most studies have shown encouraging results, but more studies including larger numbers of adrenal masses of varying aetiologies are required before definite conclusions for the utility of the technique can be drawn.

Scintigraphy

The accumulation of radiocholesterol has been introduced as a useful tool to discriminate between benign and malignant masses. Benign adrenal adenomas usually accumulate iodocholesterol and often this is accompanied by suppression of uptake in the contralateral gland, similar to non-toxic functional ('hot') nodules of the thyroid gland [40] (Fig. 37.9). The presence of iodocholesterol uptake is thus a useful index of the presence of adrenocortical tissue and therefore excludes the presence of a metastatic adrenal mass. Differentiated adrenocortical carcinomas may also demonstrate uptake of iodocholesterol, but in these cases biochemical evaluation is abnormal, and surgery will eventually be indicated. Undifferentiated adrenal carcinomas with normal biochemistry do not appear to concentrate radiocholesterol. In summary, identification of a 'cold' adrenal mass is a strong indication of malignancy. However, the spatial resolution of scintigraphy limits the sensitivity of the technique for lesions that are < 20 mm in diameter [14].

Fine-needle aspiration biopsy

CT-guided percutaneous aspiration biopsy remains the most

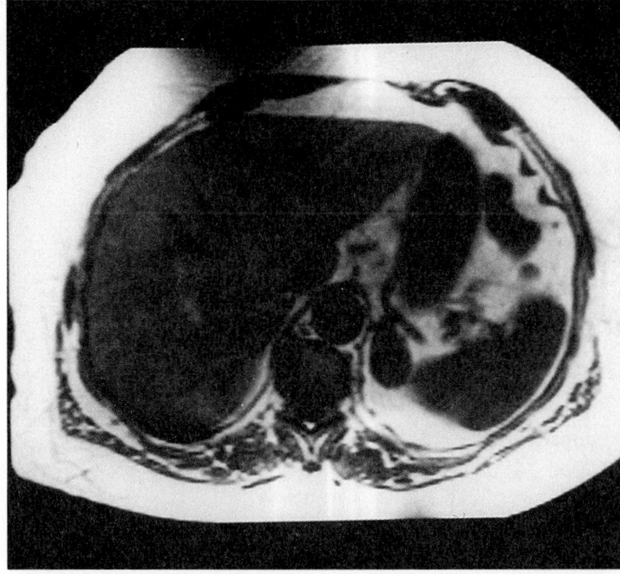

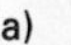

(a)

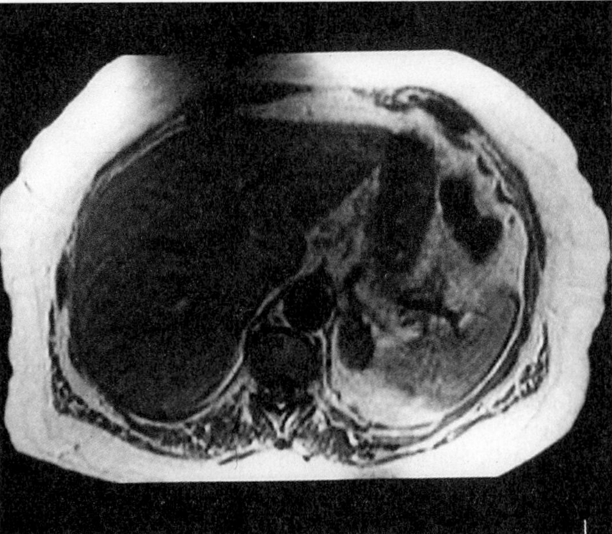

(b)

Fig. 37.8 Benign adenoma. Magnetic resonance image showing low signal intensity on both (a) T1- and (b) T2-weighted images.

definitive method to confirm or exclude adrenal metastasis with a reported accuracy of 80–100% [41]. The technique should only be reserved for suspected metastasis, since differentiation of adrenal adenomas from carcinomas is not possible. Adrenal biopsy should be used judiciously, since this is an invasive procedure with significant morbidity. Complications such as pneumothorax, septicaemia, haemorrhage and, rarely, pancreatitis, have been reported.

Integrated approach and management of adrenal incidentalomas

The clinical challenge in adrenal incidentaloma management is to define a cost-effective diagnostic and therapeutic protocol for appropriate decision making. So far, the optimal diagnostic evaluation and treatment, particularly with regard to the indications of surgical intervention, remain controversial. Our current recommendations are summarised in Fig. 37.10. However, it should be emphasised that on many occasions clinical judgement based on the patient's history, age and general condition remains the most significant determinant in final decision making.

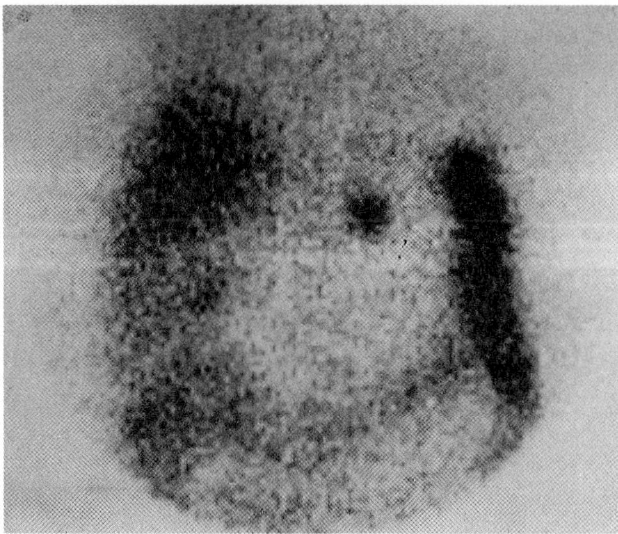

Fig. 37.9 Iodocholesterol scan showing concordant uptake of the isotope by a benign non-hyperfunctioning adrenal adenoma.

As previously mentioned, the possibility of hormonal hypersecretion should first be excluded in all patients. However, although there is general agreement that confirmation of an aldosterone- or catecholamine-producing tumour is an absolute indication for surgery, identification and management of patients with subtle glucocorticoid excess is currently an issue of much uncertainty and dispute. Our current practice is to investigate all patients with incidentally discovered adrenal masses with UFC measurements and the low-dose dexamethasone-suppression test. Until the establishment of new guidelines based on studies combining biochemical data and epidemiological data our recommendations are as follows: for those patients with consistently elevated UFC excretion and/or post-dexamethasone cortisol levels > 140 nmol/l, adrenalectomy is indicated. If surgery is undertaken, perioperative hydrocortisone cover is indicated to avoid Addisonian crisis due to suppression of the HPA axis. The adequacy of HPA function should be assessed post-surgery, and appropriate recommendations should be made depending on the results. In view of the current uncertainty regarding the natural history of functional autonomy, patients with post-dexamethasone levels in the range of 60–140 nmol/l, particularly when young, are followed by repeating HPA

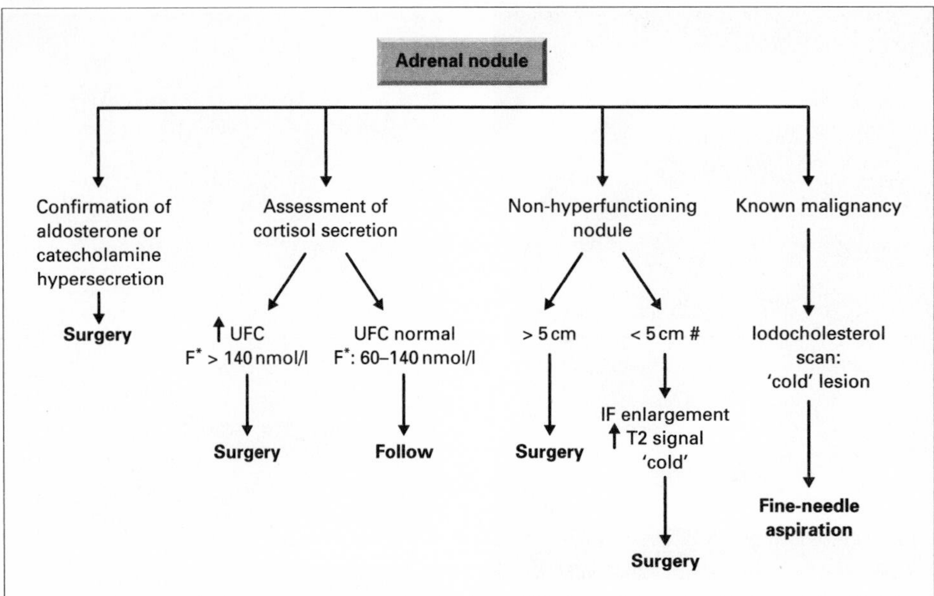

Fig. 37.10 A possible approach to the adrenal incidentaloma. F*, cortisol values following a two-day low-dose dexamethasone-suppression test. # Follow-up may be restricted to those masses with higher than zero Hounsfield attenuation values on CT scan.

testing at yearly intervals in order to exclude progression towards significant glucocorticoid excess.

Exclusion of malignancy is of primary importance only in patients with known extradrenal malignancy for whom decisions regarding the treatment of their primary malignancy will be altered by the presence of an adrenal metastasis. We currently advocate fine-needle aspiration as the investigation of choice in these patients. A more conservative approach restricts fine-needle aspiration to those lesions which appear cold on scintigraphy. Primary adrenal malignancy is fortunately very rare, and fears of missing an underlying adrenocortical carcinoma should not be overemphasised. It has been suggested that adrenal lesions > 50 mm in diameter should be removed since they carry a significant risk of primary adrenal malignancy. However, one may argue that since, even in this group of patients, benign lesions are more common than adrenal cancer, this practice will lead many patients to undergo unnecessary surgery. Our current practice is to recommend surgery to all healthy patients < 60 years of age. In older patients and those with significant operative risk we restrict surgery to those with masses indicating a high signal intensity on T2-weighted images and/or low uptake on radiocholesterol scanning. In patients with adrenal masses < 50 mm, serial imaging follow-up is recommended for those patients with attenuation values on CT scanning higher than 0. Enlargement of such a mass, however, does not prove malignancy; if it occurs, surgery is indicated if MRI or scintigraphy favours a non-benign lesion.

References

1 Kloos RT, Gross MD, Francis IR, Korobkin M, Shapiro B. Incidentally discovered adrenal masses. *Endocr Rev* 1995; **16**: 460–84.

2 Griffing GT. Editorial: A-I-D-S: The new endocrine epidemic. *J Clin Endocrinol Metab* 1994; **79**: 1530–1.

3 Prinz RA, Brooks MH, Churchill R *et al.* Incidental asymptomatic adrenal masses detected by computed tomographic scanning. Is operation required? *JAMA* 1982; **248**: 701–4.

4 Abecassis M, McLoughlin MJ, Langer B, Kudlow JE. Serendepitous adrenal masses: prevalence, significance, and management. *Am J Surg* 1985; **149**: 783–8.

5 Herrera MF, Grant CS, Van Heerden JA, Sheedy PF, Ilstrup DM. Incidentally discovered adrenal tumours: an institutional perspective. *Surgery* 1991; **110**: 1014–21.

6 Gross MD, Shapiro B. Clinically silent adrenal masses. *J Clin Endocrinol Metab* 1993; **77**: 885–8.

7 Dieckman KP, Hamm B, Pickartz H *et al.* Adrenal myelolipoma: clinical, radiologic, and histologic features. *Urology* 1987; **11**: 1–8.

8 Reznek RH, Armstrong P. Imaging in endocrinology. The adrenal gland. *Clin Endocrinol* 1994; **40**: 561–76.

9 Berliner L, Bosniak MA, Megibow A. Adrenal pseudotumors on computed tomography. *J Comput Assist Tomogr* 1982; **6**: 281–5.

10 Hedeland H, Ostberg G, Hokfelt B. On the prevalence of adrenocortical adenomas in an autopsy material in relation to hypertension and diabetes. *Acta Med Scand* 1968; **184**: 211–14.

11 Russell RP, Masi AT, Richter ED. Adrenal cortical adenomas and hypertension. A clinical pathologic analysis of 690 cases with matched controls and a review of the literature. *Medicine* 1972; **51**: 211–25.

12 Neville AM. The nodular adrenal. *Invest Cell Pathol* 1978; **1**: 99.

13 Dahia PLM, Grossman AB. The molecular pathogenesis of adrenal tumours. *Endoc Rel Cancer* 1995; **2**: 267–79.

14 Gross MD, Shapiro B, Francis IR *et al.* Scintigraphic evaluation of clinically silent adrenal masses. *J Nucl Med* 1994; **35**: 1145–52.

15 Racz K, Pinet F, Marton T *et al.* Expression of steroidogenic enzyme messenger ribunocleic acids and corticosteroid production in aldosterone-producing and 'nonfunctioning' adrenal adenomas. *J Clin Endocrinol Metab* 1993; **77**: 677–82.

16 Reincke M, Nieke J, Krestin GP *et al.* Preclinical Cushing's syndrome in adrenal 'incidentalomas': comparison with adrenal Cushing's syndrome. *J Clin Endocrinol Metab* 1992; **75**: 826–32.
17 Osella G, Terzolo M, Borretta G *et al.* Endocrine evaluation of incidentally discovered adrenal masses (incidentalomas). *J Clin Endocrinol Metab* 1994; **79**: 1532–9.
18 Ambrosi B, Peverelli S, Passini E *et al.* Abnormalities of endocrine function in patients with clinically 'silent' adrenal masses. *Eur J Endocrinol* 1995; **132**: 422–7.
19 Ross NS, Aron DG. Hormonal evaluation of the patient with an incidentally discovered adrenal mass. *N Engl J Med* 1990; **323**: 1401–5.
20 Sutton MG, Sheps SG, Lie JT. Prevalence of clinically unsuspected pheochromocytoma: review of a 50-year autopsy series. *Mayo Clin Proc* 1981; **56**: 354–60.
21 Bouloux P-M,G, Fakeeh M. Investigation of phaeochromocytoma. *Clini Endocrinol* 1995; **43**: 657–64.
22 Copeland PM. The incidentally discovered adrenal mass. *Ann Intern Med* 1983; **98**: 940–5.
23 Glomset DA. The incidence of metastasis of malignant tumors. *Am J Cancer* 1938; **32**: 57–61.
24 Abrams HL, Spiro R, Goldstein N. Metastases in carcinoma: analysis of 1000 autopsied cases. *J Urol* 1959; **81**: 711–19.
25 Young WF, Hogan MJ, Klee GG *et al.* Primary aldosteronism: diagnosis and treatment. *Myao Clin Proc* 1990; **65**: 96–9.
26 Dunnick NR. Adrenal Imaging: current status. *Am J Radiol* 1990; **154**: 927–36.
27 McKenna TJ, Sequeira SJ, Heffernan A *et al.* Diagnosis under random conditions of all disorders of the renin–angiotensin–aldosterone axis, including primary hyperaldosteronism. *J Clin Endocrinol Metab* 1991; **73**: 952–7.
28 Trainer PJ, Grossman A. The diagnosis and differential diagnosis of Cushing's syndrome. *Clin Endocrinol* 1991; **34**: 317–30.
29 Crapo L. Cushings syndrome: a review of diagnostic tests. *Metabolism* 1979; **28**: 955–77.
30 Kennedy L, Atkinson AB, Johnson H *et al.* Serum cortisol concentration during the low dose dexamethasone suppression test to screen for Cushing's syndrome. *Br Med J* 1984; **289**: 1188–91.
31 Yanovski JA, Cutler GB, Chrousos GP, Nieman LK. Corticotropin-releasing hormone stimulation following low-dose dexamethasone suppression. *JAMA* 1993; **269**: 2232–8.
32 Newell-Price J, Trainer P, Perry L *et al.* A single sleeping midnight cortisol has a 100% sensitivity for the diagnosis of Cushing's syndrome. *Clin Endocrinol* 1995; **43**: 545–50.
33 Tsagarakis S, Mihaliou D, Vasilatou E, Nikolou H, Thalassinos N. Evidence for incomplete suppression of cortisol on low-dose dexamethasone suppression test in patients with adrenal incidentalomas. *Eur J Endocrinol* 1994; **130** (Suppl. 2): 109.
34 Hussain S, Belldegrun a, Seltzer SE *et al.* Differentiation of malignant from benign adrenal masses: predictive indices on computed tomography. *Am J Roentgenol* 1985; **144**: 61–5.
35 Fishman EK, Deutch BM, Hartman DS *et al.* Primary adrenocortical carcinoma: CT evaluation with clinical correlation. *Am J Roentgenol* 1987; **148**: 531–5.
36 Lee MJ, Hahn PF, Papanicolaou N *et al.* Benign and malignant adrenal masses. CT distinction with attenuation coefficient size and observer analysis. *Radiology* 1991; **179**: 415–18.
37 Reinig JW, Doppman JL, Dwyer AJ *et al.* Adrenal masses differentiated by MR. *Radiology* 1986; **158**: 81–4.
38 Doppman JL, Reinig JW, Dwyer AJ *et al.* Differentiation of adrenal masses by magnetic resonance imaging. *Surgery* 1987; **102**: 1018–26.
39 Mitchell DG, Grovello M, Matteucci T *et al.* Benign adrenocortical masses: diagnosis with chemical shift MR imaging. *Radiology* 1992; **185**: 345–51.
40 Gross MD, Shapiro B, Bouffard JA *et al.* Distinguishing benign from malignant adrenal masses. *Ann Intern Med* 1988; **109**: 613–18.
41 Silverman SG, Mueller PR, Pinkney LP *et al.* Predictive value of image-guided adrenal biopsy: analysis of results of 101 biopsies. *Radiology* 1993; **187**: 715–18.

Part 6
The Adrenal Medulla

CHAPTER 38

The sympatho-adrenal system, phaeochromocytomas and related tumours

P.-M.G. Bouloux

Anatomy of the sympatho-adrenomedullary system

Sympathetic nervous system

The peripheral sympathetic pathways and the adrenal medulla make up the functional unit known as the sympatho-adrenomedullary system. The dominant subcortical origins of this system are in the hypothalamus (anterior hypothalamus, paraventricular nuclei, the limbic system and circumventricular organ), from which fibres travel to the brainstem. Adrenergic (phenylethanolamine-*N*-methyl transferase-containing) cells within the rostral ventrolateral medullary C1 area [1] send axons to synapse with intermediolateral (IML) cells which form the preganglionic cell bodies of peripheral sympathetic fibres. Inhibitory noradrenergic neurons of the caudal ventrolateral medullary A1 area project onto the C1 area, as well as onto the nucleus tractus solitarius and the paraventricular nuclei. Thus, hypothalamic neurons are themselves influenced by limbic and cortical inputs, as well as afferent signals from the brainstem.

Sympathetic preganglionic neurons are found in four main nuclei within the intermediate spinal grey matter [2]. The bulk of sympathetic preganglionic neurons are found within the IML cell column (in the nucleus intermediolateralis thoracolumbalis, pars principalis), located in the lateral horn of the grey matter. Another group is found extending from the IML column into the lateral funiculus. The intercalated cell group is found medial to the IML column, and a fourth group dorsolateral to the central canal is known as the central autonomic nucleus. The cell bodies of the sympathetic preganglionic neurons form a ladder-like arrangement when viewed in horizontal section. The IML cell bodies are localised between T1 and L2. The spontaneous discharge rate of these cells is low, and tonic activity depends on stimulatory input from chemoreceptor, somatic and visceral afferents. Their preganglionic axons synapse with post-ganglionic sympathetic neurons in the paravertebral, superior, middle and inferior cervical, coeliac and superior mesenteric plexuses, and lower abdominal sympathetic ganglia. Fibres that pass through the ganglia of T5 through L2 form the splanchnic nerves that innervate the adrenal medulla. The cranium is supplied by fibres from the superior cervical ganglion, while the heart is innervated by all three cervical ganglia. The upper thoracic ganglia also innervate the heart and lungs, and the viscera are supplied from the preaortic plexuses; the pelvic structures receive innervation via the sacral spinal nerves and pelvic plexuses.

The neurotransmitters at the preganglionic IML cell bodies include serotonin and possibly thyrotrophin-releasing hormone (TRH), and in the sympathetic ganglia acetylcholine, which acts predominantly at nicotinic post-ganglionic cell receptors. Opioids and other neuropeptide cotransmitters are also released from the preganglionic terminals and may modulate preganglionic transmitter release. Ganglia also contain interneurons, some of which release dopamine. Each preganglionic nerve innervates several post-ganglionic neurons. Post-ganglionic unmyelinated axons innervate blood vessels and viscera (neurotransmitter noradrenaline) and sweat glands (acetylcholine). In such sympathetically innervated tissues, each post-ganglionic axon comprises several thousand *en passage* varicosities which contain the neurotransmitter packaged in vesicles. Vascular nerve terminals thus form lattice-like networks in the adventitial and adventitiomedial layers of arterioles.

The adrenal medulla

The adrenal medulla contributes about 10% the weight of the adrenals. The chromaffin cells are irregularly shaped polyhedrons organised into cords or small clumps surrounded by nerves, connective tissue and blood vessels. It receives both direct arterial (medullary arteries) and a corticomedullary portal venous supply formed from the coalescing of capillaries from the cortical zona reticularis. These bring a high cortisol concentration to the adrenaline-secreting cells which are particularly dense at the cortico-medullary junction. The adrenal medulla synthesises and secretes adrenaline, noradrenaline and dopamine. Venous drainage is through a series of sinusoids which coalesce into a central vein, which then empties in the renal vein on the left and into the inferior vena cava on the right.

Embryology of the sympatho-adrenomedullary system

Primitive sympathetic cell precursors (sympathogonia) of neural crest origin differentiate into neuroblasts and phaeochromoblasts, which form the sympathetic ganglia and chromaffin cells, respectively, at approximately 6 weeks' gestation. Phaeochromoblasts invade the mesenchymal cells destined to form the adrenal cortex, and differentiate into adrenal medullary chromaffin cells. Some primitive phaeochromoblasts remain in close association with the neuroblasts which are destined to become ganglia. These extra-adrenal chromaffin cells are found in the abdominal preaortic sympathetic plexuses and in the paravertebral chain, but undergo degeneration post-natally. However, significant remnants may remain along the vagus nerve in the para-vertebral sympathetic ganglia, the arch of the aorta, the carotid arteries, and particularly at the origin of the inferior mesenteric artery (organ of Zuckerkandl). These extra-adrenal chromaffin cells may undergo tumour formation in later life. Maturation of adrenal chromaffin cells is only complete by 3 years after birth.

Catecholamines as neurotransmitters

Biosynthesis (Fig. 38.1)

The catecholamines have a 3,4-dihydroxyphenyl core, originally derived from a tyrosine precursor (either dietary or from hydroxylation of phenylalanine). The cytosolic tyrosine hydroxylase enzyme catalyses the conversion of tyrosine to DOPA (dihydroxyphenylalanine). Molecular oxygen and a tetrahydrobiopterin cofactor are required for its activity. This is the rate-limiting step in catecholamine biosynthesis, the catechols acting to antagonise activation of the reduced pteridine cofactor (end-product inhibition).

DOPA is a substrate for the cytosolic enzyme aromatic L-amino-acid decarboxylase, which requires a pyridoxal phosphate cofactor, and is converted to dopamine. This is then transported into the storage vesicle, where the membrane-bound dopamine β-hydroxylase (DBH) catalyses the addition of a β-hydroxyl group, forming noradrenaline. The enzyme requires oxygen and also ascorbic acid as a cofactor.

Phenylethanolamine-*N*-methyl transferase (PNMT) is present in the cytoplasm of adrenaline-producing cells (in the adrenal medulla, extra-adrenal chromaffin tissue and the central nervous system (CNS)), and methylates noradrenaline to form adrenaline using the methyl donor *S*-adenosylmethionine (SAM). Noradrenaline leaves the storage vesicle in order to be methylated to adrenaline in the cytoplasm. PNMT is inducible by high concentrations of cortisol. Adrenaline is then taken up into the vesicle for storage prior to release by exocytosis.

Subcellular storage and release

Both in the peripheral sympathetic system and in the adrenal medulla, catecholamines are taken up into 50–350-nm storage particles by an energy-requiring stereospecific, saturable, reserpine-blockable process which is competitive with respect to substrate. It has been suggested that granular uptake protects dopamine from deamination by monoamine oxidase (MAO), for which it is a preferential substrate. Neuropeptides such as somatostatin, neuropeptide Y and enkephalins are also stored in the granular vesicles within the adrenal medulla, in addition to the acidic chromogranins. Vesicles are very impermeable to H^+ and other ions, and maintain both *in vivo* and *in vitro* an intravesicular pH of about 5.5. Catecholamines are accumulated and stored in these vesicles by a chemiosmotic coupling to H^+/ATPase (adenosine triphosphatase) in the vesicle membrane. The activity of this specific proton-translocating ATPase serves to generate an electrochemical proton gradient which is coupled to carrier-mediated catecholamine uptake by an antiport mechanism. Inside the vesicles, four catecholamine molecules are complexed to every one ATP molecule, with an intravesicular catecholamine concentration of around 0.5 mol/l. About 5–10% of catecholamines are free within the cytosol.

Following nicotinic stimulation, depolarisation of the post-ganglionic cell or chromaffin cell occurs through increased sodium permeability. This stimulates influx of Ca^{2+} which then leads to movement of secretory vesicles to the plasma membrane where exocytosis takes place, the contents of the vesicle being expelled into the extracellular space. Catecholamines are complexed to ATP (in a 4 : 1 ratio) within the synaptic vesicle, and both are released during exocytosis. Synaptic vesicles also contain a number of neuropeptides, some of which are biologically active (see below).

Metabolic pathways of clearance

During adrenergic neurotransmission within the sympathetic nervous system, only a small fraction of noradrenaline binds

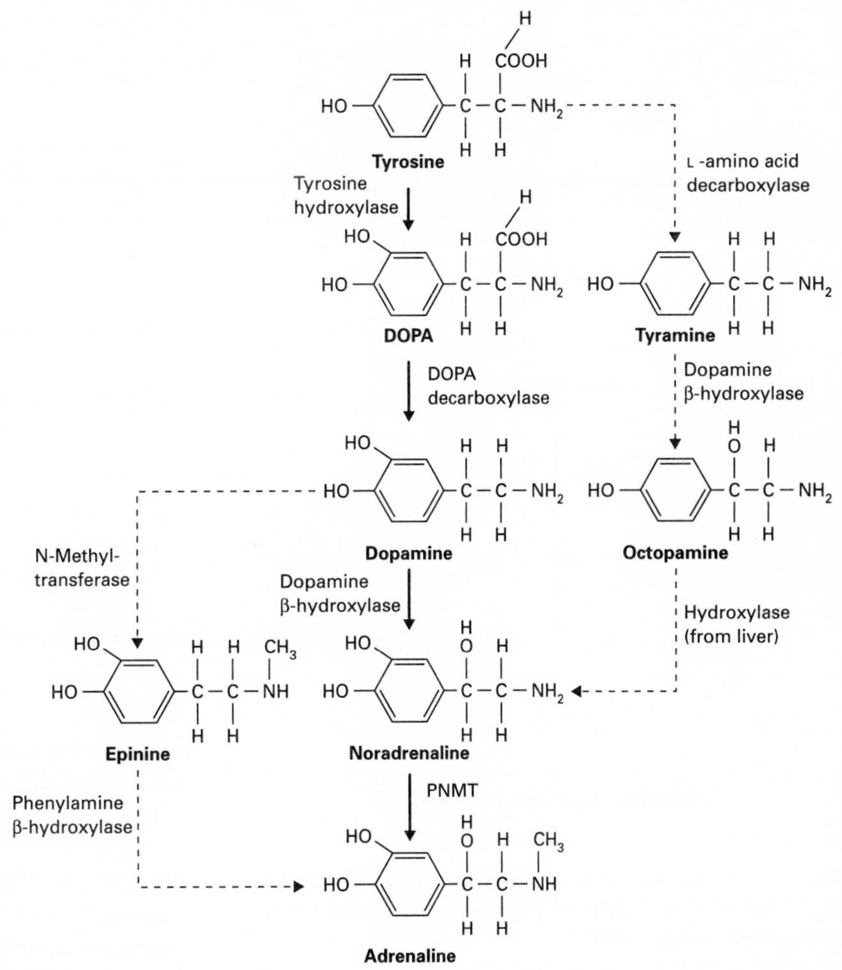

Fig. 38.1 Biosynthetic pathway for dopamine, noradrenaline and adrenaline.

to adrenoceptors. Some is metabolised at the site of release, some diffuses into the circulation, while the majority is actively transported by an energy-dependent stereospecific, saturable, sodium-dependent mechanism back into the preganglionic neuronal terminal (uptake$_1$); the relative importance of these processes depends on the individual tissues. Those that are heavily innervated use reuptake as a major inactivation mechanism. The process is blocked by cocaine, desimipramine, sympathomimetic amines and phenothiazines.

Once inside the cytoplasm, the noradrenaline is rapidly actively transported back into the storage vesicles. Any remaining cytoplasmic catecholamines are deaminated by mitochondrial MAO. Uptake$_1$ is of little importance in the adrenal medulla, where the catecholamines are rapidly transported away by blood flow. The clearance of catecholamines within blood is rapid, both adrenaline and noradrenaline having half-lives of 1–2 min. Transformation into the O-methylated and deaminated metabolites are the dominant forms of extraneuronal inactivation (uptake$_2$). Phenoxybenzamine and glucocorticoids block this pathway. There is recent evidence to suggest that, at least within the central nervous system, a post-synaptic amine transporter (uptake$_p$) may also be operative, and that this is also blockable by desimipramine [3]. It is possible that this protects the post-synaptic noradrenergic receptor from excessive exposure to noradrenaline, thereby preventing down-regulation.

Monoamine oxidase

MAO is a mitochondrial flavoprotein present in most tissues, particularly liver, kidney, intestine and stomach. It catalyses the oxidative deamination of catecholamines (and 5-hydroxytryptamine) to their corresponding aldehydes; these are in turn immediately oxidised to their carboxylic acid or alcohol by aldehyde and alcohol dehydrogenase enzymes, respectively. The action of MAO on noradrenaline and

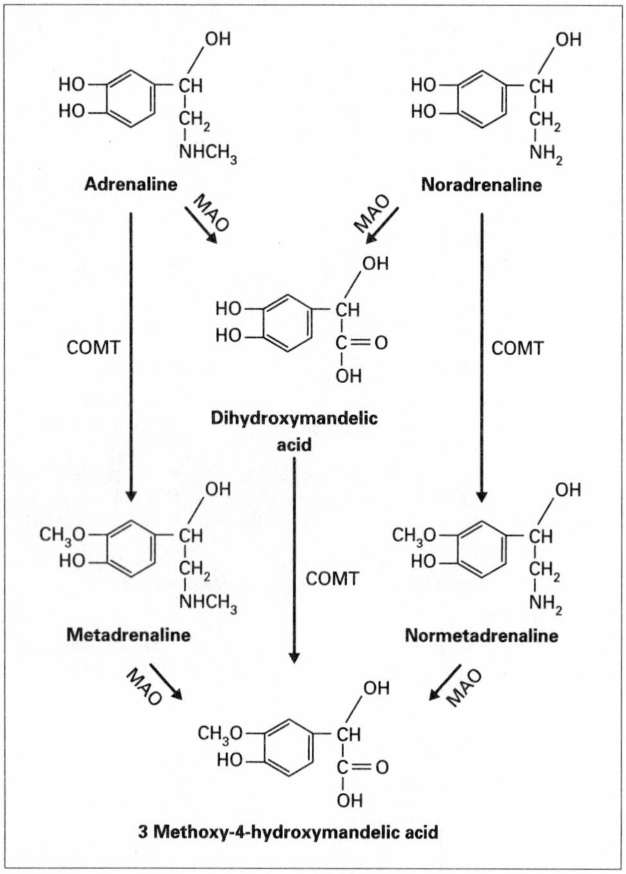

Fig. 38.2 Metabolic pathway of catecholamine degradation. MAO, monoamine oxidase; COMT, catecholamine-*O*-methyl transferase; VMA, vanillyl mandelic acid.

adrenaline is to form 3,4-dihydroxyphenylglycol (DOPEG) or the acid 3,4-dihydroxymandelic acid (DOMA). The major functions of MAO are the metabolism of ingested amines, intraneuronal metabolism of dopamine and noradrenaline, and metabolism of circulating catechols. Oxidative deamination of O-methylated derivatives (metanephrines) leads to formation of vanillyl mandelic acid (VMA or 3-methoxy-4-hydroxymandelic acid) (Fig. 38.2). At least two forms of MAO are present, one predominating within the gastrointestinal tract, the other within the CNS.

Catecholamine-*O*-methyl transferase

COMT is found in the cytosolic fraction of liver and kidney predominantly, and uses SAM as methyl donor. It produces normetanephrine and metanephrine from noradrenaline and adrenaline, respectively, and methoxytyramine from dopamine. Some of the enzyme is intraneuronal. In humans, normetanephrine and metanephrine are converted to 3-methoxy-4-hydroxymandelic acid (MHMA) by MAO and

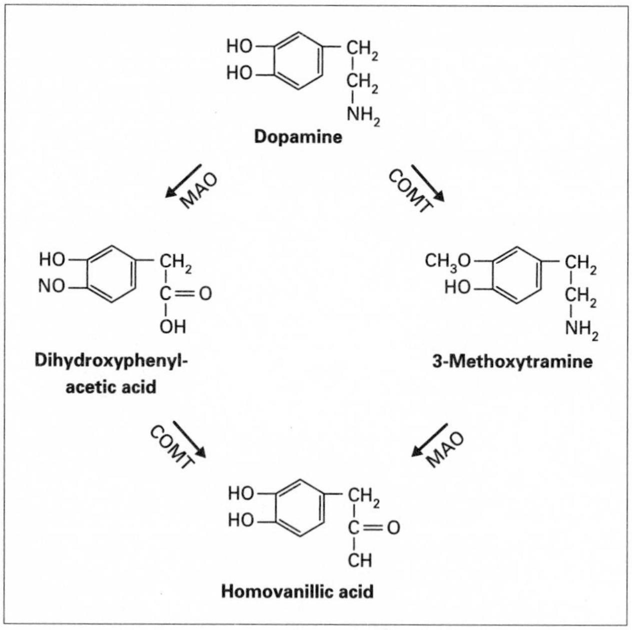

Fig. 38.3 Metabolic pathway for degradation of dopamine.

aldehyde oxidase. An alternative reaction sequence is the oxidative deamination of adrenaline and noradrenaline to 3,4-dihydroxymandelaldehyde, followed by conversion to 3,4-dihydroxymandelic acid by aldehyde oxidase, and final conversion to VMA by O-methylation. The final product of dopamine metabolism is 3-methoxy-4-hydroxyphenylacetic acid (homovanillic acid, HVA) (Fig. 38.3). The daily excretion rate for VMA is up to 35-µmol/24 hours; metanephrines <5 µmol/24 hours; HVA <45 µmol/24 hours. As noted above, the extraneuronal metabolism of catecholamines by MAO and COMT is called uptake$_2$ and is inhibited by corticosteroids.

Sulpho- and glucurono-conjugation

The liver and gut can sulpho- and glucuronoconjugate the hydroxy group of catechols, these conjugates being excreted in the urine in severalfold higher concentrations compared with free catecholamines.

Urinary free catecholamines

Both unmetabolised noradrenaline and adrenaline are excreted in the urine in approximately the same relative proportions as found in plasma. Urinary dopamine appears to be synthesised within the kidney from DOPA, and its concentration in the urine is approximately 10-fold that of noradrenaline. The normal ranges for urinary free noradrenaline, adrenaline and dopamine, based on high-performance liquid chromatography (HPLC) coupled with electrochemical detection (ECD) measurements, are approximately <560, <150 and <3200 nmol/24 hours, respectively.

Plasma catecholamines

Plasma noradrenaline

Under most physiological conditions, noradrenaline acts primarily as a neurotransmitter in the peripheral sympathetic nervous system, being released from the axon terminals of post-ganglionic neurons and deposited directly at innervated target cells. Although most is taken back up into the presynaptic terminal (uptake$_1$), a small fraction spills over into the blood. Supine plasma levels of noradrenaline are 0.5–3 nmol/l in most laboratories. With severe exercise, plasma concentrations may exceed 10–30 nmol/l; at these levels, extrasynaptic adrenoceptors may be stimulated, and a more classical hormonal action of noradrenaline demonstrable. About 50–60% of noradrenaline is loosely bound to albumin in the circulation. Only a small proportion (2%) of noradrenaline is estimated to be of adrenomedullary origin under basal conditions. Much of the plasma noradrenaline is derived from innervation of small arteries and arterioles, which are the primary determinants of peripheral resistance and therefore crucially influence blood pressure. Noradrenaline also comes from venous capacitance vessels. The extent of noradrenaline spillover from the synaptic cleft to the general circulation depends on the cleft width. Perisynaptic noradrenaline concentrations are relatively low for narrow gaps (6×10^{-9} mol/l) but high for wide gaps, where the concentration approaches those attained in the synapse (10^{-6} mol/l) [4]. Vascular intramural synapses have wide gaps, and it seems likely that their proportional contribution to circulating noradrenaline is large.

The level of circulating noradrenaline represents the result of the amount entering the circulation from the synaptic cleft, and the amount leaving it by either uptake$_1$ or uptake$_2$ (extraneuronal metabolism). Urinary excretion and platelet uptake (with conjugation) also play a part in clearance. If the proportion of transmitter overflowing were constant and metabolism and renal elimination were unchanged, plasma noradrenaline would directly reflect changes in neurotransmitter release and therefore nerve impulse traffic in sympathetic neurons. However, as tissue blood flow, reuptake and excretion are unlikely to remain constant under many conditions in which sympathetic activity changes, plasma noradrenaline provides only a rather indirect measure of sympathetic activity [5].

Further, responses of the autonomic nervous system are highly differentiated, and independent changes may occur in muscle, cutaneous or splanchnic beds. Thus, small but highly significant changes in sympathetic tone to splanchnic resistance vessels may occur without significant changes in plasma venous noradrenaline, when the diluting effects of haemodynamically unimportant tissues (i.e. those with a low density of sympathetic innervation) and hepatic extraction of noradrenaline are taken into consideration. The site of sampling for noradrenaline is critical. For example, it has been calculated that about 45% of arterial noradrenaline reaching the forearm muscle is extracted in one passage through the forearm under basal conditions, and that about half the plasma noradrenaline appearing in the antecubital venous plasma is derived from the forearm tissues, reflecting forearm muscle sympathetic activity [5].

Despite these considerations, burst activity recordings in humans from sympathetic fibres still show a significant correlation between muscle sympathetic activity and plasma noradrenaline obtained from antecubital vein sampling [6]. Skeletal muscles appear to be the most important contributors to noradrenaline in mixed venous blood. At present, arterial levels of noradrenaline are probably the best 'sum total' of sympathetic nervous activity.

Plasma adrenaline

Plasma adrenaline is a true hormone in the classical sense, being released solely from the adrenal medulla. A large number of stimuli including hypoglycaemia, heavy exercise, cigarette smoking, pain and fear stimulate adrenaline release. Levels in venous plasma (0.05–1.08 nmol/l) are about one-tenth those of noradrenaline under basal conditions. In pathological states, such as myocardial infarction and circulatory shock states, levels may rise 100-fold. Infusions of adrenaline to generate venous levels of 0.5–2 nmol/l are associated with subtle but definite cardiovascular and metabolic changes. Thus, effects on heart rate, systolic blood pressure, and plasma glycerol at *venous* plasma adrenaline levels of 0.5 nmol/l or less are demonstrable, whilst increases in plasma glucose and lactate, and reductions in diastolic blood pressure occur at approximately 1 nmol/l. The threshold for the stimulation of thermogenesis is similar to that for lipolysis (0.6 nmol/l), and that for lowering plasma potassium approximately 1 nmol/l. Elevations in arterial levels of adrenaline in the range 0.40–0.88 nmol/l have been found in one mental stress paradigm (Stroop colour-word test).

Plasma dopamine

Dopamine is a relatively minor neurotransmitter in the autonomic nervous system, and circulating levels are about those of adrenaline. Most dopamine in plasma is sulphoconjugated (about 99%), and thus inactive.

Table 38.1 Drugs that influence the level of circulating catecholamines.

Drug	Classification	Noradrenaline (change from baseline) (%)	Adrenaline (change from baseline) (%)	Time
α-Methyldopa	α_2-Agonist	−20–30	–	Rapid
Amphetamine	Indirect-acting amine	+29–34	–	3 hours
Atenolol	β_1-Antagonist	0	0	2–24 hours
Bromocriptine	Dopamine agonist	−20	−4	2 h
		−63	−65	1 week
Caffeine	Adenosine receptor agonist	+75	+207	1–3 hours
Clonidine	α_2-Agonist	−80 total catecholamines		2–3 hours
Dexamethasone	Glucocorticoid	−48	–	3 days
Fenfluramine	Anorectic	−30–73	–	3 days
Fentanyl	Opiate (μ)	−30	−48	minutes
Hydralazine	Vasodilator	+43	–	1 hour
Hydrochloro-thiazide	Diuretic	+55–65	–	1–6 weeks
Insulin	Hormone	+60	Depends on glycaemia	45 min
Isoprenaline	β_1-Agonist	+	–	
L-DOPA	Dopamine precursor	−55	–	1 hour
Marijuana	Cannabinoid	+85	–	0.5–1 hour
Minoxidil	Vasodilator	+33–140	–	2–26 months
Nifedipine	Calcium antagonist	+47–93	–	1 hour–3 weeks
Oxprenolol	Agonist-antagonist	+50–60	–	6 weeks
Phenoxy-benzamine	α-Blocker	+85	–	6 weeks
Pindolol	β-Blocker	−41	–	16 weeks
Prazosin	α-Blocker	+65	–	4 weeks
Propranolol	β-Blocker	−50	–	24 hours
		+13–50	+25–108	6–8 weeks
Saralasin	Angiotensin-II antagonist	+46–256	–	5 min
Tobacco	Nicotine	+43	+156	10–15 min

Pharmacological agents that influence the level of circulating catecholamines are summarised in Table 38.1.

Physiological actions of catecholamines

Catecholamines act by binding to specific cell-surface receptors. These are divided into (α_1, α_2, β_1, β_2) adrenoceptors, and in the case of dopamine D1 and D2 receptors. Receptors are classified on the basis of their affinities to agonists and antagonists, as well as their location (presynaptic or post-synaptic). Presynaptic receptors (α_2, inhibitory; β_2, stimulatory) autoregulate the amount of catecholamine released from the axon terminal, whereas post-synaptic receptors are located on the effector cell. Extrajunctional receptors occur at sites of non-innervation, and are the target of circulating catecholamine action.

Cardiovascular effects

The sympathetic nervous system regulates cardiac output and the peripheral circulation (both general and regional). In particular, sympathetically mediated adjustments in peripheral resistance provide adequate perfusion of vital organ systems in the face of changing circulatory and metabolic demands. The sympathetic nervous system responds to changes in circulatory volume and pressure which are detected by afferent activity from high- and low-pressure baroreceptors.

Thus, small increments or decrements in volume or pressure are detected by afferent receptors, and impulses are conducted to the nucleus tractus solitarius and then finally on to the rostral ventrolateral medulla, which is responsible for generating sympathetic tone. A decrease in afferent activity causes a reciprocal increase in sympathetic efferent activity. Thus, small decrements in venous return, such as those induced by alterations in position, will stimulate efferent sympathetic activity to the heart, arterioles and veins. The α-mediated venoconstriction will increase venous return, and peripheral resistance is increased by α-mediated vasoconstriction in the subcutaneous, mucosal, splanchnic and renal vascular beds. Increase in heart rate and force of contraction is mediated by β_1-adrenoceptors.

Visceral effects

In general, catecholamines relax smooth muscle by a β_2 action and cause contraction by α_1 actions. Dopaminergic receptors mediate relaxation in the gut and vascular smooth muscle. Catecholamines diminish acetylcholine release from the gastrointestinal myenteric plexus. Thus, intestinal relaxation may be consequent upon either direct β-receptor-induced relaxation or α_2-mediated suppression of acetylcholine release. Catecholamines modulate fluid and electrolyte transport in the intestine, gallbladder, trachea, cornea and renal epithelium, as well as stimulating the secretion of peptides into biological fluids such as saliva and tears. They also stimulate cell growth and division. For example, in the intestine they stimulate intestinal crypt growth by an α_2 effect, and inhibit it by α_1 and β mechanisms. Erythroid colony formation is stimulated via the β_2-receptor. Adrenaline promotes platelet aggregation by an α_2-mediated mechanism.

Metabolic effects

Infusion of catecholamines induces increased oxygen consumption by a β-receptor mechanism, and the sympathetic nervous system regulates thermogenesis in response to cold exposure (non-shivering thermogenesis) and to dietary intake (diet-induced thermogenesis). Catecholamines also stimulate breakdown of stored fuels from liver, adipose tissue and skeletal muscle into utilisable substrates either locally (e.g. glycogenolysis in the heart) or for systemic distribution. Both circulating adrenaline and direct tissue sympathetic neural activity are involved in these processes, which also involve interactions with insulin and glucagon release.

Catecholamines promote net glucose efflux from the liver by activating β-mediated glycogenolysis. This occurs through stimulation of cyclic adenosine monophosphate (cAMP) formation, which in turn activates a protein kinase which phosphorylates both phosphorylate kinase and glycogen synthase. Phosphorylation activates the former and inactivates the latter, thereby enhancing glycogen breakdown. Catecholamines also suppress insulin secretion and provoke glucagon release, and these augment the actions of catecholamines on the liver. The hepatic effects of catecholamines are mediated in part by direct hepatic neural innervation and partly by circulating catecholamines.

Effects on lipoproteins

In adipose tissue, catecholamines stimulate β_1, cAMP-mediated lipolysis by activating triacylglycerol lipase, the enzyme that cleaves triglycerides into fatty acids and glycerol, and promote α_1- and β-mediated glucose uptake. In humans, infusion of adrenaline within the physiological range can be shown to increase lipolysis. Catecholamines also stimulate glycogenolysis in muscle by a β-adrenoceptor mechanism. Infusions of catecholamines will lead to short-term increases in both cholesterol and triglyceride levels. In the latter case, part of this effect is secondary to lipolysis-stimulated increased free fatty acid levels which serve as substrate for hepatic triglyceride synthesis.

Water and electrolyte metabolism

Catecholamines directly influence sodium excretion by an effect on the renal tubule, and, in animals, renal denervation or reflex suppression of renal sympathetic activity acutely increases sodium excretion. They also influence renal sodium handling by vascular and hormonal effects. Thus, intense renal sympathetic discharge will reduce the glomerular filtration rate and stimulate sodium reabsorption. Catecholamines also stimulate renin release (β-adrenoceptor effect) from the juxtaglomerular apparatus, thus stimulating the renin–angiotensin–aldosterone system and inducing distal sodium reabsorption. Dopamine, when infused in low doses in humans (0.5 μg/kg/min), produces renal vasodilatation and a natriuresis. Endogenous dopamine is largely formed by intrarenal conversion of DOPA. Urinary dopamine increases in response to sodium loading and diminishes with salt deprivation. Adrenaline transiently increases plasma potassium by an α-receptor-mediated hepatic effect, but then causes hypokalaemia by β_2-mediated stimulation of muscle Na^+/K^+ ATPase activity which drives potassium intracellularly [7]. Serum magnesium levels also fall in response to adrenaline infusion. In humans, β-blockade potentiates the increase in potassium during exercise.

Effect on hormone secretion

One role of the sympatho-adrenal system may be to regulate the sensitivity of endocrine cells to stimulation by their usual secretagogues, in addition to a pure secretagogue action.

Renin secretion

Renal sympathetic nerve stimulation or infusion of catecholamines increases renin secretion independent of changes in renal blood flow or in filtered sodium load. The juxtaglomerular apparatus is innervated by sympathetic fibres, and the cells have β-receptors on their surface. Catecholamine stimulation of renin release is part of the physiological response to volume depletion and hypotension, and deficient renin release in response to postural challenge is a not infrequent accompaniment of autonomic neuropathy.

Insulin and glucagon release

β_2-Adrenoceptor activation in the pancreas transiently increases secretion of both insulin and glucagon, but the α_2 suppression of insulin release is the more important physiological response. Increased glucagon release is frequently coincidental with sympatho-adrenal activation, but whether catecholamines cause the rise in glucagon secretion is not established.

Other hormones

Catecholamines have been shown to increase levels of several hormones: these include somatostatin, pancreatic polypeptide, thyroxine (T_4), triiodothyronine (T_3), parathyroid hormone, gastrin, erythropoietin and progesterone. However, as adrenoceptor blockade is without major effects on any of these hormones, the physiological function of this control is unclear.

Pattern of sympathetic activity

Both sympathetic and parasympathetic activity respond in a highly differentiated manner to stresses. There are several situations in which sympathetic and adrenomedullary activity are dissociated. For example, during mild exercise and orthostasis, rises in plasma noradrenaline are not accompanied by significant changes in adrenaline. During hypoglycaemia, adrenaline is preferentially released with only slight changes in noradrenaline. Furthermore, sympathetic responses are themselves highly selective and differentiated with regard to activity in particular vascular beds.

Measurement of plasma catecholamines

Plasma noradrenaline represents spillover from nerve endings, and only about 5% of noradrenaline released at nerve endings finds its way into the circulation. Adrenaline, on the other hand, is a hormone in the classical sense. The origin of circulating dopamine is presently unclear, although some may be renal in origin. Catecholamines circulate in low nanomolar concentrations, and although their quantification has posed many problems in the past, they are now readily measurable.

Currently HPLC–ECD is preferred to radioenzymatic assays (REA), which transfer a labelled methyl group (using *S*-adenosyl-methionine) to the 3-hydroxy position of the catechol ring using the enzyme COMT. In the former, catecholamines are adsorbed from plasma onto acidified alumina under alkaline conditions in the presence of an internal standard. Desorption of catecholamines from the alumina is effected with a small volume of acid (e.g. phosphoric acid) which is then loaded onto a reversed phase HPLC column, and the separated catecholamines quantified by electrochemical oxidation [8]. In REA, labelled methoxy derivatives are extracted and separated by thin layer chromatography prior to oxidation to VMA before counting. REA offers greater sensitivity and precision at the lower ends of the physiological range than HPLC–ECD, but the convenience and relative simplicity of the latter makes it the analytical method of choice clinically.

Other methods of measuring sympathetic activity

Kinetic techniques

Radiotracer techniques for studying the rate of noradrenaline release to, and removal from, plasma in humans have been described [9]. The method involves the infusion of tritiated noradrenaline at a constant rate to reach a plateau concentration of 10–15 fmol/l. Noradrenaline clearance can then be calculated from the relationship:

$$\text{NA clearance} = \frac{\text{NA-}^3\text{H infusion rate}}{\text{Plasma NA-}^3\text{H concentration}}$$

Noradrenaline spillover rate can be estimated by the relationship:

$$\text{NA spillover} = \frac{\text{NA-}^3\text{H infusion rate}}{\text{Plasma NA specific radioactivity}}$$

These measurements give a better guide to overall sympathetic activity, but the disadvantage, besides the complexity, is that the technique does not identify the source of released noradrenaline, unless individual beds are investigated. However, using these tracer techniques, several examples of mismatch between noradrenaline concentrations in plasma and the calculated plasma noradrenaline spillover caused by alterations in clearance have been documented. These include drugs (desimipramine, propranolol), increasing age (which diminishes noradrenaline clearance), and autonomic insufficiency, where plasma noradrenaline clearance is slowed.

Plasma dopamine β-hydroxylase

Dopamine β-hydroxylase (DBH) and catecholamines are released from the storage vesicle together during exocytosis. Given the long half-life of plasma DBH (3 hours), ease of assay and absence of neuronal reuptake, it was thought that DBH would be a good surrogate for plasma noradrenaline and hence evaluation of sympathetic activity [10]. However, several discrepancies between plasma noradrenaline and plasma DBH have been documented. This may be in part due to the fact that the release of DBH is under genetic control, with some individuals not releasing DBH during exocytosis.

Plasma chromogranin

Chromogranins are coreleased with catecholamines during exocytosis, and their measurement in plasma has been advocated as an index of sympathetic activity [11] and used as a surrogate marker in the diagnosis of tumorous catecholamine excess. Neither its secretion nor its measurement is influenced by drugs commonly used in the treatment of phaeochromocytoma. Chromogranin A (CgA) has poor diagnostic specificity in ruling out the disease; this is because renal elimination plays a large part in its clearance, such that relatively minor falls in creatinine clearance lead to significant rises in chromogranin A [12]. The overall specificity of CgA in diagnosis is approximately 74%; when creatinine clearance falls below 80 ml/min, diagnostic specificity drops to 50% [12]. Furthermore, chromogranins are released by several tissues secreting hormones, and those present in plasma cannot be assumed to be solely sympathetic in origin.

Platelet catecholamine content

Catecholamines are taken up into platelets, and the platelet catecholamine content has in several studies been shown to reflect recent plasma catecholamine levels.

Physiological factors influencing plasma catecholamine levels

Emotional stimuli

Numerous emotional stimuli such as anxiety, pain and anger elicit sympathetic responses, with predominant rises in adrenaline. Several studies have shown that venepuncture and its anticipatory emotional stress result in small but significant elevations of plasma catecholamines. Interestingly, the use of laboratory staff to generate a normal range for catecholamines may not be appropriate; they may have lower catecholamine levels than other control groups due to familiarisation with the procedures involved. Thus, comparative studies should preferably recruit patients and controls from as similar populations as possible.

Time courses for catecholamine responses

More-or-less stable stimulated catecholamine levels can be obtained at 6–8 min for lower body negative pressure and isometric contralateral handgrip, as well as submaximal exercise. During mental stress, peak responses occur at approximately 3 min.

Posture

As the primary neurotransmitter, noradrenaline is involved in the sympathetic response to upright posture. Thus, standing is accompanied by a rapid two- to threefold rise in noradrenaline and, less significantly, in adrenaline, within 2–5 min.

Circadian variation

Noradrenaline secretion exhibits a circadian variation under normal sleep/wake conditions. It appears to be secreted in an episodic manner, with most peaks occurring between 0600 hours and 1800 hours. The lowest levels occur during sleep, when there is a paucity of secretory peaks [13].

Age and sex

Age also influences catecholamine levels. Day-time basal supine noradrenaline levels have been shown to display an age-related increase. Further, it has been shown that noradrenaline levels associated with upright posture and isometric exercise are increased to a greater extent with advancing age than are supine noradrenaline concentrations. This age-related increase in plasma noradrenaline appears to be greater at night, and reflects in part diminished clearance. It is also known that there is an age-related decrease in the sensitivity to catecholamines. In premenopausal women, there is significant variation of plasma noradrenaline concentration during the menstrual cycle.

Exercise

Vigorous exercise markedly increases plasma noradrenaline and adrenaline, but concentrations of these hormones rapidly decline with rest. Age and obesity have both been shown to exaggerate exercise-induced increases in plasma catecholamine levels.

Obesity

Increases in sympathetic activity have been associated with overfeeding, and diminished sympathetic activity has been associated with starvation or hypocaloric feeding. Sympathetic nervous overactivity has been implicated in the pathogenesis of hypertension in obese individuals. Basal supine plasma noradrenaline concentrations and levels achieved after upright posture are greater in obese subjects than in non-obese controls matched for age, sex and race. The mechanism by which obesity increases sympathetic activity is unknown. Noradrenaline turnover is reduced in pancreatic, hepatic and cardiac tissues in animals with starvation, and reversed by sucrose feeding. Marked carbohydrate restriction has been shown to reduce blood pressure in the spontaneously hypertensive rat, consistent with a reduction in sympathetic activity. Conversely, increased plasma noradrenaline levels occur in humans following glucose ingestion. It seems, therefore, that carbohydrate intake alters sympathetic activity at the hypothalamic level or peripherally. Stimulation of insulin secretion is a possible mechanism, as the latter has been shown to increase sympathetic activity.

Sodium intake

Resting plasma noradrenaline and adrenaline are significantly increased in response to a low sodium diet and the ensuing sodium and volume depletion. The plasma noradrenaline response to upright posture has also been found to be significantly augmented by sodium restriction compared with either normal or high sodium intake [13].

Cardiac status

It has been shown that resting supine plasma noradrenaline levels are related to prognosis, those patients having the highest concentrations showing the greatest increase in mortality.

Thyroid status

Numerous studies have shown that basal muscle sympathetic activity is increased in the hypothyroid state. This is the likely cause of the elevated plasma noradrenaline level seen in untreated hypothyroid patients. By contrast, plasma noradrenaline levels are within the normal range in the hyperthyroid state, where upregulation of β-adrenoceptors is known to occur.

Sympathetic pharmacology

Several classes of drug are capable of interfering with the function of the sympathetic nervous system.

1 α-Methylparatyrosine is a false substrate for the rate-limiting enzyme tyrosine hydroxylase, and blocks catecholamine biosynthesis. It has been used clinically in the medical treatment of phaeochromocytoma.

2 α-Methylnoradrenaline (derived from α-methyldopa), clonidine and guanfacine act predominantly centrally at post-synaptic α_2-adrenoceptors to reduce sympathetic discharge. Carbidopa inhibits peripheral, but not central, L-aromatic amino-acid decarboxylase, and thus prevents the metabolism of L-DOPA in the periphery.

3 Cocaine and the tricyclic antidepressants block the uptake_1 pathway, leading to increased noradrenaline concentrations in the synaptic cleft. The uptake of noradrenaline into storage vesicles is inhibited by reserpine and guanethidine: this leads to gradual catecholamine depletion at the nerve ending.

4 Tyramine, amphetamine and ephedrine are indirectly acting amines that act by stoichiometric displacement of cytosolic and vesicular catecholamine stores out of the cell. They are taken up into the cell by uptake_1 mechanisms, and are thus competitive inhibitors of noradrenaline uptake. These effects are independent of extracellular Ca^{2+} concentration, and are not inhibited by colchicine.

5 The adrenergic neuron blockers bretylium, debrisoquine, guanethidine and bethanidine act by blocking the coupling of the action potential to catecholamine release, and are thus associated with a fall in circulating plasma noradrenaline.

6 MAO inhibitors prevent the oxidative deamination of catecholamines and thus increase the intracellular stores of catecholamines.

7 The phosphodiesterase inhibitors theophylline, aminophylline and caffeine attenuate cAMP degradation, and thus accentuate those effects of catecholamines mediated through adenyl cyclase activation. Some of their actions are, however, mediated through blockade of purinergic (adenosine) receptors.

General characteristics and classification of adrenoceptors

Catecholamines exert their biological actions by binding to specific membrane recognition sites known as adrenoceptors. This interaction initiates a number of membrane and intracellular events ending as a biological response, a process known as signal-transduction coupling (see also Chapter 4).

Until recently, two major subclasses of adrenoceptors were defined on the basis of differential agonist potencies and responses to antagonists: α-adrenergic and β-adrenergic; for each, two subclasses, α_1 and α_2 and β_1 and β_2, have been

Table 38.2 Properties of adrenoceptors.

	α_1	α_2	β_1	β_2
Agonist potency series	ADR > NA > PE > I	ADR > NA > PE > I	I > ADR > NA > PE	I > ADR > NA > PE
Selective agonists	Methoxamine Phenylphrine	Clonidine, Guanfacine α-Methyl NA	Dobutamine	Albuterol Fenoterol Terbutaline Salbutamol
Specific antagonists	Thymoxamine Prazosin Terazosin Trimazosin Doxazosin	Yohimbine Idazoxan	Propranolol Alprenolol Pindolol Metoprolol Betaxolol Acebutolol Atenolol	Propranolol Alprenolol Pindolol
Physiological response	Vasoconstriction Intestinal relaxation Uterine contraction Pupillary dilatation Stimulation of hepatic glycogenolysis	Inhibition of presynaptic NA release Platelet aggregation Inhibition of insulin secretion, lipolysis, renin release	Stimulation of heart rate and contraction Lipolysis Intestinal relaxation Stimulation of renin release	Bronchodilatation Vasodilatation Presynaptic NA release

ADR, adrenaline; NA, noradrenaline; PE phenylephrine; I, isoprenaline.

recognised on the basis of pharmacological properties and binding studies with radiolabelled antagonists. Data from recent radioligand binding, combined with studies of the second messengers, formed when different types and subtypes of receptors are activated, suggest that the α-receptors can be further subclassified into α_{1A}, α_{1B}, α_{2A} and α_{2B}. Table 38.2 summarises the properties of the main classes of adrenoceptors.

Three of the four subtypes of adrenergic receptors are linked to the enzyme adenylate cyclase, which generates the second messenger cAMP. The enzyme is stimulated by β_1- and β_2-receptors and inhibited by α_2-receptors. The α_1-receptor is coupled to intracellular phosphoinositol pathways (see below).

Structure of adrenoceptors

All adrenoceptors are integral membrane proteins containing seven stretches of 20–28 hydrophobic amino acids which represent membrane-spanning regions (Fig. 38.4). Amino-acid identities are concentrated within these transmembrane domains. The first two cytoplasmic loops (CI, CII) are fairly well conserved, but the extracellular domain and the putative third cytoplasmic loop (CIII) and the cytoplasmic terminal tail are all quite divergent, and contain potential sites of regulatory phosphorylation. The conserved membrane spanning regions play an important role in the binding of adrenergic ligands. The main function of the cytoplasmic domain is coupling to guanine nucleotide regulatory proteins, and the third cytoplasmic loop seems most important in this process. The carboxy terminal and third cytoplasmic domain contain two consensus cAMP-dependent kinase phosphorylation sites.

Signal/transduction mechanism (see also Chapter 4)

Adrenergic receptors are members of a large superfamily of receptors linked to guanine nucleotide-binding proteins (G-proteins). All G-protein-coupled receptors share a number of features in common: extracellular amino-acid terminals with sites for N-linked glycosylation, seven a-helical domains that are each thought to span the plasma membrane, and intracellular carboxy-terminals containing amino-acid sequences that indicate probable sites of phosphorylation by one or more kinases. The superfamily of G-protein-coupled receptors, comprising several hundred members, include in addition to adrenoceptors, receptors for acetylcholine, dopamine, histamine, prostaglandins as well as peptides (such as vasopresin, oxytocin and angiotensin) and proteins (such

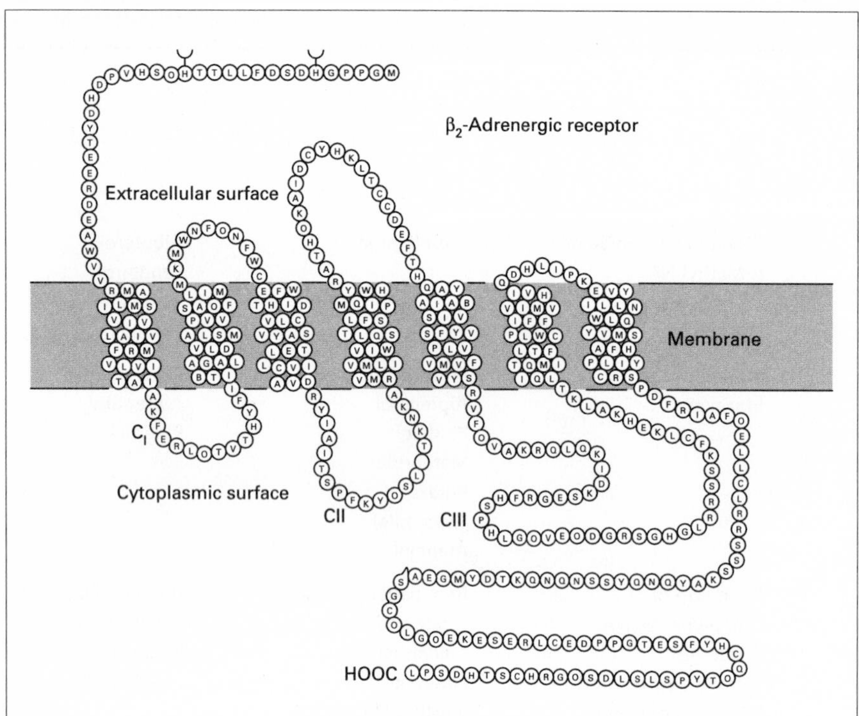

Fig. 38.4 Proposed topology of the β_2-adrenergic receptor with respect to the plasma membrane bilayer. The ligand binds to external domain. Three intracytoplasmic loops (CI, CII, CIII) are shown.

as glucagon, follicle-stimulating hormone (FSH), luteinising hormone (LH) and thyroid-stimulating hormone (TSH). G-proteins are made up of α-, β- and γ-subunits. Each is part of a family consisting of multiple members: approximately 20 α-subunits (which have been divided into four families: α_s, α_i, α_q, α_{12}), at least five β-subunits (β_{1-5}), and at least six γ-subunits (γ_{1-6}). Although several hundred heterotrimeric complexes are theoretically possible, the combination of G proteins used for signalling by a particular receptor is limited.

Each type of G-protein can be used for signalling by more than one type of receptor, and many receptors that stimulate adenylate cyclase activity can activate G_s. Each adrenoceptor preferentially couples to a different subfamily of G_α proteins: β-adrenoceptors to $G_{\alpha s}$, α_1-adrenoceptors to $G_{\alpha q}$ and α_2-adrenoceptors to $G_{\alpha i}$. In turn, each of these G_α proteins can link to numerous effector molecules. For example, β-adrenoceptors are preferentially coupled by G_s to activation of adenylate cyclase (and Ca^{2+} channels in some tissues) α_1-adrenoceptors by G_q to the activation of phospholipases, especially phospholipase C, and α_2-adrenoceptors by G_i to adenylate cyclase inhibition. Each of these linkages leads to the changes in intracellular concentrations of second messengers such as cAMP, Ca^{2+}, diacylglycerol and inositol 1,4,5-triphosphate. These second messengers modulate cellular events, regulating the phosphorylated states of cell proteins by activating protein kinases. cAMP stimulates phosphokinase A (PKA), diacylglycerol and Ca^{2+} activate PKC, and Ca^{2+} and calmodulin activate calmodulin-dependent kinases.

Catecholamines, although hydrophilic, bind not to the highly charged extracellular domains of the receptors but to the more hydrophobic membrane-spanning domains. When an agonist binds to the receptor, conformational changes within the receptor occur, causing in particular the third intracellular loop to interact with G-protein. Under basal conditions, G-proteins are inactive, and the guanine nucleotide-binding site on the G_α is occupied by inactive guanosine diphosphate (GDP). When agonist binds to the receptor, guanosine triphosphate (GTP) displaces GDP from the G_α, causing the latter to dissociate from the βγ-subunits which are tightly bound and appear to function as a dimer. Both G_α and $G_{\beta\gamma}$ subunit dimer can regulate the activity of effector molecules and second-messenger formation. The G-protein is activated until such time as the GTP is hydrolysed to form GDP, facilitating reassociation of the subunits.

Subunit dissociation of G_s by β-adrenoceptor activation is the principal mechanism method of amplification of β-adrenoceptor signalling; the number of adenylate cyclase molecules limits the response to activated G_s. Each β-adrenoceptor can activate several G_s-proteins; and the number of G_s proteins far exceeds the number of receptors and effector molecules.

Enzymes in the adrenergic systems

Adrenoceptor numbers are regulated by biosynthesis, processing and plasma membrane insertion. Glucocorticoids, thyroid hormones and other hormones regulate the expression of several adrenoceptors through transcriptional and in some cases post-translational modification.

At least four enzymes are involved in the catecholamine-modulated effects on cells: adenylate cyclase, which is stimulated (β_1 and β_2) or inhibited (α_2) to produce cAMP; β-adrenergic receptor kinase (β-ARK) which phosphorylates the agonist-occupied form of the receptor; GTPase, which hydrolyses GTP into GDP once the GTP-loaded α-subunit of the G_s-protein has activated adenylate cyclase; and finally phosphodiesterase which breaks down cAMP.

The regulation of adrenoceptors by agonists (desensitisation) is a multistep process involving several discrete events. These include the rapid phosphorylation of receptors, receptor sequestration in a cellular compartment not readily accessible from outside the cell, uncoupling of the receptor so that ligand binding still occurs but second-messenger formation is decreased, and the internalisation of the receptor to intracellular sites. Loss of receptors can also occur with persistent exposure of agonist to receptor through degradation, but this is a relatively slow process.

Desensitisation of adrenoceptors

Desensitisation is a general adaptive process whereby prolonged exposure of an effector tissue to a stimulus of constant intensity leads to a diminishing response. It is known that prolonged exposure of agonists to α- and β-adrenoceptors leads to a reduction in adrenoceptor numbers [14]. Similarly, absence of an agonist leads to increased receptor number and the phenomenon of up-regulation. In the regulation of hormone responsiveness, homologous desensitisation refers to a situation in which, after stimulation of a system by a specific agonist, sensitivity is lost only to stimulation by that agonist; responsiveness to other diverse types of agonists is maintained. In heterologous desensitisation, stimulation by one agonist leads to decreased responsiveness to a whole series of structurally unrelated agonists working through distinct receptors, and even to stimulants that may bypass normal receptor mechanisms.

Receptor phosphorylation

Original studies focused on the action of PKA and PKC, but at present it is likely that G-protein receptor kinases (previously known as β-adrenoceptor kinase) are predominantly implicated in receptor phosphorylation. In the resting state, these are cytosolic enzymes, but some bind to βγ subunits derived from dissociated G-proteins. At least six types of G-protein-receptor kinases with unique tissue distribution and localisation have been identified. G-protein-receptor kinases work in concert with arrestins (β-arrestins) which together with receptors phosphorylated by G-protein-receptor kinases blunt the interaction of the adrenoceptors with G-proteins, thereby causing uncoupling [14].

The α_1-receptor

α_1-Adrenoceptors appear to control cytosolic Ca^{2+} levels through effects on inositol phospholipid metabolism. Like other Ca^{2+}-mobilising receptors, activation of α_1-adrenoceptors increases the hydrolysis of the specific membrane lipid phosphatidyl inositol. This is unique among membrane lipids in that it occurs in two or more highly phosphorylated forms, phosphaditylinositol-4-monophosphate (PIP) and phosphatidyl inositol 4,5-bisphosphate (PIP_2). Stimulation of α_1-adrenoceptors leads to activation of membrane-bound phospholipase C which catalyses PIP_2 breakdown to release diacylglycerol and inositol (1,4,5)P_3. The latter releases intracellular Ca^{2+} which is responsible for initiating the effector mechanism. Diacylglycerol also appears to act as a second messenger and activates protein kinase C by reducing its requirements for Ca^{2+}.

Adrenoceptor variants and human disease

There is a high degree of polymorphism at certain loci in the β_2-adrenoceptors. In particular, one polymorphism that leads to an amino-acid change from arginine to glycine at codon 16 is significantly more prevalent in patients who have a history of nocturnal asthma [15]. Experimentally, this mutant receptor appears more sensitive to a down-regulating response to adrenoceptor agonists. In contrast, substitution of glutamic acid for glutamine at codon 27 yields a receptor that has decreased down-regulation, and this is associated with a decrease in bronchoconstriction. A polymorphism at codon 64 of the β_3-adrenoceptor (see below) converts tryptophan to arginine. This polymorphism is more frequent in Pima Indians and in morbidly obese French patients, and when homozygous, is associated with morbid obesity.

Dopamine receptors

These are currently classified into D1 and D2 subtypes in terms of their ability to activate (D_1) or inhibit (D_2) adenylate cyclase. Apomorphine and bromocriptine are typical ligands at these receptors. Dopamine receptors are widely distributed throughout the CNS (especially the nigrostriatal pathway and the lactotroph of the anterior pituitary), as well as in the periphery (gut: inhibition of motility, mesenteric vasodilatation) and kidney (vasodilatation of renal vessels with natriuresis).

Clinical conditions associated with altered adrenoceptors

Prolonged adrenoceptor agonist treatment (or phaeochromocytoma) is associated with desensitisation of both α- and β-adrenoceptors, whereas conversely abrupt antagonist withdrawal is associated with super-sensitisation and up-regulation of receptors. In myocardial ischaemia, there is some evidence for up-regulation and uncoupling of β-receptors, and enhanced α_1-adrenoceptor coupling. In essential hypertension up-regulation and altered coupling of α-adrenoceptors may occur together with down-regulation of β-adrenoceptors. In congestive cardiac failure, there may be down-regulation of β_1-adrenoceptors, and β_2-receptor uncoupling, possibly due to an increase in G-protein-receptor kinases. In asthma, certain β_2-adrenoceptor polymorphisms predispose to desensitisation.

β_3-Adrenoceptors

An atypical adrenoceptor (β_3) has been cloned, and the mRNA found in humans in pancreas, colon, stomach, gall-bladder, brown and white adipose tissue, placenta and brain (temporal, frontal and posterior cortex). β_3-Adrenoceptors differ structurally from β_1- and β_2-receptors in the C-terminal intracellular domain, whereby β_3-receptors lack sites for phosphorylation [16]. This may render these receptors less susceptible to down-regulation. Stimulation of β_3-receptors in rodents leads to increased energy expenditure, whereas the β_3-agonist BRL 26830A, when administered to obese people, increased both resting metabolic rate and the thermic response to a glucose load. Although any β_3-agonists lack specificity and also react with β_2-adrenoceptors (CL 316243, ICI D7114, BRL 35135), a newer class of β_3-agonists, the phenylethanolaminotetralines, demonstrate greater receptor specificity. Potential clinical applications of β_3-agonists are in the sphere of obesity and type 2 diabetes mellitus, where there is some evidence they may increase insulin sensitivity.

Catecholamine-deficiency states

The most important cause of catecholamine deficiency is autonomic neuropathy, which most frequently supervenes in the context of diabetes mellitus. Inherited conditions such as the Shy–Drager syndrome are also associated with dysautonomia. The Guillain–Barré syndrome is also associated with autonomic dysfunction.

Although rare, congenital deficiency of dopamine β-hydroxylase has been reported [17] and is associated with undetectable circulating adrenaline and noradrenaline, but with increased dopamine and DOPA levels. Patients give a life-long history of severe orthostatic hypotension, ptosis, nasal stuffiness and a failure to show increases in heart rate and cardiac output with stimulation. Treatment with DL-*threo*-3,4-dihydroxyphenylserine (DL-DOPS) has been shown to be effective in such patients; this compound is taken up by the nerve endings, and is decarboxylated into noradrenaline, thus bypassing the enzymatic defect. Normal noradrenergic function may be restored with treatment.

Catecholamine-secreting tumours

Catecholamine-secreting tumours are rare, and account for 0.1–1% of all cases of hypertension. In a series from the Mayo Clinic, 76% of 54 autopsy proven were clinically unsuspected during life, and only 17% correctly diagnosed during life [18]; 7% were incidentally discovered at laparotomy for unrelated conditions [18,19]. Tumours originate from within the adrenal medulla (phaeochromocytoma) or from extra-adrenal neural crest derivatives (paraganglioma) such as the sympathetic chain. A classification is given in Table 38.3. The extensive distribution of neural crest derivatives underlies the diverse localisation of such tumours which can occur at the base of the skull, the pericardium, the atria, the para-aortic area (classically the organ of Zuckerkandl), as well as the urinary bladder and the testicle (Table 38.4). Given the potential multicentric origin of tumours, malignant behaviour is difficult to predict from histology alone, and depends upon the demonstration of metastatic disease, usually within lymph nodes, liver and bone. The 'rule of 10' usefully summarises many features of chromaffin tumours (Table 38.5). Although mainly sporadic, hereditable lesions are recognised in association with the multiple endocrine neoplasia (MEN) and neurocutaneous syndromes [20,21] (Table 38.6). In familial cases, there is a higher incidence of bilaterality, multiplicity and multicentricity.

Phaeochromocytomas

Macroscopic and microscopic features

Tumours are usually slow growing, and vary in size from a

Table 38.3 Classification of catecholamine secreting tumours.

Tumour	Cell or origin
Phaeochromocytoma Paraganglioma	Chromaffin cell
Ganglioneuroma Ganglioneuroblastoma	Ganglion cell
Sympathoblastoma	Sympathogonia
Neuroblastoma	Sympathoblast

Table 38.4 Classification of sites of origin of extra-adrenal tumours (paragangliomas).

Branchiomeric
Intercarotid
Jugulotympanic
Orbital
Laryngeal
Subclavian
Aorticopulmonary
Coronary
Pulmonary
Intravagal
Aorticosympathetic
Neck
Thoracic
Abdominal
Visceral–autonomic
Atria of heart
Urinary bladder
Liver hilum
Mesenteric vessels

Table 38.5 *Aide-mémoire* to important features of phaeochromocytomas.

Six Hs	Hypertension Headache Hyperhidrosis Hypomotility of gut Hyperglycaemia Hypermetabolism
Rule of 10	10% hypermetabolism 10% hyperglycaemia 10% malignant 10% extra-adrenal 10% occur in children
Four Cs	Cholelithiasis Cutaneous lesions Cerebellar haemangioblastoma Cushing's syndrome

few grams to over 1 kg. They are most often solitary, and the cut surface usually shows areas of haemorrhage and necrosis. Microscopically, the tumours are composed of large pleomorphic chromaffin cells. Electron microscopy reveals typical dense core chromaffin granules, somewhat larger than those found in normal chromaffin cells. Malignant tumours (3–14%) are difficult to diagnose because there are no specific histological appearances, and diagnosis relies therefore on the demonstration of unequivocal metastatic disease. It has been suggested that ploidy of tumour cells, as gleaned from flow cytometry studies, may predict malignant behaviour.

Table 38.6 Disorders associated with phaeochromocytomas.

Multiple endocrine neoplasia (MEN) syndromes
MEN-2A
Medullary carcinoma of thyroid
Hyperparathyroidism (hyperplasia)
Phaeochromocytoma
MEN-2B
As above +
Marfanoid phenotype
Visceral neuromas
Neurocutaneous syndromes
Neurofibromatosis
von Hippel–Lindau disease
Ataxia telangiectasia
Tuberose sclerosis
Sturge–Weber syndrome
Multiple neoplasia triad syndrome
Extra-adrenal paragangliomas
Gastric epithelioid leiomyosarcoma
Pulmonary chondromas

Thus, 30–40% of tumours demonstrating an abnormal DNA flow histogram (suggesting aneuploidy) were malignant [22] in one series; analysis of other reports does not, however, support the contention that diploidy necessarily predicts benign behaviour [23].

Molecular genetics

Germline mutations in the *ret* proto-oncogene, which codes for a receptor tyrosine kinase, cause MEN-2. Mutation in one of five cysteine codons (609, 611, 618 and 620 in exon 10, and 634 in exon 11), which codes for part of the extracellular cysteine-rich domain, are found in the majority of families with MEN-2A. In contrast, the phaeochromocytoma associated with MEN-2B is associated with a single codon mutation (918; exon 16) which lies within the substrate recognition pocket of the tyrosine kinase catalytic core [24]. Von Recklinghausen's neurofibromatosis occurs in 5% of patients, the incidence of phaeochromocytoma in these patients being about 1%. Other molecular genetic characteristics have been identified for the Von Hippel–Lindau (VHL) disease tumour suppression gene which is located on chromosome 3p24–25. The incidence of phaeochromocytoma in VHL disease is very variable ranging from 0 to 92% in affected families. Missense mutations (in particular, in codon 238) have been recognised as the major abnormality of the VHL gene in patients harbouring a phaeochromocytoma.

Neurofibromatosis (NF-1) is also associated with phaeochromocytoma. The defective gene, encoding the neurofibromin protein, possesses GTPase activity. Defective or absent neurofibromin induces constitutive activity of adenylate cyclase. Indeed, reduced expression of neurofibromin may occur in other familial phaeochromocytomas, including MEN-2A, MEN-2B and VHL. These tumours show a predominant expression (60–75%) of a shorter form of the protein, resulting from alternative splicing. This isoform lacks 63 nucleotides corresponding to exon 23a of the NF-1 gene. The shorter form of neurofibromin may be related to a more intensely proliferative state of adrenal tissue, thereby contributing to tumour development. Interestingly, this protein acts as a negative regulator of $p21^{RAS}$ under normal conditions, and it is possible that loss of reduced expression of neurofibromin may enhance $p21^{RAS}$ activity, contributing to cell proliferation [25].

Catecholamine storage in phaeochromocytoma

Tumour chromaffin granules do not differ significantly from those of the normal adrenal medulla, although in some tumours the catecholamine/ATP ratio exceeds the normal 4 : 1. The *in vitro* rate of catecholamine synthesis is, however, substantially greater than normal, and in some tumours this is associated with an increase in tyrosine hydroxylase activity which is not subject to feedback inhibition by catechols. Similarly, turnover of catecholamines is increased, and intratumour metabolism is rapid.

Clinical features (Table 38.7)

Hypertension is intermittent in 50% of patients (when it can occur on a background of normotension) and constant in the remainder [18,26,27]. In those patients with persistent hypertension, the normal circadian blood pressure variation (with nocturnal falls, caused largely by decreased sympathetic tone to resistance vessels and a fall in cardiac output) is retained. This strongly suggests that despite pathological circulating catecholamine levels, underlying sympathetic nervous regulation of the cardiovascular system is still operative. The unexpected fall in blood pressure following clonidine administration in patients with phaeochromocytoma, as well as appropriate increases in heart rate and diastolic pressure with 60° head-up tilt, further support the contention that neurally mediated increases in noradrenaline release at the synaptic sympatho-effector junction remain functionally important in patients with phaeochromocytoma. In one study of circulating catecholamine levels in phaeochromocytoma [29], it was found that despite having 10-fold higher catecholamine levels, phaeochromocytoma patients had haemodynamic characteristics similar to patients with essential hypertension, and that in individual patients the ratio of circulating noradrenaline to adrenaline showed no relation to the haemodynamic profile. In both groups, increased total peripheral resistance was primarily responsible for maintenance of hypertension [25]. Occasionally, a paradoxical rise in blood pressure occurs on introducing a β-blocker in the treatment regimen, thus alerting the physician to the possibility of underlying phaeochromocytoma (see below).

Table 38.7 Clinical features of phaeochromocytomas.

Symptoms	Signs
Headache	Hypertension (sustained and/or paroxysmal)
Hyperhidrosis	Orthostatic hypotension
Palpitations	Bradycardia, tachycardia
Anxiety	Postural tachycardia
Tremulousness	Pallor and flushing
Nausea, vomiting	Tremor
Chest and abdominal pain	Raynaud's phenomenon
Weight loss	Thyroid swelling (intermittent)
Dyspnoea	Pyrexia
Heat intolerance	Signs of complications
Constipation	Left ventricular failure
Acroparaesthesiae	Pulmonary oedema
Seizures	Circulatory shock
	Cerebrovascular accident
	Paralytic ileus

Patients with phaeochromocytoma usually present with a history of poorly controlled and occasionally accelerated hypertension; detailed history then reveals superimposed episodes of headache, palpitations, pallor and profuse sweating; other presentations are listed in Table 38.5. There is a large differential diagnosis to such symptoms, however (Table 38.8). Occasionally, patients present with acute myocardial infarction, or acute renal failure and stroke due to massive catecholamine release; presentations with pseudo-obstruction of the bowel and chronic constipation are well recognised. The 'crises' are usually of uniform composition in individual patients, although they may vary in duration and intensity. The onset is usually sudden, with severe pounding headache, palpitations and intense pallor, associated with sweating and often a feeling of impending death; the peak severity is reached within a few minutes, with a slower offset and a total duration usually less than 15 min, and shorter than 60 min in 80% of cases [29]. Crises may occur from several times a day to less frequently (e.g. weekly). Flushing is rare, but urticaria-like reactions have been reported.

Catecholamine excess may cause cardiac hypertrophy and eventual failure secondary to sustained hypertension. Myocardial infarction is frequently diagnosed in these patients due either to myocarditis or coronary spasm, both of which cause release of cardiac enzymes and produce electrocardiographic patterns strongly resembling those of myocardial

Table 38.8 Differential diagnosis: causes of pseudo-phaeochromocytoma.

Anxiety state
Hyperadrenergic essential hypertension
Menopausal vasomotor instability
Hyperventilation
Excess caffeine intake
Alcohol withdrawal syndrome
Diencephalic seizures (autonomic epilepsy)
Autonomic hyperreflexia
Thyrotoxicosis
Other causes of paroxysmal hypertension
Acute intermittent porphyria
Acute or chronic lead poisoning
Tabetic crisis
Clonidine, methyldopa withdrawal
Tetanus
Guillain–Barré syndrome
Cord section

infarction [30]. Acute pulmonary oedema may also occur, and in one case known to the author was the presenting complication. A dilated catecholamine cardiomyopathy is occasionally seen, and usually recovers following successful extirpation of the tumour. Cardiac tachyarrhythmias resistant to treatment and reversible changes of transmural myocardial infarction on electrocardiography may also suggest the presence of phaeochromocytoma.

Early diagnosis of phaeochromocytoma is of considerable importance. Patients harbouring such tumours are at risk of severe hypertensive crises, often unpredictable, and caused by massive tumour catecholamine release. The mechanism of such uncontrolled catecholamine release is uncertain, but is episodic in some individuals and continuous in others. Activity of the enzymes tyrosine hydroxylase, aromatic amino-acid decarboxylase and dopamine-β-hydroxylase is markedly enhanced in these tumours, whereas the activity of enzymes involved in catecholamine metabolism are reduced. Thus, excessive amounts of newly synthesised noradrenaline that cannot be stored in granules may escape metabolism and diffuse from the tumour into the circulation. The pressor crises have a significant morbidity and occasional mortality. Although frequently spontaneous, they may be precipitated by a number of stimuli (Table 38.9).

Postural hypotension

Orthostatic hypotension occurs in about 50% of patients with phaeochromocytoma [31]. Potential mechanisms include hypovolaemia, decreased stroke volume and impaired adaptation of peripheral resistance during tilt (implying inadequate arteriolar and venous responsiveness). It is unclear whether neuropeptides released from phaeochromocytoma (see below) may precipitate orthostatic hypotension.

Metabolic abnormalities in phaeochromocytoma

Lactic acidosis in the absence of a shock state should evoke suspicion of phaeochromocytoma. Adrenaline increases the concentrations of lactic acid by stimulation of glycogenolysis and glycolysis, and the associated increased oxygen utilisation coupled with decreased oxygen delivery leads to lactate accumulation [32]. Adrenaline secretion also antagonises the effects of insulin, leading to glucose intolerance of frank diabetes mellitus [33].

Tumour secretory products

The dominant tumour secretory products are noradrenaline, adrenaline, dopamine and their precursor DOPA. These vasoactive biogenic amines produce their effect by interacting with α_1, α_2, β_1 and β_2 or dopamine (D_1, and D_2) receptors which are widely distributed in vascular tissues. Many, but not all, biological actions of catecholamines account for the characteristic symptoms and signs of phaeochromocytoma. The manifestations in individual cases depend to some extent on the dominant type of catecholamine it produces, the site and size of the tumour, as well as the amount and pattern

Table 38.9 Factors known to precipitate catecholamine release from phaeochromocytomas.

Spontaneous secretion
Exercise
Bending over
Urination, defaecation
Pressure on the abdomen
Induction of anaesthesia
Tumour palpation
Straining, as during parturition
Drugs, injection of:
histamine
tyramine
guanethidine
glucagon
naloxone
metoclopramide
droperidol
ACTH
cytotoxic drugs
saralasin
Tricyclic antidepressants
Phenothiazines

ACTH, adrenocorticotrophic hormone.

of release. Predominantly noradrenaline-secreting tumours (e.g. extra-adrenal tumours) activate peripheral α_1- and α_2-receptors (extrasynaptic) with widespread cutaneous effects (pallor) and splanchnic vasoconstriction, territories dense in α-receptors. Associated pressor crises are accompanied by baroreflex-mediated bradycardia. Adrenaline-secreting tumours (usually, although not invariably, of intra-adrenal origin), cause both α and β stimulation; pressor crises are associated with increased pulse pressure and tachycardia [32]. Glucose intolerance is particularly associated with adrenaline-secreting tumours [33]. Dopamine and DOPA secretion may contribute to occasional cases of hypotension seen in phaeochromocytoma. Postural hypotension is more usually due to shrinkage of the intravascular volume secondary to vasoconstriction, with concomitant failure to compensate fully on orthostatic stimulation.

There is no correlation between tumour size and symptomatology. Indeed, the larger tumours are characterised by intratumour catecholamine metabolism and thus release proportionately fewer active amines. Paradoxically, small tumours (< 50 g) are capable of producing devastating pressor crises. Tumours classified in the small tumour group in one series had a mean rate of catecholamine turnover that was eight times greater than that of tumours in the large tumour group.

Dopamine-secreting tumours

Pure dopamine-secreting tumours are rare. Those reviewed by Proye *et al.* [34] were all malignant, and no patient was hypertensive. All patients had an 'inflammatory syndrome' with high erythrocyte sedimentation rate, weight loss and fever. They were being investigated for suspected hypernephromas. Mixed noradrenaline and dopamine-secreting tumours are commoner, but also tend to portend malignancy, although not invariably so.

Non-catecholamine tumour products

Catecholamines are not the sole secretory products of phaeochromocytomas. Table 38.10 details neuropeptides that have been extracted from phaeochromocytomas and found in significant circulating concentrations, particularly during crises. They have diverse biological actions capable of directly or indirectly causing many non-catecholamine-mediated effects of phaeochromocytoma. For example, calcitonin gene-related peptide (CGRP) and some opioids may cause hypotension and constipation, respectively; tachykinins may account for sweating; and neuropeptide Y will provoke pressor crises partially refractory to α-adrenoceptor blockade. Parathormone may lead to hypercalcaemia, and ACTH secretion from phaeochromocytomas is a recognised cause of ectopic Cushing's syndrome. Catecholamines are costored with chromogranin A in secretory vesicles; the cosecreted chromogranin A has a longer half-life than catecholamines (1–2 min), and its measurement has been advocated as an aid in the detection of phaeochromocytoma. Adrenomedullin was discovered in 1993 in extracts of human phaeochromocytoma, and found to elevate cAMP levels in platelets and to exert profound hypotensive effects when injected into animals [35]. Adrenomedullin shares structural homology with CGRP and amylin, and is a 52-amino-acid peptide with a single internal disulphide bond: the mRNA for adrenomedullin is found in normal adrenal medulla as well as human lung, cardiac ventricle, kidney and brain, and pituitary. Plasma levels of adrenomedullin have been reported in the 10–20 pg/ml range, and levels rise in renal failure, cardiac failure and severe hypertension. Thus, it may act as a physiological antipressor agent, and its release from phaeochromocytomas could blunt surges in blood pressure.

Table 38.10 Biologically active non-catecholamine tumour secretory products.

Substance	Biological action
Vasoactive intestinal peptide	Flushing
Substance P and tachykinins	Sweating, hypotension
Opioids	Constipation
Somatostatin	
Neuropeptide Y	Pallor, vasoconstriction
Endothelin	Vasoconstriction
Calcitonin gene-related peptide	Flushing, hypotension
Bombesin	
Gastrin	
Serotonin	
Histamine	Hypotension
Melatonin	
Adrenocorticotrophic hormone	Hypertension, Cushing's syndrome
Thyrotrophin-releasing hormone	Hypertension
Insulin	Hypoglycaemia
Calcitonin	
Cholecystokinin	
Renin	Hypertension
Angiotensin-converting enzyme	Hypertension
Vasopressin	Hypertension
Growth hormone-releasing hormone	
Parathormone	Hypercalcaemia
Chromogranin A, DBH	

Diagnosis

Patients requiring investigation

There is considerable controversy as to which hypertensive patients should be investigated biochemically for exclusion of phaeochromocytoma [36]. Young hypertensives, those with a positive family history of phaeochromocytoma or MEN-2, or those with refractory or extremely labile hypertension (especially if accompanied by phaeochromocytoma-associated symptomatology, see above) clearly require investigation. Similarly, patients with hypertension and a neurocutaneous syndrome such as neurofibromatosis, Sturge–Weber syndrome or VHL disease should be screened for catecholamine-secreting tumours. Hypertension with evidence of glucose intolerance should also prompt an investigation for a phaeochromocytoma.

Biochemical diagnosis

Use of catecholamine metabolites

The diagnosis of phaeochromocytoma has traditionally depended on the biochemical demonstration of elevated 24-hour (or overnight) urinary catecholamine metabolites, VMA and metanephrines measured by the Pisano method [37]; more recently, analysis of a 24-hour urinary free-catecholamine estimation (using HPLC fractionation into noradrenaline, adrenaline and dopamine) has become more generally available, with comparable sensitivity and specificity to urinary metanephrines (sensitivity, 90%; specificity, 90%). Since VMA measurements have only about 60% sensitivity, at the very least metanephrines should replace VMA excretion as the urinary screening test of choice. For VMA and metanephrine estimations, patients should be on vanilla and phenolic acid-free diets for 72 hours before collection to reduce the likelihood of false-positive estimations. It should be noted that methylglucamine, a component of many iodinated contrast media, destroys a reagent in the Pisano assay. Elevated homovanillic acid excretion is classically seen in cases of neuroblastoma and malignant phaeochromocytomas. The MEN syndromes deserve special mention. It has been found that either a 24-hour urinary free adrenaline level or the calculated ratio of adrenaline to noradrenaline is a relatively sensitive screening test for a lesion which invariably starts off as adrenomedullary hyperplasia with relative excess adrenaline secretion.

Plasma catecholamine estimations

Highly sensitive and specific plasma catecholamine estimations (radioenzymatic assays and HPLC–ECD) have recently become more widely available in many laboratories. Blood samples need to be taken under standardised conditions (venous cannulation 30 min before sampling supine), and heparinised blood separated by cold centrifugation and plasma stored at −80°C prior to assay. Plasma noradrenaline levels consistently exceeding 10 nmol/l (normal range 1.1–3.07 nmol/l) and adrenaline levels exceeding 1.5 nmol/l (normal range 0.05–1.07 nmol/l) give a diagnostic specificity of about 95%, and a sensitivity of 85%, particularly when other causes of plasma catecholamine elevation have been ruled out. When blood is sampled during a crisis, plasma catecholamine levels are usually diagnostic. Noise, stress, discomfort, position of body, the use of coffee, caffeine, nicotine and food may raise plasma catecholamines. Because of the potential overlap between plasma noradrenaline levels in essential hypertension and phaeochromocytoma, from a study of 19 patients with phaeochromocytoma, Brown [38] has advocated the use of the ratio of 3,4-dihydroxyphenylethylene glycol (DHPG, a noradrenaline metabolite formed in noradrenergic neurons) to noradrenaline in plasma, and found a ratio <0.5 in phaeochromocytomas and >2.0 in essential hypertension (Fig. 38.5). DHPG reflects mainly nervous release of noradrenaline, whereas noradrenaline released directly into the bloodstream (as in a phaeochromocytoma) is not converted into DHPG (Fig. 38.6). Elevated plasma adrenaline or increased urinary metanephrine excretion generally suggests a tumour of adrenal origin, whereas exclusively noradrenaline-secreting tumours suggest either a very large adrenal tumour or a paraganglioma.

Platelet catecholamine estimation

Platelets take up and store catecholamines, and the determination of platelet catecholamines may assist in phaeochromocytoma diagnosis when plasma levels are equivocal [39]. However, this diagnostic method is seldom used.

Urinary free catecholamines

This is a sensitive indicator of phaeochromocytoma [40], and may be determined on a 24-hour, a 12-hour overnight, or a timed collection during crisis. However, a correction for renal function is required. Measurement of urinary noradrenaline, adrenaline and dopamine by reverse-phase HPLC coupled with electrochemical detection has increased the sensitivity of phaeochromocytoma diagnosis to 95%, but with some loss of specificity. In general, only 50–70% of tumours produce elevated adrenaline levels (these are invariably adrenal or Zuckerkandl tumours), whereas 85% produce elevated noradrenaline levels. The measurement of urinary adrenaline levels is of greatest value in the screening of families for MEN-2 and adrenomedullary hyperplasia.

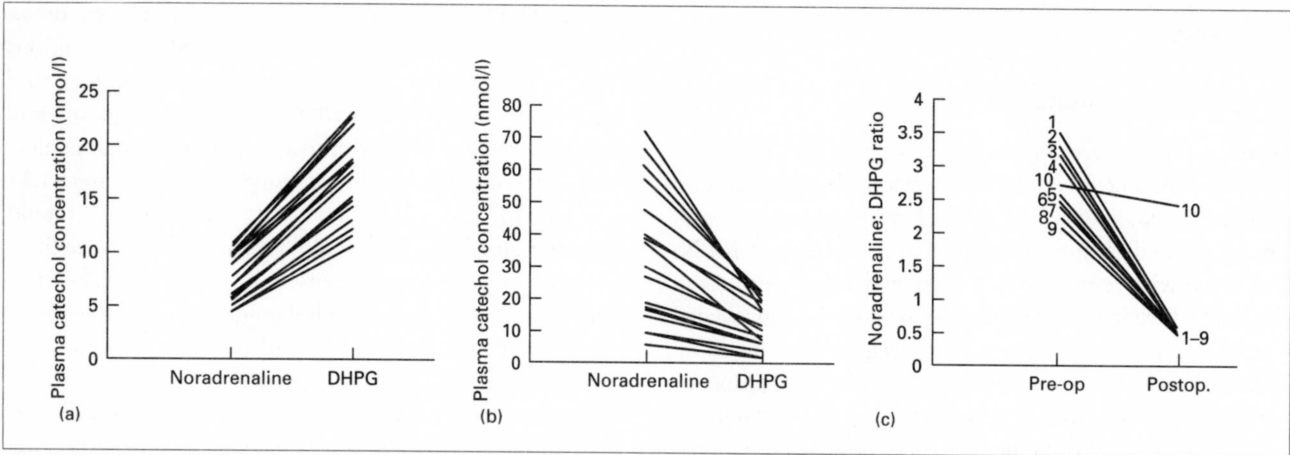

Fig. 38.5 (a) Plasma noradrenaline and dihydroxyphenylglycol (DHPG) concentration in 19 non-phaeochromocytoma patients. (From [22].) (b) Plasma noradrenaline and DHPG concentrations in 17 patients with phaeochromocytoma. (c) Reversal of noradrenaline to DHPG ratio after removal of a phaeochromocytoma in nine patients. In patient no. 10, a further tumour remained.

Diagnosis of small adrenal lesions

Suppression tests

Very small lesions pose a problem, and minor elevations of circulating adrenaline under basal conditions may be the only indicator of the presence of small intra-adrenal tumours. Catecholamine levels may be sited in an intermediate 'grey' zone, and therefore not 'diagnostic' (Fig. 38.7). A suppression test to see whether these represent physiological elevations or genuinely represent autonomous adrenaline tumour secretion is then indicated. The ganglion-blocking agent pentolinium can help distinguish between these two possibilities [41]; 2.5–5 mg pentolinium i.v. will suppress plasma catecholamines into the normal range in patients with a 'physiological' elevation of adrenaline or noradrenaline, but has no effect in cases of tumorous catecholamine elevation, since these lesions are devoid of nicotinic cholinergic neural innervation (Fig. 38.8). The centrally acting α_2-agonist clonidine has also been used to demonstrate autonomous noradrenaline production by these tumours. Oral clonidine (0.3 mg) suppresses plasma noradrenaline into the low normal range in

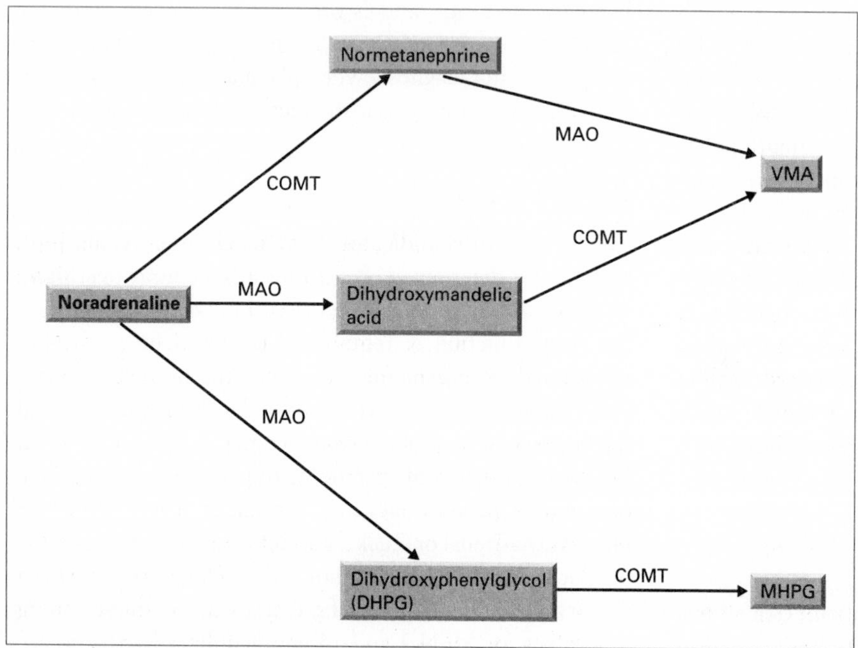

Fig. 38.6 Simplified scheme of noradrenaline metabolism. MAO, monoamine oxidase; COMT, catecholamine-*O*-methyl transferase; MHPG, methoxyphenylglycol. COMT is present in extraneuronal tissue only. MAO is present in nerve endings and in extraneuronal tissue.

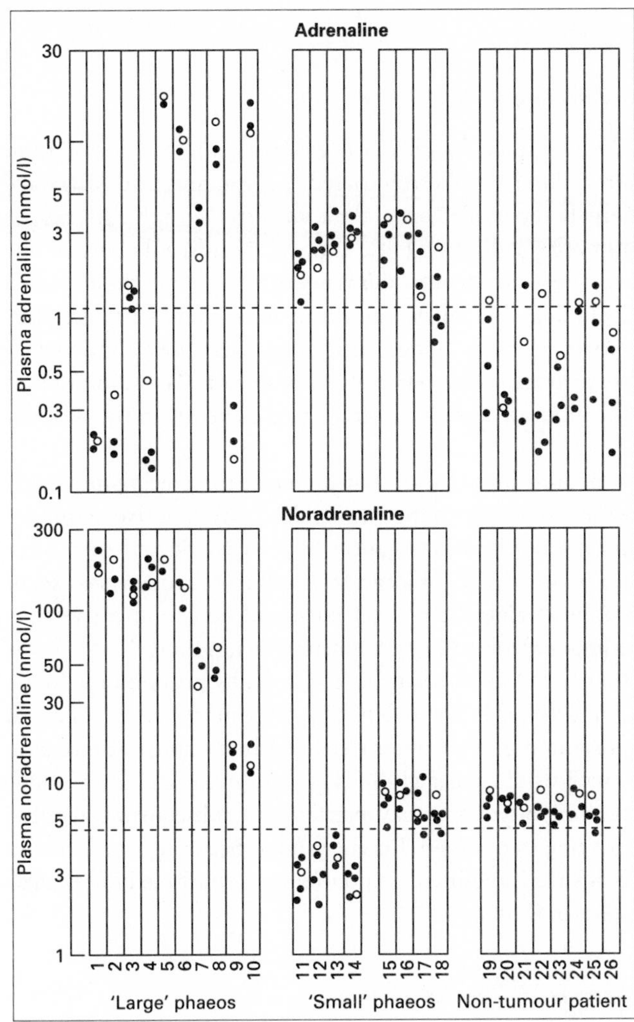

Fig. 38.7 Distribution of noradrenaline and adrenaline levels in patients with large and small phaeochromocytomas and in non-tumour patients. Small adrenal tumours almost invariably have elevated plasma and adrenaline levels, but the values may overlap with those found in non-tumour patients.

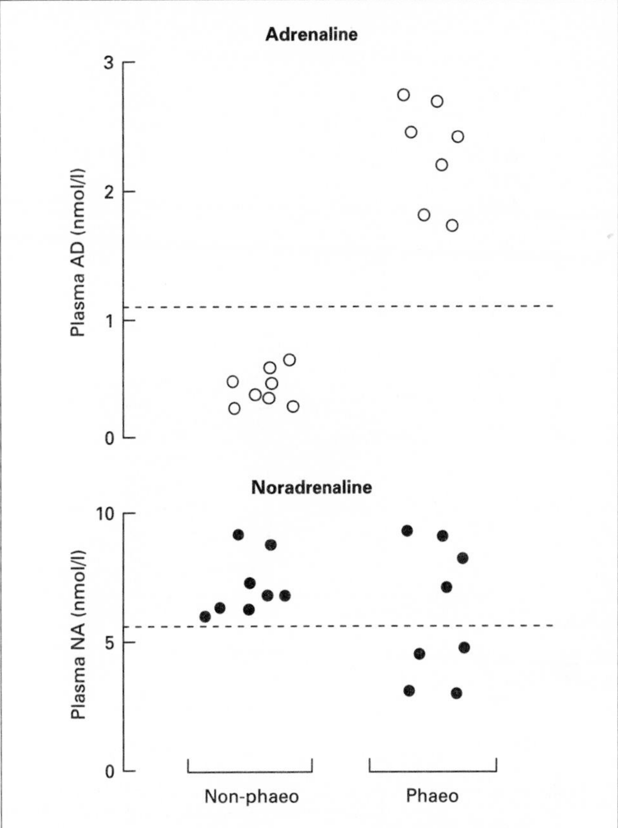

Fig. 38.8 Response of noradrenaline and adrenaline to iv pentolinium (2.5 mg) in non-phaeochromocytoma patients and those with small phaeochromocytomas. The 10-min adrenaline value in non-phaeochromocytoma patients is fully suppressed into the normal range, whereas those of phaeochromocytoma patients remain outside the normal range.

normal and essential hypertensive individuals, but not in patients with tumorous noradrenaline secretion [42] (Fig. 38.9).

By contrast, plasma catecholamines are invariably raised in hypertensive patients harbouring a phaeochromocytoma. This is because in the presence of persistently raised catecholamines, adrenergic receptors down-regulate (desensitisation); in order to produce hypertension under these circumstances, plasma catecholamines have to be elevated severalfold.

Episodic catecholamine secretors

Episodic catecholamines secretors with a background of normotension pose a difficult problem. If sampling is carried out during normotension, plasma catecholamines may be normal; although 24-hour urinary catecholamine metabolites or timed urinary samples may be elevated under these instances, definitive biochemical of catecholamine secretion in such cases may require sampling during a symptomatic crisis. Where symptomatology strongly suggests the presence of an underlying phaeochromocytoma, but the biochemistry is normal, a provocative test with pharmacological agents such as intravenous tyramine (1 mg), histamine (10 μg), glucagon (1 mg) or naloxone (10 mg) [43] may be justified, although this should only be carried out under effective α- and β-blockade with plasma catecholamine measurement rather than blood pressure as the response parameter. The glucagon test using blood pressure and plasma catecholamine measurement is generally considered to be the safest and most accurate provocation test of all. A threefold increase in plasma noradrenaline concentration over the basal level is considered diagnostic, provided blood is sampled at the time of blood pressure rise.

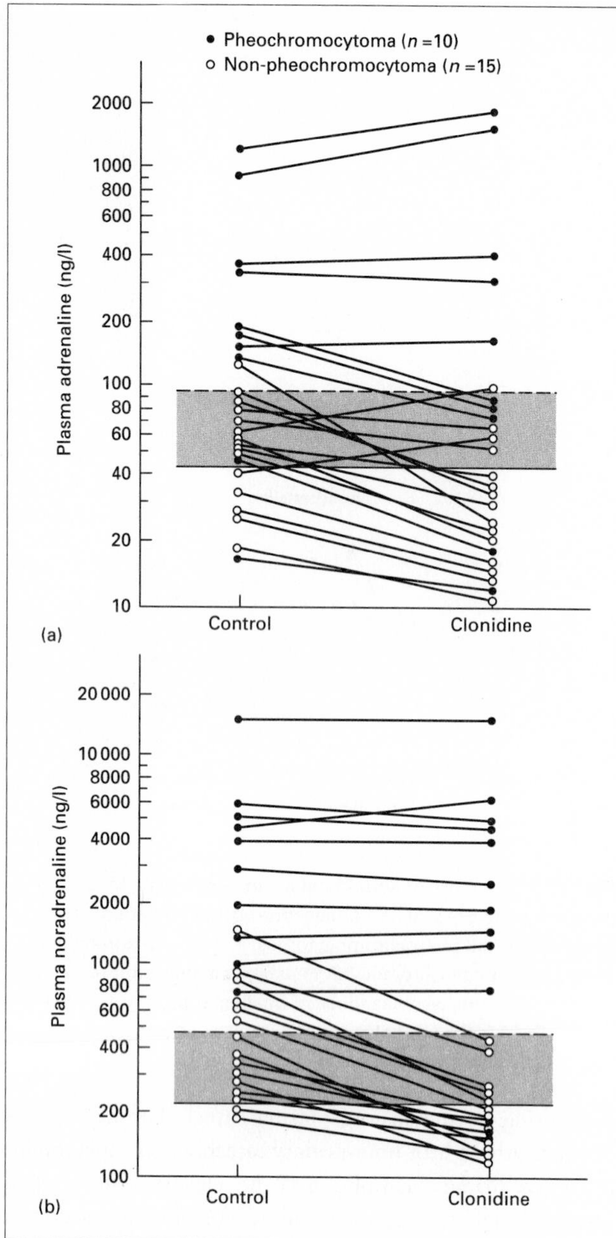

Fig. 38.9 Response of plasma noradrenaline (a) and adrenaline (b) to 0.3 mg oral clonidine in 10 patients with phaeochromocytoma and 15 non-phaeochromocytoma patients. Neither adrenaline nor noradrenaline levels were suppressed by clonidine in the patients with phaeochromocytoma.

Echocardiography

The performance of an echocardiogram is the final step in the diagnostic evaluation and will yield important information as to the presence of underlying catecholamine-induced dilated cardiomyopathy.

Localisation

CT scanning

On obtaining biochemical evidence, tumour localisation procedures should be initiated. CT scanning and MRI have largely superseded urographic and arteriographic studies for tumour localisation [44]. Initially, the adrenal glands alone may be scanned, but if this is negative the rest of the abdomen including the pelvis, chest and neck should be included. However, most modern helical scanners may allow for all these areas in one relatively brief session. The resolution of the most advanced CT scanners is currently in the order of 5 mm.

Because intravenous contrast media can precipitate pressor crises, the examination (as indeed any invasive radiographic procedure) has generally been conducted only after adequate α- and β-blockade. A suitable regimen consists of administering the non-selective and non-competitive $\alpha_{1/2}$-adrenoceptor antagonist phenoxybenzamine, 10–20 mg 6-hourly followed, after the first dose, by propranolol 40 mg 8-hourly [45]. The α-blocking drug must be given first to prevent potential unopposed α-adrenoceptor stimulation which would rise if a β-blocker were given first. Intravenous phenoxybenzamine may interfere with subsequent and mIBG imaging (see below). Recently, it has been suggested that no blockade is required if a non-ionic contrast medium such as iohexol is used.

Magnetic resonance imaging

MRI allows some degree of tissue characterisation. Most phaeochromocytomas give high T2-weighted signal intensity [46,47]. The technique is particularly useful in the imaging of tumours in close proximity to major vessels—including intracardiac lesions—because of the signal void from flowing blood. CT and MRI are about equally sensitive (98–99%).

Venous catheterisation

This is particularly valuable in patients with strong clinical and biochemical evidence of a phaeochromocytoma, but negative CT examination [48,49]. Blood is sampled from the internal jugular veins, the subclavians, brachiocephalic, thymic, superior intercostals, azygous, right atrium, coronary sinus, inferior vena cava, hepatic renal, adrenal, renal, gonadal and internal and external iliac veins. The presence of a noradrenaline 'hotspot' but normal adrenaline in such instances strongly suggests an extra-adrenal tumour. The technique is also of value in the investigation of possible bilateral or multiple lesions. Because of the frequently multicentric origin of tumours, several sites may need to be sampled (see Table 38.4). Provided all likely sites have been sampled (including the coronary sinus), venous sampling is a good way of refuting the diagnosis, particularly when levels of noradrenaline are elevated during sampling.

The interpretation of catheter data is not straightforward, especially when dealing with adrenal venous samples. As such, there are no 'diagnostic levels' of catecholamines to indicate the presence of a phaeochromocytoma. Levels generated are critically dependent on the adrenal blood flow rate at the time of sampling, the position of the catheter tip, and direct mechanical stimulation of release by the catheter. The degree of stress experienced by the patient also has an important bearing on interpretation. The absolute levels of noradrenaline and adrenaline are not, therefore, as helpful as the ratio between the two. Adrenaline is the dominant catecholamine secreted from the adrenal medulla both basally and following stress. Under basal sampling conditions, the adrenaline/noradrenaline ratio is between 4 and 10:1. A reversal of this ratio (i.e. more noradrenaline than adrenaline released) is highly significant and indicates the presence of an adrenal tumour. It is useful to measure the cortisol level in adrenal venous effluent to confirm the validity of the sampling site.

Radionuclide scanning

More recently, the radionuclide meta-iodo (^{123}I or ^{131}I) benzylguanidine (mIBG) [50,51], a guanethidine analogue (Fig. 38.10) taken up by chromaffin cells and incorporated into vesicles, has been used to assist in tumour localisation, and is of special value in the localisation of extra-adrenal paragangliomas and metastases, the demonstration of bilateral lesions, and multifocal disease (Fig. 38.11). Normal adrenomedullary tissue can also be visualised in 80–90% of cases using ^{123}I-mIBG. About 22% of tumours are not demonstrable (false negative) by this technique, but false positives are rare (1–3%). Specificity is 100% in malignant lesions and in familial tumours. Since mIBG is actively concentrated in sympathomedullary tissue through the catecholamine pump, the administration of drugs that block the reuptake mechanism may result in a false-negative test. The tricyclic antidepressants, guanethidine and labetalol may interfere with the test. However, prazosin, propranolol, oral phenoxybenzamine and calcium antagonists do not interfere with mIBG uptake.

Intraoperative localisation with ^{123}I-mIBG

Where there are discrepancies between CT scanning of the abdomen and radionuclide imaging (e.g. mIBG shows uptake, but there is no corresponding mass on CT scanning), a preoperative 4-mCi dose of mIBG may be administered and direct measurement of tissue activity carried out intra-operatively, allowing surgical removal of labelled tumour tissue. A flow chart giving a strategy for the diagnosis, localisation and treatment of suspected phaeochromocytoma is given in Fig. 38.12.

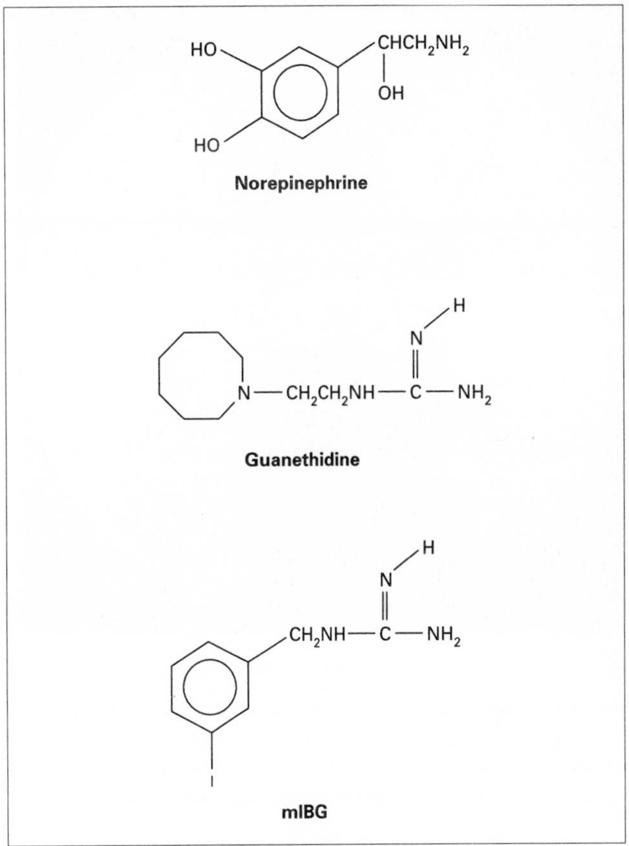

HO, HO, $CHCH_2NH_2$, OH

Norepinephrine

H, N, N — CH_2CH_2NH — C — NH_2

Guanethidine

H, N, CH_2NH — C — NH_2, I

mIBG

Fig. 38.10 Structural similarities between noradrenaline, guanethidine and meta-iodobenzylguanidine (mIBG).

Other localising modalities

Somatostatin-receptor imaging with ^{123}I-labelled Tyr^{3}-octreotide [52] and positron-emission tomography with hydroxyephedrine [53] may be positive where ^{123}I-mIBG has proven negative.

Treatment

Most phaeochromocytomas are benign; complete excision leads to normotension in 75% of cases.

Medical therapy of phaeochromocytoma

Once the diagnosis is confirmed, or if there is strong clinical suspicion, but biochemical confirmation is not yet available,

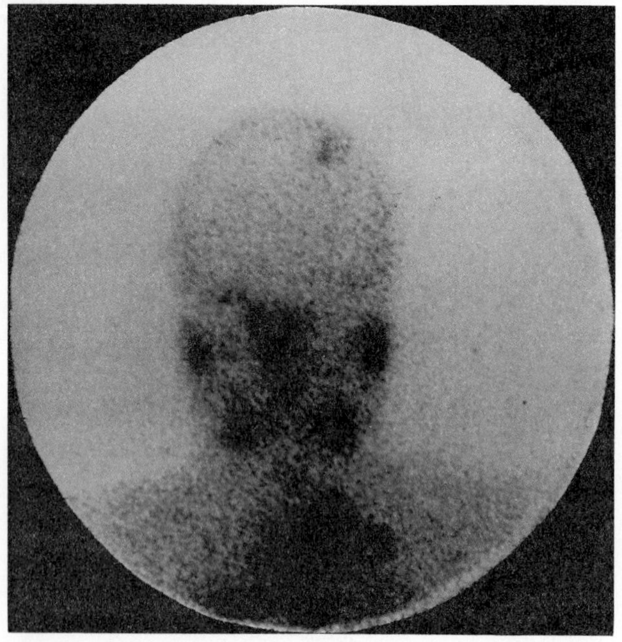
(a)

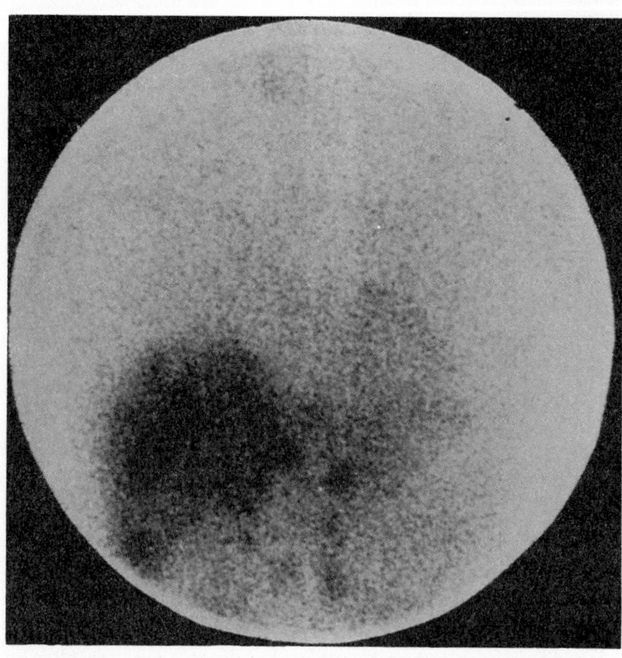
(b)

Fig. 38.11 Meta-iodobenzylguanidine (mIBG) scans of upper mediastinum and skull (a) and liver (b) of patients with disseminated paragangliomas. The symmetrical uptake of radionuclide in the skull represents (normal) uptake into the salivary glands. There is a small skull deposit, as well as multiple primary intrathoracic lesions. The liver (b) is full of tumour deposits.

the patient should be commenced on the mixed non-competitive α_1/α_2 antagonsit phenoxybenzamine. The starting dose is 5–10 mg b.d. orally, and the does titrated upwards until satisfactory blood pressure control is achieved. Some patients may require doses as high as 240 mg t.d.s. of phenoxybenzamine. Twenty-four hours after starting the phenoxybenzamine, propranolol 40 mg t.d.s. should be started. It is important to give these drugs in the above order to avoid precipitating an exacerbation of blood pressure were the β-blocker used first (leading to unopposed α-adrenoceptor stimulation). The patient should be warned of postural hypotension, nasal stuffiness and drowsiness. It is not unusual for the haematocrit to fall on treatment (expansion of intravascular volume, and partially dilutional), and indeed a patient may need a preoperative blood transfusion on occasion.

Competitive α-antagonists (e.g. doxazosin, prazosin)

It is not the author's practice to use competitive antagonists in the medical management of phaeochromocytoma, although there have been several reports of their efficacy. Doxazosin, terazosin and prazosin are specific α_1-antagonists, and therefore may cause first dose postural hypotension. They suffer from the disadvantage that they are selective for α_1-receptors, are competitive (and may therefore be displaced from the α-adrenoceptors surges of circulating catecholamines) and do not block post-synaptic α_2-adrenoceptors, which are also the target of circulating catecholamines.

Labetalol

This is a theoretically attractive drug for the management of hypertension in phaeochromnocytoma, being an α- and β-adrenoceptor-blocking drug. However, it has a 1 : 4–6 ratio of α- to β-adrenoceptor antagonist activity, and this will lead to inadequate α-blockade at a dose when significant cardiac slowing may occur. It also suffers from the disadvantage of being a competitive antagonist, as well as interfering with the HPLC-ECD estimation of adrenaline both in plasma and urine.

Metyrosine (α-methyl para tyrosine)

This drug competitively inhibits the enzyme tyrosine hydroxylase, the rate-limiting step in catecholamine biosynthesis. The starting dosage is 250 mg 6-hourly, and the dose can be titrated upwards to a maximum dose of 4 g daily. It may causes sedation and more rarely Parkinsonian features (it crosses the blood–brain barrier).

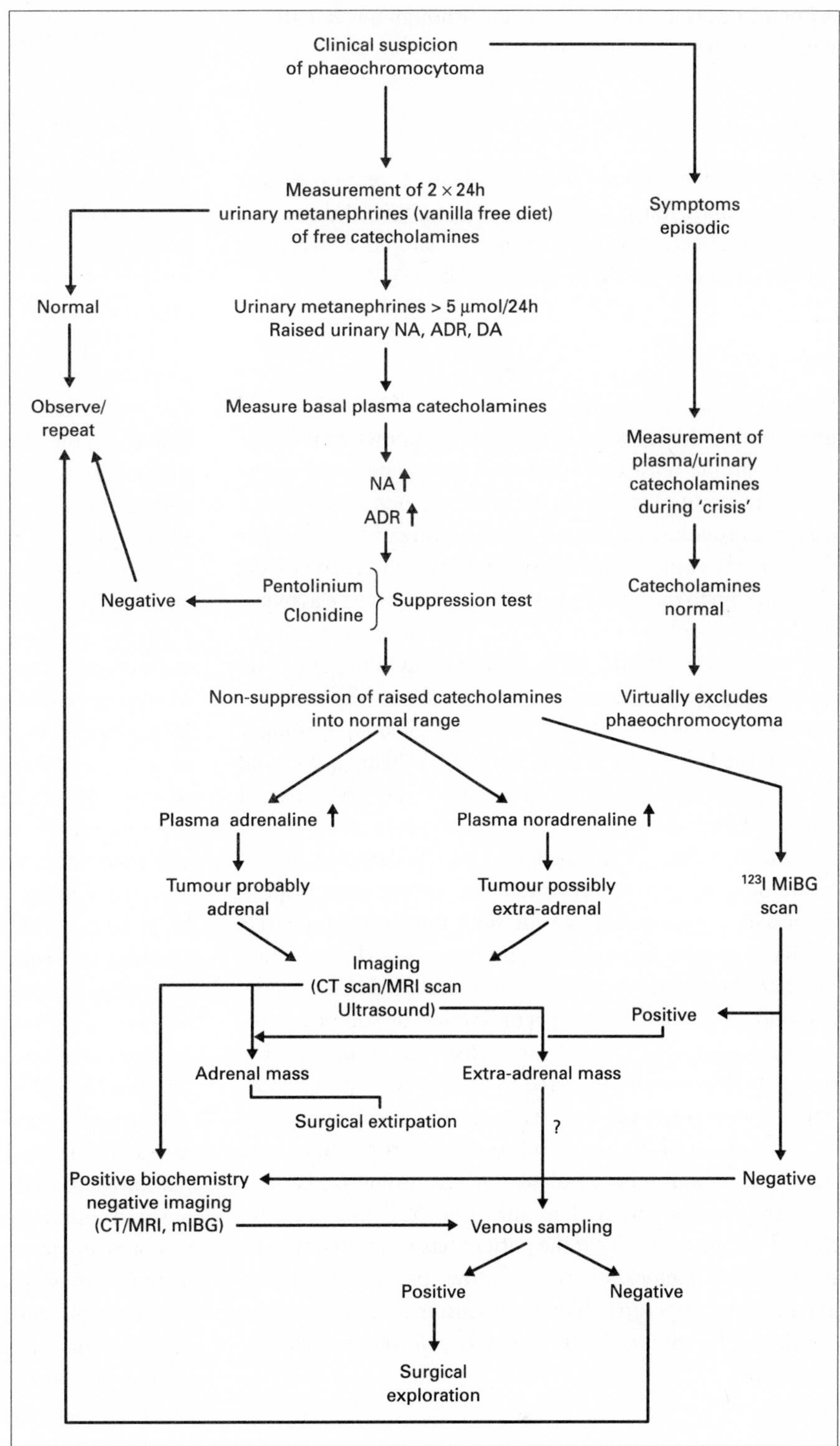

Fig. 38.12 A suggested strategy for the diagnosis and treatment of phaeochromocytoma. NA, noradrenaline; ADR, adrenaline; DA, dopamine.

Calcium antagonists

Nifedipine (and other dihydropyridine calcium channel blockers) has been used effectively to control infrequent spikes in blood pressure in patients with phaeochromocytoma. It is rapidly absorbed in the stomach, and is a potent vasodilator, as well as blocking calcium entry into the cell. Tumour cell calcium blockade may reduce catecholamine secretion. Experience of use of calcium antagonists is nowhere as extensive as with phenoxybenzamine, but this group of drugs appears promising, although not in patients with very severe hypertension.

Premedication

Droperidol (inhibition of catecholamine reuptake) and phenothiazines, morphine (release of histamine) and atropine (vagolytic effect, causing tachycardia) should be avoided; benzodiazepines are the drugs of choice.

Intraoperative

Surgery should be elective wherever possible, and should not use anaesthetic agents or manoeuvres known to provoke catecholamine release [54]. Vecuronium appears to be the muscle relaxant of choice, as it has no autonomic effects and does not provoke catecholamine release directly or indirectly through histamine release. Hypoxia, which sensitizes the myocardium to the effects of catecholamines, is to be avoided. Isoflurane or enflurane are the inhalational agents of choice as they are associated with a smaller arrhythmogenic risk. Continuous intraoperative blood pressure and electrocardiogram monitoring is mandatory. In general, phenoxybenzamine is given for 1–2 weeks in oral doses of 10–20 mg q.d.s., and 40 mg propranolol t.d.s. is given after the first dose of phenoxybenzamine. Intravenous phenoxybenzamine is then infused at a dose of 0.5 mg/kg iv in 5% dextrose over 2 hours on 2 successive days and 1 day before surgery [45]. Even with complete α-blockade with this non-competitive inhibitor, pressor crises may still be precipitated by induction of anaesthesia and tumour manipulation. These usually respond to bolus doses of phentolamine or sodium nitroprusside infusions. The recommended dose of the latter is 0.5–10 μg/kg/min administered by an intravenous infusion. Phenoxybenzamine has the advantage that it is an antagonist at both α_1, and α_2 sites. Intravenous propranolol and lignocaine should be available in the event of cardiac arrhythmias. Noradrenaline infusion (for hypotension) should not be necessary if the patient has been prepared by preoperative α-blockade, which allows plasma volume re-expansion. Preoperative blood transfusions are occasionally required if haematocrit falls excessively during preparatory treatment.

General principles of phaeochromocytoma surgery

Certain rules apply to lesions irrespective of the site. There should be wide exposure of tumours, meticulous attention to haemostasis, early isolation of vascular supply, minimal tumour manipulation, delivery of tumour with capsule intact, and exploration of all accessible sites of second primary or metastatic lesions.

Abdominal tumours

Eighty to ninety per cent of lesions are intra-abdominal and intra-adrenal, and a posterior approach is not recommended, since exposure is suboptimal. A transabdominal approach allows the inspection of a wide area of the retroperitoneum, allowing removal of any suspicious lesions and early control of adrenal veins. A bilateral subcostal (chevron) incision provides better superior and lateral access to the adrenal gland and is preferable for orthotopic adrenal tumours. Large tumours, particularly on the right may prompt a thoraco-abdominal incision. Medial rotation of the right lobe of the liver after dividing the falciform and right triangular ligaments may preclude the use of a thoraco-abdominal incision in some cases. The shortness of the right adrenal vein, and its retrocaval anatomy, may necessitate mobilisation of the superior and inferior vascular pedicles of the right adrenal gland before the adrenal vein can be secured. The entire adrenal and surrounding areolar tissue should be removed *en bloc*, and a thorough abdominal exploration with examination of the contralateral gland and palpation of the paraaortic sympathetic chains into the pelvis should be performed to check for previously unidentified tumours or metastatic disease. Tumour extension into the renal vein or inferior vena cava may require venotomy.

An extraperitoneal approach has been advocated by some, although there are inadequate data to assess the risk of recurrence using this approach. A posterior approach may be indicated for small tumours (< 50 mm), although less vascular control is possible and there is poorer exposure. However, postoperative recovery is more rapid. The newer techniques of laparoscopic adrenalectomy should only be performed by surgeons with considerable experience, small tumours being the most appropriate for laparoscopic removal.

Bilateral lesions require total adrenalectomy. A difficulty arises in cases of MEN-2, when one adrenal is clearly pathological and the other looks normal. The latter may harbour adrenomedullary hyperplastic tissue, and since tumours in this syndrome may be bilateral (even though metachronous), given the risks of a second operation and the effective replacement regimens for adrenocortical insufficiency, total adrenalectomy might seem appropriate. However, it should be stated that the latency to tumour development in a macroscopically normal adrenal gland in MEN-2 may be considerable, and during this interval patients are at minimal cardiovascular and oncological risk. On this basis, if unilateral adrenalectomy is performed, patients will require regular surveillance to monitor any clinical, radiological or biochemical changes that would prompt intervention.

Thoracic tumours

Most lesions are sited in the posterior mediastinum, arising from the sympathetic ganglia. These are approached by a posterior thoracotomy. Pericardial and cardiac lesions pose a great challenge, and cardiac bypass surgery may be required before evaluating operability. Bleeding from the arterial tumour site may be life-threatening.

Pelvic lesions

Bladder lesions may be exophytic and protrude into the bladder lumen, or infiltrate the bladder wall. Hypertensive crises may result from bladder distension; partial cystectomy with reimplantation of the ureter may be necessary.

Phaeochromocytoma during pregnancy

If the diagnosis is made in early pregnancy, termination is recommended. Should the condition be discovered late in the pregnancy, α-blockade with phenoxybenzamine is recommended, and elective caesarean section should be performed via a vertical lower abdominal incision. This may then be extended, and the abdomen explored at the time of delivery.

Post-operative management

Particular attention needs to be paid to volume status following resection. Hypovolaemia may ensue, particularly in the presence of α-blockade and blood loss. Central venous pressure measurement will assist in fluid repletion therapy. Preoperative blood transfusions, given if the haematocrit has fallen significantly following α-blockade, significantly lessens the severity of hypovolaemia. Slow emergence from anaesthesia and persistent lethargy and somnolence after surgery should arouse suspicion of underlying hypoglycaemia. This has been ascribed to rebound hyperinsulinism that occurs when the inhibitory effect of noradrenaline on insulin secretion is suddenly withdrawn. Preoperative depletion of glycogen stores from previous stimulation of glycogenolysis and lipolysis by catecholamines may also contribute to the problem. Further, residual β-adrenoceptor antagonism may mask some of the noradrenergic responses to neuroglycopenia, and impair recovery from hypoglycaemia.

Complete normalisation of plasma and urinary free catecholamines may take several days after the operation. This presumably reflects the uptake of and storage of catecholamines of phaeochromocytomal origin in sympathetic neurons. Residual hypertension is present in up to 33% of patients, but this is not paroxysmal and is usually 'essential'. Other causes for residual hypertension are incomplete extirpation of tumour and inadvertent ligation of a renal artery.

Treatment of inoperable or metastatic lesions

The occurrence of tumour deposits in sites normally devoid of chromaffin tissue is diagnostic of metastatic disease. This may occur from apparently benign primary lesions. Seeding during the resection of the primary tumour may occur. The overall mortality rate at 5 years is 40–50%, but a significant proportion of patients with overt metastatic disease survive for many years with good quality of life.

Treatment of malignant phaeochromocytoma/paraganglioma

Disseminated malignancy frequently occurs several years after benign tumour resection, and thus there is a need for long-term follow up of these lesions. Paragangliomas and lesions presenting in younger patients are particularly prone to increased risk of malignancy.

Over the past 15 years, there has been some progress made in the management of metastatic lesions that were formerly treatable only symptomatically, using long-term α- and β-blockade or the tyrosine hydroxylase inhibitor α-methylparatyrosine. While external-beam irradiation continues to have a role in relief of pain from osseous metastases—though not controlling tumour growth—the results of single- or multiple-agent chemotherapy have in general been disappointing, with only occasional reports of partial remissions being induced by cyclophosphamide, vincristine and dacarbazine [55]. Clinical experience with these chemotherapeutic agents is limited; thus, in one series of 14 patients, this triple regimen produced a complete or partial response rate of 54% with a mean duration of 21 months [55]. When patients are symptomatic despite full α- and β-blockade, the production of catecholamines may be reduced by α-methyl-*p*-tyrosine. This drug can reduce circulating catecholamines by up to 80% and alleviate some of the clinical manifestations of the disease. The initial daily dose is 500–1000 mg in divided doses, with gradual incremental rises of 250–500 mg to a total dose of 4 g daily. However, control of blood pressure may remain incomplete and serious side-effects, including extrapyramidal signs, diarrhoea, anxiety and crystalluria, have been reported.

^{131}I-mIBG therapy

Labelled mIBG has been used in the treatment of malignant lesions [56]. The current model of mIBG action is one of so-called type 1 specific, high-affinity, energy and sodium-dependent uptake into the intravesicular compartment. In all tissues, there is some non-specific uptake which is diffusional and non-energy dependent, contributing to the general background activity, but tissue retention is transient

Table 38.11 Drugs which may potentially reduce meta-iodobenzylguanidine uptake.

Drugs	Mechanism
Tricyclics	$Uptake_1$ inhibition
Phenylephrine	
Phenylpropanolamine	Depletion of storage vesicles
Pseudo-ephedrine	
Ephedrine	
Cocaine	$Uptake_1$ inhibition
Labetalol	$Uptake_1$ inhibition
Reserpine	Depletion of storage vesicle content

Table 38.12 Commonly used drugs with no effect on meta-iodobenzylguanidine uptake.

Antihypertensive drugs
α-Adrenergic blockers (clonidine, oral phenoxybenzamine, phentolamine, prazocin)
α-Methyldopa
ACE inhibitors
β-Adrenergic blockers (except labetalol)
Digitalis glycosides
Diuretics
Analgesics
Morphine and other opioids
Aspirin, paracetamol
Hypnotics and minor tranquillisers
α-Methyl paratyrosine

ACE, angiotensin-converting enzyme.

Table 38.13 Selection criteria for ^{131}I meta-iodobenzylguanine (mIBG) therapy. Adapted from [59].

	Phaeochromocytoma	Neuroblastoma
Histological diagnosis	Yes	Yes
Tumour location	Metastatic Primary but locally invasive or otherwise unresectable	Recurrent or or residual despite standard therapy
Anticipated survival	12 months	3 months
mIBG uptake	All known tumour sites	All known tumour sites
Dosimetric studies	Whole body Tumour (where possible)	Whole body Tumour (where possible)
Informed consent	Yes	Parent or guardian if < 18 years of age

and diminishes over time more rapidly than in tissues with specific uptake and storage. Drugs which may potentially interfere with mIBG uptake are shown in Tables 38.11 and 38.12. Within 24 hours, 55% of the injected radioactivity is excreted in the urine, rising to 90% by 4 days, except in renal failure where clearance is markedly reduced. Most radioactivity is excreted as unchanged mIBG, with 2–16% in the form of free iodine, metaiodobenzoic acid and 4-hydroxy-3-iodobenzylguanidine. A small fraction of activity (< 5%) appears in the faeces. The prominent hepatic uptake appears to be due to metabolism and not to $uptake_1$.

The intense and prolonged uptake and retention of tracer doses of mIBG by many malignant and otherwise irresectable tumours has provided the rationale for the therapeutic use of large doses of ^{131}I-mIBG, an approach well established in the treatment of thyroid cancer. The criteria for patient selection for ^{131}I-mIBG treatment of phaeochromocytoma and neuroblastoma are shown in Table 38.13. After whole-body, blood and tumour radiation dosimetric determinations performed over 5–7 days using a tracer dose of ^{131}I-mIBG, a therapeutic dose of high specific activity (33–50 Ci/mg) ^{131}I-mIBG is infused over 90 min; blood pressure and electrocardiogram are monitored continuously for the duration of the infusion, and thereafter at regular intervals for 24 hours. The patient should stay in a restricted specially prepared room until the body burden of ^{131}I is below 30 mCi, at which time the distribution of the therapy dose is confirmed by scintigraphy, and the patient discharged for a follow-up protocol which examines bone marrow, liver kidney, thyroid, adrenocortical and autonomic neuronal function and tumour response. Thyroid blockade with potassium perchlorate is continued for at least 4 weeks. Therapy doses of 200–300 mCi are administered to adults and doses calculated to deliver 100–200 cGy whole-body radiation to children. Calculated tumour doses have ranged from 2550 to 34 000 cGy per dose, although tumour uptake and retention of mIBG should be sufficient to deliver an absorbed tumour radiation dose of at least 5.4 Gy per GBq. Extensive bone-marrow infiltration is a contraindication to treatment.

Minimal patient preparation is required before therapy, other than withdrawal of drugs known to inhibit uptake of the radionuclide. The patient should be in a stable clinical state so as to avoid major medical, surgical or nursing intervention while the patient is radioactive.

Because mIBG may induce catecholamine release from the tumour, slow intravenous infusion is recommended (over at least 30 min) with continuous blood pressure and pulse monitoring. Exacerbation of hypertension is controlled by reducing the infusion rate, and intravenous phentolamine available for emergency intravenous use. Nausea may occur for up to 48 hours after mIBG administration, but responds to ondansetron, which may be given prophylactically and has advantages over metoclopramide and domperidone in not precipitating pressor crises in phaeochromocytoma.

Post-therapy γ-camera imaging is used to evaluate tumour extent, which may not be fully apparent from mIBG tracer studies. Therapy doses have been repeated at variable intervals to cumulative doses of 900–2300 mCi, usually using 3–6 month dosage schedules, based on the experience for papillary carcinoma. More recently, it has been recognised that shorter dosing intervals may be more appropriate for metabolically active tumours. Ideally, 6-weekly treatment intervals are advisable, but this may need to be longer if bone marrow recovery is delayed [57,58].

Little pharmacological toxicity has been noted, though mild radiation sickness results in anorexia, nausea and vomiting in some patients. Myelosuppression is more likely to occur in children receiving treatment for neuroblastoma, and is occasionally permanent in this group although seldom in adults receiving treatment. Prior bone-marrow transplantation may sensitise patients to this type of response. Hypothyroidism may also occur.

Dosimetry

The absorbed radiation dose delivered to the tumour is influenced by uptake and retention of radiopharmaceutical by tumour, renal clearance and the administered activity. The accuracy of the radiation dose is limited by the unreliability of tumour volume measurements. It has been estimated that absorbed radiation doses in the order of 200 cGy may be necessary to achieve objective responses in malignant phaeochromocytoma. Despite repeated cycles of ^{131}I-mIBG, the cumulative absorbed dose to tumour is often disappointingly low. Methods of improving the efficacy of treatment by pharmacological intervention or substitution of alternative radiolabels require further investigation. mIBG labelled with the Auger cascade emitter ^{125}I has been used for neuroblastoma but the range of electrons within the cell may be too short to achieve DNA damage. ^{211}Astatine, which emits α-particles with higher linear energy transfer, may have an advantage in a hypoxic environment.

Complete response after therapy is the exception, and more commonly partial remissions occur, which may last for many years. The relatively high-energy β-particles emitted by ^{131}I-mIBG can penetrate several millimeters and are thus not suited to micrometastases, which in neuroblastoma are frequently present in the bone marrow and which may be responsible for relapses. The lower-energy non-penetrating Auger electrons of ^{125}I may be better suited to these lesions.

Response assessment

The primary aim of treatment is tumour eradication, although in practice, arrest of tumour growth may be a more realistic aim. mIBG uptake may decrease following treatment, indicating a reduction of functioning tumour mass. This may not necessarily correlate with anatomical site, and it is essential that apparent tumour shrinkage, shown by γ-camera imaging, is confirmed by CT or ultrasound scanning. Because reduction in tumour volume occurs slowly over many months, CT is most useful after two or three treatments.

The second aim of treatment is symptomatic palliation, achieved by reducing the metabolic function and catecholamine output of the tumour. This objective is particularly relevant for patients whose survival is likely to be prolonged, but who are distressed by the effects of raised catecholamines or bone pain.

Results

Several protocols have been used for treatment worldwide making comparison of treatment protocols particularly difficult. Overall, > 50% patients improved on treatment, and a number of complete responses have been noted. Tumour response is associated with a fall in plasma catecholamines and easier control of blood pressure. Although metastatic bone pain responds well to mIBG therapy, control of soft tissue disease is more effective than osseous metastases. Recalcification of lytic bone lesions can occur after therapy.

Other toxicity associated with ^{131}I-mIBG therapy

23% patients develop temporary leucopenia or thrombocytopenia, and the risk of myelosuppression is cumulative. As a precautionary measure, some departments now routinely harvest and store bone marrow from all new patients for marrow rescue if necessary. Mild tenderness over liver metastases, transient alopecia overlying a skull metastasis, and, after multiple treatments, hypothyroidism, has occurred in some patients. No change in the function of salivary glands, adrenals, liver, kidney, heart, or bladder, and no autonomic dysfunction has been observed hitherto, but long-term vigilance for these potential complications is warranted.

Follow-up

It is recommended that patients who have had phaeochromocytomas successfully resected should have periodic blood-pressure measurements, and when appropriate, urinary catecholamine estimations, at yearly intervals. This is because risk of recurrence (about 10%) or malignant behaviour may be difficult to predict. Follow-up is particularly indicated in patients with paraganglioma, MEN-2, and neurocutaneous syndromes where tumours may be metachronous and multicentric. Where there is suspicion of recurrence, mIBG scanning may be a useful early investigation to locate the lesion.

Screening of family members at risk

Familial phaeochromocytoma is rare and may occur as part of an autosomal dominant condition. It is important to the first-degree relatives of patients who give a positive family history of phaeochromocytoma in whom blood-pressure measurement and urinary catecholamine estimation should be performed. In MEN-2 patients and relatives, the use of urinary adrenaline estimation appears to be the best indicator as to the presence of adrenomedullary hyperplasia, the precursor to phaeochromocytoma in these patients. The use of provocative testing with glucagon in asymptomatic normotensive at-risk subjects has also been advocated. More recently, genetic testing of family members has become increasingly available.

Neuroblastoma

This is a tumour of infancy and childhood which usually arises from the adrenal medulla but occasionally from the sympathetic chain; about 25% arise within the thorax. The tumour can occur prenatally, but usually presents during the first 2 years of life, commonly in males. The adrenal variety may be unilateral or bilateral, and unicentric or multicentric. The tumour is highly vascular, and red in colour with necrotic areas. Histologically, tissues vary between being poorly differentiated and highly malignant to a relatively benign and mature ganglioneuroma. Both histologies may occur within the same tumour. Characteristically, cells are arranged in a pseudo-rosette formation. The malignant form spreads by bloodstream to liver, bone, brain and skull, particularly the orbits; direct spread to the kidney occurs. Often the condition presents with an abdominal mass, or perhaps as the result of a secondary deposit.

Diagnosis

Radiologically, the presence of scattered calcification within the tumour may suggest the diagnosis. When intra-abdominal, intravenous urography usually shows distortion of the renal calyces with the affected kidney pushed down. CT is now the imaging modality of choice, and is particularly useful for establishing the extent and size of the lesion. The tumour can elaborate and secrete significant quantities of catecholamines. A proportion of cases present with features of catecholamine excess with hypertension, sweating attacks, pallor and diarrhoea. Traditionally, the diagnosis is established by demonstrating pathological levels of homovanillic acid in the urine (raised in 75–80% of cases), but now more often relies on elevated urinary catecholamines.

Treatment

This depends on staging. Localised disease generally responds to surgical removal, with a cure rate of 75%. More extensive disease is first treated by combination chemotherapy, and then by surgery if there has been a response. Drugs in common use include cyclophosphamide, vincristine, cisplatinum and teniposide. Only about 10% of patients with advanced disease respond to this treatment. Administration of large doses of ^{131}I-mIBG is playing an increasingly important role in the management of these tumours, and prolonging useful life.

References

1 Ross CA, Ruggiero DA, Park DH *et al*. Tonic vasomotor control by the ventrolateral medulla: effect of electrical or chemical stimulation of the area containing C1 adrenaline neurons on arterial pressure, heart rate, and plasma catecholamines and vasopressin. *J Neurosci* 1984; **4**: 474–80.

2 Gilbey MP, Spyer KM. Essential organization of the sympathetic nervous system. *Baillière's Clin Endocrinol Metab* 1993; **7**: 259–78.

3 Al Damluji S, Kopin I. Functional properties of the uptake of amines in immortalized peptidyl neurones. *Br J Pharmacol* 1996; **117**: 111–18.

4 Bevan JA, Su C. Variation of intra and perisynaptic adrenergic transmitter concentrations with width of synaptic cleft in vascular tissues. *J Pharmacol Exp Ther* 1974; **190**: 30–8.

5 Hjemdahl P. Plasma catecholamines—analytical challenges and physiological limitations. *Baillière's Clin Endocrinol Metab* 1993; **7**: 307–53.

6 Wallin BG, Sundlof G, Eriksson B-M, Dominiak P, Grobecker H, Lindblat LE. Plasma noradrenaline correlates with sympathetic muscle nerve activity in normotensive man. *Acta Physiol Scand* 1971; **111**: 69–73.

7 Struthers AD, Reid JL, Whitesmith R, Rodger JC. Effect of intravenous adrenaline on electrocardiogram, blood pressure and serum potassium. *Br Heart J* 1983; **49**: 90–3.

8 Bouloux PMG, Perrett D, Besser GM. Methodological considerations in the determination of plasma catecholamines by high performance liquid chromatography coupled to electrochemical detection. *Ann Clin Biochem* 1986; **22**: 194–203.

9 Esler MD. Catecholamines and essential hypertension. *Baillière's Clin Endocrinol Metab* 1993; **7**: 415–38.

10 Planz G, Wiethold G, Appel E, Bohmer D, Palm D, Grobecker H. Correlation between increased dopamine beta hydroxylase activity and catecholamine concentration in plasma: determination of acute changes in sympathetic activity in man. *Eur J Clin Pharmacol* 1975; **8**: 181–8.

11 O'Connor DT, Bernstein KN. Radioimmunoassay of chromogranin

A in plasma as a measure of exocytotic sympathoadrenal activity in normal subjects and patients with phaeochromocytoma. *N Engl J Med* 1984; **311**: 764–70.

12 Canale MP, Bravo EL. Diagnostic specificity of serum chromogranin A for phaeochromocytoma patients with renal dysfunction. *J Clin Endocrinol Metab* 1994; **78**: 1139–44.

13 Steve M, Panagliotis N, Tuck ML *et al.* Plasma norepinephrine levels are influenced by sodium intake, glucocorticoid administration and circadian changes in normal man. *J Clin Endocrinol Metab* 1980; **51**: 1340–5.

14 Perkins JP, Hausdorff WP, Lefkowitz RJ. Mechanisms of ligand induced desensitisation of β-adrenoceptors. In: The β-adrenergic receptors. JP Perkins (ed.). Clifton NJ: Humana Press, 1991: 73–124.

15 Turki J, Pak J, Gren SA, Martin RJ, Liggett SB. Genetic polymorphisms of the beta-2 adrenergic receptor in nocturnal and non nocturnal asthma. Evidence that Gly16 correlates with the nocturnal phenotype. *J Clin Invest* 1995; **95**: 1635–41.

16 Liggett SB, Raymond JR. Pharmacology and molecular biology of adrenergic receptors. *Baillière's Clin Endocrinol Metab* 1993; **7**: 279–306.

17 Man in't Veld AJ, Boomsla F, Moleman P, Schalekamp MADH. Congenital dopamine-beta-hydroxylase deficiency. A novel orthostatic syndrome. *Lancet* 1987; i: 183–7.

18 Manger WM, Gifford RW, Jr, Hoffman BB. Phaeochromocytoma: a clinical and experimental overview. *Curr Probl Cancer* 1985; **9**: 1.

19 Bittar DA. Unsuspected phaeochromocytoma. *Can Anaesth Soc J* 1982; **29**: 183–4.

20 Humble RM. Phaeochromocytoma, neurofibromatosis and pregnancy. *Anaesthesia* 1967; **22**: 296–303.

21 Carney JA, Sizemore GW, Tyce GM. Bilateral adrenal medullary hyperplasia in multiple endocrine neoplasia, type 2: the precursor of bilateral phaeochromocytoma. *Proc Mayo Clin* 1975; **50**: 3–10.

22 Hosaka Y, Rainwater LM, Grant CS. Phaeochromocytoma: nuclear deoxyribonucleic acid patterns studied by flow cytometry. *Surgery* 1986; **100**: 1003–10.

23 Pattarino F, Bouloux PMG. Diagnosis of malignant phaeochromocytoma. *Clin Endocrinol* 1996; **44**: 239–41.

24 Mulligan LM, Kwok JBJ, Healey CS *et al.* Germ-like mutations of the RET proto-oncogene in multiple endocrine neoplasia. *Nature* 1993; **363**: 458–60.

25 Dahia PLM, Grossman AB. The molecular pathogenesis of adrenal tumours. *Endocr Rel Cancer* 1995; **2**: 267–79.

26 Bravo EL. Evolving concepts in the pathophysiology, diagnosis, and treatment of phaeochromocytoma. *Endocr Rev* 1994; **15**: 356–68.

27 Modlin IM, Farndon JR, Shepherd A *et al.* Phaeochromocytoma in 72 patients: clinical and diagnostic features, treatment and long term results. *Br J Surg* 1979; **66**: 456–56.

28 Bravo EL, Tarazi RC, Fouad FM, Textor SC, Gifford RW, Vidt DG. Blood pressure regulation in phaeochromocytoma. *Hypertension* 1982; **4** (Suppl. II): 193–9.

29 Thomas JE, Rooke ED, Kvale WF. The neurologist's experience with phaeochromocytoma: a review of 100 cases. *JAMA* 1966; **197**: 754–8.

30 Cohen CD, Dent DM. Phaeochromocytoma and acute cardiovascular death (with special reference to myocardial infarction). *Post Med J* 1984; **60**: 111–115.

31 Levenson JA, Safar ME, London GM, Simon AC. Haemodynamics in patients with phaeochromocytoma. *Clin Sci* 1980; **58**: 349–56.

32 Page LB, Raker JW, Berberich FR. Phaeochromocytoma with predominant epinephrine secretion. *Am J Med* 1969; **47**: 48–52.

33 Duncan LE, Semans JH, Howard JE. Case report. Adrenal medullary tumour (phaeochromocytoma) and diabetes mellitus: disappearance of disease and removal of the tumour. *Ann Intern Med* 1944; **20**: 815–78.

34 Proye C, Fossati P, Wemeau JL, Cecat P, Marmousez TH, Lagache G. Le phéochromocytome dopamino-sécrétant. *Chirurgie* 1984; **110**: 304–8.

35 Schell DA, Vari RC, Samson WK. Adrenomedullin: a newly discovered hormone controlling fluid and electrolyte homeostasis. *Trends Endocrinol Metab* 1996; **7**: 7–13.

36 Plouin PF, Degoulet P, Tagaye A *et al.* Le dépistage du phéochromocytome: chez quels hypertendus? Etude sémiologique chez 2885 hypertendus dont 11 ayant un phéochromocytome. *Nouv Presse Med* 1981; **10**: 869–71.

37 Freier DT, Harrison TS. Rigorous biochemical criteria for the diagnosis of phaeochromocytoma. *J Surg Res* 1973; **14**: 177–81.

38 Brown MJ. Simultaneous assay to noradrenaline and its deaminated metabolite, dihydroxyphenylglycol, in plasma: a simplified approach to the exclusion of phaeochromocytoma in patients with borderline elevation of plasma noradrenaline concentration. *Eur J Clin Invest* 1984; **14**: 67–72.

39 Zweifer AJ, Julius S. Increased platelet catecholamine content in phaeochromocytoma: a diagnostic test in patients with elevated plasma catecholamines. *N Engl J Med* 1982; **306**: 890–3.

40 Ganguly A, Henry DP, Yung HY *et al.* Diagnosis and localisation of phaeochromocytoma. Detection by measurement of urinary norepinephrine excretion during sleep, plasma norepinephrine concentration and computerised axial tomography. *Am J Med* 1979; **67**: 21–4.

41 Brown MJ, Allison DJ, Lewis PJ *et al.* Increased sensitivity and accuracy of phaeochromocytoma diagnosis achieved by plasma adrenaline estimations and a pentolinium suppression test. *Lancet* 1981; i: 174–5.

42 Bravo EL, Tarazi RC, Fouad FM *et al.* Clonidine suppression test: a useful aid in the diagnosis of phaeochromocytoma. *N Engl J Med* 1981; **305**: 623–6.

43 Bouloux PMG, Grossman A, Besser GM. Naloxone releases catecholamines from phaeochromocytomas and paragangliomas. *Clin Endocrinol* 1986; **26**: 154–61.

44 Sheedy PF II, Hattery RR, Stephens DH *et al.* Computed tomography of the adrenal gland. In: Hagga JR, Alfidi FJ, eds. *Computed Tomography of the Whole Body*, Vol. 2. St Louis: CV Mosby, 1983: 681–97.

45 Ross EJ, Prichard BNC, Kaufmann L *et al.* Preoperative and operative management of patients with phaeochromocytoma. *Anesth Analg Reanimation* 1967; 63: 142–51.

46 Doppman JL, Reinig JW, Dwyer AJ *et al.* Differentiation of adrenal masses by magnetic resonance imaging. *Surgery* 1987; **102**: 1018–26.

47 Fink IJ, Reinig JW, Dwyer AJ *et al.* MR imaging of phaeochromocytoma. *J Comput Assist Tomogr* 1985; **9**: 454–6.

48 Allison DJ, Brown MJ, Jones DH *et al.* Role of venous sampling in locating a phaeochromocytoma. *Br Med J* 1983; **286**: 1122–6.

49 Jones DH, Allison DJ, Hamilton CA *et al.* Selective venous sampling in the diagnosis and localisation of phaeochromocytoma. *Clin Endocrinol* 1979; **10**: 179–83.

50 Gasnier B, Rosin MP, Scherman D *et al.* Uptake of meta-iodobenzylgaunidine by bovine chromaffin granule membranes. *Mol Pharm* 1986; **29**: 275–9.

51 Guilotteau D, Baulieu J-L, Huguet F *et al.* Metaiodobenzylguanidine

adrenal medulla localisation: autoradiographic and pharmaceutical studies. *Eur J Nucl Med* 1984; **9**: 278–82.

52 Lamberts SWJ, Bakker WH, Reubi JC. Somatostatin-receptor imaging in the localization of endocrine tumours. *N Engl J Med* 1990; **305**: 12–17.

53 Shulkin BL, Wieland DM, Schwaiger M *et al.* PET scanning with hydroxyephedrine: an approach to the localization of phaeochromocytoma. *J Nucl Med* 1992; **33**: 1125–31.

54 Desmonts JM, Marty J. An anaesthetic management of patients with phaeochromocytoma. *Br J Anaesth* 1984; **56**: 781–9.

55 Averbuch SD, Steakley CS, Young RC *et al.* Malignant phaeochromocytoma: effective treatment with a combination of cyclophosphamide, vincristine and decarbazine. *Ann Intern Med* 1988; **109**: 267–73.

56 Krempf M, Lumbroso J, Mornex R. Use of m-131I-MB in the treatment of malignant phaeochromocytoma. *J Clin Endocrinol Metab* 1991; **72**: 455–61.

57 Lewington VJ, Zivanovic MA, Tristam M, McEwan M, Ackery DM. Radiolabelled metaiodobenzylguanidine targeted radiotherapy for malignant phaeochromocytoma. *J Nucl Biol Med* 1991; **35**: 280–3.

58 Shapiro B, Sisson JC, Wieland DM *et al.* Radiopharmaceutical therapy of malignant phaeochromocytoma with 131I-metaiodobenzylguanidine: results from 10 years experience. *J Nucl Biol Med* 1991; **35**: 269–276.

59 Shapiro B. Imaging of catecholamine-secreting tumours: uses of MIBG in diagnosis and treatment. *Ballière's Clin Endocrinol Metab* 1993; **7**: 491–507.

Part 7
Pancreatic Islet Cells

CHAPTER 39

Insulinoma

V. Marks

Introduction

Though rare, insulinomas are the commonest form of hormone-secreting tumour of the pancreas. They invariably manifest themselves through their ability to produce hypoglycaemia, and occur with a frequency of one case per million of the population per year. Some estimates, however, put it four times higher.

Women outnumber men by 6:4 for benign, but not for metastatic tumours, which account for some 10% of all cases. This situation is unlike that of most other pancreatic endocrine tumours, where malignancy is the rule.

Insulinomas are generally small, between 10 and 20 mm in diameter in most cases, and usually sporadic. They may also occur, however, as one of the commonest lesions in families with multiple endocrine neoplasia 1 (MEN-1) syndrome (see Chapter 46). Insulinoma is not generally a feature of MEN-2. Regardless of their size, insulinomas, whether single or multiple, are evenly distributed throughout the pancreas, and are exceedingly rarely found in ectopic sites.

Symptoms caused by insulinomas are almost invariably intermittent, except in the elderly, in whom they may resemble those of dementia or depression [1,2]. The median duration of symptoms before diagnosis has decreased, from an average of 44 months prior to 1950, to <10 months in a series of cases reported from the Mayo Clinic [3]. Occasionally, tumours are diagnosed within days of the onset of symptoms, but sometimes not for as long as 30 years afterwards. Remissions lasting many years are far from unknown, and may be due to necrosis in a tumour which has outgrown its blood supply.

Classifications of hypoglycaemia

Many classifications of hypoglycaemia are possible. One of the commonest and most useful is separation into fasting or non-fasting hypoglycaemia. Similarly, hypoglycaemia may be classified into ketotic or non-ketotic [4], insulinaemic or non-insulinaemic varieties. Another possible classification is based on aetiology; each classification has its uses, but none is either exclusive or all inclusive.

Whereas a diagnosis of insulinoma can only be entertained if, and when, hypoglycaemia has been established as the cause of a patient's symptoms, it is none the less a comparatively rare cause of proven non-iatrogenic hypoglycaemia. Spontaneous, or seemingly spontaneous, hypoglycaemia, is less often due to insulinoma than to one of the hundred or so other conditions—including accidental poisonings—in which hypoglycaemia occurs with a severity ranging from life-threatening to little more than a barely symptomatic epiphenomenon.

It is for this reason that the differentiation of hypoglycaemia due to insulinoma from that secondary to other disease is so important. Fortunately this is comparatively simple by judicious use of plasma hormone assays so that it is seldom necessary nowadays to subject patients to the rigors of the past [5,6].

It is no longer necessary to insist that the blood glucose level falls below 2.2 mmol/l providing that inappropriate insulin (and/or proinsulin) secretion can be demonstrated in the fasting subject when the blood glucose concentration is 3.0 mmol/l or less.

Diagnosis

Diagnosis of insulinoma takes place in four essential and usually sequential stages [7]. The first and most difficult is the recognition of hypoglycaemia as the cause of the patient's symptoms. The second is determining, on the basis of the history and physical examination, its most likely aetiology, and the third is using hormone and other laboratory procedures to confirm it. The fourth and final stage is localisation of the lesion. This is usually best done at operation—the treatment of choice for insulinoma.

Stages I and II

The symptoms produced by an insulinoma are invariably due to spontaneous hypoglycaemia and are many, varied, and usually intermittent [1–3]. In the elderly, symptoms of chronic neuroglycopenia may be confused with dementia, and sometimes patients present in hypoglycaemic coma or precoma with no preceding history. Usually, however, the patient will not be hypoglycaemic when first seen and, unless hypoglycaemia is suspected in everyone and anyone whose complaint is of intermittent episodes of altered consciousness or behaviour, delays in diagnosis are inevitable.

Symptoms are often remarkably mild. They may take the form of, or be accompanied by, changes in personality—of which the patient is unaware—or gradual deterioration of work performance. Seventy-five percent of patients are unaware of any relationship between symptoms and fasting until their attention is drawn to it, and very few recognise any relationship to exercise. Hunger is complained of by only 14% of patients and obesity is very rarely a cause of presentation, although it is a variable feature of some 30% of cases in all.

Contrary to common belief, symptoms of acute neuroglycopenia and panic attacks are comparatively uncommon although, because of their florid nature and intrusiveness, they are often the immediate cause of presentation. Only a meticulous history, coupled with a physical examination, can point to the correct differential diagnosis and consequently which tests are likely to yield the most clinically useful information. Symptoms of hypoglycaemia sometimes remit in women who become pregnant only to recur when the pregnancy ends. More commonly, however, pregnancy uncovers a previously unsuspected insulinoma by precipitating hypoglycaemia.

Stages III and IV

There is nothing specific about the symptoms caused by hypoglycaemia except their relief by intravenous glucose. The diagnosis must therefore be made by demonstrating a low blood glucose concentration when the patient is suffering spontaneously from symptoms (or by demonstrating inappropriate hyperinsulinaemia in the fasting subject).

In the past it was common to admit patients to hospital for observation and fasting for up to 72 hours. It is, however, comparatively simple to teach the close family or friends, or even patients themselves, how to collect blood during spontaneous symptomatic episodes whilst the patient is going about his or her everyday life. Fingerprick blood can be collected onto prepared pieces of filter paper or preferably into a sodium-fluoride containing capillary tube which can then be sent to the laboratory for measurement of its glucose content. Glucose-oxidase impregnated glucose test strips and other devices—which are designed for self-monitoring of diabetes—should not be used for this purpose as they are unreliable in the hypoglycaemic range [8] and could not reasonably be expected to be read properly by someone whilst suffering from neuroglycopenia [9].

Table 39.1 Plasma proinsulin, insulin, C-peptide and blood glucose levels in various subject groups after an overnight fast (or, in the case of stimulative hypoglycaemia, during the hypoglycaemia).

Patients	Glucose (mmol/l)	Proinsulin (pmol/l)	Insulin (pmol/l)	C-peptide (pmol/l)	Insulin/proinsulin
Controls (n = 17)	5.12 ± 0.4	6.7 ± 1.7	38.0 ± 5	370 ± 30	6:1
Insulinoma patients (n = 21)	1.67 ± 0.48	255 ± 479	245 ± 236	1126 ± 828	1:1
Sulphonylurea-induced hypoglycaemic patients (n = 3)	1.6 ± 0.23	15.7 ± 2.3	173 ± 125	963 ± 405	10:1
Glucose-induced 'reactive' hypoglycaemic patients (n = 10)	2.0 ± 0.52	7.4 ± 8.8	36.8 ± 25.8	196 ± 82.6	5:1
Non-insulin-dependent diabetics (n = 11)	9.36 ± 3.1	14.2 ± 2	48.0 ± 20	530 ± 200	3.4:1

Values expressed as mean ± SD.

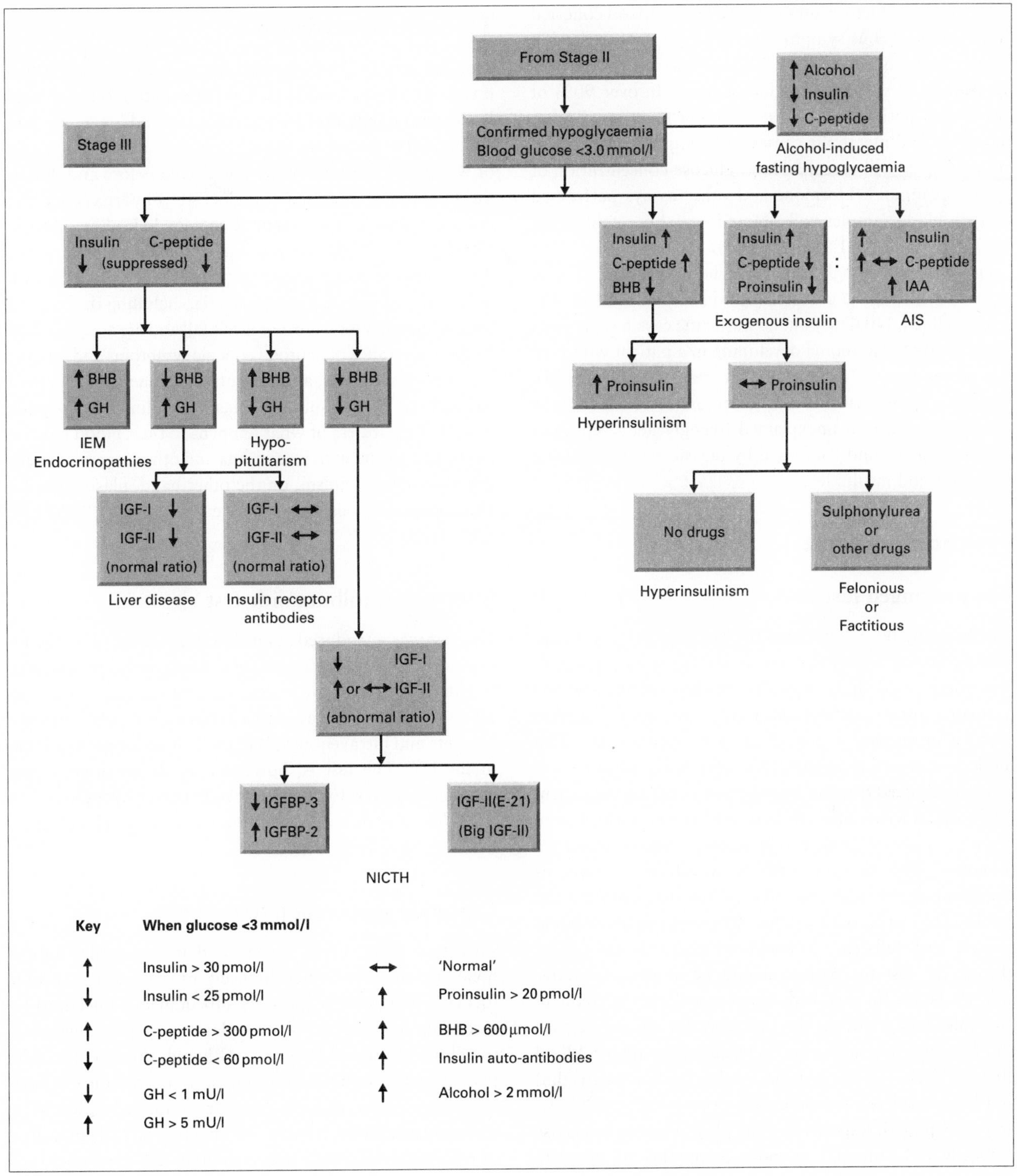

Fig. 39.1 Algorithm for testing blood samples taken after a 12-hour fast. IEM, inborn errors of metabolism; IAA, insulin autoantibodies; AIS, autoimmune insulin syndrome; BHB, β-hydroxybutyrate; GH, growth hormone.

A blood glucose concentration of 4.0 mmol/l at the beginning, or early in the course, of a typical spontaneous symptomatic episode virtually excludes hypoglycaemia as its cause, and one of 2.5mmol/l or less makes it almost certain.

As a less satisfactory alternative to testing blood collected during spontaneous symptomatic hypoglycaemic episodes, blood can be collected after a 12-hour fast on at least three occasions and subjected to glucose assay. In over 90% of insulinoma patients and those suffering from most other endocrine and metabolic causes of hypoglycaemia, one or more samples will reveal a blood glucose concentration of below 3.0 mmol/l. Hormone and other assays performed on such blood samples will almost invariably establish the diagnosis (Table 39.1 and Fig. 39.1).

Insulinomas, though rare, have been recorded [10] in patients with type 2 diabetes (non-insulin dependent diabetes mellitus, NIDDM) but no authentic case has yet been established of insulinoma developing in a patient with type 1 diabetes (insulin-dependent diabetes mellitus, IDDM). Factitious hypoglycaemia must therefore be considered the most likely cause of unexplained hypoglycaemic episodes in such patients and confirmed by measuring their plasma C-peptide and insulin levels.

Provocative tests

The prolonged fast test

This has long been considered the 'gold standard' for confirming fasting hypoglycaemia as the cause of a patient's symptoms [1–3]. It is, however, neither specific for any particular disease, for example insulinoma, nor is it always positive in surgically proven cases of insulinoma. With modern methods of diagnosis it is very rarely required.

The prolonged fast test is performed by taking the patient into hospital where they can be strictly supervised and given nothing to eat or drink except water or unsweetened tea or coffee. This prevents caffeine withdrawal symptoms complicating the issue and does not interfere with the test results. The fast is continued for 72 hours or until the blood glucose level falls to 3.0 mmol/l, whichever is the earlier. During the test the patient should be moderately active and not be confined to bed. Blood is collected at frequent intervals throughout the day and night for glucose, ketone and hormone measurements. In insulinoma patients, blood glucose levels fall but plasma insulin (and/or proinsulin) and C-peptide levels remain inappropriately high (>30pmol/l and > 100 pmol/l, respectively), and plasma ketone levels rise modestly (< 1.5 mmol/l) at most. Symptoms of subacute neuroglycopenia may or may not develop.

Asymptomatic hypoglycaemia, with blood glucose levels as low as 1.5 mmol/l, is said to be comparatively common in young and middle-aged women subjected to a 72-hour fast. Plasma insulin and C-peptide levels are, however, suppressed appropriately and β-hydroxybutyrate levels are raised. The electroencephalogram is unaltered.

The rigorous exercise test

This test, unlike the prolonged fast test, can be performed on an out-patient basis [11]. The patient attends the clinical investigation unit after an overnight fast and is exercised on a treadmill or stationary bicycle until they are no longer able or willing to continue. Blood is collected before and during the test and is analysed for glucose, β-hydroxybutyrate, insulin, proinsulin and C-peptide content. In healthy subjects, blood glucose levels may rise, fall or remain stationary, but do not appear to influence performance. In patients with most types of fasting hypoglycaemia, including that caused by insulinoma, blood glucose levels fall and are accompanied by the appearance of neuroglycopenic symptoms and fatigue.

In healthy subjects, and patients with illnesses other than endogenous hyperinsulinism, plasma insulin and C-peptide levels fall regardless of what happens to their blood glucose levels. In patients with insulinoma and other causes of endogenous hyperinsulinism, on the other hand, plasma insulin and C-peptide levels remain above 30 pmol and 300 pmol/l, respectively.

Intravenous tolbutamide test

This test was introduced as an alternative to the oral glucose tolerance test for the diagnosis of diabetes, but gained greater popularity as a test for insulinoma until modern hormone assays became readily available. It has now become virtually obsolete and intravenous tolbutamide is no longer available in the UK. The test is, however, just as sensitive as the prolonged fast test for the diagnosis of fasting hypoglycaemia providing it is done and interpreted correctly [2,12]. It is, however, equally non-specific.

C-peptide suppression test

This test relies upon the fact that ordinarily during hypoglycaemia—whether induced by exogenous insulin (0.1 U/kg bodyweight given by subcutaneous injection) or secondary to some pathology—plasma C-peptide levels fall to below 300 pmol/l (1 ng/ml). Although this is unusual in patients with autonomous insulin-secreting tumours, it does sometimes occur making the test of limited value as a screening procedure. Its main use now is as an early indicator of recurrence following resection of an apparently solitary insulinoma [13].

Other provocative tests

Many other procedures have been used to provoke hypoglycaemia in patients suspected of suffering from spontaneous hypoglycaemia. Whilst some, for example glucagon,

L-leucine, calcium infusion and mixed meal tests, still have a role to play in the recognition and differential diagnosis of hypoglycaemia due to causes other than an insulinoma, none has any role in the initial recognition of hypoglycaemia.

The oral glucose load (tolerance) test, which has probably been responsible for more misdiagnosis than any other test currently in the clinical chemistry repertoire, has no role to play in either the diagnosis or differential diagnosis of spontaneous hypoglycaemia [14], and its use should be confined to research and as an infrequently required test for diabetes.

Chemical pathology

In most respects there is nothing about the chemical pathology of hypoglycaemia produced by insulinomas that distinguishes it from other types of fasting hypoglycaemia. Its immediate cause is inhibition of hepatic glucose release at a time when absorption of glucose from the gut is either zero, or is too slow to meet the loss of glucose from the body glucose pool.

The most characteristic feature of the hypoglycaemia produced by insulinoma is its provocation by fasting and the coexistence of inappropriately high plasma insulin (and/ or proinsulin) and C-peptide levels [1].

Soon after the introduction of immunoassay for the measurement of insulin in peripheral blood it became evident that hypoglycaemia produced by insulinomas was a consequence of inappropriate rather than of excessive insulin secretion. Indeed, many insulin secreting tumours fail to release insulin in response to hyperglycaemia and this, when coupled with peripheral insulin insensitivity—itself a common finding in patients with insulinoma—can result, paradoxically, in impaired glucose tolerance (IGT).

Failure to suppress insulin release in response to hypoglycaemia is the distinguishing feature and *sine qua non* of insulinoma. Other abnormalities of insulin secretion, such as increased sensitivity to L-leucine and glucagon, and reduced sensitivity to somatostatin [15], are too variable to be of diagnostic value.

A characteristic feature of the hypoglycaemia caused by insulinomas is its association with normo- or even hypoketonaemia (i.e. plasma β-hydroxybutyrate level < 0.5 mmol/l) except after prolonged fasting [4]. This, like the hypoglycaemia itself, is a consequence of inappropriate insulin action and in virtually all other illnesses (apart from insulin-like growth factor 2 (IGF-2)-secreting tumours [16], autoimmune hypoglycaemia, cachexia (including anorexia nervosa), some drugs and, of course, endogenous and exogenous hyperinsulinism) plasma ketone levels exceed 0.5 mmol/l during spontaneous hypoglycaemic episodes.

A special feature of the β-cells of insulinomas is their relative incompetence in cleaving proinsulin into insulin and C-peptide prior to release into the circulation [5,6]. This fact can be utilised in both the diagnosis and differential diagnosis of hypoglycaemia (Table 39.1 and Fig. 39.1), some so-called insulinomas secreting exclusively proinsulin.

Differential diagnosis

The differential diagnosis of insulinoma from other causes of fasting hypoglycaemia takes place in three stages. The first is the differentiation of hyperinsulinaemic from other causes of fasting hypoglycaemia. The second is differentiation of endogenous from factitious hyperinsulinism especially that caused by sulphonylurea ingestion. The third is differentiation of solitary insulinoma from other causes of β-cell dysfunction including multiple or diffuse adenomatosis, MEN-1, nesidioblastosis, metastatic and mixed endocrine-cell tumours. This is desirable, but not always possible preoperatively, since their optimal management is not only different from other causes of hypoglycaemia but also from one another [1].

Endogenous hyperinsulinism

Inappropriate insulin secretion

Spontaneous or fast-provoked hypoglycaemia is associated with inappropriately high immunoreactive insulin (including proinsulin and proinsulin metabolites) and C-peptide levels in patients with endogenous hyperinsulinism, but in virtually no other illness apart from certain types of drug misuse [17]. Exactly what constitutes inappropriateness has caused some confusion in the past possibly due to unrecognised problems with the specificity of the assays used. With the introduction of assays specific for native insulin which do not cross-react with proinsulin the difficulty has been exacerbated since some 'insulinomas' secrete only proinsulin and its cleavage products. These, though having reduced hypoglycaemic potency, may nevertheless produce hypoglycaemia even in the absence of insulin itself. It is therefore necessary when investigating a patient with hypoglycaemia to measure proinsulin in addition to insulin and C-peptide if errors of diagnosis are to be avoided.

Causes of hyperproinsulinaemia other than 'insulinoma' do occur but none, apart from sulphonylurea overdose [17], is known to be associated with fasting hypoglycaemia.

Endogenous versus exogenous hyperinsulinism

Most cases of factitious hypoglycaemia are due to exogenous insulin, and may mimic that caused by insulinoma very closely.

They no longer present any difficulty in differentiation from insulinoma since plasma C-peptide levels are invariably low in the former and inappropriately high in the latter (Table 39.1). Insulin antibodies are also often present in patients with factitious hyperinsulinism and were, at one time, almost the only way of distinguishing them from patients with insulinoma.

Nowadays it is important to distinguish factitious hypoglycaemia from the autoimmune insulin syndrome in which insulin antibodies are the cause rather than a consequence of the patient's illness. Difficulties may arise if too much reliance is placed upon the insulin/C-peptide molar ratio during hypoglycaemia since this may be abnormally high in both conditions.

Sulphonylurea abuse, though less common than insulin abuse, may be difficult to distinguish from endogenous hyperinsulinism unless a drug screen for sulphonylurea metabolites in blood or urine is carried out on every patient in whom the diagnosis of insulinoma is made [17]. One such drug-abusing patient known to us underwent laparotomy on at least two occasions before the correct diagnosis was eventually made.

Solitary insulinoma versus multicentric β-cell dysfunction

Whilst a preoperative diagnosis of endogenous hyperinsulinism can now be made with high precision, differentiation between the anatomical and functional varieties is much more difficult and can only be made with certainty by anatomical and histological examination of the pancreas after surgery [1,18].

As a group, insulinomas show variable staining with immunohistological agents which generally serve as markers of neuroendocrine tumours or APUDomas. Solitary insulinomas are composed largely or wholly of seemingly normal β-cells, though meticulous examination of tumours by electron microscopy or immunocytochemistry generally reveals a small and variable number of other pancreatic endocrine cell types. The atypical β-granules found in insulinoma cells correspond to the coated β-granules which are present in small numbers in normal β-cells. Their presence indicates impaired conversion of proinsulin to insulin and C-peptide and their increased numbers in insulinomas equates with the increased content of proinsulin of insulinomas compared with normal pancreatic islets.

A classification of insulinomas based on functional rather than histological characteristics was proposed by Berger *et al.* [18]. Group A tumours are characterised by almost complete suppressibility of insulin and proinsulin secretion by diazoxide and somatostatin, and by an abundance of well-granulated β-cells with a trabecular arrangement within the tumour. Group B tumours show a marked resistance to the suppressant effects of diazoxide and somatostatin and have fewer, less well-granulated β-granules and a medullary type of histological appearance. A substantially greater proportion of the total plasma insulin is due to proinsulin in group B patients, in whom it represents 46% of total insulin rather than in group A patients in whom it represents only 20%.

Histological appearances of insulinomas give no indication as to their ability to metastasise, nor whether more than one tumour is present in the pancreas. A suggestion that expression of the α-chains of human chorionic gonadotrophin was confined to malignant or metastatic tumours and might therefore be useful in differentiating solitary benign from malignant insulinomas has not, unfortunately, been confirmed [19].

MEN 1 should be suspected in all cases of familial or multiple insulinoma and plasma Ca^{2+} measurements should be part of the regular work-up of patients with endogenous hyperinsulinism. Genetic markers for MEN-1 are available and should be used to confirm or refute the diagnosis in suspicious cases.

Material with the histological properties of amyloid and currently known as amylin is discernible in many insulinomas. Amylin was at one time thought to represent a breakdown product of insulin, but this is now known not to be so; it is a distinct peptide which is comanufactured with insulin in the β-cells of normal islets as well as of insulinomas. Its physiological role, if any, is currently unknown.

Nesidioblastosis and islet hyperplasia

Although insulinomas occur at any age, they are extremely rare before the age of 4 years. In 1970, Brown and Young suggested that hyperinsulinaemic hypoglycaemia in infants and young children was due to disruption of the normal architecture of the endocrine pancreas. They called the distinctive anatomical features they observed in these children, nesidioblastosis.

Features that they considered characteristic of the condition include gross enlargement of the islet-cell mass due to an increase both in the number and size of recognisable islets of Langerhans, and the presence of multifocal ductulo-insular proliferation dispersed throughout much or all of the pancreas. Subsequently, age and case-controlled studies of the pancreas showed that nesidioblastosis, far from providing a unique anatomical basis for infantile hyperinsulinaemic hypoglycaemia, is a natural stage of the development of the endocrine pancreas [20]. Clinically, the condition of infantile hyperinsulinism is indistinguishable from insulinoma, except that it tends to remit when the child reaches adolescence.

Comparatively little information is available about non-tumour-associated hyperinsulinaemic hypoglycaemia in adults. Most reports relate to a single case, or are so poorly documented as to provide little useful data. The topic, which has recently been reviewed [21], continues to be controversial. Some authorities believe that it accounts for up to 5% of all adult cases of endogenous hyperinsulinism, whilst others find it extremely rarely, if at all [22].

Generalised islet hyperplasia is common in proven cases of insulinoma, as well as in many other endocrine and non-endocrine disorders. Histological features that were previously described as characteristic of nesidioblastosis are also common in people who never experienced hypoglycaemia in life. Therefore, whilst some adults with severe intractable hypoglycaemia who have been described in the literature as having nesidioblastosis or islet hyperplasia probably did have a purely functional derangement of the pancreatic β-cell similar, if not identical, to that observed in infants; others probably had a small but occult insulinoma that was overlooked at operation or during examination of the resected pancreas, or were surreptitiously taking sulphonylureas [23].

Infants with hyperinsulinaemic hypoglycaemia due to a functional, rather than tumorous, lesion of the β-cells are just as likely to have disproportionately high plasma proinsulin to insulin levels as adults with insulinomas. This is probably also true of adults with functional hyperinsulinism due to islet hyperplasia, though because of its rarity data are not yet available to support this belief. In any event it is unlikely, as was once suggested [21], that this type of hyperinsulinism can be differentiated preoperatively from insulinoma purely on the basis of plasma proinsulin measurements [23].

Localisation

The role of physical methods for localising insulinomas, once the diagnosis has been made on clinical and laboratory grounds, is still far from clear, being advocated by some authors in every case of established hyperinsulinism and by others only for those cases in which surgical exploration has already been unsuccessful. The older methods of localisation including selective coeliac axis or pancreatic arteriography, contrast radiography, scintiscanning with isotopic selenium or ^{131}I-labelled toluidine blue, as well as computerised tomography (CT), have all had their proponents. None, in my opinion, has proved sufficiently reliable to make them more than of questionable value except in the hands of their developers and a few enthusiasts [24]. All have comparatively high false-positive and -negative rates and, at best, only help a surgeon localise a tumour within the pancreas once the decision to operate has been taken. No physical localisation technique is sufficiently reliable, at the present time, to be used to dismiss a diagnosis of insulinoma that has been made on sound clinical and biochemical grounds [24,25]. However, there is some evidence that radionuclide scanning with labelled octreotide may localise tumours in 50% of cases, and may be useful in assessing sensitivity to octreotide therapy.

Probably the most valuable tumour localisation techniques are those that employ selective blood sampling and insulin assay, and can be undertaken preoperatively by percutaneous transhepatic portal venography (PTPV) or, intraoperatively, under direct vision [26,27]. PTPV is not without risk, is costly and depends heavily upon the skills and experience of the radiologist. It should probably be reserved for use in cases in which difficulties have already been encountered at a previous operation [28] or where they might reasonably be expected to occur because of coexisting disease. For maximum benefit, access to a rapid insulin assay with a turn-around time of less than 1 hour is required [27].

Intraoperative ultrasonography (IOUS) is the most recently developed technique for localising intrapancreatic tumours and has the same sensitivity as a skilled surgeon using his or her fingers [29,30]. In a recent series [29] of 28 cases the tumour could not be felt by the surgeon in four but was correctly located by IOUS. There were, on the other hand, some tumours that could be felt but were not visualised ultrasonographically. IOUS may, therefore, be a useful addition to palpation, especially in cases where multiple tumours are thought likely.

Treatment of hyperinsulinism

Solitary or multiple tumours

The treatment of choice for all types of insulinoma is surgical ablation [22]. This confers an excellent prognosis unless metastasis has occurred, which is rare. Even then, removal of the primary and as many secondaries as possible may add many years of useful life.

Early collected results, which revealed cure rates of 63% with an operative mortality of 11% and persistence or recurrence of hypoglycaemia in a further 16% of cases, are still sometimes quoted. They do not represent current experience in which cure rates for non-malignant tumours of up to 95% with perioperative mortalities of $< 5\%$, except in the very elderly, are commonplace [2,3]. Long-term prognosis in patients in whom straightforward removal of a benign insulinoma has been accomplished is no different from that of healthy people of similar age but is substantially reduced in those who undergo blind pancreatectomy as the only way of preventing them becoming hypoglycaemic [22].

In patients over the age of 70 years operative mortality increases and medical alternatives to surgery should be considered. In patients with metastatic disease, in whom surgical treatment is not possible, survival for up to 10 years can sometimes be achieved with return to a full and active life, providing that death from hypoglycaemia can be prevented.

Various medical treatments have been employed but combined therapy with diazoxide and chlorothiazide (or certain other thiazides) is the most effective [1]. If, or—in the case of malignant tumours—when, combined therapy fails to be effective, other treatments, including the use of β-adrenergic antagonists, Ca^{2+}-channel blockers and long-acting somatostatin and its analogues are worth trying [31–33]. In particular, subcutaneous octreotide can often be extremely useful when diazoxide has failed, but tumours initially sensitive may eventually become refractory.

Attempts at curative therapy using cytotoxic agents such as streptozotocin, 5-fluorouracil and other specific antitumour drugs may be made at the outset but, in my opinion, should be reserved for treatment of the intractable hypoglycaemia that heralds impending demise. In favourable cases such therapy may produce a further remission for up to 5 years [33]. Hepatic arterial embolisation is also worthy of trial and may produce worthwhile remissions of up to several years, as may cryotherapy.

Nesidioblastosis and islet hyperplasia

In infants with hyperinsulinism due to the 'nesidioblastotic' syndrome and adults with islet hyperplasia, and in whom there is no focal source of inappropriate insulin secretion, treatment should be instituted with diazoxide and chlorothiazide or with long-acting somatostatin. Only if this medical treatment fails to remedy the abnormality of glucose homeostasis should surgery be undertaken [34].

Surgery should be confined, in the first instance, to removal of some 80% of the pancreas as this is generally sufficient to bring the condition under control, either with or without continuing medication. Total pancreatectomy should be used only as the last resort since the dangers and difficulties of life-long IDDM and pancreatic insufficiency are great [32].

References

1 Marks V, Rose FC. *Hypoglycaemia*, 2nd edn. Oxford: Blackwell Scientific Publications, 1981.
2 Service FJ. *Hypoglycemic disorders. N Engl J Med* 1995; **332**: 1144–52.
3 Service FJ, Dale AJD, Elveback LR, Jiang N-S. Insulinoma—clinical and diagnostic features of 60 consecutive cases. *Mayo Clin Proc* 1976; **51**: 417–29.
4 Teale JD, Pearse AG, Marks V. The measurement of insulin- C-peptide and B-hydroxybutyrate in the differential diagnosis of spontaneous hypoglycaemia. In: Andreani D, Marks V, Lefebvre PJ, eds. *Hypoglycemia.* New York: Raven Press, 1987: 281–2.
5 Hampton SM, Beyzavi K, Teale D, Marks V. A direct assay for proinsulin in plasma and its applications in hypoglycaemia. *Clin Endocrinology* 1988; **29**: 9–16.
6 Cohen RM, Camus F. Update on insulinomas or the case of the missing (pro)insulinoma. *Diabetes Care* 1988; **11**: 506–8.
7 Marks V, Teale JD. Investigation of hypoglycaemia. *Clin Endocrinol* 1996; **44**(2): 133–6.
8 Southgate HJ, Marks V. Measurement of hypoglycaemia by reflocheck. *Pract Diabetes* 1986; **3**: 206–7.
9 Snorgaard O, Binder C. Monitoring of blood glucose concentration in subjects with hypoglycaemic symptoms during everyday life. *Br Med J* 1990; **300**: 16–18.
10 Kane LA, Grant CS, Nippoldt TB, Service FJ. Insulinoma in a patient with NIDDM. *Diabetes Care* 1993; **16**: 1298–1300.
11 Jarhult J, Ericsson M, Holst J, Ingemansson S. Lack of suppression of insulin secretion by exercise in patients with insulinoma. *Clin Endocrinol* 1981; **15**: 391–4.
12 McMahon MM, O'Brien PC, Service FJ. Diagnostic interpretation of the intravenous tolbutamide test for insulinoma. *Mayo Clin Proc* 1989; **64**: 1481–8.
13 Argoud GW, Schade DS, Eaton RP, Sterling WA. C-peptide suppression test and recurrent insulinoma. *Am J Med* 1989; **86**: 335–7.
14 Service FJ. Hypoglycemia and the postprandial syndrome. *N Engl J Med* 1989; **321**: 1472–3.
15 Gama R, Marks V, Wright J, Teale JD. Octreotide exacerbated fasting hypoglycaemia in a patient with a proinsulinoma: the glucostatic importance of pancreatic glucagon. *Clin Endocrinology* 1995; **43**: 117–20.
16 Teale JD, Marks V. Inappropriately elevated plasma insulin-like growth factor II in relation to suppressed insulin-like growth factor I in the diagnosis of non-islet cell tumour hypoglycaemia. *Clin Endocrinol* 1990; **33**: 87–98.
17 Teale JD, Starkey BJ, Marks V *et al.* The prevalence of factitious hypoglycaemia due to sulphonylurea abuse in the UK: a preliminary report. *Pract Diabetes* 1989; **6**: 177–8.
18 Berger M, Bordi C, Cuppers H-J *et al.* Functional and morphologic characterisation of human insulinomas. *Diabetes* 1983; **32**: 921–31.
19 Graeme-Cook F, Bell DA, Compton CC. Immunocytochemical staining for human choriogonadotrophin does not predict malignancy in insulinomas. *Am J Clin Pathol* 1990; **93**: 273–6.
20 Gregory JW, Aynsley-Gree A. Hypoglycaemia in the infant and child. *Ballière's Clin Endocrinol Metab* 1993; **7**: 683–704.
21 Fong T-L, Warner NE, Kumar D. Pancreatic nesidioblastosis in adults. *Diabetes Care* 1989; **12**: 108–14.
22 Thompson GB, Service FJ, van Heerden JA *et al.* Reoperative

insulinomas, 1927 to 1992: an institutional experience. *Surgery* 1993; **114**: 1196–1206.

23 Marks V. Hypoglycaemia—real, unreal, lawful and unlawful: the 1994 Banting Lecture. *Diabet Med* 1995; **12**: 850–64.

24 Marks V, Teale JD. Hypoglycaemia in the adult. *Ballière's Clin Endocrinol Metab* 1993; 7: 705–29.

25 Bottger TC, Junginger T. Is preoperative radiographic localisation of islet cell tumors in patients with insulinoma necessary? *World J Surg* 1993; **17**: 427–32.

26 Glaser B, Valtysson G, Fajans SS *et al.* Gastrointestinal/pancreatic hormone concentrations in the portal venous system of nine patients with organic hyperinsulinism. *Metabolism* 1981; **30**: 1001–10.

27 Stringel G, Dalpe-Scott M, Perelman AH, Heick HMC. The occult insulinoma operative localisation by quick insulin radioimmunoassay. *J Ped Surg* 1985; **20**: 734–6.

28 Fonseca V, Ames D, Ginsburg J. Hypoglycaemia for 26 years due to an insulinoma. *J Roy Soc Med* 1989; **82**: 437–8.

29 Norton JA, Cromack DT, Shawker TH *et al.* Intraoperative ultrasonographic localization of islet cell tumors: a prospective comparison to palpation. *Ann Surg* 1988; **207**: 160–8.

30 Galiber AK, Reading CC, Charboneau JQ *et al.* Localization of pancreatic insulinoma: comparison of pre- and intraoperative US with CT and angiography. *Radiology* 1988; **166**: 405–8.

31 Eriksson B, Oberg K, Andersson T, Lundqvist G, Wide L, Wilander E. Treatment of malignant endocrine pancreatic tumors with a new long-acting somatostatin analogue, SMS 201–995. *Scand J Gastroenterol* 1988; **23**: 508–12.

32 Boden G, Ryan IG, Shuman CR. Ineffectiveness of SMS 201–995 in severe hyperinsulinemia. *Diabetes Care* 1988; **11**: 664–8.

33 Kvols LK, Buck M. Chemotherapy of endocrine malignancies: a review. *Semin Oncol* 1987; **14**: 343–53.

34 Soltesz G, Aynsley-Green A. Hyperinsulinism in infancy and childhood. In: Frick H von P *et al.*, eds. *Advances in Internal Medicine and Pediatrics*. Berlin: Springer-Verlag, 1984: 51.

CHAPTER 40

Islet-cell tumours (excluding insulinomas and carcinoids)

D. O'Shea, D. Wynick and S.R. Bloom

Introduction

The hormones of the pancreas are secreted by specialised cells lying within the pancreatic islet. Our understanding of these endocrine cells and their relationship to various clinical syndromes has greatly increased during the past two decades: this is particularly due to advances in immunocytochemistry and radioimmunoassay. Immunocytochemistry allows us to localise and differentiate the different types of secretory granule that characterise endocrine cells, while radio-immunoassay permits measurement of the various peptides secreted by such cells. It has been proposed that all endocrine cells share certain features of amine metabolism. This gave rise to the term APUD (*a*mine content *p*recursor *u*ptake and *d*ecarboxylation), and the term APUDoma was used to describe dysfunction of endocrine cells such as hyperplasia, adenomas and carcinoma which secreted various hormones to excess. We now know, however, that not all neuro-endocrine cells fit the APUD concept. Pancreatic endocrine tumours are more simply and accurately referred to as islet-cell tumours.

Islet-cell tumours of the pancreas may produce a large number of peptides normally found in the adult pancreas (orthotopic secretion, e.g. insulin, glucagon and somatostatin) and substances normally only found in other glands and tissues (ectopic secretion, e.g. gastrin and vasoactive intestinal polypeptide, VIP). Islet-cell tumours may be single or multiple in the pancreas and associated with hyperplastic and/or neoplastic lesions in other tissues as part of the syndrome of multiple endocrine neoplasia (MEN).

Clinical features of pancreatic islet-cell tumours

The first pancreatic islet-cell tumour was observed by W.J. Mayo in 1927 in a physician with recurrent hypoglycaemia [1]. A tumour found within the pancreas at laparotomy was subsequently shown to contain a factor that reproduced the symptoms of hypoglycaemia when injected into rats. In the intervening years many more clinical syndromes have been discovered. It was initially believed that each tumour had only a single peptide product, but it is now apparent that most pancreatic tumours secrete more than one peptide of varying biological activity and that for each peptide secreted differing molecular weight forms are produced [2]. The various hormonal syndromes are usually named after the secretory peptide whose biological activity can be linked to the major clinical features of each case.

Islet-cell tumours have several clinical features in common: they tend to be slow growing and are often lethal because of systemic effects of peptide hypersecretion rather than local tumour bulk until a very late stage in the disease [3]. With the exception of the insulinoma, most of the tumours tend to be malignant and metastases within the abdominal cavity have frequently occurred by the time of diagnosis. Excision of a solitary lesion within the pancreas is often curative in the case of insulinoma and may give many years of symptom-free life in the case of the other neuroendocrine pancreatic tumours. With metastatic tumours surgical debulking, systemic or local cytotoxic chemotherapy and hepatic artery embolisation are the mainstays of therapy aimed at reducing tumour bulk. However, it is now possible to reduce secretory products from tumours by use of one of the long acting somatostatin analogues. These may keep the disease process and the systemic effects of the peptide hypersecretion under control for long periods of time, often years, thus allowing patients to return to fully active lives.

The clinical features associated with pancreatic endocrine tumours are listed in Table 40.1, and the more important tumours are considered individually below. Each individual tumour syndrome is dealt with as a separate entity though it is well recognised that simultaneous multiple

Table 40.1 Clinical features associated with pancreatic islet-cell tumours.

Clinical features	Pancreatic islet cell tumour
Hypoglycaemia	Insulinoma
Hyperglycaemia	Glucagonoma Somatostatinoma Corticotrophinoma Phaeochromocytoma
Diarrhoea	Carcinoid tumour Gastrinoma VIPoma
Peptic ulceration	Gastrinoma (and other tumours in MEN syndromes)
Hypokalaemia:	
Acidotic	VIPoma
Alkalotic	Corticotrophinoma
Necrolytic migratory dermatitis	Glucagonoma
Flushing and other vasomotor manifestations	VIPoma Carcinoid Phaeochromocytoma

hypersecretion is very common, with either one syndrome predominating or with a mixed clinical picture.

Gastrinoma

Gastrinomas have up to now been the second most commonly diagnosed type of pancreatic islet-cell tumour. Up to 60% are malignant and have hepatic metastases at the time of diagnosis, though that figure is higher when associated with MEN-1. Five-year survival is directly related to the presence or absence of metastases; those presenting with multiple metastases to the liver and extra abdominal sites have a 20% survival rate at 5 years. Those who present with a single resectable lesion have >80% survival rate. With the increasing availability of radioimmunoassay for gastrin as part of the supraregional assay service in the UK, plasma gastrins are being measured earlier in patients with duodenal and gastric ulceration; this should lead to earlier diagnosis in patients with gastrinoma. We have found that up to 17% of patients with abnormal gastrin levels are not investigated further despite the absence of a known cause for the hypergastrinaemia. This will lead to the tumours being missed in a number of subjects at a curable stage.

Simple peptic ulceration is common, and the problem is to detect the relatively rare cases of the gastrinoma. The common perception is that the higher the gastrin, the more likely a tumour is the cause. However, the highest gastrin levels, 50–100-fold above the upper limit of normal (40 pmol/l), are usually associated with hypo- or achlorhydria or chronic renal failure rather than a gastrinoma. Acid output studies must be performed in *all* subjects with raised gastrin levels. The presence of both an elevated gastrin and a high basal acid output (> 10 mmol/hour with a blunted response to pentagastrin stimulation) is diagnostic of a gastrinoma.

Many centres use the secretin test as a further confirmatory test but it is doubtful whether its use adds significantly to the diagnosis in that false positives and negatives are frequent. We would thus suggest that if a patient has both an elevated gastrin and a high acid output they should be considered to have a gastrinoma, and a search undertaken for the source. This search should include selective visceral angiography with a secretin-provocation test to attempt to regionalise the tumour. If no tumour is found, then treatment with omeprazole, a proton-pump inhibitor, should be instituted, and localisation investigations repeated at 2- or 3-year intervals.

Since gastrin stimulates gastric acid secretion, the clinical presentation is usually that of recurrent peptic ulceration; indeed, this was the clinical pattern originally described by Zollinger and Ellison in 1955 [4]. It is now recognised that diarrhoea and malabsorption due to a combination of acid inactivation of digestive enzymes and acid-induced mucosal damage of the upper small bowel may be a part of the syndrome, or even the major presenting feature, in 10% of patients. Indeed, with early diagnosis the classical picture of severe ulceration or perforated ulcers is rare, and many patients are clinically indistinguishable from those with simple duodenal ulceration.

Glucagonoma syndrome

The cardinal clinical feature of the glucagonoma syndrome is the necrolytic migratory erythematous rash which occurs in nearly 75% of patients [5], thus making it the only pancreatic endocrine tumour that can be diagnosed with reasonable reliability on clinical criteria alone. The rash usually starts in the groin but often affects the thighs, buttocks and perineal area and may well spread to almost anywhere within the body (Figs. 40.1 and 40.2). The rash is often associated with angular stomatitis and glossitis. The cause of the rash is unknown, and it is unlikely that the increased glucagon concentration in the blood is directly responsible although the hypocatabolic state, low plasma and skin zinc concentrations and hypoproteinaemia that are all induced by the raised glucagon level may well play a large part in the aetiology.

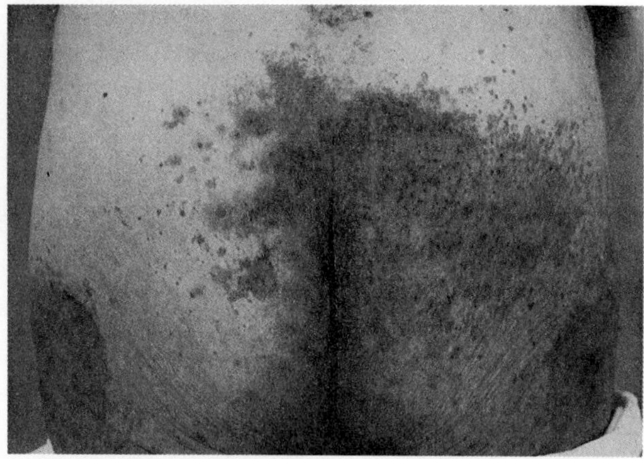

Fig. 40.1 Buttocks of a patient with the glucagonoma syndrome.

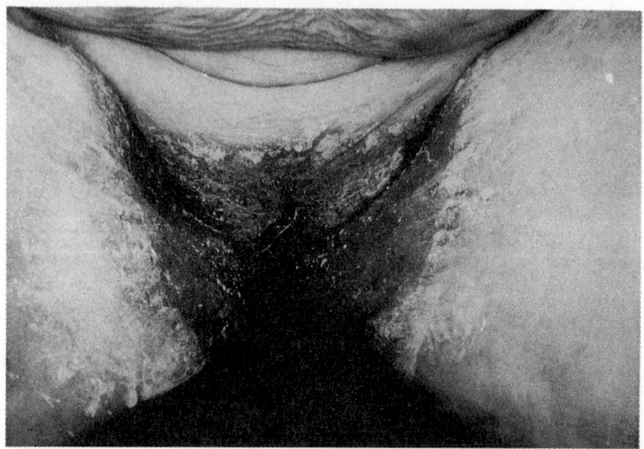

Fig. 40.2 Groin of the patient in Fig. 40.1 demonstrating severe painful excoriation associated with the glucagonoma syndrome.

The other clinical features accompanying the hyperglucagonaemia include weight loss, normochromic normocytic anaemia, psychiatric disturbance (depression is particularly common) and an increased risk of venous thrombosis which often proves fatal [6]. Glucagon levels in the plasma are considerably elevated, and thus a single blood sample will usually confirm or refute the diagnosis since the only other causes are acute hypoglycaemia, chronic renal failure and treatment with the androgenic steroid danazol. Glucagonomas often present relatively late, and permanent surgical cure is possible in < 5% of patients since liver metastases are usually present at the time of diagnosis.

VIPoma syndrome

The descriptive title of WDHA syndrome (*w*atery *d*iarrhoea, *h*ypokalaemia and *a*chlorhydria) and pancreatic cholera are used synonymously with the Verner–Morrison syndrome [7]. It is now known that peptide–histamine–valine (PHV) and peptide–histamine–methionine (PHM), two cosynthesised peptides derived from the same prepro-VIP, are also active in stimulating secretion from the bowel [8], but recent work has shown that VIP is the predominant factor in the aetiology of the VIPoma syndrome. Most VIP-secreting tumours are pancreatic in origin; however, VIP may also be secreted by ganglioneuroblastomas, which most commonly occur in childhood, and by adrenal phaeochromocytomas. Patients have profuse watery diarrhoea but without steatorrhoea, and stool volume may be up to 20 litres a day. Hypokalaemic acidosis occurs due to specific loss of bicarbonate and potassium into the bowel and is a major life-threatening feature of the disease. Death, if it occurs, is due to a combination of dehydration and cardiac standstill. Although achlorhydria was emphasised as a classical feature of the disease, it is often absent but if present does help to differentiate the VIPoma from the gastrinoma. The diagnosis of a VIPoma is dependent upon the clinical setting and the demonstration of an elevated VIP in the plasma. PHM, the flanking peptide of VIP which is cosecreted with it, is often elevated in the same plasma sample.

Other peptides secreted by neuroendocrine tumours

The islets of Langerhans contain α-cells (which secrete glucagon) and β-cells (which secrete insulin) and two other cell types; the D cells which produce somatostatin and the PP cells which produce pancreatic polypeptide. It is not surprising, therefore, to find some pancreatic endocrine tumours producing large quantities of somatostatin, PP or both. About half the patients with the somatostatinoma syndrome have diabetes mellitus, gallstones, low acid output and weight loss. These tumours are thought to be the slowest growing of all pancreatic endocrine tumours, and their natural history may be in excess of 25 years [9]. At presentation the tumour bulk may be considerable, making resection difficult. Tumours producing PP alone are not associated with a clinical syndrome [10]; indeed, elevation of plasma PP is usually detected as an incidental finding in patients suffering from one of the other pancreatic tumour syndromes [11] (Table 40.2). PP elevation is thus useful as a general marker [12] for the presence of pancreatic endocrine tumours (as is the enzyme neuron-specific enolase [13] and the proteins chromogranin and 7B2 [14]), and its presence often helps to confirm the diagnosis of an islet-cell tumour.

Ten per cent of VIPomas also have an elevated neurotensin, and even more rarely patients may be found to have a pure neurotensin-secreting tumour [15], but in neither case are symptoms currently attributable to the elevated neurotensin. It is noteworthy that fibrolamellar carcinomas of the liver, a rare endocrine type of tumour, also produce large quantities

Table 40.2 Number and percentage of patients with islet-cell tumours who have coincidental elevation of pancreatic polypeptide (PP). Adapted from Bloom SR, Polak JM (eds): *Gut Hormones* (2nd edn.). Edinburgh: Churchill Livingstone, 1981.

Primary clinical diagnosis	Number studied	Number (%) with PP > 300 pmol/l
Gastrinoma	169	96 (57)
Insulinoma	86	15 (18)
Glucagonoma	42	18 (44)
VIPoma	47	29 (61)
PPoma	5	5 (100)
Somatostatinoma	3	2 (66)
Neurotensinoma	4	2 (50)
All pancreatic endocrine tumours	326	167 (51)
Carcinoid syndrome	115	54 (47)

of neurotensin but have no associated clinical endocrine syndrome.

A whole range of other peptides secreted by neuroendocrine pancreatic tumours with appropriate clinical syndromes have been described in the literature including adrenocorticotrophic hormone (ACTH)- or corticotrophin-releasing hormone (CRH)-secreting tumours with associated Cushing's syndrome [16], growth hormone-releasing hormone (GHRH)-secreting tumours with secondary acromegaly, parathyroid hormone-related peptide (PTHRP) with associated hypercalcaemia and hypophosphataemia. The latter, which is seen fairly frequently in specialised centres, can be confusing initially as endocrinologists are attuned to MEN patients and thus suspect parathyroid hyperplasia. However, plasma PTH itself is very low, indicating another cause of the hypercalcaemia.

Long-term follow-up

Follow-up of patients with pancreatic endocrine tumours over a 5-year period [17] has revealed that, subsequent to their initial diagnosis, up to 7% of patients will develop elevation of other hormone levels with new associated clinical symptoms. Over 50% of these patients will develop hypergastrinaemia with the clinical features of a gastrinoma.

It is now recognised that with the advent of improved palliative techniques, patients may thus live long enough to develop a second or even third hormone syndrome with associated new and potentially fatal clinical symptoms. Awareness of this possibility will allow prompt therapy and decrease morbidity and mortality in patients who develop hypergastrinaemia as their second or third hormonal elevation. We therefore recommend that once the diagnosis of a pancreatic endocrine tumour (be it secretory or non-secretory) has been made, the patient should have their gut hormones monitored at regular intervals (ideally every 6 months) for life.

Investigation and localisation of islet-cell tumours

Modern radioimmunoassay and biochemical methods for measuring hormone levels are specific and accurate. The normal ranges for plasma and urinary values for most of the clinically important hormones and their degradation products have now been established. Significant elevation of particular hormones in the presence of an appropriate clinical syndrome establishes the existence of an islet-cell tumour. Once the presence of an islet tumour is suspected, every effort should be made to localise the tumour. Surgical removal is curative in the case of benign lesions, while in the case of malignant lesions surgery may reduce the risk of secondary spread. Where spread has occurred the patient may obtain excellent palliation for many years as a result of debulking surgery.

Imaging techniques (see also Chapter 65)

Centres that have expertise in a particular technique tend to use and report their experience with it. Hence the literature is full of series making claims about success rates that other centres have difficulty matching.

Ultrasound

Ultrasound imaging does not require the use of ionising radiation, is widely available, non-invasive and relatively cheap. Published success rates for the detection of small insulinomas vary widely from 25 to 60%, whilst the results for gastrinomas are worse, averaging about 20%. In centres that have experience in the use of transoesophageal ultrasound, detection rates for pancreatic and duodenal tumours are high. Intraoperative ultrasound is excellent for the detection of tumours not found prior to surgery. At surgery, however, systematic palpation by an experienced surgeon is as good as most techniques described.

Computed tomography scanning

Computed tomography (CT) scanning is relatively non-invasive, and modern scanners produce very high resolution images (Fig. 40.3). Short-time scans decrease problems due to respiratory movement, and the performance of rapid dynamic scanning following a bolus injection of contrast increases the likelihood of detecting a small vascular en-

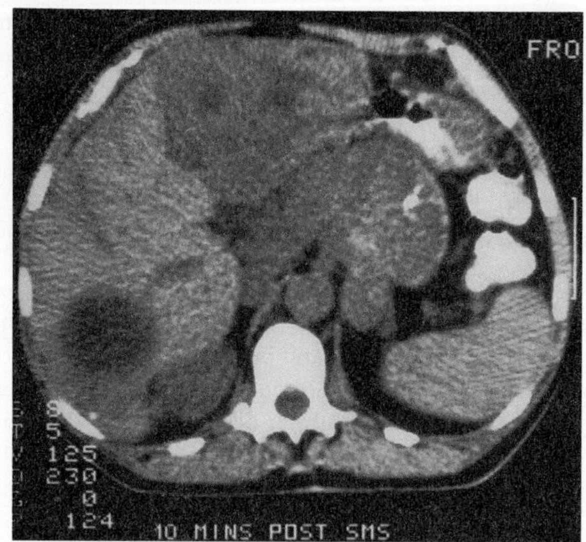

Fig. 40.3 Computed tomography scan of the abdomen of a patient with the vasoactive intestinal polypeptide (VIP)oma syndrome, demonstrating multiple hepatic metastases in both lobes of the liver.

hancing tumour. Detection rates are between 80 and 90% [18], though the gastrinoma is by far the most difficult to localise since it is frequently extrapancreatic and often very small at the time of presentation, up to 40% being < 10 mm in diameter.

Angiography [19]

Angiography and arteriography have now become the yardstick for assessment of pancreatic endocrine tumours, often used in combination with portal venous sampling. The highest rates of tumour localisation are achieved when meticulous arteriography technique is combined with skilled radiography. With this, localisation is achieved in up to 92% of cases. Combining angiography with local arterial tumour stimulation and simultaneous venous sampling, a simpler procedure, gives localisation rates of up to 100% [20].

Radiolabelled somatostatin-analogue scans

In this technique radiolabelled somatostatin is injected intravenously and the subject scanned to see if an abnormal population of somatostatin receptors exists. Most islet-cell tumours express an excess of these receptors, and in extensive disease can be easily detected. However, the role of this kind of scanning in detecting the smaller primary tumour may be disappointing. A recent development is the use of the intraoperative injection of radiolabelled somatostatin, and a hand-held γ detecting probe. This technique appears useful for the identification of extent of spread and may help delineate the margins for resection at the time of surgery. Other peptides are being labelled and used for scanning also, in particular chromogranin and VIP. Tumours that express somatostatin receptors in general respond to somatostatin-analogue therapy [21].

Therapy of pancreatic endocrine tumours

Since islet-cell tumours are slow growing, morbidity and even mortality are usually initially caused by the metabolic disturbance induced by the secreted peptide(s) rather than by tumour bulk alone. It is therefore worthwhile to actively treat such tumours and reduce peptide secretion or neutralise its effect even when multiple metastases exist. This can achieve long-term palliation in many instances of metastatic disease.

Surgery

Complete surgical excision is the only means of cure of islet-cell tumours. This is feasible in the insulinoma in up to 90% of cases and may occasionally occur in the VIP-oma and glucagonoma [22]. However, even when at laparotomy one single lesion is found with no evidence of macroscopic metastases, hepatic metastases often manifest themselves many years later. As the majority of tumours present with metastases, debulking surgery is the only operative option available [23]. This consists of excising the primary tumour and metastases where possible, since a decrease in tumour bulk in turn will reduce peptide production and hence relieve symptoms.

Hepatic artery embolisation [24–26]

Good palliation may result from embolizing the hepatic artery supplying the liver metastases. This requires considerable expertise and the portal vein must be fully patent (Fig. 40.4). All patients become pyrexial and have a dramatic alteration in their liver function tests during the first week following embolisation, as the tumour literally infarcts. Duration in response to successful embolisation ranges from 3 to 10 months, with a median of 5 months (Fig. 40.5). The procedure may be repeated a number of times when symptoms recur, providing the portal vein remains patent. Large doses of somatostatin analogues in the period immediately following embolisation are usually needed. This decreases the symptoms resulting from the 'rush' release of tumour products that occurs with infarction of the tumour.

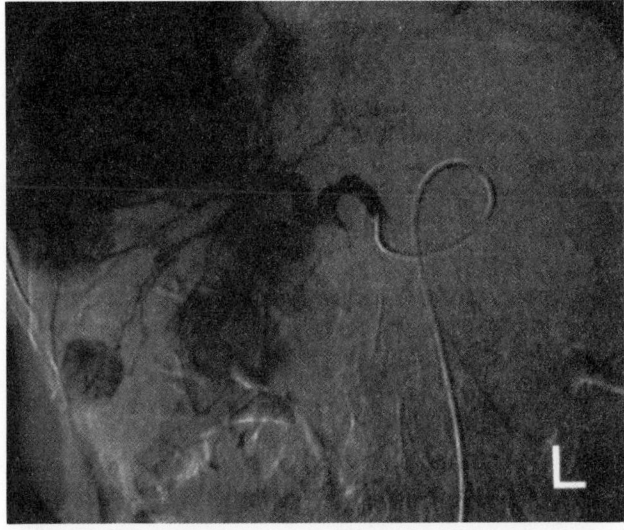

(a)

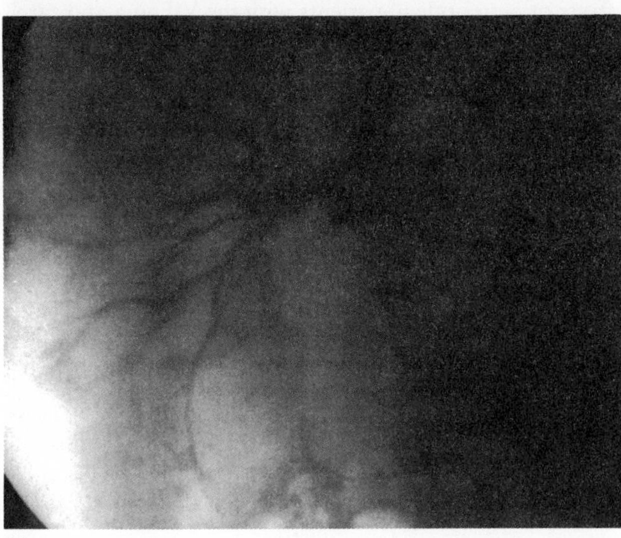

(b)

Fig. 40.4 Angiogram demonstrating multiple, vascular, hepatic metastases in a patient with the glucagonoma syndrome, before (a) and after (b) embolisation.

Cytotoxic chemotherapy [27–31]

Initial reports of chemotherapy in carcinoid from Moertel [32] using 5-fluorouracil and streptozotocin were encouraging with a response rate for the islet-cell tumours of 63%. However, while 63% 'responded' the *magnitude* of the response is often small. Further studies since then using different dosage regimens of streptozotocin and 5-fluorouracil, with or without the addition of vincristine or adriamycin, have shown little improvement on these figures. The regime we use is 500 mg/m^2 of streptozotocin and 400 mg/m^2 of 5-fluorouracil infusion, on alternate days for 10 days with close monitoring of renal, hepatic and bone-marrow function. Courses are given at 2–3-month intervals, and we

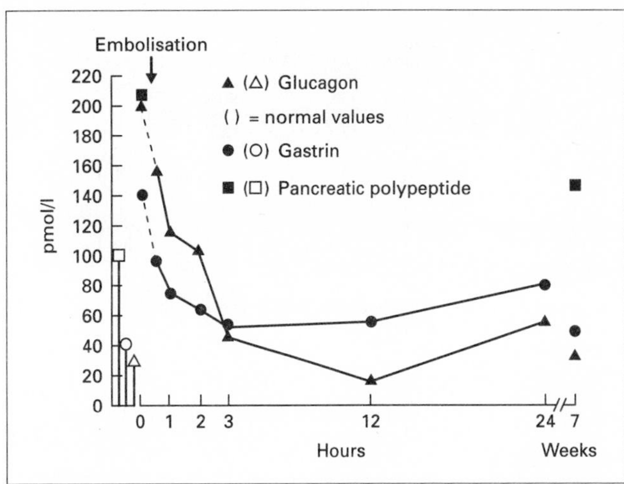

Fig. 40.5 Follow-up of a patient with a mixed islet-cell tumour secreting gastrin and glucagon. Response to hepatic artery embolisation.

would give at least three to four courses before concluding that there is no tumour response. Since most patients do not benefit significantly and the treatment is unpleasant and nephrotoxic, it should be not be used as first-line therapy. The exception is VIPomas, which are particularly sensitive to chemotherapy, the response rate being as high as 90%. Gastrinomas respond less well, the response rate of 20% being similar to that of the carcinoid syndrome. Mean duration of palliation is between 11 and 18 months.

Use of recombinant α-interferon has been proposed, with reported excellent response rates in terms of a reduction in peptide secretion; however, the number of patients who actually show a decrease in tumour bulk was not more than 25%. Recent studies have supported the poor response rates and highlighted the many side-effects, including autoimmune haemolytic anaemia and leukopenia with associated flu-like symptoms. We do not currently advocate the use of interferon for the average patient as the adverse effects of the treatment exceed the symptoms of the disease.

Long-acting somatostatin analogues

Varying doses of somatostatin analogues [33] (Fig. 40.6) have been shown to significantly lower basal plasma levels of PP, glucagon, insulin, VIP and gastrin and also suppress post-prandial release of VIP and gastrin in patients with pancreatic endocrine tumours. Clinical symptoms caused by the hormonal secretion have also diminished or even abolished in the majority of patients with pancreatic endocrine and carcinoid tumours treated with these analogues. The cloning of the five distinct receptor subtypes for somatostatin has opened the way for potentially more selective analogues to target symptom control in this tumour group [21].

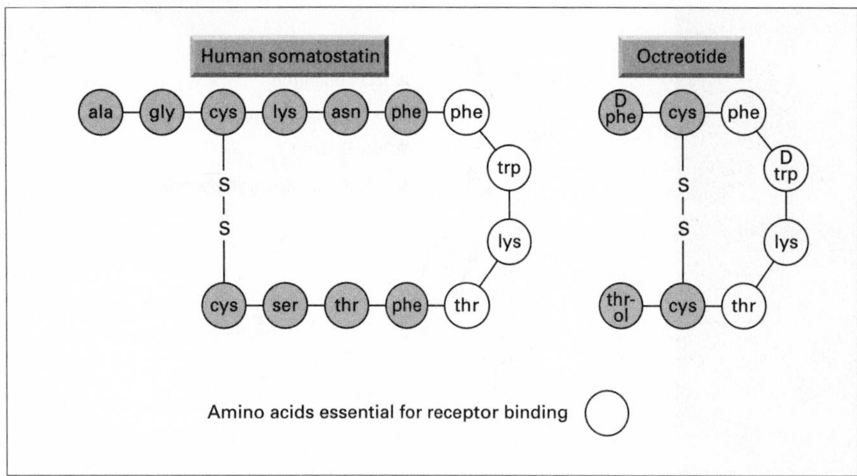

Fig. 40.6 Structure of native somatostatin and the long-acting octapeptide analogue octreotide (Sandostatin). Note the identical amino-acid residues at the receptor-binding site.

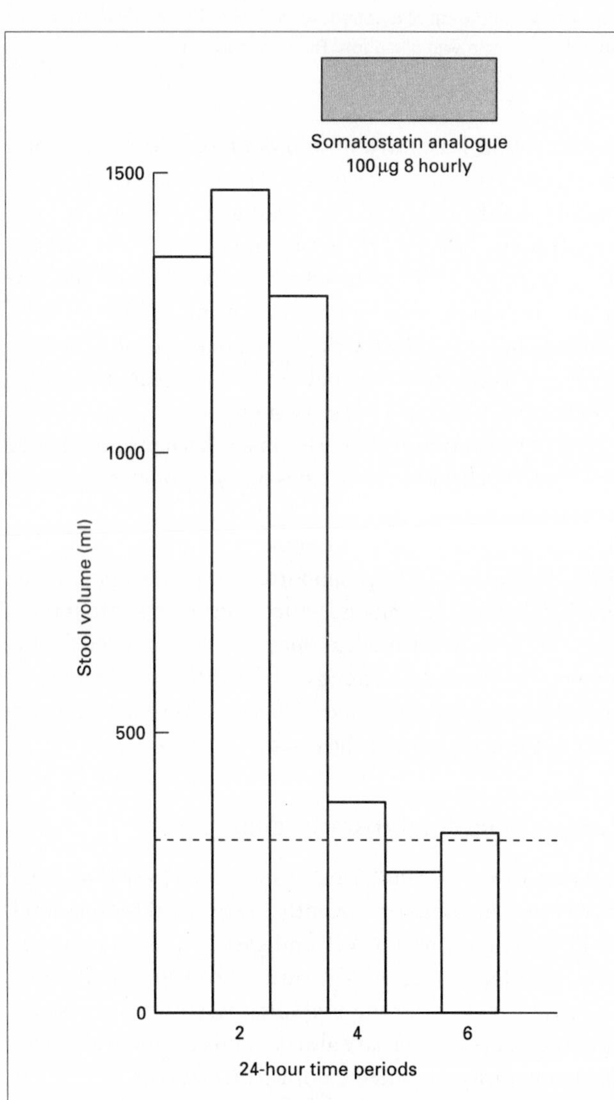

Fig. 40.7 Response in a vasoactive intestinal polypeptide (VIP)oma patient to the introduction of octreotide. Note a profound and sustained fall in the daily stool volume.

A number of case studies have demonstrated the life-saving effects of octreotide in patients with the VIPoma and carcinoid syndromes who were having acute crises. Diarrhoea was reduced within 24 hours to almost normal and major electrolyte imbalance resolved within 48 hours (Figs. 40.7 and 40.8). Studies have also shown that the length and severity of the glucagonoma rash exacerbation is reduced with chronic analogue therapy [34].

We have now treated patients with glucagonomas and VIPomas over an 8-year period with these analogues. Treatment is initially very effective in all cases, symptoms being improved or alleviated with an associated reduction in hormonal levels. Escape from symptom control may occur as early as 5 months after the start of therapy (100 μg twice daily) but can be countered by increasing the dose of octreotide over the next 6–12 months to a maximum of 500 μg t.d.s. This dose is rarely needed. If complete resistance emerges, patients tend to die within a 6-month period once this phase of their illness had been reached [35,36]. One of the problems even with the long-acting analogues has been their required three times a day administration. We and others have been studying several very-slow-release preparations of somatostatin analogues. They appear to provide equivalent or better symptom control and require injection from once a week to once a month. This development will undoubtedly further improve the quality of life in these patients. Several of these subtypes of somatostatin receptors activate tyrosine phosphatases and thus might be expected to reduce cell growth rates. There is some clinical evidence to confirm slower tumour growth with somatostatin-analogue therapy.

Other treatments

Gastrinoma

Omeprazole and lanoprazole, substituted benzimidazoles,

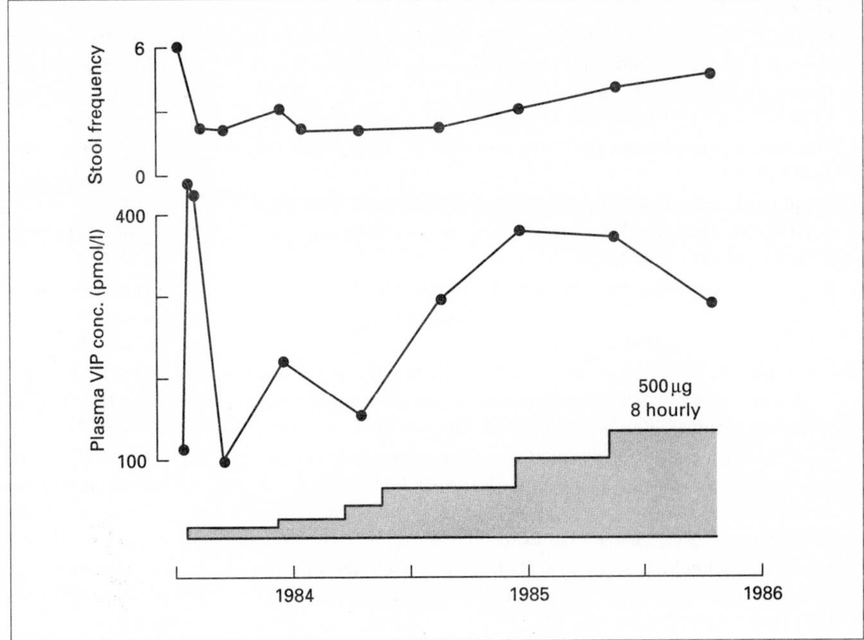

Fig. 40.8 Two-year follow-up of another patient with the vasoactive intestinal polypeptide (VIP)oma syndrome on octreotide demonstration that the analogue maintains the stool volume within normal limits despite the elevation of VIP to prediagnosis level, implying a direct effect of the analogue on the bowel.

are highly effective, non-competitive inhibitors of the gastric hydrogen potassium adenosine triphosphatase (ATPase) ('proton pump'), and are thus referred to as inducing a 'medical gastrectomy'. Acid inhibition is almost absolute at doses of 80–120 mg/day [37], and will reduce the basal acid output to <5 mmol/hour after 2 days of treatment. Ninety-five per cent of ulcers will heal within 2 weeks of therapy, and all heal within 1 month. Providing therapy is maintained long term, symptoms and ulcers do not recur.

Glucagonoma

Apart from non-specific chemotherapy, hepatic artery embolisation and use of somatostatin analogues, ofther therapeutic measures particularly for the rash include tight control of the diabetes (with insulin), oral and topical zinc, and amino-acid and blood transfusions during an acute exacerbation.

VIPoma

Once again chemotherapy (which is very effective for VIPomas), hepatic artery embolisation and octreotide are the main treatment modalities; other palliative measures include electrolyte support during an acute exacerbation when many litres of intravenous saline will be required. High-dose steroid (40–60 mg prednisolone/day) is effective, if other measures to control the diarrhoea have failed. The steroid common of symptoms is generally a temporary phenomenon and escape usually occurs within 6 months.

Summary

Radioimmunoassay and immunocytochemistry for a large range of peptides has allowed the diagnosis of an increasing number of different tumour types and associated clinical syndromes. Peptide secretion from many tumours is mixed. When exception of the insulinoma, most islet-cell tumours are malignant, and metastases at the time of diagnosis makes surgical cure rare. Effective palliative regimes with cytotoxic agents, hepatic artery embolisation and recently developed long-acting somatostatin analogues have allowed a reasonable quality of life in previously terminal situations.

References

1 Wilder R, Allen FR, Power MH, Robertson HE. Carcinoma of the islets of the pancreas. Hyperinsulinism and hypoglycaemia. *JAMA* 1987; **89**: 348–61.
2 O'Shea DB, Bloom SR. Gastrointestinal polypeptides as tumour markers. *TMU* 1994; **6**: 107–10.
3 Friessen SR. Tumours of the endocrine pancreas. *N Engl J Med* 1982; **306**: 580–90.
4 Zollinger RM, Ellison EH. Primary peptide ulceration of the jejunum associated with islet cell tumours of the pancreas. *Ann Surg* 1955; **142**: 709–73.
5 Sweet D. A dermatosis specifically associated with a tumour of pancreatic alpha cells. *Br J Dermatol* 1984; **90**: 301–8.
6 Mallinson CN, Bloom SR, Warin AP, Salmon PR, Cox B. A glucagonoma syndrome. *Lancet* 1974; **ii**: 1–5.
7 Verner JV, Morrison AB. Islet cell tumour and a syndrome of refractory, watery diarrhoea and hypokalemia. *Am J Med* 1958; **25**: 374–80.

8 Yiangou Y, Williams SJ, Bishop AE, Polak JM, Bloom SR. Peptide–Histidine–Methionine-Immunoreactivity in plasma and tissue from patients with VIP secreting tumours and watery diarrhoea. *J Clin Endocrinol Metab* 1987; **64**: 131–9.
9 Krejs GJ, Orci L, Conlon JM *et al.* Somatostatinoma syndrome: biochemical, morphologic and clinical features. *N Engl J Med* 1979; **301**: 285–92.
10 Tomita T, Friesen S, Kimmel JR, Doull V, Pollock HG. Pancreatic polypeptide secreting islet cell tumours: a study of three cases. *Am J Pathol* 1983; **113**: 134–42.
11 Adrian TE, Uttenthal LO, William SJ, Bloom SR. Secretion of pancreatic polypeptide in patients with pancreatic and endocrine tumours. *N Engl J Med* 1986; **315**: 287–91.
12 Polak JM, Bloom SR, Adrian TE, Heitz PH, Bryant MG, Pearse AGE. Pancreatic polypeptide in insulinomas, gastrinomas, VIPomas and glucagonomas. *Lancet* 1976; **i**: 328–30.
13 Polak JM, Marangos PJ. Neuron-specific enolase: a marker for neuroendocrine cells. In: Falkmer S, Hakanson R, Sundler F, eds. *Evolution and Tumour Pathology of the Neuroendocrine System.* Amsterdam: Elsevier Science Publishers, 1984.
14 Suzuki H, Ghatei MA, Williams SJ *et al.* Product of pituitary protein 7B2 I-R by endocrine tumours and its possible diagnostic value. *J Clin Endocrinol Metab* 1986; **63**: 758–65.
15 Blackburn AM, Bryant MG, Adrian TE, Bloom SR. Pancreatic tumours produce neurotensin. *J Clin Endocrinol Metab* 1981; **52**: 820–2.
16 Lokich J, Bothe A, O'Hara C, Fedamen D. Metastatic islet cell tumour with ACTH, gastrin and glucagon secretion clinical and pathological studies with multiple therapies. *Cancer* 1987; **59**: 2053–8.
17 Wynick D, Williams SJ and Bloom SR. Symptomatic secondary hormone syndromes in patients with established malignant pancreatic endocrine tumours. *N Engl J Med* 1988; **319**: 599–604.
18 Galiber AK, Reading CC, Charboneau JW *et al.* Localisation of pancreatic insulinoma: comparison of pre- and intraoperative US with CT and angiography. *Radiology* 1988; **166**: 405–8.
19 Rossi P, Allison DJ, Bezzi M *et al.* Endocrine tumors of the pancreas. *Radiol Clin North Am* 1989; **27**: 129–61.
20 O'Shea D, Rohrer-Theus A, Lynn JA, Jackson JA, Bloom SR. Localisation of insulinomas by selective intraarterial injection of calcium. *J Clin Endocrinol Metab* 1996; **81**: 1623–7.
21 O'Shea D, Bloom SR. Somatostatin in the diagnosis and treatment of neuroendocrine tumors. *Curr Opin Endocrinol Diabetes* 1995; **2**: 177–81.
22 Thompson GB, van Heerden JA, Grant CS, Carney JA, Ilstrup DM. Islet cell carcinomas of the pancreas: a twenty-year experience. *Surgery* 1988; **104**: 1011–17.
23 McCarthy DE. The place of surgery in the Zollinger Ellison syndrome. *N Engl J Med* 1980; **302**: 1344–7.
24 Ajani JA, Carrasco CH, Charnsangavej C, Samaan NA, Levin B, Wallace S. Islet cell tumors metastatic to the liver: effective palliation by sequential hepatic artery embolization. *Ann Intern Med* 1988; **108**: 340–4.
25 Alison DM, Modlin IM, Jenkins WJ. Treatment of carcinoid liver metastases by hepatic artery embolisation. *Lancet* 1977; **2**: 1323–5.
26 Alison DM. Therapeutic embolisation. *Br J Hosp Med* 1978; **20**: 707–15.
27 Broder LE, Carter SK. Pancreatic islet cell carcinoma. II. Results of therapy with streptozotocin in 52 patients. *Ann Intern Med* 1973; **79**: 108–18.
28 Frame J, Kelsen D, Kemeny N *et al.* A phase II trial of streptozotocin and adriamycin in advanced APUD tumors. *Am J Clin Oncol* 1988; **11**: 490–5.
29 Hansen R, Helm J, Wilson JF, Wilson S. Nonfunctioning islet cell carcinoma of the pancreas. Complete response to continuous 5-fluorouracil infusion. *Cancer* 1988; **62**: 15–17.
30 Kvols LK, Moertel CG, O'Connell MJ, Schutt AJ, Rubin J, Hahn RG. Treatment of the malignant carcinoid syndrome. Evaluation of a long-acting somatostatin analogoue. *N Engl J Med* 1986; **315**: 663–6.
31 Lee SM, Forbes A, Williams R. Metastatic islet cell tumour with clinical manifestations of insulin and glucagon excess: successful treatment by hepatic artery embolisation and chemotherapy. *Eur J Surg Oncol* 1988; **14**: 265–8.
32 Moertel CG, Hanley JA, Johnson LA. Streptozotocin alone compared with 5-flourouracil in treatment of advanced islet cell carcinoma. *N Engl J Med* 1980; **303**: 1189–94.
33 Bauer W, Brimer U, Doepfner W *et al.* SMS 201–995: a very potent and selective octapeptide analogue of somatostatin with prolonged action. *Life Sci* 1982; **31**: 1133–41.
34 Anderson JV, Bloom SR. Neuroendocrine tumours of the gut: long-term therapy with the somatostatin analogue SMS 201–995. *Scand J Gastroenterol* 1986; **21** (Suppl. 119): 115–28.
35 Lamberts SW, Pieters GF, Metselaar HJ, Ong GL, Tan HS, Reubi JC. Development of resistance to a long-acting somatostatin analogue during treatment of two patients with metastatic endocrine pancreatic tumours. *Acta Endocrinol (Copenh)* 1988; **119**: 561–6.
36 Wynick D, Anderson JV, Williams SJ, Bloom SR. Resistance of metastatic pancreatic endocrine tumours after long term treatment with the somatostatin analogue octreotide (SMS 201–995). *Clin Endocrinol* 1988; **30**: 385–8.
37 McArthur J, Collen MJ, Maton PN *et al.* Omeprazole: Effective, convenient therapy for Zollinger–Ellison syndrome. *Gastroenterology* 1985; **88**: 939–44.

Part 8
Disorders of Calcium Metabolism

CHAPTER 41

Regulation of calcium metabolism: hypercalcaemia

D.A.Heath

Introduction

Calcium metabolism is carefully regulated by a series of hormonal factors resulting in fine control of serum calcium and skeletal calcium. The normal range of serum calcium concentration is usually between 2.2 and 2.6 mmol/l (8.8–10.4 mg/100 ml), but in the individual patient it varies by a much smaller amount.

Calcium in serum exists as ionised (Ca^{2+}), protein-bound and complexed forms, all of which are measured by the standard 'total' calcium methods. Complexed calcium represents a small percentage of total calcium, usually $<5\%$, while the remainder is usually equally divided between ionised and protein-bound forms. Only the ionised form is physiologically active but it is much more difficult to measure, and to date no automated method has been developed. Protein-bound calcium is mainly associated with albumin and, to a lesser degree, globulins. Changes in serum protein concentrations markedly influence protein-bound calcium without affecting ionised calcium and hence alter total calcium levels (Fig. 41.1). It is therefore advisable always to measure serum albumin (and possibly globulin) at the same time as serum calcium.

While it is customary to state that blood for serum calcium estimation should be taken from an uncuffed arm, this is impractical and unnecessary. Only prolonged venous stasis increases serum calcium concentration and this is accompanied by an increase in the levels of serum proteins and hence can easily be detected. No disease state has been described whereby there is an overproduction of albumin, and an elevated serum albumin level is due to either venous stasis or dehydration. Many diseases are associated with hyperglobulinaemia. Because the various globulins bind calcium differently it is very difficult to interpret total calcium changes in hyperglobulinaemic states. Many disease states are associated with hypoalbuminaemia and this will cause a reduced total calcium concentration.

Serum calcium concentration is regulated by controlling the passage of calcium from the intestine, bone and kidneys (Fig. 41.2). Absorption from the intestine is under the control of 1,25-dihydroxyvitamin D but probably plays little part in the minute-to-minute control of serum calcium levels. Provided the patient has an adequate calcium intake a further increase in oral calcium does not lead to a significant increase in net calcium absorption but merely an increase in faecal calcium excretion.

The skeleton consists of a large reservoir of calcium which imparts great mechanical strength to the bones. In addition, it provides a source of calcium to help maintain the serum calcium. Normal calcification of bone requires adequate concentrations of 1,25-dihydroxyvitamin D, which probably acts by allowing appropriate concentrations of calcium and phosphate to be produced in the vicinity of the calcification front. Vitamin D deficiency is associated with rickets in children and osteomalacia in adults. While being essential for normal bone formation, vitamin D in excess, by a direct action on bone, increases bone resorption and causes hypercalcaemia. Although bone formation appears to be normal in parathyroid hormone (PTH) deficiency states, PTH has a very important action on bone, increasing bone resorption. While osteoclasts are the cells responsible for resorption and are increased in number in hyperparathyroid states, PTH acts directly on osteoblasts, the bone-forming cells. By mechanisms that are not yet understood, but almost certainly involve paracrine factors, the osteoblasts stimulate increased osteoclastic activity. For this reason most disorders associated with increased bone resorption are also associated with increased bone formation. Under normal circumstances, the amount of calcium entering and leaving bone is the same, and this is essential to maintain the integrity of the skeleton.

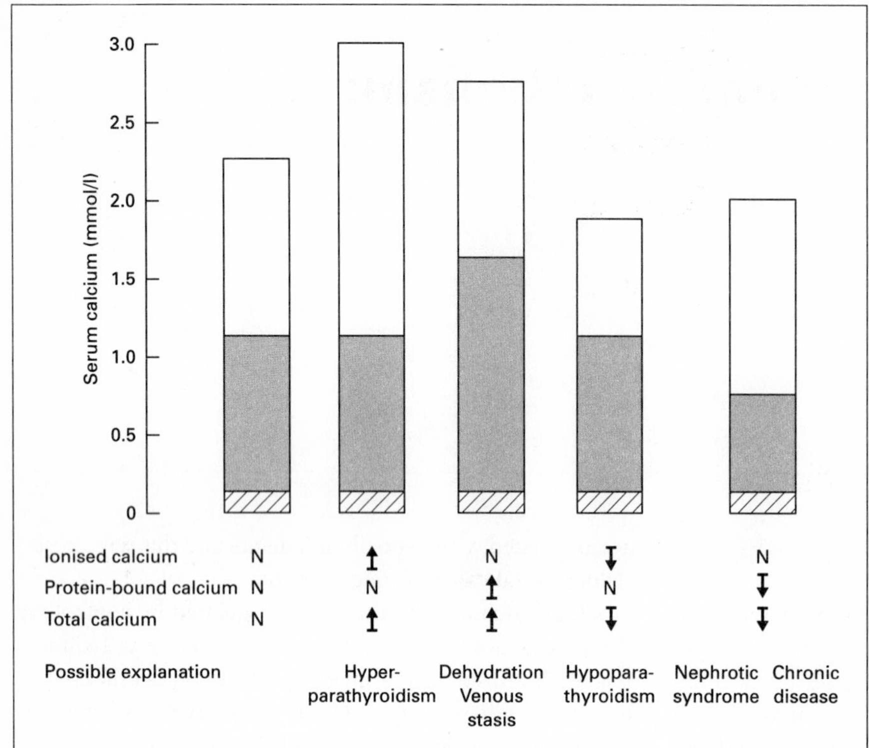

Fig. 41.1 Diagrammatic representation of the influences of changes in serum protein concentration on total serum calcium levels. Open bars represent ionised calcium; grey bars represent protein-bound calcium; and hatched bars represent complexed calcium.

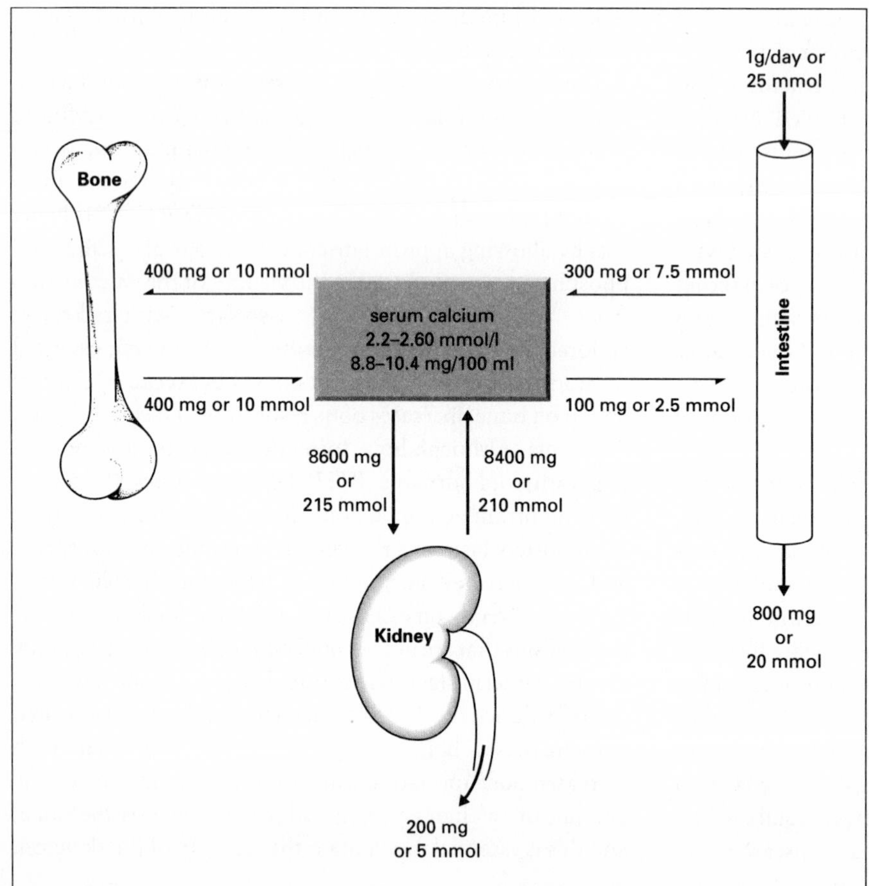

Fig. 41.2 Diagrammatic representation of calcium balance in an adult who is in zero balance. The figures represent typical amounts exchanged by the major organs.

Mobilisation of skeletal calcium takes time, and the minute-to-minute regulation of serum calcium concentration is unlikely to be due to rapid changes in bone resorption.

Large amounts of calcium are filtered by the kidney every day, with the vast majority being reabsorbed in the proximal and distal tubules. Very small changes in the fractional reabsorption of calcium have the potential to cause rapid, large changes in serum calcium concentration. For this reason it is likely that the regulation of renal calcium handling is the most important factor in controlling serum calcium levels. Renal calcium handling is affected by many factors including PTH, 1,25-dihydroxyvitamin D and renal sodium status.

Parathyroid hormone

Like many peptide hormones, PTH is initially synthesised as a larger precursor, prepro-PTH, in membrane-bound ribosomes. The amino-terminal portion of the molecule is termed the leader sequence, and allows the protein to be transported to the rough endoplasmic reticulum (RER); the leader sequence is then cleaved to yield pro-PTH. Pro-PTH passes from the RER to the Golgi apparatus, during which the pro sequence is removed. PTH is subsequently stored in secretory vesicles. The major regulator of PTH secretion is extracellular calcium and, to a lesser degree, magnesium (Fig. 41.3). Low calcium concentration stimulates PTH secretion while a high calcium concentration inhibits but does not completely suppress secretion. Magnesium has similar but weaker effects, although marked magnesium deficiency can inhibit PTH secretion and cause hypocalcaemia. In addition, 1,25-dihydroxyvitamin D inhibits PTH secretion by a direct action on the parathyroid gland. The regulation of PTH secretion by Ca^{2+} involves an extracellular Ca^{2+}-sensing receptor (CaR) situated in the wall of the parathyroid cell [1]. The receptor is present in other tissues including renal cortex and medulla. Abnormalities of this receptor can lead to a resetting of the 'calciostat' resulting in either hypercalcaemia (familial benign hypercalcaemia) or hypocalcaemia (familial hypocalcaemia). CaR is a member of the superfamily of G-protein-coupled receptors. Stimulation of the receptor leads to an increase in phospholipase-C activity and the intracellular accumulation of inositol 1,4,5-trisphosphate. This, in turn increases cytosolic calcium and decreases PTH release from the parathyroid cell. The regulation of PTH gene transcription, as well as PTH secretion, is regulated by calcium and vitamin D, and the upstream region of the PTH gene contains a specific promoter element which interacts with 1,25-dihydroxyvitamin D and inhibits transcription as well as sequences responsive to the level of extracellular calcium [2].

Secreted PTH consists of 84 amino acids of which the first 34 are responsible for all the known biological actions

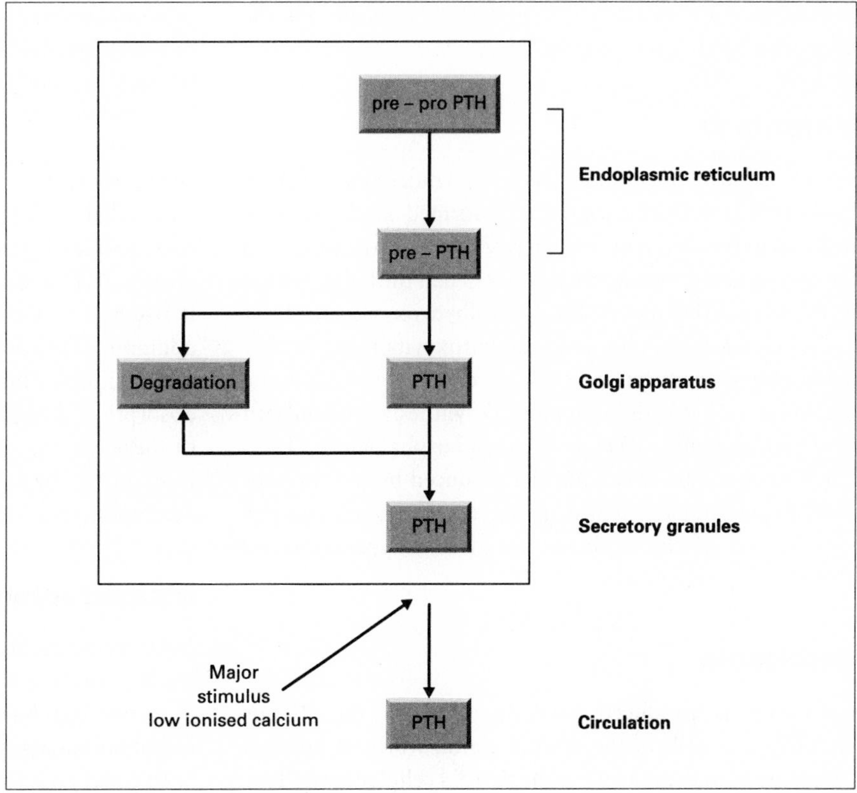

Fig. 41.3 Diagrammatic representation of parathyroid hormone synthesis and secretion within the parathyroid gland.

of PTH. The function of the remaining 50 amino acids is unknown. Either during circulation or after binding to its receptors, a proportion of the intact PTH is cleaved yielding biologically inactive fragments. The half-life of PTH is about 8 min but the carboxy-terminal fragments have a longer half-life and can accumulate, especially in renal failure.

The main target organs for PTH action are bone and kidney. Both are thought to contain transmembrane receptors for PTH which are linked by intermediary G-proteins to a classical adenylate cyclase system. Stimulation of the receptor by PTH results in the production of cyclic adenosine monophosphate (cAMP). In addition, PTH is now known to influence the phosphoinositide system, and both mechanisms can influence cytosolic calcium concentrations.

The action of PTH on bone is to increase bone resorption, although there is also experimental evidence that, under certain circumstances, bone formation can be increased. On the kidney, PTH increases calcium resorption while at the same time increasing phosphorus excretion. It also increases 1,25-dihydroxyvitamin D synthesis. Other actions of PTH include actions on vascular smooth muscle causing vasodilatation and stimulation of plasminogen activator activity.

Although there is abundant evidence that PTH-related protein messenger RNA (PTHrP-mRNA) is present in parathyroid tissue and that small amounts can be extracted from parathyroid adenomas, there is no evidence that this protein plays any role in the regulation of serum calcium or in causing hypercalcaemia in hyperparathyroidism. (For the actions of PTHrP, see Chapter 74).

Vitamin D

The metabolism of vitamin D is covered more extensively in Chapter 42. Basically, vitamin D, formed in the skin or ingested in the diet, is converted to 25-hydroxyvitamin D in the liver, and this metabolite is converted in the kidney either to the very active metabolite 1,25-dihydroxyvitamin D or to the inactive metabolite 24,25-dihydroxyvitamin D. Which metabolite is produced is dependent on a variety of factors. Increased 1,25-dihydroxyvitamin D synthesis is stimulated by hypocalcaemia, PTH and hypophosphataemia. 1,25-Dihydroxyvitamin D can also be produced by certain non-renal tissues, in particular activated macrophages, and this may be one of the explanations for the hypercalcaemia complicating sarcoidosis.

Calcitonin

Calcitonin is produced predominantly by the 'C' or parafollicular cells of the thyroid gland, which in humans constitute a small minority of the thyroid cellular mass. Two calcitonin genes have been recognised which both encode two proteins, calcitonin and calcitonin gene-related peptide (CGRP). By a process of differential splicing, either calcitonin or CGRP mRNA is produced (see also Chapter 3). Translation of the mRNA produces prohormones which are processed to yield either calcitonin or CGRP together with flanking amino- and carboxy-terminal fragments (Fig. 41.4). In the second gene, the region encoding the calcitonin-like protein is not expressed. As a result, humans produce one form of calcitonin but two forms of CGRP which differ by three amino acids. The processing is tissue dependent with calcitonin mRNA predominating in the thyroid gland and CGRP mRNA in neural tissue. Both forms of CGRP can be demonstrated in neuronal cells, and receptors for it have been identified in both the central and peripheral nervous system. Calcitonin, although mainly restricted to the thyroid gland, has also been identified in small amounts in neural tissue.

Calcitonin has hypocalcaemic actions in experimental animals but in humans this is clearly apparent only in states of increased bone turnover (e.g. Paget's disease). The hypocalcaemic action is due to an inhibition of osteoclastic bone resorption. Osteoclasts contain surface receptors for calcitonin. To date, no clear-cut role for calcitonin has emerged and in medullary thyroid carcinoma, where circulating concentrations of calcitonin may be extremely high, serum calcium level is normal.

Although CGRP has weak hypocalcaemic actions, it has very potent vasodilatory actions. Its role in normal neurophysiology is currently unknown. The flanking amino- and carboxy-peptides which are produced by the processing of both the calcitonin and CGRP precursors have not yet been shown to have any specific actions.

In summary, the control of calcium homeostasis is mainly controlled by PTH and 1,25-dihydroxyvitamin D. If the extracellular ionised calcium level falls, PTH secretion increases. PTH acts on the bones to increase calcium resorption; it also acts on the kidney to increase calcium resorption. In addition, PTH increases 1,25-dihydroxyvitamin D production in the kidney. This acts on the intestine to increase calcium absorption. A high extracellular calcium level has the reverse of these effects, and as 1,25-dihydroxyvitamin D synthesis is inhibited, the production of 24,25-dihydroxyvitamin D is increased.

Measurement of PTH

Measurements of PTH play a very important part in the study of disorders of calcium metabolism. Recent advances in technology have seen the replacement of the standard radioimmunoassays by two-site radioimmunometric assays. Such assays involve the use of two antibodies to different

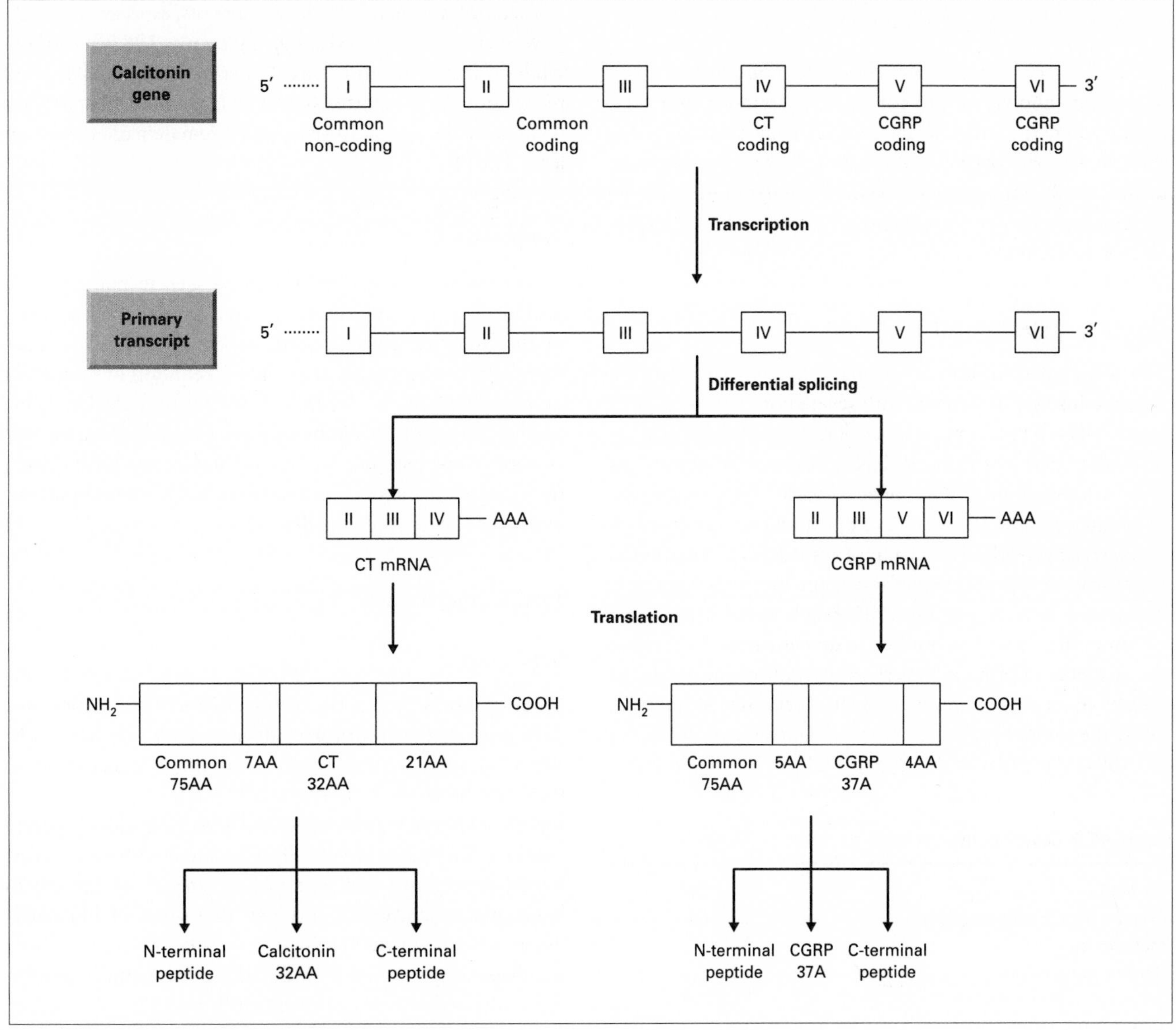

Fig. 41.4 Derivation of calcitonin and calcitonin gene-related peptide from a common gene.

regions of the PTH molecule. Only fragments containing regions recognised by both antibodies are detected. As a result, 'intact' PTH is thought to be measured and smaller biologically inactive fragments, usually detected by previous radioimmunoassays, do not get measured.

Indirect measurements of PTH action

Many indirect assessments of PTH action have been described. They include changes in serum phosphate and renal phosphate handling, renal calcium measurements and cAMP excretion. With the development of sensitive and accurate PTH assays, none is now routinely indicated.

Hypercalcaemia

The symptoms of hypercalcaemia are quite non-specific and mimic many other disorders; mild hypercalcaemia may be completely asymptomatic. Common symptoms are nausea, thirst, polyuria, constipation and malaise. With increasing hypercalcaemia, vomiting and epigastric discomfort may occur. Later, mental confusion and impaired consciousness may develop.

Hypercalcaemia can never be diagnosed with certainty from the history or physical examination. It is often brought to light by a biochemical profile which includes a calcium measurement. Where biochemical profiles are not performed, it has been suggested that a serum calcium measurement should be included in the investigation of most symptomatic patients.

Causes of hypercalcaemia

The causes of hypercalcaemia are listed in Table 41.1; they have been subdivided into common, uncommon and rare. Primary hyperparathyroidism and malignancy account for the vast majority of cases seen in clinical practice. Hospitals dealing with patients with chronic renal failure will see hypercalcaemia not infrequently. Other causes of hypercalcaemia are uncommon except in specialised clinics.

Primary hyperparathyroidism

The initial descriptions of primary hyperparathyroidism were exclusively of patients with severe bone disease and/or renal stones. At the time, serum calcium measurements were difficult to perform and were basically restricted to patients with suspected bone and renal disease. With improved techniques serum calcium measurements were performed on an increasingly broad spectrum of disorders culminating in the biochemical profile whereby calcium measurements were performed on most patients attending hospital irrespective of symptoms. This has resulted in an enormous increase in the incidence of primary hyperparathyroidism and a marked change in its presenting features. In Rochester, Minnesota, USA, the annual incidence in the diagnosis rose from 7.8 per 100 000 population in 1965 to 51.1 per 100 000 in 1974.

Table 41.1 Causes of hypercalcaemia.

Common
Primary hyperparathyroidism
Malignancy
Chronic renal failure
Uncommon
Familial benign hypercalcaemia
Thyrotoxicosis
Sarcoidosis
Milk–alkali syndrome
Vitamin D poisoning
Rare
Immobilisation
Recovery phase of acute renal failure
Phaeochromocytoma
Vasoactive intestinal peptide-secreting tumours
Lithium
Addison's disease
Idiopathic hypercalcaemia of childhood
Coccidioidomycosis
Berylliosis
Vitamin A poisoning
Benign breast hyperplasia
Hypereosinophilic syndrome

The change was mainly in elderly patients, especially women. In women aged over 60 years the figure was 188 per 100 000, while in men over 60 it was 92 per 100 000 [3]. All other recent series have reported similar changes, with most patients being over the age of 50 years and a female/male ratio of at least 3 : 1 [4].

Symptoms

A wide variety of symptoms can be seen in patients with primary hyperparathyroidism, ranging from complications of the hyperparathyroid state or symptoms of hypercalcaemia to no symptoms at all. The likelihood of symptoms or complications is dependent on the population being studied. Screening of healthy subjects is most likely to identify asymptomatic patients, while screening in specialist clinics, for example urology clinics, is most likely to find patients with complications of the disease.

Specific complications

Bone disease

Osteitis fibrosa cystica, the classic disease of bone associated with primary hyperparathyroidism, is now rare in the UK. When present, patients may complain of generalised or localised bone pain. The presence of brown tumours in superficial bones may be associated with a clinically apparent swelling. Such cases are usually associated with more severe hypercalcaemia so that many of the specific symptoms of hypercalcaemia are often present. In a series of 111 newly diagnosed patients with primary hyperparathyroidism, with the diagnosis being made following a biochemical profile, there was not one case of osteitis fibrosa [5].

Renal stones

Renal stones were the commonest presentation of hyperparathyroidism until recently. Of patients presenting with renal colic, about 1–2% will be shown to have primary hyperparathyroidism. Of the same 111 patients mentioned above, only 7% had a renal stone. Once a patient with hyperparathyroidism has had a renal stone, they are at greater risk of further stones. The reason for the increased incidence of stones is unclear as there is no difference in urinary calcium excretion in those complicated by stones as opposed to those who are not. Patients with hyperparathyroidism and renal stones often have serum calcium values which are not particularly high; if the value is close to the upper limit of normal, then repeated measurements of the calcium level will often reveal values that are within the normal range. A serum calcium level that is repeatedly around the upper limit of normal is likely to be abnormal and to indicate hyperparathyroidism.

Chondrocalcinosis

There is a well-recognised association between primary hyperparathyroidism and chondrocalcinosis. Clinically, chondrocalcinosis may present as pseudo-gout with an acute monoarthritis and this may lead to the recognition of the hyperparathyroid state. Less well recognised is precipitation of pseudo-gout shortly after a successful parathyroidectomy. Such patients who previously may never have had joint problems develop an acute arthritis. This may involve several joints and be associated with fever and malaise. A pyrexia, with a high white count and elevated erythrocyte sedimentation rate (ESR), may also be found. These features almost invariably coincide with the lowest serum calcium level and hence are usually noted 2–3 days after surgery. Unless recognised, alternative diagnoses, such as septicaemia, may be considered. There is a good response to non-steroidal anti-inflammatory drugs.

Hypertension

Hypertension has been noted in about one-third of patients. It is seldom influenced by parathyroidectomy.

Pancreatitis

Acute pancreatitis may be a presenting feature of hyperparathyroidism. As serum calcium often falls shortly after a severe attack of pancreatitis, the underlying condition can be missed unless calcium measurements are repeated after recovery.

Non-specific symptoms of hyperparathyroidism

Tiredness and fatigue

The commonest symptoms now seen in primary hyperparathyroidism are those of tiredness and fatigue [6]. These are usually attributed by the patient to ageing. Often associated with these symptoms, and perhaps causing them, is a proximal muscle weakness. Patients generally feel tired and may have to rest after physical activity. Walking, especially uphill, becomes more difficult, as does getting out of low chairs or baths.

Other non-specific symptoms of hypercalcaemia

Increased thirst, polyuria and constipation may be noted. The polyuria and polydipsia may be so marked as to suggest diabetes mellitus. Nausea and vomiting may occur with more severe hypercalcaemia.

Although 'abdominal groans' have long been claimed to be a feature of hyperparathyroidism, they are rare. The incidence of peptic ulceration is probably no higher than a control population. General abdominal discomfort may be complained of.

Vague musculoskeletal aches are not infrequently complained of. Generalised headaches, which can be severe, have been noted in a number of reported series. Itching may occur in severe hypercalcaemia, but is much more common if renal function is impaired.

Diagnosis

The diagnosis of primary hyperparathyroidism is usually simple. The presence of hypercalcaemia associated with an elevated PTH level measured in a modern two-site assay is usually sufficient to make the diagnosis. With mild hypercalcaemia the PTH value may be within the high side of the normal range. Other non-specific tests of parathyroid function are rarely, if ever, indicated. Radiological bone disease is uncommon and is virtually never seen when the serum calcium level is below 3.0 mmol/l. When present, the changes are most frequently seen on hand radiography.

Pathology

Eighty to ninety per cent of cases of primary hyperparathyroidism are due to a single parathyroid adenoma. Occasionally two adenomas may be present. Parathyroid hyperplasia affecting all four glands is present in around 10% of cases, and may indicate a familial syndrome. Parathyroid carcinoma is rare; when present it is usually locally invasive and rarely metastatic.

Management

There is currently only one effective treatment for primary hyperparathyroidism—parathyroidectomy. Medical treatment to lower serum calcium values does not reduce PTH concentrations and cannot be recommended as a long-term treatment. It may rarely be indicated when hypercalcaemia is severe to prepare the patient for subsequent surgery. Until recently most patients with hyperparathyroidism were recommended for parathyroidectomy. The identification of significant numbers of elderly, asymptomatic patients has led to a reappraisal of that policy. There is universal agreement that all patients with the complications of bone disease and/or renal stones, and patients with clear-cut symptoms of hypercalcaemia, should be offered surgery. Most would recommend surgery for all younger patients irrespective of symptoms. Older patients, for instance those over 50 years of age if asymptomatic or those with very mild symptoms, are being followed conservatively by an increasing number of clinicians [7]. If such a policy is adopted, then patients should be kept under long-term review to ensure that there is no deterioration of renal function or significant worsening of the hypercalcaemia [8]. There is a concern that mild, untreated hyperparathyroidism may accentuate bone loss in post-menopausal women. Immediately after successful parathyroidectomy, there is an increase in bone density [9]. However, short- and long-term follow-up of mild cases who have been managed conservatively do not show an increased loss of bone mass [10,11]. Furthermore, long-term follow-up has not shown any evidence of increased fracture risk [12].

Surgical management

Once the diagnosis of hyperparathyroidism has been made and a decision taken to advise a parathyroidectomy, the operation should be performed only by an experienced parathyroid surgeon [13]. Such a surgeon is likely to be performing at least 20 such operations per year. Preoperative localisation of the abnormal parathyroid glands should be undertaken only if requested by the surgeon; most experienced surgeons do not require it for the first neck exploration, reserving it for cases needing re-exploration after unsuccessful surgery [14]. Localisation techniques should never be performed in order to try to confirm a diagnosis, nor should they be considered if surgery is not envisaged. All available techniques are most successful with larger parathyroid glands which are most readily found at surgery anyway. Ultrasonographic examination in skilled hands will identify about 60% of tumours. A slightly higher proportion will be found by thallium–technetium subtraction isotope scanning, computed tomographic scanning and magnetic resonance imaging. Such techniques have not been shown to reduce operating time or to improve surgical results.

More recent studies suggest that radionucleotide scanning with ^{99m}Tc-sestamibi is the best technique for the preoperative identification of abnormal parathyroid glands. This technique is reported to have a sensitivity of around 90% with high specificity. It also appears to be the best technique for identifying mediastinal tumours. Despite these claims, it is still unnecessary to recommend routine preoperative localisation, but it can be extremely helpful following failed surgery. [15,16].

At surgery a single adenoma is looked for and removed. Confirmation that it is a parathyroid tumour should always be made using frozen sections. Three normal parathyroid glands should wherever possible be identified, although formal biopsy of all three glands significantly increases the risk of permanent postoperative hypoparathyroidism. Parathyroid hyperplasia affecting all four glands has traditionally been treated in the past by three-and-a-half-gland removal, but is frequently complicated by recurrent hyperparathyroidism. Currently one of two alternative policies can be used. All four glands can be removed and the resulting hypoparathyroidism controlled with long-term vitamin D therapy. Alternatively, all four glands can be removed and one can be cut into small slices and embedded in the muscles of the forearm. Such glands function well and, should they become overactive, they can be treated by simple local surgery rather than further neck surgery.

Following successful surgery the serum calcium concentration should have fallen into the normal range within 24 hours. Mild hypocalcaemia may then occur but is usually asymptomatic and self-correcting within 24–48 hours. In the presence of severe preoperative hypercalcaemia, especially in the presence of radiological bone disease, there may be a prolonged period of postoperative hypocalcaemia which may last for several weeks before correcting itself. When significant, it requires treating with constant intravenous calcium sufficient to maintain an adequate serum calcium concentration until the depleted bone stores have been replaced. Occasionally, permanent hypoparathyroidism develops. This is particularly likely if previous parathyroid surgery has been undertaken or if more than one parathyroid gland is removed. Such cases require long-term vitamin D therapy. Other complications of parathyroid surgery are rare. Damage to the recurrent laryngeal nerve should occur in $<1\%$ of cases.

Familial hyperparathyroidism [17]

Familial hyperparathyroidism may occur in the context of multiple endocrine neoplasia type 1 (MEN-1) and type 2 (MEN-2). In MEN-1, hyperparathyroidism is the most commonly occurring abnormality. In MEN-2, hyperparathyroidism is less common than medullary thyroid carcinoma (for further details on MEN-1 and MEN-2, see Chapters 46 and 47). Occasionally hyperparathyroidism, without other endocrine disorders, may be inherited in an autosomal dominant way. In all these familial forms of hyperparathyrodism, affected individuals are not hypercalcaemic at birth and this rarely develops before the age of 12 years (cf. familial benign hypercalcaemia).

Hypercalcaemia in chronic renal failure

Calcium disturbance is common in chronic renal failure, and hypercalcaemia can occur for a variety of different reasons [18]. Because of the failure to produce 1,25-dihydroxyvitamin D in the kidney, hypocalcaemia occurs and stimulates secondary hyperparathyroidism. To prevent this, potent vitamin D analogues—1,25-dihydroxyvitamin D or 1α-hydroxyvitamin D—may be given. Treatment with both may be complicated by hypercalcaemia.

The prolonged secondary hyperparathyroidism associated with chronic dialysis leads to parathyroid hyperplasia. In some patients the hypertrophied glands become autonomous and lead to the development of hypercalcaemia—so-called tertiary hyperparathyroidism.

In order to reduce phosphate retention in chronic renal failure, aluminium hydroxide has traditionally been given orally to bind phosphate in the gut. Small amounts of aluminium can be absorbed, leading to deposition of aluminium in the bone—so-called aluminium bone disease. Such cases are more frequently associated with hypercalcaemia even if PTH concentrations are not elevated. To avoid aluminium retention, aluminium hydroxide has in part been replaced by calcium salts, especially calcium carbonate, which itself may cause hypercalcaemia.

Hypercalcaemia of malignancy

This is considered more extensively elsewhere (see Chapter 74). Briefly, it is usually associated with disseminated malignancy. Patients rarely, if ever, develop complications such as renal stones. The patients are usually unwell with evidence of the malignant process. If confusion with hyperparathyroidism exists, the finding of a low PTH concentration would eliminate hyperparathyroidism. Malignancy and hyperparathyroidism are both common conditions in the elderly and the two may coincide. It is particularly important to realise that the patient who has a previous history of malignancy which has been thought to be cured and who develops hypercalcaemia without evidence of malignancy is most likely to have hyperparathyroidism rather than occult, recurrent malignancy. Such patients should always initially have PTH measurements rather than extensive screening for malignancy.

Familial benign hypercalcaemia [19]

Familial benign hypercalcaemia (FBH), or familial hypocalciuric hypercalcaemia (FHH), is a condition that has become increasingly recognised over the past 15 years. It emerged as an entity with the recognition that among patients initially diagnosed as having primary hyperparathyroidism, and who had undergone an unsuccessful parathyroidectomy, were some patients in whom multiple family members were hypercalcaemic. In such families parathyroidectomy was almost invariably unsuccessful in curing the hypercalcaemia. Biochemical studies revealed the tendency for a low urinary calcium excretion rate which gave rise to one of the names for the condition—FHH. FBH is a dominantly inherited condition with almost complete penetrance. Affected individuals are hypercalcaemic from birth, which is in marked contradistinction to familial hyperparathyroidism. The affected members appear to have few or no symptoms or complications of their hypercalcaemia. Consequently, they are at no greater risk of renal stones than unaffected family members. Very rarely, affected neonates can have severe hypercalcaemia at birth which is life-threatening and which may be helped by total parathyroidectomy. Only a small number of such cases have been described. Within some kindreds several cases of pancreatitis have been reported, but it remains unclear as to whether this is a real association. Because of its benign nature, the hypercalcaemia of FBH is almost invariably found by chance. If the patient is not a member of a known family with FBH there is a high risk of an erroneous diagnosis of primary hyperparathyroidism being made.

The cause of FBH has now been shown to be due to an inherited defect of the CaR (see above). A variety of mutations of the CaR gene have now been reported in families with FBH. Most affected family members are heterozygous for the mutation while those rare cases of severe neonatal disease have the homozygous form of the disorder. The occurrence of hypercalcaemia from birth and the failure of parathyroidectomy to cure the hypercalcaemia clearly separates it from primary hyperparathyroidism. Clinically, it requires identification in order that neck surgery can be avoided. Biochemically in FBH, there is a tendency for the serum magnesium concentration to be high to normal, whereas in primary hyperparathyroidism it tends to be low to normal. The urine calcium level tends to be low. Serum PTH values are variable and may vary with different assays; usually they are normal but even in the 'intact' PTH assays, mildly elevated values may occur.

None of these tests, individually or together, will unequivocally separate FBH from primary hyperparathyroidism. Because multiple, different mutations of the CaR gene have been found, it is not yet possible to use molecular biological techniques to diagnose new index cases of the condition. The best method of making a diagnosis is to identify other affected family members. If both parents can be shown to be normocalcaemic, then this should exclude the diagnosis unless new mutations are common. If a parent is affected, the finding of affected children among other family members separates the condition from familial hyperparathyroidism. It is impracticable and unnecessary to screen the families of all patients with suspected hyperparathyroidism. It should be mandatory for all asymptomatic patients who are being considered for parathyroid surgery.

Once FBH has been diagnosed, a positive decision should be taken to avoid parathyroid surgery and the patient should be reassured as to the benign nature of the disease.

Vitamin D poisoning

Vitamin D poisoning is a well-recognised cause of hypercalcaemia. It is a risk in all patients being treated with large doses of vitamin D (e.g. 100 000 U daily or more) and those on 1–2 μg/day of the active metabolites, 1,25-dihydroxyvitamin D and 1α-hydroxyvitamin D. As a consequence, all patients on such treatment should have periodic serum calcium measurements. Virtually all patients seen with vitamin D poisoning are aware that they are receiving and taking vitamin D preparations. Provided patients are asked about vitamin D therapy, the diagnosis is usually obvious and the measurement of vitamin D concentration is rarely required. Once diagnosed, it is usually sufficient to stop the vitamin D preparation and wait for the hypercalcaemia to resolve. If the hypercalcaemia is more severe, then intravenous fluids and prednisolone, 20 mg/day, should be given. Failure of the hypercalcaemia to resolve on this treatment should lead to investigations to seek other possible causes for the hypercalcaemia.

Sarcoidosis

Hypercalcaemia is a well-recognised but infrequent complication of sarcoidosis, perhaps occurring in no more than 1–2% of cases. It is usually intermittent and hence is an unlikely cause of hypercalcaemia known to have been present for a long time. In some patients it can be recurrent and associated with sun exposure.

The mechanism of the hypercalcaemia in sarcoidosis is an inappropriate overproduction of 1,25-dihydroxyvitamin D, probably in the abnormal granulomatous cells constituting the sarcoid lesion. Whilst hypercalcaemic, serum 1,25-dihydroxyvitamin D concentrations are elevated and they fall to normal when the calcium returns to normal [20]. The hypercalcaemia of sarcoidosis is responsive to steroid therapy. In most cases encountered the sarcoid process is clinically apparent, either on chest radiography or because of the presence of other clinical features of sarcoidosis. Occasionally, however, there may be no evidence: such cases are easily missed. In sarcoidosis, serum PTH concentrations are suppressed. Therefore, the finding of a suppressed PTH level in the absence of obvious malignancy or other non-parathyroid causes of hypercalcaemia should raise the possibility of sarcoidosis. In this situation a steroid suppression test is very useful. Hydrocortisone, 40 mg 8-hourly for 10 days, will completely control the hypercalcaemia of sarcoidosis. Very few other conditions will respond in this way apart from haematological malignancies. If such a response is seen, a liver biopsy should be performed and this will usually confirm the diagnosis.

Once diagnosed, hypercalcaemia is a clear indication for the use of corticosteroids. A starting dose of 20 mg prednisolone is usually sufficient and this should be reduced rapidly to the minimum dose necessary to maintain a normal serum calcium concentration. After a period of normocalcaemia, attempts should be made to withdraw the steroids as the hypercalcaemia is usually self-limiting.

Thyrotoxicosis

Thyrotoxicosis is infrequently complicated by hypercalcaemia. In thyrotoxicosis there is increased bone turnover and the mean serum calcium concentration is higher than in euthyroid controls. When hypercalcaemia occurs, the thyrotoxicosis is very severe. Treatment of the thyrotoxicosis with carbimazole and β-blockers will control the hypercalcaemia but it may take a number of weeks for the serum calcium to become normal. If normocalcaemia does not develop, concomitant hyperparathyroidism should be suspected and confirmed by finding an elevated PTH concentration.

Milk–alkali syndrome

Although rare, the milk–alkali syndrome is easily missed. This is because excessive milk ingestion is rarely part of the syndrome and the antacids causing them are rarely prescribed by doctors but are more likely to be over-the-counter preparations. Consequently, a routine drug history may fail to pick up the tablet-taking. The commonest preparation involved in the UK is 'Rennies', with affected patients ingesting at least a packet a day. Clues to the diagnosis are mild impairment of renal function with suppressed PTH concentrations. It is likely that this condition will become increasingly rare as 'H_2-blockers' also become available without prescription.

Acute renal failure

Acute renal failure is associated with hypocalcaemia and hyperphosphataemia. During the recovery phase, a polyuric period may be experienced, which may be associated with hypercalcaemia. This is particularly true when the acute renal failure follows extensive muscle trauma and rhabdomyolysis. The pathogenesis of the condition is unclear but it is self-limiting.

Other endocrine tumours

Hypercalcaemia associated with other endocrine tumours should raise the possibility of associated hyperparathyroidism as part of the MEN syndromes (see Chapters 46 and 47). Hypercalcaemia may be associated with vasoactive intestinal polypeptide-secreting tumours (VIP)omas and otherwise non-functioning islet-cell tumours, with phaeochromocytomas, and with carcinoid tumours. PTH concentrations are suppressed and the hypercalcaemia is due to production of PTHrP by the tumours.

Immobilisation

Immobilisation is occasionally associated with hypercalcaemia. Typically it occurs in patients with increased bone turnover, especially rapidly growing teenagers who develop tetraplegia or who are immobilised in hip spicas. The mechanism is presumably excessive bone resorption. PTH concentrations are low. The condition usually develops a number of weeks after immobilisation and is cured by active mobilisation and weight bearing.

Lithium

Hypercalcaemia very occasionally complicates lithium therapy, even though the lithium concentrations are within the therapeutic range. PTH concentrations are usually elevated and, when the lithium is stopped, both serum calcium and PTH levels often return to normal. Further challenge with lithium may cause a recurrence of the hypercalcaemia. Such patients appear to have a mild form of hyperparathyrodism which is brought to light by the lithium therapy. If the lithium therapy is necessary to control the associated psychiatric state then a parathyroidectomy is indicated.

Other possible causes of hypercalcaemia

Although thiazide diuretics and Paget's disease are often listed as causes of hypercalcaemia, it is more likely that concomitant primary hyperparathyroidism is the true explanation.

Idiopathic hypercalcaemia of childhood is a rare disorder which may be associated with characteristic facies, mental retardation and supravalvular aortic stenosis. The hypercalcaemia is often transient and in many cases unconfirmed. Hypercalcaemia has been reported in association with tuberculosis, possibly only when vitamin D supplementation is also given. Parenteral nutrition, Addison's disease, various infective granulomatous diseases, berylliosis, vitamin A poisoning and the hypereosinophilic syndrome have all been reported to cause hypercalcaemia. Massive benign breast hyperplasia may cause hypercalcaemia due to the local overproduction of PTHrP.

An approach to the diagnosis of hypercalcaemia

The first encounter with a hypercalcaemic patient will enable the likely diagnosis to be made in the vast majority of patients. The history will reveal whether the patient is known to have current malignancy, is taking vitamin D or antacids, or has renal failure. Having excluded these cases, if the patient is well, primary hyperparathyroidism is most likely and a serum PTH estimation should be requested. If the patient is unwell, malignancy is most likely and evidence of this is usually found after initial investigation. If malignancy is not found, PTH levels should be measured, an elevated value confirming the unusual case of hyperparathyroidism with marked hypercalcaemia. A low PTH level, with no evidence of malignancy in a patient who is well or ill, should have thyrotoxicosis excluded and the patient should then be considered for a steroid suppression test. If complete suppression occurs, sarcoidosis is likely and a liver biopsy should be performed. The other rare causes of hypercalcaemia usually give some evidence of the underlying diagnosis.

Approached in this way, most cases of hypercalcaemia can be diagnosed in out-patients using the minimum of investigations.

Management of hypercalcaemia

In the vast majority of cases, the treatment, when indicated, is of the underlying condition when this is possible. Only when the hypercalcaemia is severe is it necessary to give urgent non-specific therapy to control the hypercalcaemia. With severe hypercalcaemia the initial treatment involves adequate rehydration. Intravenous fluids are essential with 3–4 litres being given within the first 24 hours. Diuretics are not routinely required. Calcitonin is of very limited efficacy and is probably best avoided. Steroid therapy is ineffective in the vast majority of cases except when the hypercalcaemia is due to vitamin D toxicity or to a haematological malignancy. If drug therapy is indicated, then almost without exception, this should involve the use of a bisphosphonate drug intravenously.

With mild to moderate hypercalcaemia, treatment depends on the underlying cause. If due to hyperparathyroidism, medical treatment is not indicated. If treatment is thought to be necessary, it should be a parathyroidectomy. Hypercalcaemia due to vitamin D therapy requires a reduction in vitamin D dosage. If due to malignancy, treatment is advised, as unless the underlying disease can be rapidly controlled, the severity of the hypercalcaemia may well worsen. Except in haematological malignancies, oral steroids are rarely effective. Oral bisphosphonates may be effective, especially sodium clodronate 800 mg twice daily on an empty stomach. Alternatively, short infusions of an intravenous bisphosphonate can be given on an outpatient basis every 2–4 weeks. A low dietary calcium is ineffective and inconvenient to the patient. Further details of specific therapies are given in Chapter 74.

References

1 Pearce SHS, Brown EM. Calcium-sensing receptor mutations: insights into a structurally and functionally novel receptor. *J Clin Endocrinol Metab* 1996; **81**: 1309–11.

2 Kronenberg HM, Igarashi T, Freeman MW *et al.* Structure and expression of the human parathyroid hormone gland. *Recent Prog Horm Res* 1986; **42**: 641–63.

3 Heath HW III, Hodgson SF, Kennedy MA. Primary hyperparathyroidism: incidence, morbidity and potential economic impact on the community. *N Engl J Med* 1980; **302**: 189–93.

4 Heath DA. Primary hyperparathyroidism. Clinical presentation and factors influencing clinical management. *Endocrinol Metab Clin North Am* 1989; **18**: 631–46.

5 Mundy GR, Cove DH, Fisken R *et al.* Primary hyperparathyroidism; changes in the pattern of clinical presentation. *Lancet* 1980; **i**: 1317–20.

6 Mallette LE, Bilezikian JP, Heath DA *et al.* Primary hyperparathyroidism: clinical and biochemical features. *Medicine (Baltimore)* 1974; **53**: 127–46.

7 Potts JT Jr. Management of asymptomatic hyperparathyroidism (editorial). *J Clin Endocrinol Metab* 1990; **70**: 1489–93.

8 Heath DA, Heath EM. Conservative management of primary hyperparathyroidism. *J Bone Miner Res* 1991; **6** (Suppl. 2): 117–24.

9 Silverberg SJ, Gartenberg F, Jacobs TP *et al.* Increased bone mineral density after parathyroidectomy in primary hyperparathyroidism. *J Clin Endocrinol Metab* 1995; **80**: 729–34.

10 Silverberg SJ, Gartenberg F, Jacobs TP *et al.* Longitudinal measurements of bone density and biochemical indices in untreated primary hyperparathyroidism. *J Clin Endocrinol Metab* 1995; **80**: 723–8.

11 Elvius M, Lagrelius A, Nygram A *et al.* Seventeen year follow-up study of bone mass in patients with mild asymptomatic hyperparathyroidism, some of whom were operated on. *Eur J Surg* 1995; **161**: 863–9.

12 Larssen K, Ljunghall S, Kirusema UB, Naessen T, Lindl E, Persson I. The risk of hip fracture in patients with primary hyperparathyroidism: a population-based cohort study with a follow-up of 19 years. *J Intern Med* 1993; **234**: 585–93.

13 Barnes AD. The changing face of parathyroid surgery. *Ann Roy Coll Surg Engl* 1984; **66**: 77.

14 Eisenberg H, Pallotta J, Sacks B *et al.* Parathyroid localisation, three-dimensional modelling and percutaneous ablation techniques. *Endocrinol Metab Clin North Am* 1989; **18**: 659–700.

15 Heath DA. Localisation of parathyroid tumours. *Clin Endocrinol* 1995; **43**: 523–4.

16 Mitchell BK, Kinder BK, Corneluis E, Stewart AS. Primary hyperparathyroidism: pre-operative localisation using technetium-sestamibi scanning. *J Clin Endocrinol Metab* 1995; **80**: 7–9.

17 Marx SJ, Brandi ML. Familial primary hyperparathyroidism. *Bone Miner Res* 1987; **5**: 375–407.

18 Malluche H, Faugere MC. Renal bone disease 1990: an unmet challenge for the nephrologist (editorial). *Kidney Int* 1990; **38**: 193–211.

19 Heath DA. Familial hypocalciuric hypercalcaemia In: Bilizikian JP, Marcus R, Levine MA, eds. *The Parathyroids. Basic and Clinical Concepts*. New York: Raven Press 1994: 699–710.

20 Papapoulos SE, Clemens TL, Fraher LJ *et al.* 1,25-dihydroxy cholecalciferol in the pathogenesis of the hypercalcaemia of sarcoidosis. *Lancet* 1979; **1**: 627–30.

CHAPTER 42

Defects of the parathyroid–vitamin D axis: hypocalcaemia, hypoparathyroidism, rickets and osteomalacia

M.-L. Brandi, A. Falchetti, L. Masi and T.C.B. Stamp

Introduction

Homoeostasis of calcium and phosphorus is maintained by the combined, interdependent activity of the parathyroid and vitamin D endocrine systems through their respective hormones, parathyroid hormone (PTH) and 1,25-dihydroxyvitamin D_3 (1,25$(OH)_2D)_3$. The effect of both hormones is to raise the level of ionised calcium (Ca^{2+}) in extracellular fluid.

As discussed in Chapter 41, PTH may mobilise calcium from bone and increase resorption via the kidney. The former involves both transfer of calcium from the bone extracellular fluid [1,2] and stimulation of osteoclasts, via osteoblasts as intermediaries [3]. In the kidney, PTH diminishes renal tubular phosphate resorption in both the proximal and distal tubules, with similar proximal tubular effects on sodium and bicarbonate reabsorption [4,5]. PTH also stimulates calcium reabsorption in the distal tubule. It is also the major stimulus to the enzyme 25-hydroxyvitamin D (25-OHD) 1α-hydroxylase situated in the proximal renal tubule which converts 25-OHD to 1,25-$(OH)_2D_3$, calcitriol [6–10].

1,25-$(OH)_2D_3$ stimulates active intestinal calcium transport largely by a genomic action which results in production of calcium-binding protein (calbindins) [11]. Part of its activity appears to be too rapid to involve DNA transcription, and is probably a direct brush-border effect on membrane lipid configuration. Experimentally, calcitriol also resorbs bone with rapid calcium release *in vitro* (see above), but any net *in vivo* effect is less obvious and difficult to evaluate. Parathyroid activity is regulated by a long-loop feedback involving inhibition by calcium, and a short-loop feedback by 1,25-$(OH)_2D_3$ which itself suppresses every stage from parathyroid gene transcription to PTH release [10,12]. A wide range of mammalian cells possess calcitriol receptors, suggesting a broad permissive function in intracellular calcium transport, the intestinal effect being only the most obvious, and certain microendocrine or paracrine systems involving 1,25-$(OH)_2D_3$ are becoming clarified [9,10,13,14]. The molecular endocrinology of PTH is considered further in the section on pseudo-hypoparathyroidism, and that of 1,25-$(OH)_2D_3$ is expanded in the section on rickets and osteomalacia.

Both hormones, PTH and 1,25-$(OH)_2D_3$, are liable to hereditary or acquired deficiencies; target-organ resistance to their effects may also be inherited or acquired. All such defects produce hypocalcaemia by reversal of their activities, thereby reducing mobilisation of Ca^{2+} from bone and diminishing intestinal calcium absorption and renal tubular calcium reabsorption. However, 'hypocalcaemia' is a term that needs to be defined and understood in relation both to physiology and to methodology.

Hypocalcaemia

Changes in total serum calcium are important only to the extent that they reflect a disturbance in Ca^{2+}, the latter being difficult to measure accurately for routine purposes. As previously noted (see Chapter 41), just under half of the total serum calcium is ionised, a similar fraction is bound to albumin, while a small amount is complexed with citrate and protein. Major changes in total calcium may therefore result from changes in albumin which have nothing to do with calcium homoeostasis—haemoconcentration due to a tight tourniquet, upright posture or albumin deficiency associated with liver disease, nephrotic syndrome and protein-losing enteropathies. In order to employ measurements of *total* calcium as an index of *ionised* calcium, all calcium measurements should therefore be corrected to a standard mean albumin concentration (or total protein, provided the globulin concentration is normal). Ideally, all laboratories should set their own range. In practice, a mean albumin of 41 g/l is often used; for every 6 g/l above or below this, a

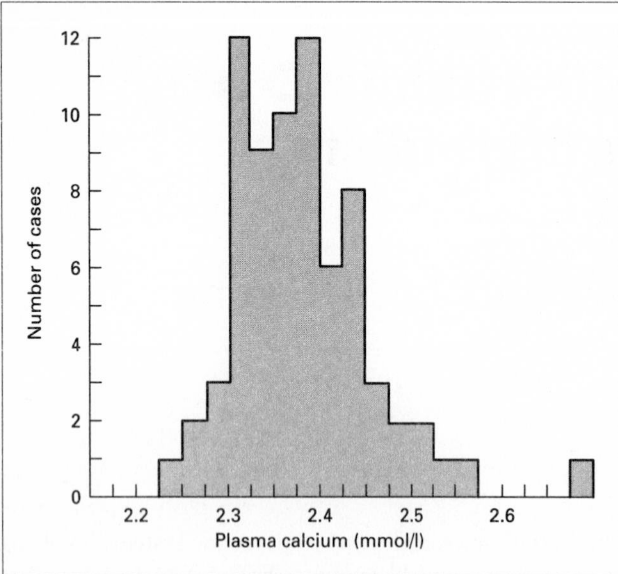

Fig. 42.1 Distribution of fasting plasma calcium in 73 normal volunteers measured by atomic absorption spectrophotometry. The values are corrected for changes in plasma specific gravity. From [15].

calcium value of 0.1 mmol/l is respectively substracted or added and intermediate values are corrected *pro rata*. The resulting normal range for serum (or plasma) calcium lies within a range of 0.35 mmol/l [15] (Fig. 42.1). The exact limits depend on the method used, the reference being atomic absorption spectrophotometry which is the most accurate [16]. Even so, the required use of SI units to two decimal places to give a normal range for corrected calcium of 2.22–2.57 mmol/l (equivalent to the normal range of 8.9–10.3 mg/dl) implies laboratory accuracy which is, in fact, unattainable. In addition, binding of calcium to albumin is pH dependent and reduced in systemic acidosis: Ca^{2+} in chronic renal failure may be higher than suggested by 'corrected' total calcium.

The causes of hypocalcaemia are listed in Table 42.1. Hypoparathyroid disorders, rickets and osteomalacia are considered in detail below. The remainder fall largely outside the scope of an endocrinological textbook and are described only in outline. Hypocalcaemia is common in premature infants, and is due to a variable combination of deficient intake and immaturity of the vitamin D–endocrine system [17]. Excessive phosphate intake, usually through feeding cow's milk, suppresses serum calcium in neonates. Maternal hypercalcaemia also suppresses neonatal parathyroid responsiveness, and may give rise to neonatal tetany.

Magnesium deficiency usually results from severe small bowel disease (e.g. chronic diarrhoea, extensive surgical ileal resection), but also occurs in a familial form associated with defective intestinal transport. Magnesium is required both for PTH release, through the magnesium-dependent parathyroid gland adenosine triphosphatase (ATPase), and for target-organ expression of PTH activity both in the kidney and in bone; both mechanisms are important clinically. Hypomagnesaemia occasionally complicates both hypoparathyroidism and pseudo-hypoparathyroidism [1,15,18].

Table 42.1 Causes of hypocalcaemia.

Spurious (i.e. normal ionised Ca^{2+})
Due to lack of correction for low serum albumin levels
Systemic acidosis
Neonatal
Prematurity
Maternal hypercalcaemia
Excessive phosphate intake, especially feeding cow's milk
Hypoparathyroid disorders
Acquired hypoparathyroidism, especially surgical
Idiopathic hypoparathyroidism
Pseudo-hypoparathyroidism
Rickets and osteomalacia (most, but not all, forms)
Hypomagnesaemia
Acute pancreatitis
Drugs
e.g. gentamicin
certain cytotoxic drugs, eg. *cis*-platinum
Osteosclerotic, osteoblastic skeletal disease, e.g. metastases

Hypocalcaemia may complicate acute pancreatitis and indicates serious disease: locally released free fatty acids chelate calcium, while other contributing factors include vomiting, hypoalbuminaemia and hypomagnesaemia. Critically ill patients with many serious diseases may develop hypocalcaemia associated with many factors including Gram-negative septicaemia, rhabdomyolysis or tumour lysis with hyperphosphataemia, especially when renal function is poor. Hypocalcaemia also results from a toxic effect on renal tubules from some antitumour drugs, for example *cis*-platinum, and from gentamicin. It is a manifestation of massive fluoride intoxication. L-Asparaginase, a cytoxic drug, has caused hypoparathyroidism in experimental animals (only). Some other drugs also lower serum calcium levels, for example calcitonin, mithramycin, glucocorticoids, bisphosphonates and oestrogens (in post-menopausal women), but hypocalcaemia is rarely a clinical problem.

Symptoms and signs

The main symptoms and signs of hypocalcaemia are those due to increased neuromuscular excitability. Paraesthesiae may be felt around the mouth and fingertips. Tetany is manifest by carpopedal spasms (hands and feet) producing the *main d'accoucheur* (Fig. 42.2). This may be elicited as Trousseau's sign by inflating a sphygmomanometer cuff to just above systolic pressure for 3 min. Just how much 'spasm' constitutes a positive response may be uncertain; muscle tone

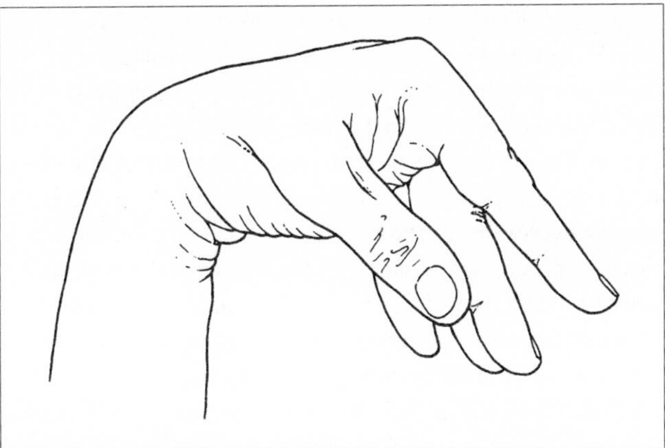

Fig. 42.2 Carpal spasm is hypocalcaemic tetany, which may be elicited clinically as Trousseau's sign (*le main d'accoucheur.*) There is flexion at the wrist and metacarpophalangeal joints with extension of the interphalangeal joints and adduction of the thumb.

in the thenar eminence and resistance to passive abduction of the thumb by the examiner, are probably the best guide. Chvostek's sign is elicited by light percussion with the tip of the middle finger over the area where the branches of the facial nerve emerge in front of the parotid gland, from above downwards; this produces twitches from each of the facial muscles in turn. Some healthy people may show a single flicker. These changes may also be produced in susceptible, anxious patients by hyperventilation: when severe this condition has been termed spasmophilia; *le spasmophilie* is more widely diagnosed on the European subcontinent than in the UK, where many do not recognise it as a separate entity.

Epileptic seizures are the most severe manifestation of hypocalcaemia, and simple epilepsy is all too frequently a mistaken diagnosis in long-standing hypoparathyroidism. Hypocalcaemia may produce papilloedema for uncertain reasons, and cataract if prolonged. Intestinal hurry may occur; the electrocardiogram shows prolongation of the QT interval. Dry skin and hair loss are other manifestations. Lastly, emotional depression may occur, especially during acute hypocalcaemia following parathyroidectomy for primary hyperparathyroidism; it vanishes with intravenous calcium administration.

Hypocalcaemia is rarely severe enough to require parenteral calcium except following parathyroidectomy in the presence of osteitis fibrosa, when 10–20 ml 10% calcium gluconate may be administered intravenously over at least 10 min. Oral calcium supplements providing 800–1000 mg elemental calcium daily are sensible during the 4–6 months it may take to heal a severe skeletal deficit in hyperparathyroidism or osteomalacia, together with vitamin D derivatives. Still higher doses of oral calcium, 2–6 g daily, may rarely be indicated after operation in severe osteitis fibrosa. The mildest degree of chronic hypoparathyroidism may be controlled by oral calcium alone, but a vitamin D derivative is generally preferable; thiazides are sometimes used. It may be essential to correct hypomagnesaemia with large oral supplements of magnesium hydroxide or glycerophosphate. Rarely, intestinal disease may require regular intramuscular magnesium sulphate, and the intravenous route is occasionally needed for acute control of hypomagnesaemia. More specific details of treatment are given below.

Parathyroid disorders

Hypocalcaemic disorders may be classified into two main groups of conditions: parathyroid- and non-parathyroid-dependent disorders. Both groups encompass several different diseases, which will be described below. Many acquired or inherited diseases can account for hypoparathyroidism that can depend on either decrease of PTH synthesis and secretion and/or peripheral tissue resistance.

Primary hypoparathyroidism

Among the idiopathic disorders, autoimmune hypoparathyroidism, either alone or associated with the polyglandular autoimmune syndrome type I (PGA-I), is the most common type (Table 42.2) In the latter condition hypoparathyroidism has a prevalence of 89%, being associated with chronic mucocutaneous candidiasis (75% of cases) and primary adrenal insufficiency or Addison's disease (60% of cases).

Table 42.2 Variable constituents of the polyglandular autoimmune syndrome.

Type	
Hypoparathyroidism	(HAM syndrome)
Addison's disease	
Moniliasis (candidiasis)	
Hypothyroidism	
Diabetes mellitus	
Early menopause	
Pernicious anaemia	
Liver disease	
Alopecia (partial or total)	
Steatorrhoea	
Type II	
As above, but without hypoparathyroidism	
Type III	
As above, but with neither hypoparathyroidism nor Addison's disease	

Other autoimmune features can also be present, such as primary hypogonadism, diabetes mellitus, pernicious anaemia, vitiligo and thyroid diseases. Clinical signs generally appear in early childhood, before age 15 and these include hypoparathyroidism. In 50% of cases PGA-I is described as a familial form, inherited in an autosomal recessive fashion. No linkage disequilibrium with any particular human leucocyte antigen (HLA) haplotype has been described. Frequently, organ-specific antibodies have been found in plasma from affected subjects [19].

The DiGeorge syndrome is the most common form of hypoparathyroidism due to branchial dysembryogenesis, and is associated with other branchial cleft abnormalities such as an absent thymus, defective cell-mediated immunity, facial abnormalities and defects of the aortic arch or the heart (Fallot's tetralogy). The responsible gene has been mapped to chromosome 22q11 [20].

Congenital hypoparathyroidism can occur in more than 50% of patients with the Kenney–Caffey syndrome, where it is associated with several abnormalities such as short stature, osteosclerosis and cortical thickening of the long bones, delayed closure of the anterior fontanelle, basal ganglia calcification, nanophthalmos and hyperopia [21]. It is likely that the hypoparathyroidism may be due to an embryological defect of parathyroid development, and indeed no parathyroid tissue was found during autopsy of an affected patient [22].

PTH gene abnormalities have been described in isolated hypoparathyroidism in both autosomal dominant and recessive forms, with mutations involving different parts of the PTH gene (exon 2 (autosomal dominant) and exon 2–intron 2 boundary (autosomal recessive)) [23,24]. X-linked recessive hypoparathyroidism has also been reported in the literature [25,26], with linkage studies mapping the responsible gene to Xq26–q27 [27].

PTH-resistance syndromes

This group of disorders is increasing in size, with the recognition of the clinical conditions parallelling our knowledge of the molecular basis underlying these defects. Two main subgroups can be recognised, pseudo-hypoparathyroidism (PHP) and pseudo-pseudo-hypoparathyroidism (pseudo-PHP).

The term PHP describes a heterogeneous group of syndromes characterised by biochemical hypoparathyroidism (hypocalcaemia and hyperphosphataemia), increased circulating PTH levels, and the absence of a peripheral response to the biological actions of PTH. Most of the disorders can be classified as type I, characterised by lack of responsivity to PTH, in terms of urinary cAMP and phosphate excretion. The type I form can in turn be subdivided into type Ia, associated with multihormonal resistance, mental retardation, ophthalmic defects and Albright's hereditary osteodystrophy (AHO), and type Ib, with isolated PTH resistance in the absence of the clinical features of Albright's osteodystrophy. The disorders appear to be transmitted in an autosomal manner. Type Ic represents a heterogeneous group of disorders, with lack of responsivity to PTH manifest only as a decreased urinary excretion of phosphates, but a maintained urinary cAMP excretion response to PTH. No familial form for this latter type has been described [28]. Pseudo-PHP represents a normocalcaemic variant syndrome with normal hormonal responses, including normal responsivity to PTH.

Subdividing the molecular mechanisms of PTH action into prereceptor, receptor and post-receptor [29,30] should allow us to correlate the recognised molecular defects of the PTH-resistance syndromes with their varied clinical manifestations.

Prereceptor defects

The pathogenesis of this syndrome may be due to the existence of a circulating PTH inhibitory factor or a currently unknown PTH antagonist. These factors could be responsible for the apparent dissociation between plasma levels of endogenous PTH, both immunoreactive and bioactive, and the capacity of the plasma of the affected patients to decrease the *in vitro* biological activity of exogenous PTH [31]. It has been noted that prolonged hypercalcaemia can significantly reduce the level of inhibitory activity in the plasma of patients with PHP: this suggests that the parathyroid glands could be the source of the inhibitor(s). High-performance liquid chromatography (HPLC) analysis has revealed the presence of abberrant forms of immunoreactive PTH in plasma from these patients [32]. However, it is probable that the PTH-like activity of circulating antagonists may be the *result* of the sustained secondary hyperparathyroidism resulting from the primary biochemical defect.

Receptor defects

These patients do not exhibit any features of AHO, but demonstrate PTH resistance limited to target organs with normal activity of the subunit α of the G_s-protein [29] (Fig. 42.3). A PTH-receptor defect could be responsible for this resistance syndrome. A possible example of this type of defect is PHP-Ib, where patients do not exhibit features of AHO. Although patients affected by PHP-Ib do not respond to PTH in terms of nephrogenic cyclic adenosine monophosphate (cAMP), they frequently exhibit skeletal lesions similar to those of hyperparathyroid patients [33]. This suggests that at least one intracellular signalling pathway coupled to the PTH receptor may be intact. In addition, fibroblast cultures of subjects affected by PHP-Ib

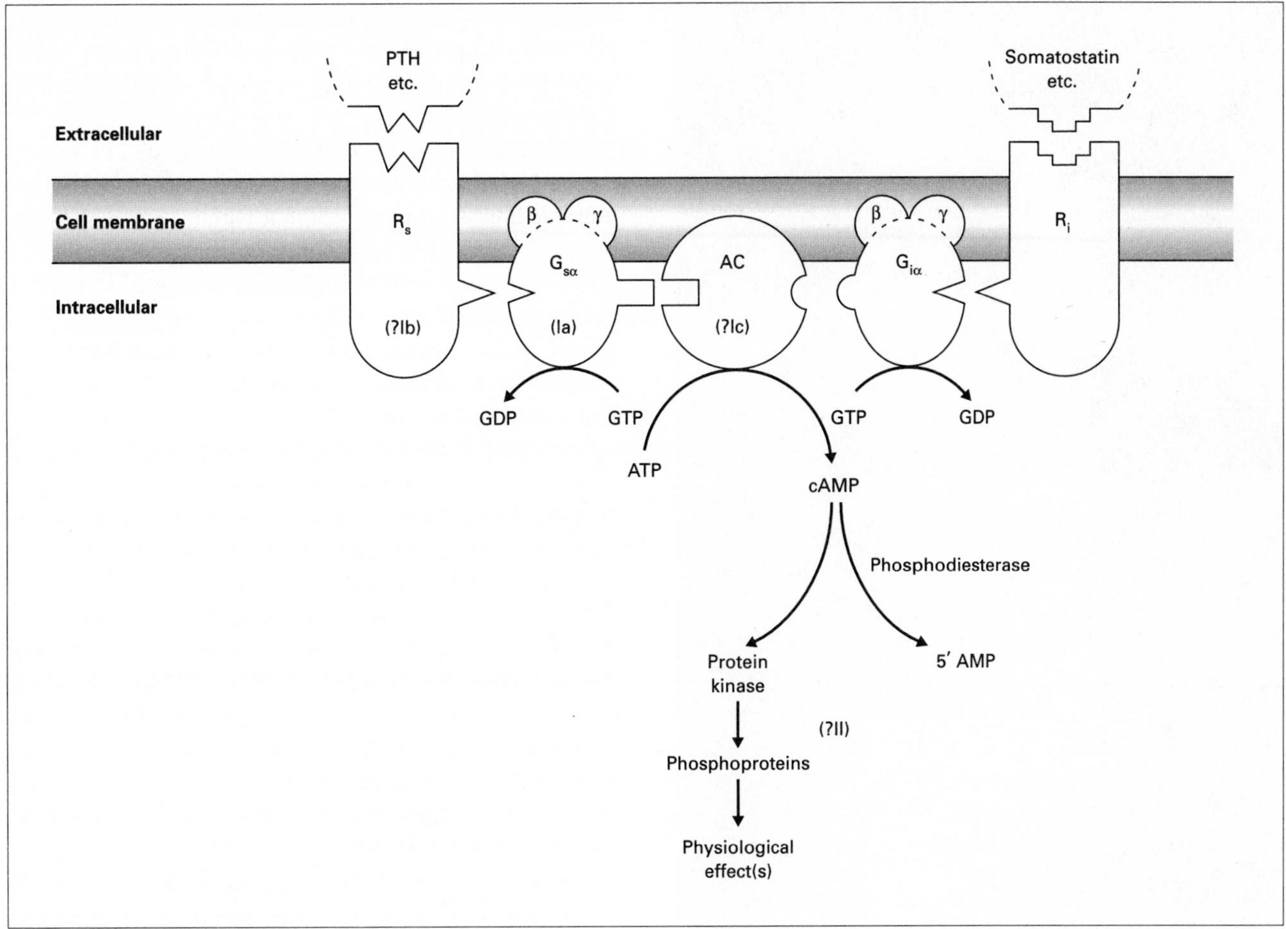

Fig. 42.3 Hormone–receptor coupling and activation of the adenylate cyclase/cyclic adenosine monophosphate (cAMP) system. R_s and R_i, stimulatory and inhibitory receptors; G_s and G_i, stimulatory and inhibitory guanosine nucleotide binding proteins (with α-, β- and γ-subunits); AC, catalytic unit of adenylate cyclase; (?I_{a-c}, II), putative site of defect in the different types of pseudo-hypoparathyroidism (see text).

show deficient cAMP response to PTH stimulation, but normal responses to other agonists, such as prostaglandin E_1 (PGE_1) and forskolin [34]. Indeed, the receptor can effectively couple to two different signal transduction pathways, both adenyl cyclase and phospholipase C. For these reasons, defect uncoupling adenyl cyclase from the PTH receptor, leaving the phospholipase C pathway intact, may explain the clinical findings. The molecular basis for reduced PTH-receptor activity has so far not been unravelled, and to date no mutations of the human PTH receptor have been demonstrated in such patients.

Post-receptor defects

A good example of this type of disorder is shown by PHP-Ia, where patients exhibit the clinical features of AHO (short stature with short neck, round face, flattened nasal bridge, reduced IQ, heterotopic ossification of soft tissues or skin (osteoma cutis), brachydactyly, shortening of the distal phalanx of the thumb—the so-called 'potter's thumb'—and shortening of the third to the fifth metacarpals) [35] (Figs. 42.4–6). Endocrine alterations consequent on resistance to other hormones and neurotransmitters coupled to adenyl cyclase may also be associated (i.e. PTH , thyroid-stimulating hormone (TSH), luteinising hormone (LH), follicle-stimulating hormone (FSH), glucagon) [30]. In such patients the existence of a generalised deficiency of $G_{s\alpha}$, associated with decreased responsiveness of target tissues to hormonal stimuli, has been clearly demonstrated.

The $G_{s\alpha}$ gene mutations described so far are missense mutations, point mutations in effective splicing sites, and small deletions [36–39]. In AHO, inherited mutations in the G_s gene lead to decreased expression or to reduced function of the G_s protein. In addition, patients affected by pseudo-PHP also exhibit a reduction in $G_{s\alpha}$ activity, without showing any clinical features of a hormone-resistance condition.

It is important to note that kindreds with hypocalcaemia secondary to the AHO syndrome encompass family members with clinical features of both PHP-Ia and pseudo-PHP,

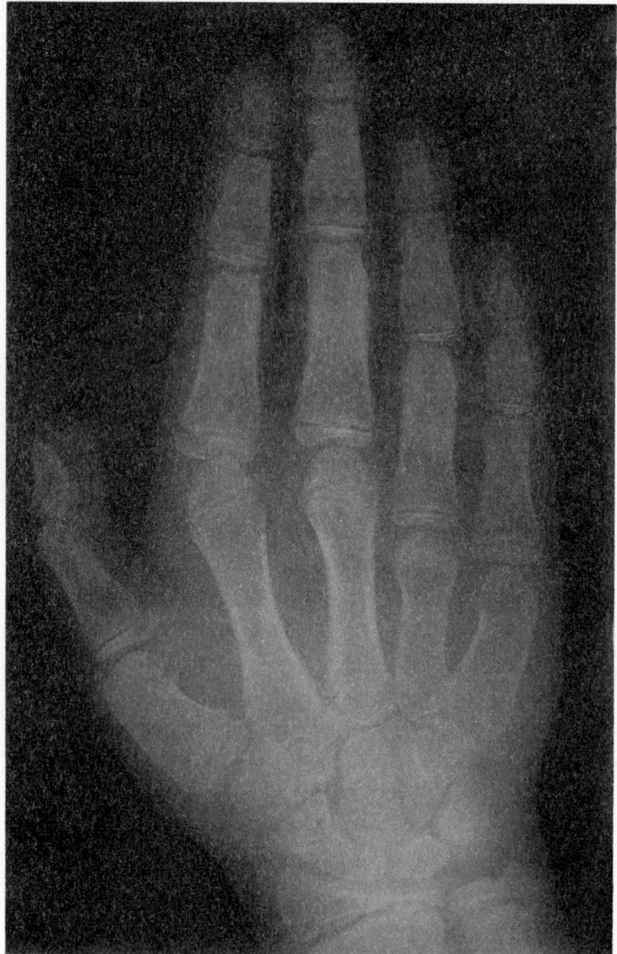

Fig. 42.4 Hand radiograph of a 13-year-old boy with pseudo-hypoparathyroidism and Albright's hereditary osteodystrophy. Note the typically shortened first, fourth and fifth metacarpals. The phalanges are abnormally modelled. The distal radial and ulnar growth plates are normal.

with similar G_s gene mutations and reductions in $G_{s\alpha}$ levels. However, comprehensive review of the inheritance of AHO indicates that neither PHP-Ia nor pseudo-PHP occur in the same generation.

Among the post-receptor defects one should include those which characterise the AHO syndrome associated with multiple hormonal resistance, but without a demonstrable defect of G_s or G_i proteins [40]. The nature of the molecular abnormality in these patients has not been well established, but it may be linked to a different component of the receptor–adenyl cyclase system, such as the catalytic subunit [41]. Mutations at different levels in the signal transduction pathway may also need to be considered.

A decrease in the phosphaturic response to PTH in PHP type II is also present in patients with severe vitamin D deficiency-dependent hypocalcaemia [42], suggesting an inability of intracellular cAMP to initiate the metabolic events that lead to PTH activity. For example, a defect of the cAMP-dependent protein kinase A has been proposed, even though no clear demonstration to support this hypothesis is available. Alternatively, a defect in other PTH-sensitive signal transduction pathways could explain the absence of the phosphaturic response. A potential candidate might therefore be the PTH–sensitive phospholipase C, which modulates the increase of intracellular inositol 1,4,5-trisphosphate, diacylglycerol and cytosolic calcium [43,44]. It is of interest to note that in some PHP type II patients the phosphaturic response to PTH is restored by normalisation of plasma calcium levels or by calcium infusion or vitamin D therapy [45].

Vitamin D metabolism

Vitamin D is a seco-steroid in which the B ring of the

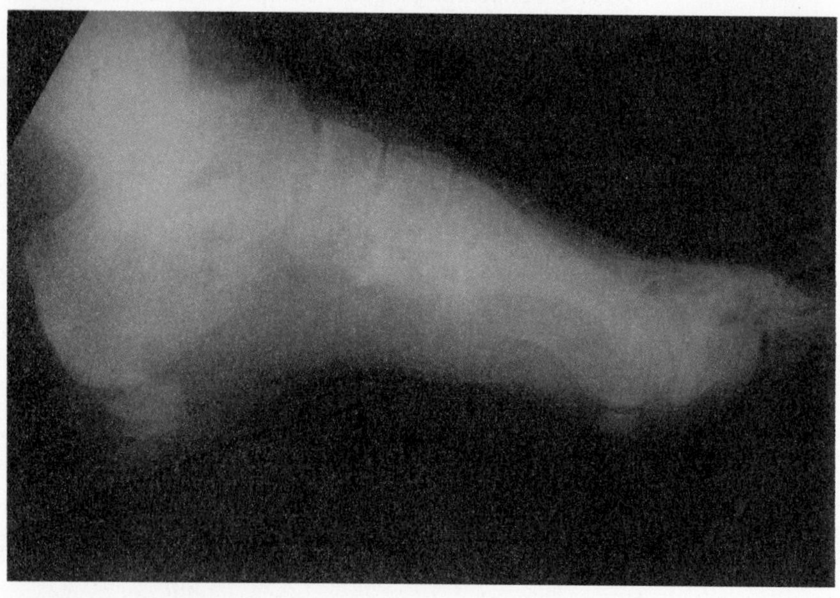

Fig. 42.5 Pseudo-hypoparathyroidism and Albright's hereditary osteodystrophy showing subcutaneous calcification beneath the calcaneum (same case as in Fig. 42.3); the patient presented with a painful heel.

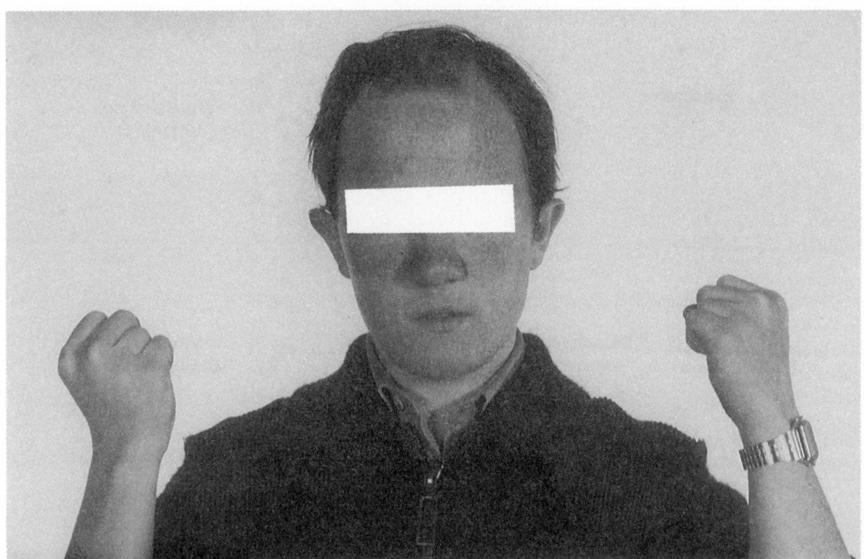

Fig. 42.6 Pseudo-hypoparathyroidism with Albright's hereditary osteodystrophy (same patient as in Figs 42.3 and 42.4, some years later aged 19 years). Note the clinically shortened knuckles and premature hair loss.

cyclopentanoperhydrophenanthrene structure is cleaved. It is obtained from the diet or is produced in the skin from 7-dehydrocholesterol which is restored in the Malpighian layer of the epidermis. Vitamin D circulates in the blood primarily bound with vitamin D-binding protein (DBP). Three enzymes are responsible for the production of the vitamin D metabolites: one of these, indicated as 25-hydroxylase, is present in the liver and converts the vitamin D_2 (ergocalciferol from diet) and vitamin D_3 (cholecalciferol from skin and diet after irradiation) into 25-OHD_3 (Fig. 42.7). Accordingly, circulating 25-OHD_3 concentrations represent the best indicator of vitamin D_3 levels and availability. Subsequently, the renal 1α-hydroxylase enzyme converts the 25-OHD_3 into 1,25-$(OH)_2D_3$ which is the biologically active form of the hormone. This enzyme is located in the proximal convoluted tubules and pars recta of the proximal tubules. The 1α and 25-(OH) groups are required for the full biological activity of the hormone. Many factors control renal 1α-hydroxylase activity; in particular, PTH and low inorganic phosphate levels directly up-regulate 1α-hydroxylase activity [46]. In addition, oestrogens, growth hormone (GH) and prolactin are able to modulate 1α-hydroxylase activity. Under conditions of adequate plasma calcium levels, 25-OHD_3 is alternatively converted to 24,25-$(OH)_2D_3$ by the 24-hydroxylase enzyme; 24,25-$(OH)_2D_3$ is a metabolite whose physiological role is unclear in humans [47].

The 1,25-$(OH)_2D_3$ form exerts its biological effects through specific intracellular receptors (Fig. 42.8) which are transcription factors of the steroid receptor gene superfamily [48,49]. The 1,25-$(OH)_2D_3$ receptor (VDR) is an intracellular protein, its mechanism of action involving interactions of the receptor zinc-finger regions with specific nucleotide sequences (hormone response elements). VDRs are localised not only in the gut, kidney and bone, which are the classical vitamin D targets, but also in many other tissues. The most important activity of the 1,25-$(OH)_2D_3$ on the classical target tissues is to elevate plasma calcium. VDRs also stimulate transepithelial calcium transport across the gut, from the renal tubular lumen into the bloodstream, and cooperate with PTH in stimulating short-term bone calcium mobilisation. In addition, vitamin D increases the number of osteoclastic cells derived from bone-marrow precursors in the long term. However, the osteoblasts, which express 1,25-$(OH)_2D_3$-receptors, are the recognised major bone targets for vitamin D. Osteoblastic responses to the hormone include increased synthesis of osteocalcin and down-regulation of type I collagen production. In addition, 1,25-$(OH)_2D_3$ increases the levels of several vitamin-D calcium binding proteins (CaBP-Ds or calbindins) [50] and reduces PTH synthesis and secretion from the parathyroids [51].

Cytosolic receptor proteins for 1,25-$(OH)_2D_3$ are also present in tissues not involved in calcium homeostasis. For instance, 1,25-$(OH)_2D_3$ alters inactivated lymphocyte proliferation and cell function by decreasing sensitivity to many cytokines and/or by influencing lymphocytic cytokine production. In addition, 1,25-$(OH)_2D_3$ induces macrophage differentiation, activation and fusion. In vascular smooth muscle, several investigators have found the presence of VDR through which 1,25-$(OH)_2D_3$ appears to stimulate the proliferation of vascular smooth muscle cells and so increase their contractile responses to adrenaline or serotonin [52]. Finally, 1,25-$(OH)_2D_3$ decreases cardiac contractility independently of plasma calcium levels; moreover, vitamin D-deficient rats demonstrate cardiac hypertrophy [53]. Taken together, these data are important in establishing the direct effects of 1,25-$(OH)_2D_3$ on cardiac muscle physiology.

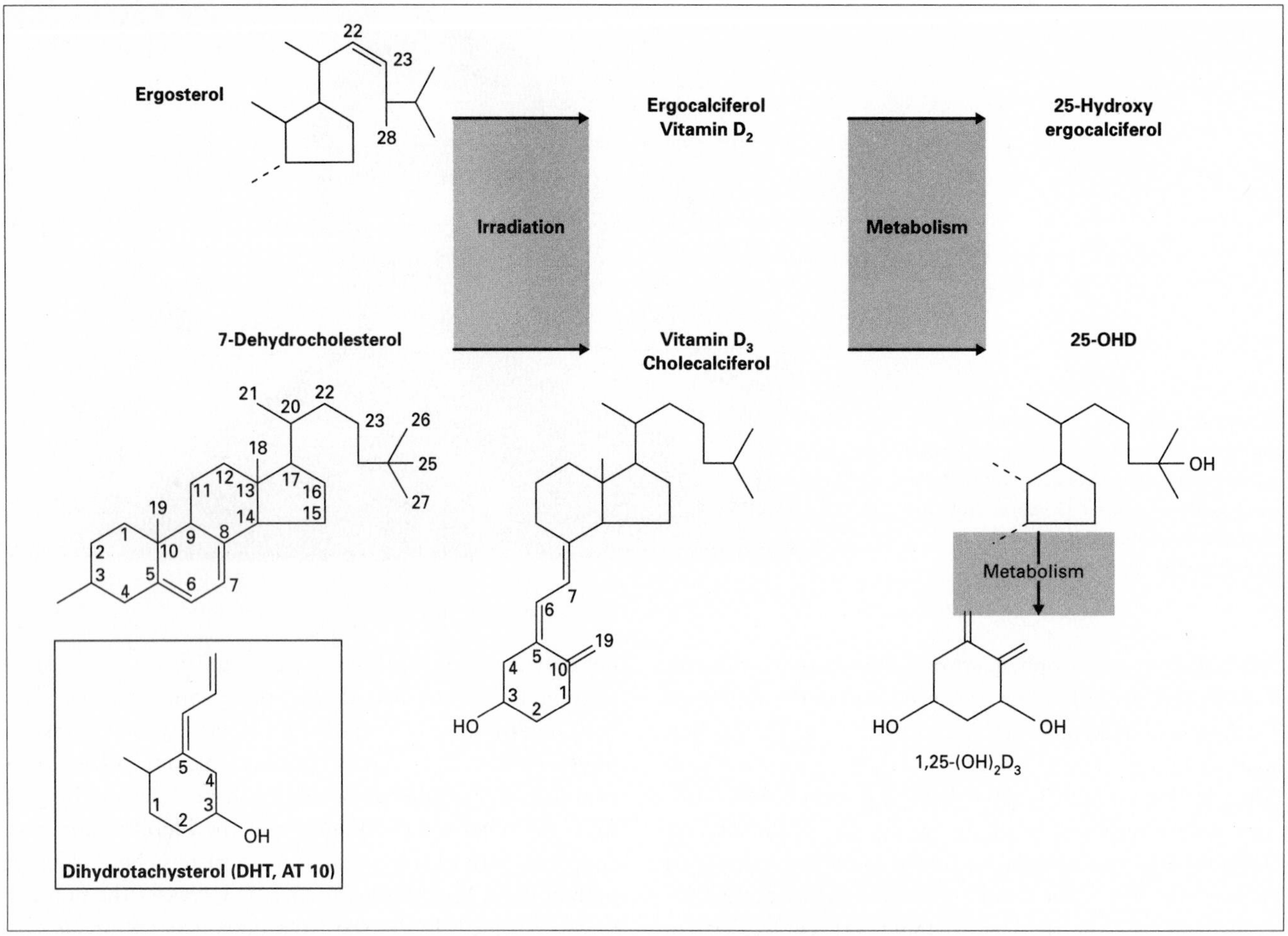

Fig. 42.7 Chemical transformation of vitamins D_2 and D_3 and their major metabolites. Vitamin D_2 (ergosterol) differs only in its side-chain form 7-dihydrocholesterol and only this side chain is shown. Similar changes are produced in both molecules by ultraviolet irradiation. Only the side chain of 25-hydroxyvitamin D (25(OH)D_3) and the A ring of 1,25-dihydroxyvitamin D (1,25(OH)$_2D_3$) are shown.

Many studies have reported the presence of VDRs in skeletal muscle or myoblast cells where the effects of 1,25-(OH)$_2D_3$ include increases in 24-hydroxylase activity and of intracellular calcium levels. Boland *et al.* showed that 1,25-(OH)$_2D_3$ has effects on skeletal muscle via both genomic and non-genomic mechanisms [54]. Recent studies have also demonstrated that vitamin D is important for normal reproductive activity in rats; the levels of VDRs in the testis are low in immature rats and increase during puberty. In addition, stimulation of the testis with FSH increases VDR levels. Finally, VDRs are found also in the pancreas [53], and calcium homeostasis has been shown to be altered in diabetes mellitus in humans. The effect of 1,25-(OH)$_2D_3$ on β-cells is specific, since neither glucagon nor somatostatin secretion are affected by 1,25-(OH)$_2D_3$ challenge. Insulin is also important in modulating PTH stimulation of the renal

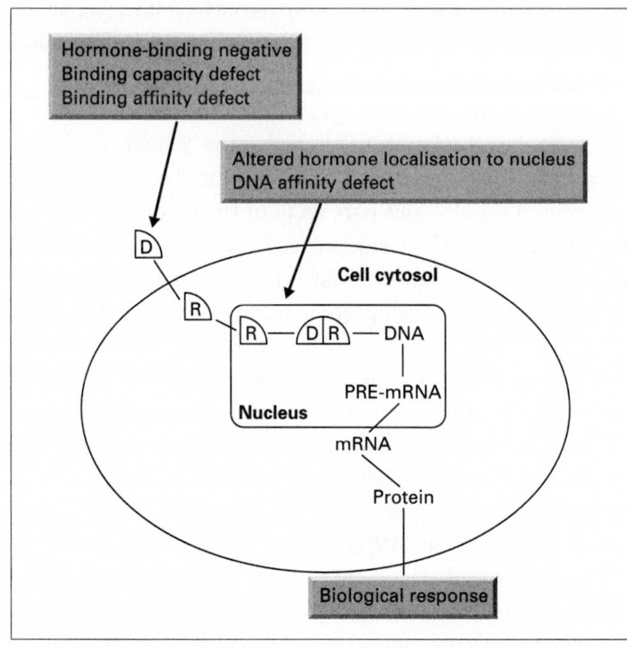

Fig. 42.8 Vitamin D interactions with its intracellular receptor and induction of biological responses. Five classes of defects in the intracellular interactions are recognised to cause vitamin D-dependent rickets. D, vitamin D; R, receptor.

1α-hydroxylase enzyme *in vivo*, as insulin therapy is able to reverse the typical alterations of calcium homeostasis seen in diabetic patients.

Vitamin D nutrition

The historical designation of cholecalciferol (vitamin D_3) as a 'vitamin' was based on its alternative availability within certain animal foods, among which oily fish is the only prominent source (or as vitamin D_2, ergosterol, from irradiated yeast sterol), together with the potential shortage of necessary ultraviolet irradiation [8,55]. Before the development of radiostereoassays for 25-OHD in 1971 [56] all information on vitamin D content was derived solely from tedious bioassays of antiricketic activity in rats, leading to expression of potency in international units (iu) and promulgation of recommended intakes in these terms. One iu is contained in 0.025 μg vitamin D (i.e. 1 μg vitamin D contains 40 iu). In terms of receptor affinity, however, the iu is almost meaningless; vitamin D has essentially no affinity and must be converted to 25-OHD, whose affinity in turn is about two orders of magnitude less than that of 1,25-$(OH)_2D_3$ [6,7,10]. The receptor affinity of 25-OHD, however low, nevetheless explains why pharmacological doses of vitamin D (and 25(OH)-D) are effective substitutes in the virtual absence of 25-OHD 1α-hydroxylase (e.g. in renal failure, the anephric state, vitamin D-dependent rickets type 1 and hypoparathyroidism).

Because sunshine is the major determinant of vitamin D nutrition, recommended daily vitamin D intakes (e.g. 400 iu for adults) are valid only when adequate solar exposure is in jeopardy. Nutrition is best evaluated in individuals by measurement of circulating 25-OHD. Winter sunshine is inadequate for vitamin D synthesis in temperate latitudes. Plasma levels of 25-OHD therefore show marked seasonal variation with a roughly log-normal distribution [57]. The mean maximum level of approximately 20–25 ng/ml is achieved in the UK in September, and a mean minimum of about 10 ng/ml is associated with deficiency disease, although assumptions regarding previous nutritional status are not necessarily valid. Figure 42.9 shows the relationships

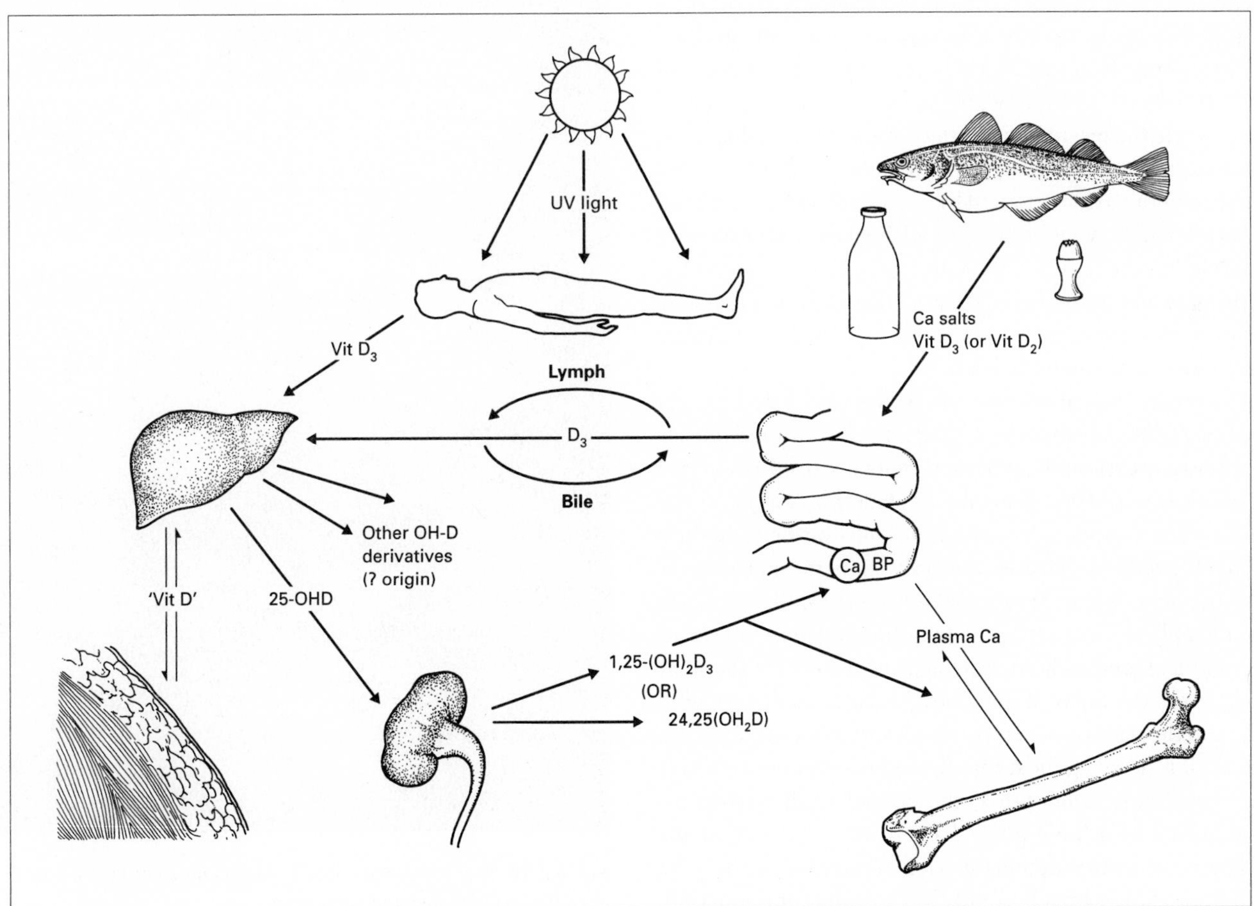

Fig. 42.9 Major pathways of vitamin D metabolism through skin, small intestine, liver, kidney, bone and storage organs (muscle and adipose tissue). 25-OHD, 25-hydroxyvitamin D; 1,25$(OH)_2D_3$, 1,25-dihydroxyvitamin D; CaBP, calcium binding protein(s).

between serum 25-OHD, oral vitamin D (and 25-OHD) intake and ultraviolet irradiation. Evolution of vitamin D metabolism seems to have ensured a mechanism for abundant synthesis and storage in summer, followed by slow metered release and utilisation in winter.

The normal range of serum 1,25-$(OH)_2D_3$ is broad, numerous laboratories reporting a lower limit of 15–19 pg/ml and an upper limit of 45–58 pg/ml [2]. Normal levels are higher among children and adolescents. Persistently low levels characterise some forms of 'vitamin D-resistant', hypophosphataemic osteomalacia. In privational disease, levels rise so briskly after a small amount of administered vitamin D that they are of no diagnostic significance; in this situation the renal 1α-hydroxylase is so primed by hyperparathyroidism that one Multivite tablet daily (11 μg vitamin D_3) may produce 1,25- $(OH)_2D_3$ levels more than double those achieved by 1 μg 1,25-$(OH)_2D_3$ daily.

Rickets and osteomalacia

Rickets and osteomalacia are the respective childhood and adult diseases that result from inadequate vitamin D activity, and are manifest by defective mineralisation of the cartilaginous growth plate and bone, respectively. Centuries separated their original clinical descriptions from their histopathology in the late 19th century, their radiographic delineation early in the 20th century, and their biochemical profiles from the 1920s onward; many accounts are available [15]. While the broadening of these terms may be disputed, more recent descriptions of their histopathology have included other conditions characterised by apparently defective mineralisation which have little to do with vitamin D: excessive fluoride ingestion, aluminium and gallium nitrate toxicity, etidronate therapy and even Paget's disease. Aluminium toxicity is important in the pathogenesis of bone disease during long-term renal haemodialysis.

The main clinical features of rickets and osteomalacia are bone pain and tenderness, skeletal deformity and muscle weakness, occasionally with signs of tetany from associated hypocalcaemia. They generally provide no clue as to the cause. Rickets occurs, by definition, only during growth; it is characterised by defective mineralisation, most prominent in those areas where bone growth is most rapid, usually in the metaphyseal region of the long bones. Hence, many of the physical (and radiological) signs of rickets are found at these sites. The areas of most rapid bone growth vary with age, and the signs of rickets therefore vary similarly. At birth, the skull is growing most rapidly and neonatal rickets may therefore show craniotabes, the cranial vault having the consistency of a 'ping-pong' ball. In the first year of life rickets becomes manifest in the swollen epiphyses at the wrist and in swelling ('breading') of the costochondral junction, the so-called 'ricketty rosary'. The inward pull of the diaphragm produces a groove in the rib cage, Harrison's sulcus. Rickects in the toddler tends to produce bow-leg deformities, while knock-knees are characteristic of rickets in later childhood. Both occasionally occur as 'wind-swept legs' (Fig. 42.10).

Ricketty myopathy is part of the differential diagnosis of the 'floppy baby'. If muscle weakness is severe enough to prevent walking, it may limit deformity of the lower limbs. Conversely, one form of childhood rickets which is not associated with myopathy, the X-linked dominant hypophosphataemic syndrome, tends to produce early severe bow legs. A variable degree of dwarfism is another obvious feature of rickets. Pathological fractures in the shafts of long bones occur only in very severe forms.

Symptoms of osteomalacia in the adult may be more vague. Bone pains usually occur in the axial skeleton—spine,

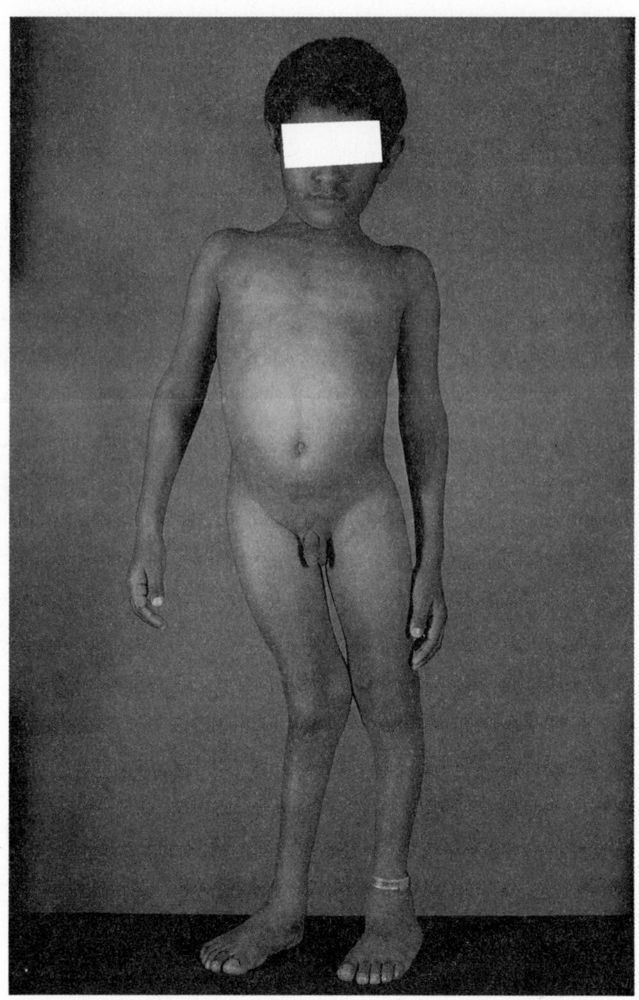

Fig. 42.10 The 'windswept' legs of rickets presenting in a boy aged 8 years with Fanconi syndrome.

shoulders, ribs and pelvis. Localised pain, for example in the groin, may be due to an undisplaced femoral neck fracture, or may be associated with an underlying radiological Looser zone (see below), although the latter does not usually produce symptoms. Tenderness may be elicited by spinal percussion or by sternal and lateral rib compression; the most painful bones are generally those with the thinnest cortices. When adult osteomalacia occurs as a recrudescence of childhood rickets, stigmata of previous dwarfism, deformity or even scars of long-forgotten osteotomies may be a helpful sign in the differential diagnosis. In severe cases, vertebrae become compressed.

Osteomalacia myopathy has a characteristic proximal distribution, the reason for which is unknown. Possible results of distributed vitamin D metabolism in muscle include defective Ca^{2+} transport, which is necessary for contraction. It may be difficult clinically to ascertain myopathy in the presence of pain; even when it is undoubtedly present, electromyographic abnormalities are non-specific and may be absent. Symptoms of tetany from associated hypocalcaemia are occasionally present. The often vague nature of osteomalacia pain and muscle weakness can easily lead to a missed diagnosis.

Histopathology

Rickets is characterised by elongation and distortion of the normal columnar arrangement of chondrocytes in the zone of hypertrophy of cartilaginous growth plate. In the underlying zone of maturation, provisional calcification is delayed or absent, and vascularisation via defective or obliterated channels is impaired and irregular (Fig. 42.11). The primary spongiosa is also grossly abnormal; detailed reviews are available [55,58–61].

The diagnosis of osteomalacia in adults may be confirmed by trephine biopsy of the iliac crest. It is often unnecessary, however, since the diagnosis is frequently clear from the combination of clinical features, biochemical abnormalities, and radiographic and scintigraphic appearances. Coverage of trabecular bone surfaces by unmineralised osteoid is normally <27% and can rise to 100% in osteomalacia. Osteoid thickness, or 'volume', may be measured; another rule of thumb is the number of osteoid 'light lines', birefringent lamellae under polarised light, four being the normal maximum. There is usually evidence of increased resorption (secondary hyperparathyroidism). More sophisticated research techniques may be employed including prior *in vivo* labelling of the mineralisation front by oral tetracycline, which then shows as fluorescent lines under ultraviolet light [60–63].

Radiology

Radiological assessment may vary from being pathognomonic to, in osteomalacia, being entirely non-contributory. The ricketic growth plate is always widened, splayed and cupped (concave, towards the diaphysis) frayed and ragged (Figs 42.12 and 42.13). In the adult, however, the skeleton may appear normal or it may show one or more characteristic Looser zones—ribbon-like areas of decalcification similar to stress fractures (Fig. 42.14); when accompanied by subperiosteal resorption due to secondary hyperparathyroidism

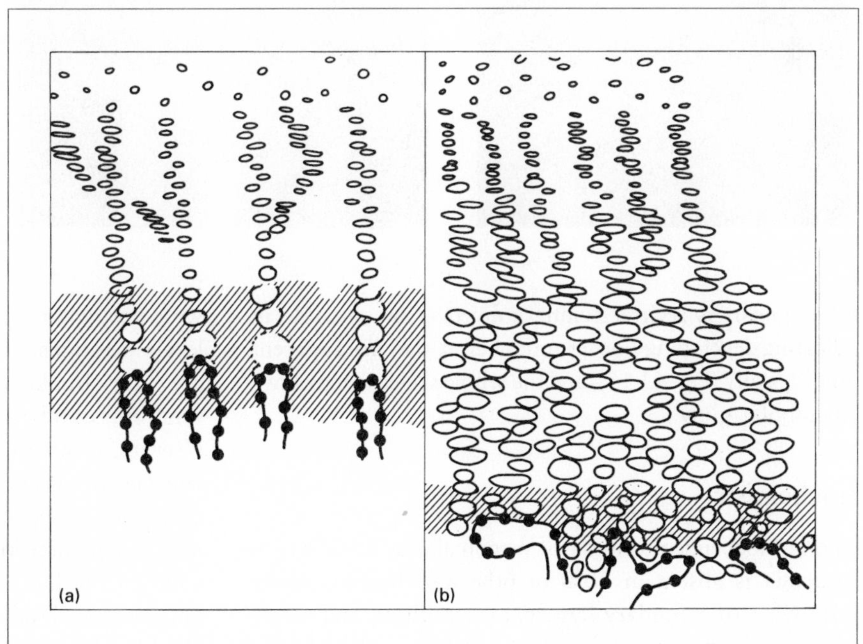

Fig. 42.11 Diagrammatic representation of the cartilaginous growth plate (a) in health and (b) in rickets. The top of the diagram faces toward the epiphysis and the bottom towards the diaphysis. The main features of the disturbance are the elongation and distortion of the normal columnar arrangement of chondrocytes and the resulting barrier to capillary vascularisation [39].

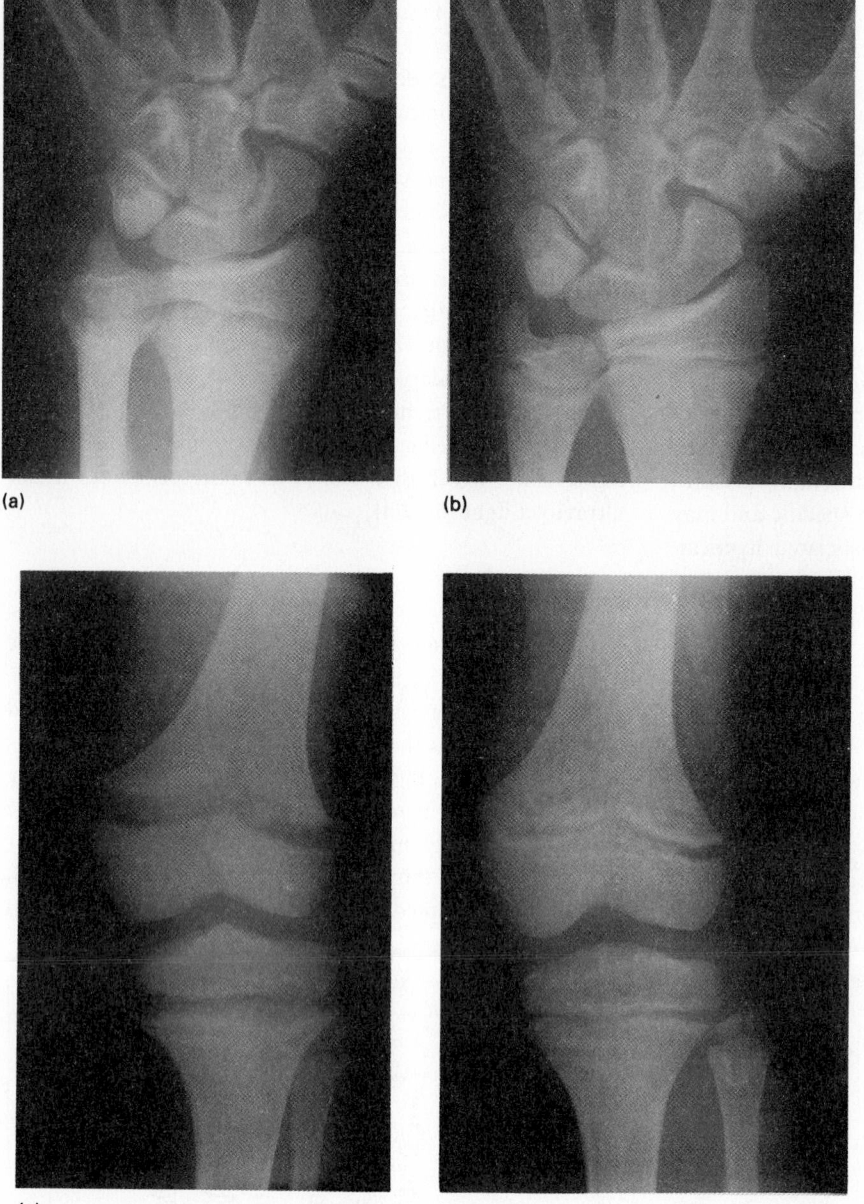

(a) (b)

Fig. 42.12 Radiographs of the wrist of a 14-year-old Asian boy resident in the UK taken (a) in June, showing privational rickets (see text for description), and (b) in October, following a 4-month holiday in India, having received no medication showing spontaneous healing.

(a) (b)

Fig. 42.13 Radiographs of the knee of a 9-year-old girl with X-linked hypophosphataemic rickets: (a) before treatment; (b) after 7 weeks' treatment in hospital with alfacalcidol 10μg daily and microcrystalline hydroxyapatite compound 6g daily. Rickets had almost healed without development of hypercalcaemia or hypercalciuria, despite the massive alfacalcidol dosage which was five times higher than that required for ultimate maintenance (see text for discussion).

the diagnosis is secure. Scintigraphy may be valuable in indicating developing Looser zones before they are apparent radiologically (Fig. 42.15), and the whole skeleton may have a metabolic 'glow'.

Biochemistry

Among biochemical criteria of osteomalacia, frank hypocalcaemia is absent in 50% of otherwise healthy adults [64] owing to secondary hyperparathyroidism, and rarely occurs in the hypophosphataemic syndromes. Within the wide normal limits, loosely assigned to serum phosphorus, levels are almost always towards the lower limit of normal, are only frankly abnormal in the hypophosphataemic syndromes, and may be paradoxically high if hypocalcaemia is severe, as can occur in infancy. Serum alkaline phosphatase concentration is generally high, but it must be remembered that levels in healthy adolescents at peak height velocity may reach three times the upper normal adult limits; in addition, one in 15 affected adults may have a serum alkaline phosphatase level within the strict normal adult range [45,64]. Urinary total hydroxyproline excretion, an index

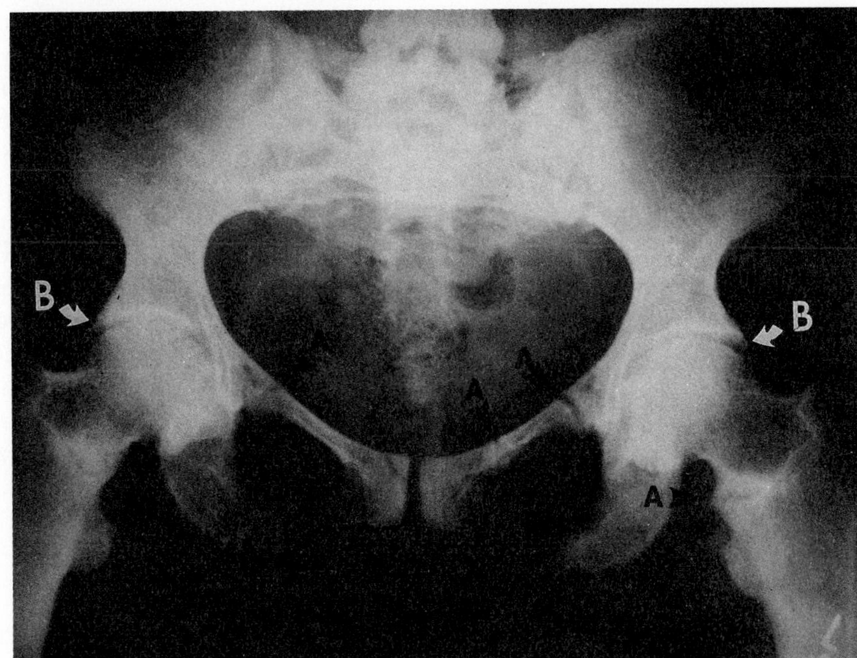

Fig. 42.14 Radiograph of the pelvis showing multiple Looser zones (arrowed) in an asymptomatic woman with X-linked hypophosphataemia. The arrows point to early heterotopic ossification around the hip joint which is not a feature of other forms of osteomalacia (see text).

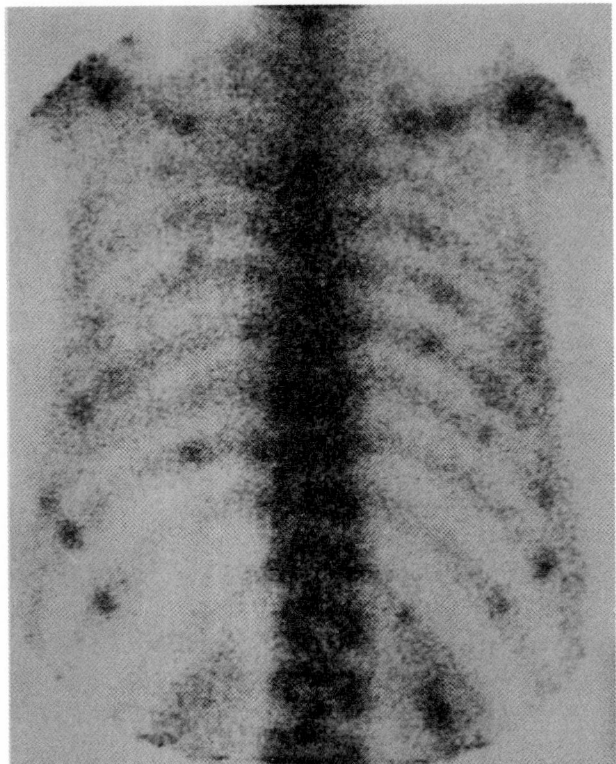

Fig. 42.15 Isotope bone scan in a 37-year-old man with severe osteomalacia associated with an intestinal malabsorption syndrome (hereditary immunoglobulin deficiency). The majority of the 'hot spots' were not evident as Looser zones radiologically.

of bone resorption, may be high; immunoreactive PTH levels are most invariably raised, except in the hypophosphataemic syndromes, and a high PTH level is often associated with mild metabolic acidosis owing to enhanced renal bicarbonate excretion and with mild generalised aminoaciduria.

Vitamin D disorders

Abnormalities in vitamin D metabolism can be classified in three main categories:

1 vitamin D deficiency;
2 acquired or inherited disorders of vitamin D metabolism;
3 resistance to vitamin D action.

Vitamin D deficiency

The recommended dietary intake of vitamin D in infants and adults is about 400 iu. A reduction in vitamin D intake during the day may result in rickets or osteomalacia in children and adults, respectively.

The causes of vitamin D deficiency are represented by inadequate sunlight exposure or insufficient dietary intake. Another important cause of vitamin D deficiency is represented by vitamin D malabsorption that may occur in patients with severe gastrointestinal disorders (i.e. non-tropical sprue, Crohn's disease, pancreatic insufficiency, etc.). Because the gastrointestinal tract is the major area of nutrient absorption it is not surprising to find alterations of absorption of vitamin D and calcium in these disorders [65]. In vitamin D deficiency due to malabsorption, the dose of vitamin D therapy must be adjusted depending on serum levels of phosphorus, calcium and alkaline phosphatase. On the other hand, for patients with a deficiency of vitamin D from lack of exposure to sunlight, either increased exposure to sunlight or to artificial ultraviolet light is useful. In addition, the consumption of cereals and other grain products high in phytate may lead to intraluminal calcium malabsorption. Finally, calcium deficiency may also be seen with total parenteral nutrition. The response of the skeleton to alterations in calcium homeostasis can vary in these patients, from mild osteopenia to severe osteomalacia.

Modifications of vitamin D metabolism

The acquired group of diseases comprises patients with cholestatic liver disorders, patients with advanced renal insufficiency, and patients on chronic therapy with anticonvulsants, particularly phenytoin and carbamazepine. In the first, patients can develop osteomalacia and secondary hyperparathyroidism as a consequence of reduced hepatic vitamin D hyroxylation. In these patients, circulating levels of 25-OHD are reduced and hypocalcaemia is usually modest. On the other hand, patients with renal insufficiency have low plasma calcium levels as a consequence of reduced 1α-hydroxylase activity. Rickets may appear earlier when tubular damage predominates over glomerular destruction, for example in hereditary or acquired Fanconi syndromes.

An important inherited abnormality of vitamin D metabolism is the vitamin-D dependent rickets type I (VDDR-I), which is a rare autosomal recessive disorder presenting in children with hypocalcaemia. The pathogenesis of this disorder appears to be a selective defect in 1α-hydroxylase activity with a lack of ability to convert 25-OHD to 1,25-$(OH)_2D_3$. These patients may be treated with physiological dose of $1,25(OH)_2D_3$ (0.25–1 mg/day).

Vitamin D-resistance syndromes

The VDDR type II (VDRR-II) is an inherited vitamin D disorder described for the first time by Brooks, and characterised by end-organ resistance to the actions of vitamin D. Affected children are usually normal at birth, with rickets occurring before the age of 2 years, although cases of presentation later in life have been reported. In contrast to VDDR-I, hypocalcaemia in VDDR-II is accompanied by a dramatic increase in circulating 1,25-$(OH)_2D_3$. Serum 25-OHD concentrations are normal and alkaline phosphatase levels are elevated. In about two-thirds of children alopecia is present which is probably a direct consequence of resistance to 1,25-$(OH)_2D_3$. In the same patients, ectodermal anomalies as multiple milia, epidermoid cysts and oligodontia appear as well [66]. At least five phenotypically distinct intracellular defects have been found (Fig. 42.8) In one type, hormone binding is negative [49]; this is the most common form and is characterised by the absence of 1,25-$(OH)_2D_3$ binding to the cytosolic binding protein owing to a deletion of a large portion of the 1,25-$(OH)_2D_3$-binding domain. Defects may also affect the hormone binding capacity and affinity. Altered nuclear translocation of the 1,25-$(OH)_2D$–VDR complex has also been described [67]. Finally, patients may also exhibit a decreased affinity of the hormone-receptor complex to heterologous DNA.

In VDDR-II, therapy must be initiated with high doses of vitamin D analogues in order to maintain high serum concentrations of 1,25-$(OH)_2D_3$. In addition, calcium supplementation (3 g elementary calcium/day) should be administered; the duration of this therapy is 3–5 months, sufficient to mineralise depleted bones and allow recovery from the 'hungry bone' syndrome.

Hypophosphataemia

The commonest cause of hypophosphataemic rickets in childhood is X-linked, the abnormal gene having been mapped to the short arm. Males are generally affected more severely than females, who may occasionally show hypophosphataemia without ever developing rickets. About one-third of cases appear as a spontaneous mutation. The typical toddler is sturdy, strong and thriving, but bow legs and a decreased height velocity are progressive. The disease is almost unique in two respects; first, there is an absence of myopathy (unless the child has been immobilised), and secondly, there is a progressive thickening of bone cortices which continues throughout adult life, associated with variably progressive calcification of paraspinal ligaments and tendon insertions (this disorder being known as enthesopathy) [55] (Fig. 42.16). Dental root hypoplasia is not uncommon and apical abscesses are a complication. Serum calcium concentration is almost always normal and secondary hypoparathyroidism is absent.

The nature of the renal tubular phosphate leak at the cellular level is uncertain; 1,25-$(OH)_2D_3$ levels are inappropriately normal or low and do not respond to further phosphate depletion. PTH infusions invoke a cAMP response, but evidence concerning changes in serum calcium, 1,25-$(OH)_2D_3$ and tubular phosphorus reabsorption are currently conflicting [68,69]. The progressive skeletal changes clearly indicate an intrinsic abnormality of bone turnover, the nature of which is unclear. Treatment requires calcitriol ($1,25(OH)_2D_3$) or alfacalcidol in doses similar to those given in hypoparathyroidism, and it is sensible to begin with higher doses to arrest progressive deformity, after which the long bones will tend to straighten progressively. A high calcium intake, with calcium supplements if necessary for

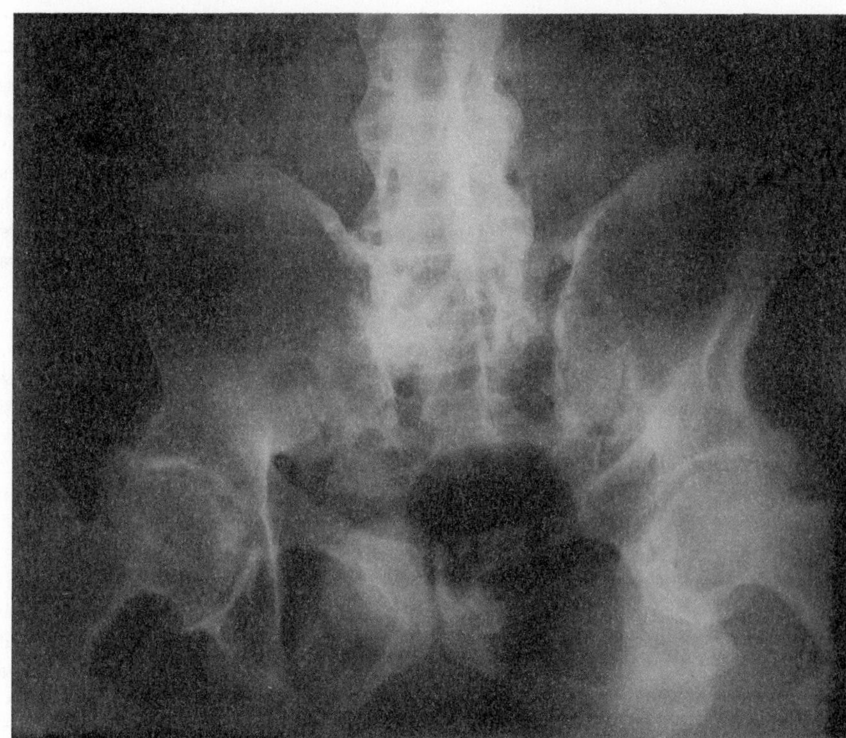

Fig. 42.16 Radiograph of the pelvis of a 63-year-old man with X-linked hypophosphataemia (transmitted to daughter and granddaughter). Note the gross enthesopathy, i.e.calcification and ossification in paraspinal ligaments ('bamboo spine'), periarticular region of the hips, etc. These patients are negative for the histocompatibility antigen HLA-B27.

3–4 months, is also advisable. Patients should then grow normally along the centiles obtaining at diagnosis. Phosphate supplements should be added if there is any uncertainty over adequate control; Phosphate-Sandoz is convenient, in an initial dose of half a tablet thrice daily for toddlers, increasing to one tablet thrice daily. Treatment must be continued until growth ceases at the end of adolescence; it is no use reducing, or stopping, treatment in the hope that the rickets may remain cured. Hypophosphataemia is life long and virtually uninfluenced by treatment, final height correlating poorly with mean serum phosphorus levels. Occasionally, the disease recrudesces in adult life; such patients may show gross, asymptomatic Looser zones (see Fig. 42.14) and occasionally present with a pathological fracture through one. These Looser zones are indolent and refractory to treatment. On the other hand an osteotomy, and even leg lengthening, generally heals well. Deafness and spinal cord compression are additional, rare complications. Dominant and autosomal recessive forms of this phenotype have been reported. A different form of autosomal recessive hypophosphataemic rickets has been reported among widely intermarried Bedouin tribespeople [70]. It is characterised by hypercalciuria which is expressed in heterozygotes.

Acquired, adult-presenting hypophosphataemic osteomalacia is either idiopathic or associated with mesenchymal tumours, which are usually benign. The natural history of both forms is identical [71], and both are very different from hereditary X-linked disease. Patients develop osteomalacia with severe skeletal demineralisation, widespread bone pains and severe myopathy, and become chair-bound without treatment. Careful search for a tumour should be undertaken, with computed tomographic scanning at least of the head and neck if necessary. Hypophosphataemic rickets and osteomalacia may also appear, at any age, in association with neurofibromatosis, polyostotic fibrous dysplasia, or linear sebaceous naevus [72]. These variants, forming a spectrum from fibrous dysplasia to fibromatous neoplasia, are of obvious theoretical interest, but causal relationships, if any, are obscure. Serum calcium concentration is almost always normal. Production of $1,25\text{-}(OH)_2D_3$ is often disturbed but low levels are not invariable. Rarely, glycosuria may occur, or a mildly abnormal urine amino-acid pattern, for example isolated excess glycine. Resection of apparently single tumours usually, but not always, cures the disease with its associated hypophosphataemia, but relapse is possible. Necessary doses of calcitriol, etc., are similar to those for hypoparathyroidism, with higher doses initially advisable, together with calcium supplements, to heal the skeleton as quickly as possible.

Phosphate supplements are mandatory throughout. Even after successful tumour resection aided by the above medication, long-term follow-up is necessary lest hypophosphataemia should recur. The responsible tumours have been classified into several types [73] but are usually described

Table 42.3 Causes of rickets and osteomalacia.

Privational
- Classic deficiency
  - Immigrant children: infants and puberty ('late') rickets
  - Immigrant adults
  - Indigenous elderly and other institutionalised groups
  - Food faddists

Gastrointestinal
- Partial gastrectomy
- Small-bowel malabsorption syndromes
  - Gluten-sensitive enteropathy (coeliac disease)
  - Purgative addition
  - Visceral scleroderma
  - Amyloidosis
  - Regional enteritis
  - Mesenteric tuberculosis
  - Surgical resection or bypass
  - Hereditary γ-globulin deficiency
- Chronic pancreatic insufficiency
- Hepatobiliary disturbance
  - Prematurity
  - Biliary atresia
  - Neonatal hepatitis
  - Primary biliary cirrhosis
  - Ascending cholangitis
  - Chronic active hepatitis
  - Anticonvulsant drugs (?multifactorial)

Hereditary renal disease (usually renal phosphate 'leaks' with high phosphate clearances)
- Hypophosphataemia
  - X-linked dominant; also, rarely
  - Autosomal dominant
  - Autosomal recessive
  - Dominant with neurofibromatosis
  - Hypophosphataemic hypercalciuric autosomal recessive
- Vitamin D-dependent rickets type I
- Vitamin D-dependent rickets type(s) II
- Fanconi syndromes
  - Cystinosis: infantile form, late childhood form
  - Fanconi syndrome without cystinosis
    - Childhood form
    - Adult form with and without diabetes mellitus

Hereditary renal disease (*cont.*)
  - Oculocerebrorenal (Lowe's) syndrome
    - Wilson's disease (hepatolenticular degeneration)
  - Hereditary tyrosinaemia
  - Glycogenosis with abnormal galactose metabolism
  - Familial nephrosis (Fanconi 'tubule' without rickets: hereditary fructose intolerance, galactosaemia)
- Distal renal tubular acidosis (renal rickets with nephrocalcinosis and dwarfism)

Acquired renal disease
- Azotaemic renal osteodystrophy (any form)
- Hypophosphataemic syndromes
  - Idiopathic
  - Mesenchymal tumours
    - Benign
    - Malignant
  - Linear sebaceous naevus
  - Neurofibromatosis
  - Polyostotic fibrous dysplasia
  - Hypercalciuric hypophosphataemic
- Fanconi syndromes
  - Obstructive uropathy
  - Ureterosigmoidostomy and ileal bladder
  - Gammopathies including idiopathic varieties, paraproteinaemia and myelomatosis
  - Primary amyloidosis
  - Sjögren' syndrome
  - Heavy metal poisoning: calcium, lead, gold, uranium, mercury
  - Outdated tetracycline and other poisons
  - Renal homotransplantation
  - Idiopathic Fanconi syndromes
    - Adult forms, with and without diabetes mellitus
    - Pancreatic carcinoma
    - ?Associated with chronic pancreatic insufficiency

Miscellaneous forms
- Phosphate depletion (intestinal P binders)
- Calcium depletion
- ?Magnesium depletion
- Primary hyperparathyroidism
- Diphosphonates
- ?Axial osteomalacia

as non-ossifying or ossifying fibromas, or haemangiopericytomas; they are vascular tumours frequently containing islets of cartilage, which may be calcified, and osteoclast-like giant cells. Studies of tumour extracts and parabiosis have shown in some instances that hypophosphataemia and depressed 1,25-$(OH)_2D_3$ production may be experimentally transmitted [74].

The Fanconi syndrome

The term Fanconi syndrome, the only surviving eponym among the names of De Toni, Lignac and Debré, is used to define the coexistence of multiple proximal tubular reabsorptive defects chiefly involving phosphate, glucose, amino acids and bicarbonate but extending to calcium, potassium, urate and water in this and other parts of the tubule. Although original descriptions were probably those of cystinosis, they date prior to the introduction of amino-acid chromatography when only 'non-urea nitrogen' was measurable. Their causes are listed in Table 42.3. All cases of rickets and osteomalacia are associated with variable combinations of hypophosphataemia, acidosis and defective production of 1,25-$(OH)_2D$. Tubular damage may be associated with a specific form of 'tubular' proteinuria including β-microglobulinuria; a rare, specific form of 'hypercalciuric rickets' with β-microglobulinuria has recently resurfaced [75].

Treatment involves supplementation as required with sodium bicarbonate (2.4 g three times daily may be necessary), potassium (given as Effercitrate tablets up to three times daily which also provides alkali) and phosphate. Giving vitamin D alone, or with inadequate supplements, may worsen hypercalciuria and produce or worsen renal calcification. Coexistent nephrogenic diabetes insipidus necessitates a high fluid intake.

Renal tubular acidosis

There are two main types of renal tubular acidosis [76]. Type I ('distal' or 'gradient', see below) was originally described graphically as 'nephrocalcinosis with renal rickets and dwarfism', which denotes its cardinal features. It is due to defective hydrogen-ion secretion in the distal tubule, in other words an inability to maintain a pH gradient between the cell and the tubular lumen (hence the alternative names). In the 'complete' form, urine pH remains at or above 5.6 despite systemic acidosis; in the 'incomplete' form, systemic acidosis is absent despite symptoms. Diagnosis is established by administering an acid load in the form of ammonium chloride 0.1 g/kg bodyweight and following hourly urine pH; urine pH in the range 5.2–5.6 may be regarded as a partial defect. The reabsorptive threshold for bicarbonate in the proximal tubule is normal. The disease is either inherited by autosomal dominant gene or acquired, usually in association with a polyclonal gammopathy. Other conditions include Sjögren's syndrome and the autoimmune vasculitides, Calcium and potassium are excreted in excess. Urinary citrate excretion, perhaps the chief guardian against renal calcification, is low. Acquired renal tubular acidosis may on occasion show simultaneous evidence of proximal tubular damage, for example aminoaciduria.

The disease may present clinically in one of three disparate ways: as rickets (or osteomalacia), as urolithiasis (or nephrocalcinosis), or as hypokalaemic paralysis which may be life-threatening. The same patient has been known to present, years apart, first with osteomalacia and then with paralysis. Treatment with sodium bicarbonate alone normally restores all abnormalities and vitamin D needs to be given only to ensure adequate nutritional status. The effect of acidosis on production of 1,25-$(OH)_2D$ is variable and remains unclear. Children need bicarbonate in a daily dose of 4–5 mmol/kg bodyweight daily, while adults may need at least 7.2 g daily. Effercitrate is a potassium-containing alternative. If nephrocalcinosis has progressed to cause significant renal glomerular failure, higher doses of vitamin D derivatives may be required, but vitamin D alone is dangerous, worsening hypercalciuria and renal calcification. Progression of nephrocalcinosis, if present, is usually but not always halted by alkali therapy; this outcome may hinge on the extent to which alkali therapy increases urinary citrate excretion.

Type II, proximal renal tubular acidosis, is characterised by partial failure of bicarbonate reabsorption in the proximal tubule with excretion of at least 15% of the filtered load. Urine is normally alkaline, but severe acidosis may reduce bicarbonate excretion to the point where urine pH falls, indicating that hydrogen ion secretion in the distal tubule remains intact. Proximal renal tubular acidosis may be isolated, but it is often part of a complete or partial Fanconi syndrome; it occurs in vitamin D deficiency where there is evidence that it is not due to secondary hyperparathyroidism alone. Production of 1,25-$(OH)_2D_3$ in type II renal tubular acidosis is variable.

Other hypocalcaemic conditions

Among the other types of hypocalcemia, five conditions deserving particular mention are:

1 magnesium deficiency;
2 pancreatitis;
3 hyperphosphataemia;
4 drugs;
5 neonatal hypocalcaemia.

Hypocalcaemia secondary to hypomagnesaemia

In chronic and severe magnesium deficiency, PTH secretion is impaired. Patients with hypocalcaemia due to hypomagnesaemia exhibit both renal and skeletal resistance to exogenous PTH [77]. Magnesium therapy can reverse this resistance. Clinically, these patients are also resistant to parenteral calcium and to vitamin D therapy.

Hypocalcaemia secondary to pancreatitis

Several mechanisms have been proposed to explain this type of hypocalcaemia. The damaged pancreas generates free fatty acids into the peritoneum which chelate calcium from extracellular fluids [78]. In addition, hypomagnesaemia resulting from complications typical of pancreatitis, such as poor oral intake, alcohol abuse and vomiting, can contribute to the development of severe hypocalcaemia.

Hypocalcaemia secondary to hyperphosphataemia

Hyperphosphataemia determines hypocalcaemia only if severe and rapid in onset. The four causes of hyperphosphataemia accounting for hypocalcaemia are as follows.

Enteral or parenteral excessive phosphate administration

In this condition, calcification of soft tissues is observed, as described in diabetic ketoacidosis and acute alcoholism. Infants fed with ' humanised' cow's milk, rich in phosphate, can also become hypocalcaemic.

Tumour-lysis syndrome and hypocalcaemia associated with malignant diseases

In the tumour-lysis syndrome the release of intracellular phosphates is massive with consequent hyperphosphataemia [79]. Breast and prostate cancers are frequently complicated by osteoblastic metastases, which can induce hypocalcaemia secondary to accelerated bone formation.

Rhabdomyolisis-induced acute renal failure

This occurs after an important traumatic event or alcohol abuse following an early oliguric phase. The mechanism for hypocalcaemia appears to be similar to that of the tumour-lysis syndrome [80].

Advanced renal insufficiency

In the course of chronic renal failure, hypocalcaemia may be secondary to both the hyperphosphataemia (due to tubular phosphate retention) and to the reduction in 1,25(OH)$_2$-D$_3$ production secondary to reduced tubular 1-hydroxylase activity [80].

Drug-induced hypocalcaemia

A wide variety of drugs can lead to a hypocalcaemic state, such as bisphosphonates, calcitonin, gallium nitrate, plicamycin, phosphates, etc. However, treatment with inhibitors of bone resorption generally causes only a moderate hypocalcaemia, while the use of anticonvulsants may induce severe hypocalcaemia consequent on the altered metabolism of vitamin D. Phenobarbital enhances the catabolism of vitamin D and 25-OHD$_3$ in liver. Phenytoin appears to act by impairing the calcium release from bone and reducing its intestinal absorption [81].

Ethylenediamine tetra-acetate and/or citrate present in blood transfusions and radiographic contrast may also cause calcium chelation with consequent hypocalcaemia. Fluoride excess may cause hypocalcaemia [82]. Foscarnet, a pyrophosphate analogue used to treat cytomegalovirus infections, causes hypocalcaemia by chelating extracellular fluid calcium and by inducing hypomagnesaemia [83]. Ketoconazole and pentamidine also have hypocalcaemic potential [84].

Neonatal hypocalcaemia

Clinical symptoms of neonatal hypocalcemia do not substantially differ from those of adults. One can classify these according the time of onset: after birth results in: (i) early onset, within the first 3–4 days, possibly associated with the DiGeorge syndrome, with diabetes in infants or in their mothers, with perinatal asphyxia and with pre-eclampsia; and (b) late onset, at 5–10 days of life, frequently present in winter, in infants of a mother with limited vitamin D intake or in the presence of dietay phosphate load [85]. Other conditions can be classified as congenital hypoparathyroidism, as 'late-late' hypocalcaemia in premature infants with inadequate dietary mineral and/or vitamin D intake, as hypocalcaemia in infants of a hyperparathyroid mother (frequently undiagnosed), and as hypocalcaemia in infants with alkalosis [85].

Summary of therapeutic consideration

A diagnosis of privational osteomalacia is occasionally equivocal on clinical, biochemical and radiological grounds, for example in an elderly housebound subject who may have suffered a proximal femoral fracture; on another occasion rickets may be obvious but the differential diagnosis uncertain. At such times a short diagnostic trial of vitamin D replacement in a physiological dosage of 1500–3000 U daily is a valid approach. The diagnosis of vitamin D deficiency will be confirmed by a brisk rise in serum phosphorus occurring in the first 2–3 weeks of treatment. Alkaline phosphatase levels show a frequent temporary rise, or 'flare', during this period. Failure to respond to physiological vitamin D replacement indicates a 'metabolic' (i.e. vitamin D-resistant) cause.

As mentioned above, small doses of vitamin D may produce very high levels of 1,25-(OH)$_2$D$_3$ (at least 150 pg/ml) in privational disease (see Fig. 42.17), associated with a profound fall in faecal calcium excretion. The oral dosage of calcitriol required to achieve such levels is uncertain, but there is a good argument for treating severe vitamin D-resistant disease with high doses of calcitriol to achieve similar levels, 2–5 μg daily in the early stages. The dosage can then be reduced over 3–4 months to maintenance levels. Calcium supplements are sensible when the initial mineral

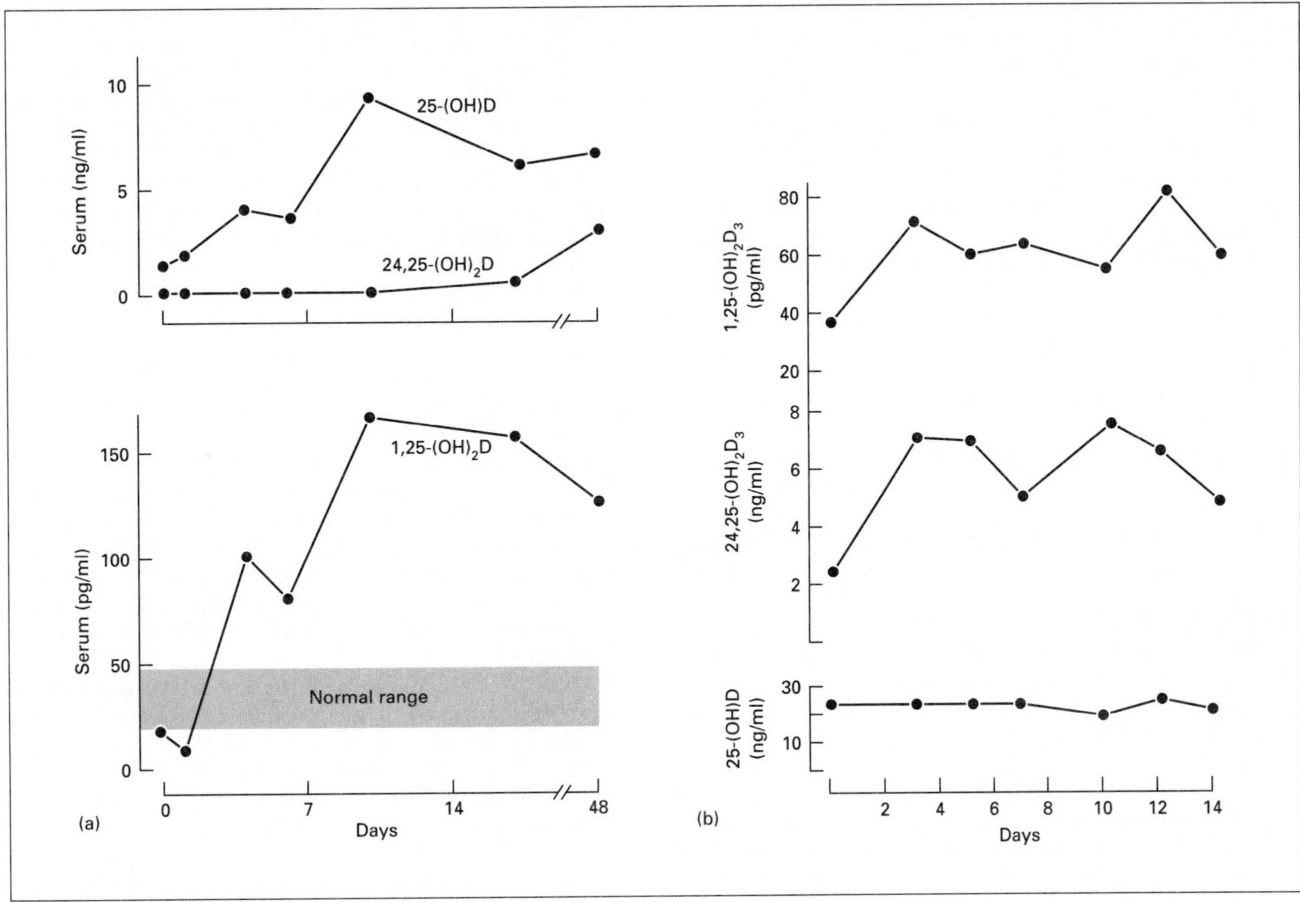

Fig. 42.17 (a) Vitamin D metabolites in the serum of a young woman with osteomalacia treated from day 0 with 450 iu vitamin D daily. Note the relationship between low or low-normal 25-hydroxyvitamin D (25-OHD$_3$) throughout and the rapid development of markedly raised 1,25-dihydroxyvitamin D (1,25-(OH$_2$D$_3$). (b) Vitamin D metabolites in the serum of a healthy control subject given 1 μg 1,25(OH)$_2$D$_3$ daily from day 0 [86].

deficit is large. Long-term phosphate supplements are often advisable in X-linked hypophosphataemia and are mandatory in adult-onset hypophosphataemic osteomalacia. Alkali therapy is mandatory in renal tubular acidosis. Effective therapy often produces transient worsening of bone pains in the first few days or week, the 'stirring-up phenomenon', and patients should be forewarned and reassured of this effect.

Conclusions

Hypocalcaemia is a disorder whose treatment is now well recognised by clinicians. Prevention of hypocalcaemic conditions is very important in children, during skeletal growth of the young and also in the elderly. The pathogenic role of hypocalcaemia is well recognised in several disorders of different organs and tissues. Physicians are therefore becoming increasingly aware of this condition and of the needs for prevention and therapy.

Recent advances in molecular genetics have made possible the characterisation of the pathogenic basis of many of the disorders of the PTH–vitamin D axis. The identification of additional defects will help to elucidate the pathogenesis of these disorders of calcium homeostasis, and will also undoubtedly increase our understanding of the function of vitamin D and PTH in normal physiology.

References

1 Parfitt AM, Kleerekoper M. Clinical disorders of calcium, phosphorus and magnesium. In: Maxwell MH, Kleeman CR, eds. *Clinical Disorders of Fluid and Electrolyte Metabolism*. New York: McGraw-Hill, 1987: 947.

2 Drezner MK, Neelon FA. Pseudohypoparathyroidism. In: Stanbury JB, Wyngaarden JB, Fredrickson JS, Goldstein JL, Brown MS, eds. *The Metabolic Basis of Inherited Disease*, 5th edn. New York: McGraw-Hill, 1990: 1508–27.

3 McSheeny PMJ, Chambers TJ. Osteoblastic cells mediate osteoclastic responsiveness to parathyroid hormone. *Endocrinology* 1986; **118**: 824–8.

4 Klahr S, Hruska K. Effects of parathyroid hormone on the renal reabsorption of phosphorus and divalent actions. In: Peck WA, ed. *Bone and Mineral Research*, Annual 2. Amsterdam: Elsevier, 1984: 64–124.

5 Aurbach GD. Calcium-regulating hormones: parathyroid hormone and calcitonin. In: Nordin BEC, ed. *Calcium in Human Biology*. London: Springer-Verlag, 1988: 43–68.

6 De Luca HF, Schnoes HK. Vitamin D: recent advances. *Ann Rev Biochem* 1983; **52**: 411–39.

7 Bell NH. Vitamin D-endocrine system. *J Clin Invest* 1985; **76**: 1–6.

8 Fraser DR. Regulation of the metabolism of vitamin D. *Physiol Rev* 1980; **60**: 551–613.

9 Fraser DR. Calcium-regulating hormones: vitamin D. In: Nordin BEC, ed. *Calcium in Human Biology*. London: Springer-Verlag, 1988: 27–41.

10 Reichel H, Koeffler HP, Norman AW. The role of the vitamin D endocrine system in health and disease. *N Engl J Med* 1989; **320**: 980–91.

11 Bronner F. Vitamin D-dependent active calcium transport: the role of calcium binding protein. *Calcif Tiss Int* 1988; **43**: 183–7.

12 Silver J, Naveh-Many T, Mayer H, Schmeizer JH, Popovtzer M. Regulation by vitamin D metabolites of PTH gene transcription *in vivo* in the rat. *J Clin Invest* 1986; **78**: 1296–301.

13 Haussler MR, Mangelsdorf DJ, Komm BS *et al*. Molecular biology of the vitamin D hormone. *Recent Prog Horm Res* 1988; **44**: 263–305.

14 Merke J, Milde P, Lewicka S *et al*. Identification and regulation of 1,25-dihydroxyvitamin D receptor activity and biosynthesis of 1,25-dihydroxyvitamin D. Studies in cultured bovine aortic endothelial cells and human dermal capillaries. *J Clin Invest* 1989; **83**: 1903–15.

15 Davies DR, Dent CE, Watson L. Idiopathic hypercalciuria and hyperparathyroidism. *Br Med J* 1971; **i**: 108.

16 Favus MJ, ed. *Primer on the Metabolic Bone Disease and Disorders of Mineral Metabolism*. Kelseyville, California: American Society for Bone and Mineral Research, 1990.

17 Editorial. Metabolic bone disease of prematurity. *Lancet* 1987; **i**: 200.

18 Stamp TCB. Mineral metabolism. In: Dickerson JWT, Lee HA, eds. *Nutrition in the Clinical Management of Disease*, 2nd edn. London: Edward Arnold, 1988: 290–325.

19 Neufeld M, Blizzard RM. Polyglandular autoimmune disease. In: Pinchera A, Doniach D, & Fenzi GF, eds. *Symposium on Autoimmune Aspects of Endocrine Disorders*. New York: Academic Press, 1980: 357–65.

20 Driscoll DA, Budfart ML, Emanuel BS. A genetic etiology of DiGeorge syndrome: consistent deletions and microdeletions of 22q11. *Am J Hum Genet* 1992; **50**: 924–33.

21 Franceschini P, Testa A, Bogetti G. Kenney–Caffey syndrome in two sibs born to consanguineous parents: evidence for an autosomal recessive variant. *Am J Hum Genet* 1992; **42**: 112–16.

22 Boyonton JR, Pheasant TR, Johnson BL, Levin DB, Streeten BW. Ocular findings in Kenny's syndrome. *Arch Ophthalmol* 1979; **97**: 896–900.

23 Arnold A, Horst SA, Gardella TJ, Baba H, Levine MA, Kronenberg HM. Mutation of the signal peptide-encoding region of the pre-proparathyroid hormone gene in familial isolated hypoparathyroidism. *J Clin Invest* 1990; **86**: 1084–7.

24 Parkinson DB, Thakker RV. A donor splice site mutation in the parathyroid hormone gene is associated with autosomal recessive hypoparathyroidism. *Nature Genet* 1992; **1**: 149–52.

25 Peden VH. True idiopathic hypoparathyroidism as a sex-linked recessive trait. *Am J Hum Genet* 1960; **12**: 323–37.

26 White MP, Weldon VV. Idiopathic hypoparathyroidism presenting with seizures during infancy: X-linked recessive inheritance in a large Missouri kindred. *J Pediatr* 1981; **99**: 608–11.

27 Thakker RV, Davies KE, Whyte WP, Wooding C, O'Riordan JHL. Mapping the gene causing X-linked recessive idiopathic hypoparathyroidism to Xq26–Xq27 by linkage studies. *J Clin Invest* 1990; **86**: 756–8.

28 Van Dop C. Pseudohypoparathyroidism: clinical and molecular aspects. *Semin Nephrol* 1989; **9**: 168–78.

29 Levine MA, Downs RW, Jr, Moses AM *et al*. Resistance to multiple hormones in patients with pseudohypoparathyroidism. Association with deficient activity of ganine nucleotide regulatory protein. *Am J Med* 1983; **74**: 545–56.

30 Levine MA, Schwindinger WF, Downs RW, Jr, Moses AM. Pseudohypoparathyroidism. Clinical, biochemical and molecular features. In: Bilezikian J, Levine, MA & Marcus R eds. *The Parathyroids*. New York: Raven Press, 1994: 781–800.

31 Loveridge N, Fischer JA, Nagant de Deuxchaisens C *et al*. Inhibition of cytocromical bioactivity of parathyroid hormone by plasma in pseudohypoparathyroidism type I. *J Clin Endocrinol Metab* 1982; **54**: 1274–5.

32 Mitchell J, Goltzman D. Examination of circulating parathyroid hormone in pseudohypoparathyroidism. *J Clin Endocrinol Metab* 1985; **61**: 328–334.

33 Kidd GS, Schaaf M, Adler RA, Lassman MN, Wray HL. Skeletal responsiveness in pseudohypoparathyroidism: a spectrum of clinical disease. *Am J Med* 1980; **68**: 772–81.

34 Silve C, Santora A, Breslau N, Moses A, Spiegel A. Selective resistance to parathyroid hormone in cultured skin fibroblasts from patients with pseudohypoparathyroidism type Ib. *J Clin Endocrinol Metab* 1986; **62**: 640–4.

35 Poznanski AK, Werder WA, Giedon A. The pattern of shortening of the bones of the hand in PHP and PPHP:a comparison with brachydactyly in Turner syndrome, and acrodysostosis. *Radiology* 1977; **123**: 707–18.

36 Patten JL, Johns DR, Valle D. Mutation in the gene encoding the stimulatory G protein of adenylylate cyclase in Albright hereditary osteodystrophy. *N Engl J Med* 1990; **322**: 1412–19.

37 Weinstein LS, Gejman PV, Friedman E *et al*. Mutations of the Gs alpha subunit gene in Albright hereditary osteodystrophy detecting by denaturing gradient gel electrophoresis. *Proc Natl Acad Sci USA* 1990; **87**: 8287–90.

38 Schwindinger WF, Miric A, Levine MA. Identification of a novel missense mutation in the gene encoding the alpha subunit of the stimulatory G protein of adenyl cyclase in a subject with Albright hereditary osteodystrophy. In: *Program and Abstracts, 74th Annual Meeting of the Endocrine Society*, San Antonio, Texas, 1992: 35.

39 Weinstein LS, Gejman PV, de Mazancourt P, American N, Spiegel AM. A heterozygous 4-bp deletion mutation in the Gsα gene (GNAS1) in a patient with Albright hereditary osteodystrophy. *Genomics* 1992; **13**: 1319–21.

40 Izraeli S, Metzker A, Horev G, Karmi D, Merlob P, Farfel Z. Albright hereditary osteodystrophy with hypoparathyroidism, normocalcemia, and normal Gs protein activity. *Am J Med* 1992; **43**: 764–7.

41 Barret D, Breslau NA, Wax MB, Molinoff PB, Downs RW, Jr. New form of pseudopseudohypoparathyroidism with abnormal catalytic adenylylate cyclase. *Am J Physiol* 1989; **257**: E277–83.

42 Rao DS, Parfitt AM, Kleerekoper M, Pumo BS, Frame B. Dissociation between the generation and phosphate reabsorption in hypocalcaemia due to vitamin D depletion: An acquired disorder resembling pseudohypoparathyroidism type II. *J Clin Endocrinol Metab* 1995; **61**: 285–90.

43 Reid ID, Civitelli R, Halstead LR, Avioli LV, Hruska KA. Parathyroid hormone acutely elevates intracellular calcium in osteoblast-like cells. *Am J Physiol* 1987; **253**: E45–51.

44 Yamaguchi DT, Hahn TJ, Iida-Klein A, Kleeman CR, Muallem S. Parathyroid hormone-activated calcium channels in an osteoblast-like clonal osteosarcoma cell line. *J Biol Chem* 1987; **262**: 7711–18.

45 Kruse K, Kracht U, Wohlfart K, Kruse U. Biochemical markers of bone turnover, intact serum parathyroid hormone and renal calcium excretion in patients with pseudohypoparathyroidism and hypoparathyroidism before and during vitamin D treatment. *Eur J Pediatr* 1989; **148**: 535–9.

46 Portale AR. Physiologic regulation of the serum concentration of 1-25-dihydroxyvitamin D by phosphorus in normal men. *J Clin Invest* 1989; **83**: 1494–9.

47 Reichel H, Norman AW. Systemic effects of vitamin D. *Ann Rev Med* 1989; **40**: 71–73.

48 Haussler MR. Molecular biology of the vitamin D hormone. *Recent Prog Horm Res* 1988; **44**: 263.

49 Pike JW, Dokoh S, Haussler MR, Liberman UA, Marx SJ, Eil C. Vitamin D-resistant fibroblasts have immunoassayable 1,25 dihydroxyvitamin D_3 receptors. *Science* 1984; **224**: 879–81.

50 Gross M, Kumar R. Physiology and biochemistry of vitamin D-dependent calcium binding proteins. *Am J Physiol* 1990; **259**: F195.

51 Russel J, Lettieri D, Adler J, Sherwood LM. 1,25-Dihydroxyvitamin D_3 has opposite effects on the expression of parathyroid secretory protein and parathyroid hormone genes. *Mol Endocrinol* 1990; **4**: 505–9.

52 Bukoski RD, Wang D, Wagman DW. Injection of 1-25 $(OH)_2$ vitamin D_3 enhances resistance artery contractile properties. *Hypertension* 1990; **16**: 523.

53 Walters MR. Hormonal regulation of bone and mineral metabolism. In: Negro-Vilar, A., ed. *Endocrine Reviews Monographs*. USA: Endocrine Society Press 1995: 1–46.

54 Boland R. Role of vitamin D in skeletal muscle function. *Endocr Rev* 1986; **7**: 434.

55 Stamp TCB. The clinical endocrinology of vitamin D. In: Parsons JA, ed. *Endocrinology of Calcium Metabolism*. New York: Raven Press, 1982: 363–422.

56 Haddad JG, Chyu KJ. Competitive protein-binding radio-assay for 25-hydroxycholecalciferol. *J Clin Endocrinol Metab* 1971; **33**: 992–4.

57 Stamp TCB, Round JM. Seasonal changes in human plasma levels of 25-hydroxycholecalciferol. *Nature (Lond)* 1974; **247**: 563–5.

58 Mankin HJ. Rickets, osteomalacia and renal osteodystrophy. *J Bone Joint Surg* 1974; **56A**: 101–28.

59 Peacock M. Osteomalacia and rickets. In: Nordin BEC, ed. *Metabolic Bone and Stone Disease*. London: Churchill-Livingstone, 1986: 71–111.

60 Aaron JE. Histological aspects of vitamin D and bone. In: Lawson DEM, ed. *Vitamin D*. London: Academic Press, 1978: 201–65.

61 Byers PD. The diagnostic value of bone biopsies. In: Avioli LV, Krane SM, eds. *Metabolic Bone Diseases*, Vol. 1. New York: Academic Press, 1977: 183–236.

62 Recker RR, ed. *Bone Histomorphometry: Techniques and Interpretations*. Boca Raton, Florida: CRC Press, 1983.

63 Parfitt AM, Drezner MK, Glorieux FH *et al.* Histomorphometry: standardization of nomenclature, symbols and units. *J Bone Miner Res* 1987; **2**: 595–610.

64 Stamp TCB, Walker PG, Perry W, Jenkins MV. Nutritional osteomalacia (and late rickets) in Greater London, 1974–79. Clinical and metabolic studies in 45 patients. *Clin Endocrinol Metab* 1980; **9**: 81–105.

65 Klein GL. Nutritional rickets and osteomalacia. In: Favus MJ, ed. *Primer on the Metabolic Bone Diseases and Disorders of Mineral metabolism*, 2nd edn. New York: Raven Press, 1993: 264–73.

66 Liberman UA, Samuel R, Halabe A *et al.* End-organ resistance to 1,25 dihydroxy cholecalciferol. *Lancet* 1989; **1**: 504–6.

67 Liberman UA, Marx SJ. Vitamin D dependent rickets. In: Favus MJ, ed. *Primer on the Metabolic Bone Diseases and Disorders of Mineral Metabolism*, 2nd edn. New York: Raven Press, 1993: 274–8.

68 Insogna KL, Broadus AE, Gertner JM. Impaired phosphorus conservation and 1,25-dihydroxyvitamin D generation during phosphorus deprivation in familial hypophosphataemic rickets. *J Clin Invest* 1983; **71**: 1562–9.

69 McElduff A, Posen S. Parathyroid hormone sensitivity in familial X-linked hypophosphataemic rickets. *J Clin Endocrinol Metab* 1989; **69**: 386–9.

70 Teider M, Modia D, Shaked U *et al.* Idiopathic hypercalciuria and hereditary hypophosphataemic rickets: two phenotypic expressions of a common genetic defect. *N Engl J Med* 1987; **316**: 129–9.

71 Dent CE, Stamp TCB. Hypophosphataemic osteomalacia presenting in adults. *Q J Med* 1971; **40**: 303–29.

72 Carey DE, Drezner MK, Hamolan JA *et al.* Hypophosphataemic rickets/osteomalacia in linear sebaceous nevus syndrome: a variant of tumour-induced osteomalacia. *J Paediatr* 1987; **111**: 855–7.

73 Weidner N, Santa Cruz D. Phosphaturic mesenchymal tumours. A polymorphous group causing osteomalacia or rickets. *Cancer* 1987; **59**: 1442–54.

74 Meyer RA. Parabiosis suggest a humoral factor is involved in X-linked hypophosphataemia in mice. *J Bone Miner Res* 1988; **4**: 493–500.

75 Carey DE, Hopfer SM. Hypophosphataemic rickets with hypercalciuria and microglobulinuria. *J Paediat* 1987; **111**: 860–3.

76 Morris RC, Jr. Renal tubular acidosis. *N Engl J Med* 1982; **304**: 418–20.

77 Rude RK. Magnesium metabolism and deficiency. *Endocrinol Metab Clin North Am* 1993; **22**: 377–95.

78 Stewart AF, Longo W, Kreutter D, Jacob R, Burtis WJ. Hypocalcemia due to calcium soap formation in a patient with a pancreatic fistula. *N Engl J Med* 1986; **315**: 496–8.

79 Zusman T, Brown D, Nesbit M. Hyperphosphatemia, hyperphosphaturia and hypocalcemia in acute lymphoblastic leukemia. *N Engl J Med* 1973; **289**: 1335–40.

80 Llach F, Felsenfeld A, Haussler M. The pathophysiology of altered calcium metabolism in rhabdomyolysis-induced acute renal failure. *N Engl J Med* 1981; **305**: 117–23.

81 Tjellesen L, Gotfredsen A, Christiansen C. Different actions of vitamin D_2 and D_3 on bone metabolism in patients treated with phenobarbitone/phenytoin. *Calcif Tissue Int* 1985; **37**: 218–22.

82 Gessner BD, Beller M, Middaugh JP, Withford GM. Acute fluoride poisoning from a public water system. *N Engl J Med* 1994; **330**: 95–9.

83 Jacobson MA, Gambertoglio JG, Aweeka FT, Causey DM, Portale

AA. Foscarnet-induced hypocalcemia and effects of foscarnet on calcium metabolism. *J Clin Endocrinol Metab* 1991; **72**: 1130–5.
84 Grinspoon SK, Bilezikian JP. HIV disease and the endocrine system. *N Engl J Med* 1992; **327**: 1360–5.
85 Cole DEC, Carpenter TO, Goltzman D. Calcium homeostasis and disorders of bone and mineral metabolism. In: Collu R, ed. *Pediatric Endocrinology Comprehensive Endocrinology Series*. New York: Raven Press, 1988: 509–80.
86 Mawber EB. Clinical implications of measurements of circulating vitamin D metabolites. *Clin Endocrinol Metab* 1980; **9**: 63–79.

CHAPTER 43

Osteoporosis

J. Compston

Definition and prevalence

Osteoporosis is characterised by a reduction in bone mass and disruption of cancellous bone structure, leading to reduced bone strength and an increase in fracture risk [1]. The resulting fractures are now widely recognised as a major cause of morbidity and mortality in elderly populations in the western world and impose a huge financial burden on the health services. In the UK approximately 60 000 hip fractures, 50 000 fractures of the distal radius and 40 000 clinically diagnosed vertebral fractures occur annually, with an estimated total cost to the health services of £742 million [2]. The remaining lifetime risk of fragility fracture for a 50-year-old British Caucasian woman has been estimated at 14%, 11% and 13% for the hip, spine and radius, respectively [3]; the corresponding figures in North American women are slightly higher, being 17.5%, 15.6% and 16%, respectively, whilst in men, the estimated remaining lifetime risk of any fragility fracture at age 50 approaches 13% [4].

The morbidity and mortality resulting from osteoporosis are solely attributable to fragility fracture. Fractures of the femoral neck occur mainly in the very elderly, the peak incidence being in the ninth decade; the mortality of these fractures is around 20% at 6 months and the majority of survivors exhibit increased dependency. Although the secular increase in hip fracture incidence reported from a number of countries may now be stabilising, increasing life expectancy and the resulting increase in the number of elderly individuals in many populations will lead to a sharp rise in the number of hip fractures over the next few decades.

Vertebral fractures are a significant although as yet largely unquantified cause of morbidity in late middle-aged and elderly women. Because the majority of these fractures do not come to medical attention, their true incidence is uncertain and the figure of 40 000 occurring annually is likely to represent only one-third or less of all vertebral fractures [5]. Their morbidity is attributable to both the direct and indirect effects of fracture; pain, although not invariable, may be severe and persistent and reduction in vertebral height leads to spinal deformity, loss of height and disability. Fractures of the distal radius have a peak incidence in the seventh decade of life and, although causing less morbidity than hip and vertebral fractures, may be associated with significant long-term discomfort and disability. Finally, fragility fractures at other sites, particularly the humerus and pelvis, number around 70 000 annually in the UK and contribute to the morbidity resulting from osteoporosis.

Lifetime changes in bone mass

Bone mass increases during childhood and adolescence to reach its peak during the third decade of life. This increase is due mainly to linear and transverse growth of the bones; after linear growth ceases, bone width continues to increase throughout life by periosteal appositional growth [6]. The age at which bone loss begins is uncertain, some studies demonstrating premenopausal bone loss, but during the menopause there is an acceleration in the rate of bone loss (Fig. 43.1). There is increasing evidence that bone loss continues well into old age both in women and men; overall, it is estimated that approximately 35% and 50% of cancellous bone are lost over a lifetime in women, the loss in men being approximately two-thirds of this amount [7]. Rates of bone loss in normal subjects show considerable heterogeneity, at least over relatively short periods of time, although whether there is a distinct population of 'fast losers' remains controversial. Both the onset and rate of bone loss differ between skeletal sites and between cortical and cancellous bone; because of the much greater surface area of the latter, rates of bone loss are generally greater than in cortical bone.

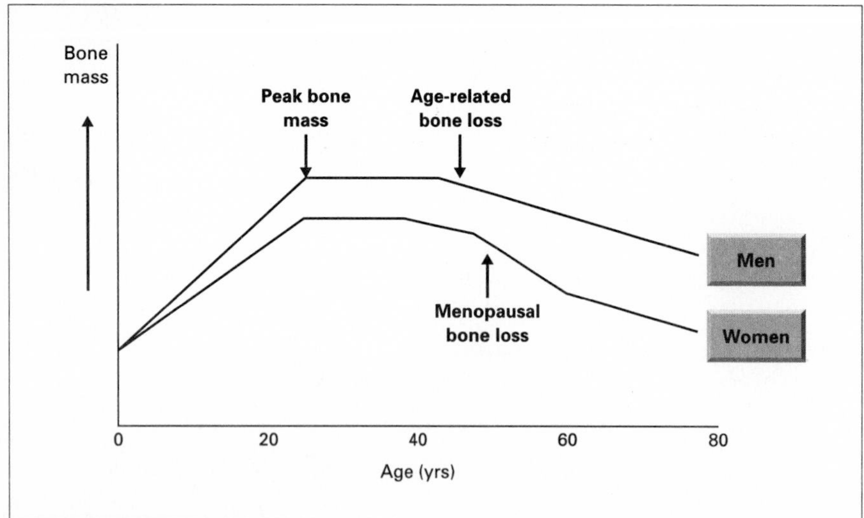

Fig. 43.1 Diagrammatic representation of lifetime changes in bone mass. From [55].

Diagnosis

Assessment of bone mass

In recent years new techniques have been developed which enable reasonably accurate and precise measurement of bone mass at potential fracture sites. These techniques are summarised in Table 43.1; at present, dual energy X-ray absorptiometry (DXA) is the method of choice because of its low radiation dose, good precision and applicability to both the axial and appendicular skeleton [8]. In common with all the other techniques, other than quantitative computed tomography, DXA generates an areal bone mineral density (BMD) in units of g/cm^2 rather than a true volumetric density and is therefore influenced, to some extent, by bone size [6]. The latest generation of DXA systems can perform bone density measurements within a few minutes and also possess the potential to produce high-grade lateral images of the thoracic and lumbar spine, thus obviating the need for conventional radiology in the assessment of vertebral deformity.

Absorptiometric techniques are subject to some limitations. In particular, measurements of BMD in the lumbar spine may be affected by extraskeletal calcification, osteophytes, scoliosis and vertebral deformity, all of which become increasingly common in the elderly [9]. It should also be noted that a low bone mineral density is not specific to osteoporosis but also occurs in osteomalacia. Finally, the distribution of osteoporosis within the spine may be heterogeneous and thoracic spine fractures sometimes occur in patients with a normal lumbar spine as assessed by bone densitometry and radiology.

The rationale for bone densitometry in clinical practice is based on the demonstration, in a number of prospective studies, of the relationship between bone mass and subsequent fracture risk [10–13]. These studies, which have been

Table 43.1 Measurement of bone mineral density.

Method	Site	Accuracy (%)	Precision (%)
Dual-energy X-ray absorptiometry	Spine	5–10	1
	Femur	5–10	2–3
	Whole body	1–2	1
Single X-ray absorptiometry	Radius	2–5	1–2
Single photon absorptiometry	Radius	2–5	1–2
Quantitative computed tomography	Spine	5–10	2–4
	Radius	5–10	2–4
Broad-band ultrasonic attenuation	Os calcis	Uncertain	2–4

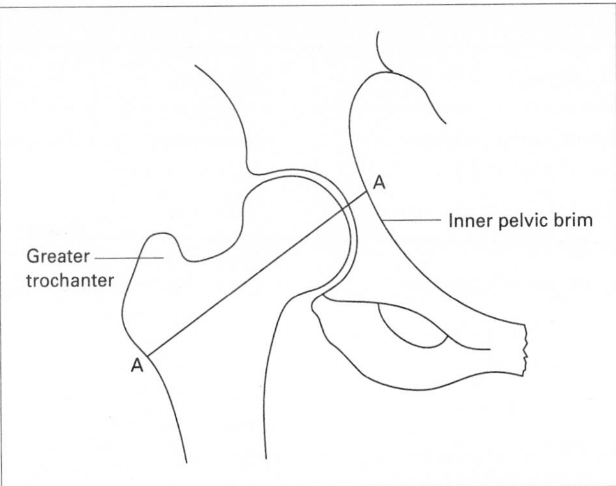

Fig. 43.2 Diagram to show the hip axis length (line A–A). This can be measured automatically by the dual energy X-ray absorptiometry (DXA) software during measurement of femoral bone mineral density. From [38].

conducted only in women, have shown an increasing gradient of fracture risk with decreasing bone mass, a decrease in BMD of 1 SD being associated with a two- to threefold increase in subsequent fracture risk. Although measurement of bone mass at any of the skeletal sites commonly assessed appears to be of predictive value, there is some evidence, at least for the hip, that the best prediction is obtained if BMD is assessed at the potential fracture site [14]. The majority of these studies have been performed in women in the seventh and eighth decades of life, and more data are required to establish the relationship between bone mass and fracture risk in perimenopausal women.

Three other important predictors of fracture risk have recently been identified. The first relates to the geometry of the femoral neck (Fig. 43.2); the hip axis length is positively related to hip-fracture risk, an effect which is independent of bone density, height or weight [15]. Secondly, a past history of fragility fracture and/or the presence of a prevalent vertebral fracture significantly increases the risk of further fracture, an effect which is also independent of BMD; thus, the presence of one or two prevalent vertebral fractures will increase future fracture risk approximately sevenfold [16]. Finally, as might be expected, risk factors for falling are an important determinant of hip fracture in the elderly, and morbidity-related risk factors such as visual or cognitive impairment, reduced mobility and low bodyweight significantly increase hip fracture risk at any given BMD [17].

Densitometric criteria for the diagnosis of osteopenia and osteoporis

Since the gradient of increasing fracture risk with decreasing bone mass is continuous, there is no cut-off point below which fracture will always occur and above which it will not. Nevertheless, for diagnostic purposes it is helpful to define densitometric criteria for osteoporosis; a World Health Organization Study Group has recently proposed two such thresholds, based on the relationship between bone mass and fracture risk [18]. Because absolute values for any given BMD may vary by as much as 12% between different DXA systems, T scores, which represent the number of standard deviations above or below the mean reference value for healthy premenopausal women, are used to define the following diagnostic categories:

Normal:	T score above –1
Osteopenia:	T score between –1 and –2.5
Osteoporosis:	T score below –2.5
Severe or established osteoporosis:	T score below –2.5 + one or more fractures

Included within this definition of osteoporosis are the majority of those women who will sustain a fracture in the future; this may therefore be regarded as an indication for intervention in most cases. The presence of osteopenia constitutes a relative indication for prevention, dependent upon a number of factors including the age of the woman and risks and benefits of the proposed treatment. These thresholds apply only to women and appropriate criteria for men are not presently available.

Although the above categories are useful in clinical practice, several limitations should be noted. The diagnostic classification of an invidual will depend critically upon the absolute values, pattern of age-related bone loss and variance of the reference data used; unfortunately there are significant differences between the reference data supplied by different manufacturers and there may also be true geographical variations in bone mass and age-related bone loss. Appropriate and standardised reference data are therefore essential for accurate classification by densitometric criteria. Secondly, the classification as outlined above does not include those patients who have a history of peripheral fragility fractures or prevalent thoracic spine fractures in the presence of normal lumbar spine and hip BMD. Thirdly, osteopenia thus defined covers a wide range of BMD and will include nearly all elderly women; the therapeutic implications of this diagnosis are thus less clear than in the case of osteoporosis.

Radiology

Radiological osteopenia is a relatively insensitive sign of osteoporosis although its presence constitutes an indica-

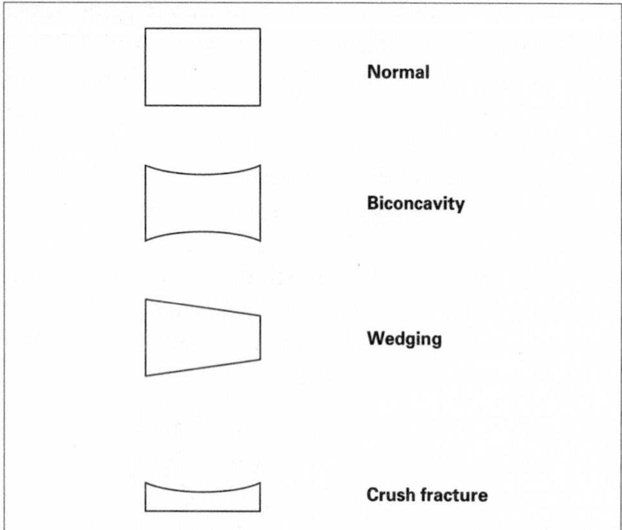

Fig. 43.3 Vertebral deformities associated with osteoporosis.

tion for further investigation. Radiology does, however, play an important role in the diagnosis of vertebral fractures (Fig. 43.3), and in recent years quantitative approaches to the assessment of vertebral deformity have been described which take into account inter- and intra-individual variations in vertebral shape in the normal population [19]. These are based on measurements of the anterior, middle and posterior heights of each vertebra and expressed in terms of percentage reduction of height or as number of standard deviations below reference mean values. There is some evidence that back pain, disability and height loss are only significantly associated with vertebral deformities involving a 25% or greater reduction in vertebral height (approximately 4 SD below the reference mean); however, the contribution of lesser degrees of deformity to morbidity requires further research.

Biochemical markers

A number of biochemical markers of bone resorption and formation have been identified [20] (Table 43.2). These provide indices of whole-body bone turnover and may be used to assess rates of bone loss over relatively short periods of time. They do not, however, indicate absolute levels of bone mass, and their ability to reflect site-specific changes in bone mass is uncertain. The large biological variability in these markers restricts their value in clinical practice although serial measurements may be useful in monitoring short-term responses to therapy in clinical trials. There is some evidence that the addition of selected biochemical markers to measurements of BMD may significantly improve prediction of fracture risk in perimenopausal and elderly women.

Table 43.2 Biochemical markers of bone turnover.

Resorption	Formation
Serum tartrate-resistant acid phosphatase	Serum alkaline phosphatase bone isoenzyme
Urinary pyridinoline and deoxypyridinoline	Serum osteocalcin
Urinary hydroxyproline	Serum Type 1 procollagen C-terminal propeptide (P1CP)
Urinary N-terminal cross-linked telopeptide (NTx)	Serum Type 1 procollagen N-terminal propeptide (P1NP)
Urinary crosslaps	
Serum type 1 collagen C-terminal telopeptide	

Risk factors

Many risk factors for osteoporosis have been identified, both endogenous and exogenous [21] (Table 43.3). Although combinations of these have been shown to have relatively poor specificity and sensitivity in predicting either bone density or fracture risk in population-based studies, this partly reflects the varying strength and prevalence of the risk factors used. Thus, common but relatively weak risk factors such as cigarette smoking and physical inactivity will have a greater influence on risk factor scores in the general population than strong risk factors, for example premature menopause and corticosteroid therapy. However, in clinical practice, identification of risk factors plays an important role in the detection and subsequent management of high-risk subjects.

Clinical indications for bone densitometry

In clinical practice, bone densitometry is used both to assess fracture risk in individuals with strong risk factors for osteoporosis and to confirm or refute a diagnosis of osteoporosis

Table 43.3 Major risk factors for osteoporosis.

Endogenous	Exogenous
Caucasian/Asian race	Premature menopause
Female sex	Secondary amenorrhoea
Advanced age	Primary hypogonadism
Small body build	Corticosteroid therapy
Maternal history of hip fracture	Previous or prevalent fragility fracture
	Intestinal disease

Table 43.4 Clinical indications for bone densitometry.

Presence of strong risk factors
Premature menopause
Prolonged secondary amenorrhoea
Primary hypogonadism
Corticosteroid therapy (>7.5 mg daily for 1 year or more)
Anorexia nervosa
Malabsorption
Primary hyperparathyroidism
Post-transplantation
Chronic renal failure
Myelomatosis
Hyperthyroidism
Prolonged immobilisation
Radiological osteopenia and/or vertebral deformity
Previous or prevalent fragility fracture
Monitoring of therapy
Patients with secondary osteoporosis
Treatment with newer drugs, e.g. bisphosphonates, calcitonin, vitamin D metabolites/analogues, sodium fluoride

in patients with radiological osteopenia and/or a previous or prevalent fragility fracture. Clinical indications for bone densitometry are shown in Table 43.4; assessment of bone mass is only justified in those cases in which the result obtained will influence management. Thus, in women with a premature menopause, hormone replacement therapy should be given routinely and bone densitometry is only required in those cases where there are strong contra-indications to treatment or if demonstration of low bone mass is required to gain compliance with therapy. Similarly, if multiple vertebral deformities have been demonstrated radiologically, bone densitometry is not usually required for diagnostic purposes. Bone densitometry is also used in the monitoring of some treatments; the frequency of measurements depends on the precision error of the technique and the expected rate of bone loss in the absence of treatment, but in individual patients, significant benefits of treatment may often be demonstrated within 1–2 years in the lumbar spine and within 3 years in the femoral neck.

Pathogenesis of osteoporosis and differential diagnosis

Primary osteoporosis has traditionally been divided into post-menopausal and senile or type I and type II osteoporosis. Although these classifications may have some merit, however, the dominance of oestrogen deficiency as a pathogenetic factor in women is increasingly recognised, and many now regard primary osteoporosis in post-menopausal and elderly women as a single entity, whilst recognising that the proportional contribution of different pathogenetic factors may vary according to age. In men, the pathogenesis of primary osteoporosis is poorly understood.

Many secondary causes of osteoporosis have been described (Table 43.5). Some of these may be detected on clinical examination or history taking, but in the absence of obvious secondary causes, routine investigations are recommended in all cases to exclude the commoner conditions which may be associated with osteoporosis. These include full blood count, calcium, phosphate and alkaline phosphatase, liver function tests, thyroid function tests, serum protein immunoelectrophoresis and urinary Bence–Jones proteins. In primary osteoporosis, serum calcium and phosphate are normal; alkaline phosphatase is also usually within normal limits although it may rise transiently after fracture. If not already performed, lateral X-rays of the thoracic and lumbar spine should also be obtained to detect vertebral deformity. Other investigations may be indicated where there is a high index of clinical suspicion and/or abnormalities revealed by routine tests, and it should be noted that in a small proportion of patients with myeloma, serum and urinary proteins may be normal and bone-marrow

Table 43.5 Secondary causes of osteoporosis.

Endocrine
Primary and secondary hypogonadism
Thyrotoxicosis
Hyperparathyroidism
Cushing's syndrome
Hyperprolactinaemia
Malignant disease
Myelomatosis
Leukaemia
Lymphoma
Mastocytosis
Drug-related
Glucocorticoids
Heparin
Alcohol
Connective-tissue disorders
Osteogenesis imperfecta
Marfan's syndrome
Ehlers–Danlos syndrome
Homocystinuria
Others
Malabsorption/bowel disease
Post-gastrectomy
Chronic liver disease
Chronic renal disease
Post-transplantation
Rheumatoid arthritis

trephine is required to establish the diagnosis. Isotope bone scanning is useful in cases of suspected malignancy, although increased uptake may occur at the site of a recent fracture. If osteomalacia is suspected, bone biopsy may be required to confirm the diagnosis.

In men with osteoporosis, secondary causes may be present in up to 50 or 60% of cases and more thorough investigation is required. Hypogonadism is a common secondary cause and measurement of serum testosterone and gonadotrophins should be routine; in cases with low testosterone but normal gonadotrophins, serum prolactin levels should be assessed. Alcohol abuse and glucocorticoid treatment are also relatively common causes of secondary osteoporosis in men.

Pathophysiology

Bone remodelling

In the adult human skeleton the mechanical integrity of bone is preserved by the process of bone remodelling, in which a quantum of old bone is removed and subsequently replaced by newly formed bone [22]. This process takes place on the cancellous bone surface and around Haversian systems in cortical bone, and consists of the resorption of bone by osteoclasts followed by the formation, by osteoblasts, of new bone. Under normal circumstances the temporal sequence is always that of resorption followed by formation (coupling), and in the young adult skeleton the amounts of bone resorbed and formed within a remodelling unit are quantitatively similar (balance). The new packet of bone thus formed is referred to as a bone structural unit; the time required to complete one remodelling cycle is around 3–6 months, most of this period being occupied by the formation of osteoid and its subsequent mineralisation.

The initiation of bone remodelling at any given site is poorly understood and is unlikely to be random in either time or space. Mechanical stresses, transmitted to the lining cells via the osteocyte–canalicular network, are believed to be responsible for site-specific activation in both cortical and cancellous bone [23]. Many other factors play a role in the regulation of bone remodelling; these include systemic hormones, locally produced cytokines and growth factors, prostaglandins, nitric oxide and free oxygen radicals. Many of the effects of systemic hormones and mechanical strain are believed to be mediated by the release of these local factors which are produced by bone cells or matrix and by cells in the bone microenvironment, and act on bone in an autocrine or paracrine manner [24].

Mechanisms of bone loss in osteoporosis

In osteoporosis, an increase in the activation frequency of new bone remodelling units provides quantitatively the most important mechanism of bone loss. This results in high bone turnover with an increase in the percentage of the bone surface occupied by resorption cavities. In addition, the amount of bone formed within remodelling units may be less than that resorbed, leading to remodelling imbalance. These two mechanisms of bone loss both operate in postmenopausal osteoporosis.

Changes in bone structure in osteoporosis

The changes in bone remodelling responsible for bone loss in osteoporosis determine the accompanying alterations in cancellous bone microstructure. Increased activation frequency, with or without an increase in resorption depth, favours trabecular penetration and erosion, leading to loss of connectivity, whereas remodelling imbalance due to reduced bone formation predisposes to trabecular thinning with relative preservation of bone architecture [25]. These changes have important mechanical and therapeutic implications; loss of connectivity is associated with a greater reduction in bone strength for any given bone mass than is trabecular thinning. Furthermore, whereas trabecular thickening can be achieved therapeutically, it is unlikely that the structural integrity of bone, once disrupted, can be restored.

Prevention and treatment of osteoporosis

General considerations

Agents used in the prevention and treatment of osteoporosis are generally classified as antiresorptive and anabolic (Table 43.6). Drugs in the former category preserve bone mass, often with a small and transient increase in bone mass which is attributable to in-filling of the remodelling space created by high turnover. Anabolic agents, such as sodium fluoride and parathyroid hormone, lead to an increase in cancellous bone mass which is sustained throughout the duration of therapy. At present, all the agents commonly used in the prevention and treatment of osteoporosis act primarily as antiresorptive agents.

Management of patients with osteoporosis should be aimed not only at improving bone mass but also at providing symptomatic relief, increasing mobility and restoring confidence. In patients with acute vertebral fracture who present with severe pain, immobilisation should be restricted to a minimum and strong analgesics are usually required. A course of daily calcitonin injections given over 2–3 weeks is often effective in reducing the pain associated with vertebral fracture.

Table 43.6 Drugs used in the treatment of osteoporosis.

Inhibitors of resorption	Stimulators of formation
Oestrogens	Sodium fluoride
Progestogens	Parathyroid hormone peptides
Bisphosphonates	
Calcitonin	
Calcium	
Vitamin D and calcitriol	
Anabolic steroids	

Hormone-replacement therapy

The role of oestrogen deficiency in the pathogenesis of post-menopausal osteoporosis and the beneficial effects of oestrogen replacement on bone mass are well established. Oestrogen replacement at or after the menopause prevents bone loss at the radius, spine and femur [26–29], and observational studies indicate that it is also associated with a reduction in fracture of the radius, hip and spine [30–33]. However, the latter studies are biased by factors related to differences in health status between women who choose to take oestrogens and those who do not, and the 50–75% reduction in fracture risk reported in many studies is almost certainly an overestimate.

There is considerable uncertainty about the duration of hormone-replacement therapy required to protect against osteoporosis. Observational studies indicate that the greatest protection is seen in current users, suggesting some reduction in efficacy after withdrawal of treatment. Central to this issue is the question as to whether bone loss accelerates after cessation of treatment; the available data are conflicting and further studies are required. Nevertheless, it seems unlikely that 5–10 years' hormone-replacement therapy at the time of the menopause will provide significant protection against the development of hip fracture two to three decades later, and there is a growing belief that life-long treatment after the menopause may be necessary for maximum protection against fracture, particularly of the hip.

A number of hormone-replacement formulations are licensed for the prevention and treatment of osteoporosis. The skeletal effects of combined (oestrogen plus progestogen) and unopposed (oestrogen only) preparations appear to be similar and oral, parenteral and transdermal preparations are effective. Combined continuous preparations, which theoretically avoid breakthrough bleeding and 84-day cycle (3-monthly bleed), may be useful in some cases. Tibolone, which possesses oestrogenic, progestogenic and androgenic properties, appears to have similar effects on bone mass to conventional hormone-replacement preparations and does not stimulate the endometrium.

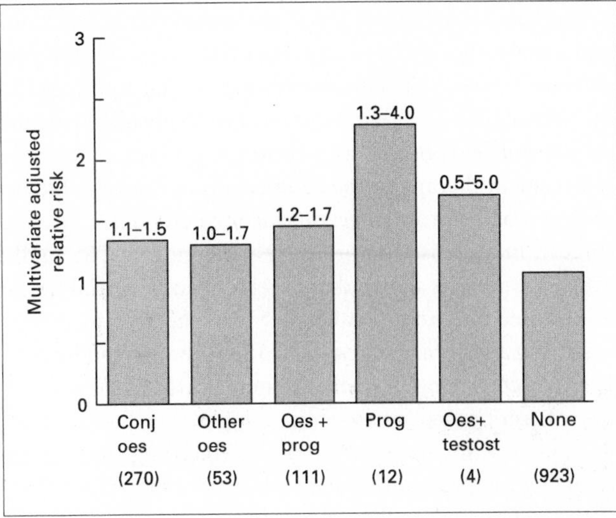

Fig. 43.4 Adjusted relative risk of breast cancer according to type of hormone-replacement therapy. The figures on top of the columns give the 95% confidence intervals and the figures beneath the columns show the number of women in each group with breast cancer. From [35].

Evaluation of the therapeutic use of long-term hormone replacement in osteoporosis must include a consideration of the extraskeletal risks and benefits of this treatment [34]. There is evidence that long-term therapy is associated with an increase in the risk of breast cancer; overall, the magnitude of this increase appears to be around 30%. A recent prospective study has shown that the increase in risk is similar for women taking combined or oestrogen-only preparations (Fig. 43.4), and that a significant increase in risk was evident after 5 years of treatment, particularly in older women [35]. An increase in the relative risk of death from breast cancer was also shown in this study, indicating that the increased number of cases diagnosed could not be attributed to greater surveillance and screening.

In contrast, there is evidence that menopausal oestrogen use confers significant protection against cardiovascular disease [36]. Observational studies suggest a reduction of 50% or more, although this is likely to be an overestimate because of the confounding factors mentioned earlier. It is uncertain whether this beneficial effect is influenced by the addition of progestogens in combined preparations; although theoretical considerations suggest possible adverse cardiovascular effects of progestogens, a recent study indicates that both unopposed and combined hormone-replacement formulations are protective against coronary heart disease [37]. Overall, current evidence does not support a significant protective effect of hormone replacement therapy against stroke [37]; however, a recent report suggests that oestrogen use in post-menopausal women may delay the onset and decrease the risk of Alzheimer's disease [56].

Recently, two other risks associated with hormone replacement therapy have been described. A two- to threefold increase in venous thromboembolism has been reported [57]; this translates into only a small increase in absolute risk and should not be regarded as a contraindication to hormone replacement therapy in the absence of predisposing factors such as a past history of venous thromboembolism, obesity, surgery, immobilisation or severe varicose veins. Secondly, a recent study has shown that the risk of endometrial cancer is increased two- to threefold after five years treatment with oestrogen and cyclic progestogen [58]. Although this increase in risk is considerably smaller than that associated with the use of unopposed oestrogens, it highlights the need for prompt investigation of irregular bleeding in women receiving long-term hormone replacement therapy.

Evaluation of the risks and benefits of long-term hormone-replacement therapy is thus extremely complex. On the one hand, it seems likely that life-long treatment after the menopause is required to provide optimal protection against osteoporosis, but few physicians or patients will be prepared to recommend this in the face of the increased risk of breast cancer. Current practice, which is to prescribe between 5 and 10 years' hormone replacement therapy at the menopause, is likely to continue but may have relatively little impact on hip fracture risk [38]. Finally, if the benefits of oestrogens on cardiovascular disease morbidity and mortality are confirmed in prospective studies and extended to combined preparations, this will be an important factor in reaching decisions about the risks and benefits of long-term hormone-replacement therapy, since coronary heart disease far outweighs both osteoporosis and breast cancer as a cause of death in post-menopausal women. The development of selective oestrogen-receptor modulators, such as raloxifene and droloxifene, provides a means by which the beneficial effects of oestrogens may be retained whilst avoiding unwanted effects on the endometrium, liver and breast; these drugs offer an exciting prospect for the future.

Bisphosphonates

The bisphosphonates are synthetic analogues of pyrophosphate which inhibit bone resorption. Bisphosphonates are non-biodegradable and appear to be absorbed, excreted and stored unchanged. Intestinal absorption is poor, varying between <1% and 10%, with a rapid plasma clearance and rapid uptake of 20–60% of the absorbed fraction into the skeleton, the rest being excreted in the urine. The skeletal half-life of bisphosphonates is very long, release only occurring after resorption of bone into which the compounds have been taken up [39]. A number of bisphosphonates have been synthesised, with varying antiresorptive potency. Two of these, etidronate and alendronate, are licensed for the treatment of post-menopausal osteoporosis in the UK and some other parts of the world (Fig. 43.5). Etidronate is given in a cyclic intermittent regime with calcium whereas alendronate is administered as a continuous, once-daily regimen.

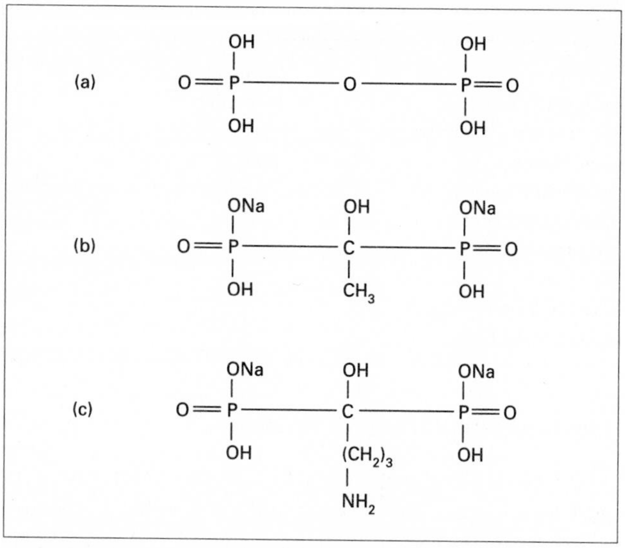

Fig. 43.5 Chemical structure of pyrophosphate and some bisphosphonates. (a) Pyrophosphate; (b) etidronate; (c) alendronate.

Both these treatments have been shown to preserve spinal and femoral neck bone mass in women with post-menopausal osteoporosis [40–42]; as in the case of oestrogens, small increases in bone mass are seen at both sites consistent with in-filling of the remodelling space. For both etidronate and alendronate, the increase at the spine is greater than that observed at the femoral neck. Although small decreases in vertebral fracture rate were claimed in the phase III studies of etidronate, the statistical power of these studies to demonstrate this was inadequate and its antifracture efficacy thus remains unproven. In the Fracture Intervention Trial [59], alendronate therapy was shown to result in a significant reduction in vertebral fracture risk in women with established postmenopausal osteoporosis and a significant reduction in hip and wrist fractures was also seen.

Bisphosphonates are generally well tolerated although gastrointestinal symptoms, particularly nausea and diarrhoea, may occur and severe oesophagitis has been reported in a small number of patients taking alendronate [60]. The aminobisphosphonates, particularly pamidronate, may cause transient fever with leucopenia and increased C-reactive protein levels. Intestinal absorption of bisphosphonates is reduced even further in the presence of calcium-containing foods or medications, or other bivalent ions such as iron. It is therefore essential that oral bisphosphonates are taken at least 2 hours before or after food or calcium supplements.

The optimum duration of treatment with bisphosphonates is uncertain but a minimum of three years is recommended.

Vitamin D and its metabolites/analogues

Evidence that vitamin D deficiency and secondary hyperparathyroidism contribute to age-related bone loss suggests that vitamin D repletion, either as the native vitamin or a more potent metabolite or analogue, may have a role in the prevention and treatment of osteoporosis. A recent study from New Zealand demonstrated that the major active metabolite of vitamin D, 1,25-dihydroxyvitamin D_3, in a dose of 0.25 μg twice daily for 3 years, reduced vertebral fracture rate in women with post-menopausal osteoporosis [43], and this treatment is now licensed for use for osteoporosis in the UK and some other parts of the world. Although problems due to hypercalcaemia and hypercalciuria were reportedly uncommon, they are a potential concern particularly in the elderly and careful monitoring of serum calcium levels is mandatory in treated patients. The analogue of 1,25-dihydroxyvitamin D_3, 1α-hydroxyvitamin D_3, is also used in the treatment of osteoporosis in some parts of the world, particularly Japan.

Native vitamin D may also be effective in preventing osteoporotic fractures. In a recent study from France, a daily regime of 800 iu vitamin D_3 plus 1.2 g calcium was shown significantly to reduce hip and other non-vertebral fractures in elderly women living in residential care [44,45]. The mean age of this cohort was 84 years and significant effects on fracture were observed after a mean treatment period of only 12–18 months and subsequently confirmed at 3 years (Fig. 43.6). These results indicate that even in the very elderly with low bone mass, relatively short-term treatment may be beneficial in terms of fracture reduction, an effect which may be explained on the basis of continuing bone loss in this age group and the mechanical benefits induced in cancellous bone by reducing bone turnover. Whether the results of the French study can be extended to free-living elderly populations requires further study, as do the relative roles of vitamin D and calcium in contributing to the observed effects.

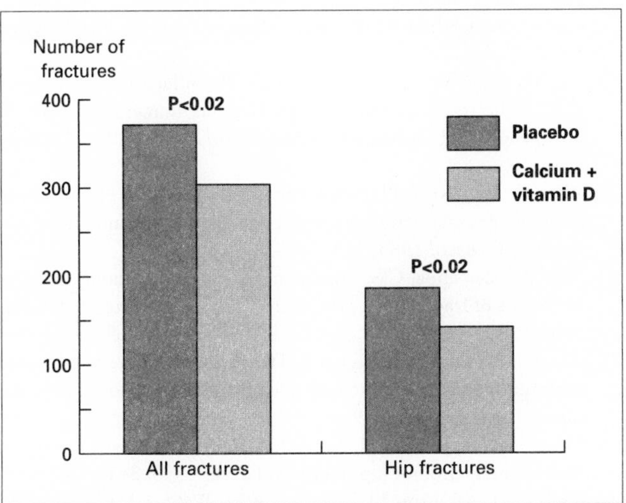

Fig. 43.6 Effect of 3 years' treatment with calcium and vitamin D supplementation (1200 mg and 800 iu/day, respectively) on non-vertebral fracture rate in elderly women in residential care. From [45].

Calcitonin

Calcitonin inhibits bone resorption by a direct action on osteoclasts. The majority of studies indicate preservation of bone mass both in healthy perimenopausal women and in women with post-menopausal osteoporosis, but as yet reduction in vertebral or other fracture rates has not been convincingly demonstrated [46]. Calcitonin can be administered parenterally or intranasally. Side-effects associated with parenteral calcitonin are relatively common and include nausea, flushing, diarrhoea and paraesthesiae.

Calcium

The ability of calcium supplementation to reduce bone loss in post-menopausal women has been demonstrated in many studies [47]. Its effects are most marked in cortical bone and there is evidence that benefits in cancellous vertebral bone may be transient. Beneficial effects on bone mass are observed in women over a broad range of dietary calcium intakes, although there is some evidence that larger doses are required in those women with higher intakes. A large range of calcium supplements are available and have been shown to be effective. However, in most studies of women during and immediately after the menopause, calcium supplementation has been shown to attenuate rather than prevent bone loss and hence it should be regarded as an adjunct to treatment rather than as definitive therapy [48]. Calcium supplements should ideally be prescribed three to four times daily to optimise the absolute amount absorbed and daily doses of between 1 and 1.5 g are recommended if dietary intakes around this level cannot be achieved. Dairy products provide the most efficient form of dietary intake, 1 pint of milk containing approximately 0.75 g.

Exercise

The beneficial effects of weight-bearing exercise on the skeleton are well documented, whilst immobilisation leads to rapid bone loss. However, excessive exercise may result in oestrogen deficiency and bone loss, as seen in elite female athletes and ballet dancers. A number of studies have investigated the effects of exercise regimes on post-menopausal bone loss; overall, although some have demonstrated attenuation of bone loss, most indicate that this effect is partial and bone loss is not totally prevented [49]. In the elderly, exercise may reduce the frequency of falling and improve the protective response to falls through an increase in muscle strength.

Sodium fluoride

Sodium fluoride produces large increases in vertebral cancellous bone mass but has neutral or even negative effects on cortical bone in the femoral neck. The effects on vertebral and non-vertebral fracture rate are controversial; some evidence suggests a significant reduction in vertebral fracture rate in treated patients although other studies have failed to demonstrate such an effect [50,51]. These differences may be explained by the narrow therapeutic window of sodium fluoride in bone; doses of over 60 mg daily do not appear to reduce vertebral fracture risk despite large increases in spinal bone mass whereas favourable effects on fracture rate of lower doses (40–50 mg/day) have been reported. However, increased risk of non-vertebral fracture, including hip fracture, have been reported in patients treated with moderate and high doses of sodium fluoride [52], and painful stress fractures in the lower limbs may also occur. Gastrointestinal symptoms are relatively common and a significant proportion of patients fail to respond to treatment. The role of sodium fluoride in the treatment of osteoporosis thus remains uncertain; its use requires careful monitoring and should be confined to specialist centres.

Anabolic steroids

Despite their name, the effect of anabolic steroids on bone is predominantly antiresorptive. In post-menopausal women they have been shown to preserve cortical and cancellous bone mass but their effect on fracture rate has not been established. Because of their hepatotoxic and virilising side-effects they are now rarely used in the treatment of osteoporosis.

Prevention and treatment of glucocorticoid osteoporosis

Glucocorticoid-induced osteoporosis is commonly encountered in clinical practice but relatively few studies have investigated the use of preventive or therapeutic interventions. Hormone-replacement therapy, vitamin D, 1,25-dihydroxyvitamin D_3, calcitonin and the bisphosphonates etidronate and pamidronate have been shown to prevent or reduce glucocorticoid-induced bone loss, but many of these studies have been relatively short-term and the effects of these regimens on fracture rate is unknown [53,54].

Restriction of the dose of glucocorticoids to the minimum required, with constant revision and reduction of the dose where possible, should be exercised since there is evidence that the adverse skeletal effects of glucocorticoids are, to some extent, dose dependent. The use of bone-sparing steroids such as deflazacort may reduce bone loss although this remains unproven. Most available evidence suggests that glucocorticoid-induced bone loss is most rapid during the first few months of treatment, emphasising the need for intervention in the early stages of treatment.

References

1 Anonymous. Consensus Development Conference: diagnosis, prophylaxis and treatment of osteoporosis. *Am J Med* 1993; **94**: 646–50.
2 Compston JE, Cooper C, Kanis JA. Bone densitometry in clinical practice. *Br Med J* 1995; **310**: 1507–10.
3 Cooper C. Epidemiology and public health impact of osteoporosis. *Clin Rheumatol* 1993; **7**: 459–77.
4 Melton LJ, Chrischilles EA, Cooper C, Lane AW, Riggs BL. Perspective. How many women have osteoporosis? *J Bone Miner Res* 1992; **7**: 1005–10.
5 Cooper C, Melton LJ. Vertebral fractures. How large is the silent epidemic? *Br Med J* 1992; **304**: 793–4.
6 Compston JE. BMC, BMD, or corrected BMD? *Bone* 1995; **16**: 261–7.
7 Compston JE. Osteoporosis. *Clin Endocrinol* 1990; **33**: 653–82.
8 Mazess RB, Collick B, Trempe J, Barden H, Hanson J. Performance evaluation of a dual-energy X-ray bone densitometer. *Calcif Tissue Int* 1989; **44**: 228–32.
9 Reid IR, Evans MC, Ames R, Wattie DJ. The influence of osteophytes and aortic calcification on spinal bone mineral density in postmenopausal women. *J Clin Endocrinol Metab* 1991; **72**: 1372–4.
10 Wasnich RD, Ross PD, Heilbrun LK, Vogel JM. Prediction of postmenopausal fracture risk with bone mineral measurements. *Am J Obstet Gynecol* 1985; **153**: 745–51.
11 Hui SL, Slemenda CW, Johnston CC. Age and bone mass as predictors of fracture in a prospective study. *J Clin Invest* 1988; **81**: 1804–9.
12 Gärdsell P, Johnell O, Nilsson B. The predictive value of bone loss for fragility fractures in women: a longitudinal study over 15 years. *Calcif Tissue Int* 1991; **49**: 90–4.
13 Cummings SR, Black DM, Nevitt MC *et al.* Bone density at various sites for prediction of hip fractures. *Lancet* 1993; **341**: 72–5.
14 Melton LJ, Atkinson EJ, O'Fallon WM, Wahner HW, Riggs BL. Long-term fracture prediction by bone mineral assessed at different skeletal sites. *J Bone Miner Res* 1993; **8**: 1227–33.
15 Faulkner KG, Cummings SR, Glüer CC, Palermo L, Black D, Genant HK. Simple measurement of femoral geometry predicts hip fracture. *J Bone Miner Res* 1993; **8**: 1211–17.

16 Wasnich RD, Davis JW, Ross PD. Spine fracture risk is predicted by non-spine fractures. *Osteoporosis Int* 1994; **4**: 1–5.

17 Cummings SR, Nevitt MC, Browner WS *et al.* Risk factors for hip fracture in white women. *N Engl J Med* 1995; **332**: 767–73.

18 World Health Organisation. Assessment of fracture risk and its application to screening for postmenopausal osteoporosis. *WHO Technical Report Series 843*. Geneva: WHO, 1994.

19 Smith-Bindman R, Cummings SR, Steiger P, Genant HK. A comparison of morphometric definitions of vertebral fracture. *J Bone Miner Res* 1991; **6**: 25–34.

20 Delmas PD. Biochemical markers of bone turnover: methodology and clinical use in osteoporosis. *Am J Med* 1991; **91** (Suppl. 5B): 59–63S.

21 Compston JE. Risk factors for osteoporosis. *Clin Endocrinol* 1992; **36**: 223–4.

22 Parfitt AM. The cellular basis of bone remodelling. The quantum concept re-examined in light of recent advances in cell biology of bone. *Calcif Tissue Int* 1984; **36**: S37–45.

23 Lanyon LE. The success and failure of the adaptive response to functional load-bearing in averting vertebral fracture. *Bone* 1992; **13** (Suppl. 2): S17–21.

24 MacDonald BR, Gowen M. Cytokines and bone. *Br J Rheumatol* 1992; **31**: 149–55.

25 Compston JE, Mellish RWE, Croucher PI, Newcombe R, Garrahan NJ. Structural mechanisms of trabecular bone loss in man. *Bone Miner* 1989; **9**: 330–50.

26 Lindsay R, Hart DM, Forrest C, Baird C. Prevention of spinal osteoporosis in oophorectomised women. *Lancet* 1980; **ii**: 1151–3.

27 Nachtigall LE, Nachtigall RH, Nachtigall RD, Beckman EM. Estrogen replacement therapy 1: a 10-year prospective study in the relationship to osteoporosis. *Obstet Gynecol* 1979; **53**: 277–81.

28 Ettinger B, Genant HK, Cann CE. Long-term oestrogen replacement therapy prevents bone loss and fractures. *Ann Intern Med* 1985; **102**: 319–24.

29 Quigley MET, Martin PL, Burnier AM, Brooks P. Estrogen therapy arrests bone loss in elderly women. *Am J Obstet Gynecol* 1987; **156**: 1516–23.

30 Hutchinson A, Polansky SM, Feinstein AR. Post-menopausal estrogens protect against fractures of the hip and distal radius: a case control study. *Lancet* 1979; **ii**: 705–9.

31 Weiss NS, Ure CL, Ballard JH, Williams AR, Daling JR. Decreased risk of fractures of the hip and lower forearm with postmenopausal use of estrogens. *N Engl J Med* 1980; **303**: 1195–8.

32 Paganini-Hill A, Ross RK, Gerkins VR, Henderson BE, Arthur M, Mack TM. Menopausal estrogen therapy and hip fractures. *Ann Intern Med* 1981; **95**: 28–31.

33 Kiel DP, Felson DT, Anderson JJ, Wilson PWF, Moskowitz MA. Hip fracture and the use of estrogens in postmenopausal women: the Framingham study. *N Engl J Med* 1987; **317**: 1169–74.

34 Grady D, Rubin SM, Petitti DB *et al.* Hormone therapy to prevent disease and prolong life in postmenopausal women. *Ann Intern Med* 1992; **117**: 1016–37.

35 Colditz GA, Hankinson SE, Hunter DJ *et al.* The use of estrogens and progestins and the risk of breast cancer in postmenopausal women. *N Engl J Med* 1995; **332**: 1589–93.

36 Barrett-Connor E, Bush TL. Estrogen and coronary heart disease in women. *JAMA* 1991; **265**: 1861–7.

37 Grodstein F, Stampfer MJ, Manson JE *et al.* Postmenopausal estrogen and progestin use and the risk of cardiovascular disease. *N Engl J Med* 1996; **335**: 453–61.

38 Compston JE. Hormone replacement therapy for osteoporosis: clinical and pathophysiological aspects. *Rep Med Rev* 1994; **3**: 209–24.

39 Compston JE. The therapeutic use of bisphosphonates. *Br Med J* 1994; **309**: 711–15.

40 Storm T, Thamsborg G, Steiniche T, Genant HK, Sorensen OH. Effect of intermittent cyclical etidronate therapy on bone mass and fracture rate in women with postmenopausal osteoporosis. *N Engl J Med* 1990; **322**: 1265–71.

41 Watts NB, Harris ST, Genant HK *et al.* Intermittent cyclical etidronate treatment of postmenopausal osteoporosis. *N Engl J Med* 1990; **323**: 73–9.

42 Harris ST, Watts NB, Jackson RD *et al.* The effects of four years of intermittent cyclical etidronate treatment for postmenopausal osteoporosis. *Am J Med* 1993; **95**: 557–66.

43 Tilyard MW, Spears GFS, Thomson J, Dovey S. Treatment of postmenopausal osteoporosis with calcitriol or calcium. *N Engl J Med* 1992; **326**: 357–62.

44 Chapuy MC, Arlot ME, DuBoeuf F *et al.* Vitamin D_3 and calcium to prevent hip fractures in elderly women. *N Engl J Med* 1992; **327**: 1637–42.

45 Chapuy MC, Arlot ME, Delmas PD, Meunier PJ. Effect of calcium and cholecalciferol treatment for three years on hip fractures in elderly women. *Br Med J* 1994; **308**: 1081–2.

46 Burckhardt P, Burnand B. The effect of treatment with calcitonin on vertebral fracture rate in osteoporosis. *Osteoporosis Int* 1993; **3**: 24–30.

47 Cumming RJ. Calcium intake and bone mass: a quantitative review of the evidence. *Calcif Tissue Int* 1990; **47**: 194–201.

48 Compston JE. The role of vitamin D and calcium supplementation in the prevention of osteoporotic fractures in the elderly. *Clin Endocrinol* 1995; **43**: 393–405.

49 Mosekilde L. Osteoporosis and exercise. *Bone* 1995; **17**: 193–5.

50 Mamelle N, Meunier PJ, Dusan R *et al.* Risk–benefit ratio of sodium fluoride treatment in primary vertebral osteoporosis. *Lancet* 1988; **ii**: 361–5.

51 Riggs BL, Hodgson SF, O'Fallon WM *et al.* Effect of fluoride treatment on the fracture rate in postmenopausal women with osteoporosis. *N Engl J Med* 1990; **322**: 802–9.

52 Hedlund LR, Gallagher JC. Increased incidence of hip fracture in osteoporotic women treated with sodium fluoride. *J Bone Miner Res* 1989; **4**: 223–5.

53 Gennari C. Glucocorticoid induced osteoporosis. *Clin Endocrinol* 1994; **41**: 273–4.

54 Eastell R. Management of corticosteroid-induced osteoporosis. *J Intern Med* 1995; **237**: 439–47.

55 Compston JE. Osteoporosis, corticosteroids and inflammatory bowel disease. *Aliment Pharmacol Ther* 1995; **9**: 237–50.

56 Tang M-X, Jacobs D, Stern Y et al. Effect of oestrogen during menopause on risk and age at onset of Alzheimer's disease. *Lancet* 1996; **348**: 429–32.

57 Gutthann SP, Rodriguez LAG, Castellsague J, Oliart AD. Hormone replacement therapy and risk of venous thromboembolism: population based case-control study. *Br Med J* 1997; **314**: 796–800.

58 Beresford SAA, Weiss NSA, Voigt LF, McKnight B. Risk of endometrial cancer in relation to use of oestrogen combined with cyclic progestagen therapy in postmenopausal women. *Lancet* 1997; **349**: 458–61.

59 Black DM, Cummings SR, Karpf DB *et al.* Randomised trial of effects of alendronate on risk of fracture in women with existing vertebral fracture. *Lancet* 1996; **348**: 1535–41.

60 De Groen PC, Lubbe DF, Hirsch LJ *et al.* Esophagitis associated with the use of alendronate. *N Engl J Med* 1996; **335**: 1016–21.

CHAPTER 44

Paget's disease of bone

P.C. Richardson and D.C. Anderson

Paget's disease of bone is neither an endocrine nor a metabolic disease. It is a condition that often presents to clinical endocrinologists, lying as it does between the disciplines of rheumatology, metabolism, orthopaedics and endocrinology—not to speak of geriatrics. Each of these branches of medicine has something to contribute and something to learn from this enigmatic disease; it is an exciting time for those interested in this extremely common condition, with major advances in treatment and the promise of real understanding of its aetiology. Paget's disease may be defined as a chronic, slowly progressive, focal disorder of bone characterised by excessive and abnormal osteoclastic and secondary osteoblastic activity in affected bones. To a first approximation the rest of the skeleton appears to be entirely normal, while bone turnover is increased 20-fold or more in diseased areas.

History and epidemiology

Although Czerny [1] had described the condition some 30 years earlier, the distinguished London surgeon Sir James Paget [2] gave the first authoritative and clear description of the disorder based on cases seen at St Bartholomew's Hospital, in 1876. He named the disease osteitis deformans, and clinical photographs as well as some of the bones from his most severe cases are on display in the hospital's pathology museum to this day (Fig. 44.1). These cases are of what we loosely describe as 'mega-Paget's' disease, with advanced disease in multiple bones; these account for 10–20% of cases presenting to specialist units, and probably for 1–2% of all cases, although obviously they constitute a high proportion of patients with major problems.

Information on the epidemiology of the condition worldwide is patchy. Paget's disease has a particularly high incidence in people of Anglo-Saxon descent; the highest incidence in the world appears to be in the north-west of England, where it was found to be as high as 8% of the elderly in some towns [3]. This was based on the appearance on plain abdominal radiographs taken for reasons unconnected with Paget's disease (Fig. 44.2). Elsewhere in Europe the incidence is highly variable, with levels of 3% in France and as low as 0.5% in Sweden. The incidence in Australia and New Zealand approaches that in the UK, with moderately high levels in the USA, and vanishingly low levels in Japan. In the UK there is often a positive family history, with about 20% of cases having an affected first-degree relative; this is thought to be accounted for equally as well by exposure to a common environmental agent as by inheritance.

Various theories to explain the disease have been proposed. Our observation of an apparent link with a high incidence of previous dog ownership in two case–control studies [4,5], has been confirmed in New Zealand [6], although here an independent association with cat ownership was found. The evidence for a viral aetiology is discussed below, and the observations relating to dog ownership suggest that a canine virus such as canine distemper merits further examination. If an infectious cause is responsible, the pace of development of the established case suggests that initial exposure must usually have taken place in childhood, adolescence or early adult life.

Pathophysiology

Observations of the histopathology of Paget's disease largely result from observations of biopsy specimens from affected iliac bones. Provided coagulation function is normal, a transiliac bone biopsy of an 8-mm diameter core of bone can be obtained safely and simply under local anaesthesia from such patients. This usually reveals the end-product of many years of remodelling, in which the architecture of the bone matrix is highly abnormal, showing the classical

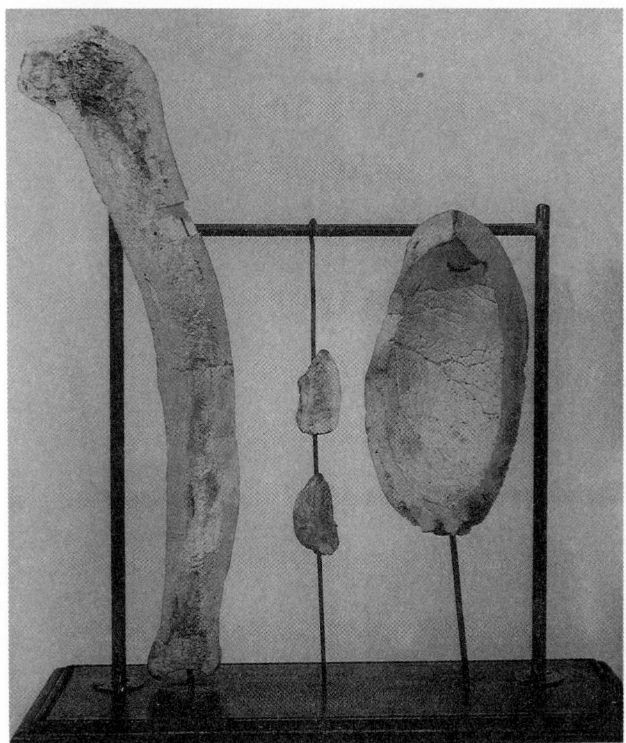

Fig. 44.1 Bones from one of Sir James Paget's original cases held in the museum at St Bartholomew's Hospital. (Courtesy of the Department of Medical Illustration, St Bartholomew's Hospital, London.)

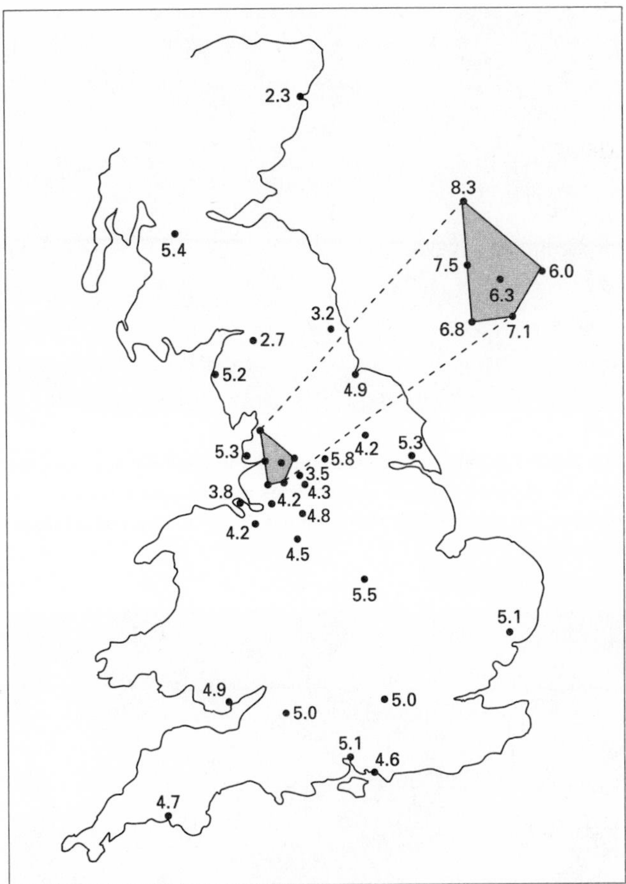

Fig. 44.2 Prevalence (%) of Paget's disease of bone in British towns. From [3], with permission.

mosaic pattern that results from repeated cycles of disordered osteoclastic bone resorption followed by new osteoblastic bone formation (Figs 44.3 and 44.4). The volume of mineralised and unmineralised (osteoid) bone matrix is increased, as are the number of surfaces undergoing osteoclastic bone resorption and bone formation. The osteoclasts are strikingly increased in number, size and degree of multinuclearity; counts of 100–200 times normal are commonplace, and since these cells are much bigger than normal, the osteoclast volume is even higher. Osteoblasts are also highly active, but appear to function normally; at least they lay down organised lamellar bone once bone resorption is effectively inhibited with a bisphosphonate. Other typical features include an increase in periosteal new bone, which may be buried deep below the surface; marrow fibrosis, which is generally very extensive; increased vascularity; increased numbers of mast cells; and *de novo* bone formation visible within areas of marrow fibrosis.

Several studies have reported an abnormal morphology of Pagetic osteoclasts, with the presence of prominent nucleoli, and nuclear inclusion bodies [7]. Electron-microscopic studies have reported the regular occurrence of paracrystalline structures within both osteoclast nuclei and cytoplasm, which have been attributed to viral nucleocapsids [8,9]. The messenger RNA (mRNA) from the nucleocapsid protein is the first to be transcribed by the viral RNA polymerase of paramyxoviruses, and has the property of binding to viral genomic RNA, which is probably of importance in preventing its intracellular degradation. Further studies have reported the apparent detection by immunocytochemistry of viral antigens to a range of viruses including measles, although the specificity of this technique in bone is open to question. One study reported detection of the mRNA for measles nucleocapsid protein [10] by *in situ* hybridisation using DNA probes. In contrast, our group [11] found evidence by the same technique, but using the more specific RNA probes, for canine distemper virus (two separate genes) in nearly half of the cases tested. We also found evidence of viral RNA from canine distemper by polymerase chain reaction [12], although this has not been confirmed by others [13,14]. Clearly the issue is not yet settled, and more work remains to be done.

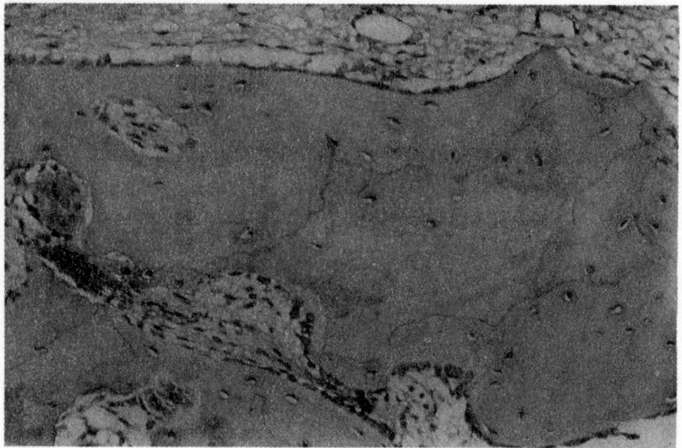

Fig. 44.3 Typical histological picture of untreated Paget's disease of bone, showing irregular cement lines and the typical mosaic pattern. The cement lines represent the line of advance of previous osteoclasts.

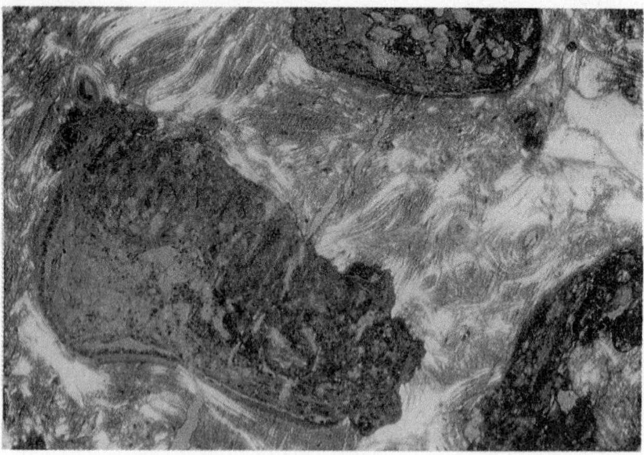

Fig. 44.4 Paget's disease of bone viewed under polarised light showing the chaotic mixture of woven and lamellar bone. The marrow is darker, and much of the bone surface is irregular due to osteoclastic bone resorption.

How might a virus cause the changes seen in Paget's disease?

Paramyxoviruses code for a fusion protein which is incorporated into the cell membrane, and which leads to fusion of cells to form syncytia. The osteoclast is a cell that fuses with other cells of the same lineage, so one possibility is that the viral fusion protein acts as a surrogate for the normal osteoclast fusion protein. If cell fusion leads to production of more precursors, the stage would be set for a self-perpetuating process. Intact virus would never need to leave the cell, since osteoclasts can break up as well as fuse, and the process could spread through bone slowly as infected osteoclasts advanced.

There is ample clinical, radiological and histological evidence that osteoclasts in Paget's disease advance through unaffected bone at about 1 cm per year as a so-called 'lytic front' [15]; behind this all osteoclastic cells appear abnormal in form and activity. The changes in *osteoblastic* activity appear to result from the stimulatory effect that osteoclasts have on osteoblastic function, an essential component of normal bone remodelling whereby formation is coupled to resorption at a local level. In fact, in most cases there is a marked and progressive increase in bone formation as the disease progresses; this is particularly evident when bone resorption is inhibited and a backlog of formation occurs as committed osteoblast precursors complete the process.

Natural history and clinical features

Nothing is known about the natural history of very early Paget's disease. Indeed, what is known overall has been derived from fragmentary observations of the progression of disease in individual cases. We believe that the pattern of disease fits best with a single point-in-time infection of osteoclast precursors, which would then take the agent into a proportion of osteoclasts undertaking bone resorption; this would set up a focus of disease, initially microscopic, from which the process might be propagated progressively. In long bones the disease appears usually to start at one or other end of the bone, probably at the epiphysial plate. The disease appears to select bones at random. If one bone is affected there is approximately a two in three chance that a second will be affected, and so on, at least up to seven bones [16]. Occasional cases are observed where a new focus of disease appears to arise after many years, suggesting blood-borne spread.

One possibility to account for the very high prevalence in the north-west of England might be the high incidence of rickets during the 1920s and 1930s, especially in industrial towns. The resulting increased osteoclasts may be presumed to increase the chance of infection taking hold.

The disease typically passes through a *lytic phase*, to a phase of progressively increased bone turnover and new bone growth (*sclerotic phase*). The lytic phase is, by definition, seen only when the disease is sufficiently early not to have involved the whole of the bone, for example as in osteoporosis circumscripta in the skull (Fig. 44.5) and as a 'blade of grass' appearance in long bones. Progressively thereafter bones become expanded and distorted, in ways that appear to be determined by the forces to which the bone is normally subjected. The distortions themselves lead to progressively abnormal transmission of forces through the bone. The phase of expansion and distortion is most obvious on superficial inspection in bones of the lower limb, notably tibia, and to a lesser extent femur (Fig. 44.6). The

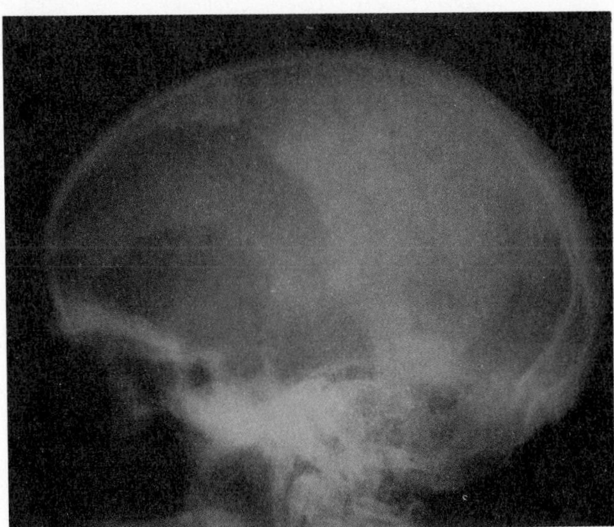

Fig. 44.5 Classical picture of osteoporosis circumscripta of the skull, showing clearly demarcated area of osteolysis with lytic edge proceeding through the skull.

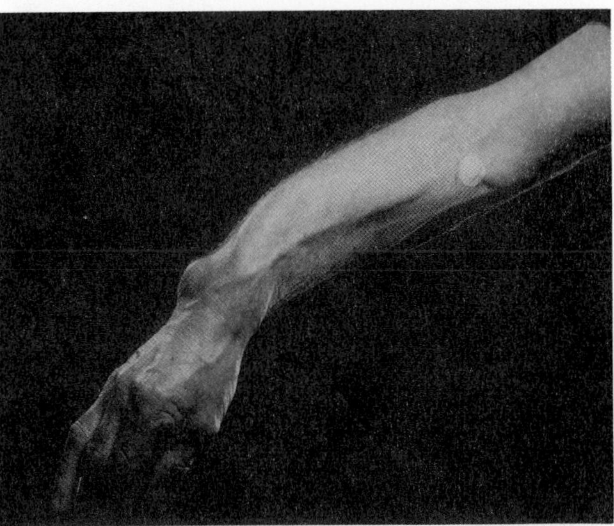

Fig. 44.7 Characteristic expansion and distortion occurring in a Pagetic radius with forearm fixed in pronation.

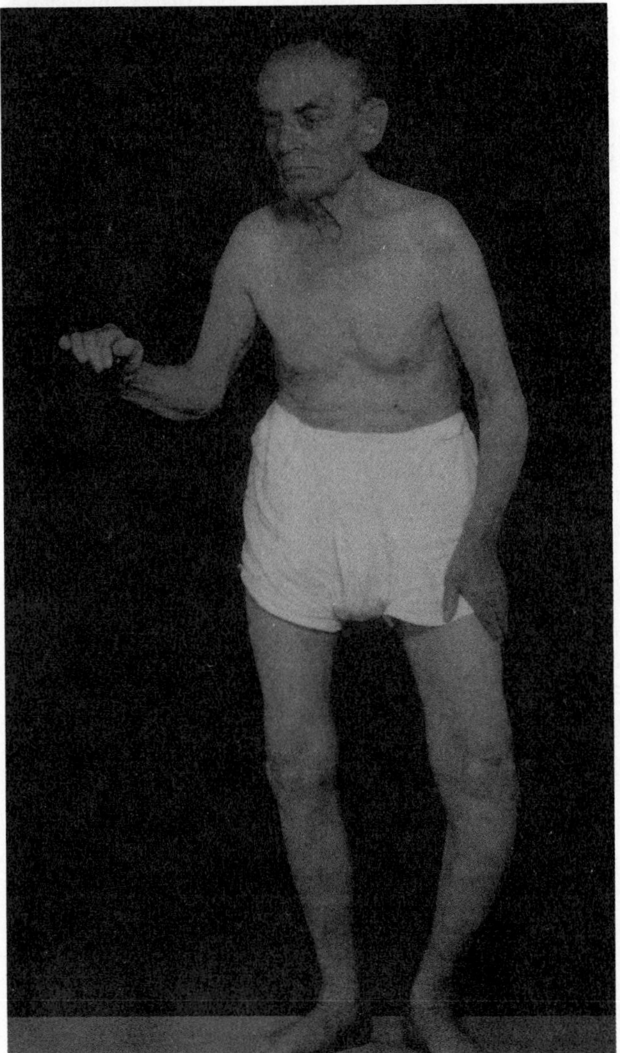

radius also distorts in a characteristic way, such that the forearm becomes fixed in pronation (Fig. 44.7). The skull also changes shape, with invagination of the spinal column into the base of the skull, and collapse of the back and sides of the skull. There may be marked focal new bone growth giving rise to the distorted expanded and 'bumpy' skull. If the disease starts on one side of the skull, expansion may be asymmetrical. The pelvis commonly becomes distorted with the acetabulum being pushed progressively inwards.

The final phase of Paget's disease is the phase of late complications. The disease is probably asymptomatic in most cases until this stage. Complications may result from a number of processes. Expansion of bone is accompanied by soft-tissue swelling; since the bone is highly vascular it is also very warm and surrounding soft tissues are vasodilated. Pressure on nerves may be evident; deafness is extremely common with skull involvement, and is in part due to pressure on the auditory nerves (giving rise to nerve deafness) and in part due to involvement of the ossicles and the structures of the inner ear. Another important structure that may be involved is the spinal cord, where there is vertebral involvement; nerve root involvement is also common.

Secondary skeletal problems include the development of incremental fractures which have a typical appearance; they are often 'stacked up' on the inner aspect of the outer cortex of an affected lower limb long bone (Fig. 44.8). Paget's disease doses not generally cross joints, even fibrous ones; it

Fig. 44.6 Severe long-standing Paget's disease showing skull enlargement, multiple involvement of vertebrae, tibial and femoral bowing on left, and left radial deformity. Note the hearing aid.

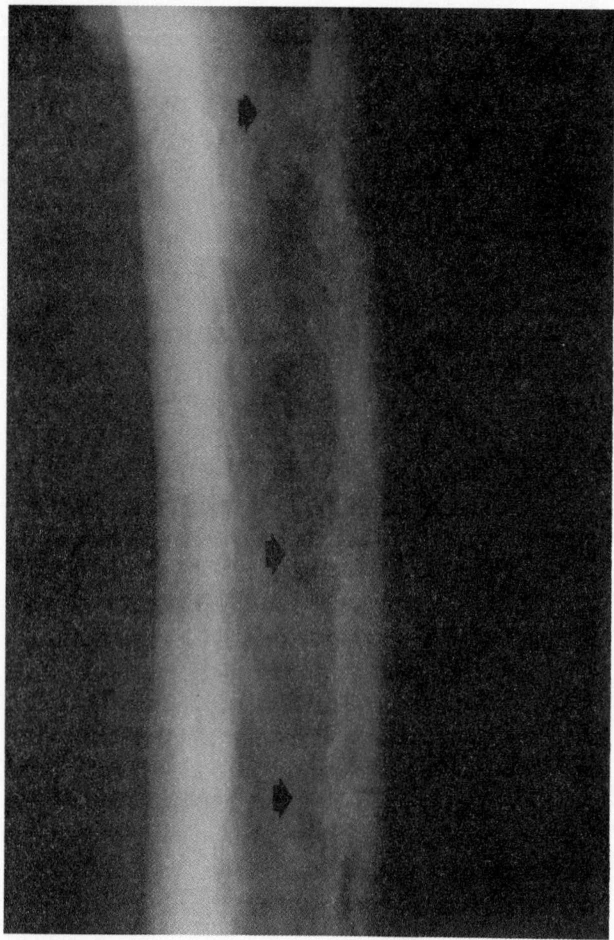

Fig. 44.8 Typical stacks of incremental fractures occurring in a Pagetic femur. These are always in the convex side of the bone.

undoubtedly predisposes to the development of osteoarthritis in joints when the disease reaches the articular cartilage.

Diagnosis and investigation

The diagnosis is most commonly made fortuitously: some unrelated problem or relevant symptom such as bone pain leads to radiography, from which the diagnosis is made. Sometimes a 'biochemical screen' reveals an isolated elevation of serum alkaline phosphatase level, the result of increased osteoblastic activity. Here, the level is roughly proportional to the product of the extent and severity of the disease. Typically, since bone formation and resorption are in balance, there is no abnormality of serum calcium and phosphate levels. A more direct, but in our experience less useful, biochemical marker, which directly reflects osteoclastic activity, is the urinary hydroxyproline level; since this is affected by dietary intake of gelatin, it is best assessed by measuring the ratio of hydroxyproline to creatinine in a fasting morning urine specimen (the second specimen passed before breakfast). The ratio correlates roughly with the serum alkaline phosphatase level.

Biochemical tests are of little value in assessing local activity when Paget's disease is confined to one small bone, such as a vertebra. Here, the most useful test is the ^{99}Tc-labelled bisphosphonate bone scan, where late-phase (3-hour) scans indicate focal areas of bone uptake. Typically, Paget's disease is easily distinguished on bone scan from other focal bone disorders such as metastases; because of its long-standing nature, the disease is generally much more extensive in a given bone than is metastatic disease. On bone scans, anything from one to 20 bones may be involved. As expected, bones close to the surface, such as limb bones, skull and spine, are most easily scanned, with different regional views being most suitable to detect and monitor disease activity in particular bones. The disease appears to select bones at random, although small avascular bones seem generally to be less frequently affected than larger ones.

Whatever the mode of diagnosis, the correct approach is to ensure that in each case baseline biochemistry (notably measurement of serum alkaline phosphatase levels) and a bone scan are undertaken, with radiography being confined to 'hot' bones. Other biochemical measurements such as serum level of osteocalcin are of little additional value. The main purpose of investigation is to establish the extent of disease, and to determine appropriate levels of baseline markers to establish what follow-up investigations will be most informative in assessing the response to treatment in each case.

Treatment [17,18,19]

There can be few common and crippling diseases in which the past 25 years has seen such advances in the potential for treatment.

The three major phases of recent development of effective treatment are:
1 calcitonin;
2 first-generation bisphosphonates;
3 second- and third-generation bisphosphonates.

In addition, other treatments, notably the drug mithramycin, have been used, but are now superseded because of their toxic effects. Because of the efficacy and safety of the second-generation bisphosphonates, pamidronate and clodronate and a multitude of third-generation bisphosphonates, earlier treatment regimens should soon be of purely historical interest.

Calcitonin

This polypeptide hormone is produced by the C-cells of the

thyroid gland in humans and by the ultimobranchial bodies of fish and birds. Its physiological role in mammals is uncertain; its principal action is to inhibit osteoclastic bone resorption by acting upon cell-surface receptors which function through coupling to adenylate cyclase and elevation of cellular cyclic adenosine monophosphate (cAMP) levels. The principal therapeutic forms are the synthetic salmon and porcine forms; salmon calcitonin has a higher potency on a weight-for-weight basis, and a relatively long half-life. It is given by subcutaneous injection and causes acute inhibition of osteoclastic bone resorption, with a consequent fall in serum calcium and phosphate levels. When used from daily to three times weekly administration, its use is associated with a modest fall in disease activity, reflected in a fall in urinary hydroxyproline/creatinine ratio, serum alkaline phosphatase, and sometimes by radiological improvement. There may be some symptomatic benefit. The drug is expensive (£1000–3000 per year currently in the UK) and does not exert any significant long-term effect on the disease. It is often responsible for side-effects, notably headaches and flushing shortly after injection. Antibodies are regularly produced, and progressive resistance may develop over the first year of therapy.

Bisphosphonates

The bisphosphonates (diphosphonates) are drugs of simple structure which are analogues of pyrophosphate; in place of a phosphate–oxygen–phosphate bond, the oxygen is replaced by carbon (Fig. 44.9). This bond is resistant to enzymatic cleavage by phosphatases. As with pyrophosphate itself, the bisphosphonates bind strongly to hydroxyapatite; their properties are further altered by varying the two side chains off the central carbon. Bisphosphonates have effects on osteoclastic bone resorption, which they inhibit by mechanisms that are still not completely clear; they also inhibit the mineralisation of newly formed bone matrix. Unfortunately the therapeutic margin between these two effects for etidronate is very low; for clodronate it is intermediate, and for pamidronate bone resorption is inhibited at levels 10^3–10^4 times lower than those that inhibit mineralisation. The more potent bisphosphonates appear to bind with high affinity to bone surfaces exposed by osteoclasts [18], possibly by binding to partially degraded collagen, and inhibit further osteoclastic bone resorption.

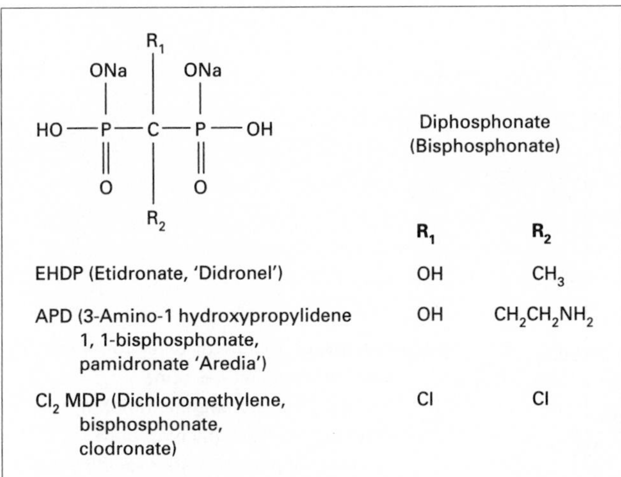

Fig. 44.9 The structure of the presently available bisphosphonates.

Route of administration and dose regimens

All the bisphosphonates are poorly and variably absorbed when given by mouth and have the potential to cause oesophageal irritation and ulceration. Furthermore, until recently there were no suitable methods for assay, and those now developed are not available for routine clinical use. If it is given orally, < 1% of a dose of APD (3-amino 1-hydroxypropylidene 1,1-bisphosphonate) is absorbed; the drug must be given on an empty stomach and without food or calcium-containing liquids.

We have opted for a regimen of intravenous administration; the drug is dissolved in 250–500 ml saline, and infused over 2–6 hours. Most of the administered drug is taken up by bone, while the rest is excreted in the urine over the 6–8 hours following the end of infusion. A satisfactory regimen for the initial treatment which we have evolved is as follows. An initial infusion of 30 mg is given intravenously over 2 hours, followed 1 week later by the first infusion of 60mg intravenously over 4 hours [19]. If the alkaline phosphatase level is < 500 U/l three infusions of 60 mg each are given and, if more, six such infusions are given. The initial lower dose is given because where febrile reactions occur this is usually only after the first dose, and clinical impression suggests that they may be milder after 30 mg than after 60mg. Other centres have adopted different approaches; the important thing is that 200–400 mg is given over a period of a few weeks [20].

Response to pamidronate therapy

There is an immediate fall in the urinary hydroxyproline/creatinine ratio within 24–48 hours as osteoclastic bone resorption is inhibited, and a more gradual fall in serum alkaline phosphatase concentration, as osteoblastic activity declines in parallel. There is an acute decline in serum calcium concentration, which is seldom marked as the parathyroid glands are activated. Serum levels of 1,25-dihydroxyvitamin D increase, gastrointestinal calcium absorption is promoted, and the serum phosphate level declines as parathyroid hormone induces phosphaturia through its action on the renal tubule.

The most cost-effective and efficient way to treat patients with Paget's disease is to administer a course, and then to evaluate the need for further treatment after at least 6 months. Objective evaluation is best achieved at that stage by measuring the serum alkaline phosphatase level, and by repeating the bone scan. Figure 44.10 shows a typical satisfactory biochemical response to a total of 180 mg i.v. pamidronate over 6 weeks and Fig. 44.11 gives the result of repeated courses of treatment in a more resistant case. Figure 44.12 illustrates the type of improvement that may be seen in bone scan. Radiography likewise may show dramatic responses, particularly in lytic lesions (Fig. 44.13). In approximately 90% of patients taking one or more courses of pamidronate, it is possible to achieve complete biochemical remission. This is paralleled by a marked improvement in bone histology, with normal lamellar bone overlying the mosaic of mixed lamellar and woven bone typical of active Paget's disease. Current evidence suggests that in a significant proportion of cases of prolonged remission, cure may have been achieved. It seems likely that the drug by inhibiting osteoclastic access to, and resorption of, bone, prevents the recruitment of further precursors, while the affected (and presumably infected) cells eventually die out.

These indicators of response are accompanied by variable but often marked improvement in pain and general well-being, which may be dramatic.

Future developments

It is to be hoped that by applying molecular biology techniques, and further epidemiological studies, over the next

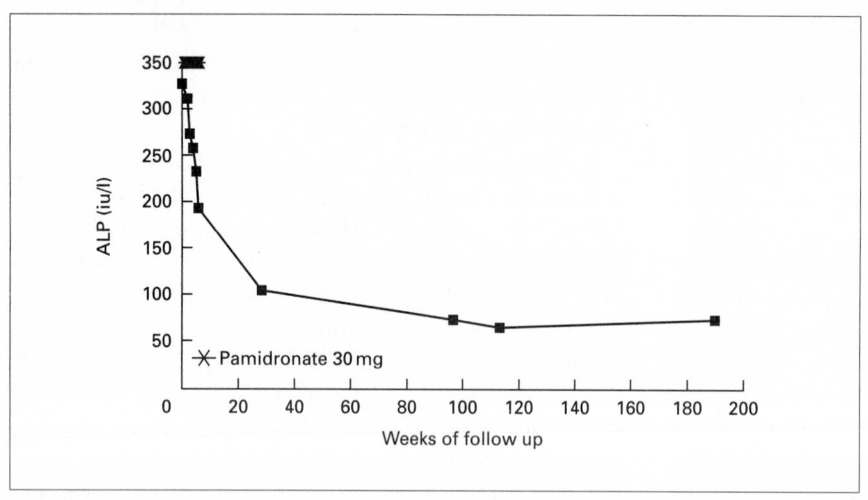

Fig. 44.10 Response to a single course of intravenous pamidronate (six 30-mg infusions given at weekly intervals) which have resulted in full biochemical and bone-scan remission for nearly 4 years.

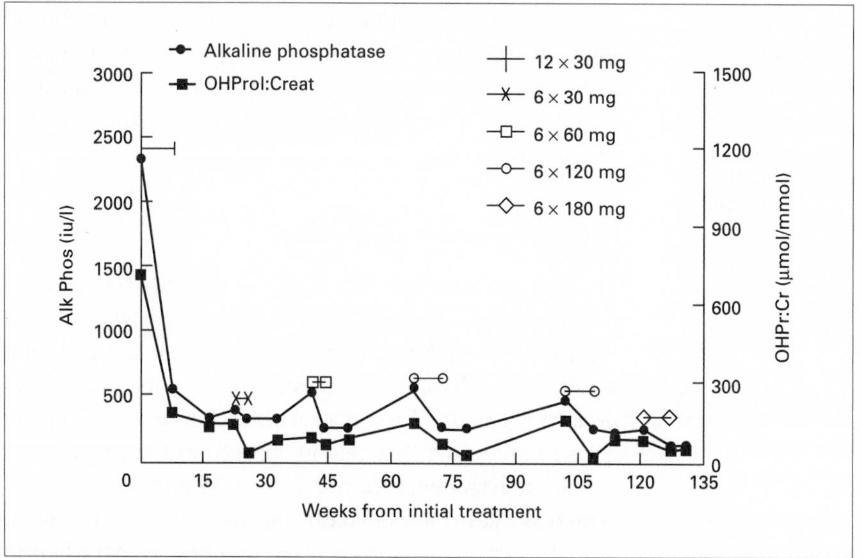

Fig. 44.11 Biochemical response (serum alkaline phosphatase, urine hydroxyproline/creatinine ratio) to repeated, increasingly high-dose, infusions of pamidronate over 2.5 years in a patient with extensive symptomatic Paget's disease.

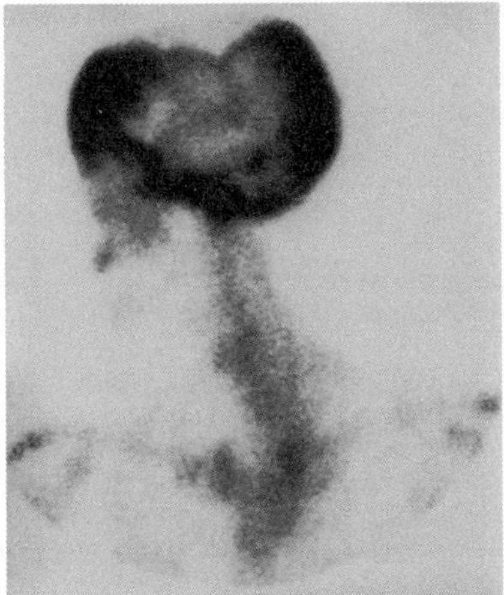

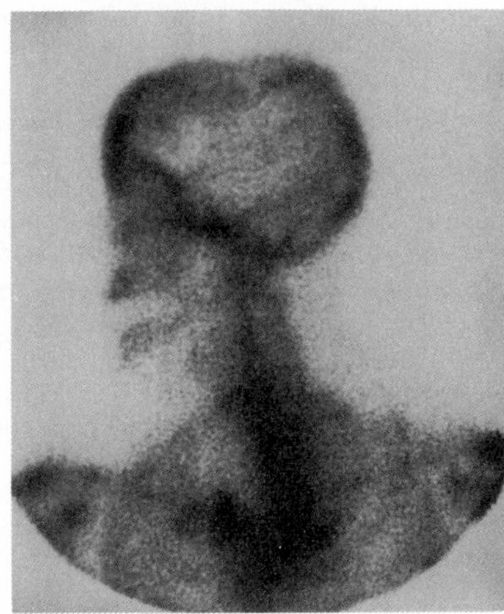

Fig. 44.12 Improvement in bone scan following treatment with intravenous pamidronate (right).

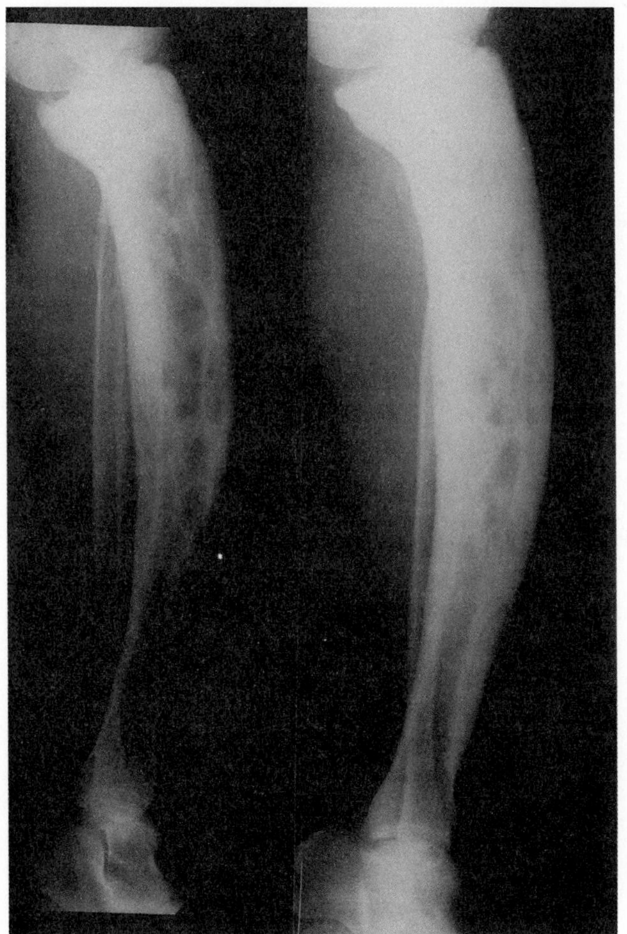

Fig. 44.13 Improvement in lytic lesions in a patient with long-standing tibial Paget's disease following treatment with intravenous pamidronate (right).

10 years the cause of Paget's disease will be established beyond reasonable doubt. This in turn is likely to throw light on the mechanism whereby bone resorption and bone formation are normally coupled. On the treatment side, effective therapy is now available, with the development of pamidronate and clodronate. A major challenge presents itself to all those concerned with health care, including doctors, drug companies and politicians, to ensure that these agents are made available to the enormous backlog of severely affected patients. Meanwhile, it appears that even more potent bisphosphonates (such as alendronate) will be yet more effective, provided they are administered in sufficiently high a dose. Early studies with the early form of this agent are encouraging, particularly in comparison to etidronate, using a total daily dose of 40 mg [20,21]. We believe that to assess relative efficacies against the best licensed drug (pamidronate) the best strategy will be to use short courses of these drugs intravenously. Greater potency should allow prolonged remission and cure to be achieved in a higher percentage of cases.

References

1 Czerny V. Eine lokale Malacie des Unterschenkels. *Wiener Medizinische Wochenschrift* 1873; **23**: 295.

2 Paget J. On a form of chronic inflammation in bones (osteitis deformans). *Med Chir Trans* 1877; **60**: 37–63.

3 Barker DJP, Chamberlain AT, Guyer PB, Gardner MJ. Paget's disease of bone: the Lancashire focus. *Br Med J* 1980; **280**: 1105.

4 O'Driscoll JB, Anderson DC. Past pets and Paget's disease. *Lancet* 1985; ii: 919–21.

5 O'Driscoll JB, Buckler HM, Jeacock J, Anderson DC. Dogs, distemper and osteitis deformans: a further epidemiological study. *Bone Miner* 1990; **11**: 209–16.

6 Holdaway IM, Ibbertson AK, Wattre D, Scragg R, Graham P. Previous dog ownership and Paget's disease. *Bone Miner* 1990; **8**: 53–8.

7 Mills BG, Singer FR. Nuclear inclusions in Paget's disease of bone. *Science* 1976; **194**: 201–2.

8 Harvey L, Gray T, Beneton MNC, Douglas DC, Kanis JA, Russell RGG. Ultrastructural features of osteoclasts from Paget's disease

of bone in relation to a viral aetiology. *J Clin Pathol* 1982; **35**: 771–9.

9 Gherardt G, Lo Cascio V, Bonucci E. Fine structure of nuclei and cytoplasm in Paget's disease of bone. *Histopathology* 1980; **4**: 63–74.

10 Rebel A, Basle MF, Fournier JG, Rozenblatt S, Bouteille M. Measles virus RNA detected in Paget's disease bone tissue by *in situ* hybridization. *J Gen Virol* 1986; **67**(5): 907–13.

11 Gordon MG, Anderson DC, Sharpe P. Canine distemper virus localised in bone cells of patients with Paget's disease. *Bone* 1991; **12**: 195–201.

12 Gordon MT, Mee A, Anderson DC, Sharpe PT. Canine distemper virus transcripts sequenced from Pagetic bone. *Bone Miner* 1992; **19**: 159–74.

13 Ralston SH, Digione SS, Gallagher SJ, Boyle IT, Duff GW. Failure to detect paramyxovirus sequences in Paget's disease of bone using the polymerase chain reaction. *J Bone Miner Res* 1991; **6**: 1243–8.

14 Birch MA, Taylor W, Fraser WD, Ralston SH, Hart CA, Gallagher JA. Absence of paramyxovirus RNA in cultures of Pagetic bone cells and in Pagetic bone. *J Bone Miner Res* 1994; **9**: 11–16.

15 Maldague B, Malghem J. Dynamic radiologic patterns of Paget's disease of bone. *Clin Orthop* 1987; **217**: 126–51.

16 Harinck HI, Bijvoet OLM, Blauksma HJ, Vellenga CJLR, Frijlinck WB. The relation between signs and symptoms in Paget's disease of bone. *Q J Med* 1986; **226**: 133–51.

17 Cantrill J, Anderson DC. Treatment of Paget's disease of bone. *Clin Endocrinol* 1990; **32**: 507–18.

18 Sato M, Grasser W, Endo N *et al.* Bisphosphonate action; alendronate localisation in rat bone and effects on osteoclast ultrastructure. *J Clin Invest* 1991; **88**: 2095–105.

19 Anderson DC, Richardson PC, Kingsley Brown J *et al.* Intravenous pamidronate: evolution of an effective treatment strategy. *Sem Arthr Rheum* 1994; **23**: 273–5.

20 Proceedings of the First International Symposium on Paget's disease of bone. *Semin Arth Rheum* 1994; **23**: 215–86.

21 Siris E, Weinstein RS, Altman R *et al.* Comparative study of alendronate versus etidronate for the treatment of Paget's disease of bone. *J Clin Endocrinol Metab* 1996; **81**: 961–7.

Part 9
Cranial Syndrome and Multiple Endocrine Neoplasia

CHAPTER 45

Carcinoid syndrome

K. Öberg

Introduction

The term *Karzinoid* was introduced in 1907 by Oberndorfer to describe intestinal tumours with a less aggressive course than more common intestinal adenocarcinomas. However, the first clinical and histopathological description of carcinoid tumours was made by Otto Lubarsch in 1888, who described the multicentric origin of carcinoid tumours of the gastrointestinal tract, while 2 years later Ranson reported a patient with ileal carcinoma with liver metastases who experienced diarrhoea and dyspnoea induced by eating. It was subsequently generally accepted that the carcinoid tumour was a very slowly growing, benign neoplasm with no potential for invasiveness and little tendency to give rise to metastases. This myth of 'benignity' has survived to the present day, even though in 1949 Pearson and Fitzgerald described a large series of metastasising carcinoid tumours.

In 1914, Gosset and Masson using silver impregnation techniques demonstrated that carcinoid tumours might develop from enterochromaffin cells, the 'Kulchitsky cell' in the glands of Lieberkühn, and the argentaffinity of these tumour cells was further established 10 years later. In 1953, Lembeck demonstrated the presence of serotonin in carcinoid tumours, and in 1954 Thorsson *et al.* first described a series of patients with small intestinal carcinoids and hepatic metastases producing serotonin and causing the typical symptoms of diarrhoea, flushing asthma, cyanosis and right heart failure, the so-called carcinoid syndrome.

During the past decade the rapid progression in immunohistochemical and radioimmunoassay techniques, as well as molecular biology, has enabled researchers to demonstrate the content of various peptide hormones, such as the tachykinins, and other agents kallikrein (bradykinin) and prostaglandins, which might be involved in the symptomatology of the carcinoid syndrome.

Classification of carcinoid tumours

Carcinoid tumours constitute about 2% of all malignant tumours of the gastrointestinal tract. The incidence is similar in men and women, and the condition is usually diagnosed between the ages of 25 and 80 years with a median of 58 years. The incidence of carcinoid tumours found at autopsy is 2.1 per 100 000 population [1]. However, the incidence of patients presenting with the carcinoid syndrome is estimated at 0.5 per 100 000 population [2].

Carcinoid tumours derive from so-called APUD cells of the diffuse endocrine system. These cells show characteristic light microscopic and histochemical features such as argentaffin and argyrophil reactions. These cells have the capacity for amine precursor uptake and decarboxylation (APUD). The so-called enterochromaffin cells (EC) belong to the group of APUD cells and are said to be the origin of the carcinoid tumours. These cells occur throughout the whole gastrointestinal tract except the oesophagus, and are numerous in distal parts of small intestine. They are somewhat more sparsely distributed in the large bowel and stomach. The appendicial carcinoids develop from another cell type which is more related to the peripheral nervous system. This might also explain the benign clinical features of this type of carcinoid [3].

In 1963 Williams and Sandler [4] introduced a new classification of gastrointestinal endocrine tumours based on embryonic origin and histological and biochemical features, and divided them into three groups: foregut, midgut and hindgut carcinoids (Table 45.1). Foregut tumours include neuroendocrine tumours of the thymus, bronchial, gastric and duodenal mucosa and pancreatic carcinoids. The midgut tumours are primarily located in jejunum, ileum and proximal colon, whereas hindgut tumours are those of distal colon and rectum. Nowadays, such a classification might seem

Table 45.1 Classification of gastrointestinal endocrine tumours. From [3].

Origin	Organ	Silver staining	Hormone production*	Clinical symptoms
Foregut†	Thymus	Argyrophil	CRH, ACTH, GHRH (5-HT)	Cushing's syndrome Acromegaly
	Lung	Argyrophil Sevier–Munger (Argentaffin)	CRH, ACTH, GHRH PP, hCG-α, neurotensin 5-HTP, 5-HT, histamine	Cushing's syndrome Acromegaly Carcinoid syndrome
	Stomach (ECLoma)	Argyrophil Sevier–Munger	CRH, ACTH, GHRH, gastrin	Cushing's syndrome Pernicious anaemia Acromegaly, Zollinger–Ellison syndrome
	Duodenum	(Argentaffin) (Argyrophil)	Gastrin, somatostatin, neurotensin, tachykinins, 5-HT	Somatostatinoma syndrome, carcinoid syndrome, Zollinger–Ellison syndrome
Midgut ('classical carcinoid')	Ileum	Argyrophil	Tachykinins, bradykinins	Carcinoid syndrome
	Jejunum	Argentaffin	CGRP	
	Proximal colon		5-HT	
	Appendix	Argyrophil	(Tachykinins), (5-HT)	Not hormone related
Hindgut	Distal colon	Argyrophil	PP, HCG-α, PYY	Not hormone related
	Rectum	Sevier–Munger	Somatostatin	

* All carcinoids produce peptides from the chromogranin family (A, B).
† Endocrine pancreatic tumours are not included among carcinoids. CRH, corticotrophin-releasing hormone; ACTH, adrenocorticotrophic hormone; GHRH, growth hormone-releasing hormone; PP, pancreatic polypeptide; hCG, human chorionic gonadotrophin; CGRP, calcitonin gene-related peptide; PYY, peptide YY; ECL, enterochromaffin-like; 5-HTP, 5-hydroxytryptophan; 5-HT, 5-hydroxytryptamine, serotonin.

inappropriate, but from the clinical point of view it is very useful because tumours included in these main groups present different clinical features and produce different combinations of hormones.

About 86% of carcinoid tumours develop in the gastrointestinal tract, 10% in the lung, and the rest in various organs such as thymus, kidney, ovary, testes and prostate. The most frequent location in the gastrointestinal tract is the appendix, followed by the small intestine and rectum (Table 45.2). Carcinoids constitute about 34% of all tumours in the small intestine, but only 1% of all neoplasms in the stomach, colon or rectum [5].

Table 45.2 Percentage distribution of 1867 carcinoids by site.* From [5].

Site	%
Lung and bronchi	10
Stomach	2
Duodenum	2
Jejunum	1
Ileum	11
Small intestine (not specified)	5
Caecum	3
Appendix	44
Colon	5
Rectum	15

* Only frequencies of at least 1% are listed.

Histological appearance

By light microscopy, carcinoid tumours are easily identified with their uniform round-cell nuclei and regular growth pattern (insular, trabecular or glandular, or a mixture of these three types) (Plate 45.1, opposite p. 332). These growth patterns are not related to the site of origin (foregut, midgut or hindgut), even if midgut carcinoids predominantly show an insular growth pattern. Foregut carcinoids exhibit an argyrophil reaction with the Grimelius silver staining method and are often positive with the Sevier–Munger staining technique. Almost all midgut carcinoids are Grimelius-positive (Plate 45.2), but also show an argentaffin reaction (Masson staining) indicating their content of serotonin. Serotonin-positive cells can also be demonstrated by immunohistochemical methods. Hindgut carcinoid tumours demonstrate mainly positive reactions with Grimelius and Sevier–Munger silver staining [6].

Neuroendocrine properties of carcinoid tumours can further be shown by immunohistochemical methods, utilising antibodies against chromogranin A and B, and neuron-specific enolase (NSE). Extensive immunohistochemical investigations have revealed that, in particular, foregut and hindgut tumours are multihormonal (Table 45.1), whereas midgut carcinoids demonstrate a more uniform pattern of hormone production, especially tachykinins and serotonin.

Electron microscopy has demonstrated the presence of both amines and peptides within the same tumour cells, for example serotonin and substance P. The neurosecretory granules within tumour cells are dependent on the origin of the primary tumour; foregut carcinoid tumours have small, round, regular cytoplasmic granules, whereas midgut carcinoids contain large pleomorphic granules, and hindgut tumours contain round neurosecretory granules.

Macroscopically the gastrointestinal carcinoids, particularly midgut carcinoids, present very small primary tumours (5–10 mm diameter) (Plate 45.2), being multiple in one-third of patients. Lymph node and liver metastases may be fairly large (100–150 mm diameter).

Biochemistry

While serotonin (5-hydroxytryptamine, 5-HT) had been isolated from a carcinoid tumour by Lembeck in 1953, and it had been shown that blood 5-HT concentrations were increased in the carcinoid syndrome and that there was an increase in urinary excretion of 5-hydroxyindoleacetate (5-HIAA), 5-HT still remains the most important diagnostic biochemical feature of the carcinoid syndrome [2,7].

5-HT is synthesised in the carcinoid tumour by two enzymatic steps. First, tryptophan is 5-hydroxylated to form 5-hydroxytryptophan (5-HTP), which is then decarboxylated to form 5-HT. Tumour arising from the lung, pancreas and stomach may have a relative lack of 5-HTP decarboxylase whereby the tumour fails to decarboxylate all the 5-HTP. The tumour then excretes 5-HTP, 5-HT and 5-HIAA in the urine. This may be of diagnostic relevance in certain patients. The high 5-HT levels in blood are mainly due to the increased amount of 5-HT bound to blood platelets rather than to a marked rise in plasma 5-HT *per se*. 5-HT released from hepatic metastases into the hepatic veins is largely taken up by the lung. The 5-HT released is oxidatively deaminated to 5-HIAA, which is excreted in the urine.

However, 5-HIAA may also be produced within the tumour; thus, urinary 5-HIAA reflects not only circulating 5-HT oxidatively deaminated but also 5-HIAA produced and released from the tumour [7]. 5-HT is suggested to be a mediator of the carcinoid diarrhoea.

Oates *et al.* [8], some 20 years ago, provided evidence that kinins are released in patients with the carcinoid syndrome. Carcinoid tumours contain the enzyme kallikrein, which after incubation with purified human kininogen produces lysyl-bradykinin which is converted within the circulation to bradykinin. This polypeptide produces vasodilatation, and may be involved in the flush seen in some patients with carcinoid syndrome. However, not all patients have increased plasma bradykinin during flushes and intravenous bradykinin does not produce a typical carcinoid flush.

Histamine, found particularly in patients with foregut carcinoid tumours, is known to give rise to a very vivid red patchy flushing ('geographically'). Several investigators have found increased histamine and histamine metabolites in the urine, particularly in patients with gastric carcinoid tumours [7].

Blood levels of prostaglandins E and F have also been found to be elevated in some patients with the carcinoid syndrome [9]. However, no correlation between clinical symptoms and blood levels has been demonstrated. The role of prostaglandins in carcinoid symptoms has yet to be further evaluated.

Several members of the tachykinin peptide family have been demonstrated in carcinoid tumours and are secreted *in vivo* and *in vitro* from carcinoid tumour cells [10]. Tachykinins represent a peptide family which share an identical C-terminal amino-acid sequence (Fig. 45.1), with a widespread distribution from vertebrate to invertebrate animals. The prototypic member of the family, substance P, was isolated from the mammalian gastrointestinal tract and brain by von Euler and Gaddum as early as 1931. The occurrence of substance P in carcinoid tumours was first demonstrated by Håkansson *et al.* in 1977.

Until recently, substance P was regarded as the only tachykinin occurring in mammalian species. However, we have been able to demonstrate production and secretion of several members of the tachykinin family, including neuropeptide K (NPK), and neurokinins A and B (NKA and NKB). There exist at least two larger molecular forms of the tachykinins α- and β-preprotachykinin, of which β-preprotachykinin is mainly found in the gut (Fig. 45.2). This prohormone contains substance P, NPK and NKA amino-acid sequences, and these peptides can be cleaved at specific cleavage sites. This might explain the ability of carcinoid tumours to secrete different molecular forms of

Substance P	Arg-Pro-Lys-Pro-Gln-Gln-Phe-Phe-Gly-Leu-Met-NH_2
Neurokinin A	His-Lys-Thr-Asp-Ser-Phe-Val-Gly-Leu-Met-NH_2
Neurokinin B	Asp-Met-His-Asp-Phe-Val-Gly-Leu-Met-NH_2
Eledoisin	Pyr-Pro-Ser-Lys-Asp-Ala-Phe-Ile-Gly-Leu-Met-NH_2
Kassinin	Asp-Val-Pro-Lys-Ser-Asp-Glu-Phe-Val-Gly-Leu-Met-NH_2
Physalemin	Pyr-Ala-Asp-Pro-Asn-Lys-Phe-Tyr-Gly-Leu-Met-NH_2
Neuropeptide K	Arg-His-Lys-Thr-Asp-Ser-Phe-Val-Gly-Leu-Met-NH_2
	-Lys-His-Ser-Ile-Gln-Gly-His-Gly-Tyr-Leu-Ala-Lys
	Asp-Ala-Asp-Ser-Ser-Ile-Glu-Lys-Gln-Val-Ala-Leu-Leu

Fig. 45.1 Amino-acid sequences of some members of the tachykinin peptide family. Note the similar C-terminal amino-acid sequences.

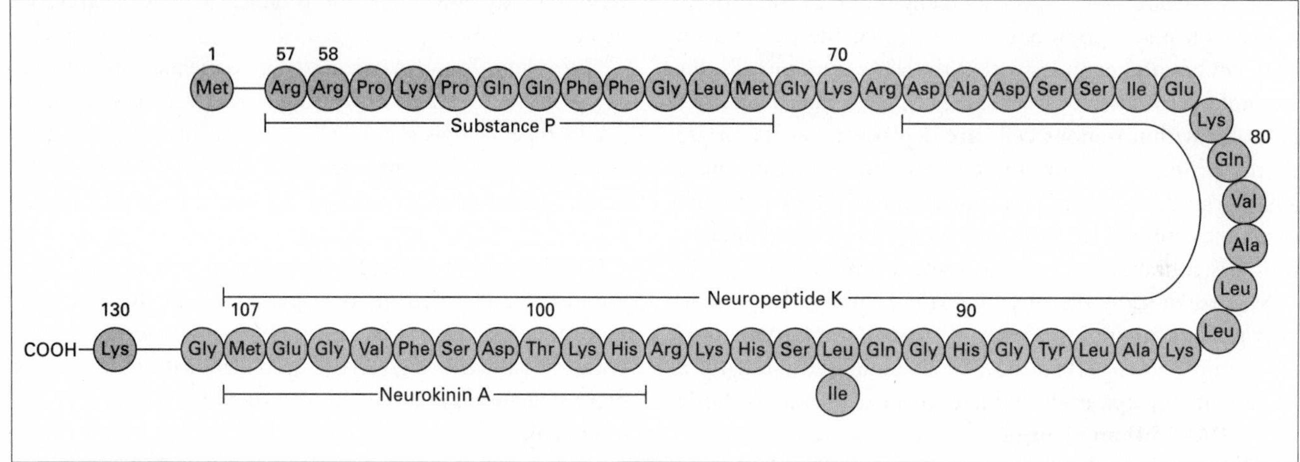

Fig. 45.2 The β-preprotachykinin amino-acid sequence. Typical enzymatic cleavage sites are between the amino acids Lys and Arg.

tachykinins. We have furthermore been able to demonstrate a release of tachykinins during spontaneous and pentagastrin-induced flushing reactions (Fig. 45.3). The tachykinins are very strong vasodilators, and are strong candidates for the flush reaction in carcinoid patients [11].

Chromogranin A (CgA) is the major member of a family of acidic glycoproteins, the chromogranin/secretogranin proteins, found ubiquitously in the soluble matrix of dense-core secretory granules in neurons and endocrine cells. Mature CgA (molecular weight 50 kDa) contains 439 amino-acid residues (human) and contains 10 basic amino-acid residues which may serve as targets for endoproteolytic attack by processing enzymes. Several biologically active peptides are cleaved off, for example pancreastatin, β-granin, chromostatin, vasostatin and parastatin (Fig. 45.4). CgA is a high-capacity calcium-binding protein and has the ability to sort peptide hormones and neurotransmitters and package them into secretory granules. Proteolytic processing of CgA occurs both intracellularly and extracellularly in the circulation. It is released from the cells together with costored peptides. The precise role of circulating CgA is unknown, but some of its cleavage products are biologically active. Pancreastatin inhibits glucose-stimulated insulin secretion whereas vasostatin (1–76) inhibits arterial smooth muscle contraction *in vitro* [12]. Elevated circulating immunoreactive CgA levels have been found in many patients with a variety of neuroendocrine neoplasms (Fig. 45.5). Particularly high plasma levels have been noticed in patients with carcinoid tumours, where it also reflects tumour mass [13,14]. Furthermore, recent data indicate that CgA is an independent marker of poor prognosis in patients with carcinoid tumours which might indicate a growth-promoting role for CgA or its spliced smaller fragments [14]. Other peptide hormones secreted by carcinoids are pancreatic polypeptide (PP), human chorionic gonadotrophin α- and β-subunits (HCG-α/β), calcitonin gene-related peptide (CGRP), calcitonin, gastrin, somatostatin, neurotensin,

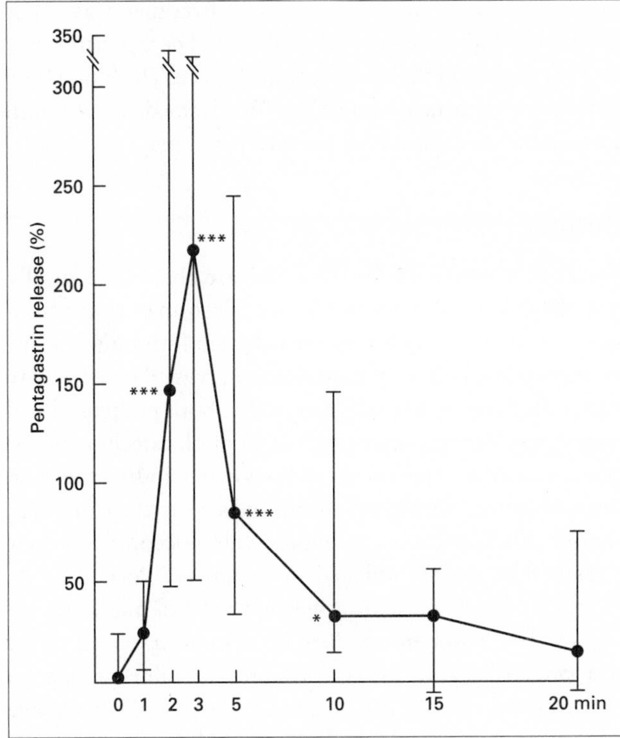

Fig. 45.3 Pentagastrin-induced release of tachykinins in patients with carcinoid tumours. Maximal release after 3 min (median and interquartile ranges). *** $P < 0.0001$; * $P < 0.05$.

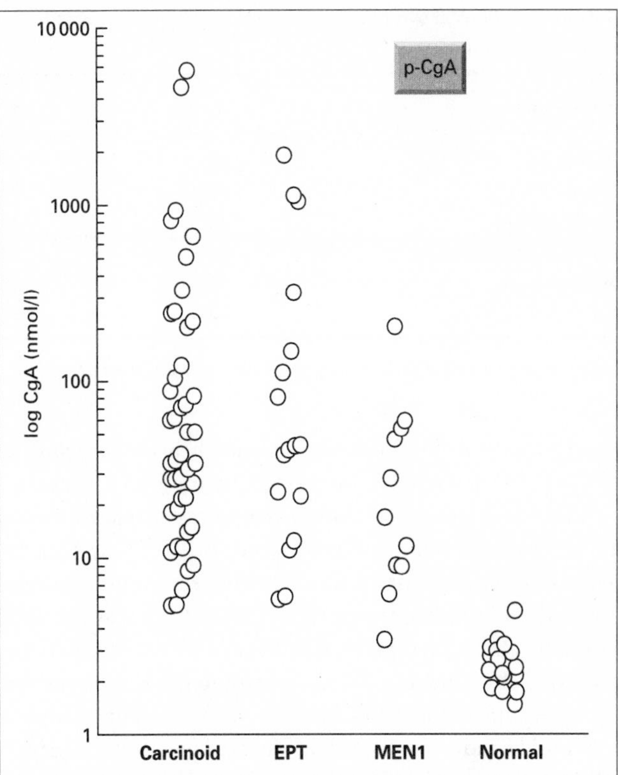

Fig. 45.5 Plasma levels of chromogranin A in patients with carcinoids, endocrine pancreatic tumours, multiple endocrine neoplasia type 1 and compared with healthy controls.

corticotrophin-releasing hormone (CRH or CRH-41) and growth hormone-releasing hormone (GHRH).

Clinical presentation (Table 45.3)

Carcinoid tumours are known to contain and secrete a large number of hormones and amines. Despite this fact, the majority of the tumours do not present with any hormone-related clinical symptoms. The reason for this is not fully understood, but might depend on secretion of biologically inactive forms of hormones, release of only small amounts of active peptides into the bloodstream, or rapid degradation of secreted agents within the tumour itself, in the blood or in the liver or lungs. Carcinoids with little tendency to metastasise, for example carcinoids of the appendix, will rarely present with hormone-related clinical symptoms, but rather with symptoms such as abdominal pain and intestinal obstruction. Rectal carcinoids secrete hormones that do not cause any specific clinical syndromes, such as PP, PYY, HCG-α/β subunits and CgA and the most common clinical presentation is abdominal pain, intestinal obstruction, bleeding or liver enlargement. The majority of midgut carcinoids will, however, metastasise and present with the classical carcinoid syndrome which includes flushing,

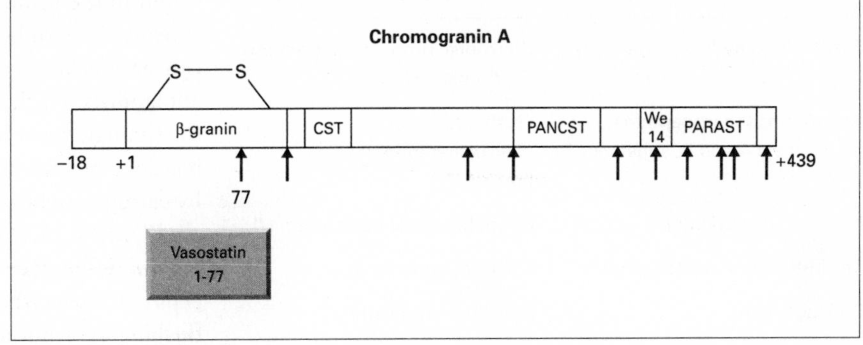

Fig. 45.4 Schematic drawing of the glycoprotein chromogranin A. Arrows indicate dibasic cleavage sites. CST, chromostatin; PANCST, pancreastatin; PARAST, parastatin.

Table 45.3 Clinical symptoms at referral in 103 patients with carcinoid tumours.

Symptoms	*n*	%
Diarrhoea	86	84
Flush	77	75
Ileus/subileus	45	44
Cardiac insufficiency	34	33
Asthma	15	15
Carcinoid syndrome*	69	67

*Both flushing and diarrhoea together with increased 5-HIAA.

diarrhoea, bronchial constriction, right heart failure and, as the original description, increased urinary 5-HIAA levels.

Table 45.3 shows the clinical symptoms at referral found in 103 patients with carcinoid tumours [2]. These patients were referred because of metastasising carcinoid tumours, the majority of midgut type (87%). Diarrhoea was the most common clinical symptom, occurring in 84% of the patients followed by flushing 75%, gastrointestinal obstruction in 44% and cardiac insufficiency in 33%. The complete carcinoid syndrome, including elevated levels of urinary 5-HIAA, was found in 67% of the patients. Other less common features of the carcinoid syndrome are pellagra-like skin lesions and arthropathy of large joints. A recent update of our patient material of 301 carcinoid patients revealed the carcinoid syndrome in 74% of the patients.

The carcinoid syndrome (Table 45.4)

Almost all patients with the carcinoid syndrome and gastrointestinal carcinoids have metastatic disease, mainly liver metastases. Some bronchial carcinoids may present with the syndrome without recognised metastases, which might depend on the liberation of causing agents directly into the systemic circulation. A small proportion of patients with midgut carcinoid tumours do not have liver metastases, but still present with the carcinoid syndrome. These patients may have metastases in the retroperitoneal space. The blood flow from these metastases might then be drained directly into the systemic circulation via prevertebral veins.

Table 45.4 Carcinoid syndrome: suggested pathophysiology.

Secretory product	Clinical symptoms
Serotonin (5-hydroxytryptamine)	Diarrhoea, bronchoconstriction (?), fibrosis (??)
Tachykinins (neuropeptide K, neurokinins A and B, substance P)	Flush, bronchial obstruction (oedema), fibrosis (??)
Kallikrein (bradykinin)	Flush, bronchial obstruction (?)
Calcitonin gene-related peptide	Flush (?), oedema (?)
Prostaglandins	Diarrhoea (?), flush (?)

Flushing

The mechanisms of the flush reaction are pharmacologically and physiologically heterogeneous. Flush may result from agents acting directly on the vascular smooth-muscle cells, or may be mediated by vasomotor nerves; the latter may lead to flushing as a result of events at both peripheral and central sites. Several agents such as alcohol, catecholamines, calcium and pentagastrin are well known to induce the flush reaction in patients with the carcinoid syndrome. Carcinoid tumour cells are known to express adrenoceptors on their surface. The alcohol-induced flush can be blocked by α-adrenergic blockade, indicating that alcohol might act via release of catecholamines. Pentagastrin is suggested to act in a similar way via release of catecholamines acting on the carcinoid tumour cells, causing a release of vasoactive substances such as 5-HT, tachykinins, kallikrein and CGRP. Adrenalectomy in cats seems to prevent pentagastrin-induced release of 5-HT into the portal circulation, indicating involvement of an adrenal mechanism.

There is growing evidence that vasodilatation is responsible for the flush reaction seen in the carcinoid syndrome. Agents released from the tumour cells are involved, and the observed flush might be a result of combination effects of coreleased mediators, such as members of the tachykinin family (NKA, NKB, NPK and substance P), kallikrein, bradykinin, histamine and CGRP. The pentagastrin as well as alcohol-induced flush closely resembles a spontaneous flush reaction, and a maximum release of tachykinins is seen within 3–5 min from induction (Fig. 45.3). The occurrence of the flush, however, does not correlate with the release of serotonin. Pretreatment with a somatostatin analogue (octreotide) blocks the release of tachykinins and concomitantly decreases the flush reaction. Another mediator of the carcinoid flush might be histamine, which has been found in the urine and circulation of patients with mainly foregut carcinoids. The flushing reaction in these patients can be blocked by a combination of H_1- and H_2-receptor antagonists. Furthermore, pentagastrin has also been shown to stimulate histamine release from gastric carcinoids, and it is quite possible that some of the flushing reactions induced by eating may be mediated via gastrin release. For reviews, see [7,10,11,15,16].

Four different clinical subsets of flush have been described [7]. A diffuse erythematous flush affects not only the normal flushing area but also the skin of the back, abdomen and palms; it is paroxysmal, usually lasting for 2–5 min (Plate 45.3). Another more violaceous flush associated with dilated cutaneous facial veins, telangiectases, watery eyes and conjunctival suffusion, is very often seen in patients with long-standing carcinoid syndrome (Plate 45.4). A bright-red patchy flush associated with gastric carcinoids and excess of histamine release is a third type. Bronchial carcinoids are sometimes associated with a flush lasting for hours with facial skin swelling, lacrimation, swelling of the salivary glands, hypotension, exacerbation of diarrhoea and palpitations. This is the most severe type of flush reaction and it might sometimes be a part of a 'carcinoid crisis' (Plate 45.5).

Precipitating factors of flush are heat, spicy foods, hot drinks, exercise, alcohol, physical and psychiatric excitement, defaecation and postural changes. Many patients feel the strongest flush reactions are first thing in the morning when having breakfast after a night's sleep. Patients with chronic flushes experience decreasing symptoms with time and even if they are constantly flushing they no longer experience any discomfort.

Diarrhoea

Diarrhoea may occur without flushing and vice versa, and the relationship between the two symptoms is variable. Often there is no definite temporal relationship between diarrhoea and flushing, which might lead to the conclusion that these two symptoms are not related to the same humoral secretion. Watery stools, accompanied by 'colicky' abdominal pain and urgency of defaecation is common. Some patients might experience passage of fluid stools as often as 20 times a day. Usually the diarrhoea appears to be dependent on increased intestinal motility. Serotonin (5-HT) stimulates small-bowel motility and increased fluid secretion. This can be shown experimentally by infusion of serotonin in humans and animals. Diarrhoea can be successfully treated by serotonin antagonists such as methysergide, cyproheptadine and ketanserin. The same serotonin antagonists do not influence symptoms of flush. Occasionally, the diarrhoea may be associated with intestinal obstruction by a primary tumour, and may also occur postoperatively as a 'short-bowel syndrome' after resection of a primary carcinoid tumour together with a long portion of the small bowel. Steatorrhoea occurs very rarely, but malabsorption might develop due to vascular insufficiency, small-bowel resection and bile-salt malabsorption. Other causes are bacterial overgrowth and obstruction of the mesenteric lymphatics. The pellagra-like skin lesion, which nowadays occurs very rarely, is thought to be due to nicotinamide deficiency induced by tryptophan deficiency, which in turn arises from utilisation of tryptophan by the tumour in making 5-hydroxyindoles.

Abdominal pain

Abdominal pain is, for some reason, a rather common clinical symptom associated with carcinoid tumours of the gastrointestinal tract. About 40% of the patients are referred to hospital due to symptoms of gastrointestinal obstruction. This obstruction might be due to the primary tumour itself, although in most situations it is very small. On the other hand, intestinal obstruction might also depend on tumour-associated fibrosis causing a rosette-like kinking of the mesentery (Fig. 45.6). Pain related to intestinal infarction is very rare, but in patients with long-standing disease intestinal entrapment is recognised. Some patients experience a colicky pain which is associated with increased intestinal motility and diarrhoea.

Pain arising from hepatic metastases is rather uncommon and is predominantly noticed in patients with large metastases with grossly enlarged livers. Tension of the liver capsule might lead to tenderness and pain. Some patients experience periods of metastatic infarction with fever and abdominal pain, which is quite common in patients with rectal carcinoids and large liver metastases.

Bronchial constriction

Symptoms of bronchoconstriction are less common than other features of the carcinoid syndrome, constituting about 15–20%. Asthma-like episodes are associated with flush attacks and might be related to the same mediators, tachykinins and/or bradykinin. Bronchospasm *per se* is rather rare, and in most situations lung symptoms might depend

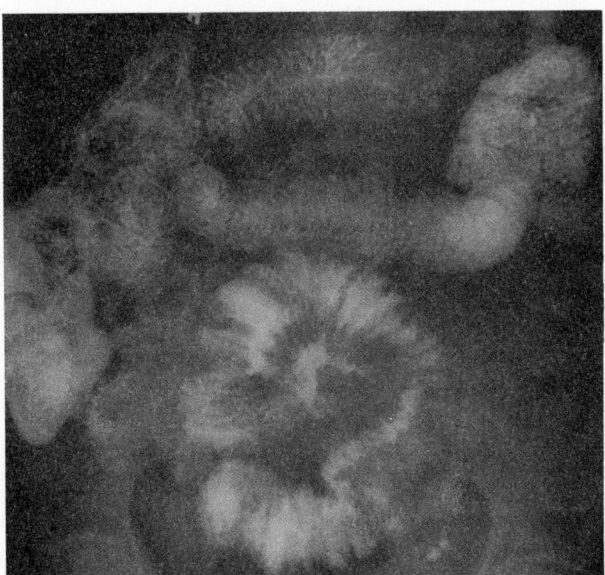

Fig. 45.6 Barium enema in a patient with a carcinoid tumour. A 'rosette'-like kinking of the small bowel is noticed.

on hyperventilation which is observed during flush episodes. Bronchoconstriction can be seen during anaesthesia, and catecholamines should not be given systemically because they may worsen the symptomatology. Nowadays, treatment with somatostatin analogues has solved most of the anaesthetic problems.

Carcinoid heart disease

It is unique for a malignant tumour to be associated with a pathognomonic cardiac disease which is also of great importance in the morbidity and mortality of the carcinoid syndrome. The frequency of carcinoid heart disease based on autopsy diagnosis in patients with carcinoid syndrome has been reported as 35–50%. However, in a recent study we demonstrated (by means of echocardiography) that about 70% of consecutively referred patients with the carcinoid syndrome presented signs of carcinoid heart disease [17]. The most frequent pathological findings were morphological and functional abnormalities of the tricuspid valve. The carcinoid heart lesions are 'plaque-like' or diffuse pearl-grey endocardial thickening. They are almost invariably found on the right side of the heart. The papillary muscles and cordae tendineae of the tricuspid valves are often shortened and enclosed in a fibrous white 'capping', which reduces the amplitude of the valve motion, or totally immobilises the cusps (Plate 45.6). The tricuspid leaflets themselves, as well as the pulmonary cusps, are frequently thickened and retracted by a fibrotic process (Plate 45.7). Microscopically, the lesions are mainly composed of an elastin-deficient stroma rich in acid mucopolysaccharides and collagen intermingled with a moderate number of cells. The two most frequent cell types have ultrastructural characteristics of the usual type of smooth-muscle cells and some fibroblast characteristics, so-called 'myofibroblasts'. The aetiology of carcinoid heart disease remains obscure. The tumours release vasoactive substances which might be involved in pathogenesis, and there exists a correlation between the degree of heart involvement and circulating levels of tachykinins and serotonin [17]. Recent findings indicate increased expression of growth factors of the transforming growth factor-β (TGF-β) family [18]. These growth factors are involved in stromal formation and stimulate matrix production in tumours.

Miscellaneous manifestations

Retroperitoneal fibrosis is found in patients with lymph-node metastases located to the retroperitoneal space, and might occasionally cause ureteric obstruction and renal failure. Similar to the fibrosis in the right heart, fibrosis of great veins and large abdominal arteries can be seen which might cause abdominal pain, discomfort and even intestinal infarction. Very rarely, a carcinoid tumour might cause paraneoplastic polyneuropathy, myopathy or arthropathy.

Gastrointestinal bleeding may occur from carcinoid tumours throughout the gastrointestinal tract. Foregut carcinoid tumours occasionally present with symptoms of common endocrine disease such as the syndrome of inappropriate antidiuretic hormone secretion (SIADH), Cushing's syndrome and acromegaly. These tumours ectopically secrete vasopressin, adrenocorticotrophic hormone (ACTH), CRH and GHRH. A very few patients have been reported with hypoglycaemic symptoms due to production of insulin-like growth factors 1 and 2 (IGF-1 and IGF-2). The occurrence of psychiatric disturbances in the carcinoid syndrome is disputed. There are a few observations of patients who developed severe mental depression concomitant with the discovery of a carcinoid tumour. Treatment with oral L-tryptophan reversed the mental depression, suggesting a tryptophan deficiency which might perhaps have been causing brain 5-HT deficiency. Carcinoids of foregut origin are associated with the multiple endocrine neoplasia type 1 syndrome (MEN-1) with autosomal dominantly inherited predisposition to develop pituitary, parathyroid, endocrine pancreatic and adrenocortical tumours (adenomas). A specific genetic defect has been localised to chromosome band 11q13 (see Chapter 46). Recently, the gene for MEN-1 has been cloned, coding for a protein called menin without known function [35]. Duodenal carcinoids and carcinoids of the ampulla of Vater have been reported to be associated with von Recklinghausen's disease (for review see [3,15]). Simultaneous occurrence of other malignant tumours in carcinoid patients is fairly frequent, about 5% in our own material [2]. Such tumours include breast and colonic cancer occurring simultaneously with the carcinoid.

Diagnosis of the carcinoid syndrome
(Table 45.5)

A large number of gastrointestinal carcinoids do not present any particular clinical features or hormone-related symptoms but may show up with different kinds of liver enlargement, intestinal obstruction or gastrointestinal bleeding. Common use of abdominal computed tomographic (CT) scanning might incidentally demonstrate liver and lymph node metastases in patients with diffuse abdominal symptoms of discomfort, pain, borborygmus, gastritis and diarrhoea. The problem is then to find out the true nature of such lesions. When a midgut carcinoid has metastasised to the liver, the majority of the patients present with the carcinoid syndrome and the diagnosis might be quite easy to establish.

Table 45.5 Suggested diagnosis scheme for gastrointestinal carcinoid tumours.

Biochemical diagnosis

p-Chromogranin A

Urinary 5-hydroxyindoleacetic acid (U-5HIAA)

p-Neuropeptide K (substance P), (s-pancreatic polypeptide, s-human chorionic gonadotrophin-α/β, s-gastrin, p-corticotrophin-releasing hormone, growth hormone-releasing hormone)

Urinary histamine metabolites

Flush provocation (pentagastrin 0.6 μg/kg bodyweight i.v. bolus)
P-Neuropeptide K at –15, 0, 1, 3, 5, 15, 30 min

Histopathology and immunocytochemistry

Argyrophil staining (Grimelius)

Argentaffin staining (Masson)

Chromogranin A + B

Synaptophysin
PGP 9.5

Neuron-specific enolase

5-Hydroxytryptamine

Other neuroendocrine peptides

Electron microscopy

Radiology

Abdominal (thoracic) computed tomography, ultrasonography and magnetic resonance imaging

Angiography
(barium enema)

Lung radiography

^{111}In-DTPA-D-Phe^{1}-octreotide scintigraphy

Positron-emission tomography
(^{11}C-5-HTP)

Other investigations

Echocardiography of the heart

Gastroscopy (foregut origin)

Colonoscopy (hindgut origin)

Bone scintigraphy

Endoscopic ultrasound (duodenal, pancreatic carcinoids)

p, plasma; s, serum.

Biochemical diagnosis (Table 45.6)

As soon as suspicion about a gastrointestinal carcinoid tumour has emerged, one should analyse urinary 5-HIAA; normally, 5-HIAA excretion should not exceed 50 μmol (10 mg)/24 hours. False positives may occur in patients taking drugs such as chlorpromazine or eating bananas, avocado, pineapples and walnuts; also, chocolate and coffee should be avoided. It is important to be aware of the paroxysmal nature of carcinoid symptoms and release of agents; thus, it is important to perform several 24-hour urine collections, particularly in the early stages of the disease [7]. Another important screening marker for carcinoid tumours is determination of plasma CgA. Plasma CgA was elevated in all patients with verified carcinoid tumours ($n = 44$) (Fig. 45.5) [13]. This marker is also particularly useful for demonstrating small tumours and even 'hyperplastic' lesions, and is also of great value in determining response to treatment. About 60% of patients with the carcinoid syndrome show elevated plasma levels of the tachykinins, particularly NPK, the larger molecular form (Fig. 45.2) of which has a longer half-life in circulation than NKA or substance P [11]. Other useful markers for gastrointestinal carcinoids are PP, HCG-α and -β subunits. Determination of plasma ACTH, CRH or GHRH might be of importance if the patient presents with symptoms of Cushing's disease or acromegaly.

Flush reactions can be provoked in a standardised manner by injection of pentagastrin (0.6 μg/kg bodyweight) administered as an intravenous bolus injection. Blood samples are drawn before, during and after the flush for analysis of plasma tachykinins [11]. A flush reaction could also be provoked by ingestion of alcohol or food [11,16].

Table 45.6 Tumour markers in patients with carcinoid tumours.*

Marker	Increase in circulation (%)
p-Chromogranin A + B	100
Urinary 5-hydroxyindoleacetate	88
p-Neuropeptide K	66
s-Pancreatic polypeptide	43
s-Human chorionic gonadotrophin-α	28
s-Gastrin	15
s-Human chorionic gonadotrophin-β	12

p, Plasma; s, serum.
* Includes 130 patients with metastasising carcinoid tumours (87% of midgut origin).

Histology and immunocytochemistry

Specimens obtained from tumour tissue either at surgery or by coarse-needle biopsies from liver and lymph-node metastases should be screened for neuroendocrine properties on histology. Staining with both argyrophil (Grimelius) and argentaffin stains (Masson) not only confirms the diagnosis of a gastrointestinal carcinoid, but a positive argentaffin reaction also suggests a midgut offspring. Other useful neuroendocrine markers for screening purpose are immunohistochemical staining with antibodies against CgA, synaptophysin, PGP 9.5 and NSE [3,6,15,16]. The diagnosis of a midgut carcinoid can be established by immunohistochemical investigation with an antiserotonin antibody. Carcinoid tumours can be further characterised immunohistochemically by using antisera against multiple peptides, for example PP, gastrin, HCG-α/β and CGRP. Only exceptionally has one to perform electron microscopy to identify secretory granules, and in rare cases *in situ* hybridisation with a radiolabelled probe hybridising with mRNA for a peptide for example, CgA or β-preprotachykinin.

Radiology

Ultrasound investigation of the abdomen and CT scans are efficient for detecting liver metastases, provided that these metastases are more than 0.5 cm in diameter. Magnetic resonance imaging (MRI) has not proved to be of any advantage compared with contrast-enhanced CT scanning or ultrasound investigations in detecting carcinoid tumours and metastases. Furthermore, ultrasonography can be combined with guided coarse-needle biopsies to obtain tissue specimens for histochemical and immunocytochemical investigation. Primary tumours of the small bowel are very difficult to visualise in most patients, but sometimes one may find a 'positive' barium enema (Fig. 45.6). The primary tumour *per se* is not visualised by this procedure, but due to a fibrotic reaction surrounding the local metastases, localisation of the primary can be obtained. Angiography of the superior and inferior mesenteric arteries is more reliable, enabling localisation of primary tumours, regional lymph-node and liver metastases. A typical 'corkscrew' appearance of the blood vessels leading to the tumours may be noted.

Scanning with the agent ^{131}I-meta-iodobenzylguanidine (mIBG) can be utilised to detect rather small carcinoids, particularly in uncommon locations [15]. Recently, a radiolabelled somatostatin analogue (octreotide) has been used to localize carcinoid tumours [19]. ^{111}In-DTPA-D-Phe^1-octreotide (Plate 45.8) has a favourable half-life (2.8 days) and is excreted through the kidneys. ^{111}In-DTPA-D-Phe^1-octreotide binds to somatostatin receptor subtype 2 and 5 (sst_2, sst_5; see below). Several reports on the usefulness of scintigraphy with this isotope in patients with carcinoids have been published during the past few years [20,21]. Positive scans have been obtained in 80–90% of patients with the carcinoid tumours and liver metastases. Small primary tumours of about 5 mm diameter can sometimes be visualised and somatostatin receptor scintigraphy produces a more accurate staging of the carcinoid disease than CT or ultrasound. Every patient with a carcinoid tumour should now be scanned with somatostatin-receptor scintigraphy.

Positron-emission tomography (PET) using short-lived isotopes coupled to 5-HTP can also be used. C^{11}-5-HTP is able to visualise all tested patients with the carcinoid syndrome [22] (Plate 45.9). However, the method is limited to centres with the ability to generate short-lived radioisotopes and a cyclotron. ^{11}C-5-HTP-PET is an excellent method to monitor treatment (Plate 45.9) and almost every substance can be labelled.

Other diagnostic procedures

All patients with signs of the carcinoid syndrome should be investigated concerning heart involvement by means of transthoracic echocardiography. In some very rare situations, one can perform transhepatic catheterisation of the portal vein and superior mesenteric vein, taking blood samples from different sites for analysis of peptides such as chromogranins and tachykinins, in order to localise primary tumours and regional metastases. Concomitant pentagastrin stimulation can further enhance the sensitivity of such procedure. Bone scintigraphy should be performed, particularly in patients with a long history of carcinoid disease complaining of skeletal pain. Somatostatin-receptor scintigraphy has nowadays mostly replaced traditional bone scintigraphy. Gastroscopy and colonoscopy may be of great value in patients with foregut and hindgut carcinoids, respectively. Endoscopic ultrasonography has recently come into clinical use and is particularly useful to localise small tumours in the duodenal wall and pancreas (B. Wiedenmann, personal communication). Pulmonary radiography, thoracic CT and bronchoscopy are of value in the diagnosis of bronchial carcinoids.

Metastatic spread

In a group of 103 patients with carcinoid tumours referred for medical treatment, the distribution of metastatic spread is indicated in Table 45.7. All patients revealed local metastases, and $>90\%$ of the patients had liver metastases. The skeleton was involved in about 13% of patients. The majority of the patients had a midgut origin for the primary tumour [2,10].

Treatment

Surgical therapy should be considered in every patient with a carcinoid tumour. In cases with local disease, primary tumour and only local metastases, surgery can be curative.

Table 45.7 Localisation of metastases in 103 patients with carcinoid tumours.

Metastases	*n*	%
Local	103	100.0
Liver	96	93.2
Skeleton	14	13.6
Peripheral lymph nodes	7	6.8
Ovaries	4	3.9
Lung	2	1.9
Skin	1	1.0
Pancreas	1	1.0
Pleural	1	1.0
Pituitary gland	1	1.0

However, even in patients with 'bulky' disease, liver and mesenteric metastases, an aggressive surgical approach may be of clinical benefit [23]. The reduction of tumour mass by surgical intervention might enhance a favourable outcome for further medical treatment. Appendiceal carcinoids with a diameter of <20 mm are always considered to be benign, and these patients are cured by surgical resection. When liver metastases are confined to one lobe, one may perform a liver segmental resection. Furthermore, surgery should always be considered during the clinical course of gastrointestinal carcinoid tumour. Intestinal obstruction may occur during medical treatment, and 'conservative' resections of the intestine and fibrotic areas may alleviate clinical symptoms [36].

The majority of patients with midgut carcinoid tumours presenting with the carcinoid syndrome have multiple liver metastases and cannot be cured surgically. In these situations, hepatic artery occlusion has been attempted with palliation of clinical symptoms for a median of 6–12 months [24]. Due to development of collateral blood supply, this treatment is very rarely curative, but the procedure can be repeated several times. The effect of the procedure, however, diminishes with the number of performed occlusions. Lower dearterialisation can be performed with either gelfoam powder (Ivalon, Spongostan) injected into the hepatic artery or ligation of the artery.

External radiotherapy has been tried in a number of patients with metastatic gastrointestinal carcinoids. The results have so far been dismal, with only a small number of short-term clinical responses [25]. External radiotherapy is nowadays mostly utilised for treatment of bone metastases in order to obtain pain relief. ^{111}In-DTPA-D-Phe^{1}-octreotide using high doses has very recently been applied in a small number of patients with advanced disease. Preliminary data are promising but very few patients have been treated so far [37]. Partial responses have been reported with ^{131}I-mIBG where scanning uptake has been positive (26).

Definitive medical treatment

Chemotherapy in different combinations has been attempted for the past two decades in the treatment of malignant carcinoid tumours, demonstrating rather low response rates in most series. The most promising combination of cytostatic drugs has so far been streptozotocin plus 5-fluorouracil, giving rather short-lasting responses in 10–30% of patients [27,28]. Natural somatostatin (SOM-14) was used in the 1970s to control hormone-related clinical symptoms in carcinoid patients. From the clinical point of view it was a problem because of its short half-life (2–3 min) in the circulation necessitating continuous infusions. During the last decade somatostatin analogues with longer half-life (4–6 hours), which can be given subcutaneously, have been developed. They are all octapeptides (octreotide (Sandostatin), octastatin (RC-160)), lanreotide (Somatuline), octreotide being the most commonly used. All three analogues bind to somatostatin receptors 2 and 5 (sst_2,sst_5) with similar affinity [29]. Both the antitumour effect and inhibition of hormone release seem to be mediated through sst_2. In the future more receptor subtype-specific analogues will delineate these mechanisms in more detail.

Octreotide is approved in most countries for the treatment of the carcinoid syndrome. Maximum biochemical response occurs in a dose range of 0.2–0.3 mg/dl in two or three divided doses (for review see [30]). The biochemical response rate is 50–70% whereas antitumour response is <10%. Recently we have been able to show that high-dose therapy (9–12 mg/dl) induces apoptosis in carcinoid tumours and might generate greater antitumour response [38]. Long-acting formulations (LAR) of somatostatin analogues with injection every 2–4 weeks intramuscularly are currently being evaluated in clinical trials. Such long-acting formulation will further improve the quality of life in carcinoid patients.

Over the last decade another new treatment has been introduced for carcinoid tumours, α-interferon therapy, which might control tumour growth, reduce tumour-secreted agents and clinical symptoms. The obtained objective clinical response rates are about 50% with clinical improvement in about 70% of patients [28,31]. α-Interferon exerts a direct effect and causes a block in cell division in G_0–G_1 phase. It decreases the production of different peptide hormones and growth factors by blocking intracellular mRNA formation. α-Interferon is also a strong immunomodulator and induces class I antigens on tumour cells. The treatment can be continued for several years without the development of 'resistance', and patients have been treated continuously for more than 12 years with low doses (3–6 million units subcutaneously three times per week). The somatostatin analogues and α-interferon can be combined for an even more effective treatment in patients with severe carcinoid syndrome [32]. The precise role of this combination is currently explored in several randomised multicenter studies.

Symptomatic medical treatment

Several agents have been tried to relieve the symptoms of the carcinoid syndrome over the years: α-adrenergic blocking agents such as clonidine, phentolamine, methyldopa and propranolol; inhibition of serotonin synthesis by para-chlorophenylalanine; peripheral serotonin antagonists such as cyproheptadine, methysergide and ketanserin; histamine-receptor antagonists such as cyproheptadine and cimetidine, as well as steroids and chlorpromazine. Almost all these symptomatic drugs have now been replaced by somatostatin analogues, and only in exceptional cases (some biochemical carcinoids) does one have to consider any of the other drugs. Diarrhoea in patients with the carcinoid syndrome can very often be controlled by use of loperamide, and patients presenting with diarrhoea alone should first try this drug before considering the somatostatin analogues. One reason for this is that the analogue has to be given two or three times per day as subcutaneous injection, which is reducing the quality of life and might in some patients cause pain at the site of injection; moreover, somatostatin inhibits exocrine pancreatic function which might cause diarrhoea *per se*, although this is rarely a problem in practice.

Anaesthetic considerations

During anaesthesia of patients with carcinoid tumours and the carcinoid syndrome, adrenergic drugs should be avoided. The somatostatin analogues have replaced most other drugs for controlling the carcinoid syndrome during anaesthesia. Pre- and intraoperative infusion of octreotide at doses of 50–100 μg/hour will control carcinoid symptoms. There have not been any serious perioperative complications during surgery in any of our patients since using it. Another favourable effect might be in reducing effects on splanchnic and liver blood flow, thus diminishing bleeding during surgical procedures.

Carcinoid crisis

Carcinoid crisis is a rare complication following surgery, chemotherapy or tumour devascularisation, and is due to massive release of the mediators of the carcinoid syndrome. The patients experience hyperthermia, severe flush, low blood pressure, tachycardia and bronchoconstriction. The carcinoid crisis can be completely reversed by intravenous infusion of octreotide.

Prognosis and survival

There is a myth that carcinoid tumours are quite benign, that liver metastases grow very slowly, and that the patient might live for 10–15 years after occurrence of metastatic disease. In a review by Godwin [5], the 5-year survival rate for patients with carcinoids by different sites were the following: stomach 52%, small intestine 54%, appendix 99%, colon 52%, rectum 83%, lung 87%. These data might indicate a relatively good prognosis. However, when liver metastases are present, the 5-year survival rate decreased to 18–38% in different patient groups, and the median survival time has been calculated as about 23 months in patients with liver metastases and increased urinary 5-HIAA levels [33].

In our own series of 301 patients with carcinoid tumours the overall median survival was 90 months from diagnosis. There was a significant difference in survival from the start of treatment between patients with foregut carcinoids, median 26 months, and midgut carcinoids, median 67 months ($P = 0.004$), indicating differences in tumour biology (Fig. 45.7). The 5-year survival from diagnosis among midgut carcinoid patients with extensive liver disease was 47% while it was 73% in patients with only lymph-node metastases ($P = 0.002$) (Fig. 45.8) [34]. These survival data are considerably better than historical data and might be a result of better management of these patients, including more aggressive surgery in combination with biotherapy.

Since most patients present with metastatic disease at diagnosis, earlier diagnosis is mandatory. When we reviewed our patient material for the first time im 1985 (103 patients) and 10 years later (301 patients) the age at diagnosis, delay from first symptom until diagnosis or until start of treatment had not significantly changed [14]. Increasing use of the tumour marker CgA in patients complaining about various symptoms from the gastrointestinal tract might enable earlier diagnosis and curable surgery. In planning future therapy studies of carcinoid tumours aspects of tumour biology must be considered and included in the randomisation procedure. The type of carcinoid and the extent of tumour disease (stage) are important factors. We have also recently found bad prognostic factors in carcinoid tumours, such as high proliferation index (Ki-67), expression of PDGF-α receptor and the adhesion molecule CD44 as well as high levels of circulating levels of chromogranin A. These factors have to be considered together with somatostatin receptor content in the therapy decision. The future treatment will be more individualised and 'tailor-made' for the patient.

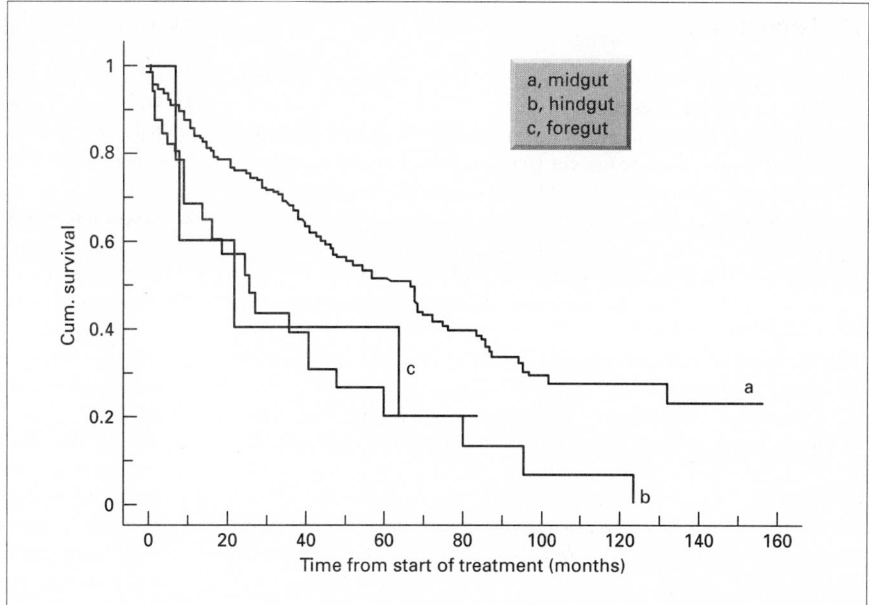

Fig. 45.7 Survival analysis of 301 patients with carcinoid tumours. There is a significant difference in the survival between midgut carcinoids and foregut carcinoids ($P = 0.004$) from start of treatment.

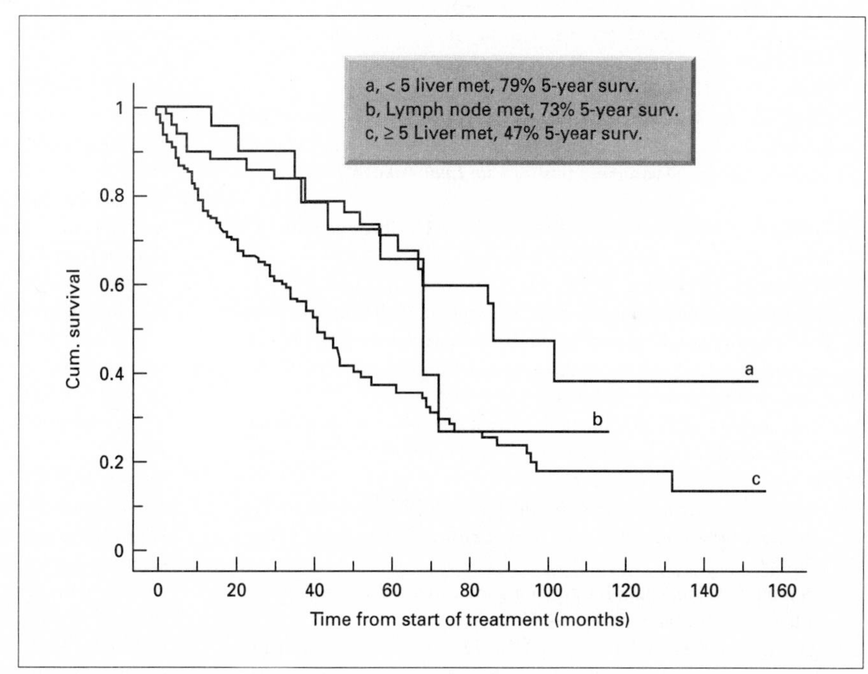

Fig. 45.8 Survival analysis of 301 patients with regard to tumour stage and the extent of liver involvement. There is a significant difference between extensive liver disease (more than five liver metastases) compared with those with only lymph node metastases and limited number of liver metastases ($P = 0.002$).

References

1 Berge T, Linell F. Carcinoid tumours. *Acta Path Microbial Scand Sect A* 1976; **84**: 322–30.

2 Norheim I, Öberg K, Theodorsson-Norheim E *et al.* Malignant carcinoid tumors: an analysis of 103 patients with regard to tumour localization, hormone production and survival. *Ann Surg* 1987; **206**: 115–25.

3 Wilander E, Lundqvist M, Öberg K. Gastrointestinal carcinoid tumours. Prog Histochem Cytochem 1989; **19**: 1–85.

4 Williams ED, Sandler M. The classification of carcinoid tumours. *Lancet* 1963; **i**: 238–9.

5 Godwin DJ. Carcinoid tumours; an analysis of 2,837 cases. *Cancer* 1975; **36**: 560–9.

6 Grimelius L, Wilander E. Silver impregnation and other non-immunocytochemical staining methods. In: Polak JM, Bloom SR, eds. *Endocrine Tumours*. Edinburgh: Churchill Livingstone, 1985: 95–115.

7 Grahame-Smith DG. The carcinoid syndrome. In: de Groot LJ, ed. *Endocrinology*, Vol 3. New York: Grune and Stratton, 1979: 1721–31.

8 Oates JA, Melmon K, Sjoerdsma M, Gillespie L, Mason DT. Release of a kinin peptide in the carcinoid syndrome. *Lancet* 1964; **ii**: 514–17.

9 Sandler M, Karim SM, Williams ED. Prostaglandins in aminepeptide-secreting tumours. *Lancet* 1968; **ii**: 1053–5.

10 Norheim I. Carcinoid tumors: clinical studies and the use of tachykinins as tumor markers. *Acta Univ Upsaliensis* 1986; Doctoral thesis.

11 Norheim I, Theodorsson-Norheim E, Brodin E, Öberg K. Tachykinins in carcinoid tumors: their use as a tumor marker and possible role in the carcinoid flush. *J Clin Endocrinol Metab* 1986; **63**: 605–12.

12 Hendy NG, Bevan S, Maltei M-G, Mouland AJ. Chromogranin A; review. *Clin Invest Med* 1995; **18**: 47–65.

13 Stridsberg M, Öberg K, Li Q, Engström U, Lundqvist G. Measurements of Chromogranin A, Chromogranin B (secretogranin I), Chromogranin C (secretogranin II) and pancreastatin in plasma and urine from patients with carcinoid tumours and endocrine pancreatic tumours. *J Endocrinol* 1995; **144**: 49–59.

14 Tiensuu Janson E, Holmberg L, Stridsberg M *et al.* Carcinoid tumors; analysis of prognostic factors and survival in 301 patients from a referral center. (In press).

15 Harris AL. Carcinoid tumours. In: Fielding JWL, Priestman TJ, eds. *Gastrointestinal Oncology*. Castle House Publications, 1986: 256–79.

16 Creutzfeld W, Stöckman F. Carcinoids and carcinoid syndrome. *Am J Med* 1987; **82** (Suppl. 5B): 4–16.

17 Lundin L, Norheim I, Landelius J, Öberg K, Theodorsson-Norheim E. Carcinoid heart disease: relationship of circulating vasoactive substances to ultrasound-detectable cardiac abnormalities. *Circulation* 1988; 77: 264–9.

18 Waltenberger J, Lundin L, Öberg K *et al.* Involvement of transforming growth factor-β in the formation of fibrotic lesions in carcinoid heart disease. *Am J Pathol* 1993; **142**: 71–8.

19 Krenning EP, Bakker WM, Breemar WAP *et al.* Localization of endocrine related tumours with a radiolabelled analogue of somatostatin. *Lancet* 1989; **i**: 242–5.

20 Kwekkebom DJ, Krenning EP, Bakker WH, Oei HY, Kooij PPM, Lamberts SWJ. Somatostatin analogue scintigraphy in carcinoid tumours. *Eur J Nucl Med* 1993; **20**: 283–92.

21 Westlin JE, Tiensuu Janson E, Arnberg H, Ahlström H, Öberg K, Nilsson S. Somatostatin receptor scintigraphy of carcinoid tumours using the [^{111}In-DTPA-D-Phe-I-octreotide]. *Acta Oncol* 1993; **32**: 783–6.

22 Eriksson B, Bergström M, Lilja A, Ahlström H, Långström B, Öberg K. Positron emission tomography (PET) in neuroendocrine gastrointestinal tumors. *Acta Oncol* 1993; **32**: 189–96.

23 Makridis C, Öberg K, Juhlin C *et al.* Surgical treatment of midgut carcinoid tumors. *World J Surg* 1990; **14**: 377–85.

24 Marlink RG, Lakich JJ, Robins JR, Clouse ME. Hepatic arterial embolization of metastatic hormone secreting tumors. *Cancer* 1991; **65**: 2227–30.

25 Shupak KP, Wallner KE. The role of radiation therapy in the treatment of locally unresectable or metastatic carcinoid tumors. *Int J Radiol Oncol Biol Phys* 1991; **20**: 489–93.

26 Bomanji J, Britton KE, Ur E, Hawkins L, Grossman AB, Besser GM. Treatment of malignant phaeochromocytoma, paraganglioma and carcinoid tumours with ^{131}I-metaiodobenzyl-guanidine. *Nucl Med Commun* 1993; **14**: 856–61.

27 Kvols LK, Buch M. Chemotherapy of metastatic carcinoid and islet cell tumours; a review. *Am J Med* 1987; **82** (Suppl. 5B): 77–83.

28 Öberg K. Endocrine tumors of the gastrointestinal tract: systemic treatment. *Anti-Cancer Drugs* 1994; **5**: 503–19.

29 Reisine T, Bell GJ. Molecular biology of somatostatin receptors. *Endocr Rev* 1995; **16**: 427–42.

30 Haris A-G, Redfam JS. Octreotide treatment of carcinoid syndrome: analysis of published dose titration data. *Aliment Pharmacol Ther* 1995; **9**: 387–94.

31 Öberg K, Norheim I, Lind E *et al.* Treatment of malignant carcinoid tumours with human leukocyte interferon. Long-term results. *Cancer Treat Rep* 1986; **70**: 1297–304.

32 Tiensuu Janson E, Ahlström H, Andersson T, Öberg K. Octreotide and interferon alfa: a new combination for the treatment of malignant carcinoid tumours. *Eur J Cancer* 1992; **28A**: 1647–50.

33 Moertel CG, Sauer WG, Dockerty MB, Baggentoss AM. Life history of the carcinoid tumour of the small intestine. *Cancer* 1961; **14**: 901–12.

34 Tiensuu Janson E. *Carcinoid tumors: clinical aspects and the use of somatostatin analogues for characterization and treatment.* Thesis, Uppsala University, 1995.

35 Chandiasckharappa SC, Guth SC, Manichan P *et al.* Positional cloning of the gene for multiple endocrine neoplasia-type 1. *Science* 1997; **276**: 404–6.

36 Goldstone NP, Scott-Coombes DM, Lynn JA. Surgical management of gastrointestinal endocrine tumours. In: O'Shea D, Bloom SR eds. *Ballière's Clinical Gastroenterology* Vol 10; 1994: 707–36.

37 Krenning EP, Kooij PPM, Pawels S *et al.* Somatostatin receptor: scintigraphy and radionucleotide therapy: Digestion 1996 (suppl. 1): 57–61.

38 Eriksson B, Janson ET, Bax ND *et al.* The use of new somatostatin analogues, lanreotide and octastatin in newoendocrine gastro-intestinal tumours. *Digestion* 1966; **57** (suppl. 1): 77–80.

CHAPTER 46

Multiple endocrine neoplasia type 1

R.V. Thakker

Introduction

Multiple endocrine neoplasia [1,2] is characterised by the occurrence of tumours involving two or more endocrine glands within a single patient. The disorder has previously been referred to as multiple endocrine adenopathy (MEA) or the pluriglandular syndrome. However, glandular hyperplasia and malignancy may also occur in some patients and the term multiple endocrine neoplasia (MEN) is now preferred. There are two major forms of MEN referred to as type 1 and type 2, and each form is characterised by the development of tumours within specific endocrine glands (Table 46.1). Thus, the combined occurrence of tumours of the parathyroid glands, the pancreatic islet cells and the anterior pituitary is characteristic of MEN-1, which is also referred to as Wermer's syndrome. In addition to these tumours, adrenal cortical, carcinoid and lipomatous tumours have also been described in patients with MEN-1. However, in MEN-2, which is also called Sipple's syndrome, medullary thyroid carcinoma (MTC) occurs in association with phaeochromocytoma, and three clinical variants referred to as MEN-2A, MEN-2B and MTC-only are recognised. In MEN-2A, which is the most common variant, the development of MTC is associated with phaeochromocytoma and parathyroid tumours. However, in MEN-2B parathyroid involvement is absent and the occurrence of MTC and phaeochromocytoma is found in association with a marfanoid habitus, mucosal neuromas, medullated corneal fibres and intestinal autonomic ganglion dysfunction leading to a megacolon. In the variant of MTC only, medullary thyroid carcinoma appears to be the sole manifestation of the syndrome. Although MEN-1 and MEN-2 usually occur as distinct and separate syndromes as outlined above, some patients occasionally may develop tumours which are associated with both MEN-1 and MEN-2. For example, patients suffering from islet-cell tumours of the pancreas and phaeochromocytomas, or from acromegaly and phaeochromocytoma, have been described and these patients may represent an 'overlap' syndrome. All these forms of MEN may either be inherited as autosomal dominant syndromes, or they may occur sporadically, i.e. without a family history. However, this distinction between sporadic and familial cases may sometimes be difficult as in some sporadic cases the family history may be absent because the parent with the disease may have died before developing symptoms. In this chapter, the main clinical and biochemical features of MEN-1 and its pathogenesis will be discussed. MEN-2 is discussed in Chapter 47.

Clinical findings, biochemical abnormalities and treatment

The incidence of MEN-1 has been estimated from randomly chosen autopsy studies to be 0.25%, and to be 18% amongst patients with primary hyperparathyroidism. The disorder affects all age groups, with a reported age range of 5–81 years, and 80% of patients have developed clinical manifestations of the disorder by the fifth decade. The clinical manifestations of MEN-1 are related to the sites of tumours and to their products of secretion. In addition to the triad of parathyroid, pancreatic and pituitary tumours, which constitute the major components of MEN-1, adrenal cortical, carcinoid and lipomatous tumours have also been described.

Parathyroid tumours

Primary hyperparathyroidism is the most common feature of MEN-1 and occurs in more than 95% of all MEN-1 patients [2,3]. Patients may present with asymptomatic hypercalcaemia, nephrolithiasis, osteitis fibrosa cystica, or vague symptoms associated with hypercalcaemia, for example polyuria, polydipsia, constipation, malaise or

Table 46.1 The major forms of multiple endocrine neoplasia (MEN).

Type	Tumour sites	Inheritance
MEN-1	Parathyroid Pancreatic islets Pituitary (anterior) (Associated tumours of: adrenal cortex carcinoids lipoma)	Autosomal dominant
MEN-2A	Thyroid C cells Adrenal medulla Parathyroids	Autosomal dominant
MEN-2B	Thyroid C cells Adrenal medulla (Associated abnormalities: Mucosal neuromas Marfanoid habitus Medullated corneal nerve fibres Megacolon)	Autosomal dominant
Overlap syndrome	Pancreatic islets + Adrenal medulla or Pituitary (anterior) + Adrenal medulla	Autosomal dominant

occasionally with peptic ulcers. Biochemical investigations reveal hypercalcaemia usually in association with raised circulating parathyroid hormone (PTH) concentrations. No effective medical treatment for primary hyperparathyroidism is generally available, and surgical removal of the abnormally overactive parathyroids is the definitive treatment. However, all four parathyroid glands are usually affected with multiple adenomas or hyperplasia, although this histological distinction may be difficult, and parathyroidectomy for primary hyperparathyroidism in patients with MEN-1 has been associated with a high failure rate. Subtotal parathyroidectomy has resulted in persistent or recurrent hypercalcaemia in 50% of patients and in hypocalcaemia, which required long-term therapy with vitamin D or its active metabolite calcitriol, in 10% of patients with MEN-1 [4]. These rates are markedly higher than those observed for parathyroidectomies in patients who do not have MEN-1, in whom recurrent hypercalcaemia occurs in 4–16% and hypocalcaemia in 1–8% of patients. In order to avoid neck re-exploration, which is difficult, and to improve the treatment of primary hyperparathyroidism in patients with MEN-1, total parathyroidectomy with autotransplantation of parathyroid tissue in the forearm has been performed [5,6,7]. Both fresh and cryopreserved parathyroid tissue have been used for autotranplantation. The use of cryopreserved parathyroid tissue allows the confirmation of hypoparathyroidism in the patient prior to autotransplantation, but unfortunately only 50% of parathyroid grafts survive cryopreservation. The use of fresh parathyroid tissue for autotransplantation in the forearm results in viable grafts which secrete parathyroid hormone. However, the presence of functioning autotransplanted parathyroid tissue leads to recurrent hypercalcaemia in more than 50% of patients with MEN-1, and surgical removal of transplanted grafts has been required. Thus, the management of primary hyperparathyroidism in patients with MEN-1 is difficult; parathyroid surgery in these patients is associated with a higher prevalence of persistent or recurrent hypercalcaemia. Total parathyroidectomy, which would prevent this, has therefore been proposed as the definitive treatment for primary hyperparathyroidism in MEN-1, with the resultant life-long hypocalcaemia being treated with oral calcitriol (1,25-dihydroxyvitamin D_3). It is recommended that such total parathyroidectomy should be reserved for the symptomatic hypercalcaemic patient with MEN-1, and that the asymptomatic hypercalcaemia MEN-1 patient should not have parathyroid surgery but have regular assessments for the onset of symptoms and complications, when total parathyroidectomy should be undertaken.

Pancreatic tumours (see also Chapter 40)

The incidence of pancreatic islet-cell tumours in MEN-1 patients varies from 30 to 80% in different series [1,2]. The majority of these tumours produce excessive amounts of hormone, for example gastrin, insulin, glucagon or vasoactive intestinal polypeptide (VIP), and are associated with distinct clinical syndromes.

Gastrinomas

These gastrin-secreting tumours represent over 50% of all pancreatic islet-cell tumours in MEN-1, and are the major cause of morbidity and mortality in MEN-1 patients. This is due to the recurrent severe multiple peptic ulcers which may perforate. This association of recurrent peptic ulceration, marked gastric acid production and non-β-islet-cell tumours of the pancreas is referred to as the Zollinger–Ellison syndrome. Additional prominent clinical features of this syndrome include diarrhoea and steatorrhoea.

The diagnosis is established by demonstration of a raised fasting serum gastrin concentration in association with an increased basal gastric acid secretion [8]. Occasionally, intravenous provocative tests with either secretin (2 U/kg) or calcium infusion (4 mg Ca^{2+}/kg/hour for 3 hours) are required to distinguish patients with Zollinger–Ellison syndrome from other patients with hypergastrinaemia, as, for example, in antral G-cell hyperplasia. However, in patients with MEN-1, the Zollinger–Ellison syndrome does not appear to occur in the absence of primary hyperparathyroidism, and hypergastrinaemia has also been reported to be associated with hypercalcaemia. Thus, the diagnosis of Zollinger–Ellison syndrome may be difficult in some MEN-1 patients.

Medical treatment of MEN-1 patients with the Zollinger–Ellison syndrome is directed towards reducing basal acid output to <10 mmol/l, and this may be achieved by large doses of the histamine H_2-receptor antagonists cimetidine and ranitidine. More recently, the parietal cell H^+/K^+ adenosine triphosphatase (ATPase) inhibitor, omeprazole, has proved efficacious, and has become the drug of choice for gastrinomas. Surgical treatment with total gastrectomy is recommended only for persistently non-compliant patients. The ideal treatment for a non-metastastic gastrinoma is surgical exision of the gastrinoma. However, in patients with MEN-1 the gastrinomas are frequently multiple or extrapancreatic and surgery has not been successful [9,10]. The use of transhepatic selective venous gastrin sampling to preoperatively localise the gastrinomas in MEN-1 patients has been reported to improve the surgical outcome [11]; venous sampling in this study revealed that the MEN-1 patients with Zollinger–Ellison syndrome had either diffuse gastrin secretion from multiple pancreatic sites or localised gastrin secretion from a single region. The patients in whom gastrin secretion was localised benefited from resection of the gastrinoma by partial pancreatectomy, and required no drug therapy postoperatively. Other tumour-localisation studies using ultrasonography, computed tomography (CT), magnetic resonance imaging (MRI), selective abdominal angiography or venous sampling have demonstrated that these techniques are not often useful and do not improve the surgical success rate [12]. The treatment of disseminated gastrinomas is difficult and chemotherapy with streptozotocin and 5-fluorouracil, hormonal therapy with octreotide, hepatic artery embolisation, administration of human leucocyte interferon, and removal of all resectable tumour have all occasionally been successful.

Insulinoma

These β-islet-cell tumours secreting insulin represent one-third of all pancreatic tumours in MEN-1 patients [1,2]. Insulinomas also occur in association with gastrinomas in 10% of MEN-1 patients, and the two tumours may arise at different times. Patients with an insulinoma present with hypoglycaemic symptoms which develop after a fast or exertion and improve after glucose intake. Biochemical investigations reveal raised plasma insulin concentrations in association with hypoglycaemia. Circulating concentrations of C-peptide and proinsulin, which are also raised, may be useful in establishing the diagnosis, as may an insulin suppression test. Medical treatment, which consists of frequent carbohydrate feeds and diazoxide, is not always successful, and surgery may be required. Most insulinomas are multiple and small, and preoperative localisation with CT scanning, coeliac axis angiography and pre-/perioperative percutaneous transhepatic portal venous sampling is difficult and success rates have varied. Surgical treatment, which ranges from enucleation of a single tumour to a distal pancreatectomy or partial pancreatectomy, has been curative in some patients. Chemotherapy, usually streptozotocin or octreotide, is used for metastatic disease.

Glucagonoma

These α-islet-cell, glucagon-secreting pancreatic tumours have been reported in only five MEN-1 patients [1,2]. The characteristic clinical manifestations of a skin rash (necrolytic migratory erythema), weight loss, anaemia and stomatitis may be absent, and the presence of the tumour is indicated only by glucose intolerance and hyperglucagonaemia. The tail of the pancreas is the most frequent site for glucagonomoas; surgical removal of these is the treatment of choice. However, treatment may be difficult as 50% of patients have metastases at the time of diagnosis. Medical treatment of these with octreotide, or with streptozotocin or dimethyltriazenolmidazole carboxamide (DTC), has been successful in some patients.

VIPoma

Patients with VIPomas, which are VIP-secreting pancreatic tumours, develop watery diarrhoea, hypokalaemia and achlorhydria (the WDHA syndrome). This clinical syndrome has also been referred to as the Verner–Morrison syndrome or the VIPoma syndrome. VIPomas have been reported in only a few MEN-1 patients and the diagnosis is established by documenting a markedly raised plasma VIP concentration. Surgical management of VIPomas, which are mostly located in the tail of the pancreas, has been curative. However, in patients with unresectable tumour treatment with streptozotocin, octreotide, corticosteroids, indomethacin, metoclopramide and lithium carbonate has proved beneficial.

PPoma

These tumours, which secrete pancreatic polypeptide (PP), are found in a large number of patients with MEN-1. No pathological sequelae of excessive PP secretion are apparent and the clinical significance of PP is unknown, although the use of serum PP measurements has been suggested for the detection of pancreatic tumours in MEN-1 patients.

Pituitary tumours

The incidence of pituitary tumours in MEN-1 patients varies from 15 to 90% in different series [1,2]. Approximately 60% of MEN-1-associated pituitary tumours secrete prolactin, 25% secrete growth hormone (GH), 3% secrete adrenocorticotrophic hormone (ACTH) while the remainder appear to be non-functioning. The clinical manifestations depend upon the size of the pituitary tumour and its product of secretion. Enlarging pituitary tumours may compress adjacent structures such as the optic chiasm or normal pituitary tissue and cause bitemporal hemianopia or hypopituitarism, respectively. The tumour size and extension are radiologically assessed by CT scanning and MRI imaging. Treatment of pituitary tumours in MEN-1 patients is similar to that in non-MEN-1 patients and consists of medical therapy or selective hypophysectomy by the transsphenoidal approach if feasible, with radiotherapy being reserved for residual unresectable tumour.

Associated tumours

Patients with MEN-1 may have tumours involving glands other than the parathyroids, pancreas and pituitary [13]. Thus, carcinoid, adrenal cortical, thyroid and lipomatous tumours have all been described in association with MEN-1.

Carcinoid tumours, which occur more frequently in patients with MEN-1, may be inherited as an autosomal dominant trait in association with MEN-1. The carcinoid tumour may be located in the bronchi, the gastrointestinal tract, the pancreas or the thymus. Most patients are asymptomatic and do not suffer from the flushing attacks and dyspnoea associated with the carcinoid syndrome, which usually only develops after the tumour has metastasised to the liver.

The incidence of asymptomatic *adrenal cortical tumours* in MEN-1 patients has been reported to be as high as 40%. The majority of these tumours are non-functioning. However, functioning adrenal cortical tumours in MEN-1 patients have been documented to cause hypercortisolaemia and Cushing's syndrome, as well as primary hyperaldosteronism as in Conn's syndrome.

Thyroid tumours, consisting of adenomas, colloid goitres and carcinomas, have been reported to occur in over 25% of MEN-1 patients. However, the prevalence of thyroid disorders in the general population is high, and it has been suggested that the association of thyroid abnormalities in MEN-1 patients may be incidental and not significant.

Molecular genetics

Models of tumour development
(see also Chapter 73)

The development of tumours may be associated with mutations or inappropriate expression of specific normal cellular genes, which are referred to as *oncogenes* (reviewed in [1,2]). Two types of oncogenes referred to as *dominant* and *recessive* oncogenes have been described. An activation of dominant oncogenes leads to transformation of the cells containing them, and the genetic changes which cause this activation have recently been elucidated. For example, chromosomal translocations affecting such dominant oncogenes are associated with the occurrence of chronic myeloid leukaemia and Burkitt's lymphoma. In these conditions, the mutations which lead to activation of the oncogene are dominant at the cellular level, and therefore only one copy of the mutated gene is required for the phenotypic effect. Such dominantly acting oncogenes may be assayed in cell culture by first transferring them into recipient cells and then scoring the numbers of transformed colonies, and this is referred to as the *transfection assay*. However, in some inherited neoplasms which may also arise sporadically, such as retinoblastoma, tumour development is associated with two recessive mutations which inactivate oncogenes, and these are referred to as recessive oncogenes. In the inherited tumours, the first of the two recessive mutations is inherited via the germ-cell line and is present in all the cells. This recessive mutation is not expressed until a second mutation, within a somatic cell, causes loss of the normal dominant allele (Fig. 46.1). The mutations causing the inherited and sporadic tumours are similar but the cell types in which they occur are different. In the inherited tumours the first mutation occurs in the germ cell, whereas in the sporadic tumours both mutations occur in the somatic cell. Thus, the risk of tumour development in an individual who has not inherited the first germ-line mutation is much smaller, as both mutational events must coincide in the same somatic cell. In addition, the apparent paradox that the inherited cancer syndromes are due to recessive mutations but dominantly inherited at the level of the family is explained because, in individuals who have inherited the first recessive mutation, a loss of a single remaining wild-type allele is almost certain to occur in at least one of the large number of cells in the target tissue. This cell will be detected because it forms a tumour, and almost all individuals who have inherited the germ-line mutation will express the disease, even though they inherited a single copy of the recessive gene. This model involving two (or more) mutations in the development of tumours is known as the 'two-hit' hypothesis. The normal function of these recessive oncogenes

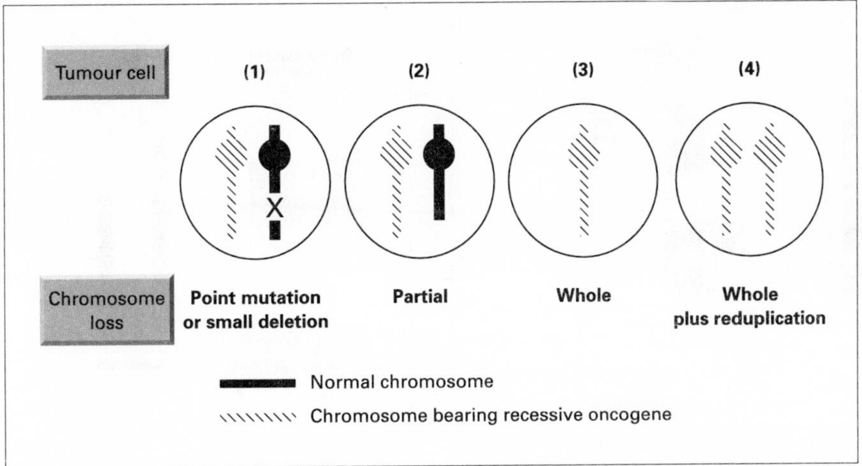

Fig. 46.1 Chromosomal mechanisms involved in the 'second hit' of Knudson's hypothesis. A pair of chromosomes, one normal and the other bearing the recessive oncogene, are schematically represented in each of four tumour cells (1–4). Four main forms of the 'second hit' involving the normal chromosome, i.e. the normal dominant allele, are shown. In tumour cell (1), there has been a point mutation or a small deletion, whereas in tumour cells (2) and (3), partial and complete losses of the normal chromosomes have respectively occurred. A complete loss of a chromosome, resulting in autosomal monosomy, may be disadvantageous to cell growth, and reduplication of the chromosome bearing the recessive oncogene may occur, as shown in tumour cell (4). These 'second hits' involving the normal dominant allele would lead to an unmasking of the recessive oncogenic mutation and thereby result in tumour development. From [14] with permission.

appears to be in regulating cell growth and differentiation, and these genes have also been referred to as *anti-oncogenes* or *tumour-suppressor genes*. An important feature which has facilitated the investigation of these genetic abnormalities associated with tumour development is that the loss of the remaining allele, which occurs in the somatic cell and gives rise to the tumour, often involves a large-scale loss of chromosomal material (Fig. 46.1). This represents a much larger target than the inherited mutation, which may be a small deletion or point mutation, in the search for the genetic loci involved in the development of different inherited tumours.

The investigation of the genetic abnormalities involved in tumour development and the search for these inherited cancer genes has become possible as a result of advances in molecular biology (reviewed in [14]) which have provided cloned human DNA sequences to detect these mutations (Fig. 46.2). These cloned DNA probes identify restriction fragment length polymorphisms (RFLPs), which are the result of variations in the primary DNA sequence of individuals and may be due to either single base changes, deletions, additions, or translocations. These changes in DNA sequence occur frequently (approximately once every 250 bp) in the non-coding regions, do not usually affect gene function, and are often at a distance away from the disease gene. These polymorphisms may, however, lead to the presence or absence of a cleavage site for a restriction enzyme, which cleaves DNA in a sequence-specific manner. The information obtained from these cloned DNA probes may sometimes be limited as many of them are often not highly polymorphic. In order to gain maximal genetic information, highly polymorphic genetic markers are required and the polymerase chain reaction (PCR) is utilised to directly detect DNA-sequence polymorphisms which are length variations in microsatellite tandem repeats, for example $(CA)_n$, where $n = 10–60$. In addition to tandem repeats in the sequence (CA), microsatellite tandem repeats consisting of $(AT)_n$, $(GA)_n$, $(ATT)_n$, $(ATTT)_n$ and the hexanucleotide $[T(Pu)T(Pu)T(Pu)]_n$ have also been reported. These tandem repeats, which are highly polymorphic and are inherited in a Mendelian manner, are estimated to occur once in every 50–100 kbp. Thus, these microsatellite polymorphisms and the PCR represent valuable techniques in obtaining a detailed genetic map around a disease locus, for example MEN-1 [14]. In this approach oligonucleotide primers are synthesised on either side of the repeat, and PCR is used to amplify the repeat sequence (Fig. 46.3). The smaller and larger fragment length polymorphisms in these repetitive sequences are detected by separation, either on a polyacrylamide sequencing gel or an agarose gel, respectively. These DNA-sequence polymorphisms, due to either RFLPs or variations in the tandem repeat of microsatellites, were used in two complementary approaches to identify the genetic abnormalities involved in the development of tumours in MEN-1. In one approach, RLFPs and microsatellite polymorphisms obtained from a patient's leucocyte DNA were compared with those obtained from tumour DNA, and differences were sought. In the second approach, these

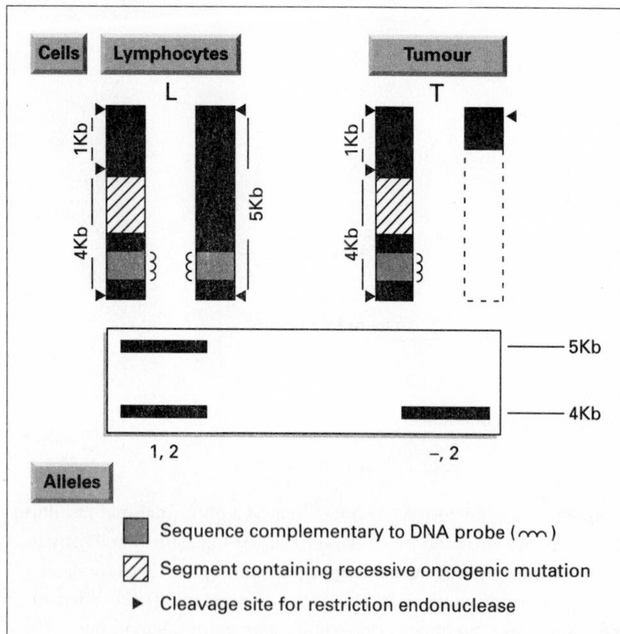

Fig. 46.2 Schematic representation of the use of restriction fragment length polymorphisms (RFLPs) to investigate the chromosomal mechanisms involved in the 'second hit'. This example is a partial loss of the normal chromosome in the tumour, i.e., tumour cell (2) in Fig. 46.1. RFLPs obtained from the leucocyte (L) and tumour (T) DNA of a patient are compared to detect deletions in the tumour tissue. The leucocytes are heterozygous (alleles 1, 2), and one of the pair of chromosomes in the leucocytes contains the segment containing the recessive oncogenic mutation, whereas the other chromosome contains the normal dominant allele. In the example illustrated, there has been a partial loss of the normal chromosome in the tumour, i.e. tumour cell (2) in Fig. 46.1, and this is detected by a loss of one of the RFLPs, which have been designated alleles. This abnormality in the tumour cells has been referred to as loss of heterozygosity, loss of alleles, or allelic deletions. From [14], with permission.

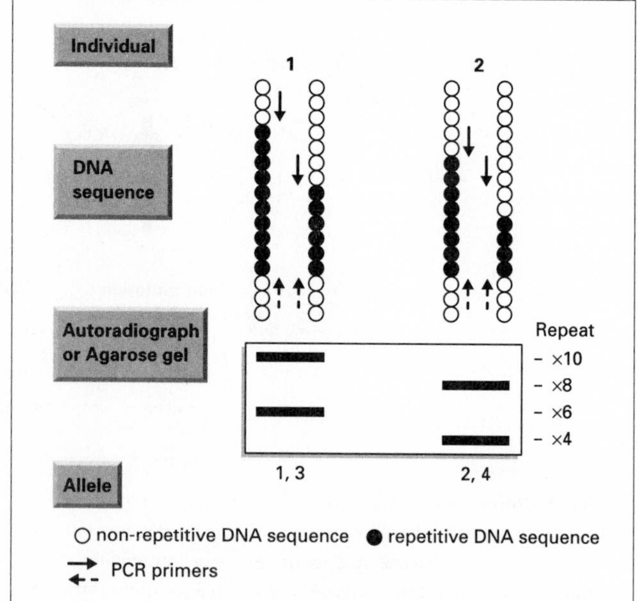

Fig. 46.3 Schematic representation of polymorphisms in microsatellite tandem repetitive DNA sequences, which may consist, for example, of the dinucleotide CA, or the trinucleotide ATT, or the tetranucleotide ATTT, or the hexanucleotide TATATG. Oligonucleotide primers corresponding to the non-repetitive sequences on either side of the repetitive DNA sequence are synthesised and the polymerase chain reaction (PCR) is utilised to amplify the repeat in genomic DNA obtained from different individuals. The resulting PCR products are separated either by polyacrylamide gel or agarose gel electrophoresis, and the polymorphisms are revealed by autoradiography or by viewing of an ethidium bromide-stained agarose gel under ultraviolet light. Thus, of the pair of chromosomes from individual (1), one has 10 repeats and the other has six repeats, whereas of the pair of chromosomes from individual (2) one has eight repeats and the other has four repeats. Following PCR amplification and separation by gel electrophoresis, these variations in the length of the repeats will be revealed by the differences in the size of the bands, which have been designated alleles; for example, the larger band consisting of 10 repeats is designated allele 1, and those consisting of 8, 6 and 4 repeats are designated alleles 2, 3 and 4, respectively. These microsatellite tandem repetitive sequences, which are highly polymorphic, show Mendelian inheritance (see Fig. 46.5) and can be used as genetic markers in multiple endocrine neoplasia type 1 families. From [14], with permission.

polymorphisms were used as genetic markers in linkage studies of affected families to localise the gene causing MEN-1.

Tumour deletion mapping studies

A two-stage genetic mutational model has been proposed for the development of tumours in MEN-1, and this is analogous to that reported for retinoblastoma. A comparison of the alleles obtained from leucocyte DNA and tumour DNA using either RFLPs or microsatellite polymorphisms can facilitate the detection of the chromosomal abnormalities associated with the 'second hit' in tumour DNA, and this is illustrated in Fig. 46.2. A restriction enzyme is used to cleave leucocyte and tumour DNA, and the resulting DNA fragments are separated according to size by agarose gel electrophoresis and transferred by Southern blotting to a nylon membrane, which is hybridised with a single-stranded radiolabelled DNA probe. The labelled DNA probe will anneal to any fragments which have a complementary sequence, and these restricted fragments of varying lengths (RFLPs) are revealed by autoradiography. The exact number and size of RFLPs will vary in relation to the number of recognition sites for the restriction enzyme, as shown in Fig. 46.2. In this example, the two chromosomes from the leucocytes differ in the number of restriction enzyme cleavage sites; one chromosome has three cleavage sites and the other has two cleavage sites. Following digestion and hybridisation, two fragments will be revealed at autoradiography. The chromosome bearing the recessive oncogenic mutation has three cleavage sites, and although two fragments of 4 kb and 1 kb will result from the enzymatic cleavage, only the 4 kb fragment will be visualised at autoradiography as it contains the complementary sequence to the radiolabelled DNA probe. However, the normal chromosome, i.e. the one not containing the recessive oncogenic mutation, has a loss of one restriction enzyme cleavage site, due to a change in the DNA sequence, and following digestion only restriction fragments of 5 kb in size will result. A single 5-kb RFLP is observed at autoradiography. Alleles can be designated to these RFLPs; for example, the larger, 5-kb RFLP is designated allele 1 and the smaller, 4-kb RFLP is designated allele 2. Thus, the leucocytes in this example are heterozygous (alleles 1, 2) and the chromosome bearing the recessive oncogenic mutation has allele 2, whilst the normal chromosome with the dominant allele has allele 1. A partial loss of the normal chromosome, i.e, the 'second hit' (Fig. 46.1), associated with the development of the tumour, would be detected by the loss of the 5-kb RFLP (allele 1). Thus, the tumour cells would be hemizygous (allele –, 2) as illustrated in Fig. 46.2, or they may be homozygous (allele 2, 2) if a reduplication of the chromosome bearing the recessive oncogenic mutation had occurred (Fig. 46.1). This type of analysis, involving paired leucocyte and tumour DNA, which has been referred to as the detection of a loss of alleles, allelic deletions, or a loss of heterozygosity in tumours, has been used in localising the tumour suppressor gene causing MEN-1. Microsatellite polymorphisms can also be used in a similar way to detect loss of heterozygosity in tumour DNA, and this is illustrated in Fig. 46.4. A loss of alleles involving the whole of chromosome 11 is observed in the parathyroid tumour of a patient with familial MEN-1. This loss of alleles in the tumour results from the loss of chromosomal regions containing the marker loci; the complete absence of alleles suggests that this abnormality has occurred within all the tumour cells studied and indicates a monoclonal origin of the tumour. In addition, combined pedigree and tumour studies have demonstrated that such tumour-related allelic deletions of chromosome 11 occur on the chromosome inherited from the normal parent and not the one from the affected parent [15,16]. Thus, the second mutation involves the normal dominant allele, and these studies provided additional evidence for the proposed two-stage recessive mutation model for the development of tumours in MEN-1.

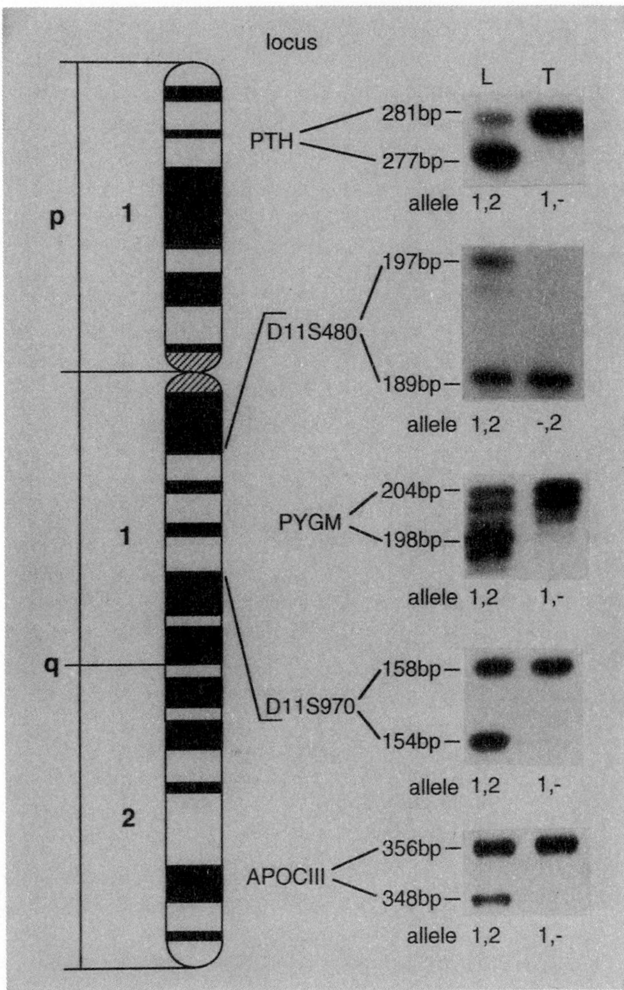

Fig. 46.4 Loss of alleles on chromosome 11 in a parathyroid tumour from a patient with familial multiple endocrine neoplasia type 1 (MEN-1). The microsatellite polymorphisms obtained from the patient's leucocyte (L) and parathyroid tumour (T) DNA at the PTH, D11S480, PYGM, D11S970 and APOCIII loci are shown. These microsatellite polymorphisms have been identified using specific primers or sequence tagged sites (STSs) for each of the loci which have been localised to chromosome 11, and are shown juxtaposed to their region of origin on the short (p) and long (q) arms of chromosome 11. The microsatellite polymorphisms are assigned alleles (see Fig. 46.3). For example, D11S480 yielded a 197-bp product (allele 1) and a 189-bp product (allele 2) following PCR amplification of leucocyte DNA, but the tumour cells have lost the 197-bp product (allele 1) and are hemizygous (alleles –, 2). Similar losses of alleles are detected using the other DNA markers, and an extensive loss of alleles involving the whole of chromosome 11 is observed in the parathyroid tumour of this patient with MEN-1. In addition, the complete absence of bands suggests that this abnormality has occurred within all the tumour cells studied, and indicates a monoclonal origin for this MEN-1 parathyroid tumour. From [17], with permission.

Studies of MEN-1 and non-MEN-1 parathyroid tumours, insulinomas and anterior pituitary tumours have revealed that allelic deletions on chromosome 11 are also involved in the monoclonal development of these tumours. A detailed examination of such tumours has revealed allele loss within tumours involving smaller regions of chromosome 11, and these studies have mapped the MEN-1 locus to the region within chromosome band 11q13 (reviewed in [2]). These results indicate that the *MEN1* gene is telomeric to the PYGM locus, which encodes human muscle glycogen phosphorylase, and centromeric to the locus D11S146 [18]. In addition, these studies have demonstrated that allelic deletions of chromosome 11 are involved in the development of sporadic non-MEN-1 parathyroid tumours, gastrinomas, prolactinomas and somatotrophinomas, and thus the region 11q13 appears to be involved in the development of non-MEN-1 and MEN-1 endocrine tumours [18,19].

Family linkage studies

In order to localise the gene causing MEN-1, family linkage studies were used as a parallel and complementary approach to the deletion mapping studies. This investigation of the tumour suppressor gene involved in the MEN-1 syndrome was facilitated by the use of RFLPs and microsatellite polymorphisms as genetic markers in studies of affected families. These polymorphisms are inherited in a Mendelian manner and their inheritance can be followed together with a disease in an affected family. The consistent inheritance of a polymorphic allele with the disease indicates that the

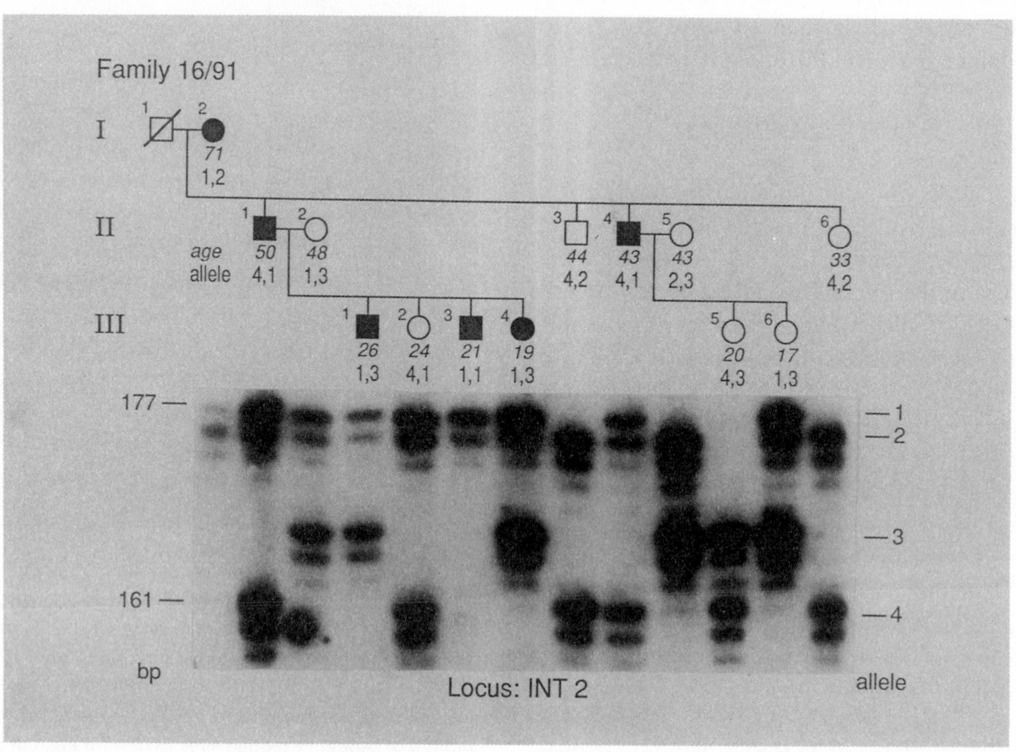

Fig. 46.5 Segregation of INT-2 and multiple endocrine neoplasia type 1 (MEN-1) in family 16/91. Genomic DNA from the family members (upper panel) was used with γ^{32} P adenosine triphosphate (ATP) for polymerase chain reaction (PCR) amplification of the polymorphic repetitive element $(TG)_n$ at this locus. The PCR amplification products were detected by autoradiography on a polyacrylamide gel (lower panel). PCR products were detected from the DNA of each individual; these ranged in size from 161 to 177 bp. Alleles were designated for each PCR product and are indicated on the right. For example, individuals II.1 and II.4 reveal two pairs of bands on autoradiography. The upper pair of bands is designated allele 1 and the lower pair of bands is designated allele 4; and these two individuals are therefore heterozygous (alleles 1, 4). A pair of bands for each allele is frequently observed in the PCR detection of microsatellite repeats. The upper band in the pair is the 'true' allele and the lower band in the pair is its associated 'shadow' which results from slipped-strand mispairing during the PCR. The segregation of these bands and their respective alleles together with the disease can be studied in the family members whose alleles and ages are shown. In some individuals, the inheritance of paternal and maternal alleles can be ascertained; the paternal allele is shown on the left. Individuals are represented as unaffected male (□), affected male (■), unaffected female (○), and affected female (●). The MEN-1 phenotypes in this family were determined by biochemical screening and the age-related penetrance values derived from Fig. 46.5 were used in linkage analysis, as described in the text. Individual II.1 is affected and heterozygous (alleles 4, 1) and an examination of his affected children (III.1, III.3 and III.4) and his mother (I.2) and sibling (II.4) reveals inheritance of allele 1 with the disease. The unaffected individuals II.3, II.6, III.2 and III.5 have not inherited this allele 1. However, the daughter (III.6) of individual II.4 has inherited allele 1, but remains unaffected at the age of 17 years; this may either be a representation of age-related penetrance, or a recombination between the disease and INT-2 loci. From [24], with permission.

two genetic loci are close together, i.e. *linked*. Genes that are far apart do not consistently cosegregate but show recombination because of the crossing-over during meiosis. By studying recombination events in family studies, the distance between two genes and the probability that they are linked can be ascertained [1]. The distance between two genes is expressed as the *recombination fraction* (θ), which is equal to the number of recombinants divided by the total number of offspring resulting from informative meioses within a family. The value of the recombination fraction (θ) can range from 0 to 0.5. A value of zero indicates that the genes are very closely linked, while a value of 0.5 indicates that the genes are far apart and not linked. The probability that the two loci are linked at these distances is expressed as a 'LOD score', which is $\log_{10}$ of the odds ratio favouring linkage. The odds ratio favouring linkage is defined as the likelihood that two loci are linked at a specified recombination (θ) versus the likelihood that the two loci are not linked. A LOD score of +3, which indicates a probability in favour of linkage of 1000 : 1, establishes linkage between two loci, and a LOD score of –2, indicating a probability against linkage of 100 : 1, is taken to exclude linkage between two loci. LOD scores are usually evaluated over a range of recombination fractions (θ), thereby enabling the genetic distance and the maximum (or peak) probability favouring linkage between two loci to be ascertained. This is illustrated in Fig. 46.5 for family 16/91 which suffers from MEN-1.

In family 16/91, shown in Fig. 46.5, the disease and INT-2 loci are cosegregating in nine out of the 10 children, but in one individual (III.6), assuming a 100% penetrance (see below) in early childhood, recombination is observed. Thus, MEN-1 and INT-2 are cosegregating in 9/10 of the meioses and not segregating in 1/10 meioses, and the likelihood that the two loci are *linked* at (θ) = 0.10 is $(9/10)^9 \times (1/10)^1$. If the disease and the INT-2 loci were not linked, then the disease would be associated with allele 1 in one-half (1/2) of the children and with allele 2 in the remaining half (1/2) of the children, and the likelihood that the two loci are *not linked* is $(1/2)^{10}$. Thus, the odds ratio in favour of linkage between the MEN-1 and INT-2 loci at θ = 0.10, in this family, is therefore $(9/10)^9 \times (1/10)^1 \div (1/2)^{10} = 39.67 : 1$, and the LOD score = 1.60 (i.e. $\log_{10}$ 39.67). Additional studies from other families have also demonstrated positive LOD scores between MEN-1 and the INT-2 locus. LOD scores from individual families can be summated, and the peak LOD score between MEN-1 and the INT-2 locus has exceeded +3, thereby establishing linkage between MEN-1 and INT-2 loci.

This segregation analysis relies on an accurate assignment of the MEN-1 phenotype (i.e. affected or unaffected) and this depends on the methods used to detect MEN-1 and the age of the individual (Fig. 46.6). The age-related onset, which helps in the estimation of the penetrance of MEN-1 and is detailed below in screening studies, was used in the phenotypic assessment of individuals in MEN-1 families, and linkage was established (i.e. LOD score > +3) between MEN-1 and the 11q13 loci, PYGM and INT-2 [15,16]. Recombinants between INT-2 and MEN-1 have been observed, and this indicates that the oncogene INT-2 is not the MEN-1 gene itself. No recombinants between MEN-1 and PYGM have been observed in affected individuals from studies of 33 families with MEN-1 [20,21]. The genetic map of this region (11q13) has been defined with polymorphic markers to be 11cen-PGA-PYGM-D11S97-D11S146-INT-2-11qter, and linkage between MEN-1 and these markers has been established (Table 46.2). In addition, the MEN-1

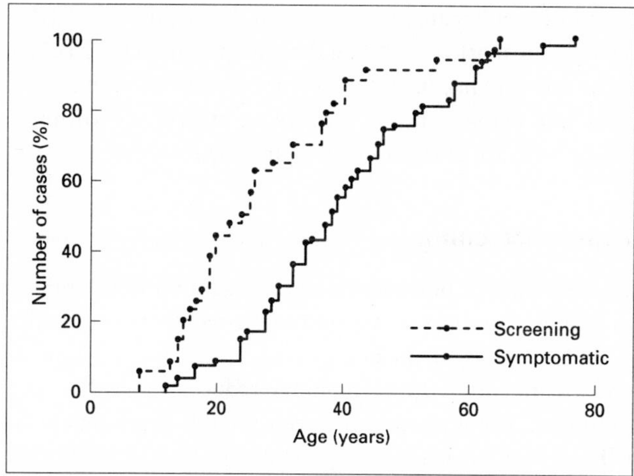

Fig. 46.6 Age-related onset of familial multiple neoplasia type 1 (MEN-1). The ages for diagnosis in 87 patients with familial MEN-1 were found to range from 8 to 76 years. The patients were subdivided, depending on the method used to detect MEN-1, into two groups. The symptomatic group consisted of 53 patients and the age-related onset for MEN-1 in these members at 20, 35 and 50 years of age was 9%, 43% and 75%, respectively. In another 34 asymptomatic patients, MEN-1 had been detected by biochemical screening and the respective age-related onset for MEN-1 in these members increased to 44%, 74% and 91%. Thus, biochemical screening detected an earlier onset of MEN-1 in all age groups. From [14], with permission.

Table 46.2 LOD scores for linkage of chromosome 11 markers and multiple endocrine neoplasia type 1. From [21], with permission.

Locus	Peak LOD score	Recombination fraction (θ)
PGA	7.78	0.023
PYGM	13.71	0.047
D11S97	13.76	0.076
D11S146	8.27	0.000
INT-2	7.04	0.059

gene has been located to a region in the vicinity of PYGM. The genetic markers defining the region around the MEN-1 locus are proving useful in further studies of cloning the gene (see below) and in identifying individuals within a family who are at risk of developing the disorder.

Family screening

The detection by biochemical screening for the development of MEN-1 tumours in asymptomatic members of families with MEN-1 is of great importance, as earlier diagnosis and treatment of these tumours reduces morbidity and mortality. The attempts to screen for the development of MEN-1 tumours in the asymptomatic relatives of an affected individual have depended largely on measuring the serum concentrations of calcium, gastrointestinal hormones and prolactin (reviewed in [2]). Parathyroid overactivity causing hypercalcaemia is invariably the first manifestation of the disorder [22] and this has become a useful and easy screening investigation. Pancreatic involvement in asymptomatic individuals has previously been detected by estimating the fasting plasma concentrations of gastrin and PP. However, one recent study has reported that a stimulatory meal test is a better method for detecting pancreatic disease in individuals who have no demonstrable pancreatic tumours by CT scanning. An exaggerated increase in serum gastrin and/or PP proved to be a reliable early indicator for the development of pancreatic tumours in these individuals [23]. Some asymptomatic pituitary tumours may be detected by the demonstration of hyperprolactinaemia.

Screening in MEN-1 is difficult because the clinical and biochemical manifestations in members of any one family are not uniformly similar, and because the age-related penetrance (i.e. the proportion of gene carriers manifesting symptoms or signs of the disease by a given age) has not been established. The proportion of affected individuals who have been detected at a certain age by clinical symptoms or biochemical screening in different series has ranged from 11 to 47% at 20 years of age, 52 to 94% at 35 years and 83 to 100% at 50 years; biochemical screening, which detects asymptomatic patients, increased the proportion of affected individuals at all ages [2]. Thus, the likelihood of wrongly

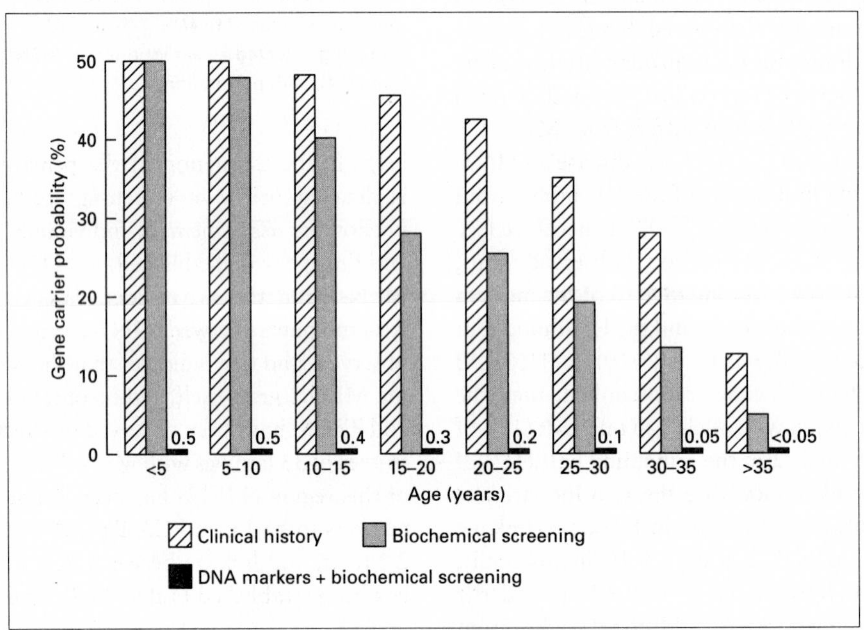

Fig. 46.7 Probabilities for gene carriers of multiple endocrine neoplasia type 1 (MEN-1). The probabilities (shown as per cent) for a child of an affected MEN-1 parent being a gene carrier following negative screening results using clinical history, biochemical screening, i.e. serum calcium, prolactin and gastrointestinal hormone concentrations, and/or DNA marker studies (Fig. 46.5) are shown for eight age groups. The risk, assessed clinically at birth, of having inherited this autosomal dominant disorder is 50%, and biochemical estimations are not useful in reducing this risk factor. In contrast, DNA marker studies using flanking DNA probes can markedly reduce the risk of being a carrier to 0.5%. With increasing age, the clinically assessed risk for the unaffected child of an affected parent declines gradually from 50% to only 28% at the age of 35 years. However, the risk as assessed by biochemical tests declines more rapidly from 50% at birth to 25% by age 25 years, and to 12.5% by age 35 years. These risks can be further decreased by the combined use of flanking DNA markers and the significantly lower 0.5% risk of being a gene carrier at birth is reduced to 0.05% at the age of 35 years. Thus, the use of DNA markers can help considerably in reassuring those individuals who are not gene carriers for MEN-1 and in identifying those individuals who are *MEN-1* gene carriers and who therefore require regular screening. From [2], with permission.

attributing an 'unaffected' status to an individual with no manifestations of the disease at the age of 35 years may be as high as 1 in 2, or as low as 1 in 20, and depends on whether clinical symptoms alone or biochemical screening methods are used to detect the disease. In order to improve this situation, further biochemical screening and systematic family studies have been undertaken. Results from two studies in which 87 patients with familial MEN-1 were investigated are shown in Fig. 46.6. This reveals that the age-related onset for MEN-1 detected by clinical manifestations (symptomatic group), at 20, 35 and 50 years of age is 9, 43 and 75% respectively. The respective age-related onset for MEN-1 detected by biochemical screening is markedly improved to 44, 74 and 91%. However, the identification of individuals at risk in an affected family can still be difficult (Fig. 46.7), although the recent availability of DNA markers for MEN-1, together with the identification of the *MEN-1* gene itself (see below), has helped to reduce these problems [24].

The use of DNA markers, which may enable carriers of the mutant MEN-1 gene to be detected within a family, may help to identify those individuals who need to undergo repeated screening tests for the development of tumours. This is illustrated in Fig. 46.5 for a family suffering from MEN-1. The alleles of each individual at the INT-2 locus which reveals a < 6% recombination rate with MEN-1 (Table 46.2) are shown. Individual I.2 is an affected female who is heterozygous (allele 1, 2) and is the mother of four children; her affected children, II.1 and II.4, indicate segregation of allele 1 and the disease. Her other children II.3 and II.6, who are 44 and 33 years old, respectively, are biochemically normal and this indicates that they have a low probability (5 and 13%, respectively) of being gene carriers (Fig. 46.7). In addition, the results of genetic marker analysis reveal that II.3 and II.6 have inherited allele 2 which is not associated with the disease in this family, and this indicates a low probability (< 6%) for these being gene carriers.

The use of a closer flanking marker, for example PYGM, would help to reduce this probability to < 1%, and the combined use of flanking DNA markers and biochemical screening in this age group helps to reduce further the risk for these individuals being carriers to < 0.05%. The two daughters (III.5 and III.6) of the affected male II.4 who is heterozygous (alleles 4, 1) are in a younger age group (17–20 years) and have not developed the disease. The finding of normal serum biochemistry in these individuals still indicates a residual 40% risk of their being gene carriers. However, individuals III.5 has inherited allele 4 from her affected father II.4, and this indicates a low probability (< 6%) of her being a gene carrier. The combined use of flanking DNA markers and biochemical screening in this individual, who is 20 years old, reduces this risk to 0.3%. In contrast, individual III.6 has inherited allele 1 from her affected father and is at high risk of developing the disease, as the probability of being a gene carrier exceeds 94%. The use of a closer flanking marker such as PYGM (Table 46.2) would help to confirm and increase this probability to 99.5%; this individual should undergo regular biochemical screening. Thus, the application of DNA markers has helped to determine the carrier risk status of many individuals, and this has substantially altered the screening strategy (Fig. 46.7) and clinical management of these patients. It is suggested that DNA analysis should now be introduced in the screening programme of MEN-1 families [2].

The advantages of DNA analysis are that it requires a single blood sample and does not need to be repeated, unlike the biochemical screening tests [1]. This is because the analysis is independent of the age of the individual and provides an objective result. The limitations of DNA analysis are that blood samples for DNA analysis must be available from two or more affected family members to conclude which allele of the marker is inherited with the *MEN-1* gene. In addition, DNA analysis may be subject to a small but significant error rate because of recombination between the marker and the gene. This error rate can be minimised by the use of flanking DNA markers. The recent cloning of the gene itself (see below) will help to identify mutations directly and thereby remove this limited uncertainty. At present, an integrated programme of both DNA screening, to identify gene carriers, and biochemical screening, to detect the development of tumours, is recommended [24]. Thus, a DNA test identifying an individual as a mutant gene carrier is likely to lead not to immediate medical or surgical treatment but to earlier and more frequent biochemical screening, whereas a DNA result that leaves an individual with a residual carrier risk of < 1% will lead to a decision for either infrequent or no screening.

At present it is suggested that individuals at high risk of developing MEN-1 should be screened once per annum. Screening should commence in early childhood, as the disease has developed in some individuals by the age of 8 years, and should continue for life as some individuals have not developed the disease until the eight decade. Screening history and physical examination should be directed towards eliciting the symptoms and signs of hypercalcaemia, nephrolithiasis, peptic ulcer disease, neuroglycopaenia, hypopituitarism, galactorrhoea and amenorrhoea in women, acromegaly, Cushing's disease, visual field loss and the presence of subcutaneous lipomas [1]. Biochemical screening should include serum calcium and prolactin estimations in all individuals; measurement of gastrointestinal hormones and more specific endocrine function tests should be reserved for individuals who have symptoms or signs suggestive of a clinical syndrome [1]. Thus, the recent advances in molecular biology which have enabled the localisation and identification of the gene causing MEN-1 have helped in the clinical management of patients and their families with this disorder.

Molecular genetics of non-MEN-1 parathyroid tumours

PRAD1

The molecular basis of non-MEN-1 parathyroid tumours has been investigated and a structural defect within the parathyroid hormone (PTH) gene itself identified. The human PTH gene has been localised to the short arm of chromosome 11 by using rodent–human hybrid cell lines and its nucleotide sequence determined. Further analysis of the organisation of the prepro-PTH gene revealed that it consists of three exons and two intervening sequences (introns). The first exon, at the 5′ end, encodes an untranslated regulatory domain, the second exon encodes the signal peptide and part of the 'prohormone' sequence, while the third exon encodes the remainder of the 'prohormone' sequence together with the PTH peptide and the 3′ untranslated region (reviewed in [1]). Structural abnormalities within the organisation of the PTH gene have been identified in two non-MEN-1 parathyroid adenomas [25]. These abnormalities involved a separation of the first exon from the fragment containing the second and third exons together with a rearrangement in which the PTH regulatory elements became juxta-opposed with 'new' non-PTH DNA, which was referred to as D11S287. Investigation of D11S287 localised it to the long arm of chromosome 11, band 11q13, a region which contains the *MEN1* gene. Detailed analysis revealed that D11S287 contained a sequence that was highly conserved in different species and that was expressed in normal parathyroids and in parathyroid adenomas. This expressed sequence from D11S287 was designated *PRAD1*, but further mapping studies revealed that the *PRAD1* gene was not the *MEN1* gene. However, the combination of the clonal rearrangement of one copy of the *PRAD1* gene and the altered gene expression indicated that *PRAD1* is a dominant oncogene whose activation is associated with the development of parathyroid tumours. Similar activation of cellular oncogenes through analogous rearrangements (reviewed in [1]) has been implicated in the pathogenesis of several tumours, for example Burkitt's lymphoma and chronic myeloid leukaemia. The *PRAD1* complementary DNA (cDNA) was isolated from a human placental cDNA library, and an analysis revealed that this cDNA encoded a protein of 295 amino acids which had similarities to the cyclin family of proteins [26]. Cyclins were first identified in the dividing cells of clams and sea urchins, in which they were associated with a cell cycle-regulated proteolysis in the immediate period preceding the onset of anaphase. Cyclins have also been identified in humans, in whom they also have an important role in regulating progress through the cell cycle (reviewed in [17]). Thus, *PRAD1*, which appears to encode a novel cyclin, referred to as cyclin D1 (CCND1), may also be a regulator of the cell cycle, and an overexpression of *PRAD1* may be an important event in the development of parathyroid tumours. In addition, studies of lymphomas have revealed that *PRAD1* is likely to be the B-cell lymphoma type 1 (BCL-1) oncogene and to be involved in breast carcinomas and squamous cell carcinomas of the head and neck. A further characterisation of the role of the *PRAD1* gene in regulating the cell cycle and in mitosis will help to elucidate the aetiology of these and parathyroid tumours.

Retinoblastoma gene

The proliferation of parathyroid cells in the aetiology of tumours is likely to involve regulators of the cell cycle, for example *PRAD1* [26]. Another such gene regulating the cell cycle is the retinoblastoma tumour-suppressor gene (*RB*), whose protein product normally inhibits cell growth by a possible interaction with cyclin D1, which itself is a product of the *PRAD1* gene. An analysis of the *RB* gene in parathyroid carcinomas, by examining for allelic deletions in these tumours, revealed that inactivation of the *RB* gene was common in parathyroid carcinomas [27] and that this was likely to be an important component in the progression to these malignant tumours.

Circulating growth factors in MEN-1

A factor with high parathyroid mitogenic activity has been identified in the plasma of MEN-1 patients by *in vitro* studies, which used bovine parathyroid cells maintained in a long-term culture system [28]. Plasma from MEN-1 patients stimulated these bovine parathyroid cells to rapidly incorporate ^{3}H-thymidine and to proliferate. This plasma mitogenic activity was markedly reduced by heat, acid and dithiothreitol treatment, indicating that the stimulatory properties may be due to a protein containing disulphide bonds. Gel-filtration analysis demonstrated the mitogenic activity to be within a single peak in a region between bovine serum albumin and ovalbumin, thereby indicating that the protein has a molecular weight in the range 50 000–55 000. This mitogenic factor was demonstrated to be a distinct factor from other growth factors such as epidermal growth factor (EGF), platelet-derived growth factor (PDGF), nerve growth factor (NGF), fibroblast growth factor (FGF), insulin-like growth factor 1 (IGF-1) or transforming growth factor (TGF), and was shown not to be an autocrine product from the parathyroid glands themselves. This plasma mitogenic factor appeared to be specific for parathyroid cells and did not stimulate activity in anterior pituitary or pancreatic islet cells. More recent studies [29] have revealed that a basic fibroblast growth factor (bFGF) or a closely related factor is present in the plasma of patients with MEN-1; the role of this mitogenic factor in MEN-1 patients needs to be further elucidated.

Animal model for MEN-1

An animal model for MEN-1 would greatly facilitate studies into the pathogenesis, gene expression and pharmacological therapies for this disorder. A mouse model with multiple endocrine tumours which has similarities to the human MEN-1 disorder has been described [30]. Animal models for human diseases have been produced by the introduction of cloned recombinant DNA sequences into the germ cells of mice. The inserted gene, which is stably transmitted from generation to generation, is referred to as a transgene. These advances have enabled animal models to be produced for human genetic diseases and thereby permitted further study of these disorders. For example, the introduction of a recombinant oncogene containing the insulin gene promoter into fertilised mouse eggs resulted in an inherited form of insulinoma in transgenic mice. The introduction by microinjection of a hybrid oncogene consisting of the promoter region of the bovine arginine vasopressin (AVP) gene fused to the DNA sequence coding for the large T antigen of simian virus 40 (SV40) into fertilised one-cell mouse eggs resulted in transgenic mice with anterior pituitary and pancreatic tumours [30]. The pancreatic tumours consisted of insulin-producing cells, but those of the pituitary appeared to be non-functioning. Hypercalcaemia and parathyroid tumours were not detected in preliminary studies. This intriguing transgenic mouse model may prove useful in investigating the pathogenesis of MEN-1 in humans.

Note added in proof

Identification of the *MEN-1* gene

Combined tumour deletion and family linkage studies defined the location of the MEN-1 gene to be in an interval bounded centromerically by PYGM and telomerically by D11S1783. This interval is <300 kbp in size and an investigation of genes from this region has identified the MEN-1 gene [31,32] which is referred to as *MENIN*. *MENIN* is ubiquitously expressed as a 2.9 kbp transcript [31,32] and an additional transcript of 4.2 kbp has been observed in pancreas and thymus [32]. The *MENIN* gene consists of 10 exons that encode a 610 amino-acid protein, which has no known homologies, or identifiable motifs, or nuclear localisation signal or signal peptide. Thus, the role of *MENIN* as a putative tumour suppressor gene, which usually encodes a growth factor, receptor, signal transducer, or nuclear factor, remains to be elucidated. However, inactivating *MENIN* mutations, which consist mainly of nonsense, deletional or insertional frameshift mutations, have been identified in MEN-1 families [31,32], and this is consistent with the role of *MENIN* as a tumour suppressor gene.

References

1 Thakker RV, Ponder BAJ. Multiple endocrine neoplasia. In: Sheppard MC, ed. *Clinical Endocrinology and Metabolism*, Vol. 2, No. 4. *Molecular Biology of Endocrinology*. London: Baillière Tindall, 1988: 1031–68.

2 Thakker RV. Multiple endocrine neoplasia type 1 (MEN 1). In: DeGroot LJ, Besser GK, Burger HG, Jameson JL, Loriaux DL, Marshall JC, Odell WD, Potts JT, Rubinstein AH, eds. *Endocrinology*. Philadelphia: WB Saunders, 1995: 2815–31.

3 Marx SJ, Spiegel AM, Levine MA *et al.* Familial hypocalciuric hypercalcaemia: the relation to primary parathyroid hyperplasia. *N Engl J Med* 1982; **307**: 416–26.

4 Rizzoli R, Green J, Marx SJ. Primary hyperparathyroidism in familial multiple endocrine neoplasia Type 1. Long term follow-up of serum calcium levels after parathyroidectomy. *Am J Med* 1985; **78**: 467–74.

5 Wells SA, Jr, Farndon JR, Dale JK, Leight GS, Dilley WG. Long-term evaluation of patients with primary parathyroid hyperplasia managed by total parathyroidectomy and heterotopic autotransplantation. *Ann Surg* 1980; **192**: 451–8.

6 Saxe AW, Brennan MF. Re-operative parathyroid surgery for primary hyperparathyroidism caused by multiple-gland disease: total parathyroidectomy and autotransplantation with cryopreserved tissue. *Surgery* 1982; **91**: 616–21.

7 Mallette LE, Blevins T, Jordan PH, Noon GP. Autogenous parathyroid grafts for generalised primary hyperplasia: Contrasting outcome in sporadic versus multiple endocrine neoplasia Type I. *Surgery* 1987; **101**: 738–45.

8 Wolfe MM, Jensen RT. Zollinger–Ellison syndrome. Current concepts in diagnosis and management. *N Engl J Med* 1987; **317**: 1200–9.

9 Delcore R, Hermreck AS, Friesen SR. Selective surgical management of correctable hypergastrinemia. *Surgery* 1989; **106**: 1094–102.

10 Sheppard BC, Norton JA, Dopmann JL, Maton PN, Gardner JD, Jensen RT. Management of islet cell tumours in patients with multiple endocrine neoplasia: a prospective study. *Surgery* 1989; **106**: 1108–18.

11 Thompson NW, Bondeson AG, Bondeson L, Vinik A. The surgical treatment of gastrinoma in MEN1 syndrome patients. *Surgery* 1989; **106**: 1081–6.

12 Wise SR, Johnson J, Sparks J, Carey LC, Ellison EC. Gastrinoma: The predictive value of preoperative localisation. *Surgery* 1989; **106**: 1087–93.

13 Marx SJ, Vinik AI, Santen RJ, Floyd JC, Mills JL, Green J. Multiple endocrine neoplasia type 1: assessment of laboratory tests to screen for the gene in a large kindred. *Medicine* 1986; **65**: 226–41.

14 Thakker RV. The molecular genetics of the multiple endocrine neoplasia syndromes. *Clin Endocrinol* 1993; **38**: 1–14.

15 Larsson C, Skogseid B, Oberg K, Nakamura Y, Nordenskjold MC. Multiple endocrine neoplasia type I gene maps to chromosome 11 and is lost in insulinoma. *Nature* 1988; **332**: 85–7.
16 Thakker RV, Bouloux P, Wooding C *et al.* Association of parathyroid tumors in multiple endocrine neoplasia type 1 with loss of alleles on chromosome 11. *N Engl J Med* 1989; **321**: 218–24.
17 Pang JT, Thakker RV. Multiple endocrine neoplasia type 1. *Eur J Cancer* 1994; **30A**: 1961–8.
18 Byström MC, Larsson C, Blomberg C *et al.* Localisation of the MEN1 gene to a small region within chromosome 11q13 by deletion mapping in tumours. *Proc Natl Acad Sci* 1990; **87**: 1968–72.
19 Thakker RV, Pook MA, Wooding C, Boscaro M, Scanarini M, Clayton RN. Association of somatotrophinomas with loss of alleles on chromosome 11 and with *gsp* mutations. *J Clin Invest* 1993; **91**: 2815–21.
20 Thakker RV, Wooding C, Pang J, Farren B and MEN1 Collaborative Group. Linkage analysis of 7 polymorphic markers at chromosome 11p11.2-11q13 in 27 multiple endocrine neoplasia type 1 families. *Ann Human Genet* 1993; **57**: 17–25.
21 Pang JT, Lloyd SE, Wooding C *et al.* Genetic mapping studies of 40 loci and 23 cosmids in chromosome 11p13-11q13, and exclusion of u-calpain as the multiple endocrine neoplasia type 1 gene. *Human Genet* 1996; **97**: 732–41.
22 Benson L, Ljunghall S, Akerstrom G, Oberg K. Hyperparathyroidism presenting as the first lesion in multiple endocrine neoplasia Type 1. *Am J Med* 1987; **82**: 731–7.
23 Skogseid B, Oberg K, Benson L *et al.* A standardized meal stimulation test of the endocrine pancreas for early detection of pancreatic endocrine tumours in Multiple Endocrine Neoplasia Type 1 syndrome: Five years experience. *J Clin Endocrinol Metab* 1987; **64**: 1233–40.
24 Thakker RV. Molecular mechanisms of tumor formation in hereditary and sporadic tumors of the MEN1 type: the impact of genetic screening in the management of MEN1. In Gagel RF, ed. *Endocrinology and Metabolism Clinics of North America.* Philadelphia: WB Saunders, 1994: 117–35.
25 Arnold A, Kim HG, Gaz RD *et al.* Molecular cloning and chromosomal mapping of DNA rearranged with the parathyroid hormone gene in a parathyroid adenoma. *J Clin Invest* 1989; **83**: 2034–40.
26 Motokura T, Bloom T, Kim HG *et al.* A novel cyclin encoded by a *bcl1*-linked candidate oncogene. *Nature* 1991; **350**: 512–15.
27 Cryns VL, Thor A, Xu H-J *et al.* Loss of the retinoblastoma tumor-suppressor gene in parathyroid carcinoma. *N Engl J Med* 1994; **330**: 757–61.
28 Brandi ML, Aurbach GD, Fitzpatrick LA *et al.* Parathyroid mitogenic activity in plasma from patients with familial multiple endocrine neoplasia Type I. *N Engl J Med* 1986; **314**: 1287–93.
29 Zimering MB, Brandi ML, de Grange DA *et al.* Circulating fibroblast growth factor like substance in Familial Multiple Endocrine Neoplasia Type 1. *J Clin Endocrinol Metab* 1990; **70**: 149–54.
30 Murphy D, Bishop A, Rindi G *et al.* Mice transgenic for a vasopressin-SV40 hybrid oncogene develop tumours of the endocrine pancreas and the anterior pituitary. *Am J Pathol* 1987; **129**: 552–66.
31 Chandrasekharappa SC, Guru SC, Manickan P *et al.* Positional cloning of the gene for multiple endocrine neoplasia type 1. *Science* 1997; **276**: 404–7.
32 The European Consortium on MEN1. Identification of the multiple endocrine neoplasia type 1 (MEN1) gene. *Hum Mol Genet* 1997 (in press).

CHAPTER 47

Multiple endocrine neoplasia type 2 and medullary thyroid carcinoma

C. Eng and B.A.J. Ponder

Introduction

Medullary carcinoma of the thyroid (MCT) is an uncommon cancer which arises from the parafollicular C cells which produce calcitonin. About 75% of cases are probably non-hereditary, but the remaining 25% occur as part of the dominantly inherited cancer syndrome, multiple endocrine neoplasia type 2 (MEN-2) in which MTC is associated in some individuals with phaeochromocytoma and with hyperplasia or adenoma of the parathyroid. In both forms of MTC, surgery of the localised disease is the only curative treatment, although useful responses may be gained with radiotherapy and rarely with chemotherapy. The best prospects for improved quality and duration of survival probably rest with more thorough attempts to evaluate and surgically remove local disease in the neck and mediastinum, and with better recognition and screening, both genetic and biochemical, of family members at risk of the heritable disease.

Classification of MEN-2 and 'sporadic' MTC

Three varieties of MEN-2 are distinguished on clinical grounds (Table 47.1). Current evidence indicates that all three are due to mutations of the *RET* proto-oncogene on chromosome sub-band 10q11.2 (see below).

Multiple endocrine neoplasia type 2A

This is the commonest form of MEN-2. Fig. 47.1 gives the age-incidence curves for presentation of MEN-2A with clinical disease and for detection by biochemical screening [1,2]. Note that an estimated one-third of individuals who inherit the *MEN2A* gene have not developed disease sufficiently to lead them to seek medical help by the age of 70 years. This has implications for the recognition and management of families, discussed below.

Multiple endocrine neoplasia type 2B

This accounts for about 5% of MEN-2. Points of difference from MEN-2A [3–5] include:

1 associated developmental abnormalities in other tissues (Table 47.2);

2 rare or absent parathyroid involvement [6];

3 younger age at onset of tumours;

4 possibly a more aggressive natural history of thyroid tumours, although this is controversial [7–9];

5 low reproductive success due probably to a combination of impaired survival, low marriage rates, and impotence due to neurological problems and infertility, with the result that the majority of cases are apparently isolated new mutations.

MTC only

A small number of very extensive pedigrees have been described in which MTC alone (familial MTC, FMTC) is inherited as an autosomal dominant trait with incomplete penetrance; there is no associated adrenal or parathyroid involvement. The MTC presents, on average, later than in MEN-2A, and is rarely if ever the cause of death [10].

MTC without a family history—'sporadic' MTC

The incidence of MTC is about one per 1000000 per year (about 60–80 cases in the UK). About 10% of these will give a family history clearly suggestive of MEN-2; a

Table 47.1 Clinical varieties of multiple endocrine neoplasia type 2 (MEN-2).

	MTC	Phaeochromocytoma	HPT	Other features
MEN-2A	+	+	+	Commonest form Usually no associated abnormalities
MEN-2B	+	+	–	Less common Earlier onset Associated developmental abnormalities especially mucosal neuromas
FMTC	+	–	–	Late onset Indolent course

MTC, medullary thyroid carcinoma; FMTC, familial MTC; HPT, hyperparathyroidism.

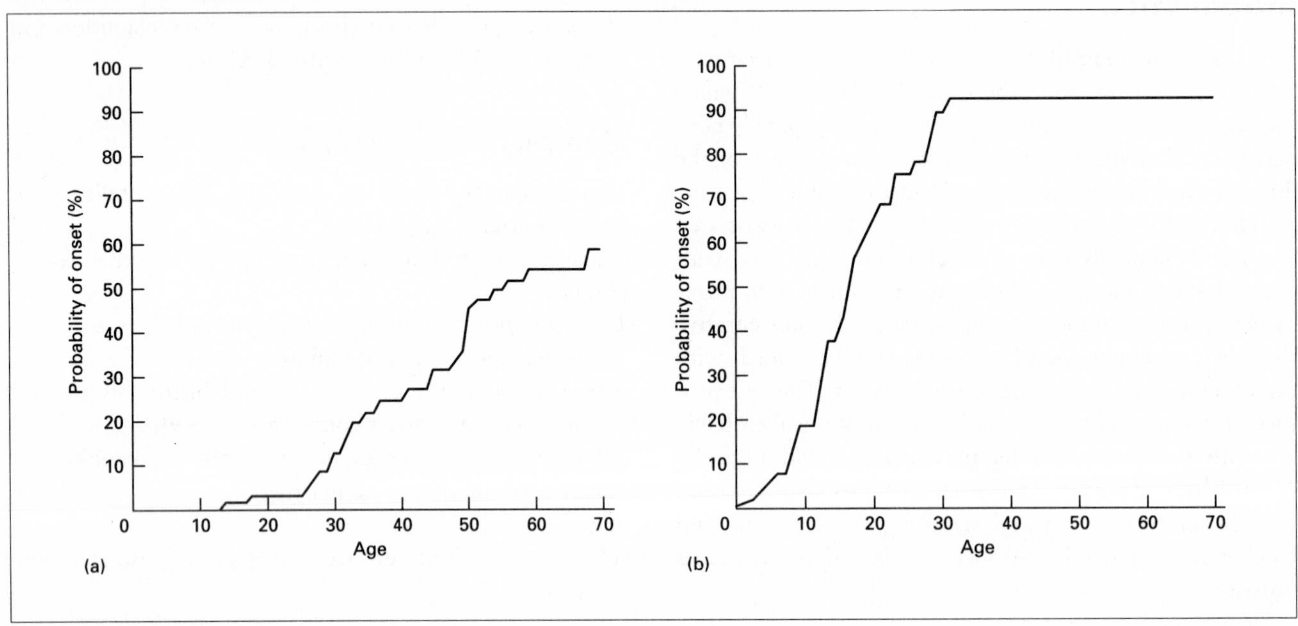

Fig. 47.1 Age-related probability of detection of disease in multiple endocrine neoplasia type 2A (MEN-2A): probability that an individual with the MEN-2A gene will (a) have presented to medical attention, and (b) be detectable by a pentagastrin stimulation test (see text) by a given age. From [2], with permission.

further 10–15% will be found to have evidence of familial involvement after further investigation (more careful history; family screening) [11,12]. A further unknown (but small) proportion of apparently isolated cases are new mutations to heritable disease (see below). Overall, therefore, about 25% of cases are of the heritable type. The remaining 75% are non-hereditary.

It is important to bear in mind that the hereditary form is not always recognisable by family history. A patient with no family history could still have hereditary disease either because he or she has inherited the gene from a parent who did not develop clinically evident disease (30–40% of gene carriers have no symptoms by the age of 70 years) or because of a new mutation to MEN-2. The commonly used description 'sporadic MTC' or apparently sporadic MTC should be a shorthand which means 'having no evident family history, an isolated case'. It does not mean that the case is necessarily non-hereditary. Many series of MTC reported in the literature prior to the isolation of the *MEN2* susceptibility gene are a mixture of hereditary and non-hereditary cases, some diagnosed by family screening and others when they presented with symptoms.

Table 47.2 Features of multiple endocrine neoplasia type 2B and their recognition [3,53].

Pathology	Recognition
Musculokeletal abnormalities	Clinical features
Marfanoid body habitus but no lens, palate or cardiac anomalies	
Pes cavus	
Pectus excavatum	
Hypotonia, proximal muscle weakness	Electromyogram c/w chronic neurogenic atrophy
Neuromas of lips, anterolateral surface of tongue, conjunctiva	Typical facies Biopsy of nodule
Medullated corneal nerve fibres	Slit-lamp examination
Ganglioneuromatosis of intestine	Constipation and diarrhoea Failure to thrive in childhood Barium studies Rectal biopsies

Pathology

Gross

MTC is typically a circumscribed rounded tumour which occurs within the middle or upper third of the thyroid lobe, where the concentration of C cells is greatest. Calcification of primary or metastatic tumour may occur. Multiple or bilateral foci of tumour are typical of MEN-2, where the inherited predisposition may result in several independent primaries.

Histology

A variety of cellular and morphological patterns are seen [13]. Tumours are typically composed of nests or trabeculae of cells separated by septae of connective tissue, and often containing amyloid deposits. Distinct follicular structures may be seen within sheets of tumour cells. The cells may have a polygonal, spindle-shaped or round-cell morphology.

Because of the variable morphology, diagnosis should be confirmed with special stains. Amyloid positivity is strongly suggestive of MTC, but MTC has been reported in which amyloid was lacking [13]. Calcitonin immunostaining is the best diagnostic criterion. Rarely, however, less well-differentiated tumours, especially metastases, may show weak or absent calcitonin staining.

'Mixed' follicular and C-cell tumours have been reported. The evidence that they contain elements of thyroid follicular differentiation is based on morphology but also on thyroglobulin staining, while the C-cell component is identified by calcitonin staining. They may arise from a cell of branchial pouch origin which has the capacity for follicular cell or parafollicular (C-cell) differentiation [14,15].

Metastases

MTC disseminates by direct and lymphatic spread within the neck and upper mediastinum, and by haematogenous spread to distant sites. The sites most commonly involved are liver, bone and lung.

C-cell hyperplasia

C-cell hyperplasia (CCH) is characteristic of the hereditary forms of MEN-2 [16]. The recognition of CCH in a thyroid resected from an apparently isolated case of MTC is therefore of great importance because it implies familial disease, and therefore the need to consider family screening.

The recognition of CCH is not, however, always straightforward. There appears to be a grey area between the extremes of physiological variation of C cells, and hyperplasia indicative of MEN-2. C cells normally lie between the epithelium of the thyroid follicles and the basement membrane. The criteria of abnormality are:

1 increased number of C cells;
2 the arrangement of the C cells in clusters or nodules;
3 the position of the C cells in relation to the follicle;
4 cytological atypia.

More than 10 C cells per low-power microscope field was originally proposed as a criterion for hyperplasia, but studies of autopsy thyroids from individuals without thyroid disease [17,18] show that there is a great range in C-cell numbers in the normal population (the numbers being highest in the elderly). A cut-off based only on numbers is likely to be unsound. Discrete nodules of C cells, especially if they displace or are associated with degeneration of the follicular epithelium, are strongly suggestive of pathological hyperplasia, as is cytological atypia [17,18]. Breach of the follicular basement membrane may be taken as the criterion of carcinoma: in practice, the distinction between CCH and early carcinoma is hard to make and of little practical significance.

Because of the possible overlap with normal, CCH on its own is rarely a completely reliable indicator of heritable disease in an otherwise isolated case (although it certainly carries weight); conversely, because of the uneven distribution of C cells throughout the thyroid and the possibility of sampling errors, the absence of CCH cannot completely exclude heritable disease.

Clinical features and diagnosis

MTC may present clinically with:
1 local or metastatic tumour masses;
2 the effects of biologically active substances secreted from the tumour; or
3 presentation of other components of the MEN-2 syndrome.

A few cases are incidental findings at thyroidectomy for other disease, and an increasing proportion of familial cases are diagnosed by screening (see below). By far the commonest presentation is a painless lump in the neck; the next most common is diarrhoea, due to an unidentified tumour product.

Tumour masses

Local disease presents in the thyroid, cervical lymph nodes and mediastinum. The commonest sites of metastatic presentation are liver and lung. The primary or the metastasis may show radiological calcification.

Paraneoplastic syndromes

MTC may synthesise a number of hormonal and non-hormonal substances. The known ones include:
1 polypeptide hormones—adrenocorticotrophic hormone (ACTH), β-endorphin, somatostatin, vasoactive intestinal polypeptide (VIP);
2 bioactive amines and enzymes—dopamine, dopa-decarboxylase, histaminase, serotonin;
3 miscellaneous—carcino-embryonic antigen (CEA), melanin, nerve growth factor, prostaglandins.

Diarrhoea, due to an unidentified tumour product, is often an indication of a large tumour burden. Any of the bioactive substances which may be secreted by MTC will produce their typical associated syndrome. One of the more common is Cushing's syndrome due to ACTH secretion. Families have been described in which MEN-2A was associated with localised amyloid of the skin [19].

Presentation with other components of the MEN-2 syndrome

Multiple endocrine neoplasia type 2A

MTC is the commonest clinical presentation, but occasional patients present first with phaeochromocytoma or with renal stones or hypercalcaemia due to parathyroid disease. In these cases, if indeed the patient has MEN-2, a stimulated calcitonin screening test will almost certainly be positive [20]. The proportion of patients with MEN-2A who present with parathyroid adenoma or unilateral phaeochromocytoma is not sufficient to justify screening for MTC in these patients unless there are other indications, for example a suggestive family history, multiple foci of parathyroid, adrenal hyperplasia or a proven germline mutation in the *RET* proto-oncogene (see below).

Multiple endocrine neoplasia type 2B

The clinical features of MEN-2B are listed in Table 47.2. The characteristic facial appearance (Fig. 47.2), the mucosal neuromas, and constipation or diarrhoea with failure to thrive caused by ganglioneuromatosis of the intestine should lead to the diagnosis at an early age; however, many cases are missed, or are realised to be abnormal but not diagnosed as MEN-2B. Failure to take food and the 'floppy baby' syndrome in the neonatal period, while, of course, not specific to MEN-2B, are common features. The characteristic facies is probably overdiagnosed, but the diagnosis can be confirmed by biopsy of a mucosal neuroma, or by slit-lamp examination for thickened corneal nerves. Suspicion of the diagnosis should lead to biochemical testing for MTC and genetic (DNA-based) testing (see below).

Differential diagnosis

MTC has been widely recognised only since the late 1960s, and it is certain that many cases in the past have been missed. The differential diagnosis includes all other tumours, the morphology of which on routine pathology slides can resemble MTC. These include especially lymphomas and anaplastic thyroid epithelial cancers. Staining for calcitonin and for amyloid will give the correct diagnosis in most cases.

Genetics

Mode of inheritance; variation in expression

MEN-2 has an autosomal dominant pattern of inheritance, i.e. any child of an affected parent has a 50:50 chance of inheriting the gene. Transmission is equal through males

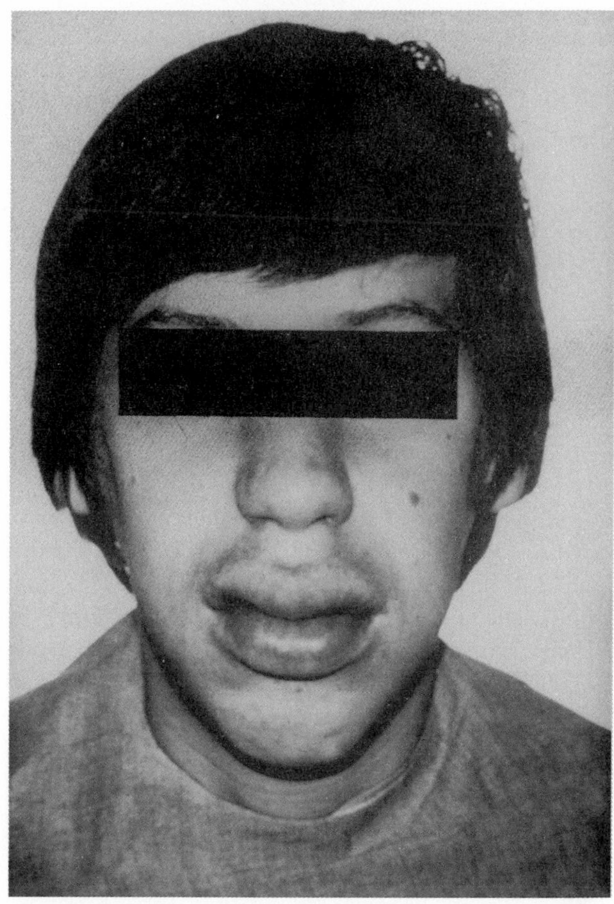

Fig. 47.2 Patient with multiple endocrine neoplasia type 2B. Note the characteristic facies. (Courtesy of Professor J. Farndon, Bristol Royal Infirmary.)

and females, and there is no evidence that the disease differs in severity in males or females, or according to the parent from whom it was inherited. There is considerable variation between and within families in the age at which the tumours develop (Fig. 47.1), and in the incidence of adrenal and parathyroid involvement. At present, there is no evidence that in MEN-2A families, the likely severity of the manifestations in one family member can be predicted from the pattern of the disease in the rest of that family.

The *MEN2* mutation

The predisposing gene for MEN-2 has been mapped to the region near the centromere of chromosome 10 by genetic linkage [21–23]. Only one previously identified gene, the *RET* proto-oncogene, which codes for a receptor tyrosine kinase expressed in neural crest-derived tissues (see below), was known to lie within the 480-kb *MEN2A* region at 10q11.2 [24].

Analysis of this candidate gene led to the identification of different mutations in the *RET* proto-oncogene which predispose to the MEN-2 syndromes. The identification of these mutations in MEN-2 has made genetic diagnosis and management of families possible (see below).

RET encodes a receptor tyrosine kinase

The *RET* proto-oncogene encodes a receptor tyrosine kinase (RTK) [25,26]. RTKs are transmembrane proteins mediating cell to cell signalling. If RET is like other RTKs, then its intracellular tyrosine kinase is activated by ligand interaction with the extracellular domain (reviewed in [27–29]). This ligand binding induces receptor dimerisation. Consequently, dimerisation activates intracellular signal transduction pathways by inducing autophosphorylation of the receptor's intracellular domain and phosphorylation of cytoplasmic substrates. The ligand(s) of RET has yet to be identified.

Germline mutations of the *RET* proto-oncogene in MEN-2

Missence mutations of the *RET* proto-oncogene have been found in the germline DNA of the majority of patients with MEN-2A, FMTC and MEN-2B [30–36]. A detailed compilation of known *RET* mutations can be found in the preliminary report of the International *RET* Mutation Consortium [37].

In MEN-2A and FMTC, the majority of mutations alter one of five cysteine residues in exons 10 (codon 609, 611, 618 and 620) and 11 (codon 634 and in only one example, codon 630) within the cysteine-rich domain of *RET* (Fig. 47.3). There is a correlation between the particular cysteine residue which has been mutated and the spectrum of tissues involved. Mutation at cysteine 634, which accounts for over 75% of mutations, is more frequent in families with MEN-2A, whereas mutation at the other cysteine codons is more frequent in families with FMTC [37,38]. Mutation at codon 634 is associated with the presence of phaeochromocytoma and hyperparathyroidism in a given family [38,39]. In addition, a particular mutation, which alters cysteine (TGC) to arginine (CGC), is highly significantly associated with parathyroid involvement (but not with phaeochromocytoma *per se*) in one series [38] but not in two others [39,40]. A founder effect to explain this association has been excluded by examining the haplotypes on which codon 634 cysteine → arginine mutations have occurred [41]. Interestingly, three FMTC families have been identified in which codon 768 (glutamate) in the intracellular tyrosine kinase domain is mutated to aspartate and a further three FMTC families have a codon 804 mutation where a leucine is altered to a valine (Fig. 47.3) [35,36]. To date, no MEN-2A or MEN-2B families have these two tyrosine kinase domain codon mutations.

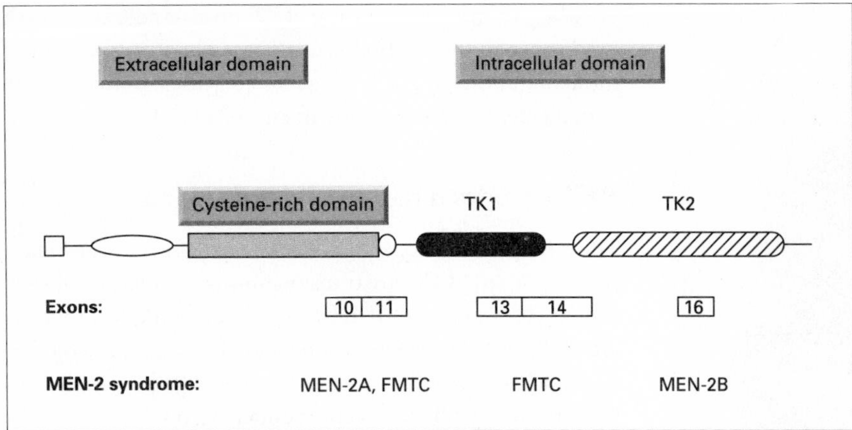

Fig. 47.3 Schematic representation of the *RET* proto-oncogene. Germline mutations within the exons shown cause multiple endocrine neoplasia type 2 (see text).

A single missense mutation affecting codon 918, altering a methionine (ATG) to a threonine (ACG), has been found in >93% of patients with MEN-2B [33,37,42]. The patients without the codon 918 mutation appeared to have classic MEN-2B and did not differ clinically from the rest of the patients with mutations [33,42,43]. *De novo* mutation in MEN-2B has been shown to occur on the paternal chromosome much more frequently than the maternal chromosome [44].

Somatic mutations of the *RET* proto-oncogene in sporadic tumours

Although MTC and phaeochromocytoma are component tumours of the MEN-2 syndromes, they also occur as sporadic, i.e., non-inherited, tumours. By analogy with other inherited cancer syndromes, one might expect that somatic *RET* mutations corresponding to the germline mutations observed in MEN-2A and MEN-2B would be involved in the tumorigenesis of these sporadic tumours.

A search for somatic mutations in sporadic MTC has revealed approximately one-third with *RET* mutations, the majority of which are somatic MEN-2B-type mutations (codon 918, changing ATG to ACG) at codon 918. Of 157 sporadic MTC, 61 had this mutation [32,33,45–50]. In contrast, exon 10 and 11 MEN-2A-type cysteine codon mutations are rare. Examples include only one of an unknown number of sporadic MTC to have a 6-bp deletion which removed cysteine 630, and three of 77 apparently sporadic MTC with MEN-2A-type cysteine codon mutations [31,45,47]. Of these latter three cases, two were occult germline mutations and germline DNA was not available for the third. The rare germline codon 768 FMTC mutation was initially thought to be more common in sporadic MTC, occurring in four of the first 10 (40%) tumours initially analysed [35]. However, no codon 768 mutations have been detected in the subsequent 62 sporadic MTC analysed and thus, no more than 10% of sporadic MTC have somatic codon 768 mutations [50] (C. Eng, B.A.J. Ponder, unpublished). In contrast to sporadic MTC, MTC from MEN-2 cases rarely have somatic codon 918 mutations [51].

Unlike sporadic MTC, only six of 112 (5%) apparently sporadic phaeochromocytoma had a somatic mutation of codon 918, two (1.5%) had proven somatic missense mutations affecting the cysteine-rich region, and three others had novel somatic mutations affecting the splice junction of exon 9, codon 632–633 and codon 925 [33,52–55]. Since only some of the 21 *RET* exons [56] have been analysed for somatic mutations in these tumours, it is possible that mutations elsewhere in *RET* (other exons, introns or promoter) or in another gene may also play a role in tumorigenesis.

Tumour progression in MEN-2 and related tumours

Multiple genetic events are recognised in the progression of MEN-2 type tumours. *RET* mutations identified in MEN-2 are activating and thus loss or inactivation of the normal *RET* allele is not required for tumorigenesis [57,58]. Allele loss on chromosome 10 is rare in MEN-2-related tumours and generally represents loss of an entire chromosome copy [57]. In fact, the majority of tumours examined express both the normal and disease copy of *RET* [30,33].

Allele losses, presumably reflecting the involvement of multiple tumour-suppressor loci, have been identified in tumour progression of MTC and phaeochromocytoma. In general, loss of heterozygosity occurs in a greater proportion of tumours and for more chromosomal regions in phaeochromocytoma than in MTC. The most frequently affected region in both MEN-2-type tumours is chromosome 1p which is lost in 25% MTC and 60–100% phaeochromocytoma [57]. Interestingly, in tumours from patients with MEN-2 these events involve the entirely of the short arm of the chromosome plus the centromere, and do not appear to be a consequence of isochromosome 1q formation [57]. Other regions of consistent chromosome loss include chromosome arms 3p and 22q [57].

Despite the identification of several genetic events in MTC tumour progression (above), none can yet be confidently used to predict the behaviour of the tumour.

Mutations of the *RET* proto-oncogene in Hirschsprung disease

Hirschsprung disease (HSCR) is not an inherited cancer syndrome but a congenital developmental disorder characterised by intestinal obstruction resulting in megacolon. The intestinal obstruction is caused by the absence of ganglion cells within Meissner's and Auerbach's plexuses of the intestine [59]. This is in contrast to the overgrowth of these ganglion cells sometimes observed in MEN-2B.

A susceptibility locus for HSCR was mapped to chromosome 10q11.2 [60,61], the region which also contained the *MEN2* locus. Subsequently, it was shown that mutations scattered along the length of *RET* proto-oncogene can also predispose to HSCR [62–65]. Unlike the role of *RET* mutations in MEN-2, *RET* mutations in HSCR are likely to be inactivating or loss of function [66].

Eight families with MEN-2 and HSCR have been reported to have cysteine codon 618 or 620 mutations [64,67,68] (International *RET* Mutation Consortium, unpublished). Both MEN-2 and HSCR appear to cosegregate in seven of these families; in one, both phenotypes segregated with different chromosome 10 haplotypes [67]. No other disease-associated mutations could be detected within exons 2–20 of the gene (exon 21 had not been discovered at that time). Mechanistically, it is difficult to explain how a cysteine codon alteration, typical of MEN-2A/FMTC, can cause a syndrome postulated to result from a gain of function of *RET* [58] and also cause HSCR, which is believed to be secondary to a loss of function [66]. None the less, from a clinical point of view, individuals diagnosed with HSCR in the first few years of life who are found to have cysteine codon 618 or 620 mutations, particularly if these are TGC to CGC, may be at subsequent risk for MEN-2A or FMTC [67].

Investigation and management

An outline of investigation and management is given in Table 47.3.

Investigation after primary surgery

Ideally, the diagnosis of MTC should be made before surgery, either by needle biopsy of the thyroid nodule or because of a known family history. Preoperative investigations for phaeochromocytoma and parathyroid disease should then be carried out, and the extent of neck surgery planned after investigation of the extent of local disease. More often, however, the diagnosis of MTC is made only after thyroid surgery when the pathology is available. In such a case, the steps in investigation are as follows.

1 Is this the heritable form (MEN-2)? Take a careful family history; check the patient for evidence of phaeochromocytoma (see Chapter 38) or hyperparathyroidism (serum calcium); although CCH is not always pathognomonic for heritable disease, review the thyroid pathology for CCH using systematic sampling and calcitonin immunostains. If MEN-2 is likely, examination of germline DNA for *RET* mutations should be performed (see above). If a mutation is found, then other at-risk individuals (first-degree relatives of the mutation-positive person) should be tested for the presence or absence of mutations (see family screening below). Continue to screen the patient for phaeochromocytoma at yearly intervals. Consider total thyroidectomy if the first operation was incomplete.

If no *RET* mutation can be identified and a meticulous family history (to second- and ideally, third-degree relatives) and a search for CCH and multifocal disease within the thyroid specimen have been performed, then it is less likely (but not impossible) that the patient has MEN-2.

2 Investigate the extent of residual disease. Plasma calcitonin levels are the most sensitive measure of residual tumour. The use of calcitonin measurements in follow-up is discussed on p. 644. If elevated calcitonin levels suggest residual disease, local and distant disease should be investigated as for any other cancer.

Computed tomography scanning

Computed tomography (CT) scanning is probably the most sensitive technique for the delineation of disease within the thyroid and in the neck and upper mediastinum. Ultrasonography is less sensitive, but occasionally useful [69]. Magnetic resonance imaging (MRI) may prove useful in the near future.

Radionuclide scans

Two new scanning agents are reported to show uptake in MTC. The most promising is ^{99m}Tc-DMSA (dimercaptosuccinic acid), which in one series gave 95% sensitivity of detection of bony and soft tissue lesions, without false positives [70]. ^{131}I-MIBG (metaiodobenzylguanidine) was developed as an agent for imaging phaeochromocytoma, but has been shown to accumulate in tumour in some patients with MTC. It does not have a primary diagnostic role, but in tumours which show uptake it may have therapeutic potential.

Table 47.3 Outline of management after diagnosis of medullary thyroid carcinoma.

Management of family	Management of patient
1 Is the family history positive? • If not, estimate probability that patient has heritable disease. Consider DNA testing (see text) • If family history positive, construct accurate family tree and estimate risks to each member. Contact clinical geneticist or endocrinologist and proceed with DNA testing	1 Does the patient have MEN-2? Check: • MEN-2B phenotype • careful family history at least to second-, if not third-, degree relatives • CCH—immunostains of thyroid • urinary catecholamines/clinical evidence of phaeochromocytoma • serum calcium Probably familial disease: 2 DNA testing (see text) 3 Was a total thyroidectomy done (if technically feasible)? If no: consider further surgery unless MEN-2 is very unlikely and postoperative CT normal • normal basal CT and CEA: consider CT-stimulation test to search for minimal residual disease if surgeon would reoperate (e.g. if only limited neck dissection so far) • elevated but stable CT/CEA, patient well: consider localising tests before further surgery especially if neck/mediastinum not fully explored at previous surgery. If no prospect of further surgery for local residual disease, do nothing • rising CT or CEA: vigorous search for local disease for possible surgery/local radiotherapy. If disseminated disease, try ^{131}I-MIBG uptake for possible therapy. Use chemotherapy with reluctance if clinical picture demands it

MEN, multiple endocrine neoplasia; CCH, C-cell hyperplasia; CT, calcitonin; CEA, carcinoembryonic antigen; mIBG, metaiodobenzylguanidine.

Occasional positives are obtained with thallium-201; and ^{99m}Tc methylene diphosphonate will image about 50% of bony metastases from MTC. For the assessment of local disease in the neck and mediastinum, DMSA is likely to be a useful adjunct to CT scanning.

Selective venous catheterisation

Transfemoral catheterisation of the neck veins and selective sampling for calcitonin assay has been proposed as a logical means of locating small or diffuse deposits of residual disease, which are unlikely to show on scans, before secondary surgery. Although successful in the hands of the group that did the initial work [71], informal and published reports suggest that others have found the technique either difficult to use or of uncertain value (see for example [72]).

Metastatic disease

The common sites are liver, lung and bone. Since there is no effective systematic treatment, and the disease is often indolent, a detailed search for asymptomatic deposits may not be clinically justified. Knowledge of metastatic disease is useful: (i) if an attempt at cure by radical removal of local disease is contemplated; (ii) if there are symptoms that might be related to metastases; (iii) at sites at which complications might be foreseen and averted by early treatment, for example bone deposits in the femora; and (iv) if objective evidence is needed to judge response to therapy.

A large tumour burden, and hence the probability of metastatic disease, is suggested by a very high level of calcitonin or CEA, and the symptom of diarrhoea (see above).

Staging

There is no generally used staging system for MTC. The tumour node metastasis (TNM) and Union Internationale Contre le Cancer (UICC) classifications are almost never used in published series, suggesting that they do not meet practical needs. In cases detected by screening, the preoperative level of basal and stimulated calcitonin is probably the best staging criterion by which to assess the results of primary surgery. The postoperative level of basal and stimulated calcitonin is the best measure of residual disease and therefore the best short-term indicator of the probable success or otherwise of surgery in securing long-term cure.

Staging based on description of the extent of disease does not take account of the rate of progression of the disease, which in MTC may be extremely variable, and is probably the strongest prognostic factor. The most complete staging of disease after thyroidectomy would therefore contain three elements:

1 clinical/pathological evidence of spread;
2 the level of basal or stimulated calcitonin;
3 the change of that level over the immediate past.

Preoperative investigation of a patient with suspected MTC

Family screening or some clinical feature (MEN-2B phenotype, diarrhoea associated with a thyroid nodule) may point to the diagnosis of MTC before thyroid surgery.

The diagnosis of MTC will be confirmed by finding an elevated plasma calcitonin level and possibly by needle biopsy. The level of calcitonin will give an approximate indication of tumour burden and thus of the likelihood of local or distant spread beyond the thyroid.

The absence of phaeochromocytoma should be fully checked before thyroid surgery in every case.

In cases where biochemical screening indicates CCH, but there is some residual uncertainty, confirmation may be sought by CT scanning of the thyroid using iodide contrast or MRI scanning. This allows C-cell nodules as small as 2–3 mm to be demonstrated as low-density areas (or high-density areas on MRI T2-weighted scans) within the thyroid (although of course, similar appearances could be given by other structures of non-follicular origin). For the CT with iodide contrast technique, the patient is given two or three capsules of potassium iodide (180 mg), with a large glass of milk to minimise gastric irritation, 24 hours before the scan. Although sometimes helpful in cases detected by screening, the calcitonin abnormality is borderline, this is mandatory preoperative investigation.

If disease outside the thyroid is suspected, CT scanning or DMSA radionuclide scanning may be helpful in identifying sites of disease, especially in the mediastinum.

Screening

Who should be screened?

Decisions in a known MEN-2 family

If the family has a known *RET* mutation (see above), all first-degree relatives of any affected/mutation-positive individual should have their DNA checked for the presence of the family-specific mutation. Mutation-positive family members should be screened for the presence of MTC/CCH (or have prophylactic thyroidectomy) and phaeochromocytoma annually. If genotype–phenotype correlations (see above) can be confirmed in large studies, then the presence of a codon 634 mutation in a family should alert the clinician to the high likelihood of the development of phaeochromocytoma and parathyroid disease. Similarly, the presence of a codon 634 TGC → CGC mutation could be a genotypic marker for the likelihood of developing parathyroid disease although this has to be reconfirmed in a consortium analysis.

Decisions in the family of an apparently isolated case

Here, the need is to estimate the probability that the patient has familial disease. If we ignored any DNA mutation data, the risk calculations are as follows.

1 The prior risk is now the risk that a patient with MTC presenting at a given age will have familial disease, regardless of the family history.
2 The conditional risk takes account of the family history: if this is positive, the final risk becomes 1; if negative, the final risk is less than the prior risk by an amount dependent on the ages and numbers of apparently unaffected relatives.

In practice, only the parents are usually considered. An explanation and worked example is given in Ponder *et al.* [1]; illustrative risks are shown in Table 47.4. Note that a young patient with no evident family history is still at significant risk of having hereditary disease. The presence or absence of CCH in the thyroid specimen can also be taken into account, although the data are insufficient to do this in a quantitative way. The presence of CCH is an indication to screen the family but is not pathognomonic [73,74]. Because of sampling problems, absence of CCH should not carry much weight unless the thyroid has been examined with unusual care.

If a germline *RET* mutation is detected in an apparently sporadic case of MTC, then it is obvious that the case represents an occult or *de novo* case of MEN-2, and appropriate genetic (see above) and clinical screening can be instituted. However, absence of germline mutation in *RET* does not always exclude MEN-2. Approximately 5% of classic MEN-2A cases and 30% of 'small' FMTC families (three or fewer affected individuals) do not have mutations detected in the codons usually screened. While absence of mutation does suggest the absence of classic MEN-2A to a high probability, there is still a small but finite probability that the individual might still have heritable disease.

Table 47.4 Probability of a patient presenting with medullary thyroid carcinoma (MTC) at a given age with no history of multiple endocrine neoplasia type 2 (MEN-2) in the parents.

Age, Patient at diagnosis	Age at which parents were apparently unaffected				
	30 and 70	40 and 70	50 and 70	60 and 70	70 and 70
30	0.29	0.27	0.25	0.22	0.21
45	0.15	0.14	0.13	0.11	0.10
60	0.06	0.06	0.05	0.04	0.04
70	0.03	0.03	0.02	0.02	0.02

The age at which the parents were known to have had no symptoms suggestive of MEN-2 modifies the risk (30 and 70 means that one parent was known symptom-free aged 70, the other aged 30). For example, a patient diagnosed with MTC aged 30, whose parents are both well at 70 years of age, and in whom there is no other family history, has a 21% chance of having MEN-2. Note that C-cell hyperplasia, the possibility of new mutation (see text) and the results of *RET* mutation testing (see text) are not taken into account in this table. The risk calculations and the assumptions on which they are based are given in [1].

The possibility of a new mutation

Even if the risk calculations from family history are low, there is always the possibility that an isolated case of MTC could be the start of a new MEN-2 family. The proportion of MTC cases which fall into this category is not precisely known, but is probably <5%. Even so, it may be wise to consider looking for germline *RET* mutations in the patient, especially those presenting young and/or those whose thyroid specimen contains CCH.

Screening procedure

General considerations

A careful family history is the first essential, with review of the thyroid pathology for CCH where hereditary disease is in doubt.

Choice of screening test

All screening should be preceded by a simple clinical examination, to include palpation of the neck and measurement of blood pressure.

The simplest biochemical screen is a basal calcitonin level. However, this is not sufficiently sensitive either to detect all MTC at a stage when surgical cure is possible, or to exclude the possibility that a family member is a gene carrier. A stimulated calcitonin test (see below) and direct DNA testing is preferable.

Biochemical screening: stimulated calcitonin tests

Types of stimuli

A variety of stimuli has been proposed, but the principle in each is similar. The C cells are induced to release their stored calcitonin into the circulation, and the size of the calcitonin peak following the stimulus is a measure of the C-cell mass, and hence of CCH. The stimuli most commonly used are intravenous pentagastrin [75,76], intravenous calcium [76] or ethanol [77] (as vodka or whisky) by mouth. Procedures are given in Table 47.5. Pentagastrin (Peptavlon) is the most widely used. Its advantages are that more data are available to aid interpretation of the results, and it probably is more discriminatory than ethanol. The disadvantage is that it causes unpleasant side-effects of tightness in the chest, paresthesiae in the limbs, nausea, flushing or stomach cramps, which although tolerable in most subjects, are occasionally severe. Children seem to tolerate pentagastrin better than adults, and they much prefer it to ethanol.

Calcium infusion is also being used, and may be as discriminatory as pentagastrin with fewer side-effects. These consist of flushing or an unpleasant feeling of warmth and nausea.

Interpretation

The history of calcitonin radioimmunoassay has been plagued by a variable number of 'false positives' in most assays [73,74,78]. This problem should be less, but likely still present, with the newer two-site assays. Nevertheless, it is wise: (i) not to accept a small elevation of basal calcitonin as indicating CCH unless at least a twofold increment can be obtained on stimulation; (ii) to store duplicate aliquots of plasma for measurement in a different assay with different characteristics in cases of doubt; and (iii) to get to know the characteristics of the assay that you will use, and discuss the interpretation of results with the assay team.

Table 47.5 Procedure and stimuli for calcitonin tests. (Note: procedures used by different groups vary in detail from those given.)

	Stimulus	Blood samples
Ethanol	50 ml whisky or vodka by mouth in 1-2 min	Before, 5, 10, 15 and 30 min after stimulus
Pentagastrin	0.5 µg/kg i.v. Dilute in 5-10 ml sterile saline and inject i.v. over 5–15 seconds	Before, 1, 2, 5, 10 min after stimulus
Calcium	2 mg/kg of Ca^{2+} as 10% Ca gluconate i.v. over 1 min	Before, 1, 2, 5, 10 min after stimulus
Calcium + pentagastrin	2 mg/kg Ca^{2+} as 10% Ca gluconate i.v. over 1 min followed by 0.5 µg/kg pentagastrin i.v. over 5–15 sec	Before, 1, 2, 5, 10 min after final stimulus

The subject need not be fasting, but only a light food intake and no alcohol in the hours before the test are advisable. The subject lies on a couch, and a cannula is inserted in an arm vein. Blood is withdrawn for one or two baseline samples; the stimulus is given (pentagastrin or calcium can be given through the same cannula); the cannula is flushed with dilute heparin; and blood samples withdrawn at the times shown. The side-effects of the stimuli are discussed in the text.

Each blood sample should be 5–10 ml, taken into heparin tubes precooled in an ice bucket. The sample tubes are labelled and replaced on ice, and centrifuged to separate plasma immediately after the test is completed. Two to three 1-ml aliquots of plasma from each sample should be immediately frozen in dry ice and placed in a –70°C freezer. One aliquot is sent on dry ice for assay; the others are kept in reserve in case the first samples are thawed in transit or the assay results require to be confirmed.

Age and frequency of screening

The age-onset curve in Fig. 47.1 indicates that the first positives to pentagastrin screening in MEN-2A can be expected at or before 5 years of age, and about 90% of gene carriers are detected by the age of 30 years. Reported instances of conversion from negative to positive after the age of 40 years are very rare (but perhaps few have been tested). The time taken for CCH to progress from first detection to MTC not curable by surgery, which would determine screening interval, is not known. A consensus screening strategy for MEN-2A might be: pentagastrin or pentagastrin/Ca^{2+} stimulation yearly from the age of 5 years. For MEN-2B, there is no published consensus. In view of the sometimes early onset and aggressive tumour, screening for MTC in the child of a patient with MEN-2B or a *RET* codon 918 mutation-positive child should start in early childhood, probably at the age of 1 year. In this situation, some clinicians would advocate thyroidectomy on the basis of the phenotype alone or the phenotype together with demonstrated presence of the codon 918 mutation. In cases with no family history, it should start as soon as the phenotype is suspected.

Screening for other components of the MEN-2 syndrome

Phaeochromocytoma

Screening usually consists of annual blood-pressure measurement and plasma or urinary catecholamines. In MEN-2A, however, it is very uncommon for a family member who presents with symptoms from phaeochromocytoma not to have also an unequivocal abnormality on stimulated calcitonin screening [20]. In addition, an occult or *de novo* case of MEN-2 rarely presents as an apparently sporadic case of phaeochromocytoma [55]. The presence of a codon 634 mutation in an MEN-2A family should alert the physician to the likelihood of phaeochromocytoma in that family [37–39]. Probably, therefore, screening for phaeochromocytoma is unnecessary as a routine until the calcitonin tests are abnormal. An exception should be made in cases at particular risk, for example women of child-bearing age, and those about to undergo general anaesthesia.

Pending confirmation, it might be arguable to suggest that individuals who are at-risk in families that have the codon 634 TGC to CGC (Cys → Arg) mutation [38] be followed for the development of parathyroid involvement as well.

DNA screening

Since germline mutations in the *RET* proto-oncogene have been identified in ≥90% of cases with MEN-2A, MEN-2B and classic FMTC (four or more affected individuals in a family), it is possible to determine if one of the mutations is present in a given family (see above). Thus, using DNA-based genetic testing, it is possible to identify gene carriers (mutation-positive individuals) and non-carriers (mutation-negative individuals). In an MEN-2 family with a known *RET* mutation, mutation-negative individuals do not have to be subjected to any screening tests. Carriers of the mutation can then be targeted to receive serial biochemical screening and/or prophylactic thyroidectomy.

DNA screening for MEN-2 families

The consensus for DNA-based testing for MEN-2 reached at the Fifth International Multiple Endocrine Neoplasia Workshop (Stockholm, Summer, 1994) was that the specific mutation segregating with each MEN-2 kindred should be initially determined. Direct DNA sequence analysis of *RET* exons 10, 11, 13, 14 and 16 should be performed on DNA from a known clinically affected individual. If a mutation is detected, then subsequent DNA-based diagnosis, whether by sequence analysis or, more practically, by differential restriction digestion (see for example [79]), for asymptomatic individuals at risk belonging to the same family would be possible and is 100% accurate. This mutation analysis should be repeated on DNA extracted from newly drawn blood samples to avoid sample mix-up. Individuals who test negative twice do not need to be screened and can also be reassured. Individuals who test positive should be considered candidates for prophylactic thyroidectomy. Since metastatic MTC has been reported to occur as early as 6 years of age [80], the Workshop consensus was to perform thyroidectomies between the ages of 5 and 6 years. This should only be performed by endocrine surgeons with expertise in these operations. Theoretically, 95% of gene carriers will be cured by undergoing prophylactic thyroidectomies. Subsequent serial biochemical screening for the presence of phaeochromocytoma should then be instituted. Extramural to the Workshop consensus, however, it is still controversial whether prophylactic thyroidectomy or serial pentagastrin-stimulated calcitonin screening should be instituted in individuals who are *RET* mutation-positive.

The steps to follow to obtain DNA testing for a family are as follows.

1 Take a full family history, including affected and unaffected individuals, their ages and screening status.

2 Discuss with the family the probability that prediction will or will not be possible, and the likely accuracy (especially in apparently sporadic MTC presentations).

3 Collect the blood (usually 20–30 ml EDTA-anticoagulated), taking great care that each sample is correctly and unambiguously labelled (it is surprising how easily mistakes can be made).

RET mutation testing in apparently sporadic MTC

It is important to recognise, if possible, those apparently sporadic MTC that are certainly sporadic and those which are likely to be heritable so that screening can be directed only at those who need it. Since over 96% of families with typical MEN-2A have a mutation in one of exons 10 or 11 [37,38], very few *de novo* or occult MEN-2A cases will have a mutation outside these exons. Hence, it appears that few apparently sporadic MTC (strictly defined as no first- or second-degree relatives with MTC or phaeochromocytoma or known MEN-2; and no multifocality within the gland) are in fact true cases of classic MEN-2A or classic FMTC [81]. A *RET* mutation screen of exons 10 and 11 would identify the majority of apparently sporadic cases as MEN-2A or classic FMTC. Adding exons 13, 14 and 16 to the screen would pick up additional cases of MEN-2B and rare cases of FMTC due to exon 13 and 14 mutations [35,36]. There is, however, an unknown percentage of apparently sporadic MTC cases who do not have a *RET* mutation in the screened exons and who will turn out to have heritable MTC. This is related to the fact that there are as many as one-third of 'small' FMTC families that do not have obvious mutations in exons 10, 11, 13, 14 or 16 [37–39].

With the current available data, the evaluation of a patient with apparently sporadic MTC may be as follows [81].

1 Take a meticulous family history with reference to the features suggestive of MEN-2A or MEN-2B.

2 Evaluate the thyroid specimen for evidence of C-cell hyperplasia although it is no longer thought to be pathognomonic for heritable disease. However, CCH in a specimen would be a persuasive indication for genetic and biochemical screening of the family.

3 Analyse germline DNA for known mutations of *RET* associated with MEN-2/FMTC (currently, exons 10, 11, 13, 14 and 16).

Surgical treatment

Surgery is the only proven curative treatment for MTC. The proper extent of primary surgery is controversial. For all patients with MTC, total thyroidectomy is advised. This is because of the possibility of inherited (and so bilateral) disease, and of intrathyroidal metastasis. For all patients, even those detected only by stimulated calcitonin screening and without macroscopic tumour, dissection of the nodes in the central compartment of the neck is advisable with intraoperative frozen sections to look for metastasis. Some surgeons advocate a more extensive dissection, extending into the lateral compartments, mediastinum and including removal of the thymus. Others extend the dissection only if there is gross or frozen section evidence of node involvement [82].

Postoperatively, the patient must be followed with measurement of calcitonin and CEA. Reoperation is advised if the levels show a rising trend and there is evidence or reasonable suspicion of resectable disease in the neck or mediastinum. More controversial is what to do if the calcitonin and/or CEA levels are elevated postoperatively, but stable. The decision will be influenced by the extent of primary surgery, and the likely-site and extent of residual disease, judged by calcitonin level and by clinical and radiological evidence. If primary surgery was limited, reoperation with dissection of remaining nodes may be advisable [83]. Even if not curative, it may postpone distressing symptoms of local disease, and surgery may be easier than at a later stage when the anatomy is distorted.

Tisell *et al.* [84] have claimed that in patients in whom the only evidence of residual disease is a raised level of calcitonin after stimulation, a super-radical neck dissection may provide a chance of cure. The evidence for benefit so far is based on conversion of a marginally raised calcitonin to an undetectable level; much longer follow-up is needed to see whether this translates to cure. If this approach is to be taken, patients with undetectable basal calcitonin postoperatively must be followed at regular intervals with stimulation tests, and action taken as soon as an abnormality (in practice, a rising peak calcitonin level) is detected.

Whenever technically feasible, surgery is the first line of treatment for local disease which is causing or about to cause symptoms.

Radiation therapy

External-beam radiation

The use and timing of radiation therapy in patients with known local residual disease is controversial, but a consensus is probably as follows.

1 There is no place for radiation as an adjunct to apparently successful primary surgery.

2 For a patient with clinical or biochemical evidence of residual disease, further surgery is the preferred treatment.

3 Radiotherapy should usually be reserved until there is either clear evidence of disease progression not amenable to surgery or symptomatic local disease.

4 In some instances, for example threatened tracheal or oesophageal compression, a combination of 'debulking' surgery and radiotherapy is likely to be appropriate.

5 Radiation is of course, to be used for metastatic deposits, for example painful bony metastases, as in any cancer.

Radioiodine

Attempts have been made to use ^{131}I to ablate C cells in the thyroid remnant following incomplete thyroidectomy for MEN-2, and so prevent second tumour formation. These were apparently unsuccessful [85], and complete thyroidectomy is to be preferred.

^{131}I-mIBG (see above), a scanning agent, is taken up by a small number of MTCs. In cases where systemic treatment is needed, it is worth testing uptake with a scanning dose and, if positive, considering therapy.

Chemotherapy

MTC is generally unresponsive. Chemotherapy should therefore be reserved for patients with rapidly progressing or symptomatic disease, in whom other measures have failed.

In small series, responses have most often been reported with adriamycin and *cis*-platinum (separately or in combination) and with etoposide [86,87].

Prognosis

Non-hereditary MTC is detected, on average, at a later stage than hereditary MTC. If age and extent of disease at presentation are taken into account, there is probably little difference in mortality from MTC between patients with hereditary and non-hereditary disease [11]. Overall, 10-year survival figures reported by Samaan *et al.* [9] were: disease confined to thyroid gland, 90%; involving local nodes, 70%; nodes and soft tissue, 60%; distant metastases, 20%. Many patients with hereditary and non-hereditary MTC coexist with metastatic tumour for many years with minimal or no symptoms. Treatment of such patients is probably meddlesome. Once the disease is clearly progressive, palliation can sometimes be obtained by combination of surgery, radiotherapy and/or chemotherapy, usually for a few weeks or months, but occasionally for longer, but death from metastatic disease is very probable. Rising CEA levels with stable or falling calcitonin may indicate an evolution of the tumour or to a less well-differentiated state, and are often associated with a particularly poor prognosis.

Acknowledgements

We thank the many clinicians and scientists, especially members of the Cancer Research Campaign Medullary

Thyroid Group and the International *RET* Mutation Consortium,* with whom we have worked on MTC and MEN-2. The authors are supported by the Cancer Research Campaign (CRC) Dana–Farber Cancer Institute Fellowship, the Lawrence and Susan Marx Investigatorship in Cancer Genetics in the Division of Cancer Epidemiology and Control, Dana–Farber Cancer Institute, the Markey Charitable Trust and Charles A. Dana Foundation (to CE), and core and programme grants from the CRC (to BAJP). BAJP is a Gibb Fellow of the CRC.

Note added in proof

The International *RET* Mutation Consortium has completed analyses of 477 independent MEN-2 families for genotype–phenotype correlations [88]. Any mutation at codon 634 is associated with the development of phaeochromocytoma and HPT in a given MEN-2A family. The codon 634 cysteine to arginine mutation was found to be associated with HPT. However, FMTC families have thus far never been shown to harbour the 634 cysteine to arginine mutation. New correlations of codon 768 and 804 mutations and FMTC were found. From a clinical point of view, the results of the pooled analyses would suggest that any family carrying a codon 634 mutation should be carefully screened for the development of phaeochromocytoma and HPT. If a family carries a 634 cysteine to arginine mutation yet appears to have only members with MTC, then the clinician should initiate a meticulous search for phaeochromocytoma and HPT. Finally, if reconfirmed with larger numbers and longer follow-up, it might be possible to streamline surveillance for families with codon 768 or 804 mutation.

A ligand for RET, glial cell line-derived neurotrophic factor (GDNF), was discovered in mid-1996 [89–92]. Unlike other classic receptor tyrosine kinases, however, GDNF was shown to bind a novel co-receptor, GDNFR-α, before this GDNF–GDNFR-α complex could bind RET. Whether mutations in the genes encoding the receptor and co-receptor of RET can account for those MEN-2 families without *RET* mutations are being investigated.

* The International *RET* Mutation Consortium was convened at the Fifth International Multiple Endocrine Neoplasia Workshop (Stockholm, Summer, 1994) and is maintaining an active database of *RET* mutations in MEN-2. It is dedicated to examining genotype–phenotype correlations in the expanding dataset and plans to collect submissions on *RET* mutations in sporadic MTC and phaeochromocytoma in the near future. In addition, the collaborating centres in the Consortium will be working together, and in conjunction with EuroMEN, to examine the entire sequence of *RET* in those MEN-2 and MEN-2-like families who do not have the classic mutations. If you are interested in the Consortium, please contact Charis Eng, MD, PhD, fax + 1 617 632 4280, e-mail charis_eng @macmailgw.dfci.harvard.edu or Lois M. Mulligan, PhD, fax + 1 613 548 1348, e-mail mulligal @ qucdn.queensu.ca. The Consortium would especially like to welcome centres from South America and Africa.

References

1 Ponder BAJ, Ponder MA, Coffey R *et al.* Risk estimation and screening in families of patients with medullary thyroid carcinoma. *Lancet* 1988; **i**: 397–400.

2 Easton DF, Ponder MA, Cummings T *et al.* The clinical and screening age-at-onset distribution for the MEN-2 syndrome. *Am J Hum Genet* 1989; **44**: 208–15.

3 Dyck PJ, Carney A, Sizemore GW, Okazaki H, Brimijoin WS, Lambert E. Multiple endocrine neoplasia type, type 2B: clinical recognition. *Ann Neurol* 1979; **6**: 302–14.

4 Carney JA, Sizemore GW, Hayles AB. C-cell disease of the thyroid in multiple endocrine neoplasia, type 2b. *Cancer* 1979; **44**: 2173–83.

5 Gorlin RJ, Sedano HO, Vickers RA, Cervenka J. Multiple mucosal neuromas, phaeochromocytoma and medullary carcinoma of the thyroid—a syndrome. *Cancer* 1968; **22**: 293–9.

6 Cance WG, Wells SA, eds. *Current Problems in Surgery*, MM Ravitch, ed. Vol. XXII. *Multiple Endocrine Neoplasia Type IIa.* 1985: 7–56.

7 Kullberg BJ, Nieuwenhuijzen-Kruseman AC. Multiple endocrine neoplasia type 2b with a good prognosis. *Arch Intern Med* 1987; **147**: 1125–7.

8 Norton JA, Froome LC, Farrell RE, Wells SA. Multiple endocrine neoplasia type IIb, the most aggressive form of medullary thyroid carcinoma. *Surg Clin North Am* 1979; **59**: 109–18.

9 Samaan NA, Schultz PN, Hickey RC. Medullary thyroid carcinoma: prognosis of familial versus sporadic disease and the role of radiotherapy. *J Clin Endocrinol Metab* 1988; **67**: 801–5.

10 Farndon JR, Leight GS, Dilley WG *et al.* Familial medullary thyroid carcinoma without associated endocrinopathies: a distinct clinical entity. *B J Surg* 1986; **73**: 278–81.

11 Ponder BAJ, Finer N, Coffey R *et al.* Family screening in medullary thyroid carcinoma presenting without a family history. *Q J Med* 1988; **67**: 299–308.

12 Sizemore GW, Carney JA, Heath HI. Epidemiology of medullary carcinoma of the thyroid gland: a 5-year experience (1971–76). *Surg Clin North Am* 1977; **57**: 633–45.

13 Socinski MA. Endocrine tumors and malignancy. In: Skarin AT, ed. *Dana–Farber Cancer Institute Atlas of Diagnostic Oncology.* Philadelphia: JB Lippincott, 1991: 7.1–35.

14 Ljungberg O, Bondeson L, Bondeson A-G. Differentiated thyroid carcinoma, intermediate type: a new tumour entity with features of follicular and parafollicular cell carcinoma. *Hum Pathol* 1984; **15**: 218–28.

15 Ljungberg O, Nilsson PO. Hyperplastic and neoplastic changes in ultimobranchial remnants in parafollicular (C) cells in bulls: a histologic and immunohistochemical study. *Vet Pathol* 1985; **22** 95–103.

16 Block MA, Jackson CE, Greenawald KA, Yott JB, Tashjian AH. Clinical characteristics distinguishing hereditary from sporadic medullary thyroid carcinoma. *Arch Surg* 1980; **115**: 142–8.

17 Gibson WGH, Peng T-C, Croker BP. Age-associated C-cell hyperplasia in the human thyroid. *Am J Pathol* 1982; **106**: 388–93.

18 O'Toole K, Fenoglio-Preiser C, Pushparaj N. Endocrine changes

associated with the aging process. III. Effect of age on the number of calcitonin immunoreactive cells in the thyroid gland. *Hum Pathol* 1985; **16**: 991–1000.

19 Gagel RF, Levy ML, Donovan DT, Alford BR, Wheeler T, Tschen JA. Multiple endocrine neoplasia type 2a associated wtih cutaneous lichen amyloidosis. *Ann Intern Med* 1989; **111**: 802–6.

20 Gagel RF, Tashjian AH, Cummings T *et al.* The clinical outcome of prospective screening for multiple endocrine neoplasia type 2a. *N Engl J Med* 1988; **318**: 478–84.

21 Mathew CGP, Chin KS, Easton DF *et al.* A linked genetic marker for multiple endocrine neoplasia type 2A on chromosome 10. *Nature* 1987; **328**: 527–8.

22 Simpson NE, Kidd KK, Goodfellow PJ *et al.* Assignment of multiple endocrine neoplasia type 2A to chromosome 10 by linkage. *Nature* 1987; **328**: 528–30.

23 Gardner E, Papi L, Easton DF *et al.* Genetic linkage studies map the multiple endocrine neoplasia type 2 loci to a small interval on chromosome 10q11.2. *Hum Mol Genet* 1993; **2**: 241–6.

24 Mole SE, Mulligan LM, Healey CS, Ponder BAJ, Tunnacliffe A. Localisation of the gene for multiple endocrine neoplasia type 2A to a 480-kb region in chromosome band 10q11.2. *Hum Mol Genet* 1993; **2**: 247–52.

25 Takahashi M, Buma Y, Hiai H. Isolation of ret proto-oncogene cDNA with an amino-terminal signal. *Oncogene* 1989; **4**: 805–6.

26 Takahashi M, Buma Y, Taniguchi M. Identification of ret proto-oncogene products in neuroblastoma and leukemia cells. *Oncogene* 1991; **6**: 297–301.

27 Pawson T, Schlessinger J. SH2 and SH3 domains. *Curr Biol* 1993; **3**: 434–42.

28 Pazin MJ, Williams LT. Triggering signaling cascades by receptor tyrosine kinases. *Trend Biochem Sci* 1992; **17**: 374–8.

29 Resh MD. Interaction of tyrosine kinase oncoproteins with cellular membranes. *Biochim Biophys Acta* 1993; **1155**: 307–22.

30 Mulligan LM, Kwok JBJ, Healey CS *et al.* Germline mutations of the *RET* proto-oncogene in multiple endocrine neoplasia type 2A. *Nature* 1993; **363**: 458–60.

31 Donis-Keller H, Dou S, Chi D *et al.* Mutations in the *RET* proto-oncogene are associated with MEN 2A and FMTC. *Hum Mol Genet* 1993; **2**: 851–6.

32 Hofstra RMW, Landsvater RM, Ceccherini I *et al.* A mutation in the *RET* proto-oncogene associated with multiple endocrine neoplasia type 2B and sporadic medullary thyroid carcinoma. *Nature* 1994; **367**: 375–6.

33 Eng C, Smith DP, Mulligan LM *et al.* Point mutation within the tyrosine kinase domain of the *RET* proto-oncogene in multiple endocrine neoplasia type 2B and related sporadic tumours. *Hum Mol Genet* 1994; **3**: 237–41.

34 Carlson KM, Dou S, Chi D *et al.* Single missence mutation in the tyrosine kinase catalytic domain of the *RET* proto-oncogene is associated with multiple endocrine neoplasia type 2B. *Proc Natl Acad Sci USA* 1994; **91**: 1579–83.

35 Eng C, Smith DP, Mulligan LM *et al.* A novel point mutation in the tyrosine kinase domain of the *RET* proto-oncogene in sporadic medullary thyroid carcinoma and in a family with FMTC. *Oncogene* 1995; **10**: 509–13.

36 Bolino A, Schuffenecker I, Luo Y *et al. RET* mutations in exons 13 and 14 of FMTC patients. *Oncogene* 1995; **10**: 2415–19.

37 Mulligan LM, Marsh DJ, Robinson BG *et al.* Genotype-phenotype correlation in MEN 2: Report of the International *RET* Mutation Consortium. *J Intern Med* 1995; **238**: 343–6.

38 Mulligan LM, Eng C, Healey CS *et al.* Specific mutations of the *RET* proto-oncogene are related to disease phenotype in MEN 2A and FMTC. *Nature Genet* 1994; **6**: 70–4.

39 Schuffenecker I, Billaud M, Calender A *et al. RET* proto-oncogene mutations in French MEN 2A and FMTC families. *Hum Mol Genet* 1994; **3**: 1939–43.

40 Frank-Raue K, Höppner W, Frilling A *et al.* Mutations of the *RET* proto-oncogene in German MEN families: relation between genotype and phenotype. *J Clin Endocrinol Metab* 1996; **81**: 1780–3.

41 Gardner E, Mulligan LM, Eng C *et al.* Haplotype analysis of MEN 2 mutations. *Hum Mol Genet* 1994; **3**: 1771–4.

42 Rossel M, Schuffenecker I, Schlumberger M *et al.* Detection of a germline mutation at codon 918 of the RET proto-oncogene in French MEN 2B families. *Hum Genet* 1995; **95**: 403–6.

43 Toogood AA, Eng C, Smith DP, Ponder BAJ, Shalet SM. No mutation at codon 918 of the *RET* gene in a family with multiple endocrine neoplasia type 2B. *Clin Endocrinol* 1995; **43**: 759–62.

44 Carlson KM, Bracamontes J, Jackson CE *et al.* Parent-of-origin effects in multiple endocrine neoplasia type 2B. *Am J Hum Genet* 1994; **55**: 1076–82.

45 Zedenius J, Wallin G, Hamberger B, Nordenskjöld M, Weber G, Larsson C. Somatic and MEN 2A *de novo* mutations identified in the RET proto-oncogene by screening of sporadic MTCs. *Hum Mol Genet* 1994; **3**: 1259–62.

46 Blaugrund JE, Johns MM, Eby YJ *et al. RET* proto-oncogene mutations in inherited and sporadic medullary thyroid cancer. *Hum Mol Genet* 1994; **3**: 1895–7.

47 Eng C, Mulligan LM, Smith DP *et al.* Mutation of the *RET* proto-oncogene in sporadic medullary thyroid carcinoma. *Genes Chrom Cancer* 1995; **12**: 209–12.

48 Komminoth P, Kunz EK, Matias-Guiu X *et al.* Analysis of *RET* proto-oncogene point mutations distinguishes heritable from non-inheritable medullary thyroid carcinomas. *Cancer* 1995; **76**: 479–89.

49 Dou S, Chi D, Carlson KM, Moley JA, Wells SAJ, Donis-Keller H. RET proto-oncogene mutations associated with sporadic cases of medullary thyroid carcinoma. *The Fifth International Workshop on Multiple Endocrine Neoplasia* 1994: 73 (abstract).

50 Marsh DJ, Learoyd DL, Andrews SD *et al.* Somatic mutations in the *RET* proto-oncogene in sporadic medullary thyroid carcinoma. *Clin Endocrinol* 1996; in press.

51 Marsh DJ, Andrew SD, Eng C *et al.* Germline and somatic mutations in an oncogene—*RET* mutations in inherited medullary thyroid carcinoma. *Cancer Res* 1996; **44**: 249–57.

52 Lindor NM, Honchel R, Khosla S, Thibodeau SN. Mutations in the *RET* proto-oncogene in sporadic phaeochromocytomas. *J Clin Endocrinol Metab* 1995; **80**: 627–9.

53 Beldjord B, Desclaux-Arramond F, Raffin-Sanson M *et al.* The *RET* proto-oncogene in sporadic pheochromocytomas: frequent MEN 2-like mutations and new molecular defects. *J Clin Endocrinol Metab* 1995; **80**: 2063-8.

54 Komminoth P, Kunz E, Hiort O *et al.* Detection of *RET* proto-oncogene point mutations in paraffin-embedded pheochromocytoma specimens by nonradioactive single-strand conformation polymorphism analysis and direct sequencing. *Am J Pathol* 1994; **145**: 922–9.

55 Eng C, Crossey PA, Mulligan LM *et al.* Mutations of the *RET* proto-oncogene and the von Hippel–Lindau disease tumour suppressor gene in sporadic and syndromic phaeochromocytoma. *J Med Genet* 1995; **32**: 934–7.

56 Myers SM, Eng C, Ponder BAJ, Mulligan LM. Characterization of *RET* proto-oncogene 3′ splicing variants and polyadenylation sites:

a novel C-terminal for RET. *Oncogene* 1995; **11**: 2039–45.

57 Mulligan LM, Gardner E, Smith BA, Mathew CGP, Ponder BAJ. Genetic events in tumour initiation and progression in multiple endocrine neoplasia. *Genes Chrom Cancer* 1993; **6**: 166–77.

58 Santoro M, Carlomagno F, Romano A *et al.* Activation of *RET* as a dominant transforming gene by germline mutations of MEN 2A and MEN 2B. *Science* 1995; **267**: 381–3.

59 Okamoto E, Ueda T. Embryogenesis of intramural ganglia of the gut and its relation to Hirschsprung disease. *J Pediatr Surg* 1967; **10**: 437–43.

60 Lyonnet S, Bolino A, Pelet A *et al.* A gene for Hirschsprung disease maps to the proximal long arm of chromosome 10. *Nature Genet* 1993; **4**: 346–50.

61 Angrist M, Kauffman E, Slaugenhaupt SA *et al.* A gene for Hirschsrpung disease (megacolon) in the pericentromeric region of human chromosome 10. *Nature Genet* 1993; **4**: 351–6.

62 Edery P, Lyonnet S, Mulligan LM *et al.* Mutations of the *RET* proto-oncogene in Hirschsprung's disease. *Nature* 1994; **367**: 378–80.

63 Romeo G, Ronchetto P, Luo Y *et al.* Point mutations affecting the tyrosine kinase domain of the *RET* proto-oncogene in Hirschsprung's disease. *Nature* 1994; **367**: 377–8.

64 Angrist M, Bolk S, Thiel B *et al.* Mutation analysis of the RET receptor tyrosine kinase in Hirschsprung disease. *Hum Mol Genet* 1995; **4**: 821–30.

65 Attié T, Pelet A, Edery P *et al.* Diversity of *RET* proto-oncogene mutations in familial and sporadic Hirschsprung disease. *Hum Mol Genet* 1995; **4**: 1381–6.

66 Pasini B, Borrello MG, Greco A *et al.* Loss of function effect of *RET* mutations causing Hirschsprung disease. *Nature Genet* 1995; **10**: 35–40.

67 Mulligan LM, Eng C, Attié T *et al.* Diverse phenotypes associated with exon 10 mutations of the *RET* proto-oncogene. *Hum Mol Genet* 1994; **3**: 2163–7.

68 Borst MJ, van Camp JM, Peacock ML, Decker RA. Mutation analysis of multiple endocrine neoplasia type 2A associated with Hirschsprung's disease. *Surgery* 1995; **117**: 386–9.

69 Schwerk WB, Grun R, Wahl R. Ultrasound diagnosis of C-cell carcinoma of the thyroid. *Cancer* 1985; **55**: 624–30.

70 Clarke SEM, Lazaro CR, Wright P, Sampson C, Maisey MN. Pentavalent [99mTc] DMSA, [131I] MIBG, and [99mTc]msp—an evaluation of three imaging techniques in patients with medullary thyroid carcinoma of the thyroid. *J Nucl Med* 1988; **29**: 33–8.

71 Wells SA, Baylin SB, Johnsrude IS *et al.* Thyroid venous catheterisation in the early diagnosis of familial medullary thyroid carcinoma. *Ann Surg* 1982; **196**: 505–11.

72 Rougier P, Parmentier C, Laplanche A *et al.* Medullary thyroid carcinoma: prognostic factors and treatment. *Int J Radiat Oncol Biol Phys* 1983; **9**: 161–9.

73 Lips CJM, Landsvater RM, Höppener JWM *et al.* Clinical screening as compared with DNA analysis in families with multiple endocrine neoplasia type 2A. *N Engl J Med* 1994; **331**: 828–35.

74 Marsh DJ, McDowall D, Hyland VJ *et al.* The identification of false positive responses to the pentagastrin stimulation test in RET mutation negative members of MEN 2A families. *Clin Endocrinol* 1996; **44**: 213–20.

75 Telenius-Berg M, Almqvist S, Berg B *et al.* Screening for medullary carcinoma of the thyroid in families with Sipple's syndrome: evaluation of new stimulation tests. *Eur J Clin Invest* 1977; **7**: 7–16.

76 Wells SA, Baylin SB, Linehan WM, Farrell RE, Cox EB, Cooper CW. Provocative agents and the diagnosis of medullary carcinoma of the thyroid gland. *Ann Surg* 1978; **188**: 139–41.

77 Dymling JF, Ljungberg O, Hillyard CJ, Greenberg PB, Evans IMA, MacIntyre I. Whisky: a new provocative test for calcitonin secretion. *Acta Endocrinol* 1976; **82**: 500–9.

78 Body JJ, Heath H. "Nonspecific" increases in plasma immunoreactive calcitonin in healthy individuals: discrimination from medullary thyroid carcinoma by a new extraction technique. *Clin Chem* 1984; **30**: 511–14.

79 McMahon R, Mulligan LM, Healey CS *et al.* Direct, non-radioactive detection of mutations in multiple endocrine neoplasia type 2A families. *Hum Mol Genet* 1994; **3**: 643–6.

80 Wells SA, Chi DD, Toshima D *et al.* Predictive DNA testing and prophylactic thyroidectomy in patients at risk for multiple endocrine neoplasia type 2A. *Ann Surg* 1994; **200**: 237–50.

81 Eng C, Mulligan LM, Smith DP *et al.* Low frequency of germline mutations in the *RET* proto-oncogene in patients with apparently sporadic medullary thyroid carcinoma. *Clin Endocrinol* 1995; **43**: 123–7.

82 Russell CF, van Heerden JAV, Sizemore GW *et al.* The surgical management of medullary thyroid carcinoma. *Ann Surg* 1983; **197**: 42–8.

83 Block MA, Jackson CE, Tashjian AH. Management of occult medullary thyroid carcinoma. *Arch Surg* 1978; **113**: 368-72.

84 Tisell L-E, Hansson G, Jansson S, Salander H. Reoperation in the treatment of medullary thyroid carcinoma. *Surgery* 1985; **99**: 60–6.

85 Nieuwenhuijzen-Kruseman AC, Bussemaker JK, Frolich M. Radioiodine in the treatment of hereditary medullary carcinoma of the thyroid. *J Clin Endocrinol Metab* 1984; **59**: 491–4.

86 Hoskin PJ, Harmer CJ. Chemotherapy for thyroid cancer. *Radiother Oncol* 1987; **10**: 187–94.

87 Pertursson S. Metastatic medullary thyroid carcinoma. Complete response to combination therapy with dacarbazine and 5-fluorouracil. *Cancer* 1988; **62**: 1899–1903.

88 Eng C, Clayton D, Shuffenecker I *et al.* The relationship between specific *RET* proto-oncogene mutations and disease phenotype in multiple endocrine neoplasia type 2. International *RET* Mutation Consortium analysis. *JAMA* 1996; **276**: 1575–9.

89 Jing S, Wen D, Yu Y *et al.* GDNF-induced activation of the Ret protein tyrosine kinase is mediated by GDNFR-α, a novel receptor for GDNF. *Cell* 1996; **85**: 1113–24.

90 Trupp M, Arenas E, Fainzilber M *et al.* Functional receptor for GDNF encoded by the *c-ret* proto-oncogene. *Nature* 1996; **381**: 785–9.

91 Durbec P, Marcos-Gutierrez CV, Kilkenny C *et al.* GDNF signalling through the Ret receptor tyrosine kinase. *Nature* 1996; **381**: 789–93.

92 Treanor JS, Goodman L, de Sauvage F *et al.* Characterization of a multicomponent receptor for GDNF. *Nature* 1996; **382**: 80–3.

Part 10
Hypothalamo-Pituitary–Gonadal Axis

CHAPTER 48

Basic physiology of the hypothalamo-pituitary–gonadal axis

W.G. Rossmanith

The endocrine basis of human reproduction

The primary organs involved in the endocrine control of human reproductive function are the brain, the pituitary and the gonads. Optimal function of each constituent is essential for successful procreation. An orchestrated interplay of interrelated interactions between these organs is required to ensure activation of the reproductive axis. To this end, their functions are integrated into multifaceted connections in order to coordinate release of humoral substances. Reproductive processes ultimately cumulate in the production and excretion of mature gametes from the gonads and in the establishment of appropriate secretion of gonadal hormones.

Control of human reproduction: anatomical and physiological premises

It is generally accepted that the brain is the command centre which initiates all events required for successful reproduction. It integrates various inputs from inside and outside the central nervous system into an efferent signal that travels to distant sites. The question of how the brain translates hormonal inputs that it receives into an output that supports reproduction is still unresolved. Therefore, understanding of the physiology of reproduction starts with analysis of central nervous function.

The hypothalamus (see also Chapters 5 and 6)

The hypothalamus is the area which integrates cerebral (cortex, limbic system), environmental (light, temperature) and metabolic cues (steroid feedback) from close and distant sites, and thus represents the final common pathway for communication between the brain and the gonads. This structure lies at the base of the diencephalon and extends from the mamillary bodies to the optic chiasm (tuber cinereum). The infundibular stalk protrudes from the mid-line, and the portion of this stalk that interfaces with the hypothalamus represents the median eminence. The external zone of the median eminence contains the short capillary loops that form part of the portal plexus. This area is rich with a variety of different types of nerve endings, some glial cells and ependymal processes, but few neuronal cell bodies. A variety of neurotransmitters are concentrated in this region. The internal zone of the median eminence contains fibre tracts with hypothalamic connection to the neurohypophysis. The diverse population and the complex interconnections of neuronal cell types that the hypothalamus contains reflect the range of physiological functions that it serves. Most neurons aggregate in clusters with a primary location in the medial part of the hypothalamus. The hypothalamic area with particular importance for human reproduction is the arcuate nucleus [1], which is situated ventrally along the side of the third ventricle in the region of the infundibular recess in direct vicinity to the median eminence. This nucleus comprises a brain region outside of the blood–brain barrier, and can therefore be influenced by blood-borne factors. Relevant to reproductive function is the ventromedial nucleus (dorsal to the arcuate nucleus) which acts to relay extrahypothalamic connections for the regulation of feeding and sexual behavior. The medial preoptic area is not strictly limited to the hypothalamus and acts to control sexual behaviour and secretion of anterior pituitary hormones. The suprachiasmatic nucleus (SCN) as a small nucleus on the top of the optic chiasm receives inputs from fibers from the retina and serves to coordinate biological rhythms.

Hypothalamic releasing and inhibiting hormones are mostly peptides derived from larger precursor molecules that are cleaved and processed to the mature hormones. These hypothalamic hormones not only regulate pituitary hormone release, but most of them also act as neurotransmitters elsewhere in the nervous system. One of the first releasing hormones to be identified was gonadotrophin-releasing hormone (GnRH), also known as luteinising hormone-releasing hormone (LHRH). GnRH-containing neurons originate in the olfactory placode from which they migrate during embryonic development into the preoptic area and arcuate nucleus [2]. Most GnRH-containing neurons are concentrated in the arcuate nucleus. As neurosecretory cells, they terminate with their axons on fenestrated capillaries of a portal system which represents the non-nervous connection with cells of the anterior pituitary. When GnRH neurons become activated, they release GnRH into the portal system from where it travels to the anterior pituitary to exert its biological action on cells that show surface-bound cell receptors. Although the majority of GnRH neurons project to the median eminence where GnRH can be released into the portal vasculature, there are currently no anatomical or cellular characteristics that indicate the identity of these GnRH neurons.

GnRH has been characterised as a decapeptide [3], its active form being derived from precursors of high molecular weight. The biological half-life of GnRH is limited to 4–6 minutes; the compound is then rapidly cleared by specific hypothalamic endopeptidase regulated, among other factors, by ovarian sex steroids. GnRH binds to specific receptors on the cell surface whose density is also regulated by sex steroids. Binding to the receptor provokes a series of intracellular events involving calcium, cyclic adenosine monophosphate (cAMP) and arachnidonic acid [4]. GnRH regulates the gene expression for, and synthesis and secretion of, the pituitary gonadotrophins, and thus controls the release of both luteinising hormone (LH) and follicle-stimulating hormone (FSH) from the anterior pituitary. How one releasing hormone can independently regulate the release of two pituitary hormones is still a matter of debate, but may occur via distinct changes in the pattern of GnRH release [5]. A wide variety of neurotransmitters have been found in terminals making synaptic contacts with GnRH neurons. Many hypothalamic neurosecretory neurons that synthesise releasing and inhibiting hormones also secrete additional neurotransmitters, which possibly exert autocrine or paracrine influence directly at the GnRH-containing neurons [6].

Pituitary

Hypophysial cells that synthesise and secrete the gonadotrophins have been identified by their cytochemical and ultrastructural features. These cells are found scattered in the pars distalis of the adenohypophysis and store and secrete the gonadotrophins LH and FSH. In contrast to other adenohypophysial hormones produced by their particular cell types, LH and FSH are produced in one single cell type, the gonadotrophs. LH and FSH are glycoproteins composed of a common α-chain and a β-subunit unique for each glycoprotein. The messenger RNA (mRNA) encoding for the unique β-subunit appears to be differentially regulated, dependent on the stimulation mode of GnRH [7]. The capacity of the gonadotrophs to synthesise, store and release gonadotrophins is controlled by hypothalamic GnRH, local factors within the pituitary and circulating steroid hormones from the gonads [8]. In this system, sex steroids act by increasing GnRH receptors in number and density on the gonadotrophs. In the gonadotrophs, the LH and FSH concentrations vary in accordance with the menstrual cycle, reaching peak concentrations around the mid-cycle gonadotrophin surge. An increased synthesis of gonadotrophins in excess of release occurs in the preovulatory phase and ensures that the reservoir of pituitary gonadotrophins is replenished for the mid-cycle surge.

LH and FSH bind to specific cell-surface receptors at various targets, in particular at the gonads. Binding initiates a whole cascade of intracellular events, involving G-protein coupling, activation of adenyl cyclase, and coupling of cAMP to protein kinases for the promotion of steroidogenesis [9]. In the female, FSH acts primarily on the granulosa cells and promotes follicular maturation. LH dominates the secretory activity of theca interna cells in regulating androgen production and is indispensable for the maintenance and optimal function of the human corpus luteum [10]. In the male, FSH acts to promote production of mature sperms within the seminiferous tubules, while LH regulates production and release of androgens by the testes.

The human gonads

The human gonads serve two principal functions for reproductive physiology. They produce and release mature gametes (sperms, oocytes) as a requirement for fertilisation, and they also have the capacity to synthesise and release adequate quantities of steroid hormones with diverse endogenous functions. While gonads are indispensable for the production of gametes, production of sex steroids is not strictly confined to the gonads, but is also found in other tissues, such as in the adrenal gland and adipose tissue. The two major functions of the gonads are supported by structural compartments within the testes or the ovaries. In the testes, production and release of mature sperms occurs in the seminiferous tubules, while the major production site of androgens are the Leydig cells. In the ovaries, the immature gametes grow to full maturity in follicles, and the two principal sex steroids 17β-oestradiol and progesterone are derived from granulosa cells within the growing follicle and from the luteinised cells of the corpus luteum.

The human gonads are paired spheroid structures that originate from the genital ridges. At about the third gestational week, primordial germ cells migrate from the ectoderm of the yolk sac to the genital ridges and are incorporated into the developing gonads by 6 weeks. During fetal development, the female gonads descend, but stay intra-abdominally with a retroperitoneal location; they are attached to the posterior aspect of the uterine broad ligament by the mesovarium. In the male, the testes remain intra-abdominally for the majority of fetal life, but migrate shortly before birth to the scrotum, an extra-abdominal pouch derived from the labioscrotal folds. This mechanism of extra-abdominal placement serves to maintain a testicular temperature lower than intra-abdominally, which is required for optimal spermatogenesis.

Testes

The testes (average weight, 25 g; length, 4 cm) are protected by thick fibrous layers, the tunica albuginea and the tunica vaginalis. They contain coiled seminiferous tubules which account for the majority of testicular mass. The seminiferous tubules drain into the epididymis attached posteriorly to the upper pole of the testes. The vas deferens enters the abdominal cavity and opens into the ejaculatory duct in the prostatic portion at the base of the bladder. Blood supply for the testes is provided by testicular branches of the abdominal aorta. Veins from the testes form a plexus (plexus pampiniformis) and drain into the testicular veins of which the left testicular ends in the renal vein and the right directly in the inferior vena cava.

The seminiferous tubules consist of germ and Sertoli cells which cover the thickness of the tubule wall and separate it into a basal and adluminal compartment. They rest on the basal lamina and are attached to one another by specialised junctional complexes near the basal portion of each cell. Stem germ cells in the basal compartment are known as spermatogonia and are continuously replenished by mitotic division; spermatogonia migrate to the luminal compartment where a series of divisions takes place. This process yields the production of mature spermatids that carry the haploid human chromosomal set. Spermatids undergo transformation into spermatozoa, a process of spermatogenesis that takes approximately 80 days to complete. Sertoli cells in this system supply the nutrients for the maturational process to the spermatids; they also secrete a variety of protein factors which regulate and coordinate sperm development and the release of mature sperm into the lumen. They release an androgen-binding protein which can concentrate testosterone in the lumen thus providing high concentrations of androgens to the developing gametes. Spermatogenesis is under the control of FSH which acts on Sertoli cells to modulate the production of local factors. Semen is composed of mature spermatids as well as the accumulated products from several locations of the male genital tract. It is rich in fructose that sperms, with their lack of cellular metabolic machinery, have to rely on. The volume of semen produced in each ejaculation varies between 2 and 4 ml, with an average sperm content between 10 and 80×10^6/ml (see also Chapter 50).

Production of androgens, another principal function of the testes, is achieved by a specialised cell system. The interstitial Leydig cells (about 10% of the total testicular volume) are situated within the connective tissue stroma of the testes and represent lipid-rich cells which cluster within the intertubular tissue. The production of their hormones and local factors is under primary control of pituitary LH which binds to specific high-affinity glycoprotein receptors at the cell surfaces. By activating an intracellular cascade of events involving coupling to G-proteins, production of cAMP and activation of protein kinase A, LH is capable of stimulating the production of testosterone and other testicular androgens.

Ovaries

The female gonads represent a pair of retroperitoneal organs (average weight, 40 g; length, 3 cm). As ever-changing tissue, it varies from the male gonads in its ability to intermittently produce mature gametes, mostly just one oocyte at a time. Many features of the ovarian reproductive cycle compare with the conditions found in the male, but additional mechanisms add on to cyclical phenomena. Ovarian function ensures cyclic germ-cell production and the maintenance of an appropriate sex steroid environment in support of possible fertilisation. Folliculogenesis with the production of gametes and the concomitant release of sex steroids occur in structurally distinct compartments, which are functionally interrelated for optimal tuning. Primary oocytes are found at about 12 weeks of gestation and arrest at this stage of their development. The primordial follicles surrounding these oocytes are characterised by a flat layer of granulosa cells which originate from the sex cords. The number of oocytes in the ovaries reach a maximum at mid-gestation (4 million) when the number gradually declines to about 1 million at birth. At puberty, approximately 40 000 primordial follicles are discerned, and just 400 are destined to ovulate in a woman's fertile period, which underlines the redundancy of the reproductive system.

Primary follicles are surrounded by cubic granulosa cells in several layers, but do not show any blood supply. The growth and development of early follicular forms is continuous from fetal life to childhood and occurs independent of the cyclical ovarian changes. Thus, even during anovulatory periods such as in pregnancy, during the post-partum period or use of oral contraceptives, primary follicles continue to grow. Under the influence of FSH, these follicles develop into secondary follicles characterised by a multilayer of granulosa cells, which are separated by a basal membrane from the theca cells. The capacity of a follicle to thrive is limited by its initial maturational stage, the hormonal environment and its ensuing vascularisation. Secondary follicles start to produce oestradiol by an action of FSH on its receptors on the granulosa cells. FSH induces the activity of aromatase in the granulosa cells with the ability to aromatise androgens into oestrogens. Thus, the fate and future of any given follicle is critically dependent on its capacity to convert the androgenic into an oestrogen-dominated follicular micromilieu [11]. Only a small minority of follicles undergoes all these structural changes and grows to a preovulatory tertiary (or Graafian) follicle. The majority of follicles shows atretic changes at various sizes and developmental stages. Among the cohort of follicles recruited in the preceding cycle, the dominant follicle alone is destined to become fully mature and to ovulate.

A tertiary or Graafian follicle is characterised by the development of a large fluid-filled cavity, the antrum. Within this structure, the oocyte resides on a stalk of granulosa cells (cumulus oophorus). At this follicular stage, a maximal density of LH receptors is induced by FSH on the cells, providing optimal conditions for the luteinisation of the follicle after rupture. In the preovulatory period, the meiotic division of the oocyte is finalised. Granulosa cells in immediate contact with the oocyte produce and secrete a peptide known as oocyte maturation inhibitor (OMI). Production of this factor is inhibited by LH, and its suppression by high levels of LH in the preovulatory period ensures completion of meiosis. Follicular rupture and expulsion of the oocyte is accomplished by combined effects of various intrafollicular factors, amongst them prostaglandins and relaxin [11]. Activation of plasminogen activators in the follicular wall by gonadotrophins, prostaglandins and progesterone initiates a whole cascade of events, ultimately leading to formation of collagenases and rupture of follicular membrane. Follicular fluid is released together with the oocyte, thus providing nutrients and a high concentration of sex steroids. After rupture, the oocyte migrates into the Fallopian tubes where it may be fertilised. The ruptured follicle is then transformed by vascular and cellular proliferation into the corpus luteum. This formation is not an isolated endocrine event, but the consequence of normal follicular maturation and ovulation.

The corpus luteum is an organ with a predetermined lifespan of 12–14 days. It accumulates large quantitites of cholesterol giving it the yellowish appearance and covering the biological demand for enhanced steroidogenesis. The main luteal steroid is progesterone from luteinised granulosa cells, whose synthesis by far surpasses the amount of oestradiol in this organ. Progesterone serves to transform the endometrium in preparation for the blastocyst to implant. As a luteotrophic hormone, LH is essential in the maintenance of the endocrine function of the human corpus luteum, and its absence causes premature luteal demise. Luteal function may be sustained by the presence of human chorionic gonadotrophin (hCG) produced by the early blastocyst. This glycoprotein, with structural and biological similarities to LH, binds to identical membrane receptors on luteinised granulosa cells of the corpus luteum and maintains its function, such that the endometrium is not shed and implantation of the blastocyst can occur. In the absence of fertilisation, the corpus luteum begins to involute towards the end of the menstrual cycle, presumably by factors endogenous to the organ [9], and menstruation ensues as consequence of progesterone withdrawal.

Steroidogenesis

The principal sex steroids produced by the follicular apparatus are oestrogens (oestradiol, oestrone), progesterone (in the corpus luteum) and androgens (particularly androstenedione and testosterone), whereas the testes produce mainly testosterone. All these steroids share a common pathway for their synthesis in that they derive from cholesterol. This compound is converted to pregnenolone; the key enzyme cholesterol desmolase is under control of LH. In the stepwise cascade of conversions during steroidogenesis, progesterone and androgens are mandatory precursors of oestrogens; their conversion into oestrogens is catalysed by an FSH-dependent enzyme, aromatase. The capacity of an endocrine organ to produce predominantly androgens or oestrogens is determined by the activity of aromatase the organ is endowed with. In the human, oestradiol is the major steroid; it is produced mainly in the growing follicle and the corpus luteum, but also stems from other sources such as adipose tissue. Steroidogenesis in the growing follicle is compartmentalised and occurs within two distinct structures in the secundary and tertiary follicles (Fig. 48.1). In the theca cell layer, androgens are synthesised and released under the control of pituitary LH and passively diffuse through the basal membrane of the follicle into the fluid surrounding the granulosa cells. After uptake in the granulosa cells, androgens are aromatised to oestrogens. Theca cells do not only produce androgens, but also progesterone, which may serve, amongst other purposes, as precursor for the synthesis of androgens in the theca interna. In addition, granulosa cells are the source of a variety of products such as peptides like inhibin and activin (see below), vasopressin and prostaglandins. The physiological function

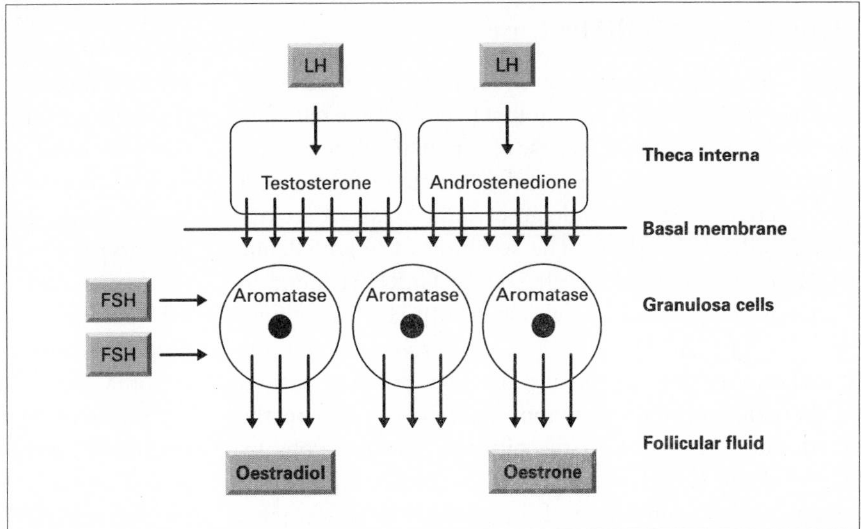

Fig. 48.1 Concept of compartmentalised synthesis and release of sex steroids from the human follicle.

of these products is at present unresolved, but may relate to a paracrine control of ovarian function, to the local regulation of ovulation and luteolysis [9].

When serum concentrations of FSH are low or the bioavailability of this hormone is decreased, the catalysing effects of aromatase are compromised and androgens accumulate in the follicular fluid. Growing follicles become atretic, when androgens dominate the follicular micromilieu. When a follicle is richly endowed with FSH receptors and exposed to increasing FSH concentrations, it has the capacity to grow. For this purpose, oestradiol from the growing follicle induces not only its own, but also FSH receptors in secondary follicles. This process is further self-perpetuated by induction of FSH and LH receptors through FSH itself. Thus, the FSH-dependent induction of LH receptors establishes the basis for LH-induced processes around the mid-cycle surge and for luteinisation of the tertiary follicle. From about day 8 of the menstrual cycle, serum concentrations of oestradiol steadily increase, signalling growth of the dominant follicle. Increasing LH secretion raises the production of androgens in the theca cells, which, with the exception of the growing dominant follicle, is deleterious to the remaining cohort of recruited follicles. The mechanisms by which one single follicle is selected to ovulate are far from being understood. In the preovulatory phase maximal oestradiol concentrations are attained, setting a signal for the initiation of the mid-cycle LH surge. At this stage, LH acts at the dominant follicle through FSH-induced LH receptors and induces luteinisation of the granulosa cells. This is reflected by a small but discernible increase in progesterone levels at mid-cycle, and serves to facilitate the timing and magnitude of a gonadotrophin surge [12]. Collectively, the growing follicle and *not* the hypothalamo-pituitary unit sets the biological signal for impending ovulation.

In the human male, testosterone and other androgens are produced in testicular Leydig cells under the influence of LH. Most circulating testosterone is bound to albumin and sex hormone-binding globulin (SHBG), leaving a small fraction of biologically active free testosterone. Androgenic effects at various target organs are mediated by cytosolic steroid receptors which bind to nucleoproteins and initiate DNA transcription. Androgen-sensitive tissue is capable of converting testosterone to dihydrotestosterone (DHT), a far more potent ligand for the androgen receptors. Androgens are necessary in fetal life for the differentiation of the internal and external genitalia, and during puberty for the development of the secondary sexual characteristics and for growth and body composition. In the adult male, they maintain sexual characteristics and imprint several patterns of male psychosocial behaviour.

Ontogeny of the pulsatile gonadotrophin signal

One of the fundamental observations in the chronobiology of gonadotrophin release in humans is the orchestrated interplay of multiple biological rhythms. Pituitary hormones are secreted in a rhythmic fashion, as during the human menstrual cycle, when the periodic secretion of gonadotrophins serves as an example of a monthly rhythm. In addition, hormone secretion may be synchronised to the time of day by circadian (daily) variations. Finally, most hormones are released in discrete secretory episodes or pulses (ultradian rhythm). The secretion patterns of anterior pituitary hormones usually consist of a complex combination of several interrelated rhythms.

Hypothalamic GnRH release

Most ultradian rhythms are thought to be a pituitary response to the pulsatile secretion of hypothalamic releasing and inhibiting hormones. Release of hypothalamic hormones in discrete pulses into the portal circulation suggests that neurosecretory neurons undergo periodic bursts of activity in a coordinated fashion. The secretion of hypothalamic GnRH occurs discontinuously so that GnRH is found in secretory episodes in the portal system [13]. This intermittent hypothalamic GnRH release is required to ensure episodic stimulation of gonadotrophins [1]. The ultradian pattern in the gonadotrophin secretion apparently relates to the intermittent activation of the pituitary gonadotrophs by hypothalamic (GnRH) inputs. As a direct reflection of intermittent GnRH stimulation of the pituitary gonadotrophs, episodic fluctuations have been discerned in the serum levels of gonadotrophins (Fig. 48.2). They are more prominent for the secretion of LH than for FSH, due to the shorter half-life of this compound. These secretory episodes occur at a frequency of a pulse approximately every 90 min ('circhoral activity')[14]. Close temporal and functional links between the hypothalamic GnRH secretion, its release into the portal system and the pituitary gonadotrophin response have been demonstrated [15]. Thus, a characteristic increase in neuronal electrical activity coincides with the episodic discharge of GnRH into the portal blood. Therefore, the episodic secretion of GnRH relates to a synchronisation of the electrical activity in neurosecretory neurons within the arcuate nucleus [16].

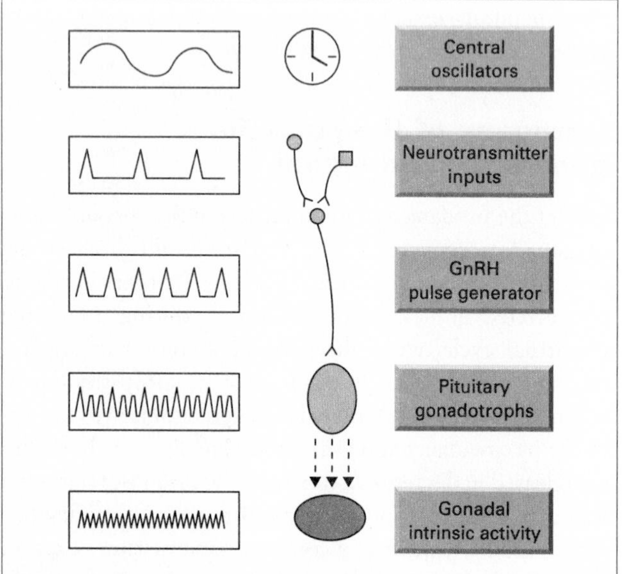

Fig. 48.2 Ontogeny of the pulsatile gonadotrophin and sex steroid release.

Since the disconnected mediobasal hypothalamus is capable of generating these pulses independent of external sources, pulsatility of GnRH release has been thought to represent an intrinsic property of GnRH neurons within the mediobasal hypothalamus [17]. There must be a network of interconnections between GnRH neurons to synchronise their activity. In the human, this pattern of LH release appears to be profoundly modulated by factors from outside the hypothalamus. The GnRH pulse generator activity is subject to feedback actions by gonadal steroids which have both stimulatory and inhibitory effects at the level of the hypothalamus. Therefore, the human hypothalamus plays a permissive, but necessary, role in generating LH peaks or 'pulses', since the character of LH pulsatile secretion is differentially regulated by the neuronal feedback of ovarian sex steroids on the central 'pulse generator'. Thus, the 'biological clock' for orchestrated LH pulsatile release presumably resides within the ovary and *not* in the hypothalamus [1].

Although the pulsatile release of pituitary hormones has been known for more than two decades, the physiological significance of pulsatile hormone release is unknown at present. It appears that at least some hormones are more effective when secreted in a pulsatile fashion. Pulsatile secretion may be required to maintain the response of the pituitary to hypothalamic hormones, so that the sensitivity of the system to the patterning of GnRH secretion is preserved. GnRH given continuously to radiolesioned monkeys increases gonadotrophin levels initially, but then this rise is followed by a sustained decrease of gonadotrophin levels (desensitisation). The pituitary response to GnRH can be restored by shifting from a continuous to a pulsatile mode of administration [18]. The frequency of hormone administration may transduce additional information to the gonadotrophs. Another possibility is that GnRH as a single hormone could differentially control the release of two different hormones in that changes in the stimulation frequencies evoke an elective release of one gonadotrophin [18]. Finally, pulsatile gonadotrophin release as reflection of intermittent GnRH stimulation may be required to economise the magnitude of the signal and help the gonads to distinguish the signal from the noise.

Neurotransmitter regulation of GnRH release

The dispersal of GnRH neurons permits regulation of these cells by a wide range of other neuronal systems. Indeed, a whole array of neurotransmitters have been implicated in the regulation of pulsatile GnRH secretion [8]. In most instances, it is not known whether a neurotransmitter system acts directly on the GnRH neuron or at a distant site that ultimately influences GnRH secretion. The innervation of

GnRH neurons is relatively sparse, but several direct inputs from transmitter systems have been demonstrated. Classical neurotransmitter such as endogenous opioid peptides, bioamines (serotonin, dopamine), *N*-methyl-D-aspartate (NMDA) and γ-aminobutyric acid (GABA) are believed to have synaptic contacts directly on GnRH neurons. Since GnRH neurons are not thought to display oestrogen receptors and do not accumulate oestradiol in themselves [19], other neuronal systems may be interposed to transduce the steroid signal into the hypothalamic neurons. One candidate may be the endogenous opiates known to exert chronic inhibition on hypothalamic GnRH release [20]. In humans, amplitudes and frequencies of LH pulsatile release can be suppressed by opiates and opioid analogues, while opiate antagonists have opposite effects [21]. The LH response to opioidergic blockade is greatest during the late follicular and luteal phase of the cycle and is absent in post-menopausal women, indicating steroid hormone regulation of endogenous opiate activity [22]. While noradrenergic neurons have been shown to mediate oestradiol feedback to hypothalamic neurons in animals, little evidence suggests a similar role for this catecholamine for the regulation of GnRH release in humans. Dopamine or dopaminergic compounds inhibit gonadotrophin release in humans, while perifusion of isolated human hypothalami clearly increases GnRH secretion [23], indicating a differential GnRH response to dopamine dependent on the conditions. In addition to these neurotransmitter systems, an increasing number of neuropeptides have been identified as colocalised with GnRH in identical neurons. These substances are cosynthesised and released from the same neurons, possibly serving as autocrine or paracrine regulators in the fine-tuning of episodic GnRH activity [6]. The large number of inputs indicates the complexity of the GnRH neuronal regulation, which also ensures the redundancy of this system.

Control of gonadotrophin secretion

Sex steroid feedback

Gonads respond to stimulation by releasing sex steroids into the circulation. These hormones serve to relay information about the status of the target tissue back to the hypothalamus and pituitary. This feedback arrangement allows hypothalamic neurosecretory neurons and endocrine cells in the pituitary to adjust their output to the demands of their gonadal organs (Fig. 48.3). Increased levels of sex steroid hormones cause the hypothalamus and pituitary to reduce their stimulation on the target tissues, a process referred to as long-loop negative feedback. Negative feedback is the most common type and acts to stabilise endocrine homeostasis. In the absence of any target tissue response, negative feedback may occur directly from the pituitary to the hypothalamus. In fact, after release from the nerve terminals, GnRH is thought to feed back to its own neurons in order to reduce further GnRH release thus establishing an ultra-short loop negative feedback system [24].

Because steroids are lipophilic, they easily cross the blood–brain barrier to act at hypothalamic sites and on the basal forebrain. Steroids affect cellular activity by binding to intracellular receptors which, in turn, attach to specific genomic sites to influence gene transcription. GnRH containing cells are thought not to have oestrogen receptors themselves nor to concentrate oestradiol [19]. Therefore, the feedback effects of oestradiol appear to be transferred by other interposed neuronal systems impinging on GnRH-containing neurons. Besides their action in the hypothalamus to control the secretion of releasing and inhibiting hormones, steroids also have direct effects on the pituitary gonadotrophs of the pars distalis [25]. While steroids by themselves do not directly alter pituitary hormone secretion, they modify the response of pituitary gonadotrophs to hypothalamic hormones. In the male, negative-feedback control of LH and FSH secretion is effected by testosterone at the hypothalamus to reduce the release frequency and amplitude of GnRH [26]. Feedback is also exerted at the pituitary to inhibit gene expression of the glycoprotein subunits in the gonadotrophs and also reduces the sensitivity of gonadotrophs to respond to hypothalamic GnRH. Some of these effects appear to be mediated by aromatisation of testosterone to oestradiol [27].

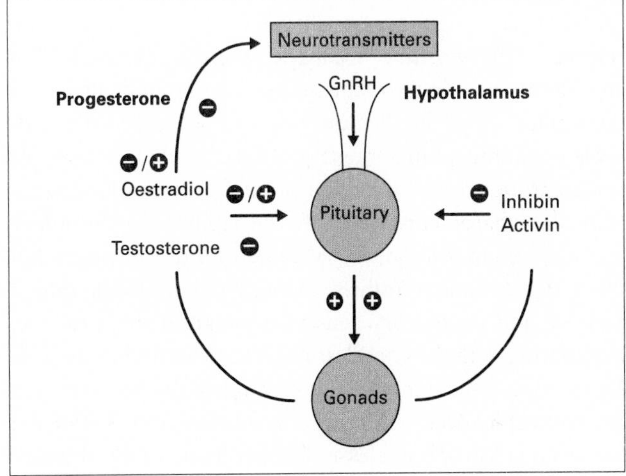

Fig. 48.3 Diagrammatic presentation of interrelations in the hypothalamo-pituitary–gonadal axis, as exemplified in the female reproductive system. Dark arrows represent stimulatory and inhibitory effects. GnRH, gonadotrophin-releasing hormone; LH, luteinising hormone.

Changing steroid feedback in the female: the human menstrual cycle

The principle of negative-feedback control of gonadotrophins by sex steroids also applies to the regulation of the human menstrual cycle. Yet, while many features of the regulation of the ovarian cycle compare to those found in the control of the male gonads, additional complex control mechanisms ensure cyclical reproductive phenomena in the female. Oestradiol from the mature follicle and from the corpus luteum represents the primary component of this inhibitory feedback. It decreases the activity of mRNA encoding the α- and β-subunits of gonadotrophins in the gonadotrophs. Synthesis and release of FSH is particularly sensitive to negative feedback by oestradiol. Secondary and tertiary follicles produce large quantities of oestradiol which, in turn, acts on granulosa cells to promote expression of FSH receptors. In the late follicular phase of the cycle, high levels of oestradiol, in concert with a rise in inhibin (see below), act to suppress further FSH secretion. This indicates the time of the selection of a dominant follicle; it occurs within a time frame ('window') when one follicle is selected to grow and ovulate while the remainder of recruited follicles become atretic. Undoubtedly, the inability of the non-dominant follicles to survive relates, at least in part, to the fall in circulating levels of FSH which occurs in the mid-follicular phase in response to negative oestrogen feedback.

In the late follicular phase, a unique shift in the feedback control of gonadotrophin secretion occurs. When rising serum titres of oestradiol exceed a threshold level (usually 600–700 pmol/l) for a critical duration (more than 36 hours), the inhibitory influence of oestradiol on gonadotrophin secretion is switched to facilitate further gonadotrophin release. This *positive* feedback exerted by oestradiol cumulates in a massive discharge of LH and also in a coincident, albeit smaller, increase of FSH, called the mid-cycle gonadotrophin surge (Fig. 48.4). While low levels of follicular oestradiol exert *negative* feedback during the follicular phase, as reflected by the inhibition of pituitary gonadotrophin release, the sustained release of oestradiol from the dominant follicle changes the feedback into a *positive* and facilitatory action on gonadotrophin release, cumulating with the gonadotrophin surge at mid-cycle [12]. During the follicular phase, gonadotrophins are stored in gonadotrophs, due to *de novo* synthesis in excess of the actual gonadotrophin release. The sensitivity of the pituitary gonadotrophs to respond to GnRH is enhanced, as oestradiol induces GnRH receptors in the pituitary [28]. A preovulatory increase in GnRH secretion reflects the GnRH secretory activity unrestrained from inhibitory neurotransmitter influences [29]; this acts to amplify the trophic effects of GnRH on the gonadotrophs. The mid-cycle gonadotrophin surge in humans implies a changing capacity of the pituitary gonadotrophs to synthesise, store and release gonadotrophins, but may also entail altered hypothalamic GnRH release as consequence of a short-lasting switch in feedback activity.

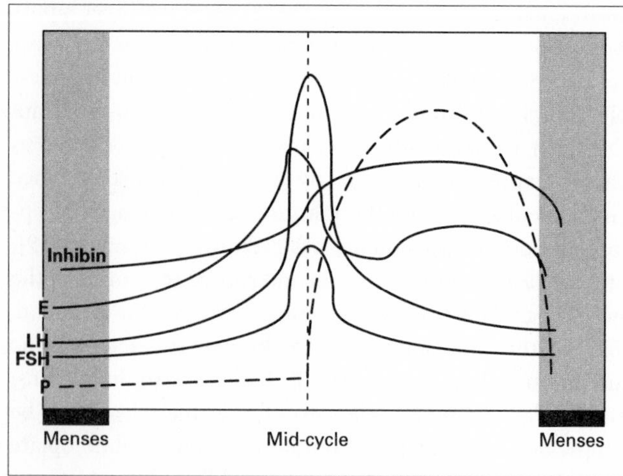

Fig. 48.4 Schematic presentation of the circulating levels of gonadotrophin (luteinising hormone (LH), follicle-stimulating hormone (FSH)), inhibin and sex steroid (oestradiol (E), progesterone) across the human menstrual cycle.

Although endocrine function of the corpus luteum is maintained by LH stimulation, the luteal production of oestradiol and progesterone starts to inhibit this LH release. While oestradiol feeds back at both the hypothalamus and pituitary [30], progesterone acts mainly at the hypothalamic site by increasing opioidergic inhibition on GnRH release [21]. Negative feedback on gonadotrophin release ultimately leads to insufficient LH to maintain production of luteal sex steroids. Clearly, luteal demise does not require a central gonadotrophin signal; local factors within the corpus luteum (prostaglandins, oxytocin) are produced under the control of oestradiol and provoke luteolysis to occur. At the time of the luteal–follicular transition, the inhibitory influences of sex steroids on the secretion of LH and FSH are virtually absent, and consequently, LH and FSH secretion may increase to facilitate recruitment of follicles and appropriate follicular production of sex steroids.

Gonadotrophin pulsatility and sex steroids

Since close temporal and functional links have been demonstrated between the hypothalamic activity and the pituitary gonadotrophin response, it is possible to determine serum gonadotrophin patterns as indirect measures of hypothalamo-pituitary activity in humans. As a result, sex steroids from the ovaries and testes have emerged as major determinants in the regulation of gonadotrophin pulsatility.

Conversely, gonadotrophin pulsatility with its corresponding pulse frequency and amplitude is unrestrained, when any significant ovarian sex steroid feedback is absent or markedly reduced.

In the human male, secreted testosterone exerts its negative feedback on pulsatile LH secretion, since serum gonadotrophin concentrations are elevated in hypogonadal men, a consequence of increased pulse frequency and amplitude [26]. Conversely, injections of testosterone restore LH pulse frequency and amplitude and return gonadotrophin levels to normal. Testosterone can block the action of GnRH at the pituitary gonadotroph, in that it reduces sensitivity presumably by receptor-mediated processes. Some of testosterone's suppressive effects may be conveyed indirectly by aromatisation to oestradiol [27].

In the female, the character of episodic LH secretion depends on the prevailing sex steroid environment (Fig. 48.5). LH pulses of high frequency, but of low amplitude are observed during periods of increasing oestradiol exposure, as in the follicular phase of the cycle. This pulse pattern is instantaneously changed to low frequency and high amplitude, when progesterone slows the hypothalamo-pituitary pulse generator during the luteal phase of the cycle. Highest LH pulse amplitude and presumably frequency are attained during the mid-cycle surge [31]. In the early follicular phase, a characteristic slowing of the LH pulse frequency is exhibited during sleep, concomitant with a rise in pulse amplitude. This slowing of frequency presumably relates to a sleep-associated increase of hypothalamic opioidergic activity. Significant ovarian steroid feedback is absent in hypogonadal women, and therefore, in this hypogonadal state, LH pulsatility may constitute the unrestrained pulse rhythm at its maximal rate [32]. As for LH pulse amplitude, this increases from the follicular to the luteal phase of the cycle, reflecting sex steroid activity on the change of pituitary sensitivity [8]. Even during the mid-cycle LH surge when maximal positive oestrogen feedback is attained, the increase in LH pulse amplitude appears to not exceed that found in hypogonadal women, suggesting that gonadotrophin pulsatility in hypogonadal women indeed represents the maximal activity of the central nerval pulse generator. A marked slowing of LH pulse frequency coincides with large pulse amplitude during the luteal phase of the menstrual cycle, reflecting the actions of progesterone on the central pulse generator (Fig. 48.5). The tight functional and temporal coupling of the LH signal to the sex steroid response from the corpus luteum emphasises the need of the target to experience gonadotrophin stimulation [33]. During the time of luteal–follicular transition, an increase in LH pulse frequency is seen. Androgens do not appear to be important for changes in the gonadotrophin pulsatility and for the regulation of the human menstrual cycle.

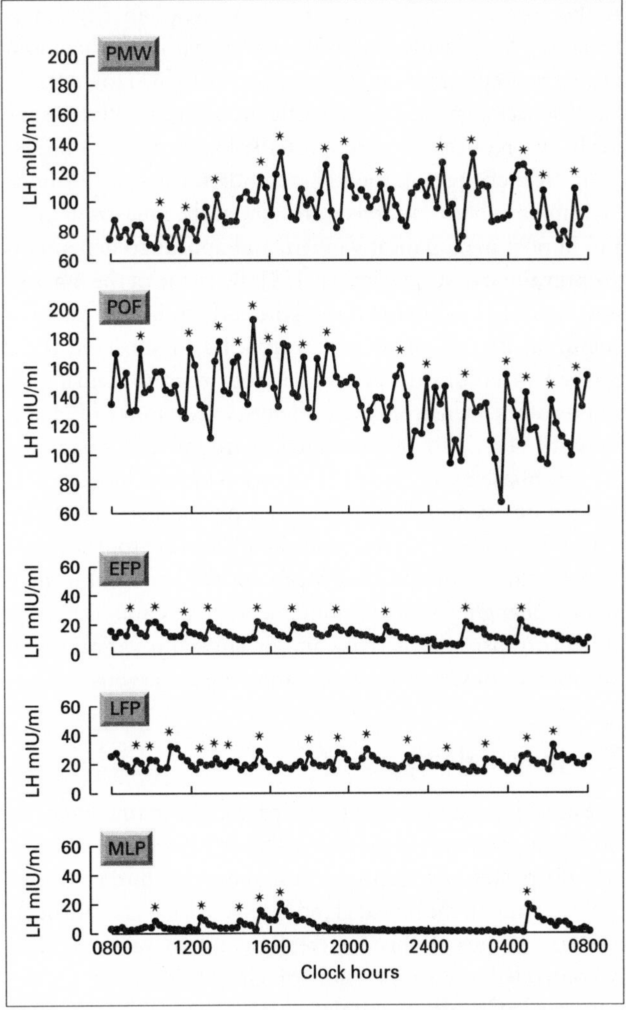

Fig. 48.5 24-hour secretory profiles of luteinising hormone (LH) during the normal menstrual cycle (early follicular phase (EFP), late follicular phase (LFP), mid-luteal phase (MLP)) and in hypogonadal women (post-menopausal woman (PMW), premature ovarian failure (POF)). Asterisks indicate significant LH secretory episodes. Note the differences in the LH scales.

Central nervous oscillators

An important circadian oscillator in the mammal resides in the SCN. While the mechanisms responsible for the generation of rhythmic activity in the SCN remain unknown, the expression of the rhythm appears to depend on action potentials within this nucleus. The generation of a circadian rhythm is distributed across cells in the nucleus. The SCN receives direct input from the eye through axons from the optic chiasm and fibres from the retina. These connections are involved in synchronising the rhythm to the light–dark cycle. The SCN makes efferent connections with neurons throughout the hypothalamus and limbic system. These connections appear to be important for maintaining rhythms in the secretion of LH and FSH. A circadian rhythm is generated by an endogenous oscillator that is synchronised to external cues such as temperature or light. However, in the absence of environmental influences, this oscillator runs freely at a natural frequency, usually longer than 24 hours.

Discrete changes in the LH secretion during the 24-hour rhythm have been observed throughout the menstrual cycle and in post-menopausal women, and appear to depend on the prevailing oestrogen milieu [34]. By virtue of the marked slowing of LH exhibited during the early follicular phase, a nocturnal decline in mean LH appears to subserve these marked variations during the 24-hour rhythm. During all phases of the menstrual cycle, highest excursions of LH and highest LH amplitudes are found at around mid-day, while the acrophase times in the LH secretion of post-menopausal women are generally observed during the early morning hours. The underlying mechanisms accounting for the circadian rhythm in LH pulsatility are not yet known, but may involve changing activity within the SCN, circadian changes in neurotransmitter activity and/or circadian variations in the number of receptors within the central nervous units.

The pineal gland

The pineal gland may also participate in the maintenance of circadian or longer periodicities. This small organ is situated near the posterior commissure just above the third ventricle. In the mammal, the pineal gland receives visual cues through complex routes. Reproductive function in many species is controlled via suppression of GnRH secretion by the influence of a pineal indoleamine, melatonin, on GnRH release. This hormone is released on a circadian basis, with the greatest secretion occurring at night [35]. Synthesis and release of melatonin is governed by a day–night rhythm, and therefore light exposure at various intensity and duration may influence reproductive function. Melatonin is thought to diffuse passively into the general circulation and travels across the blood–brain barrier to act on receptors located in the pituitary (pars tuberalis) and on the SCN. Although the function of the human gonads does not appear to be directly affected by pineal melatonin, this compound may indirectly modulate gonadal function via influences exerted at central sites. Such an assumption is suggested by the functional and temporal links observed between pituitary hormone and melatonin secretion [36]. Furthermore, nocturnal rises of melatonin are highest during the follicular phase, at about the time when the nocturnal suppression of LH secretion is most pronounced [35].

Inhibin

The existence of a non-steroidal factor from the gonads which specifically inhibits pituitary FSH production and release has been postulated for many years. A novel glycoprotein heterodimer composed of two dissimilar disulphide-linked subunits α (20 kDa) and β (12 kDa) was identified from preparations of ovarian follicular fluid preparations and subsequently characterised as selectively inhibiting the secretion of FSH at the pituitary level [37]. Both LH and FSH stimulate inhibin production by the granulosa cells. The action of inhibin appears to be largely confined to the reproductive system. The inhibin β-subunit exists in two highly homologous forms, β_A and β_B, yielding two inhibin heterodimers inhibin A ($\alpha\beta_A$) and inhibin B ($\alpha\beta_B$). Cloning of the subunit genes revealed that the inhibin β-subunit belongs to a family of structurally related molecules. An additional member of this family, activin, was also isolated from follicular fluid, and is a dimer composed of two inhibin β-subunits ($\beta\beta$). Activin stimulates FSH release from pituitary cells, but is also important in other function such as differentiation of the mesoderm in the early embryo. Inhibin and activin act directly on the pituitary gland to regulate the levels of FSH subunit mRNA and the release of intact FSH. In the human ovary, the developing follicle is the major source of inhibin for the circulation, but inhibin is also produced in the luteinised granulosa cells of the corpus luteum [37]. Inhibin has also been shown to act in a paracrine fashion at the level of the ovary by promoting LH-induced androgen production in theca interna cells. Serum levels rise in parallel with oestrogens during the follicular phase of the cycle, a phenomenon which correlates with the coincident fall in FSH (Fig. 48.4). This inhibition is clearly overrun at the time of the preovulatory gonadotrophin surge. In the male gonads, Sertoli cells in the seminiferous tubules are known to secrete inhibin, where it is under the stimulatory control of FSH and growth factors. Serum inhibin levels rise in parallel with increasing levels of LH and FSH during gonadal development, as it occurs at puberty. Serum inhibin levels also rise markedly during pregnancy, when the main source is the placenta. Although inhibin appears to have a physiological role in the differential regulation of gonadotrophins in the female, the situation in the male is far less clear [38]. Here, androgens appear to be more important than inhibin in the feedback control of FSH secretion in the adult male.

Interdependent secretory autonomy rather than functional hierarchy?

Our current understanding of the mechanism leading to pulsatile gonadotrophin release is based on the fundamental premise that the hypothalamus represents a major pacemaker in the generation of gonadotrophin pulsatility and, subsequently, of steroid release from the gonads. This view of the hypothalamus as the sole pacemaker for hormone pulsatility has recently been challenged (Fig. 48.2). The pituitary may have an inherent property to release gonadotrophins in an episodic fashion, independent of hypothalamic inputs [39]. In fact, the gonads by themselves are capable of secreting steroid hormones in an episodic fashion, and do so without gonadotrophin stimulation [40]. This spontaneous hormone secretion suggests secretory autonomy in various tissues, at least within close temporal and functional limits. Thus, a new concept of hormonal regulation is emerging, in which the perception of a hierarchic dominance may be gradually replaced by a wider functional autonomy of individual endocrine organs. These 'pulse generators' in organs of the human reproductive axis may function independently, but appear to be rather entrained to one another by mechanisms that coordinate their activities. Hence, the observations of episodic release of GnRH from the mediobasal hypothalamus, autonomous pulsatile gonadotrophin secretion from the human pituitary and of sex steroids from the gonads, demonstrate that episodic hormone discharge is a common release phenomenon, but also indicates some degree of functional autonomy within the interdependent system of reproductive hormone release.

Hypothalamo-pituitary–gonadal activity during physiological states

Puberty

Puberty is a complex process of mental and somatic steps, leading to the development of secondary sexual characteristics, fertility and psychosexual maturity. Initiation of puberty reflects the activation of GnRH neurons whose secretory activity awaken the entire reproductive axis. In the human, puberty is a brain-driven event which can occur in the absence of the gonads. Although hypothalamic GnRH neurons have the capacity to synthesise and secrete GnRH long before onset of puberty, they do so in a non-orchestrated fashion [41]. Levels of gonadotrophins are very low in prepubertal children, but the release of gonadotrophins is already pulsatile [42], indicating the functional integrity of the neuroendocrine system. This view is supported by the observations that pharmacological manipulation of central neurotransmitter activity or pulsatile administration of GnRH [43] is capable of inducing pubertal changes. The activity of the hypothalamo-pituitary axis appears to be restrained by central mechanisms inhibiting GnRH release ('gonadostat'). A number of brain factors have been implicated in this pubertal disinhibition of neuroendocrine activity, among them impaired hypothalamic activity of endogenous opioid peptides or increase in the concentrations of excitatory amino-acid concentrations [41]. The biosynthetic potential of generating GnRH within the neurons is unlikely to be a mandatory step, since cellular levels of GnRH message remain relatively constant across transition from juvenile life to adulthood. Increased expression of cotransmitters localised within GnRH neurons has been assumed to subserve this pubertal activation [6].

Pubertal maturation is indicated by a gradual rise in gonadotrophin secretion with subsequent stimulation of the gonads. Secretion of gonadotrophins begins with sleep-entrained release episodes at night. A preferential release of FSH, then also of LH, occurs in peaks. At the later stages of puberty, pulsatile gonadotrophin secretion extends to the day, finally displaying the pulsatility of gonadotrophins across the 24-hour clock with appropriate gonadal stimulation. In the male, puberty begins at the age of about 11 years with the stimulation of seminiferous tubules by FSH, which results in increased testicular size. LH begins to stimulate the production of androgens from Leydig cells which mediates the development of sexual characteristics and sexual behaviour. In the female, thelarche (development of breasts) is the earliest manifestation of increased gonadal oestrogen synthesis and usually occurs around the age of 10 years [44]. This is followed by steroid-induced changes in the shape of the pelvis and by menarche as the onset of menstruation at mean age of 12 years. Menstrual cycles remain anovulatory or with luteal phase defects in adolescent girls until full ovarian activity is established a year or two later.

Pregnancy and the post-partum period

When fertilisation and implantation of the blastocyst occurs, the endocrine function of the corpus luteum is maintained by the influence of hCG on its receptors. Rising levels of oestradiol and progesterone provide a signal for the neuroendocrine axis to be inactivated. The massive increase in sex steroids from the developing early placenta leads to hypothalamic GnRH suppression and to hypogonadotrophic ovarian inactivity. This state extends into the post-partum period, when recovery of the reproductive axis follows a sequence of predictable events. Several weeks after delivery, a sleep-entrained release of FSH, then also of LH, is observed. Resumption of GnRH secretory activity resulting from diminished hypothalamic inhibition accounts for the gradual recovery from post-partum amenorrhoea to full reproductive competence. These observations closely resemble those neuroendocrine events known to drive puberty; therefore, the concept of the post-partum period as a 'miniature puberty' has emerged [45].

Menopause and ageing (see also Chapter 56)

The menopausal transition is characterised by a progressive loss of follicles in the ovaries, subsequently leading to diminished sex steroid release. The menopause is indicated by amenorrhoea and usually occurs in women at a mean age of 52 years. The progressive loss of ovarian sex steroids becomes manifest in several features of hypo-oestrogenism, including atrophy of the external and internal genitalia and loss of pubic hair, but also a progressive reduction in bone mass particularly in trabecular bone structures. One prominent symptom is hot flushes, presumably resulting from withdrawal of oestrogens from hypothalamic thermogenic sites. Primary ovarian failure leads to lack of negative-feedback control by ovarian sex steroids after the onset of the menopause, and therefore gonadotrophin release is invariably enhanced—a prolonged state of hypergonadotrophic hypogonadism ensues [14]. As FSH secretion is more sensitive to oestrogen feedback, concentrations of FSH rise initially, indicating early perimenopausal years. This is followed by an increase in LH levels while the menopause progresses. The secretion of gonadotrophins is episodic, and these LH pulse characteristics become very prominent in the post-menopausal period (Fig. 48.5). The gonadotrophin pulsatility of post-menopausal hypogonadal women is unrestrained by any sex steroid feedback, and thus represents the maximal activity of the hypothalamo-pituitary axis [32]. Gonadotrophin release in post-menopausal women is also characterised by circadian variability, and this rhythm is preserved even at old age, in keeping with the notion that the neuroendocrine system remains responsive despite advanced age. Episodic gonadotrophin secretion declines during ageing in post-menopausal women, presumably a reflection of hypothalamic functional decay rather than pituitary hypofunction [46].

In men, a rapid loss of gonadal function is not observed, but rather a subtle attenuation of testicular function with age. This is usually not manifested before the age of 70 years. At this time, a gradual increase of gonadotrophin levels with distinct changes in the gonadotrophin pulsatile patterns indicates a decrease in testicular androgen production with subsequent attenuation of androgen feedback control [47]. However, full reproductive competence may continue even into very old ages.

Stress

The term stress covers a variety of psychological and physical stimuli and entails rapid or chronic adaptation of the endocrine system to environmental, nutritional and endogenous cues. The impact of stress on reproductive hormones depends on variables such as age, sex, endocrine status and time of day. Most stress effects are thought to be mediated by affecting the secretory capacity of hypothalamic neurosecretory neurons, presumably in response to inputs from higher brain centres [48]. All forms of stress including food deprivation, severe physical exercise, increased energy expenditure, malnutrition or severe mental and physical challenges share the common feature in that they suppress pulsatile GnRH release from the hypothalamus leading to a loss of gonadotrophin pulsatility. Stress activates the adrenal axis with a resulting increased release of corticotrophin-releasing hormone (CRH) from the hypothalamic paraventricular nucleus. This peptide causes a prompt cessation of the electrophysiological activity of the hypothalamic GnRH pulse generator, consequently leading to attenuation of hypothalamic GnRH release [49]. The effects of CRH on hypothalamic GnRH release appear to be mediated by increased opioidergic inhibition of GnRH release, independent of hypercortisolism, and this effect is reversed by administration of opiate antagonists [50]. Thus, reproductive dysfunction in response to stress is a hypothalamic functional decline resulting from mechanisms dependent or independent of the activation of the adrenal axis which interfere with coordinated GnRH release.

References

1 Knobil E. The neuroendocrine control of the menstrual cycle. *Rec Prog Horm Res* 1980; **36**: 53–88.

2 Schwanzel-Fukuda M, Pfaff DW. Origin of luteinizing hormone releasing hormone neurons. *Nature* 1989; **338**: 161–4.

3 Matsuo H, Baba Y, Nair RMG, Arimura A, Schally AV. Structure of the porcine LH and FSH releasing factor. I. The proposed amino acid sequence. *Biochem Biophys Res Commun* 1971; **43**: 1334–8.

4 Conn PM. The molecular basis of gonadotropin-releasing hormone action. *Endocr Rev* 1986; **7**: 3–30.

5 McCann SM, Mizunuma H, Samson WK. Differential hypothalamic control of FSH secretion: a review. *Psychoneuroendocrinology* 1983; **8**: 299–308.

6 Rossmanith WG, Clifton DK, Steiner RA. Galanin gene expression in GnRH neurons of the rat: a model for autocrine regulation. *Horm Metab Res* 1996; **8**: 248–61.

7 Kirk SE, Dalkin AC, Yasin M, Haisenleder DJ, Marshall JC. Gonadotropin-releasing hormone pulse frequency regulates expression of pituitary follistatin messenger ribonucleic acid: a mechanism for differential gonadotrope function. *Endocrinology* 1994; **135**: 876–80.

8 Yen SSC. The hypothalamic control of pituitary hormone secretion. In: Yen SSC, Jaffe RB, eds. *Reproductive Endocrinology*. Philadelphia: WB Saunders, 1991: 65–104.

9 Adashi EY. The ovarian life cycle. In: Yen SSC, Jaffe RB, eds. *Reproductive Endocrinology*. Philadelphia: WB Saunders, 1991: 65–104.

10 Rossmanith WG. Contemporary insights into the control of the corpus luteum function. *Horm Metab Res* 1993; **25**: 192–8.

11 Lippner H. Mechanism of mammalian ovulation. In Knobil E, Neill J, eds. *The Physiology of Reproduction*. New York: Raven Press, 1988: 447–76.

12 Liu JH, Yen SSC. Induction of midcycle gonadotropin surge by ovarian steroids in women: a critical evaluation. *J Clin Endocrinol Metab* 1983; **57**: 797–802.

13 Antunes JL, Carmel PW, Housepian EM, Ferin M. Luteinizing hormone-releasing hormone in human pituitary blood. *J Neurosurg* 1978; **49**: 382–6.

14 Yen SSC, Tsai CC, Naftolin F, Vandenberg G, Ajabor L. Pulsatile pattern of gonadotropin release in subjects with and without ovarian function. *J Clin Endocrinol Metab* 1972; **34**: 671–5.

15 Clarke IJ, Cummins JT. The temporal relationship between gonadotropin releasing hormone (GnRH) and luteinizing hormone (LH) secretion in ovariectomized ewes. *Endocrinology* 1982; **111**: 1737–9.

16 Wilson RC, Kesner JS, Kaufman JM, Uemura T, Akena T, Knobil E. Central electrophysiologic correlates of pulsatile luteinizing hormone secretion in the rhesus monkey. *Neuroendocrinology* 1984; **39**: 256–60.

17 Ferin M, Antunes JL, Zimmerman E *et al.* Endocrine function in female rhesus monkeys after hypothalamic disconnection. *Endocrinology* 1977; **101**: 1611–18.

18 Wildt L, Häussler A, Marshall G *et al.* Frequency and amplitude of gonadotropin releasing hormone stimulation and gonadotropin secretion in the rhesus monkey. *Endocrinology* 1981; **109**: 376–85.

19 Shivers BD, Harlan RE, Morrell JI, Pfaff DW. Absence of oestradiol concentration in cell nuclei of LHRH-immunoreactive neurones. *Nature* 1983; **304**: 345–47.

20 Rasmussen DD, Gambacciani M, Swartz WJ, Tueros VS, Yen SSC. Pulsatile GnRH release from the human mediobasal hypothalamus in vitro: opiate receptor mediated suppression. *Neuroendocrinology* 1989; **49**: 150–6.

21 Rossmanith WG. Opioid regulation of LH secretion in women. In: Negri M, Lotti G, Grossman A, eds. *Clinical Perspectives of Opioid Peptide Production*. London: Wiley and Sons, 1992: 154–95.

22 Grossman A. Brain opiates and neuroendocrine function. *J Clin Endocrinol Metab* 1983; **12**: 725–46.

23 Rasmussen DD, Liu JH, Swartz WH, Tueros VS, Wolf PL, Yen SSC. Human fetal hypothalamic GnRH neurosecretion: dopaminergic regulation in vitro. *Clin Endocrinol* 1986; **65**: 127–32.

24 Sarkar DK. In vivo secretion of LHRH in ovariectomized rats is regulated by a possible auto-feedback mechanism. *Neuroendocrinology* 1987; **45**: 510–13.

25 Karsch F. Central actions of ovarian steroids in the feedback regulation of pulsatile secretion of luteinizing hormone. *Ann Rev Physiol* 1987; **49**: 365–82.

26 Matsumoto AM, Bremner WJ. Modulation of pulsatile gonadotropin secretion by testosterone in man. *J Clin Endocrinol Metab* 1984; **58**: 929–35.

27 Bagatell CE, Dahl KD, Bremner WJ. The direct pituitary effect of testosterone to inhibit gonadotropin secretion in men is partially mediated by aromatization to estradiol. *J Androl* 1994; **15**: 15–21.

28 Adams TE, Norman RL, Spies HG. Gonadotropin-releasing hormone receptor binding and pituitary responsiveness in estradiol-primed monkeys. *Science* 1981; **213**: 1388–91.

29 Rossmanith WG, Mortola JF, Yen SSC. Role of endogenous opioid peptides in the initiation of the midcycle luteinizing hormone surge in normal cycling women. *J Clin Endocrinol Metab* 1988; **67**: 695–700.

30 Fink G. Oestrogen and progesterone interactions in the control of gonadotrophin and prolactin secretion. *J Steroid Biochem* 1988; **30**: 169–78.

31 Filicori M, Santoro N, Merriam GR, Crowley WF. Characterization of the physiological pattern of episodic gonadotropin secretion throughout the human menstrual cycle. *J Clin Endocrinol Metab* 1986; **62**: 1136–44.

32 Rossmanith WG, Liu CH, Laughlin GA, Mortola JF, Suh BY, Yen SSC. Relative changes in LH pulsatility during the menstrual cycle: using data from hypogonadal women as a reference point. *Clin Endocrinol* 1990; **32**: 667–80.

33 Rossmanith WG, Laughlin GA, Mortola JF, Johnson ML, Veldhuis JD, Yen SSC. Pulsatile co-secretion of estradiol and progesterone by the midluteal phase corpus luteum: temporal link to luteinizing hormone pulses. *J Clin Endocrinol Metab* 1990; **70**: 990–5.

34 Rossmanith WG, Lauritzen C. The luteinizing hormone pulsatile secretion: diurnal variations in normally cycling and postmenopausal women. *Gynecol Endocrinol* 1991; **5**: 249–65.

35 Wetterberg L, Arendt J, Paunier L, Sizonenko PC, von Donselaar W, Heyden T. Human serum melatonin changes during the menstrual cycle. *J Clin Endocrinol Metab* 1976; **42**: 185–8.

36 Bispink G, Zimmermann R, Weise HC, Leidenberger FA. The effects of wakefulness and light exposure upon nighttime levels of melatonin, prolactin and luteinizing hormone in ovulatory women. *J Pineal Res* 1990; **8**: 97–102.

37 McLachan RI, Cohen NL, Vale WW *et al.* The importance of luteinizing hormone in the control of inhibin and progesterone secretion by the corpus luteum. *J Clin Endocrinol Metab* 1989; **68**: 1078–85.

38 De Kretser DM, Robertson DM, Risbridger GP. Recent advances in the physiology of human inhibin. *J Endocrinol Invest* 1990; **13**: 611–31.

39 Gambacciani M, Liu JH, Swartz WH, Tueros VS, Yen SSC, Rasmussen DD. Intrinsic pulsatility of luteinizing hormone release from the human pituitary in vitro. *Neuroendocrinology* 1987; **45**: 402–6.

40 Rossmanith WG, Schick M, Benz R, Lauritzen C. Autonomous progesterone secretion from the bovine corpus luteum *in vitro*. *Acta Endocrinol* 1991; **124**: 179–87.

41 Urbanski HF, Ojeda SR. Neuroendocrine mechanisms controlling the onset of female puberty. *Reprod Toxicol* 1988; **1**: 129–38.

42 Apter D, Butzow TL, Laughlin GA, Yen SSC. Gonadotropin-releasing hormone pulse generator activity during pubertal transition in girls: pulsatile and diurnal patterns of circulating gonadotropins. *J Clin Endocrinol Metab* 1993; **76**: 940–49.

43 Wildt L, Marshall G, Knobil E. Experimental induction of puberty in the infantile female rhesus monkey. *Science* 1980; **207**: 1373–4.

44 Styne DM. Physiology of puberty. *Horm Res* 1994; **41**: 3–6.

45 Liu JH, Rebar RW, Yen SSC. Neuroendocrine control of the postpartum period. *Clin Perinatol* 1983; **10**: 723–31.

46 Rossmanith WG. Gonadotropin secretion during aging in women. *Exp Gerontol* 1995; **30**; 369–81.

47 Deslypere JP, Kaufman JM, Vermeulen T, Vogelaers D, Vandalem JL, Vermeulen A. Influence of age on pulsatile luteinizing hormone release and responsiveness of the gonadotropins to sex hormone feedback in men. *J Clin Endocrinol Metab* 1987; **64**: 68–76.

48 Ferin M, van Vugt DA, Wardlaw S. The hypothalamic control of the menstrual cycle and the role of endogenous opioid peptides. *Rec Prog Horm Res* 1984; **40**: 441–85.

49 Gambacciani M, Yen SSC, Rasmussen DD. GnRH release from the mediobasal hypothalamus: *in vitro* inhibition by corticotropin-releasing factor. *Neuroendocrinology* 1986; **43**: 533–8.

50 Wildt L, Leyendecker G. Induction of ovulation by the chronic administration of naltrexone in hypothalamic amenorrhea. *J Clin Endocrinol Metab* 1987; **64**: 1334–5.

CHAPTER 49

Male hypogonadism

P. Belchetz

Historical background

The castration of farm animals and humans has been performed in many societies for thousands of years. The uses for which this act was undertaken imply a clear understanding of the function of the testicles. These range from fattening animals in farming to manipulation of humans to produce a trustworthy caste of high officials who would not threaten the ruling line and thus could act as civil servants, generals and court advisers. Varying degrees of hypogonadism could be induced, so that some eunuchs had physical relations with members of the harem in the Ottoman Court. The loss of libido and fertility underlay the use of castration as a punishment—recorded as early as the 2nd millenium BC in Assyria—and in various religious sects such as the Skopzes of Russia. The castration of young boys to produce adult male sopranos (castrati) was performed in Italy until 1878, when it was banned by Pope Leo XIII.

The great Muslim Empires from 750 AD, and the ancient Chinese, not only established an important role for eunuchs in their courts, but also advocated the use of testicular extracts. Mesue the Elder (777–837 AD) in Baghdad recommended them as an aphrodisiac, while Hsu Shu-Wei (1132 AD) used desiccated pig testicles for the treatment of hypogonadism and impotence. Between the 11th and 17th centuries the Chinese iatro-chemists developed techniques for extracting hormones, including androgens, from urine.

The major impetus towards our modern understanding of testicular function came with John Hunter's celebrated experiments involving the transplanting of spurs in fowls and testes in cocks in the late 18th century. In 1849, Berthold reported his classical demonstration that transplantation of a cock's testes to an ectopic site prevented atrophy of the comb which is the usual consequence of such castration. Berthold's contribution to our current understanding was to recognise that testes act by means of a product released into the bloodstream, thus affecting the rest of the body. Much of the recognition of his work was, however, delayed for almost a century.

These animal experiments provided a theoretical basis for much of what was to emerge as the science of endocrinology. With the advent of clinical experimentation, raffish and even scandalous elements were attracted to the field. The ageing Brown-Séquard developed the concept of organotherapy, announcing to his audience at the Society of Biology in Paris, in 1889, the remarkable effects that injections of aqueous testicular extracts had produced in himself. Sceptical British attitudes stood in marked contrast to the wild and uncritical responses which were seen in the USA [1]. A number of dubious exponents flourished, culminating in the widely publicised activities of Serge Voronoff in Algiers, who practised 'monkey gland' grafts for 'rejuvenation' using chimpanzee or baboon implants. Scientific investigation reasserted itself, and in 1927 McGee produced the first authentic androgen extract. Testosterone was finally crystallised by Laqueur in 1935, and within a couple of years the use of testosterone implants had entered clinical practice [2].

Physiology and biochemistry of androgen action

The wide-ranging impact of androgens includes crucial actions in male fetal development. This section will briefly summarise the overall basis for androgen activity as a necessary setting for the description of various types of hypogonadism, and the therapeutic approaches which can be adopted.

The male phenotype results from the activity of the fetal testis (Fig. 49.1). The early bipotential gonad is programmed to develop into a testis in the sixth to seventh week of gestation by the action of the testis-determining gene carried on the short arm of the Y chromosome [3] (see

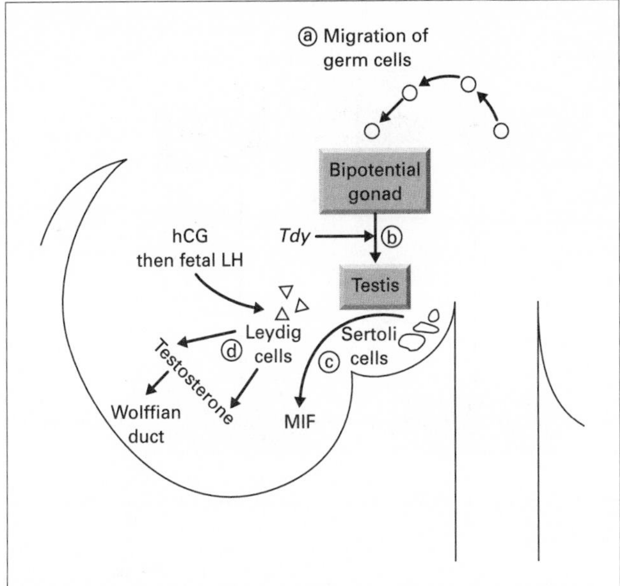

Fig. 49.1 Stages in the development of the male phenotype. (a) Migration of germ cells from the yolk sac to the bipotential gonad during fourth week of fetal life. (b) Development of definitive testis under influence of testis-determining gene (*Tdy*), during sixth to seventh weeks. (c) Secretion of Müllerian inhibitory factor (MIF) from Sertoli cells. (d) Induction of Wolffian duct structures by testosterone from Leydig cells from day 60, initially stimulated by human chorionic gonadotrophin (hCG) but later fetal pituitary luteinising hormone (LH) secretion.

also Chapter 57). The differentiated testis secretes Müllerian inhibitory factor from the Sertoli cells. Leydig cells appear by day 60 (32–35 mm crown–rump length) and are initially stimulated by human chorionic gonadotrophin (hCG). The early production of testosterone organises the development of the Wolffian duct structures. This is a direct effect of testosterone diffusing locally to act in a paracrine fashion. Later, by the 16th week of gestation, testosterone levels rise transiently to match adult male levels. By this time the fetal pituitary gonadotrophins are taking over from the waning levels of hCG. The latter part of fetal life is characterised by the development of the male external genitalia with scrotal fusion, further phallic development with the scrotal fusion development of the corpus spongiosum, and forward development and enlargement of the phallus with the penile urethra. The development of the prostate is induced and vesicovaginal septum inhibited, preventing development of the vagina. These are responses to the target organs' production of dihydrotestosterone (DHT) from the high circulating levels of testosterone, mediated by the local tissue activity of the enzyme 5α-reductase [4].

Apart from the earliest weeks of fetal life, testosterone production is dependent on pituitary luteinising hormone (LH) secretion, which in turn depends on the pulsatile release of gonadotrophin-releasing hormone (GnRH). The quiescence of childhood gonadal activity appears due to the inhibition of the hypothalamic 'pulse generator' responsible for driving the pulses of GnRH into the portal hypophysial system (see also Chapter 48). The disinhibition at puberty involves initially the appearance of nocturnal pulsatile LH secretion which subsequently stretches throughout the 24 hours during sexual maturity [5]. Gonadal steroids exert a negative feedback on gonadotrophin secretion, and thus loss of testosterone production during adult life leads to raised levels of LH. The feedback actions of testosterone are quite complex. There is a clear-cut action at the hypothalamic level, with slowing of the frequency of LH pulses. A direct action of testosterone and antiandrogens has been demonstrated on the pulsatile release of GnRH from hypothalamic explants *in vitro*. Testosterone is known to be extensively metabolised in brain tissue to both oestradiol and dihydrotestosterone, which may each have separate feedback actions.

LH stimulates Leydig cells via specific plasma membrane receptors. It seems likely that several second messengers may be involved, including cyclic adenosine monophosphate (cAMP) and Ca^{2+}. Synthesis of testosterone involves a series of enzymatically catalysed steps involving cytochrome P-450 enzymes. The cholesterol side-chain cleavage to yield pregnenolone occurs in mitochondria, and the transfer of cholesterol from outer to inner mitochondrial membranes appears to be rate limiting. The further metabolism of pregnenolone occurs in the endoplasmic reticulum. The human testis preferentially utilises the Δ5 as opposed to the Δ4 pathway (Fig. 49.2). Rare biosynthetic defects are described. 17-ketoreductase deficiency affects the testes alone, with marked pubertal virilisation and variable gynaecomastia. 5α-reductase deficiency is also associated with ambiguous genitalia, but with virilisation at puberty [4]. The latter indicates which tissues are testosterone responsive. It raises the question, however, of how differential responses to testosterone and DHT occur, since both apparently bind to the same receptor, although perhaps with different affinities. The pubertal partial development of external genitalia probably indicates some induction of 5α-reductase activity.

The action of androgen on target tissues is mediated by a specific androgen receptor (Fig. 49.3). This has been characterised and belongs to the superfamily of nuclear receptors, to which belong other steroid hormone receptors, vitamin D receptors and thyroid hormone receptors; they may also include the proto-oncogene c-*erb* A, which shows marked homologies between the DNA-binding domains with zinc-finger structures, and the steroid-binding domains as well as the N-terminal regions thought to be involved in transcriptional activation [6]. Varying types and degrees of abnormality in androgen-binding receptors are associated

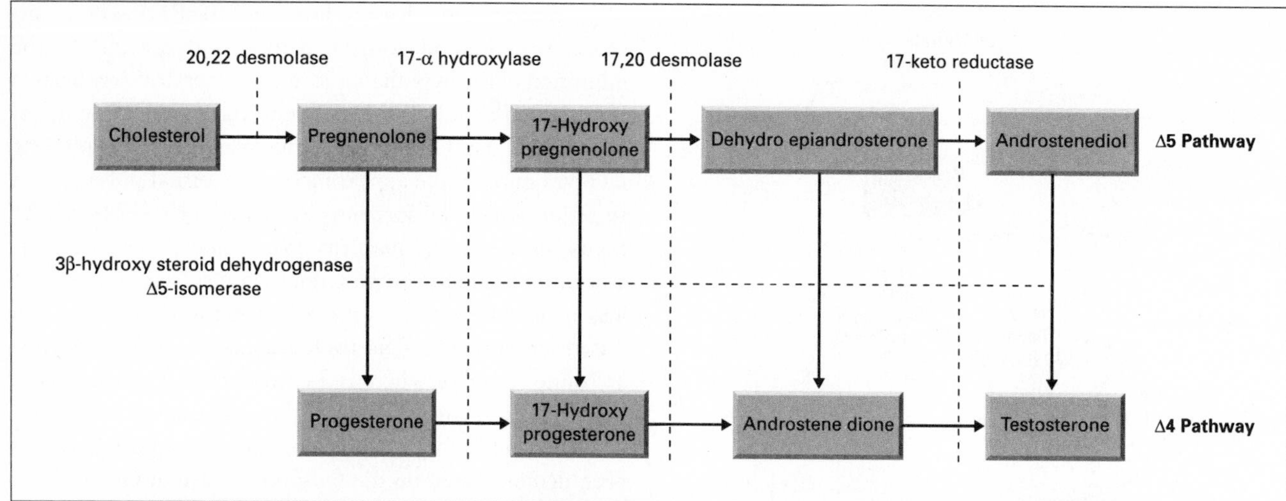

Fig. 49.2 Diagram of biosynthetic pathways leading to testosterone; note Δ5 pathway favoured in humans, indicated by large arrows.

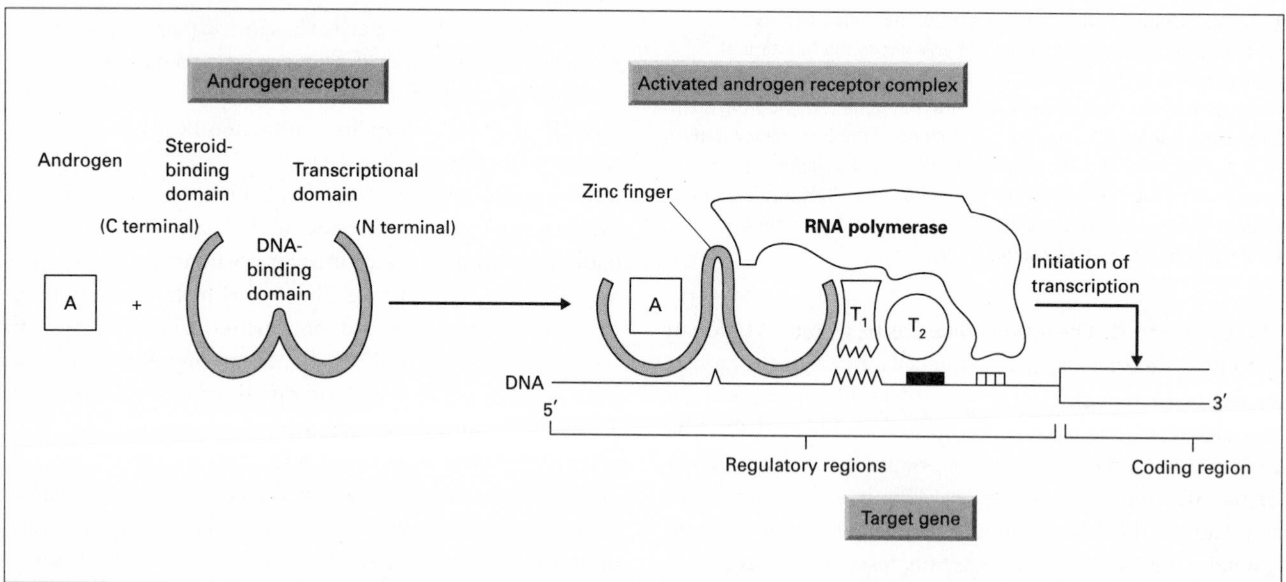

Fig. 49.3 Androgen–nuclear receptor interactions. The binding of androgen to the steroid-binding domain causes conformational changes exposing the zinc finger DNA-binding region and allowing the transcriptional domain to initiate transcription of the target gene.

with clinical syndromes ranging from complete androgen insensitivity (testicular feminisation) to a variety of more minor defects associated with male pseudo-hermaphroditism. The type I familial incomplete male pseudo-hermaphroditism is inherited as an X-linked recessive. A whole range of virilisation can be expressed even within a single family with presumably the same genetic defect, but with the constant feature of infertility [7]. A variety of receptor abnormalities have been described including reduced binding of labelled DHT, discordant findings at 37°C and 42°C, and post-receptor defects. Following the characterisation of the androgen receptor and the elucidation of the corresponding X-chromosome located gene, two patients with testicular feminisation have had distinct abnormalities described in the steroid-binding domain of the androgen receptor [8].

Clinical features of male hypogonadism

As will be clear from the foregoing introductory remarks, the features associated with male hypogonadism are highly dependent on whether they are congenital, or if acquired, at what age, as well as the severity of the deficiency.

Major congenital defects, especially affecting the early stages of sexual differentiation, are covered in Chapter 57. As has already been emphasised, however, disorders causing relatively minor effects can have a genetically determined basis. Disorders presenting before and thus preventing or retarding pubertal development have several features in common. These include microphallus, which indicates the importance of early androgen exposure for penile development. The lack of pubertal androgen delays epiphysial closure with consequent excessive growth of long bones. This in turn leads to the eunuchoidal proportions whereby span exceeds vertical height by 5 cm or more (Fig. 49.4). When there is cryptorchidism the persistent exposure to body temperature, as opposed to the considerably lower scrotal temperature, impairs spermatogenesis and also induces a markedly increased susceptibility to malignant change [9].

Secondary sexual characteristics

During the course of normal puberty the rapid rise in testosterone secretion from the testes evokes characteristic changes. Post-pubertal androgen deficiency reverses some of these changes, but to strikingly varying degrees in different individuals.

Fig. 49.4 Development of eunuchoidal proportions. In the normally virilised male androgen secretion advances epiphysial fusion so that height (2A) equals span (2A). The protracted growth of long bones in hypogonadism adds an extra length (X) to the limbs so that with the legs growing in parallel height = 2A + X, but the span has the addition of both arms in series, i.e. span = 2A + 2X: span exceeds height by X which may be considerably greater than 5 cm.

Hair growth and skin

Androgen-dependent hair growth occurs with two patterns: ambisexual, which is common to men and women involving growth of a flat topped pubic hair pattern and axillary hair growth, and masculine hair growth. This involves facial hair, upward extension of pubic hair, body hair on the chest and back, and increased limb hair growth. In addition, there is androgen-induced reversion from terminal pattern hair growth to vellus hair on the scalp to varying degrees but invariably with some temporal hair recession. The degree of masculine-pattern hair growth is highly dependent on genetic factors, with well-recognised and marked racial variations despite similar androgen levels. The pattern of pubic hair growth in boys during puberty has been studied and classified; it forms an integral part of the assessment of pubertal development. Loss of androgen function in adults is associated with very wide variations in the degree to which facial and body hair is lost, or more commonly growth softened and retarded. Once established, male-pattern baldness undergoes little reversal even with castration. The differences between secondary sexual hair patterns in men and women are not simply due to the quantitative differences in circulating testosterone. The evidence

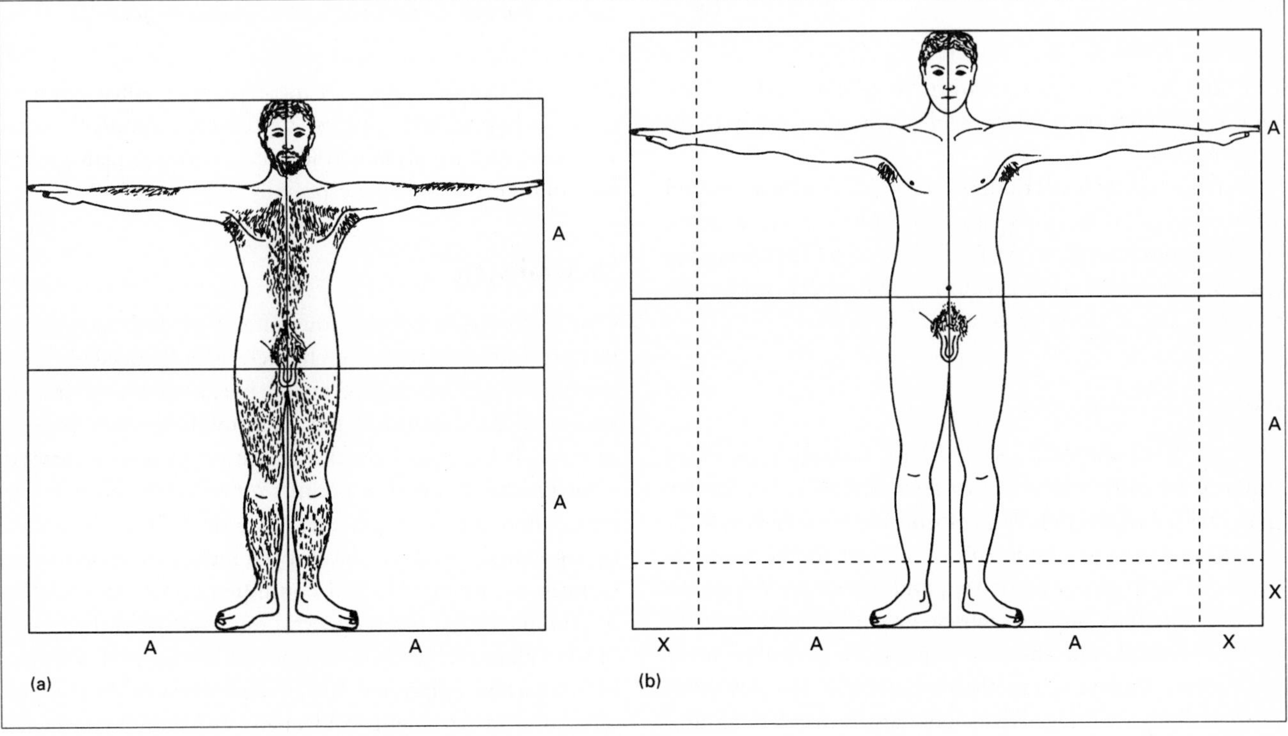

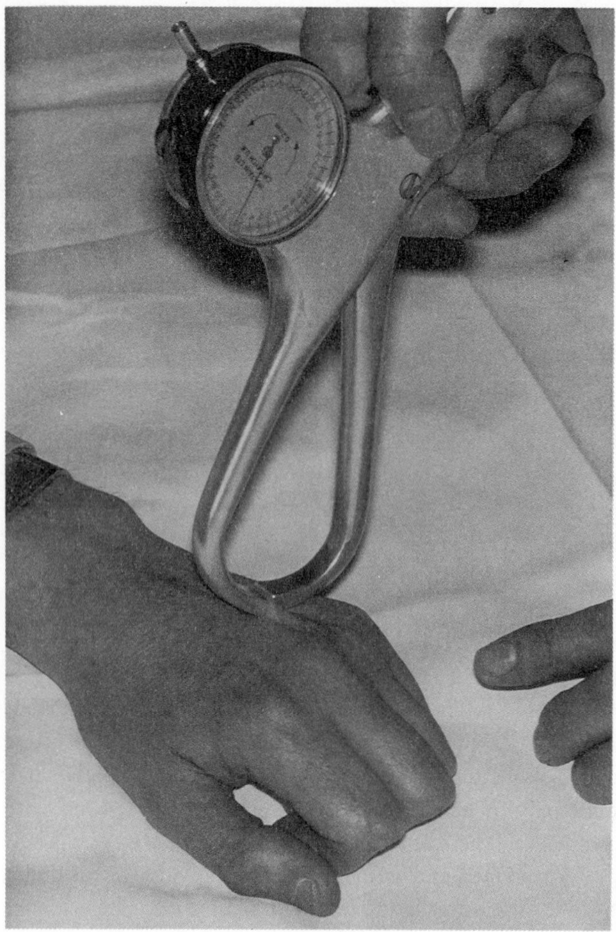

Fig. 49.5 Use of calipers to measure skin thickness on dorsum of the hand.

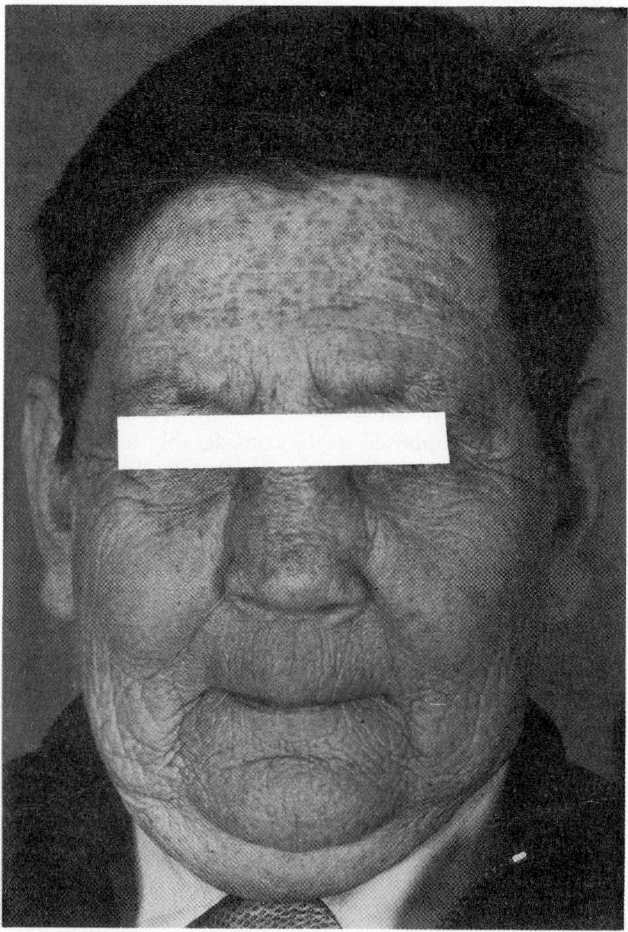

Fig. 49.6 Facies of a hypogonadal male showing finely wrinkled hairless face with conspicuous vertical creases on upper lip.

provided by male subjects with 5α-reductase deficiency indicates an important role for DHT in the masculine pattern of hair growth.

Hypogonadism leads to thin skin which can be measured with calipers on the dorsum of the hand—a site without subcutaneous fat (Fig. 49.5). Finely wrinkled facial skin gives the appearance of 'ageing youth'—vertical creases on the upper lip are particularly notable (Fig. 49.6).

Muscle development

In contrast to secondary sexual hair, skeletal muscle appears to be fully responsive to testosterone *per se* rather than DHT. Skeletal muscle constitutes approximately 40% of body mass and is considerably responsible for the powerful action of androgens on nitrogen and phosphate retention. There is an effect on most muscle groups, but the muscles of the pectoral and shoulder region are probably most responsive. Efforts to synthesise anabolic steroids with relatively little virilising activity have largely met with failure.

The action of androgens is most marked when administered to hypogonadal males. Optimum responses require an otherwise normal endocrine milieu, with adequate growth hormone secretion being especially important.

Skeletal system

One of the most conspicuous effects of androgens is on laryngeal growth with the characteristic 'breaking' of the voice. This is clearly an irreversible phenomenon. Androgens appear to be responsible for the growth spurt of puberty in boys. It hastens skeletal maturation as well as growth velocity, and its absence permits a protracted growth pattern, often into the patient's twenties. This allows the hypogonadal youth to develop eunuchoidal proportions. Conversely, premature and continued androgen secretion or administration in prepubertal boys can yield the typical 'pocket Hercules' pattern, with accelerated growth followed by premature epiphysial fusion and irreversible compromise of ultimate height. Androgens undoubtedly influence patterns of growth hormone secretion, especially amplitude of pulses of growth hormone. The growth spurt in boys tends to be a late pubertal process compared with girls, it is said to occur when the testicular volume reaches 10–12 ml, but in fact wide variations are seen in normal boys [10].

In the wake of widespread interest in post-menopausal osteoporosis, it is now widely recognised that hypogonadal men are also susceptible to developing severe osteoporosis. This has been demonstrated in a variety of hypogonadal states, most graphically after castration [11]. Preliminary data suggest that, in some situations, correction of hypogonadism prevents further bone loss and may even increase bone mineral density. The mechanisms by which androgens affect bone are unknown, but may involve DHT receptors, although aromatisation to oestrogens may also play a role. Earlier data regarding calcitonin and generation of 1,25-dihydroxyvitamin D levels remain unconfirmed.

Psychological effects of testosterone

Testosterone has major psychological effects, most obviously on sexuality, but also on aggression, activity, cognition and emotional state. Hypogonadism is associated with loss of libido and impotence. The variation between individuals is large and depends partly on the age, speed and degree to which testosterone falls, as well as independent confounding factors of a primarily psychological nature. In general, where there is a straightforward endocrine cause for low testosterone secretion, suitable replacement therapy improves all aspects of sexual behaviour from sexual thoughts and interest to erections, orgasm and ejaculation. The level of plasma testosterone below which sexual function fails varies quite markedly between men, in one study ranging from 7 to 15 nmol/l [12] and in another from 5 to 11 nmol/l [13]. The administration of exogenous testosterone to impotent, but ostensibly endocrinologically normal men, is generally reported to have little effect. Self-reporting studies reveal either no or only a weak association between sexual function and plasma testosterone levels. By contrast, objective measures of penile tumescence correlate positively with circulating testosterone concentration in men whose levels fall within the normal range. Cyproterone acetate, which acts both as an antiandrogen and, probably by virtue of its progestational properties, lowers gonadotrophins, has been used to lower libido and sexual activity in sexual offenders. Testosterone is not the sole hormone to affect libido; hyperprolactinaemia is clearly associated with impotence. This may in part be by hypothalamic suppression of the GnRH pulse generator. An independent action is indicated by the failure of testosterone replacement to correct impotence when prolactin remains high, but treatment with prolactin-lowering drugs such as bromocriptine may then prove effective [14]. However, suppression of prolactin without correcting testosterone deficiency is also ineffective.

Inconsistent results have attended efforts to relate testosterone levels to aggressive behaviour. Various aspects of cognition, especially spatial ability, are reported to relate positively to plasma testosterone levels. Although less fully investigated than other aspects of endocrine function, studies of testosterone levels in various emotional states suggest that high testosterone levels are associated with states of relaxation and joyfulness and negatively correlated with anxiety and depression. Subjects with high levels of testosterone also seem to show lesser degrees of response to emotional stress.

Spermatogenesis

The twin functions of the testis, testosterone secretion and spermatogenesis, are often dealt with as distinct processes. There is ample evidence of necessary and intimate relationships between them (Fig. 49.7). It is highly likely that follicle-stimulating hormone (FSH) not only affects spermatogenesis but also Leydig-cell function by means of Sertoli-cell products acting in a paracrine manner [15]. Conversely, there is no doubt about the important role of intratesticular testosterone

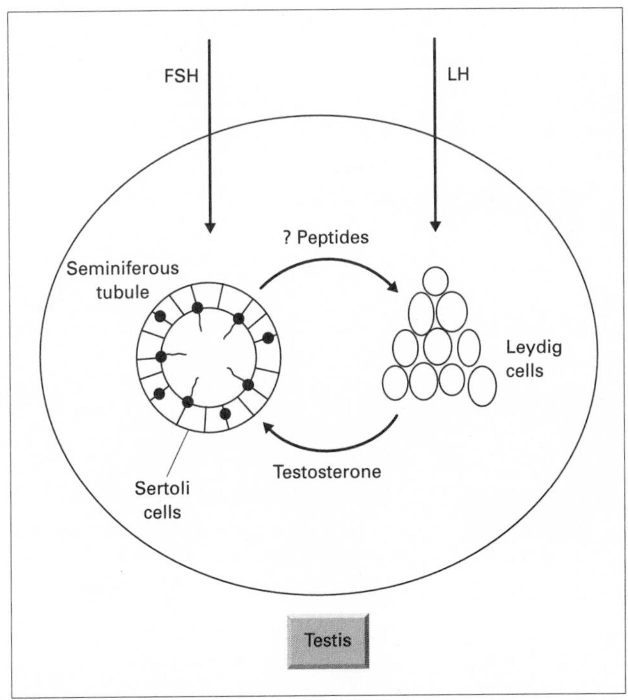

Fig. 49.7 The seminiferous tubules and Leydig cells appear able to communicate with each other by means of paracrine secretion. The exact nature and significance remains to be elucidated.

in the maintenance of spermatogenesis. Precise details are not easily come by since most information relates to the laboratory rat, which undoubtedly differs in several important respects from primate species and humans in particular [16]. Nevertheless, the relative roles of FSH, which acts on the spermatogenic tubules, and testosterone in relation to spermatogenesis show marked species variations. It is clear that raised concentrations of testosterone are important. In humans, the occurrence of Leydig-cell tumours in prepubertal boys is clearly associated with spermatogenesis in the vicinity of the tumours, where presumably testosterone concentrations are locally raised. The modulation of intratesticular testosterone levels, over and above the control exerted by pituitary LH secretion, has been attributed to various paracrine factors, though the evidence is incomplete and again more readily applicable to the rat than primates. The Leydig cells, in turn, are also considered to be under the paracrine influence of seminiferous tubules or germ cells with a host of candidate agents suggested by *in vitro* experiments.

Gynaecomastia

Feminising features are common in many hypogonadal states and may present with female patterns of hair growth, fat deposition and most strikingly with gynaecomastia. This is dealt with in detail separately in Chapter 55. However, a few points about it deserve brief mention in this context. Hypergonadotrophic hypogonadism may be associated with frankly elevated oestradiol concentrations, but more subtle endocrine imbalances may also lead to the same effect. These include relatively low testosterone/oestradiol ratios, where the latter lies within the normal adult range, and also raised sex hormone-binding globulin (SHBG). The latter is a not infrequent consequence of parenchymal liver disease, for example cirrhosis, and may also occur in thyrotoxicosis. It has been postulated that this is because SHBG has a relatively higher affinity for testosterone than oestradiol 17β, and thus when SHBG is elevated relatively more testosterone is bound to it than oestradiol [17]. The latter is therefore relatively higher in the unbound state, which is generally held to correspond to biological activity (Fig. 49.8). There are situations such as puberty where the circulating hormone levels are apparently normal but the breast tissue has a raised aromatase enzymatic activity leading to locally enhanced oestrogen production. It is not uncommon in 17-ketoreductase deficiency but, as would be predicted, absent in 5α-reductase deficiency. With increasing degrees of androgen insensitivity, gynaecomastia becomes a more conspicuous feature.

Aetiology

Hypogonadism can be caused by primary testicular dis-

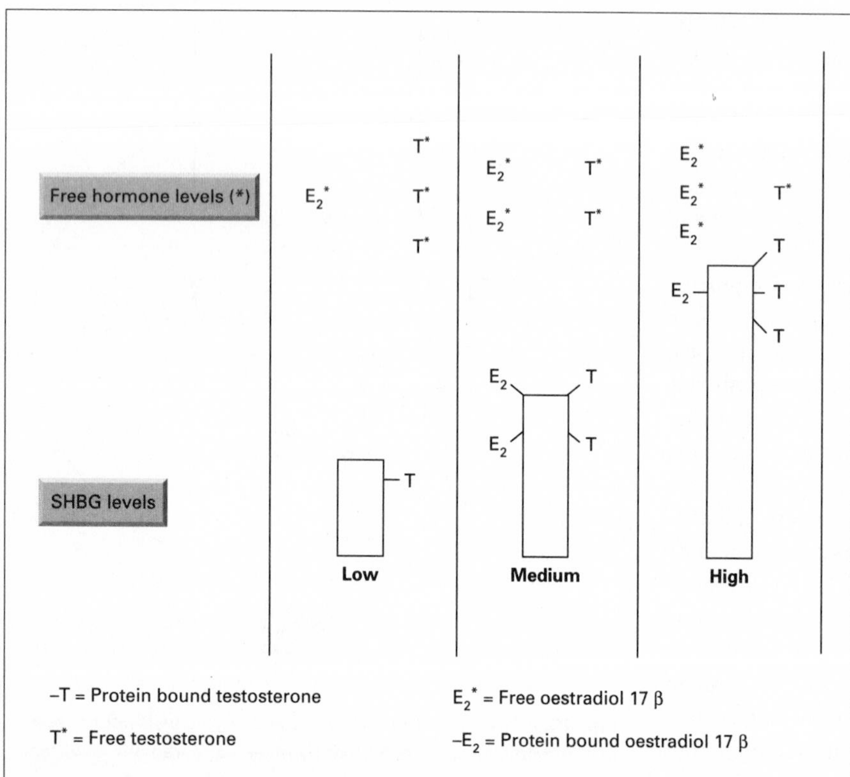

Fig. 49.8 Effects of varying SHBG levels on the relative distribution of bound/free testosterone to oestradiol ratios resulting from the greater affinity of SHBG for testosterone than oestradiol 17β.

ease or disorders of the hypothalamo-pituitary-regulating mechanisms. Biosynthetic and androgen insensitivity disorders will not be dealt with further, as details can be found elsewhere in this volume.

Primary gonadal failure

Trauma

Surgical castration has been studied where it is still used in some societies, especially for the punishment of sexual offenders. The reduction of libido, spontaneous erections and sexual potency follows, but marked variations exist between individuals. Somatic changes in hair growth, muscle fat and bone occur more slowly and to very different degrees. The sudden fall in circulating testosterone levels may be accompanied by hot flushes, as with menopausal women. Unlike women, however, the restoration of normal testosterone levels in some subjects may be relatively ineffective in abolishing the vasomotor disturbances. Surgical hypogonadism is sometimes induced as part of a block resection for treatment of carcinoma of the penis. Testicular damage has been recorded after attempted sterilisation when the testicular arteries have been inadvertently ligated as well as, or even instead of, the vasa deferentia. Torsion of the testes may similarly lead to testicular atrophy. While physical trauma may lead to acute inflammation, lasting some weeks, long-term atrophy is an infrequent but well-recognised sequela.

Irradiation

The seminiferous tubules are considerably more susceptible to damage by ionising radiation than the Leydig cells. Nevertheless, along with the regular and anticipated induction of severe oligospermia or azoospermia, varying degrees of Leydig-cell dysfunction with ensuing impairment of sexual function are not uncommon (see Chapter 75). The latter seems disproportionate to measured change in hormone levels which may give apparently normal readings for both LH and testosterone concentrations, though characteristically FSH will be raised. The explanation of this discrepancy is unclear, especially as the psychological contribution to sexual dysfunction cannot readily be quantified.

Concealed within such apparently normal indices of pituitary–Leydig cell axis function may be altered levels of SHBG and also changes in the ratios of biological to immunological reactivity. The most readily discernible deviation from normal is the so-called 'compensated Leydig cell failure', where a rise in LH maintains circulating testosterone within the normal reference range. Since the homeostatic set points within individuals are tight, this may be a misleading term as the testosterone level may be reduced compared to pre-irradiation values and thus low for that individual.

Drugs

The use of drugs, especially alkylating agents and particularly cyclophosphamide, in the chemotherapy of malignant disease may also impair testicular function [18]. Efforts have been made to spare testicular damage based on the premise that the prepubertal testis may be more resistant to irradiation and drugs. These approaches have attempted to provide protection by inducing a state of reversible hypogonadotrophic hypogonadism during treatment by means of gonadotrophin superagonists; the outcome of these trials has generally been disappointing.

A large number of drugs and toxins damage tubular function, and by means of subtle paracrine effects they also affect Leydig-cell function. Several specific antiandrogens have been introduced, mainly as part of the therapeutic armamentarium used in androgen dependent prostatic carcinoma. These include flutamide and cyproterone acetate. The latter also has progestational properties which lower gonadotrophin secretion. It has long been used in the treatment of sexual offenders [19]. Spironolactone has multiple actions: while principally employed as a mineralocorticoid antagonist, it is also a powerful antiandrogen and additionally acts as a weak oestrogen. High doses of spironolactone reduce testosterone biosynthesis. Gynaecomastia, which is usually unpleasantly tender, is a frequent side-effect in men treated with spironolactone. Feminising side-effects have been reported in patients on digitalis glycosides, and appear to be due to digitoxin rather than digoxin. Cimetidine is also antiandrogenic and may be associated with gynaecomastia. Earlier reports suggested that cimetidine caused hyperprolactinaemia, thus providing another mechanism for impairing sexual function; subsequent studies suggest this is not a feature associated with the oral use of cimetidine in conventional doses although transient elevation in prolactin follows intravenous injection of the drug [20]. Ketoconazole has a short-lived action on testosterone biosynthesis but in daily doses exceeding 400 mg prolonged suppression can be achieved, and the drug has been used in various forms of male precocious puberty especially familial testotoxicosis [21]. Short-term tetracycline use has been associated with modest declines in testosterone levels. Several drugs of abuse have been associated with impaired gonadal and sexual function. These include opiates which act centrally, but cannabis probably has a direct action on the testis as well as centrally. Alcohol has multiple antigonadal sites of action, apart from causing liver dysfunction; it causes both acute and chronic depression of testosterone production (see Chapter 77) [22].

Infections, inflammation and infiltration

Viral infections are the commonest cause of testicular failure in adult life. Many viruses have been implicated but by far the most frequent is mumps. One in four adult men with mumps develop orchitis, which is bilateral in about one-third of cases. During the acute phase, testosterone falls and gonadotrophins rise. In the long term, testicular atrophy occurs in one-third of men following mumps orchitis and in 10% it is bilateral. Bilateral atrophy is commonly associated with some degree of seminiferous tubule failure and Leydig-cell dysfunction, but with normal oestrogen production as gonadotrophins rise; hypogonadism and gynaecomastia result in many cases. Use of glucocorticoids during the acute illness has not been demonstrated to prevent the long-term consequences of testicular damage caused by mumps.

Testicular damage is seen in granulomatous conditions and formerly was a not uncommon feature of syphilis. It is also seen in lepromatous leprosy. Tuberculosis often causes epididymitis but rarely affects the testis.

Testicular damage can occur as part of an autoimmune process. It is particularly seen in patients with Addison's disease who have a generalised autoantibody directed against steroid-producing cells [23]. In acutely ill patients with Addison's disease there may be several accompanying hormonal abnormalities which correct on recovery with the institution of appropriate corticosteroid therapy. These include raised LH and depressed testosterone suggesting Leydig-cell dysfunction, and transient hyperprolactinaemia may be seen. Sarcoidosis may affect many systems and cause hypogonadism by involvement of the hypothalamo-pituitary region, but it can also produce the picture of primary testicular failure; liver involvement is also common.

Iron overload can similarly disrupt pituitary, liver and testicular functions. It is a feature not only of primary haemochromatosis but also other iron overload states, especially chronic anaemias requiring repeated blood transfusion. A prime example is thalassaemia major, which can cause irreversible infertility even if vigorous chelation with desferrioxamine is used. The brunt of the damage appears to be borne by the testis but androgen replacement can provide adequate virilisation (see Chapter 81).

Chromosomal abnormalities

Klinefelter's syndrome is the commonest chromosomal abnormality associated with male hypogonadism. In the classical type with 47XXY karyotype, which occurs in one in 1000 newborn males [24], a wide range of clinical features, ranging from marked feminisation to full virilisation is found (Fig. 49.9). Small firm testes are a constant feature, and hence it is necessary to measure testis size accurately.

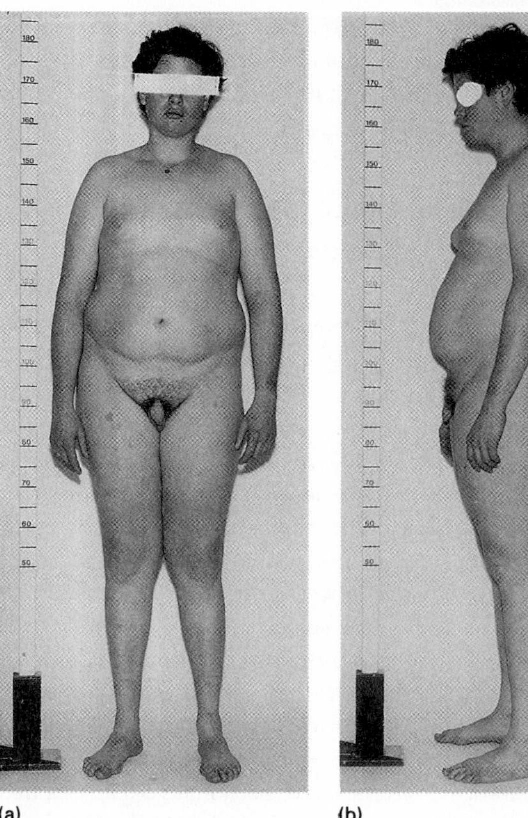

(a) (b)

Fig. 49.9 Klinefelter's syndrome, showing gynaecomastia, partial virilisation and small testes.

The seminiferous tubules are severely affected with hyalinisation, and infertility is the rule, despite the very rare claim that motile spermatozoa can be demonstrated in the ejaculate. The condition is not usually suspected prepubertally, although long limbs may already be a feature [25]. Thereafter, eunuchoidal proportions and feminine fat contours, together with gynaecomastia and diminished secondary sexual hair on the face and body, contribute to the classical picture. Characteristically, marked elevation in FSH is found at all stages but LH may range from normal adult to markedly elevated levels depending on Leydig-cell function. Because of the severity of seminiferous tubular atrophy occurring in post-pubertal life, there is an illusion of Leydig-cell hyperplasia which quantitative studies have disproved [26]. LH levels are frequently raised, even in the 25% with normal testosterone levels, indicating failing Leydig-cell reserve. This is confirmed by the markedly impaired testosterone rise following administration of hCG to patients with Klinefelter's syndrome [27]. Testosterone levels diminish rapidly from the third decade on in many subjects. In late teenage life, however, when testosterone secretion is usually at its highest, oestradiol is also raised, then both tend to fall with passing years. At all times there is, therefore, a raised oestradiol/testosterone ratio, which, together with the raised SHBG, is probably responsible for the frequently occurring gynaecomastia. Without androgen replacement there is a propensity for older patients with Klinefelter's syndrome to develop expanded pituitary fossae, presumably due to deficient sex steroid feedback.

Patients with Klinefelter's syndrome may display other features. The bones are liable to develop osteoporosis which may be disproportionate to the degree of hypogonadism, though clearly exacerbated by it. Similar considerations apply to the skeletal musculature. There is a tendency for patients with Klinefelter's syndrome to have reduced verbal intelligence and also psychosocial problems which may present with delinquent behaviour. As well as relatively tall stature, obesity (in 30–50%) and gynaecomastia, there is a 20-fold increase in the incidence of breast cancer compared with normal men. Varicose veins, pulmonary disease, diabetes mellitus and thyroid dysfunction occur with increased frequency.

Klinefelter's syndrome classically arises from meiotic non-disjunction—40% arising from the spermatozoon and 60% during oogenesis; this is often associated with advanced maternal age. In about 10% of Klinefelter's syndrome 46XY/47XXY mosaicism occurs as a result of mitotic non-disjunction in either 46XY or 47XXY zygotes. Mosaics show less marked features, testis volumes may be larger and fertility has been reported. Patients with the 48XXYY karyotype tend to be taller, mentally retarded and more disturbed than patients with classical Klinefelter's syndrome. They have a marked tendency to peripheral vascular abnormalities and show unusual dermatoglyphic patterns. With increasing supernumerary chromosomes more profound mental retardation and other congenital, especially bony, defects are found.

The XX male syndrome is related to Klinefelter's syndrome. It has an incidence of approximately one in 20 000 live male births. The underlying mechanisms allowing male phenotypic development and the apparent absence of a Y chromosome is not fully explained. The clinical features differ from Klinefelter's syndrome in that these patients tend to be shorter, intelligence is unaffected and hypospadias occurs in about 10%.

Cryptorchidism

Cryptorchid testes are primarily associated with infertility, and there is clear evidence that early orchidopexy improves the outlook. Nevertheless, the results are often disappointing even when only one testis was cryptorchid, suggesting a bilateral defect in addition to that conditioned by the raised temperature the intra-abdominal testis is exposed to. Varying degrees of Leydig-cell dysfunction have been reported [28]. Primary endocrine disorders are exceptional, but include various male pseudo-hermaphrodite conditions and also disorders of the hypothalamo-pituitary complex.

Varicocele (see also Chapter 50)

Although epidemiological surveys have disclosed how often varicoceles may coexist with fully normal fertility, sex function and endocrinology, it does seem that varicocele can act as an aetiological agent in some cases of infertility. Again, the rise in testicular temperature, caused by abnormality of the cremasteric venous plexus, may be pathogenetic. Leydig-cell function tends to fall with age, but symptoms and biochemistry respond to surgical correction [29].

Systemic diseases

Primary testicular damage is common in paraplegia, possibly because of failure of mechanisms maintaining the testicular temperature sufficiently low. Myotonic dystrophy is an autosomal dominant condition characterised by progressive muscular weakness, myotonia, mental retardation, frontal baldness and cataracts (Fig. 49.10). There is damage to the seminiferous tubules, accompanied by raised FSH

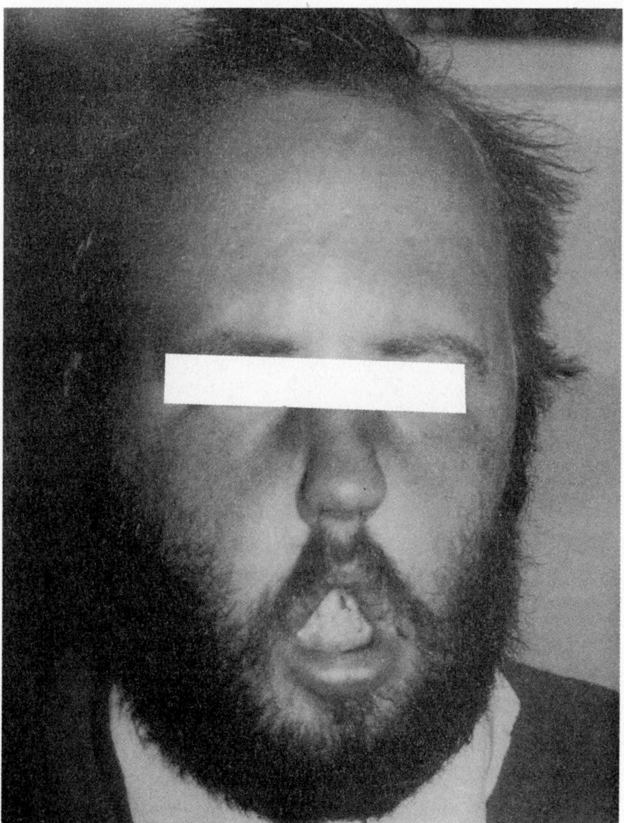

Fig. 49.10 Myotonic dystrophy. Note frontal balding and loss of wrinkles on forehead. Cataracts and variable mental retardation as well as myotonia may be present.

levels, but less well marked Leydig-cell dysfunction may be seen with low testosterone and exaggerated LH responses to GnRH [30].

Renal failure is commonly associated with testicular failure affecting both spermatogenesis and testosterone production, leading to increased plasma LH and FSH levels. Hyperprolactinaemia is not uncommon. This situation is little improved by haemodialysis but is generally much better after successful renal transplantation.

Hepatic cirrhosis is commonly accompanied by hypogonadism and feminisation. Multiple factors probably operate including altered rates of steroid hormone metabolism, enhanced production of oestrogens, particularly oestrone but also oestradiol, and increased levels of SHBG [31]. Particular effects of specific disorders with hepatic complication found in iron-overload states, ethanol abuse and sarcoidosis have been mentioned above.

In adult male patients with untreated coeliac disease infertility is not uncommon, and this has been associated with an endocrine profile suggestive of partial androgen insensitivity with elevation of both LH and testosterone levels; in fact, the resemblance is closest to 5α-reductase deficiency since there is a concomitant reduction of DHT [32].

Thyrotoxicosis may cause impotence and gynaecomastia. The mechanism may be via the elevation in SHBG secretion that hypethyroidism induces, since there is a shift to a relatively lower free testosterone/free oestradiol ratio. The sexual dysfunction is not often a presenting complaint, and may need precise but tactful questioning to distinguish it from the general lassitude and depression that often accompanies thyrotoxicosis.

Secondary gonadal failure

This results from deficient secretion of pituitary gonadotrophins, particularly LH. The abnormality may reside in the pituitary itself or may be due to deficient hypothalamic action. This in turn may be due to faulty synthesis or secretion of GnRH , while chronic unremitting exposure to GnRH paradoxically desensitises the pituitary gonadotrophs. Hyperprolactinaemia can impair the pulsatile release of GnRH and thus induce secondary hypogonadism.

Pituitary tumours

Non-functioning pituitary adenomas may gradually encroach on normal pituitary reserve. There is a surprising consistency in the progression of hormonal deficits, with growth hormone loss occurring early but this is of relatively minor effect in adults. At about the same time, reduction in gonadotrophin secretion occurs with LH proving particularly vulnerable [33]. The conventional explanation is pressure exerted by the growing mass of tumorous tissue on the remaining normal gland. While this may seem plausible in the case of massive tumours, secondary hypogonadism may occur with

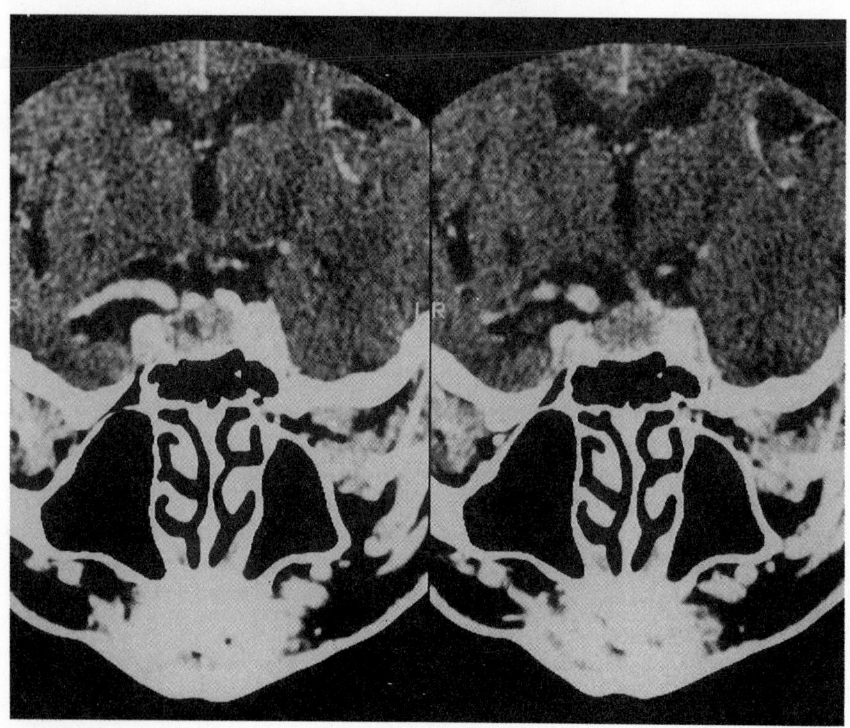

Fig. 49.11 Computed tomography through an intrasellar pituitary microadenoma (right-sided hypodense area on left-hand image, causing displacement of pituitary stalk to the left). This was associated with acquired hypogonadotrophic hypogonadism.

relatively small microadenomas (Fig. 49.11). The pressure hypothesis is also inconsistent with the remarkable paucity of endocrine effects in many patients with benign cranial hypertension, where the pituitary fossa is often greatly expanded with pituitary tissue flattened thinly against the floor at the bottom of an empty sella. Hypogonadism can complicate hypersecreting tumours of various types for different reasons. Thus, it is not uncommon in Cushing's syndrome of any aetiology because of the hypercortisolism. In some patients with pituitary-dependent Cushing's disease, corticotroph hyperplasia is found rather than a discrete adenoma; this may indicate a primary hypothalamic overproduction of corticotrophin-releasing hormone which in experimental models has been shown to have antigonadotrophic properties. Hyperprolactinaemia can induce hypogonadism, when due to either a pituitary prolactin-secreting adenoma or secondarily associated with a non-secretory tumour causing distortion of the pituitary stalk, which impairs delivery of prolactin inhibitory factors such as dopamine. The distinction between the two causes of hyperprolactinaemia is largely based on the level of prolactin secretion; high levels (over 6000 mU/l) are invariably from true prolactinomas as determined by immunostaining [34]. As mentioned above, the antigonadal action of prolactin is largely mediated by inhibiting the neural mechanism which drives the pulsatile secretion of GnRH. There may also be some impairment by prolactin of the action of LH on Leydig cells (Fig. 49.12). Many substances other than the classical anterior pituitary hormones have been localised to the adenohypophysis. Much interest in the paracrine effects between one pituitary cell type and another has arisen, and this may be a means by which hypogonadotrophic hypogonadism can arise. Hypogonadism commonly follows pituitary damage as may occur with pituitary surgery, irradiation or infarction; the latter may be silent or occur in acute pituitary apoplexy. Primary deficiency in gonadotroph reserve appears to underly the rare Laurence–Moon–Biedl syndrome; it also adds to the damage in iron-overload as in haemochromatosis.

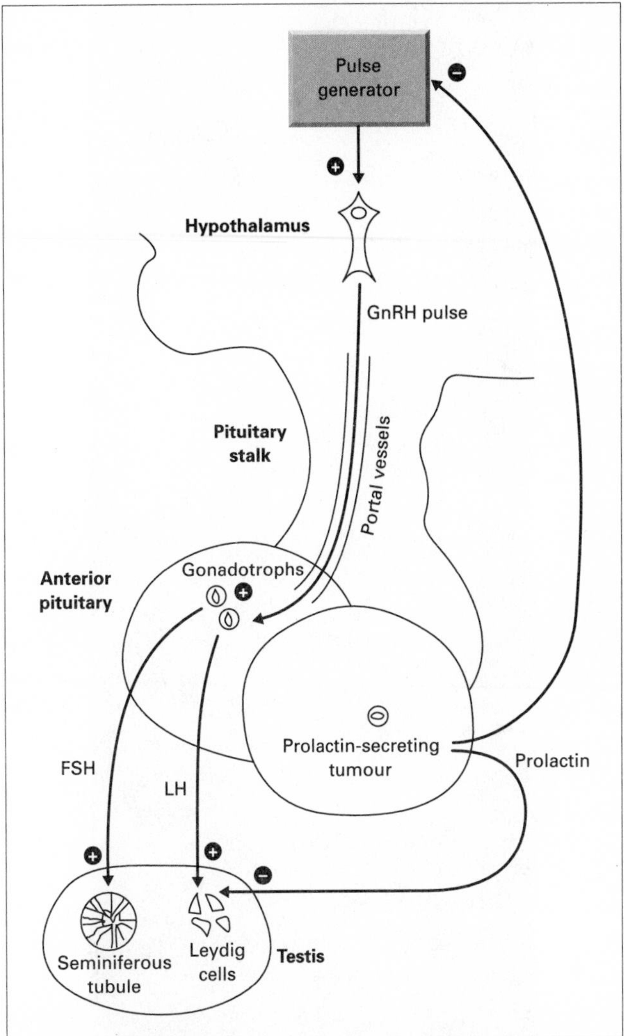

Fig. 49.12 Hyperprolactinaemia causes hypogonadism by inhibiting and slowing the hypothalamic pulse generator which drives the coordinated pulsatile release of gonadotrophin-releasing hormone into the portal vessels. It is also suggested that prolactin inhibits the action of gonadotrophins on the testis.

Hypothalamic disorders

Craniopharyngiomas may present at any time from infancy to old age and although mass effects, especially leading to visual loss, are the predominant features at the extremes of childhood and old age, there is characteristically hypogonadotrophic hypogonadism in most patients [35] (Fig. 49.13).

Isolated gonadotrophin deficiency may occur without any obvious additional features, or it may be associated with anosmia or hyposmia in Kallmann's syndrome where there is failure of olfactory lobe development. Consistent with this is the demonstration that GnRH neurons apparently originate from the olfactory placode in early fetal life rather than in the central nervous system. Several other features may be found such as centrally situated 'hare lip' and cleft palate, increased incidence of colour blindness (this has been disputed), neural deafness, cryptorchidism and abnormalities of the renal tract [36]. Absent septum pellucidum and corpus callosum have been described in some patients. In other patients there is a specific LH deficiency, variable spermatogenesis and gynaecomastia which has been labelled the 'fertile eunuch' syndrome (Fig. 49.14). Other patients combine growth hormone with gonadotrophin deficiency; the former presents in childhood, but microphallus is a marked feature.

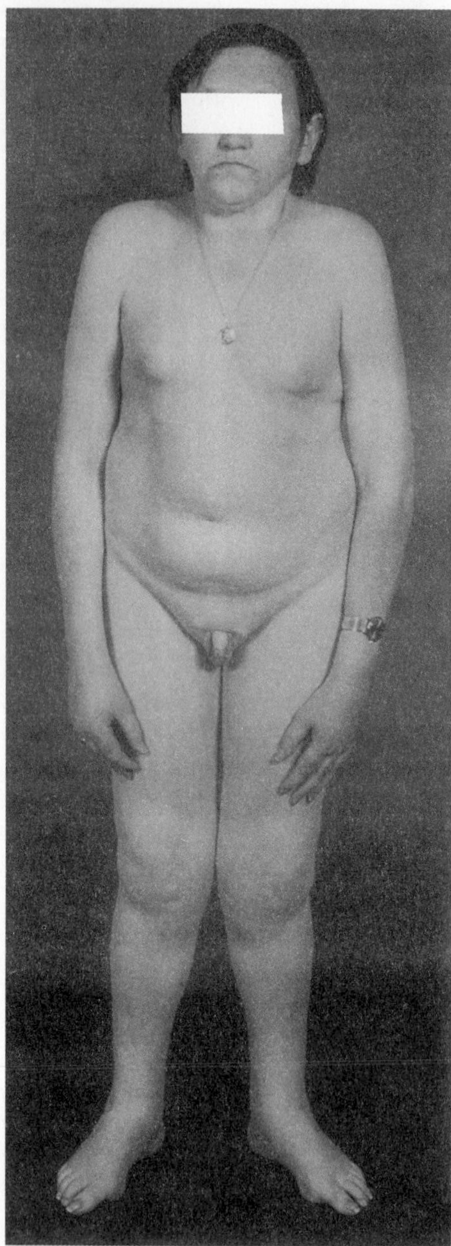

Fig. 49.13 A 53-year-old male with a calcified craniopharyngioma causing left-sided blindness, right temporal hemianopia, panhypopituitarism including sexual infantilism.

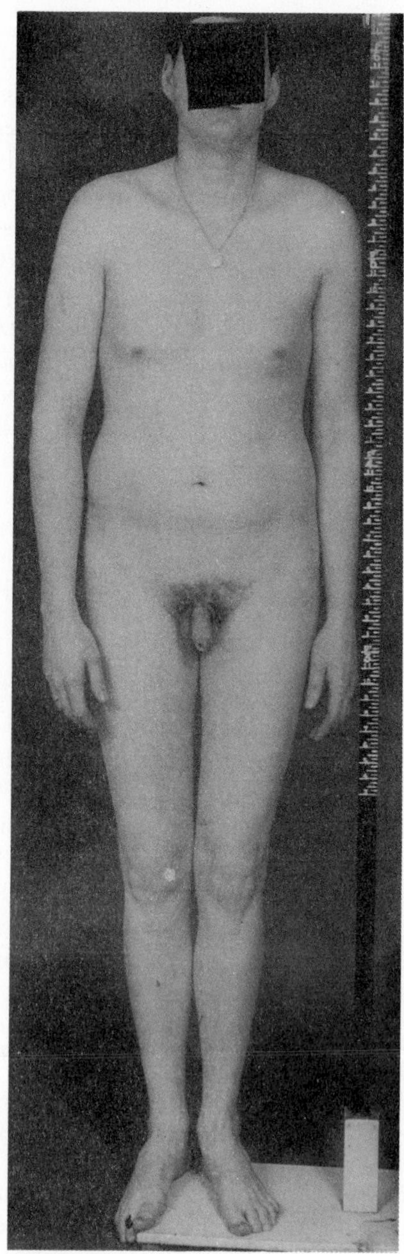

Fig. 49.14 Fertile eunuch. Note hypogonadal features, eunuchoidal proportions and gynaecomastia.

Constitutional delay in growth and development may be difficult to distinguish confidently from hypogonadotrophic hypogonadism; although several methods have been suggested, none has proved totally reliable. This is a self-limiting condition and the patients have delayed bone age and generally short stature. In these patients there is often a family history of delayed puberty. While the mechanism imposing sexual quiescence in childhood remains unknown, it does not appear to be due to absence of GnRH, but rather inhibition by some means of the pulse generator (although small amplitude LH pulses have been documented in prepubertal children) [37]. In non-human primates the pulsatile administration of excitatory amino acids such as *N*-methyl-D-aspartate (NMDA) immediately releases GnRH and LH may activate the whole hypothalamo-pituitary–gonadal axis [38].

The pulsatile release of GnRH is required for maintained gonadotrophin release. Unremitting exposure of the pituitary to GnRH eventually inhibits LH secretion (Fig. 49.15). The desensitisation of gonadotroph function has been facilitated

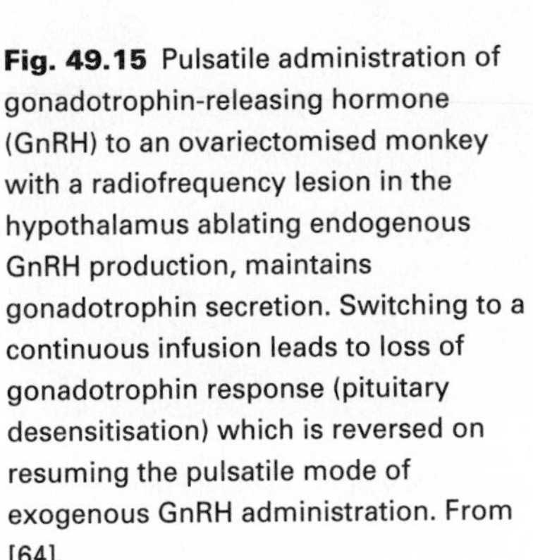

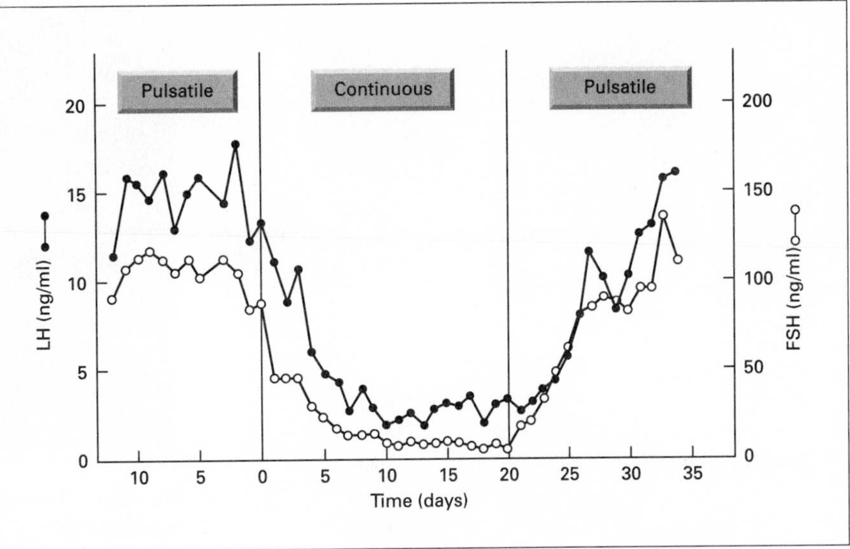

Fig. 49.15 Pulsatile administration of gonadotrophin-releasing hormone (GnRH) to an ovariectomised monkey with a radiofrequency lesion in the hypothalamus ablating endogenous GnRH production, maintains gonadotrophin secretion. Switching to a continuous infusion leads to loss of gonadotrophin response (pituitary desensitisation) which is reversed on resuming the pulsatile mode of exogenous GnRH administration. From [64].

by the development of so-called GnRH superagonists, which after initial stimulation cause long-term suppression especially of LH secretion. These analogues of GnRH usually contain D-amino acids in position 6 of the decapeptide in place of the glycine residue in the native molecule, and *N*-ethylamide in place of glycine-amide in position 10 [39]. They bind more avidly and are degraded much more slowly, leading to marked enhancement in biological half-life, while incorporation into depot preparations allows administration at monthly intervals. The induced hypogonadism so achieved has been most widely used in the treatment of carcinoma of the prostate (see Chapter 76). GnRH antagonists have also been synthesised. The use of early examples was hindered by their marked histamine-releasing properties but later generations of compounds seem free of this unwanted effect. GnRH antagonists have yet to establish a safe therapeutic role for themselves, although several compounds show considerable promise [40].

Testicular enlargement

Testicular enlargement may have many causes, which in turn may be associated with a variety of endocrine disturbances. The most important cause of testicular enlargement is neoplastic. Several hormonal abnormalities may be seen, for example interstitial tumours quite frequently secrete excessive amounts of oestrogen and can thus be associated with gynaecomastia and hypogonadism. Seminomas of the testis may be associated with excessive oestradiol production. A variety of granulomatous conditions may affect the testes—in the past, gumma of the testes was a well-recognised cause of testicular enlargement and impaired function.

The primary endocrine disorder most often associated with testicular enlargement is acromegaly—another example of organomegaly caused by growth hormone hypersecretion; testosterone secretion is, however, quite often reduced in adult male acromegalics. A rare, curious phenomenon is marked testicular enlargement associated with elevated inhibin secretion in FSH-secreting pituitary macroadenomas [41].

Macro-orchidism is found in the majority of patients with the fragile X syndrome which is one of the commonest forms of mental retardation. The testes have additional interstitial fluid, increased number of tubules, decreased tubular diameter and a first spermatogenic arrest [42].

Diagnosis

The diagnosis and assessment of male gonadal function is necessarily clinical in the first instance. These features have been summarised, but the importance of quantitative estimation of testicular volume demands emphasis. Linear dimensions can be measured with calipers but this is less satisfactory than assessing testis volume since this increases as a cube function of length (Fig. 49.16). Volume is easily and accurately estimated by comparing each testis with a series of appropriately shaped and accurately made ellipsoids ranging from 1 to 25 ml (Fig. 49.17), as suggested by Prader [43]. The circadian rhythm of testosterone merits some consideration; highest levels are usually found in the morning, but the amplitude is only about 30% and is thus much less important than in the measurement of cortisol or other adrenocortical steroid hormones or metabolites. Measurement of SHBG is not a first-line requirement in assessment of most male patients—far less important than with women—but examples where it is helpful have been mentioned, for example liver disease and thyrotoxicosis. It is particularly helpful to measure LH in conjunction with testosterone, bearing in mind the pulsatile pattern of LH

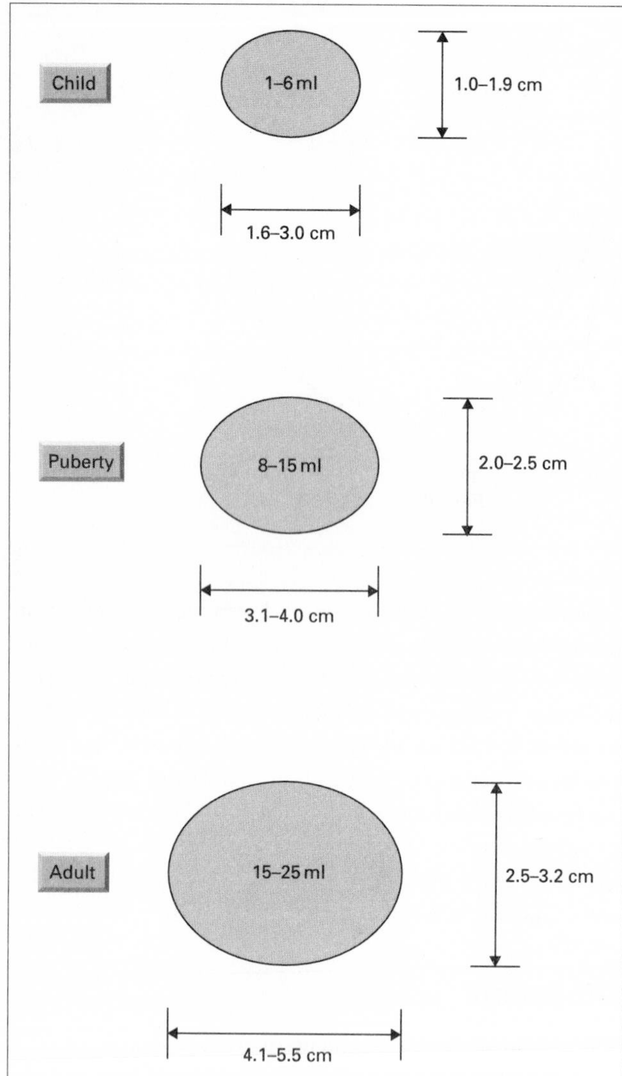

Fig. 49.16 Linear and volumetric dimensions of the testis at different stages of development.

release which is seen in an amplified form in many conditions of primary gonadal failure when basal LH levels are raised. The use of GnRH is a simple test involving blood samples at 0, 20 and 60 min after intravenous injection of 100 μg of exogenous GnRH (see Chapter 83). Its diagnostic value is, in fact, relatively limited. The use of the antioestrogen clomiphene has passed its vogue; it is a protracted test lasting several days and the results are often difficult to interpret. By contrast, the use of exogenous hCG is very helpful in various clinical situations: to ascertain the presence of testicular tissue in cryptorchid individuals, to distinguish them from the vanishing testis syndrome and to demonstrate the magnitude of Leydig-cell reserve [44]. Apart from these diagnostic functions, hCG has been widely used to accelerate pubertal development in constitutional delay,

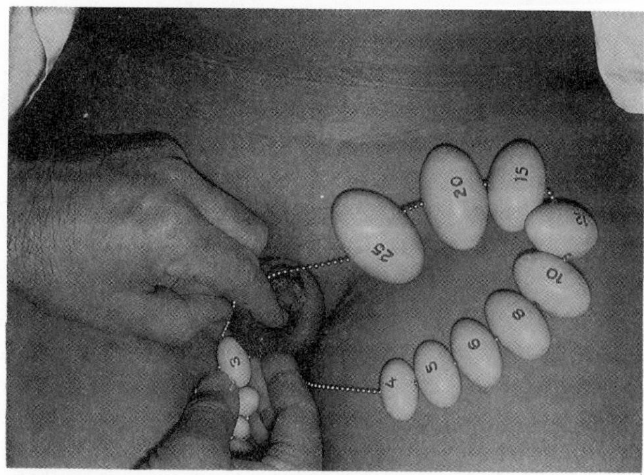

Fig. 49.17 Assessment of testicular volume using a Prader orchidometer.

while there are some advocates of its use in attempting to treat cryptorchidism; but it is not certain whether in supposedly successful cases marked retractility of the testis has always been excluded.

Treatment

Modern treatment of male hypogonadism is largely confined to various testosterone preparations. A variety of analogues, particularly 17α-alkylated derivatives, have been withdrawn from use despite their efficacy orally as exemplified by methyltestosterone. This was on account of hepatotoxicity leading to raised liver enzymes, cholestasis, peliosis hepatis and liver tumours. Mesterolone is a derivative of DHT, methylated at position 1 which confers resistance to hepatic metabolism enabling oral use but freedom from hepatotoxicity. Its structure precludes aromatisation to oestrogens but it is too weak to be useful as an androgen. Mesterolone has enjoyed a vogue in the treatment of oligospermia but most trials have been inadequately controlled and there is no convincing evidence for its effectiveness [45].

Testosterone preparations

Four major routes of testosterone administration have been explored: intramuscular, oral, subcutaneous and transdermal.

Intramuscular testosterone

Free testosterone has a half-life of only 10 min but injection of various testosterone esters provides the most frequently used mode of administration of testosterone. In the UK Sustanon 250, a mixture of esters, is most commonly used, partly because it is the cheapest preparation. It consists of

30 mg testosterone proprionate, 60 mg testosterone phenylproprionate, 60 mg testosterone isocaproate and 10 mg of testosterone decanoate. It is erroneously supposed to give a better (more constant) profile of circulating concentration of testosterone than using 250 mg of a single long-acting ester such as oenanthate, cypionate or cyclohexanecarboxylate. In fact, the peak testosterone concentration after injecting 250 mg testosterone oenanthate is reached very rapidly—by 10 hours after injection. The addition of testosterone proprionate which has a biological half-life of < 1 day simply distorts the early peak (Fig. 49.18).

Studies of multiple-dose pharmacokinetics have been conducted with various testosterone esters, and the optimum frequency with testosterone oenanthate 250 mg is about 2-weekly [46]. There is also a report of very constant levels being obtained by weekly injections of 100 mg. When the frequency decreases to three-weekly there are subnormal testosterone levels for the third week, and with four-weekly administration the nadir of testosterone reached prior to each injection is right down to basal levels. Since sexual function closely follows testosterone levels in hypogonadal men on replacement treatment [47], it follows that the commonly adopted practice of administering testosterone oenanthate or comparable esters at four-weekly intervals is significantly suboptimal. Occasional patients find one preparation consistently painful and even associated with systemic symptoms suggesting hypersensitivity, but can usually be transferred satisfactorily to alternative forms. Efforts are underway to evaluate the usefulness and safety of an extremely long-acting ester, testosterone-*trans*-4-*n*-butylcyclohexyl-carboxylate. A further development has been to incorporate testosterone into biodegradable poly (DL-lactide-co-glycolide) microspheres.

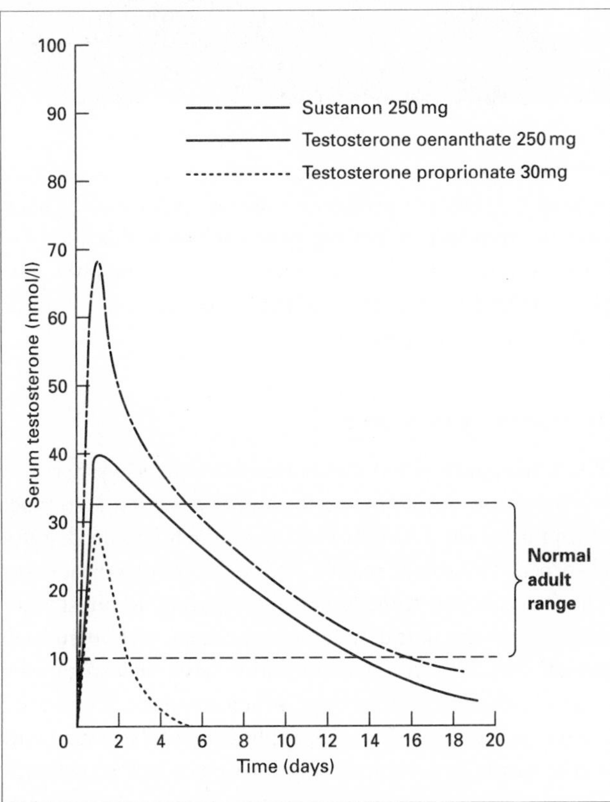

Fig. 49.18 Time course of plasma testosterone levels after the intramuscular injection of Sustanon 250, testosterone oenanthate 250 mg, testosterone proprionate 30 mg.

Oral testosterone

Testosterone is rapidly inactivated on its first pass through the liver after oral ingestion. Over 200 mg daily must be taken to outstrip this, and if such large (and uneconomic) doses are taken there is the risk of hepatotoxicity or at least excessive effect on hepatic metabolism, possibly affecting various lipoproteins, clotting factors and hormone-binding globulins, especially SHBG. Sublingual administration of testosterone in a variety of vectors has not been developed to the point of usefulness. The one major advance has been testosterone undecanoate, where the steroid is esterified at the 17β position with the long aliphatic undecanoic acid; this modification permits absorption via the lymphatics. The peak testosterone levels are high but reached at variable times after administration and, most importantly, are only very briefly maintained requiring at least twice- and probably thrice-daily or even more frequent administration. The clinical results with testosterone undecanoate are thus variable and often both costly, inconvenient and still suboptimal [46]. It is also difficult to monitor the dose as testosterone levels tend to be low when DHT levels are normal or even supranormal.

Subcutaneous testosterone

Subdermal implants of testosterone were first used in 1937—just 2 years after its characterisation and synthesis; few scientific investigations were reported. Initial use of cholesterol as an excipient with testosterone produced pellets with undesirable properties. Thereafter, pellets were made by heating testosterone above its melting point and compressing it into a long cylindrical mould. The pellets are cylinders of 4.5 mm diameter cut into 6 or 12 mm lengths to give 100 and 200 mg implants with 117 and 202 mm^2 surface area, respectively. They are implanted subcutaneously in any of a number of regions but usually in the lower abdomen using local anaesthesia, a small scalpel incision and a trocar and cannula under strictly aseptic conditions (Fig. 49.19). The wound may or may not need closure with a suture or otherwise adhesive strip and covered with a simple dressing.

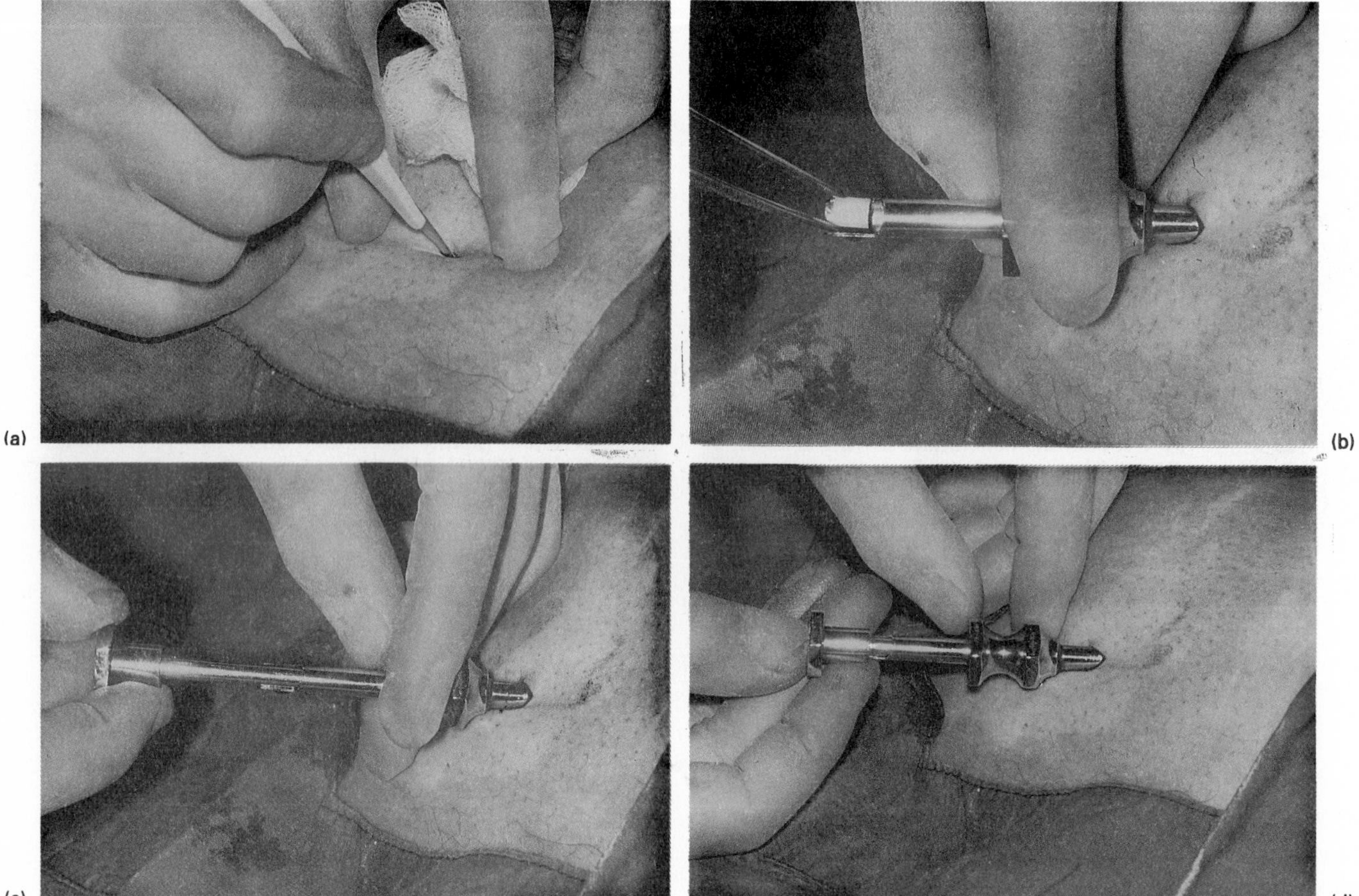

Fig 49.19 Technique for implanting testosterone pellets, after injecting area with local anaesthetic. (a) A small incision is made through which trocar and cannula are inserted. (b) After trocar is withdrawn pellet of testosterone is placed in groove at proximal end of side-loading cannula. (c) Trocar used to move pellet forward. (d) Pellet pushed out of distal end of cannula in subcutaneous site.

This technique has recently undergone renewed popularity (in spite of the British National Formulary declaring that the technique has been largely superseded). This is primarily due to the work of Anderson's group [48] and more recently Handelsman *et al.* in Australia [49]. The latter have studied the weight of pellets extruded at various times after implantation (this is a regrettably not uncommon occurrence). There is approximately 1.5 mg of testosterone absorbed daily from each 200 mg pellet or 0.65 mg/day/100 mg pellet. The bioavailability is almost complete. Studies of three regimens: 6 × 100 mg, 3 × 200 mg and 6 × 200 mg pellets showed the third protocol produced markedly higher levels and the testosterone levels were still slightly elevated above baseline at 6 months compared with the first two regimens where baseline levels were reached. The peak values are found between 2 and 4 weeks after implantation. The dynamics are such that it is predictably possible to replicate the daily 3–9 mg testosterone production of eugonadal men by using between two and six 200 mg pellets which will last for 4–6 months (Fig. 49.20). Testis-shaped large implants have been devised to double as testicular prostheses for use in orchidectomised patients.

Transdermal testosterone

The development of transdermal testosterone-delivery systems has been slower than for oestradiol, as the latter is so much more potent on a weight basis that much less needs to be absorbed. This can be readily achieved through normal skin. The feasibility of transdermal testosterone administration depends on the uniquely high absorbency of human male genital skin. The ALZA Corporation have devised a means of administering testosterone which involves dry shaving the scrotum every 1–2 weeks, application of the system with warm hands and compressing into place for 10 seconds. The use of this technique involving wearing a device for 22 hours each day has given generally excellent endocrine and biological effects. The Testoderm-TTS 3.6 mg system gives excellent physiological levels, whereas the 2.4 mg system was

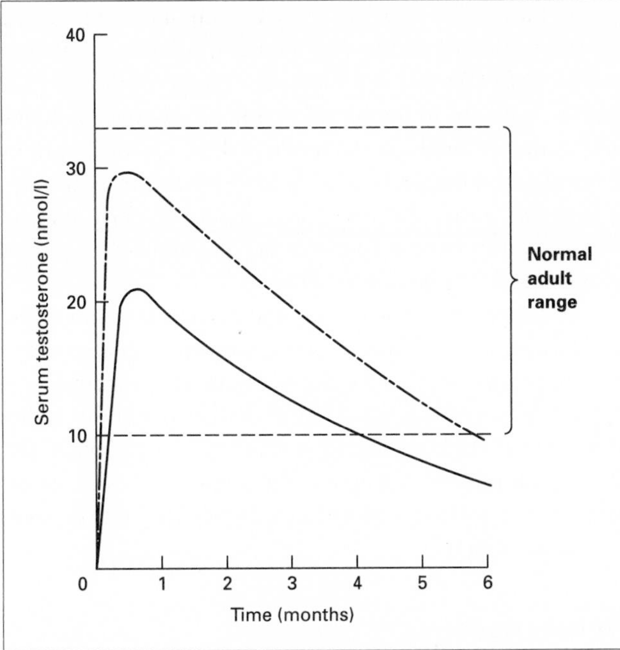

Fig. 49.20 Time course of serum testosterone levels following the subcutaneous implantation of 600 mg testosterone (——) (either 3 × 200 mg or 6 × 100 mg pellets) which produce testosterone levels in the normal range for approximately 4 months or 1200 mg (—-—) (6 × 200 mg) which keep the testosterone levels within the normal range for approximately 6 months.

conspicuously inferior. Numerous patients have evaluated these devices, including 62 for more than 1 year and 50 patients for more than 2 years. Of these, 11 discontinued their use: two because of intercurrent illness, three because the participating centre withdrew and six because of perceived lack of efficacy. Minor scrotal discomfort occurred in several patients occasionally but not sufficient to merit discontinuation in a total of more than 90 000 patient-days [50]. This route remains still at the stage of evaluation but certainly holds much promise.

A second-generation system of testosterone patches has been developed which uses permeation enhancers, enabling sufficient testosterone to be absorbed when applied to non-scrotal skin. Two patches applied to the back each night raised testosterone levels in hypogonadal men to within the normal adult male range during the trial of their application. In addition, the levels of DHT also remain normal while the patches are *in situ*, in contrast to the supraphysiological levels produced by scrotal patches, which are the result of the higher 5α-reductase activity of genital skin. Oestradiol levels also remain within the male range, contrasting to the higher levels which frequently follow the intramuscular injection of testosterone esters [51].

Alternative androgens

Dihydrotestosterone gel applied daily to a large area of abdominal skin and then washing off the application after 10 minutes has been evaluated in France [52]. The DHT appears to be readily absorbed and active as evidenced by the enhanced plasma levels of DHT and its principal metabolite 3α-androstanediol glucuronide. There appears to be no adverse effect on lipids or, as yet, on the prostate, while virilisation, muscular development and sexual function all improve. The pulsatile release of gonadotrophins is slowed by DHT administration to normal men, but is without effect on the LH and FSH responses to GnRH. Percutaneous DHT has been advocated for the treatment of idiopathic gynaecomastia, but with variable response.

Anabolic steroids

The use of anabolic steroids is probably still widespread in body-building fanatics, though hopefully it is diminishing in most sports especially power athletes because of the intensive and sophisticated monitoring that has been introduced. The risks of anabolic steroids, as used illicitly and certainly largely off prescription from the 'black market', are necessarily difficult to assess. There is potential added danger because of the popularity of using multiple anabolic steroids, orally and by injection as well as testosterone both serially and in combination: so called 'stacking the pyramid'. There is *no* evidence that improved strength or athletic performance follows. There are clearly potential dangers, but these might be mitigated by the use of these agents cyclically with wash-out periods of varying lengths of time in between. Gynaecomastia and feminising effects are paradoxically common, as is infertility.

Adverse cardiovascular effects mediated by changes in lipid profiles are a major long-term risk. 17α-alkylated androgens are still widely used with all their hepatotoxic hazards [53]. One 40-year-old man presented to us with an aggressive carcinoma of the prostate having abused anabolic steroids in this fashion for many years; the link is circumstantial but highly suggestive.

Other uses of androgens

Androgens are still being evaluated as part of the package providing effective, safe and acceptable male contraception.

Their use in children is limited, but is well established in managing constitutional delay in growth and development. Treatment courses generally are limited to no more than 3 months, but can be repeated if necessary. The ultimate height when used in this way is not compromised but the growth acceleration and virilisation are very beneficial, especially psychologically (see Chapter 62). The limited course approach allows discernment of true hypogonadotrophic hypogonadism when it occurs—which may be difficult to differentiate. Another, probably under-used, indication for testosterone in early childhood is in the treatment of micro-phallus [54]. When the course is again brief there are no adverse long-term sequelae, although the development of the penile shaft may be most effectively achieved. Catch-up growth, as ever, cannot be adequately achieved if treatment is postponed too late. Very occasionally androgens have been used to control excessive skeletal growth.

Androgens have been used in a variety of refractory anaemias including aplastic anaemia, with varying but occasionally dramatic responses. In several types, especially that associated with chronic renal failure, the advent of recombinant erythropoietin has made this use of androgens redundant.

Androgen deficiency and replacement in elderly men

Androgen production falls variably with age [55]. The sometime postulated 'andropause' is neither as inevitable, nor so rapid and large in scale, as the changes seen in the female menopause. Nevertheless, plasma levels below the normal range occur in 7% of men aged 40–60, 20% in the age group 60–80 and 35% in men over 80 years of age [56].

Age-related changes in body composition which may be associated with falling testosterone levels are seen in bone, with 50% of elderly men sustaining femoral neck fractures being hypogonadal biochemically though the clinical features may not be overt [57]. In addition, central fat develops while muscle mass diminishes, although this may relate in part to growth hormone 'deficiency'. Sexual function and general vigour also lessen with advancing age.

The potential role of androgen replacement reversing these changes remains to be established. Testosterone therapy in elderly men with low testosterone appears to reduce urinary excretion of hydroxyproline, increases lean body mass and tends to reduce body fat [58]. Muscle strength also increases [59]. These desirable changes have to be weighed against possible risks of cardiovascular disease and prostate cancer.

Surveillance of patients on testosterone

The remarkable safety of testosterone replacement in young adults means that routine monitoring is not needed provided an approved preparation and schedule is employed. In elderly men receiving testosterone more care is mandatory. The most significant risk is prostate cancer. Although cogent arguments have been levelled against population screening with measurements of prostatic-specific antigen (PSA) [60], if only for medico-legal prudence PSA should be measured before starting treatment and after 3–6 months of therapy in men aged 50 years and older. The concentration of PSA may be expected to double on treating hypogonadal males [61]. Conventional cut-off levels of PSA should apply in determining whether further investigations are indicated. Subsequent measurements of PSA should be performed at biannual intervals or of course earlier if symptoms suggestive of possible prostatic disease develop.

Less certain is whether lipids and haematocrit should be regularly monitored. Short-term treatment with androgens in elderly men may cause the haematocrit to increase by up to 7% [58,59]. Total cholesterol does not show major changes but there is usually a small fall in plasma HDL cholesterol which is of unknown significance [62]. Sleep apnoea may develop with or be exacerbated by testosterone replacement [63].

References

1 Wilson JD. Charles-Edouard Brown-Séquard and the centennial of endocrinology. *J Clin Endocrinol Metab* 1990; **71**: 1403–9.
2 Medvei VC. *A History of Endocrinology*. Lancaster: MTP, 1982.
3 Belchetz PE. Disorders of sexual differentation. In: Dawson AM, Compston ND, Besser GM, eds. *Recent Advances in Medicine*, Vol. 19. Edinburgh: Churchill Livingstone, 1984: 97–124.
4 Imperato-McGinley J, Guerrero L, Gautier T, Peterson RE. Steroid 5 Alpha-reductase deficiency in man: an inherited form of male pseudohermaphroditism. *Science* 1974; **186**: 1213–15.
5 Boyar RM, Rosenfeld RS, Kapen S *et al.* Human puberty. Simultaneous augmented secretion of luteinizing hormone and testosterone during sleep. *J Clin Invest* 1974; **54**: 609–18.
6 Evans RM. The steroid and thyroid hormone receptor superfamily. *Science* 1988; **240**: 889–95.
7 Wilson JD, Harrod MJ, Goldstein JL *et al.* Familial incomplete male pseudohermaphroditism, Type I. Evidence for androgen resistance and variable clinical manifestation in a family with the Reifenstein syndrome. *N Engl J Med* 1974; **290**: 1097–103.
8 Schweikert H-U, Romalo G. Syndromes caused by androgen resistance. In: Nieschlag E, Behre HM, eds. *Testosterone—Action, Deficiency, Substitution.* Berlin: Springer-Verlag, 1990: 72–91.
9 Whitaker RH. Management of the undescended testis. *Br J Med* 1970; **4**: 25–37.
10 Buckler J. *A Longitudinal Study of Adolescent Growth*. London: Springer-Verlag, 1990.
11 Stepan JJ, Lachman M, Zverina J *et al.* Castrated men exhibit bone loss: effect of calcitonin treatment on biochemical indices of bone remodeling. *J Clin Endocrinol Metab* 1989; **69**: 523–7.
12 Salmimies P, Kockott G, Pirke KM *et al.* Effects of testosterone replacement on sexual behaviour in hypogonadal men. *Arch Sex Behav* 1982; **11**: 345–53.
13 Gooren LJ. Androgen levels and sex functions in testosterone-treated hypogonadal men. *Arch Sex Behav* 1987; **16**: 463–73.
14 Nagulesparen M, Ang V, Jenkins JS. Bromocriptine treatment of males with pituitary tumours, hyperprolactinaemia and hypogonadism. *Clin Endocrinol* 1978; **9**: 73–9.
15 Sharpe RM. Intratesticular control of steroidogenesis. *Clin Endocrinol* 1990; **33**: 787–807.

16 Weinbauer GF, Nieschlag E. The role of testosterone in spermatogenesis. In: Nieschlag E, Behre HM, eds. Testosterone-action, deficiency, substitution. Berlin: Springer-Verlag, 1990: 23–50.

17 Burke CW, Anderson DC. Sex-hormone-binding globulin is an oestrogen amplifier. *Nature* 1972; **240**: 38.

18 Sherrins RJ, De Vita VT. Effect of drug treatment for lymphoma on male reproductive capacity. *Ann Intern Med* 1973; **79**: 216–20.

19 Bancroft J, Temment T, Loncas K, Cass J. Control of deviant sexual behaviour by drugs and behavioural effects of oestrogens and antiandrogens. *Br J Psychiatr* 1974; **125**: 310–15.

20 Delitala G, Stubbs WA, Wass JAH *et al.* Effects of the H_2 receptor antagonist cimetidine on pituitary hormones in man. *Clin Endocrinol* 1979; **11**: 161–7.

21 Holland FJ, Fishman L, Bailey JD, Fazekas ATA. Ketoconazole in the management of precocious puberty not responsive to LHRH-analogue therapy. *N Engl J Med* 1985; **312**: 1023–8.

22 Van Thiel DH, Lester R. Sex and alcohol. *N Engl J Med* 1974; **291**: 251–3.

23 Irvine WJ, Barnes EW. Adrenocortical insufficiency. *Clin Endocrinol Metab* 1972; **1**:549–94.

24 Chandley AC. The chromosomal basis of human infertility. *Br Med Bull* 1979; **35**: 181–6.

25 Schibler D, Brook CGD, Kind HP *et al.* Growth and body proportions in 54 boys and men with Klinefelter's syndrome. *Helv Paediat Acta* 1974; **29**: 325–33.

26 Ahmad KN, Dykes JRW, Ferguson-Smith MA *et al.* Leydig cell volume in chromatin positive Klinefelter's syndrome. *J Clin Endocrinol Metab* 1971; **33**: 517–20.

27 Anderson DC, Marshall JC, Young JL, Russell Fraser T. Stimulation of pituitary Leydig cell function in normal male subjects and hypogonadal males. *Clin Endocrinol* 1972; **1**: 127–40.

28 Bramble FJ, Houghton AL, Eccles S *et al.* Reproductive and endocrine function after surgical treatment of bilateral cryptorchidism. *Lancet* 1974; **ii**: 311–14.

29 Comhaire F, Vermeulen A. Plasma testosterone in patients with varicocele and sexual inadequacy. *J Clin Endocrinol Metab* 1975; **40**: 824–9.

30 Sagel J, Distiller LA, Morley JE, Isaacs H. Myotonia dystrophica: studies on gonadal function using luteinizing-releasing hormone (LRH). *J Clin Endocrinol Metab* 1975; **40**: 1110–13.

31 Galvoá-Teles A, Anderson DC, Burke CW *et al.* Biologically active androgens and oestradiol in men with chronic liver disease. *Lancet* 1973; **i**: 173–7.

32 Green JRB, Goble HL, Edwards CRW, Dawson AM. Reversible insensitivity to androgens in men with untreated gluten enteropathy. *Lancet* 1977; **i**: 280–2.

33 Belchetz PE. Hypopituitarism. In: Belchetz PE, ed. *Management of Pituitary Disease*. London: Chapman and Hall, 1984; 103–15.

34 Ross RJM, Grossman A, Boulouz P *et al.* The relationship between serum prolactin and immunocytochemical staining for prolactin in patients with pituitary macroadenomas. *Clin Endocrinol* 1985; **23**: 227–35.

35 Jenkins JS, Gilbert CJ, Ang V. Hypothalamic-pituitary function in patients with craniopharyngiomas. *J Clin Endocrinol Metab* 1976; **43**: 394-9.

36 Santen RJ, Paulsen CA. Hypogonadotrophic hypogonadism. I. Clinical study of the mode of inheritance. *J Clin Endocrinol Metab* 1973; **36**: 47–54.

37 Jacacki RI, Kelch RP, Sauder SE *et al.* Pulsatile secretion of luteinizing hormone in children. *J Clin Endocrinol Metab* 1982; **55**: 453–8.

38 Gay VL, Plant TM. *N*-Methyl-D, L-aspartate elicits hypothalamic gonadotrophin releasing hormone release in prepubertal male rhesus monkeys. *Endocrinology* 1987; **120**: 2289–96.

39 Belchetz PE. Gonadotrophin regulation and clinical applications of GnRH. *Clin Endocrinol Metab* 1983; **12**: 619–40.

40 Conn PM, Crowley WF, Jr. Gonadotropin-releasing hormone and its analogues. *N Engl J Med* 1991; **324**: 93–103.

41 Heseltine D, White MC, Kendall-Taylor P *et al.* Testicular enlargement and elevated serum inhibin concentrations occur in patients with pituitary macroadenomas secreting follicle stimulating hormone. *Clin Endocrinol* 1989; **31**: 411–23.

42 Rudelli RD, Brown WT, Wisniewski K *et al.* Adult fragile X syndrome. Clinicopathological findings. *Acta Neuropathol* 1985; **67**: 289–96.

43 Prader A. Delayed adolescence. *Clin Endocrinol Metab* 1975; **4**: 143–55.

44 Belchetz PE. Endocrine factors in male gonadal function. In: Hendry WF, ed. *Recent Advances in Urology/Andrology*, Vol. 3. Edinburgh: Churchill Livingstone, 1981: 291–323.

45 World Health Organisation Task Force on the Diagnosis and Treatment of Infertility. Mesterolone and idiopathic male infertility: a double-blind study. *Int J Androl* 1989; **12**: 254–64.

46 Behre HM, Oberpenning F, Nieschlag E. Comparative pharmacokinetics of androgen preparations: application of computer analysis and simulation. In: Nieschlag E, Behre HM, eds. *Testosterone—Action, Deficiency, Substitution.* Berlin: Springer-Verlag, 1990: 115–35.

47 Davidson JM, Camargo CA, Smith ER. Effects of androgen on sexual behavior in hypogonadal men. *J Clin Endocrinol Metab* 1979; **48**: 955–8.

48 Cantrill JA, Dewis P, Large DM *et al.* Which testosterone therapy? *Clin Endocrinol* 1984; **21**: 97–107.

49 Handelsman DJ, Conway AJ, Boylan LM. Pharmacokinetics and pharmacodynamics of testosterone pellets in man. *J Clin Endocrinol Metab* 1990; **71**: 216–22.

50 Place VA, Atkinson L, Prather DA. Transdermal testosterone replacement through genital skin. In: Nieschlag E, Behre HM, eds. *Testosterone—Action, Deficiency, Substitution.* Berlin: Springer-Verlag, 1990: 165–81.

51 Meikle AW, Mazer NA, Moellmer JF *et al.* Enhanced transdermal delivery of testosterone across non-scrotal skin produces physiological concentrations of testosterone and its metabolites in hypogonadal men. *J Clin Endocrinol Metab* 1992; **74**: 623–8.

52 Schaison G, Renoir M, Lagogney M, Mowszowicz I. On the role of dihydrotestosterone in regulating luteinizing hormone secretion in man. *J Clin Endocrinol Metab* 1980; **51**: 1133–7.

53 Wilson JD. Androgen abuse by athletes. *Endocr Rev* 1988; **9**: 181–99.

54 Burstein S, Grumbach MM, Kaplan SL. Early determination of androgen-reponsiveness is important in the management of microphallus. *Lancet* 1979; **ii**: 983–6.

55 Bremner WJ, Vitiello MV, Prinz PN. Loss of circadian rhythmicity in blood testosterone levels with ageing in normal men. *J Clin Endocrinol Metab* 1985; **56**: 1278–81.

56 Vermeulen A, Kaufman JM. Ageing of the hypothalamo-pituitary–testicular axis in men. *Horm Res* 1995; **43**: 25–8.

57 Stanley HL, Schmitt BS, Poses RM, Deiss WP. Does hypogonadism contribute to the occurrence of minimal trauma fractures in men? *J Am Geriatr Soc* 1991; **39**: 766–71.

58 Tenover JS. Effects of testosterone supplementation in the ageing male. *J Clin Endocrinol Metab* 1992; **75**: 1092–8.

59 Morley JE, Perry HM III, Kaiser FE *et al.* Effects of testosterone replacement therapy in old hypogonadal males: a preliminary study. *J Am Geriatr Soc* 1993; **41**: 149–52.
60 Woolf SH. Screening for prostate cancer with prostate-specific antigen. *N Engl J Med* 1995; **333**: 1401–5.
61 Behre HM, Bohmeyer J, Nieschlag E. Prostate volume in testosterone-treated and untreated hypogonadal men in comparison to age-matched normal controls. *Clin Endocrinol (Oxf)* 1994; **40**: 341–9.
62 Bagatell CJ, Bremner WJ. Androgens in men—uses and abuses. *N Engl J Med* 1996; **334**: 707–14.
63 Matsumoto AM, Sandblom RE, Schoene RB *et al.* Testosterone replacement in hypogonadal men: effects on obstructive sleep apnoea, respiratory drives, and sleep. *Clin Endocrinol (Oxf)* 1985; **22**: 713–21.
64 Belchetz PE, Plant TM, Nakai Y *et al.* Hypophysial responses to continuous and intermittent delivery of hypothalamic gonadotrophin-releasing hormone (GnRH). *Science* 1978; **202**: 631–3.

CHAPTER 50

Male infertility: diagnosis, anti-sperm antibodies and surgical treatment

W.F. Hendry

Introduction

The easiest factor to check in a childless marriage is the seminal analysis, and it is the easiest factor to criticise. Too few spermatozoa, too slow, too abnormal, the blame is easy to shift onto the male with little or no effort made to define the underlying cause. The 'male factor' is all-too-often made the culprit for otherwise unexplained infertility; there it remains in many cases, unexamined, uninvestigated and untreated, considered by many to be beyond serious therapeutic endeavour. In fact, investigation of male infertility [1] requires detailed clinical examination, with measurement of endocrinological and immunological factors, as well as assessment of local thermoregulatory mechanisms and, in selected cases, definition of the patency of the sperm-conducting passages. Over and over again a correctable factor can be found in men who have been referred for assisted fertilisation or dismissed as hopeless, even consigned to the easy option of donor insemination. A responsible approach to the infertile couple should include methodical and systematic investigation of the male partner.

Investigations

The clinical history

This should cover the age, occupation and religion of the patient and his partner, the length of time that they have been trying to produce a family, together with the frequency and success of sexual intercourse. Present medical conditions, especially endocrine disorders, and any current drug therapy or exposure to toxic chemicals are reviewed [2]. Relevant past history may include tuberculosis, adult mumps, venereal disease, maldescended testes or hernia repairs. In the social history, intake of tobacco, alcohol and drugs may be relevant.

Examination

The general body build, hair distribution, and type of underpants worn are checked. The patient is examined standing in a good light to search for possible varicocele. The penis, foreskin and external meatus are checked. Attention is then turned to the testicles, noting their size and consistency; it is helpful to record the volume of each testis, looking particularly for any asymmetry, using ultrasound scanning [3] or Prader's orchidometer. The epididymes and vasa are palpated individually, searching for distension or tenderness that may indicate obstruction [4]. The scrotal skin is examined for signs of irritation due to eczematous dermatitis that may lead to thickening and hyperaemia of the dermis [5]. Finally, the patient should be placed in the left lateral position to examine the prostate gland and seminal vesicles; if tenderness suggestive of prostatovesiculitis is present, prostatic fluid should be expressed by gentle massage and sent in transport medium for microbiological examination, including bacterial culture and sensitivities.

Transrectal ultrasound

This is a useful supplement to digital rectal examination, and will accurately identify congenital malformations such as a Müllerian duct cyst, as well as showing acquired obstructions to the ejaculatory ducts [6].

Scrotal thermography

The scrotum is normally about 5°C cooler than the rest of the body (Fig. 50.1) and a significant varicocele can be detected by the thermographic abnormality it produces. Thermography [7] can be very helpful in settling doubts about the possible presence of a small varicocele or about the significance of any residual veins persisting after surgery

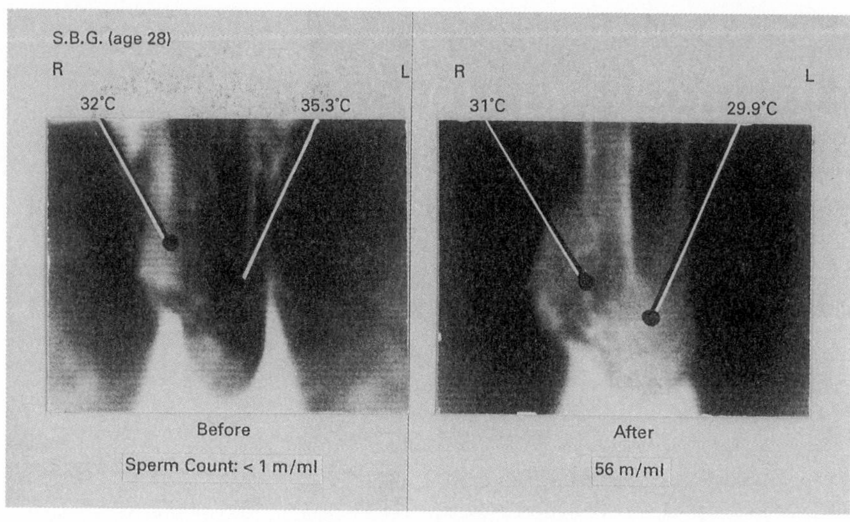

Fig. 50.1 Scrotal thermography before and after varicocele ligation.

or embolisation, and in deciding whether they are unilateral or bilateral.

Seminal analysis

It is generally accepted that normal sperm concentration should exceed 20 million/ml, of which more than 30% should be moving actively within 4 hours of production, in a seminal fluid volume of at least 1.5 ml. Irrespective of the findings reported in previous tests, it is always wise to check two more specimens in a known and trusted laboratory (for details of accepted seminology techniques see WHO Manual). The patient is instructed to produce the specimen by masturbation, after at least 3 days abstinence, directly into a suitable plastic container which should be marked with the time of production. A condom should not be used unless it is specially made for the purpose of sperm collection—this is sometimes necessary for Orthodox Jewish patients. Analysis should be performed within 2 hours, with measurement of volume, sperm concentration and motility, together with an assessment of the proportion of abnormal forms.

The number and type of cells in the ejaculate should be noted; an increased number of polymorphonuclear leucocytes may indicate prostatitis, and there is evidence that this may be related to defective sperm function [8]. Biochemical analysis of seminal plasma has shown few differences in electrolyte content between fertile and infertile patients. However, measurement of pH and zinc content in prostatic secretions or split ejaculate semen specimens may be informative in patients with poor sperm motility or prostatitis.

Fructose is absent in cases with absence of the vasa or vesicles, or ejaculatory duct obstruction; the volume of the ejaculate is usually small (< 1 ml) in these cases, and the pH is acid (< 7.0). Detailed assessment of problems with sperm motility requires examination of semen samples freshly produced at the hospital and examined immediately in the seminology laboratory. Facilities must be provided to enable patients to produce such samples in reasonable security. Liquefaction of semen, detailed bacteriological examination and electron microscopy can then be done. Occasionally abnormalities in microtubules or absence of the dynein arms in the sperm tails will be detected [9]. Agglutination of sperm may be observed, but this is a non-specific phenomenon and it should *not* be interpreted as evidence of agglutinating sperm antibodies.

Antisperm antibodies

These are most readily detected bound to the patient's own spermatozoa, using as a marker either sensitised red blood cells in the direct mixed antiglobulin reaction (MAR test) [10] or, after washing thoroughly to get rid of unbound immunoglobulin in seminal plasma, by addition of immunobeads (direct IB test) [11]. Whilst the former test has the advantage of being quick, reliable and easy to read [12], it is really only useful for detection of IgG, whereas with class-specific IB, the class of antibody on the spermatozoa can be defined. Thus, although the MAR test is an excellent screening test, positive results should be studied further with IB tests [13]. In addition, the amount of unbound antibody should be measured in the patient's serum and seminal plasma by the tray agglutination test (TAT) [14], which uses donor spermatozoa and micro-quantities of reagents; this has replaced the older macroscopic gelatin agglutination test (GAT) (see below).

Post-coital test

In order to establish a man's potential fertility, it should be demonstrated that his spermatozoa can produce an adequate post-coital test (PCT) in his partner's ovulatory cervical mucus—this is usually defined as more than five *motile* sperms per high-power field. Of course, the PCT might be poor for a number of reasons, but the coexistence of a normal sperm count and a persistently poor PCT strongly suggests the existence of sperm antibodies, and these most commonly occur in the husband [15]. The partner with the antibodies can be identified by direct testing for sperm antibodies, and their significance should be confirmed by sperm–cervical mucus testing using donor sperm and mucus as controls [16] (see below).

Hormone studies

Normal spermatogenesis requires both luteinising hormone (LH) and follicle-stimulating hormone (FSH), together with a high testosterone environment within the testicle. Normal spermatogenesis provides the negative feedback for FSH, while a normal level of circulating testosterone controls LH production. Failure of spermatogenesis due to gonadotrophin deficiency is uncommon, but these cases are important to recognise as they respond well to replacement therapy. Much more often, the cause is a primary defect in spermatogenesis, which may be recognised because the FSH level is usually elevated. Indeed, the combination of azoospermia, small testes and a grossly elevated FSH level is diagnostic of absent or grossly impaired spermatogenesis for which there is no treatment [17]. The situation is more complex when one or both testes are of reasonable size and the FSH level is normal or only slightly elevated [18]; scrotal exploration and testicular biopsy is needed to assess spermatogenesis and exclude obstruction. With oligozoospermia, the obstruction may be unilateral, and it should be remembered that one atrophic testis can raise the serum FSH even though there is normal spermatogenesis on the other side. There are considerable diurnal and other variations in both gonadotrophin and testosterone levels, and these should always be repeated if there is any doubt about their significance.

The coexistence of impotence with infertility calls for full endocrinological investigation. If the testosterone level is low, the gonadotrophin levels, with LH-releasing hormone (LHRH) stimulation if necessary, will indicate whether the cause is primarily hypothalamic, pituitary or testicular. An elevated prolactin level should be interpreted with great care—it can be raised by stress and by drugs such as phenothiazines (see also Chapter 9). However, a persistently elevated serum prolactin on serial testing, especially if it is associated with relative impotence, may indicate a pituitary tumour.

Thyroid and adrenal cortical hormone levels should be checked if there is any clinical suspicion of abnormality.

Chromosome studies

These studies are of interest in patients with infertility. Somatic chromosomes may be checked in buccal smears or blood, and cases of Klinefelter's syndrome or examples of balanced translocation may be found in subfertile males. Meiotic chromosome studies show considerable variations from normal, including translocations, low chiasma frequency and asynapsis, and supernumerary chromosomes [19]. Patients with such abnormalities respond poorly to treatment, although some pregnancies may be produced; patients with demonstrable chromosome abnormalities should therefore be offered genetic counselling, and any pregnancy that is produced should be checked for prenatal diagnosis of abnormality.

Other tests

Any systemic disease may affect male fertility, and it is sensible to check full blood count, blood urea, fasting blood sugar, liver function tests and folic acid, and perform routine urinalysis as part of the general work-up. Sickle status should be established in patients of African descent.

Testicular biopsy

In carefully selected cases, it is important to exclude unilateral or bilateral testicular obstruction at the same time as spermatogenesis is assessed; testicular biopsy is, therefore, usually combined with exploration of the scrotum so that the epididymes can be examined and vasography performed if indicated. The testicular biopsy is best done under general anaesthetic and the tissue should be fixed in Bouin's solution (*not* formalin). The Johnsen mean score count system [20] rates spermatogenesis from 0 to 10: patients who respond well to treatment have significantly higher scores than those who do not; however, pregnancies can be produced by patients with mean scores as low as 6.0 [1], which includes most patients with moderate or severe oligozoospermia, indicating that the result has limited value for the individual patient as an accurate prognostic index. Biopsy is unnecessary in patients with small testes and grossly elevated FSH levels.

Subsequent care

Once these investigations are completed, the patient and his partner can be advised as to whether there is a specific abnormality which requires attention, or whether non-specific measures would be more appropriate. This decision is seldom simple; if specific abnormalities are present, therapeutic options can be detailed. Adverse factors should be identified and removed: these include excessive indulgence in alcohol or smoking, and adverse effects of drugs which may be taken by the patient or administered therapeutically [21]. The temperature of the testes is critically important for normal function, and correction of defects which interfere with normal scrotal heat regulation can lead to significant improvement in sperm quality. Varicocele is the commonest abnormality which may produce such problems, especially when the right testis is atrophic [22]. Genital infection is associated with impairment of sperm motility, possibly due to release of superoxide radicals, and prolonged treatment with an appropriate antibiotic may correct this defect. Anti-spermatozoal antibodies lead to poor sperm penetration of cervical mucus, and may produce oligozoospermia if there is an associated autoimmune orchitis; these phenomena can interfere with fertility, but may be responsive to appropriate therapy with corticosteroids (see below).

Testicular obstruction may reduce sperm output if unilateral and stimulate the production of anti-sperm antibodies, or produce sterility if bilateral: modern microsurgical operative techniques permit accurate surgical reconstruction with a high degree of functional success (see below).

There are many couples where a specific defect cannot be identified; this does not mean that a careful search should not be made for one, since its correction can provide a long-lasting and cost-effective solution to their infertility problem. In others, modern methods of assisted reproduction now provide real hope where previously there was none.

Anti-sperm antibodies

Autoimmunity to spermatozoa can occur spontaneously, after genital infection or associated with testicular obstruction, either unilateral or bilateral. The resulting anti-sperm antibodies can impair spermatozoal penetration of cervical mucus, interfere with sperm–egg fusion, and lead to oligozoospermia. These antibodies are highly complex and may affect sperm function differently in different individuals.

Many laboratory tests have been devised for the detection of anti-sperm antibodies, and all have an apparently sound immunological basis. Unfortunately, the results obtained by some tests have not correlated well with those obtained by others, and this has led inevitably to confusion and some incredulity as to the significance of autoimmunity as a cause of human infertility. Mindful of these difficulties, a World Health Organization reference bank was organised, the tests were standardised [23] and the results of an international workshop were published [24]. The GAT [25] and TAT [14] gave consistent and reproducible results with samples distributed to many laboratories in different parts of the world. Likewise, the complement-dependent sperm-immobilisation test (SIT) devised by Isojima [26] gave reproducible results which correlated well with infertility. These tests all used normal donor sperm as the substrate, and the agglutination or immobilisation titre was defined by serial dilution of patients' serum or seminal plasma.

Tests carried out on the patients' own spermatozoa are more difficult to interpret. The MAR test [10] uses group O Rh-positive red blood cells sensitised with anti-D as the indicator, mixed with patients' spermatozoa and anti-human IgG—a positive response being indicated by the formation of mixed agglutinates. This test is applicable to most human semen samples and correlates well with GAT and TAT results [12].

IB can be used directly to detect surface antibody on patients' spermatozoa, or indirectly to measure antibody titres in the patients' serum or seminal plasma [11]. However, correlation with the classical agglutination tests has not always been good, and this is largely due to the exquisite sensitivity of IB testing, estimated at eight times that of the TAT [27]. Inevitably, some false-positive results must be expected and these have led to difficulties.

Immunofluorescence or radioimmunoassay demonstration of antibody on patients' spermatozoa has given results which show little or no correlation with the results of the classic agglutination tests [28]. This is probably because fixation of spermatozoa prior to testing reveals subsurface antigen to which antibody becomes non-specifically attached. As a general rule, it seems that *live* spermatozoa must be used as the substrate for anti-sperm antibody testing if valid results are to be obtained.

Antibody on the man's spermatozoa leads to impaired penetration of cervical mucus. This occurs irrespective of whether the mucus is from his partner or a donor—the phenomenon of 'cervical hostility' is a result of abnormality of the *spermatozoa*, rather than of the cervical mucus. The sperm–cervical mucus contact (SCMC) test and the crossed-hostility test provide an opportunity to directly study the reaction between spermatozoa and the new environment in which they have to make forward progress. This test is of fundamental importance, and provides a reference point against which the results of other tests can checked for significance. Many men with anti-sperm antibodies after vasectomy reversal are fertile and have spermatozoa that penetrate cervical mucus well, whereas this is exceptionally uncommon in spontaneously (i.e. non-vasectomised) infertile males. Most of the former have predominantly IgG on their spermatozoa, whereas the latter have both IgG and IgA (with secretory piece, thus confirming its local origin) [29]. It is likely that IgA is a mucosal antibody, locally produced in the genital tract, whereas IgG is its circulating systemic counterpart.

Several points should be noted about the critical path through the various tests that have been described, leading eventually to treatment. The MAR and PCT are merely screening tests: these should be supplemented by serum testing for antibodies to provide a baseline titre; and since serum antibodies are not always accompanied by seminal plasma antibodies and IgA on the spermatozoa (e.g. after vasectomy reversal), their presence or absence should be defined as well. Ultimately, the significance of the antibodies can be established by SCMC testing, and ideally treatment should not commence until this has been done.

Treatment

Any effective therapy for subfertility due to anti-sperm antibodies is demanding on the time of clinical and laboratory staff, and requires great patience and perseverance from the couple concerned. It can also produce serious adverse effects. It is, therefore, essential to make sure, before starting treatment, that the anti-sperm antibodies are making a significant contribution to the infertility, that the husband's sperm output is as good as possible, and that the wife is normally fertile. In addition, every care should be taken to be as sure as possible that the treatment will not cause problems. With these aims in mind we have established the following treatment protocol.

Patients

Males who have been trying unsuccessfully to produce a pregnancy for at least 1 year and satisfying the following criteria.

1 The female partner has patent tubes (preferably demonstrated by laparoscopy) and has been documented to be ovulating adequately. If she is not ovulating adequately, then she should be appropriately treated and no therapy given to the husband until this has been shown to have been effective by repeating the measurement of progesterone levels.

2 Some spermatozoa are present in the ejaculate in at least two samples (MAR test should be positive if it is technically possible to do this test).

3 There is an abnormal PCT (less than five progressively (motile sperms per high-power field) done between the 12th and 14th day of cycle after intercourse 8–12 hours previously.

4 Serum GAT or TAT are positive at titre of 32 or more and/or seminal plasma GAT or TAT are positive at titre of 4 or more.

5 SCMC test is abnormal with sperm 'shaking' on 12th-14th day of cycle.

If these criteria are satisfied, it is reasonable to conclude that autoimmunity to spermatozoa in the male partner is a significant factor in the couple's infertility. Various methods of treatment have been tried, but in our experience prednisolone has been the most effective. Various regimens have been used, and the results will be described, but before starting treatment various general medical checks should be carried out.

Pretreatment work-up

Diastolic blood pressure should be <90 mmHg, and chest X-ray and liver-function tests should be normal. The blood sugar 2 hours after food should be <8.9 mmol/l, and there should be no glycosuria. There should be no first-degree family history of diabetes; if there is, then a glucose tolerance test should be performed and shown to be normal. Finally, there should be no significant history of dyspepsia. If these criteria cannot be fulfilled, the patient should be referred for detailed medical assessment before treatment is commenced.

Informed consent

Both partners should be interviewed together and the details of treatment explained in full. Precautions to be followed whilst on steroid therapy, and possible side-effects are detailed on an information sheet which is given to the couple to take away and keep. Mention of possible serious complications is made, and the final decision on whether to proceed or not is left to the couple. If necessary a further consultation is arranged to give the couple time to consider their decision and, if they wish, discuss it with their general medical practitioner.

Steroid regimens

Three steroid regimens have been used: long-term, low-dose prednisolone; intermittent, high-dose methylprednisolone; and intermediate, graduated-dose prednisolone.

Long-term, low-dose prednisolone

Fifteen patients with average pretreatment sperm counts of <20 million/ml received prednisolone 5 mg t.d.s. daily for 3–12 (average 6) months. The sperm counts rose to normal levels in 10 (67%) and two partners became pregnant. Fourteen patients with normal sperm counts also received prednisolone 5 mg t.d.s. for a similar period: pronounced variation in the quality of the seminal analysis in six cases became consistently normal, but only two pregnancies were produced [30].

In seven males with severe oligozoospermia (<1 million/ml) or azoospermia, and very high anti-sperm antibody titres (serum TAT >512), continuous prednisolone (5 mg T.D.S.

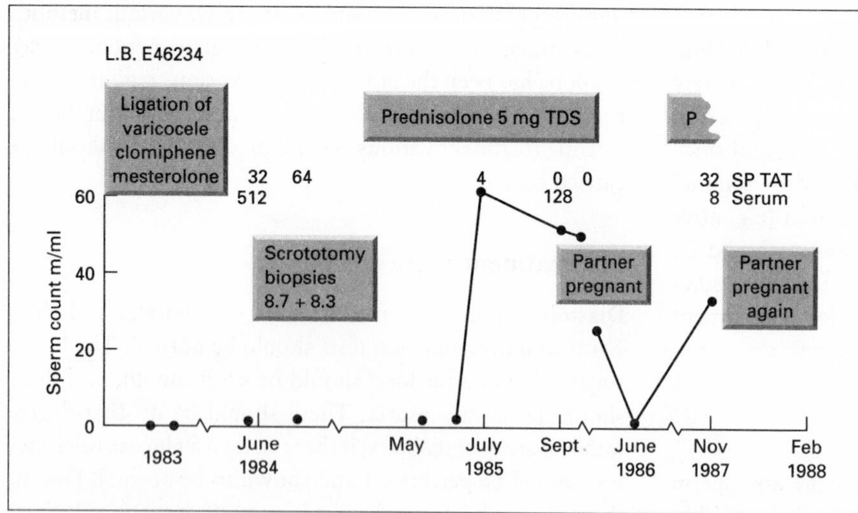

Fig. 50.2 Response to prednisolone of a patient with severe oligozoospermia and high sperm antibody titres.

for 6 months) produced normalisation of the sperm count and one partner became pregnant (Fig. 50.2). Testicular biopsies in three of these cases showed focal mononuclear cell infiltration of the seminiferous tubules indicating autoimmune orchitis (see below).

Intermittent, high-dose methylprednisolone

Shulman *et al.* recommended repeated courses of methylprednisolone (MP) 96 mg/day for 7 days, given to the man from day 21–28 of his female partner's menstrual cycle [31]. This was based on the observation that in 17 normal men it produced a significant reduction in circulating IgG (in 86%) and IgA (in 43%) which reached a maximum depression in the third week after therapy [32]. With Shulman's regime, this would coincide with the anticipated time of the female partner's next ovulation.

We treated 45 men with this regimen and 14 female partners became pregnant in the cycle after treatment in their men, two after one course, six after the second and six after the third or subsequent courses [33]. Unfortunately, one man developed bilateral aseptic necrosis of the hips 1 year later, requiring bilateral replacement of the hip joints [34]. This complication was also encountered by Shulman and Shulman [35]. As a result, this regimen was abandoned.

Intermediate, graduated-dose prednisolone

This regimen was developed as a result of the side-effects experienced with the Shulman regime. Soluble prednisolone 20 mg was taken twice daily with meals from day one to 10 of the female partner's cycle, followed by 5 mg daily on days 11 and 12 [36]. Alcohol was avoided during this period. After three courses the antibody titres were remeasured in serum and seminal plasma, and seminal analysis was checked. If the antibody titres were falling, two more 3-monthly courses were given. If the titres did not drop, the dose was increased to 40 mg twice daily for the remainder of the treatment cycles. Not more than nine courses were given, although an occasional additional course was permitted, for example linked with a cycle of *in vitro* fertilisation (IVF). Seventy-six males were treated, and 25 (33%) of the partners became pregnant during a treatment cycle. Comparison of serum TAT result before and after treatment showed no evidence that titres fell more profoundly in men whose partners became pregnant compared with those who did not. No serious complications occurred, although mood change including irritability and sleeplessness were not uncommonly encountered and couples are now warned specifically about this effect which can damage the relationship.

A randomised, double-blind, cross-over trial was then completed comparing this prednisolone regime with placebo [37]. Twenty-seven couples completed the 18-month period of study, and nine produced pregnancies whilst receiving prednisolone compared with only one on placebo. This result indicated a highly significant benefit from the prednisolone therapy (by Fisher's exact test $P < 0.05$). No serious side-effects were encountered, and mood change was also reported with placebo.

This treatment regimen continues to be useful in the management of infertile couples where the male partner has anti-sperm antibodies, although it should be recognised that IVF now offers an alternative form of therapy. It is difficult to predict which men are going to respond to prednisolone, and so it is probably reasonable to try this form of treatment for 3–6 months, and if pregnancy does not occur spontaneously then IVF can be done in the last trimester.

Other treatments

Artificial insemination and sperm washing

Kremer recommended intrauterine artificial insemination by husband (AIH) to get beyond the barrier created by the cervical mucus, and obtained three pregnancies in 15 women whose husbands had spermag-glutinin titres of 32 or more [38]. Artificial insemination can be combined with sperm washing, using either phosphate-buffered saline or sterile 4% human serum albumin. We treated 30 couples with this technique for one to 13 (average four to five) cycles with the production of only three pregnancies. Analysis showed that in all three cases where the wife became pregnant, the husband had previously received steroid therapy, and no other pregnancies occurred. There are good grounds for doubting whether antibodies (especially IgA) can be removed from spermatozoa by simply washing them and we have long since abandoned this treatment.

In vitro fertilisation

The precise effect of anti-sperm antibodies on sperm–ovum interaction is not known, but experimentally they have been shown to be generally inhibitory both in animals [39] and in humans [40]. In subfertile couples these antibodies can be shown to interfere with fertilisation[41]; however, once fertilised there is no reduction in the implantation and subsequent pregnancy rate. Since anti-sperm antibodies impair sperm motility, it is possible that this may also interfere with ovum fertilisation. In some couples in whom pregnancy does not occur spontaneously with prednisolone therapy, successful ovum fertilisation and pregnancy can be produced by combining a course of prednisolone (given as described above) with one or more cycles of IVF. The possibility of anti-sperm antibodies on husband's spermatozoa should be kept in mind in IVF assessments where sperm quality seems inadequate, since sperm count and motility can be significantly improved by prednisolone therapy. Alternatively, IVF can be combined with intracytoplasmic sperm injection (ICSI) [42].

Antibiotics

Prostatitis has been noted in 37% of men with anti-sperm antibodies [43]. We found that 55% of patients with antibodies had positive semen cultures, compared with only 15% of unselected patients without such antibodies [44]. In our experience with 290 patients, however, pregnancies occurred with equal frequency with or without positive semen cultures, irrespective of whether the organisms were treated with antibiotics or not (unpublished observations). Furthermore, electron microscopic studies in 57 patients with large numbers of cells in the ejaculate showed that in 60% the leucocytes contained spermatozoa, and in only 28% were bacteria seen within the cells [45]. Nevertheless, prostatitis can be associated with anti-sperm antibodies, and a positive culture in expressed prostatic secretions should probably be treated by long-term, low-dose antibiotics before and during prednisolone therapy [46].

Anti-sperm antibodies and testicular obstruction

The immunological response to testicular obstruction was first studied in a large group of infertile men by Rumke and Hellinga [47], who noted that anti-sperm antibodies occurred much more frequently in those with occlusion of the vas deferens or epididymis than in those without obstruction. This reaction was thought to be stimulated by extravasation of highly immunogenic spermatozoa in the interstitium, lymphatics and even the capillaries of the testis as a result of the occlusion. This phenomenon was studied experimentally by vasectomy in rams and boars [48], and confirmed clinically in man by the finding of spermatozoa in an abdominal lymph node 1 year after vasectomy [49]. Although patchy local obstructive changes are commonly observed in the epididymis at autopsy, especially in the ductuli efferentes [50], relatively few men develop anti-sperm antibodies [51], suggesting that there is normally a degree of local tolerance to extravasated spermatozoa. Complete obstruction to the outflow, however, seems to produce antigenic overload with stimulation of anti-sperm antibody production in immunologically responsive individuals [52].

Rumke and Titus [53] studied the association between testicular obstruction and anti-sperm antibody formation by subcutaneous injection of sperm, unilateral vasectomy and vasoligation in rats. A brisk antibody response was dependent upon the injection of adequate numbers of sperm, and was observed more often after vasectomy than vasoligation, presumably because more sperm were extravasated. Antibody titres fell significantly after removal of the obstructed testis in all animals. Kessler *et al.* [54] used inbred DBA/1J mice, which are known to be high antibody formers; unilateral vasectomy consistently induced an antibody response and significantly reduced fertility, whereas sham operation or unilateral orchiectomy did not.

Bilateral testicular obstruction inevitably causes sterility as a result of the ensuing azoospermia, and the individual may or may not form anti-sperm antibodies depending on his immunological responsiveness and the cause of the blockage [55]. With unilateral obstruction, on the other hand, sperm output is maintained from the unobstructed testis and impairment of fertility therefore depends on the strength of the antibody response. This was illustrated graphically in our study of 30 men who had had obstructive genital tract injuries in childhood, comparing those with unilateral and bilateral damage; anti-sperm antibody titres were significantly higher in those with unilateral blocks [56]. Thus, there are likely to be men with unilateral obstruction who retain their fertility because they do not produce a significant antibody response.

It is not known how often unilateral or incomplete testicular obstruction exists in subfertile men with anti-sperm antibody formation. Rumke [57] reviewed the past histories of 64 men with anti-sperm antibodies and found a history of previous genital infection, surgery or injury in just over half, while we found such a history in 40% [44].

Surgical treatment

The recent technical advances in microscopic epididymal sperm aspiration (MESA) and in IVF now permit production of pregnancy without the need for correction of genital outflow tract obstruction, although total reconstruction undoubtedly allows more natural and more cost-effective reproduction. The choice of treatment depends on the underlying cause of the obstruction, whether it is affecting one or both testicles, the success rate of the repair procedure and, perhaps most important, the requirements of the couple concerned; it is essential to consider the man and his partner as a single reproductive unit. In advising them, the physician must be familiar with the detailed anatomy of the male genital tract, and the pathological processes that may affect its various parts, as well as the treatment options that are available.

The outflow passages from the testicle become obstructed at different sites due to a variety of aetiological factors, and yet the exact site involved is generally related to the underlying cause. As a result, it is possible to classify descriptively testicular obstruction according to the site of the blockage, and still take into account the different pathophysiological processes involved. This is of practical importance since supplementary medical treatment may be required in addition to surgery. A classification based upon the external appearance of the epididymis, testicular biopsy results and vasography findings at exploratory scrototomy in 370 patients with azoospermia and normal serum FSH levels [58] is shown in Table 50.1. The incidence of each type of obstruction is shown, and the commonly related aetiological factors are indicated. In some cases the lesions may be asymmetrical, and this is emphasised when it appears to be a common feature. Although this descriptive classification was developed in patients with azoospermia, it is equally applicable to unilateral testicular obstruction since its basis is anatomical.

Table 50.1 Classification of testicular obstruction based on findings in 370 azoospermic males with normal serum follicle-stimulating hormone levels (excluding vasectomy reversals). From [58].

Group	Incidence (%)	Aetiology	Biopsy	Vasogram
Caput epididymis	106 (29%)	Young's syndrome	Normal	Normal
Cauda epididymis	70 (19%)	Post infective	Normal	May be blocked
Empty epididymis	49 (13%)	Defective spermatogenesis	Sertoli cell only (14) Maturation arrest (31)	Not done
		Immune orchitis	Normal +/– mononuclear cells(4)	Not done
Blocked vas	40 (11%)	Post-infective Post-surgical	Normal	Blocked
Absent vas bilateral	67 (18%)	Congenital	Normal	—
unilateral	19 (5%)	Various		—
Ejaculatory duct	14 (4%)	Congenital Traumatic Neoplastic	Normal	Abnormal

Epididymal obstruction

Incomplete epididymis

In a few cases part or all of the epididymes may be missing, usually as a result of previous surgical excision of epididymal cysts or painful nodules. Rarely, there may be congenital lack of continuity, usually between the head and midpiece, and sometimes this is associated with maldescent. Surgical reconstruction by epididymovasostomy may be successful [58].

Caput epididymis

This was the commonest group seen in the UK, and the results of surgery in this group were bad. Capital blocks are associated with chronic chest disease in three-quarters of the patients, an association known as Young's syndrome. The lesions are symmetrical and the transition zone between distended and empty tubules coincides with the change from ductuli efferentes in the head of the epididymis, lined by ciliated columnar epithelium, to ductus epididymis in the body, lined by stratified columnar epithelium with microvilli. The epithelial lining of the ductuli efferentes and the nasal and respiratory passages are similar. Since the cilia are ultrastructurally normal, with normal beat frequency, increased viscosity seems the most likely explanation for the demonstrably impaired mucociliary clearance in these patients. In Young's syndrome there is excess lipid in the epithelial cells and in the lumina of the ductuli efferentes with abnormal accumulation of lipid; this appears to impair flow in the ductuli efferentes and respiratory passages [58].

There was a definite past history of Pink disease (mercury intoxication) in childhood in 10% of our patients with Young's syndrome. Both Pink disease and Young's syndrome became much less common in men born after 1955, when mercury-containing teething powders were withdrawn in the UK. It is, therefore, quite likely that exposure to mercury in childhood may have played a part in the aetiology of this condition [59].

Cauda epididymis

These blocks occur in the ductus epididymis, and may be situated anywhere in the body or tail of the epididymis (Fig. 50.3). Most of these men give a history of infection—epididymitis, urethritis or smallpox, although the history may not be forthcoming in all individuals. Coexisting vasal blocks are commonly present, and the lesions may be asymmetrical, for example a caudal epididymal block on one side and a vasal block on the other side; vasography is therefore mandatory. The results of surgery are much better than with capital blocks.

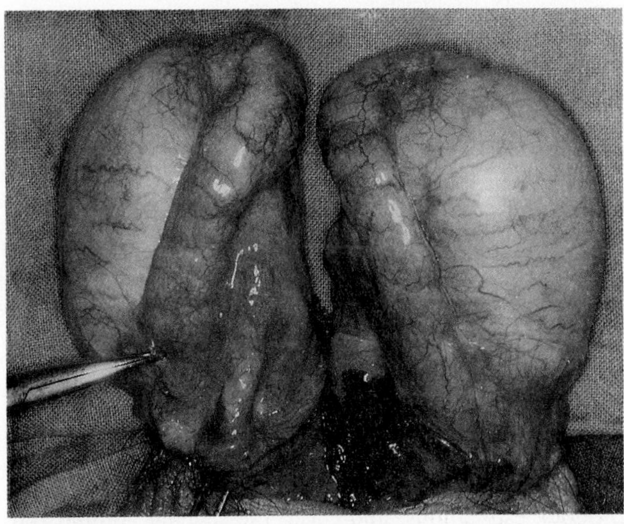

Fig. 50.3 Bilateral caudal epididymal blocks.

Unilateral caudal blocks may be found after epididymitis: the appearances at exploration are characteristic and easy to recognise.

Empty epididymes

The finding of an empty epididymis is an unfavourable sign which usually indicates defective spermatogenesis, which will be demonstrated by testicular biopsy. Occasionally the histology shows maturation arrest associated with gonadotrophin deficiency, and this may respond to gonadotrophin therapy.

Empty epididymes can be seen occasionally in men with azoospermia and normal spermatogenesis. There are two rather rare conditions in which this occurs: first, with very high levels of anti-sperm antibodies (the serum TAT is usually >512), there may be focal mononuclear cell infiltration in and around seminiferous tubules, with maximal cell infiltration around the rete testis—the weakest part of the blood–testis barrier. This is strong evidence of autoimmune orchitis; however, as a result of its patchy distribution, the absence of this mononuclear cell infiltration on testicular biopsy should not be interpreted as evidence that this condition is not present. This is important because appropriate steroid therapy may lead to normalisation of the sperm output. Since spermatogenesis in most tubules is reasonably normal, the severe oligozoospermia or azoospermia presumably must be due to the autoimmune orchitis and hold-up due to cellular infiltrate at the rete testis [58]. This mechanism may also play a part in the production of oligozoospermia sometimes seen with unilateral testicular obstruction associated with normal spermatogenesis and positive anti-sperm antibodies [60].

The second possible cause of the paradoxical finding of azoospermia with normal spermatogenesis and empty epididymes is a Müllerian duct cyst which causes obstruction but absorbs most of the pressure, making the epididymes appear empty. The volume, pH and fructose content of the semen should always be measured prior to exploration and if they are abnormal, transrectal ultrasound scanning should be done. If the seminal vesicles are distended, vasography should be done to define the site of the block [6].

In most cases with empty epididymes, however, vasography can be omitted until the results of the testicular biopsy are available. As a general rule, if the epididymes are empty it is best to take a biopsy, obtain the results of anti-sperm antibody estimations, and check the seminal volume and biochemistry, then await histology results before proceeding further. The epididymes and vasa must not be damaged in these cases by needless anastomosis.

Vasal obstruction

Blocked vas

This occurs in its simplest form after vasectomy. Vasal blocks also occur following infections such as gonorrhoea or non-specific urethritis, when they may coexist with caudal epididymal blocks, either on the same or on the other side. Ipsilateral epididymal block is excluded by finding a good flow of milky fluid containing spermatozoa on incising the vas. The most common sites affected are at the neck of the scrotum and at the internal inguinal ring, where the vas changes direction sharply. Totally impenetrable blocks are occasionally encountered, which generally turn out to be tuberculous. The vas may be obstructed following groin surgery such as hernia repair in infancy or childhood [60]. The level of the block may be defined by vasography, which should also confirm patency of the vas beyond the block.

Absent vas

Bilateral absence of the vas is found in about 18% of patients with azoospermia and normal serum FSH levels [58]. If seminal analysis indicates that this is the likely diagnosis (small volume, low pH, absent fructose) and the vasa are impalpable, the patient can be spared surgical exploration unless it is linked with IVF. Transrectal ultrasound scanning will define the presence or absence of the seminal vesicles. Unilateral absence of the vas is found in about 5% of patients with azoospermia, and this may be associated with a variety of problems on the other side such as testicular atrophy, or post-infective blocks. Alternatively, there may be other congenital anomalies, and urological abnormalities such as pelvic kidney or renal agenesis are commonly associated with these complex Wolffian duct abnormalities.

Ejaculatory duct obstruction

Problems were found in this area in 4.5% of the author's series of 370 azoospermic men [58]. These blocks can be diagnosed preoperatively by looking at the seminal volume and biochemistry—if the volume is <1 ml, the pH <7 and fructose absent, and if the vasa are palpable, then there must be ejaculatory duct obstruction. Transrectal ultrasound scanning clearly shows dilatation of the seminal vesicles, and in many cases will show the ejaculatory ducts and may define the site of the block. More accurate localisation will be obtained by seminal vesiculography which can be done by perineal needle puncture under transrectal ultrasound control, or by vasography at the time of operation. Familiarity with the normal appearances on vasography allows congenital anomalies such as Müllerian duct cysts (Fig. 50.4) or Wolffian duct abnormalities to be recognised. Obstruction may also occur after urethral injury, excision of the rectum, correction of imperforate anus or excision of seminal vesicle cysts; in later life carcinoma of the prostate can cause obstruction in this region. Sometimes, grossly dilated vesicles may be encountered in men with patent ejaculatory ducts as demonstrated by vasography or injection of methylene blue dye; such 'megavesicles' are the equivalent of megaureters, and may be considered part of a spectrum of conditions leading to functional impairment of ejaculation [6].

Results of surgery

The surgical techniques of genital tract reconstruction have

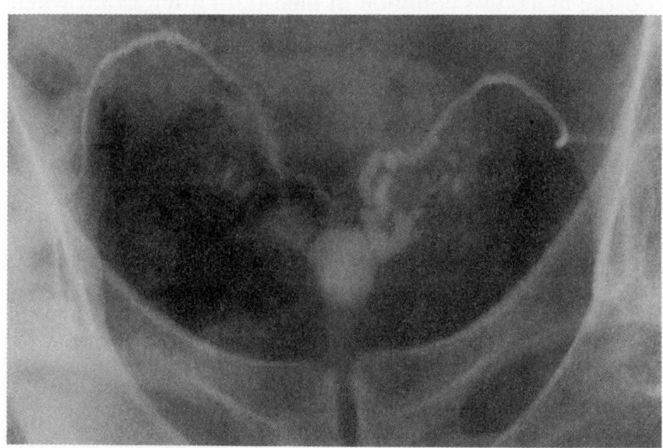

Fig. 50.4 Vasogram showing Müllerian duct cyst causing vasal obstruction.

been described in detail and critically reviewed elsewhere [61]. The success rate of surgical reconstruction for testicular obstruction depends primarily on the underlying cause, and to a lesser extent on the surgical technique. This is illustrated by the results of the author's experience collected in Table 50.2, using a standard side-to-side one-layer anastomosis with 6.0 prolene throughout. It may be seen that vasectomy reversal is much the most successful [62], even when done for a second or subsequent time as a 'redo' procedure, either as vasovasostomy or epididymovasostomy as indicated by the findings at exploration [63]. These results can be compared with those obtained elsewhere (Table 50.3). Experience with 1469 men from five institutions in the USA over a 9-year period showed that there was a direct relationship between time since vasectomy and success rate, the pregnancy rates being 76% after <3 years, 53% after 3–8 years, 44% after 9–14 years and 30% after >15 years [64]. Couples can be advised that the chances of success in terms of producing a pregnancy after vasectomy reversal are around 'fifty-fifty', but somewhat less if the interval has been prolonged to more than 10 years since the vasectomy was done. Nevertheless, even a one-in-three chance provides most couples with a good reason to go ahead with surgery.

Anti-sperm antibodies develop in the serum of 60–80% of men following vasectomy. We found antibodies in the sera of 79% of 130 men presenting for vasectomy reversal; they were present in seminal plasma in 9.5% before, rising to 29.5% after the vasovasostomies [62]. Overall, 44% impregnated their partners, and we could show no statistically significant fall off in fertility until very high serum titres (512 or more) were reached, and even then 25% were fertile. Meinertz *et al.* [65] used the mixed antiglobulin reaction to define the percentage of spermatozoa with IgG or IgA bound to the sperm membrane; they found that following vasectomy reversal the conception rate fell from 86% in a subgroup with a pure IgG response to 43% when IgA was present on the sperm as well, to 22% when 100% of sperm were covered with IgA, and ultimately to zero when there was IgA on all the sperm and a strong immune response as shown by a serum TAT titre of 256 or more.

It may be seen from Table 50.2 that side-to-side vasovasostomy provides good results with post-inflammatory vasal blocks that may be encountered when operating for obstructive azoospermia [58]. Transvasovasostomy offers a temptingly easy alternative to total anatomical reconstruction, but the results are significantly less good (Table 50.2).

Side-to-side epididymovasostomy for post-inflammatory caudal epididymal blocks gives results which are only marginally less good than vasectomy reversal (Table 50.2). Tubule-to-tubule anastomosis is preferred by some surgeons, and claims have been made for the superiority of this method [66]. In fact, detailed review of the recent literature (Table 50.4) provided little support for this view, as compared with the results obtained by the traditional method of side-to-

Table 50.2 Results of surgical treatment of testicular obstruction (author's experience).

Surgical procedure	Reference	Number followed up	Patency (%)	Pregnancies (%)
Vasectomy reversal	[62]	104	93	45
Redo vasectomy reversal	[63]	23	87	37
Vas-vas (+/– ep-vas)	[58]	11	73	27
Trans-vas-vas	[58]	11	9	0
Ep-vas (caudal)	[58]	60	43	30
Redo ep-vas (caudal)	[58]	10	50	50
Ep-vas (capital)	[58]	90	12	3

Table 50.3 Some recent results of vasectomy reversal.

Reference	Number of cases	Patency (%)	Pregnancy (%)
Lee and McLoughlin [78]	41 26*	90 96	46 54
Fallon *et al.* [79]	36	74	57
Fitzpatrick [80]	14	90	64
Middleton *et al.* [81]	73	81	49
Amelar and Dubin [82]	26	88	53
Kessler and Freiha [83]	83	92	45
Urquhart-Hay [84]	50	84	52
Cos *et al.* [85]	87*	75	46
Soonawalla and Lal [86]	194 339*	81 89	44 63
Belker *et al.* [64]	1012*	86	52
Silber [66]	282*†	91	81
Meinertz *et al.* [65]	145	90	53
Fox [87]	103*	84	48
Kabalin and Kessler [88]	111	79	36

* Microsurgical technique.
† Excluding 44 patients with no sperm in vas fluid.

Reference	Number of cases (%)	Patency (%)	Pregnancy (%)
Dumin and Amelar [89]	69	20	10
	46*	39	13
Jequier [90]	24	12.5	4
Fogdestam *et al.* [91]	41*	85	37
Schoysman and Bedford [92]	565	–	18
Lee [93]	97	31	12
	158*	37	20
Thomas [94]	50*	66	42
Silber [95]			
Corpus	139*	78	56
Caput	51	73	31
Matsuda *et al.* [96]	24	81	42
Niederberger *et al.* [97]	21	48	18

* Microsurgical technique.

Table 50.4 Recent results of epididymovasostomy.

side anastomosis, the method still favoured by the author. If the operation fails, it is not difficult to re-enter the scrotum and redo the anastomosis between epididymis and vas, which have already been approximated by the first procedure.

Blocks in the head of the epididymis, on the other hand, produce poor results. Failure of flow through the ductuli efferentes is now recognised as the basis cause of the problem, part of the failure of mucociliary clearance reflected in the high incidence of nasal and respiratory disease in these men. Some improvement in the results of surgery, and in nasal and respiratory symptoms has been observed with adjuvant therapy using carbocisteine (Mucodyne) 375 mg t.d.s. for 6–12 months [58].

Ejaculatory duct obstruction is easily missed unless the seminal biochemistry is checked preoperatively, and either a transrectal ultrasound scan done preoperatively or vasography carried out at the time of scrotal exploration. Among 87 cases recently reviewed [6] the most successful group were those with Müllerian duct cysts; this diagnosis is particularly easy to miss since the epididymes may not be distended, and since saline injected up the vas may easily be accommodated. Endoscopic incision of the cyst leads to significant improvement in sperm output in most cases.

Unilateral testicular obstruction

Among subfertile men with unilateral testicular obstruction, the causes may be defined by surgical exploration as post-infective, post-traumatic or congenital; among 125 such men, two-thirds had oligozoospermia or azoospermia, and half had significantly raised serum anti-sperm antibody titres. The outflow tracts were either reconstructed or the obstructed testis was removed and replaced with a prosthesis depending on the exact findings in each particular man. Reconstruction produced significant improvement in sperm concentration in the ejaculate, but little change in anti-sperm antibody titres. Orchidectomy lowered seminal plasma antibody titres and had no effect on sperm output. Although sperm output was improved by reconstruction, the stimulus to antibody production was more reliably eliminated by orchidectomy, and orchidectomy plus prednisolone was most effective in terms of pregnancies produced in the female partners. However, testicular biopsies showed that spermatogenesis was normal on the side of the block in 90% of cases, whereas it was impaired in the contralateral testis in 40% of men [60]. Sperm concentration, anti-sperm antibody titres and bilateral testicular biopsy results must therefore be taken into account before making a final therapeutic recommendation in these men with unilateral testicular obstruction. They are a favourable group amongst subfertile men, in whom the diagnosis of testicular obstruction should not be missed if careful clinical examination is coupled with critical review of the results of seminal analysis and anti-sperm antibody testing.

Varicocele

Varicocele occurs in about 10% of the normal male population and in about 20% of men attending a subfertility clinic. Retrograde caval venography has shown that the basic abnormality is reversed blood flow due to incompetence of valves in the testicular vein [67] which results in pooling of blood around the testicles and an increase in temperature of the scrotum [68,69], the extent of which depends on the size of the varicocele [70]; this is probably the cause of the depression of spermatogenesis that accompanies this condition. Most varicoceles only involve the left side, although bilateral varicoceles have been described in up to 15% of cases; the right side is affected alone very rarely, when a search should be made for situs inversus. A careful search, with the patient standing in good light, is certainly worthwhile, since there is evidence that improvement in seminal analysis is equally good after ligation of small or large varicoceles [71]. In cases of doubt it is worth arranging for scrotal thermography to confirm or refute the diagnosis; this examination should be repeated 2–3 months after surgery to make sure that the operation has been successful in correcting the scrotal temperature [7].

The reported results of surgical treatment are excellent—improvement in seminal analysis occurs in about 70% of patients, and up to 40% of the female partners become pregnant within 2 years (Table 50.5). The author's experience was less sanguine—42 (24%) of 173 patients produced pregnancies after ligation of varicocele, but nine (21%) of 42 did so without surgery, mostly while waiting for operation after having been advised to wear loose-fitting underwear [72]. Two prospective trials have shown similar pregnancy rates produced by men with varicoceles, irrespective of whether they were operated on or not. However, other studies have shown significant benefit [73], and it is the author's practice to correct a varicocele if it is associated with demonstrably abnormal scrotal thermography. Among 15 men with left varicoceles and atrophic or absent right testes, all except one showed marked improvement in seminal analysis after high ligation, and nine (60%) of the female partners became pregnant [22].

Embolisation is the treatment of choice at the present time, provided that adequate radiological expertise is available [74,75]. Alternatively, few complications occur if the veins are ligated at or above the internal ring, although hydrocele formation is seen occasionally. Testicular atrophy is very uncommon with this approach, whereas it occurs in up to 10% of cases following multiple scrotal ligation or scrotal excision [76]. Recurrence of varicocele occasionally needs reoperation. Defects in hormonal synthesis and spermatogenesis seen in some men with varicoceles have been shown to be reversible [77].

Table 50.5 Reported results of ligation of varicocele.

Reference	Number of cases	Semen improved (%)	Pregnancies (%)
Tulloch [98]	30	66	30
Charny [99]	36	64	39
Scott and Young [100]	166	70	22–36
Hanley and Harrison [101]	60	70	30
Brown *et al.* [102]	185	55–60	43
Macleod [103]	108	74	40
Dubin and Amelar [104]	986	70	53

References

1 Hendry WF, Sommerville IF, Hall RR, Pugh RC. Investigation and treatment of the subfertile male. *Br J Urol* 1973; **45**: 684–92.

2 Beeley L. The unwanted effects of drugs on the male reproductive system. In: Whitfield HN, Hendry WF, eds. *Textbook of Genito-urinary Surgery*. Edinburgh: Churchill Livingstone, 1985: 1198–203.

3 Lenz S, Giwercman A, Elsorg A *et al.* Ultrasonic testicular texture and size in 444 men from the general population: correlation to semen quality. *Eur Urol* 1993; **24**: 231–8.

4 Hendry WF, Parslow JM, Stedronska J, Wallace DM. The diagnosis of unilateral testicular obstruction in subfertile males. *Br J Urol* 1982; **54**: 774–9.

5 Hendry WF, Munro DD. Wash leather scrotum (scrotal dermatitis): a treatable cause of male infertility. *Fertil Steril* 1990; **53**: 379–81.

6 Pryor JP, Hendry WF. Ejaculatory duct obstruction in subfertile males: analysis of 87 patients. *Fertil Steril* 1991; **56**: 725–30.

7 Jones CH, Hendry WF. Thermographic examination of the scrotum. *Acta Thermographica* 1979; **4**: 38–43.

8 Aitken RJ, Buckingham DW, Brindle J, Gomez E, Baker HWG, Irvine DS. Analysis of sperm movement in relation to the oxidative stress created by leukocytes in washed sperm preparations and seminal plasma. *Human Reprod* 1995; **10**: 2061–71.

9 Ryder TA, Mobberley MA, Hughes L, Hendry WF. A survey of ultrastructural defects associated with absent or impaired human sperm motility. *Fertil Steril* 1990; **53**: 556–60.

10 Jager S, Kremer J, Van Slochteren-Draaisma T. A simple method of screening for antisperm antibodies in the human male. *Int J Fertil* 1978; **23**: 12–21.

11 Clarke GN, Elliott PJ, Smaila C. Detection of antibodies in semen using the immunobead test; a survey of 813 consecutive patients. *Am J Reprod Immunol* 1985; **7**: 118–23.

12 Stedronska J, Hendry WF. The value of the mixed antiglobulin reaction (MAR test) as an addition to routine seminal analysis in the evaluation of the subfertile couple. *Am J Reprod Immunol* 1983; **3**: 89–91.

13 Rajah SV, Parslow JM, Howell RJ, Hendry WF. Comparison of mixed antiglobulin reaction and direct immunobead test for detection of sperm-bound antibodies in subfertile males. *Fertil Steril* 1992; **57**: 1300–3.

14 Friberg J. A simple and sensitive micro-method for demonstration of sperm agglutinating antibodies in serum from infertile men and women. *Acta Obstet Gynecol Scand* 1974; **36** (Suppl): 21–9.

15 Kremer J, Jager S, Van Slochteren-Draaisma T. The 'unexplained' poor post coital test. *Int J Fertil* 1978; **23**: 277–81.

16 Morgan H, Stedronska J, Hendry WF, Chamberlain GF, Dewhurst CJ. Sperm/cervical-mucus crossed hostility testing and antisperm antibodies in the husband. *Lancet* 1977; **1**: 1228–30.

17 Pryor JP, Pugh RCB, Cameron KM, Newton JR, Collins WP. Plasma

gonadotrophic hormones, testicular biopsy and seminal analysis in men of infertile marriages. *Br J Urol* 1976; **48**: 709–17.

18 Martin-du-Pan RC, Bischof P. Increased follicle stimulating hormone in infertile men: is increased plasma FSH always due to damaged germinal epithelium? *Human Reprod* 1995; **10**: 1940–50.

19 Hendry WF, Polani PE, Pugh RC, Sommerville IF, Wallace DM. 200 infertile males: correlation of chromosome, histological, endocrine and clinical studies. *Br J Urol* 1976; **47**: 899–908.

20 Johnsen SG. Testicular biopsy score count. A method for registration of spermatogenesis in human testis: normal values and results in 335 hypogonadal males. *Hormones* 1970; **1**: 1–24.

21 Hendry WF. Iatrogenic damage to male reproductive function. *J Roy Soc Med* 1995; **88**: 579–84.

22 Hendry WF. Effects of left varicocele ligation in subfertile males with absent or atrophic right testes. *Fertil Steril* 1992; **57**: 1342–3.

23 Rose NR, Hjort T, Rumke P, Harper MJK, Vyazov O. Techniques for detection of iso and autoantibodies to human spermatozoa. *Clin Exp Immunol* 1976; **23**: 175–99.

24 World Health Organisation. Auto- and iso-antibodies to antigens of the human reproductive system; I. Results of an international comparative study. *Clin Exp Immunol* 1977; **30**: 173–80.

25 Kibrick S, Belding DL, Merrill B. Methods for the detection of antibodies against mammalian spermatozoa. II A gelatin agglutination test. *Fertil Steril* 1952; **3**: 430–8.

26 Isojima S, Li TS, Ashitaka Y. Immunologic analysis of sperm-immobilizing factor found in sera of women with unexplained sterility. *Am J Obstet Gynec* 1968; **101**: 677–83.

27 Adeghe JHA, Cohen J, Sawers SR. Relationship between local and systemic autoantibodies to sperm, and evaluation of immunobead test for sperm surface antibodies. *Acta Eur Fertil* 1986; **17**: 99–105.

28 Stedronska-Clark J, Clark DA, Hendry WF. Antisperm antibodies detected by ZER enzyme-linked immunosorbent assay kit are not those detected by tray agglutination test. *Am J Reprod Immunol Microbiol* 1987; **13**: 76–7.

29 Parslow JM, Poulton TA, Besser GM, Hendry WF. The clinical relevance of classes of immunoglobulins on spermatozoa from infertile and vasovasostomized males. *Fertil Steril* 1985; **43**: 621–7.

30 Hendry WF, Stedronska J, Hughes L, Cameron KM, Pugh RC. Steroid treatment of male subfertility caused by antisperm antibodies. *Lancet* 1979; **2**: 498–501.

31 Shulman S, Harlin B, Davis P, Reyniak JV. Immune infertility and new approaches treatment. *Fertil Steril* 1978; **29**: 309–13.

32 Butler WT, Rossen RD. Effects of corticosteroids on immunity in man. *J Clin Invest* 1973; **52**: 2629–40.

33 Hendry WF, Stedronska J, Parslow J, Hughes L. The results of intermittent high dose steroid therapy for male infertility due to antisperm antibodies. *Fertil Steril* 1981; **36**: 351–5.

34 Hendry WF. Bilateral aseptic necrosis of femoral heads following intermittent high-dose steroid therapy (letter). *Fertil Steril* 1982; **38**: 120.

35 Shulman JF, Shulman S. Methylprednisolone treatment of immunologic infertility in the male. *Fertil Steril* 1982; **38**: 591–9.

36 Hendry WF, Treehuba K, Hughes L *et al.* Cyclic prednisolone therapy for male infertility associated with autoantibodies to spermatozoa. *Fertil Steril* 1986; **45**: 249–54.

37 Hendry WF, Hughes L, Scammell G, Pryor JP, Hargreave TB. Comparison of prednisolone and placebo in subfertile men with antibodies to spermatozoa. *Lancet* 1990; **335**: 85–8.

38 Kremer J, Jager S, Kuiken J. Treatment of infertility caused by antisperm antibodies. *Int J Fertil* 1978; **23**: 270–6.

39 Tzartos SJ. Inhibition of in vitro fertilisation of intact and denuded hamster eggs by univalent antisperm antibodies. *J Reprod Fertil* 1979; **55**: 447–55.

40 Tsukui S, Noda Y, Fukuda A, Matsumoto H, Tatsumi K, Mori T. Blocking effect of sperm immobilising antibodies on sperm penetration of human zonae pellucidae. *J In Vitro Fert Embryo Transf* 1988; **5**: 123–8.

41 Rajah SV, Parslow JM, Howell JR, Hendry WF. The effects on in-vitro fertilisation of autoantibodies to spermatozoa in subfertile men. *Human Reprod* 1993; **8**: 1079–82.

42 Nagy ZP, Verheyen G, Liu J *et al.* Results of 55 intracytoplasmic sperm injection cycles in the treatment of male-immunological infertility. *Human Reprod* 1995; **10**: 1775–80.

43 Fjallbrant B, Obrant O. Clinical and seminal findings in men with sperm antibodies. *Acta Obstet Gynec Scand* 1968; **47**: 451–68.

44 Hendry WF, Morgan H, Stedronska J. The clinical significance of antisperm antibodies in male subfertility. *Br J Urol* 1977; **49**: 757–62.

45 Hughes L, Ryder TA, McKenzie ML, Pryse-Davies J, Stedronska J, Hendry WF. The use of transmission electron microscopy to study non-spermatozoal cells in semen. In: Frajese G, ed. *Oligozoospermia*. New York: Raven Press, 1981: 65–75.

46 Fjallbrant B, Nilsson S. Decrease of sperm antibody titer in males, and conception after treatment of chronic prostatitis. *Int J Fertil* 1977; **22**: 255–6.

47 Rumke P, Hellinga G. Autoantibodies against spermatozoa in sterile men. *Am J Clin Path* 1959; **32**: 357–63.

48 Ball RY, Setchell BP. The passage of spermatozoa to regional lymph nodes in testicular lymph following vasectomy in rams and boars. *J Reprod Fertil* 1983; **68**: 145–53.

49 Ball RY, Naylor CPE, Mitchinson MJ. Spermatozoa in an abdominal lymph node after vasectomy in a man. *J Reprod Fertil* 1982; **66**: 715–16.

50 Ball RY, Mitchinson MJ. Obstructive lesions in the genital tract in men. *J Reprod Fertil* 1984; **70**: 667–73.

51 Rumke P. Autoantibody formation against spermatozoa caused by extravasation of spermatozoa into the interstitium of the epididymis of aged men. *Int J Fertil* 1972; **17**: 86–8.

52 Rumke P. Spermagglutinating autoantibodies in relation to male infertility. *Proc Roy Soc Med* 1968; **61**: 275–8.

53 Rumke P, Titus M. Spermagglutinin formation in male rats by subcutaneously injected syngeneic epididymal spermatozoa and by vasoligation or vasectomy. *J Reprod Fertil* 1970; **21**: 69–79.

54 Kessler DL, Smith WD, Hamilton MS, Berger RE. Infertility in mice after unilateral vasectomy. *Fertil Steril* 1985; **43**: 308–12.

55 Flickinger CJ, Howards SS, Herr JC, Carey PO, Yarbro ES, Sisak JR. Factors that influence fertility after vasovasostomy in rats. *Fertil Steril* 1991; **56**: 555–62.

56 Parkhouse H, Hendry WF. Vasal injuries during childhood and their effects on subsequent fertility. *Br J Urol* 1991; **67**: 91–5.

57 Rumke P. Autospermagglutinins: a cause of infertility in men. *Ann NY Acad Sci* 1965; **124**: 696–701.

58 Hendry WF, Levison DA, Parkinson MC, Parslow JM, Royle MG. Testicular obstruction: clinicopathological studies. *Annals of the Royal College of Surgeons of England* 1990; **72**: 396–407.

59 Hendry WF, A'Hern RP, Cole PJ. Was Young's syndrome caused

by exposure to mercury in childhood? *Br Med J* 1993; **307**: 1579–82.
60 Hendry WF, Parslow JM, Parkinson MC, Lowe DG. Unilateral testicular obstruction: orchidectomy or reconstruction? *Human Reprod* 1994; **9**: 463–70.
61 Hendry WF. Testicular obstruction: causes, evaluation and the results of surgery. In: Webster G, Kirby RS, Goldwasser B, King L, eds. *Reconstructive Urology*. Oxford: Blackwell Scientific Publications, 1993: 1031–48.
62 Parslow JM, Royle MG, Kingscott MM, Wallace DM, Hendry WF. The effects of sperm antibodies on fertility after vasectomy reversal. *Am J Reprod Immunol* 1983; **3**: 28–31.
63 Royle MG, Hendry WF. Why does vasectomy reversal fail? *Br J Urol* 1985; **57**: 780–3.
64 Belker AM, Thomas AJ, Fuches EF, Konnak JW, Sharlip ID. Results of 1469 microsurgical vasectomy reversals by the vasovasostomy study group. *J Urol* 1991; **145**: 505–11.
65 Meinertz H, Linnet L, Andersen PF, Hjort T. Antisperm antibodies and fertility after vasovasostomy: a follow-up study of 216 men. *Fertil Steril* 1990; **54**: 315–21.
66 Silber SJ. Pregnancy after vasovasostomy for vasectomy reversal: a study of factors affecting long-term return of fertility in 282 patients followed for 10 years. *Human Reprod* 1989; **4**: 318–22.
67 Ahlberg NE, Bartley O, Chidekel N, Fritjofsson A. Phlebography in varicocele scroti. *Acta Radiol (Diagn) (Stockh)* 1996; **4**: 517–28.
68 Goldstein M, Eid JF. Elevation of intratesticular and scrotal skin surface temperature in men with varicocele. *J Urol* 1989; **142**: 743–5.
69 Ali JI, Weaver DJ, Weinstein SH, Grimes EM. Scrotal temperature and semen quality in men with and without varicocele. *Arch Androl* 1990; **24**: 215–19.
70 Kormano M, Kahanpaa K, Svinhufvud U, Tahti E. Thermography of varicocele. *Fertil Steril* 1970; **21**: 558–64.
71 Kiszka EF, Cowart GT. Treatment of varicocele by high ligation. *J Urol* 1960; **83**: 713–15.
72 Stanwell-Smith RE, Hendry WF. The prognosis of male subfertility: a survey of 1025 men referred to a fertility clinic. *Br J Urol* 1984; **56**: 422–8.
73 Okuyama A, Fujisue H, Matsui T *et al.* Surgical repair of varicocele: effective treatment for subfertile men in a controlled study. *Eur Urol* 1988; **14**: 298–300.
74 Thomas AJ, Geisinger MA. Current management of varicoceles. *Urol Clin North Am* 1990; **17**: 893–907.
75 Braedel HV, Steffens J, Ziegler M, Polsky MS. Outpatient sclerotherapy of idiopathic left sided varicocele in children and adults. *Br J Urol* 1990; **65**: 536–40.
76 Fritjofsson A, Ahlberg NE, Bartley O, Chidekel N. Treatment of varicocele by division of the internal spermatic vein. *Acta Chir Scand* 1966; **132**: 200–10.
77 Hudson RW, Perez-Marrero RA, Crawford VA, McKay DE. Hormonal parameters of men with varicoceles before and after varicocelectomy. *Fertil Steril* 1985; **43**: 905–10.
78 Lee L, McLoughlin MG. Vasovasostomy: a comparison of macroscopic and microscopic techniques at one institution. *Fertil Steril* 1980; **33**: 54–5.
79 Fallon B, Jacob E, Bunge RG. Restoration of fertility by vasovasostomy. *J Urology* 1978; **119**: 85–6.
80 Fitzpatrick TJ. Vasovasostomy: the flap technique. *J Urol* 1978; **120**: 78–9.
81 Middleton RG, Smith JA, Moore MH, Urry RL. A 15-year follow up of a non microsurgical technique for vasovasostomy. *J Urol* 1987; **137**: 886–7.
82 Amelar RD, Dubin L. Vasectomy reversal. *J Urol* 1979; **121**: 547–50.
83 Kessler R, Freiha F. Macroscopic vasovasostomy. *Fertil Steril* 1981; **36**: 531–2.
84 Urquhart-Hay D. A low power magnification technique for reanastomosis of the vas. *Br J Urol* 1981; **53**: 446–69.
85 Cos LR, Valvo JR, Davis RS, Cockett AJK. Vasovasostomy: current state of the art. *Urology* 1983; **22**: 567–75.
86 Soonawalla FB, Lal SS. Microsurgery in vasovasostomy. *Indian J Urol* 1984; **1**: 104–8.
87 Fox M. Vasectomy reversal—microsurgery for best results. *Br J Urol* 1994; **73**: 449–53.
88 Kabalin JN, Kessler R. Macroscopic vasovasostomy re-examined. *Urology* 1991; **38**: 135–8.
89 Dubin L, Amelar RD. Magnified surgery for epididymovasostomy. *Urology* 1984; **23**: 525–8.
90 Jequier AM. Obstructive azoospermia: a study of 102 patients. *Clin Reprod Fertil* 1985; **3**: 21–36.
91 Fogdestam I, Fall M, Nilsson S. Microsurgical epididymovasostomy in the treatment of occlusive azoospermia. *Fertil Steril* 1986; **46**: 925–9.
92 Schoysman RJ, Bedford JM. The role of the human epididymis in sperm maturation and sperm storage as reflected in the consequences of epididymovasostomy. *Fertil Steril* 1986; **46**: 293–9.
93 Lee HY. A 20-year experience with epididymovasostomy for pathologic epididymal obstruction. *Fertil Steril* 1987; **47**: 487–91.
94 Thomas AJ. Vasoepididymostomy. *Urol Clin North Am* 1987; **14**: 527–38.
95 Silber SJ. Results of microsurgical vasoepididymostomy: role of epididymis in sperm maturation. *Human Reprod* 1989; **4**: 298–303.
96 Matsuda T, Horii Y, Muguruma K, Komatz Y, Yoshida O. Microsurgical epididymovasostomy for obstructive azoospermia: factors affecting postoperative fertility. *Eur Urol* 1994; **26**: 322–6.
97 Niederberger C, Ross LS. Microsurgical epididymovasostomy: predictors of success. (Review). *J Urol* 1993; **149**: 1364–7.
98 Tulloch WS. Varicocele in subfertility: results of treatment. *Br. Med J* 1955; **2**: 356–8.
99 Charny CW. Effect of varicocele on fertility: results of varicocelectomy. *Fertil Steril* 1962; **13**: 47–56.
100 Scott LS, Young D. Varicocele: a study of its effects on human spermatogenesis, and of the results produced by spermatic vein ligation. *Fertil Steril* 1962; **13**: 325–34.
101 Hanley HG, Harrison RG. Nature and surgical treatment of varicocele. *Br J Surg* 1962; **50**: 64–7.
102 Brown JS, Dubin L, Hotchkiss RS. The varicocele as related to fertility. *Fertil Steril* 1967; **18**: 46–56.
103 Macleod J. Further observations on role of varicocele in human infertility. *Fertil Steril* 1969; **20**: 545–63.
104 Dubin L, Amelar RD. Varicocelectomy: 986 cases in a twelve year study. *Urology* 1996; **10**: 446–9.

CHAPTER 51

Hypogonadism in women

D.F. Wood and S. Franks

Introduction

Hypogonadism in the female presents clinically with disorders of menstrual function in the form of oligomenorrhoea or amenorrhoea. Oligomenorrhoea is defined as an intermenstrual interval of greater than 6 weeks. Amenorrhoea, the complete absence of menses for 6 months or more, is traditionally divided into two groups: primary and secondary amenorrhoea. Thus, women with primary amenorrhoea are those who have never menstruated whilst secondary amenorrhoea describes the absence of menses in patients who have menstruated before. Whilst the conventional classification will be followed in this chapter, it is important to note that the distinction is artificial, so that many of the common causes of secondary amenorrhoea may present with primary amenorrhoea [1] whereas rarely patients with congenital disorders may menstruate.

Primary amenorrhoea

The causes of primary amenorrhoea are listed in Table 51.1. Primary amenorrhoea is an uncommon disorder, with about 60% of cases being due to developmental abnormalities of the ovaries, genital tract or external genitalia. Syndromes of gonadal dysgenesis account for about half of these cases, with one-third being due to abnormalities of genital tract development.

In all women with primary amenorrhoea, assessment of pubertal development should be made [2]. Many patients will have delayed puberty, and it is important to identify those girls with disorders not directly related to the hypothalamo-pituitary–gonadal axis. There is a wide variation in the age of onset of puberty [3,4] with menarche being a late event, usually occurring after a girl has reached peak growth velocity. Age at the menarche is related to bone age and is influenced by a number of genetic and environmental factors [5]. Thus, the definition of delayed menarche is somewhat arbitrary. An important pointer to an underlying endocrine disorder is deviation from the normal consonance of pubertal development, for example breast development in the absence of pubic and axillary hair growth may suggest an androgen-resistance syndrome as the cause of primary amenorrhoea. Constitutional delay is a less common cause of delayed puberty in girls than in boys [6]. Gonadal dysgenesis and other developmental abnormalities should be actively considered as more likely causes of delayed puberty in girls, as should the effects of low weight and exercise seen, for example, in ballet dancers and athletes [7,8].

Clinical assessment

The history should include detailed questions about the age of onset, progression and synchrony of pubertal development. A history of chronic childhood illness and in particular chemotherapy or radiotherapy to the hypothalamo-pituitary–gonadal axis should be sought. Symptoms of other endocrine disorders such as diabetes and hypothyroidism may be present. Growth failure, anosmia, congenital deafness, musculoskeletal anomalies and cutaneous lesions should be enquired after. Visual field abnormalities may be caused by tumours in the hypothalamo-pituitary region. Psychological assessment is essential, as emotional and social deprivation are important causes of delayed or arrested pubertal development and amenorrhoea. Family history is important; a number of abnormalities of gonadal and genital development are familial and a family history of sexual immaturity and infertility may be obtained. Furthermore, the age at which the parents entered puberty is relevant in determining the predicted age of onset in children with delayed puberty.

Examination should start with accurate measurement of height and weight and these should be plotted onto Tanner

Table 51.1 Causes of primary amenorrhoea.

Gonadal dysgenesis
Turner's syndrome
Mixed gonadal dysgenesis
Pure gonadal dysgenesis
Genital tract (Müllerian) dysgenesis
Disorders of genital differentiation
Female pseudo-hermaphroditism
Male pseudo-hermaphroditism
True hermaphroditism
Ovarian insensitivity
17α-hydroxylase deficiency
'Resistant ovary syndrome'
Gonadal irradiation/chemotherapy
Hypothalamo-pituitary disease
Hypogonadotrophic hypogonadism
Combined pituitary hormone deficiency
Radiotherapy/chemotherapy
Hypothalamo-pituitary tumours
Delayed puberty
Constitutional delay
Chronic illness
Psychogenic
Polycystic ovary syndrome

growth charts where appropriate. For example, normal or excess weight in a small girl with primary amenorrhoea suggests combined growth hormone (GH) and gonadotrophin deficiency, whereas low weight may suggest chronic illness. Girls with isolated gonadotrophin deficiency are of normal height or are tall. The genitalia and secondary sexual characteristics should be examined and classified according to Tanner's stages [4]. Special attention should be paid to ambiguous genitalia, inguinal herniae, palpable masses in the labia or hernial orifices and a blind-ending vaginal canal suggesting intersex abnormalities or genital tract dysgenesis. Neurological examination should include assessment of the visual fields and determination of anosmia or deafness. Finally, other dysmorphic body features associated with gonadal dysgenesis should be noted (see below).

Investigation

Relevant investigations should be dictated by the physical findings. For example, in girls of low weight and with primary amenorrhoea, investigations of malabsorption may be most appropriate. Measurement of bone age and thyroid function tests are essential in girls with delayed puberty. Basal gonadotrophin concentrations should be measured to distinguish primary from secondary hypogonadism. Ultrasound scan of the pelvis will reveal the presence or absence of ovarian tissue, and ovarian morphology can be examined. Ovarian follicular development occurs throughout childhood, so that by the age of 8 years multifollicular ovaries occur in normal girls [9]. A multifollicular morphology is the ovarian response to increasing amplitude of gonadotrophin pulses, and when found in girls with delayed puberty and primary amenorrhoea suggests that eventually puberty will progress normally. Ultrasound scanning will also identify patients with polycystic ovaries, which occasionally present with primary amenorrhoea [10]. Finally, chromosome analysis should be undertaken in patients with dysmorphic body features and in all short girls with delayed puberty as Turner mosaics may be phenotypically normal (see below).

Treatment

It is clear from the above that there are many causes of primary amenorrhoea and treatment must therefore depend upon the underlying diagnosis. The treatment of individual syndromes is considered below.

Gonadal dysgenesis: Turner's syndrome and its variants

Turner's original description of seven phenotypic females with short stature, sexual immaturity, webbing of the neck and cubitus valgus was made in 1938 [11]. Subsequent investigations revealed characteristic increased urinary gonadotrophin excretion and the presence of bilateral 'streak' gonads lacking all germ cells. The 45XO karyotype associated with the disorder was described in the late 1950s [12].

The complete absence of a second sex chromosome is associated with the typical features of Turner's syndrome, namely female phenotype, short stature, sexual infantilism and a variety of somatic malformations. However, these may be modified in the presence of other patterns of sex chromosome deficiency, so that the clinical syndromes of gonadal dysgenesis range from the typical Turner profile through patients with ambiguous genitalia to phenotypically normal females or males. The most useful classification depends upon the X-chromatin pattern which identifies X-chromosome material in addition to the monosomic X. Generally, those patients with additional X-chromatin fall within the phenotypic spectrum of sexually infantile to normal females, whereas X-chromatin-negative patients range between sexually infantile females and hypogonadal males.

Typical Turner's syndrome (45XO gonadal dysgenesis)

The typical features of 45XO Turner's syndrome are shown in Table 51.2. The somatic manifestations are highly variable between patients, but short stature is always present. Growth retardation in Turner's syndrome starts during intrauterine life and becomes more apparent during childhood, culminating in loss of the pubertal growth spurt [13]. The reasons for this abnormal growth pattern remain unclear. Alterations in the dynamics of GH secretion in children with Turner's syndrome have been sought, but no typical abnormality has been established. GH pulsatility may be normal, or there may be reduced pulse frequency or amplitude; peak plasma GH concentrations in response to pharmacological stimuli have been reported as normal or impaired [14]. Furthermore, there is no obvious abnormality of insulin-like growth factor 1 (IGF-1) secretion [15]. It appears that the relationship between GH release and growth is less clear in patients with Turner's syndrome than in normal children. The contribution of end-organ resistance to GH, possibly due to skeletal dysplasia, remains to be clarified.

Sexual infantilism with normal female genitalia is the second hallmark of Turner's syndrome. The term 'streak gonads' is used to describe the streaks of connective tissue located in the mesosalpinges. These consist of fibrous stroma arranged in whorls similar to those found in ovarian stroma but lacking primordial follicles. The pattern of gonadotrophin secretion in these children is similar to that seen in normal girls although the absolute levels are higher. Elevated plasma levels of follicle-stimulating hormone (FSH) and luteinising hormone (LH) are seen between the ages of 0 and 4 years; these concentrations fall into the high normal range between 5 and 10 years of age and subsequently rise to castrate levels [16]. Rarely, ovarian function may be preserved in some Turner patients and there are isolated reports of normal fertility [17]. Ultrasonography has revealed 'non-streak' gonads in up to one-third of girls with Turner's syndrome; these findings are highly correlated with spontaneous breast development and preservation of the long arm of the second X-chromosome [18]. Ovarian ultrasound scanning may thus be helpful in the identification of those patients with a greater chance of spontaneous pubertal development, although accurate prediction of future fertility is doubtful.

Table 51.2 Clinical features of typical Turner's syndrome (45XO).

Short stature
Sexual infantilism
Dysmorphic features
Micrognathia, epicanthal folds
Low set ears
'Carp-like' mouth
Ptosis
Broad chest
Widely spaced nipples
Short, webbed neck (in 25–40%)
Cutaneous abnormalities
Multiple pigmented naevi
Hypoplastic nails
Cardiovascular abnormalities
Coarctation of the aorta
Aortic stenosis/bicuspid aortic valve
Dissecting aortic aneurysm
Congenital lymphoedema
Musculoskeletal
Cubitus valgus (in 50%)
Short 4th metacarpal (in 50%)
High arched palate
Vertebral hypoplasia
Genu valgum
Renal
Horse-shoe kidney
Other structural abnormalities

The dysmorphic body features associated with Turner's syndrome are shown in Table 51.2. Cardiovascular abnormalities, in particular coarctation of the aorta with or without aortic stenosis or bicuspid aortic valve, occur in 10–20% of patients. Congenital lymphoedema occurs in about one-third of cases with the eponym Bonnevie–Ullrich syndrome used to describe female infants with *gross* lymphoedema of the extremities, loose folds of skin over the back of the neck and gonadal dysgenesis. Musculoskeletal abnormalities are common with a wide-carrying angle (cubitus valgus) and short fourth metacarpal being seen most frequently. Renal abnormalities occur in at least 30% of cases, although they are not necessarily associated with the hypertension seen in some patients, which remains unexplained. Otological abnormalities are very common and deafness may occur either following recurrent otitis media or in association with a congenital sensorineural deficit. Turner's syndrome is associated with a number of other abnormalities including autoimmune thyroid disease, rheumatoid arthritis and inflammatory bowel disease. Impaired glucose tolerance and non-insulin dependent diabetes mellitus occur in adult Turner's patients. Finally, it should be noted that the incidence of mental retardation is not increased, but the patients may show abnormalities in spatial orientation.

Treatment of Turner's syndrome (see also Chapter 62)

Treatment of patients with Turner's is aimed at achieving maximum stature, inducing secondary sexual characteristics and correcting somatic abnormalities. Initial attempts to treat short stature in Turner patients with pituitary-derived GH were disappointing, but studies using recombinant human GH preparations suggest that this therapy may induce increased growth velocity in advance of bone maturation

[19,20]. Studies of the optimum dosage and frequency of administration suggest that once-daily injections of GH are adequate to induce growth in these patients [21]. The anabolic steroid oxandrolone also increases growth velocity and may be of value in combination with GH [15]. However, the dose-related side-effects of oxandrolone such as virilisation and insulin resistance may preclude its use in the long term. Low-dose ethinyl oestradiol has also been used to accelerate growth velocity in Turner's syndrome, both alone and in conjunction with GH [13,19]. However, the advancement of bone maturation induced by ethinyl oestradiol causing premature epiphysial fusion means that the final height is not increased. The early onset of growth failure in Turner's syndrome and its worsening in mid-childhood mean that treatment should be commenced as early as possible and preferably under the age of 10 years. This strategy has psychological as well as physiological benefits.

Secondary sexual characteristics may be induced in girls with Turner's syndrome by appropriate sex hormone replacement. Oestrogen therapy is best started between the ages of 13 and 14 years, and low doses should be used initially in an attempt to allow maximal height to be attained. Treatment with ethinyl oestradiol, 2 μg daily, should be replaced with a low-dose combined oestrogen/progestogen preparation once growth has ceased.

Variants of gonadal dysgenesis

The features associated with classical 45XO Turner's syndrome may be modified by sex chromosome mosaicism or a partial sex chromosome monosomy. In mosaic patients the ratio of 45XO to 46XX primordial germ cells in the gonad probably determines whether the ovary becomes streak, hypoplastic or normal. Furthermore, the quantitative relationship between 45XO and 46XX cells in peripheral tissues may also determine the degree of somatic abnormality [22]. In patients with a single cell line the clinical features are related to the nature and degree of deletion of the second X or Y chromosome.

Chromatin-positive variants of gonadal dysgenesis. Those patients with the most common chromatin-positive mosaicism (45XO/46XX) may be of normal height and demonstrate ovarian activity in the form of menses and, rarely, fertility. However, the majority lack normal menstrual cycles and detailed chromosome analysis should be considered in women with primary amenorrhoea for no obvious cause. Deletions of the second sex chromosome are generally associated with short stature and streak gonads, often with only minor stigmata of Turner's syndrome.

Chromatin-negative variants of gonadal dysgenesis. Patients with chromatin-negative mosaicism, structural abnormalities of the Y chromosome or occult Y chromosome material detected by screening for the SRY gene [23] have a modified Turner phenotype with varying degrees of masculinisation of the genital tract. Patients with 45XO/46XY, 45XO/47XYY and related forms of mosaicism have a highly variable phenotype with short stature and somatic abnormalities being inconsistent features. The term 'mixed gonadal dysgenesis' is used to describe those patients where a streak gonad and Fallopian tube are associated with a contralateral testis. These patients usually have the karyotype 45XO/46XY, with phenotypic development of the external genitalia being dependent upon the extent of testicular differentiation. Gonadal tumours are more common in patients with Y-chromatin material, and prophylactic removal of streak gonads or undescended testes should be undertaken in phenotypic females.

Pure gonadal dysgenesis. Patients with pure gonadal dysgenesis are phenotypic females with a 45XX or 45XY karyotype who have streak gonads, sexual infantilism and primary amenorrhoea. Varying degrees of masculinisation and genital ambiguity may occur, and these determine the sex of rearing of children with such abnormalities. Treatment of patients with the variant forms of gonadal dysgenesis depends upon assignation of gender. Surgical removal of dysgenetic gonads and remnants of inappropriate internal genitalia and plastic reconstruction of external genitalia should be undertaken. The appropriate sex hormone replacement therapy should then be instituted. Detailed explanations and counselling, including expert psychological assistance, are essential parts of the treatment of patients with all forms of gonadal dysgenesis.

Genital tract (Müllerian) dysgenesis

Developmental abnormalities of the genital tract form the second most common cause of primary amenorrhoea. Congenital absence of the vagina has been reported in one in 5000 female births [24]. Clinically, patients with genital tract dysgenesis have a history of primary amenorrhoea and normal pubertal development. They may give a history of cyclical abdominal pain. Examination reveals normal secondary sexual characteristics with an absent or hypoplastic vagina. The uterus may be absent, may be bicornuate or may be normal. The syndrome is sometimes associated with musculoskeletal and renal abnormalities. Treatment involves surgical reconstruction appropriate to the lesion and haematocolpos may be prevented if surgery is undertaken early in puberty.

Disorders of genital differentiation
(see also Chapters 57 and 58)

The intersex disorders produced by errors of fetal genital differentiation are classified into three main groups: female pseudo-hermaphroditism, male pseudo-hermaphroditism and true hermaphroditism. All are rare and may present as phenotypic females with primary amenorrhoea.

Female pseudo-hermaphroditism

Female pseudo-hermaphroditism occurs in individuals with a 46XX karyotype with normal internal genitalia and ambisexual external genitalia. The female fetus becomes masculinised by extragonadal androgens; in the majority of cases this is produced by virilising congenital adrenal hyperplasia. These inborn errors of steroid biosynthesis are considered in Chapter 58. A similar picture of female pseudo-hermaphroditism may be produced by excess maternal androgens, either ingested or endogenously produced by virilising ovarian and adrenal tumours, or by congenital adrenal hyperplasia in the mother.

Male pseudo-hermaphroditism

Male pseudo-hermophroditism describes any condition in which the gonads are testes but the external genitalia and genital tracts are incompletely masculinised. There is a spectrum of phenotypes ranging from female to cryptorchidism with minimal genital ambiguity in a phenotypic male. The causes of male pseudo-hermaphroditism are shown in Table 51.3 [25,26]. In all cases, treatment of male pseudo-hermaphroditism depends upon the degree of genital abnormality and upon the gender identity of the patient. Gonadectomy is advisable in 46XY individuals reared as females, with appropriate sex hormone replacement.

Table 51.3 Causes of male pseudo-hermaphroditism.

Dysgenetic
X-chromatin negative gonadal dysgenesis
XY gonadal dysgenesis and variants
Leydig-cell agenesis or hypoplasia
Errors of testosterone biosynthesis
With defective corticosteroid synthesis
Congenital adrenal hyperplasia
3β-hydroxysteroid dehydrogenase deficiency
17α-hydroxylase deficiency
With normal corticosteroid synthesis
17–20-lyase deficiency
17-ketosteroid reductase deficiency
Androgen-resistance syndromes
Receptor/post-receptor defects
Testicular feminisation and variants
Reifenstein's syndrome
Defective testosterone metabolism
5α-reductase deficiency
Persistent Müllerian duct syndrome
Maternal ingestion of oestrogen/progestogen

True hermaphroditism

True hermaphrodites are patients with both ovarian and testicular tissue in the same or opposite gonads. It is most commonly seen in those with a 46XX karyotype, with a 46XX/46XY mosaic or 46XY pattern being rarely found. The gonads are usually ovotestes with the majority of subjects being reared as males due to the size of the phallus. However, most patients possess a uterus, and breast development is common during puberty. Clinical management depends upon the age at diagnosis and the functional capacity of the genitalia. Surgical and endocrine therapy should then be directed towards the appropriate gender assignation.

Ovarian resistance syndromes

Ovarian resistance syndromes are rare disorders where primary amenorrhoea occurs because the ovary is unable to respond to gonadotrophin stimulation. Biochemically, patients with ovarian resistance have hypergonadotrophic hypogonadism with low plasma oestrogen and elevated LH and FSH concentrations.

Resistant ovary syndrome

Resistant ovary syndrome is part of the spectrum of primary ovarian failure where elevated gonadotrophin levels are associated with multiple ovarian antral follicles. Primary ovarian failure of this type generally presents with secondary amenorrhoea and is discussed below.

17α-hydroxylase deficiency

Hypergonadotrophic hypogonadism occurs in patients with 17α-hydroxylase deficiency due to impaired synthesis of 17-hydroxyprogesterone and 17-hydroxypregnenolone and hence of cortisol, oestradiol and testosterone. Sexual infantilism and hypergonadotrophic primary amenorrhoea is associated with increased adrenocorticotrophic hormone (ACTH) levels (secondary to reduced cortisol release). Hypertension with hypokalaemic alkalosis is secondary to increased deoxycorticosterone and 18-hydroxycorticosterone production. Treatment is by glucocorticoid and sex steroid replacement.

Gonadal irradiation and chemotherapy
(see also Chapter 75)

Bone-marrow transplantation (BMT) is now an established treatment for haematological malignancies and other neoplastic and immunological disorders in young people. Prior to BMT, immunosuppressive therapy is given as chemotherapy, often in combination with total-body irradiation. Recovery of ovarian function is age related, such that the older the patient at transplantation, the less likely the recovery of function. Treatment of prepubertal girls is thus more likely to result in restored ovarian function, although this is seen only in the minority of cases and most will present with primary ovarian failure [27]. However, as the majority of patients receive BMT after puberty most women present with secondary amenorrhoea (see below).

Hypothalamo-pituitary disease

Any of the causes of hypothalamo-pituitary disease which present with secondary amenorrhoea may occur in childhood. Thus, primary amenorrhoea, usually with signs of delayed puberty or other anterior pituitary deficiency, may be the presenting feature of tumours in the region of the hypothalamus and pituitary, in particular craniopharyngiomas [28]. Childhood irradiation to the hypothalamus or cytotoxic chemotherapy may also cause hypothalamic primary amenorrhoea.

Hypogonadotrophic hypogonadism

Isolated gonadotrophin deficiency occurs in both sporadic and familial forms and is caused by congenital gonadotrophin-releasing hormone (GnRH) deficiency. Classical Kallmann's syndrome involves isolated GnRH deficiency with anosmia and other mid-line abnormalities [29] and may be inherited in autosomal dominant, autosomal recessive or X-linked patterns (in males). Whilst the gene responsible for the more common X-linked form of the disease has been identified, the genetic defects in the autosomally inherited forms of the syndrome are as yet unknown [30]. Typically, patients are of normal height or tall, with eunuchoid body proportions and delayed puberty. However, the spectrum of clinical presentation of GnRH deficiency is wide and in its mildest form in females may present simply with primary (or even secondary) amenorrhoea.

Gonadotrophin deficiency may be associated with other anterior pituitary hormone deficiencies, in particular GH deficiency due to absent growth hormone-releasing hormone deficiency [1].

Secondary amenorrhoea

The majority of women with amenorrhoea present with secondary amenorrhoea, reflecting a wide range of underlying pathology. The causes of secondary amenorrhoea are listed in Table 51.4 and can be broadly divided into primary and secondary ovarian failure, genital tract abnormalities and functioning ovarian tumours. Many of the causes of secondary amenorrhoea are rare; the relative frequency of the more common diagnoses is shown in Table 51.5.

Clinical assessment

Clinical assessment of women with secondary amenorrhoea should begin with a detailed menstrual history. Many women with 'regular' menstrual cycles may be found to have variable or prolonged intermenstrual intervals, and a long history of irregular cycles is strongly suggestive of the polycystic ovary syndrome. Previous pregnancies, miscarriages or post-partum haemorrhage should be noted, as should a history of therapeutic abortion, pelvic infection or surgery. Symptoms of oestrogen deficiency or galactorrhoea may be present and headaches and visual disturbance should be

Table 51.4 Causes of secondary amenorrhoea.

Primary ovarian failure
Premature menopause
Resistant ovary syndrome
Post-irradiation/chemotherapy
Post-infection (mumps)
Postoperative
Gonadal dysgenesis (rare)
Secondary ovarian failure
Hypothalamo-pituitary dysfunction
Hyperprolactinaemia
Hypothalamo-pituitary tumours
Sheehan's syndrome
Post-CNS irradiation
Postoperative
Functional disorders
Weight loss/anorexia nervosa
Exercise
Psychogenic
Severe acute/chronic illness
Idiopathic hypogonadotrophic hypogonadism
Polycystic ovary syndrome
Genital tract disorders
Asherman's syndrome
Ovarian tumours
Producing oestrogens
Producing androgens

CNS, central nervous system.

Table 51.5 Diagnosis in 570 consecutive patients with secondary amenorrhoea attending the endocrine clinic at the Middlesex Hospital. From [72], with permission.

Diagnosis	Percentage of patients
Polycystic ovary syndrome	37
Primary ovarian failure	24
Hyperprolactinaemia	17
Weight loss	10
Hypogonadotrophic hypogonadism	6
Hypopituitarism	4
Exercise related	3

enquired after. Careful questioning may be required to identify eating disorders, periods of rapid weight loss or excess physical exercise. Symptoms of other endocrine disorders may be present. A past history of radiotherapy or chemotherapy is important.

Examination should begin with the height and weight and calculation of the body mass index (BMI = weight (kg)/ height^2 (m^2); normal range 20–25 kg/m^2). It should be noted that patients with weight loss-related amenorrhoea may not necessarily appear underweight at the time of presentation. Hirsutism, acne or more severe signs of virilisation may be found. Breast examination should be performed—galactorrhoea may occur on expression only. Signs of other endocrine disorders such as hypothyroidism or Cushing's syndrome may be present. The visual fields should be assessed.

Investigation

Initial investigations should include measurement of serum gonadotrophin and prolactin concentrations and an assessment of oestrogen production. Measurement of serum FSH will specifically distinguish primary from secondary ovarian failure. In primary ovarian failure serum LH levels will be elevated, but basal LH is also elevated in 60–70% of women with the polycystic ovary syndrome [31]. Measurement of serum prolactin levels will identify those patients with hyperprolactinaemia, and suggest further relevant investigations such as thyroid function tests and pituitary radiology. Serum oestradiol measurements are unreliable because there is considerable overlap between serum oestradiol concentrations in women with biological evidence of oestrogen deficiency and in normal women in the early follicular phase of the menstrual cycle [9]. Assessment of oestrogen production is best performed by monitoring the response to a progestagen challenge. Vaginal bleeding after a short course of an oral progestagen (e.g. medroxyprogesterone acetate, 5 mg daily for 5 days) is a biological marker of oestrogen activity [32]. Other endocrine function tests should be performed if dictated by the clinical findings. Thyroid function testing has been routinely recommended in patients with amenorrhoea but the true prevalence of oligomenorrhoea or amenorrhoea in such patients is unknown. However, primary hypothyroidism may be associated with hyperprolactinaemia, so it is important to assess thyroid function in hyperprolactinaemic women. Thyroid hormone replacement in this situation lowers serum prolactin levels and restores ovulatory menstrual cycles [33]. The use of the GnRH test is of limited value in individual patients with secondary amenorrhoea and should not be used routinely. Although the mean LH response to 100 μg GnRH administered intravenously is slightly lower in women with hypothalamic amenorrhoea, the test provides poor discrimination between groups of patients and normal women (Fig. 51.1).

Pelvic ultrasonography is an important investigation to reveal ovarian size and morphology, in particular polycystic and multifollicular ovaries. Furthermore, assessment of uterine dimensions and endometrial thickness provides useful information about endogenous oestrogen production [34].

Primary ovarian failure

Women with primary ovarian failure present with amenorrhoea often associated with symptoms of oestrogen deficiency such as hot flushes, loss of libido and vaginal dryness. The diagnosis is established by finding an elevated serum FSH concentration.

Resistant ovary syndrome and premature ovarian failure

The terms resistant ovary syndrome and premature ovarian failure (POF) describe the clinical findings in women with primary ovarian failure depending on the presence or absence of primordial follicles on ultrasound or biopsy. Women with resistant ovary syndrome are those in whom high serum gonadotrophin concentrations are associated with an apparently normal ovarian follicular apparatus [35]. The aetiology of POF remains unknown in the majority of cases although a familial tendency has been reported [36]. In one study of affected families a mutation in the FSH receptor (FSH-R) gene has been identified; this causes an amino-acid substitution in the extracellular ligand-binding domain of the receptor producing a reduction in binding capacity and signal transduction at the FSH-R [37]. However, in another study of sporadic POF, the FSH-R gene was noted to be polymorphic in both patients and normal controls and no causative genetic defect was identified [38]. Furthermore, abnormalities of the FSH-β gene producing a dysfunctional

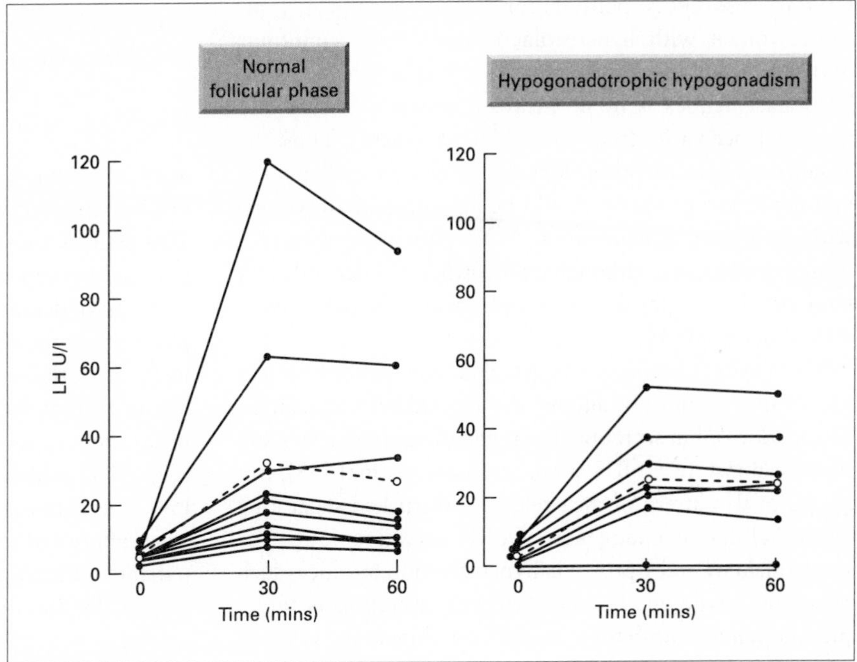

Fig. 51.1 Response to gonadotrophin-releasing hormone (GnRH) in normal women in the follicular phase of the menstrual cycle (left-hand panel) and in women with hypogonadotrophic hypogonadism (right-hand panel). 100 μg GnRH was administered intravenously at time 0 min and blood collected for measurement of luteinising hormone (LH) at 30 and 60 min. Individual responses are shown by the unbroken lines and black circles, with the mean responses shown by the dotted lines and open circles. From [73], with permission.

protein have not been detected in women with POF [39], although one family has been described with isolated FSH *deficiency* due to a frame-shift deletion in the FSH-β gene resulting in hypogonadism and amenorrhoea in the homozygotes [40]. Other genetic defects may yet be identified.

There is an association between premature ovarian failure and other autoimmune endocrine diseases [41] with up to 50% of women having evidence of other autoantibodies [42]. Anti-gonadotrophin-receptor antibodies, analogous to those seen in autoimmune hypothyroidism and myasthenia gravis, have thus been postulated as a cause of premature menopause. This suggestion is supported by occasional reports of the restoration of ovarian function following immunosuppressive therapy [43]. However, in a study using highly specific recombinant human gonadotrophin receptors, no antibodies blocking the actions of human FSH or LH were detected [44], suggesting that antibodies in this condition are directed against targets other than the hormone receptor. Further work is required to identify the exact nature of the autoimmunity associated with premature ovarian failure.

Gonadal irradiation

The improved survival rates after chemotherapy and/or radiotherapy for the treatment of malignant disease or prior to BMT mean that the endocrine consequences of such therapies are increasingly seen. The ovarian consequences of such therapy depend both upon the nature of the drug and radiotherapy regimens used and upon the age of the patient at treatment [45]. In young women (under 26 years) receiving cytotoxic chemotherapy alone the prospect for resumption of normal menstrual cycles is good, but this recovery is much less in those women treated at a later age. However, after total-body irradiation prior to BMT, loss of ovarian function occurs rapidly, particularly in patients treated with fractionated therapy rather than a single dose [46].

Other causes of primary ovarian failure

These include infection, especially mumps and rarely gonadal dysgenesis presenting as secondary amenorrhoea. Previous surgery for benign or malignant disease of the ovaries or elsewhere in the pelvis may also be responsible.

Secondary ovarian failure

Secondary ovarian failure is caused by intrinsic hypothalamo-pituitary dysfunction, by functional disorders of the regulation of gonadotrophin secretion and by the polycystic ovary syndrome. The latter, an important cause of secondary amenorrhoea, is discussed in detail in Chapter 54, and will not be considered further here.

Hypothalamo-pituitary dysfunction

Hyperprolactinaemia

Hyperprolactinaemia accounts for up to 20% of all cases of secondary amenorrhoea and is the most common specific pituitary disorder responsible for amenorrhoea [47]. Typically, women with hyperprolactinaemia have symptoms of oestrogen deficiency associated with galactorrhoea [48], but galactorrhoea is by no means a constant feature and its prevalence varies from 30 to 90% of patients. Thus, the absence of galactorrhoea does not exclude the diagnosis, and the serum prolactin should be measured in all women with secondary amenorrhoea. Most patients will have a pituitary adenoma, although its identification depends to a large extent upon the degree of sophistication of the imaging techniques used [49].

Much evidence exists to suggest that hyperprolactinaemia causes amenorrhoea by altering the hypothalamic regulation of gonadotrophin secretion. Basal gonadotrophin levels and their response to GnRH stimulation are normal [48], but the pulsatile pattern of their release is disturbed suggesting abnormalities of endogenous GnRH secretion [50]. The mechanism whereby prolactin hypersecretion produces such effects is unknown. Normal prolactin secretion is under predominantly inhibitory control by dopamine released by hypothalamic tuberoinfundibular neurons [51]. A short-loop feedback system exists to regulate this system and dopamine turnover in the hypothalamus is increased in hyperprolactinaemic states. This alteration in dopamine activity may be responsible for the change in GnRH pulsatility, with the effects being mediated within the hypothalamus by endogenous opiates [52]. Treatment of hyperprolactinaemia with dopamine-agonist therapy restores normal gonadotrophin secretion and ovarian function (see below).

Other hypothalamo-pituitary disorders

Secondary amenorrhoea may occur in association with other hypothalamo-pituitary disorders via a number of different mechanisms. Gonadotrophin deficiency may occur with any large tumour in the region of the hypothalamus and pituitary. Such tumours may cause hyperprolactinaemia and hence amenorrhoea due to compression of the pituitary stalk and interference with dopamine secretion or transport. Menstrual disorders in acromegaly may be secondary to gonadotrophin deficiency, to concurrent hyperprolactinaemia or to associated polycystic ovaries. Pituitary-dependent Cushing's disease is associated with amenorrhoea, possibly due to the development of polycystic ovaries as a consequence of adrenal androgen hypersecretion [31], although recent evidence suggests that it is more likely to be a direct effect of cortisol at the hypothalamus. Other lesions of the pituitary gland such as Sheehan's syndrome, lymphocytic hypophysitis and granulomatous infiltration cause secondary amenorrhoea. Previous surgery or central nervous system irradiation may also be responsible.

Functional disorders of the regulation of gonadotrophin secretion

Weight loss-related amenorrhoea

Marked weight loss, resulting in a BMI of less than 16 kg/m^2, is associated with profound gonadotrophin deficiency. This reflects impaired GnRH secretion producing a prepubertal pattern of gonadotrophin release [53]. In women with lesser degrees of weight loss or during the recovery phase of weight-related amenorrhoea, the pattern of activity in the hypothalamo-pituitary–ovarian axis is exactly analogous to that seen during normal puberty. Thus, ovarian ultrasonography shows a multifollicular morphology [9] (Fig. 51.2) which is identical to that seen during puberty [54]. This pattern represents the response of the normal ovary to an abnormal (or immature) gonadotrophin stimulus. In patients with weight loss the gonadotrophin pulse pattern is typically that of reduced-frequency LH pulses of normal

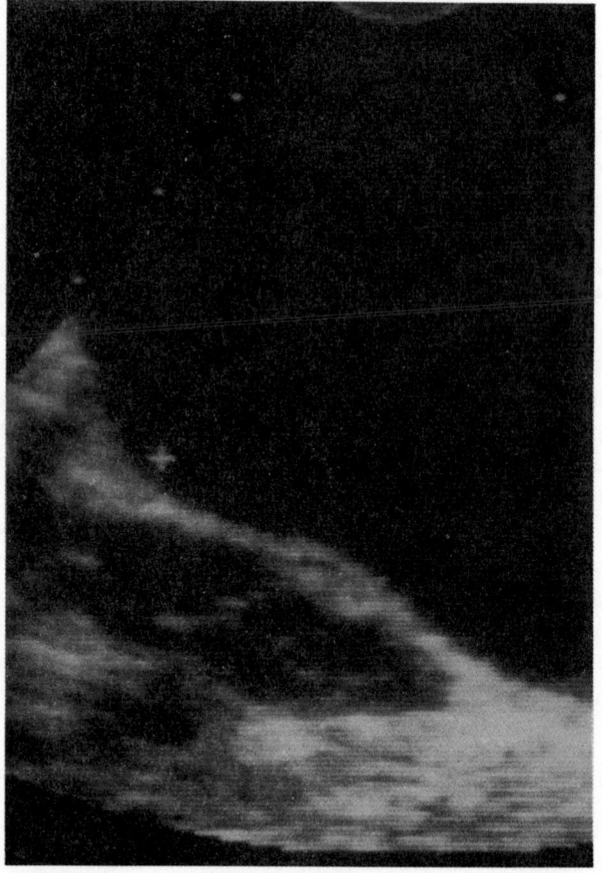

Fig. 51.2 Ovarian ultrasound scan showing a multifollicular morphology in a women with weight-related amenorrhoea. The ovary contains more than six cysts of greater than 4-mm diameter. (Courtesy of J. Adams, Reproductive Endocrinology Unit, Massachusetts General Hospital.)

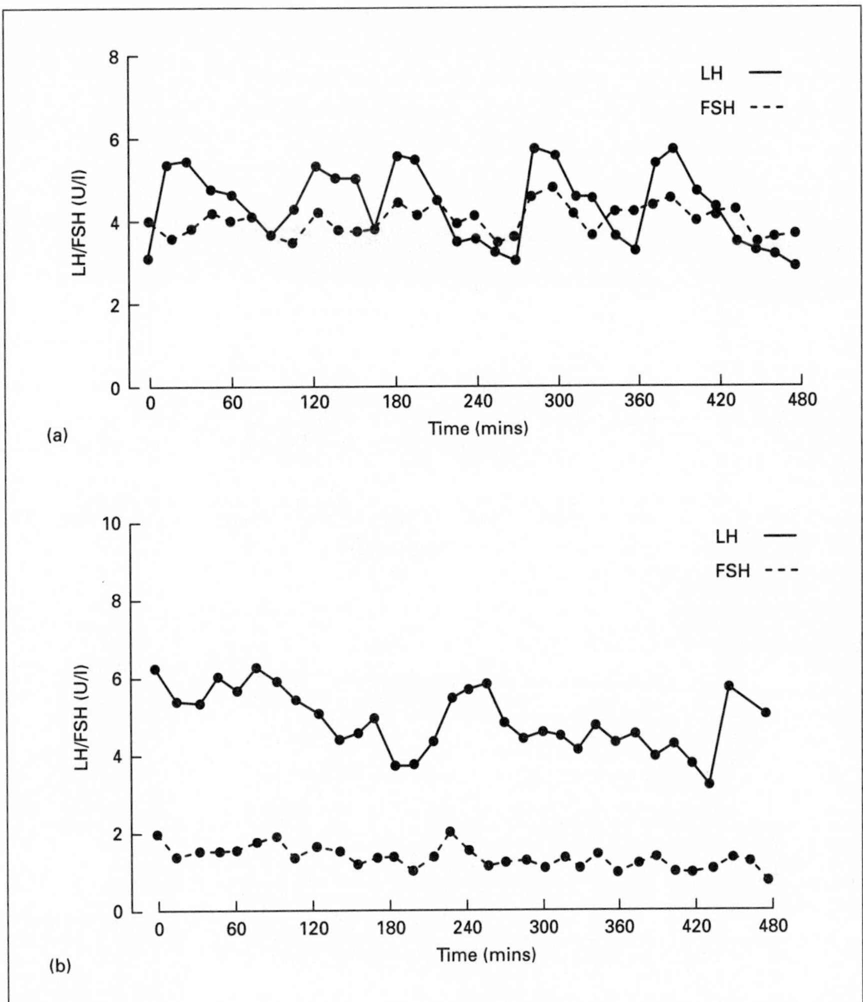

Fig. 51.3 Representative 8-hour hormone profiles to show luteinising hormone (LH; unbroken lines) and follicle-stimulating hormone (FSH; dotted lines). Hormone profiles are shown in a normal subject (a) and a woman with weight-related amenorrhoea (b).

amplitude [55] (Fig. 51.3). However, in about 20% of cases the only abnormality is high-amplitude pulses which lack the characteristic nocturnal slow frequency observed in normal cycles (Fig. 51.4). This pattern is virtually identical to that seen in late puberty [5]. Circulating leptin concentrations are known to decrease in healthy adults with diet-induced weight loss [74]. A possible role for leptin in modulating gonadotrophin secretion in women with weight loss-related amenorrhoea remains to be elucidated.

Exercise-related amenorrhoea

The patterns of gonadotrophin secretion and ovarian morphology seen in patients with amenorrhoea induced by strenuous physical exercise are similar to those seen in weight-related amenorrhoea. Clearly, psychological factors may play a role in the development of amenorrhoea in both these groups of women. However, it appears that body-weight itself (or body composition) may be the most important factor, as the same abnormalities can be identified in women who are underweight as a result of chronic illness [56].

Psychogenic amenorrhoea

Disturbed menstrual function is commonly reported at stressful times in women's lives. The endocrine abnormalities underlying this phenomenon have not been clearly identified.

Idiopathic hypogonadotrophic hypogonadism

This term is used to describe women with hypothalamic amenorrhoea of unknown cause. The condition is characterised by marked abnormalities of gonadotrophin secretion in the absence of any of the recognised associated disorders.

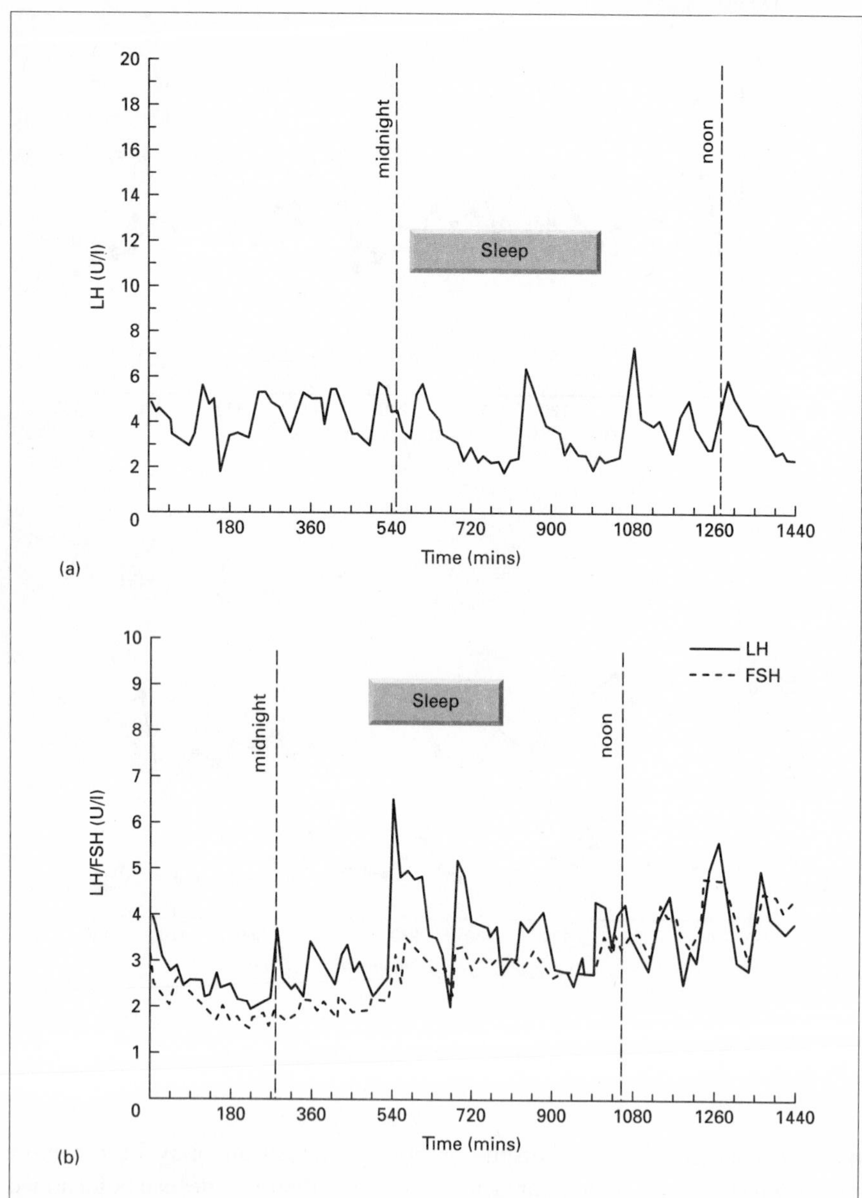

Fig. 51.4 Hormone profiles to show luteinising hormone (LH) and follicle-stimulating hormone (FSH) concentrations during waking hours and sleep. A representative LH profile firom a normal subject is shown in (a) and LH and FSH profiles from a patient with weight-related amenorrhoea in (b).

Genital tract abnormalities

Asherman's syndrome describes secondary amenorrhoea caused by intrauterine adhesions resulting in virtually complete obliteration of the uterine cavity. Endocrine function is normal. The syndrome usually follows post-partum or post-abortion endometritis, or myomectomy. Normal menstrual function is restored by surgical division of the adhesions, although subsequent miscarriages or intrauterine deaths are not uncommon [57].

Ovarian tumours

Rarely, secondary amenorrhoea may result from functioning ovarian tumours producing oestrogens or androgens, although it is not a feature of the more common epithelial ovarian carcinomas [58]. Of the functioning tumours, oestrogen-secreting granulosa theca-cell tumours are the most frequent, accounting for 5–10% of all solid ovarian tumours. Androgen-secreting dysgerminomas, gonadoblastomas, lipoid-cell and hilar cell tumours are much less common and present with a short history of severe virilisation and amenorrhoea.

Treatment of secondary amenorrhoea

The principles of treatment of secondary amenorrhoea in young women are to treat oestrogen-deficiency symptoms in those who do not wish to become pregnant and to induce ovulation in those who do. A further reason for treatment is to prevent the long-term complications of hypo-oestrogenaemia, in particular osteoporosis and adverse changes in plasma lipoprotein patterns associated with an increased risk of cardiovascular disease [59]. As bone mass reaches its peak before the age of 30, adolescents and young women with hypothalamic amenorrhoea of any cause are at particular risk for osteoporosis in later life [60]. Whilst bone mineral density can be improved with appropriate oestrogen therapy, the reversal of bone changes may be slow, emphasising the need for rapid diagnosis and treatment in young women [61]. The effects of synthetic progestogens, given in a cyclical manner with oestrogen for endometrial protection may antagonise the beneficial effects of oestrogen on plasma lipids. This unwanted effect is not seen with the preparations of natural progesterone being developed, although the best method of delivery of the natural hormone remains to be identified [59].

Primary ovarian failure

Treatment of primary ovarian failure is symptomatic as there is no therapy which specifically increases the chance of ovulation although spontaneous ovulation occasionally occurs in these women. There is no clear evidence that attempts to induce 'rebound ovulation' following gonadotrophin suppression with gonadal steroids or GnRH analogues provide any increased chance of ovulation over and above that seen in untreated women [62]. The use of embryo donation in the context of an *in vitro* fertilisation programme is now able to offer some hope of fertility to young women with primary ovarian failure [63]. For the majority of women with primary ovarian failure, treatment should be by hormone-replacement therapy in the form of a cyclical combined oestrogen/progestogen preparation.

Secondary ovarian failure

Management of patients with secondary ovarian failure is determined by the underlying diagnosis. Thus, pituitary tumours may require surgery with subsequent appropriate hormone replacement, hypothyroidism should be treated with thyroxine etc. Certain specific problems are considered here.

Hyperprolactinaemia (see also Chapter 9)

Reduction of circulating prolactin concentration allows recovery of the hypothalamo-pituitary–ovarian axis and the resumption of normal menstrual cycles. Treatment is with long-acting dopamine agonists, and the semisynthetic ergot derivative bromocriptine has been in use for over 20 years. Bromocriptine suppresses prolactin secretion in the majority of cases, irrespective of the initial serum prolactin concentration. It is useful in the management of large prolactinomas in addition to microadenomas, as it also causes significant tumour shrinkage [64]. Bromocriptine is safe for use in pregnancy and has been widely used for the induction of ovulation in hyperprolactinaemic women prior to conception [65]. Bromocriptine in therapeutic doses is generally well tolerated although the side-effects, in particular nausea, postural hypotension and giddiness, are dose related and may be intolerable in a small group of patients. Adverse effects may be minimised by starting treatment with a small dose, for example 1.25 mg at night with food, and slowly increasing the dose in a stepwise fashion until the serum prolactin level is normalised and menstrual function returns. However, a significant proportion of patients are unable to tolerate bromocriptine, even when the dose is built up slowly. Two alternative dopamine agonists, quinagolide and cabergoline, have become available recently for the treatment of hyperprolactinaemia [66,67]. These have longer biological half-lives than bromocriptine and may have fewer side-effects and are thus useful in the treatment of women intolerant of bromocriptine. Finally, in a small group of patients medical therapy fails, either due to intolerable side-effects or ineffectiveness in reducing serum prolactin levels or tumour size, and in these women transsphenoidal surgery may be required.

Weight-related amenorrhoea

The treatment of weight-related amenorrhoea is weight gain, which is specific therapy and may require the additional expertise of dietitians and psychologists. Induction of ovulation by exogenous gonadotrophins or pulsatile GnRH therapy should be avoided in underweight women who may be psychologically unable to cope with a pregnancy. Furthermore, women who conceive whilst significantly underweight have a greater risk of having an underweight baby [68]. It is worth considering induction of ovulation in women who have regained and maintained their normal bodyweight but not restarted ovulatory menstrual cycles.

Women with exercise-related amenorrhoea such as athletes and ballet dancers may be reluctant or unable to reduce their amount of physical activity. It is advisable to assess oestrogen status in such women. Those who do not respond to a progestogen challenge should be treated with replacement therapy in the form of a cyclical combined oestrogen/progestogen preparation. Such therapy should also be discussed with amenorrhoeic women who have a positive response to progestogen, in view of the increased risk of osteoporosis in these subjects [61].

Hypogonadotrophic hypogonadism

Women with Kallmann's syndrome or idiopathic hypogonadotrophic hypogonadism should be treated with sex hormone replacement unless fertility is required. Induction of ovulation can then be achieved with pulsatile GnRH therapy or gonadotrophins.

Pulsatile gonadotrophin-releasing hormone therapy. Pulsatile GnRH therapy allows the normal ovarian–pituitary feedback mechanism to function and can therefore be regarded as the most 'physiological' method of ovulation induction in women with hypothalamic amenorrhoea. In early studies GnRH was delivered by the intravenous route using an automatic pulsatile infusion pump but subsequently the efficacy of subcutaneous delivery has been established. This treatment restores normal fertility to women with hypothalamic amenorrhoea and also to a proportion of those with intrinsic pituitary disease, suggesting adequate gonadotrophin reserves in at least some of these patients [69]. The major side-effect of pulsatile GnRH therapy is an increase in the rate of multiple pregnancy, although this has usually been found to be lower than that seen with gonadotrophin treatment. Multiple pregnancies occur more frequently when conception occurs during the first treatment cycle so the problem can be largely overcome by careful ultrasound monitoring and appropriate advice to the patient.

Human menopausal gonadotrophin and recombinant FSH

Prior to the development of pulsatile GnRH therapy, exogenous gonadotrophins derived from urine had been used successfully in the treatment of hypothalamic amenorrhoea. This form of treatment remains acceptable, but has a higher risk of multiple pregnancy. The availability of recombinant human FSH means that a readily available supply of hormone is now present, although it is unlikely to prove more effective in treatment induction of ovulation regimens [70]. Treatment should start with low-dose therapy and increase in a stepwise fashion according to the ovarian response. Recent work suggests that the addition of short-term low-dose growth hormone may reduce the requirement for exogenous gonadotrophins but, as yet, no significant effects on ovulation and pregnancy rates have been shown in women who are resistant to gonadotrophins [71].

References

1 Franks S. Primary and secondary amenorrhoea. In: *Gynaecology Clinical Algorithms*. London: BMJ Publications, 1989: 41–5.

2 Wood DF, Franks S. Delayed puberty. *Br J Hosp Med* 1989; **4**: 223–30.

3 Marshall WA, Tanner JM. Variation in the pattern of pubertal changes in girls. *Arch Dis Child* 1969; **44**: 291–303.

4 Tanner JM. *Growth at Adolescence*. Oxford: Blackwell Scientific Publications, 1962.

5 Styne DM. The physiology of puberty. In: Brook CGD, ed. *Clinical Paediatric Endocrinology*. Oxford: Blackwell Science, 1995: 234–52.

6 Bridges NA, Brook CGD. Disorders of puberty. In: Brook CGD, ed. *Clinical Paediatric Endocrinology*. Oxford: Blackwell Science, 1995: 253–73.

7 Warren MP. Amenorrhea in endurance runners. *J Clin Endocrinol Metab* 1992; **75**: 1393–7.

8 Warren MP. The effects of exercise on pubertal progression and reproductive function in girls. *J Clin Endocrinol Metab* 1980; **51**: 1150–7.

9 Adams JM, Franks S, Polson DW *et al.* Multifollicular ovaries: clinical and endocrine features and response to pulsatile gonadotrophin releasing hormone. *Lancet* 1985; **2**: 1375–9.

10 Canales ES, Zarate A, Castelazo-Ayala L. Primary amenorrhoea associated with polycystic ovaries. Endocrine, cytogenetic and therapeutic considerations. *Obstet Gynaecol* 1971; **37**: 205–10.

11 Turner HH. A syndrome of infantilism, congenital webbed neck and cubitus valgus. *Endocrinology* 1938; **23**: 566–74.

12 Ford CE, Jones KW, Polani PE *et al.* A sex chromosome anomaly in a case of gonadal dysgenesis (Turner's syndrome). *Lancet* 1959; **1**: 711–13.

13 Lyon AJ, Preece MA, Grant DB. Growth curve for girls with Turner syndrome. *Arch Dis Child* 1985; **60**: 932–5.

14 Saenger P. The current status of diagnosis and therapeutic intervention in Turner's syndrome. *J Clin Endocrinol Metab* 1993; **77**: 297–301.

15 Massarano AA, Brook CGD, Hindmarsh PC *et al.* Growth hormone secretion in Turner's syndrome and influence of oxandrolone and ethinyl oestradiol. *Arch Dis Child* 1989; **64**: 587–92.

16 Conte FA, Grumbach MM, Kaplan SL. A diphasic pattern of gonadotrophin secretion in patients with the syndrome of gonadal dysgenesis. *J Clin Endocrinol Metab* 1975; **40**: 670–4.

17 Muram D, Jolly EE. Pregnancy and gonadal dysgenesis. *J Obstet Gynaecol* 1982; **3**: 87–8.

18 Massarano AA, Adams JA, Preece MA, Brook CGD. Ovarian ultrasound appearances in Turner syndrome. *J Pediatr* 1989; **114**: 568–73.

19 Vanderschueren-Lodeweyckx M, Massa G, Maes M *et al.* Growth promoting effect of growth hormone and low-dose ethinyl estradiol in girls with Turners syndrome. *J Clin Endocrinol Metab* 1990; **70**: 122–6.

20 Rongen-Westerlaken C, Wit JM, Drop SLS *et al.* Methionyl human growth hormone in Turner's syndrome. *Arch Dis Child* 1988; **63**: 1211–17.

21 Van Teunenbroek A, De Muinck Keizer-Schrama SMPF, Stijnen T *et al.* Dutch Working Group on Growth Hormone. Effect of growth hormone administration frequency on 24 hour growth hormone profiles and levels of other growth related parameters in girls with Turner's syndrome. *Clin Endocrinol* 1993; **39**: 77–84.

22 Morishima A, Grumback MM. The inter-relationship of sex chromosome constitution and phenotype in the syndrome of gonadal dysgenesis and its variants. *Ann New York Acad Sci* 1968; **155**: 695–715.

23 Medlej R, Lobacarro JM, Berta P. Screening for Y-derived sex determining gene SRY in 40 patients with Turner syndrome. *J Clin*

Endocrinol Metab 1992; **75**: 1289–92.

24 Griffin JE, Edwards C, Madden JD, Harrod MJ, Wilson JD. Congenital absence of the vagina. The Mayer–Rokitanski–Kuster–Hauser syndrome. *Ann Intern Med* 1976; **85**: 224–36.

25 Quigley CA, De Bellis A, Marschke KB, El-Awady MK, Wilson EM, French FS. Androgen receptor defects: historical, clinical and molecular perspectives. *Endocr Rev* 1995; **16**: 271–321.

26 Wilson JD, Griffin JE, Russell DW. Steroid 5 alpha-reductase 2 deficiency. *Endocr Rev* 1993; **14**: 577–93.

27 Sanders JE, Pritchard S, Mahoney P *et al.* Growth and development following bone marrow transplantation for leukaemia. *Blood* 1986; **68**: 1129–35.

28 Banna M. Craniopharyngioma: based on 160 cases. *Br J Radiol* 1976; **49**: 206–23.

29 Kallmann FJ, Schoenfeld WA, Barrera SE. The genetic aspects of primary eunuchoidism. *Am J Mental Def* 1944; **48**: 203–36.

30 Rugarli EI, Ballabio A. Kallmann syndrome from genetics to neurobiology. *JAMA* 1993; **270**: 2713–16.

31 Franks S. Polycystic ovary syndrome: a changing perspective. *Clin Endocrinol* 1989; **31**: 87–120.

32 Hull MGR, Knuth UA, Murray MAF, Jacobs HS. The practical value of the progestagen challenge test, serum oestradiol estimation or clinical examination in assessment of the oestrogen state and response to clomiphene in amenorrhoea. *Br J Obstet Gynaecol* 1979; **86**: 799–805.

33 Semple CG, Beastall GH, Teasdale G, Thomson JA. Hypothyroidism presenting with hyperprolactinaemia. *Br Med J* 1983; **286**: 1200–1.

34 Tan SL, Jacobs HS. Recent advances in the management of amenorrhoea. *Clin Obstet Gynaecol* 1985; **12**: 725–47.

35 Starup J, Sele V, Henrikson B. Amenorrhoea associated with increased production of gonadotrophins and a morphologically normal ovarian follicular apparatus. *Acta Endocrinologica* 1971; **66**: 248–56.

36 Coulam CB, Stringfellow S, Hoefnagel D. Evidence for a genetic factor in the etiology of premature ovarian failure. *Fertil Steril* 1983; **40**: 693–5.

37 Aittomaki K, Lucena JLD, Pakarinen P *et al.* Mutation in the follicle-stimulating hormone receptor gene causes hereditary hypergonadotropic ovarian failure. *Cell* 1995; **82**: 959–68.

38 Whitney EA, Layman LA, Chan PJ, Lee A, Peak DB, McDonough PG. The follicle-stimulating hormone receptor gene is polymorphic in premature ovarian failure and normal controls. *Fertil Steril* 1995; **64**: 518–24.

39 Layman LC, Shelley ME, Huey LO, Wall SW, Tho SPT, McDonough PG. Follicle-stimulating hormone beta gene structure in premature ovarian failure. *Fertil Steril* 1993; **60**: 852–7.

40 Matthews CH, Borgato S, Beck-Peccoz P *et al.* Primary amenorrhoea and infertility due to a mutation in the beta-subunit of follicle stimulating hormone. *Nature Genet* 1993; **5**: 83–6.

41 La Barbera AR, Miller MM, Ober C, Rebar RW. Autoimmune etiology in premature ovarian failure. *Am J Reprod Immunol* 1988; **16**: 115–22.

42 Hague WM, Tan SL, Adams JA. Hypergonadotrophic amenorrhoea: aetiology and outcome in 93 young women. *Int J Obstet Gynaecol* 1987; **25**: 121–5.

43 Cowchock FS, McCabe JL, Montgomery BB. Pregnancy after corticosteroid administration in premature ovarian failure (polyglandular endocrinopathy syndrome). *Am J Obstet Gynecol* 1988; **158**: 118–19.

44 Anastasi JN, Flack MR, Froehlich J, Nelson LM. The use of human recombinant gonadotropin receptor to search for immunoglobulin G-mediated premature ovarian failure. *J Clin Endocrinol Metab* 1995; **80**: 824–8.

45 Shalet SM. Cancer therapy and gonadal dysfunction. In: Sheaves R, Jenkins P, Wass JA, eds. *Clinical Endocrine Oncology*. Oxford: Blackwell Science, 1994: 510–13.

46 Shalet SM, Didi M, Ogilvy-Stuart AL, Schulga J, Donaldson MDC. Growth and endocrine function after bone marrow transplantation. *Clin Endocrinol* 1995; **42**: 333–9.

47 Sarapura V, Schlaff WD. Recent advances in the understanding of the pathophysiology and treatment of hyperprolactinaemia. *Curr Opin Obstet Gynaecol* 1993; **5**: 360–7.

48 Jacobs HS, Franks S, Murray MAF, Hull MGR, Steele SJ, Nabarro JD. Clinical and endocrine features of hyperprolactinaemic amenorrhoea. *Clin Endocrinol* 1976; **5**: 439–54.

49 Elster AD. Modern imaging of the pituitary. *Radiology* 1993; **187**: 1–14.

50 Moult PGA, Dacie JE, Rees LH, Besser GM. Prolactin pulsatility in patients with gonadal dysfunction. *Clin Endocrinol* 1981; **14**: 387–94.

51 Wood DF, Johnston JM, Johnston DG. Dopamine, the dopamine receptor and pituitary tumours. *Clin Endocrinol* 1991; **35**: 455–66.

52 Grossman A, Moult PGA, McIntyre H *et al.* Opiate mediation of amenorrhoea in hyperprolactinaemia and in weight-loss related amenorrhoea. *Clin Endocrinol* 1982; **17**: 379–88.

53 Nillius SJ, Wide L. The pituitary responsiveness to acute and chronic administration of gonadotrophin releasing hormone in acute and recovery stages of anorexia nervosa. In: Vigersky RA, ed. *Anorexia Nervosa*. New York: Raven Press, 1977: 225–41.

54 Stanhope R, Adams J, Jacobs HS, Brook CGD. Ovarian ultrasound assessment in normal children, idiopathic precocious puberty and during low dose pulsatile gonadotrophin releasing hormone treatment of hypogonadotrophic hypogonadism. *Arch Dis Child* 1985; **60**: 116–19.

55 Mason HD, Sagle M, Polson DW *et al.* Reduced frequency of luteinizing hormone pulses in women with weight-loss related amenorrhoea and multifollicular ovaries. *Clin Endocrinol* 1988; **28**: 611–18.

56 Stead RJ, Hodson ME, Batten JC, Adams J, Jacobs HS. Amenorrhoea in cystic fibrosis. *Clin Endocrinol* 1987; **26**: 187–95.

57 March CM, Israel R. Gestational outcome following hysteroscopic lysis of adhesions. *Fertil Steril* 1981; **36**: 455–9.

58 Scully RE. Ovarian tumors with endocrine manifestations. In: DeGroot LJ, ed. *Endocrinology*. Philadelphia: WB Saunders 1995: 2113–27.

59 Schachter MD, Shoham MD. Amenorrhoea during the reproductive years—is it safe? *Fertil Steril* 1994; **62**: 1–16.

60 Hergenroeder AC. Bone mineralization, hypothalamic amenorrhoea and sex steroid therapy in female adolescents and young adults. *J Pediatr* 1995; **126**: 683–9.

61 Guleki B, Davies MC, Jacobs HS. Effect of treatment on established osteoporosis in young women with amenorrhoea. *Clin Endocrinol* 1994; **41**: 275–81.

62 Baird DT. Amenorrhea, anovulation and dysfunctional uterine bleeding. In: DeGroot LJ, ed. *Endocrinology*. Philadelphia: WB Saunders, 1995: 2059–79.

63 Lutjen P, Trounson A, Leeton J, Wood C, Renon P. The establishment and maintenance of pregnancy using *in vitro* fertilization and embryo donation in a patient with primary ovarian failure. *Nature* 1984; **307**: 174–5.

64 Bevan JS, Webster J, Burke CW, Scanlon MF. Dopamine agonists and pituitary tumor shrinkage. *Endocr Rev* 1992; **13**: 220–40.

65 Turkalj I, Braun P, Krupp P. Surveillance of bromocriptine in pregnancy. *JAMA* 1982; **247**: 1589–91.

66 Webster J, Piscitelli G, Polli A, Ferrari CI, Ismail I, Scanlon MF. A comparison of cabergoline and bromocriptine in the treatment of hyperprolactinaemic amenorrhoea. *N Engl J Med* 1994; **331**: 904–9.
67 Homburg R, West C, Brownell J, Jacobs HS. A double-blind study comparing a new, non-ergot, long acting dopamine agonist, CV 205–502, with bromocriptine in women with hyperprolactinaemic amenorrhoea. *Clin Endocrinol* 1990; **32**: 565–71.
68 Van der Spuy Z, Steer PJ, McCusker M, Steele SJ, Jacobs HS. Outcome of pregnancy in underweight women after spontaneous and induced ovulation. *Br Med J* 1988; **296**: 962–5.
69 Martin KA, Hall JE, Adams JM, Crowley WF. Comparison of exogenous gonadotropins and pulsatile gonadotropin releasing hormone for induction of ovulation in hypogonadotropic amenorrhoea. *J Clin Endocrinol Metab* 1993; **77**: 125–9.
70 Franks S, Gilling-Smith C. Advances in induction of ovulation. *Curr Opin Obstet Gynaecol* 1994; **6**: 136–40.
71 Katz E, Ricciarelli E, Adashi EY. Review: the potential relevance of growth hormone to female reproductive physiology and pathophysiology. *Fertil Steril* 1993; **59**: 8–34.
72 Kyei-Mensah AA, Jacobs HS. The investigation of female infertility. *Clin Endocrinol* 1995; **43**: 251–5.
73 Franks S. Diagnostic uses of LHRH. In: Shaw RW, Marshall JC, eds. *LHRH and its Analogues*. London: Wright, 1989: 80–91.
74 Consadine RV, Sinha MK, Heiman ML *et al.* Serum immunoreactive leptin concentrations in normal-weight and obese humans. *N Engl J Med* 1996; **334**: 292–5.

CHAPTER 52

The oral contraceptive

D.J. Hemrika and J. Schoemaker

Introduction

Since the introduction of the first birth control pill in 1960, oral contraceptives (OCs) have gained a prime position in the array of methods that are available to prevent the occurrence of unwanted pregnancy. At present, more than 50 million women worldwide depend on OCs for reliable contraception [1]. Although the currently available contraceptive formulations contain only a fraction of the steroid dose used in the initial preparations, there is constant concern in the lay community as well as in the medical profession with regard to the safety of contraceptive steroids. In contradistinction to the problem of unwanted side-effects, the use of OCs provide unquestionable health benefits, such as protection against gynaecological cancers and certain sexually transmitted diseases.

Faced with this dilemma of risks and benefits, medical practitioners must choose from a wide range of different contraceptive formulations to best suit the needs of the individual patient. This chapter will focus on the currently available OCs, their steroid composition and inherent properties. A discussion of contraindications, side-effects, and common problems with OCs will provide guidelines for patient management.

Contraceptive steroids

History

Native ovarian steroids are rapidly inactivated by enzymatic degradation in the digestive tract and through the enterohepatic circulation when administered orally. Natural oestrogens, like 17β-oestradiol and conjugated equine oestrogens, have to be administered in very high dosages to achieve inhibition of ovulation. The inevitable side-effects that occur with these high dosages of oestrogens, such as nausea, make these compounds impractical for incorporation into contraceptive formulations. In 1938 it was discovered that addition of an ethinyl group ($-C \equiv CH$) at the 17 position of 17β-oestradiol resulted in an orally active and potent oestrogenic compound (17α-ethinyl-17β-oestradiol, ethinyl oestradiol). Similarly, addition of an ethinyl group to testosterone produced ethisterone, a compound that could be administered orally but principally behaved as an androgen. In 1951, removal of the 19 carbon from ethisterone resulted in the synthesis of norethisterone (17α-ethinyl-19-nortestosterone) [2]. The most important result of this remodelling was that it changed the major biological effect from an androgen into a progestogen.

The first clinical trials with oral contraceptive preparations started in 1952 and were conducted by Gregory Pincus, a consultant at the Searle laboratories. In November 1959, Enovid (Searle) was the first commercially available oral contraceptive, containing 0.15 mg mestranol (the 3-methyl ether of ethinyl oestradiol) and 9.85 mg norethinodrel, to be followed in 1962 by Ortho-Novum (Syntex), containing 0.6 mg mestranol and 10 mg norethisterone. The synthesis of more potent progestational agents with reduced androgenic action has resulted in a dramatic dose reduction of both the oestrogenic and gestagenic component of modern contraceptive preparations, resulting in a significant reduction of side-effects without compromising contraceptive reliability.

Chemistry of synthetic steroids

At present ethinyloestradiol (EE) is the most commonly used oestrogenic compound in oral contraceptives. It is synthesised by addition of an ethinyl group at the C-17 position of the 17β-oestradiol molecule (Fig. 52.1). It is a more potent oestrogen than oestradiol. The other synthetic oestrogen that has been used in oral contraceptives, mestranol, is the 3-methyl ether of EE. Mestranol is a prohormone and is converted

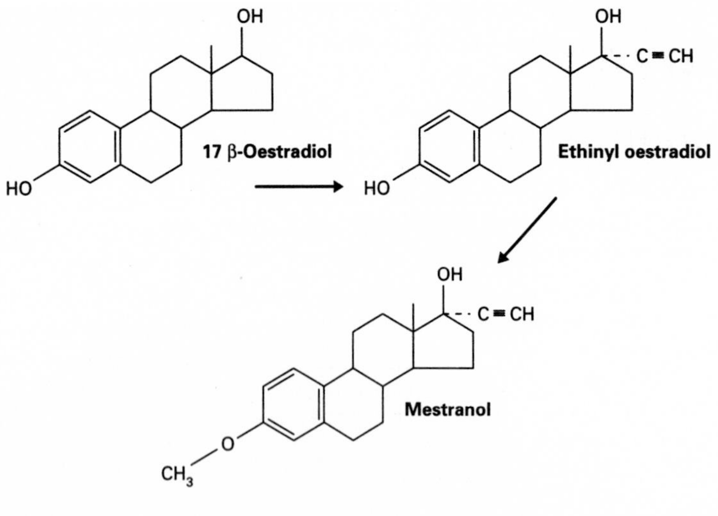

Fig. 52.1 Chemical structure of oestrogens.

in the liver into the active compound, EE. The efficacy of this enzymatic conversion is approximately 65%, resulting in a weaker oestrogenic effect of mestranol as compared with EE at identical dosages.

The synthetic progestogens used in oral contraceptives are all derivatives of testosterone. As was already stated in the previous section, addition of an ethinyl group at the C-17 position produced the orally active compound ethisterone, while deletion of the C-19 carbon resulted in the progestational compound norethisterone (Fig. 52.2). These progestins are known as 19-nortestosterone derivatives, referring to the absent carbon at the 19 position. Addition of another methyl group at the C-18 position produces norgestrel, of which the laevo-rotatory enantiomer is the biologically active molecule, hence the name levonorgestrel. The new progestogens, like norgestimate, desogestrel and gestodene, have resulted from modifications of the norgestrel molecule. These new compounds are almost completely devoid of androgenic side-effects and produce minimal changes in blood lipid composition, coagulation parameters or carbohydrate metabolism [34].

Pharmacokinetics of synthetic steroids

Ethinyloestradiol is absorbed from the small intestine either as a free steroid or conjugated to a sulphate group. In the liver, EE can be conjugated to a sulphate or to a glucuronide group. In addition, the A-ring may undergo hydroxylation, resulting in a biologically inactive compound. Hydroxylated EE is secreted in the bile and passed on to the intestine. From there EE may be excreted in the faeces, or, after hydrolysation by the intestinal bacterial flora, may be reabsorbed into the enterohepatic circulation [5]. After oral administration approximately 60% of the EE dose is inactivated by this enterohepatic degradation, so the bioavailability of orally administered EE is 40% [6]. In serum, EE is almost exclusively bound to albumin (±97%), with virtually no binding to sex hormone-binding globulin (SHBG). After oral administration, serum EE levels peak after 1–2 hours, and show a steady decline in the following 22 hours. There are great interindividual differences in the EE serum level after ingestion of the same EE dose [7]. To date, the reasons for these differences remain largely unexplained [8]. Some authors found evidence that the gestagenic component of the oral contraceptive can influence the pharmacokinetics of EE, possibly by interfering with hydroxylation in the liver [9], although this is disputed by others [10].

Progestogens are absorbed from the intestine and bound initially to albumin, and to a lesser extent to SHBG. The EE-induced increase in SHBG after multiple dosing results in a larger proportion of gestagens being bound to SHBG during chronic OC ingestion. In the liver, inactivation occurs through hydroxylation at the 3 or 5 position. There are, however, differences in metabolism between various gestagens: norethisterone has a bioavailability of ±65%, while norgestrel and gestodene do not undergo a first-pass effect in the liver, resulting in a 100% bioavailability [5]. Desogestrel is transformed in the intestinal mucosa and in the liver into 3-ketodesogestrel, which is the biologically active compound, resulting in a bioavailability of 60–80%. In analogy with the situation for EE as discussed above, serum levels of synthetic gestagens show a wide variation among individuals [5].

A better understanding of the pharmacokinetics of these compounds is important, since the large interindividual differences in serum levels result in differences in bioavailability

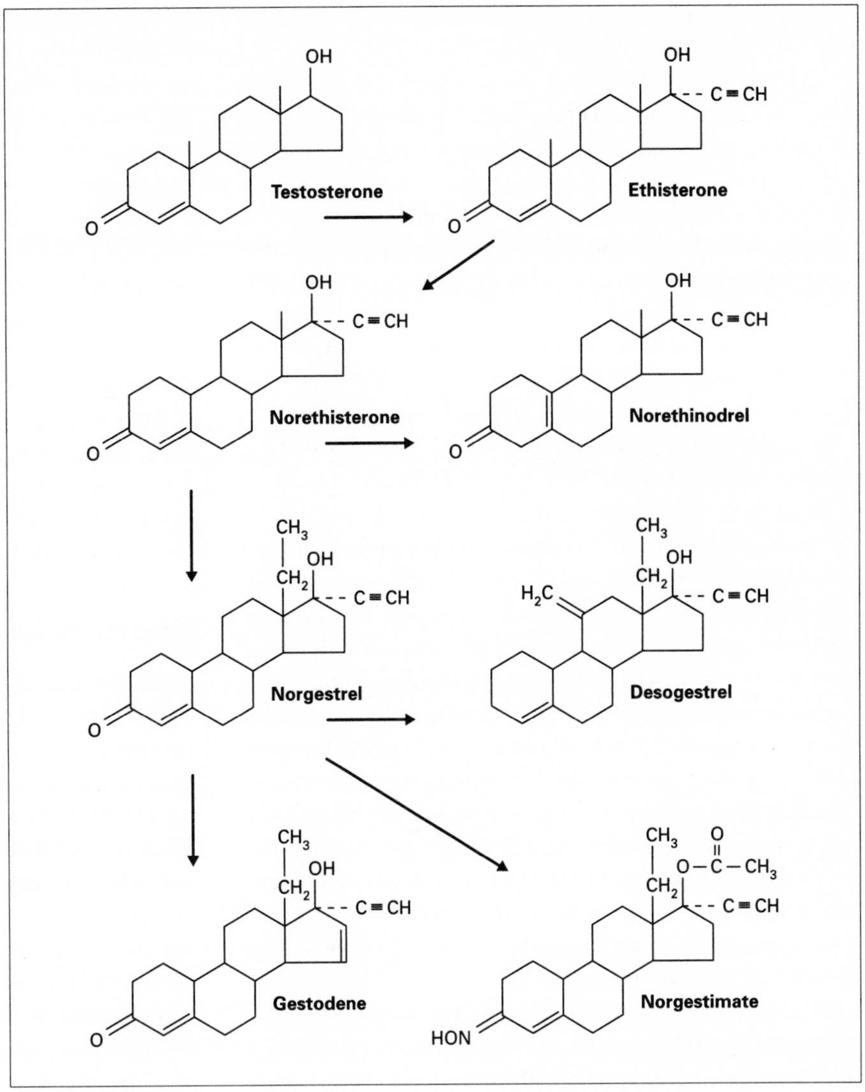

Fig. 52.2 Chemical structure of progestogens.

of the steroids, which may have consequences for the reliability of contraceptive action as well as for the occurrence of side-effects.

Mode of action of oral contraceptives

Although oral contraceptives are commonly designated as inhibitors of ovulation, they essentially suppress folliculogenesis. The suppression of pituitary release of gonadotrophins, predominantly follicle-stimulating hormone (FSH), prevents the growth and maturation of a dominant follicle, thereby abolishing the mid-cycle rise of oestradiol, which is the principal trigger for the preovulatory surge of luteinising hormone (LH). Suppression of serum levels of FSH, as well as the sensitivity of the pituitary to release FSH in response to a gonadotrophin-releasing hormone (GnRH) challenge, is most probably accomplished by negative feedback of EE at the pituitary [11]. This suppression of FSH is accomplished within a few days after the start of the OC cycle, and is as effective in first cycles as in long-term OC users [12].

The suppression of serum LH levels during OC ingestion is mediated by the gestagenic component of the pill, and caused by a gestagen-induced slowing down of the hypothalamic pulse generator. The result of this feedback effect of gestagens is a progressive decrease in LH pulse frequency, which is both dose and time dependent and differs with the chemical structure of various synthetic gestagens [11–13]. The amplitudes of LH pulses are not decreased, probably due to the EE-induced priming of the pituitary to release LH in response to a GnRH bolus. The result of these gestagen-induced effects is a low-frequency, high-amplitude pulse pattern which resembles the pulse pattern seen in the luteal phase of the normal menstrual cycle. It is generally believed that the low frequency of LH pulses (and by inference of GnRH pulses) block the LH surge mechanism, although firm experimental data for this supposition are not available for the gestagens and the dosages at which they are used in OC formulations.

Although several authors in the past were concerned that the profound suppression of the hypothalamo-pituitary axis by oral contraceptives would increase the risk of 'post-pill amenorrhoea', normal gonadotrophin release is quickly reinstated after discontinuation of the pill. After the 7-day pill-free interval, basal and GnRH-stimulated gonadotrophin levels have returned to normal early follicular phase levels [11,14], although synthetic steroids are still measurable in serum. This is further substantiated by the observation that the first preovulatory LH surge occurs 21–28 days after discontinuation of oral contraceptives [15].

In spite of the effective suppression of gonadotrophins, ovarian activity is not completely abolished by OCs. Development of follicles in the ovary during the use of OCs containing 0.02–0.035 mg EE has been demonstrated by several authors using serial ovarian ultrasonography. In approximately 50% of cycles, follicle-like structures appear in the ovaries, and in 30% these follicles grow to a diameter of 18 mm [16–18]. Usually these follicles regress spontaneously and disappear within 14 days [18]. Consequently, this finding does not support the fear of some investigators that low-dose OCs increase the risk of ovarian cyst formation. Whether these follicle-like structures detected by ultrasound reflect true follicle growth, which would question contraceptive reliability, is unlikely, since in a majority of cases a concomitant increase in oestradiol levels does not occur, and progesterone elevation or ultrasound-proven ovulation virtually never takes place.

In addition to suppressing ovarian follicle growth, OCs exert additional effects on the reproductive tract which interfere with fertility. The continuous administration of gestagens results in a pseudo-decidualized endometrium with atrophic glands, in which successful implantation is unlikely to occur. Sperm transport is theoretically impeded by the effects of progestational compounds on the composition of cervical mucus. The contractility of the oviductal muscular layer, the beat of the cilia, and the secretory activity of the tubal mucosa are all influenced by ovarian steroids in the normal ovulatory cycle. Contraceptive steroids could therefore interfere with gamete transport through the oviduct and with fertilization.

Contraceptive reliability of OCs

The efficacy of a contraceptive method is expressed as the failure rate per 100 women-years of exposure (Pearl index). The theoretical failure rate for OCs is less than one pregnancy per 100 women-years of use (Pearl index 0.1–0.4) [19]. Modern, low-dose OCs have a similar efficacy as the older products [20]. In real life, however, failure rates as high as two pregnancies per 100 women-years are reported. Although disturbances in the resorption (vomiting and diarrhoea) or metabolism (drug interactions) of contraceptive steroids can sometimes attribute to pill failure, poor patient compliance is a major factor in limiting the effectiveness of oral contraception; in a survey performed in the UK, 25% of women admitted forgetting one or more pills per cycle on a regular basis [21]. In view of the complete recovery of the endocrine system of steroid feedback effects in the 7-day pill-free interval, omitting pills at the end or at the beginning of the pill cycle, and thereby prolonging the pill-free interval, is potentially most hazardous [22]. Studies addressing this issue directly by prolonging the pill-free interval to 9 and even 11 days, did show an increase in ovarian follicular development, but ovulations did not occur [23,24]. These observations confirm that even with the modern low-dose OCs, safety margins are reassuringly broad.

Contraceptive formulations

Oral contraceptives are generally administered in a 21-day cycle, with a 7-day pill-free interval. The sequential dose regimens, where the first seven pills of the pill pack contain oestrogens only and the subsequent 14 pills a combination of oestrogens and progestins, have largely been replaced by the combined-dose regimen. This regimen can be monophasic, with each pill containing the same amount of the oestrogenic and gestagenic component, or bi- or triphasic, where the dose of the gestagenic component is increased stepwise during the pill cycle in one or two incremental steps, often accompanied by a temporary dose increase in the oestrogenic component at approximately 'mid-cycle'. Although manufacturers of contraceptive formulations like to state that these phasic regimens more closely mimic the hormonal events in the normal cycle and are therefore more 'physiological', this claim is difficult to maintain when one realises that the simultaneous administration of synthetic steroids in pharmacological dosages for a period of 21 days is far removed from the events in the normal ovulatory cycle. The advantage of a phased-dose regimen lies in the reduction of the total amount of gestagens ingested during the 21-day pill cycle, which is accomplished in some, but not in all, bi- or triphasic formulations. This reduction in total gestagen dose may have beneficial effects on carbohydrate and lipid metabolism, although the chemical structure of the gestagenic compound used plays an important additional role.

Compared with the first OCs, marketed in the early 1960s, the dosage of the oestrogenic component has been gradually reduced, initially from 0.08–0.1 to 0.05 mg of EE, resulting in a dramatic decline in thromboembolic complications [25]. Modern OCs contain 0.02–0.035 mg of EE. This reduced amount of oestrogens is adequate to ensure contraceptive reliability, while at the same time the effect on the endometrium suffices to prevent breakthrough bleeding, although in some women this low amount of oestrogens results in the absence of withdrawal bleeding.

In contemporary OCs progestogens of the second generation (levonorgestrel) or the third generation (desogestrel, gestodene and norgestimate) are most commonly used. It is often stated that these new progestogens have a greater potency than norethisterone. However, potency is a confusing term, since the biological effect depends on the bioavailability of the compound, its pharmacokinetics and particularly the type of progesterone-receptor involved. Selectivity is probably a better designation, since the new-generation progestogens have a higher progestogenic activity relative to androgenic activity compared to the older progestogens [26]. This high selectivity has consequences for the safety profile of OCs, in particular with respect to the androgen-induced adverse effects on, for example, carbohydrate and lipid metabolism. Based on endometrial bioassays, the progestational potency of the currently employed progestogens can be arranged as follows (on a milligram-to-milligram basis): gestodene/norgestimate > desogestrel > levonorgestrel > norethisterone. With regard to other effects of these steroids, for example on the hypothalamo-pituitary axis or on metabolic parameters, the sequence is not necessarily identical.

In daily clinical practice the choice of an OC is often hampered by the bewildering variety of different formulations available from various pharmaceutical companies. Table 52.1 summarises the currently available contraceptive formulations, grouped by oestrogen dose, type of progestogen and dose regimen. Since all OCs share an equally good contraceptive efficacy, the choice for a particular preparation should be based on its safety profile and the probability of side-effects.

Risk factors

Thromboembolic disease

Shortly after the introduction of OCs in the early 1960s an association was found between OC use and deep venous thrombosis [27]. During OC ingestion there is a slight increase in thrombin formation, partially compensated for by an increase in fibrinolytic activity. This subtle alteration in the intricate balance between clotting factors, fibrinolysis and natural anticoagulants, is induced by EE (possibly modified by the gestagenic component of the OC), and is strictly dose dependent. Therefore, the reduction of the EE dosage in modern OCs (0.1 mg in the old preparations versus 0.035–0.02 mg in the newer ones) has resulted in a dramatic decline of the risk for thrombotic complications. In a large cohort study of 200 000 women enrolled in the Michigan Medicaid population the relative risk of venous thrombosis in women taking oestrogen preparations containing < 0.05 mg, 0.05 mg and > 0.05 mg was 1, 1.5 and 1.7, respectively [25]. The absolute incidence for thromboembolism can be estimated at 8.0 per 10 000 women-years in women using OCs containing 0.050 mg EE, and at 4.1 per 10 000 women-years in women using OCs with 0.030–0.035 mg EE, while the incidence in non-users is approximately 2.3 per 10 000 women-years [25,28–29].

Newer epidemiological studies have come up with a lower incidence of venous thrombosis of 1.5–2/10 000 in second generation OCs, and suggested a higher incidence of 3–4 in users of third generation OCs [60–62]. Although the authors of these studies were circumspect in their conclusions, licensing authorities in some countries (e.g. UK, Germany) immediately took action to restrict the use of third generation OCs and initiated a 'pill scare' within the general public. Potential sources of bias in the study design and confounding factors may have influenced the results (e.g. the lower incidence of thrombosis in users of second generation OCs may be due to the long duration of use, known as 'the healthy-user effect', while third generation OCs may have been selectively prescribed to women at high risk, because practitioners experience these OCs as safer). Most importantly, there is no plausible biological explanation as to why third generation OCs, even those preparations containing 0.020 mg of EE, would increase the risk of thromboembolism. Finally, the European Agency for the Evaluation of Medicinal products (CPMP) and the US Food and Drug Administration concluded that further studies have to be awaited and issued no specific advice regarding third generation OCs. These events, however, once more stress the importance of careful patient selection and identification of additional risk factors.

In addition to dose reduction, the recognition of specific risk factors, like age, smoking habits, obesity, pre-existent coagulation disorders (like the factor V Leiden mutation), have changed prescription habits and helped to decrease the incidence of thromboembolic complications in OC users. Women over the age of 35 years who smoke are at increased risk and should seek alternative methods of contraception. OCs are contraindicated in women with a history of deep venous thrombosis or thrombophlebitis. In contrast, women on anticoagulant therapy can safely use OCs; reliable contraception is important in these women, considering the potential teratogenic effects of oral anticoagulants.

Cardiovascular disease

Synthetic steroids influence the metabolism of lipoproteins, which are significantly associated with the risk of coronary heart disease. Oestrogens increase the level of high-density

Table 52.1 Composition of currently available oral contraceptives.

Preparation	Composition
SEQUENTIAL FORMULATIONS WITH 0.05mg EE	
Ovanon	EE 7 × 0.05 mg/day + lynestrenol/EE 15 × 2.5/0.05 mg/day
Fysioquens	EE 7 × 0.05 mg/day + lynestrenol/EE 15 × 1.0/0.05 mg/day
Ovidol	EE 7 × 0.05 mg/day + desogestrel/EE 15 × 0.125/0.05 mg/day
COMBINED FORMULATIONS WITH 0.05 mg EE	
Monophasic	
Ovulen 50	ethynodioldiacetate/EE 21 × 1.0/0.05 mg/day
Demulen	
Lyndiol	lynestrenol/EE 22 × 2.5/0.05 mg/day
Ovostat	lynestrol/EE 22 × 1.0/0.05 mg/day
Pregnon 28	lynestrol/EE 22 × 1.0/0.05 mg/day + 6 × placebo
Ortho-Novin 1/50	norethisterone/mestranol 21 × 1.0/0.05 mg/day
Norinyl 1 + 50	
Neogynon	levonorgestrel/EE 21 × 0.25/0.05 mg/day
Eugynon	
Stederil-d	
Ovran	
Microgynon 50	levonorgestrel/EE 21 × 0.125/0.05 mg/day
Eugynon 50	
Neo-Stederil	
Ovranette	
Biphasic	
Binordiol	levonorgestrel/EE 11 × 0.05/0.05 + 10 × 0.125/0.05 mg/day
COMBINED FORMULATIONS WITH <0.05 mg EE	
Monophasic	
Ministat	lynestrenol/EE 22 × 0.75/0.0375 mg/day
Mini Pregnon	lynestrenol/EE 22 × 0.75/0.0375 mg/day + 6 × placebo
Neocon	norethisterone/EE 21 × 1.0/0.035 mg/day
Loestrin	
Modicon	norethisterone/EE 21 × 0.5/0.035 mg/day
Ovysmen	
Diane 35	cyproteronacetate/EE 21 × 2.0/0.035 mg/day
Dianette	
Stederil 30	levonorgestrel/EE 21 × 0.15/0.03 mg/day
Ovran 30	
Microgynon 30	
Eugynon 30	
Marvelon	desogestrel/EE 21 × 1.5/0.03 mg/day
Minulet	gestodene/EE 21 × 0.075/0.03 mg/day
Femodene	
Gynera	
Cilest	norgestimate/EE 21 × 0.25/0.035 mg/day
Biphasic	
Gracial	desogestrel/EE 7 × 0.025/0.04 + 15 × 0.125/0.03 mg/day
Triphasic	
Trinordiol	levonorgestrel/EE 6 × 0.05/0.03 + 5 × 0.075/0.04 + 10 × 0.125/0.03 mg/day

(Continued)

Table 52.1 *Continued.*

Preparation	Composition
Trigynon	
Logynon	
Trinovum	norethisterone/EE 7 × 0.50/0.035 + 7 × 0.75/0.035 + 7 × 1.0/0.035 mg/day
Synphase	
Triminulet	gestodene/EE 6 × 0.05/0.03 + 5 × 0.07/0.04 + 10 × 0.1/0.03 mg/day
Triadene	
Trigynera	
Tricilest	norgestimate/EE 7 × 0.18/0.035 + 7 × 0.215/0.035 + 7 × 0.25/0.035 mg/day
COMBINED FORMULATIONS WITH <0.03 mg EE	
Mercilon	desogestrel/EE 21 × 0.15/0.02 mg/day
PROGESTOGEN-ONLY FORMULATIONS	
Exluton	lynestrenol 0.50 mg
Femulen	ethynodioldiacetate 0.5 mg
Microval	levonorgestrel 0.003 mg

EE, ethinyl oestradiol.

lipoprotein cholesterol (HDL-C) and decrease the level of low-density lipoprotein cholesterol (LDL-C), a situation resulting in a protective effect against atherosclerosis. Progestogens, through their androgenic properties, have opposite effects on these lipoproteins, thereby increasing the risk of atherosclerotic disease. The net effect of an oestrogen–progestogen combination depends predominantly on the extent to which the progestogen antagonises the beneficial oestrogen-induced changes.

With the old 19-nortestosterone derivatives, used at high dosages in the first-generation OCs, a 40% increase in cardiovascular mortality was initially reported [30]. This study, however, did not correct for known risk factors for arterial disease, like smoking, hypertension, diabetes, obesity, etc. In the Nurses Health Study, encompassing more than 1 million women-years of follow-up of OC use from 1976 to 1988, no increased risk for cardiovascular death was found [31]. Recent studies show no increased risk for myocardial infarction during or after OC use [32,33], while smoking seems the single most important risk factor in OC users [34]. In addition, no increased risk for cerebrovascular accidents can be ascribed to the use of OCs [28]. Modern low-dose OCs, containing progestogens with minimal androgenic and glucocorticoid action, cause no alteration in lipid metabolism, expressed predominantly by the absence of a decrease in HDL-C (for review see [4]) and can safely be prescribed to non-smoking women up to the age of menopause. Women with a history of myocardial infarction and those with known risk factors for cardiovascular disease should not use OCs. However, in a young patient with coronary artery disease the benefits of adequate contraception have to be balanced against the risks of pregnancy.

Hypertension

The occurrence of hypertension has been reported in 5% of women who used the older high-dose OCs. Even with modern, low-dose OCs subtle elevations in blood pressure can be observed, although they are hardly ever of clinical significance. The elevation of angiotensinogen serum levels found in OC users, together with the sodium-retaining effect of oestrogens, has been implicated as the mechanism that causes hypertension. In most women, however, a compensatory decrease in plasma renin levels prevents the occurrence of significant vasoconstriction, and hence hypertension [19]. Blood-pressure measurements should be a part of regular follow-up examinations during OC use and women who develop hypertension during OC ingestion should discontinue their use.

Pre-existing hypertension is a relative contraindication to the use of OCs. However, in patients with adequately controlled hypertension, low-dose OCs can be prescribed under close monitoring. In hypertensive patients the increased risk of thrombosis is the most important factor to consider before prescribing OCs. Again, smoking is an additional risk factor and would preclude the use of OCs in these patients.

Diabetes mellitus

During OC use, glucose tolerance is mildly impaired due to

an increase in peripheral resistance to the action of insulin which in normal women is compensated for by an increase in insulin secretion. These changes are so minimal that fasting glucose and insulin levels are normal. Furthermore, changes induced by low-dose OCs are completely reversible and never lead to overt diabetes. The changes in carbohydrate metabolism are traditionally ascribed to the progestational component of the OC, whereas a recent study implicated the oestrogenic component as the cause for the increased insulin resistance [35]. Progestogens probably play a modulating role, since levonorgestrel has a greater impact on carbohydrate metabolism than, for instance, norethisterone and desogestrel [4].

Low-dose OCs may be prescribed for overt diabetics. The influence on insulin requirement is unpredictable, but usually minimal. In diabetics over the age of 35, particularly in cigarette smokers, the risk of thrombosis is likely to be increased and alternative methods of contraception should be employed.

Breast cancer

The relationship between the use of contraceptive steroids and the risk of breast cancer has been the subject of over 30 studies since 1980. From the available data [31,36–38] it is safe to conclude that the overall risk of breast cancer in OC users is *not* increased as compared with never-users, nor does the duration of OC use seem to influence breast cancer risk. In some studies an increased risk was found in women diagnosed with breast cancer before the age of 35, and women who started OCs at a young age (<20 years) [39–41]. Relative risk estimates of 1.2 for never-users and 1.4 for long-term users seem to indicate a slightly increased risk for the development of breast cancer in this young age group. These studies regrettably are of a retrospective nature and subject to bias. Known risk factors for mammary carcinoma, like nulliparity and late age at first pregnancy, may be confounding factors in an era where women decide to postpone their first pregnancy to a later age (full maturation of breast tissue only occurs during pregnancy). A definitive answer to the question of whether juvenile breast tissue is more vulnerable to cellular transformation (induced by exogenous or endogenous steroids) can only be given when the results of prospective studies will become available. As yet, the benefits of OCs in this young age group (prevention of unwanted pregnancy and teenage abortion) seems to outweigh the currently scarce evidence for an alleged increased risk of breast cancer.

The incidence of benign breast disease, most commonly diagnosed in women between 35 and 45 years of age, is not increased in OC users. In contrast, OCs seem to exert a protective effect against the development of benign lesions of the breast [42,43]. Women who suffer from benign cysts or fibrocystic disease can safely use birth control pills.

Miscellaneous

In the past an association between prolonged OC use and an increased risk for the development of cervical neoplasia has been suggested [44]; other studies failed to corroborate these data [45]. Known risk factors for cervical cancer, such as age at first coitus, the number of sexual partners, exposure to certain types of human papillomavirus and smoking are but a few confounding factors, that make interpretation of these studies difficult. In addition, women on OCs tend to have Papsmears more regularly [46] adding to the problem of detection bias. The incidence of premalignant lesions of the cervix uteri (cervical intraepithelial neoplasia, CIN) is not increased in OC users and the continued use of OCs in women diagnosed with CIN does not influence the rate of progression [47].

Liver function is affected in many ways by contraceptive steroids. Oestrogens induce changes in the synthesis of liver-cell enzymes, binding globulins (SHBG and the carrier proteins of cortisol and thyroxine, CBG and TBG) and lipoproteins. A clinically significant effect of EE, potentiated by progestogens, is the impairment of bile transport; occasionally cholestatic jaundice and pruritus can occur during OC use. Acute and chronic cholestatic liver disease is an absolute contraindication to OCs. The incidence of gallstones or cholecystitis, however, is not increased by OCs. An extremely rare complication of OC use is the occurrence of liver adenomas. These adenomas, which are always benign, are induced by oestrogens, an effect that is dose related. With the modern low-dose OCs they are even more rare than with the older preparations. Their only clinical relevance is the chance of intraperitoneal haemorrhage.

Patients with classic migraine (of the vascular type, accompanied by neurological symptoms) often experience an increase in frequency of attacks, and are usually not good candidates for OCs. Women with non-vascular migraine or 'tension' headache can safely use OCs, sometimes resulting in relief of symptoms.

Epilepsy is no contraindication to the use of OCs. However, hepatic enzyme induction by antiepileptic drugs can decrease sex steroid concentrations and consequently affect contraceptive reliability. Women on antiepileptic drugs should use contraceptive pills containing 0.05 mg of EE.

Sickle-cell disease is often mentioned in the list of contraindications for the use of OCs. The effect of contraceptive steroids, oestrogens in particular, on the incidence of sickling, thrombosis and infarction are uncertain. The clinical course of sickle-cell disease seems not to be adversely affected by the use of OCs [48], while adequate contraception in these women is important in view of the serious risks of pregnancy to both the mother and fetus.

Beneficial effects of OCs

As was stated in the introductory section of this chapter, adverse effects and risks of OCs receive considerably more attention than the health benefits that they provide. Apart from clear contraceptive benefits, such as reducing the incidence of sequelae of induced abortion and ectopic pregnancy, a number of non-contraceptive beneficial effects of OCs are worth mentioning.

Menstrual disturbances

Typical hormone-related problems of adolescence, for example irregular and sometimes heavy menstrual periods, dysmenorrhoea and acne, are all favourably influenced by the use of OCs. Women in the fourth decade of life often suffer from conditions such as irregular bleeding, menorrhagia, dysmenorrhoea, fibroids, etc. The favourable effect of OCs on these troublesome conditions could prevent hysterectomy in a substantial number of cases. In particular, it should be stressed that the presence of uterine leiomyomas does not constitute a contraindication for prescribing low-dose OCs; menstrual disorders caused by uterine myomas often improve as a result of the pill and growth of myomas is virtually never observed during low-dose OCs. As was stated in the previous section, practitioners need not be reluctant to prescribe low-dose OCs to women over 35 years of age who do not smoke and otherwise are in good health [49].

Endocrine disorders

Polycystic ovary syndrome (PCOS) is a common cause of menstrual disturbance, characterised by oligoamenorrhoea and hirsutism. In PCOS patients not desirous of pregnancy, OCs comprise a near ideal treatment modality [50]. Hyperandrogenaemia is decreased by OCs through suppression of LH-stimulated ovarian androgen production, while the increased level of SHBG induced by low-dose OCs has a favourable effect on free testosterone levels. Reversal of the hyperandrogenic state may be important to reduce the increased risk of PCOS patients for long-term sequelae such as cardiovascular complications. The impact of the progestogen component of the OC results in regular withdrawal bleeding and protects against the development of endometrial carcinoma caused by unopposed oestrogen stimulation of the endometrium. Obviously, in these cases an OC with a favourable androgenic profile should be selected, preferably those with third-generation progestogens.

Hyperprolactinaemia, caused by a pituitary microadenoma, often results in a hypoestrogenic state, which puts the patient at risk of bone demineralisation and osteoporosis. Treatment with dopamine-agonists is highly successful but may occasionally be associated with substantial side-effects. In addition, as soon as menstrual regularity and ovulation is established during treatment, additional contraception is necessary. Although oestrogens can theoretically stimulate the growth of prolactin-secreting pituitary tumours, low-dose OCs have been shown to be safe in these women, without changing the usually low tendency of microadenomas to progress in size [50]. OCs provide a combination of adequate substitution treatment and contraception in these patients as long as they are under regular medical supervision. Women with macroadenomas need definitive treatment and should not be treated with OCs.

Patients with hypogonadotrophic amenorrhoea, often caused by hypothalamic dysfunction, are mostly in a hormonal state of severe hypo-oestrogenism and therefore at risk of osteoporosis. Although formal oestrogen-replacement therapy is a good choice in these subjects, OCs protect against the occasional unintended pregnancy when hypothalamo-pituitary function is restored spontaneously, as it often does, especially in young women with stress- or weight-related amenorrhoea. In the past, concern existed as to whether OCs might negatively influence amenorrheic conditions. The occurrence of 'post-pill amenorrhoea' was the prime reason for this concern. Since it has now been unequivocally established that there is no cause-and-effect relationship between OC use and the occurrence of amenorrhoea, these concerns are no longer valid and the term 'post-pill amenorrhoea' should no longer be used except as a descriptive category.

Gynaecological neoplasms

The progestin component of OCs offers a protection against endometrial cancer. The risk of development of endometrial cancer is reduced by 50% in OC users [45,46]. The risk of ever acquiring ovarian cancer, the most lethal of all gynaecological malignancies, is reduced in OC users by at least 40%. With longer duration (>10 years) and an early start (<25 years) of OC use, the risk for ovarian cancer is reduced by as much as 80% [46,51]. It must be kept in mind, however, that these epidemiological data largely reflect the impact of OCs containing at least 0.05 mg EE. Although theoretically low-dose OCs are expected to have the same effects, the extent to which they protect against these malignancies awaits further study [52]. In addition to these beneficial effects on the incidence of ovarian cancer, there is an important reduction in functional ovarian cysts of up to 90% [53], thereby avoiding ovarian surgery that may interfere with future fertility.

Sexually transmitted disease

The thick, viscous cervical mucus plug, which is the result of the progestational effect of combined OCs on the endocervical glands, prohibits microorganisms from ascending to the upper genital tract. As a result, the use of OCs reduces the risk of salpingitis as well as the degree of severity, with a 50% reduction in hospitalisation for pelvic inflammatory disease [54]. Whether the same protection exists for asymptomatic tubal infection with *Chlamydia trachomatis* is uncertain. Adequate protection from the human immunodeficiency virus (HIV) can only be accomplished by the additional use of condoms. In particular, adolescents and women with multiple sexual partners should be advised to use condoms in addition to OCs.

Practical aspects of oral contraceptives

Patient selection

Before prescribing OCs a thorough evaluation of contraindications must be made in every individual case. Although the majority of risks and possible adverse effects have been discussed in previous parts of this chapter, the major contraindications are repeated here for reference. The US Food and Drug Administration lists the following absolute contraindications:

1 thrombophlebitis or thromboembolic disorders;
2 a past history of deep venous thrombosis or thromboembolic disorders;
3 cerebrovascular or coronary artery disease;
4 known or suspected carcinoma of the breast;
5 known or suspected oestrogen-dependent neoplasia, especially endometrial carcinoma;
6 undiagnosed abnormal genital bleeding;
7 cholestatic jaundice of pregnancy or jaundice with prior pill use;
8 hepatic adenomas or carcinomas;
9 congenital hyperlipidaemia;
10 smokers (>15 cigarettes/day) who are over age 35;
11 known or suspected pregnancy.

In addition, there are a number of conditions which are relative contraindications for OC use and require clinical judgement in the individual case. These relative contraindications are:

1 significant hypertension (160/100 and above)—young women whose blood pressure is controlled by medication can elect to use the pill;
2 vascular migraine;
3 sickle-cell disease;
4 gallbladder disease;
5 severe impairment of liver or renal function.

Choosing the type of OC formulation

Since there are no differences in contraceptive efficacy between the older OCs and the new low-dose pills, a formulation containing 0.020–0.035 mg of EE should initially be chosen in most cases. Triphasic formulations usually have the lowest total progestogen dose and may therefore induce less metabolic effects. However, the dose schedule of triphasics is more complicated and may lead to more mistakes in pill taking [55].

Selecting the time for starting OC

Starting the OC on the first day of the menstrual period will ensure full contraceptive reliability in the first cycle and obviates the need for additional contraception. When switching OCs, for example from a 0.05 mg EE formulation to a low-dose pill, the new preparation can be started after the usual 7-day pill-free interval without compromising contraceptive efficacy.

The resumption of OCs after delivery is usually undertaken after 6 weeks. However, in women who do not breast feed, the first ovulation can occur as early as 4 weeks post-partum. Starting OCs 3 weeks post-partum is preferable. When lactation is suppressed by bromocriptine, contraception should be commenced even earlier. In women who breast feed, OCs may interfere with milk production and these women should be advised to use alternative methods of contraception. After an abortion, both spontaneous and induced, OCs can be started immediately.

Before starting an OC preparation, the possibility of an existing pregnancy should always be excluded, since inadvertent administration of contraceptive steroids in early pregnancy has been associated with congenital malformations of the VACTREL group (vertebral, anal, cardiac, tracheoesophageal, renal and limb).

Patient monitoring

A first return visit after the initiation of OC treatment is usually scheduled after 3 months. This is a good time to question the patient regarding cycle control and side-effects and to check for changes in blood pressure. Thereafter, yearly follow-up visits suffice in otherwise healthy patients. Measurement of blood pressure and a breast examination should be done on these occasions. A cervical Papsmear should be performed at the usual intervals. Routine laboratory surveillance is unnecessary and not cost-effective and should only be used when indicated in high-risk subjects.

Drug interactions with OCs

A variety of drugs have been implicated as diminishing the contraceptive efficacy of OCs. The mechanism usually is liver-enzyme induction, resulting in an increased metabolism of contraceptive steroids. In addition to contraceptive failure, lower plasma levels of EE and progestogens may increase the incidence of breakthrough bleeding. Antibiotics, for example penicillin and tetracycline, are often incriminated in cases of pill failures, but sound evidence as to their deleterious effect is lacking. Since broad-spectrum antibiotics sometimes induce gastrointestinal side-effects, vomiting and diarrhoea may cause pill failure.

Table 52.2 summarises the drugs that affect liver metabolism and are known to interfere with OC reliability. Patients who use these medications should be prescribed an OC containing at least 0.05 mg of EE or should be advised to use alternative methods of contraception [56]. Women who use antiepileptic medication can safely use a 0.05 mg EE OC. Since the pill-free interval is the most vulnerable period in the OC cycle, patients can be advised to shorten the pill-free interval to 4–5 days, or to decrease the frequency of a pill-free interval to once every 3–4 months.

Common problems with OCs

Side-effects of OCs are mostly limited to the first cycles and reflect adaptation of the body to the new hormonal environment. The occurrence of side-effects often prompts patients to discontinue the use of OCs, leading to the use of less efficient methods of contraception. Anxiety about possible harmful effects and risks associated with the use of OCs make women alert to minor complaints. Reassurance as to the transient nature of side-effects and adequate counselling with regard to the risks and benefits of OCs by an emphatic doctor can resolve these issues and enhance compliance. In general, switching to another preparation within 3 months because of side-effects is inadvisable since most problems will disappear spontaneously, and introducing a new formulation is likely to prolong the period of adaptation.

Table 52.2 Drugs reported to reduce the efficacy of oral contraceptives. From [56].

Drug	Mechanism of action	Documentation level
Hydantoins	Liver-enzyme induction	Established
Barbiturates		
Primidone		
Carbamazepine		
Rifampicin	Liver-enzyme induction	Established
Griseofulvin	Liver-enzyme induction	Suspected
Penicillins	Enterohepatic circulation	Doubtful
Tetracycline		

Breakthrough bleeding

The incidence of breakthrough bleeding and spotting is higher with modern low-oestrogen preparations in comparison to the older formulations. Breakthrough bleeding very often occurs in the first cycles and women should be encouraged to persist for at least 3 months as it usually resolves in subsequent cycles. Breakthrough bleeding occurring after many months or years of OC use is a consequence of the pseudo-decidualization and atrophy of the endometrium induced by long-term exposure to progestogens. Advising the woman to temporarily take two pills per day will not resolve the problem, since doubling the oestrogen dose will also double the progestin dose, and the dominating effect on the endometrium will still be progestational. A 7-day course of additional oestrogens, for example 0.02 mg EE or 2.5 mg of conjugated oestrogens, while continuing the OC,

Table 52.3 Oestrogen/progestogen balance of combined oral contraceptives (total dose per cycle in micrograms).

Preparation	Oestrogen	Progestogen	E/P balance
Levonorgestrel			
Neogynon	1050	5250	1:5
Stederil-d			
Microgynon 50	1050	2625	1:2.5
Binordiol	1050	1800	1:1.7
Microgynon 30	630	3150	1:5
Stederil 30			
Trigynon	680	1925	1:2.8
Trinordiol			
Desogestrel			
Mercilon	420	3150	1:7.5
Marvelon	630	3150	1:5
Gracial	730	2050	1:2.8
Ovidol	1100	1875	1:1.7
Gestodene			
Femodene	630	1575	1:2.5
Minulet			
Triadene	680	1650	1:2.4
Tri-Minulet			
Norgestimate			
Cilest	735	5250	1:7.1
Tri-Cilest	735	4550	1:6.2

will usually stop the bleeding. If breakthrough bleeding persists, a 7-day course of oestrogens in the pill-free interval may be helpful to give a proliferative impulse to the endometrium in the absence of progestogens. Switching to a low-dose formulation with a higher EE/progestogen ratio may be indicated (Table 52.3). When all these measures fail, a 0.05 mg EE-containing OC can be prescribed. Finally, it must be kept in mind that irregular bleeding during the use of OCs may have other reasons, and gynaecological evaluation should be considered.

Amenorrhoea

The low oestrogen content and the dominating progestational effect on the endometrium of modern OCs result in the absence of withdrawal bleeding in up to 5% of women. Although benign in nature, it frequently causes anxiety with regard to the possibility of pregnancy. In addition, many women experience the monthly withdrawal bleeding as a reassuring sign that 'the system will works'. Even though this is an erroneous interpretation of what is really happening, most women will not accept amenorrhoea while on the pill. Switching to a more oestrogen-dominant preparation will usually resolve the problem (Table 52.3).

Effects on bodyweight

Control of bodyweight is an important issue to many women and OC users commonly associate weight gain with the use of the pill. Fluid retention caused by the oestrogenic component of the OC and androgenic effects of the progestational compound, such as an increase in appetite, can theoretically account for a small increase in bodyweight. However, in placebo-controlled studies a statistically significant increase in bodyweight or a change in body fat distribution has never been substantiated [57,58].

Nausea and vomiting

The occurrence of nausea is related to the oestrogen content of the OC and usually is a transient feature in the woman who first starts with an OC. If the problem persists, taking the pill during a meal or at bedtime can reduce discomfort. When nausea and vomiting is the result of gastrointestinal disturbance, adequate resorption of steroids may not be guaranteed and the woman should be advised to temporarily use additional barrier contraception.

Effects on acne and hirsutism

Although the older OCs, through androgenic side-effects of the first generation progestogens, sometimes induced or aggravated these conditions, modern low-dose OCs have a beneficial effect on sebum production and hair growth. Suppression of gonadotrophin-stimulated ovarian androgen production and an increase in SHBG synthesis in the liver are the prime mechanisms by which low-dose OCs decrease the level of free androgens available to the androgen receptors.

Effects on breast symptoms

Breast tenderness, mastodynia, is related to the oestrogen content of the OC. It can be relieved by switching to a preparation that is more progestogen-dominant. In addition, avoiding methylated xanthines in the diet (coffee, tea, chocolate) may prove helpful.

Effect on libido

Loss of libido is observed infrequently and mostly affects women taking OCs with a relatively high progestogen dominance. Although many factors are to be considered as a possible cause, a more oestrogenic OC may be tried.

Missed pills

The omission of one or more pills from a pack occurs far more often than is appreciated by most practitioners. As was stated earlier, more than 25% of OC users admit to forget taking the pill regularly [21]. Advice given to women who seek medical help after omission of one or more pills should be based on a thorough understanding of the mechanisms by which OCs inhibit follicular growth and ovulation. The '7-day rule' introduced by Guillebaud [22] provides an easy guide to the appropriate action to be taken in individual cases. This 7-day principle involves the following: 7 days of continuous pill ingestion results in complete suppression of follicular growth [59]; within 7 days of the last pill ovulation will not take place; after 7 days follicular growth and ovulation may occur.

In daily practice this leads to the following advice.

1 When a pill is missed and the patient discovers the omission within 36 hours, the omitted pill should be taken and the pillstrip continued as usual. Contraceptive reliability is not impaired.

2 When a pill is missed and more than 36 hours have elapsed since the last pill, the action to be taken depends on the part of the pill cycle in which the omission occurred.

(a) First week: complete the pill cycle and use additional contraception for 7 days. When intercourse occurred within 48 hours before or after the omitted pill, morning-after contraception is to be advised.

(b) Second week: complete the pill cycle as usual. Additional contraception is unnecessary.

(c) Third week: complete the pill cycle, and continue with a new pillstrip without the usual 7-day pill-free interval.

In general, contraceptive failure is most likely to occur when pills are omitted at the end of a pill cycle or at the beginning of a new cycle, since in these cases the 7-day pill-free interval is likely to be prolonged. When withdrawal bleeding does not occur after a defective pill cycle, a urinary pregnancy test is mandatory.

An alternative to combined OCs: progestin-only preparations

A progestin-only preparation, or the 'mini-pill', contains a small dose of a potent synthetic progestogen which should be taken continuously on a daily basis. The contraceptive action of the 'mini-pill' largely depends on changes in cervical mucus composition and endometrial effects, since ovulation is inhibited in only 10% of cycles. Contraceptive efficacy is lower than with combined OCs: the Pearl index is reported to be between 2–4 with optimal use. Due to the low dose of progestogens side-effects are minimal, but unpredictable breakthrough bleeding occurs in 40% of cycles and adds significantly to patient dissatisfaction. In certain clinical situations, in general in women in whom there is a contraindication to the use of oestrogens, the progestogen-only pill may be considered as an alternative to regular combined OCs.

References

1 Forrest DJ, Fordyce RR. U.S. women's contraceptive attitudes and practice: How have they changed in the 1980's? *Fam Plann Perspect* 1988; **20**: 112.

2 Djerassi C, Miramontes L, Rosenkranz G. 17α ethinyl-19-nortestosterone. *American Chemical Society Meeting*, 1952, Abstract 18J.

3 Robinson GE. Low-dose combined oral contraceptives. *Br J Obstet Gynaecol* 1994; **101**: 1036–41.

4 Newton JR. Classification and comparison of oral contraceptives containing new generation progestogens. *Hum Reprod Update* 1995; **1**: 231–63.

5 Kuhl H. Pharmacokinetics of oestrogens and progestogens. *Maturitas* 1990; **12**: 171–97.

6 Foster DC. Low-dose monophasic and multiphasic oral contraceptives: a review of potency, efficacy, and side effects. *Sem Reprod Endocrinol* 1989; **7**: 205–12.

7 Zacur HA, Burkman RT, Kimball AW, Kwiterovich P, Bell WR. Existence of multiple peaks in plasma ethinylestradiol and norethindrone after oral administration of a contraceptive pill. *J Clin Endocrinol Metab* 1992; **75**: 1268–72.

8 Goldzieher JW. Selected aspects of the pharmacokinetics and metabolism of ethinyl estrogens and their clinical implications. *Am J Obstet Gynecol* 1990; **163**: 318–22.

9 Jung-Hoffmann C, Kuhl H. Interaction with the pharmacokinetics of ethinylestradiol and progestogens contained in oral contraceptives. *Contraception* 1989; **40**: 299–312.

10 Orme M, Back DJ, Ward S, Green S. The pharmacokinetics of ethinylestradiol in the presence and absence of gestodene and desogestrel. *Contraception* 1991; **43**: 305–16.

11 Hemrika DJ, Slaats EH, Kennedy JC, de Vries Robles-Korsen TJM, Schoemaker J. Pulsatile luteinizing hormone patterns in long-term oral contraceptive users. *J Clin Endocrinol Metab* 1993; **77**: 420–6.

12 Hemrika DJ, Slaats EH, Kennedy JC, de Vries Robles-Korsen TJM, Schoemaker J. Pulsatile luteinizing hormone secretion during the first and the fourth cycle on two different oral contraceptives containing gestodene. *Acta Endocrinol* 1993; **129**: 229–36.

13 Hemrika DJ, Slaats EH, Kennedy JC, de Vries Robles-Korsen TJM, Schoemaker J. The effects of levonorgestrel, desogestrel and gestodene on the pulsatile release of luteinizing hormone in oral contraceptive users. *Gynaecol Endocrinol* 1993; **7**: 191–200.

14 Van der Spuy ZM, Sohnius U, Pienaar CA, Schall R. Gonadotropin and estradiol secretion during the week of placebo therapy in oral contaceptive pill users. *Contraception* 1990; **42**: 597–609.

15 Klein TA, Mishell DR. Gonadotropin, prolactin and steroid hormone levels after discontinuation of oral contraceptives. *Am J Obstet Gynecol* 1977; **127**: 585–9.

16 Van der Vange N. *Seven low dose oral contraceptives and their influence on metabolic pathways and ovarian activity*. PhD thesis, University of Utrecht, The Netherlands, 1986.

17 Hamilton CJCM, Hoogland HJ. Longitudinal ultrasonographic study of the ovarian suppressive activity of a low-dose triphasic oral contraceptive during correct and incorrect pill intake. *Am J Obstet Gynecol* 1989; **161**: 1159–62.

18 Young RL, Snabes MC, Frank ML, Reilly M. A randomized, double-blind, placebo-controlled comparison of the impact of low-dose and triphasic oral contraceptives on follicular development. *Am J Obstet Gycenol* 1992; **167**: 678–682.

19 Henzl MR. Contraceptive hormones and their clinical use. In: Yen SSC, Jaffe RB, eds. *Reproductive Endocrinology*. Philadelphia: WB Saunders 1991; 807–29.

20 Speroff L, DeCherney A. Evaluation of a new generation of oral contraceptives. *Obstet Gynecol* 1993; **81**: 1034–47.

21 Finlav IG, Scott MBG. Patterns of contraceptive pill-taking in an inner city practice. *Br Med J* 1986; **293**: 601–2.

22 Guillebaud J. The forgotten pill and the paramount importance of the pill-free week. *Br J Fam Plann* 1987; **12**: 35–43.

23 Killick SR, Bancroft K, Oelbaum S, Morris J, Elstein M. Extending the duration of the pill-free interval during combined oral contraception. *Adv Contraception* 1990; **6**: 33–40.

24 Letterie GS, Cho GE. Effect of missed pills on oral contraceptive effectiveness. *Obstet Gynecol* 1992; **79**: 979–82.

25 Gerstman BB, Piper JM, Tomita DK, Ferguson WJ, Stadel BV, Lundin FE. Oral contraceptive estrogen dose and the risk of deep venous thromboembolic disease. *Am J Epidemiol* 1991; **133**: 32–7.

26 Kloosterboer HJ, Vonk-Noordegraaf CA, Turpijn EW. Selectivity in progesterone and androgen receptor binding of progestagens used in oral contraceptives. *Contraception* 1988; **38**: 325–32.

27 Royal College of General Practitioners. Oral contraception and thromboembolic disease. *J Roy Coll Gen Pract* 1967; **13**: 267–79.

28 Ramcharan S, Pellegrin FA, Ray R, Hsu JP, Vessey MP. *The Walnut Creek Contraceptive Drug Study*, Vol. III. Bethesda, MD: Center for Population Research, 1981.

29 Royal College of General Practitioners. Oral contraceptives, venous thrombosis, and varicose veins: Royal College of General Practitioners' Oral Contraception Study. *J Roy Coll Gen Pract* 1978; **28**: 393–9.

30 Beral V. Mortality among oral contraceptive users. Royal College

of General Practitioners' Oral Contraception Study. *Lancet* 1977; **ii**: 721–33.

31 Colditz GA, The Nurses Health Study Research Group. Oral contraceptive use and mortality during 12 years of follow-up: the Nurses' Health Study. *Ann Intern Med* 1994; **120**: 821–6.

32 Thorneycroft IH. Oral contraceptives and myocardial infarction. *Am J Obstet Gynecol* 1990; **163**: 1393–7.

33 Rosenberg L, Palmer JR, Lesko SM, Shapiro S. Oral contraceptive use and the risk of myocardial infarction. *Am J Epidemiol* 1990; **131**: 1009–16.

34 Thorogood M, Mann J, Murphy M, Vessey M. Is oral contraceptive use still associated with an increased risk of fatal myocardial infarction? Report of a case-control study. *Br J Obstet Gynaecol* 1991; **98**: 1245–53.

35 Godsland IF, Walton C, Felton C, Proudler A, Patel A, Wynn V. Insulin resistance, secretion, and metabolism in users of oral contraceptives. *J Clin Endocrinol Metab* 1991; **74**: 64–70.

36 Romieu I, Berling JA, Colditz G. Oral contraceptives and breast cancer. Review and meta-analysis. *Cancer* 1990; **66**: 2253–63.

37 Thomas DB. Oral contraceptives and breast cancer: review of the epidemiologic literature. *Contraception* 1991; **43**: 597–642.

38 Malone KE, Daling JR, Weiss NS. Oral contraceptives in relation to breast cancer. *Epidemiol Rev* 1993; **15**: 80–97.

39 White E, Malone KE, Weiss NS, Daling JR. Breast cancer among young US women in relation to oral contraceptive use. *J Natl Cancer Inst* 1994; **86**: 505–14.

40 Rookus MA, van Leeuwen FE. Oral contraceptives and risk of breast cancer in women aged 20–54 years. Netherlands oral contraceptives and breast cancer study. *Lancet* 1994; **344**: 844–51.

41 Collins JA. Hormonal contraception and breast cancer: accounting for age at diagnosis. *J Soc Obstet Gynecol Canada* 1995; **17**: 33–42.

42 Hislop TG, Threfall WJ. Oral contraceptives and benign breast disease. *Am J Epidemiol* 1984; **120**: 273–80.

43 Charreau I, Plu-Bureau G, Bachelot A, Contesso G, Guinebretiere JM, Le MG. Oral contraceptive use and risk of benign breast disease in a French case-control study of young women. *Eur J Cancer Prev* 1993; **2**: 147–54.

44 Vessey MP, Lawless M, McPherson K, Yeates D. Neoplasia of the cervix uteri and contraception: a possible adverse effect of the pill. *Lancet* 1983; **ii**: 930–4.

45 Thomas DB. The WHO collaborative study of neoplasia and steroid contraceptives: the influence of combined oral contraceptives on risk of neoplasms in developing and developed countries. *Contraception* 1991; **43**: 695–710.

46 The Cancer and Steroid Hormone Study of the Centers for Disease Control and the National Institute of Child Health and Human Development. Combination oral contraceptive use and the risk of endometrial cancer. *JAMA* 1987; **257**: 796–800.

47 Brinton LA. Oral contraceptives and cervical neoplasia. *Contraception* 1991; **43**: 581–95.

48 Lutcher CL, Milner PP. Contraceptive-induced vascular occlusive events in sickle cell disorders: Fact or fiction? *Clin Res* 1986; **34**: 217A.

49 Casper RF, Senoz S, Ben-Chetrit A. The use of oral contraceptives in women over 35 years. *Reprod Med Rev* 1995; **4**: 115–20.

50 Loriaux DL, Wild RA. Contraceptive choices for women with endocrine complications. *Am J Obstet Gynecol* 1993; **168**: 2021–26.

51 Whittemore AS, Harris R, Itnyre J. Characteristics relating to ovarian cancer risk: collaborative assessment of oral contraceptive use and risk of ovarian cancer. *Am J Epidemiol* 1992; **136**: 1184–203.

52 Goldzieher JW. Are low-dose oral contraceptives safer and better? *Am J Obstet Gynecol* 1994; **171**: 587–90.

53 Vessey M, Metcalfe A, Wells C, McPherson K, Westhoff C, Yeates D. Ovarian neoplasms, functional ovarian cysts and oral contraceptives. *Br Med J* 1987; **294**: 1518–20.

54 McGregor JA, Hammill HA. Contraception and sexually transmitted diseases: interactions and opportunities. *Am J Obstet Gynecol* 1993; **168**: 2033–41.

55 Ketting E. The relative reliability of oral contraceptives. Findings of an epidemiological study. *Contraception* 1988; **37**: 343–8.

56 Geurts TBP, Goorissen EM, Sitsen JMA. *Summary of Drug Interactions with Oral Contraceptives.* Carnforth, UK: The Parthenon Publishing Group, 1993.

57 Goldzieher JW, Moses LE, Averkin E. A placebo-controlled double-blind cross-over investigation of the side-effects attributed to oral contraceptives. *Fertil Steril* 1971; **22**: 609–23.

58 Litchfield RE, Grunewald KK. Oral contraceptives and fat patterning in young adult women. *Hum Biol* 1988; **60**: 793–800.

59 Smith SK, Kirkman RJE, Arce BB, McNeilly AS, Loudon NB, Baird DT. The effect of deliberate omission of Trinordiol or Microgynon on the hypothalamic-pituitary–ovarian axis. *Contraception* 1986; **34**: 513–22.

60 Spitzer WO, Lewis MA, Lothar AJ, Heinemann LA, Thorogood M, MacRae KD (on behalf of the Transnational Research Group of Oral Contraceptives and the Health of Young Women). Third generation oral contraceptives and risk of venous thromboembolic disorders: an international case-control study. *Br Med J* 1996; **312**: 83–8.

61 WHO Collaborative Study of Cardiovascular Disease and Steroid Hormone Contraception. Effect of different progestogens in low oestrogen oral contraceptives on venous thromboembolic disease. *Lancet* 1995; **346**: 1582–8.

62 Jick H, Jick SS, Gurewich V, Wald Meyers M, Vasilakis C. Risk of idiopathic cardiovascular death and nonfatal venous thromboembolism in women using oral contraceptives with different progestogen components. *Lancet* 1995; **346**: 1589–93.

CHAPTER 53

Premenstrual tension and the premenstrual syndrome

R.J. Hart and A.L. Magos

Introduction

There is little doubt that cyclical premenstrual complaints are increasingly being recognised as a source of distress, sometimes *in extremis*, of women during their reproductive years. Few women report a total absence of symptoms in the days leading up to menstruation, minor physical and psychological symptoms being the norm rather than the exception; it is when these mild symptoms become distressing, disruptive or incapacitating that the term 'premenstrual syndrome' is commonly used as a diagnostic label. This is, however, a considerable oversimplification of this complex syndrome, our current understanding being characterised by a universal lack of consensus concerning definition, diagnostic criteria, pathogenesis and treatment [1].

Terminology

Although premenstrual malaise has been recognised as a distinct entity since ancient times, it was only in 1931 that the term 'premenstrual tension' was introduced into the medical language when Frank described a group of women with typical cyclical symptoms appearing in the second half of the menstrual cycle and relieved by menstruation [2]. The terminology was later changed to 'premenstrual syndrome' by Greene and Dalton in 1953 as the multisymptom and indeed multisystem nature of the condition became appreciated; some authorities have subsequently combined the two into 'premenstrual tension syndrome' [3]. More recently, Studd (personal communication) suggested that 'ovarian cyclical syndrome' may be an even more meaningful description, highlighting two of the few absolutes known about the condition, namely the incidental role of menstruation, and the fundamental role of cyclical ovarian activity in pathogenesis. The term 'late luteal phase dysphoric disorder' has been introduced in the USA as a classification within the 3rd edition of *The Diagnostic and Statistical Manual of Mental Disorders* published by the American Psychiatric Association (DSM-III). Currently, however, premenstrual syndrome (PMS) remains the most widely accepted term used by both professionals and patients.

Symptoms

In 1969 Moos noted more than 150 symptoms that can regularly fluctuate with the menstrual cycle [4]. Clinical experience suggests that virtually *any* symptom, be it psychological, physical or behavioural, involving *any* body system can fluctuate with the ovarian cycle.

Physical symptoms

The most common and severe physical symptoms tend to be mastalgia and breast swelling, abdominal bloating and weight gain, although the latter is often more subjective than real [5]. However, it may well be that the bloatedness is due to a redistribution of fluid from the intravascular compartment to the extracellular compartment; this is supported by the observed increase in capillary filtration coefficient in the luteal phase [6] and a decrease in luteal atrial natriuretic peptide in women with premenstrual syndrome [7]. Less frequent complaints include reduced coordination, headaches and altered bowel habit.

Psychological symptoms

These symptoms generally cause the most distress for patients, particularly in the case of irritability, tension, tiredness, mood swings and depression. Altered appetite, often characterised by overeating and cravings, are other commonly reported complaints. It is interesting that most women with PMS notice a reduction in their sexual urges premenstrually, whereas one of the early reports of the condition by Israel in 1938 commented on nymphomania [8].

Behaviourial symptoms

Studies over the past 30 years have suggested that a wide range of activities can alter during the menstrual cycle, causing criminal behaviour, suicide attempts, hospital and psychiatric admissions, absenteeism from work, accidents, and affecting sleep and even cognitive performance. The situation is, however, far from clear, contradictory evidence for some of these observations having recently been presented. It is known that stress itself exerts an important influence on the menstrual cycle and may precipitate menstruation, a relationship which may thus falsely perpetuate the link between behavioural phenomena and the premenstrual phase of the cycle [9].

As an example, the relative prevalence and severity of the commoner symptoms taken from our audit of 150 women with a convincing history of PMS are shown in Figs. 53.1 and 53.2. Most women were found to have a mix of complaints, with only 10.3% being affected by purely physical and 3.5% by only psychological/behaviourial premenstrual symptoms [10]. Our analysis did not support the hypothesis that the majority of women complaining of PMS can be divided into several symptom-based subtypes.

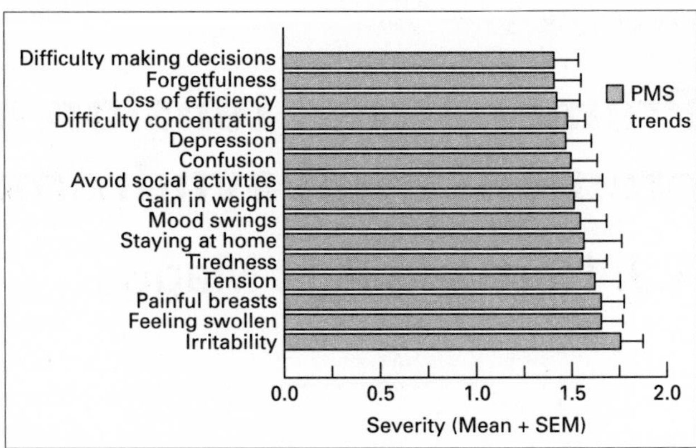

Fig. 53.2 The 15 most severe symptoms associated with premenstrual syndrome as assessed by trend analysis of daily self-ratings based on a modified menstrual distress questionnaire.

Definition

With such multiplicity of symptomatology, any definition of PMS has to rely more on the severity of symptoms and their timing rather than the symptoms themselves. In this setting, severity is of course a subjective phenomenon and one that is difficult to quantify, but the degree of disruption to everyday life can act as a useful index. As for timing, symptoms typically commence during the second half of the cycle and come to a peak on the day preceding menstruation, abating with the onset of the menses; rarely, symptoms may also be noticed at other times, often around the time of presumed ovulation. Classically, symptoms are confined to these times with complete absence of complaints during the remainder of the cycle; however, the majority of women experience an exaggeration of chronic symptomatology in the premenstruum, and there is no evidence that different aetiological mechanisms are involved in these cases.

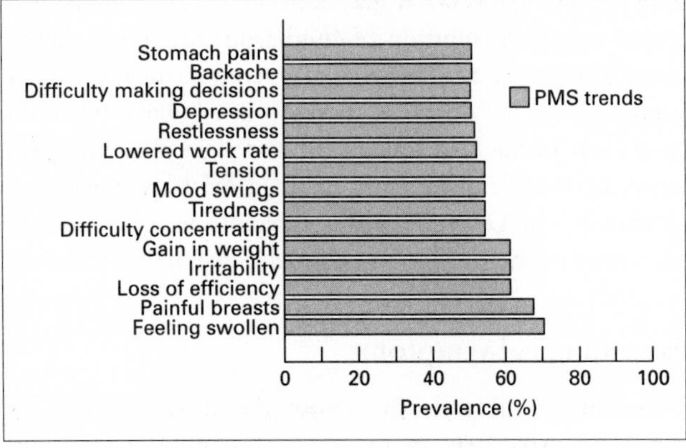

Fig. 53.1 The 15 most common symptoms associated with premenstrual syndrome as assessed by trend analysis of daily self-ratings based on a modified menstrual distress questionnaire.

As noted earlier, menstruation is not a prerequisite for the diagnosis as cyclical symptoms continue after hysterectomy, provided ovarian function continues [11]. In contrast, natural ovarian activity is essential and the adverse cyclical symptoms that can affect women taking the contraceptive pill or menopausal hormone-replacement therapy [12,13] should be considered pharmacological side-effects rather than true PMS. Similarly, it is generally agreed that symptoms secondary to organic disease such as dysmenorrhoea should not be included in the definition of the syndrome, although the two may coexist.

Based on these considerations, PMS can be defined as:

> Distressing physical, psychological and behaviourial symptoms, not caused by organic disease, which regularly recur during the same phase of the menstrual (ovarian) cycle, and which significantly regress or disappear during the remainder of the cycle.

Diagnosis

While it may seem that application of the above definition would make diagnosis an easy matter, particularly as patients often come with their own self-made diagnosis, this is unfortunately not so. Certainly, careful questioning may immediately exclude the diagnosis in favour of conditions such as dysmenorrhoea, anxiety state, chronic depression or cyclical oedema, but there is controversy as to how reliable a positive history of PMS should be considered. Evidence suggests that there can be relatively poor correlation between retrospective recall of menstrual cycle symptomatology and prospective recordings, symptoms typically being exaggerated by those who are only mildly affected by them [14,15], a phenomenon that highlights the important influences of learnt beliefs, attitudes and expectations [16]. In contrast, women with marked premenstrual symptoms appear to be more reliable historians as confirmed by prospective monitoring [17,18]. For instance, we found that over 96% of women with a convincing history of severe PMS produced daily symptom records consistent with the syndrome for at least one of the six symptom clusters studied, with almost one-third being affected premenstrually by all symtoms being monitored (Fig. 53.3).

This diagnostic uncertainty stems from the fundamental absence of a reliable biological marker for the syndrome. It is therefore generally agreed that a diagnosis of PMS can only be made with any degree of confidence by some form of objective-structured symptom assessment, particularly in doubtful cases or in women who do not appear to be severely affected. Although detailed retrospective questionnaires have been developed [19,20] and detailed guidelines have been issued in the DSM-III, daily prospective symptom recordings must be considered to be the 'gold-standard' in this field [21–23]. In recent years, computer-based mathematical models and analyses have been developed with the aim of increasing diagnostic accuracy [24–28] but their complexity means that they are only suitable for specialist clinics. As a simple alternative for general use but with good sensitivity and specificity compared with trend analysis, a form of time series analysis, we developed the 'PMT-Cator' to differentiate cyclical from non-cyclical symptoms [29] (Fig. 53.4).

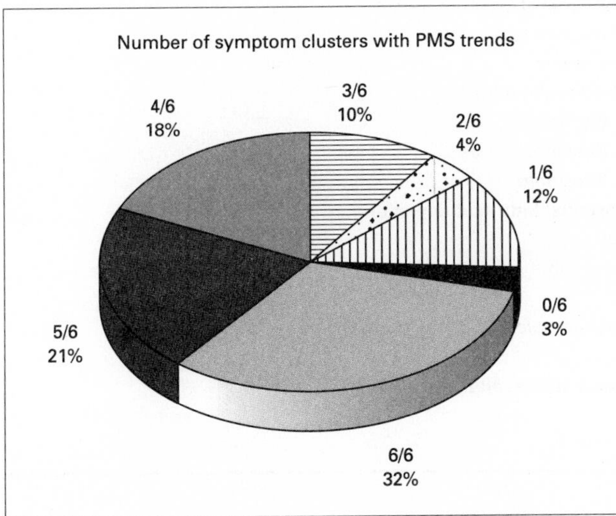

Fig. 53.3 The number of symptom clusters of a modified menstrual distress questionnaire consistent with premenstrual syndrome as assessed by trend analysis.

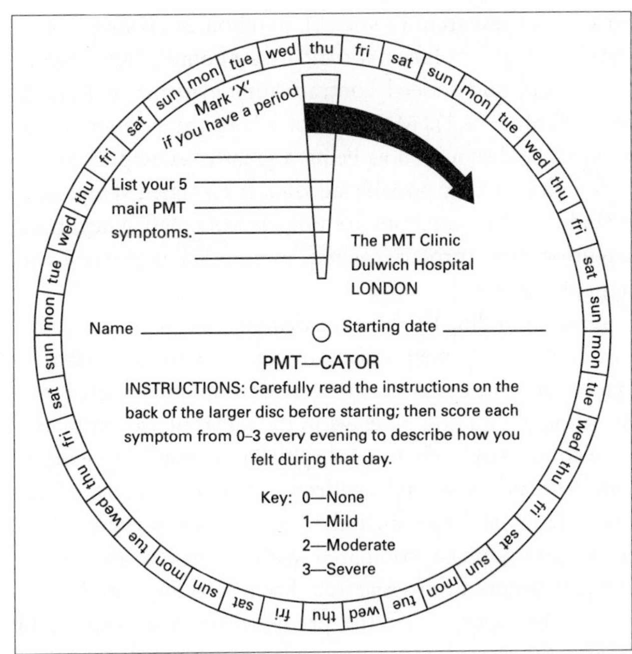

Fig. 53.4 The PMT-Cator (manufactured by Rocked of London, Watford WD2 4XX, UK).

Prevalence

Appreciating the problems with diagnosis, the need for prospective confirmation of cyclical symptomatology in all but severely affected cases, and above all differentiation of premenstrual symptoms which are distressing from those which are mild and can be considered normal, it is not surprising that estimates of the prevalence of PMS vary from 5 to 95%! It would seem that most women experience mild adverse symptoms premenstrually, often physical in nature [30], whereas psychological symptoms tend to be more sporadic [31]. Reid summarised it as follows: 10–15% of women are relatively asymptomatic, 50% have mild and 30% moderate premenstrual symptoms, and 5–10% suffer from severe premenstrual distress [32]. He further suggested that 'moderate' and 'severe' symptom categories should be considered as PMS, as these represent those women who are sufficiently troubled to seek medical help.

Pathogenesis

The precise cause of PMS remains unknown despite over

60 years of research. Biological, psychological, social, genetic and even evolutionary theories abound, but none is convincing and indeed contradictory evidence exists for many (Table 53.1). Most, if not all, of the popular theories can be discounted as being a great oversimplification, although they may possibly account for isolated symptoms; included in this category are progesterone deficiency, fluid retention, hyperprolactinaemia, pyridoxone deficiency and hypoglycaemia.

A recent finding has been the demonstration of abnormalities in serotonin metabolism in women with premenstrual syndrome, characterised by decreased uptake of serotonin by whole blood and platelets in the luteal phase compared with controls [33–35]. Cerebrospinal fluid samples of women with the premenstrual syndrome also demonstrated an abnormality of serotonin and other monoamine metabolites in the luteal phase compared with control women [36]. It has therefore been suggested that serotonin is implicated in the pathogenesis of the premenstrual syndrome, and treatment with serotonin-uptake inhibitors may be an effective way of managing the condition when tension, irritability and dysphoria are the main symptoms.

Psychosocial factors are also important in modulating the manifestations of PMS, and certainly psychological distress usually accounts for much morbidity, but there is no evidence that they are primary to the development of the syndrome. While it is entertaining to consider that post-ovulatory hostility and rejection of the male leads to increased ardour during the following fertile period, and that recurrent hostility following repeated unsuccessful conception would lead to the breakdown of infertile relationships, such theories are difficult to prove. Similarly, there is circumstantial evidence for a genetic background to PMS but this has to be untangled from learnt responses and expectations, which are so important in this area.

The conclusion from the mass of available data is that it is unlikely that a single aetiological factor can be responsible for the great diversity of symptoms associated with PMS. Much more plausible is the theory that PMS is not a homogeneous condition but one made up of interrelated symptom complexes, each with its own pathophysiology [37] a concept which is consistent with the unique nature of each woman's symptomatology. It now seems that the common denominator in pathogenesis is cyclical ovarian activity as first recognised by Studd in 1979 [38]. Whether a single factor produced by the corpus luteum and yet to be identified is involved, as suggested by Hammarback and Backstrom in 1988 [39], or whether symptoms are the end result of the influence of the many physiological changes that normally accompany cyclical ovarian activity on susceptible women, remains to be determined. It is certainly well documented that a wide range of physical, psychological and behaviourial variables normally fluctuate during the menstrual cycle, and these can exert a profound influence on disease processes such as epilepsy, arthritis, asthma, etc.

Table 53.1 Aetiological theories for the premenstrual syndrome.

Biological
Female sex hormones
Oestrogen excess
Progesterone deficiency
Oestrogen/progesterone ratio
Oestrogen/progesterone withdrawal
Glucocorticoids
Androgens
Prolactin
Fluid retention
Sex hormones
Renin–angiotensin–aldosterone axis
Prolactin
Reduced atrial naturetic protein
Vasopressin
Dietary factors
Renin–angiotensin–aldosterone axis
Prolactin
Antidiuretic hormone
Vitamin deficiency
A
B_6
Tryptophan deficiency
Elemental abnormality
Calcium deficiency
Magnesium deficiency
Zinc/manganese ratio
Reactive hypoglycaemia
Endogenous hormone allergy
Prostaglandins
Excess
Deficiency
Hypersensitivity to prolactin
Endogenous opioid peptides
Mid-luteal increase
Premenstrual withdrawal
Menstrual toxin
Melatonin
Neurotransmitters
Cholinergic
Catecholamines
Serotonin
Essential fatty acid depletion
Tea
Infection
Psychological
Social and evolutionary
Genetic

[40]. PMS would seem to be yet another condition modulated by the complex events surrounding ovulation.

Treatment

There are two fundamental considerations regarding medical treatment of PMS. First, in the absence of a well-defined single causative agent, it should not be unexpected that therapies aimed at correcting specific and theoretical abnormalities are doomed to fail, at least in a pharmacological sense. Secondly, it has become evident that women complaining of PMS demonstrate a considerable response to placebo, as much as 89% to oral medication [41] and up to 94% to surgical implants [42], which means that uncontrolled assessments of therapy, typical of the majority of early therapeutic studies, become meaningless, particularly with respect to psychological symptoms [43].

The list of suggested treatments for PMS parallels the numerous (and usually purely unfounded) theories relating to aetiology, but few have proved themselves in the setting of a placebo-controlled study for anything other than isolated symptoms (Table 53.2). Many of the traditional and popular treatments fall into this category, including progesterone and progestogens, diuretics, bromocriptine, pyridoxine (vitamin B_6) and psychotrophic drugs [44].

One therapeutic strategy which has consistently been shown by independent investigators to be effective for the management of PMS is one aimed at inhibiting cyclical ovarian activity. Such a blunderbuss approach to therapy may seem crude, but until we understand the precise sequence of events that generate premenstrual distress, it is the best we can do; suppression of *all* luteal phase changes may well involve many metabolic processes which are not relevant to the syndrome, but equally, this is the only means we have to guarantee inhibition of those which are, and hence control of symptoms. The same logic extends to the management of other cyclical disorders which are exacerbated premenstrually such as catamenial epilepsy [45], acute intermittent porphyria [46], systemic lupus erythematosus [47] and even periodic hypersomnia [48].

Suitable agents for the inhibition of ovarian activity include oestrogens, danazol and luteinising hormone-releasing hormone (LHRH) agonists. Although there is considerable incidental evidence that the combined contraceptive pill can ameliorate premenstrual distress, a proper prospective placebo-controlled study has yet to be published. In contrast, several careful studies have demonstrated the efficacy of treatment with natural oestrogen implants (Fig. 53.5) or patches combined with cyclical oral progestogen (necessary to prevent the development of endometrial hyperplasia from unopposed oestrogen therapy) [10,49], danazol [50,51], and LHRH agonists [39,52,53]. However, the use of LHRH agonists is a form of 'medical oophorectomy' and so treatment should not be continued for more than a few months due to the undesirable effects of bone demineralisation and

Table 53.2 Treatments for the premenstrual syndrome.

Pharmacological
Sex hormones
Progesterone
Progestogens
Combined oral contraceptive pill
Oestradiol implants and patches
Danazol
LHRH analogues
Androgens
Diuretics
Bromocriptine
Vitamins
B_6
A
E
Prostaglandin mediators
Prostaglandin synthetase inhibitors
γ-linolenic acid
Psychoactive drugs
Tranquillisers
Anti-depressants
Lithium
'Bellergal'
Serotonin-uptake inhibitors
Magnesium
Calcium
Tryptophan
Desensitisation
Diet
Miscellanous drugs
Atenolol
Clonidine
Doxycycline
Ca^{2+} supplement
Naltrexone
Surgical
Bilateral oophorectomy
Endometrial ablation
Psychological and social support
Miscellaneous
Physical activity
Hypnosis
Meditation
Yoga
Acupuncture
Radiation menopause
Bright lights
Reflexology

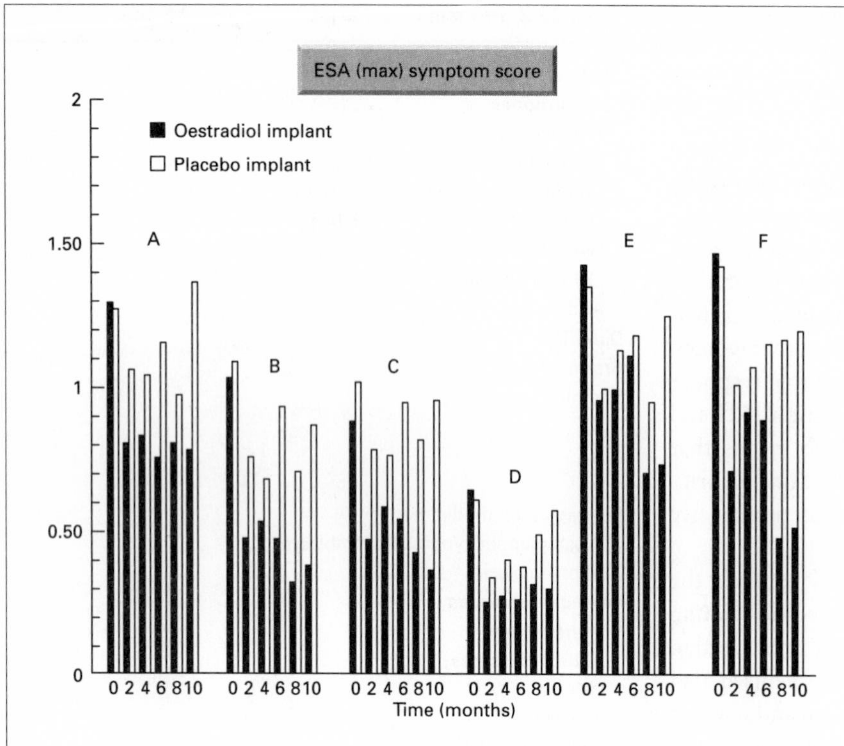

Fig. 53.5 Comparison of treatment with subcutaneous oestradiol implants combined with cyclical oral norethisterone and placebo in 68 women with premenstrual syndrome. Response assessed by trend analysis of a modified menstrual distress questionnaire, symptoms being scored on a scale of 0–3 (none–severe) and expressed as the maximum exponentially smoothed average symptom rating.

the alteration of the blood lipid profile. Therefore 'low-dose add-back therapy' with continuous oestrogen and a cyclical progestogen has been employed to reduce these undesirable effects and does not significantly reduce the beneficial effects of the analogue [54]. This therapy has been shown to have no significant effect on bone density and the blood lipid profile [55]. However, of these treatments, oestrogen/progestogen combinations appear to be best tolerated and most suitable for long-term treatment.

Currently the most successful non-hormonal treatment for the premenstrual syndrome appears to be with serotonin uptake inhibitors. D-Fenfluramine, for instance, reduced premenstrual depression scores by 60% as opposed to 30% in placebo-treated patients [56]. It was also noted to significantly suppress the premenstrual rise in kilocalorie uptake, and carbohydrate and fat intake, which are well documented forms of self-medication in patients with the PMS [57]. The most frequently used serotonin-uptake inhibitor is fluoxetine [58,59], and indeed the long-term effectiveness of fluoxetine has been demonstrated [60].

Evening primrose oil has been reported to have beneficial effects in women with the premenstrual syndrome [61], but Khoo found no difference compared with placebo [62].

There are occasional exceptions to successful treatment with agents other than those previously mentioned, but almost all represent isolated reports which have not been replicated by other workers. In this category are included an alkaloid/ergotamine/barbiturate mixture [63], desensitisation with gammaglobulin/histamine complex [64], α-tocopherol [65], the prostaglandin synthetase inhibitor mefenamic acid [66], conditioning exercise [67], the benzodiazepine derivative alprazolam [68,69], the opiate antagonist naltrexone [70], doxycycline [71], the non-sedating, non-benzodiazepine anxiolytic buspirone [72], clonidine [73], calcium supplementation [74], magnesium supplementation [75], a diet high in calcium but low in manganese [76], tryptophan supplementation [77], and the use of hand and foot reflexology [78]. Methodological and other considerations suggest the need for confirmatory data before any of these treatments can be widely recommended.

A model for PMS and plan of management

Although several theoretical models have been proposed to explain the development of PMS [79], fundamental to the development of PMS must be cyclical ovarian activity. This is generally associated with mild symptoms, but in a certain subgroup increased sensitivity to these 'normal' changes leads to an exaggerated response and distressing symptoms. Why this should be remains an unknown, but it seems likely that central pathways and psychosocial conditions are involved (Fig. 53.6).

Based on such a model, what is a logical approach to management? Initially, it is important to confirm the diagnosis, particularly in milder cases and this is best done using

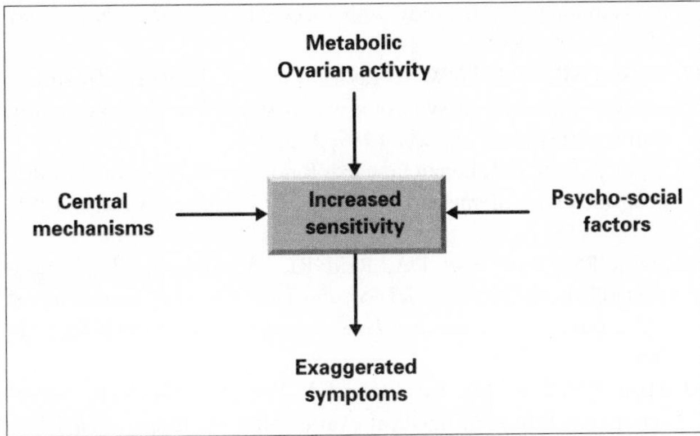

Fig. 53.6 Model for the premenstrual syndrome.

one of the prospective symptom questionnaires. Treatment should then reflect the severity of symptoms and the degree of disruption to everyday living. Women with mild symptoms may be satisfied with an explanation, coupled to reassurance, and advice concerning the avoidance of obvious aggravating factors and stresses. Moderate symptoms generally warrant medical treatment, and it would not be unreasonable to try one of the traditional if 'unproven' treatments because of their simplicity, even if nothing more than a placebo response is elicited. Rarely, women with isolated symptoms may respond to a specific therapy (e.g. premenstrual mastalgia has been shown to respond to tamoxifen [80], bromocriptine or evening primrose oil [81]). Severe cases as well as those who fail to respond to simpler measures require more definitive treatment, and here one of the anovulatory agents should be used.

Conclusions

In many ways, PMS remains as much of an enigma today as in 1931 when Frank first described the syndrome. Our knowledge is characterised by much negative information and a lot of misapprehension particularly concerning treatment. Despite this confusion, our current understanding is sufficient to be able to manage our patients with a considerable degree of success. Lest we get too despondent, it has been shown that the premenstruum can also be a time of positive feelings and creativity [82]!

References

1 Smith S, Schiff I. The premenstrual syndrome—diagnosis and management. *Fertil Steril* 1989; **52**: 527–43.

2 Frank RT. The hormonal basis of premenstrual tension. *Arch Neurol Psychiatr* 1931; **26**: 1053–7.

3 Greene R,Dalton K. The premenstrual syndrome. *Br Med J* 1953; **i**: 1007–14.

4 Moos RH. Typology of menstrual cycle symptoms. *Am J Obstet Gynecol* 1969; **103**: 390–402.

5 Faratian B, Gaspar A, O'Brien PMS, Johnson IR, Filshie GM, Prescott P. Premenstrual syndrome: weight, abdominal swelling, and perceived body image. *Am J Obstet Gynecol* 1984; **150**: 200–4.

6 Tollan A, Oian P, Fadnes HO, Maltau JM. Evidence for altered transcapillary fluid balance in women with the premenstrual syndrome. *Acta Obstet Gynecol Scand* 1993; **72**: 238–42.

7 Hussain SY, O'Brein PM, De Souza V, Okonofua F, Dandona P. Reduced atrial naturetic peptide concentrations in the premenstrual syndrome. *Br J Obstet Gynaecol* 1990; **97**: 397–401.

8 Israel SL. Premenstrual tension. *JAMA* 1938; **110**: 1721–3.

9 Parlee MB. The psychology of the menstrual cycle: biological and physiological perspectives. In: Friedman RC, ed. *Behavior and the Menstrual Cycle*. New York: Marcel Dekker, 1982: 77–99.

10 Magos AL, Brincat M, Studd JWW. Treatment of the premenstrual syndrome by subcutaneous oestradiol implants and cyclical oral norethisterone: placebo controlled study. *Br Med J* 1986; **i**: 1629–33.

11 Backstrom T, Boyle H, Baird DT. Persistence of symptoms of premenstrual tension in hysterectomized women. *Br J Obstet Gynaecol* 1981; **88**: 530–6.

12 Hammarback S, Backstrom T, Holst J, von Schoultz B, Lyrenas S. Cyclical mood changes as in the premenstrual tension syndrome during sequential estrogen–progestagen postmenopausal replacement therapy. *Acta Obstet Gynecol Scand* 1985; **64**: 393–7.

13 Magos AL. Premenstrual syndrome. *Contemp Rev Obstet Gynaecol* 1988; **1**: 80–92.

14 McCance RA, Luff MC, Widdowson EM. Physical and emotional periodicity in women. *J Hygiene* 1937; **37**: 571–611.

15 Ablanalp JM, Donnelly AF, Rose RM. Psychoendocrinology of the menstrual cycle: I. Enjoyment of daily activities and mood. *Psychosom Med* 1979; **41**: 587–604.

16 Ruble DN. Premenstrual symptoms: a reinterpretation. *Science* 1977; **197**: 291–2.

17 Haskett RF, Steiner M, Osmun JN, Carroll BJ. Severe premenstrual tension: deliniation of the syndrome. *Biol Psychiatr* 1980; **15**: 121–39.

18 Magos AL Brincat M, Studd JWW. Trend analysis of the symptoms of 150 women complaining of the premenstrual syndrome. *Am J Obstet Gynecol* 1986; **155**: 277–82.

19 Steiner M, Haskett RF, Carroll BJ. Premenstrual tension syndrome: the development of research diagnostic criteria and new rating scales. *Acta Psychiat Scand* 1980; **62**: 177–90.

20 Halbreich U, Endicott J, Schacht S, Nee J. The diversity of premenstrual changes as reflected in the Premenstrual Assessment Form. *Acta Psychiatr Scand* 1982; **65**: 46–65.

21 O'Brien PMS, Craven D, Selby C, Symonds EM. Treatment of premenstrual syndrome by spironolactone. *Br J Obstet Gynaecol* 1979; **86**: 142–7.

22 Rubinow DR, Roy-Byrne P, Hoban C, Gold PW, Post RM. Prospective assessment of menstrually related mood disorders. *Am J Psychiat* 1984; **141**: 684–6.

23 Magos AL, Studd JWW. The premenstrual syndrome—a review. In: Studd JWW, Whitehead MI, eds. *The Menopause*. Oxford: Blackwell Scientific Publications, 1988: 271–88.

24 Sampson GA, Jenner FA. Studies of daily recordings from the Moos menstrual distress questionnaire. *Br J Psychiat* 1977; **130**: 265–71.

25 Magos AL, Studd JWW. Assessment of menstrual cycle symptoms by trend analysis. *Am J Obstet Gynecol* 1986; **155**: 271–7.

26 Schnurr PP. Some correlates of prospective defined premenstrual syndrome. *Am J Psychiat* 1988; **145**: 491–4.

27 Livesey JH, Wells JE, Metcalf MG, Hudson SM, Bates RH. Assessment of the significance of premenstrual tension. I. A new model. *J Psychosom Res* 1989; **33**: 269–79.

28 Severino SK, Hurt SW, Shindledecker RD. Spectral analysis of cyclic symptoms in late luteal phase dysphoric disorder *Am J Psychiat* 1989; **146**: 1155–60.

29 Magos AL, Studd JWW. A simple method for the diagnosis of the premenstrual syndrome using a self-assessment disc. *Am J Obstet Gynecol* 1988; **158**: 1024–8.

30 Taylor JW. The timing of menstruation-related symptoms assessed by a daily symptom rating scale. *Acta Psychiat Scand* 1979; **60**: 87–105.

31 Metcalf MG, Livesey JH, Wells JE, Braiden V. Mood cyclicity in women with and without the premenstrual syndrome. *J Psychosom Res* 1989; **33**: 407–18.

32 Reid RL. Premenstrual syndrome. In: Leventhal JM, ed. *Current Problems in Obstetrics, Gynecology and Fertility*, Vol. VIII. Chicago: Year Book Medical Publishers, 1985: 1–57.

33 Taylor DL, Mathew RH, Ho BT. Serotonin levels and platelet uptake during premenstrual tension. *Neuropsychobiology* 1984; **12**: 16–18.

34 Rapkin AJ, Edelmuth E, Chong LC *et al.* Whole blood serotonin in premenstrual syndrome. *Am J Obstet Gynecol* 1987; **70**: 553–7.

35 Ashby CR, Carr LA, Cook CL, Steptoe MM, Franks DD. Alteration of platelet serotonergic mechanisms and monoamine oxidase activity on premenstrual syndrome. *Biol Psychiat* 1988; **24**: 225–33.

36 Eriksson E, Alling C, Andersch B, Andersson K, Berggen U. Cerebrospinal fluid levels of monoamine metabolites. A preliminary study of their relation to menstrual cycle phase, sex steroids and pituitary hormones in healthy women and in women with premenstrual syndrome. *Neuropsychopharmacology* 1994; **11**: 201–13.

37 Coppen A, Kessel N. Menstruation and personality. *Br J Psychiat* 1963; **109**: 711–21.

38 Studd JWW. Premenstrual tension syndrome. *Br Med J* 1979; **i**: 410.

39 Hammarback S, Backstrom T. Induced anovulation as treatment of premenstrual tension syndrome. A double-blind cross-over study with GnRH-agonist versus placebo. *Acta Obstet Gynecol Scand* 1988; **67**: 159–66.

40 Magos AL, Studd JWW. Effects of the menstrual cycle on medical disorders. *Br J Hosp Med* 1985; **33**: 68–77.

41 Mattsson B, von Schoultz B. A comparison between lithium, placebo and a diuretic in premenstrual tension. *Acta Psychiat Scand* 1974; 255 (Suppl.): 75–84.

42 Magos AL, Brewster E, Singh R, O'Dowd T, Brincat M, Studd JWW. The effects of norethisterone in postmenopausal women on oestrogen replacement therapy: a model for the premenstrual syndrome. *Br J Obstet Gynaecol* 1986; **93**: 1290–6.

43 Metcalf MG, Hudson SM. The premenstrual syndrome: selection of women for treatment trials. *J Psychosom Med* 1985; **29**: 631–8.

44 Magos AL. Advances in the treatment of the premenstrual syndrome. *Br J Obstet Gynaecol* 1990; **97**: 7–10.

45 Rossi NP, Goplerud CP. Recurrent catamenial pneumothorax. *Arch Surg* 1974; **109**: 173–6.

46 Pelroth MG, Marver HS, Tschudy DP. Oral contraceptive agents and the management of acute intermittent porphyria. *JAMA* 1965; **194**: 1037–42.

47 Morley KD, Parke A, Hughes GRV. Systemic lupus erythematosus: two patients treated with danazol. *Br Med J* 1982; **i**: 1431–2.

48 Sachs C, Persson HE, Hagenfeldt K. Menstruation-related periodic hypersomnia: a case study with successful treatment. *Neurology* 1982; **32**: 1376–9.

49 Watson NR, Studd JWW, Savvas M, Garnett T, Baber RJ. Treatment of severe premenstrual syndrome with oestradiol patches and cyclical oral norethisterone. *Lancet* 1989; **2**: 730–2.

50 Watts JF, Butt WR, Logan Edwards R, Holder G. Hormonal studies in women with premenstrual tension. *Br J Obstet Gynaecol* 1985; **92**: 247–55.

51 Hahn PM, Van Vugt DA, Reid RL. A randomized, placebo-controlled, crossover trial of danazol for the treatment of premenstrual syndrome. *Psychoneuroendocrinology* 1995; **20**: 193–209.

52 Muse KN, Cetel NS, Futterman LA, Yen SSC. The premenstrual syndrome. Effects of 'medical ovariectomy'. *N Engl J Med* 1984; **311**: 1345–9.

53 Bancroft J, Boyle H, Fraser HM. An LHRH agonist, administered by nasal spray, as a long-term treatment for premenstrual syndrome. An exploratory study. *Br J Clin Practice* 1987; **48** (Suppl.): 53–7.

54 Mortola JF, Girton L, Fischer U. Successful treatment of severe premenstrual syndrome by combined use of gonadotrophin-releasing hormone agonist and estrogen/progestin. *J Clin Endocrinol Metab* 1991; **72**: 250–1.

55 Mezrow G, Shoupe D, Spicer D, Lobo R, Leung B, Pike M. Depot leuprolide acetate with estrogen and progestin add-back for long-term treatment of premenstrual syndrome. *Fertil Steril* 1994; **62**: 932–7.

56 Brezezinski AA, Wurtman RJ, Wurtman RJ, Gleason R, Greenfield J, Nader T. D-Fenfluramine suppresses the increased calorie and carbohydrate intakes and improves the mood of women with premenstrual depression. *Obstet Gynecol* 1990; **76**: 296–301.

57 Wurtman JJ, Brezezinski AA, Wurtman RJ, Laferrere B. Effect of nutrient intake on premenstrual depression. *Am J Obstet Gynecol* 1989; **161**: 1228–34.

58 Stone AB, Pearlstein TB, Brown WA. Fluoxetine in the treatment of premenstrual syndrome. *Psychopharmacol Bull* 1990; **26**: 331–5.

59 Steiner M, Steinberg S, Steward D *et al.* Fluoxetine in the treatment of premenstrual dysphoria. *N Engl Med J* 1995; **332**: 1529–34.

60 Pearlstein TB, Stone AB. Longterm fluoxetine treatment of late luteal phase dysphoric disorder. *J Clin Psychiat* 1994; **55**: 201–13.

61 O'Brien PMS, Massil H. Premenstrual syndrome: clinical studies on essential fatty acids. In: Horrobin DF, ed. *Omega-6 Essential Fatty Acids. Pathophysiology and Notes in Clinical Medicine.* New York: Wiley–Liss, 1990: 523–45.

62 Khoo SK, Munro C, Battistatta D. Evening primrose oil and treatment of premenstrual syndrome. *Med J Aust* 1990; **153**: 189–92.

63 Robinson K, Huntington KM, Wallace MG. Treatment of the premenstrual syndrome. *Br J Obstet Gynaecol* 1977; **84**: 784–8.

64 Atton-Chamla A, Favre G, Goudard J-R *et al.* Premenstrual syndrome and atopy: a double-blind clinical evaluation of treatment with a gamma-globulin/histamine complex. *Pharmatherapeutica* 1980; **2**: 481–6.

65 London RS, Sundaram GS, Murphy L, Goldstein PJ. The effect of alpha-tocopherol on premenstrual symptomatology: a double-blind study. *J Am Coll Nutr* 1983; **2**: 115–22.

66 Mira M, McNeil D, Fraser IS, Vizzard J, Abraham S. Mefenamic acid in the treatment of premenstrual syndrome. *Obstet Gynecol* 1986; **68**: 395–8.

67 Prior JC, Vigna Y, Sciarreta D, Alojado N, Schulzer M. Conditioning exercise decreases premenstrual symptoms: a prospective, controlled 6-month trial. *Fertil Steril* 1987; **47**: 402–8.

68 Smith S, Rinehart JS, Ruddock VE, Schiff I. Treatment of premenstrual syndrome with alprazolam: results of a double-blind, placebo-controlled, randomized crossover clinical trial. *Obstet Gynecol* 1987; **70**: 37–43.

69 Freeman EW, Rickels K, Sanheimer SJ, Polansky M. A double-blind trial of oral progesterone, alprazolam and placebo in treatment of severe premenstrual syndrome. *JAMA* 1995; **274**: 51–7.

70 Chuong CJ, Coulam CB, Bergstralh EJ, O'Fallon WM, Steinmetz GI. Clinical trial of naltrexone in premenstrual syndrome. *Obstet Gynecol* 1988; **72**: 332–6.

71 Toth A, Lesser ML, Naus G, Brooks C, Adams D. Effect of doxycycline on premenstrual syndrome: a double-blind randomized clinical trial. *J Int Med Res* 1988; **16**: 270–9.

72 Rickels K, Freeman E, Sondheimer S. Buspirone in treatment of premenstrual syndrome. *Lancet* 1989; i: 777.

73 Giannini AJ, Sullivan B, Sarachene J, Loiselle RH. Clonidine in the treatment of premenstrual syndrome.: a subgroup study. *J Clin Psychiat* 1988; **49**: 62–3.

74 Thys Jacobs S, Ceccarelli S, Bierman A, Weisman H, Cohen MA, Alvir J. Calcium supplementation in premenstrual syndrome: a randomized crossover trial. *J Gen Intern Med* 1989; **4**: 183–9.

75 Facchinetti F, Borella P, Sances G, Fiorini L, Nappi RE, Genazzi AR. Oral magnesium successfully relieves premenstrual mood changes. *Obstet Gynecol* 1991; **78**: 177–81.

76 Penland JG, Johnson PE. Dietary calcium and manganese effects on menstrual cycle symptoms. *Am J Obstet Gynecol* 1993; **168**: 1417–23.

77 Sayeh R, Schiff I, Wurtman J, Spiers P, McDermott J, Wurtman R. The effect of a carbohydrate-rich beverage on mood, appetite and cognitive function in women with the premenstrual syndrome. *Obstet Gynecol* 1995; **86**: 520–8.

78 Oleson T, Flocco W. Randomized controlled study of premenstrual symptoms treated with ear, hand and foot reflexology. *Obstet Gynecol* 1993; **82**: 906–11.

79 Rubinow DR, Schmidt PJ. Models for the development and expression of symptoms in premenstrual syndrome. *Psychiatr Clin North Am* 1989; **12**: 53–68.

80 Messinis I, Lolis D. Treatment of premenstrual mastalgia with tamoxifen. *Acta Obstet Gynecol Scand* 1988; **67**: 307–9.

81 Mansel RE, Pye JK, Hughes LE. Effects of essential fatty acids on cyclical mastalgia and non cyclical breast disorders. In: Horribin DF, ed. *Omega-6 Essential Fatty Acids. Pathophysiology and Notes in Clinical Medicine*. New York: Wiley–Liss, 1990: 557–66.

82 Stewart DE. Positive changes in the premenstrual period. *Acta Psychiatr Scand* 1989; **79**: 400–5.

CHAPTER 54

Hirsutism and the polycystic ovary syndrome

T.J. McKenna

Introduction

Hirsutism can be defined as the occurrence in a woman of male-type sexual hair in the characteristic distribution for an adult man. This disorder is due in the majority of instances to a mild excess of androgens, or to the abnormal metabolism of androgens in the hair follicle giving rise to an excessive androgenic stimulus to hair growth. On relatively rare occasions a clearly defined pathological entity such as congenital adrenal hyperplasia (see Chapter 35) or an androgen-secreting adrenal or ovarian tumour is the cause of the androgen excess. However, in the majority of instances there is mild androgen excess causing hirsutism with or without disruption of regular ovulation and in the absence of virilisation.

Controversy surrounds the mechanisms involved in the development of this mild androgen excess and the sequence of events that may lead to the commonly associated disorders for which the terms idiopathic hirsutism (IH) and polycystic ovary syndrome (PCOS) will be used here. These are probably closely related clinical presentations, with PCOS representing a more severe disorder than IH.

These terms need to be clearly defined; unfortunately, there is no consensus on the definitions used so that similar terms may be used to convey slightly different concepts by different authors, rendering exact comparisons between texts difficult to achieve.

Definitions

Idiopathic hirsutism (IH). This condition is characterised by the occurrence of hirsutism in a woman who continues to menstruate and ovulate regularly. IH does not imply the absence of cystic changes within the ovaries detectable by ultrasound examination.

Polycystic ovary syndrome (PCOS). This disorder is characterised by disruption of the normal menstrual pattern, frequently associated with oligomenorrhoea in patients who may also be hirsute and/or obese. Ultrasound and laparoscopic examination usually reveal the typical appearances of cystic lesions in the ovaries. The histological picture of the ovaries is characterised by a thickened capsule, theca-cell hyperplasia and poorly developed granulosa cells with atretic follicles.

Undoubtedly these terms are not entirely satisfactory. A recent international meeting which addressed this problem failed to arrive at a generally accepted definition [1]. The most favoured terms included 'chronic hyperandrogenaemic anovulation', but this excludes the many IH patients who continue to ovulate regularly and who undoubtedly have a closely related problem. An alternative term that avoids exclusion of the IH group of patients is 'chronic essential hyperandrogenism'. However, the use of the word 'essential' might appear to exclude those with demonstrated cystic changes in the ovaries.

Incidence

The exact incidence of IH or PCOS has not been established. Various estimates have been made, varying between 1% of all women to 30% of infertile women. However, using ultrasound examination polycystic ovaries were noted in 22–23% of normal women [2,3]. Based on admittedly limited databases, the incidence of PCOS and of IH can be estimated to be approximately 2% for each condition. Approximately 10–20% of women are subfertile with ovulation failure accounting for one-third; of that group approximately 40% have PCOS [4], while in the author's experience there are approximately equal numbers of women with IH and PCOS.

Aetiology

The aetiology of IH and of PCOS is unknown. In those situations in which there is a clearly associated disorder such as congenital adrenal hyperplasia [5,6] or an androgen-secreting adrenal [7] or ovarian [8] tumour, the mechanism whereby PCOS develops has not been determined. Indeed, the precise sequence in which ovarian and hormonal abnormalities occur has not been established. These abnormalities include the classical morphological changes in the ovaries associated with increased ovarian androgen secretion, abnormal gonadotrophin secretion, obesity, insulin resistance and hyperinsulinaemia, increased adrenal sensitivity to stimulation and elevated oestrone levels: these are all the subjects of intense scrutiny, speculation and debate that have been extensively reviewed [9–12].

Approximately one-quarter of women demonstrate polycystic ovaries. However, less than 5% of women present with IH of whom approximately 90% demonstrate polycystic ovaries [13] or with PCOS. It appears that there is a familial incidence of polycystic ovaries which may be inherited as an autosomal dominant trait [14]. Therefore, approximately 75% women with polycystic ovaries do not come to clinical attention. Associated disorders such as obesity, adrenal androgen excess and insulin resistance have a more variable association with IH and PCOS. Subjects with PCOS tend to have a higher body mass index than do IH patients [15], while insulin resistance is only seen in PCOS [16]. These associations suggest that in most instances the possession of polycystic ovaries is not sufficient for the clinical expression of either IH or PCOS. However, if an individual with polycystic ovaries coincidentally has one or more of a group of disorders which predispose independently to the development of hyperandrogenism and/or menstrual disturbances, then IH or PCOS may emerge. Indeed, it is possible that in some instances the predisposing additional factor may not be abnormal *per se*, for example body mass index falling within the upper 10% for the normal population, adrenal androgen levels which are within the upper 10% of the normal population or insulin sensitivity which falls within that of the lower 10% of the normal population. When one or more of these features are coincident with polycystic ovaries the combination may be sufficient to trigger the evolution of a clinical disorder, IH or PCOS. When an unequivocal abnormality such as an elevated body mass index, raised adrenal androgen secretion or insulin resistance is present, it is easier to identify the precipitating factor. We will now examine some of those conditions which are associated with IH and PCOS and explore their possible roles in the pathogenesis and evolution of the disorders.

Ovarian and extraovarian abnormalities

The primary abnormality may be an inherited vulnerability to the development of PCOS manifest by the presence of polycystic ovaries in almost a quarter of women during the reproductive phase of their life. A hormonal marker of this may be excessive ovarian responsiveness to stimulation as indicated by an exaggerated steroidogenic response to the exhibition of a gonadotropin-releasing hormone (GnRH) agonist in PCOS subjects when compared with that occurring in normal subjects. The clearest distinction is seen when the 17-hydroxyprogesterone and androstenedione responses are examined [10]. The suggestion has been made that in PCOS the steroidogenic pathways are hyperresponsive, and that the enzymes responsible for 17-hydroxyprogesterone and androstenedione production, 17-hydroxylase and 17,20-lyase, respectively, are induced. These enzymes are controlled by a common enzyme cytochrome P-450_{c17}. However, the generalised hyperresponsiveness which also affects the adrenal may be due to an earlier defect such that cholesterol side-chain cleavage is abnormally responsive to stimulation and provides precursors for all subsequent steroidogenic pathways. These abnormalities may then lead variably to a subclinical disorder (polycystic ovaries only), or IH or PCOS depending upon the extent to which the inherited condition is expressed and the coincidental occurrence of aggravating conditions and their severity.

Primary and secondary abnormalities in gonadotrophin secretion

The ovarian abnormalities in IH/PCOS may be secondary to extraovarian disturbances including abnormal gonadotrophin secretion. An unusual feature of the anovulation associated with PCOS is the association with normal or elevated oestrogen levels. Oestrogen may arise from the ovary but may also arise from adipose tissue. Oestradiol mainly arises from the ovary directly, while oestrone is derived from the predominantly adrenal androgen androstenedione in adipose tissue. PCOS is characterised by elevated oestrone levels in blood. This may create an abnormal oestrogen environment which feeds back on gonadotrophin secretion leading to the relative excess of luteinising hormone (LH) secretion and the raised LH/FSH (follicle-stimulating hormone) ratio which is a feature of PCOS [17]. The abnormal gonadotrophin pattern may lead to failure of ovulation as the developing Graafian follicle depends upon stimulation from FSH, whose levels may be depressed. FSH stimulates the conversion of androgens to oestrogen by inducing the enzyme aromatase in granulosa cells. Androgen in the ovary arises from the outer layer of theca cells in the Graafian follicle. Androgen production is controlled by LH. Thus, in PCOS there is a shift in ovarian steroidogenesis which favours androgen production while in the periphery there is a shift in steroidogenesis which favours oestrogen production. Chronic exposure of the ovary to the resulting abnormal hormonal milieu may lead to the development of the typical picture of PCOS. However, evidence also exists that when anovulation occurs with normal or elevated oestrogen levels, LH secretion becomes abnormal with increased LH pulses; this may be due to the absence of the normal regular luteal phase surges in progesterone levels [18].

The possibility exists that a primary abnormality of neurotransmitters involved in the control of gonadotrophin secretion may lead to increases in the frequency and amplitude of LH secretory pulses. It has been suggested that dopaminergic activity, which normally has a suppressive effect on gonadotrophin secretion, may be diminished in this disorder [19]. While certainly these abnormalities in LH secretion exist, it is likely that they are secondary phenomena, since they can be reversed by intervention such as low-dose glucocorticoid treatment to suppress adrenal androgen secretion [20], weight loss [21], or by inhibition of oestrogen action by clomiphene citrate treatment [22].

Insulin and obesity

Insulin may also play an important aetiological role in the development of PCOS [9,23]. The hyperinsulinaemia which occurs in insulin-resistance states may bring about increased androgen production by direct ovarian stimulation [24]. Insulin resistance has been demonstrated in PCOS in excess of that attributable to obesity; insulin resistance is also seen in lean PCOS subjects. However, whether the hyperinsulinaemia develops as a *consequence* of androgen excess or is *responsible* for it has not been definitively established, although the latter appears more likely [25]. *In vitro* studies demonstrate that insulin may stimulate androgen secretion from the theca cells. Extreme insulin resistance has been associated with the development of PCOS associated with profound hyperandrogenaemia. The association of lesser degrees of insulin resistance with mild/moderate hyperandrogenaemia may have a qualitatively similar association. To explain the paradoxical occurrence of insulin-mediated events in an insulin-resistant state it is necessary to postulate that not all insulin receptors are affected; while those involved in glucose transfer into cells may be unresponsive to stimulation, insulin receptors mediating other responses, for example androgen production from the ovary, function normally, and are exposed to excessive stimulation due to the hyperinsulinaemia. Alternatively, the androgen-stimulating effect of insulin may be mediated through insulin-like growth factor (IGF) receptors which have significant affinity for insulin. It is pertinent to recall that the most frequently encountered insulin-resistant state is obesity. Therefore, the obese subject is in double jeopardy; in addition to generating excess oestrogen and thereby perturbing gonadotrophin secretion causing ovarian androgen overproduction, hyperinsulinaemia may directly stimulate ovarian androgen biosynthesis. If insulin resistance exists in association with polycystic ovaries, PCOS may develop.

Adrenal androgen excess

The possibility that adrenal androgen excess may be pathogenetically associated with the development of PCOS is suggested by the following observations:

1 Unequivocal disorders of adrenal androgen excess are associated with the development of PCOS, for example congenital adrenal hyperplasia [6], and androgen-secreting adrenal tumours [7] are also associated with the secondary development of PCOS.

2 The uniquely adrenal androgen dehydroepiandrosterone sulphate (DHEAS) is found to be elevated in approximately 30% of patients with PCOS [26,27].

3 Suppression of adrenal activity with near-physiological doses of glucocorticoid is associated with correction of the hormonal and clinical features of PCOS in some subjects [19].

4 Excessive adrenal androgen and glucocorticoid responsiveness to stimulation with exogenous or endogenous adrenocorticotrophic hormone (ACTH) is characteristic of PCOS [19].

The underlying adrenal disorder in PCOS has not been definitively established, but a number of different mechanisms have been proposed [28]. Mild adrenal enzymatic defects associated with impaired cortisol secretion which is compensated for by raised ACTH levels result in elevated androgen production, and this may be associated with the development of PCOS [5]. Congenital adrenal hyperplasia appears to have a high incidence rate in some races, for example Ashkenazi Jews, Hispanics, Italians and Inuits (Eskimos), while the disorder is relatively rare in the Anglo-Saxon population [29]. In contrast, many patients with PCOS demonstrate excessive cortisol responsiveness to stimulation with ACTH, although elevated levels of precursors such as 17-hydroxyprogesterone, 17-hydroxypregnenolone and androstenedione indicate a generalised adrenal androgen responsiveness rather than accumulation of a product proximal to impaired enzymatic activity. The possibility that a stimulator of adrenal androgen production other than ACTH exists has much to support it but has not been proven [30]; non-ACTH pro-opiomelanocortin (POMC) fragments such as 'joining peptide' and β-endorphin have been implicated [28,30,31]. If such a factor does exist, it is possible that a mild excess could lead to elevated adrenal androgen production and, either directly or following conversion to oestrogen, this could result in disruption of normal function of the hypothalamo-pituitary–ovarian axis to bring about the development of PCOS.

Another recently suggested mechanism whereby adrenal androgen excess may occur includes over activity of enzymes responsible for the metabolism and clearance of cortisol including 5α-reductase and 11β-hydroxysteroid dehydrogenase [32,33]. As a consequence of excessively rapid clearance of cortisol there is a tendency for cortisol levels to fall; a compensatory increase in ACTH secretion occurs in order to maintain normal blood levels of cortisol. While the compensatory increase in ACTH brings cortisol levels back to normal, androgen levels become elevated. It is also theoretically possible that increased adrenal androgen secretion may occur as a consequence of the effect of ovarian androgen excess. While evidence exists to suggest that male androgen levels may be associated with greater adrenal androgen production than normal female androgen levels [34], the relatively mild androgen excess seen in IH/PCOS is unlikely to influence adrenal androgen production [35].

Cigarette smoking has been reported to stimulate adrenal androgen production in normal premenopausal and postmenopausal women. In a group of hirsute patients, smokers were found to have higher androgen levels than non-smokers [15]. However, the occurrence of IH and PCOS was similar in the cigarette smokers and non-smokers. While no report exists on the frequency of the development of hirsutism amongst smokers and non-smokers, it is certainly likely that cigarette smoking may convert mild to more severe androgen excess and may thereby facilitate crossing the threshold leading to clinically significant androgen excess and PCOS.

Prolactin

Prolactin levels have been found to be elevated in approximately 25% of patients with PCOS, but the role of prolactin in the disorder is unknown [36]. A generalised decrease in dopaminergic tone in the hypothalamus may be responsible not only for the increased LH release but also for increased prolactin secretion in PCOS [37]. Since oestrogen stimulates prolactin secretion it is possible that hyperoestronaemia may provoke hyperprolactinaemia in PCOS. However, some investigators have suggested that prolactin may play a primary role in PCOS, i.e. it may directly stimulate adrenal androgen excess. While elevated DHEAS levels are frequently seen in hyperprolactinaemic patients, a clinically significant role for prolactin in the stimulation of adrenal androgens has never been convincingly demonstrated [38].

Although some patients with hyperprolactinaemia associated with PCOS respond to treatment with the prolactin-lowering agent bromocriptine [39], it is unlikely that hyperprolactinaemia plays an important role in the development of PCOS.

Summary

IH and PCOS probably belong to a spectrum extending from totally normal subjects to subjects with no clinical expression of PCOS but who will be seen on ultrasound examination to harbour polycystic ovaries, through to subjects who present with hirsutism while continuing to ovulate regularly although the ovaries will demonstrate polycystic changes, to subjects with anovulation, hirsutism and polycystic ovaries.

Whether or not PCOS can develop in anyone affected by a predisposing disorder, or only in those who have a genetic susceptibility, is not known. Table 54.1 lists disorders associated with the development of PCOS. Figure 54.1 provides a model where cystic ovaries are necessary but not sufficient for the development of PCOS. The emergence of PCOS may depend upon the coexistence of polycystic ovaries with other clinical features which facilitate the full evolution of the disorder, for example insulin resistance and/or obesity and/or adrenal androgen excess, etc.

The model is qualitative and not quantitative. Figure 54.2 suggests a sequence with several potential starting points whereby the abnormalities characteristic of PCOS may be interrelated. The development of the hormonal abnormalities in PCOS may be at least in part secondary to anovulation

Table 54.1 Disorders associated with the development of idiopathic hirsutism and polycystic ovary syndrome.

- Congenital polycystic ovaries
- Ovarian androgen excess
  - Ovarian overresponsiveness (induced 17-P450/SCC-P45 enzymes)
  - Ovarian tumour
- Adrenal androgen excess
  - Idiopathic—possibly due to mild excess of specific cortical androgen stimulating hormone
  - Congenital adrenal hyperplasia
  - Accelerated cortisol metabolism
  - Generalised adrenal hyperresponsiveness (induced 17-P450/SCC-P45 enzymes)
  - Adrenal tumour
- Hyperinsulinaemia and insulin resistance
- Obesity
- Raised luteinising hormone/follicle-stimulating hormone ratio
  - Reduced central dopamine tone
  - Oestrogen excess (obesity, ovarian/adrenal tumour)
- Cigarette smoking
- Hyperprolactinaemia

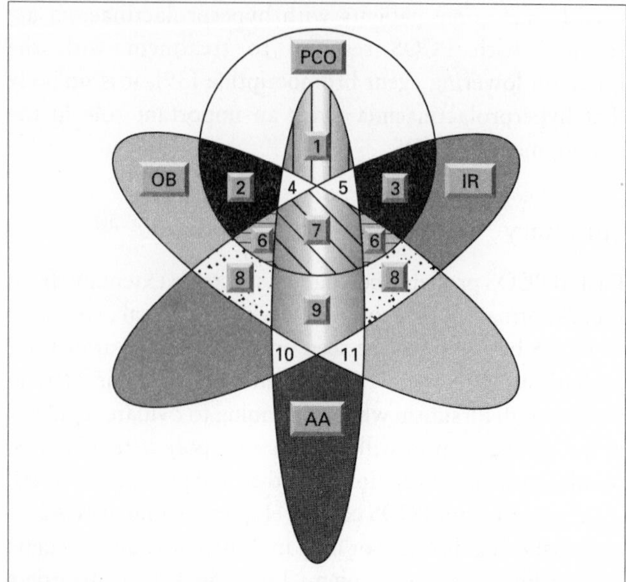

Fig. 54.1 This is a schematic representation of the coincidence of abnormalities occurring within the general population. The circle represents approximately 25% of young women who demonstrate polycystic ovaries (PCO). Some of these will also be found to be obese (OB), and/or to have insulin resistance (IR) and/or to have elevated adrenal androgen levels (AA). The postulate is that where insulin resistance, obesity or elevated adrenal androgen levels exist there is an increased likelihood of those women with PCO evolving to demonstrate polycystic ovary *syndrome* (PCOS). The numbers indicate the variable combinations which may occur. Thus, 1,2 and 3 indicate the coincidence of PCO and adrenal androgen excess, obesity and insulin resistance, respectively. Subsets 6 and 7 indicate the coincidence of obesity and insulin resistance and obesity, insulin resistance and adrenal androgen excess respectively. These are the subgroups which may be most at risk of developing diabetes mellitus. Of course obesity, insulin resistance and adrenal androgen excess may also occur in individuals who do not have polycystic ovaries and are represented in the sections 8, 9, 10 and 11.

rather than being causal. Thus, the absence of cyclical luteal phase surges of progesterone associated with normal or elevated oestrogen levels, irrespective of the cause, may bring about abnormal gonadotrophin secretion from the pituitary gland characterised by an increase in the LH/FSH ratio [18]. In this model the problem of ovulation is compounded, and ovarian androgen secretion is enhanced leading to the full-blown clinical expression of PCOS.

Ovarian morphology

Typically, the polycystic ovaries are enlarged and irregular with cysts obvious on cross-section. However, PCOS may be present in patients with ovaries of normal size; multiple small cysts are usually apparent on section of the ovaries. The cysts tend to be distributed subcapsularly, and there is an apparent increase in stroma [39,40]. However, corpus luteum formation is rare and there is a decreased number of corpora albicans, testimony of decreased frequency of previous ovulation. Graaffian follicle development is diminished but some atretic follicles are apparent. Theca-cell hyperplasia is evident and the capsule of the ovaries is thickened. These morphological findings are consistent with the most obvious clinical features of the syndrome: ovulation disturbance, hyperandrogenaemia (derived from theca cells) and enlarged cystic ovaries frequently identified on ultrasonographic examination.

Presentation

Patients with IH present because of hirsuties, while patients with PCOS frequently also present because of a gradual worsening of hirsutism and/or decreasing frequency and increasing irregularity of menstrual bleeding (11,40–42). Typically, these features have been developing gradually for more than a year prior to the point at which medical advice is sought. This usually reflects the relative mildness of the features and their slow progression. The onset of these features almost always occurs in the decade between 15 and 25 years. The advent of these symptoms outside these age limits prompts diligent evaluation for other disorders, for example congenital adrenal hyperplasia, Cushing's syndrome or androgen-secreting adrenal or ovarian tumours [43]. Differential clinical features are summarised in Table 54.2.

Hirsutism is present in 60–70% of patients with PCOS. It usually affects the face with the greatest severity. The upper lip, side-burn regions, the skin immediately lateral to the mid-point of the chin and overlying the more anterior aspect of the mandible, and the neck are the usual sites affected. However, the face may be relatively unaffected while the trunk and limbs demonstrate moderate to severe hirsutism. The principal non-facial areas affected include the periareolar regions, the central chest, the lower abdominal wall (taking on the typical male, inverted V-shaped hair pattern running from the pubic hair up to the umbilicus) and on the upper inner aspects of the thighs. In patients with severe hirsutism the upper arms and lower portions of the back may also be affected. Hirsutism is accompanied by acne affecting the face and skin over the upper thorax, particularly on the dorsal surface in approximately 25% of patients [11,42]. However, significant hyperandrogenaemia may exist without the development of hirsutism [44]. This probably reflects the lower end of the normal distribution of hair-follicle sensitivity to stimulation by androgens. Indeed, the same phenomenon is seen within individuals who may have severe hirsutism affecting one part of their body while other areas, which typically contain androgen-responsive hair follicles, are unaffected. Table 54.3 and Fig. 54.3 outline a scoring method

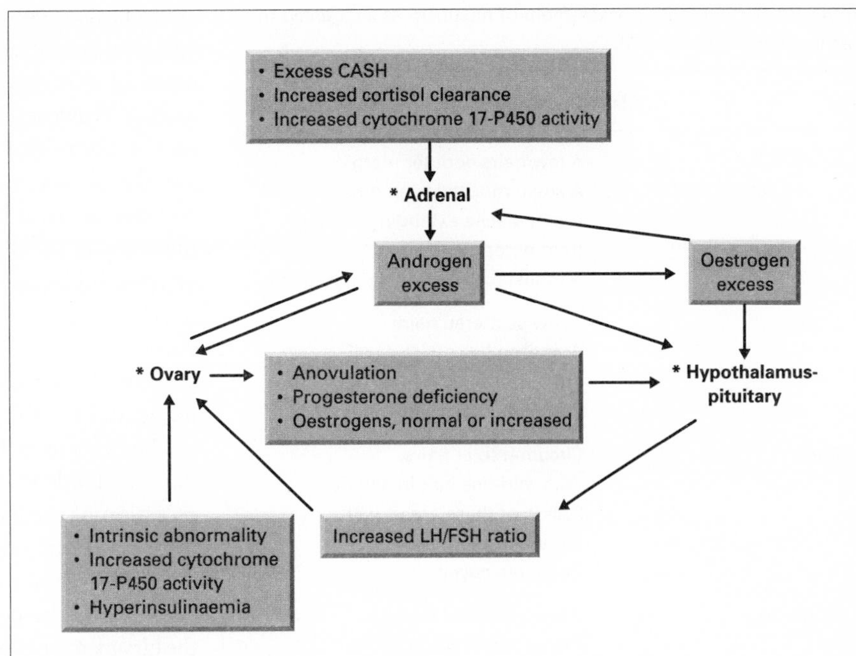

Fig. 54.2 Schematic representation of interrelating hormonal abnormalities identified in polycystic ovary syndrome. The asterisks indicate sites where the initiating abnormality may arise. The figure assumes that some and not all abnormalities depicted will be operative in an individual patient. The arrows indicate the source from which a hormonal abnormality arises and the direction of the impact of that abnormality. CASH, cortical androgen-stimulating hormone. From [108], with permission.

Table 54.2 Presenting clinical features of polycystic ovary syndrome in patients with hirsutism of various aetiologies.

Diagnosis	Time of onset	Time of onset to medical presentation	Hirsutism	Menstrual disturbances	Virilisation	Comment
Idiopathic hirsutism	15–25 years	Years	+	–	–	Acne may be present
Polycystic ovary	15–25 years	Years	+	+	Rare	Obesity 40%; enlarged ovaries may be palpable
Congenital adrenal hyperplasia	Congenital	May be present at birth, in adolescence or in adulthood	+	+	+	Small stature, evidence of intrauterine androgen excess, e.g. labial fusion; usually primary amenorrhoea
Cushing's syndrome	Any time	Months–years	+	+	Unusual	Coexisting evidence of glucocorticoid excess
Androgen-secreting tumour	Any time	Weeks–months	+	+	+	Palpable mass may be present
Hyperthecosis ovarii	Any time outside childhood	Months–years	+	+	+	Ovaries may appear to be normal

described by Ferriman and Gallwey which is useful in providing an objective and quantitative assessment of hirsutism [45]. This is more useful in assessing response to treatment than in establishing the diagnosis of hirsutism. However, a cut-off score of 7 can be accepted as an arbitrary distinction between patients with significant hirsutism and those who probably demonstrate an extreme of the normal hair growth in women. It is useful to assess the Ferriman and Gallwey score at the first opportunity, and to reassess it on a 6-monthly basis during treatment.

As a result of the ovulatory disturbance, infertility is a frequent symptom which prompts the patient with PCOS to seek medical advice. While the usual symptom in PCOS is infrequent and irregular menstrual bleeding, some patients demonstrate prolonged frequent but anovulatory bleeding. Anovulatory bleeding is usually not associated with

Table 54.3 Quantitative assessment of hirsutism as suggested by Ferriman and Gallwey [45].

Site	Grade	Definition
1 Upper lip	1	A few hairs at outer margin
	2	A small moustache at outer margin
	3	A moustache extending halfway from outer margin
	4	A moustache extending to midline
2 Chin	1	A few scattered hairs
	2	Scattered hairs with small concentrations
	3 and 4	Complete cover, light and heavy
3 Chest	1	Circumareolar hairs
	2	With mid-line hair in addition
	3	Fusion of these areas, with three-quarter cover
	4	Complete cover
4 Upper back	1	A few scattered hairs
	2	Rather more, still scattered
	3 and 4	Complete cover, light and heavy
5 Lower back	1	A sacral tuft of hair
	2	With some lateral extension
	3	Three-quarter cover
	4	Complete cover
6 Upper abdomen	1	A few mid-line hairs
	2	Rather more, still midline
	3 and 4	Half and full cover
7 Lower abdomen	1	A few midline hairs
	2	A midline streak of hair
	3	A midline band of hair
	4	An inverted V-shaped growth
8 Upper arm	1	Sparse growth affecting not more than a quarter of the limb surface
	2	More than this: cover still incomplete
	3 and 4	Complete cover, light and heavy
9 Thigh	1,2,3,4	As for arm

Grade 0, absence of coarse hair growth. Total scores above 5 are seen in 9.9% of the general population while scores above 7 are found in 4.3% of women [45].

dysmenorrhoea or a sensation of fullness or tenderness of the breasts, and usually lasts for less than 3 days during which only spotting may occur. While many women with PCOS never establish regular menstrual cycles, some may have a normal ovulatory pattern prior to the emergence of the disturbance. Some subjects, particularly those who are obese, may have an early menarche. Obesity is seen in approximately 40% of PCOS patients. This may be present from early childhood, or may develop immediately before the onset of the other clinical abnormalities. Some obese subjects also demonstrate acanthosis nigricans. This dermatological condition is characterised by raised, dark, velvety areas of skin frequently occurring on the neck or in the axillae. However, acanthosis nigricans can occur anywhere on the body. The areas involved are discrete and may be variable in size, i.e. from approximately 1 cm in diameter to large areas in excess of 10 cm in diameter. Acanthosis nigricans is usually associated with insulin resistance, and affected subjects frequently have diabetes mellitus [46]. The development of diabetes mellitus, hyperlipidaemia and coronary artery disease are all more common in PCOS than in unaffected women, even in the absence of acanthosis nigricans [47–49].

The occurrence of virilisation in association with PCOS is unusual. Evidence of virilisation includes scalp-hair thinning, recession of the hairline in the temporal regions giving rise to a male-type hair line, enlargement of the larynx with deepening of the voice, increase in muscle mass in an android pattern and the development of clitoral enlargement. Like the hirsutism or oligomenorrhoea occurring outside the decade of 15–25 years, the presence of virilisation should also prompt extensive evaluation for the possibility of other underlying disorders (Table 54.2).

Differential diagnosis

Abundant normal hair

Some ethnic groups have more body hair growth, particularly facial, than others. This may be a cause of cosmetic embarrassment but is not a medical disorder. Subjects descended from Mediterranean races frequently have conspicuous fine dark hair on the upper lip and on the sideburn region extending down on to the neck. This fine hair lies along the skin and, unlike androgen-dependent hair, it does not grow away from the skin, become coarse or curl. Androgen abnormalities are not found in association with this type of hair growth pattern which will not respond to systemic treatment, for example antiandrogens. Normal women presenting with hair of this type should be reassured that they do not have a hormonal disorder and advised to utilise any local cosmetic forms of treatment that prove successful for them.

Congenital adrenal hyperplasia (Tables 54.2 and 54.4, see also Chapter 35)

In the classical or severe type of congenital adrenal hyperplasia, usually 21-hydroxylase deficiency or the 3β-ol-dehydrogenase $\Delta_{4,5}$-isomerase deficiency, the disorder usually presents at birth or early childhood and is associated with adrenal failure and virilisation [50]. However, non-classical or mild

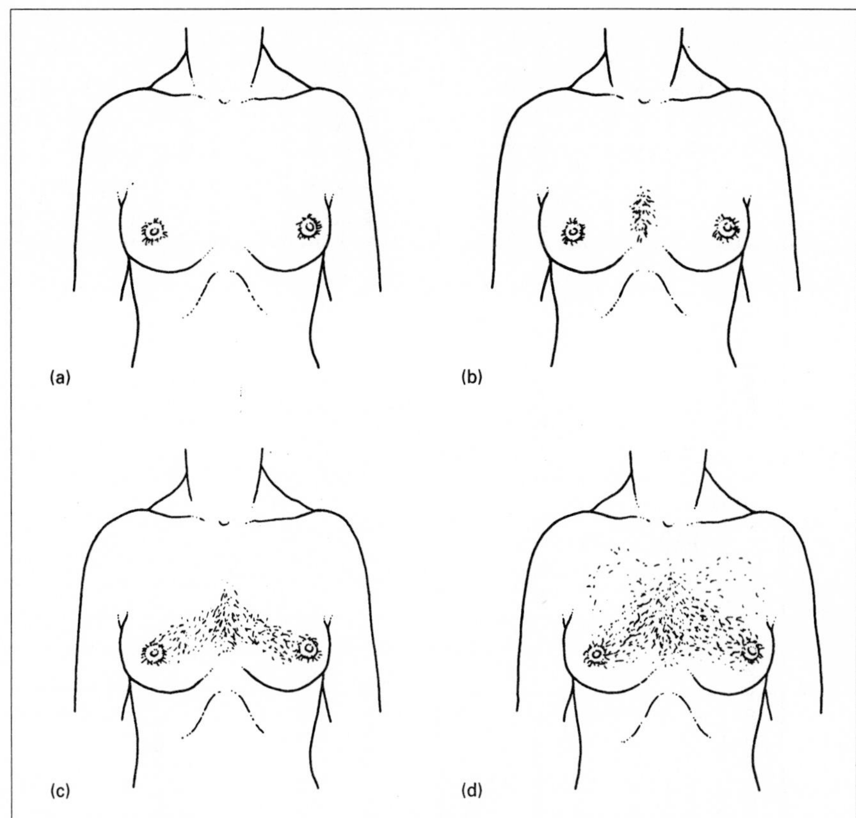

Fig. 54.3 Diagrammatic representation of Ferriman and Gallwey scoring system for hirsutism affecting the chest ranging from mild, (a), to severe, (d). From [45].

forms of the disorder have been reported to present in the second or third decades of life because of hirsutism, and/or acne, and/or oligomenorrhoea [5]. This disorder is usually seen in Hispanics, Ashkenazi Jews and Inuits (Eskimos). It is relatively rare in white Anglo-Saxons. Because a diurnal rhythm persists in patients with congenital adrenal hyperplasia, unremarkable plasma levels of 17-hydroxyprogesterone, 17-hydroxypregnenolone, DHEA, androstenedione and testosterone levels may be found in the afternoon. However, if basal blood sampling is performed in the morning, i.e. before 10.00 hours, markedly elevated plasma concentrations of these steroids will be noted if a clinically significant enzyme defect is present. The possibility of congenital adrenal hyperplasia is also suggested because of race, a strong familial incidence of the symptoms, the precocious development of pubic hair, an unusual somatic growth pattern characterised by rapid early linear growth and general development but short adult height, and the occasional occurrence of virilisation including partial labial fusion, an index of intrauterine androgen excess.

Under these circumstances, and in the absence of diagnostic information available from basal steroid levels, an ACTH test may be indicated. Dr. Maria New and her colleagues have described a nomogram which categorises 17-hydroxyprogesterone responses 10, 30 or 60 min after intravenous injection of $\alpha_{1\text{-}24}$-ACTH, 250 μg, in relationship to the basal 17-hydroxyprogesterone level [5,50]. Using the nomogram, the intersection for these two values will identify classical and non-classical forms of 21-hydroxylase deficiency in addition to values typical of the general population, and therefore of individuals who may be heterogeneous for the disorder. However, clinically significant congenital adrenal hyperplasia requires homogeneous occurrence of the autosomal recessive genetic abnormality, or the coincidence of the genetic abnormality for the mild and severe forms of the disorder (see Chapter 35).

Administration of dexamethasone leads to prompt suppression of all steroids, and is helpful in distinguishing congenital adrenal hyperplasia from androgen-secreting tumours (Table 54.4).

Androgen-secreting tumours (Tables 54.2 and 54.4)

Androgen-secreting tumours may occur at any age, and demonstrate rapid progression of symptoms and signs including hirsutism, acne, scalp-hair thinning, oligomenorrhoea, clitoromegaly, breast atrophy and other signs of virilisation which usually come to medical presentation within months of their first appearance [43,51]. Androgen levels and androgen and glucocorticoid precursor values tend to be markedly elevated, for example androstenedione, testosterone, 11-deoxycortisol and, in the case of adrenal tumours,

Table 54.4 Hormonal features in patients presenting with hirsutism of various aetiologies.

Diagnosis	Plasma testosterone and/or androstenedione	Plasma 17α-hydroxyprogesterone	Cortisol following dexamethasone administration	Luteinising hormone	Follicle-stimulating hormone	Miscellaneous
Idiopathic hirsutism	↑ in about 50%	N	Suppressed	N	N	Ultrasonography may show enlarged ovaries with cysts
Polycystic ovary syndrome	↑ in about 75% of patients	N/↑	Suppressed	N	N	Ultrasonography may show enlarged ovaries with cysts
Congenital adrenal hyperplasia ‡	↑↑*	↑↑*	Suppressed	N/↑	N/↓	
Cushing's syndrome	↑	N/↑†	Not suppressed	N/↑	N/↓	May have evidence of pituitary or adrenal tumour: measure adrenocorticotrophic hormone
Androgen-secreting tumours						Adrenal and ovarian ultrasonography, computed tomography, arteriography, selective venous sampling, adrenal radiocholesterol scanning: will all yield localising information
Adrenal	↑↑	N/↑†	Variable	↓	↓	
Ovarian	↑↑	N/↑	Suppressed	↓	↓	
Hyperthecosis ovarii	↑↑	↑↑	Suppressed	N	N	Ovaries enlarged or normal on ultrasound examination; cysts not seen typically

↑, Elevated; ↓, suppressed.

* Suppresses on treatment with replacement doses of glucocorticoids taken at night.

† Progesterone and other precursors, e.g. 11-deoxycortisol, 17-OH-pregnenolone, may be elevated in patients with an adrenal adenocarcinoma.

‡ Congenital adrenal hyperplasia represented here is of the 21-hydroxylase deficiency type—see relevant chapter for characteristics of 11-hydroxylase and 3β-ol-dehydrogenase, $\Delta_{4,5}$ isomerase deficiencies.

DHEAS, although the absence of elevated DHEAS does not exclude the adrenals as the site of the tumour [52]. In the majority of patients there may also be evidence of cortisol excess with features of Cushing's syndrome including a rounded plethoric face, hypertension and glucose intolerance, but the anabolic effect of androgens may protect against the occurrence of the usual catabolic features of cortisol excess, for example easy bruising, striae formation, myopathy and osteoporosis.

Androgen, cortisol and precursor levels do not respond to the normal suppressive effects of dexamethasone. Adrenal tumours are usually detectable on computed tomography examination [53]. Ultrasound examination of the ovaries will frequently also detect the presence of an androgen-secreting tumour [54]. However, ovarian tumours may be undetectable by all imaging procedures. If the clinical presentation is suggestive of an androgen-secreting tumour when imaging procedures have not identified its location, i.e. adrenal or ovary, there is a good case to proceed to an exploratory laparotomy where it may be necessary to section the ovaries before the presence of a small tumour can be identified. Venous sampling from adrenal and ovarian veins with a view to detecting the venous drainage area in which the tumour exists may be undertaken preoperatively. However, the procedure is technically demanding; sometimes it is not possible to catheterise the four veins sought and it is almost certain that a laparotomy will eventually be required. Nevertheless, in experienced hands venous sampling studies may supply some helpful preoperative information [55].

Cushing's syndrome (Tables 54.2 and 54.4)

While hirsutism and oligomenorrhoea occur in women of reproductive age affected by the disorder, presentation of Cushing's syndrome is usually dominated by features of glucocorticoid excess (see Chapter 33). The syndrome may present at any age, and may include the rapid progress of symptoms such that they come to medical attention 6–12 months after their initial appearance. Features of cortisol excess include the occurrence of abdominal skin striae, myopathy, easy bruising, truncal weight gain and a plethoric appearance related to an androgen-induced increase in red-cell mass. Cortisol and androgen levels are resistant to the normal suppressive effects of dexamethasone [56].

Hyperthecosis ovarii

Hyperthecosis ovarii is a benign disorder of the ovaries which may be a severe extension of PCOS or a distinct disorder in its own right. It is characterised histologically by the presence of nests of luteinised theca cells in a hyperplastic ovarian stroma and is manifest clinically as masculinisation including marked balding and menstrual disturbances, which may occur at any age [57,58] (Table 54.2). Hyperthecosis should be suspected in any patient who presents with severe hyperandrogenaemia in the absence of evidence of Cushing's syndrome, congenital adrenal hyperplasia or an adrenal or ovarian tumour. While there is considerable clinical overlap with PCOS, patients with hyperthecosis differ in that they tend to be virilised as well as severely hirsute, gonadotrophin levels are normal, and while morphologically the ovaries are usually enlarged they are not typically polycystic. Administration of an oestrogen/progestogen anovulant is not associated with suppression of androgen levels, although treatment with long-acting GnRH analogues may be effective [58]. Ovarian resection provides the best form of long-term treatment for the disorder: the induction of ovulation may not be possible.

Investigations

Hormonal

Steroid measurements (Table 54.4)

The majority of patients with IH or PCOS demonstrate mild to moderately elevated serum testosterone levels, although measurement of the free fraction may be required to identify the abnormality. While direct assays for free testosterone are generally not available outside research settings, measurement of sex hormone-binding globulin (SHBG) and the calculation of a testosterone/SHBG (T/SHBG) ratio provides an index of free testosterone levels which will increase the identification of abnormal values in patients with IH and PCOS [59]. More precise formulae utilising serum protein concentrations in addition to T/SHBG are available whereby a 'calculated free testosterone' level can be derived, but the added complexity is probably not justified in routine clinical situations [60]. On rare occasions, androstenedione levels are elevated where the T/SHBG ratio is normal [59]. In contrast to IH and PCOS, measurements of androgen blood levels yield markedly elevated values in androgen-secreting tumours, hyperthecosis ovarii and also in congenital adrenal hyperplasia when measured in morning samples (Table 54.4). DHEAS levels are sometimes elevated in patients with IH and PCOS [27,28]; this may indicate the presence of a significant adrenal contribution to the development of the disorders. However, excessive androgen responsiveness to stimulation with ACTH may be present in IH and PCOS patients with normal DHEAS values [61,62]. Because androgen levels are not inevitably elevated in patients with IH or PCOS, an index of intracellular androgen activity has also been utilised. Testosterone is converted to 5α-dihydrotestosterone intracellularly in order to express its biological activity;

5α-dihydrotestosterone is then metabolised further to 3α,5α-androstanediol and its glucuronide, which have been reported to provide good indices of intracellular androgen activity [63]. However, not all investigators have been able to demonstrate a clear separation between hirsute and non-hirsute women on the basis of these measurements [64]. The possible reasons for this include differences in assay technique or differences in the populations studied. Thus, the presence of a clinical feature indicating androgen excess, for example hirsutism, is the most useful assay of androgen bioactivity. Androgens may be elevated in amenorrhoeic women who do not demonstrate hirsutism [44]; this may be explained by reduced androgen-receptor sensitivity. Basal 17-hydroxyprogesterone levels may be mildly elevated in patients with IH or PCOS, and probably indicate increased production rather than impaired utilisation of the steroid as occurs in congenital adrenal hyperplasia. In IH and PCOS, the 17-hydroxyprogesterone levels are significantly different from those occurring in unaffected women, but the mean level is only trivially elevated and is quite different from the values usually seen in congenital adrenal hyperplasia [27,62]. Where a strong suspicion of congenital adrenal hyperplasia exists, either on the basis of clinical presentation, family or ethnic background, it is advisable to measure the 17-hydroxyprogesterone response to ACTH in the rare instances where the early morning value does not prove to be diagnostic and where clinical doubt still exists. In patients with 3β-ol-dehydrogenase and $\Delta_{4,5}$-isomerase enzyme system deficiency, elevated 17-hydroxypregnenolone and DHEA values are associated with elevated 17-hydroxypregnenolone/17-hydroxyprogesterone and DHEA/androstenedione ratios [50].

Gonadotrophins

A single blood sample obtained for measurement of LH and FSH may not identify any abnormality. Gonadotrophins are secreted in a pulsatile manner, and three samples obtained over 30–90 min are more likely to identify an abnormal LH/FSH ratio. An elevated LH/FSH ratio may be the most frequently detected abnormality in PCOS [27]. Since the characteristics of gonadotrophin assays vary greatly, it is necessary for investigators to identify the normal range for LH/FSH ratios in the assays that they are using. In general, ratios in excess of 3 are certainly abnormal, although ratios above 2 may be abnormal in some assays. In addition to finding an elevated LH/FSH ratio, the LH response to GnRH is almost inevitably markedly elevated in PCOS. In IH, the GnRH-stimulated LH level is intermediate between values seen in non-hirsute women and in those with PCOS [19]. Mild prolactin excess may be identified in approximately 25% of patients with PCOS [36].

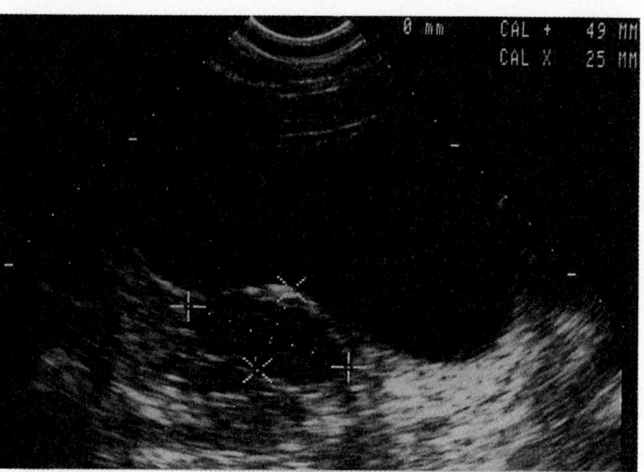

Fig. 54.4 Example of ultrasonographic appearance of polycystic ovaries. The cysts are distributed peripherally and there is an increase in stroma above that seen in normal ovaries. The ovary is enlarged, being approximately 23.2 ml. (Courtesy of Dr J. Masterson, St Vincent's Hospital, Dublin.)

Ultrasonography of the ovaries

Ultrasonographic examination of the ovaries frequently demonstrates the presence of multiple, small, peripherally distributed cysts in enlarged ovaries in patients with IH or PCOS, an example of which is shown in Fig. 54.4 [13,27]. Ovaries demonstrating the occurrence of dense stroma and the presence of more than 10 peripherally distributed cysts in any plane are typical of PCOS. Adams *et al.* [65] make a distinction between the polycystic ovaries described above and multicystic ovaries, in which cysts are plentiful but distributed throughout the ovaries where they are not associated with an increase in stroma. The latter appearances are associated with any amenorrhoeic state, for example prepuberty, hyperprolactinaemia or hypothalamic hypogonadism. Ultrasonographic detection of the polycystic ovaries is a sensitive method, but may be 'too sensitive'. Twenty-three per cent of an unselected population of normal young women demonstrate a picture characteristic of polycystic ovaries [2,3]. Patients with IH, who by definition continued to ovulate regularly, have been reported to demonstrate cystic changes in the ovaries in over 80% of those examined. Therefore, ultrasonographic examination appears to be a highly sensitive method for the identification of polycystic ovaries, but their presence is not specific for PCOS.

Practical approach to the investigation of IH/PCOS

The clinical presentation of IH/PCOS is so characteristic, with mild symptoms arising in the decade between 15 and

25 years and with gradual progression usually requiring years before coming to medical attention (Table 54.2), that it can be argued that investigations for diagnostic purposes are not necessary. However, measurement of androgen levels, particularly testosterone in association with SHBG, is helpful for at least two reasons. First, the finding of only mildly elevated androgen values provides the investigator and the patient with an assurance that other disorders such as a tumour or congenital adrenal hyperplasia are not lurking in a cryptic form. Secondly, a baseline androgen value against which to compare subsequent values is necessary to assess the early impact of treatment, as suppression of androgen levels will precede by months the emergence of any clinical change, particularly in hirsutism. A case may also be made for measurement of LH and FSH and for undertaking ultrasonographic examination of the ovaries. However, the author does not believe that all of these investigations are necessary in all patients, or that additional investigations for the presence of congenital adrenal hyperplasia, hyperprolactinaemia, androgen-secreting tumours, etc. should be undertaken unless a specific clinical indication exists, for example the development of hirsutism and oligomenorrhoea outside the decade of 15–25 years, or the finding of a markedly elevated testosterone value or the presence of virilisation [43]. Each investigator must be familiar with the testosterone assay utilised, but levels 100% above the normal range or T/SHBG ratios three times above the normal range should certainly be regarded as highly suspicious and warrant additional investigation.

Treatment

Ovulation induction

General approach

In very rare instances it may be possible to identify a specific underlying disorder associated with PCOS, for example congenital adrenal hyperplasia or an androgen-secreting tumour; under these circumstances treatment is directed towards the underlying disorder. In the vast majority of patients presenting with PCOS no specific associated disorder will be identified. Non-specific but important treatment measures listed in Table 54.5 and discussed in detail in the following section should supplement other strategies utilised to induce ovulation. These general strategies include weight loss for the overweight patient [20,66,67] and the cessation of cigarette smoking where applicable [15]. Before entering into treatment with the aim of inducing ovulation for patients who wish to become pregnant, it is important that seminal analysis is performed on the patient's partner so that his fertility status is also established.

Table 54.5 Treatment of anovulation in polycystic ovary syndrome.

Weight loss (for obese patients)
Anti-oestrogen (clomiphene citrate)
Adrenal suppression
Anti-oestrogen and adrenal suppression
Follicle stimulating hormone
Gonadotrophin-releasing hormone long-acting analogues plus follicle-stimulating hormone
Pulsatile gonadotrophin-releasing hormone with or without preceding analogue treatment
Ovarian resection (electrocautery)

Clomiphene citrate

It is generally accepted that failure of ovulation in PCOS is due to suppression of FSH levels; FSH facilitates both the development of the Graafian follicle and oestrogen biosynthesis. Although the precise mechanisms by which FSH secretion is restrained in PCOS has not been established, it is clear that negative feedback from oestrogen on the hypothalamo-pituitary unit is involved. Clomiphene citrate is an anti-oestrogen which can interrupt the negative feedback from oestrogen and thereby allow FSH secretion and ovulation to occur [68], and has been useful in the induction of ovulation in PCOS [69,70]. The increase in FSH is analogous to the follicular phase rise in FSH secretion which occurs in the normal menstrual cycle. When clomiphene citrate is successful in initiating the development of the Graafian follicle in this way, oestrogen biosynthesis subsequently results in positive feedback on gonadotrophin secretion; this is associated with the mid-cycle surge in LH secretion which is responsible for ovulation. Before administering clomiphene citrate it is conventional to induce withdrawal bleeding by administration of a progestogen. Medroxyprogesterone acetate, 10 mg daily for 5 days, is administered to subjects with oligomenorrhoea. Since PCOS is characterised by normal or elevated oestrogen levels, withdrawal bleeding almost always occurs following this short course of the progestogen. This confirms that the patient is not pregnant; in addition, treatment with progestogen prior to administration of clomiphene citrate is associated with a decline in LH and androgen levels [18] and an improved ovulation rate than when clomiphene is used without exposure to exogenous or endogenous progestogen [71]. Clomiphene citrate is administered from the fifth day of menstrual bleeding in a dose commencing with 50 mg daily for 5 days. Occasionally, this may be associated with some vaginal spotting, probably a manifestation of the anti-oestrogenic effect of the clomiphene citrate. When treatment is successful, ovulation usually occurs approximately 7–10 days following the fifth day of administration of clomiphene citrate [69]. Amenorrhoeic patients are encouraged to keep a careful record of all menstrual bleeding, to note changes in vaginal mucus, and to obtain basal body temperature readings to provide indices of ovulation. Measurement of plasma progesterone levels may also be useful. Blood for measurement of progesterone values should be obtained at the estimated mid-point of the luteal phase of the menstrual cycle, i.e. 19–22 days from the commencement of treatment with clomiphene citrate, or preferably serial levels may be obtained. Alternatively, progesterone levels in saliva can be measured. The patient collects saliva each day or on alternate days until a menstrual bleed occurs; then appropriate samples are chosen, i.e. those from approximately 7 days before the onset of bleeding, to check progesterone levels as an index of corpus luteum function and presumably ovulation. Failure of ovulation to occur is signalled in most patients by absence of menstrual bleeding. However, the possibility of pregnancy should always be checked under these circumstances. Where ovulation does not occur, the dosage of clomiphene citrate can be increased by 50 mg daily for each 5-day course in successive treatment cycles. The use of high doses of clomiphene citrate, i.e. 150–200 mg day, should be carefully monitored for the possible occurrence of the hyperstimulation syndrome [72,73]. In this condition large ovarian cysts develop and a generalised state of increased vascular permeability occurs. This is associated with development of ascites and pleural effusions, vascular collapse, oliguria and liver dysfunction and may be life-threatening. Ultrasonographic examination before the administration of clomiphene citrate in high dosage is indicated, and where there is evidence of increasing ovarian cyst size, treatment should be interrupted. Measurement of urinary or plasma oestrogens, which rise markedly in the patient with hyperstimulation syndrome, should also be monitored under these circumstances. If severe hyperstimulation syndrome occurs then vascular collapse should be treated immediately using plasma expanders and the correction of electrolyte abnormalities and paracentesis of ascitic and pleural effusions [73].

Where clomiphene citrate is effective in inducing ovulation but pregnancy is not achieved, treatment with clomiphene citrate at the same dosage should be repeated commencing on the fifth day of menstrual bleeding. This cyclical treatment may be continued for 6–12 months. On occasion it has been found helpful to combine dexamethasone treatment with clomiphene citrate as the yield of ovulation induction is higher using combined treatment than when using either agent alone [74]. For conception to occur in normal women it is necessary that intercourse takes place during the 72 hours before or on the day of ovulation [75].

Approximately 80% of PCOS women treated with clomiphene citrate ovulate and approximately 40% become pregnant [70, 110]. However, there is a high miscarriage rate, approximately 40%, which may be a result of the high androgen levels present. When conception occurs following treatment with clomiphene citrate, it is associated with a higher than normal incidence of multiple births i.e. approximately 10% of clomiphene-induced pregnancies will be associated with twins and approximately 1% with three or more viable fetuses [70].

Adrenal suppression

Many patients with PCOS will respond by establishing regular ovulation when treated with glucocorticoids [61,76,77]. The basis for the use of these agents has been outlined on pp. 742–743 and the theoretical response to adrenal suppression is depicted in Fig. 54.5. The steroid should be used only once daily and administered before sleep in a near physiological dosage. For the glucocorticoid to be effective in preventing the early morning surge in the secretion of ACTH and other

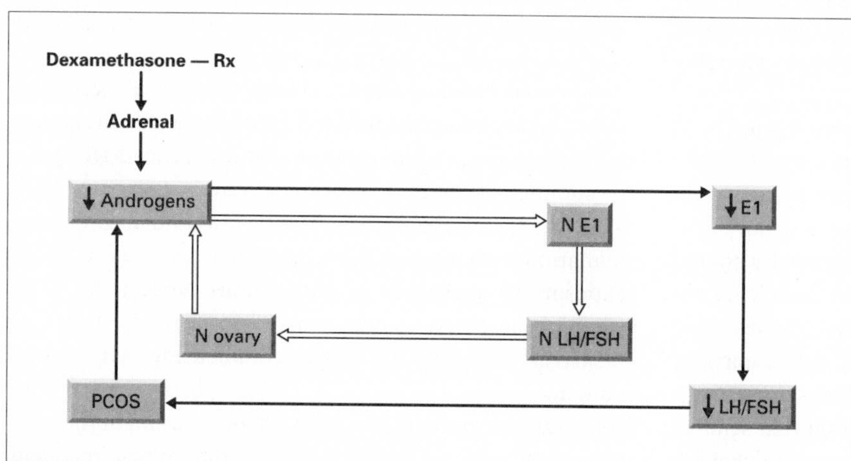

Fig. 54.5 Schematic representation for the proposed impact of adrenal suppression therapy on the cycle of events leading to the development of polycystic ovary syndrome (PCOS). E1, oestrone; ↑, increased; ↓, decreased; N, normal. From [109], with permission.

POMC fragments, it is necessary to use a steroid with a relatively long half-life. Dexamethasone, 0.25–0.5 mg taken prior to sleep has been found to be useful for this purpose. Approximately 60–70% of patients respond with a fall in androgen levels and a correction of the gonadotrophin abnormalities [61]. Obese subjects tend to be very sensitive to the appetite-stimulating effect of even small doses of glucocorticoids. If used at all in these subjects, only a very low dose of dexamethasone, 0.25 mg, should be employed, and patients should be alerted to the possibility of an increase in their appetite. Dietary advice obtained at the onset of treatment is also helpful. Patients should understand that at least 3 months of treatment, if not longer, will be required before it is clear whether or not success has been achieved. If after 3 months of treatment with dexamethasone an increase in the frequency of ovulation has not occurred, then alternative therapy should be explored.

Gonadotrophin therapy

The forms of treatment outlined above, dexamethasone and clomiphene citrate, are designed to stimulate endogenous secretion of FSH either by administering an anti-oestrogen and thus decreasing oestrogen feedback or by reducing the availability of the oestrogen precursor. An alternative form of therapy is to use exogenous FSH to stimulate Graafian follicle development [69,70,78]. FSH is available in a highly purified form or as a preparation of FSH and LH extracted from the urine of menopausal women; both preparations are similarly potent [78]. FSH, 75–150 U/day, is administered intramuscularly. Changes in the developing follicle are assessed primarily by ultrasonography of the ovaries and endometrium and/or measurement of urinary or plasma oestrogen concentrations [79]. The endometrial thickness enables the investigator to monitor the functional capacity of the ovaries. The granulosa cells in the follicle synthesise oestrogen which may provide a positive-feedback signal for LH secretion [80]. This results in the induction of ovulation in the normal menstrual cycle. A spontaneous surge of LH secretion may occur during the FSH treatment cycles, but it is usual to administer human chorionic gonadotrophin (hCG) as surrogate LH to bring about rupture of the follicle when it has reached an appropriate size as seen on ultrasonography and/or when oestrogen levels indicate functional maturity of the follicle. In this way it is possible to bypass the impact of disturbed endogenous gonadotrophic secretion on the ovary by superimposing a more favourable gonadotrophin environment from exogenous sources. Gonadotrophin induction of ovulation is more complex than treatment with either dexamethasone or clomiphene citrate, and for that reason is usually reserved for patients who fail to respond to other forms of therapy [78]. In such circumstances, FSH administration is a useful option for non-responders: when undertaken by experienced clinicians it may offer a 50% possibility of pregnancy. As in the case of induction of ovulation in PCOS using clomiphene citrate, the hyperstimulation syndrome may occur, and indeed is most likely to occur, during the use of exogenous gonadotrophins.

Because sensitivity to gonadotrophins may vary, the dose must be titrated according to the response of the individual patient. Treatment may be commenced using 75 U FSH and increased by 75 U every 3 days if oestradiol levels have not doubled or follicle size is not increasing [69]. Once follicle size is 15–18 mm, hCG 5000 U should be administered. Treatment with hCG should be withheld if oestradiol levels exceed 5500 pmol/l, if more than four dominant follicles are present, or if follicle size is greater than 18 mm. Following these guidelines the risk of significant ovarian hyperstimulation is minimised. The risk of multiple pregnancy correlates with the numbers of dominant follicles present at the timing of hCG administration, so that it is approximately 4% when two dominant follicles are present increasing to 18% in the presence of three to four dominant follicles [70]. The pregnancy rate for gonadotrophin therapy in clomiphene-resistant PCOS is approximately 20%. This low success rate may reflect release of endogenous gonadotrophins from the pituitary in response to rising oestrogen levels leading to an early LH surge before the follicles reach maturity. Pretreatment with a GnRH agonist to suppress endogenous gonadotrophic secretion, and thus prevent premature luteinisation, has been associated with a higher conception rate [81].

The incidence of spontaneous miscarriage following gonadotrophin therapy may be as high as 30% [82]. In an effort to overcome the problems associated with conventional gonadotrophin therapy in PCOS, namely the low pregnancy rate and increased risk of miscarriage, multiple pregnancy and ovarian hyperstimulation, alternative gonadotrophin regimens have been proposed. The use of low-dose gonadotrophins with a starting dose of 52.5 iu, which may be maintained for up to 14 days, has been proposed [83]. A variation of the low-dose regimen, the so-called step-down protocol, attempts to mimic the FSH profile seen in the early and the mid-follicular phases of the normal cycles [84]. In this protocol, which starts with a conventional high dose of gonadotrophin, the dose is gradually reduced as follicles develop. Following the low-dose regimen the incidence of multiple pregnancy was only 7% and there were no cases of severe hyperstimulation syndrome. However, the pregnancy and miscarriage rates were disappointingly similar to those observed with conventional-dose gonadotrophin therapy.

Gonadotrophin-releasing hormone

GnRH is a decapeptide first synthesised in 1971. Its clinical efficacy is dependent on pulsatile administration delivered either subcutaneously or intravenously by a small portable programmable infusion pump. Under physiological conditions GnRH is secreted from the hypothalamus in a pulsatile fashion, about every 60–90 min, and stimulates LH and FSH secretion from the pituitary gland. However, when GnRH is administered continuously, inhibition of gonadotrophin release occurs by a process termed 'down-regulation' following a brief period of stimulation. GnRH analogues which have a long duration of activity achieve similar biological effects to the continuous administration of short-acting naturally occurring GnRH and suppress gonadotrophin secretion. When attempting to induce ovulation, GnRH 5–10 μg i.v. or 10–20 μg s.c. is administered in pulses every 60–90 min, i.e. 90-min intervals for the first week of folliculogenesis, increasing to 60-min intervals in the mid-follicular phase until ovulation occurs [85]. The frequency of GnRH administration is then slowed to every 90 min for 1 week after ovulation and thereafter to every 4 hours for the remainder of the luteal phase until either menstruation or pregnancy ensues. As an alternative to continuing GnRH therapy, luteal phase support may be provided by administering hCG 2000 U every third day over 6 days. The ovulatory rate achieved with pulsatile GnRH therapy in PCOS does not generally exceed 40–50%, with a pregnancy rate of approximately 16% per cycle [86]. However, treatment with a GnRH analogue for 6–8 weeks prior to the initiation of pulsatile GnRH therapy increases the ovulatory rate to approximately 80% and the pregnancy rate to approximately 30%. Because endogenous feedback mechanisms are still operative during pulsatile GnRH therapy, the degree of monitoring required is considerably less than for gonadotrophin therapy. In addition, the incidence of multiple pregnancy is lower at 5–8%, and severe ovarian hyperstimulation has never been reported [85].

Encouraging results in the induction of ovulation have been reported when FSH has been used following suppression of endogenous gonadotrophin achieved using long-acting GnRH analogues [86,87]. The precise role of combined GnRH analogue/FSH and hCG treatment in the induction of ovulation in PCOS has yet to be determined.

Ovarian resection

Before the availability of medical treatment for PCOS, wedge resection of the ovaries was frequently undertaken and was associated with a subsequent transient phase during which ovulation occurred. The mechanism whereby ovarian resection may bring about ovulation has not been established: the most likely explanation is that resection of a mass of hormone-secreting tissue reduces blood levels of androgens and oestrogens and leads to correction of gonadotrophin values. If electrocautery is applied to only one ovary, ovulation may occur in the contralateral ovary. However, after about 2 years of ovulatory cycles, the previous abnormalities usually re-emerge. Ovarian resection can now take place without the necessity for a laparotomy by using a laparoscope. The results of ovarian electrocautery are similar to those achieved using exogenous gonadotrophins for patients with clomiphene-resistant PCOS [88–90]. The hyperstimulation syndrome does not occur, and the incidence of singleton pregnancies improves with electrocautery. The treatment response and frequent occurrence of adhesions dictate that the procedure should be used only when immediate pregnancy is desired. Under these circumstances, ovarian electrocautery offers an effective and relatively inexpensive form of therapy which does not require intensive hormonal monitoring.

Hirsutism

General approach

The treatment of hirsutism falls broadly into three categories:
1 general considerations;
2 drug treatment summarised in Table 54.5;
3 local cosmetic measures listed in Table 54.6.

General considerations include similar advice to that provided for patients with PCOS wishing to ovulate, for example weight loss. Although the serum testosterone levels tend to be normal in obese subjects, the associated SHBG levels are suppressed, resulting in elevated free testosterone levels. Weight loss is associated with correction of this abnormality and correction of the hormonal abnormalities of PCOS and the resumption of regular ovulation and improvement of hirsutism [20,66,67]. We have previously noted that androgen levels are higher in hirsute women who smoke cigarettes than in those who do not smoke [15]. Therefore, cessation of cigarette smoking should also lead to an improvement in the general androgenic milieu.

Table 54.6 Treatment of hirsutism.

Non-androgenic oestrogen/progestogen anovulant reduces ovarian and adrenal androgen secretion)
Antiandrogens (cyproterone acetate, spironolactone)
Anovulants and antiandrogen
Adrenal suppression
Gonadotrophin-releasing hormone analogues
5α-reductase inhibitors

Drug treatment

Anovulants

The combined oestrogen/progestogen anovulants usually used for contraceptive purposes theoretically provide a near ideal form of treatment for the hirsutism of PCOS. The oestrogen/progestogen combination therapy is used to suppress gonadotrophin secretion, and thereby removes the stimulus to increase ovarian androgen secretion [91]. In addition, there is a reduction in the cortisol production rate due to changes in the metabolic clearance of cortisol [92]. This results in a decreased requirement for ACTH secretion and thereby reduces adrenal androgen production. As an epiphenomenon, SHBG levels will rise. However, this is unlikely to be of therapeutic significance as an isolated event, since an increase in SHBG levels in the absence of alterations in androgen production or clearance will not be associated with more than a fleeting reduction in the free fraction of androgens. None the less, the reduction in ovarian and adrenal androgen secretion is associated with a fall in free testosterone levels in anovulant-treated PCOS patients. Much concern has been expressed about the potentially deleterious effects of utilising a progestogen with androgenic properties. This concern is well founded, as the suppression of endogenous androgen secretion could be largely offset by the effects of an exogenous androgenic progestogen. Indeed, non-hirsute subjects occasionally become mildly hirsute when taking an anovulant containing the more usual androgenic progestogen. However, this problem can be circumvented by the use of non-androgenic progestogens, and indeed the availability of an antiandrogenic progestogen. Desogestrel and ethynodiol diacetate are non-androgenic progestogens, while cyproterone acetate is antiandrogenic, particularly when used in high dosage [93]. However, when used in low dosage, i.e. 2 mg, if not antiandrogenic it is certainly non-androgenic. Clinicians should be careful to prescribe only anovulants containing non-androgenic progestogens for the treatment of hirsutism. However, recently there have been surprising reports that the low-dose oestrogen preparations combined with some non-androgenic progestogens may be associated with an excess of venous thromboembolic events [94–96]. Anovulant therapy should be undertaken for a minimum of 1–2 years in the treatment of hirsutism. A clinically obvious impact of anovulant treatment on hirsutism will require 4–6 months to emerge. Patients may notice a decrease in the number of hairs or, more frequently, a longer interval between those occasions when local cosmetic measures are required. All forms of hormonal treatment will benefit from the supplemental use of the wide variety of cosmetic measures available. While the cosmetic measures provide only transient benefit (with the exception of electrolysis), they provide an immediate effect while the impact of long-term hormone treatment is awaited.

Anovulant treatment should bring about involution of theca-cell hyperplasia. Following withdrawal of the anovulant the likelihood of inducing ovulation may be greater than before the onset of treatment in patients with PCOS. Simultaneous correction of an underlying disorder, for example obesity, adrenal androgen excess, etc., will further enhance the likelihood of re-establishing normal ovulatory cycles on the withdrawal of anovulant treatment in PCOS.

Low-dose oestrogen, i.e. equivalent to ethinyl oestradiol 30 μg, is effective in treatment. The clinician must be aware of the usual side-effects associated with the use of anovulants, such as the possibility of thromboembolic disease and hypertension: these are much more likely to occur in women aged over 35 years, in obese women and in women who smoke. The role of anovulant treatment in the subsequent development of breast cancer, if any, has not been established [97]. It is probably prudent to avoid use of anovulants in women with an immediate family history of breast cancer. While on treatment with the anovulant pill, regular checking for the emergence of varicose veins, hypertension or breast lumps should be undertaken. The recent reports of deep venous thrombosis with 'modern' combination anovulants should be borne in mind [94–96]. Some women have difficulty tolerating anovulants because of the development of nausea, easy weight gain, malaise or decreased libido.

Antiandrogen therapy

Cyproterone acetate. Cyproterone acetate is an antiandrogen in addition to being a progestogen. This agent has been used successfully in the treatment of hirsutism when combined with an anovulant to ensure contraception [98,99]. A male fetus conceived during treatment with an antiandrogen will develop feminised external genitalia. For this reason, concurrent treatment with an anovulant is usually regarded as an essential component when using antiandrogens; this also ensures regular withdrawal bleeding. When used in high dose the effect of cyproterone acetate is prolonged. To ensure withdrawal bleeding on interrupting treatment used with the usual 21 days-on/7 days-off cyclical oestrogen regimen, cyproterone acetate should be used for the first 10–12 days, rather than in the conventional manner where the progestogen is employed either continuously in combined treatment or on the last 11 days of sequential anovulant therapy.

This form of treatment has been termed 'reverse sequential' by Hammerstein [99]. Cyproterone acetate 50–200 mg is usually taken for the first 11 days of a 21-day treatment cycle with ethinyl oestradiol 30–50 μg daily, or for the first 11 days of treatment with a non-androgenic combined anovulant.

Treatment with cyproterone acetate, 50–100 mg, has been associated with 'a definite' improvement in even severe hirsutism in 50% of patients by 6 months and in 70% at 1 year, while a 50% success rate in treating hirsutism was achieved in approximately 1 year using a much lower dose, 2 mg/day in a combined anovulant [99]. In contrast, a carefully conducted study failed to establish a significant advantage of high-dose cyproterone therapy [100]. This raises the possibility that the oestrogen component in the treatment schedule may have been a more active agent than cyproterone acetate in the treatment of hirsutism [101]. In addition, side-effects associated with cyproterone acetate, including headache, nausea, weight gain and loss of libido, may be more frequently associated with high-dose treatment. Undoubtedly, there is an important role for cyproterone acetate in the treatment of hirsutism, although its superiority to other agents may have been exaggerated.

Spironolactone. Spironolactone is a widely used anti-mineralocorticoid which also has less well-appreciated anti-androgenic properties [102,103]. Spironolactone is widely used in the USA in the treatment of hirsutism, where cyproterone acetate has not yet been approved for this use by the Food and Drug Administration. Spironolactone competes with testosterone for the androgen receptor and thereby blocks the biological action of testosterone in a manner similar to that of cyproterone acetate. Spironolactone is not as powerful an antiandrogen as cyproterone acetate. However, it is a useful form of treatment, particularly where anovulant therapy may be contraindicated.

Spironolactone has a special role to play in hypertensive subjects where its use may be associated with a lowering of blood pressure. Spironolactone in a dosage of 50-100 mg/day has been associated with significant improvement in the majority of hirsute patients after 6 months. Menstrual bleeding may become irregular on this treatment, and spironolactone may be combined with an anovulant in those patients where no contraindication exists in order to increase the therapeutic effectiveness, to regularise menstrual bleeding, and to ensure contraception; similar constraints exist concerning pregnancy as when using cyproterone acetate.

Adrenal suppression

The underlying mechanism whereby adrenal suppression brings about lowering of androgen levels has been outlined in Fig. 54.5. Suppression of adrenal androgen secretion is associated with lowering of oestrone levels, normalisation of gonadotrophin secretion, and reduced ovarian androgen secretion and thereby correction of the cycle of events underlying PCOS in some patients [61]. Adrenal androgen excess present in patients with IH has been demonstrated to benefit also from low-dose treatment with dexamethasone as outlined for the induction of ovulation [60]. Dexamethasone 0.25–0.5 mg is given before sleep each night. Adrenal suppression is the only form of treatment for hirsutism which also addresses the ovulatory disturbance underlying PCOS. All other forms of treatment involve suppression of ovarian activity. In addition, some forms of treatment used in the induction of ovulation, for example clomiphene citrate, are associated with increasing androgen levels. In contrast, the establishment of regular ovulation while suppressing androgen levels and thereby providing treatment for hirsutism makes adrenal suppression an ideal form of therapy for some patients. Approximately 40–50% of patients with PCOS treated in this way achieve definite improvement in hirsutism within 6 months. It is best to avoid glucocorticoid treatment in obese subjects in whom the appetite centre appears to be particularly sensitive to glucocorticoid treatment. Weight gain is not seen in normal-weight or underweight women treated with low-dose glucocorticoid. As with all forms of hormonal treatment, the most satisfactory results are achieved when cosmetic measures are used in combination with dexamethasone treatment. When successful, this treatment should be used for 1–2 years. Following cessation of treatment, androgen abnormalities fail to recur in some patients.

GnRH analogues

Although GnRH analogues have been used in the treatment of prostatic cancer, there is only limited experience with GnRH analogues in the treatment of hirsutism. Long-acting GnRH analogues [104] suppress LH and FSH secretion and reduce ovarian androgen secretion. This also produces an oestrogen-suppressed state with a possible effect on bone density. In the long term, this leads to a reduction in hirsutism. However, this can probably be more effectively achieved using an anovulant, thus avoiding an oestrogen-deficiency state and the potential of osteoporosis.

5α-reductase inhibitors

In order for testosterone to stimulate the hair follicle to grow, it must be converted to 5α-dihydrotestosterone. The hair follicle is rich in the enzyme required, 5α-reductase. Finasteride is a potent inhibitor of 5α-reductase activity which has been used in the treatment of benign prostatic hyperplasia. Finasteride has also been used in the treatment of hirsutism. Following 6 months in a comparative trial, approximately the same lessening of hair growth was achieved by spironolactone 100 mg daily, and finasteride 5 mg daily.

This was achieved despite the observation that testosterone levels rose significantly during treatment. However, the circulating levels of dihydrotestosterone and its breakdown product 3α-androstane-3α,17α-diol glucuronide fell significantly [105]. The place of finasteride in the treatment of hirsutism has yet to be established, and it is not clear that it has advantages over other less expensive agents of proven safety.

Cosmetic treatment

The widespread belief that the removal of hair other than by electrolysis is associated with deterioration in hirsutism is ill-founded. This appears to be based on the observation that when hair is removed more hair subsequently appears than had been present at the time of removal. This merely reflects the natural progress of the condition and is not an effect of the intervention. Cosmetic measures have an important role to play in the management of hirsutism [106]. Severe psychological trauma is inflicted by well-intentioned but misguided advice not to remove hair. Patients should be encouraged to complement any hormonal treatment undertaken with the simple cosmetic measures listed in Table 54.7.

Overview

It is important that patients have realistic expectations for the outcome to be achieved from both hormonal and cosmetic treatments. It is unlikely that hormonal treatment will bring about an obvious change in hair growth before 3 months of treatment; the effectiveness of treatment increases upon to approximately 2 years. Cosmetic measures should be used as frequently as is required to achieve the cosmetic endpoint with which the patient is comfortable. Many patients require encouragement and reassurance from the clinician before undertaking hair removal procedures of any type. It is therefore important that the clinician outlines carefully what the patient can reasonably anticipate at the start of the treatment for hirsutism. Too often, the poorly informed patient abandons treatment, which in the long term would have been effective, after only a few weeks because no change in hair growth has been seen, on the assumption that improvement should have occurred. To be successful, the treatment of hirsutism requires patience and stamina from both clinician and patient.

Table 54.7 Cosmetic treatment of hirsutism.

Depilatory creams
Plucking/shaving/waxing
Bleaching
Electrolysis

Complications and prognosis

The long-term outlook for patients with PCOS may be compromised by the increased incidence of oestrogen-dependent tumours, for example endometrial and breast cancers [107]. There appears to be clear evidence that these disorders are more likely to occur in patients with PCOS than in the general population. It is likely that early treatment intervention will lessen the likelihood of the occurrence of these complications. In addition, insulin resistance, frequently seen in patients with PCOS is associated with increased cardiovascular risk and the development of diabetes mellitus in some patients [46–48]. In the absence of oestrogen-dependent tumours and diabetes mellitus, only obesity, frequently seen in PCOS patients, should significantly compromise the long-term outlook of these patients when compared with the general population.

References

1 Zawadski JK, Dunaif A. Diagnostic criteria for polycystic ovary syndrome: towards a rational approach. In: Dunaif A, Givens JR, Merriam G, Haseltine F, eds. *Current Issues in Endocrinology and Metabolism: The Polycystic Ovary Syndrome.* Boston, MA: Blackwell Scientific Publications, 1992; 377–84.

2 Poslon DW, Adams J, Wadsworth J, Franks S. Polycystic ovaries—a common finding in normal women. *Lancet* 1988; i: 870–2.

3 Clayton RN, Ogden V, Hodgkinson J *et al.* How common are polycystic ovaries in normal women and what is the significance for the fertility of the population? *Clin Endocrinol* 1992; **37**: 127–34.

4 Hull MGR, Glazener CMA, Kelly NJ *et al.* Population study of causes, treatment and outcome of infertility. *Br Med J* 1985; **291**: 1693–7.

5 New MI. Polycystic ovarian disease in congenital and late-onset adrenal hyperplasia. *Endocrinol Metab Clin North Am* 1988; **17**: 637–48.

6 Hague WH, Adams J, Rodda C *et al.* The prevalence of polycystic ovaries in patients with congenital adrenal hyperplasia and their close relatives. *Clin Endocrinol* 1990; **33**: 501–10.

7 Case N, Kowal J, Perloff W, Soffer LJ. *In vitro* production of androgens by virilising adrenal adenoma and associated polycystic ovaries. *Acta Endocrinol* 1953; **44**: 15–19.

8 Dunaif A, Scully RE, Andersen RN, Chapin DS, Crowley WF, Jr. The effects of continuous androgen secretion on the hypothalamic-pituitary axis in women: evidence from a luteinized thecoma of the ovary. *J Clin Endocrinol Metab* 1984; **59**: 389–93.

9 Futterweit W. Pathophysiology of polycystic ovary syndrome. In: Redmond GP, ed. Androgenic disorders. New York: Raven Press, 1995; 77–166.

10 Ehrmann DA, Barnes RB, Rosenfield RL. Polycystic ovary syndrome as a form of functional ovarian hyperandrogenism due to dysregulation of androgen secretion. *Endocr Rev* 1995; **16**: 322–53.

11 Franks S. Polycystic ovary syndrome. *N Engl J Med* 1995; **333**: 853–61.
12 McKenna TJ, Hayes FJ. Recent advances in diagnosis and treatment of polycystic ovary syndrome. In: Bonnar J, ed. *Recent Advances in Obstetrics and Gynaecology*, Vol. 19. Edinburgh: Churchill Livingstone, 1995: 121–38.
13 Adams J, Polson DW, Franks S. Prevalence of polycystic ovaries in women with anovulation and idiopathic hirsutism. *Br Med J* 1986; **293**: 355–9.
14 Kerri AH, Chan KL, Shortt F, White DM, Williamson R, Franks S. Evidence for a single gene defect causing polycystic ovaries and male pattern baldness. *Clin Endocrinol* 1993; **18**: 653–8.
15 Byrne B, Cunningham SK, Igoe D, Conroy R, McKenna TJ. Sex steroids, adiposity and smoking in the pathogenesis of idiopathic hirsutism and polycystic ovary syndrome. *Acta Endocrinol* 1991; **124**: 370–4.
16 Robinson S, Kiddy D, Gelding SV *et al.* The relationship of insulin insensitivity to menstrual pattern in women with hyperandrogenism and polycystic ovaries. *Clin Endocrinol* 1993; **39**: 351–5.
17 McKenna TJ. Pathogenesis and treatment of polycystic ovary syndrome. *N Engl J Med* 1988; **318**: 558–62.
18 Fiad TM, Cunningham, SK, McKenna TJ. The role of progesterone deficiency into the development of luteinizing hormone and androgen abnormalities in polycystic ovary syndrome. *Eur J Endocrinol* 1996; **135**: 335–9.
19 Hall JE. Polycystic ovarian disease as a neuroendocrine disorder in the female reproductive axis. *Endocrinol Metab Clin North Am* 1993; **22**: 75–92.
20 McKenna TJ, Cunningham SK, Loughlin T. The adrenal cortex and virilisation. *J Clin Endocrinol Metab* 1985; **14**: 997–1020.
21 Guzick DS, Wing R, Smith D *et al.* Endocrine consequences of weight loss in obese hyperandrogenaemic anovulatory women. *Fertil Steril* 1994; **61**: 598–604.
22 Lopez-Lopez E, Nogeura Mc, Fuente T *et al.* Response to clomiphene citrate in polycystic ovary syndrome according to different LH:FSH ratios. *Human Reprod* 1987; **2**: 635–8.
23 Poretsky L, Piper B. Insulin resistance, hypersecretion of LH, and a dual defect hypothesis for the pathogenesis of polycystic ovary syndrome. *Obstet Gynaecol* 1994; **64**: 61–21.
24 Poretsky L, Kalin NF. Gonadotrophic function of insulin. *Endocr Rev* 1987; **8**: 132–41.
25 Nestler JE, Clore JN, Blackard WG. Effects of insulin on steroidogenesis *in vivo*. In: Dunaif A, Givens JR, Merriam G, Haseltine F, eds. *Current Issues in Endocrinology and Metabolism: The Polycystic Ovary Syndrome*. Boston, MA: Blackwell Scientific Publications, 1992: 265–78.
26 Hoffman DI, Kleve K, Lobo RA. Prevalence and significance of elevated dehydroepiandrosterone sulphate in anovulatory women. *Fertil Steril* 1984; **42**: 76–81.
27 Obhrai M, Lynch SS, Holder G, Jackson R, Tang L, Butt WR. Hormonal studies on women with polycystic ovaries diagnosed by ultrasound. *Clin Endocrinol* 1990; **32**: 467–74.
28 McKenna TJ, Cunningham SK. Adrenal androgen production in polycystic ovary syndrome. *Eur J Endocrinol* 1995; **133**: 383–9.
29 New MI. Clinical and endocrinological aspects of 21-hydroxylase deficiency. *Ann NY Acad Sci* 1985; **458**: 1–27.
30 McKenna TJ, Cunningham SK. The control of adrenal androgen secretion. *J Endocrinol* 1991; **129**: 1–3.
31 Aleem FA, McIntosh T. Elevated plasma levels in β-endorphin in a group of women with polycystic ovarian disease. *Fertil Steril* 1984; **42**: 686–9.
32 Stewart PM, Shackleton CHL, Bestall DH, Edwards CRW. 5α-reductase activity in PCOS. *Lancet* 1990; **335**: 431–3.
33 Rodin A, Thakkar H, Taylor N, Clayton R. Hyperandrogenism in polycystic ovary syndrome; evidence of dysregulation of 11β-hydroxysteroid dehydrogenase. *N Engl J Med* 1994; **330**: 460–5.
34 Polderman KH, Gooren LJ, van der Veen EA. Effects of gonadal androgens and oestrogens on adrenal androgen levels. *Clin Endocrinol* 1995; **43**: 415–21.
35 McKenna TJ. Polycystic ovary syndrome. *N Engl J Med* 1988; **319**: 229–34.
36 Corenblum B. Hyperprolactinaemic polycystic ovary syndrome. In: Mahesh VB, Greenblatt RB, eds. *Hirsutism and Virilism: Pathogenesis, Diagnosis and Management*. Boston, MA: John Wright, 1983: 239–46.
37 Del Pozo ES, Falaschi P. Prolactin and cyclicity in polycystic ovary syndrome; role for oestrogens and the dopaminergic system. *Prog Reprod Biol* 1980; **6**: 252–9.
38 Parker LN. Control of adrenal androgen secretion. In: Parker LN. *Adrenal Androgens in Clinical Medicine*. San Diego: Academic Press, 1989: 30–57.
39 Pehrson JJ, Vaitukaitis J, Longcope C. Bromocriptine, sex steroid metabolism and menstrual patterns in the polycystic ovary syndrome. *Ann Intern Med* 1986; **105**: 129–30.
40 Goldzieher JW, Green JA. Polycystic ovary syndrome. 1. Clinical and histological features. *J Clin Endocrinol Metab* 1962; **22**: 325–38.
41 Greenblatt RB, Mahesh B. The androgenic polycystic ovary. In: Mahesh VB, Greenblatt RB, eds. *Hirsutism and Virilism: Pathogenesis, Diagnosis and Management*. Boston, MA: John Wright, 1983: 213–37.
42 Conway GS, Honour JW, Jacobs HS. Heterogeneity of the polycystic ovary syndrome: clinical, endocrine and ultrasound features in 556 patients. *Clin Endocrinol (Oxf)* 1989; **30**: 459–70.
43 McKenna TJ. Screening for sinister causes of hirsutism. *N Engl J Med* 1994; **331**: 1015–16.
44 McKenna TJ, Moore A, Magee F, Cunningham S. Amenorrhoea with cryptic hyperandrogenaemia. *J Clin Endocrinol Metab* 1983; **56**: 893–6.
45 Ferriman DM, Gallwey JD. Clinical assessment of body hair growth in women. *J Clin Endocrinol Metab* 1961; **21**: 144–7.
46 Dunaif A. Diabetes mellitus and polycystic ovary syndrome. In: Dunaif A, Givens JR, Haseltine FP, Merriam GR, eds. *Current Issues in Endocrinology and Metabolism: The Polycystic Ovary Syndrome*. Boston, MA: Blackwell Scientific Publications, 1992: 347–58.
47 Dahlgren E, Janson PO, Johansson S, Lapidus L, Odena. Polycystic ovary syndrome and risk for myocardial infarction; evaluated from a risk factor model based on a perspective study of women. *Acta Obstet Gynecol Scn* 1992; **71**: 599–604.
48 Conway GS, Jacobs HS. Clinical implications of hyperinsulinaemia in women. *Clin Endocrinol (Oxf)* 1993; **39**: 623–32.
49 Wild RA. Hyperandrogenism: implications for cardiovascular disease. In: Redmond GP, ed. *Androgenic Disorders*. New York: Raven Press, 1995: 261–78.
50 White PC, New MI, Dupont B. Congenital adrenal hyperplasia. *N Engl J Med* 1987; **316**: 1519–24, 1580–6.
51 Derksen J, Nagesser SK, Meinders AE, Haak HR, van de Velde CJH. Identification of virilizing adrenal tumours in hirsute women. *N Engl J Med* 1994; **331**: 968–73.
52 McKenna TJ, O'Connell Y, Cunningham SK, McCabe M, Culliton M. Steroidogenesis in an oestrogen-producing adrenal tumour

in young woman: comparison with steroid profiles associated with cortisol and androgen-producing tumours. *J Clin Endocrinol Metab* 1990; **70**: 28–34.
53 Chan FL, Wang C. Imaging for adrenal tumours. *Baillière's Clin Endocrinol Metab* 1989; **3**: 153–89.
54 Neiman HC, Mendelson EB. Ultrasound evaluation of the ovary. In: Callen PW, ed. *Ultrasonography in Obstetrics and Gynaecology*. Philadelphia: WB Saunders, 1988: 423–46.
55 Gabrilove JL, Seman AT, Sebet R, Mitty HA, Nicolis GL. Virilizing adrenal adenoma with studies on the steroid content of the adrenal venous effluent and a review of the literature. *Endocr Rev* 1981; **21**: 462–70.
56 Montwill J, Igoe D, McKenna TJ. The overnight dexamethasone test is the procedure of choice in screening for Cushing's syndrome. *Steroids* 1994; **59**: 296–8.
57 Nagamani M, Lingold JC, Gomez LG, Garza JR. Clinical and hormonal studies in hyperthecosis of the ovaries. *Fertil Steril* 1981; **36**: 326–32.
58 Pascale MM, Pugeat M, Roberts M *et al.* Androgen suppressive effect of Gn-RH agonist in ovarian hyperthecosis and virilizing tumours. *Clin Endocrinol* 1994; **41**: 571–6.
59 Cunningham SK, McKenna TJ. Plasma sex hormone-binding globulin and androgen levels in the management of hirsute patients. *Acta Endocrinol* 1983; **104**: 365–71.
60 Nanjee MN, Wheller MJ. Plasma free testosterone—is an index sufficient? *Ann Clin Biochem* 1985; **22**: 387–90.
61 Moore A, Magee F, Cunningham S, Culliton M, McKenna TJ. Adrenal abnormalities in idiopathic hirsutism. *Clin Endocrinol (Oxf)* 1983; **18**: 391–9.
62 Loughlin T, Cunningham S, Moore A, Smyth PPA, McKenna TJ. Adrenal abnormalities in polycystic ovary syndrome. *J Clin Endocrinol Metab* 1986; **62**: 142–7.
63 Horton R, Lobo RA. Peripheral androgens and the role of androstanediol glucuronide. *Clin Endocrinol* 1986; **15**: 293–306.
64 Wudy SA, Wachter UA, Homoki J, Teller WM. 5α androstane-3α, 17β-diol, and 5α-androstane-3α, 17β-diol-glucuronide in plasma of normal children, adults and patients with idiopathic hirsutism: a mass spectrometric study. *Eur J Endocrinol* 1996; **134**: 87–92.
65 Adams J, Franks S, Polson DW *et al.* Multicystic ovaries: clinical and endocrine features and response to pulsatile gonadotrophin releasing hormone. *Lancet* 1985; ii: 1375–9.
66 Pasquali R, Antenucci D, Casimirri F *et al.* Clinical and hormonal characteristics of obese amenorrhoeic hyperandrogenic women before and after weight loss. *J Clin Endocrinol Metab* 1989; **68**: 173–9.
67 Kiddy DS, Hamilton-Fairley D, Bush A *et al.* Improvement in endocrine and ovarian function during dietary treatment of obese women with polycystic ovary syndrome. *Clin Endocrinol* 1992; **36**: 105–11.
68 Wu CH. Plasma hormones in clomiphene citrate therapy. *Obstet Gynecol* 1977; **49**: 443–8.
69 Blacker CM. Ovulation stimulation and induction. *Endocrinol Metab Clin North Am* 1992; **21**: 57–84.
70 Kelly KJ, Adashie EY. Ovulation induction. *Obstet Gynaecol Clin North Am* 1987; **14**: 831–8.
71 Homburg R, Weissglas L, Goldman J. Improved treatment of anovulation in polycystic ovary disease untilizing the effect of progesterone on the inappropriate gonadotrophin release and clomiphene response. *Human Reprod* 1988; **3**: 285–8.
72 Borenstein R, Elhalah U, Lunenfeld B, Schwartz ZS. Severe ovarian hyperstimulation syndrome: a re-evaluated therapeutic approach. *Fertil Steril* 1989; **51**: 791–5.
73 Aboulghar M, Mansour RT, Serour GI. Management of ascites and pleural effusions in ovarian hyperstimulation syndrome. *Fertil Steril* 1995; **64**: 1228.
74 Fayez JA. Selection of patients for clomiphene citrate therapy. *Obstet Gynecol* 1976; **47**: 671–6.
75 Wilcox AJ, Weinberg CR, Baird DD. Timing of sexual intercourse in relation to ovulation; effects the probability of conception, survival of pregnancy, and sex of baby. *N Engl J Med* 1995; **333**: 1517–21.
76 Steinberger E, Smith KD, Rodriguez-Rigau LJ. Hyperandrogenism and female infertility. In: Crossignani PG, Rubin BL, eds. *Endocrinology of Human Fertility: New Aspects*. London: Academic Press, 1981; 327–42.
77 McKenna TJ, Cunningham SK. Testing for adrenal abnormalities in polycystic ovary syndrome. In: Filicori M, Flamigni C, eds. *The Ovary: Regulation, Dysfunction and Treatment*. Excerpta Medica International Congress Series 1106. Amsterdam: Elsevier Science, 1996; 295–301.
78 McFaul PB, Traub AL, Thompson W. Treatment of clomiphene citrate-resistant polycystic ovary syndrome with pure follicle-stimulating hormone or human menopausal gonadotrophin. *Fertil Steril* 1990; **53**: 792–7.
79 Shoham Z, Di Carlo C, Patel A, Conway GS, Jacobs JS. Is it possible to run a successful ovulation induction programme based solely on ultrasound monitoring? The importance of endometreal measurements. *Fertil Steril* 1991; **56**: 836–41.
80 Taylor AE, Whitney H, Hall JE, Martin K, Crowley WF. Midcycle levels of sex steroids are sufficient to recreate the follicular-stimulating hormone but not luteinizing hormone mid-cycle surge; evidence for the contribution of other ovarian factors to the surge in normal women. *J Clin Endocrinol Metab* 1995; **80**: 1541–7.
81 Dodson WC, Hughes CI, Whiteslider DB, Haney AF. The effect of leuprolide acetate on ovulation induction with human menopausal gonadotrophins in polycystic ovary syndrome. *J Clin Endocrinol Metab* 1987; **65**: 95–100.
82 Ginsburg J, Hardiman P. The response to gonodotrophin therapy in infertile women with polycystic ovaries. In: Shaw RW, ed. *Polycystic Ovaries—a Disorder or Symptom?* New Jersey: Parthenon Publishing Company, 1991: 165–78.
83 Kiddy D, Watson H, Sagle M, Franks S. Low dose gonadotrophin therapy for induction of ovulation in 100 women with polycystic ovary syndrome. *Human Reprod* 1991; **6**: 1095–9.
84 Fauser BCMJ. Step-down follicle-stimulating hormone regimens in polycystic ovary syndrome. In: Filicori M, Flomigni C, eds. *Ovulation Induction: Basic Science and Clinical Advances*. Amsterdam: Excerpta Medica, 1994: 153–62.
85 Martin K, Santoro N, Hall J, Filicori M, Wierman M, Crowley WF. Management of ovulatory disorders with pulsatile gonadotrophin-releasing hormone. *J Clin Endocrinol Metab* 1990; **71**: 1081A–G.
86 Filicori M, Flamigni C, Dellai P *et al.* Treatment of anovulation with pulsatile gonadotrophin-releasing hormone: prognostic factors and clinical results in 600 cycles. *J Clin Endocrinol Metab* 1994; **76**: 1215–20.
87 Fleming R, Jamieson ME, Hamilton MPR, Black WP, MacNaughton MC, Coutts JRT. The use of Gn-RH analogues in combination with exogenous gonadotrophins in infertile women. *Acta Endocrinol* 1988; **119** (Suppl.): 77–84.
88 Cohen MB. Surgical management of infertility and polycystic

ovarian syndrome. In: Givens JR, ed. *The Infertile Female*. Chicago: Yearbook Medical Publishers, 1979; 273–300.
89 Donesky BW, Adashi ET. Surgically induced ovulation in the polycystic ovary syndrome: wedge resection revisited in the age of laproscopy. *Fertil Steril* 1995; **63**: 439–63.
90 Abdel Gadir A, Mowafi RS, Alnarer HMI, Alrashid AH, Alonezi OM, Shaw RW. Ovarian electrocautery versus human menopausal gonadotrophins and pure follicular stimulating hormone therapy in the treatment of patients with polycystic ovarian disease. *Clin Endocrinol* 1990; **33**: 585–92.
91 Derman RJ. Androgens and oral contraceptives. In: Redmond GP, ed. *Androgenic Disorders*. New York: Raven Press, 1995: 301–23.
92 Wild RA, Umstot ES, Andersen RN, Givens JR. Adrenal function in hirsutism. II. Effect of oral contraceptive. *J Clin Endocrinol Metab* 1982; **54**: 676–81.
93 Humpel M, Nieuweboer B, Dusterberg B, Wendt H. The pharmacokinetics of cyproterone acetate in man. In: Hammerstein J, Lachnit-Fixson U, Neumann F, Plewig G, eds. *Androgenization in Women: Acne, Seborrhoea, Androgenetic Alopecia and Hirsutism*. Amsterdam: Excerpta Medica, 1980: 209–20.
94 World Health Organisation Collaborative Study of Cardiovascular Disease and Steroid Hormone Contraception. Venous thromboembolic disease and combined oral contraceptives: results of international multicentre case-control study. *Lancet* 1995; **346**: 1575–82.
95 Jick H, Jick S, Gurewich V, Myers MW, Vasilakis C. Risk of idiopathic cardiovascular death and non-fatal venous thromboembolism in women using oral contraceptives with differing progestagen components. *Lancet* 1995; **346**: 89–1593.
96 Weiss N. Commentary: third-generation oral contraceptives: how risky? *Lancet* 1995; **346**: 1570.
97 Editorial. Oral contraceptives and breast cancer. *Lancet* 1986; **328**: 665–6.
98 Miller JA, Jacobs HS. Treatment of hirsutism and acne with cyproterone acetate. *J Clin Endocrinol Metab* 1986; **15**: 373–89.
99 Hammerstein J. Cyproterone acetate (the European experience). In: Greenblatt RB, Mahesh BB, Gambrell RD, eds. *The Cause and Management of Hirsutism*. Carnforth: The Parthenon Publishing Group, 1987: 147–59.
100 Barth JH, Cherry CA, Wojnarowska F, Dawber RPR. Cyproterone acetate for severe hirsutism: results of a double-blind dose-ranging study. *Clin Endocrinol* 1991; **35**: 1–3.
101 McKenna TJ. Cyproterone acetate in the treatment of hirsutism. *Clin Endocrinol* 1991; **35**: 5–10.
102 Tremblay RR. Treatment of hirsutism with spironolactone. *J Clin Endocrinol Metab* 1986; **15**: 363–71.
103 Barth JH, Cherry CA, Wojnarowska F, Dawber RPR. Spironolactone is effective and well tolerated systemic antiandrogen therapy for hirsute women. *J Clin Endocrinol Metab* 1989; **68**: 966–70.
104 Adashi EY. Potential utility of gonadotropin-releasing hormone antagonists in the management of ovarian hyperandrogenism. *Fertil Steril* 1990; **53**: 765–9.
105 Wang JL, Morris RS, Chang L, Spohn M-A, Stanczyk FZ, Lobo RA. A prospective randomized trial comparing finasteride to spironolactone in the treatment of hirsute women. *J Clin Endocrinol Metab* 1995; **80**: 233–8.
106 Weigner RF. Local removal of facial and body hair. In: Redmon GP, ed. *Androgenic Disorders*. New York: Raven Press, 1995; 325–9.
107 Coulam CB, Annegers JF, Kranx JS. Chronic anovulation syndrome and associated neoplasia. *Obstet Gynaecol* 1983; **61**: 403–7.
108 McKenna TJ, Cunningham SK. Adrenal androgen production in polycystic ovary syndrome. *Eur J Endocrinol* 1995; **133**: 383–9.
109 McKenna TJ, Cunningham S. Adrenal abnormalities in PCOS and the impact of their correction. In: Dunaif A, Givens JR, Merriam G, Haseltine F, eds. *Current Issues in Endocrinology and Metabolism: The Polycystic Ovary Syndrome*. Boston, MA: Blackwell Scientific Publications, 1992; 183–93.
110 Issacs JD, Lincoln MD, Cowan BD. Extended clomiphene citrate (CC) and prednisone for the treatment of chronic anovulation resistant to CC alone. *Fertil Steril* 1997; **67**: 641–3.

CHAPTER 55

Gynaecomastia

P.C. Sizonenko

Introduction

Gynaecomastia is defined as a benign hyperplasia of the breast tissue in men. Most frequently, it appears as a physiological event, in particular at some stages of life. Gynaecomastia is generally the clinical consequence of an imbalance between androgens and oestrogens, the decreased secretion or action of testosterone and/or the excessive production of oestrogens. It may be the symptom of a disease which should be recognised, revealing an endocrine disease or an occult secreting tumour, or it may be associated with chronic disease.

Embryology

Identical development of breast tissue is observed in the male and the female fetus. However, the mammary bud remains rudimentary in males, probably under the influence of androgens [1]. The mammary gland consists of a system of lobuloalveolar glands constituting the acini, which are responsible for the synthesis of the milk products and which in turn are linked to the galactophoric ducts; both structures are surrounded by a stroma consisting of loose connective tissue [2].

Physiology and pathophysiology

Development of the breast tissue requires the synergistic action of female sex steroids (oestrogens, progesterone), and of growth hormone, insulin and growth factors, prolactin, thyroid hormones and cortisol which play permissive and regulatory roles [3] (Fig. 55.1). Prolactin primarily acts on the differentiated breast acini to stimulate milk protein synthesis: its effect requires the presence of oestrogens [4]. Testosterone exerts a generalised inhibitory effect on the development of the mammary gland through a specific anti-oestrogen action [5]. The reduction of testosterone into 5α-dihydrotestosterone is not a prerequisite for its action. Oestradiol stimulates the cellular growth and proliferation of parenchymal epithelium to form ductal elements. In addition, oestradiol induces vascularisation of the stroma, and hypertrophy and oedema of the connective tissue through oestrogen receptors. These receptors have not been found in every case of gynaecomastia [6]. In addition to the presence of androgen receptors, aromatase activity has been found in breast tissue suggesting that androstenedione and testosterone can be converted *in situ* into oestrone and oestradiol [7]. Oestrogens have a triple origin in men: adrenal glands, adipose tissue and the testes; 10% of the total production of oestradiol and 5% of oestrone are probably produced in the testes [8–10]. The zona reticularis of the adrenal gland is able to synthesise 5–10% of the total amount of oestrone produced, while 80% of the production of oestradiol and oestrone results from the peripheral aromatisation of testosterone and androstenedione [11]. Aromatisation takes place in the splanchnic system and in adipose tissue, and increases with obesity and age [12]. Oestrogens circulate mainly bound to sex hormone-binding globulin (SHBG), which circulates at approximately half the level in the male compared with the female. The affinity of SHBG is double that for testosterone as compared with oestradiol [13]. Elevation of the concentration of SHBG induces a relative decrease of free testosterone and a relative increase in oestrogens, with increased conversion of androgens to oestrogens and consequently an increased free oestradiol/free testosterone ratio. Such a situation is probably able to induce development of breast tissue in males.

Histology

Proliferation of the stroma and of the epithelium of the excretory ducts induces hyperplasia of the mammary gland.

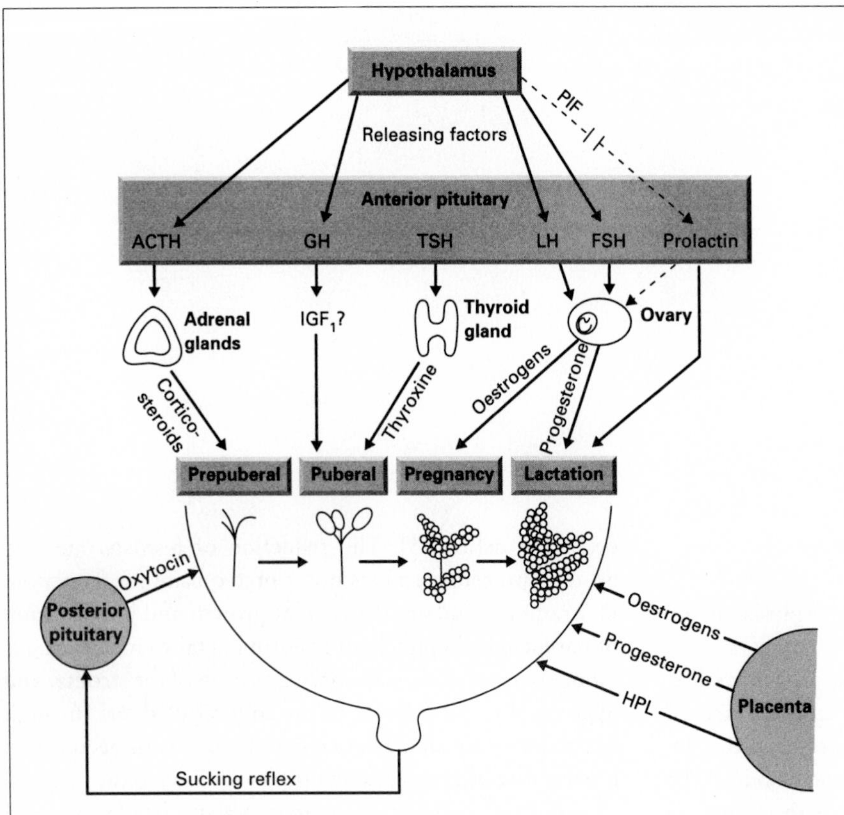

Fig. 55.1 Hormonal control of mammary growth. PIF, prolactin-inhibiting factor; ACTH, adrenocorticotrophic hormone; GH, growth hormone; IGF-1, insulin-like growth factor 1; TSH, thyroid-stimulating hormone; LH, luteinising hormone; FSH, follicle-stimulating hormone; HPL, human placental lactogen. Galactorrhea results from increased levels of prolactin and oestrogens. Suckling reflex with milk ejection has been provoked in men after administration of these hormones [4].

Two features are observed, depending on the duration of the gynaecomastia. In early diagnosed gynaecomastia, hyperplasia of the ducts is associated with periductal oedema and fibroblastic proliferation of the stroma; in gynaecomastia of longer duration, the stroma appears fibrotic, acellular, even hyalinised, and ductal hyperplasia is rare [14]. In absence of progesterone production there is no development of the acini. There is a progressive variation of the histological appearance depending on the duration of the gynaecomastia, but no correlation with any specific aetiology. Therefore, biopsy of breast tissue is a useless procedure in the diagnosis of the cause of the gynaecomastia.

Clinical features

The diagnosis of gynaecomastia is relatively easy. Clinical examination should evaluate whether the breast development is unilateral or bilateral, symmetrical or asymmetrical. The vertical and horizontal diameters of the breast should be measured for future comparison. Changes of the areolae may be present: an increase in size, hyperpigmentation and overdevelopment of the Montgomery tubercles are signs of hyperoestrogenism. On palpation, the gland is recognised by its firm and rubbery consistency compared with the soft surrounding adipose tissue. It is located behind the areola. Spontaneous galactorrhea may be present; it should be sought by firmly pressing the gland. Gynaecomastia can be painful, particularly when the gland is pressed. A malignant tumour of the breast is usually a hard nodule, or has irregular and very firm zones inside the tumour. Breast carcinoma is rare in males and not usually clinically confused with gynaecomastia. Mammography and ultrasonography of the breast are useful for recognising these conditions. Gynaecomastia must also be differentiated from excess fat as in obesity and lipoma. Examination of genitalia, and secondary sex characteristic, and palpation and measurement of the testes, should always be performed.

A directed clinical examination includes a careful drug history, identification of the presence of systemic, liver, kidney, heart or lung disease, evaluation of signs of chronic alcoholism and previous malnutrition, and of hyperthyroidism. The history of gynaecomastia should reveal the date of onset, its degree and its rate of progression. Clinical signs of oestradiol, prolactin, growth hormone, cortisol, thyroxine excess or androgen deficiency should be noted.

Clinical judgement dictates which laboratory or radiological tests should be performed. Hormonal evaluation includes measurements of plasma testosterone, oestradiol, oestrone, luteinising hormone (LH) and follicle-stimulating hormone (FSH), prolactin, and other androgens (androstenedione, dehydroepiandrosterone and its sulphate), β-human chorionic gonadotrophin (β-hCG) and SHBG. Liver, renal and thyroid function tests should be assessed in some cases, depending on physical examination. Buccal smear and karyotype may be useful for the diagnosis of chromosomal abnormalities, as well as radiography of the chest and the sella turcica, and computed tomography (CT) and magnetic resonance imaging (MRI) techniques for suspected malignant secretory tumours.

Aetiology

The aetiology of gynaecomastia is very varied; its differential diagnosis depends very much on the age of the patient, particularly for so-called 'physiological' gynaecomastia. This should be separated from gynaecomastia due to pathological causes. Two possible approaches to the aetiological diagnosis of gynaecomastia are useful for the clinician: consideration of various disorders on the basis of pathophysiology (Table 55.1) or practical attention to the most frequent causes [15,16,17].

Table 55.1 Pathophysiological causes of gynaecomastia.

PATHOLOGICAL CAUSES
Deficiency of androgen secretion or action
Hypergonadotrophic syndromes
Klinefelter syndrome
Other XY chromosome abnormalities
Primary testicular diseases
Androgen-resistance syndrome
Complete testicular feminisation
Partial: Reifenstein, Rosewater, Lubbs, Dreyfuss syndromes
Non-virilising congenital adrenal hyperplasia
17β-hydroxysteroid dehydrogenase
3β-hydroxysteroid dehydrogenase
17α-hydroxylase
Hypogonadotrophic syndromes
Fertile eunuch syndrome
Isolated gonadotrophic deficiency
Panhypopituitarism
Excessive production of oestrogens
Adrenal carcinoma
Leydig-cell tumour
Sertoli-cell tumour
Testicular and adrenal tumour
Excessive production of peptide hormones
hCG-producing tumours (testis, lung, colon, etc.)
Hyperprolactinemia
Hypothyroidism
Pituitary adenoma
Alterations of the testosterone/oestradiol ratio
Systemic chronic illnesses
Acromegaly
Cushing's syndrome
Hyperthyroidism
Liver disease
Renal disease, haemodialysis
Starvation and refeeding
Increased peripheral aromatase activity
Heredity
Iatrogenic causes
Oestrogens, oestrogen analogues and precursors
Androgen-antagonist drugs
Catecholamine antagonists or depleters
Cytotoxic drugs
Radiotherapy of the testes
PHYSIOLOGICAL CAUSES
Newborn period
Pubertal
Transient
Persistent pubertal macromastia
Old age
IDIOPATHIC

Table 55.1 *Continued.*

hCG, human chorionic gonadotrophin.

Pathological causes

Many drugs and several chronic diseases can induce breast hyperplasia, and such conditions should be first recognised before investigating pathological situations which are much less frequent (Table 55.2).

Iatrogenic causes

Iatrogenic gynaecomastia is among the most common diagnoses (Table 55.3). Oestrogen therapy for prostate cancer, cosmetics containing oestrogens and chemicals contaminated with oestrogens can induce breast development. Preparations for percutaneous or vaginal administration of oestrogens in menopausal women can be the source of gynaecomastia in the male partner. Administration of androgens such as long-acting esters of testosterone (oenanthate, proprionate) at adolescence or in hypogonadism can induce gynaecomastia by peripheral aromatisation of testosterone to oestradiol; non-aromatisable preparations such as methyltestosterone or fluoxymestrone should not stimulate breast development [15]. 17α-alkylated androgens should not be used because of their liver toxicity. Among antiandrogens, spironolactone decreases testosterone synthesis and acts as a competitor

Table 55.2 Causes of gynaecomastia by frequency. Adapted from [15].

Causes	%
Drugs and systemic illnesses	33
Drugs	30
Idiopathic	15
Liver disease	7
Refeeding	5
Primary hypogonadism	3
Persistent pubertal macromastia	1.5
Hyperthyroidism	1.5
Breast sarcoma	1.5

of dihydrotestosterone at the level of the receptor [17,18]. Cimetidine has also an antiandrogen action at the receptor level [19]. Digitoxin acts as an oestrogen with low activity, while cannabinoids such as marijuana and hashish diminish plasma testosterone concentrations. Isoniazide has also been shown to cause gynaecomastia. Chemotherapy and radiotherapy to the testis can damage the Leydig-cell function with a moderate decrease in plasma testosterone and an increase in plasma LH and FSH, inducing the development of breast hyperplasia (see Chapter 75). Several antidopaminergic drugs may also induce hyperprolactinemia and gynaecomastia (Table 55.3), frequently associated with galactorrhea; such gynaecomastia should disappear after discontinuation of the suspected drug (see also Chapter 9).

Table 55.3 Drug-induced gynaecomastia.

Excessive production of oestrogens
Estrogens, oestrogen analogues and precursors
Digitoxin
Oestrogens
Oestrogen analogues
Oestrogen precursors
Testosterone enenthate
Testosterone propionate
Deficiency of androgens secretion or action
Androgen antagonist drugs
Cimetidine
Cyproterone acetate
Finasteride
Flutamide
Hashish
Marijuana
o,p'DDD
Progestogens
Spironolactone
Prolactin-stimulating drugs
Catecholamine antagonists or depleters
α-Methyldopa
Domperidone
Metoclopropamide
Phenothiazines
Reserpine
Sulpiride
Tricyclic antidepressants
Alterations of the testosterone/oestradiol ratio
Cytotoxic drugs
Busulfan
Combination chemotherapy
Methotrexate
Nitrosurea
Vincristine
hCG administration
Unknown mechanism (GH receptors?)
Human GH in prepuberty

hCG, human chorionic gonadotrophin; GH, growth hormone.

Alterations in the testosterone/oestradiol ratio

These alterations are frequently observed in many chronic conditions (Table 55.2).

In cirrhosis of the liver, gynaecomastia is observed in 40% of cases [20]. It is associated with signs of hypogonadism such as impotence, loss of libido, scanty sexual hair, and hypotrophic testes with oligospermia (see also Chapter 77). Histology of the testis shows atrophic tubules with hyalinisation, fibrosis, persistent spermatogonia and spermatocytes and no spermatozoa. The most constant endocrine feature is the increased testosterone/oestradiol ratio, resulting from a decrease in the metabolic clearance of circulating oestrogens. Plasma androstenedione and oestrone are usually elevated. However, the pathophysiology of the endocrine alterations observed in cirrhosis is complex [21]. The liver metabolism of the sex steroids is altered and the enterohepatic cycle of the steroids is abnormal. Alcohol has a direct toxic effect on the pituitary and on the testis [22]; it inhibits the biosynthesis of testosterone. Protein and caloric deprivation decreases the activity of the hypothalamo-hypophysial–gonadal axis. In addition, drugs used for the treatment of liver disease may be relevant (e.g. spironolactone).

Chronic renal failure affects the hypothalamo-hypophysial–gonadal axis, causing high levels of immunologically assayable LH, low testosterone secretion, and relatively high levels of plasma oestrogens. Hyperprolactinemia is often present. Gynaecomastia occurs frequently when hemodialysis is started [23,24].

One particular form is associated with refeeding after a long period of starvation (as in concentration camps during

World War II), or after severe chronic illness when patients recover and regain weight.

Hyperthyroidism is associated with gynaecomastia in 30–40% of the cases in adults [25]. Metabolism of the sex steroids and of SHBG is altered in presence of excessive thyroid hormones. While the exact pathophysiological mechanism explaining the gynaecomastia remains unclear [26], the increase in SHBG is likely to be the most important feature.

Deficiency of androgen secretion or action
(see also Chapters 49 and 58)

Deficiencies of testosterone secretion or action are usually classified as part of disorders of sexual differentiation.

Among the hypergonadotrophic syndromes in the male, Klinefelter's syndrome or 47XXY gonadal dysgenesis is the most commonly considered in the differential diagnosis of adolescent gynaecomastia. Eighty-five per cent of patients with Klinefelter's syndrome develop gynaecomastia at puberty in association with tall stature, poor masculinisation, and small hard testes. However, the clinical spectrum is variable and such patients may have normal height and even their testicular size may be within the normal range. Diagnosis is confirmed by the karyotype; plasma LH and FSH levels are elevated, prolactin is normal. Azoospermia is almost always present. Plasma testosterone may be in the normal or low-normal range, between the normal male and female levels. Free testosterone is often decreased as is the testicular response to hCG; total and free oestradiol are usually normal but have been shown to be increased in some rare cases. There is also evidence for increased conversion of testosterone to oestradiol, with a possible relative hyperoestrogenic effect and increased oestradiol/testosterone ratio [27]. Such gynaecomastia should not be neglected as it has been suggested that it may predispose to breast cancer [15]. Many disorders of sexual differentiation, whether associated with chromosome abnormalities or not, develop gynaecomastia; such cases include XX males, mixed gonadal dysgenesis with 45X/46XY karyotypes, and true hermaphrodites. They are generally diagnosed because of the intersex problem. Patients with other syndromes such as anorchidia, rudimentary testes syndrome, vanishing testes syndrome, and congenital absence of Leydig cells may also present with gynaecomastia, usually with a low testosterone level (see also Chapter 58).

Testicular lesions can be the cause of gynaecomastia in Steinert's syndrome, Noonan's syndrome, cystic fibrosis or in acquired conditions such as orchitis and torsion.

Peripheral resistance to androgens (androgen insensitivity syndrome) is represented in its extreme version by complete testicular feminisation, which is associated with a totally female phenotype, a normal female body configuration, and breast development at puberty but only with scanty hair. The *complete* form should only be noted in order to understand the *incomplete* form or partial resistance to androgens. The incomplete form gives rise to a phenotypic spectrum ranging from a phenotypic female with some masculinisation (hypertrophy of the clitoris) to a phenotypic male who develops gynaecomastia. It includes classical syndromes such as Reifenstein's syndrome with gynaecomastia and hypospadias, and Rosewater's syndrome with gynaecomastia and infertility.

The mechanism involves androgen insensitivity at the level of hypothalamic feedback, resulting in inadequate negative feedback, increased gonadotrophin secretion and high levels of testosterone and oestradiol. Development of gynaecomastia depends on the degree of androgen resistance relative to the increased levels of oestradiol produced by the testes. Such syndromes have an X-linked recessive or sex-limited autosomal dominant transmission.

Disorders of testosterone biosynthesis are usually classified as male pseudo-hermaphroditism. Enzyme deficiencies inducing insufficient testosterone production are associated with feminisation of the male fetus which may be sufficient for the child to be reared as a female. An exception to this is 17β-hydroxysteroid dehydrogenase deficiency; in this disorder, gynaecomastia develops in a phenotypic male. As gonadotrophin levels rise at puberty, excessive amounts of androstenedione are produced which may be converted into oestrone and oestradiol. The low level of testosterone leads to an increased oestradiol/testosterone ratio and gynaecomastia. Mild forms of 3β-hydroxysteroid dehydrogenase deficiency and 17α-hydroxylase deficiency may also result in a phenotypic male who develops gynaecomastia at puberty [28]. Interestingly, gynaecomastia is not associated with 5α-reductase deficiency, as testosterone which is normally secreted acts as a repressor of oestrogen activity.

Excessive production of oestrogens

Excessive production of oestrogens is rare and usually related to a secreting tumour of the testis or the adrenal gland.

Among the testicular tumours, the Leydig-cell tumour is the most common. Most of them are benign, although they may occasionally be malignant. They may have no endocrine expression and be discovered by palpation of the testes. Secreting tumours are revealed by excessive secretion inducing gynaecomastia associated with precocious puberty in the child and gynaecomastia in the adult male. The gynaecomastia is explained by the excessive tumoural secretion of oestradiol with decreased secretion of testosterone due to the inhibition of the hypothalamo-pituitary axis. Ultrasonographic examination of the testes and catheterisation of the spermatic veins with measurement of oestradiol may be useful for the diagnosis of small tumours. Sertoli-cell tumours are exceptional. Aromatase activity of these cells may explain the excessive production of oestrogens; these are more frequently diagnosed in patients with testicular dysgenesis.

Feminising adrenal tumours are infrequent and generally malignant [29]. Gynaecomastia is the first sign of the disease in the male adult. In 50% of the cases they can be palpated. In boys there are often signs of both precocious puberty and gynaecomastia. They are either carcinomas or adenomas.

Excessive production of peptide hormones

Gynaecomastia may signify a tumour such as choriocarcinomas of the testis, liver, colon or chest secreting hCG. Plasma levels of hCG, and β-hCG and oestradiol are elevated, while concentrations of testosterone, LH (measured by specific β-LH radioimmunoassay) and FSH are decreased due to desensitisation of the pituitary by the excess of sex steroids. The most frequent secreting tumours are bronchial undifferentiated epidermoid cancers, hepatoblastomas, kidney cancer and adrenal choriocarcinomas. Some of these tumours also secrete chorionic somatomammotrophin or human placental lactogen. Its role in the development of the gynaecomastia remains obscure.

Hyperprolactinaemia is associated with gynaecomastia and impotence in a number of cases [30]. Pituitary adenomas should be looked for by CT/MRI of the pituitary. Hyperprolactinaemia induces a condition of hypogonadism with low testosterone.

Even after full evaluation, many patients remain without an aetiological diagnosis: such patients are classified as having idiopathic gynecomastia. To the general physician the most frequent causes of gynaecomastia are the use of drugs alone or in combination with the underlying systemic disease, liver disease, and regain of weight after severe nutritional restriction. Endocrinologists will see patients with possible disorders of gonadal deficiency or hormone excess. In many cases, endocrine evaluation remains normal and the patient is placed in the idiopathic category.

Physiological causes

Depending on the age, 'physiological' gynaecomastia may be seen in many male patients.

Gynaecomastia of the newborn

Most male neonates present with a palpable breast due to maternal oestrogens. It is rarely associated with galactorrhoea. It regresses spontaneously in several weeks.

Prepubertal gynaecomastia

Gynaecomastia observed before puberty is rare. Some of the cases are due to secretory tumours or to enzyme deficiencies or abnormality of sex steroid metabolism, although a number of them remain classified as idiopathic [31,32]. Very recently, growth hormone (GH) therapy in male patients has been associated in a few cases with adult or prepubertal gynaecomastia [33,34]; the mechanism underlying stimulation of breast development by hGH has not been established.

Pubertal gynaecomastia

Gynaecomastia is frequently observed in boys from the age of 11 years. By age 14, gynaecomastia is detectable in 30–65% of adolescent boys, although usually the diameter of the glandular tissue does not exceed 1 cm [35,36]. The gynaecomastia regresses spontaneously in nearly all patients, although it may occasionally persist. The prevalence decreases to 14% by age 16. During the early stages of puberty, the ratio of oestrogens to androgens is increased [35,37]. Persistent pubertal macromastia should be evaluated as it may signify a pathological cause, as described above.

Gynaecomastia of old age

Gynaecomastia appears to be frequent after 65 years, increasing with age [38,39]. Older men with gynaecomastia have higher oestradiol/testosterone ratios than those without gynaecomastia, providing further support for the oestrogen/androgen imbalance theory of gynaecomastia.

Therapy

When a cause for the gynaecomastia has been diagnosed, specific therapy should be instituted, if feasible. Drugs involved in the development of the gynaecomastia should be discontinued. In cases of therapy with oestrogens or antiandrogens for severe malignant diseases, preventive radiotherapy of the mammary gland has been proposed [40]. This preventive therapy is probably obsolete, because new antihormones (such as gonadotrophin-releasing hormone agonists) are presently available [41].

In the absence of a clear aetiology, gynaecomastia represents a symptom which may disappear spontaneously if the gynaecomastia is recent and of small volume. Boys with pubertal gynaecomastia should be generally reassured that regression usually occurs within 18–24 months in the great majority. However, persisting gynaecomastia may induce psychological disturbances and be poorly accepted. Because medical therapy for long-lasting and significant gynaecomastia is ineffective, surgical excision is required. Reduction mammoplasty is occasionally necessary in men with painful or cosmetically unacceptable lesions. Such a procedure should be performed by highly experienced surgeons because of the risks of unsightly scarring with malposition of the nipples, and formation of an abnormal emptiness in place of the breast tissue. Medical therapy has been tried, with little success, mainly in pubertal gynaecomastia. The use of anti-oestrogens such as tamoxifen (20 mg/day) or clomiphene (100 mg/day) to block the action of oestrogens, stimulate testosterone secretion and alter the testosterone/oestradiol ratio, is not usually successful [42,43]. Administration of non-aromatisable androgens, such as dihydrotestosterone percutaneously, fluoxymestrone or danazol, which lower oestrogen secretion and increase androgen concentrations in plasma, has been shown to decrease gynaecomastia in a number of cases. Trials of aromatase inhibitors such as testolactone have been suggested in order to suppress androgen conversion to oestrogens [44]. The use of any one of these drugs can be considered in pubertal boys when the gynaecomastia is severe, and in adult patients with idiopathic gynaecomastia. However, our present limited experience with these pharmacological agents suggests that the results are rather disappointing.

References

1 Turkington RE, Topper YJ. Androgen inhibition of mammary gland *in vitro*. *Endocrinology* 1967; **80**: 329–36.

2 Raynaud A. A morphogenesis of the mammary gland. In: Kon SK, Corvie AT, eds. *Milk, the Mammary Gland and its Secretion*, Vol. 1. New York: Academic Press, 1961: 3–20.

3 Moore DC, Sizonenko PC. The female reproductive system. In: Kelley VC, ed. *Practice of Pediatrics*, Hagerstown, Maryland: Harper & Row, 1979; **54**: 1–31.

4 Frantz AG, Kleinberg DL, Noel GL. Studies on prolactin in man. *Rec Prog Horm Res* 1972; **28**: 527.

5 Goldman AS, Shapiro BH, Neuman F. Role of testosterone and its metabolites in the differentiation of the mammary gland in rats. *Endocrinology* 1976; **99**: 1490–5.

6 Rajendran KG, Shah PN, Bagli NP, Ghost SN. Estradiol receptors in non-neoplastic gynecomastic tissue of phenotypic males. *Horm Res* 1976; **7**: 193–200.

7 MacIndoe JM. Estradiol formation from testosterone by continuously cultured human breast cancer cells. *J Clin Endocrinol Metab* 1979; **49**: 272–7.

8 Wilson JD, Aiman J, McDonald PC. The pathogenesis of gynecomastia. *Adv Intern Med* 1980; **25**: 1–32.

9 MacDonald PC, Madden JD, Brenner PF, Wilson JD, Siitteri PK. Origin of the estrogen in normal men and in women with testicular feminization. *J Clin Endocrinol Metab* 1979; **49**: 905–16.

10 Weinstein RL, Kelch RP, Jenner MR, Kaplan SL, Grumbach MM. Secretion of unconjugated androgens and estrogens by the normal and abnormal testis before and after hCG. *J Clin Endocrinol Metab* 1974; **53**: 1–6.

11 Longcope C, Layne DS, Tait JF. Metabolic clearance rates and interconversions of estrone and 17β-estradiol in normal male and female. *J Clin Invest* 1968; **47**: 93–106.

12 Kley HK, Debelaers T, Peerenboom M; Krusemper HL. Enhanced conversion of androstenedione to estrogens in obese males. *J Clin Endocrinol Metab* 1980; **51**: 1128–32.

13 Vigersky RA, Kono S, Sauer M, Lipsett MB, Loriaux DL. Relative binding of testosterone and estradiol to testosterone–estradiol-binding globulin. *J Clin Endocrinol Metab* 1979; **49**: 899–904.

14 Nicolis GL, Modlinger RS, Gabrilove LJ. A study of the histopathology of human gynecomastia. *J Clin Endocrinol Metab* 1971; **32**: 173–8.

15 Carlson HE. Gynecomastia: current concepts. *N Engl J Med* 1980; **303**: 795–9.

16 Santen RJ. The testis. In: Felig P, Baxter JD, Broadus AE, Frohman LA, eds. *Endocrinology and Metabolism*, 2nd edn. New York: McGraw-Hill, 1987: 886–9.

17 Glass AL. Gynecomastia. *Endocrinol Metab Clin North Am* 1994; **23**: 825–37.

18 Corvol P, Michaud A, Menard J, Freigels M, Mahoudeau J. Antiandrogenic effects of spironolactone: mechanism of action. *Endocrinology* 1975; **97**: 52–6.

19 Jensen RT, Collen MJ, Pandol SJ *et al.* Cimetidine-induced impotence and breast changes in patients with gastric hypersecretory states. *N Engl J Med* 1983; **308**: 883–7.

20 Valimaki M, Salaspuro M, Harkonen M, Ylikahri R. Liver damage and sex hormones in chronic male alcoholics. *Clin Endocrinol* 1982; **24**: 469–77.

21 Chopra IJ, Tulchinsky D, Greenway FL. Estrogen-androgen imbalance in hepatic cirrhosis. *Ann Intern Med* 1973; **79**: 198–203.

22 Van Thiel DM, Lester R, Vaitukaitis JL. Evidence for a defect in pituitary secretion of luteinizing hormone in chronic alcoholic men. *J Clin Endocrinol Metab* 1978; **47**: 499–507.

23 Sawin CT, Longcope C, Schmitt GW, Ryan RJ. Blood levels of gonadotropins and gonadal hormones in gynecomastia associated with chronic hemodialysis. *J Clin Endocrinol Metab* 1973; **36**: 988–90.

24 Distiller LA, Marley JE, Sagel J, Pokroy M, Rabkin R. Pituitary gonadal function in chronic renal failure: the effect of LHRH and the influence of dialysis. *Metabolism* 1974; **24**: 711–20.

25 Becker HL, Winnacker JL, Matthews MJ, Higgins GA. Gynecomastia and hyperthyroidism. An endocrine and histological investigation. *J Clin Endocrinol Metab* 1968; **28**: 277–85.

26 Bercovici JP, Mauvais-Jarvis P. Hyperthyroidism and gynecomastia: metabolic studies. *J Clin Endocrinol Metab* 1972; **35**: 671–7.

27 Wang C, Baker HWG, Burger HG, de Kretser DM, Hudson B. Hormonal studies in Klinefelter's syndrome. *Clin Endocrinol* 1975; **4**: 399–411.

28 Winter JSD. Sexual differentiation. In: Felig P, Baxter JD, Broadus AE, Frohman LA, eds. *Endocrinology and Metabolism*, 2nd edn. New York: McGraw-Hill, 1987: 983–1039.

29 Gabrilove JL, Sharma DC, Wotiz HH, Dorman RI. Feminizing adrenocortical tumors in the male: a review of 52 cases including a case report. *Medicine* 1965; **44**: 37–79.

30 Winters SJ. Clinical male reproductive neuroendocrinology. In: Vaitukaikis JL, ed. *Clinical Reproductive Neuroendocrinology*. New York: Elsevier, 1982: 69–95.

31 Descamps H, Chaussain JL, Job JC. Les gynécomasties du garçon avant la puberté. *Arch Fr Pediatr* 1985; **42**: 87–9.

32 Haibach H, Rosebholtz MJ. Prepubertal gynecomastia with lobules and acini; a case report and review of the literature. *Am J Clin Pathol* 1983; **80**: 252–5.
33 Rudman D, Feller AG, Cohn L, Shetty KR, Rudman IW, Draper MW. Effects of human growth hormone in body composition in elderly men. *Horm Res* 1991; **36** (Suppl. 1): 73–81.
34 Malozowski S, Stadel BV. Prepubertal gynecomastia during growth hormone therapy. *J Pediatr* 1995; **126**: 659–61.
35 Moore DC, Schlaepfer LV, Paunier L, Sizonenko PC. Hormonal changes during puberty: V. Transient pubertal gynecomastia: abnormal androgen–estrogen ratios. *J Clin Endocrinol Metab* 1984; **58**: 492–9.
36 Nydick M, Bustos J, Dale JH, Jr, Rawson RW. Gynecomastia in adolescent boys. *JAMA* 1961; **178**: 449–54.
37 Large DM, Anderson DC. Twenty-four hour profiles of circulating androgens and oestrogens in male puberty with and without gynecomastia. *Clin Endocrinol* 1978; **8**: 277–87.
38 Williams MJ. Gynecomastia. Its incidence, recognition and host characterization in 447 autopsy cases. *Am J Med* 1963; **34**: 103–5.
39 McFayden IJ, Bolton AE, Cameron EHD, Hunter WM, Raab G, Forrest APM. Gonadal pituitary hormone pituitary hormone levels in gynecomastia. *Clin Endocrinol* 1980; **13**: 77–82.
40 Gagnon JD, Moss WT, Stevens KR. Pre-estrogen breast irradiation for patients with carcinoma of the prostate: a critical review. *J Urol* 1979; **121**: 182–4.
41 Labrie F, Dupont A, Bélanger A *et al.* New hormonal therapy in prostatic carcinoma: combined treatment with a LH-RH agonist and an antiandrogen. *J Clin Invest Med* 1982; **5**: 267–75.
42 Plourde PV, Kulin HE, Santen SJ. Clomiphene in the treatment of adolescent gynecomastia. *Am J Dis Child* 1983; **137**: 1080–2.
43 Parker LN. Treatment of gynecomastia with tamoxifen: a double-blind crossover study. *Metabolism* 1986; **35**: 705–8.
44 Zachmann M, Eiholzer U, Muritano M, Prader A. Treatment of pubertal gynecomastia with testolactone. *Acta Endocrinol* 1986; **279** (Suppl.): 218.

CHAPTER 56

Management of the menopause

N. Panay, J.W.W. Studd,
N.R. Watson and E.A. MacGregor

Introduction

The menopause is a multisystem disorder involving the cardiovascular system, the skeleton and the psyche, and its management should encompass this broad view of the condition uninhibited by the constraints of specialist boundaries.

The strict definition of the menopause is the cessation of menstruation, but this is not always helpful as a basis for management because amenorrhoea is often preceded by many years of oestrogen-dependent symptoms. From a biological viewpoint it is unlikely that the ovaries are suddenly switched off, but decline gradually with the cessation of periods as an endpoint, which is reflected by the occurrence of irregular periods, decreased fertility, increasing premenstrual syndrome and climacteric depression before the amenorrhoea of the menopause.

Since the menopause is clearly a physiological occurrence, some would argue that it is a natural phenomenon and, therefore, the only management necessary is sympathy and emotional support. An alternative view, to which we strongly adhere, is that it is an endocrine disorder with profound generalised effects which should usually be treated by hormone-replacement therapy (HRT). With recent advances in patch and gel technology, no-bleed and long-cycle HRT and the hormone-releasing intrauterine systems, it should be possible to find a formulation to suit almost every woman.

Early symptoms

The classical symptoms of oestrogen deficiency are vasomotor and consist of hot flushes, night sweats, palpitations, headaches and dizziness. They affect 75% of women during a natural menopause, but are more common and severe in women experiencing an acute menopause after surgical castration or radiotherapy [1]. The mechanism of these symptoms is complex and poorly understood. Casper *et al.* [2] first reported a correlation between flushes and the pulsatile release of luteinising hormone (LH), but this is only an indirect link, and it seems likely that the flushes relate either to the pulsatile discharge of hypothalamic gonadotrophin-releasing hormone (GnRH) and/or the noradrenergic pathways controlling the hypothalamus.

The psychological symptoms associated with the menopause include difficulty in concentrating, loss of self-esteem, irritability, mood swings, decreased energy and depression. Montgomery *et al.* [3] reported these symptoms in 86% of women attending a menopause clinic, which compared with 56% in a general gynaecological clinic and 20% in a general out-patient clinic.

The origin of psychological symptoms is complex and likely to involve both biological and psychosocial factors. Epidemiological studies have confirmed an increase of psychological symptoms in women in the perimenopausal years [4], but as attempts to correlate these symptoms with hormone levels have failed, many psychiatrists have discounted a possible hormonal cause [5]. The orthodox psychiatric view is that the effect of depression is entirely environmental, related to domestic stress, loss of youth and fertility, the 'empty nest' syndrome and death of parents. There is no doubt that these psychosocial aspects are an important factor in depression, but that hormonal changes also play a part is suggested by the finding that the predominance of depression in women occurs only between puberty and the menopause, and is most common at times of greatest hormonal change such as in premenstrual, postnatal and climacteric depression. Conversely, during the last trimester of pregnancy, when hormone levels are stable, depression rarely occurs. Placebo-controlled studies in patients with premenstrual depression (see Chapter 53) have shown that symptoms may sometimes be effectively relieved by oestrogen treatment which suppresses ovarian activity [6], thus preventing the hormonal fluctuations that cause the cyclical symptoms [7,8]. Similarly, oestrogen treatment can effectively treat severe post-natal depression [9].

Intermediate symptoms

Oestrogen deficiency leads to the rapid loss of collagen which contributes to the generalised atrophy that occurs after the menopause [10]. In the genital tract this is manifested by dyspareunia and vaginal bleeding from fragile atrophic skin, and in the lower urinary tract by dysuria, urgency and frequency, commonly termed the urethral syndrome. More generalised changes are seen in the older woman as increased bruising and thin translucent skin which is vulnerable to trauma and infection. A similar loss of collagen from ligaments may cause many of the generalised aches and pains so common in post-menopausal women.

Long-term consequences

Osteoporosis and cardiovascular disease in women are the two major long-term health problems which have been linked to the menopause. Osteoporosis, or osteopenia, is a disorder of the bone matrix resulting in a reduction of bone strength to the extent that there is a significant increased risk of fracture. These fractures cause considerable morbidity in the elderly requiring prolonged hospital care and difficulties in remobilisation. The economic consequences are also considerable: in the UK osteoporosis causes more than 150 000 fractures each year with an estimated cost of £742 million per annum. With an ageing population and a real increase in the incidence of osteoporosis, this figure will rapidly rise [11] (see also Chapter 43).

Osteoporosis is predominantly a disease of women, who achieve a lower peak bone mass than men and are then subjected to an accelerated loss of bone density following the menopause. Women lose 50% of their skeleton by the age of 70 years, but men only lose 25% by the age of 90 years. The strength of bone is decreased to such an extent that, by 70 years of age, 50% of women will have sustained at least one osteoporotic fracture.

The aetiology of osteoporosis remains controversial, but central to current research has been the possibility of a dietary insufficiency of calcium or an abnormality of absorption and metabolism [12], either directly or through calcitonin [13] or parathyroid hormone. Considerable research has failed to demonstrate convincingly any such abnormality in the calcium-regulating hormones. A change in the bone matrix is a possibility which has received little attention. As early as 1941 Albright *et al.* [14] recognised the association of post-menopausal osteoporosis and thin skin, and suggested it was a generalised connective tissue disorder which is further supported by the coexistence of thin skin and osteoporosis with chronic steroid use, anorexia nervosa and osteogenesis imperfecta. Brincat *et al.* [10] have shown a significant decrease in skin collagen after the menopause which may be prevented (Fig. 56.1) or even restored to premenopausal levels with oestrogen therapy (Fig. 56.2). A similar decrease occurs in bone density which can also be restored to premenopausal levels by treatment with oestrogen (Fig. 56.3), raising the possibility of a similar mechanism.

Women are protected against cardiovascular disease before the menopause [15], after which the incidence rapidly increases, reaching a similar frequency to men by the age of 70 years (Fig. 56.4). The incidence of cardiovascular disease is reduced by up to half in women treated with oestrogen-replacement therapy compared with untreated women [16].

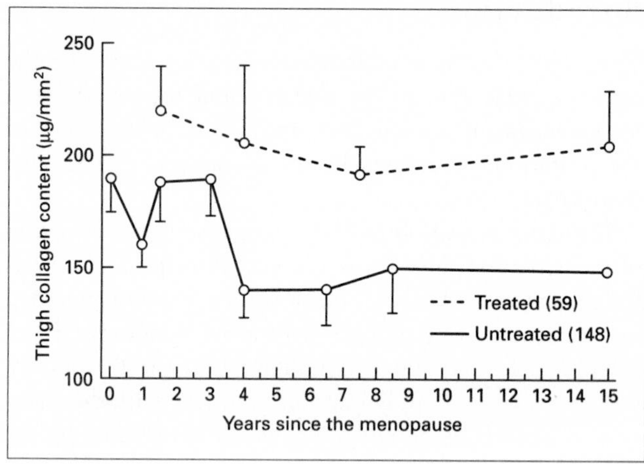

Fig. 56.1 Thigh collagen content with years after the menopause in 148 untreated post-menopausal women and 59 post-menopausal women treated with oestradiol for more than 2 years. Adapted from [10].

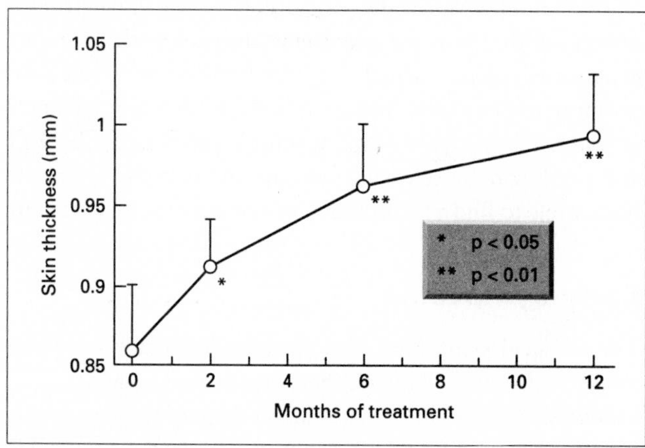

Fig. 56.2 Increase in skin thickness in 40 patients during 12 months of treatment with oestradiol implants. Adapted from [10].

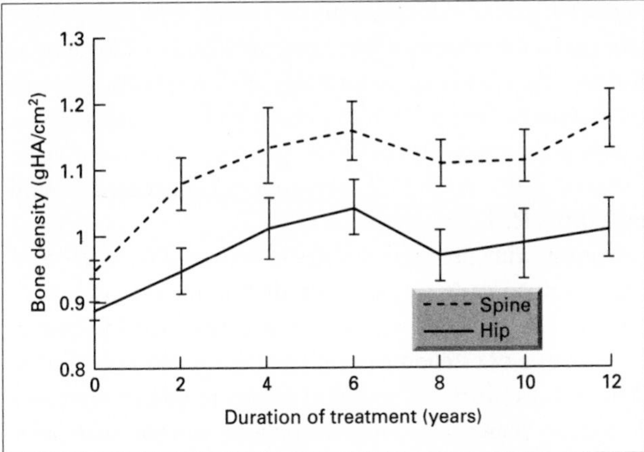

Fig. 56.3 Bone-density measurements of the hip and spine in 150 post-menopausal patients treated with oestradiol implants for up to 12 years.

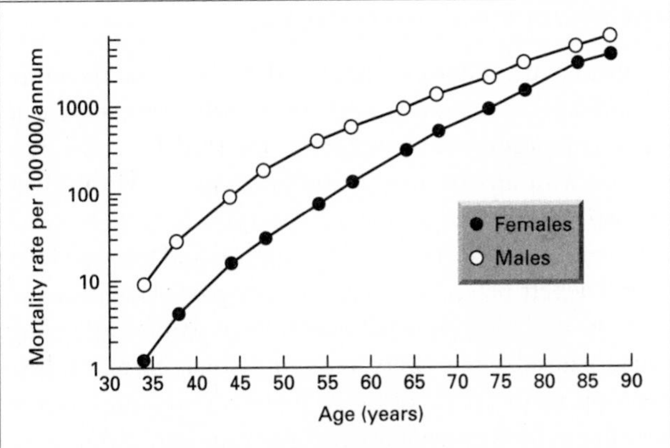

Fig. 56.4 Mortality rates from ischaemic heart disease by age and sex in England and Wales, 1982. Adapted from [15].

The protective effect of oestrogen is thought to be mediated mainly by an increase in high-density lipoprotein (HDL) and a decrease in low-density lipoprotein (LDL) which appears to be modified by the route of administration. Parenteral oestrogens will lower LDL, but do not increase HDL to the same extent as oral oestrogens [17]. However, several other mechanisms may account for this cardioprotective effect including control over release of adrenaline and noradrenaline, vasodilatation leading to increased blood flow, and a direct effect on the aorta decreasing atheroma. The oral route of administration theoretically has a greater beneficial effect on heart disease, but comparative studies are urgently required to examine this possibility.

Oestrogens also have a direct effect on the vasculature of the central nervous system. Studies have demonstrated that oestrogen replacement therapy may improve cerebral perfusion and cognition in post-menopausal women with cerebrovascular disease [18]. In the long term this may prevent diseases with a vascular aetiology such as vascular dementia [19,20]. In addition to the effect on vasculature, in Alzheimer's disease oestrogen may also intervene at the level of amyloid precursor protein as suggested by Jaffe *et al.* [21]. As well as evidence for the reduction of the relative risk of developing Alzheimer's dementia there are also data that oestrogens reduce the severity of the disease. Henderson *et al.* [22], through a case–control study, showed that not only was post-menopausal oestrogen-replacement therapy associated with a decreased risk of Alzheimer's dementia but that oestrogen replacement could improve the cognitive performance of women affected by this illness. A recently published large observational study found that the age of onset of Alzheimer's disease was significantly later in women who had taken oestrogen than in those who did not [23]. The relative risk was significantly reduced (9/156 (5.8%) oestrogen users versus 158/968 (16.3%) non-users; 0.40 (95% CI 0.22–0.85), $P < 0.01$), even after adjustment for differences in education, ethnic origin and apolipoprotein-E genotype. Further prospective studies are eagerly awaited, hopefully confirming the protective and therapeutic role of oestrogens in patients with these disorders.

Patient selection

If we support the concept that the menopause is a true endocrinopathy, all menopausal women should be offered oestrogen-replacement therapy, which should markedly reduce the incidence of depression, osteoporosis, myocardial infarction and strokes. However, the uptake of such preventive treatment will be influenced by the attitude of the prescribing doctor, the severity of the menopausal symptoms, and the patient's reluctance to return to regular menstruation. Currently the 'offer all' philosophy has little support and efforts are being made to target high-risk patients.

Preliminary investigations

The diagnosis of the menopause is simple and can usually be ascertained from a characteristic history of the vasomotor symptoms of hot flushes and night sweats and 6 months of amenorrhoea. Measurement of plasma hormone levels in patients with classical symptoms are unnecessary, expensive, time consuming and of little clinical significance. However, in the young patient or in a woman after hysterectomy, where the diagnosis is more difficult and the metabolic implications are serious, a single measurement of follicle-stimulating hormone (FSH) may be helpful, in which case a level of 15 iu or above may be regarded as climacteric.

In patients still menstruating, persistent hot flushes and night sweats are suggestive of the climacteric, but in those patients with psychological symptoms the diagnosis may be more difficult even with an elaborate psychiatric history. In such cases it may be justified to give a trial of oestrogen therapy and monitor the response before discounting a hormonal aetiology.

After the diagnosis has been established, investigations should be no more than the annual screening which is normally applicable to middle-aged women. This should include assessment of blood pressure, breast palpation, pelvic examination for ovarian disease and a routine cervical smear for cytology. Mammography should be performed as part of a national screening programme, and it is best to arrange screening before starting oestrogen therapy to identify patients with subclinical disease.

Endometrial biopsy is not a necessary prerequisite to treatment with HRT unless there are symptoms of post-menopausal bleeding or irregular perimenopausal bleeding. Attempts to decrease the morbidity of curettage by using cytology as a possible means of endometrial assessment have been found to be unhelpful [24]. In the few cases where an underlying malignancy is present, bleeding will be irregular after starting treatment, indicating the need for immediate further investigation.

There has been some enthusiasm for the implementation of a national osteoporosis screening programme by measurement of bone density, because prediction of osteoporosis from clinical risk factors and the intensity of short-term symptoms is unreliable. This judgement is premature as no studies have yet demonstrated that bone densitometry is suitable for mass screening. More importantly, osteoporosis is only one of the many consequences of oestrogen deficiency, and in terms of the number of sufferers and number of potentially avoidable deaths is less important than cardiovascular disease or strokes. Gynaecologists have an extended view that women are not merely skeletons, but expect oestrogen therapy to have a beneficial effect upon all symptoms; hence, they find it difficult to support the logic of targeting patients who need therapy by merely screening the state of the bones.

Treatment

The majority of women seeking help during the climacteric and post-menopausal years are symptomatic with a clear indication for oestrogen therapy, but an increasing number of asymptomatic women are presenting in order to prevent long-term morbidity. Treatment of these patients with no symptoms and no risk factors for osteoporosis or arterial disease is controversial but our view would be in favour of treatment, in the belief that the long-term benefits far outweigh any disadvantages. Hillner *et al.* [25] attempted to calculate the relative risks and benefits associated with HRT use in terms of quality years, taking into account the increased risk of endometrial carcinoma with unopposed oestrogen and the reduction in fractures and cardiovascular disease. He calculated an increase of 2.6 quality years of life in women taking HRT compared with non-users. These results are further supported by the studies of Hunt *et al.* [26] and Bush *et al.* [27] who found a decreased overall mortality rate in oestrogen users.

Women with premature ovarian failure, due to gonadal dysgenesis, an early surgical or radiation menopause, or an idiopathic cause, have an early and accelerated increase in the incidence of osteoporosis [28] and ischaemic heart disease [29], and are therefore a special group in whom oestrogen should be prescribed. Hysterectomised women who have not had an oophorectomy are also at increased risk as the menopause may be advanced [30] and significant bone loss can occur [31].

Non-hormonal treatment of the menopause and post-menopausal osteoporosis

The menopause is due to oestrogen deficiency, and therefore any attempts at treatment other than with oestrogen are at best a compromise and should be reserved for those few patients with an absolute contraindication to HRT. Over the years many non-hormonal therapies have been tried with limited success. Hypnotics, sedatives and tranquillisers are still widely prescribed to many menopausal women, and Cardozo *et al.* [32] reported that 40% of women attending a menopausal clinic were receiving some form of psychotropic medication, although there are no data to show any value in the treatment of oestrogen responsive symptoms. The addictive nature of these drugs should limit their administration to patients with clinically confirmed anxiety/depressive neurosis and they are best withheld from women with suspected climacteric problems until an adequate trial of oestrogen therapy has been implemented.

Clonidine, an α-adrenergic agonist, was reported to be effective in the treatment of hot flushes. This report was later supported in a multicentre, double-blind, placebo-controlled, cross-over study of 100 women which demonstrated a significant benefit for clonidine in controlling the duration and severity of hot flushes with minimal side-effects [33]. However, Lindsay and Hart [34], in a similar study, failed to find any difference between clonidine and placebo treatment. Other treatments with non-hormonal agents including ethamsylate, propranolol and prostaglandin inhibitors have been studied with conflicting results.

Considerable attention has been focused on the role of calcium in osteoporosis. Revealing that the diet of up to 59% of women is below the daily recommended dose of 800 mg calcium [35], Heaney *et al.* [36] calculated that to be in calcium balance premenopausal women need 1000 mg of elemental calcium per day, women in the perimenopause require 1200mg/day, and post-menopausal women require 1400mg/day, which is well above the average daily intake of women in this age group. Calcium supplementation in many women appears to be appropriate, but no studies have shown any benefits following calcium use in women with osteoporosis. Low-dose supplementation with calcium has been shown to reduce the daily dosage of oestrogen required to prevent osteoporosis [37], but it is by no means clear that the lowest dose of oestrogen is the desired dose for overall protection.

Studies showing a perimenopausal decline in calcitonin, superimposed on a normal age-related loss, have led to the suggestion of a link between post-menopausal bone loss and calcitonin. This link has been supported by studies which have shown that calcitonin is effective in conserving bone density [38], but the perimenopausal decline in calcitonin is likely to be a direct effect of oestrogen deficiency and plasma calcitonin levels increase in women having HRT [39]. A possible role for calcitonin in the treatment of patients with osteoporosis has been suggested, with studies demonstrating an increase in bone mass after 1 year of calcitonin therapy. However, longer-term studies have shown that this benefit is transient; bone mass was seen to decline again after 18 months of treatment, and no studies have yet shown that this increase in bone density will lead to a reduction in fracture rate.

Recently there have been many developments in the non-HRT treatment of osteoporosis including the bisphosphonates, calcitriol, ipriflavone, sodium fluoride, anabolic fragments of parathyroid hormone and growth factors. Bisphosphonates are stable, active analogues of pyrophosphate whose mechanism of action is inhibition of bone resorption allowing osteoblasts to lay down new bone, increase bone mass and reduce fracture risk. Etidronate was the prototype of this class of agent and was shown in controlled trials to prevent spinal fractures and produce a 4–5% increase in spinal bone density after 2 years of therapy [40]. Newer bisphosphonates are now available with similar anabolic bone effects. These drugs provide a useful alternative to the woman in whom HRT is truly contraindicated or who does not want to use HRT to treat osteoporosis. Unlike HRT they are not yet licensed for osteoporosis prevention and obviously do not benefit other systems.

Good nutrition and a healthy lifestyle are just as relevant after the menopause as before. Athletes, cross-country runners and ballet dancers who do not develop exercise-induced amenorrhoea have higher than average bone mass [41]. A slight 0.4% gain in bone mass in post-menopausal women has been described following 1 year of supervised thrice-weekly treadmill walking [36]. Exercise and a healthy diet have an undoubted beneficial effect on cardiovascular disease and have been claimed to reduce depression, anxiety and insomnia.

Hormonal treatment

Oestrogens

Oestrogen-replacement therapy is the logical treatment for all climacteric problems caused by ovarian failure and may be administered orally, vaginally, percutaneously as a cream or skin patch, transnasally, or subcutaneously as an implant. The pharmacodynamic and biochemical properties of exogenous oestrogens vary markedly depending upon the route used.

Oral oestrogens

Oral oestrogen therapy is the most popular form of treatment since it is both cheap and convenient. Oral preparations and dosages currently available in the UK are listed in Table 56.1. A theoretical disadvantage of oral administration is that up to 60% of the absorbed dose is converted to oestrone [42], and a significant proportion is further metabolised to the inactive oestrone-3-glucuronide by the first-pass liver effect. The principal oestrogen reaching the systemic circulation with oral preparations is oestrone, and the 2:1 ratio of oestradiol/oestrone which is normal in premenopausal women is reversed. The bolus delivery of oestrogen to the liver causes an increase in hepatic proteins including sex hormone-binding globulin, cortisol-binding globulin, renin substrate and HDLs [43].

These changes are more pronounced with the synthetic oestrogens, mestranol and ethinyl oestradiol, which are more potent and less susceptible to enzymatic degradation than the natural oestrogens [44]. They should be avoided in post-menopausal women because they increase thromboembolic disease by decreasing antithrombin III levels and increasing platelet aggregation [45]. The natural oral oestrogens also have slight effects on antithrombin III. Although this does not appear to have led to an increase in thrombosis in some studies [46], it is best to restrict their use in women with a history of clotting disorders. Despite parenterally administered oestrogens having no such effects, recent epidemiological data has suggested a two- to fourfold increase in risk of thromboembolic disease with all routes of HRT administration [87–89]. The risk of thromboembolism in an otherwise healthy woman is very small, but anyone with a past history of thromboembolic disease or clotting disorder being considered for HRT should have her individual risk/benefit ratio carefully evaluated.

In the last few years oestrogen preparations with continuous low dose progestogen have been introduced in order to provide bleed-free HRT. These preparations should be restricted to women who are at least a year post-menopausal or who have been using sequential preparations for at least a year to minimise breakthrough bleeding. A smaller dosage

Table 56.1 Currently available oral oestrogens.

Preparation	Generic name	Type of oestrogen	Dose
Oral oestrogen	Hormonin	Oestradiol Oestrone Oestriol	600 μg 1.4 mg 270 μg
	Ovestin	Oestriol	250 μg
	Premarin	Conjugated equine oestrogens	0.625 or 1.25 mg
	Progynova	Oestradiol valerate	1 or 2 mg
	Harmogen	Piperazine oestrone sulphate	1.5 mg
	Zumenon	Oestradiol	2.0 mg
	Climaval	Oestradiol valerate	1 or 2 mg
Combined sequential oral oestrogen and progestogen	Femoston	Oestradiol + Dydrogesterone Oestradiol + Dydrogesterone	1 or 2 mg 10 mg 14 days 2 mg 20 mg 14 days
	Improvera	Oestrone sulphate Medroxyprogesterone	1.5 mg 10 mg 12 days
	Nuvelle	Oestradiol valerate Levonorgestrel	2 mg 75 μg 12 days
	Climagest	Oestradiol valerate + Norethisterone	1 or 2 mg 1 mg 12 days
	Prempak-C	Conjugated equine oestrogens Norgestrel	0.625 or 1.25 mg 150 μg 12 days
	Cyclo-Progynova	Oestradiol valerate + Levonorgestrel	1 mg or 2 mg 21 days 250 μg 10 days
	Trisequens	Oestradiol (E_2) Oestriol (E_3) + Norethisterone	E_2 2 mg, E_3 1 mg 22 days E_2 1 mg, E_3 500 mg 6/7 days 1 mg 10 days
Continuous combined preparations	Kliofem	Oestradiol + Norethisterone	2 mg 1 mg
	Climesse	Oestradiol + Norethisterone	2 mg 0.7 mg
	Premique	Conjugated oestrogens Medroxyprogesterone	0.625 mg 5 mg
Long-cycle HRT	Tridestra	Oestradiol (E_2) E_2/Medroxyprogesterone Placebo	2 mg 10 weeks 2 mg + 20 mg 2 weeks 1 week

of progestogen given on a daily basis should theoretically produce fewer progestogenic side-effects and amenorrhoea with an atrophic endometrium which should be more acceptable to post-menopausal women [47]. Irregular vaginal bleeding in around 40% of women is common during the first 3 months of treatment leading to high drop-out rates, but those who continue treatment over 6–9 months can expect high rates of amenorrhoea with minimal side-effects and good rates of compliance.

Long-cycle HRT reduces to a minimum the number of progestogenic episodes, withdrawal bleeding and progestogenic side-effects. Despite there only being four cycles per year the rates of endometrial hyperplasia appear to be comparable to sequential regimens after 1 year of treatment [48]. The disadvantage of this regimen is that a relatively high dosage of progestogen is required (typically 20mg medroxyprogesterone acetate daily for 14 days) per progestogenic episode. This can lead to severe progestogenic side-effects when the episode does occur associated with heavy and/or prolonged withdrawal bleeding. Nevertheless, this regimen provides an effective regimen for some patients particularly as the prolonged unopposed oestrogenic phase allows for the beneficial effects of unopposed oestrogen on cardiovascular risk and central nervous system without the possible attenuating effects of progestogen. It is possible that this regimen may also be useful in the depressed perimenopausal women who are progesterone/progestogen intolerant.

Vaginal oestrogen creams

Vaginal oestrogens (Table 56.2) have been applied topically to the vagina for atrophic vaginitis for many years without cyclical progestogen on the assumption that they had only a local effect. However, recent studies have shown that oestrogen is rapidly absorbed into the circulation and that plasma oestradiol levels with the vaginal cream are higher than those from the same oral dose [49]. The rate of absorption of oestrogen, which depends on the base in which it is suspended and on the vascularity of the vagina, will increase with use since it increases the blood flow to the vagina. It is therefore important in patients with a uterus who regularly use vaginal creams that cyclical progestogen is added to protect the endometrium. Recently developed vaginal HRT regimens have managed to avoid the problem of endometrial stimulation. Creams using oestriol do not produce endometrial hyperplasia and the 17β-oestradiol silicone vaginal ring also provides effective relief of local symptoms without any significant endometrial effects.

Table 56.2 Currently available vaginal oestrogens.

Generic name	Type of oestrogen	Dose
Estring	Oestradiol (ring)	7.5μg/24 hours
Hormoferin	Dienoestrol	0.025%
Vagifem	Oestradiol	25μg/tablet
Ortho-Dienoestrol	Dienoestrol	0.01%
Ortho-Gynest	Oestriol	0.01%
Ovestin	Oestriol	0.1%
Premarin	Conjugated oestrogens	0.625mg/g

Oestradiol administered vaginally has advantages over the oral route, since it avoids conversion to oestrone by the intestinal mucosa and the liver, and the oestrone/oestradiol ratio remains within the premenopausal range of 1 : 2. However, at therapeutic doses significant increases in hepatic protein synthesis have been reported [50], which do not occur when the drug is delivered percutaneously.

Transdermal preparations

Lipid-soluble substances can be absorbed through the skin. They are impaired first by the stratum corneum, and then by the aqueous environment of the stratum granulosum which they can cross only if bound to an appropriate solvent such as ethanol. Passage occurs rapidly through the remainder of the epidermis to the papillary layer, where there is absorption into the capillary plexus and then into the general circulation. Initially both the percutaneous oestradiol cream and the transdermal oestradiol patch relied on an alcohol base, which led to erratic absorption and skin irritation, but alternatives with improved pharmacokinetics and fewer side-effects are now routinely used.

Transdermal patches

The first-generation oestradiol patches consist of a thin, multilayered unit containing a drug reservoir, a rate-controlling membrane and an adhesive layer, typified by the transdermal therapeutic system (TTS) (Estraderm, Ciba) (Fig. 56.5a). The reservoir contains a high dose of 17β-oestradiol, the oestrogen normally produced by the premenopausal ovary. The rate of delivery of drug is determined by the surface area of the patch. They are commercially available in three sizes, 5, 10 and 20 cm^2 which release at a controlled rate 0.025, 0.05, and 0.1 mg oestradiol per day, respectively [51]. Therapeutic levels of oestradiol are achieved within 4 hours of application of the patches and persist with continuous use if changed twice weekly. Over a 24-hour period there is significantly less fluctuation in oestradiol levels than is seen with oral treatment, and serum oestradiol concentration returns to pretreatment levels within 24 hours of stopping the patches [52]. The oestrone/oestradiol ratio is maintained within premenopausal levels, and no significant changes occur in the concentration of renin substrate, cortisol, sex hormone-binding globulin or other hepatic proteins [53]. The occlusive membrane greatly increases the diffusion of oestradiol through the stratum corneum, thus achieving therapeutic efficacy with very low doses of oestradiol.

The first-generation patches rely upon an alcohol base which can lead to erratic absorption and skin irritation. This

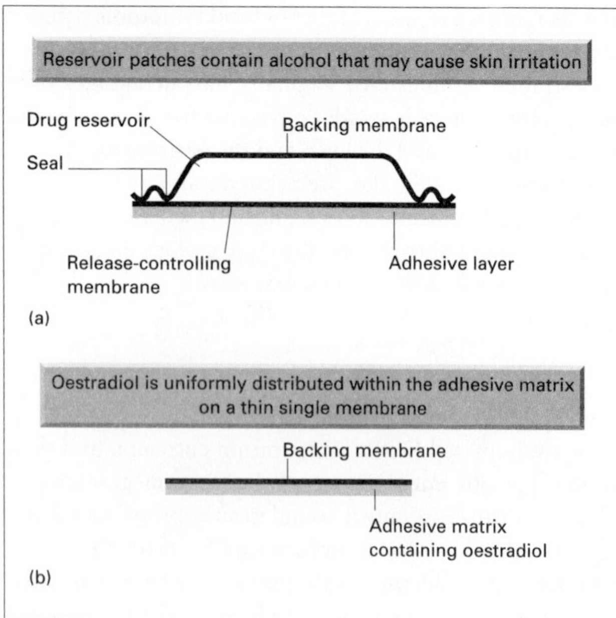

Fig. 56.5 Cross-sectional view of (a) transdermal reservoir oestrogen patch, and (b) single-membrane oestrogen patch.

led to the development of the second-generation single-membrane patches which have the oestradiol incorporated into the adhesive matrix resulting in fewer skin reactions (Fig. 56.5b) [54]. A number of single-membrane patches are now available with similar efficacies, most lasting 3–4 days but with one lasting up to a week (Table 56.3). These are available either for use on their own for hysterectomised women or prepackaged with progestogen tablets for women with a uterus. It is of course possible for the physician to vary the dosage and type of progestogen and dose of patch according to the patient's response.

Transdermal oestrogens were initially shown to significantly reduce the incidence of hot flushes, and have a positive effect on vaginal cytology, returning the maturation indices to premenopausal levels [55]. Later placebo-controlled studies showed that these improvements were significantly better than placebo [56]. Direct comparative studies of the 50-μg Estraderm patch with 0.625 mg oral conjugated equine oestrogen have shown they are equally effective in relieving symptoms [53] and conserving bone [57,58].

The rapid rise in serum oestradiol levels with transdermal patches will effectively suppress ovulation [6] (Fig. 56.6) which has been used to treat the premenstrual syndrome in premenopausal women [8]. This study also suggested a possible contraceptive role for this preparation; further work is being carried out to confirm these observations.

Percutaneous oestrogen gel

This excellent mode of delivery is particularly popular in France, and has recently become available in the UK. It uses the skin as a reservoir, providing near constant serum levels of oestradiol. Serum oestradiol levels are generally higher than those achieved with oral therapy; although serum levels rise more slowly with the gel, they are maintained for 48 hours [59].

Maximum plasma concentration is achieved within 3–5 days of starting treatment. The usual dose is 2.5 g daily applied via metered applications to the arms or inner aspect of the thighs. Percutaneous gel has been shown to induce an increase in skin collagen [60], and data are now available which demonstrate that the gel is at least as effective in preventing post-menopausal osteoporosis as oral preparations. Patients find the gel easy to use with few side-effects.

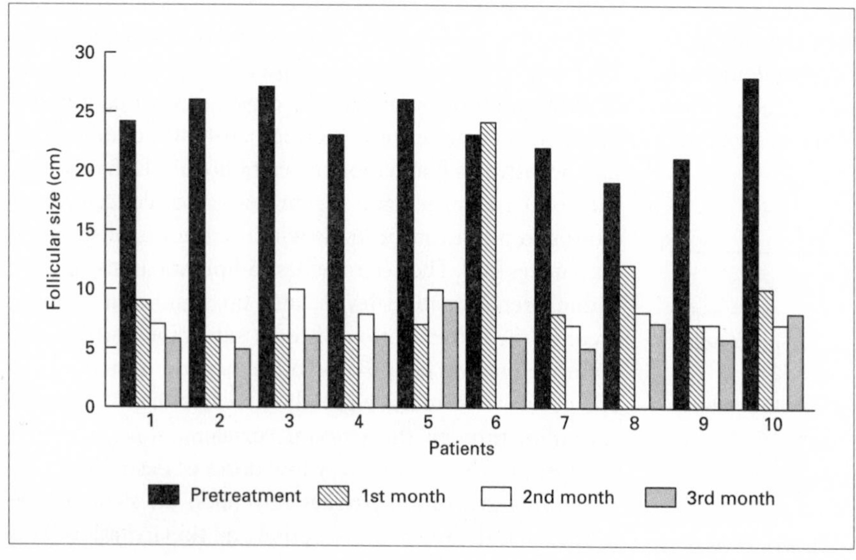

Fig. 56.6 Maximum follicular size measured by ultrasonography in patients before and during treatment with 200 μg Estraderm patches. Patient 6 ovulated during the first month of treatment. With a follicular size of < 10 mm the patient is unlikely to ovulate. Adapted from [6].

Table 56.3 Currently available transdermal oestrogens/progestogens.

Name	Constituent(s)	Dosage (μg/24 hours)/life per patch
Patch only		
Evorel	Oestradiol	25, 50, 75, 100/3–4 days
Fematrix	Oestradiol	40, 80/3–4 days
Menorest	Oestradiol	37.5, 50, 75/3–4 days
Femseven	Oestradiol	50/7 days
Estracombi	Oestradiol Norethisterone	50/3–4 days 250/3–4 days
Estraderm TTS	Oestradiol (reservoir)	25, 50, 100/3–4 days
Estraderm MX	Oestradiol (matrix)	25, 50, 100/3–4 days
Patch/tablet combinations		
Estrapak	Oestradiol Norethisterone	50/3–4 days 1 mg/12 days
Evorel-pak	Oestradiol Norethisterone	50/3–4 days 1 mg/12 days
Femapak 40	Oestradiol Dydrogesterone	40 10 mg/14 days

Subcutaneous implants

Subcutaneous implants first used to treat menopausal symptoms in 1938 [61] were later described by Greenblatt and Suran [62] to be effective in the management of many endocrine and gynaecological disorders. Several trials have now confirmed their efficacy for the treatment of menopausal symptoms. The technique of insertion is safe and simple and may be performed in an out-patient clinic under local anaesthesia using a no-touch technique [63]. The implants are convenient for patients as they need to be replaced only every 6 months, and being biodegradable they do not need to be removed.

The implants are available in the UK, as 25-, 50- and 100-mg oestradiol pellets and as 100- and 200-mg testosterone pellets. The usual dose for menopausal symptoms is a 50-mg oestradiol pellet every 6 months, to which 100 mg testosterone may be added for symptoms of decreased libido and energy. Gonadotrophin levels fall within 2 weeks of implantation to premenopausal levels and remain suppressed for approximately 6 months. Oestradiol levels peak at 2–3 months, gradually declining and by 6 months symptoms usually return, although oestradiol levels do not return to pretreatment levels [64]. Plasma oestradiol levels remain in the premenopausal range for up to 2 years from the last implant, and in women with a uterus it is important to continue with cyclical progestogens until there is no longer a withdrawal bleed produced by the progestogen.

Implants avoid the need for daily patient compliance, give good symptomatic relief, have few side-effects and rarely cause significant complications [32]. Savvas *et al.* [65] in a cross-sectional study showed that after 8 years of therapy bone density was significantly better in patients treated with implants than with oral therapy (Fig. 56.7). A 1-year prospective study of oestrogen and testosterone implants has now shown a 7% increase in bone density at the spine which occurred irrespective of the patient's age, menopausal age or pretreatment bone density, but was correlated to the oestradiol levels achieved with treatment [66] (Fig. 56.8).

Reports of tachyphylaxis in patients treated with implants have caused unnecessary anxiety. It is uncommon, occurring in 2.3% of 1388 patients. It occurs particularly in women with a previous psychiatric history, or in those with an early surgical menopause [67]. It is our experience that a pharmacological dose of oestrogen has a tonic effect on mood, thus often allowing patients on antidepressants and tranquillisers to safely stop [68]. There is no evidence that these high oestradiol levels are dangerous, and we seriously question the wisdom of the proposed management of withholding further implant therapy until oestradiol levels fall

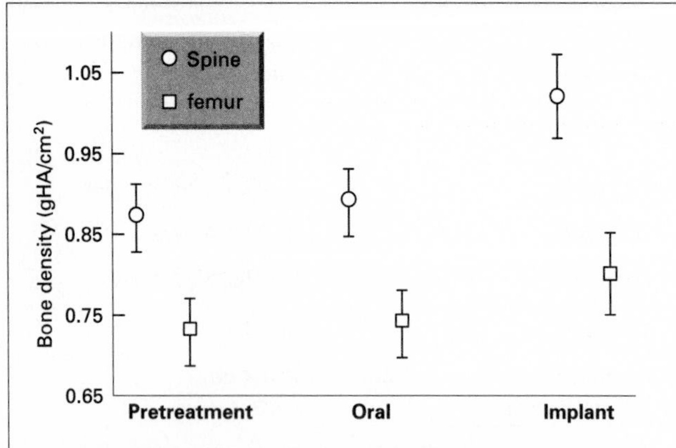

Fig. 56.7 Skeletal effects of oral oestrogen compared with subcutaneous oestrogen and testosterone in post-menopausal women. Adapted from [65].

to 200 pmol/l [69]. This is an inadequate oestradiol level for most patients, and such practice will produce recurrence of symptoms with much suffering. It may also be dangerous to women with oestrogen-responsive climacteric depression [70].

Progestogens

In 1938 Albright [71] first described the use of progestogens to produce a medical curettage and prevent endometrial pathology. Greenblatt emphasised the need to induce a regular withdrawal bleed in women using oestrogen-replacement therapy, but unfortunately was ignored until many studies in the 1970s showed an increase of early-stage endometrial cancer in women using unopposed oestrogen therapy. This could be prevented with the addition of progestogens, as shown by Sturdee *et al.* [72] in a study of 746 women where cyclical progestogen given for 13 days of each month prevented any endometrial hyperplasia (Fig. 56.9). It was also reported that cystic hyperplasia in oestrogen users could be corrected to a normal endometrium in all patients, with progestogen for 21 days of each cycle for 3 months [73].

Problems with progestogens

It is vital that we maximise compliance if patients are to receive the full benefits from HRT. One of the main factors for reduced compliance is that of progestogen intolerance. Progestogens have a variety of effects apart from the one for which their use was intended, that of secretory transformation of the endometrium. Endometrial effects vary between individuals and between different progestogens leading to bleeding problems. Symptoms of fluid retention are produced by the sodium-retaining effect on the renin–aldosterone system.

There is also concern that the addition of progestogen to oestrogen-replacement therapy will attenuate the cardioprotective effects of unopposed oestrogens. Progestogens can have a detrimental effect on carbohydrate metabolism, indirectly increasing the risk of coronary heart disease. However, these data have been derived from oral contraceptive studies, none being available from studies in post-menopausal women. Progestogens may also influence cardiovascular disease, adversely altering lipid metabolism by decreasing HDL and increasing LDL concentrations. These effects appear to be dependent on the type of progestogen used with current evidence indicating that androgenic proges-

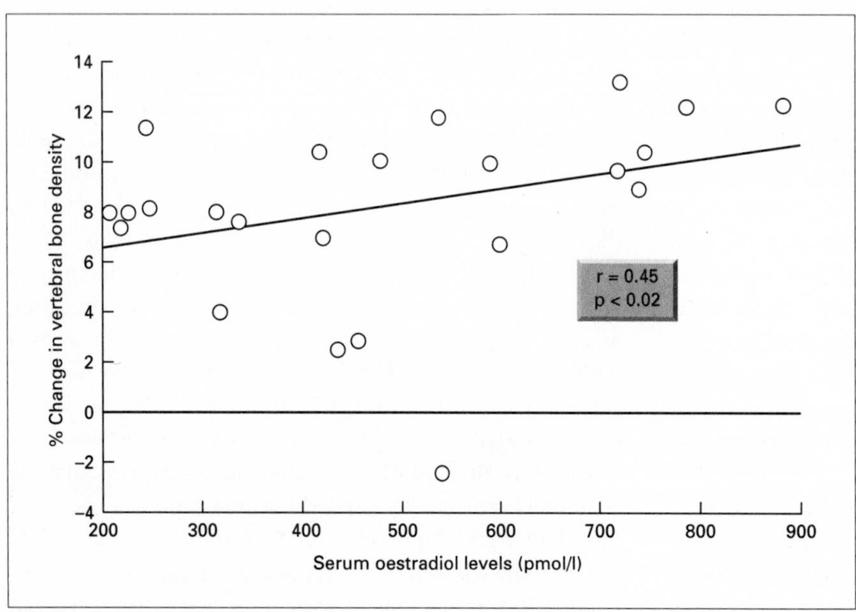

Fig. 56.8 Increase in bone density in 40 menopausal patients compared with serum oestradiol levels after 1 year's treatment with oestradiol implants. Adapted from [52].

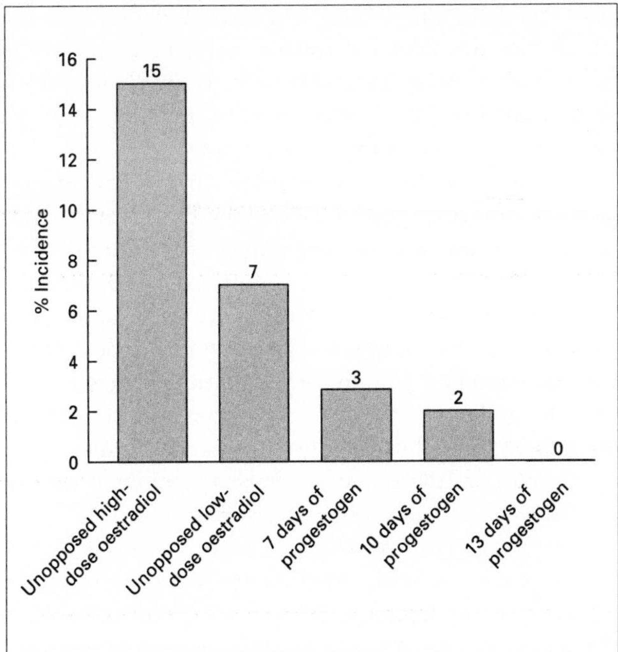

Fig. 56.9 Incidence of cystic hyperplasia in 745 women treated with oestrogen replacement therapy. Adapted from [72].

togens such as norethisterone cause the greatest change whilst progesterone derivatives, such as dydrogesterone [74], have little effect. Negative mood effects are produced by most progestogens due to the effect on neurotransmitters via central nervous system progesterone receptors [75]. These symptoms are common and seem to occur more often in patients with a past history of premenstrual syndrome. They are dose and duration dependent and may be influenced by the type of progestogen [76].

Manipulation of the dosage and duration of progestogen, continuous low-dose progestogen and a reduction in the number of progestogenic episodes can be used to improve compliance. Cyclical progestogens should always be used in the minimum dose and for the shortest possible duration [77] (Table 56.4). In an attempt to alleviate progestogenic symptoms and avoid the regular withdrawal bleed, studies of continuous oestrogen–progestogen therapy have been undertaken. Magos *et al.* [47], using oral conjugated equine oestrogen (Premarin, Wyeth) and low-dose norethisterone, eventually achieved amenorrhoea in all patients, but there was a drop-out rate of 34.7% from spotting particularly during the early part of the study. Therapy was even less successful in patients treated with oestradiol implants, as all patients invariably suffered from irregular bleeding.

A recent approach has been to give continuous oestrogens to women using the levonorgestrel- and progesterone-releasing coils and vaginal progesterone gel (Fig. 56.10). Studies with these coils have shown that although bleeding may be irregular in the first 3–6 months, approximately 70% of patients achieve complete amenorrhoea after a year [78,79] with no endometrial hyperplasia. The predominantly local action of these systems minimises systemic side-effects but, at the time of writing they are not yet licensed for use as progestogenic opposition for oestrogen therapy. Adverse effects can also be avoided by making use of the progesterone receptor-specific progestogens such as the pregnanes, for example cyproterone, norpregnanes, nomegestrol and progesterone itself. Hysterectomy remains an option for the severely progestogen-intolerant woman. In women without a uterus there has been a suggestion that the addition of cyclical progestogen will protect the breast, but there is no evidence to support such a view and the consensus is that women without a uterus do not need cyclical progestogen. In the future, progestogen intolerance may not be an issue. Selective oestrogen-receptor modulators (SERMS), agonistic to the cardiovascular, skeletal and central nervous system and antagonistic to endometrium and breast, may provide a complete alternative to HRT. These are currently in development and will probably be on the market in a few years' time.

Table 56.4 Minimum doses of progestogen given orally in hormone-replacement therapy as endometrial protection (taken for 12 days per month).

Progestogen type	Dose
Micronised progesterone	200 mg/day
Dydrogesterone	10 mg/day
Medroxyprogesterone	5 mg/day
Norethisterone	1 mg/day
Norgestrel	150 μg/day
Cyproterone	1 mg/day

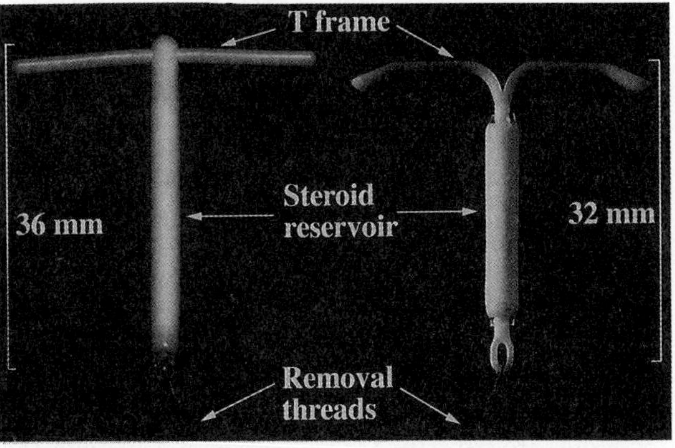

Fig. 56.10 Progesterone (left) and levonorgestrel (right) releasing intrauterine systems.

Progesterone cream

Recently interest has been generated into exploring the potential of natural progesterone cream derived from plant sources, including wild yam, where it is found in its precursor form, diosgenin. Nutritionists and some doctors claim that it is sufficient in itself to provide relief of short- and long-term menopausal problems including reversal of osteoporosis. Unfortunately, the bone data are only from a few uncontrolled cases. It certainly does appear to have minimal adverse effects and anecdotally some patients do seem to derive benefits of increased energy, libido and improved skin. However, prospective, randomised, placebo-controlled studies are necessary to confirm the claims of its benefits; these are currently being performed. It would also be interesting to see whether it could be used as progestogenic opposition for oestrogen therapy.

Contraindications

Considerable confusion has been caused by the UK Drug Licensing Board inaccurately linking the contraindications of HRT with those of the oral contraceptives, and even in the current British National Formulary for the contra-indications and side-effects of preparations for menopausal symptoms the reader is directed to the section for combined oral contraceptives. Previous myocardial infarction or angina, hypertension, varicose veins, diabetes, endometriosis, fibroids and gallstones are all linked to oral contraceptive use, but are not contraindications for oestrogen-replacement therapy.

Epidemiological studies have consistently shown an increased incidence of heart disease in women using the oral contraceptive pill but heart attacks are significantly *decreased* with oestrogen-replacement therapy [80]. Since oestrogens are protective against heart disease, it may be strongly argued that women with angina, a previous myocardial infarction and a family history of heart disease or hyperlipidaemia should be treated with HRT. Indeed, the epidemiological studies from the Leisure World retirement community support the view that oestrogens reduce heart attacks in all high-risk groups except in smokers [80].

Similarly, hypertension, because of its association with heart disease, has also been considered as a contraindication to HRT. The natural oestrogens when given to normotensive or hypertensive women do not cause an elevation in blood pressure, and when given in combination with oral progesterone may actually lower blood pressure [81]; therefore, there is no justification for withholding HRT from hypertensive women.

Fibroids are responsive to oestrogens, and involute after the menopause. HRT will continue to stimulate these benign gynaecological tumours causing some to increase in size. This can cause an increase in menstrual blood loss, but in practice this does not usually represent a problem as treatment can easily be discontinued. However, in patients with a good indication who wish to continue therapy, a hysterectomy is a possible compromise.

Endometriosis which is stimulated by cyclical ovarian activity can cause considerable pain and many patients with severe disease eventually require hysterectomy, often with bilateral oophorectomy. Unfortunately, because of a fear of using oestrogens, the ovaries are often conserved at operation and continue to stimulate the endometriosis causing continued pain in these women. Henderson *et al.* [82] have shown that 50% of women will continue to have pain until all ovarian tissue is removed, after which continuous oestrogen may safely be administered without risk of recurrence of endometriosis or pain.

Treatment of patients with a past history of endometrial cancer is controversial, but there are reports of oestrogen use without any detrimental effects [83]. Breast cancer must be regarded as the principal contraindication to oestrogen treatment, but high-risk women with a strong family history of breast malignancy or those with benign breast disease should not necessarily be denied treatment. Oestrogen therapy should be offered with advice on regular self-examination, physician examination and mammography.

Complications

The principal objection to HRT is the need for a regular withdrawal bleed in a patient with a uterus. Although this may be acceptable in a woman aged 50 years, it may be intolerable 10 years later, particularly as it may be heavy, painful and associated with cyclical premenstrual-like symptoms. Women may also develop mastalgia when starting hormones, especially if they are a few years after the menopause, but usually find all of these symptoms more tolerable if an explanation is given before starting treatment. They should be reassured that mastalgia does not indicate breast cancer and that the symptoms will decrease with time.

Unopposed oestrogen therapy is associated with an increased risk of endometrial cancer. This risk is fourfold and should be compared with the similar fourfold increase seen in women who are more than 50 lb (23 kg) overweight. The addition of cyclical progestogen therapy for 7–13 days each month will reduce this risk to less than that found in untreated women, and combined therapy should thus be offered to all women with an intact uterus.

There is no evidence to implicate HRT in the aetiology of carcinoma of the cervix or of any increase in the incidence of epithelial ovarian tumours (Table 56.5). It seems likely that cyclical opposed HRT may even confer some protective effect against ovarian cancer by decreasing levels of FSH.

The available epidemiological evidence relating to breast cancer is confusing but mostly reassuring. The studies are mostly related to the use of oral conjugated oestrogens. Although recent results from the Nurse's Health Study show a slightly increased relative risk of breast cancer after 5 or more years of oestrogen therapy [84], many meta-analyses fail to provide strong evidence for a risk increasing effect [85]. This indicates that if an adverse effect exists, it is small. It is likely that the slight excess can be explained by the increased surveillance, i.e. breast palpation and mammography, that women receiving oestrogen therapy have compared with women who are not under their physician's care for such therapy. This would lead to an increased diagnosis of early-stage tumours. There may also be a confusion of diagnosis in this hormone-dependent tissue in the same way as there was with endometrial hyperplasia and carcinoma 10 years ago. This view is supported by the finding of a significantly decreased mortality rate from breast cancer in patients receiving oestrogen therapy found in both the Hunt *et al.* [26] study (Table 56.5) and a subsequent paper from Bergkvist *et al.* [86]. Nevertheless, fear of breast cancer is the major anxiety about HRT and a question that needs urgent and precise clarification.

Conclusion

The decline in ovarian function which culminates in the menopause gives rise to a hormone-deficiency state which causes profound changes in women. Although not all women will suffer the distressing short-term symptomatic sequelae of ovarian failure, there is no doubt that all will experience the long-term oestrogen-deficient effects ranging from vaginal atrophy to an increased risk of osteoporosis and cardiovascular disease. The implications of failing to treat the increasing number of post-menopausal women early will be greater morbidity rates and considerable health-care costs; particularly as the benefits of HRT are even more extensive than once supposed, in the prophylaxis of the cardiovascular, skeletal and central nervous systems. The decision to treat a woman with HRT should therefore be considered very carefully. There are few real contraindications and a strong case can be made for the use of HRT to improve the quality of life in most women.

There has been a rapid expansion in the number of HRT preparations available over the last few years. This has led to confusion as to what should be prescribed as many of these 'new' regimens do not seem to provide a true advance in treatment. However, the development of less androgenic progestogens, continuous combined regimens, long-cycle HRT and the hormone-releasing coils have all been beneficial in providing ways of reducing progestogenic side-effects and minimising bleeding problems. This will inevitably improve uptake of HRT and compliance. Future research should focus on discovering the full extent to which HRT benefits the body systems and on the further development of HRT regimens which minimise adverse effects allowing the benefits to predominate.

References

1 Chakravati S, Collins W, Newton J, Oram D, Studd JWW. Endocrine changes and symptomatology after oophorectomy in premenopausal women. *Br J Obstet Gynaecol* 1977; **84**: 769–75.

2 Casper RF, Yen SSC, Wilkes MM. Menopausal hot flushes: a neurendocrine link with pulsatile luteinizing hormone secretion. *Science* 1979; **205**: 823–5.

3 Montgomery J, Appleby L, Brincat M *et al.* Effects of oestrogen and testosterone implants on psychological disorders of the climacteric. *Lancet* 1987; **i**: 297–9.

Table 56.5 Mortality in patients on hormone-replacement therapy by cause of death. Adapted from [26].

	Number of deaths	
Cause of death (ICD 9th revision)	Ratio observed/expected	95% confidence limits
Carcinoma of the breast	0.55	0.28–0.96
Carcinoma of the endometrium	—	0–1.78
Carcinoma of the cervix	0.71	0.08–2.56
Carcinoma of the ovary	1.43	0.62–2.82
Other neoplasms	0.69	0.48–0.96
All neoplasms	0.66	0.50–0.86
Ischaemic heart disease	0.48	0.29–0.74
Cerebrovascular disease	0.65	0.35–1.09
Suicide	2.53	0.26–4.54
All deaths due to injury	1.73	0.95–2.92
Other causes	0.34	0.19–0.57
All causes	0.59	0.49–0.70

4 Jaszman L. Epidemiology of the climacteric complaints. *Front Horm Res* 1973; **2**: 220–34.

5 Gath D, Iles S. Depression and the menopause. *Br Med J* 1990; **300**: 1287–8.

6 Watson NR, Studd JWW, Riddle AF, Savvas M. Suppression of ovulation by transdermal oestradiol patches. *Br Med J* 1988; **297**: 900–1.

7 Magos AL, Brincat M, Studd JWW. Treatment of the premenstrual syndrome by subcutaneous oestradiol implants and cyclical norethisterone in the treatment of premenstrual syndrome. *Br Med J* 1986; **i**: 1629–33.

8 Watson NR, Studd JWW, Sawas M, Garnett.T. Baber RJ. Treatment of severe premenstrual syndrome with oestradiol patches and cyclical oral norethisterone. *Lancet* 1989; **ii**: 730–4.

9 Gregoire AJP, Kumar, Everitt B, Henderson, AF, Studd JWW. Transdermal oestrogen for treatment of severe postnatal depression. *Lancet* 1996; **347**: 930–3.

10 Brincat M, Moniz C, Studd JWW, Darby A, Magos A, Embury G, Versi E. Long term effects of the menopause and sex hormones on skin thickness. *Br J Obstet Gynaecol* 1985; **92**: 256–9.

11 Compston JE, Cooper C, Kanis JA. Bone densitometry in clinical practice. *Br Med J* 1995; **310**: 1507–10.

12 Nordin BEC. Osteomalacia, osteoporosis and calcium deficiency. *Clin Orthop* 1960; **17**: 235–57.

13 Stevenson JC, White MC, Jopun GF, MacIntyre I. Osteoporosis and calcitonin deficiency. *Br Med J* 1982; **285**: 1010–11.

14 Albright F, Smith P, Richardson A. Postmenopausal osteoporosis, its clinical features. *JAMA* 1941; **116**: 2465–74.

15 Castelli W. Epidemiology of coronary heart disease: the Framingham study. *Am J Med* 1984; **76**: 4–12.

16 Stampfer MJ, Colditz GA, Willett WC *et al.* Post menopausal oestrogen therapy and cardiovascular disease: ten year follow up from the Nurse's Health Study. *N Engl J Med* 1991; **325**: 756–62.

17 Fahraeus L, Wallentin L. High density lipoprotein subfractions during oral and cutaneous administration of 17β-estradiol to menopausal women. *J Clin Endocrinol Metab* 1983; **56**: 797–801.

18 Funk JL, Mortel KF, Meyer JS. Effects of estrogen replacement therapy on cerebral perfusion and cognition amongst post-menopausal women. *Dementia* 1991; **2**: 268–272.

19 Butler RN, Aronheim H, Fillet H, Rapoport S, Tatemichi TK. Vascular dementia: stroke prevention takes on new urgency. *Geriatrics* 1993; **48**: 32–4.

20 Bueb LP, Hob PR, Bouras C *et al.* Pathological alterations of the cerebral microvasculature in *Alzheimer's* disease and related dementing disorders. 1994; **87**: 469–80.

21 Jaffe AB, Toran-Allerand D, Greengard P, Gandy SE. Estrogen regulates metabolism of Alzheimer Amyloid β precursor protein. *J Biol Chem* 1994; **269**: 13065–8.

22 Henderson VW, Paganini-Hill A, Emanuel CK, Dunn ME, Buckwalter JG. Estrogen replacement therapy in older women. *Arch Neurol* 1994; **51**: 896–900.

23 Ming-Xin T, Jacobs D, Stern Y *et al.* Effect of oestrogen during the menopause on risk and age at onset of Alzheimer's disease. *Lancet* 1996; **348**: 429–32.

24 Studd JWW, Thom M, Dische F, Driver M, Wade Evans T, Williams D. Value of cytology for detecting endometrial abnormalities in climacteric women receiving hormone replacement therapy. *Br Med J* 1979; **i**: 846–8.

25 Hillner BE, Hollenberg JP, Pauker SG. Postmenopausal estrogens in prevention of osteoporosis. Benefit virtually without risk if cardiovascular effects are considered. *Am J Med* 1986; **80**: 5–27.

26 Hunt K, Vessey MP, McPherson K, Coleman M. Long-term surveillance of mortality and cancer incidence in women receiving hormone replacement therapy. *Br J Obstet Gynaecol* 1987; **94**: 620–35.

27 Bush TL, Cowan LD, Barrett-Connor E *et al.* Estrogen use and all-cause mortality. Preliminary results from the Lipid Research Clinics Program Follow-Up Study. *JAMA* 1983; **249**: 903–6.

28 Johansson BW, Kaij L, Kullander S, Lenner H-C, Svanberg L, Astedt B. On some late effects of bilateral oophorectomy in the age range 15–30 years. *Acta Obstet Gynecol Scand* 1975; **54**: 449–61.

29 Oliver MF, Boyds GS. Effect of bilateral ovariectomy on coronary artery disease and serum lipid levels. *Lancet* 1959; **ii**: 690–4.

30 Siddle N, Sarrel P, Whitehead M. The effect of hysterectomy on the age of ovarian failure. *Fertil Steril* 1987; **47**: 94–100.

31 Watson NR, Studd JWW, Garnett T, Savvas M, Milligan P. Bone loss after hysterectomy with ovarian conservation. *Obstet Gynecol* 1995; **86**: 72–7.

32 Cardozo L, Gibb D, Tuck S, Thom M, Studd JWW, Cooper D. The use of hormone implants for climacteric symptoms. *Am J Obstet Gynecol* 1984; **148**: 336–40.

33 Clayden J, Bell J, Pollard P. Menopausal flushing: double blind trial of a non-hormonal preparation. *Br Med J* 1974; **1**: 409–12.

34 Lindsay R, Hart DM. Failure of response of menopausal vasomotor symptoms to clonidine. *Maturitas* 1978; **1**: 21–5.

35 Notelovitz M. Non-hormonal management of the menopause. In: Studd JWW, Whitehead M, eds. *The Menopause*. Oxford: Blackwell Scientific Publications, 1988: 102–15.

36 Heaney R, Gallagher J, Johnston C, Neer R, Parfitt AM, Whedon GD. Calcium nutrition and bone health in the elderly. *Am J Clin Nutr* 1982; **36** (Suppl.): 986–1013.

37 Ettinger B, Genant HK, Cann CE. Postmenopausal bone loss is prevented by treatment with low-dosage estrogen with calcium. *Ann Intern Med* 1978; **106**: 40–5.

38 Wallach S, Cohn SH, Ellis KJ, Kohberger R, Aloia JF, Zanzi I. Effect of salmon calcitonin on skeletal mass in osteoporosis. *Curr Ther Res Clin Exp* 1977; **22**: 556–72.

39 Stevenson JC, Abeyasekera G, Hillyard CJ *et al.* Regulation of calcium-regulating hormones by exogenous sex steroids in early menopause. *Eur J Clin Invest* 1983; **13**: 481–7.

40 Watts NB, Harris ST, Genant HK, Sorensen OH. Intermittent cyclical etidronate treatment of postmenopausal osteoporosis. *N Engl J Med* 1990; **323**: 73–9.

41 Dalen N, Olloson KE. Bone mineral content and physical activity. *Acta Orthopaed Scand* 1974; **45**: 170–4.

42 Lievertz RW. Pharmacology and pharmokinetics of oestrogens. *Am J Obstet Gynecol* 1987; **156**: 1289–93.

43 Silverstolpe G, Gustafson A, Samsioe G, Svanborg A. Lipid metabolic studies in oophorectomised women: effects induced by two different estrogens on serum lipids and lipoproteins. *Gynecol Obstet Invest* 1980; **11**: 161–9.

44 Mashchak C, Lobo R, Dozono-Takano R *et al.* Comparison of pharmacodynamic properties of various oestrogen formulations. *Am J Obstet Gynecol* 1982; **144**: 511–18.

45 Poller L, Thomson JM, Thomson W. Oestrogen/progestogen oral contraceptive and blood clotting: a long term follow up. *Br Med J* 1971; **4**: 648–50.

46 Rosenberg L, Amstrong B, Jick M. Myocardial infarction and oestrogen therapy in postmenopausal women. *N Engl J Med* 1976; **294**: 1256–9.

47 Magos AL, Brincat M, Studd JWW, Wardle P, Schlesinger P, O'Dowd T. Amenorrhoea and endometrial atrophy with continuous oral oestrogen and progestogen therapy in postmenopausal women.

Obstet Gynaecol 1985; **65**: 496–9.

48 Ettinger B, Selby J, Citron JT, Ettinger VM, Hendrickson MR. Cyclic hormone replacement therapy using quarterly progestin. *Obstet Gynaecol* 1994; **83**: 693–700.

49 Whitehead MI, Mirandi J, Kitchin Y, Sharples M. Systematic absorption of oestrogen from Premarin vaginal cream. In: Cooke ID, ed. *The Role of Estrogen/Progestogen in the Management of the Menopause*. Lancaster: MTP Press, 1978: 63–71.

50 Mandel FP, Geola FL, Meldrum DR *et al.* Biological effects of various doses of vaginally administered conjugated equine estrogens in post-menopausal women. *J Clin Endocrinol Metab* 1983; **57**: 133–9.

51 Sitruk-Ware R. Transdermal delivery of steroids. *Contraception* 1989; **39**: 1–20.

52 Powers MS, Shenkel L, Darley PE, Good WR, Balestra JC, Place VA. Pharmokinetics and pharmacodynamics of transdermal dosage forms of 17β-estradiol: comparison with conventional oral estrogen used for hormone replacement. *Am J Obstet Gynecol* 1985; **152**: 1099–106.

53 Chetkowski RJ, Meldrum DR, Steingold KA *et al.* Biologic effects of transdermal estradiol. *N Engl J Med* 1986; **314**: 1615–20.

54 The Transdermal HRT Investigators Group. A randomised study to compare the effectiveness, tolerability and acceptability of two different transdermal estradiol replacement therapies. *Int J Fertil* 1993; **38**: 5–11.

55 Laufer LR, De Fazio LJ, Lu JKH *et al.* Estrogen replacement therapy by transdermal estradiol administration. *Am J Obstet Gynecol* 1983; **146**: 533–40.

56 Steingold KA, Laufer L, Chetkowski RJ *et al.* Treatment of hot flashes with transdermal estradiol administration. *J Clin Endocrinol Metab* 1985; **61**: 627–32.

57 Adami S, Suppi R, Bertoldo F *et al.* Transdermal estradiol in the treatment of postmenopausal bone loss. *Bone Miner* 1989; **7**: 79–86.

58 Stevenson JC, Cust MP, Ganger KF, Hillard TC, Lees B, Whitehead MI. Effects of transdermal versus oral hormone replacement therapy on bone density in spine and proximal femur in postmenopausal women. *Lancet* 1990; **336**: 265–8.

59 Lyrenas S, Carlstrom K, Backstrom T, von Schoultz B. A comparison of serum oestrogen levels after percutaneous and oral administration of oestradiol 17β. *Br J Obstet Gynaecol* 1981; **88**: 181–7.

60 Brincat M, Versi E, O'Dowd T, Moniz C, Magos A, Kabalan S, Studd JWW. Skin collagen changes in postmenopausal women treated with oestradiol gel. *Maturitas* 1987; **9**: 1–5.

61 Bishop PMF. A clinical experiment in oestrin therapy. *Br Med J* 1938; **1**: 939.

62 Greenblatt RB, Suran RR. Indications for hormone pellets in the therapy of endocrine and gynecological disorders. *Am J Obstet Gynecol* 1949; **47**: 294–301.

63 Thom MH, Studd JWW. Procedures in practice—hormone implantation. *Br Med J* 1980; i: 848.

64 Brincat M, Magos AL, Studd JWW. Subcutaneous hormone implants for the control of climacteric symptoms. *Lancet* 1984; i: 16–18.

65 Savvas M, Studd JWW, Fogelman I, Dooley M, Montgomery J, Murby B. Skeletal effects of oral oestrogen compared with subcutaneous oestrogen and testosterone in post-menopausal women. *Br Med J* 1988; **297**: 331–3.

66 Studd JWW, Savvas M, Watson NR, Garnett T, Cooper D. Substantial increase in bone density with subcutaneous oestradiol and testosterone implants. *Am J Obstet Gynecol* 1990; **163**: 1474–9.

67 Garnett T, Studd JWW, Henderson A, Watson N, Savvas M. Hormone implants and tachyphylaxis. *Br J Obstet Gynaecol* 1990; **97**: 917–21.

68 Studd JWW, Watson NR. Oestrogens and depression. In: Belfort P, Pinotti JA, Eskes TKAB, eds. *Advances in Gynecology and Obstetrics*, Vol. 6. St Louis: Mosby Year Book 1988: 297–301.

69 Ganger K, Cust M, Whitehead MI. Symptoms of oestrogen deficiency associated with supraphysiological plasma oestradiol concentrations in women with oestradiol implants. *Br Med J* 1989; **299**: 601–2.

70 Studd JWW, Henderson A, Garnett T, Watson N, Sawas M. Symptoms of oestrogen deficiency in women with oestradiol implants. *Br Med J* 1989; **299**: 1400–1.

71 Albright F. Metropathia haemorrhagia. *J Maine Med Ass* 1938; **29**: 235–8.

72 Sturdee DW, Wade-Evans T, Paterson MEL, Studd JWW. Relations between bleeding pattern, endometrial histology, and oestrogen treatment in the postmenopausal women. *Br Med J* 1978; i: 1575–7.

73 Studd JWW, Thom M. Oestrogens and endometrial cancer. In: Studd JWW, ed. *Progress in Obstetrics and Gynaecology*, Vol. 1. Edinburgh: Churchill Livingstone, 1981: 182–98.

74 Siddle NC, Jesinger DK, Whitehead MI. Effect on plasma lipids and lipoproteins of postmenopausal oestrogen therapy with added dydrogesterone. *Br J Obstet Gynaecol* 1990; **97**: 1093–100.

75 Backstrom T, Bixo M, Seippel L, Sundstrom I, Wang M. Progestins and behaviour. In: Gennazzani AR, Petraglia F, Purdy RH, eds. *The Brain: Source and Target for Sex Steroid Hormones*. New York: The Parthenon Publishing Group, 1996: 277–91.

76 Magos AL, Brewester E, Singh R, O'Dowd T, Brincat M, Studd JWW. The effects of norethisterone in postmenopausal women on oestrogen replacement therapy: a model for the premenstrual syndrome. *Br J Obstet Gynaecol* 1986; **93**: 1290–6.

77 Consensus statement on progestin use in postmenopausal women. *Maturitas* 1988; **11**: 175–7.

78 Panay N, Studd JWW, Thomas A *et al.* The levonorgestrel intrauterine system as progestogenic opposition for oestrogen replacement therapy. *Presentation at Annual Meeting of the British Menopause Society*, Exeter, July 1996.

79 Raudaskoski TH, Lahti EI, Kauppila AJ *et al.* Transdermal estrogen with a levonorgestrel-releasing intrauterine device for climacteric complaints: clinical and endometrial responses. *Am J Obstet Gynaecol* 1995; **172**: 114–9.

80 Henderson BE, Paginini-Hill A, Ross RK. Estrogen replacement therapy and protection from acute myocardial infarction. *Am J Obstet Gynecol* 1988: **159**: 312–17.

81 Hammond CB, Jelovesk F, Leer K, Creasman W, Parker R. Effects of long-term estrogen replacement therapy. 1. Metabolic effects. *Am J Obstet Gynecol* 1976; **133**: 525–35.

82 Henderson AF, Studd JWW, Watson NR. A retrospective study of oestrogen replacement therapy after hysterectomy for endometriosis. In: *Proceedings of the ICI Symposium on Endometriosis*. Carnforth: Parthenon Press, 1989.

83 Creasman WT, Henderson D, Hinshaw W, Clarke-Pearson DL. Estrogen replacement therapy in the patient treated for endometrial cancer. *Obstet Gynecol* 1986; **67**: 326–30.

84 Colditz GA, Hankinson SE, Hunter DJ *et al.* The use of estrogens and progestins and the risk of breast cancer in postmenopausal women. *N Engl J Med* 1995; **332**: 1589–93.7

85 Steinberg KK, Smith SJ, Thacker SB, Stroup DF. Breast cancer risk and duration of estrogen use: the role of study design in meta-analysis. *Epidemiology* 1994; **5**: 415–21.

86 Bergkvist L, Adami H, Persson I, Bergstrom R, Krusemo U. Prognosis after breast cancer diagnosis in women exposed to estrogen and estrogen–progestogen replacement therapy. *Am J Epidemiol* 1989; **130**: 221–8

Part 11
Sexual Differentiation

CHAPTER 57

Sexual differentiation

N. Josso and R. Rey

Introduction

The sex of an individual results from a series of choices occurring at different times of fetal development. The first and most important event is the establishment of gonadal sex, this determines which pathway, i.e. the male or female, will be followed during subsequent steps of sex differentiation. Gender identity, also called psychological sex, is usually determined by the sex of rearing, although hormonal factors may also be involved. Emphasis in this chapter has been placed deliberately on recent developments in the field of human sex differentiation and this bias is reflected in the selection of cited references.

Establishment of gonadal sex

Testicular differentiation

In the mammalian fetus, the gonadal primordium is represented by the gonadal ridge (Fig. 57.1), a thickening of the coelomic epithelium covering the anterior surface of the mesonephros, which is progressively colonised by primordial germ cells travelling from the stalk of the allantois through the mesentery and the wall of the fetal gut. The first recognisable event of testicular differentiation is the development of a new cell type, the primordial Sertoli cells, which soon aggregate to form seminiferous tubules in which germ cells become enclosed. Spermatogonia trapped in testicular tubules do not undergo meiosis until the beginning of puberty, in contrast to extragonadal and female germ cells, which enter the prophase of the first meiotic division early in fetal life [1]. In the human fetus, the testis can be recognised as early as 7 weeks after fertilisation.

Fetal Sertoli cells are large, clear cells, with abundant cytoplasm containing vesicles of rough endoplasmic reticulum. These vesicles store, prior to secretion, a glycoprotein, anti-Müllerian hormone (AMH), which is responsible for the inhibition of the development of the Müllerian ducts in male fetuses [2]. AMH expression requires a relatively advanced differentiation of primitive Sertoli cells, its expression at 8 weeks in the human fetus coincides approximately with the formation of seminiferous tubules [3] (Fig. 57.2). Another Sertoli-cell marker, sulphated glycoprotein 2, alias clusterin, is produced somewhat later, at 17 days of gestation in the mouse, compared with 12 days for AMH [4].

Leydig cells differentiate at 8 weeks of gestation in the human fetus. Their number increases dramatically until 14–16 weeks, at which time they begin to degenerate. At birth, very few remain in the interstitial tissue. Fetal Leydig cells produce testosterone, the hormone responsible for the virilisation of Wolffian derivatives, urogenital sinus and external genital organs.

Ovarian differentiation

Initially slower than the testis to differentiate, the fetal ovary eventually reaches a more advanced stage of maturation. Up to the second month of gestation, ovogonia mix freely with somatic cells in the gonadal blastema. Later, growth of connective-tissue sheets from the medulla outwards delineates ovigerous cords, containing actively dividing ovogonia, which tend to accumulate near the ovarian surface. At 12–13 weeks some oogonia, located in the deepest layer of the cortex, have entered meiotic prophase. Maturation progresses from the centre of the gonad towards the periphery, until, at approximately 7 months gestation, all germ cells have entered or completed the meiotic prophase, and mitotic divisions are no longer seen. The X chromosome, which, in ovogonia, undergoes inactivation as in somatic cells, is reactivated at the onset of meiosis [5,6].

In parallel, the germ-cell pool is severely depleted by waves of degeneration, which preferentially affect cells undergoing

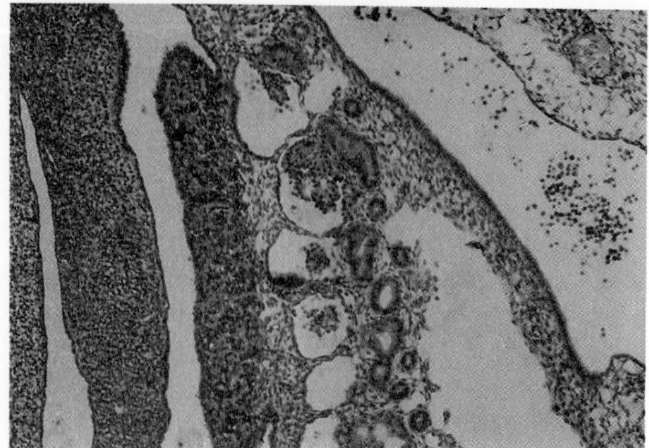

Fig. 57.1 Gonadal ridge from a 5-week human fetus. The undifferentiated gonad projects into the coelomic cavity. From [51], with permission.

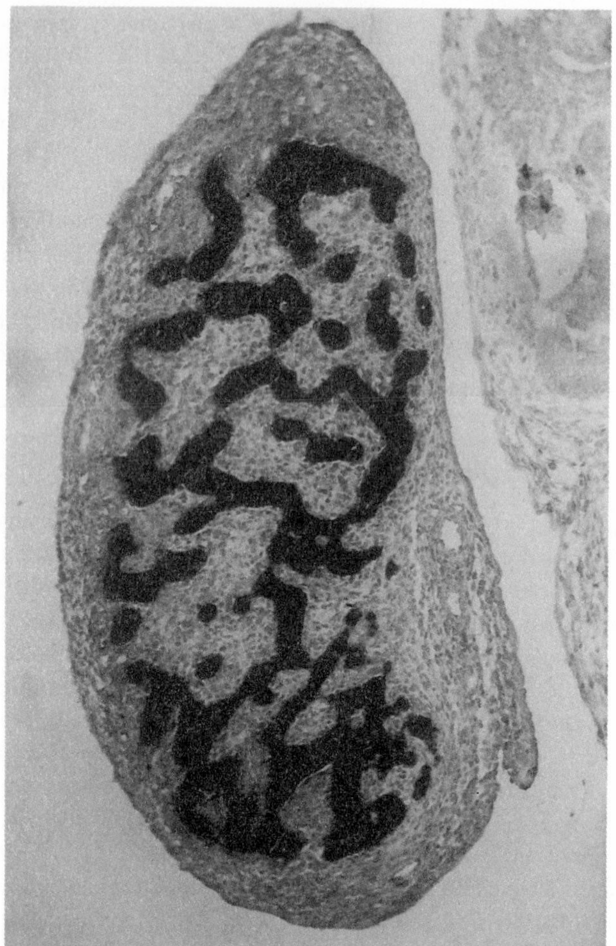

Fig. 57.2 Immunohistochemical localization of anti-Müllerian hormone (AMH) in the seminiferous tubules of a human fetal testis at 11 weeks.

mitotic divisions or in the meiotic prophase. Germ cells enclosed in follicles are relatively protected from degeneration. Primordial follicles can be recognised by 17 weeks, and Graafian follicles by 26 weeks [7]. Fetal granulosa cells produce oestrogen at the same developmental stage at which fetal testes produce testosterone [8]. In contrast, ovarian production of AMH can be demonstrated only after birth [9].

Mechanisms of sex determination

Since the gonad determines whether the male or female pathway of sex differentiation will prevail [10], the choice of gonadal sex has been called sex determination [11]. In mammals, sex determination is essentially controlled by a Y-located 'testis-determining gene', *SRY*, which interacts with autosomal and X-linked genes to induce testicular development.

The *SRY* gene

From the time the Y chromosome was first recognised as the bearer of genetic information responsible for male sex determination [12], the quest for the testis-determining factor (TDF) has been particularly eventful. The initial hypothesis that TDF was the product of a gene coding for the male-specific antigen HY was abandoned when it was realised that the loci for HY antigen and TDF are separate [13]. Human HY has now been identified as an 11-residue peptide derived from SMCY, an evolutionary conserved protein encoded on the long arm of Y chromosome [14].

Later approaches exploited genomic maps of the Y TDF, using DNA from sex-reversed individuals to narrow the search down to specific regions of the Y chromosome (Fig. 57.3). The Y chromosome is divided into pseudo-autosomal regions, shared with the X chromosome and subject to recombination at the time of meiosis, and Y-specific regions which do not normally recombine (reviewed in [11]). By definition, TDF must reside on the latter, but it may occasionally be transferred to the X chromosome in the event of abnormal recombination.

Conserved Y loci present in XX males and absent in XY females are potential candidates for the TDF title. The first serious contender was *ZFY*, located about 100 kb from the pseudo-autosomal region [15], but it was eliminated when four 46XX individuals with testicular development were found to have inherited a fragment of their fathers' Y chromosome that did not include *ZFY* [16]. Detailed genetic analysis narrowed the search to a 35-kb region, fragments of which were used to probe male and female DNA from different mammalian species. The open reading frame detected on the only fragment harbouring a conserved Y-specific sequence was christened *SRY* (for sex region Y)

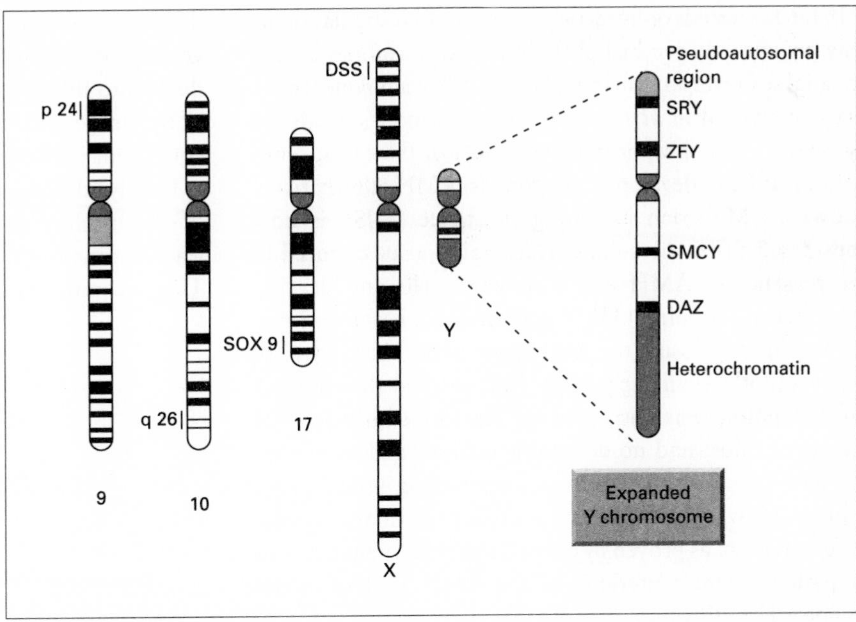

Fig. 57.3 Genes involved in sex determination and their chromosomal localisation. In mammals, testicular determination depends upon a Y-located gene, *SRY* [11], which interacts with autosomal and X-linked genes. Probable partners for *SRY* in sex determination are the X-located *DSS* [30], the autosome *SOX*-9 [27] and loci that have been located to 9p24 [28] and 10q26 [28,29]. The HY antigen, derived from *SMCY* [14] and *ZFY* [15] have been successively proposed as the testicular determining factor before *SRY*. The gene *DAZ*, although not involved in testicular determination, is necessary for normal spermatogenesis [52].

and strong evidence now equates it to the conceptual TDF. XX mice transgenic for a 14-kb DNA fragment containing the mouse *SRY* gene develop as males, albeit infertile ones [17]. The human and mouse genes are composed of a single exon and have little in common, apart from a 79 amino-acid DNA-binding domain, HMG (for high-mobility group), present in many transcription factors. *SRY* binds to a A/TAACAAT sequence [18] but this element, present in more than 10^5 sites in the human genome including the AMH and aromatase promoters [19], is not sufficient to define target genes for *SRY* [11]. The binding specificity of *SRY* is rather low, all the more since numerous substitutions in the target site are allowed and *SRY* also binds, in a non-sequence specific manner, to cruciform (four-way junction) DNA structures, which probably arise *in vivo* during transcription. Mutations of the *SRY* gene occur predominantly in the HMG box but are detectable only in 15–20% of XY sex-reversed females [20].

Autosomal and X-linked genes involved in sex determination (Fig. 57.3)

SRY requires interaction with other genes to achieve testis development. Its expression, restricted to the fetal genital ridge and later to the germ cells of the adult testis [21], is probably controlled by upstream genes which have not yet been identified. WT1, a tumour suppressor [22] and SF1, an orphan nuclear receptor [23], have been considered because both are essential to gonadal development in both sexes, but their involvement in sex determination has not been documented.

Other genes probably act in conjunction with or downstream of *SRY*. In the wood lemming *Myopus schisticolor*, a gene on the X chromosome apparently inactivates the sex-determining gene on the Y chromosome, generating a class of XY females [24]. In the mouse, normal testis determination depends on proper genetic interaction of the Y chromosome with a locus on chromosome 17, which is disrupted when the Y chromosome is bred onto the genetic background of certain inbred strains of mice [25].

In humans, the situation is even more complex. The human *SRY* gene lacks a transcriptional activator domain [26]; thus, signal transduction probably requires the cooperation of a partner protein with activating domains. Mutation of *SOX-9*, a gene located on chromosome 17, leads to failure of testicular development in XY patients with a normal *SRY* gene [27]. Monosomy of 9p [28] or 10q [28,29] is also associated with XY sex reversal. Duplication of Xp21–22 leads to sex-reversal in XY subjects. This has suggested that two active copies of a gene called *DSS*, mapping to a 160-kb region of Xp21, can override the effect of *SRY*, providing a link between the ovarian and testicular pathways [30]. However, at the present time, the mode of interaction of these autosomal or X-linked loci with *SRY* has not been elucidated.

Environmental and hormonal factors involved in sex determination

Non-genetic sex-determining mechanisms operate preferentially in lower vertebrates with no individualised sex chromosomes. In some species of reptiles, environmental factors, such as incubation temperature, drive sex differentiation along either the male or female pathway [31].

In birds, steroids or intracoelomic grafts of testicular tissue may produce sex reversal [32]. Testicular hormones induce gonadal sex reversal in mammals also. When a bovine female fetus is exposed *in utero* to testicular hormones produced by a male twin, in approximately 50% of the cases, seminiferous tubules develop in her gonads. AMH, alternatively known as Müllerian inhibiting substance (MIS), is now considered to be the culprit. Rat fetal ovaries cultured in the presence of AMH lose their germ cells and develop seminiferous tubules [33]. Construction of a transgenic mouse line expressing the AMH gene under the control of the metallothionein 1 promoter [34] showed that ovarian differentiation was disrupted in females expressing the transgene; most had no detectable ovaries, and those that did developed ovarian structures resembling seminiferous tubules. However, AMH plays no role in normal testicular differentiation, as proven by normal testicular organogenesis in patients with mutations of the AMH [35] or AMH receptor [35,36] genes.

Somatic sex differentiation

In contrast to the still unresolved problems of gonadal sex determination, the concepts regarding sex differentiation of the genital tract have undergone no major change since the ground-breaking contribution of Alfred Jost [2] indicating that masculinisation must be actively imposed upon the genital tract by the hormonal secretions of the fetal testis. Genital primordia can be masculinised only during a short, discrete developmental period, the 'critical stage', which varies for each component of the genital tract.

Morphological aspects

Shortly after gonadal differentiation, the genital tract of male or female fetuses consists of unipotential Wolffian and Müllerian ducts, and bipotential sinusal and external genital primordia.

Male development

Müllerian regression is the first step of male differentiation of the genital tract. In the human fetus, the first signs of regression appear in embyros at 8 weeks and regression is more or less complete at 10–12 weeks. Histologically, regression is characterised by loss of basement-membrane integrity, allowing close interaction between the epithelial and mesenchymal compartment [37]. The mesenchyme condenses around the duct, forming a tight fibroblastic ring around the dwindling cluster of epithelial cells.

Wolffian ducts, originally the excretory canals of the primitive kidney, become incorporated in the genital tract, developing into the vasa deferentia, epididymes and seminal vesicles. Prostatic buds develop around the opening of the ducts into the urogenital sinus, while fusion of outgrowths of the urogenital sinus forms the prostatic utricle, the male equivalent of the vagina.

Finally, closure of the labioscrotal folds and of the rims of the urethral groove, underneath the genital tubercle, lead to organogenesis of the perineal and penile urethra. This is completed at 12 weeks, but until the 16th week no

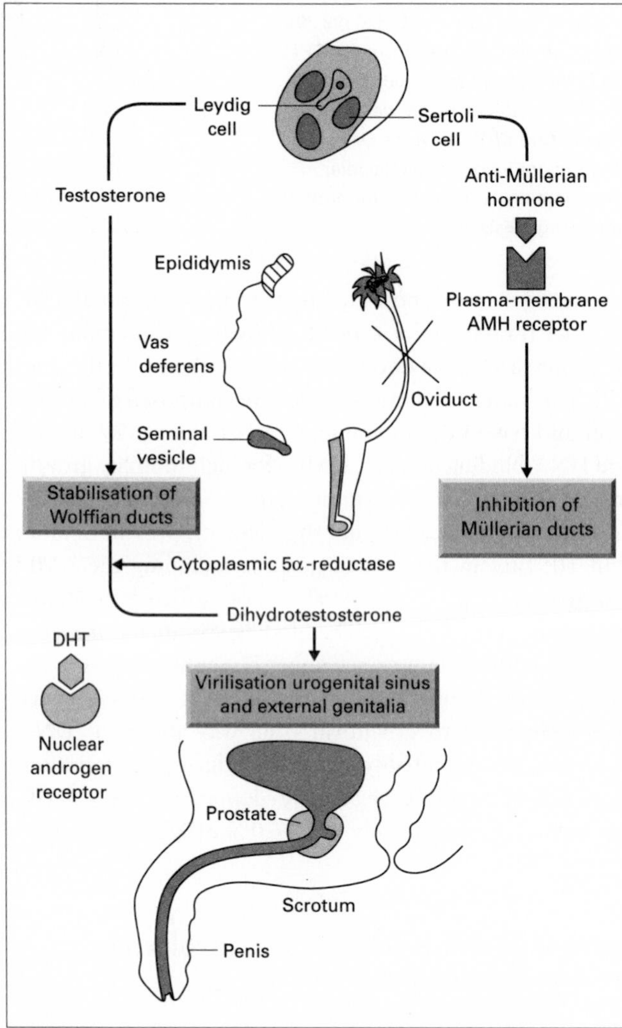

Fig. 57.4 Dual nature of fetal testicular secretion. Sertoli cells secrete anti-Müllerian hormone, a glycoprotein which induces the regression of Müllerian ducts, by acting through a plasma-membrane receptor. Leydig cells produce the steroid hormone testosterone, which binds to a nuclear receptor either as testosterone or, with greater affinity, as its 5α-reduced metabolite dihydrotestosterone (DHT). Testosterone is responsible for the maintenance of the Wolffian ducts, which give rise to the epidydimis, vas deferens and seminal vesicle. DHT induces the virilisation of the urogenital sinus and the external genitalia.

appreciable size difference exists between the penis and clitoris. Penile growth occurs between 20 weeks and term, at a time when, paradoxically, serum testosterone levels are declining.

Female development

Female sex differentiation appears to lag behind male organogenesis, although the end of the 'critical period', at which time testicular hormones no longer affect genital primordia, occurs at the same time in males and females. In the female, Müllerian ducts persist to form Fallopian tubes, uterus and upper part of the vagina; Wolffian ducts degenerate, and the vagina forms at the level of the urogenital sinus, initially between the openings of the Wolffian ducts, at the site of the Müllerian tubercle, where the prostatic utricle forms in males. The main difference between male and female organogenesis of the urogenital sinus lies in the down-growth of the vaginal plate. Whereas in males the prostatic utricle opens just beneath the neck of the bladder, in females the lower end of the vagina slides down the urethra to acquire a separate opening on the body surface. Feminisation of the external genitalia begins by the formation of the dorsal commissure, between the labioscrotal swellings, which give rise to the labia majora. The urethral folds do not fuse, and become the labia minora, and the stunted phallus develops into the clitoris.

Agents of male sex differentiation

As mentioned above, agents are required only in the event of male sex differentiation, female differentiation being constitutive in mammals. Two testicular hormones are involved, AMH, which induces the regression of Müllerian primordia, and testosterone, responsible for all other aspects of male somatic sex differentiation (Fig. 57.4).

Anti-Müllerian hormone

AMH is a 145-kDa glycoprotein homodimer synthesised by immature Sertoli cells, very soon after testicular differentiation and until puberty. It is also a product of post-natal granulosa cells. Initially, AMH was purified from incubation media of fetal bovine testicular tissue but a human recombinant product is now available. The human 2.8-kb gene (Fig. 57.5a) has been cloned [38] and mapped to chromosome 19 [39]. It consists of five exons, the last one exhibiting a 30% homology with members of a superfamily of dimeric proteins involved in growth and differentiation, the transforming growth factor β (TGF-β) family [40]. Proteolytic processing of AMH by plasmin yields a TGF-β-like fragment, which carries biological activity [41]. AMH is measurable in human serum by enzyme-linked immunosorbent assay (ELISA) and has diagnostic applications as a marker of Sertoli-cell maturation [42], testosterone insensitivity [43] and evolutivity of granulosa-cell tumours [44,45].

The gene coding for the human receptor of AMH was cloned in 1995 [36]. It is composed of 11 exons (Fig. 57.5b), maps to the long arm of chromosome 12 and encodes a serine/threonine kinase with a single transmembrane domain. It is expressed around the Müllerian duct and in granulosa and Sertoli cells. The persistent Müllerian duct syndrome, characterised by the persistence of Müllerian duct derivatives in otherwise normal males, is caused by mutations of either the AMH [35] or the AMH-receptor [36] genes. Apart from cryptorchidism and/or inguinal hernia, directly linked to the presence of uterus and tubes, the affected subjects are normal, suggesting that AMH is stringently required only for

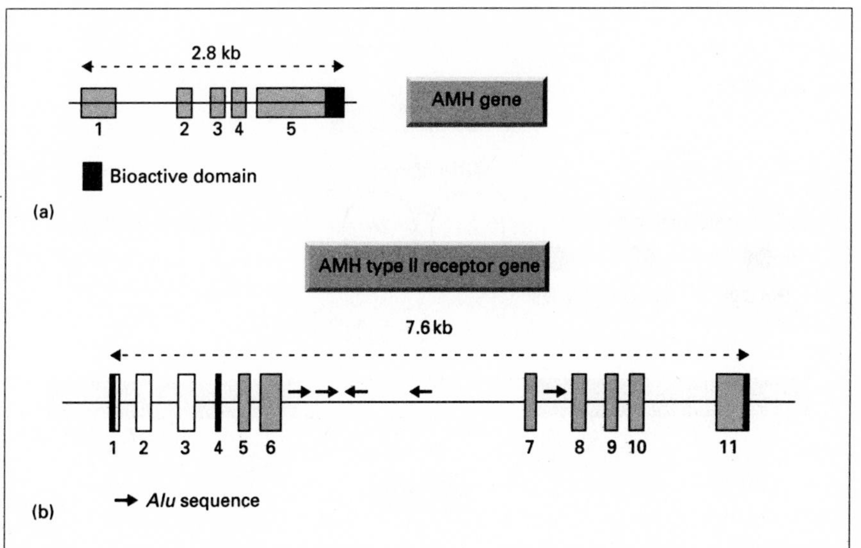

Fig. 57.5 (a) The anti-Müllerian hormone (AMH) gene is a 2.8-kb gene consisting of five exons. The biological activity of the protein resides in its C-terminal fragment [53]. (b). The AMH type II receptor gene total length is 7.6 kb. It is composed of 11 exons: exons 1–3 code for the extracellular domain, exon 4 codes for the transmembrane domain and exons 5–11 code for the intracellular serine/threonine kinase domains. *Alu* sequences that are 80–90% conserved are present in introns 6 and 7 [36].

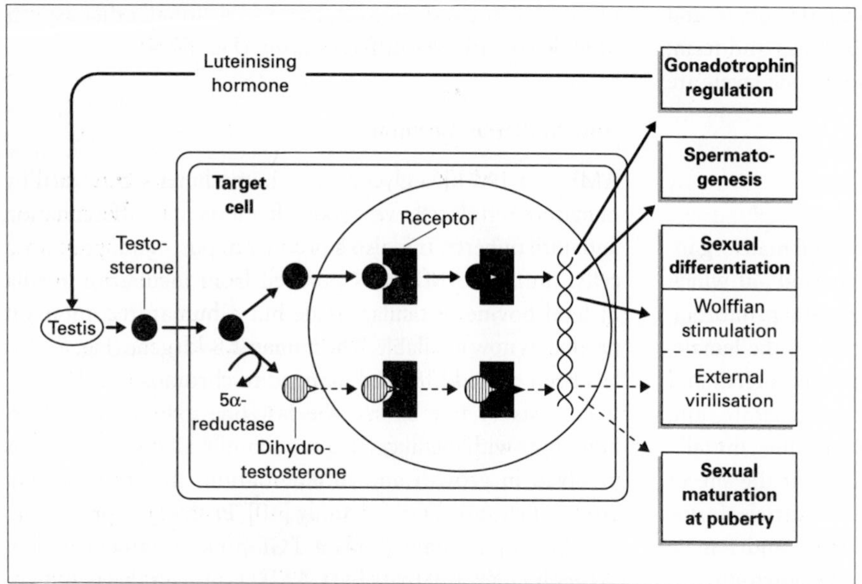

Fig. 57.6 Mechanisms of action of androgens. From ref. [54], with permission.

fetal Müllerian regression. Claims for its antiproliferative role in the female genital tract have not been substantiated [46].

Testosterone

Testosterone is produced by fetal Leydig cells from the time of their differentiation, at 8 weeks, to birth. Initiation of testosterone secretion requires no stimulation, but luteinising hormone is necessary for sustained production. Testosterone exerts its biological activity by binding to a nuclear receptor which has a much greater affinity for the reduced derivative of testosterone, dihydrotestosterone, than for testosterone itself. Therefore, in tissues such as the urogenital sinus and external genitalia, whose 5α-reductase activity enables them to generate dihydrotestosterone, the latter is the active androgen. Wolffian ducts, at the time of sex differentiation, do not express 5α-reductase activity, and consequently are the only fetal organs controlled by testosterone itself. (Fig. 57.6). This is perhaps the reason why they respond only to the high testosterone concentration achieved by local uptake in the vicinity of the testis, but cannot be maintained by systemic administration of androgen. Mutations of the gene coding for 5α-reductase type II, specifically expressed in testosterone target organs, severely impair masculine organogenesis of the genitalia while at puberty, expression of the type I isoenzyme is sufficient to promote near-normal pubertal virilisation of the affected subjects [47].

The androgen-receptor gene is a single copy gene which maps to Xq11–12 and spans 75–90 kb of genomic DNA

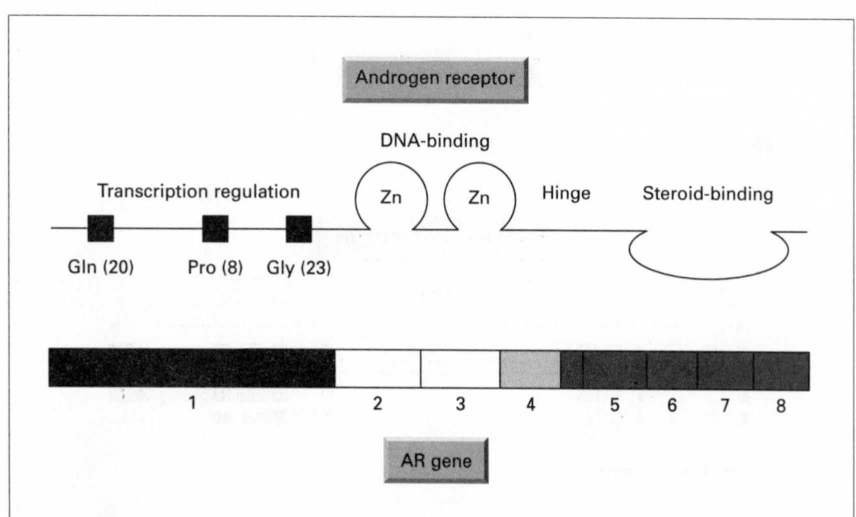

Fig. 57.7 The androgen receptor is a zinc-finger protein of the family of the nuclear steroid receptors. The androgen receptor (AR) gene is composed of eight exons; the first exon, involved in transcriptional regulation, contains polymorphic markers which are useful for genetic studies. Modified from [48], with permission.

[48] (Fig. 57.7). The first exon, which encodes half of the receptor protein, is involved in transcriptional regulation. It contains stretches of triplet repeats which serve as useful polymorphic markers for genetic studies. The number of CAG triplets coding for glutamines, normally from 11–33, is approximately doubled in patients suffering from Kennedy disease, an X-linked motor-neuron deficiency degenerative disorder [49].

Exons 2 and 3, highly conserved within the steroid receptor family, contain two zinc-finger structures involved in DNA binding, while exons 4–8 comprise the steroid-binding domain, responsible for the specific, high-affinity binding of the receptor protein to androgens. Mutations of the androgen-receptor gene lead to complete or partial androgen insensitivity exons 5 and 7, which are highly conserved between members of the steroid receptor subfamily to which the androgen receptor belongs, are highly susceptible to amino-acid substitutions (reviewed in [48]) (Fig. 57.7).

Conclusion

Because disorders of sex differentiation impair the fertility, but usually not the health, of their victims, this field offers ideal opportunities to dissect the mechanism of action of genes and hormones and invites joint efforts of physicians, molecular and developmental biologists to unravel the mystery of what Jost [50] has called a prolonged, uneasy and risky venture: becoming a male!

References

1 Upadhyay S, Zamboni L. Ectopic germ cells—Natural model for the study of germ cell sexual differentiation. *Proc Natl Acad Sci USA* 1982; **79**: 6584–8.

2 Jost A. Problems of fetal endocrinology: the gonadal and hypophyseal hormones. *Rec Progr Horm Res* 1953; **8**: 379–418.

3 Josso N, Lamarre I, Picard JY *et al.* Anti-Müllerian hormone in early human development. *Early Human Dev* 1993; **33**: 91–9.

4 Taketo T. Production of Müllerian-inhibiting substance (MIS) and sulfated glycoprotein-2 (SGP-2) associated with testicular differentiation in the XX mouse gonadal graft. In: Robaire B, ed. *The Male Germ Cell*, Vol. 637. New York: *Ann NY Academy of Science* 1991: 74–89.

5 Monk M, McLaren A. X-chromosome activity in foetal germ cells of the mouse. *J Embryol Exp Morphol* 1981; **63**: 75–84.

6 Kratzer PG, Chapman VM. X chromosome reactivation in oocytes of *Mus musculi. Proc Natl Acad Sci USA* 1981; **78**: 3093–7.

7 Pryse-Davies J, Dewhurst CJ. The development of the ovary and uterus in the foetus, newborn and infant: a morphological and enzyme histochemical study. *J Pathol* 1971; **103**: 5–25.

8 George FW, Wilson JD. Conversion of androgen to estrogen by the human fetal ovary. *J Clin Endocrinol Metab* 1978; **47**: 550–5.

9 Münsterberg A, Lovell-Badge R. Expression of the mouse anti-Müllerian hormone gene suggests a role in both male and female sex differentiation. *Development* 1991; **113**: 613–24.

10 Jost A. Recherches sur la différenciation sexuelle de l'embryon de lapin. III. Rôle des gonades foetales dans la différenciation sexuelle somatique. *Arch Anat Microsc Morphol Exp* 1947; **36**: 271–315.

11 Goodfellow PN, Lovell-Badge R. SRY and sex determination in mammals. *Ann Rev Genet* 1993; **27**: 71–92.

12 Welshons WJ, Russell LB. The Y chromosome as the bearer of male determining factors in the mouse. *Proc Natl Acad Sci USA* 1959; **45**: 560–6.

13 McLaren A, Simpson E, Tomonari K, Chandler P, Hogg H. Male sexual differentiation in mice lacking H-Y antigen. *Nature* 1984; **312**: 552–5.

14 Wang W, Meadows LR, Denhaan JMM *et al.* Human H-Y: a male-specific histocompatibility antigen derived from the SMCY protein. *Science* 1995; **269**: 1588–90.

15 Page DC, Mosher R, Simpson EM *et al.* The sex-determining region of the human Y chromosome encodes a finger protein. *Cell* 1987; **51**: 1091–104.

16 Sinclair AH, Berta P, Palmer MS *et al.* A gene from the human sex-determining region encodes a protein with homology to a conserved DNA-binding motif. *Nature* 1990; **346**: 240–4.

17 Koopman P, Gubbay J, Vivian N, Goodfellow P, Lovellbadge R. Male development of chromosomally female mice transgenic for SRY. *Nature* 1991; **351**: 117–21.

18 Harley VR, Jackson DI, Hextall PJ *et al.* DNA binding activity of recombinant SRY from normal males and XY females. *Science* 1992; **255**: 453–6.

19 Haqq CM, King CY, Donahoe PK, Weiss MA. SRY recognizes conserved DNA sites in sex-specific promoters. *Proc Natl Acad Sci USA* 1993; **90**: 1097–101.

20 Hawkins JR. Genetics of XY sex reversal. *J Endocrinol* 1995; **147**: 183–7.

21 Hacker A, Capel B, Goodfellow P, Lovell-Badge R. Expression of Sry, the mouse sex determining gene. *Development* 1995; **121**: 1603–14.

22 Kreidberg JA, Sariola H, Loring JM *et al.* WT-1 is required for early kidney development. *Cell* 1993; **74**: 679–91.

23 Luo XR, Ikeda YY, Parker KL. A cell-specific nuclear receptor is essential for adrenal and gonadal development and sexual differentiation. *Cell* 1994; **77**: 481–90.

24 Fredga K, Gropp A, Winking H, Fritz F. A hypothesis explaining the exceptional sex ration in the wood lemming. *Hereditas* 1977; **85**: 101–4.

25 Coward P, Nagai K, Chen DG, Thomas HD, Nagamine CM, Lau YFC. Polymorphism of a CAG trinucleotide repeat within Sry correlates with B6.Y^{Dom} sex reversal. *Nat Genet* 1994; **6**: 245–50.

26 Dubin RA, Ostrer H. Sry is a transcriptional activator. *Mol Endocrinol* 1994; **8**: 1182–92.

27 Foster JW, Dominquez-Steglich MA, Guioli S *et al.* Campomelic dysplasia and autosomal sex reversal caused by mutations in an SRY-related gene. *Nature* 1994; **372**: 525–30.

28 Bennett CP, Docherty Z, Robb SA, Ramani P, Hawkins JR, Grant D. Deletion 9p and sex reversal. *J Med Genet* 1993; **30**: 518–20.

29 Wilkie AOM, Campbell FM, Daubeney P *et al.* Complete and partial XY sex reversal associated with terminal deletion of 10q—report of 2 cases and literature review. *Am J Med Genet* 1993; **46**: 597–600.

30 Bardoni B, Zanaria E, Guioli S *et al.* A dosage sensitive locus at chromosome Xp21 is involved in male to female sex reversal. *Nat Genet* 1994; **7**: 497–501.

31 Pieau C, Girondot M, Richard-Mercier N, Desvages G, Dorizzi M,

Zaborski P. Temperature sensitivity of sexual differentiation of gonads in the European pond turtle: hormonal involvement. *J Exp Zool* 1994; **270**: 86–94.

32 Rashedi PM, Maraud R. Secretion of the anti-Müllerian hormone by the gonads of experimentally sex reversed female chick embryos. *Gen Comp Endocrinol* 1987; **65**: 87–91.

33 Vigier B, Watrin F, Magre S, Tran D, Josso N. Purified bovine AMH induces a characteristic freemartin effect in fetal rat prospective ovaries exposed to it *in vitro*. *Development* 1987; **100**: 43–55.

34 Behringer RR, Cate RL, Froelick GJ, Palmiter RD, Brinster RL. Abnormal sexual development in transgenic mice chronically expressing Müllerian inhibiting substance. *Nature* 1990; **345**: 167–70.

35 Imbeaud S, Carré-Eusèbe D, Rey R, Belville C, Josso N, Picard JY. Molecular genetics of the persistent Müllerian duct syndrome: a study of 19 families. *Hum Mol Genet* 1994; **3**: 125–31.

36 Imbeaud S, Faure E, Lamarre I *et al.* Insensitivity to anti-Müllerian hormone due to a spontaneous mutation in the human anti-Müllerian hormone receptor. *Nat Genet* 1995; **11**: 382–8.

37 Trelstad RL, Hayashi A, Hayashi K, Donahoe PK. The epithelial mesenchymal interface of the male rat Müllerian duct: loss of basement membrane integrity and ductal regression. *Dev Biol* 1982; **92**: 27–40.

38 Cate RL, Mattaliano RJ, Hession C *et al.* Isolation of the bovine and human genes for Müllerian inhibiting substance and expression of the human gene in animal cells. *Cell* 1986; **45**: 685–98.

39 Cohen-Haguenauer O, Picard JY, Mattei MG *et al.* Mapping of the gene for anti-Müllerian hormone to the short arm of human chromosome 19. *Cytogenet Cell Genet* 1987; **44**: 2–6.

40 Massagué J. The transforming growth factor-β family. *Ann Rev Cell Biol* 1990; **6**: 597–641.

41 Wilson CA, di Clemente N, Ehrenfels C *et al.* Müllerian inhibiting substance requires its N-terminal domain for maintenance of biological activity, a novel finding within the TGF-β superfamily. *Mol Endocrinol* 1993; **7**: 247–57.

42 Rey R, Lordereau-Richard I, Carel JC *et al.* Anti-Müllerian hormone and testosterone serum levels are inversely related during normal and precocious pubertal development. *J Clin Endocrinol Metab* 1993; **77**: 1220–6.

43 Rey R, Mebarki F, Forest MG *et al.* Anti-Müllerian hormone in children with androgen insensitivity. *J Clin Endocrinol Metab* 1994; **79**: 960–4.

44 Gustafson ML, Lee MM, Scully RE *et al.* Müllerian inhibiting substance as a marker for ovarian sex-cord tumor. *N Engl J Med* 1992; **326**: 466–71.

45 Rey R, Lhommé C, Marcillac I *et al.* Anti-Müllerian hormone as a serum marker of granulosa-cell tumors of the ovary: comparative study with serum alpha-inhibin and estradiol. *Am J Obstet Gynecol* 1996; **174**: 958–65.

46 Wallen J, Cate RL, Kiefer DM *et al.* Minimal anti-proliferative effect of recombinant Müllerian inhibiting substance on gynecological tumor cell lines and tumor explants. *Cancer Res* 1989; **49**: 2005–11.

47 Wilson JD, Griffin JE, Russell DW. Steroid 5α-reductase-2 deficiency. *Endocr Rev* 1993; **14**: 577–93.

48 Quigley CA, De Bellis A, Marschke KB, El Awady MK, Wilson EM, French FS. Androgen receptor defects: historical, clinical, and molecular perspectives. *Endocr Rev* 1995; **16**: 271–321.

49 La Spada AR, Wilson EM, Lubahn DB, Harding AE, Fischbeck KH. Androgen receptor gene mutations in X-linked spinal and bulbar muscular atrophy. *Nature* 1991; **352**: 77–9.

50 Jost A, Cressent M, Dupouy JP *et al.* Becoming a male. *Adv Biosci* 1972; **10**: 3–13.

51 Josso N. Anatomy and endocrinology of sexual differentiation. In: DeGroot L, ed. *Endocrinology*, 3rd ed, Vol. 2. Philadelphia: WB Saunders, 1994: 1888–900.

52 Reijo R, Lee TY, Salo P *et al.* Diverse spermatogenic defects in humans caused by Y chromosome deletions encompassing a novel RNA-binding protein gene. *Nat Genet* 1995; **10**: 383–93.

53 Josso N, Cate RL, Picard JY *et al.* Anti-Müllerian hormone, the Jost factor. In: Bardin CW, ed. *Recent Progress in Hormone Research*, Vol. 48. San Diego: Academic Press, 1993: 1–59.

54 Griffin JE. Androgen resistance: the clinical and molecular spectrum. *N Engl J Med* 1992; **326**: 611–18.

CHAPTER 58

Intersex states

C. Sultan and M.O. Savage

Introduction

Intersex states are characterised by an abnormality in the formation of the internal or external genital structures. This is usually due to a defect, frequently genetically determined, in the process of fetal sexual differentiation. Many intersex states are associated with an ambiguous appearance of the external genitalia resulting in disturbance of the balanced psychological and physical make-up of an individual, to which normal genital development is the key.

Over the past two decades, the study of intersex disorders moved towards the biochemical and molecular identification of the defects that cause them. If such an aetiological approach is to be used, a fundamental understanding of normal sexual differentiation, as described in the previous chapter, is required. This provides the basis for the classification, investigation and management of patients with intersex states.

Classification of intersex states

The classification which has stood the test of time and forms the basis of clinical assessment and management depends on gonadal morphology (Table 58.1). Female pseudo-hermaphroditism describes genital ambiguity resulting from abnormal virilisation of the female with normal ovaries. The male counterpart—male pseudo-hermaphroditism—is the result of incomplete virilisation of the male with differentiated testes. Finally, the true hermaphrodite possesses both ovarian and testicular tissue.

Female pseudo-hermaphroditism

Female pseudo-hermaphrodites have 46XX karyotypes with normal ovaries and Müllerian structures, but the external genitalia are virilised. The aetiology of female pseudo-hermaphroditism is given in Table 58.2. The degree of genital ambiguity can range from enlargement of the clitoris or fusion of the posterior labia to a completely male appearance (Fig. 58.1), depending on the timing of androgen production and the concentration of androgens in the fetal circulation. Virilisation may be caused by excessive production of either fetal or maternal androgens.

Virilisation by fetal androgens

Congenital adrenal hyperplasia

The commonest cause of ambiguous genitalia in the newborn female is a recessively inherited enzyme defect of cortisol synthesis, with diversion of intermediates to androgen production [1]. A reduction in steroid 21-hydroxylase or absence of 11β-hydroxylase or 3β-hydroxysteroid dehydrogenase can be the cause of congenital adrenal hyperplasia (CAH). In the absence of, or lowered potential for, cortisol production, there are high adrenocorticotrophic hormone (ACTH) levels leading to adrenal hyperplasia and excess androgen production (see Chapter 35).

21-Hydroxylase deficiency

In classical 21-hydroxylase deficiency, high plasma concentrations of androgens, due to the diversion of the precursors early in gestation, cause virilisation of the external genitalia of the 46XX female fetus. This deficiency is the most common cause of female pseudo-hermaphroditism. About 75% of patients with classic 21-hydroxylase deficiency do not correctly synthesise aldosterone which induces a potentially fatal salt-wasting state [1]. In this form of CAH, 17α-hydroxyprogesterone is not effectively converted to 11-deoxycortisol in the pathway of cortisol synthesis. The classical form of 21-hydroxylase deficiency has a frequency estimated at one in 14 000 live births. The definitive test to

Table 58.1 Classification of intersex states.

Female pseudo-hermaphrodite	Virilisation of genetic female with ovaries
Male pseudo-hermaphrodite	Incomplete virilisation of genetic male with testes
True hermaphrodite	Individual with ovarian and testicular tissue

Table 58.2 Aetiology of female pseudo-hermaphroditism.

Virilisation of fetal androgens
- Congenital adrenal hyperplasia
  - 21-Hydroxylase deficiency
  - 11β-Hydroxylase deficiency
  - 3β-Hydroxysteroid dehydrogenase deficiency
- Other causes of fetal androgen overproduction
  - Fetal adrenal adenoma
  - Nodular adrenal hyperplasia
  - Persistent fetal adrenal in preterm infants

Fetal virilisation by maternal androgens
- Ovarian tumours
- Adrenal tumours
- Aromatase deficiency: oestrogen synthetic defect

Iatrogenic fetal virilisation
- Testosterone and progestins

Female pseudo-hermaphroditism with associated congenital malformations

make the diagnosis is a standard ACTH stimulation test and measurement of plasma 17α-hydroxprogesterone. A variant of 21-hydroxylase deficiency, due to a milder defect, is the non-classical form of the disease. Affected females do not present neonatal genital ambiguity but develop other signs of androgen excess such as hirsutism.

Prenatal diagnosis is important to identify a fetus affected by the enzyme deficiency. In this way, genital ambiguity in affected females can be prevented by early dexamethasone treatment to the pregnant mother [2]. This prenatal diagnosis can be hormonal, by the measurement of amniotic fluid 17α-hydroxyprogesterone levels, or genetic after chorionic villus sampling at 9–10 weeks of gestation. Early prenatal diagnosis and treatment of 21-hydroxylase deficiency thus spares the newborn female the consequences of genital ambiguity, sex misassignment and gender confusion.

11β-hydroxylase deficiency

Female newborns usually present with signs of androgen excess such as masculinisation of external genitalia [3]. Patients may also develop signs and symptoms of aldosterone deficiency, and a small percentage develop hypertension rather than mineralocorticoid deficiency. This enzyme deficiency, which fails to convert 11-deoxycortisol to cortisol, is the second most common cause of CAH and results in a hypertensive form of the disease [4]. Humans have two isoenzymes with 11β-hydroxylase activity that are required for cortisol and aldosterone synthesis, respectively. CYP11B1, which presents the 11β-hydroxylase activity, is regulated by ACTH and CYP11B2, which presents aldosterone synthetase activity, is regulated by angiotensin II. Moreover, in addition to the 11β-hydroxylase activity, the latter enzyme has 18-hydroxylase and 18-oxidase activities and can thus synthesise aldosterone from deoxycorticosterone.

Deficiency of 11β-hydroxylase results from mutations in the CYP11B1 gene. All mutations identified in patients with the classical form abolish enzymatic activity [5]. However, there is no consistent correlation between the severity of hypertension and degree of virilisation in individuals with the same homozygous mutation. The treatment of affected children with hydrocortisone achieves a number of goals, while feminising genitoplasty must be performed at 6–12 months of age.

3β-hydroxysteroid dehydrogenase deficiency

The complete form of 3β-hydroxysteroid dehydrogenase

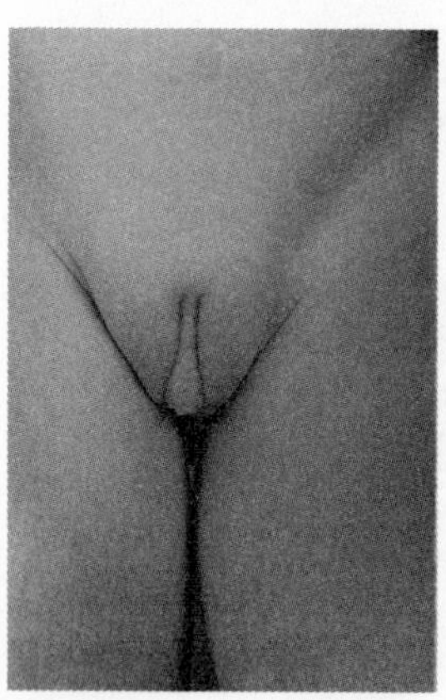
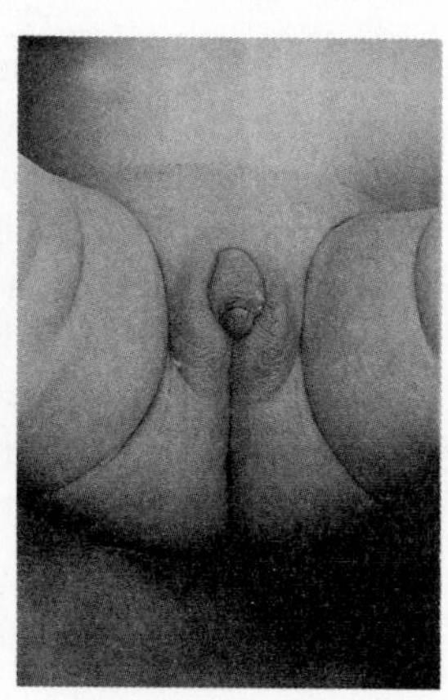
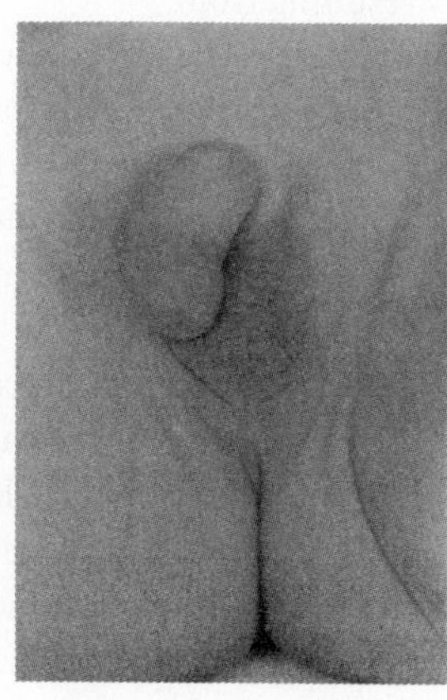

Fig. 58.1 Variation in degree of virilisation in three female infants with 21-hydroxylase deficiency.

deficiency results in partially virilised genitalia in genetic females whereas a partial form results in adolescent hyperandrogenism. Salt losing is present when the deficiency is complete. Elevated secretion of pregnenolone and 17α-pregnenolone are characteristic of this form of CAH [6]. Hydrocortisone and salt-retaining hormone replacement therapy are needed.

Oestrogen synthetic defect: aromatase deficiency

Aromatase deficiency within placental syncytiotrophoblasts is responsible for impaired or absent conversion of fetal and maternal androgens to oestrogens. It subsequently leads to the development of signs of maternal hyperandrogenism (acne, hirsutism) during the second half of pregnancy. Exposure of the female fetus to this androgen excess also causes virilisation of the infant with severe ambiguous genitalia at birth. Micropenis, hypospadias and posterior labioscrotal fusion may be present. At puberty, affected females present with pubertal failure, hypergonadotrophic hypogonadism and virilisation similar to that observed in the polycystic ovary syndrome. In aromatase deficiency oestrogen levels are exceedingly low. In both sexes it leads to delayed bone age and tall stature.

Several mutations, within the P-450 aromatase gene, have been described in the past few years [7]. The descriptions of aromatase deficiency in males and females provide new insights into the physiological roles of oestrogens in pregnancy, puberty and in bone maturation, and into the sex steroid–gonadotrophin feedback mechanism in the male.

Virilisation by maternal androgens

Virilisation of the external genitalia by a maternal ovarian or adrenal androgen-secreting tumour is a rare but well-recognised cause of female pseudo-hermaphroditism. The degree of virilisation may be striking. In a recent report and review of the literature [8], the diagnosis of female pseudo-hermaphroiditism and the causative maternal adrenal tumour (Fig. 58.2) was confirmed only when the patient, having been brought up as a boy, started to feminise at puberty.

Other causes of fetal virilisation

Female pseudo-hermaphroiditism due to maternal administration of progestogen preparations became recognised about 30 years ago. A number of dysmorphic childhood syndromes may also be associated with virilised female genitalia [9].

Male pseudo-hermaphroditism

Male pseudo-hermaphroditism arises as a result of a disturbance of normal male genital development in patients with testes and a 46XY karyotype (Table 58.3). The genital anomaly can vary from apparently female external genitalia, to male external genitalia with a small penis or perineal hypospadias. Male sexual differentiation, as described in the previous chapter, is brought about by a number of interrelated mechanisms, and failure of any of these may lead to incomplete virilisation.

Abnormalities of sex differentiation

After sex determination, the events of male sex differentiation take two pathways [10]: one inhibitory, i.e. the regression of the Müllerian ducts by action of the anti-Müllerian hormone (AMH), and the other stimulatory, which requires the two androgens, testosterone and 5α-dihydrotestosterone (DHT), and a functional androgen receptor very early in embryogenesis. It has clearly been demonstrated that androgens are essential for virilisation of Wolffian duct structures, the urogenital sinus and the genital tubercule. In

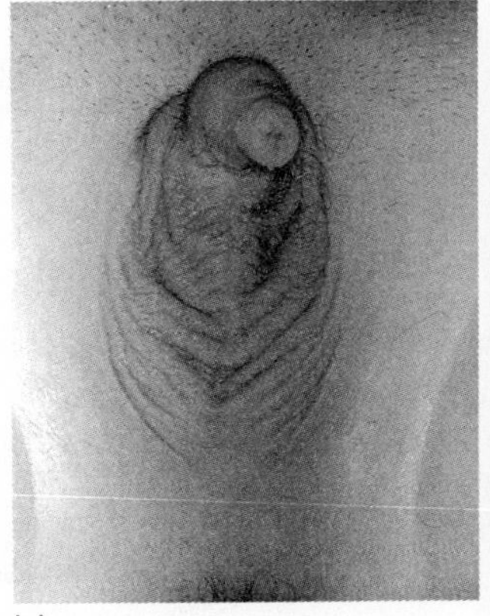

(a)

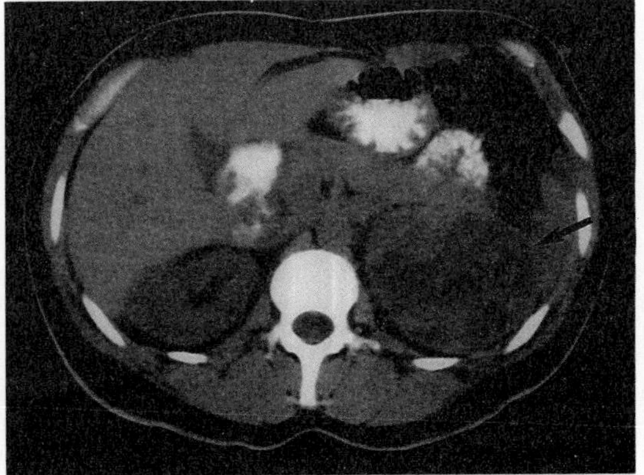

(b)

Fig. 58.2 Virilisation of a female 46XX infant during fetal life by a maternal androgen-secreting adrenal adenoma.

Table 58.3 Aetiology of male pseudo-hermaphroditism.

Impaired Leydig-cell activity
Inborn errors of testosterone biosynthesis
Congenital lipoid adrenal hyperplasia
3β-Hydroxysteroid dehydrogenase deficiency
17α-Hydroxylase deficiency
17, 20-Desmolase deficiency
Leydig-cell hypoplasia: LH receptor defect
Androgen insensitivity syndromes
Complete androgen insensitivity
Partial androgen insensitivity
5α-reductase deficiency
Incomplete differentiation of testes with deficient testosterone and anti-Müllerian hormone production
XY gonadal dysgenesis
Mixed gonadal dysgenesis
Other forms
Iatrogenic male pseudo-hermaphroditism
Associated with other congenital anomalies
Persistent Müllerian structures

LH, luteinising hormone.

the urogenital sinus and the genital tubercule, testosterone is converted to DHT by 5α-reductase; testosterone or DHT bind to a nuclear receptor to stimulate protein synthesis.

Molecular cloning and genetic, biochemical and pharmacological approaches have provided strong support for the existence of at least two steroid 5α-reductase enzymes in humans (designated as types 1 and 2 to reflect the chronological order in which the genes were isolated) [11]. Molecular genetic evidence, such as gene deletions and point mutations, demonstrated that the 5α-reductase 2 gene is the major locus for clinical 5α-reductase deficiency.

The androgen receptor belongs to the subfamily of steroid hormone receptors within a larger family of nuclear proteins which activates target gene transcription through the same hormone response elements. As a member of the nuclear receptor family (Fig. 58.3), the androgen receptor contains an NH_2-terminal region which is variable in length and has a role in transcriptional activation, a central cysteine-rich DNA-binding domain, and a carboxy-terminal ligand-binding domain [12].

Although the two physiologically active androgens, testosterone and DHT, interact directly with the androgen receptor and mediate hormonal responses, conversion of testosterone to the more potent agonist DHT in certain

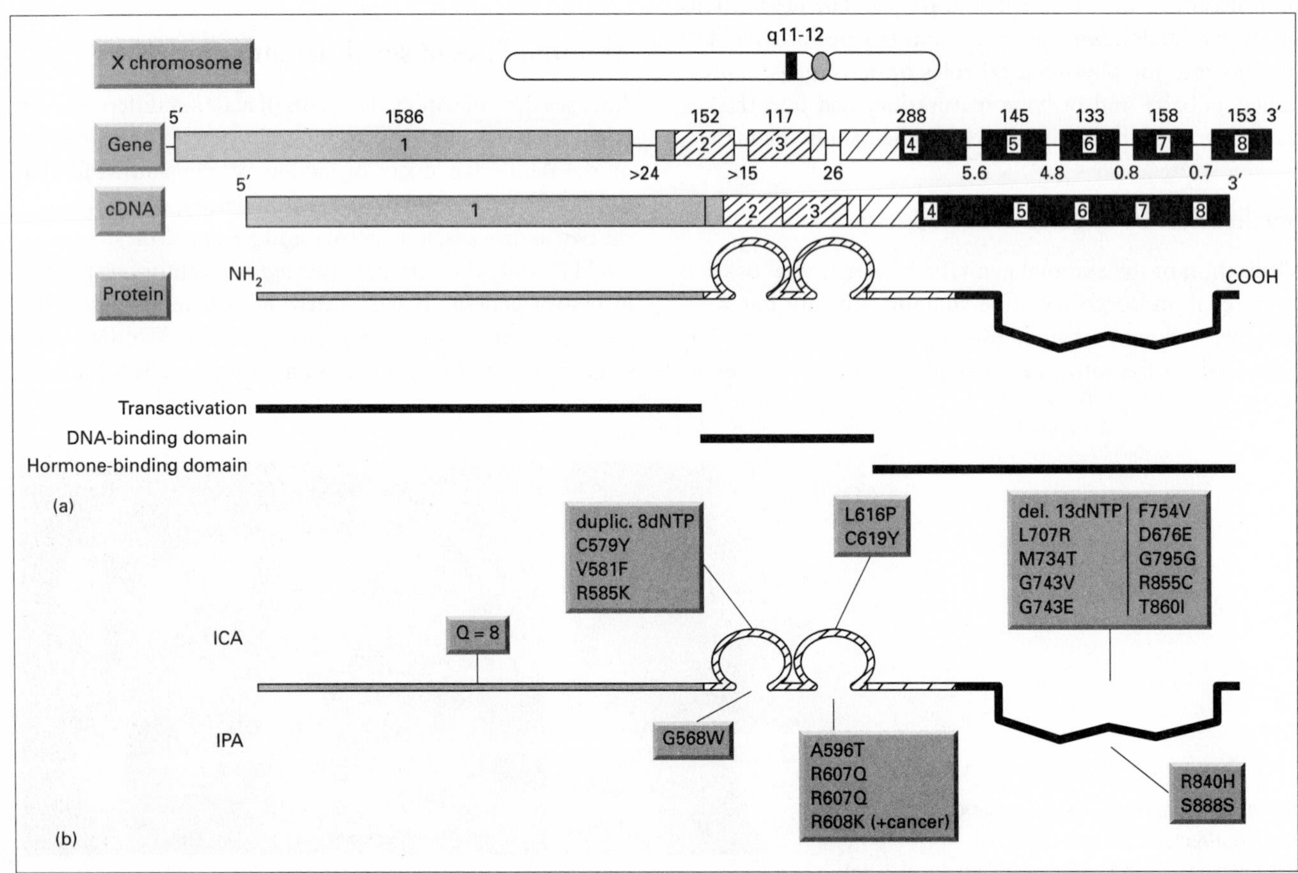

Fig. 58.3 (a) Schematic representation of the androgen-receptor gene, and protein organisation. (b) Androgen-receptor abnormalities (personal experience). The single amino-acid letter code is used.

tissues is required for androgen action to occur. This requirement is particularly clear during male sexual development, when formation of DHT is mandatory for virilisation of external genitalia and development of the prostate. Virilisation of the Wolffian duct structures is, however, thought to be mediated by testosterone. The actions of androgens on the target cell occur via the classical steroid receptor pathway (Fig. 58.4) [12]. After the binding of the androgen to its receptor, hyperphosphorylation of the N-terminal domain of the protein is observed: the androgen-activated receptor complex migrates to the nucleus and interacts as a homodimer with the androgen response elements of target genes and their flanking DNA [13]. The mechanism by which the receptor regulates gene transcription probably involves N-terminal sequences of the protein, but the molecular details of this activation process remain to be elucidated. Protein–protein interactions, probably with other transcription factors, may occur near the transcription start site of the gene. Both promoter and host-cell specificity appear to influence the requirement for the N-terminal domain in transcriptional activation, suggesting that this region interacts with cell-specific transcription factors.

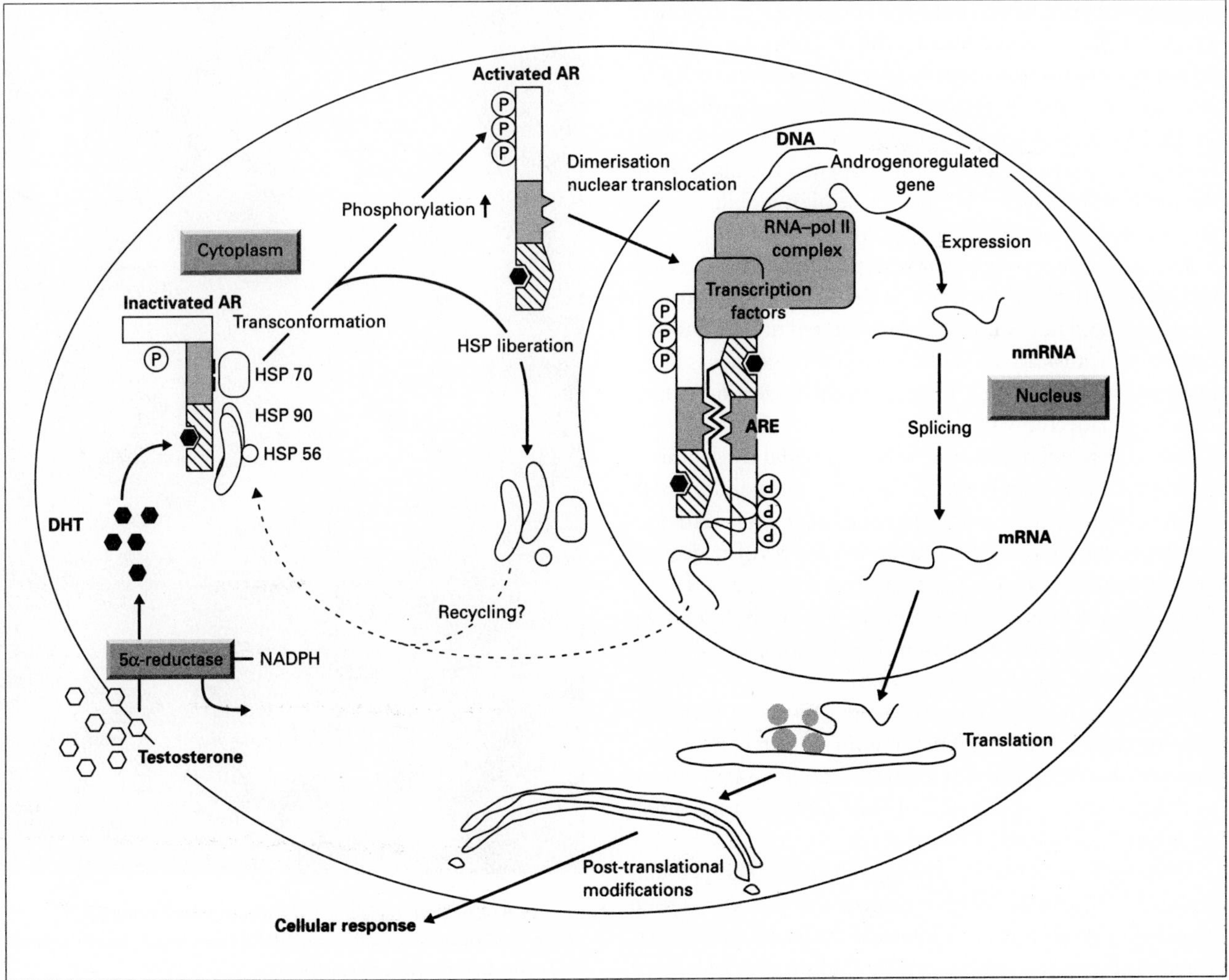

Fig. 58.4 Schematic representation of androgen action in the target cell. HSP, heat shock protein; ARE, androgen response element.

Defects of testis development

XY gonadal dysgenesis

Y-linked XY gonadal dysgenesis

XY complete gonadal dysgenesis (Swyer's syndrome). The syndrome of pure gonadal dysgenesis is characterised by the presence of bilateral streak gonads in phenotypic females with sexual infantilism and XY karyotype. Most individuals come to medical attention in their mid-teens or later for evaluation of problems related to lack of ovarian function.

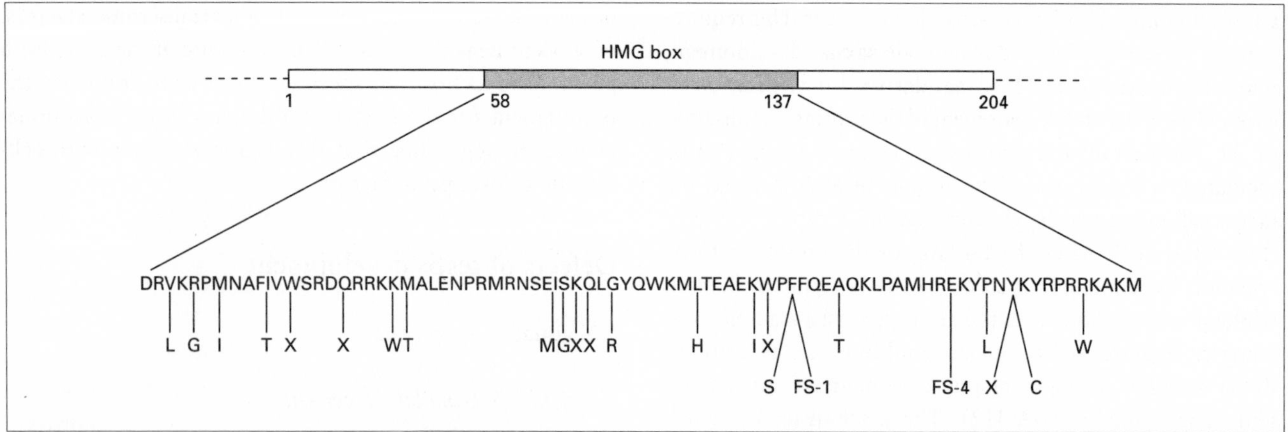

Fig. 58.5 Sex-reversing mutations in the *SRY* gene. X indicates termination codon, and FS indicates frameshift mutation. The number (n) of base pairs deleted causing frameshift is indicated as FS_n.

Most of the patients do not present with sex chromosome structural abnormalities, but some sporadic cases exist with a deletion in the short arm of the Y (Yp) or a 46 XXp resulting from translocation of an extra fragment of Xp on an otherwise normal Y chromosome. Gene abnormalities of *SRY* such as deletion and point mutations have been described in only 10–15% of the patients; the majority of the point mutations are located in the high mobility group (HMG) box of the *SRY* gene (Fig. 58.5).

The management of patients with pure gonadal dysgenesis is similar to Turner's syndrome in that long-term oestrogen therapy should be instituted at the expected time of puberty. Neoplastic transformation of the dysgenetic gonads is likely to occur in patients with XY pure gonadal dysgenesis making routine gonadectomy mandatory.

Mixed gonadal dysgenesis. Mixed gonadal dysgenesis is characterised by a unilateral testis (often intra-abdominal), a contralateral streak gonad, and persistent Müllerian duct structures, and is associated with varying degrees of inadequate masculinisation [14]. The most common karyotype is 45XO/46XY, but other mosaics have been reported with structurally abnormal or normal Y chromosome. Features of Turner's syndrome may be present (Fig. 58.6).

Patients with mixed gonadal dysgenesis are at increased risk for gonadal (and Wilms) tumour: it is recommended that they should be reared as females. This allows for removal of the gonads and avoidance of their malignant potential. As males, they would be infertile.

Dysgenetic male pseudo-hermaphroditism. This denomination encompasses wide heterogeneity and refers to a group of patients presenting with bilateral dysgenetic testes, persistent Müllerian structures, cryptorchidism and inadequate

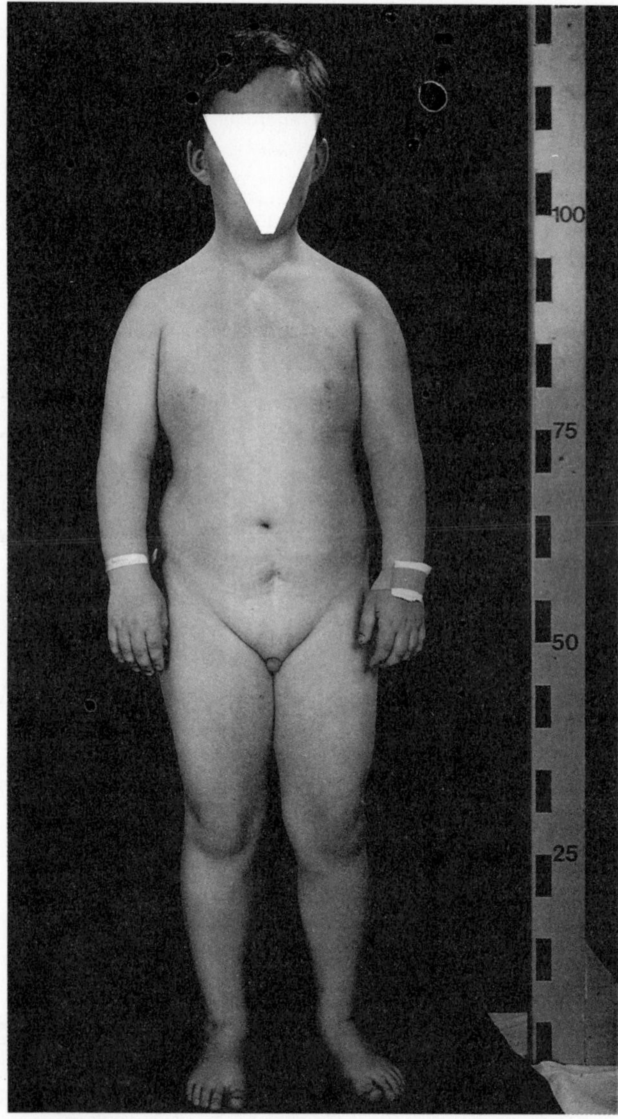

Fig. 58.6 A patient, raised as a male with mixed gonadal dysgenesis associated with a 45XO/46XY karyotype. Note the broad chest and incomplete virilisation.

virilisation [15]. Because the uterus is frequently present, the sex of rearing is often female and gonadectomy is recommended. These patients should be screened routinely for tumour formation.

X-linked 46XY gonadal dysgenesis

Sex reversal in 46XY patients with a duplication of the short arm of the X chromosome suggested the existence of a gene in the X chromosome, named *DSS* (dosage-sensitive sex reversal), which when present in two copies can override the effect of the Y chromosome [16]. In the 160-kb stretch within the Xp21 region, containing the *DSS* locus and also the locus for congenital adrenal hypoplasia, the first, and only, gene isolated is *DAX*-1. *DAX*-1 encodes a nuclear receptor related to steroidogenic factor 1 which has been shown in homozygous knock-out studies to result in the absence of gonads in both sexes. The close embryological relationship between adrenals and gonads, and their shared steroidogenic properties, support the hypothesis that *DAX*-1 might be both the *DSS* and the gene responsible for CAH. In fact, mutations of *DAX*-1 [17] do not affect testis development and no mutation has been described in XY females.

Autosomal-linked 46XY gonadal dysgenesis

Another gene has been isolated which also appears to exert its effects on sex determination in a dose-sensitive fashion. This gene, *SOX*-9 (*SRY* box-related sequence), maps to the locus known as *SRA*-1 on chromosome 17, which is associated with campomelic dysplasia and sometimes gonadal dysgenesis. *SOX*-9 belongs to the same family of HMG proteins as *SRY*. Despite similarities, it does not seem that *SOX*-9 and *SRY* would compete with each other on a target site because it is a reduction of *SOX*-9 expression [18] that leads to sex reversal from male to female.

True hermaphroditism

True hermaphroditism is defined as the simultaneous presence of testicular and ovarian tissue in a single individual in either the same or opposite gonads [19] (Table 58.4). Both external genitalia and internal duct structures of true hermaphrodites display gradations between male and female. The initial manifestations are ambiguous genitalia in 90% of cases or more rarely, isolated clitoromegaly or penile hypospadias. Two-thirds of true hermaphrodites are raised as males. Among those raised as females, most will have clitoromegaly. Virtually all patients have a urogenital sinus and in most cases a uterus is present.

The most common peripheral karyotype is 46XX but mosaicisms are observed (XX, XY). *SRY* gene is present in 10–30% of patients suggesting that true hermaphroditism is a heterogeneous condition in terms of its genetic background. The most important aspect of management of true hermaphrodites is gender assignment. Such decisions should be based upon the adequacy of the phallus and findings at laparotomy. True hermaphrodites have the potential for fertility.

XX males

These patients with no genital ambiguity develop gynaecomastia at puberty. Although they present some degree of testosterone deficiency and impaired spermatogenesis, they differ from males with XXY (Klinefelter's syndrome) in that they are not tall and show no impairment of intelligence [20]. *SRY* gene is present in some XX males. Others however, have no demonstrable Y sequences; the management of XX males is similar to that of Klinefelter's syndrome.

Leydig-cell hypoplasia

Leydig-cell hypoplasia is a form of pseudo-hermaphroditism in which Leydig-cell differentiation and testosterone production are impaired. The phenotype is female although Müllerian structures are absent. Inhibiting mutations in the sixth transmembrane domain of the luteinising hormone (LH) receptor have recently been reported in these patients [21].

Table 58.4 Gonadal distribution in 384 cases of true hermaphroditism. From van Niekerk [19].

Type of distribution			
Gonad on one side	Gonad on opposite side	Number of patients	%
Ovary	Testis	113	29.5
Ovotestis	Ovary	114	29.7
Ovotestis	Ovotestis	79	20.6
Ovotestis	Testis	40	10.4
Ovotestis	Unknown	15	3.9
Ovotestes	Variations	23	5.9

Inborn errors of testosterone biosynthesis

These rare disorders (Fig. 58.7) lead to defective testosterone secretion during the critical period of fetal sexual differentiation. The result is inadequate testosterone secretion, either locally to virilise the Wolffian ducts or peripherally to virilise the external genitalia. Lack of virilisation may be severe and many patients are raised as female. Synthesis of anti-Müllerian hormone, being a glycoprotein rather than a steroid, is unaffected. When the enzyme deficiency is situated early in the biosynthetic pathway, adrenal steroid synthesis may also be impaired. These disorders are rare and will be described only briefly as a number of reviews are available [22,23].

Congenital lipoid adrenal hyperplasia

Congenital lipoid adrenal hyperplasia (CLAH) is a rare disease characterised by a defect in the synthesis of the three classes of steroid hormones resulting in severe salt wasting and female phenotype. No mutation in humans has been found thus far in the gene encoding for P-450_{scc}, the first candidate gene, nor in the various proteins involved in the cholesterol transport, such as sterol carrier protein-2(SCP-2). Recently, the gene responsible for CLAH has been cloned and validated by the demonstration of a nonsense mutation [24]. It encodes for a protein named StAR (steroidogeneic acute regulatory protein), probably responsible for the transport of cholesterol to the inner membrane of mitochondria, and thus to the P-450_{scc} enzyme complex.

17α-hydroxylase deficiency

Defects in P-450_{c17} lead to a male pseudo-hermaphroditism with various degrees of ambiguous genitalia, most often a severe form, frequently diagnosed at puberty, associating female phenotype and hypertension. Cytochrome P-450_{c17} catalyses the transformation of progesterone and pregnenolone into 17α-hydroxyprogesterone and 17α-hydroxypregnenolone, and then into dehydroepiandrosterone and Δ_4-androstenedione.

The gene encoding for this enzyme complex, the CYP17 gene, is located on chromosome 10q24-25. Several different mutations have been reported in the CYP17 gene leading to either complete or partial form of the disease [25,26].

3β-hydroxysteroid dehydrogenase deficiency

Defects in 3β-hydroxysteroid dehydrogenase (3β-HSD) synthesis result in 46XY individuals with male pseudo-hermaphroditism, sometimes associated with salt wasting in the classical form [27]. The 3β-HSD enzyme is responsible for the conversion of Δ_5 (3β-OH) steroids into Δ_4 (3-ceto) steroids. Two different complementary DNAs (cDNAs) have

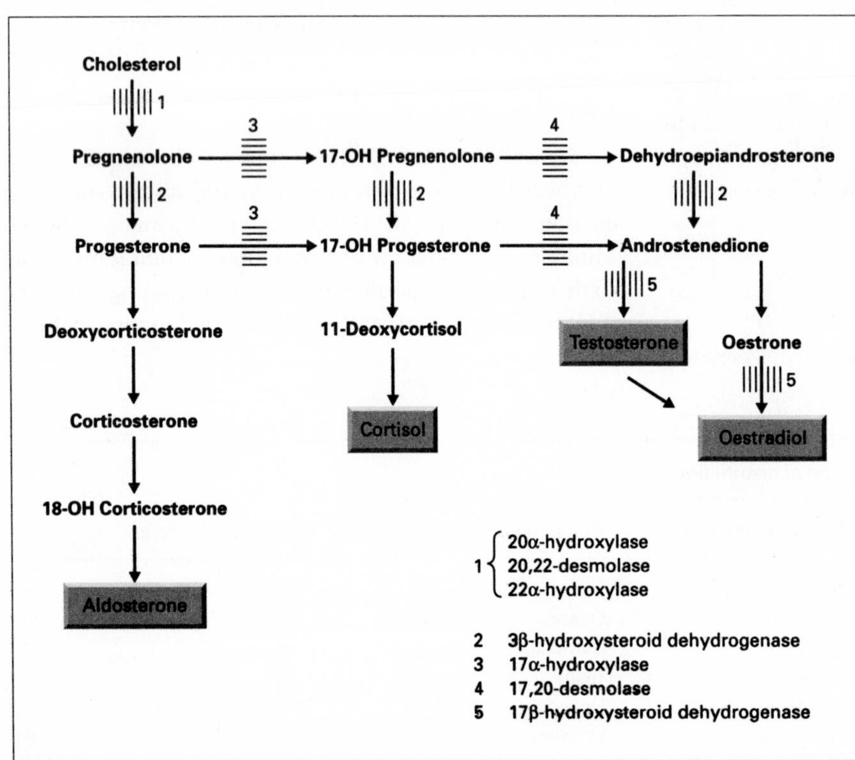

Fig. 58.7 Enzyme defects in testosterone biosynthesis.

been identified: type 1 in the placenta, and type 2 in gonads and adrenal glands. The two genes are located on chromosome 1p13.

Almost 15 mutations of the type 2 3β-HSD enzyme have been reported to date, but no mutations of type 1 have been found. This may explain the virilisation that occurs in 46XX subjects, because of a peripheral, non-steroidogenic conversion of elevated testosterone precursors. A non-classical form of 3β-HSD deficiency has been described, characterised by a late onset and less severe form of the disease. The clinical diagnosis of this form is not easy, and its existence remains controversial because no mutations of the gene have been found.

17β-hydroxysteroid dehydrogenase deficiency

17β-hydroxysteroid dehydrogenase (17β-HSD) deficiency is a rare cause of male pseudo-hermaphroditism. The typical subject is a 46XY male born with female external genitalia, the testes being located in the inguinal canals or labia majora, who virilises at the time of puberty (Fig. 58.8), associated with elevated levels of androstenedione contrasting with low or normal levels of testosterone. Two characteristics of the disorder are particularly puzzling: the defect in virilisation and the deficiency in testosterone synthesis that are usually more complete during embryogenesis than in later life, and the well-differentiated Wolffian duct structures.

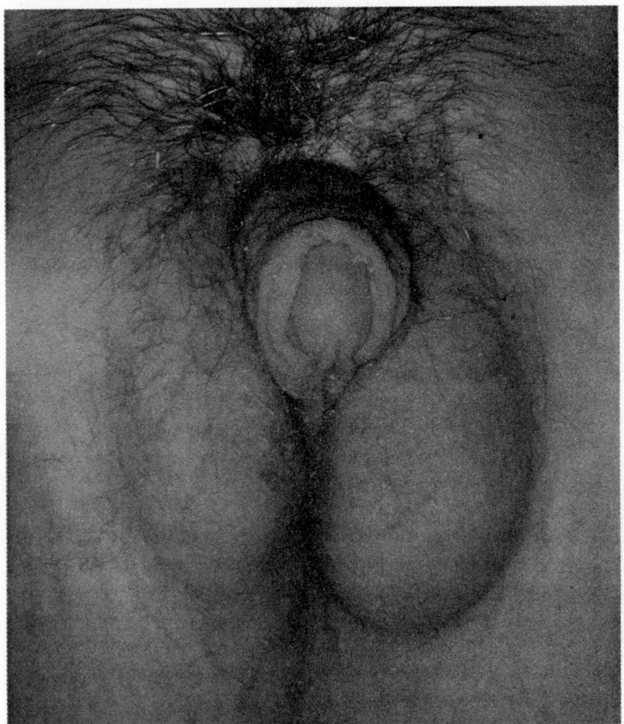

Fig. 58.8 Genital virilisation at puberty of a 46XY patient with 17β-hydroxysteroid dehydrogenase deficiency who has been raised as a female. (Courtesy of Dr D.B. Grant, Great Ormond Street Hospital.)

17β-HSD converts Δ_4-androstenedione into testosterone and dehyroepiandrosterone into androstenediol. It also acts on the interconversion of oestradiol and oestrone. This is a key enzyme leading to active androgenic compounds, and the only one of the steroidogenic pathway whose action is reversible. Four different enzymes, with tissue-specific expression, encoded by four different genes have been identified. The 17β-HSD type 1 has a peripheral activity and a specificity toward oestrogens. The 17β-HSD type 2 is mainly of placental origin and acts on both androgens and oestrogens. The 17β-HSD type 3 has a specific testicular expression and functions with nicotinamide adenine dinucleotide phosphate (NADPH) as cofactor (in contrast to the two former enzymes that utilise NADH). Finally, abnormalities of the 17β-HSD type 3 enzyme are responsible for the 17β-HSD deficiency.

Among the gene alterations, missense and nonsense mutations, splice junction abnormalities and a small deletion that resulted in a frame shift have been described [28]. Affected newborns are considered female but the sex of rearing of the patients remains questionable: the choice of sex will be influenced by the social group. We believe that during infancy or childhood, since the female sex of rearing is maintained, an orchidectomy should be carried out. If the diagnosis is not made prior to puberty, a gender change to male is acceptable [29].

Androgen insensitivity syndromes
(Table 58.5)

5α-reductase deficiency

Several investigators have reported a wide clinical, biological and biochemical spectrum associated with genetic heterogeneity in 5α-reductase deficiency. These patients are characterised at birth by the presence of a pseudo-vagina, a urogenital sinus, and testes in the inguinal canals, labia or scrotum in all cases. The clinical presentation can range from almost normal female structures, to a clear-cut male phenotype with hypospadias and normally virilised Wolffian structures that terminate in the vagina. An important characteristic of 5α-reductase deficiency is the virilisation of the external genitalia that occurs at puberty (Figs 58.9 and 58.10) along with the acquisition of male gender identity in these patients raised as female [30].

The characteristic endocrine features of 5α-reductase deficiency are normal to high male levels of testosterone and low levels of DHT, elevation in the ratio of testosterone to DHT in adulthood and after stimulation with human chorionic gonadotrophin (hCG) in childhood, and elevated

Table 58.5 Clinical phenotype of androgeninsensitivity states.

	5α-reductase deficiency	Androgen receptor disorders		
		Complete	Partial	Mild
External genitalia	Predominantly female	Female	Ambiguous	Male
Wolffian structures	Male	Absent	Hypoplastic male	Male
Urogenital sinus	Female	Female	Rudimentary male	Male
Breast	Male	Female	Gynaecomastia	±Gynaecomastia
Sexual orientation	Female→male	Female	Male/female	Male

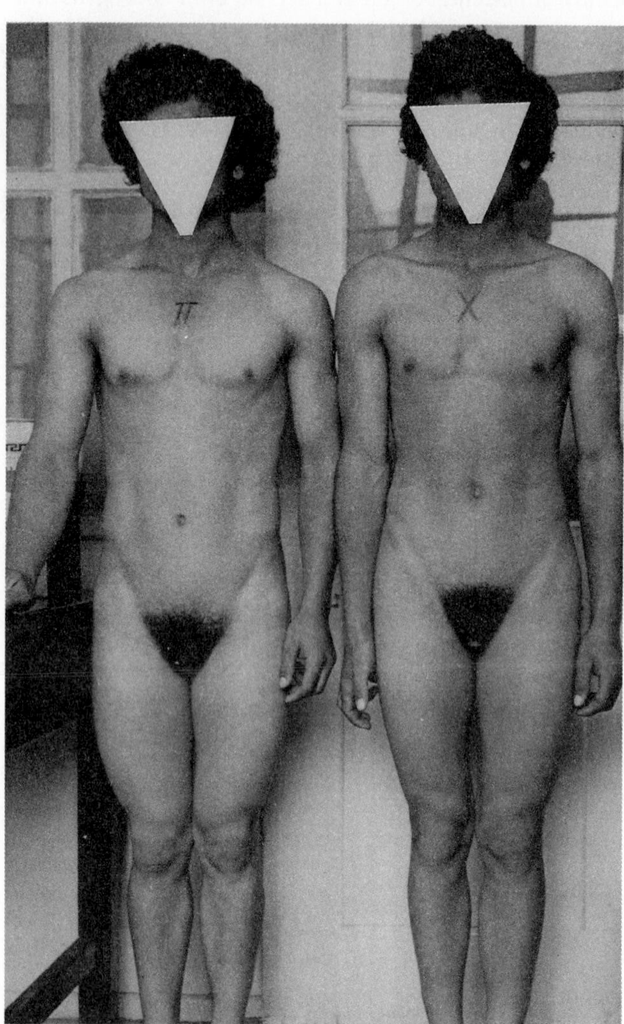

Fig. 58.9 Two Greek Cypriot brothers with 5α-reductase deficiency.

ratios of urinary 5β- to 5α-metabolites of androgen and C_{21} steroids.

From a biochemical point of view, the decrease in 5α-reductase activity in genital skin fibroblasts supports the diagnosis of 5α-reductase deficiency, but enzymatic activity is sometimes in the normal range. The decreased activity in sonicated cell extracts at acidic pH provides strong evidence that the mutation results in a loss of type 2 enzyme activity.

Isolation and sequencing of the cDNA encoding the 5α-reductase type 2 provides the molecular tools for definition of the gene abnormalities responsible for 5α-reductase deficiency. To date, only three gene deletions have been described. Indeed, when a sequence alteration is identified it is usually a point mutation, which vary greatly and are found throughout the gene; so far, the standard methods of molecular genetic analysis have revealed two nonsense mutations, one splicing defect, and 24 missense mutations [11,31,32].

The management of 5α-reductase deficiency is primarily dependent upon the phenotypic findings and gender at the time of diagnosis. Given the severe defect of the external genitalia (Fig. 58.10) most newborns are raised as female. Gonadectomy should be performed early to prevent masculinisation, along with vaginoplasty and clitoral reduction. If the diagnosis is made at puberty, one can consider raising

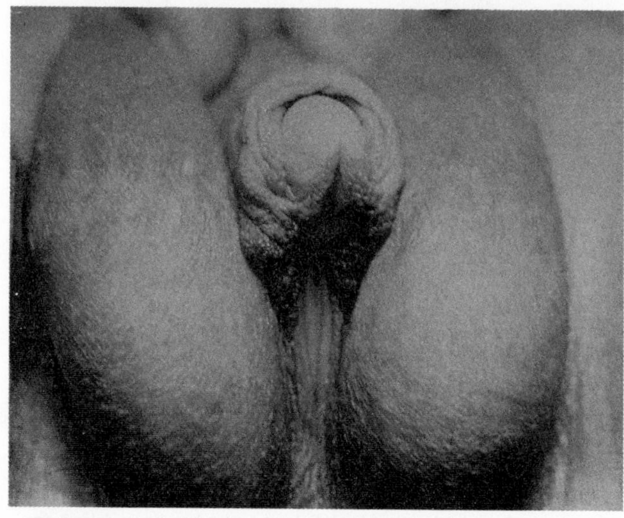

Fig 58.10 External genitalia of a pubertal patient with 5α-reductase deficiency. Note that the phallus remains small.

the patient as male. Administration of supraphysiological doses of testosterone or local application of DHT cream results in some long-term enhancement of virilisation [33].

Complete androgen insensitivity

This form of androgen insensitivity is characterised by an unambiguous female phenotype with a blind vaginal pouch and no uterus. In some cases, an underdevelopment of the clitoris and labia minora may be observed. At puberty, breast development is normal or augmented contrasting with absent or scanty axillary and pubic hair in the majority of cases. Individuals with complete androgen insensitivity come to medical attention either during infancy because of an inguinal hernia, or during puberty with primary amenorrhea.

Partial androgen insensitivity

This covers a wide spectrum of clinical phenotypes from patients with essentially female phenotype with limited virilisation such as mild clitoromegaly and/or a slight degree of posterior labial fusion, to infertile individuals who had normal responsiveness during fetal life and thus an unequivocally male phenotype with azoospermia. An X-linked pattern of inheritance may be identified (Fig. 58.11). The diagnosis may be made in infancy when the child presents with ambiguous genitalia, perineal hypospadias and palpable testes (Fig. 58.12). At puberty, virilisation and/or feminisation may occur depending upon the degree of androgen resistance.

Since the androgen-receptor gene has been cloned, molecular biology techniques have made it possible to identify mutations within the gene from patients with different phenotypes of androgen insensitivity [34]. Such techniques include restriction fragment length polymorphism analysis and enzymatic amplification of the various exons of the gene to detect large scale changes in the gene structure. Screening procedures with sequencing of the gene allow identification of subtle changes responsible for missense or nonsense mutations.

Androgen-receptor gene alterations may be classified into two groups according to the DNA and messenger RNA (mRNA) alterations:

1 loss or gain of genomic information, such as macro- and microdeletions and base-pair insertions; and

2 point mutations, responsible for nonsense, missense and splice site mutations.

A wide variety of molecular defects may underlie the clinical and biochemical heterogeneity of the androgen-insensitivity syndrome. Moreover, the same mutation can be associated with different phenotypes even within the same family. Markedly different molecular defects (major deletion, premature termination, single amino-acid substitutions in the protein) can also produce the same phenotype. The screening of carriers and prenatal diagnosis of androgen insensitivity in high-risk families is impossible unless the mutation has been identified. Thereafter, sequencing of the suspected exon of the 46XX proband or the 46XY fetus ascertains whether the affected chromosome is being carried [35].

The treatment of patients with complete androgen-insensitivity syndrome relates primarily to the optimal timing of gonadectomy. We normally perform gonadectomy before puberty and prescribe oestrogen replacement as necessary. The management of patients with partial androgen insensitivity syndrome must be individualised from the degree of genital ambiguity, the growth response of the penile size to a supraphysiological dose of testosterone, and the type of androgen receptor mutation. Although certain androgen-receptor defects may be amenable to androgen therapy,

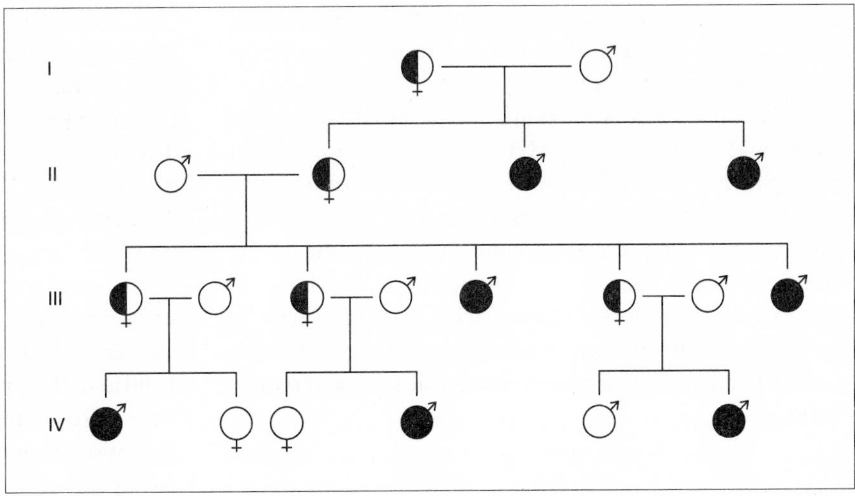

Fig. 58.11 Pedigree of a family with X-linked partial androgen insensitivity syndrome.

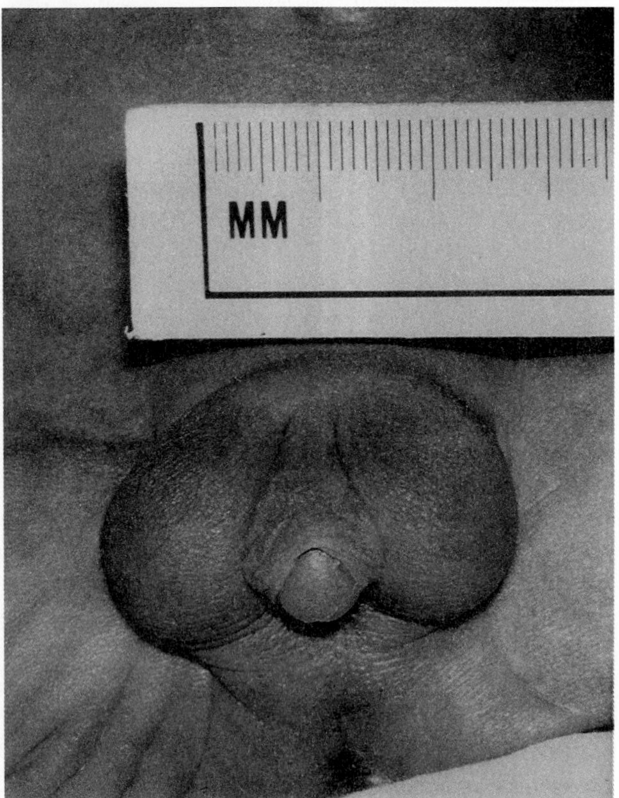

Fig. 58.12 External genitalia of a male pseudo-hermaphrodite infant with partial androgen insensitivity.

multiple reconstruction of external genitalia and azoospermia are good arguments in favour of a female sex of rearing.

Persistent Müllerian duct syndrome

Persistent Müllerian duct syndrome is usually discovered at surgery performed for cryptorchidism and/or hernia. It is a rare form of familial male pseudo-hermaphroditism characterised by persistence of uterus and Fallopian tubes in 46XY phenotypic males, and is due to defects in the synthesis or action of AMH.

To date, one homozygous mutation of the AMH receptor has been described in an AMH-positive patient out of 21 such patients [36]. This splice mutation generated two abnormal mRNAs, one missing the second exon required for ligand binding and the second mRNA coding for an abnormal protein due to an amino-acid substitution followed by the insertion of four amino acids. The treatment of persistent Müllerian duct syndrome is relatively straightforward in that all patients are phenotypic male and require orchidopexy.

Clinical and laboratory assessment of patients with intersex states

The assessment of patients with intersex states may be considered from the point of view of the paediatrician assessing an infant with ambiguous genitalia. The same principles apply to the older child or adult. It must be emphasised that the general appearance of the external genitalia, while important in deciding the appropriate gender for the child, is of very little help in defining the aetiology of the disorder.

Clinical assessment

The principles of clinical assessment are shown in Table 58.6. A history of a similar disorder in other family members may shed light on the likely diagnosis. Many of these conditions are genetically determined. Examination for other anomalies which could point to a dysmorphic syndrome known to be associated with abnormal genital development is also relevant. The most important aspect of the examination, however, is careful palpation of the gonads.

If no gonads are palpable, the most likely diagnosis is female pseudo-hermaphroditism due to CAH, and this is virtually certain if symptoms of salt loss develop. Other possible disorders are true hermaphroditism or male pseudo-hermaphroditism with intra-abdominal gonads. When *both gonads are palpable* in the scrotum or labial folds, the patient is likely to be a male pseudo-hermaphrodite, and measurement of plasma androgens will indicate whether the aetiology is a testicular or peripheral defect. A true hermaphrodite with bilateral ovotestes may also present in this way. The presence of only *one palpable gonad* or asymmetry of the perineum is suggestive of mixed gonadal dysgenesis or true hermaphroditism with asymmetrical gonads.

Laboratory assessment

A similar scheme may be devised as a guide to confirming the aetiology biochemically (Table 58.7). In all intersex patients a karyotype is indicated. *If no gonads are palpable*, determination of plasma 17α-hydroxyprogesterone will confirm or exclude 21-hydroxylase deficiency. In 11β-hydroxylase deficiency the plasma 11-deoxycortisol concentration is elevated.

The infant with *two palpable gonads* needs an hCG stimulation test to assess testicular androgen secretion. Numerous hCG regimens exist, of which two examples are 1000 iu daily for 3 days or a single injection of 1500 iu/m^2 body surface area [37]. Basal and post-stimulatory concentrations of testosterone, DHT and androstenedione should distinguish a disorder of testosterone biosynthesis from a

Table 58.6 Patient with intersex state: clinical assessment.

Family history, general examination for dysmorphic features
Examination of external genitalia
No gonads palpable
Female pseudo-hermaprodite: congenital adrenal hyperplasia (21-hydroxylase deficiency)
Male pseudo-hermaphrodite
One gonad palpable
Abnormal gonadal differentiation
Mixed gonadal dysgenesis (XO/XY)
True hermaphroditism
Two gonads palpable
Male pseudo-hermaphrodite
Impaired testosterone biosynthesis
Androgen-receptor defect
5α-reductase deficiency
True hermaphroditism

Table 58.7 Patient with intersex state: laboratory assessment.

No gonads palpable
Karyotype, plasma 17-hydroxyprogesterone, 11-deoxycortisol
One gonad palpable
Karyotype human chorionic gonadotrophin test, gonadal biopsy, pelvic ultrasonography, laparotomy
Two gonads palpable
Karyotype, human chorionic gonadotrophin test (1000 U daily × 3), plasma testosterone, dihydrotestosterone, dehydroepiandrosterone, androstenedione on days 0 and 4
In vitro androgen-binding studies
Molecular analysis
Sinography

syndrome of androgen insensitivity: molecular analysis of the androgen receptor gene may identify a mutation.

If one gonad is palpable gonadal biopsy may be helpful, particularly if ovarian tissue is suspected. Pelvic ultrasonography or exploratory laparotomy for identification of internal genital structures may also be indicated. In any patient with incomplete virilisation, urethrography should be performed to identify a vaginal cavity communicating posteriorly with the urethra.

Medical management

Choice of gender

Parents are usually shocked to learn that there is doubt as to the sex of their child; they are often under the impression that the child may grow up to be neither male or female. They often press for an early answer as to the infant's sex. Temptation to give a provisional opinion should be avoided until the nature of the disorder is known and an informed answer can be given. In the newborn the decision as to the appropriate sex-of-rearing is based mainly on the appearance of the external genitalia and on the likely pattern of secondary sexual development at puberty. This decision should be taken jointly by the paediatric endocrinologist, urologist and the parents, making use of the clinical, biochemical, cytogenetic and radiological features of the individual case. The gender should be assigned as soon as possible after birth; however, in some cases of severe ambiguity, there is a case for waiting to assess the effect of early treatment with depot testosterone (25–50 mg at monthly intervals) on phallic growth as a guide to androgen responsiveness. The karyotype has no direct bearing on the sex-of-rearing.

Virilised female infants with CAH should in general be raised as female. XY males with severe genital ambiguity due to deficient testosterone biosynthesis or androgen insensitivity are also probably best raised as females. Demonstration of absent androgen binding in cultured genital fibroblasts would add weight to this argument in the latter category. Other factors favouring female assignment are the presence of a vaginal pouch with an XO cell line. Ethnic considerations, however, which usually favour male gender assignment, may be overriding.

The concept that, once established, gender identity and role are more or less fixed has now been questioned by the studies of Imperato-McGinley *et al.* [38]. Although change of gender may be extremely difficult, the possibility of gender conversion should be viewed with an open mind in the individual subject who, because of spontaneous virilisation or feminisation at puberty, finds existence in their original gender intolerable.

Gender identity in intersex patients

Sex hormone therapy

Long-term treatment with androgens to increase phallic growth in early childhood has rightly fallen into disrepute because of the inevitable acceleration of bone maturation which leads to loss of ultimate growth potential. While standard testosterone treatment is effective for inducing pubertal development in males with androgen-responsive syndromes, it is of limited value in patients with androgen insensitivity. Induction of full masculinisation in these patients is still very unsatisfactory. It has, however, been demonstrated that some further virilisation in adult patients may be effectively induced using supraphysiological doses of depot testosterone, i.e. 500 mg weekly [33]. Effects, which were slow to appear, have been specifically seen on penile length and facial body hair growth.

In a number of intersex disorders, gender identity, i.e., the gender in which the patient perceives him- or herself, appears relatively unequivocal. For example, the female patient with virilisation of external genitalia as in CAH usually develops a predominantly female gender identity, although a number of androgen-dependent behaviour traits may be noticeable. This suggests that fetal androgen exposure influences subsequent behaviour. In complete androgen insensitivity, however, there is apparently no conflict of gender identity or role, both being unequivocally female. Patients with partial androgen insensitivity present a more complex picture. Such patients, assigned and raised as males, have been compared with those assigned and raised as females. Those raised as boys are said to have developed male gender identity, but as their pubertal development was incomplete they had difficulty in establishing male gender role. In contrast, those raised as females developed a female gender identity and role.

Recent studies of patients with 5α-reductase deficiency have rekindled the controversy of biological versus psychological origins of gender identity. Exposure to testosterone prenatally and during puberty appears to have a strong influence in converting female to male gender identity. However, no prospective studies have been performed, and the affected subjects may have been influenced by social pressures to assume a male role.

References

1 New MI. Steroid 21-hydroxylase deficiency (congenital adrenal hyperplasia). *Am J Med* 1995; **98**: 2S–8S.

2 Speicer PW, New MI. Prenatal diagnosis and treatment of congenital adrenal hyperplasia. *J Paediatr Endocrinol* 1994; **7**: 183–91.

3 Rösler A, Lieberman E. Enzymatic defects of steroidogenesis: 11β–hydroxylase deficiency congenital adrenal hyperplasia. In: New MO, Levine M, eds. *Adrenal Diseases in Childhood*. Basel: Karger, 1984: 47–71.

4 Hughes IA, Arisaka O, Perry LA, Honour JW. Early diagnosis of 11β-hydroxylase deficiency in two siblings confirmed by analysis of a novel steroid metabolite in newborn urine. *Acta Endocrinol* 1986; **111**: 349–54.

5 White PC, Curnow KM, Paseo L. Disorders of steroid 11β-hydroxylase isozymes. *Endocr Rev* 1994; **15**: 421–38.

6 Zhang L, Sakkal-Alkaddour H, Chang YT, Yang X, Pang S. A new compound heterozygous frameshift mutation in the type II 3β-hydroxysteroid dehydrogenase (3β-HSD) gene causes salt-wasting 3β-HSD deficiency congenital adrenal hyperplasia. *J Clin Endocrinol* 1996; **81**: 291–5.

7 Morishima A, Grumbach MM, Simpson ER, Fisher C, Qin K. Aromatase deficiency in male and female siblings caused by a novel mutation and the physiological role of oestrogens. *J Clin Endocrinol Metab* 1995; **80**: 3689–98.

8 Kirk JMW, Perry LA, Shand WS, Kirby RS, Besser GM, Savage MO. Female pseudohermaphroditism due to a maternal adrenocortical tumour. *J Clin Endocrinol Metab* 1990; **70**: 1280–4.

9 Rimoin DL, Schimke RN. *Genetic Disorders of the Endocrine Glands*. St Louis: CV Mosby, 1971.

10 Sultan C, Lobaccaro JM, Lumbroso S *et al.* Molecular aspects of sex differentiation applications in pathological conditions. In: Bergada C, Moguilevsky JA, eds. *Frontiers in Endocrinology. Puberty: Basic and Clinical Aspects*. Roma: Serono Symposia Publications, 1995: 21–35.

11 Wilson JD, Griffen JE, Russell DW. Steroid 5α-reductase 2 deficiency. *Endocr Rev* 1993; **14**: 577–93.

12 Brinkman AO. Steroid hormone receptors: activators of gene transcription. *J Pediatr Endocrinol* 1994; **7**: 275–282.

13 Lobaccaro JM, Poujol N, Chiche L, Lumbroso S, Brown TR, Sultan C. Molecular modeling and *in vitro* investigations of the human androgen receptor DNA-binding domain: application for the study of two mutations. *Mol Cell Endocrinol* 1996; **116**: 137–47.

14 Robboy SJ, Miller T, Donahoe PK *et al.* Dysgenesis of testicular and streak gonads in the syndrome of mixed gonadal dysgenesis: perspective derived from clinopathologic analysis of twenty-one cases. *Hum Pathol* 1982; **13**: 700–16.

15 Rajfer J, Walsh PC. Mixed gonadal dysgenesis—dysgenetic male pseudohermaphroditism. *Pediatr Acta Endocrinol* 1981; **8**: 105–15.

16 Bardoni B, Zanaria E, Guioli G *et al.* A dosage sensitive locus at chromosome Xp21 is involved in male to male sex reversal. *Nat Genet* 1994; **7**: 497–501.

17 Muscatelli F, Strom TM, Walker AP *et al.* Mutations in the DAX-I gene give rise to both x-linked adrenal hypoplasia congenital and hypogonadotrophic hypogonadism. *Nature* 1994; **372**: 672–6.

18 Wagner T, Wirth J, Meyer J *et al.* Autosomal sex reversal and campomelic dysplasia are caused by mutations in and around the SRY-related gene SOX-9. *Cell* 1994; **79**: 160–4.

19 Van Niekerk WA. True hermaphroditism. *Pediatr Adol Endocrinol* 1981; **8**: 80–99.

20 Wachtel SS, Bard J. The XX testis. *Pediatr Adol Endocrinol* 1981; **8**: 116–32.

21 Kremer H, Kraaij R, Toledo SPA *et al.* Male pseudohermaphroditism due to a homozygous missense mutation of the luteinizing hormone receptor gene. *Nature Genet* 1995; **9**: 160–4.

22 New MI, Josso N. Disorders of gonadal differentiation and congenital adrenal hyperplasia. *Endocrinol Metab Clin North Am* 1988; **17**: 339–66.

23 Forest MG. Inborn errors of testosterone biosynthesis. *Pediatr Adol Endocrinol* 1981; **8**: 133–55.

24 Lin D, Sugawara T, Staruss III JF *et al.* Role of steroidgeneic acute regulatory protein in adrenal and gonadal steroidogenesis. *Science* 1995; **267**: 1828–31.

25 Yanase T, Simpson ER, Waterman MR. 17 alpha-hydroxylase/17, 20-lyase deficiency—from clinical investigation to molecular definition. *Endocr Rev* 1991; **12**: 91–108.

26 Morel Y, Mbarki F, Portrat S. Génétique des pseudohermaphrodismes masculins par anomalies de la synthèse de la testostérone. In: Chaussain JL, Roger M, eds. *Les Ambiguïtés Sexuelles*. Paris: Publifusion; 1995; 53–75.

27 Martin F, Perheentupa, Aldercreutz E. Plasma and urinary androgens in a pubertal boy with 3β-hydroxysteroid with hypertension due to a 17α-hydroxylation deficiency. *Clin Endocrinol* 1976; **5**: 53–9.

28 Andersson S, Geissler WM, Wu L *et al.* Molecular genetics and pathophysiology of 17β-hydroxysteroid dehydrogenase 3 deficiency. *J Clin Endocrinol Metab* 1996; **81**: 130–6.

29 Gross DJ, Landau H, Kohn G *et al.* Male pseudohermaphroditism

due to 17β-hydroxysteroid dehydrogenase deficiency—a report of 3 cases. *Clin Endocrinol* 1985; **23**: 439–44.

30 Savage MO, Preece MA, Jeffcoate SL *et al.* Familial male pseudohermaphroditism due to deficiency of 5α-reductase. *Clin Endocrinol* 1980; **12**: 397–406.

31 Jenkins EP, Andersson S, Imperato-McGinley J, Wilson JD, Russell DW. Genetic and pharmacological evidence for more than one human steroid 5α-reductase. *J Clin Invest* 1991; **89**: 293–300.

32 Boudon C, Lumbroso S, Lobaccaro JM *et al.* Molecular study of the 5 alpha–reductase type 2 gene in three European families with 5 alpha-reductase deficiency. *J Clin Endocrinol Metab* 1995; **80**: 2149–53.

33 Price P, Wass JAH, Griffin JE *et al.* High dose androgen therapy in male pseudohermaphroditism due to 5α–reductase deficiency and disorders of the androgen receptor. *J Clin Invest* 1984; **74**: 1496–508.

34 Quigley CA, Debellis A, Marschke KB, Elawady MK, Wilson EM, French FA. Androgen receptor defects: historical, clinical, and molecular perspectives. *Endocr Rev* 1995; **16**: 327–32.

35 Lumbroso S, Lobaccaro JM, Belon C, Boulot P, Amram S, Sultan C. Molecular prenatal exclusion of Reifenstein syndrome. *Eur J Endocrinol* 1994; **130**: 327–32.

36 Imbeaud S, Faure E, Lamarre I *et al.* Insensitivity to anti-Müllerian hormone due to a mutation in the human anti-Müllerian hormone receptor. *Nature Genet* 1995; **11**: 382–8.

37 Smals AGH, Gerlag FFM, Pieters GFF, Drayer JIM, Benraad TJ, Kloppenborg PWC. Leydig cell responsiveness to single and repeated human chorionic gonadotrophin administration. *J Clin Endocrinol Metab* 1979; **49**: 12–14.

38 Imperato-McGinley J, Peterson RE, Gautier T, Sturla E. Male pseudohermaproditism secondary to 5α-reductase deficiency. A model for the role of androgen in both the development of the male phenotype and the evolution of a male gender identity. *J Steroid Biochem* 1979; **11**: 637–45.

Part 12
Female Infertility

CHAPTER 59

Assessment of female infertility

R. Howell

Definition

Infertility has been defined by the World Health Organization (WHO) as the inability to conceive despite cohabitation, exposure to pregnancy, and the wish to become pregnant for a period of 1 year [1].

Epidemiology

The capacity to conceive, or fecundity, may be measured by the monthly possibility of conception. The fertility of women after discontinuation of an intrauterine contraceptive device (IUCD) or barrier contraception has formed the basis of the expected fertility pattern in a group of apparently normal women [2,3]. Cumulative pregnancy rates of 0.60 and 0.88 at 3 and 12 months have been calculated, but not every couple attempting pregnancy has the same monthly fecundity. Using the life-table analysis, it has been estimated that 81% of newly married couples will have no problem with fertility, 4.8% will be sterile and 15% will have delayed conception [4]. Given an average monthly fecundity of 0.05 in the latter group, a total of 7% of couples will not have conceived within 3 years.

Over the past 20 years there has been a sharp escalation in demand for infertility services concomitant with an overall decline in fertility. Possible explanations for this are the postponement of marriage, the delayed age of childbearing, the increasing use of contraception, more liberalised abortion, more concern over environmental issues and perhaps an unfavourable economic climate [5]. The postponement of marriage and the desire for first pregnancy means that the effect of age upon fertility plays a major role. In at least 10 different populations, the decline in fertility with advancing age has been repeatedly reported [6,7]. Little is known about secular trends in the prevalence of infertility. Although some infectious causes such as tuberculosis and gonorrhoea are less common now, infertility due to *Chlamydia* infections and environmental pollution may be increasing.

About one-third of women who defer pregnancy until their mid to late 30s will have an infertility problem. Ageing has a multifactorial effect upon fertility. The increased incidence of anovulation and the effects of ageing upon oocytes and the uterus may all be acting synergistically. The older woman is also more prone to conditions such as endometriosis and fibroids, thereby reducing her fertility. There is a 50% decrease in female fecundity from the age of 25 to 35 [8]. A cumulative exposure to environmental hazards may also play a role. The increased incidence of early spontaneous abortion in the older woman is also a factor to be considered. The majority of early abortions after 35 years of age are due to chromosomal abnormalities such as autosomal trisomies and sex chromosome deletions [9]. The incidence of early abortion is about 10% up to the age of 30 years, and then increases to 18% in the late 30s and 34% in the early 40s.

The overall incidence of infertility, both primary and secondary, in one health district in England has been estimated to be 17%, or one in six couples. This represents an annual incidence of 1.2 couples for every 1000 in the population [10]. Care needs to be exercised in generalising to other health districts and countries, however, which may be different demographically and have different specialist interests and expertise.

Philosophy of infertility investigations and treatment

An alternative definition of infertility to that of the WHO is of a perceived difficulty in having a child, or difficulty in creating a relationship, that of parent and child. Medicine does not offer the only solution to this problem: there are others such as adoption. A majority will have to come to terms with involuntary childlessness. Although modern reproductive technologies permit as their end-point the techniques of 'assisted reproduction', it should not be assumed that all patients, remaining childless, will proceed along this path. Some may drop out of treatment, while others may feel reluctant or unable to proceed to these techniques for religious, ethical, financial or personal reasons.

Every clinic appointment involves counselling of patients with a full and frank discussion. Patients should be allowed to air their hopes and fears. Infertility can be a very distressing condition because parenthood is seen as a normal and desirable goal. Childlessness is stigmatised by some societies, and many patients feel ashamed, isolated and distressed by their plight. Furthermore, infertility and its medical management can take its toll on the happiest and most secure of partnerships.

Infertility is a negative experience which can have a profound effect on people's self-esteem, self-image and on their relationships. Where patients manifest symptoms of stress and depression, it should not be assumed that they are suffering from an underlying psychopathology, but rather as an outcome of the experience, investigations and treatment. The ways in which infertility is managed involve intruding into and scrutinising the most personal and private areas of people's lives, in particular their sexual relationship. Great sensitivity and understanding is required by the doctors, nurses and counsellors involved in the management. Timing is all important, and not simply because certain tests have to be carried out at the correct time in the menstrual cycle. The cause of the couple's infertility and appropriate treatment should be instigated as accurately and as quickly as possible, thereby alleviating anxiety and stress. Once a diagnosis has been reached, patients should be given a realistic assessment of their chances of becoming parents to enable them to plan and make decisions for their future. Formal counselling, other than that provided by the doctor, has been shown to enhance the quality of life, but the exact needs of the infertile couple in terms of counselling care are unknown [11]. Infertility support groups help a number of couples, but may be threatening for others as it involves a public declaration of their condition.

Aetiology of female infertility

A large number of factors may be responsible for a couple's infertility. In one-third of cases the problem is caused by one or more factors solely affecting the woman. In another 30–40% of couples requiring medical help, the aetiology is a combination of female and male factors, while in the remainder male conditions alone are responsible.

The causes of infertility may vary from one geographic and social area to another. A WHO task force [12] revealed the following causes of infertility in women: tubal factor 36%, ovulatory disorders 33%, endometriosis 6%, and no demonstrable cause 40%. A similar distribution was found in Asia, Latin America and the Middle East, whereas in Africa, most infertile women had tubal infertility. Unexplained infertility (both partners considered) has been found in 8–20% of couples [13]. Because multifactorial infertility accounts for 30–40% of the total, every couple should have a full infertility investigation.

Ovulatory failure and dysfunction

Ovulatory dysfunction plays a major treatable role in female infertility [10,14]. Ovarian, pituitary and hypothalamic factors may manifest as a spectrum of dysfunctions ranging from irregular ovulation to chronic anovulation and amenorrhoea. Several medical and psychological conditions, drug use and abuse, exercise, dieting and stress may affect ovarian function via the hypothalamus. Central nervous system tumours such as craniopharyngiomas, cysts and inflammatory and infiltrative processes may all affect the pulsatile release of gonadotrophin-releasing hormone (GnRH) or invade the sella turcica [15].

The pursuit of slenderness within western society has increased the incidence of menstrual irregularities [16]. A drastic reduction of calorie intake is associated with a change in the pattern of adult luteinising hormone (LH) secretion to a prepubertal pattern [17]. Women engaged in vigorous competitive training such as athletes and ballet dancers may suffer menstrual and ovulatory dysfunction, often becoming amenorrhoeic [18]. Bulimia, obesity and a significant weight gain may also cause hypothalamo-pituitary dysfunction. Pituitary adenomas secreting prolatin, growth hormone or adrenocorticotrophic hormone (ACTH) may all inhibit ovarian function, and obviously necessitate detailed pituitary evaluation.

Ovarian conditions that may inhibit or compromise ovulation include the polycystic ovary syndrome (PCOS), a complex multiorgan syndrome manifesting itself clinically with infertility, anovulation, obesity and hirsutism (see Chapter 54). Ovulatory dysfunction, especially oocyte entrapment, may be caused by ovarian cysts, periovarian adhesions, endometriosis and rarely malignant ovarian tumours.

The luteinised unruptured follicle syndrome (LUF) is defined as the failure to identify preovulatory follicle rupture with consequent oocyte entrapment [19].

A recent hypothesis is that hypersecretion of LH during the mid- and late follicular phase of the cycle is responsible for the impairment of fertilisation of oocytes and increased early pregnancy loss [20]. Experience from *in vitro* fertilisation (IVF) treatments indicates that high LH concentrations during the late follicular phase are associated with lower rates of fertilisation, cleavage and pregnancy. There was a significantly higher conception rate after 2 years of follow-up among 147 women who had normal follicular serum LH than in a group of 46 women with high LH concentrations (88% versus 67%) and lower frequency of miscarriage (12% versus 65%) [21].

Luteal phase defects

Luteal phase abnormalities result from a defective corpus luteum with inadequate progesterone production. The defect may refer either to a short luteal phase (<11 days) with normal levels of progesterone, or more commonly a luteal phase of normal length but with reduced progesterone levels. Both situations may cause failure of blastocyst implantation and perhaps early abortion. The luteal phase is evaluated by serial progesterone levels [22], timed endometrial biopsy, or preferably both. The histopathologist's dating of the endometrial biopsy is found to be more than 2 days out of phase with the actual day of the cycle and low progesterone levels are observed. An inadequate luteal phase can be found in up to 30% of isolated cycles from normal 'fertile' women, and only if found in at least two cycles is it thought to be a significant factor in infertility and recurrent abortion [5]. Although an inadequate luteal phase results from decreased hormone production by the corpus luteum, the underlying causes of the abnormality may be multiple [23]. Decreased follicle-stimulating hormone (FSH) levels in the follicular phase and abnormal patterns of LH and FSH secretion have been implicated. Hyperprolactinaemia may also be associated with an inadequate luteal phase. It has been found that the concentration of nuclear endometrial progesterone receptors are reduced in the proliferative phase of the cycle [23], with an inadequate luteal phase suggesting inadequate prior oestrogenic stimulation. Thus, adequacy of the luteal phase may in turn depend on factors occurring during the follicular phase.

The role of luteal phase defects in causing infertility has been challenged because the diagnosis is not predictive of recurrence in subsequent cycles and other causes of infertility have not been controlled for. Careful analysis of all published studies has also shown progesterone treatment to be of *no* benefit for luteal phase defects or early abortion [24].

Endometriosis

The cause of endometriosis is unknown. The diagnosis is frequently made because of the technical ease of modern video-laparoscopy. The easy explanation is that endometriosis follows retrograde menstruation, but much laboratory and clinical evidence suggests that endometriosis is more complex than this.

Severe endometriosis can compromise fertility by causing pelvic adhesions, distorted anatomy, and ovarian or tubal damage. In addition, the ovulatory process and ovum capture may be disturbed. The relationship between minimal endometriosis and infertility is based on indirect evidence, such as the higher fecundity of infertile women requiring donor insemination without visible endometriosis than women with endometriosis. This association is less clear than earlier believed. Firstly, the apparently high frequency (20–40%) in infertile women compared with fertile controls (<10%) may be due to observer and reporting bias [25]. Secondly, neither medical nor surgical treatment of the endometriotic foci increases the pregnancy rate. Thirdly, there are conflicting data about the monthly fecundity of women with minimal or mild endometriosis. Controlled studies have not shown any treatment-dependent improvement in fertility with medical suppression of endometriosis or surgical excision and ablation. This includes the newer endoscopic operative laparoscopy approaches. Therefore, the laparoscopic diagnosis of minimal or mild endometriosis does not necessarily mean that the cause of the infertility has been found. It may be an incidental finding and of no importance in the pathogenesis of infertility.

Tubal damage

A history of pelvic inflammatory disease (especially *Chlamydia* or *Gonoccoccus*) septic abortion, IUCD usage, ruptured appendix, pelvic surgery or ectopic pregnancy are all highly suggestive of tubal disease. However, almost 50% of women who are eventually found to have tubal disease and/or pelvic adhesions give no history of antecedent infection.

The first three bouts of acute salphingitis carry a significant risk of permanent sequelae, with a probability of doubling after each inflammatory insult [26]. Reproductive capacity is decreased when intraluminal and extraluminal disease coexist, or when both proximal and distal tubal disease are present.

Uterine abnormalities

The uterus participates in the reproductive process by allowing sperm transport and then blastocyst implantation. Acute endometritis after IUCD insertion, uterine curettage or sexually transmitted diseases may all adversely affect future fertility. Tuberculosis, intrauterine adhesions, hyperplasia, polyps, fibroids, neoplasia and congenital uterine malformations are all rarer aetiological factors.

Cervical mucus

Inadequate secretion and/or hostile cervical mucus may be

responsible for approximately 7–20% of cases of female infertility [27]. A history of previous cervical surgery such as a cone biopsy, laser therapy, repeated punch biopsies, cauterisation or cryotherapy may suggest a cervical cause. One of the commonest causes of cervical hostility is acute cervicitis and appropriate cultures from the cervix should be taken looking specifically for *Chlamydia trachomatis* and *Neisseria gonorrhoea*.

Vagina

Vaginal causes of infertility are rare. Congenital malformations of the lower genital tract such as a septum and vaginismus may lead to coital problems. Lubricants such as 'KY Jelly' and 'Surgilube' are spermicidal, and saliva, oils and glycerine may interfere with sperm transport. Acute vaginitis caused by *Candida albicans* or *Trichomonas vaginalis* both interfere with sperm viability and transport [28].

Immunological factors

Antibodies against sperm can be elicited by the antigens being placed in the vagina, cervix or uterus. The immune response is dependent on the antigen rather than the site of the inoculation. Most antigens to the female genital tract elicit a plasma cell antibody response mediated by immunoglobulin A (IgA), whereas a systemic response is mounted by IgG antibodies [29,30]. The cervical production of immunoglobulins is constant throughout the cycle but the amount of cervical mucus varies. The final IgA concentration is thus lower at mid-cycle when cervical mucus is more plentiful. Antibodies against the sperm surface may become harmful when sufficient quantities of the complement cascade are available and/or macrophages are opsonised. Phagocytosis and complement-mediated cytotoxity have been reported to affect human reproductive function. Post-coital testing in immunologically affected women usually reveals no sperm. It has also been suggested that autoantibodies to the zona pellucida contribute to female infertility [31].

Systemic disorders

Thyroid disease. Both hyper- and hypothyroidism are associated with menorrhagia, anovulation, oligomenorrhoea and amenorrhoea.

Abnormal glucocorticoid metabolism may cause menstrual abnormalities and anovulation.

Renal, hepatic and cardiovascular disorders may affect the reproductive axis with resulting ovulatory dysfunction.

Diabetes mellitus is associated with an increased incidence of anovulation [32].

Environmental factors

Cigarette smoking. A number of epidemiological studies have associated smoking with female infertility [33,34]. Smoking may directly or indirectly affect tubal and/or cervical function. Nicotine and other components of cigarettes have an adverse effect upon ciliary function. Cigarette smoke may also have direct toxic effect on oocytes which has been demonstrated in animals and the eggs of smokers show reduced fertilisation rates at IVF [35].

Marijuana, alcohol, cocaine and other mood-altering substances. These may all reduce reproductive potential. The amount of drug use, its frequency, the impurity of the ingredients, the age of the user and the length of abuse all influence potential hazardous effects upon fertility.

Pharmacological factors

Antimetabolites and chemotherapeutic agents, used to treat various neoplasias, may cause ovulatory dysfunction [36]. Greater damage may be done when women are sexually mature at the onset of therapy than if treatment is commenced prepubertally (see Chapter 75).

Antiprostaglandins may interfere with the process of ovulation, possibly causing LUF and alterations in corpus luteum function.

Central aminergic serotonin and opioid-acting drugs can all affect the function of the reproductive axis.

Congenital/genetic factors

Autosomal and sex chromosome abnormalities (deletions, insertions, etc.) and mosaicism usually present with primary ovarian failure, although they may rarely cause secondary ovulatory and menstrual dysfunction.

Psychological factors

Being infertile may generate psychological disturbances. However, do psychological factors actually have a causal or contributory role in some cases of infertility? One myth about infertility is that adoption increases the couple's fertility. Several studies have used psychological testing of large populations of infertile women compared with controls [37]. However, no consistent differences in psychological variables, such as anxiety, depression, and social adjustment, were found.

There might be an association between stress and infertility among women with ovulatory disorders or unexplained infertility, but the precise role of stress is uncertain. This does not mean that stress cannot cause infertility. Hypothalamic amenorrhoea, for instance, can be induced by stressful life events, and anorexia nervosa is clearly a psychogenic condition.

Occupational factors

Most occupational studies have examined male reproductive function, usually by measuring semen characteristics. Refinement of epidemiological research methods has enhanced the possibility of detection of environmental hazards to female fecundity. A recent example is the reporting of delayed conception in dental assistants with high exposure to nitrous oxide [37,38]. In women, occupational exposure to textile dyes, lead, mercury, and cadmium have been associated with infertility. The associations were mostly found in women classified as having unexplained infertility. In fertile women, the same exposures have been associated with delayed conceptions.

Unexplained infertility

When a couple have undergone a thorough infertility investigation and no apparent cause is found, the term 'unexplained' infertility is used. It is estimated that in up to 28% of couples with both primary and secondary infertility no cause is identifiable. The word 'unexplained' is probably a misnomer if investigations are exhaustive, and as more knowledge accumulates from assisted conception techniques this category is bound to decrease.

Table 59.1 Investigations performed at the couple's first clinic appointment.

Full history and examination of female and male
Anatomical problems (consultant discussion)
Psychosexual problems (refer to social worker or psychosexual counsellor)
Severe social problems (refer to social worker or counsellor)

Investigations on female
Haemoglobin
Blood group
Sickle (if applicable)
Rubella status
Cervical smear (if not done within 2 years)
Day 21 progesterone
Cervical swab for *Chlamydia*

If menstrual cycles are excessively long or short (<24 or >32 days) or amenorrhoeic also measure:

Luteinising hormone and follicle-stimulating hormone
Testosterone
Sex hormone-binding globulin
Oestradiol
Prolactin
Thyroid function
Androstenedione
Dehydroepiandrosterone sulphate

If a history of previous pelvic infection is given, also arrange laparoscopy and dye and hysteroscopy

Endometrial biopsy (ensure abstinence or adequate contraception in the month of operation)

Investigations on male
Semen analysis

Investigation of the infertile couple

The full range of investigations should be performed and a diagnosis made within three visits to a specialised infertility clinic. Suggested protocols for investigation are shown in Tables 59.1, 59.2 and 59.3. These are intended as guidelines for senior staff and as teaching aids for doctors in training. They are an attempt to promote uniformity of investigation and to reach a diagnosis as quickly as possible, thereby reducing the enormous stresses placed upon the couples. The uniformity of investigations and treatment also allows for better evaluation of results.

History

A comprehensive history from both female and male is a valuable aid in directing the infertility evaluation towards certain aetiological factors: for example, in the female a history of menstrual irregularity (anovulation), previous pelvic surgery, IUCD usage or pelvic infection (tubal factor), pelvic pain, secondary dysmenorrhoea or dyspareunia (endometriosis), cervical cautery or cone biopsy (cervical factor), previous abortions or curettage (uterine factor); in the male, a history of genital operations or infections, undescended testes, mumps orchitis, medications and excessive alcohol intake may all be significant.

Physical examination

Female

The general physical examination should be directed towards signs of an endocrine disorder: acne, obesity, hirsutism, skin pigmentation, galactorrhoea or thyroid abnormalities. A thorough pelvic examination is of paramount importance.

Table 59.2 Investigations to be performed at the couple's second clinic appointment.

Investigation	Management
Haemoglobin <10.0 g/dl	Ferritin Serum and red blood cell folate B_{12} Defer further investigations until results available ? Refer for specialist haematological opinion
Rubella susceptible	Vaccinate and ensure adequate contraception for 3 months
Day 21 progesterone	>30 nmol/l, arrange post-coital test (days 13 or 14) <30 nmol/l, if not done already measure: Luteinising hormone and follicle-stimulating hormone Testosterone Sex hormone-binding globulin Prolactin Oestradiol Thyroid function Androstenedione Dehydroepiandrosterone sulphate
Semen analysis	
Normal	Arrange post-coital test (day 13 or 14 if cycle regular; combine with ultrasound follicle monitoring if cycle irregular)
Abnormal	Follow protocol (not included in this chapter)
Laparoscopy and dye abnormal	Consultant discussion Arrange hysterosalpingography if tubal surgery contemplated Treat endometriosis ? *In vitro* fertilisation appropriate
If all investigations are found to be normal	Laparoscopy and dye, endometrial biopsy and hysteroscopy in the luteal phase (ensure contraception or abstinence in the month of operation) Postcoital test (day 13 or 14 of the cycle) Anti-sperm antibodies in male and female serum Serial progesterones in luteal phase days 19,21,23

The cervix should be evaluated for signs of infection and bacteriological swabs taken. A cervical smear should be taken unless recently performed. The bimanual examination may detect signs of endometriosis, fibroids, active pelvic infection or ovarian enlargement.

Male

A physical examination with particular emphasis on the penis, testes, epididymes and vasa deferens should be performed on all men at the initial consultation. Measurement of testicular size with an orchidometer and the presence of a varicocele are both important (see Chapter 50).

Initial blood tests

A full blood count should be performed as the patient may require a general anaesthetic for the laparoscopy, and also acts as a screening test for intercurrent disease. The blood group and sickle status (if appropriate) will also be required before general anaesthesia.

Rubella status is important to clarify in all women desiring pregnancy. If found to be susceptible, vaccination should be performed before any further investigations or treatment. The couple should use barrier contraception for the following 3 months.

Table 59.3 Management of the third visit to the clinic*.

Investigation	Management
Post-coital test negative (<5 motile sperm per high-power field)	Serum–cervical mucus contact test
Serial progesterone low (<30 nmol^{-1})	Clomiphene therapy
Laparoscopy and dye abnormal	Consultant discussion Arrange hysterosalpingography if tubal surgery contemplated Treat endometriosis ? *In vitro* fertilisation appropriate

* Evaluate results of second visit. By the third or very occasionally the fourth visit all couples should have a diagnosis and suitable therapy have been instigated.

Semen analysis

For a full discussion of normal semen parameters, see Chapter 50.

Post-coital test

The post-coital test (PCT) provides information regarding the 'receptivity' of cervical mucus and the ability of sperm both to reach and survive in the mucus. Just before ovulation, when oestrogen levels peak, the mucus is plentiful, clear, watery and 'stretchy'. Earlier in the cycle and 2–3 days after ovulation, when progesterone levels increase, the mucus is thick, viscid and opaque. The PCT is performed just before ovulation as determined by the length of previous cycles, if they are regular. If the cycles are irregular, vaginal ultrasound monitoring of follicular development and a timed PCT may be helpful. Ideally, the test should be performed 8–12 hours after coitus, the couple having abstained from intercourse for 48 hours before the test. The mucus is removed and examined for macroscopic and microscopic characteristics. The elasticity (Spinnbarkeit) should be at least 8–10 cm at mid-cycle. When dried on a slide it should form a distinct ferning pattern. Poor mucus at mid-cycle reduces sperm penetration and pregnancy rates, provided that the test has been timed correctly [39].

The 'normal' number of sperm in a PCT is a matter of some dispute. Estimates range from one to over 20 per high-power field (HPF), but the majority arbitrarily choose five motile sperms per HPF as the lower limit of normal. The prognostic value of the PCT is also controversial. One study found no difference in the pregnancy rates between groups having no sperm, no motile sperm, one to five motile sperm, six to 10 motile sperm and 11 or more motile sperm per HPF [39]. Another study demonstrated a statistically significant increase in pregnancies only when there were more than 20 sperm per HPF. Twenty per cent of fertile couples have been found to have no sperm or less than one sperm per HPF [40], raising doubts about the validity of the test. Others have reported that women with progressively motile sperm in the PCT have significantly higher pregnancy rates than those with no progressively motile sperm [41]. The PCT also provides information on cervical mucus quality, the adequacy of coital technique, some information on sperm number and quality, and perhaps some idea of prognosis. A poor result in the PCT may also raise the question of an immunological cause for the couple's infertility. No sperm or only dead sperm on the PCT is a difficult diagnostic problem.

It should be checked that the couple are not using any spermicidal lubricants, that the pH of the mucus is not below 7.0, and that cervical cultures are negative. Anti-sperm-antibody tests in seminal plasma and male and female sera should also be performed, especially if the sperm are seen to be 'shaking on the spot' rather than progressively motile on the PCT. A detailed discussion on anti-sperm antibodies is found in Chapter 50.

Sperm–cervical mucus contact testing

In vitro cross-testing using donor mucus and donor sperm can help elucidate whether the poor PCT is due to a defect in the mucus or the sperm. Penetration of the cervical mucus by husband and donor sperm are compared on a slide under the microscope. The sperm–cervical mucus contact (SCMC) test [42] and the crossed hostility test [43] are important in that they provide an opportunity to study directly the reaction between spermatozoa and the new environment, in which they should make forward progress.

Tests for ovulation

Symptoms

Women who have regular cycles with some premenstrual symptoms and spasmodic dysmenorrhoea are almost always ovulatory. This is reinforced by the presence of mid-cycle pain in one or other iliac fossa, and the secretion of copious clear mid-cycle mucus.

Basal body temperature

The basal body temperature (BBT) is taken immediately upon waking, before any activity. A significant rise in temperature (0.4–0.5°C) is noted 2 days after the LH peak, coinciding with the rise in progesterone. BBT records can only approximate the time of ovulation in retrospect, and they are a common source of obsession and anguish for many couples. There is also disagreement among doctors concerning the interpretation of individual charts. To be used prospectively for ovulation prediction, nearly absolute cycle regularity is needed. Their use should thus be restricted to two or three cycles before specialist clinic referral.

Endometrial biopsy

Endometrial biopsy is a reliable end-organ response of ovulation and the luteal phase. The biopsy is performed 2–3 days before the expected period and may be combined with a laparoscopy or performed as a painless out-patient procedure using modern endometrial samplers. It is now generally performed to evaluate the adequacy of the luteal phase rather than to confirm ovulation.

Serum progesterone

A single, well-timed (day 21) progesterone estimation will give highly specific information regarding ovulation [22,24]. Serial levels may be needed to confirm or refute a luteal phase defect.

Luteinising hormone

Several simple rapid monoclonal antibody assay kits for the detection of urinary LH are now commercially available to patients 'over the counter'. They are used daily beginning on days 10 or 11 of the cycle. Ovulation occurs approximately 28–36 hours after the first rise of LH so that intercourse, artificial insemination or the PCT may be properly timed to ovulation. Although they are at present expensive, they may have some value in couples with unexplained infertility, especially if combined with serial ultrasound scans. Pregnancy rates of 7–12% per cycle have been reported when vaginal ultrasonography is combined with urine LH measurements in stimulated cycles.

Serial ultrasound scans

Serial ultrasound scans starting on day 6 or 8 of the cycle, using a vaginal transducer, have become a valuable tool for monitoring follicular development. Although particularly useful for hyperstimulated cycles, scanning also plays a major role in natural cycles. Ovulation can be pinpointed to within 24 hours, enabling timed intercourse or artificial insemination to occur. The diagnosis of LUF may be confirmed or refuted when the ultrasonographic data are compared with serial progesterone estimations. It is our practice to monitor fully all couples with 'unexplained infertility' for one cycle both ultrasonographically and endocrinologically (LH and FSH on days 2 or 3 of the cycle, daily urinary LH starting on day 10, and alternate-day progesterone levels from ovulation).

Tubal and peritoneal factors

The functions of the fallopian tubes include ovum pick-up, fertilisation and transport of the ovum, sperm and embryo. The diagnostic tests of tubal function are rather crude, and the two more commonly employed are laparoscopy and hysterosalpingography.

Laparoscopy

Diagnostic laparoscopy and dye perturbation is the primary method for assessing tubal patency in most centres. In addition, this procedure allows the discovery and documentation of other pelvic pathology such as adhesions and endometriosis. Endometriosis, if found, should be accurately staged [45]. The procedure should be performed by an experienced gynaecologist to allow more accurate diagnosis, and also the option of surgical laparoscopic therapy (cautery and/or laser vaporisation of adhesions and endometriotic deposits) at the time of the diagnostic procedure.

Hysterosalpingography

Hysterosalpingography (HSG) is a simple procedure to perform and does not require a general anaesthetic, but it can be painful and poses the potential risk of infection. For these latter two reasons, many infertility specialists regard it as a second-line, albeit complementary, investigation to laparoscopy. It is, however, essential if tubal surgery is contemplated to assess intraluminal pathology, or if a uterine abnormality is suspected.

The radiographic study is performed 2–5 days after cessation of menstrual flow under image intensification fluoroscopy. A previous history of pelvic inflammatory disease necessitates antibiotic prophylaxis. A tenaculum is placed on the cervix for downward traction and a cannula is placed inside the cervical canal. Contrast medium (either oil or water-soluble radio-opaque dye) is then injected through the cannula. There are several inherent disadvantages of HSG in assessing tubal patency: (i) technical difficulties as well as tubal spasm result in a significant rate of 'false positive' proximal tubal occlusion when compared with laparoscopy; and (ii) HSG is confined to the inner architecture of the uterus and fallopian tube and 'false negatives' may occur: patent tubes on HSG are not necessarily normal laparoscopically, peritubal disease going undiagnosed. HSGs concurred with laparoscopic evaluation in only 46–78% when several series were reviewed [46].

Uterine factors

Primary infertility as a result of uterine abnormalities is rare (congenital abnormalities, adhesions, polyps and fibroids), but may contribute to recurrent pregnancy loss.

HSG is a reliable technique for assessing the uterine cavity. If filling defects are noted on HSG, then a hysteroscopy should be performed. This is a complementary investigation to HSG. The hysteroscope is good for differentiating between endometrial polyps and submucous fibroids. It permits the definitive diagnosis and treatment of intrauterine adhesions and some congenital anomalies such as a septate uterus.

References

1 World Health Organization. *Manual on the Investigation and Diagnosis of the Infertile Couple*. Geneva: WHO, 1980.

2 Tietze C. Fertility after discontinuation of intrauterine and oral contraception. *Int J Fertil* 1968; **13**: 385–9.

3 Vessey MP, Wright NH, McPherson K, Wiggins P. Fertility after stopping different methods of contraception. *Br Med J* 1978; **1**: 265–7.

4 Spira A. Epidemiology of human reproduction. *Human Reprod* 1986; **1**: 111–15.

5 Speroff L, Glass RH, Kase NG. *Clinical Gynecologic Endocrinology and Infertility*, 4th edn. Baltimore, MD: Williams and Wilkins, 1989: 514–16.

6 Tietze C. Reproductive span and rate of reproduction among Hutterite women. *Fertil Steril* 1957; **8**: 89–97.

7 Virro MR, Shewchuk AB. Pregnancy outcome in 242 conceptions after artificial insemination with donor sperm and effects of maternal age on the prognosis for successful pregnancy. *Am J Obstet Gynecol* 1984; **148**: 518–24.

8 van Noord-Zaadstra BM, Looman CWN, Alsbach H, Habbema JDF, te Velde ER, Karbaat J. Delaying childbearing: effect of age on fecundity and outcome of pregnancy. *Br Med J* 1991; **302**: 1361–5.

9 Kola I, Sathananthan H, Gras L. Chromosomal analysis of preimplantation mammalian embryos. In: Trounson A, Gardner D, eds. Handbook of *In Vitro* Fertilization. London: CRC Press, 1993: 173–93.

10 Hull MGR, Glazener CMA, Kelly NJ *et al.* Population study of causes, treatment and outcome of fertility. *Br Med J* 1985; **291**: 1693–7.

11 Edelmann RJ, Connolly KJ. Psychological aspects of infertility. *Br J Med Psychol* 1986; **59**: 209–19.

12 Cates W, Farley TMM, Rowe PJ. Worldwide patterns of infertility: is Africa different? *Lancet* 1985; **I**: 596.

13 Thonneau P, Marchand S, Tallee A *et al.* Incidence and main causes of infertility in a resident population (1850000) of three French regions (1988–1989). *Hum Prod* 1991; **6**: 811–16.

13 Pirke KM, Schweiger U, Lemmel W *et al.* The influence of dieting on the menstrual cycle of healthy young women. *Clin Endocrinol Metab* 1985; **60**: 1174–9.

14 Kim MH, Chang FE. Chronic anovulation. *Clin Obstet Gynaecol* 1984; **27**: 941–52.

15 Davajan V, Kletzky OA. Primary amenorrhoea in infertility. In: Mishell DR, Jr, Davajan V, Oradell NJ, eds. *Contraception and Reproductive Endocrinology*. New York: Medical Economics Books, 1986: 237–51.

16 Pirke KM, Schweiger U, Lemmel W *et al.* The influence of dieting on the menstrual cycle of healthy young women. *Clin Endocrinol Metab* 1985: **60**: 1174–9.

17 Schwieger U, Laessie R, Pfister H *et al.* Diet induced menstrual irregularities: effects of age and weight loss. *Fertil Steril* 1987; **48**: 746–51.

18 Shangold MM. Athletic amenorrhoea. *Clin Obstet Gynaecol* 1985; **28**: 664–9.

19 Haines CJ. Luteinised unruptured follicle syndrome. *Clin Reprod Fertil* 1987; **5**: 321–2.

20 Shohan Z, Jacobs HS, Insler V. Luteinizing hormone: its role, mechanism of action, and detrimental effects when hypersecreted during the follicular phase. *Fertil Steril* 1993; **59**: 1153.

21 Regan L, Owen EJ, Jacobs HS. Hypersecretion of luteinising hormone, infertility, and miscarriage. *Lancet* 1990; **336**: 1141–44.

22 Wathen NC, Perry L, Lilford RJ, Chard T. Luteal penetration of single progesterone measurement in diagnosis of anovulation and defective luteal phase. Observations on analysis of the normal range. *Br Med J* 1984; **288**: 7–9.

23 Jacobs MH, Balasch J, Gouzalez-Meslo JH, Vanrek JA, Wheeler C, Strauss JF III, Blasco L, Wheeler JE, Lyttle CR. Endometrial cystosolic and nuclear progesterone receptors in the luteal phase defect. *J Clin Endocrin Metab* 1987; **64**: 472–5.

24 Dawood MY. Corpus luteal insufficiency. *Curr Opin Obstet Gynaecol* 1994; **6**: 121–27.

25 Haney AF. Endometriosis associated infertility. *Baillière's Clin Obstet Gynaecol* 1993; **7**: 791–812.

26 World Health Organisation. Infections, pregnancies, and infertility: perspectives on prevention. *Fertil Steril* 1987; **47**: 964.

27 Blasco L. Consider the cervical factor in reproduction. *Contemp Ob Gyn* 1983; **22**: 187.

28 Cates W, Jr. Sexually transmitted organisms and infertility: the proof of the pudding. *Sex Transm Dis* 1984; **11**: 113–16.

29 Hass GG, Jr. Immunologic infertility. *Obstet Gynaecol Clin North Am* 1987; **14**: 1609.

30 Marshburn P, Kutten W. The role of antisperm antibodies in infertility. *Fertil Steril* 1994; **61**: 799–811.

31 Shrivers CA, Dubnbar BS. Autoantibodies to zona pellucida: a possible cause for infertility in women. *Science* 1987; **197**: 1087.

32 Poretsky L, Kalin MF. The gonodatrophic function of insulin. *Endocr Rev* 1987; **8**: 132–41.

33 Phipps WR, Cramer DW, Schiff I *et al.* The association between smoking and female infertility as influenced by cause of the infertility. *Fertil Steril* 1987; **48**: 377–82.

34 Howe G, Westhoff C, Vessey M *et al.* Effect of age, cigarette smoking, and other factors on fertility. Findings in a large prospective study. *Br Med J* 1985; **290**: 1697–700.

35 Rosevar SK, Holt DW, Lett TD, Ford CL, Wardle PG, Hull MGR. Smoking decreased fertilization rates *in vitro*. *Lancet* 1992; **340**: 1195–6.

36 Rivkees SA, Crawford JD. The relationship of gonadal activity and chemotherapy-induced gonadal damage. *JAMA* 1988; **259**: 2123–5.

37 Wright J, Allard M, Lecours A, Sabourin S. Psychological distress and infertility: a review of controlled research. *Int J Fertil* 1989; **34**: 126–42.

38 Rowland A, Baird DD, Weinberg CR, Shore DI, Shy CM, Wilcox AJ. Reduced fertility among women employed as dental assistants exposed to high levels of nitrous oxide. *N Engl J Med* 1992; **327**: 993–7.

39 Jette NT, Glass RH. Prognostic value of the postcoital test. *Fertil Steril* 1972; **23**: 29–32.

40 Kovacs GT, Newman GB, Hensen GL. The postcoital test: what is normal? *Br Med J* 1978; **1**: 818.

41 Hull MGR, Savage PE, Bromham DR. Prognostic value of the postcoital test. Prospective study based on time-specific conception rates. *Br J Obstet Gynaecol* 1982; **89**: 299–305.

42 Kremer J, Jager S. The sperm-cervical mucous contact test: a preliminary report. *Fertil Steril* 1976; **27**: 335–40.

43 Morgan H, Stedronska J, Hendry WF, Chamberlain GVP, Dewhurst CJ. Sperm/cervical mucus crossed hostility testing and antisperm antibodies in the husband. Lancet 1977; **I**: 1228–30.

44 Hull MGR, Savage PE, Bromham DR, Ismail AAA, Morris AF. The value of a single serum progesterone measurement in the midluteal phase as a criterion of a potentially fertile cycle (ovulation) derived from treated and untreated conception cycles. *Fertil Steril* 1982; **37**: 355–60.

45 American Fertility Society. Revised classification of endometriosis. *Fertil Steril* 1985; **43**: 351–2.

46 Corson SL. Use of the laparoscope in the infertile patient. *Fertil Steril* 1979; **32**: 359–69.

CHAPTER 60

Assisted reproduction

J.L. Yovich and P.L. Matson

Introduction

Prior to 1960, it appears that fewer than 20% of couples who presented with infertility subsequently conceived; in fact, those conceptions which did occur were considered to be mostly unrelated to treatment [1]. Subsequently, the prognosis improved with the introduction of effective methods for ovulation induction. This was associated with inspired discoveries and developments in understanding the hypothalamo-pituitary–ovarian axis leading to the current improved level of knowledge regarding events concerning folliculogenesis, oocyte release and luteal function in the ovarian cycle. Further significant advances during the 1960s and 1970s included: the introduction of laparoscopy as a primary investigative tool; the development of sensitive, specific and rapid hormone assays; the appreciation of the role of non-gonococcal anaerobic organisms such as *Bacteroides fragilis*, and later others such as *Chlamydia trachomatis*, in the causation of pelvic inflammatory disease; the recognition of hyperprolactinaemia and its association with infertility; the establishment of donor semen banks; the development of microsurgery (initially on the female and subsequently on the male genital tract), hysteroscopy and endoscopic procedures; and the detection of antibodies against gametes. Such advances have improved considerably the chance of patients achieving a pregnancy, and the subsequent understanding of human infertility has enabled the rational introduction of techniques to assist human reproduction.

The integration of assisted reproductive methods with the aforementioned developments in the comprehensive management of infertility has improved the potential prognosis to beyond 75% of couples who can now be successfully treated to achieve at least one live birth. In fact, the main limiting factors to the successful treatment of infertility are no longer technical but relate to the age of the female partner [2], expense, ethical considerations and certain social aspects. These latter concerns have led to certain public anxieties in many countries and a perceived need to introduce legislative constraints in both service and research aspects of assisted reproduction.

Modern treatments to assist conception may be regarded as treating specific problems (e.g. reconstructive pelvic and tubal microsurgery), general problems, which may be multifactorial or poorly understood (e.g. ovarian stimulation in women who appear to be ovulatory) or substitute (i.e. where gametes or embryos are donated). Ideally, these modes are best carried out in a single unit structured to provide a comprehensive approach to infertility management (Table 60.1). A simple assessment of the effectiveness of treatment modalities can often be difficult due to varying selection criteria of patients used by different authors, and a definite background pregnancy rate observed in the absence of treatment [3]. The systematic evaluation of treatments in controlled clinical trials is therefore vital.

Ovarian stimulation and ovulation induction

The use of drugs to either stimulate ovaries in women already ovulating spontaneously, or to induce ovulation that otherwise would not occur, has become the cornerstone of many treatments in the field of assisted reproduction. At the one extreme, the strategy to promote ovulation in women wishing to conceive by intercourse often involves the development of only a single Graafian follicle to minimise the risk of a multiple pregnancy. At the other extreme are strategies used in *in vitro* fertilisation (IVF) programmes which are designed to result in the development of several follicles to maximise the yield of oocytes, with the risk of multiple pregnancy being minimised by restricting the number of embryos returned to the uterus. The following

Table 60.1 Specific facilities required for the comprehensive management of infertility, preferably located within a single unit functioning every day.

Consultation	Both partners
Counselling	Information Emotional support
Coordination	Senior nurse Tests/instructions/results
Laboratories	Andrology Embryology Cryopreservation Hormone assays Ultrasonography and radiology
Results	Group meeting each afternoon Computer and hard-copy data registers Regular data analysis and evaluation
Treatment	Areas and facilities
Semen	Collection rooms
Theatre	Oocyte recovery/transfers Endoscopy facilities Ultrasound facility Operating microscope

section summarises the approaches, and particularly the drugs, used in improving or achieving ovulation in a range of situations.

Bromocriptine (see also Chapter 10)

Hyperprolactinaemia is an important cause of anovulatory infertility, occurring in 15–20% of patients with amenorrhoea. Up to one-third of these women may have a prolactin-secreting pituitary tumour [4] which should be identified by computed tomography (CT) scan or magnetic resonance imaging (MRI).

Treatment of infertility associated with hyperprolactinaemia is usually done by the administration of the dopamine agonist, bromocriptine, which acts by decreasing the production and secretion of prolactin by the lactotrophs. Bromocriptine causes a reduction in circulating prolactin concentrations within a few hours that can last up to 12 hours [5], and so the drug is usually given twice a day. However, recent evidence suggests that once-daily administration may be effective in many patients.

The administration of bromocriptine is usually very effective when given to carefully selected hyperprolactinaemic women with amenorrhoea, conception occurring in over 80% of cases [6,7]. The taking of bromocriptine by ovulatory infertile women reduces the serum prolactin concentrations to that below the mean for the normal population and pregnancies do ensue [8], but the empirical use of bromocriptine in the absence of clear hyperprolactinaemia is not common and is not generally recommended. Newer dopamine agonists such as quinagolide and cabergoline may be better tolerated [113], but experience of their safety for conception is more limited.

Clomiphene citrate

Clomiphene citrate is an anti-oestrogen which has been used widely in the induction of ovulation for many years, having been first introduced clinically in the early 1960s. It has no progestational, androgenic or antiandrogenic effects. However, it is not without its problems, having an apparent adverse effect upon cervical mucus quality and endometrial morphology [9] and being associated with an increased rate of pregnancy loss [10,11].

Clomiphene is usually given from the early part of the follicular phase, for example from day 2 or 5 of the menstrual cycle, for 5 days, and is thought to work predominantly by eliciting an increased secretion of endogenous follicle-stimulating hormone (FSH). Accordingly, clomiphene is less effective in patients with anovulation associated with suppressed gonadotrophin levels typical of hypothalamo-pituitary insufficiency. Interestingly, the response to clomiphene, in terms of the secretion of FSH, can be used as a bioassay of the ovarian reserve of women [12] and as a predictive marker of their ability to respond to ovarian stimulation [13].

The administration of clomiphene can be used successfully as first-line treatment for women with anovulation associated with polycystic ovary syndrome [14], with those resistant women then often gaining benefit from the use of human menopausal gonadotrophin (hMG). Oligomenorrhoeic women can often do well with treatment by clomiphene, with certain workers advocating its use as an initial therapy in cases of unexplained infertility [15]. Clomiphene can also help correct cases of luteal phase dysfunction and inadequate progesterone secretion by inducing additional luteinising hormone (LH) receptors in the corpora lutea during the mid-luteal phase [16].

There appears to be no known teratogenic effects of clomiphene given to induce ovulation, and a multiple pregnancy rate of approximately 5% is commonly reported.

Menopausal gonadotrophins

Since the initial full report on the use of FSH extracted from human menopausal urine for the treatment of anovulatory infertility [17], numerous reports have appeared in the literature showing the benefits and limitations of the drug.

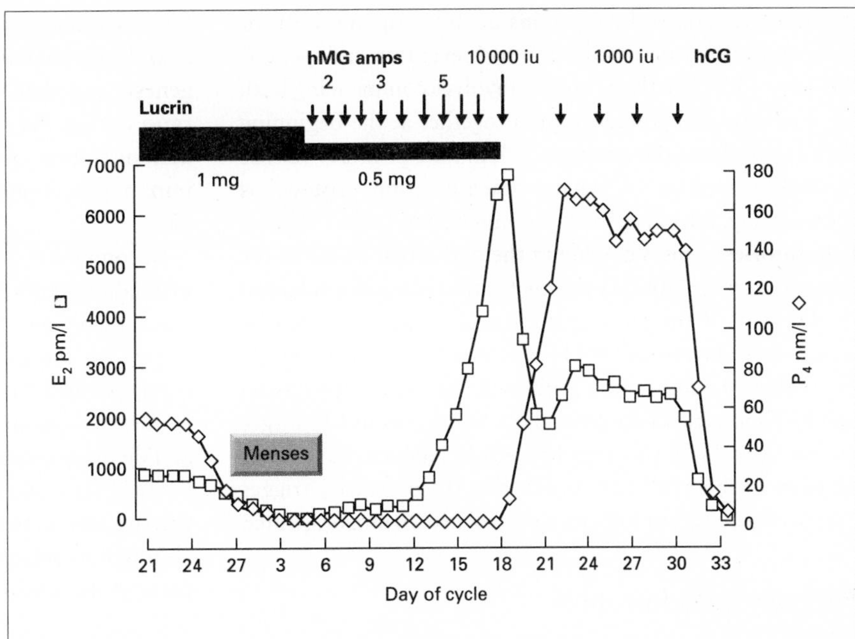

Fig. 60.1 Ovarian stimulation for *in vitro* fertilization (IVF) using leuprolide acetate (Lucrin) for pituitary desensitisation prior to human menopause gonadotrophin (hMG) stimulation. E_2 (□—□); P_4 (◇—◇).

The commercial preparations currently available contain FSH and LH in a 1 : 1 ratio, although there may be human chorionic gonadotrophin (hCG) present [18] and significant variation in the amount of bioactive FSH in different batches [19]. A major difficulty in the use of human menopausal gonadotrophin outside of an IVF programme is the controlled stimulation of a single follicle to minimise the risk of ovarian hyperstimulation and multiple pregnancy. The gonadotrophins do not exhibit a simple dose response, but are said to require a minimum 'effective daily dose' below which there is no measurable effect [20], and there is wide variation in the response of individual patients. Older reports highlight the difficulty early workers had in monitoring the response to menopausal gonadotrophins without the availability of a rapid oestrogen assay or real-time ultrasound, lamenting the fact that clinicians had to 'rely upon somewhat less reliable parameters such as ferning of cervical mucus, vaginal cytology and daily pelvic examinations' [21]. Not surprisingly, there was a significant level of hyperstimulation seen and multiple pregnancies did occur. The current availability of sophisticated monitoring facilities such as rapid oestradiol assays (often providing results within 2 hours) and real-time ovarian ultrasonography has proved of great benefit in monitoring the response of women to hMG therapy, but has not totally eliminated the occurrence of multiple pregnancies, leading to the development of procedures such as selective termination [22] with all its ethical and philosophical problems. One particularly difficult group of patients to manage are those with polycystic ovaries, usually presenting after unsuccessful attempted treatment with clomiphene citrate. These women often exhibit a higher incidence of complications associated with an exaggerated ovarian response following treatment with menopausal gonadotrophins [23]. Strategies using a low-dose regimen, commencing on 1 ampoule per day and only increasing by 1/2 an ampoule if required, appear to be effective in obtaining uniovulatory cycles and can give rise to cumulative pregnancy rates of up to 60% over 6 months [24]. However, excessive concentrations of basal LH in some of these patients can cause an increased incidence of pregnancy loss.

Anovulatory women with no endogenous follicular activity appear to do better with treatment by menopausal gonadotrophins than do those women with follicular activity but disordered ovulation [25,26]. However, the treatment of ovulatory women by menopausal gonadotrophins coupled with other procedures, such as artificial insemination [27], can yield good pregnancy rates, and may be regarded as first-line treatment before progressing to IVF or gamete intra-Fallopian transfer (GIFT).

Gonadotrophin-releasing hormone agonists

The pulsatile intravenous administration of gonadotrophin-releasing hormone (GnRH) agonists is an effective means of treating anovulation by eliciting endogenous gonadotrophin release. The use of automated pumps makes the administration of GnRH agonists much easier to manage, and the treatment has a high success rate and a low incidence of multiple pregnancy [28].

Within an IVF programme, the GnRH agonists can be used either to elicit a flare of gonadotrophins to augment the administration of exogenous gonadotrophins [29], or achieve pituitary desensitisation to prevent an endogenous LH surge [30]. The flare regimen involves commencing both the analogue and gonadotrophin together at the beginning of the cycle when the analogue will initiate pituitary release of gonadotrophins. A typical desensitisation protocol is shown in Fig. 60.1 and involves commencing Lucrin (Abbott Laboratories) 1 mg s.c. daily in the mid-luteal phase of the preceding cycle. Pituitary desensitisation is usually achieved by day 3–5 of the ensuing cycle and is demonstrated by serum concentrations of LH <5 iu/l and E_2 <200 pmol/l. Thereafter, 0.5 mg Lucrin daily will maintain suppression and hMG injections are given daily. Spontaneous LH surges do not occur with this regimen, which enables the follicles to grow to their full size by delaying the ovulatory trigger [31] until a cohort of follicles have reached 20 mm or greater.

Pituitary gonadotrophin

An early source of FSH was human pituitary glands from cadavers, utilising a range of methods to extract the gonadotrophin from the tissue. The FSH proved valuable initially with pregnancies being established in anovulatory women [32,33]. However, the subsequently transmission of Creutzfeldt–Jakob disease in patients using growth hormone preparations from the same source resulted in the suspension of clinical programmes around the world for fear of infection [34], and the occurrence of deaths following the use of the pituitary gonadotrophin have since been reported [35].

Purified and recombinant human FSH

The removal of unwanted LH from human menopausal gonadotrophin has resulted in a purified form of FSH (Metrodin; Serono Laboratories) which has been used to induce ovulation successfully in cases of polycystic ovarian disease where there is an abundance of endogenous LH relative to FSH [36] and for stimulating follicular development in normal ovulating women [37]. Furthermore, this purified FSH has been used successfully to induce multifollicular development in unselected IVF patients even when endogenous LH secretion is reduced by the administration of a GnRH agonist [38,39]. The use of a highly purified urinary FSH preparation (Metrodin HP; Serono Laboratories), which is practically devoid of LH activity [40], in cycles following pituitary desensitisation has also given good results. This has led to the conclusion that stimulation of the ovaries with exogenous FSH alone is effective, that only very low levels of endogenous LH are required in conjunction with FSH for the stimulation of follicular development and ovarian steroidogenesis, and that supplementation with exogenous LH is not needed. Studies using pituitary-desensitised rhesus monkeys have also shown that additional LH is not required for folliculogenesis and that the presence of LH with FSH in a 1 : 1 ratio during the preovulatory interval, as occurs with the administration of menopausal gonadotrophins, may even impair gametogenic events in the periovulatory period [41].

Recombinant human FSH is now available as a commercial preparation, being produced *in vitro* by genetically engineered Chinese hamster ovary cells in which the genes coding for the α- and β-subunits have been inserted. This highly purified form of FSH has very similar pharmacokinetic features to urinary FSH [42] and pregnancy rates within an IVF programme are comparable [43]. The use of recombinant FSH is likely to supersede that of any of the urinary preparations in time, given its purity and ease of production, although its relative cost will be a debatable point in many parts of the world.

Growth hormone

There is now much evidence to show that growth hormone can directly or indirectly modulate ovarian steroidogenesis. The availability of human biosynthetic growth hormone has therefore made its use as supplement feasible. The most impressive results following cotreatment with growth hormone in maximising the ovarian response and minimising the amount of gonadotrophin required to achieve that response, appear to be with amenorrhoeic patients [44,45]. However, indiscriminate administration to IVF patients showing a poor response to gonadotrophins is not useful [46], echoing the message that careful patient selection is crucial.

Artificial insemination

Male partner's semen

Currently there is a renewed interest in AIH (artificial insemination by husband) for all cases of infertility not due to tubal disease. Although the intrauterine insemination of whole semen has been reported in the past [47], the modern process of AIH is based on the intrauterine insemination of 'washed' spermatozoa [48] arising from the technical developments and improved understanding of reproductive processes involved with IVF-related procedures. The procedure has already developed an established place for the management of infertility due to cervical mucus problems (antisperm antibodies impairing sperm penetration, absence of mucus, undefined hostility and cases displaying poor sperm–mucus interaction), oligozoospermia where this is not complicated by asthenospermia, and retrograde ejaculation and psychosexual disorders which prevent normal semen deposition in the vagina.

Controlled ovarian stimulation appears to improve the chance of pregnancy and should be considered at an early stage for AIH [49], although the risk of multiple pregnancy should be minimised wherever possible. When dealing with male factor infertility, case selection is vitally important as poor results are usually obtained with reduced sperm motility [50]. Furthermore, the pretreatment of sperm with pentoxifylline can be particularly beneficial in cases in which the sperm show an impaired rate of acrosome reaction in response to a challenge by the ionophore A23187 [51].

Donated semen

The term donor insemination (DI) is preferred over the previous acronym for artificial insemination by donor (AID). The historical, clinical, technical, and ethical aspects have recently been reviewed [52]. The indications for DI include untreatable azoospermia (e.g. Klinefelter's syndrome, absent vasa, spermatogenic failure, epididymal obstructions), severe oligo/asthenospermic states and for genetic reasons (serious autosomal dominant conditions such as Huntington's disease, dystrophia myotonica, etc). However, the development of techniques such as intracytoplasmic sperm injection (ICSI), which enable the achievement of fertilisation with the male partner's sperm in cases with even the most severe impairment of spermatogenesis [53], will inevitably mean a shift in the referral patterns to DI programmes.

Because of the risk of transmission of human immunodeficiency virus (HIV) infection by the use of donated semen from an infected donor [54], accepted semen specimens in most countries are now frozen [55] and quarantined for 6 months, and can be released for clinical use only after a repeat screen of the donor (serological tests for syphilis, hepatitis B, hepatitis C and HIV) has proven negative [56]. Although not mandatory in some countries, it is generally considered to be no longer ethical to use fresh semen for DI treatments because of the risk of infection. In order to facilitate appropriate matching between donor and recipient, specific donor characteristics should be recorded including height, stature/body build, eye colour, hair colour, skin complexion, race/ethnic background and aspects of social history. However, information should be non-identifying and complete confidentiality must be maintained between donor and recipient. Notwithstanding these comments, restricted approval may be considered by some ethics committees for known-donor insemination, for example brother-for-brother donation in certain circumstances.

The cryopreservation of donated semen requires the use of an appropriate cryoprotectant to maximise the viability of thawed spermatozoa. Several cryoprotective media have been described but a particularly good one [57] contains 15% glycerol in a buffered solution of sodium citrate with glucose, fructose and streptomycin. The diluted semen is drawn into 0.5 ml coloured plastic straws which are pre-plugged at one end and then sealed with a coloured cement compound. The straws are labelled, grouped in plastic goblets with the cement ends uppermost and frozen using liquid nitrogen, with the coding system for the straws being based on their label, colour, position within the cryopreservation dewar and the particular dewar in which they are stored. Matching errors should not occur. An inexpensive hand-freezing technique, which involves precooling followed by slow freezing over nitrogen vapour prior to plunging into liquid nitrogen, may often suffice. Alternatively the straws may be frozen in a programmable freezer involving controlled rates of cooling (ranging from −1°C/min to −10°C/min down to −30°C, or even −80°C where it is held for 30 min prior to plunging into liquid nitrogen at −196°C within the storage dewar).

Inseminations are usually performed during the periovulatory phase when fertile cervical mucus is demonstrated (score ≥ 6/12). The score is maximal just prior to the LH surge, after which it falls rapidly. Generally two or three inseminations are carried out. Care should be taken to use the thawed sample as quickly as possible to minimise deterioration, and so the appropriate straw may need to be transferred from the laboratory dewar to a smaller dewar or thermos flask within the clinic. When required the straw is removed from liquid nitrogen and allowed to thaw on an aseptic area on the workbench at room temperature. The cement end of the straw is then cut off and the straw placed in an insemination gun, covered by a sterile sheath and the tip of the instrument is inserted 1–2 cm into the cervix following its exposure using a bivalve vaginal speculum with the patient in the dorsal position. The semen is injected slowly with the speculum lightly gripping the cervix where it remains for approximately 2 min. After the instruments are withdrawn the patient remains recumbent for 15–20 min and may then leave the clinic, usually without restrictions being placed on subsequent activities, such as work or sport.

Live birth rates following insemination are usually disappointing, as illustrated in Table 60.2 by the total experience in the UK for 1991 and 1992. The data was collected by the Human Fertilisation and Embryology Authority in accordance with the Human Fertilisation and Embryology Act (1990) which made the notification of all treatments mandatory. Furthermore, a clear relationship between the chance of pregnancy and the woman's age can be seen, with the rates for older women being very poor. The results can usually be improved quite dramatically by the use of spermatozoa washed through Percoll and intrauterine insemination performed close to ovulation as determined

Table 60.2 Live birth rates following *in vitro* fertilisation (IVF) or donor insemination (DI) treatment in the UK for 1991 and 1992, according to the age of the woman being treated.

Maternal	IVF		DI	
age (years)	Cycles	Live birth rate (%)	Cycles	Live birth rate (%)
<25	278	12.6	1296	7.1
25–29	3539	18.1	9157	5.6
30–34	9365	16.3	14104	5.4
35–39	8142	12.5	8400	4.1
40–44	2645	5.4	2271	1.8
≥45	210	2.4	97	1.0
Total	24179	14.0	35325	4.9

Source: 2nd and 3rd Annual Reports of the Human Fertilisation and Embryology Authority.

by the accurate identification of the endogenous LH surge [58].

Infertility surgery

Significant tubal disorders causing disturbances of the ovum pick-up mechanism or ovum transport may be present in up to 35% of infertility cases. Almost half will demonstrate complete occlusions, these being within the distal region causing fimbrial agglutination or hydrosalpinges, or in the proximal regions as a consequence of intratubal cornual obstruction or intramural isthmic obstructions due to the enigmatic condition denoted as salpingitis isthmica nodosum. Partial occlusions and limited tubal mobility usually result from peritubal adhesions. The underlying cause of most cases of pelvic disease has, in the past, been ascribed to ascending infections of the genital tract with sexually transmitted organisms such as *Neisseria gonorrhoea* and *Chlamydia trachomatis* being strongly implicated. However, the evidence remains indirect and circumstantial. The pathogenesis appears clearer for many cases arising as a consequence of ascending non-specific infections following complicated parturition, early pregnancy losses and in association with intrauterine contraceptive devices, particularly when inserted in nulligravid women. Other pelvic pathologies such as ectopic pregnancy, endometriosis and ruptured appendix cause significant secondary infertility, and even *Mycobacterium tuberculosis* and *Actinomyces israellii* have to be considered within population subsets.

The underlying aetiology should be considered in all cases of recognised pelvic disease as it is imperative to control the process prior to definitive surgery or other infertility treatments. In a disturbingly large proportion of cases, the only factor related to pelvic adhesions is past pelvic surgery performed for incidental reasons such as ovarian cystectomy, ventrosuspension, unruptured appendicectomy and paratubal cystectomy. Fortunately, such operations are performed less frequently nowadays as laparoscopic and ultrasound-directed techniques have evolved. It appears that the main offending factors in the past have been glove powder or starch irritation combined with abrasive packing techniques.

Infertility surgery has a long history but the results were universally disappointing prior to the last decade. Recent advances relate to improved understanding of the pathogenesis of pelvic adhesions and the adoption of principles of microsurgery [59]. These principles include the use of an atraumatic technique and non-reactive suture material, careful attention to haemostasis, frequent irrigation of tissues during procedures and careful washout on completion to remove fibrinous clots. Pathological tissue must be completely excised, tissue dissection is preferably by fine needle-point electrocautery or laser coagulation techniques, and bipolar electrocoagulation is required for fine vessels within and near the Fallopian tubes. Packing should be performed with moist packs only, using a non-abrasive placement technique. Magnification, preferably with a free-standing operating microscope which allows foot-controlled zoom to at least ×25, enables the use of delicate instruments and fine sutures with the precise alignment and apposition of tissue planes, and serosal reperitonealisation using free grafts if necessary. The parietal peritoneum should be everted during closure to avoid omental adhesions to the anterior abdominal wall. Individual preferences may also include the use of parenteral prophylactic antibiotics, parenteral or pelvic steroids and high-molecular-weight dextran left within the cavity on completion to minimise postoperative pelvic adhesion formation.

The current trend to laparoscopic surgery within the female pelvis already appears to be associated with a reduction in the problem of postoperative adhesions.

Myomectomy and metroplasty

Submucous fibroids, and sometimes intramural or subserous fibroids, if causing distortion of the uterine cavity or impinging on the fallopian tubes, require excision. So too do uterine synechiae and sometimes a uterine septum if indicated by a past history of recurrent pregnancy losses. Currently, an increasing proportion of such cases are proving amenable to hysteroscopically directed surgical methods using laser or diathermy resection [60]. Large intramural and subserosal fibroids are now generally resectable at laparoscopy. These endoscopic microsurgical operations should largely replace the coarse laparotomy procedures of the past with improved results and fewer complications in both short- and long-term outcomes.

Reversal of sterilisation

For re-anastomotic reversals of female sterilisation, the patency rate is better than 90% and more than 60% of women have a successful pregnancy. The results are much better for those whose final tube length is >50 mm and particularly if the ampullary/infundibular end is preserved. The prognosis for reversal is best for clip sterilisations and less so for Silastic rings, mid-tubal resections, tubal diathermy, fimbriectomy and distal salpingectomy, in descending order. Many would consider the latter two, or even three, procedures unsuitable for reversal, regarding IVF as the better option. Ectopic pregnancies are relatively low after successful reversals, being around 2%.

Post-inflammatory tubal damage

Microsurgical tubal reconstructions performed for inflammatory disorders provide pregnancy rates of 20–40% for salpingostomy, 30% for fimbrioplasty, 40% for cornual implantation, 45% for salpingolysis and up to 60% for discrete resection/re-anastomoses. When compared with conventional surgery, microsurgery confers only marginal benefits in pregnancy rates for much of this group (although markedly better for cornual implantation and discrete re-anastomoses) and this relates to the wider extent of the damage inflicted by the underlying cause [61]. The ectopic pregnancy rate following surgery for inflammatory damage is variably reported as 5–20%.

Recently, operative laparoscopy has been evolving as an increasingly viable alternative to laparotomy procedures in certain pelvic conditions, including tubal pregnancy, salpingolysis, fimbrioplasty and salpingostomy [62].

Preparation for IVF-related procedures

When ovum aspiration was universally performed by laparoscopic techniques, benefits were often obtained by preliminary pelvic surgery with extensive adhesiolysis and partial omentectomy to free the ovaries, ventrosuspend the uterus and plicate the ovarian ligaments. Subsequent laparoscopic follicle aspiration was often improved or simply made possible [63]. However, most follicle aspirations are nowadays performed by a transvaginal ultrasound-directed method and it is preferable to leave the ovaries in the pouch of Douglas, obviating the need for previous surgery.

In recent days, preliminary pelvic surgery has once again been considered to enable tethered or obstructed fallopian tubes to be made accessible for GIFT or other tubal transfer procedures. However, the results indicate that an inordinately high ectopic pregnancy rate may occur [64]. Of greater interest has been the development of preliminary pelvic surgery in preparation for IVF. It would appear to be beneficial to clear endometriotic lesions as much as possible, at least to reduce the grading down to a mild degree, as the results of IVF are inversely related to the severity of the pelvic endometriosis. Endometriomas and other endometriotic lesions can be excised laparoscopically using simple excision techniques in association with electrosurgical ablation or laser coagulation. Other considerations include laparoscopic salpingostomy or even salpingectomy in the treatment of hydrosalpinges, and ovarian drilling for polcystic ovaries associated with significant hormonal disturbance—in particular, raised androgen and LH levels.

Male microsurgery (see also Chapter 50)

The introduction of microsurgical techniques on the male genital tract has led to an improved prognosis for vasectomy reversal and other discrete obstructions of the vas [65]. Some cases of epididymal obstruction, previously not possible to consider, are now amenable to microsurgery [66]. The prognosis for patency with sperm in the ejaculate after vasovasostomy is 80% or better, but for vasoepididymostomy it is dependent upon the level (caput, body or caudal region) and ranges from only 25 to 50%. However, the likelihood of pregnancy is reduced if anti-sperm antibodies have formed, if the sterilisation was long-standing, or if long segments of vas/epididymis were missing or bypassed as spermatozoa from the caput have reduced fertilising capacity.

Of greater potential benefit is the combination of microsurgical exploration of the epididymis with IVF. Male surgery performed in IVF theatres enables the identification of the appropriate region of the epididymis where motile spermatozoa can be identified, enabling the surgeon to better select the site of anastomosis. It also provides the opportunity for IVF in a combined procedure involving subsequent ovum aspiration from the female partner, fertilisation of the recovered oocytes and subsequent transfer of embryos. In all such cases it is now recommended that sperm be recovered from the testis or the epididymis and cryopreserved for potential subsequent IVF using the ICSI technique [67,68]. Successful pregnancies have now been reported from high epididymal recoveries of spermatozoa from men with absent vasa [69] or epididymal obstruction [70], and even from cases of significant spermatogenic failure.

In vitro fertilisation

Historical aspects

Although successful embryo transfers were described in the rabbit a century ago, the process of IVF has a much shorter history with the first mammalian success producing live offspring being reported in 1959, again achieved in rabbits [71]. Interestingly, the rabbit model was not ideal with respect to spermatozoal capacitation *in vitro*, but this posed less of a problem than several other mammalian laboratory species where IVF was subsequently achieved. IVF has now been reported for a wide range of mammals, including non-human primates and domestic animals. Human IVF has proven to be relatively simple and is based on the mouse model initially described by Whittingham [72].

Crude attempts to achieve human IVF had been undertaken during the 1940s and 1950s, but it is unlikely that normal cleaving embryos were generated prior to the combined efforts of Robert Edwards (physiologist and embryologist) and the late Patrick Steptoe (gynaecologist), with contributions by Barry Bavister and the late Jean Purdy [73]. Edwards had earlier studied IVF in oocytes derived from surgical specimens of ovary and subsequently matured *in vitro*. The morphological quality of embryos was superior when preovulatory oocytes were aspirated from mature follicles at laparoscopy following stimulation with hMG and fertilised *in vitro* in a modified Tyrode's solution. They reported the first human IVF pregnancy in 1976 [74], but it proved to be an ectopic in the proximal segment of the distally occluded Fallopian tube. Interestingly, the team subsequently abandoned stimulated cycles as an ongoing pregnancy proved elusive and it was considered that such cycles were unfavourable for implantation.

The first successful pregnancies were achieved in a series of 32 cycles which reached the stage of embryo transfer (ET) after monitoring natural, unstimulated follicle development with a sensitive immunobioassay for LH performed on urine [75]. There were four pregnancies in that series and Louise Brown, a healthy female born in July 1978, became the first IVF infant [76]. A healthy male was also delivered a few months later but two other pregnancies miscarried, one in the first trimester shown to have triploidy, and another in the second trimester shown to have an inherited chromosomal anomaly [77]. The next team to report success was from Australia where IVF had been studied for almost a decade, and again this was achieved from a monitored natural cycle. However, such natural cycle pregnancies proved relatively elusive and subsequent successes were generally reported from stimulated cycles. By 1983 clinics were present in many countries around the world but most were reporting sporadic successes only amounting to a total of around 50 infants. Over the next 5 years there was a marked proliferation of service clinics and research activity leading to fairly consistent reporting of pregnancy rates in the range of 12–25%, an example of which is given in Table 60.2 from the data gathered in the UK by the Human Fertilisation and Embryology Authority.

Ovarian stimulation

The earliest workers in human IVF used hMG stimulation in order to generate several ovarian follicles when oocyte recovery techniques were relatively crude, and to counter the problems of limited fertilisation and limited developmental potential of oocytes. However, they recognized that luteal phases were shortened and the degree was directly related to the output of urinary oestrogens during the follicular phase [75]. Subsequently, when a rapid immunobioassay (Hi-Gonavis; Mochida Pharmaceutical Co., Japan) became available for LH/β-hCG detection, natural cycles were monitored and the single oocyte recovered, where possible. The first IVF pregnancies were achieved from natural cycles but the method was seen to have major limitations. These included the expense and inconvenience of prolonged hospitalisation for 8-hourly monitoring to detect the commencement of LH surge, the frustration of prolonged monitoring of disordered cycles, the difficulty of laparoscopic aspiration if the follicle was inconveniently located and inaccessible due to underlying pelvic pathology, and the need to access theatres outside a routine daytime schedule. Therefore, stimulated cycles were seen to be a requirement if IVF was to be adopted into clinical service.

The first clinic to report success with stimulated cycles [78] utilised clomiphene citrate alone for stimulation and hCG 5000 iu for the ovulation trigger. Oocytes were recovered 33–35 hours later and no luteal support was provided. Subsequently others, particularly in the USA, reported success using hMG alone for stimulation [79], triggering ovulation with hCG 10 000 iu and giving luteal support routinely in the form of progesterone 25–50 mg/day i.m. The latter was continued throughout the first trimester if pregnancy ensued. By 1986 when many IVF clinics were established worldwide, one of the most popular stimulation regimens in use combined clomiphene citrate with hMG. Generally, 50 mg clomiphene citrate was given b.d. day 2–6 or 5–9 and hMG ampoules (one to three) were given beginning a day or two after the clomiphene was commenced. Cancellation rates due to poor or inappropriate responses and premature LH surges were around 20%.

Marked improvements in IVF results have recently ensued from the diminishing use of clomiphene and the increasing use of GnRH analogues such as buserelin (Suprefact, Hoechst Laboratories) and leuprolide acetate (Lucrin, Abbott Laboratories), largely as a result of the blocking of an endogenous LH surge enabling ovarian stimulation to be continued longer and the follicles achieving a greater maturity as discussed in Chapter 48. The changing trend in ovarian stimulation regimens over the years is clearly shown in Fig. 60.2, which shows data collected on all pregnancies

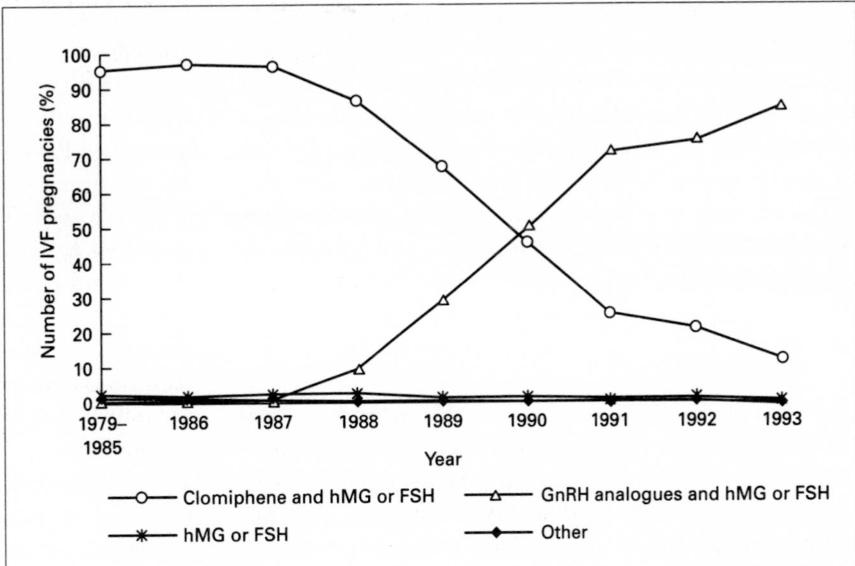

Fig. 60.2 The use of different stimulation regimens used for *in vitro* fertilisation (IVF) pregnancies achieved in Australia during 1979–93 [111].

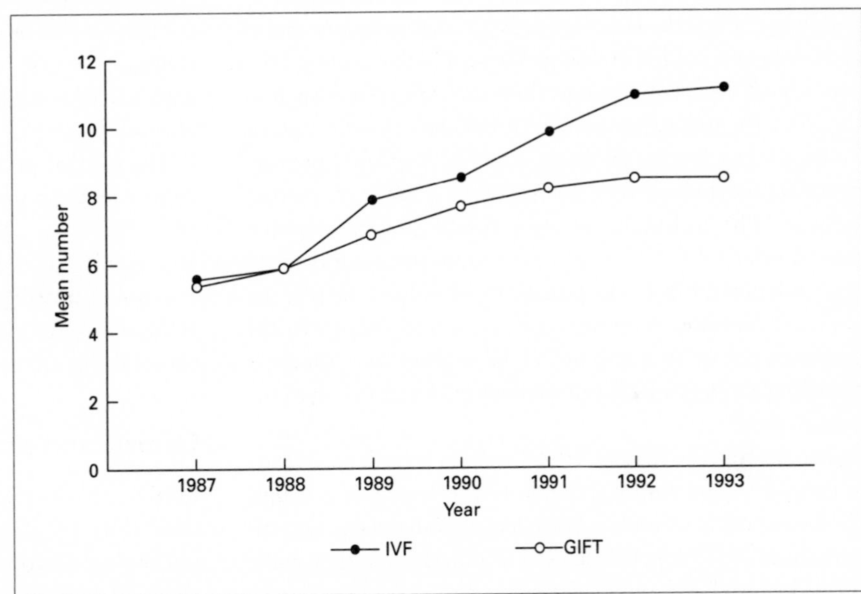

Fig. 60.3 The number of oocytes collected for *in vitro* fertilisation (IVF) and gamete intra-Fallopian transfer (GIFT) pregnancies in Australia during 1987–93 [111].

generated in Australia between 1979 and 1993. Occurring in tandem with the change in fashion in ovarian stimulation protocols has been an increase in the number of oocytes collected, as shown in Fig. 60.3.

Oocyte collection

Traditionally, oocyte recovery developed as a laparoscopic procedure but has increasingly become replaced by ultrasound-directed techniques, particularly the transvaginal approach. The optimisation of oocyte recovery has been shown to depend upon three main aspects [63]:

1 timing the recovery following LH surge or hCG induction and inducing the surge at the appropriate stage of follicle maturation;
2 the instrumentation and techniques applied for aspiration of the oocytes from follicles; and
3 accessibility of the ovaries for aspiration.

With respect to timing, the LH surge or hCG trigger should occur in cycles down-regulated with GnRH analogues when three or more follicles are 20 mm in diameter. Thereafter, follicles are aspirated 36 ± 2 hours after initiation of the LH surge or hCG trigger. Oocytes aspirated earlier than 34 hours may benefit by compensatory *in vitro* culture prior to insemination but embryo quality is poor and pregnancy rates are low if oocytes are recovered 4 or more hours earlier than optimal. Oocytes collected up to 4 hours after the optimal time remain equally suitable but the risk of spontaneous oocyte release increases although this appears to be <10% up to 42 hours in GnRH analogue cycles.

The matters of instrumentation and accessibility are considered separately for laparoscopic and ultrasound-directed recoveries.

Laparoscopic recovery

Laparoscopy requires general anaesthesia and endotracheal intubation. Access to follicles may be restricted by pelvic adhesions hence in the past preliminary pelvic adhesiolysis, ventrosuspension and plication of the ovarian ligaments has been recommended. Whilst this has significantly improved laparoscopic access, it may prejudice transvaginal access and hence is no longer encouraged.

A wide range of single- and double-lumen needles are in common use but the latter are proving increasingly popular as they enable follicle flushing. Those which enable a fine-spray flush with a continuous flow-through system such as the PIVET-Cook Laparoscopic/Ultrasound Double Lumen Ovum Pickup Needle [William A Cook, Australia] provide optimal oocyte recovery rates, being >90% of mature follicles. The technique involves needle puncture of the follicle under direct laparoscopic vision and aspiration of the contents into a 16-ml polystyrene test tube. Whilst the contents are being examined under stereomicroscopy by the embryologist in an adjacent IVF laboratory, the follicle is flushed with Hepes-buffered medium prior to moving to the next follicle.

The postoperative recovery of women after laparoscopy is sometimes uncomfortable due to the anaesthetic drugs, the laparoscopic wounds and residual abdominal gas. Serious complications among IVF cases, including deaths, are usually anaesthetic-related and occasionally due to the inadvertent puncture of bowel, bladder or vascular structures.

Ultrasound-directed recovery

The first reports using ultrasound guidance for follicle aspirations were reported from Scandinavia [80] and described a transcutaneous transvesical method. Subsequently, a transurethral method was explored briefly and finally the transvaginal method has found popular acceptance [81]. The optimisation of transvaginal ultrasound-directed aspiration requires the following [82].

1 Minimal anaesthesia, for example propofol intravenous anaesthetic or premedication combined with local anaesthesia.

2 Application of a pressure band to the lower abdomen to stabilise the ovaries and prevent them slipping away during attempts at penetration.

3 Use of very sharp needles with echo-enhanced tips which enable an efficient follicle flushing technique. The aforementioned PIVET-Cook needles were designed specifically for the purpose and are ideal.

4 Follicle aspiration and flushing is performed as previously described for laparoscopic access. It is ideal to have the theatre and IVF laboratory combined or adjacent. During follicle flushing, the follicle is only partially refilled so the flush and aspiration procedures proceed simultaneously. This requires a high-pressure fine jet to avoid 'short-circuiting' the follicle and again the PIVET-Cook needles are suitably designed.

5 The control of flow through the aspiration needles is governed by Poiseuille's Law, hence aspiration pressures require adjustment depending upon needle length (factor of ×8, e.g. 35-cm 16-FG needle requires −180 mmHg whilst 25-cm needle requires −100 mmHg) and needle diameter (inversely related to fourth power of the radius).

6 High-resolution ultrasound image is required, for example General Electric electronic phased array sector scanner with 5.0 MHz vaginal probe and needle guide is widely and effectively used.

7 The vaginal probe requires a coupling medium, such as culture medium placed in the vagina at the beginning of the procedure after saline wash-out, to maximise the contact and quality of the picture. Sterilising fluids are avoided because of possible toxic effects upon the oocytes, hence it is imperative to exclude the presence of vaginal pathogens earlier in the treatment cycle.

Gamete and embryo culture

Ideally, an IVF unit should comprise two 'embryology' laboratories—one dealing with culture-media preparation, semenology, cryopreservation, the cleaning and sterilisation of equipment, and quality-control aspects; the other as a dedicated human IVF laboratory as part of the theatre complex, which is maintained as an aseptic, quiet and low-traffic area.

Gamete preparation

From follicle aspirates and flushes, the cumulus–corona–oocyte complex is recognised as a silvery gelatinous mass which can be graded according to the overall size of the mass, number and degree of dispersal of cumulus cells, and tightness or density of the coronal cells. They are removed from the follicle flushing medium and washed twice before placing in culture medium supplemented with serum or an equivalent protein preparation. This is usually done in culture tubes or multiwell dishes. It is crucial to avoid temperature reductions as the meiotic spindles can be irreversibly damaged on cooling [83,84]. Routinely, oocytes are preincubated for 4–6 hours prior to insemination but longer periods may be required, particularly if the oocytes are immature.

Spermatozoal preparations are performed routinely by the swim-up method [114] for normospermic semen samples (Fig. 60.4). However, oligozoospermic and asthenospermic semen require the use of a discontinuous gradient separation using Percoll to achieve pure motile spermatozoal samples which are free of debris and other cells, as shown in Fig. 60.5. Current research in this area is evaluating methods of

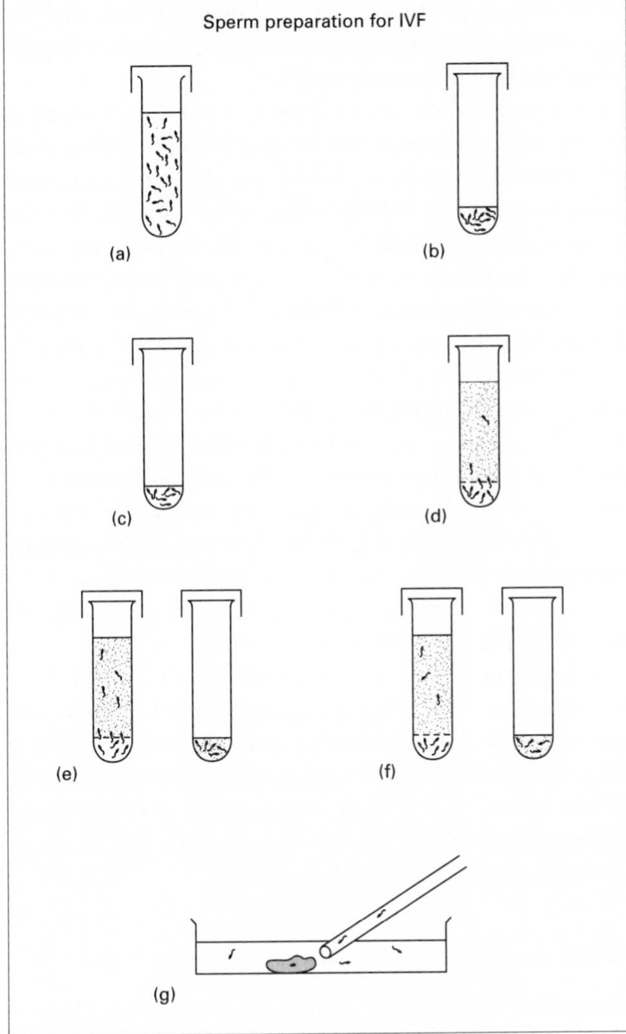

Fig. 60.4 The technique of sperm preparation by the swim-up method (with permission from Plenum Press) [86]. (a) 0.4 ml of whole semen diluted to 5 ml with medium. (b) Sample centrifuged 2–3 times at 200 ***g*** × 10 min. (c) Pellet resuspended in 0.5 ml. (d) Sample overlaid with 4.5 ml medium. (e) Top of supernatant containing motile sperm harvested. (f) Remaining supernatant removed if sperm yield poor. (g) 0.5–2.0 × 10^5 spermatozoa added per millilitre of medium containing the oocyte–cumulus mass.

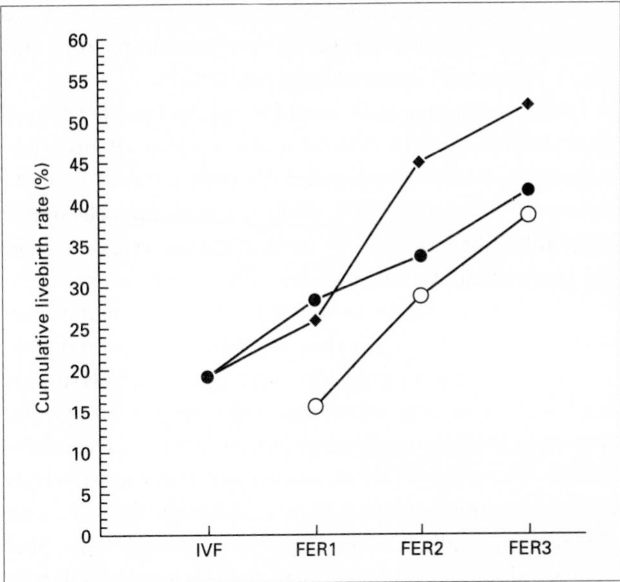

Fig. 60.5 The cumulative live birth rate in parents for the initial *in vitro* fertilisation (IVF) cycle followed by the replacement of cryopreserved embryos on one (FER1), two (FER2) and three (FER3) occasions [112]. Cases had remaining IVF embryos cryopreserved at the pronucleate (●—●) or early cleavage stage (◆—◆), or all embryos cryopreserved at the pronucleate stage because of the risk of ovarian hyperstimulation (○—○).

preparing spermatozoa which remove reactive oxygen species [85] (i.e. free hydroxyl and oxygen radicals and non-radical hydroperoxides) which damage cell membranes and sperm function. In this regard renewed interest is being paid to vitamin C and α-tocopherol, the active ingredient of vitamin E. In selected cases, sperm motility can be boosted by adding a cyclic adenosine monophosphate (cAMP) inhibitor such as pentoxifylline which will also improve the fertilisation rate [51].

Fertilisation

Spermatozoa are added to single oocytes at a concentration of 50–100 000/ml. Generally this is performed in tubes, although many units prefer to incubate in microdroplets (25–50 μl) under oil and this is beneficial when sperm numbers are low. Very small volumes can be achieved (5–10 μl) within straws. Incubation conditions must be stringently controlled [86] so the culture environment is humidified, held constant at 37°C, and gassed (ideally with 5% CO_2: 5% O_2: 90% N_2 although 5% CO_2 in air appears to suffice) to maintain the culture medium at pH 7.3. The culture medium should have an osmolarity around 285 mOsmol/l and be prepared from high-grade chemicals dissolved in highly purified water [87]. Serum additions also require stringent handling and preparation conditions, including complement deactivation.

It should satisfy strict quality-control assessment such as supporting mouse IVF or mouse embryo culture from one-cell to expanded blastocysts at a rate ≥85%.

The fertilisation process should be checked at 14–18 hours after insemination to determine the number of pronuclei within the oocyte. This involves microdissection to remove the coronal coat of cells (Fig. 60.6). The cumulus cells should have fully dispersed from hyaluronidase released from the spermatozoal acrosome cap. The check for pronuclei is important as 5–8% of seemingly normal preovulatory oocytes will contain more than two (the proportion may be much higher in poor-grade oocytes), implying polyspermy, and 1–2% may only have one, implying parthenogenetic activation. Subsequently, multipronucleate oocytes cleave rapidly into embryos which are usually, and deceptively, of the highest morphological grades, although their chromosomal abnormalities have been well defined [88]. Such oocytes should always be identified and excluded from transfer and this constitutes one of the limitations of the GIFT procedure. In addition, 25–30% of oocytes will fail to fertilise. Many will fertilise after re-insemination but resultant embryos rarely, if ever, become successfully implanting embryos resulting in live infants.

After the check for pronuclei, oocytes can be returned to short-term culture in simple medium, but some workers prefer a more complex medium such as Ham's F10 or MEM (minimal essential medium) as these have been shown to be superior for culturing through to blastocysts [89]. Human serum will also support embryo culture but current research is directed towards coculture methods, for example with endometrial or tubal cells. Embryos can be graded and scored according to morphological features, for example the regularity of blastomeres, degree of fragmentation and clarity, or granularity of the cytoplasm, as well as the cleavage times. Generally, embryos are transferred around 44–48 hours after insemination when most are at the four-cell stage.

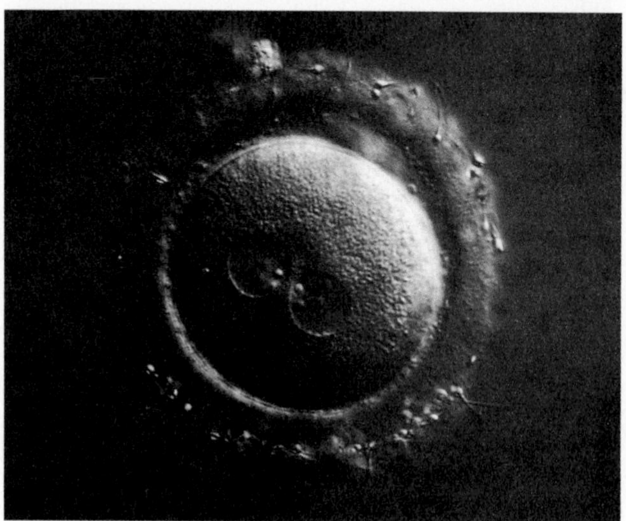

Fig. 60.6 Pronuclear oocyte after microdissection of coronal cells 14 hours after insemination.

Embryo cryopreservation

The cryopreservation and storage of human embryos remaining after an IVF cycle has proved invaluable in giving patients the opportunity to become pregnant by the subsequent replacement of thawed embryos, without the need for repeat ovarian stimulation and oocyte recovery, as shown in Fig. 60.5. Other important clinical uses of cryopreservation include the elective freezing of all embryos in cases at risk of ovarian hyperstimulation syndrome (OHSS), and the quarantine of fertilised donated oocytes to minimise the risk of infection to the recipient [90].

Cryopreservation can be done at a number of stages of embryo development using a variety of cryoprotective agents [91]. Briefly, embryos can be frozen at the pronucleate stage using propanediol, two-cell to eight-cell using propanediol or dimethylsulphoxide, or at the blastocyst stage using glycerol. Survival rates of 60–70% per embryo after thawing are commonly reported, with the initial quality of the embryo appearing to be important in determining survival [92].

The transfer of embryos is usually done in either a natural cycle, where the transfer is timed relative to the endogenous LH surge, or in cycles in which the endometrium has been prepared with exogenous oestrogen and progestogen. An example of a typical replacement cycle is shown in Fig. 60.7.

The cryopreservation of human oocytes would be extremely beneficial in an assisted conception programme. The gametes could then be fertilised upon thawing, circumventing the ethical dilemma posed when embryos are in storage and the couple separate. Also, the cryopreservation of oocytes from women, prior to undergoing chemotherapy or radiotherapy, would be helpful in maintaining their reproductive potential even though the gonads would sustain irreversible damage. Whilst advances are being made in the development of effective techniques [93], it will be a while before oocyte cryopreservation is available routinely.

Ovarian hyperstimulation syndrome

Apart from the problem of multiple pregnancies, OHSS is the main serious and life-threatening complication of ovarian stimulation. It is, therefore, an iatrogenic disorder and was first reported in 1964 in a woman who developed a wide spectrum of clinical symptoms and signs after ovulation induction. A useful classification put forward by the World Health Organization Scientific Group [94] describes three grades of severity. In its severe form there is massive ovarian enlargement, ascites, pleural effusions, haemoconcentration,

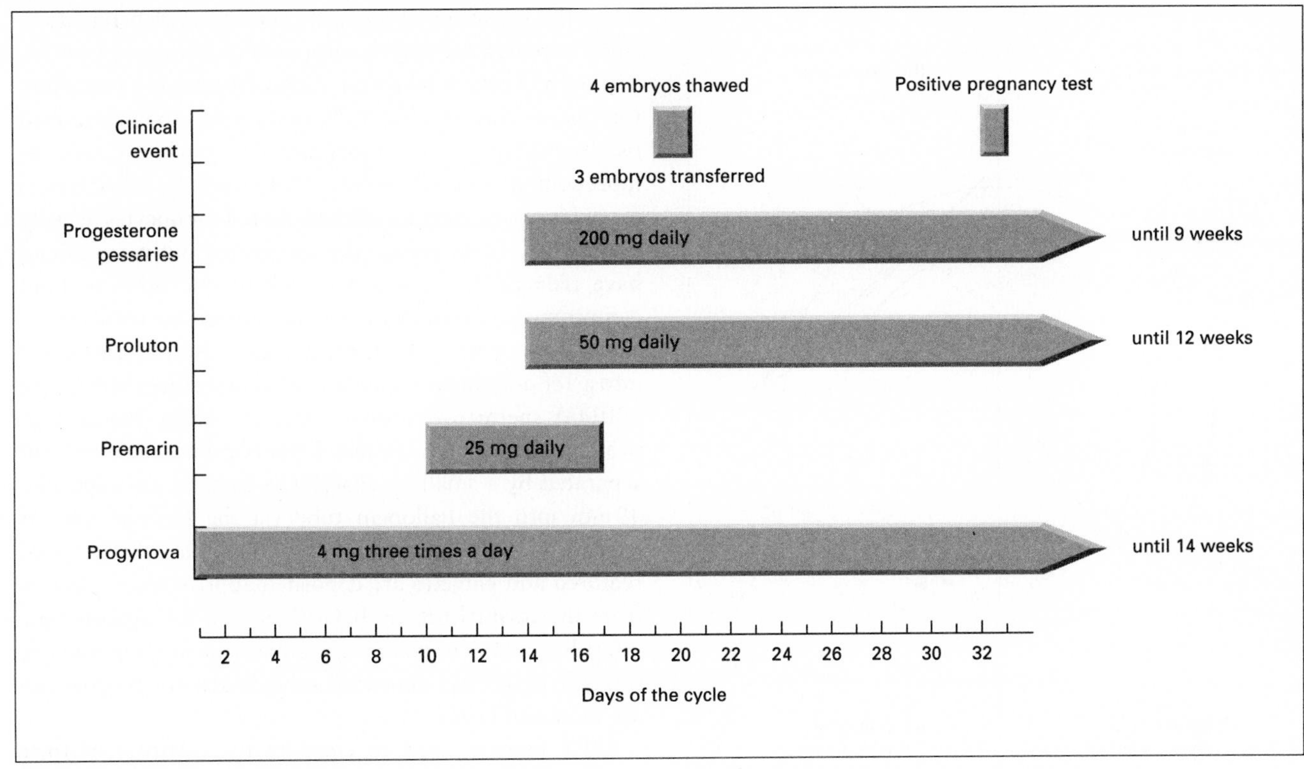

Fig. 60.7 A typical hormone-replacement cycle resulting in a viable pregnancy following the transfer of cryopreserved embryos.

oliguria, electrolyte imbalance and hypercoagulability. The main symptoms are nausea, vomiting, abdominal pain and distension, but the condition can be further complicated by rare features such as deep-vein thrombosis, cerebrovascular accidents, chronic liver disease and torsion of the ovary. To date, the pathophysiological mechanisms have not been elucidated and studies have concentrated on plasma renin activity, changes in aldosterone and the renin–angiotensin cascade [95].

OHSS requiring hospital admission is rare after clomiphene citrate alone but occurs in 1.5–3% of cycles where hMG is used. Younger women with polycystic ovary syndrome and highly responsive ovaries are most prone (conversely those women requiring very high doses of hMG are least prone) and the rates may be a little higher in cycles using GnRH analogues. Strategies used within IVF programmes to minimise the risk of symptomatic OHSS in women showing an exaggerated response to ovarian stimulation include the cancelling of the treatment cycle, the withholding of hCG as a luteal support, and the cryopreservation of all embryos generated, with thawing and replacement taking place in a subsequent cycle after the hyperstimulation has subsided [96].

Oocyte micromanipulation

Micromanipulation procedures on oocytes are undertaken to enhance fertilisation in cases of severe male factor infertility. Several techniques have been described, as shown in Fig. 60.8. The main difficulty was originally thought to be the crossing of the zona pellucida of the oocyte, and so a modification of the IVF protocol was introduced called partial zona dissection [97], in which a slit was cut through the zona with a sharp glass needle. This then acted as a gate through which the sperm could swim to gain access to the perivitelline space and interact directly with the vitelline membrane. Unfortunately, many patients still had no fertilisation, with the sperm often being unable to pass through the slit. Another difficulty was that the zona pellucida is the main block to polyspermy in the human, and so many of the oocytes became polyspermic. Subzonal insemination was then introduced [98] by which a controlled number of spermatozoa were injected directly into the perivitelline space to ensure that the zona pellucida had been bypassed. Polyspermy was still a problem, being related to the number of spermatozoa injected, but the main limitation was the persistently reduced fertilisation rate seen. This implies an inability of the spermatozoa to successfully cross the vitelline membrane. The introduction of intracytoplasmic sperm injection (ICSI) [99] appears to offer the best chance of achieving a pregnancy since excellent fertilisation and implantation rates are now being obtained by many centres

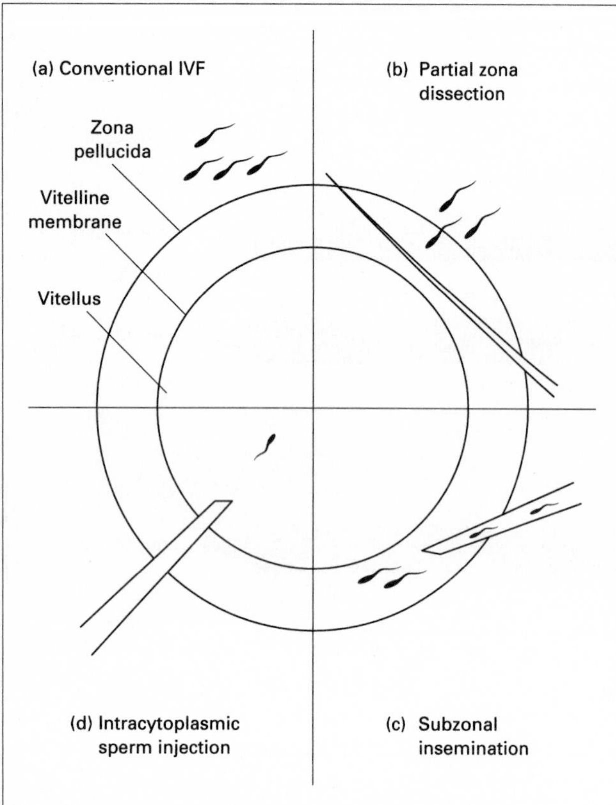

Fig. 60.8 The different *in vitro* fertilisation (IVF)-related strategies employed in the treatment of severe male factor infertility.

around the world. In this technique, a single spermatozoon is injected directly into the cytoplasm of the oocyte, bypassing both the zona pellucida and the vitelline membrane. The single sperm for ICSI can be obtained from ejaculate specimens in cases of severe oligoasthenozoospermia; epididymal aspirations for obstructive azoospermia and even testicular biopsy samples to tease spermatozoa from seminiferous tubules in cases of spermatogenic failure [115].

IVF-associated techniques

Gamete intrafallopian transfer

In many infertility clinics GIFT [100] has become established as the main procedure for non-tubal, non-male infertility. It is therefore a commonly used treatment for resistant cases of unexplained/poorly explained infertility, those with poor sperm–mucus interaction, those with pelvic endometriosis and cases of failed DI therapy. It is also a suitable option for those women likely to ovulate more than three oocytes during ovulation therapy and who should otherwise avoid conception in that cycle.

The ovarian stimulation regimen is the same as described for IVF and oocytes are recovered either by laparoscopy or by the transvaginal method. The choice depends upon surgeon preference and the proposed technique of transfer. The early workers relied on a mini-laparotomy procedure for oocyte transfer, but techniques were soon described facilitating laparoscopic tubal cannulation which is now the most commonly used method. More recently, transcervical cannulations have been explored. Up to four oocytes (usually two to each tube) are usually transferred but many clinics have reduced to three (usually all to one tube) without compromising pregnancy rates but significantly reducing the risk of high-order multiple pregnancies. Oocytes are loaded into a Teflon transfer cannula in 25 μl of medium along with 100 000 spermatozoa (male partners being required to produce their semen samples 2 hours prior)—also in 25 μl separated by a small air space. The gametes are deposited 40 mm into the Fallopian tube via the fimbrial end. If transcervical cannulation is performed, anaesthesia is not required and gametes are deposited approximately 40 mm from the cornual orifice. If GIFT is used for oligospermic infertility, higher numbers of spermatozoa are required but this is no longer recommended as blighted ovum pregnancies are increased [101].

GIFT patients need to consider the question of their supernumerary oocytes after transfer of their best three. The options for such supernumerary oocytes are to fertilise and cryopreserve them for the couple's own subsequent use, donate them for use by other infertile couples, donate them to an approved research program, or simply discard them. Supernumerary oocytes comprise those with poorer scores on grading and hence have reduced fertilisation potential [101]. Generally, it is younger women who respond sufficiently well to stimulation enabling ovum donation to be considered. Some clinics have established as stand-alone GIFT units and may consider the technique of intravaginal culture [102], enabling their patients to avail themselves of the services of a regional IVF unit for embryo cryopreservation rather than having to discard their supernumerary oocytes.

Intravaginal culture

The desire to obviate the need for an embryology laboratory led to the development of the technique of intravaginal culture [103]. The oocytes and embryos were placed into a tube containing culture medium, and the tube placed into the patient's vagina to be kept warm. The tube was then removed 48 hours later at the time of embryo transfer and the cleaved embryos selected and replaced into the uterus. After an initial following, the technique has not been used widely. The main limitations are: (i) that the only real saving is the price of an incubator since staff able to handle gametes and embryos are still required; and (ii) the omission of the check for pronuclei means that some oocytes will be polyspermic but divide to form embryos of normal appearance and so be transferred.

Transport IVF

The establishment of a good IVF laboratory is of paramount importance in obtaining good pregnancy rates in an IVF programme. The transport of oocytes collected at a peripheral unit to a central specialised laboratory for basic IVF [104] or micromanipulation [105] has therefore proved extremely valuable in increasing the access of patients to treatment. This strategic use of limited resources is an excellent way of providing IVF and is to be encouraged in areas where the establishment of a full IVF unit is not feasible.

Ovum donation

Ovum donation resulting in a successful pregnancy was first reported in 1984 [106] and was applied to a woman with primary ovarian failure. The indications have since been extended and now include cases with incipient ovarian failure, those who respond poorly to ovarian stimulation, cases with serious genetic carrier states and occasionally cases whose ovaries are inaccessible, although this is uncommon now given the wide variety of techniques available to recover oocytes. Known or anonymous donors are required to provide the oocytes and these women must undergo full ovarian stimulation, monitoring and oocyte recovery. Not surprisingly, altruistic donors are hard to find because of the practical difficulties faced [107].

The best results reported from ovum donation involve tubal transfers performed in cycles established by a hormone-replacement regimen, for example oestradiol valerate and progesterone injections or pessaries. Pregnancy rates are generally reported in the range of 35–50% per transfer indicating that around 20% of such embryos may implant [108]. This could relate to the generally younger age of donors and the benefits of a hormonally controlled cycle. The latter view has led to the use by some clinics of GnRH suppression followed by hormone replacement in cycling women having either ovum donation or their own cryopreserved embryos transferred, with improved results. Pregnancy wastage following ovum donation is low, generally being reported as 20% or less.

Surrogacy

The issue of surrogacy remains controversial such that in some locations it has been legislated against. However, a good case can be made for the concept of altruistic IVF surrogacy [109] otherwise known as 'compassionate family surrogacy'. This embodies the following four criteria:

1 an appropriate medical indication, for example absent uterus, uterine malfunction such as Asherman's syndrome or a medical condition which contraindicates pregnancy;
2 embryos are generated from the gametes of the infertile couple (or a matched anonymous donor if indicated);
3 no surrogacy fee is paid (although the surrogate's treatment expenses may be covered by the infertile couple); and
4 a relative (usually a sister) or very close friend acts as surrogate.

Such altruistic IVF surrogacy arrangements appear to have entirely satisfactory outcomes and the concern over relinquishment does not appear to arise. Children should be informed from the earliest stages of the nature of their biological backgrounds and the assistance provided by their special aunt who carried them through pregnancy on their mother's behalf. In the main, the genetic parents will be required to adopt their own children because of the common law view that a woman who delivers a child is regarded as the mother and the absence of specific supportive legislation. However, there are now parts of the world (e.g. California) with specific legislation in place to allow the commissioning parents to be regarded as the legal parents in the first instance.

Ethical and legal considerations

IVF and related areas of assisted reproduction have generated unprecedented public interest in a medical area. Certainly there are broader social, ethical, legal, religious and sometimes political issues which arise apart from the complexity of technical issues. There are four broad areas of concern:
1 standards of laboratory and clinical practice;
2 accountability to the general community;
3 protecting the welfare of children born following assisted reproduction;
4 ownership of stored gametes and embryos.

Guidelines and regulations should assist to limit the complications (e.g. high-order multiple pregnancies, ovarian hyperstimulation syndrome and anaesthetic mortalities) and ensure clinics are providing the best possible service to infertile couples, within the current limitations of knowledge. In this latter context, the need for continuing research into all aspects, including fundamental physiology as well as clinical applications, must be acknowledged and pursued. Public accountability can be incorporated within a self-regulatory mechanism by ensuring an accurate and current data reporting system which is accessible. The welfare of children, and potential children, means careful control over the disposal of gametes, avoiding mixed embryo transfers which might confuse the genetic identity of children, respecting confidentiality of donors but enabling those children who become aware of a donor background to have access to non-identifying information. Debates are current concerning access to identifying information and the question of respective responsibilities with respect to IVF surrogacy infants. Other concerns relate to ownership of stored embryos in the event of a couple's separation or death, and ensuing disputation arising over the use of these embryos. Such matters can only be resolved by specific legislation.

Conclusions

Procedures to assist reproduction have made a major impact in the area of infertility over the past decade and have been based upon wide-ranging advances in knowledge concerning reproductive physiology. This has occurred at an appropriate time as the fecundity of many industrialised communities has decreased markedly in recent years. In their turn, the procedures themselves have created the opportunity to consider providing services for the fertile population, for example in controlling genetic disease, in gamete and embryo storage for the preservation of fecundity and in new considerations for contraception. The field has excited considerable public interest and has implications for other areas of medicine such as the team approach to the management of individual cases, control by institutional ethics committees and other regulatory bodies, both voluntary and statutory. The main danger is the snowballing effect of a perceived need to introduce legislative controls, particularly in the area of embryo research, which may create an inhibitory or oppressive climate for further research [110]. Such legislation may effectively seal the current technology in its relatively inefficient state.

References

1 Jeffcoate N. Sterility and subfertility. In: *Principles of Gynaecology*. London: Butterworths, 1975: 583–607.

2 Scott RT, Opsahl MS, Leonardi MR *et al.* Life table analysis of pregnancy rates in a general infertility population relative to ovarian reserve and patient age. *Human Reprod* 1995; **10**: 1706–10.

3 Collins JA, Burrows EA, Willan AR. The prognosis for live birth among untreated infertile couples. *Fertil Steril* 1995; **64**: 22–8.

4 Jacobs H, Hull M, Murray M *et al.* Therapy-orientated diagnosis of secondary amenorrhoea. *Horm Res* 1975; **6**: 268–87.

5 Franks S, Jacobs H, Hull M *et al.* Management of hyperprolactinaemic amenorrhoea. *Br J Obstet Gynaecol* 1977; **84**: 241–53.

6 Hull M, Savage P, Jacobs H. Investigation and treatment of amenorrhoea resulting in normal fertility. *Br. Med J* 1979; **1**: 1257–61.

7 Bergh T, Nillius J, Wide L. Bromocriptine treatment of 42 hyperprolactinaemic women with secondary amenorrhoea. *Acta Endocrinologica* 1978; **78**: 435–41.

8 Lenton E, Sobowale O, Cooke I. Prolactin concentrations in ovulatory but infertile women: treatment wih bromocriptine. *Br Med J* 1977; **1**: 1179–81.

9 Massai MR, Deziegler D, Lesobre V *et al.* Clomiphene citrate affects cervical mucus and endometrial morphology independently of the changes in plasma hormonal levels induced by multiple follicular recruitment. *Fertil Steril* 1993; **59**: 1179–86.

10 Bateman BG, Kolp LA, Nunley WC *et al.* Subclinical pregnancy loss in clomiphene citrate-treated women. *Fertil Steril* 1992; **57**: 25–7.

11 Saunders DM, Lancaster PAL, Pedisich EL. Increased pregnancy failure rates after clomiphene following assisted reproductive technology. *Human Reprod* 1992; **7**: 1154–8.

12 Navot D, Rosenwaks Z, Margoliath E. Prognostic assessment of female fecundity. *Lancet* 1987; **ii**: 645–7.

13 Loumaye E, Psalti I, Billion J-M *et al.* Prediction of individual response to controlled ovarian hyperstimulation by means of a clomiphene citrate challenge test. *Fertil Steril* 1990; **53**: 295–301.

14 MacGregor A, Johnson J, Bunde C. Further clinical experience with clomiphene citrate. *Fertil Steril* 1968; **19**: 616–20.

15 Fisch P, Casper R, Brown S *et al.* Unexplained infertility: evaluation of treatment with clomiphene citrate and human chorionic gonadotropin. *Fertil Steril* 1989; **51**: 828–33.

16 Yeko T, Khan-Dawood F, Dawood M. Luteinizing hormone and human chorionic gonadotropin receptors in human corpora lutea from clomiphene citrate-induced cycles. *Fertil Steril* 1990; **54**: 601–5.

17 Lunenfeld B. Treatment of anovulation by human gonadotropins. *Int J Gynecol Obstet* 1963; **1**: 153–4.

18 Rodgers M, Mitchell R, Lambert A *et al.* Human chorionic gonadotropin contributes to the bioactivity of pergonal. *Clin Endocrinol* 1992; **37**: 558–64.

19 Rodgers M, McLoughlin J, Lambert A *et al.* Variability in the immunoreactive and bioactive follicle stimulating hormone content of human urinary menopausal gonadotrophin preparations. *Human Reprod* 1995; **10**: 1982–6.

20 Lunenfeld B, Insler V, Glezerman M. *Diagnosis and Treatment of Functional Infertility*, 3rd edn. Berlin: Blackwell Wissenschaft, 1993.

21 Taymor M, Sturgis S. Induction of ovulation with human menopausal gonadotropin. II. Probable causes of overstimulation. *Fertil Steril* 1966; **17**: 736–41.

22 Zaner R, Boehm F, Hill G. Selective termination in multiple pregnancies: ethical considerations. 1990; **54**: 203–5.

23 Wang CF, Gemzell C. The use of human gonadotrophins for the induction of ovulation in women with polycystic ovarian disease. *Fertil Steril* 1980; **33**: 479–86.

24 Hamilton-Fairley D, Kiddy D, Watson H *et al.* Low dose gonadotropin therapy for induction of ovulation in 100 women with polycystic ovary syndrome. *Human Reprod* 1991; **6**: 1095–9.

25 Dor J, Itzkowic D, Maschiach S *et al.* Cumulative conception rates following gonadotropin therapy. *Am J Obstet Gynecol* 1980; **136**: 102–5.

26 Hull MGR. Infertility treatment: relative effectiveness of conventional and assisted conception methods. *Human Reprod* 1992; **7**: 785–96.

27 Chaffkin L, Nulsen J, AA L *et al.* A comparative analysis of the cycle fecundity rates associated with combined human menopausal gonadotropin (hMG) and intrauterine insemination (IUI) versus either hMG or IUI alone. *Fertil Steril* 1991; **55**: 252–7.

28 Braat D, Schoemaker R, Schoemaker J. Life table analysis

of fecundity in intravenously gonadotropin-releasing hormone-treated patients with normogonadotropic and hypogonadotropic amenorrhea. *Fertil Steril* 1991; **55**: 266–71.

29 Macnamee MC, Taylor PJ, Howles CM *et al.* Short-term luteinizing hormone-releasing hormone agonist treatment: prospective trial of a novel ovarian stimulation regimen for in vitro fertilization. *Fertil Steril* 1989; **52**: 264–9.

30 Rutherford AJ, Subark-Sharp RJ, Dawson KJ *et al.* Improvement of in-vitro fertilization after treatment with Buserelin, an agonist of luteinising hormone releasing hormone. *Br Med J* 1988; **296**: 1765–8.

31 Conaghan J, Dimitry E, Mills M *et al.* Delayed human chorionic gonadotropin administration for in-vitro fertilisation. *Lancet* 1989; i: 1323–4.

32 Gemzell C, Diczfalusy E, Tillinger K. Clinical effect of human pituitary follicle-stimulating hormone (FSH). *J Clin Endocrinol* 1958; **18**: 1333–48.

33 Crooke A, Butt W, Palmer R *et al.* Clinical trial of human gonadotrophins: I. The effect of pituitary and urinary follicle-stimulating hormone and chorionic gonadotrophin on patients with idiopathic secondary amenorrhea. *J Obstet Gynaecol Br Commonwealth* 1963; **70**: 604–35.

34 Lazarus L. Suspension of the Australian human pituitary hormone programme. *Med J Aust* 1985; **143**: 57–9.

35 Healy DL, Evans J. Creutzfeldt–Jakob disease after pituitary gonadotrophins. *Br Med J* 1993; **307**: 517–18.

36 Seibel M, McArdle C, Smith D *et al.* Ovulation induction in polycystic ovary syndrome with urinary follicle-stimulating hormone or human menopausal gonadotrophin. *Fertil Steril* 1985; **43**: 703–8.

37 Jones G, Acosta A, Garcia J *et al.* The effect of follicle-stimulating hormone without additional luteinizing hormone on follicular stimulation and oocytes development in normal ovulatory women. *Fertil Steril* 1985; **43**: 696–702.

38 Shaw R, Ndukwe G, Imoedemhe D *et al.* Endocrine changes following pituitary desensitization with LHRH agonist and administration of purified FSH to induce follicular maturation. *Br J Obstet Gynaecol* 1987; **94**: 682–6.

39 Hull MGR, Armatage RJ, Mcdermott A. Use of follicle-stimulating hormone alone (urofillitropin(*)) to stimulate the ovaries for assisted conception after pituitary desensitization. *Fertil Steril* 1994; **62**: 997–1003.

40 Howles CM, Loumaye L, Giroud D *et al.* Multiple follicular development and ovarian steroidogenesis following subcutaneous administration of a highly purified urinary FSH preparation in pituitary desensitized women undergoing IVF—a multicentre European phase III study. *Human Reprod* 1994; **9**: 424–30.

41 Zelinskiwooten MB, Hutchison JS, Hess DL *et al.* Follicle stimulating hormone alone supports follicle growth and oocyte development in gonadotrophin-releasing hormone antagonist-treated monkeys. *Human Reprod* 1995; **10**: 1658–66.

42 le Cotonnec J-Y, Porchet H, Beltrami V *et al.* Clinical pharmacology of recombinant human follicle-stimulating hormone. I. Comparative pharmacokinetics with urinary human FSH. *Fertil Steril* 1994; **61**: 669–78.

43 Group RHFS. Clinical assessment of recombinant human follicle-stimulating hormone in stimulating ovarian follicular development before in vitro fertilization. *Fertil Steril* 1995; **63**: 77–86.

44 Homburg R, West C, Torresani T *et al.* Co-treatment with human growth hormone and gonadotropins for induction of ovulation: a controlled clinical trail. *Fertil Steril* 1990; **53**: 254–60.

45 European and Australian Multicenter Study. Co-treatment with growth hormone and gonadotropin for ovulation induction in hypogonadotropic patients: a prospective, randomized, placebo-controlled, dose–response study. *Fertil Steril* 1995; **64**: 917–23.

46 Hughes SM, Huang ZH, Morris ID *et al.* A double-blind cross-over controlled study to evaluate the effect of human biosynthetic growth hormone on ovarian stimulation in previous poor responders to in-vitro fertilization. *Human Reprod* 1994; **9**: 13–18.

47 Joyce D, Vassilopoulos D. Sperm–mucus interaction and artificial insemination. *Clin Obstet Gynaecol* 1981; **8**: 587–610.

48 Taylor PJ, Kredentser JV. Washed intra-uterine insemination—indications and success. *Int J Fertil* 1989; **34**: 378–84.

49 Dodson W, Haney A. Controlled ovarian hyperstimulation and intrauterine insemination for treatment of infertility. *Fertil Steril* 1991; **55**: 457–67.

50 Matson P. The usefulness of IVF, GIFT and IUI in the treatment of male infertility. In: Lieberman B, Matson P, eds. *Clinical IVF Forum: Current Views in Assisted Reproduction.* Manchester: Manchester University Press, 1990: 112–22.

51 Matson P, Yovich J, Edirisinghe W *et al.* An argument for the past and continued use of pentoxifylline in assisted reproductive technology. *Human Reprod* 1995; **10** (Suppl. 1): 67–71.

52 Hummel WP, Talbert LM. Current management of a donor insemination program. *Fertil Steril* 1989; **51**: 919–30.

53 Van Steirteghem A, Nagy P, Lui J *et al.* Intracytoplasmic sperm injection—ICSI. *Reprod Med Rev* 1994; **3**: 199–207.

54 Stewart G, Cunningham A, Driscoll G *et al.* Transmission of human T-cell lymphotropic virus type III (HTLV-III) by artificial insemination by donor. *Lancet* 1985; ii: 581–4.

55 Keel BA, Webster BW. Semen cryopreservation methodology and results. In: Barratt CLR, Cooke ID, ed. *Donor Insemination.* Cambridge: Cambridge University Press, 1993: 71–96.

56 Barratt C, Matson P, Holt W. British Andrology Society guidelines for the screening of semen donors for donor insemination. *Human Reprod* 1993; **8**: 1521–3.

57 Mahadevan M, Trounson A, Leeton J. Successful use of human semen cryobanking for in vitro fertilization. *Fertil Steril* 1983; **40**: 340–3.

58 Matson P, Horne G, Hamer F *et al.* Cryopreservation: sperm and embryos—results in question: In: Shaw R, ed. *Assisted Reproduction: Progress in Research and Practice.* Lancaster: Parthenon, 1995: 123–40.

59 Winston RML. Progress in tubal surgery. *Clin Obstet Gynaecol* 1981; **8**: 653–79.

60 Damewood MD, Rock JA. Reproductive uterine surgery. *Obstet Gynecol Clin North Am* 1987; **14**: 1049–68.

61 Bateman BG, Nunley WCJ, Kitchin JD. Surgical management of distal tubal obstruction—are we making progress? *Fertil Steril* 1987; **48**: 523–42.

62 Gomel V. Operative laparoscopy: time for acceptance. *Fertil Steril* 1989; **52**: 1–11.

63 Yovich JL, Matson PL, Yovich JM. The optimization of laparoscopic oocyte recovery. *Int J Fertil* 1989; **34**: 390–400.

64 Yovich JL. Tubal transfers: PROST & TEST. In: Asch RH, Balmaceda JP, Johnston I, eds. *Gamete Physiology.* Norwell, USA: Serono Symposia USA, 1990: 305–17.

65 Silber SJ, Gulle J, Friend D. Microscopic vasovasostomy and spermatogenesis. *J Urol* 1977; **117**: 299–302.

66 Silber SJ. Microsurgery for vasectomy reversal in vasoepididymostomy. *Urology* 1984; **23**: 505–24.

67 Verheyen G, De Croo I, Tournaye H *et al.* Comparison of four

mechanical methods to retrieve spermatozoa from testicular tissue. *Human Reprod* 1995; **10**: 2956–9.

68 Devroey P, Liu J, Nagy Z *et al.* Pregnancies after testicular sperm extraction and intracytoplasmic sperm injection in non-obstructive azoospermia. *Human Reprod* 1995; **10**: 1457–60.

69 Silber SJ, Ord T, Balmaceda JP *et al.* Pregnancy with sperm aspiration from the proximal head of the epididymis: a new treatment for congenital absence of the vas deferens. *Fertil Steril* 1988; **50**: 525–8.

70 Jequier AM, Cummins JM, Gearon *et al.* A pregnancy achieved using sperm from the epididymal caput in idiopathic obstructive azoospermia. *Fertil Steril* 1990; **53**: 1104–5.

71 Chang MC. Fertilization of rabbit ova *in vitro*. *Nature* 1959; **184**: 466–77.

72 Whittingham DG. Fertilization of mouse eggs *in vitro*. *Nature* 1968; **220**: 592–3.

73 Evans IE, Mukherjee AB, Schulman JD. Human *in vitro* fertilization. *Obstet Gynecol Survey* 1980; **35**: 71–81.

74 Steptoe PC, Edwards RG. Reimplantation of a human embryo with subsequent tubal pregnancy. *Lancet* 1976; **ii**: 1265.

75 Edwards RG, Steptoe PC, Purdy JM. Establishing full-term human pregnancies using cleaving embryos grown *in vitro*. *Br J Obstet Gynaecol* 1980; **87**: 737–56.

76 Steptoe PC, Edwards RG. Birth after the reimplantation of a human embryo. *Lancet* 1978; **ii**: 366.

77 Steptoe PC, Edwards RG, Purdy JM. Clinical aspects of pregnancies established with cleaving embryos grown *in vitro*. *Br J Obstet Gyn* 1980; **87**: 757–68.

78 Trounson AO, Leeton JF, Wood C. Successful human pregnancies by *in vitro* fertilization and embryo transer in the controlled ovulatory cycle. *Science* 1981; **212**: 681–2.

79 Jones HW, Jones GS, Andrews MC *et al.* The program for *in-vitro* fertilization at Norfolk. *Fertil Steril* 1982; **38**: 14–21.

80 Lenz S, Lauritsen JG, Kjellow M. Collection of human oocytes for *in vitro* fertilization by ultrasonically guided follicular puncture. *Lancet* 1981; **i**: 1163–4.

81 Wikland M, Hamberger L, Enk L *et al.* Technical and clinical aspects of ultra-sound guided oocyte recovery. *Human Reprod* 1989; **4**: 79–82.

82 Yovich JL, Grudzinskas JG. The management of infertility: a practical guide to gamete handling procedures. London: Heinemann, 1990: 276.

83 Pickering SJ, Johnson MH. The influence of cooling on the organisation of the meiotic spindle of the mouse oocyte. *Human Reprod* 1987; **2**: 207–16.

84 Johnson MH, Vincent C, Braude PR *et al.* The cytoskeleton of the oocyte: its role in the generation of normal and aberrent pre-embryos. In: Edwards RG, ed. *Establishing a Successful Human Pregnancy*. New York: Raven Press, 1990: 133–42.

85 Aitken RJ. Biochemical changes in the fertilizing spermatozoon. In: Edwards RG, ed. *Establishing a Successful Human Pregnancy*. New York: Raven Press, 1990: 87–101.

86 Purdy JM. Methods for fertilization and embryo culture *in vitro*. In: Edwards RG, Purdy JM, eds. *Human Conception In Vitro*. London: Academic Press, 1982: 135–56.

87 Yovich JL, Yovich JM, Edirisinghe WR *et al.* Methods of water purification for the preparation of culture media in an IVF-ET programme. *Human Reprod* 1988; **3**: 245–8.

88 Plachot M, Veiga A, Montagut J *et al.* Are clinical and biological IVF parameters correlated with chromosomal disorders in early life: a multicentric study. *Human Reprod* 1988; **3**: 627–35.

89 Lopata A, Hay DL. The potential of early human embryos to form blastocysts, hatch from their zona and secrete hCG in culture. *Human Reprod* 1989; **4**: 87–94.

90 Hamer FC, Horne G, Pease EHE *et al.* The quarantine of fertilized donated oocytes. *Human Reprod* 1995; **10**: 1194–6.

91 Ashwood-Smith MJ. The cryopreservation of human embryos. *Human Reprod* 1986; **1**: 319–32.

92 Mandelbaum J, Junca A, Plachot M *et al.* Human embryo cryopreservation, extrinsic and intrinsic parameters of success. *Human Reprod* 1987; **2**: 709–15.

93 Gook DA, Osborn SM, Bourne H *et al.* Fertilization of human oocytes following cryopreservation; normal karyotypes and absence of stray chromosomes. *Human Reprod* 1994; **9**: 684–91.

94 Lunenfeld B, ed. *World Health Organisation Consultation on the Diagnosis and Treatment of Endocrine Forms of Infertility*. Geneva: WHO, 1976: Technical Report Series No. 514.

95 Golan A, Ron-El R, Herman A *et al.* Ovarian hyperstimulation syndrome: an update review. *Obstet Gynecol Survey* 1989; **44**: 430–40.

96 Wada I, Matson PL, Troup SA *et al.* Does elective cryopreservation of all embryos from women at risk of ovarian hyperstimulation syndrome reduce the incidence of the condition. *Br J Obstet Gynaecol* 1993; **100**: 265–9.

97 Malter HE, Cohen J. Partial zona dissection of the human oocyte: a non-traumatic method using micromanipulation to assist zona pellucida penetration: *Fertil Steril* 1989; **51**: 139–48.

98 Fishel S, Timson J, Lisi F *et al.* Evaluation of 225 patients undergoing subzonal insemination for the procurement of fertilization *in vitro*. *Fertil Steril* 1992; **57**: 840–9.

99 Van Steirteghem AC, Nagy Z, Joris H *et al.* High fertilization and implantation rates after intracytoplasmic sperm injection. *Human Reprod* 1993; **8**: 1061–6.

100 Asch RH, Ellsworth LR, Balmaceda JP *et al.* Pregnancy following translaparoscopic gamete intrafallopian transfer (GIFT). *Lancet* 1984; **ii**: 1034.

101 Yovich JL, Cummins JM, Bootsma B *et al.* The usefulness of simultaneous IVF and GIFT in predicting fertilization and pregnancy. In: Capitanio GL, Asch RH, De Cecoo L, Croce S, eds. *GIFT: From Basics to Clinics*, Vol. 63. New York: Raven Press, 1989: 321–332.

102 Critchlow JD, Matson PL, Killick S *et al.* Pregnancy following intravaginal embryo transportation. *Br J Obstet Gynaecol* 1992; **99**: 259–60.

103 Ranoux C, Aubriot FX, Dubuisson JB *et al.* A new *in vitro* fertilization technique. *Fertil Steril* 1988; **49**: 654–7.

104 Kingsland C, Aziz N, Taylor C *et al.* Transport *in vitro* fertilization—a novel scheme for community-based treatment. *Fertil Steril* 1992; **58**: 153–8.

105 Anyaegbunam W, Biljan MM, Barker E *et al.* The first pregnancy in a transport-intracytoplasmic sperm injection (T-ICSI) scheme. *J Assist Reprod Genet* 1995; **12**: 396–8.

106 Lütjen P, Trounson A, Leeton J *et al.* The establishment and maintenance of pregnancy using *in vitro* fertilization and embryo donation in a patient with primary ovarian failure. *Nature* 1984; **307**: 174–5.

107 Horne G, Hughes SM, Matson PL *et al.* The recruitment of oocyte donors. *Br J Obstet Gynaecol* 1993; **100**: 877–8.

108 Asch RH. GIFT: Indications, results, problems and perspectives. In: Capitanio GL, Asch RH, De Cecco L, Croce S, eds. *GIFT: From Basics to Clinics*, Vol. 63. New York: Raven Press, 1989; 209–28.

109 Yovich JL, Hoffman TD. IVF surrogacy and absent uterus syndromes. *Lancet* 1988; ii: 331–2.
110 Braude P, Johnson M. Embryo research: yes or no? *Br Med J* 1989; **299**: 1349–51.
111 Lancaster P, Shafir E, Huang J. *Assisted Conception, Australia and New Zealand, 1992 and 1993*. Assisted Conception Series, Vol. 1. Sydney: AIHW National Perinatal Statistics Unit, 1995.
112 Horne G. *A retrospective and prospective evaluation of different strategies to select human embryos for cryopreservation*. MSc Thesis, University of Manchester, 1995.
113 Ferrari C, Piscitelli G, Crosignani PG. Cabergoline: a new drug for the treatment of hyperprolactinaemia. *Human Reprod* 1995; **10**: 1647–52.
114 Yovich JL, Stanger JD. The limitations of IVF from males with severe oligospermia and abnormal sperm morphology. *J Vitro Fert Embryo Transfer* 1984; **1**: 172.
115 Mansour RT, Aboulghar MA, Serour GI *et al*. Intracytoplasmic sperm injection using microsurgically retrived epididymal and testicular sperm. *Fertil Steril* 1996; **65**: 566–72.

Part 13
Disorders of Growth

CHAPTER 61

Principles of normal growth: auxology and endocrinology

M.A. Preece

The human growth curve

Most human dimensions follow a similar pattern of growth throughout childhood, and height may be used as a typical example. The height curve of an individual boy is shown in Fig. 61.1: Fig. 61.1a shows the height attained or distance curve and Fig. 61.1b shows the height-velocity curve. The distance curve represents all the height accumulated over time until the latest measurement and is, therefore, relatively insensitive to recent changes in the child's well-being. In contrast, the velocity curve represents growth over a clearly defined and relatively short period of time, which will usually be 1 year.

Study of the height-velocity curve shows a general trend for a decelerating growth rate from birth to maturity, but with two interruptions to this trend. The first, and smaller, of these occurs at between 6 and 8 years and is called the mid-growth or mid-childhood spurt. There is little difference between sexes except that it may be some 6 months earlier in girls. The mechanism of this spurt is entirely unknown although its timing is close to the initial rise in secretion of adrenal androgens.

A second and much greater interruption of the downward velocity trend is the adolescent growth spurt, which is illustrated for the average British girl and boy in Fig. 61.2. Before the onset of the growth spurt boys grow very slightly faster than girls, but the girls' growth spurt starts about 2 years before the boys and for about 4 years girls are, on average, taller than boys. However, by maturity males are 14 cm taller than females and this difference is almost entirely due to events at puberty. Males grow for 2 years longer before puberty at an average rate of 5–6 cm per year with the remainder accruing from the rather more intense male growth spurt [1].

Variation in height

The preceding descriptions are limited to the average child, both in terms of size and of the timing of events such as the adolescent growth spurt. There is, however, considerable variation in both. The magnitude of variation in size at a given age is illustrated in Fig. 61.3 which shows the new standards for height of boys in the UK [2]. Whilst the variation in size seems very straightforward, this figure to some extent obscures the variation in timing (or *tempo*, as this aspect is usually termed). This problem is of sufficient clinical importance to justify detailed consideration.

Tempo of growth

Referring to Fig. 61.4, consider initially a child, say a boy, who will ultimately reach a mature height which is exactly average for the population. If he is also exactly average in tempo then he will follow closely the mean growth curve, start the adolescent growth spurt at 12 years, reach the peak at 14 years and reach mature height at about 18 years. If on the other hand he is an early developer with a fast tempo, then he will always be rather further along his personal growth curve at any given age than average children. He will therefore seem tall at each stage until he is caught up at maturity, which he reaches early, say 16 years. In exact contrast the late developing boy, destined for average mature height, will seem short until maturity. A similar process occurs for children with all levels of mature height potential so that variation in height at any age before maturity is a combination of varying height potential and variation in tempo.

Population height standards

The construction and role of growth standards has previously

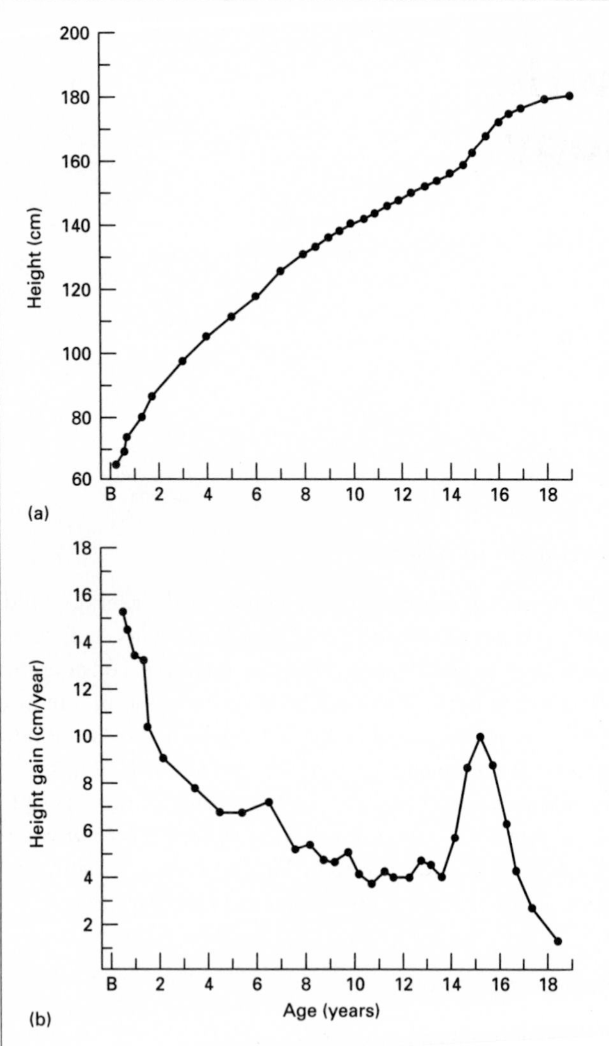

Fig. 61.1 (a) The growth curve of height of a single boy from birth to maturity. (b) The same data as above but expressed as growth velocity.

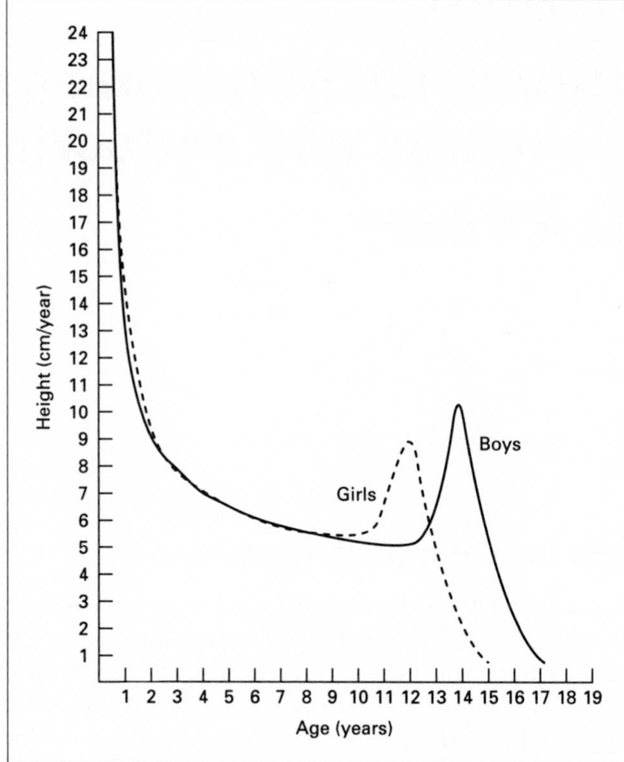

Fig. 61.2 Adolescent growth spurts of boys and girls in the UK whose peak growth spurt is reached at an average age (12 years in girls and 14 years in boys).

been reviewed in detail [3]. Much controversy exists concerning the relative merits of cross-sectional and longitudinal standards. The former are based on data from a large number of children each of which is measured on one occasion. In contrast, longitudinal standards are based on a smaller number of children measured on multiple occasions over many years. It has been argued that the latter are appropriate for clinical use because they reflect the correct shape of an individual growth curve [4,5], whereas cross-sectional curves will tend to distort the pattern of individual growth around the age of puberty because of the variability of timing of the adolescent growth spurt between individuals; see [3] for more detail. However, the analysis of longitudinal data to provide individual-type growth standards requires a number of assumptions that are not really tenable: typical is the assumption that the growth spurt has essentially the same shape in all children of the same sex, varying only in timing and intensity. In clinical practice it makes little difference which type of standard is used as long as it is remembered that normal individuals will probably cross centile lines upwards or downwards at the time of puberty, and this needs careful interpretation by the clinician. At least cross-sectional standards make no assumptions and also allow the more regular revision of data to reflect the secular trend for greater stature and earlier development of succeeding generations [6] because of the greater ease of collection of appropriate data. Fig. 61.3 shows the latest British standards for height for boys which are derived from cross-sectional data. The centile lines shown are the 0.4th, 2nd, 9th, 25th, 50th, 75th, 91st, 98th and 99.6th which are selected to allow a regular distance between adjacent centiles of 0.67 SD [7]. Children whose height falls below the 0.4th centile represent the shortest four per 1000 of the population and require immediate investigation. Those between the 0.4th and 2nd centile need careful follow-up and those above the 2nd centile a less intense evaluation.

Correction for parental heights

The above standards derive from population surveys; they

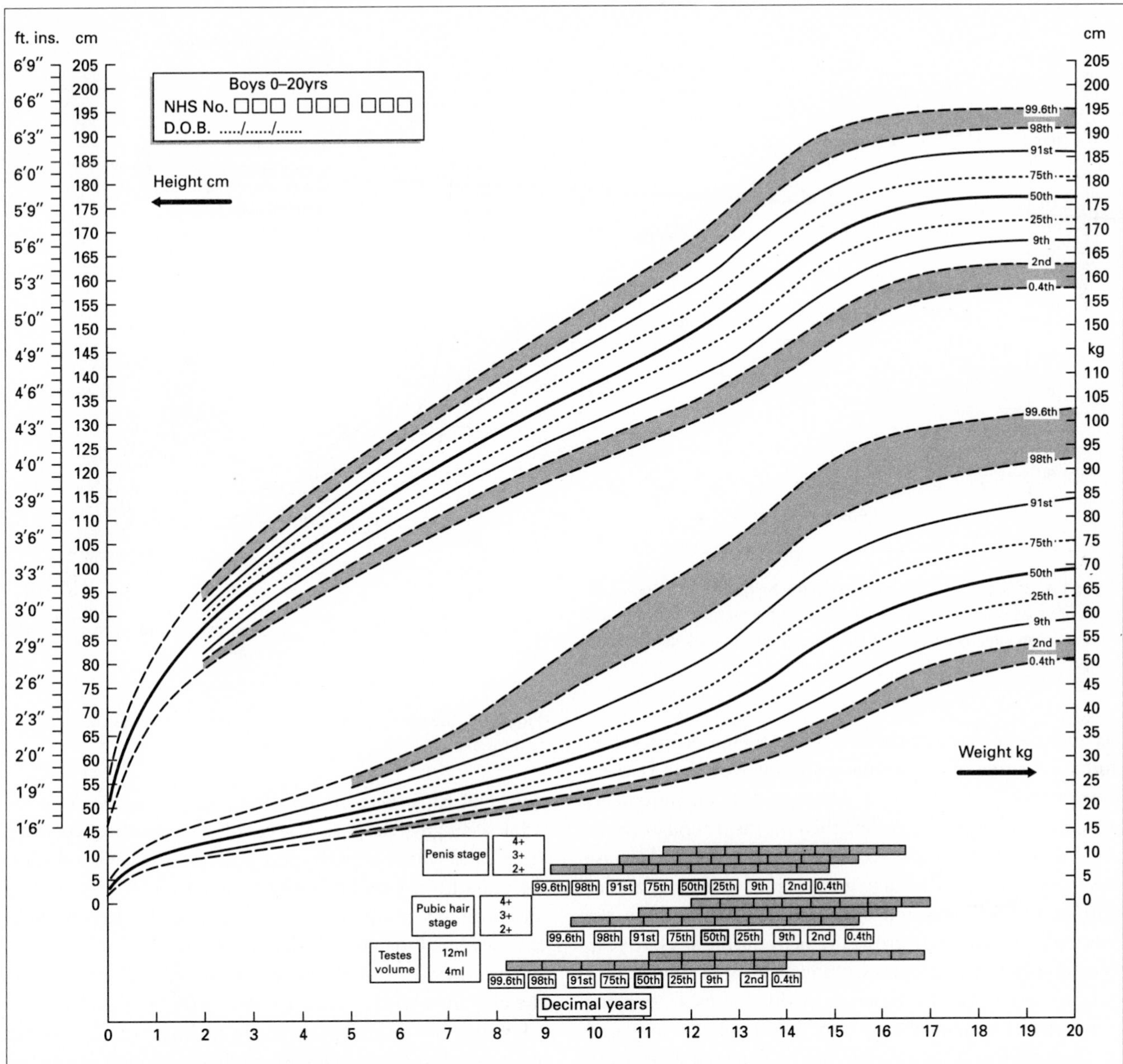

Fig. 61.3 Current standards for height and puberty for boys in the UK [2]. These charts can be obtained from Harlow Printing Company, Maxwell Street, South Shields, Tyne and Wear, NE33 4PU.

can be made more accurate for a given child if the heights of the parents are taken into account. The easiest way of doing this is to plot the parents' centiles at the right-hand edge of the chart. This is quickly done by plotting the actual height of the like-sexed parent and the father's height, minus 14 cm or the mother's height plus 14 cm, for the unlike-sexed parent. The 14 cm is the mean difference between adult men and women in the UK referred to above. This should be adjusted appropriately in other countries according to local data.

Height-velocity standards

Fig. 61.5 shows the standards for height velocity for boys. The data are based on pure longitudinal observations and the extremes of normality are indicated by centiles. It is important to make three qualifications. In the first place these standards are based on data collected before 1966 [4,5] and might not represent modern children. However, in the recent analysis of a large nationally representative sample of modern-day children [2] the *shape* of the average growth curve has changed very little except in the first 2 years of life; this implies that height velocity at any age over 2 years is also unchanged, and in the absence of any more modern data these standards remain approximately valid.

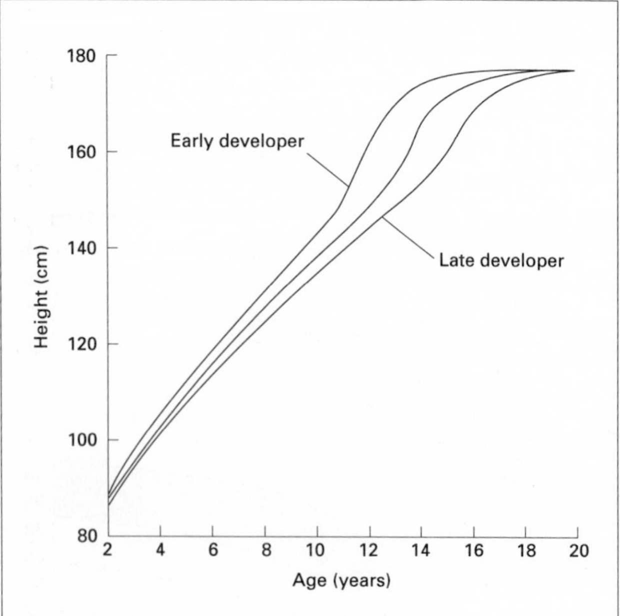

Fig. 61.4 Schematic representation of the height growth curves of three boys who all have the same potential for mature height, but who are respectively 2 years early, average and 2 years delayed in tempo.

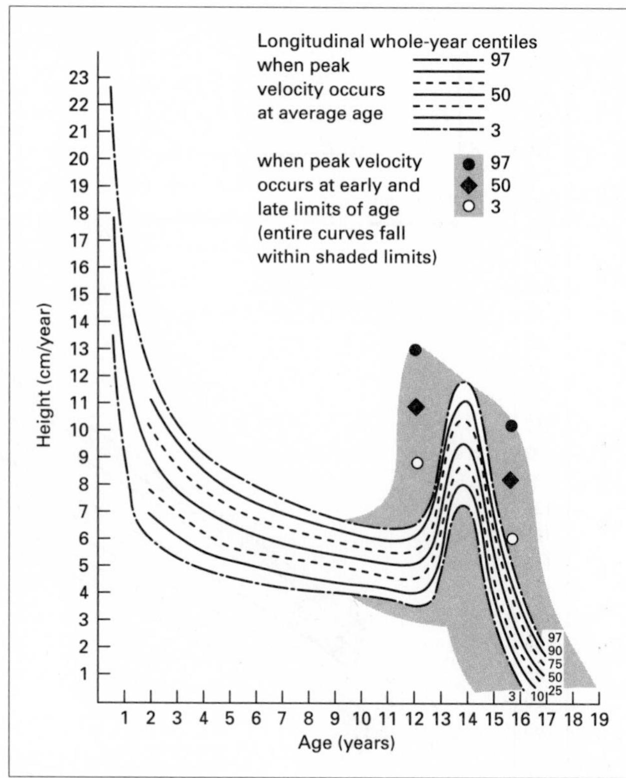

Fig. 61.5 Standard for height velocity for boys in the UK [34] (see text for explanation).

Secondly, it must be remembered that these normal values and the position of the various centiles are based on velocity measurements taken over a whole year. If measurements were taken over a shorter time then the dispersion between the 3rd and 97th centiles would be greater. This is because measurement errors assume greater importance as a proportion of the measured change and because there are substantial variations in growth velocity during any one year. It is important to interpret cautiously growth velocities in patients when they are based on periods of measurements of less than 1 year. Ideally, no velocities should be compared to these standards unless they were calculated over a full year, but in practice, of course, this often is not possible.

The final point that should be taken into account is that centiles for height velocity do have a slightly different meaning than do height centiles. On average over a year or more, any individual child who is growing normally should have a height velocity somewhere near the 50th centile for the population. If a child is to maintain his or her position on, say, the 10th centile for height, he or she should grow somewhere near the 40th centile for velocity. Similarly, a child who is maintaining height on the 90th centile will have to grow at a slightly above average velocity but only at about the 60th centile. The child persistently growing at a 10th centile velocity will steadily fall further and further behind his or her peer group and soon become distinctly short.

In Fig. 61.5 there are two large grey areas flanking the adolescent growth spurt. The centiles for the latter are those for a child whose growth spurt peaks at an average age, i.e. 14 years for a boy; however, there is considerable natural variation in this age. This is approximately ± 2 years about the mean and the grey shaded areas take this into account. In an individual case the growth spurt should occur within the grey area with a shape similar to the centile centred at 14 years. Note that, particularly in boys, earlier growth spurts tend to be more intense and later growth spurts less so. The same effect is seen in girls but to a less marked extent.

Puberty

The events of puberty

There are many skeletal and soft-tissue events that occur during puberty that are important in the development in differences in shape between the adult male and female. Proper description of these events requires a standardised method of measuring progress through puberty, and almost universally the systems in current use depend on the criteria formalised by Tanner [1]. These depend upon rating breast and pubic hair development on a five-point scale and axillary hair on a three-point scale for girls and external genitalia, pubic and axillary hair on similar scales for boys. Details of the stages are available in many standard texts [1] and will not be repeated here.

In much the same way as we discussed variation in height for age, we should also consider variation in the age of attainment of different pubertal stages; standards for achievement of puberty stages are usually included on the stature standards illustrated in Fig. 61.3. It is important to note the way in which these standards are constructed. The designation PH2, PH3, etc. represent the instant when these appearances first become visible. This is almost never observable; the doctor can only see that a child has attained PH2 but not yet PH3. We therefore describe the subject as being in PH2+ and the standards give the centiles for age of *being in* that stage. Arbitrarily the centiles are ordered such that lower ones relate to delayed pubertal progress and higher centiles to advanced progress. Thus, a boy in PH2+ and aged 13.0 years is just above the 25th centile and a little older than average for that stage, albeit quite normal. In contrast, a similar boy aged 15.0 years would be below the 0.4th centile and suspiciously delayed.

Tempo and the consonance of puberty

In general, the events of puberty, including skeletal, soft-tissue and secondary sexual characteristics, unfold in an orderly and highly integrated manner. The whole process may be advanced or delayed by up to several years, but still maintains an internal order that closely follows that of the average child [8]. Whenever this consonance is disturbed, for example with an absent growth spurt but normal pubertal progression, then pathology must be suspected. In an otherwise healthy child this will usually be an endocrinopathy.

Principles of auxological anthropometry

In the practice of clinical endocrinology the most important auxological measurements are height (or supine length in those who cannot stand), sitting height (or crown–rump length), weight and skinfolds (especially triceps and subscapular). Note that sitting height is a preferable measurement by which to assess trunk–limb proportions as opposed to the use of measurement of span or upper and lower segments. The first of these is vulnerable to positional problems as the measurement is much affected by rotation of the shoulder girdle, and the second depends upon accurate placement of the pubic symphysis which can be difficult, especially in the obese.

The basic rules for making auxological measurements should be the same as for any other endocrine parameters such as hormone measurements. There must be adequately trained technicians using properly designed equipment in a reserved area such that the measurements may be made in a conducive environment. Quality assurance is every bit as important, although this usually takes the form of repeat measurements on a series of children at appropriate intervals; the statistical analysis of assessments of reliability are discussed below. Details of measurement techniques are comprehensively described by Cameron [9].

Reliability

Good anthropometrists have standard errors of measurement (s_{meas}) ranging from 1.5 to 2.5 mm. This means that a technician with a s_{meas} of 2.0 mm (determined, say, over subjects of an age range 3.0–18.0 years) obtains a value for height which 95% of the time is within 4 mm above and 4 mm below the true value. s_{meas} can be determined by taking a series of duplicate measurements and calculating the difference *d* for each of the subjects. Provided there is no consistent change from first to second occasion (and there should not be), the $s_{meas} = s_d/\sqrt{2}$ where s_d is the standard deviation of *d*.

When we consider the precision of velocity measurements the problems are much greater. The errors of each of the component measurements are as above, but the absolute change between them may be quite small and the total error assumes a far greater proportion of the measurement of interest.

Bone age and other assessments of maturity

There are three current methods employed for assessing skeletal age although there have been earlier methods often contributing to the evolution of newer techniques. The older method still in use is of the atlas type first described in 1950 by Greulich and Pyle and subsequently revised [10]. In this method, a sequence of hand–wrist radiographs typical of children of specific chronological ages are displayed. While the authors intended the user to compare carefully each bone of the patient's X-ray with the appropriate standard and then derive a median skeletal age, the tendency is to simply find the example that most closely resembles the patient's and call that the skeletal 'age'. This is a very unsatisfactory method as the observer easily becomes focused on a few bones, especially the radius, ulna and carpal bones, leading to a biased assessment. A further problem is that the Greulich and Pyle method was based mainly on radiographs of socially advantaged children. They thus had relatively advanced skeletal maturation compared with other American children and even more so compared with European children. At present the secular trend for earlier maturation has essentially removed the social bias with respect to present-day Americans but Europeans are still, on average, 9 months delayed. Thus, an average maturing European child, assessed by the Greulich and Pyle method, will appear to have a skeletal age delay of 9 months.

Preferred methods use bone-specific scoring systems for the hand–wrist or knee. In these methods each bone is assessed according to a number of specific maturity indicators to which a score is attached. Only after scoring each indicator is it possible to derive a total maturity score which may then be translated into a skeletal 'age' by comparison with appropriate standards. Thus, it is impossible to use a short-cut as in the atlas method. The methods can be used for any population although it is wise to develop specific standards for each country by first applying the methods to X-rays of normal children of the appropriate background.

There are two bone-specific scoring methods currently used: that of Tanner *et al.* (TW2) [11], which uses the bones of the left hand and wrist, and that of Roche *et al.* [12] which uses the knee. The former is the most extensively used and also forms the basis of a mature height prediction system. The merits and demerits of these systems have been reviewed by Preece [13].

The endocrine and paracrine control of growth

Growth is controlled and modulated by many factors including hormonal mechanisms, nutrition and the environment. Sometimes the latter influences are mediated by endocrine changes, but there may also be direct effects. Many hormones influence growth including those secreted by the thyroid and the gonads, but growth hormone and its related peptides are probably the most important and these will now be described in more detail.

Growth hormone and its binding proteins

Growth hormone (GH) in its most abundant form is a peptide of 191 amino-acid residues, molecular weight 22 000 Da. There is also a shorter variant with molecular weight of 20 000 Da due to post-translational modification, but whose metabolic significance is still unclear [14]. Both GHs are synthesised and secreted by the somatotroph cells of the anterior pituitary gland. It is released in a pulsatile manner, under the influence of two opposing hypothalamic regulatory peptides, namely GH-releasing hormone (GHRH) and GH release-inhibiting hormone (or somatostatin GHRIH) which are subject to modulation by many neuronal pathways from higher centres (see also Chapter 6). These respond to a multitude of triggers of GH release such as exercise, physical and emotional stress, and high protein or carbohydrate intake to modify the underlying spontaneous rhythm of GH secretion which is linked to the sleep–wake cycle; approximately two-thirds of GH secretion occurs during the 12-hour period overnight.

Some of these cues are related more to the short-term direct actions that GH may have on intermediary metabolism, regulating avialability of glucose, fatty acids and amino-acid uptake, than to the longer-term and largely indirect effects that GH exerts on skeletal and soft-tissue growth via the insulin-like growth factors (IGFs) (see below). Pulses of GH are released with a periodicity of approximately 3–4 hours. Between pulses serum GH concentration falls, with a half-life of approximately 10–20 min, becoming undetectable by most current assay methods. The significance of this pulsatility in relation to the mechanism of GH action has long been unclear, but there is growing evidence that it may afford another level at which the actions of GH on growing tissues may be controlled.

Modulation of GH secretion is achieved physiologically by variation in the amplitude rather than the frequency of pulses, although in some pathological states there may be elevation of interpulse GH levels as an adaptive pathophysiological response, such as in diabetes mellitus, malnutrition, sepsis and catabolism [15], or intrinsic to the disease process as in acromegaly. Pulse amplitude appears to be the dominant parameter of GH secretion which can be identified as the regulator of growth rate [16].

In serum, GH is associated with specific binding proteins (GHBP) [17] in quantities approximately equimolar with interpulse levels of GH accounting for about 30% of serum GH at these levels. There are at least two GHBPs: the first is a high-affinity, low-capacity protein [18]; the second is of relatively low affinity but higher capacity [19]. The high-affinity protein is homologous with the extracellular domain of the membrane-bound GH receptor and may be derived by proteolytic cleavage during cellular processing of the receptor. Levels of the binding protein might therefore reflect expression of the GH receptor and the biological activity of GH. There is a striking age-related increase in serum GHBP levels, being very low in the neonatal period and rising through childhood.

There are a number of GH-resistance states, such as uraemia or cirrhosis, in which there may be abnormalities of the GH receptor but their impact on GHBP levels is as yet unclear [20]. There is, however, a clinical syndrome where GHBP as a mirror of GH-receptor dysfunction has a clearly defined role. 'GH-receptor deficiency', or the Laron syndrome, encompasses nearly 20 mutations in the GH-receptor gene which lead to a well-described syndrome [21], which in clinical terms mimics severe GH deficiency. The abnormality, however, resides in either the loss of GH binding by the receptor [22] or the failure to subsequently initiate the intracellular signals that are required to bring about the actions of GH actions [23]. In the former situation circulating GHBP activity is also reduced in functional assays, although in the rarer cases with normal receptor binding, GHBP activity is normal.

IGFs and their binding proteins

In 1957 Salmon and Daughaday proposed that the growth-promoting effects of GH on skeletal tissue were not direct but mediated through a secondary, GH-dependent plasma or serum factor then designated 'sulphation factor' [24]. Sulphation refers to the initial phase of proteoglycan synthesis where sulphate radicals are covalently linked to the chondroitin units: it is a marker of proteoglycan synthesis. This operational name was later changed to 'somatomedin' to denote its role as mediator of the effects of GH (somatotrophin) in promoting growth and anabolic responses in skeletal and non-skeletal tissues. Yet more recently the term insulin-like growth factors has been substituted as it more accurately reflects the function of what is clearly a group of GH-dependent peptides, of which the two major contributors to biological activity present in human serum are IGF-1 and IGF-2. IGF-1 is a basic polypeptide containing 70 amino acids, molecular weight 7469 Da; IGF-2 is slightly acidic, shares about 70% sequence homology with IGF-1, and has 67 amino acids. Both peptides share about 50% homology with human proinsulin (reviewed in [35]).

IGF-1 is more highly GH dependent than IGF-2, with IGF-1 levels rising and falling slowly after treatment of normal or GH-deficient individuals with GH, although the immunoreactive serum levels of both peptides show no significant fluctuation over 24 hours in the normal unstimulated state. This near constancy of serum IGF levels on a day-to-day basis contrasts with the pulsatility of GH and is partly accounted for by their association with specific carrier proteins which bind newly generated IGF and leave less than 1% of circulating IGF in the free form. Serum concentrations of IGF-1 in normal adults are in the range of 100–300 ng/ml, compared with concentrations of 1–20 ng/ml at which it will promote DNA synthesis and cell replication *in vivo*. Serum IGF-2 levels are two- to threefold higher than IGF-1.

There are currently six IGF-binding proteins known as IGFBP-1 to IGFBP-6. They have molecular weights in the range 23 000–31 000 Da (excluding glycosylation) and show a high degree of conservation of primary structure [26]. Each of the binding proteins has been found in the extracellular environment and in humans, apart from IGFBP-5, but the physiological role of all of them is far from understood. In the human, IGFBP-1 and -3 have been the most extensively studied.

IGFBP-3 has the greatest influence on circulating concentrations of the IGFs as it has the greatest binding capacity and longest half-life in serum. It is unique in that after the IGFs bind to gycosylated IGFBP-3 a trimeric complex is formed with a second glycoprotein, an acid-labile subunit. Both IGFBP-3 and the acid-labile subunit are dependent on GH. This intact trimer has a half-life of about 4 hours [27] compared with IGFBP-1 and -2 which have half-lives of only a few minutes. It binds more than 75% of serum IGF, and serum levels show no significant variation over 24 hours.

IGFBP-1 differs from other IGFBPs in that it follows a marked diurnal variation which appears largely due to metabolic changes. Concentrations rise dramatically during the night or during a prolonged daytime fast and fall rapidly following a meal, and are inversely related to circulating insulin concentrations [28].

The somatomedin hypothesis proposed that circulating somatomedin/IGF levels were the mediators of GH growth-promoting actions, at sites distant from the production site of IGF (probably the liver), according to classical endocrine concepts. Realisation that IGFs were synthesised *in vitro* by a number of tissues and could be shown in hypophysectomised rats to increase in concentration in tissues in response to GH treatment *before* the maximal rise in serum IGF-1 led to consideration of the role of the IGFs more as autocrine or paracrine growth factors rather than as classical hormones. Furthermore, no single organ or tissue has been shown to store IGFs in a releasable pool. Recent studies on tissue expression of IGF messenger RNA (mRNA) have shown that although the liver shows the highest level of IGF mRNA expression in most species studied, its presence can be demonstrated in almost every tissue, including the growth plate, although in some non-hepatic tissues expression may not be GH dependent [29]. Thus, the circulating levels of IGF-1 may contribute little to growth regulation of some tissues. The function of the relatively high circulating levels of the IGFs remains somewhat of a puzzle but may reflect the need for the IGFBPs to regulate IGF activity, both quantitatively and qualitatively. In contrast to the binding proteins for thyroid hormones, sex hormones and cortisol, there is *in vitro* evidence that the IGFBPs can potentiate or inhibit IGF action, probably by modification of membrane access and receptor activation [30].

The actions of growth factors at the growth plate

A paracrine mode of action for the IGFs was strongly suggested by the observation that direct injection of high doses of GH into the proximal tibial growth plate stimulated growth. This was followed by confirmation that infusion of GH into either the arterial supply to one hind limb or the

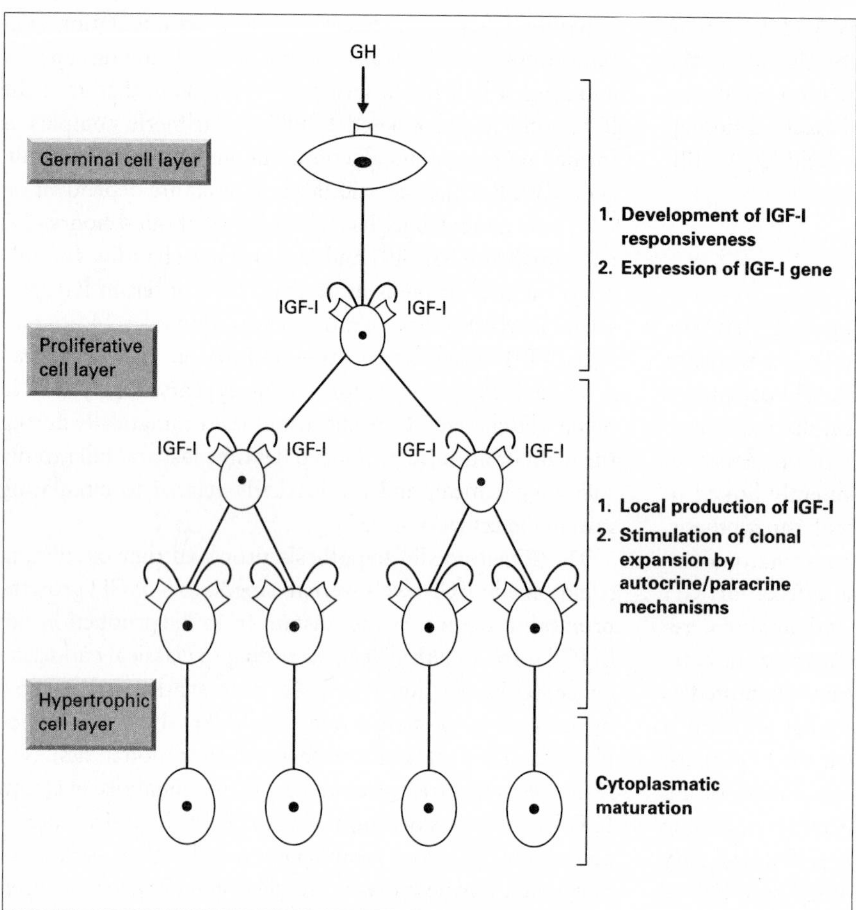

Fig. 61.6 Schematic representation of the 'dual effector' theory of the mechanism of action of growth hormone (GH) and insulin-like growth factor 1 (IGF-1) at the growth plate.

proximal tibial growth plate of hypophysectomised rats resulted in a dose-dependent, unilateral increase in width of the growth plate on the infused side. This occurred with doses of GH (1 μg/day) below that necessary to raise systemic IGF-1 levels, although when 10 μg GH/day was infused, bilateral tibial growth was stimulated. However, when rabbit antiserum to IGF-1 was co-infused into the growth plate the local effect was completely abolished, thus favouring the need for IGF-1 as mediator of the GH stimulus. However, infusion of recombinant human IGF-1 (5 μg/day) gave a smaller growth response than occurred with a lower dose of GH [31].

The response of cells to IGF-1 is mediated by specific IGF receptors which are of two types: the type 1 receptor has a structure that is very similar to, but distinct from, the insulin receptor and greatest affinity for IGF-1, while the type 2 receptor has a quite different structure with greatest affinity for IGF-2 [25]. These receptors are widely spread through many tissues, supporting the view that the IGFs have a role to play in growth and possibly function of a large number of different tissues.

In vitro studies of chondrocyte growth have better defined the respective actions of GH and IGF-1 on the subpopulations of cells within the growth plate. When epiphysial chondrocytes are cultured in stabilising medium such as agarose they yield colonies; these differ in size according to the zone of origin of the cells. Cells from the proximal portion of the growth plate have increased capacity to form colonies, which in turn are larger than those derived from the intermediate portion. When exposed to GH or IGF-1 further differences appear. GH at 10–80 ng/ml enhances colony formation from the proximal growth plate cells, with decreasing effect as the GH concentration increases. In contrast, GH has no apparent effect on colony formation from cells of the intermediate zone. IGF-1, on the other hand, stimulates a dose-dependent increase in colony formation from these cells and those from the proximal zone, with maximal effect at 100 ng/ml. Thus, whereas GH stimulates colony formation only from the most immature cells, IGF-1 enhances the proliferation to colonies of cells from both the proximal and intermediate growth plate zones. GH stimulates growth of the largest colonies and IGF-1 consistently promotes small colony formation [32].

These findings, when considered with the observations

earlier on the distribution of GH and IGF receptors within the growth plate, have led to the concept that GH acts directly on the progenitor, prechondrocyte cells of the reserve cell layer adjacent to the bony epiphysis, independent of IGF-1, to provoke development of proliferative chondrocytes. IGF-1 is then produced in the proliferative cells under the stimulatory influence of GH and acts on the more mature cells of the proliferative and hypertrophic zones (Fig. 61.6).

The mechanism of action of GH on chondrocyte proliferation and differentiation leading to longitudinal bone growth has been compared with the 'dual effector' theory [33]. Based on the concept that tissue growth occurs in two stages (differentiated cells are first formed from precursors, then young differentiated cells increase in number by limited multiplication or 'clonal expansion'), it is suggested that both these stages are promoted by GH but the first is a direct action of the hormone and the second an indirect one through a second effector, in this case IGF-1. The differentiation–clonal expansion theory now proposes that GH directly stimulates differentiation of prechondrocytes or young differentiating cells, which acquire the ability to respond to IGF-1 and express the gene for IGF-1 synthesis. IGF-1 is produced in the differentiating cells, which can be enhanced by GH, and the IGF-1 is released to interact with receptors on proliferating cells through autocrine or paracrine mechanisms. This model may well prove to be generally applicable to the growth-promoting effects of GH in skeletal and non-skeletal tissues.

References

1 Tanner JM. *Growth at Adolescence*. Oxford: Blackwell Scientific Publications, 1962.
2 Freeman JV, Cole TJ, Chinn S, Jones PRM, White EM, Preece MA. Cross-sectional stature and weight reference curves for the UK, 1990. *Arch Dis Child* 1995; **73**: 17–24.
3 Preece MA. Standardization of growth. *Acta Paediatr Scand* 1989; **349** (Suppl.): 57–64.
4 Tanner JM, Whitehouse RH, Takaishi M. Standards from birth to maturity for height, weight, height velocity, and weight velocity: British children, 1965—I. *Arch Dis Child* 1966; **41**: 454–471.
5 Tanner JM, Whitehouse RH, Takaishi M. Standards from birth to maturity for height, weight, height velocity, and weight velocity: British children, 1965—II. *Arch Dis Child* 1966; **41**: 613–35.
6 Chinn S, Rona RJ, Price CE. The secular trend in height of primary school children in England and Scotland 1972–79 and 1979–86. *Ann Human Biol* 1989; **16**: 387–95.
7 Cole TJ. Do growth chart centiles need a face lift? *Br Med J* 1994; **308**: 641–2.
8 Stanhope R, Preece MA. Management of constitutional delay of growth and puberty. *Arch Dis Child* 1988; **63**: 1104–10.
9 Cameron N. *The Measurement of Human Growth*. London: Croom Helm, 1984.
10 Greulich WW, Pyle SI. *Radiographic Atlas of Skeletal Development of the Hand and Wrist*. Stanford: Stanford University Press, 1959.
11 Tanner JM, Whitehouse RH, Cameron N, Marshall WA, Healy MJR, Goldstein H. *Assessment of Skeletal Maturity and Prediction of Adult Height (TW2 Method)*. London: Academic Press, 1983.
12 Roche AF, Wainer H, Thissen D. *Skeletal Maturity. The Knee Joint as a Biological Indicator*. New York: Plenum, 1975.
13 Preece MA. Prediction of adult height: methods and problems. *Acta Paediatr Scand* 1988; **347** (Suppl.): 4–10.
14 Lewis UJ, Singh RNP, Tutwiler GF. Hyperglycemic activity of the 20 000-dalton variant of human growth hormone. *Endocr Res Commun* 1981; **8**: 155–64.
15 Ross RJM, Buchanan CR. Growth hormone secretion: Modulation by nutritional factors. *Nutr Res Rev* 1990; **3**: 143–62.
16 Hindmarsh PC, Smith PJ, Brook CGD, Matthews DR. The relationship between height velocity and 24 hour growth hormone secretion in children. *Clin Endocrinol* 1987; **27**: 581–91.
17 Herington AC, Ymer S, Stevenson J. Identification and characterization of specific binding proteins for growth hormone in normal human sera. *J Clin Invest* 1986; **77**: 1817–23.
18 Baumann G. Growth hormone heterogeneity: Genes, isohormones, variants, and binding proteins. *Endocr Rev* 1991; **12**: 424–49.
19 Baumann G, Shaw MA. A 2nd, lower affinity growth hormone-binding protein in human plasma. *J Clin Endocrinol Metab* 1990; **70**: 680–6.
20 Baumann G, Shaw MA, Amburn K. Regulation of plasma growth hormone-binding proteins in health and disease. *Metabolism* 1989; **38**: 683–9.
21 Savage MO, Blum WF, Ranke MB *et al.* Clinical features and endocrine status in patients with growth hormone insensitivity (Laron syndrome). *J Clin Endocrinol Metab* 1993; **77**: 1465–71.
22 Amselem S, Duquesnoy P, Attree O *et al.* Laron dwarfism and mutations of the growth hormone-receptor gene. *N Engl J Med* 1989; **321**: 989–95.
23 Duquesnoy P, Sobrier ML, Duriez B *et al.* A single amino-acid substitution in the exoplasmic domain of the human growth hormone (GH) receptor confers familial GH resistance (Laron syndrome) with positive GH-binding activity by abolishing receptor homodimerization. *EMBO J* 1994; **13**: 1386–95.
24 Salmon WD, Daughaday WH. A hormonally controlled serum factor which stimulates sulfate incorporation by cartilage *in vitro*. *J Lab Clin Med* 1957; **49**: 825–36.
25 Preece MA. The insulin-like growth factors. In: Styne DM, ed. *Current Concepts in Pediatric Endocrinology*. New York: Elsevier, 1987: 155–83.
26 Baxter RC. Insulin-like growth factor binding proteins: biochemical characterization. In: Muller E, Cocchi D, Locatelli V, eds., *Growth Hormone and Somatomedins during Lifespan*. Berlin: Springer, 1993: 100–8.
27 Zapf J, Hauri C, Waldvogel M, Froesch ER. Acute metabolic effects and half-lives of intravenously administered insulin-like growth factors I and II in normal and hypophysectomised rats. *J Clin Invest* 1986; **77**: 1768–75.
28 Yeoh SI, Baxter RC. Metabolic regulation of the growth hormone independent insulin-like growth factor binding protein in human plasma. *Acta Endocrinol* 1988; **119**: 465–73.
29 Daughaday WH, Rotwein P. Insulin-like growth factors I and II. Peptide, messenger ribonucleic acid and gene structures, serum, and tissue concentrations. *Endocr Rev* 1989; **10**: 68–91.
30 Taylor AM, Dunger DB, Preece MA *et al.* The growth hormone

independent insulin like growth factor-I binding protein BP-28 is associated with serum insulin like growth factor-I inhibitory bioactivity in adolescent insulin-dependent diabetics. *Clin Endocrinol* 1990; **32**: 229–39.

31 Isgaard J, Nilsson A, Lindahl A, Jansson JO, Isaksson OGP. Effects of local administration of GH and IGF-I on longitudinal bone growth in rats. *Am J Physiol* 1986; **250**: E367–72.

32 Lindahl A, Nilsson A, Isaksson OGP. Effects of growth hormone and insulin-like growth factor-I on colony formation of rabbit epiphyseal chondrocytes at different stages of maturation. *J Endocrinol* 1987; **115**: 263–71.

33 Green H, Morikawa M, Nixon T. A dual effector theory of growth hormone action. *Differentiation* 1985; **29**: 195–8.

34 Tanner JM, Whitehouse RH. Clinical longitudinal standards for height, weight, height velocity, weight velocity and the stages of puberty. *Arch Dis Child* 1976; **51**: 170–9.

35 Jones JI, Clemmons DR. Insulin-like growth factors and their binding proteins: biological actions. *Endocr Rev* 1995; **16**: 3–34.

CHAPTER 62

Disorders of stature

A.F. Massoud, P.C. Hindmarsh and C.G.D. Brook

Introduction

The growth process is complicated, but its measurement forms the basis of the science which separates paediatrics from general medicine. Failure of physical growth is an important sign of systemic disease but it is also the hallmark of endocrine disease since pituitary, thyroid, adrenal and gonadal hormones are all involved in this process. At the other extreme, tallness in children usually presents less initial concern than shortness because being tall is socially advantageous, at least in early childhood. However, the diagnoses with which tall stature may be associated are in some ways more sinister than those causing short stature.

The extremes of stature may not only signal a disease process, but may also be a source of disability and a cause of distress in themselves, though this is largely a problem perceived by the adult carers of short children rather than the children themselves, with the exception of adolescents [1]; younger children suffer poor social or emotional adjustment as a result of their short stature [2]. This chapter discusses the endocrine causes of short and tall stature. In a text dedicated to endocrinology it is especially important to be clear that the categorisation of an individual child depends upon growth assessment and clinical examination. It does not depend, at least not in the first instance, on laboratory investigations, which should not be employed until and unless auxological data indicate them to be necessary.

The hormonal regulators of growth vary with the age of the individual. Fetal and, to a certain extent, early post-natal growth, which require cell hyperplasia and coordinated development, would be expected to have different hormonal requirements to post-natal growth, which is mainly the result of cell hypertrophy. Growth hormone (GH), thyroxine and insulin are well suited to the latter. Indeed, 65% of the growth of children aged between 4 and 12 years can be explained in terms of GH secretion [3].

Short stature

Definition

The definition of shortness is arbitrary. The general rule is that any child whose height falls below the 3rd centile for his or her community should be considered short, but this immediately raises problems over the definition of the term and the most appropriate standards for use for assessment of height. First, it is important to realise that the height standards are only a statistical description of the general population. Three per cent of children will have heights below the 3rd centile regardless whether or not there is anything wrong with them. In some countries other centiles are used for defining short stature, the 5th often in the USA. Different ethnic groups have different growth standards, for example the mean final height of the Japanese male is 6 cm less than the mean final height for the World Health Organization reference range based on growth standards developed in the USA in the 1970s. Secular trends in heights are well documented and are more marked in certain groups, for example the Japanese, and up-to-date growth charts need to be used to account for such changes. The new UK cross-sectional growth charts, in addition to providing more recent data on growth standards, follow nine equidistant centile format, allowing better growth surveillance and referral guidelines to be constructed (Table 62.1). Children should be measured at birth, 18 months, 3 years and 5 years, with possible inclusion of two further measurements at 7 and 9 years of age.

As growth is a dynamic process, merely defining abnormality on the basis of stature alone conveys little information as to the normality of the individual's growth rate. Although it is true that the further a child is away from the 50th centile the more likely that there is something wrong with them, it is not actual height which is remediable; rather, it is growth

Table 62.1 Guidelines for growth surveillance and referral.

1 Children whose heights are below the 0.4 and above the 99.6 centile

2 Any child whose height falls outside the parental target height.

3 Children under the age of 5 whose two height measurements, taken 18–24 months apart, cross two growth centiles. If only one centile is crossed, a further measurement should be taken at an interval of 18–24 months, and if during that time a further centile in height has been crossed then referral should take place

4 For children aged 5 years and over the criteria should be that over a period of 1 year, if the height crosses one centile then referral should take place. If the height crosses only half a centile then the child should be reviewed at the end of a further year and if at that time the height has crossed a further half centile the referral should take place

rate. Twenty per cent of children with a height less than the 3rd centile at the age of 5 years will have an organic reason to explain their stature. These children probably became short by growing slowly. A more appropriate assessment would be to consider the first differential of height and time, namely height velocity. This has the advantage of circumventing the secular and racial trends in height, and it simplifies the decision making of the clinician in that all that has to be decided is whether the growth rate is normal or abnormal. Needless to say, measurement techniques need to be accurate and precise in order to assess height velocity with any reliability. Even when this is accounted for, caution needs to be exercised when attempting measurements over a short period of time. Quite apart from changes in growth rates (seasonal growth) [4], errors of, say, 1 mm on measurements of height at either end of a 3-month period amount to an error of at least 1.6 cm/year if the 3-monthly velocity is corrected to an annual rate.

Using height velocity, small children can be classified into three groups: those who are small and normal, those who are small as a result of an early event or congenital anomaly which cannot be corrected, and those with short stature due to remediable conditions. A flow chart for the differential diagnosis of short stature is shown in Fig. 62.1.

Short normal children

This group of children contains at least two subgroups. The

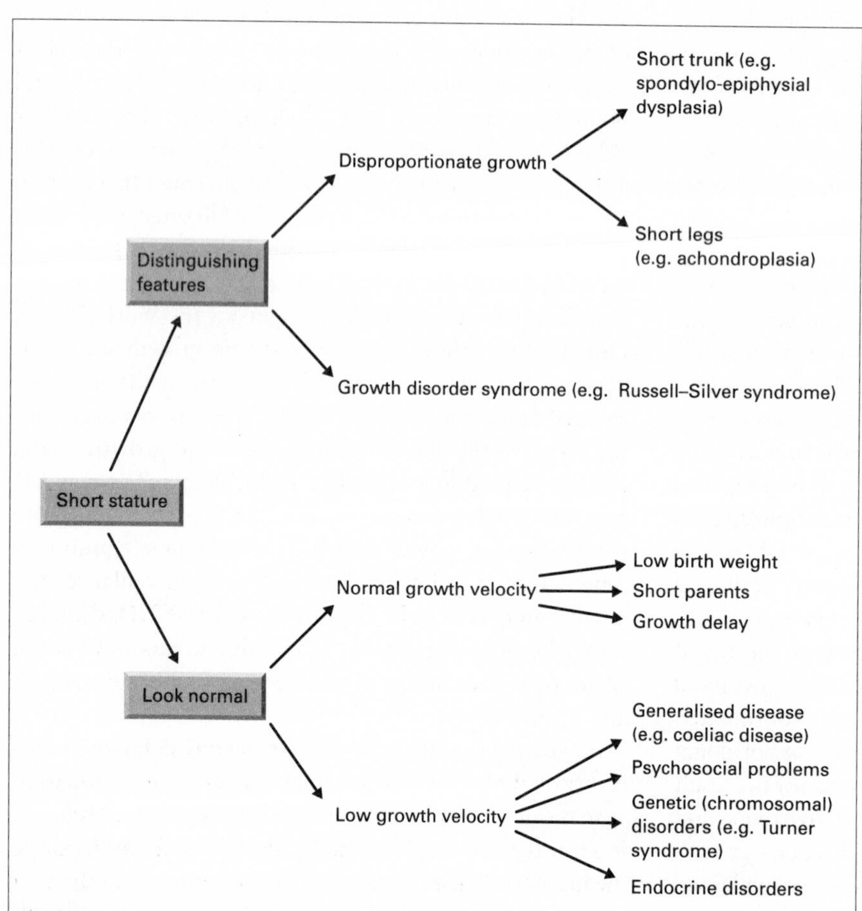

Fig. 62.1 Flow chart for use in the differential diagnosis of short stature. From [166].

first group of children are characterised by a height close to the 3rd height centile and a normal growth velocity. The height of one or both of the parents is likely to be close to the 3rd centile. The second group, which may include some children from the first, consists of children whose stature may be anywhere between the 3rd and 25th centiles and whose growth rate is normal during the childhood years, but who lose ground because of the late onset of puberty and a delayed pubertal growth spurt. Skeletal maturation becomes delayed in the children towards the end of the first decade of life and a final height appropriate for the parents is likely to ensure.

Short stature due to an earlier event

In most cases children with a syndrome who are short have been of low birth weight. The problem is not just confined to intrauterine growth retardation. Poor nutritional support of prenatal infants will produce similar effects. It is important to remember that growth in the first 6 months of life is independent of growth hormone and is largely dependent on nutrition, so poor nutritional intake during this period of rapid growth can have profound and long-lasting effects. Once GH-dependent growth becomes established, normal growth follows, but stature lost at this stage is not easily recovered.

Two syndromes deserve mention. First is the association of low birth weight and its resultant short stature with dysmorphic characteristics, the Russell–Silver syndrome [5,6]. The clinical features are a triangular-shaped facies, body asymmetry, thinness and clinodactyly of the fifth fingers (Plate 62.1, opposite p. 332). However, the most characteristic feature is the formidable difficulty encountered by the parents in feeding such children in infancy. Post-natal growth beyond 12 months of age is characteristically normal in these children. Most cases are sporadic, but familial cases have been described. Autosomal dominant and X-linked dominant forms of inheritance are most favoured [7,8]. Evidence from mice that uniparental disomy is associated with intrauterine growth retardation [9] raises the possibility that the Russell–Silver syndrome is also inherited in this form [10], and has recently been shown by Kotzot *et al.* to occur in some families with this condition [11].

The second syndrome of note is that of Turner [12] which results from abnormalities—absence, mosaicism, rings or isochromosomes—of the X chromosome. Mosaicism is common, but the effect of Turner's syndrome on growth is to add persistent low growth velocity to a prenatal growth deficit. Growth over the first 3 years of life tends to be relatively normal in terms of growth velocity, but thereafter a declining growth rate can be discerned with no obvious pubertal growth spurt [13]. The condition is common (one in 3000 female births) and there may not necessarily be the well-known dysmorphic features. Short stature is common, but the major implication of the diagnosis relates to pubertal development and reproductive capacity.

Short stature with a remediable condition

These children may or may not be short, but more importantly their growth velocity is slow. This group includes a wide spectrum of disease. An explanation for the poor growth rate needs to be found and appropriate treatment recommended. A careful history and examination may point to a remediable cause. Full investigation encompassing the renal, gastrointestinal, cardiac, respiratory, haematological and neurological systems is often required. Finally, careful attention needs to be paid to the social and family history. Psychological deprivation can take forms ranging from emotional deprivation to anorexia-by-proxy as well as the extremes of physical and sexual abuse.

Classification of growth hormone secretory disorders

The characteristic clinical picture of severe GH insufficiency is of a very short, rather plump, child with a round immature face (Fig. 62.2). Birth weight is usually normal, and poor growth is apparent from about 6 months of age. The insufficiency may be isolated or associated with other pituitary hormone deficiencies. Small genitalia are especially characteristic of associated gonadotrophin deficiency. Hypoglycaemia in the newborn period is often a feature of adrenocorticotrophic hormone (ACTH) deficiency. Prolonged neonatal jaundice, particularly a conjugated hyperbilirubinaemia, raises the question of thyroxine or cortisol deficiency.

The definition of GH insufficiency has relied heavily on the use of pharmacological tests of GH secretion. The accepted criteria in the UK were to label a child as 'severely insufficient' if the peak GH response to pharmacological stimuli was <7 mU/l and 'partially insufficient' if the values lay between 7 and 15 mU/l [14]. These values were based largely on the GH responses to pharmacological stimuli in adults. These cut-off values present many problems of interpretation: for example, a peak GH response of 25 mU/l in a 5-year-old child may be acceptable as a normal GH response, but such a value in a child at the height of the pubertal growth spurt is probably inadequate [15]. Using strict cut-off values may seem inappropriate in view of the evidence that the peak serum GH concentration response to pharmacological stimuli is continuous in a large group of short children with varying growth rates, and that clearly demarcated subpopulations do not exist [16]. The wide range of methods now available for measuring serum

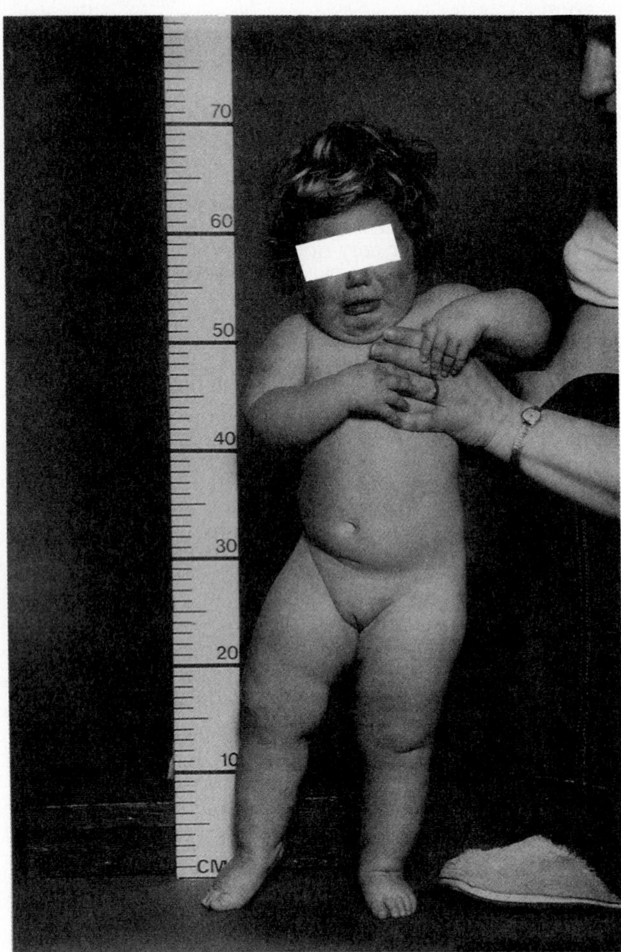

(a)

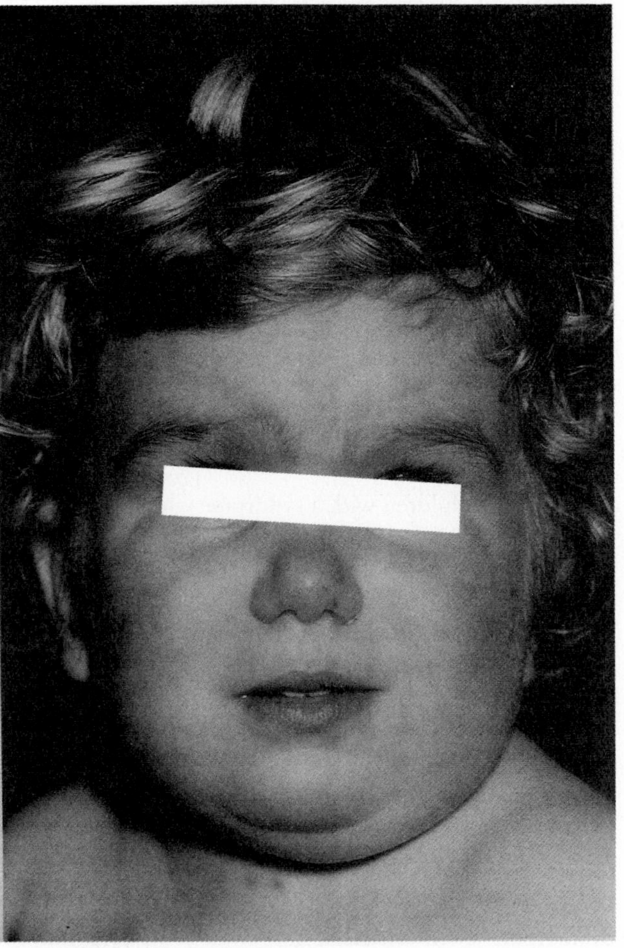

(b)

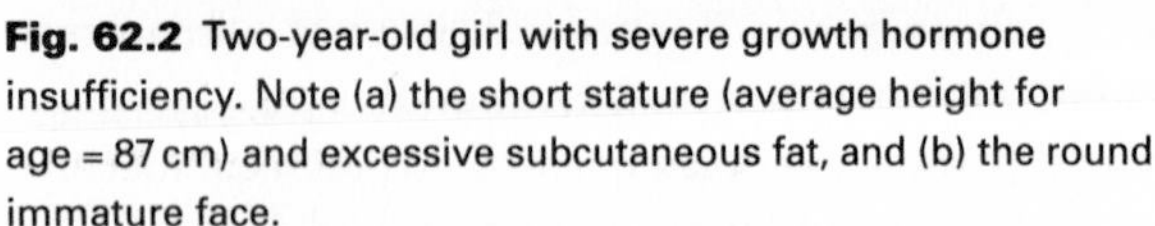

Fig. 62.2 Two-year-old girl with severe growth hormone insufficiency. Note (a) the short stature (average height for age = 87 cm) and excessive subcutaneous fat, and (b) the round immature face.

GH concentrations (radioimmunoassay, immunoradiometric assay and enzyme-linked systems) makes comparison between laboratories difficult and the use of universal cut-off values impossible [17].

As GH secretion is the final common pathway for growth promotion it is better to think of GH insufficiency/deficiency in terms of the physiology of hypothalamo-pituitary/target gland cascade rather than strict anatomical abnormalities. A schematic representation of the cascade is shown in Fig. 62.3.

Pituitary gland

The term 'GH deficiency' should be applied only to children with deletion of the GH gene. Onset of GH deficiency in children with gene deletion is extremely early, and poor growth can be detected as early as the sixth month of postnatal life. The human GH gene is located on chromosome 17 in a cluster of five genes, one coding for pituitary GH, one coding for placental GH and the remaining three coding for human chorionic somatomammotrophin. Two common mutations of the pituitary GH gene resulting from large deletions of 6.7 or 7.6 kb have been described [18]. The genetic causes of GH deficiency, in isolation or in association with multiple pituitary hormone deficiency, have been described, and are summarised in Table 62.2.

Pituitary aplasia is commonly associated with multiple pituitary hormone deficiency. Growth failure occurs early, although the effects of hypoglycaemia, hypothyroidism and the consequent persistent conjugated hyperbilirubinaemia brings the disorder to the attention of the clinician at an earlier stage. Failure of the migration of the anterior pituitary, derived embryologically from Rathke's pouch, leads to characteristic high-resolution computed tomography (CT) scan or magnetic resonance image (MRI) appearances in children with this disorder (Fig. 62.4). The pituitary fossa is very small and the neurohypophysis does not descend [19], remaining at the base of the infundibulum. This may be evident on CT and MRI as a small enhancing nodule.

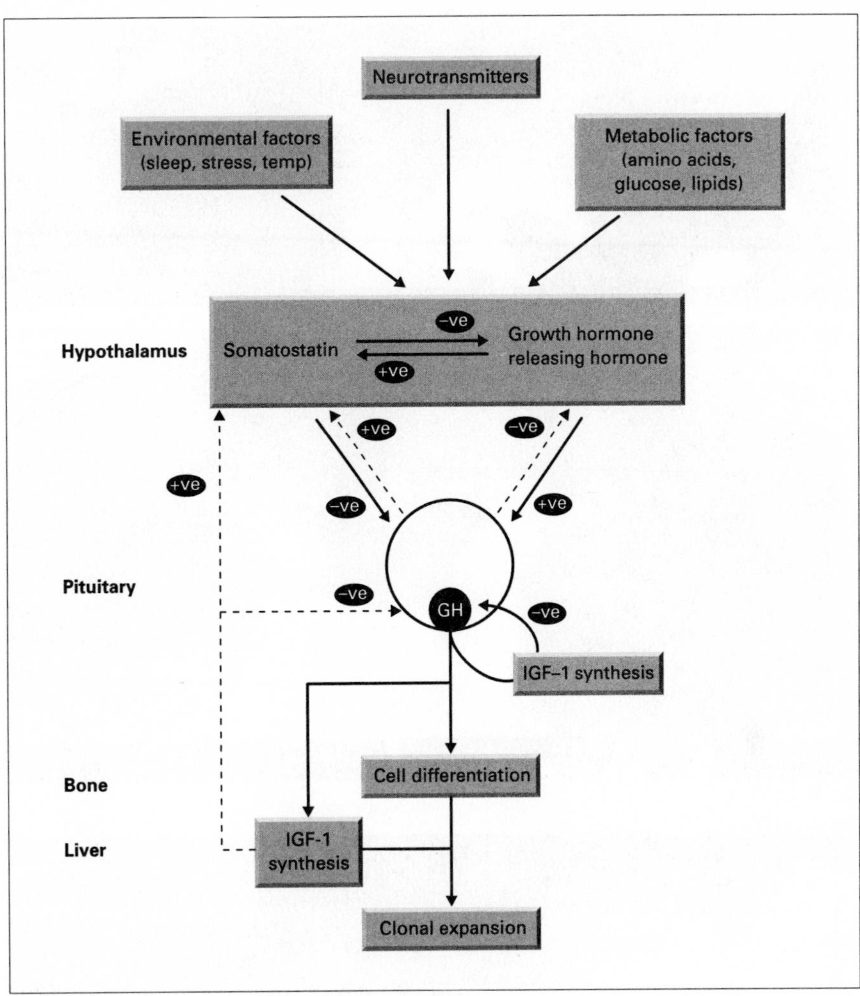

Fig. 62.3 Schematic representation of the hypothalamo-pituitary–growth hormone axis.

Table 62.2 Disorders of growth hormone (GH) synthesis.

	Type	Inheritance	GH
Primary defect: growth hormone	IA	Autosomal recessive	Absent
	IB	Autosomal recessive	Reduced
	II	Autosomal dominant	Reduced
	III	X-linked	Reduced
Multiple pituitary hormones	I (*Pit*-1 gene deletion)	Autosomal recessive	Reduced
	II	X-linked	Reduced

Hypoplastic pituitary glands are often seen on both CT scans and MRI in children with GH secretory abnormalities [20] (Fig. 62.4). The understanding of these morphological changes has been helped tremendously by the molecular and cellular findings in the studies of the GH-releasing hormone (GHRH) receptor in *little* mouse, and the earlier identification of the role of GHRH in the stimulation of GH gene transcription [21] and the induction of somatotroph cells proliferation [22]. The *little* mouse, first described in 1976 [23], transmits an autosomal recessive inherited growth defect. The final size of these mice is about 60% of age- and sex-matched control subjects. The defect has been localised to the GHRH receptor and its molecular basis determined, namely, a single nucleotide change [24,25]. The *little* mice exhibit pituitary hypoplasia, with selective loss of somatotrophs and a marked reduction

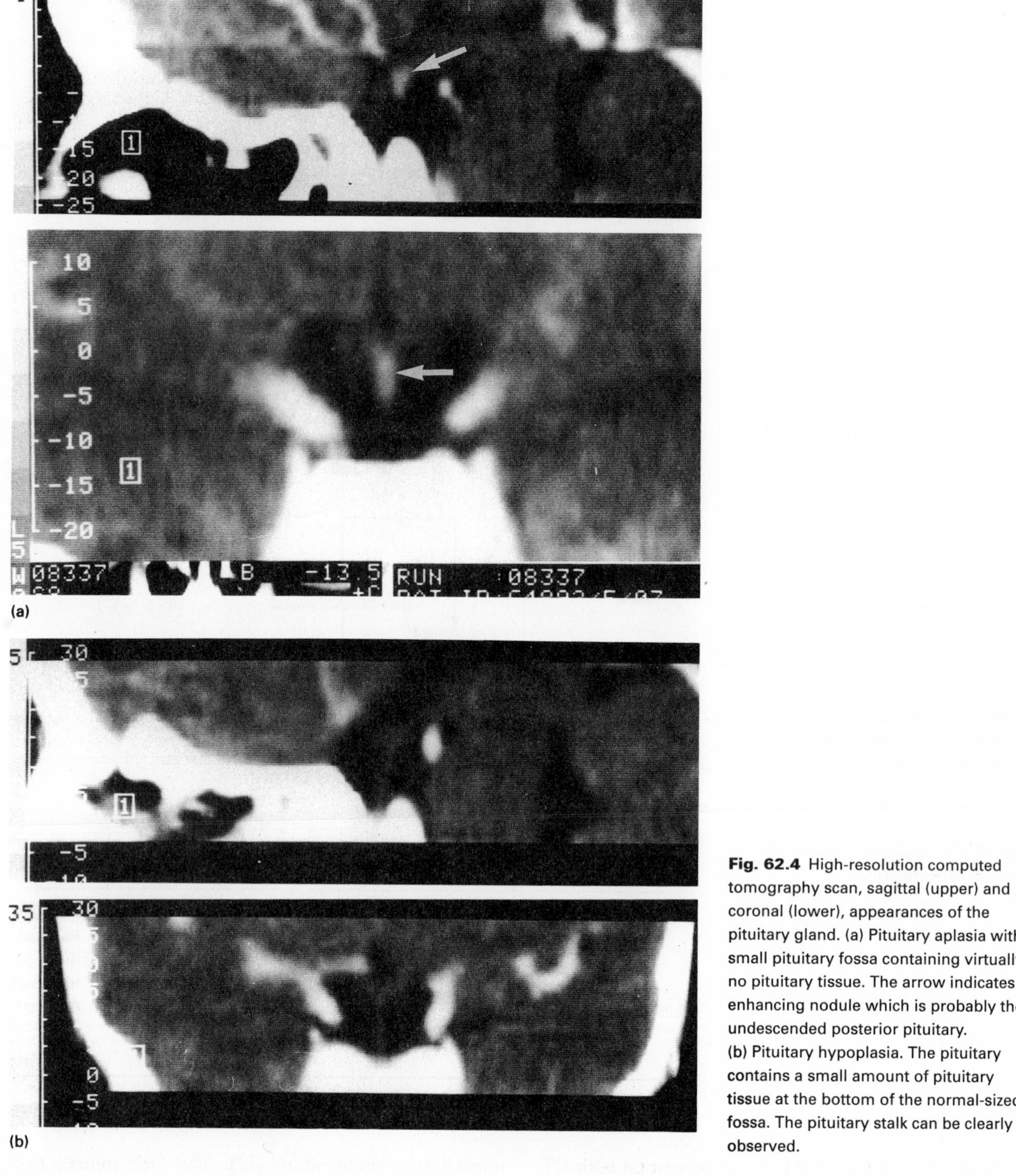

Fig. 62.4 High-resolution computed tomography scan, sagittal (upper) and coronal (lower), appearances of the pituitary gland. (a) Pituitary aplasia with a small pituitary fossa containing virtually no pituitary tissue. The arrow indicates an enhancing nodule which is probably the undescended posterior pituitary. (b) Pituitary hypoplasia. The pituitary contains a small amount of pituitary tissue at the bottom of the normal-sized fossa. The pituitary stalk can be clearly observed.

in GH messenger RNA (mRNA) and protein levels in the pituitary.

Other models of dwarfism, such as the Snell [26], Ames [27] and Pygmy [28] mice, have been studied. Dwarfism in the Snell mouse is due to a mutation of the *Pit*-1 gene, a pituitary transcription factor which is important for cell differentiation of somatotrophs and lactotrophs. Mutations of the human *Pit*-1 gene have also been described. Affected families have an autosomal recessive type of GH deficiency, associated occasionally with thyroid-stimulating hormone (TSH) and prolactin deficiency [29,30] (Table 62.2). Ames dwarf mice are known to have life-long GH deficiency, but the underlying defect remains unidentified. Pygmy mice differ from the above animal models in that their phenotype cannot be explained on the basis of aberration of the growth hormone, insulin-like growth factor (IGF-1), endocrine pathway. The defect in the pygmy mouse has been attributed to a mutation in the gene encoding an architectural transcription factor known as HMGI-C (high mobility group proteins) [31]. HMGI-C seems to be required for all cell types except those in the brain, and is especially important for adipose tissue; its inactivation perturbs the cell cycle in the developing embryo, resulting in a general reduction in growth, a disproportionately reduced content of body fat and preservation of brain size.

The clinical and auxological features of GH deficiency are also manifest in a situation where abnormal polymers of GH are secreted from the pituitary gland. Such material is bio-inactive, but measurable by immunoassay [32,33]. The situation is relatively uncommon, but the children do benefit from the administration of GH, unlike those children who have GH gene deletion in whom a transitory improvement in growth rate occurs only to be followed by growth attenuation due to the formation of high-affinity GH antibodies [34].

The phenotypic features of absent GH with severe growth failure are also seen in individuals who have mutations of the GH receptor causing GH-insensitivity syndromes [35]. Individuals with this disorder, which is inherited in an autosomal recessive pattern, have high plasma levels of GH but low levels of IGF-1.

Acquired destruction of the anterior pituitary gland is most often associated with the presence of a craniopharyngioma. Visual disturbances or headaches may be the first signs. Infiltration of the pituitary gland in histiocytosis X may result in GH deficiency (see also Chapter 18).

Transection of the pituitary stalk as a result of severe head injury is another important cause of pituitary insufficiency.

The hypothalamus and disturbances of pulsatile GH secretion

GH secretion is characterised by secretory bursts which raise the serum concentration from undetectable (by current assay) values to a peak value. Secretion then ceases and plasma values return to undetectable values. This process is regulated mainly by two hypothalamic peptides: GHRH and somatostatin (SS). In addition, a complex set of neurotransmitter pathways as well as various peripheral metabolic and hormonal factors influence GH secretion (Fig. 62.3), though their exact role in terms of the physiological control of GH secretory bursts is uncertain. In contrast, disorders in secretion of GHRH and/or SS could lead to diminished GH secretion.

In humans, and in many animal species, GH-dependent growth appears to be a pulse amplitude-modulated phenomenon [3,36]. In humans, the frequency of GH secretion is relatively fixed, with a periodicity of between 3 and 4 hours [37]. In children, little change in GH periodicity is seen between prepubertal and pubertal individuals: the major changes occur solely as a result of changes in GH pulse amplitude [37,38]. Preservation of a fixed GH frequency would appear to be the rule in physiological and pathophysiological states such as Turner's syndrome, and in the GH hypersecretion seen in adolescent diabetics.

The vast majority of short children formerly labelled as GH deficient appear to have GH *in*sufficiency on the basis of 24-hour GH secretory profiles, and the fact that they do not develop high-affinity antibodies to exogenous GH. The most likely source of pathology in these individuals probably rests in the hypothalamus rather than the pituitary gland. Disorders in secretion of GHRH would explain most of the GH pulse-amplitude problems observed. This hormone is particularly important, not only for secretion of GH, but also for regulation of the GH gene [21]. Numerous clinical studies have suggested but not proven that in the majority of children with GH insufficiency the disorder resides in the GHRH neurons. Since GHRH is also a trophic factor [22], then the abnormality seen radiologically (pituitary hypoplasia) [20] or histologically [39] may reflect an insufficiency in secretion of this hormone. Clinical studies correlating pituitary GH reserve and degree of growth failure suggest that in many children a defect in GHRH synthesis/delivery is an important factor [40,41].

GH pulse amplitude increases between the ages of 5 and 10 years [37], the changes being parallelled by plasma IGF-1 concentrations [42]. This change in GH secretion with age might represent the effects of the increasing circulating concentration of androgens that are seen towards the end of the first decade of life [43,44]. Failure to step up GH secretion during this period of time would lead to growth failure. A further important time point is the increase in GH secretion required to generate the pubertal growth spurt. It appears, therefore, that there are critical points during the development of the child where changes in GH secretion, brought about by changes in GH pulse amplitude, are essential for the maintenance of the normal pattern of growth.

Disorders of GH pulse frequency are relatively unusual. Such abnormalities can be discerned only from the performance of 24-hour GH profiles where intermittent samples have been drawn at frequent intervals. The performance of 24-hour studies of GH secretion using continuous withdrawal pumps and deriving 'integrated' concentrations of GH secretion, or the use of urinary measurements of GH, will not be able to identify such individuals. Fig. 62.5 shows

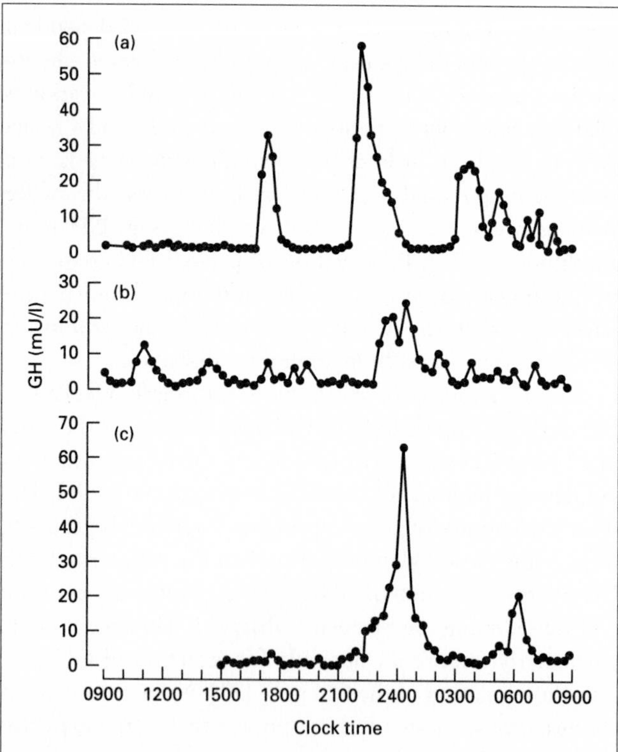

Fig. 62.5 Three different secretory patterns with similar mean concentrations. From [167].

three different patterns of GH secretion, all of which have a very similar mean GH concentration; although the mean GH concentrations are similar, the secretory patterns had a markedly different effect on growth rate. Frequency abnormalities are unusual and most commonly found in children with low birth weight. Their GH response to provocative stimuli is usually normal, but the GH profiles in such individuals either show a very fast frequency pattern or else a profile with one or two very high amplitude pulses [45].

GH secretion and GH insufficiency

GH secretion is pulsatile and during many hours of the day serum concentrations are low. As a result, provocative tests were designed to test the integrity of the hypothalamo-pituitary axis. The standard test, the insulin-induced hypoglycaemia GH stimulation test (ITT), has been the mainstay of pharmacological assessment of GH secretion. Clonidine, L-dopa, glucagon and arginine have also been used. One of the main problems in paediatrics in interpreting the response to these tests is the lack of normal data. Performing such tests on normal children is fraught with ethical problems. Furthermore, standards would also be needed for tall, normal and short children, because their GH secretion differs. If age is an important determination of GH secretion, and puberty clearly is, then values for these would have to be included as well.

In general, there is little to choose between the tests when compared with the ITT (Table 62.3). Such an analysis assumes, of course, that the ITT indicates the correct diagnosis in all cases. Where repeat ITTs have been performed, values of efficiency and sensitivity approach values given in Table 62.3. The cut-off chosen for the definition of GH deficiency/insufficiency depends on the sensitivity and specificity of the test. It will also depend, in part, on the type of assay used. Using differing cut-offs for the definition of GH sufficiency or insufficiency will determine the performance characteristics of the ITT, in this instance compared with the growth velocity as the 'gold standard'. An example of this using the Hybritech immunoradiometric assay (IRMA) is shown in Table 62.4, where optimal test performance was achieved with a serum GH concentration cut-off value of 13.5 mU/l [16].

It has been suggested that two tests of GH secretion are better than one. It has to be remembered that the response to the second test is independent of the response to the first;

Table 62.3 Performance characteristics of various tests of growth hormone (GH) secretion in the diagnosis of GH insufficiency, compared with the ITT using a cut-off value of 15 mU/l. From [165].

Test	Efficiency (%)	Sensitivity (%)	Specificity (%)
Sleep			
EEG monitored	88	86	95
Not monitored	79	67	82
Arginine	72	73	85
Clonidine	70	70	85
IGF-1	75	95	60
IGFBP-3*	96	97	95
IGFBP-3*	93	83	44

IGF, insulin-like growth factor; IGFBP, IGF-binding protein.
The efficiency of the test is how well the test identifies true positive and true negative diagnoses.
*Values quoted from two different studies.

Table 62.4 Effect of applying different peak serum growth hormone (GH) values in response to ITT for the diagnosis of GH insufficiency using height velocity as standard.

GH concentration (mU/l)	Efficiency (%)	Sensitivity (%)	Specificity (%)
10	63	50.6	79
12.5	66	60	74.6
13.5	66	63.5	70
15	67	69.4	63.4
20	68	82	49

the knowledge that a peak response has occurred on one occasion has no effect on the probability of the event in the second test. The probability of a joint event occurring can be calculated from the product law for independent events. If the likelihood of a current result is 80% and the response to the second test is independent of the response to the first, then the likelihood of the two tests giving the same result is $0.8 \times 0.8 = 0.64$ (64%).

Although great emphasis has been placed on physiological tests of GH secretion, neither sleep- nor 24-hour profile studies are easy to perform and they require a heavy manpower commitment to conduct them effectively. Urinary GH measurements may be a step forward in this situation [46] but variability is high and two or three overnight collections need to be performed to overcome this problem.

An alternative approach might be to measure the serum levels of IGFs and/or their binding proteins. The advantages of a single blood test are obvious. Serum IGF-1 is low in GH insufficiency but, because normal IGF-1 values are also low in early childhood, poor discrimination ensues. IGF-1 binding protein 3 (IGFBP-3) is largely regulated by circulating levels of GH and could be used to reflect GH status. Table 62.3 shows the performance characteristics of IGF-1 and IGFBP-3 compared with ITTs.

Physiological studies help in recognising some of the limitations of pharmacological tests of GH secretion. Children growing extremely slowly with growth velocities of <4 cm/year with normal GH response to pharmacological stimulation have been demonstrated to have very little physiological GH secretion. A variety of terms has been used to describe these individuals since the original reports of Wise *et al.* [47]. Of those, GH 'neurosecretory dysfunction' appears to be the most used [48]. This term is probably inappropriate given the available evidence [49], and it is probably simpler to accept the limitations of pharmacological testing than to construct a tangled web of neuropharmacological interactions to try to explain the results of stimuli that are unlikely to have any physiological relevance.

It is unlikely that any tests will improve on the 80–90% sensitivity and specificity reported. The reasons for false-negative results are easier to understand than the false-positives. Growth velocity of necessity is measured over a long period of time, between 6 and 12 months. The pharmacological and even the physiological tests are performed over a very short period of time, a day at the most. This must mean, in view of our knowledge of seasonal growth [4], that some stimulatory tests are performed in the period of relatively good growth but of necessity would have to be compared with the overall growth over a period of 6 months to 1 year. Explaining the false-positive results is more difficult. It is a well-recognised phenomenon that when a stimulation test is performed and the 0-min specimen is high, any further elevation in response to the stimulus is unlikely to occur during the period of the test. This has widely been ascribed to the effects of stress resulting from the insertion of the intravenous cannula, and can easily be circumvented by inserting the cannula well in advance (the night before, for example) of commencing the stimulation test. A more likely explanation is that the stimulation test has been performed upon a background of endogenous GH secretory activity. The ITT was devised for performance in adult patients in whom GH secretory episodes are unlikely to occur during the morning. This is not the case in children, where GH secretory episodes between the hours of 0900 and 1200 hours are commonplace, particularly if the individual is in puberty [50]. GH secretory bursts probably take place due to a withdrawal of SS inhibitory tone with or without a concomitant stimulation of GHRH. It is quite likely, therefore, that endogenous secretory bursts in some individuals are followed by an increase in SS tone preventing any further release in GH. This argument has been developed further by Devesa *et al.* [51], who showed that the GH response to GHRH was highly dependent on the GH secretory status during the preceding hour.

Physiological studies of GH secretion

In recent years attention has again been focused by many groups on the spontaneous GH secretion of children. A variety of methods has been used to obtain samples, ranging from continuous withdrawal pump systems to intermittent sampling techniques. The sampling interval has varied considerably between the studies, as has the duration over which the studies have been performed, the latter ranging between 5 and 24 hours. Finally, numerous methods of analysing the data have been put forward and to the uninvolved a haphazard and confused picture appears at first sight. It is important to realise that before performing such studies the investigator must have a clear idea of the precise questions that need to be answered.

Collecting the data

Sampling techniques

A variety of methods has been devised to obtain GH profiles. The first is to use discrete samples (such as 20-min sampling for 24 hours); the second involves integrated sampling where blood is withdrawn continuously. The disadvantage of the discrete method is that identification of the true peak is highly dependent on how often samples are drawn. Although two or three concentrations may be well above the level of the previous two or three, the highest need not necessarily reflect the true height of the secretory burst, unless the time interval between the samples is very short. Knowledge of the half-life of the hormone under study can help to solve this problem.

The integrated sampling method has the advantage that no peak GH concentration can occur without this being reflected in the plasma collected, but the disadvantage is that unless the interval between samples is short, the peak concentration becomes rapidly 'diluted' by the concentrations measured on the ascending and descending limbs of a pulse. Shorter 12-hour profiles with more frequent sampling might circumvent this problem but suffer from the major problem that they could quite easily start after and finish before a GH pulse, leading to a marked variation in the results obtained.

Sampling interval

To define a rhythm, sampling must take place over more than one cycle. It is important with any sampling technique also to consider the effect of the sampling interval on the possible results obtained. Inappropriately long sampling intervals can lead to spurious results and failure to detect the real oscillation of a hormone. A minimum of five or six samples per cycle is required to prevent the mismatching of infrequent sampling intervals to the predominant period of pulsatility which is being observed.

The sampling interval used determines the cycle frequency that can be detected. The lower the frequency of interest the longer the time period over which measurements need to be taken and, conversely, the higher the frequency the more frequent observations must be made. A cautious approach needs to be taken with the latter statement, however. The observation of fast frequencies may be interesting from the secretory point of view, but is probably of little relevance to the receptor if the clearance of the peptide is very long.

Analysis of profiles

The question that the investigator needs to ask at the outset of the study is whether any sophisticated form of analysis is required. A single profile requires little in the way of sophisticated analysis, since the graph contains all the information required. Where statements need to be made about populations or subpopulations or the changes within pathological states or following treatment intervention, more sophisticated techniques are required. The techniques for this fall under the general heading of 'time series analysis' which involves techniques for analysing regularly sampled data.

Estimate of the mean concentration

Routine parametric statistics can be used to establish the mean and standard deviation of the data. The area under the curve has often been used by authors. It is identical to the mean multiplied by the total duration of the sampling, and conveys little more information. It is of value when the data are not sampled at regular intervals, but as already discussed the analysis of such data leads to error.

Pulse identification

Traditional methods of pulse analysis have used blinded scorers to identify peaks by inspection and to measure and count them for analysis. The exact criteria for pulse identification are difficult to define and the interassessor variation has not been defined. However, the aim of the method is easily understood but is none the less largely subjective. Computer processing may allow rigid criteria of what constitutes a peak and improved methodology to account for biological noise [52].

Time series analysis

Several sophisticated mathematical procedures can be applied to hormone profiles. Two techniques used are autocorrelation and Fourier transformation. Autocorrelation (Fig. 62.6) is a technique for establishing whether there are regular recurring wave forms (of any shape) within a data array. The method is independent of the shape of the wave and the start point of the profile. The end result is an estimate of period and assessment of its significance. Further, the data can be pooled.

If more than one frequency or rhythm is present in the time series, these underlying frequencies may be rather difficult to assess by inspection of the autocorrelation function, because different frequencies can obscure each other. In this situation, as with any complex wave form, these can be deconvoluted into a series of sinusoids. Amplitude and frequency components of the sinusoids can be dissected, and it is this assessment which is called Fourier transformation. This method is unbiased and remarkably robust. It allows groups of data to be compared, and information is provided on frequency, frequency modulation, amplitude and amplitude modulation.

Deconvolution analysis

The concentration of a hormone measured at any point in time represents a balance between secretion from the gland of origin and clearance from the circulation. It is possible from knowledge of hormone clearance or by making *a priori* assumptions about secretion to work back from (deconvolute) the measured concentration [53,54]. The method is particularly useful for analysing hormone secretion

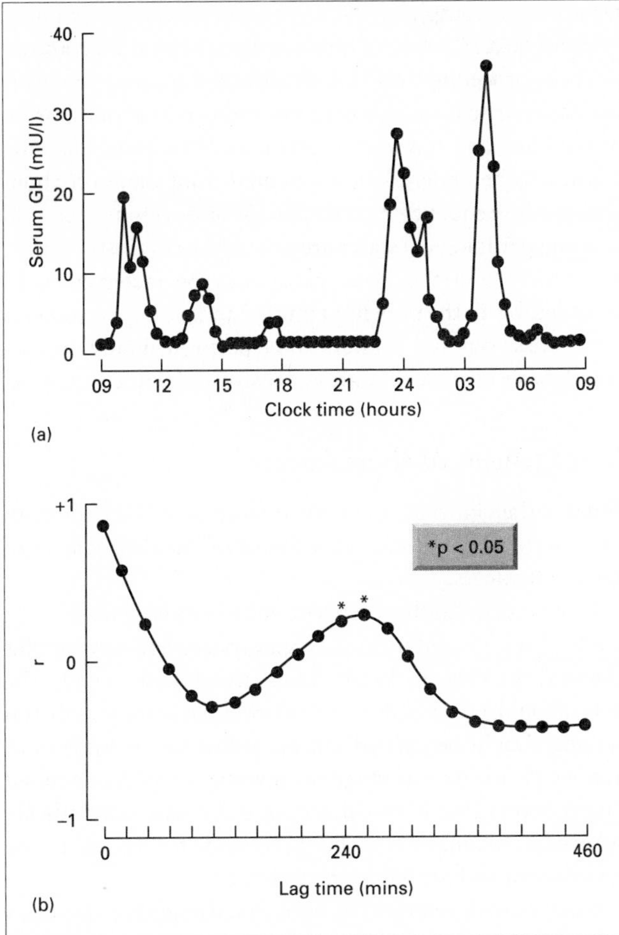

Fig. 62.6 Application of the technique of autocorrelation to a 24-hour growth hormone (GH) profile. (a) Serum GH concentration profile. (b) Autocorrelation function. Significant correlation occurs with a lag time of 240 min, suggesting that on average oscillations occur regularly with this periodicity. Examination of the concentration profile reveals pulses at 1000, 1400 and 1600 hours and at 2300, 0300 and 0700 hours.

and for understanding the physiology of that secretion. In addition, deconvolution analysis can be used to break down complex concentration wave forms into their secretory components.

Baseline occupancy

Just as estimating peak amplitude and frequency is useful, some estimate of the trough values of hormone profiles may be needed to understand pathophysiological situations, for example acromegaly and Cushing's syndrome. Trough analysis is more complex and as a compromise dwell-time at low concentrations has been used as a marker [55]. This method determines the proportion of time of the whole profile that is occupied at certain concentrations. For example, in the case of GH, the concentration at/below which the profile spent 5% of its time might be considered a marker of trough activity. In contradistinction to deconvolution analysis, baseline occupancy (and for that matter any level one chooses) gives an estimate of end organ/receptor exposure to the hormone.

Chaos

The issue of regularity and chaos arises when we try to deal with complex data arrays where regularity is less obvious. Can it be quantified and what are the implications? The traditional approach in biology is always to look for the simplest explanation. At first sight it seems inherently unlikely that biology is anything other than deterministic. Heart rate is controlled by natural pacemakers which give rise to steady regular heart beats but practical experience tells us that occasionally beats become dropped. In extremes the rhythm becomes irregular, the change in timing of one beat makes a bigger change in the next and so on; when this instability is persistent then it is termed chaos. At its extreme in the case of heart rate, survival may be threatened. Is regularity the preferred mode then? The answer appears to be 'not quite'. There have been a number of interesting studies looking at heart rates in a number of pathophysiological situations. In children who have had an aborted sudden infant death episode there is an association with regular less complex heart rate tracings [56].

Oscillating systems have a high likelihood of becoming chaotic because they possess an element of feedback. The system will always opt to make something too large smaller and something too small larger. It is sometimes useful to determine at what level the factor will settle at. Generally speaking, most people would operate for something in the middle, neither too large or too small. This is not true all of time, however.

The likelihood of chaos in the field of endocrinology must be quite high. Isolated endocrine cells have their own inherent rhythm and if an external rhythm with a different periodicity is imposed then the ensuing hormone secretion will depend on the relationship between these two periods. In some instances secretion will resume with some harmonic of the stimulus but in other cases random secretion will take place giving irregular or chaotic patterns. In endocrinology, the input and output of the control system can be measured and the two related to each other. In addition, there is latency or lag within the system and in theory if the latency is altered (e.g. gain in the feedback loop increased) then the system could become unstable and oscillate periodically. If the feedback system was made complex then periodic oscillations could ensue.

Attempts to measure these phenomena in endocrinology are in their early infancy. However, techniques have been devised for other areas of biology. Approximate entropy is one measure. This procedure attempts to quantify regularity in data in conjunction with standard measures such as the mean and root mean squared. Entropy is a concept that addresses system randomness and predictability. The greater the entropy the more the randomness and the less the system order. The models derived have been based on the Kolmogorov–Sinai entropy formula. Modifications were required because this entropy formula needs no noise and infinite amounts of data. Neither are possible in most biological systems! This is a major problem. For example, in analysing regularity in the outbreak of measles a data series of some 500 monthly points was constructed but even this was considered too short for reliable analysis.

Approximate entropy measures the logarithmic likelihood that runs of patterns that are close remain close on the next incremental comparison. The higher the value, the more random the time series [57]. The technique has been applied in a number of instances and in the endocrine field, patients with osteoporosis have been shown to have a loss of chaotic oscillations in serum levels of parathyroid hormone [58].

Fractal analysis is an important area of chaos. Fractals are geometrical shapes that are irregular all over but have the same degree of regularity on all sides. An object looks the same when examined from far away or nearby. Sometimes parts of the object are exactly like the whole. Others are more random in nature, for example maps of coastlines. Measuring the coast of a country with ever-increasing precision means that its length becomes greater because ever-smaller irregularities along the length need to be taken into account. For fractals, the counterparts of the familiar dimensions (0, 1, 2 and 3) are known as fractal dimensions. Mandelbrot described an exponent of similarity termed the fractal dimension [59] and Katz and George [60] described techniques to compute fractal dimensions from time series data.

Several algorithms exist to compute fractal dimensions. The first point to note is that the technique is not strongly related to the means and standard deviation that can be derived from the data array. A straight line has a fractal dimension equal to one as the next point is predicted from knowledge of the current situation. A single pulse has a fractal dimension close to one as there are points rising above each other (predictable) and falling below each other (predictable) but points at the apex which are less predictable, neither rising or falling. More complex shapes have higher fractal dimensions. This type of approach has been applied to a number of aspects of biology, for example blood-flow [61] and heart-rate analysis [62]. In the studies reported so far a loss of complexity or a tendency to regularity might be construed as a sign of abnormality as mentioned above.

These procedures are not straightforward and problems can easily arise from choosing the wrong period or duration of sampling and the wrong technique of analysis. Planning a study to be undertaken is essential if information about changes in frequency and amplitude or hormone secretion in many pathological states are not to be easily lost. Further, the patient and the investigator may be inconvenienced considerably in the pursuit of limited and perhaps erroneous data. These types of studies can be performed only on a research basis because they are expensive and time consuming.

Management of short stature

What is the clinician to do when faced with the child with short stature? Three elements comprise the management of such individuals.

First, careful anthropometric measurements need to be made. These should include height, triceps and subscapular skinfold thicknesses, head circumference and weight. The data should be recorded and plotted accurately. Pubertal staging should be carried out according to the method of Tanner [170]. At this stage no investigations are required unless points arise in the history or examination to indicate otherwise. Arrangements should be made for the child to be remeasured and growth rate calculated.

Once growth velocity has been calculated, then decisions can be made along the lines suggested in the algorithm. Growth-velocity charts allow the clinician to reduce to a minimum the likelihood of investigating short normal children. For example, the chances of a child growing with a height velocity over a 1-year period less than the 3rd centile and growing normally the next year is 3%, but for a child growing with a height velocity on the 10th centile a 10% chance exists that all will be well over the next year. The former child should be investigated now, but the latter should be observed for a further year. If the growth velocity over the second year is still on the 10th height velocity centile then investigations should be undertaken as there is only a 1% (10% of 10%) chance that growth is normal.

Investigation should be targeted according to the different components which comprise post-natal growth. The clinician should direct attention predominantly to nutritional factors in the first 6–12 months of life. Thereafter, GH-dependent growth predominates, and investigation should be directed along the lines outlined previously. The specificity and sensitivity of any of the tests of GH secretion is only 80%, so the clinician should expect false-positive and false-negative results. Repeat stimulation tests rarely clarify the situation. Physiological tests of GH secretion are time consuming, expensive and add little further information in the vast majority of cases. They should be performed only in exceptional circumstances. Clinicians must remember to treat the patient, not pieces of data.

The final element of the management of short stature is to target treatment. Treatment designed to augment growth in the childhood component is likely to be without effect on either the infancy or the pubertal components of growth. The next section discusses treatment options for children with short stature who present during childhood. Puberty is dealt with in Chapter 64, and the treatment of infancy growth failure is covered in paediatric textbooks.

Treatment options for children with short stature

Growth hormone

GH insufficiency

In 1932 a treatment to promote growth with crude anterior pituitary extract was reported [63], but it was not until Raben's observations in 1958 [64] and until methods of GH extraction became generally available that large studies could be conducted. These larger studies showed a beneficial effect of human GH in promoting growth in children who had the clinical features of GH deficiency [65–67]. The advent of radioimmunoassay allowed the measurement of GH concentration in blood in response to a variety of pharmacological stimuli, and these measurements provided the clinician with means of collecting children who might benefit from the limited supplies of human GH then available. Exogenous human GH promoted rapid growth in the short term, with the most dramatic response seen over the first 6 months. Subsequently, this growth rate returned slowly to normal values. A disproportionate increase in bone maturation did not accompany the therapy [68].

In general, long-term effects have not been as dramatic as the short-term studies might have suggested. Although final height has been increased compared with what would have happened if no treatment had been given to the patients, most groups found that patients with isolated GH insufficiency were still some 2 standard deviation scores (SDS) from the mean at the end of treatment [69]. Selection of patients on the basis of height achieved rather than on height velocity must have contributed a great deal, as one of the original criteria was a height of –2 SDS from the mean. However, dose of GH administered and frequency of administration may have been additional important factors.

Treatment of short children without GH insufficiency

The initial studies of Tanner *et al.* [67] included children who were short but growing normally. Numbers were small and many had the Russell–Silver syndrome. These children showed an improvement in growth velocity which was less than that seen in their GH-insufficient peers, but was none the less an improvement on the rate at which they had been growing previously. Since then, there have been many reports of GH therapy in children with 'normal' GH responses to provocative stimuli. These reports can be broadly divided into three categories: (i) the treatment of short normal children; (ii) those with Turner's syndrome; and (iii) those with intrauterine growth retardation (Russell–Silver syndrome).

The description of these individuals has ranged from those who secrete biologically inactive GH, as described originally by Hayek *et al.* [32] and Kowarski *et al.* [70], through those who have low spontaneous GH secretion [71,72], to a group described as having normal variant short stature by Rudman *et al.* [73]. Problems exist in interpreting the biologically inactive human GH studies. A major problem is the use of assay systems such as a radioreceptor assay which has poor sensitivity. Very few of the assays measuring 'bioactive' GH actually measure the known biological effects of GH. As newer assays of GH bioactivity are validated [74,75], such problems are less likely to arise in the future. In addition, it is frequently difficult to verify structurally abnormal human GH in a suspect case. The hallmark of these patients is that their growth velocities were poor and a disproportionate emphasis was placed on the result of pharmacological testing. The children were labelled as being short and normal in a very loose way, and the 'normal' part of the description is often dependent only on the biochemical response to a pharmacological stimulus.

Of the 91 children reported in the world literature who have been described as short normal, only a small percentage had height velocity SDS between 0 and –0.8 [76,77,78]. These studies are also complicated by many of the children not entering puberty at the correct time. In others, the response to exogenous GH could be ascribed to the patient's own pubertal growth spurt. Further, some groups have included a wide variety of diagnostic categories in their studies including children with dysmorphic syndromes and low birth weight [79,80]. Short-term studies have demonstrated acceleration of growth in short children following the administration of exogenous GH [81,82]. The growth response to exogenous GH was more marked in those children who secreted very little GH and grew poorly compared with those who were short but growing at a normal velocity, in whom the growth response to exogenous GH was less than that of their worse-off peers [82] (Fig. 62.7). The promising short-term response to GH treatment prompted longer-term studies. Over the first few years of observation children receiving GH did not have a disproportionate advance in skeletal maturity. This

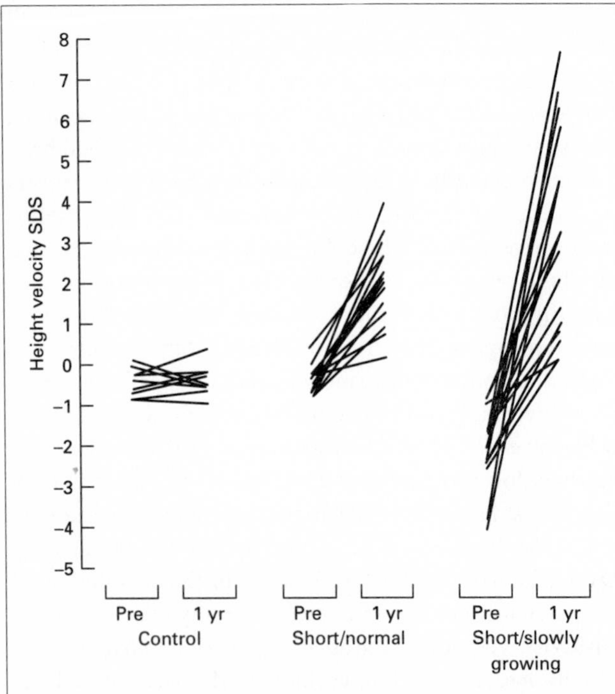

Fig. 62.7 Effect of treatment with biosynthetic human growth hormone (hGH) on growth velocity standard deviation score (SDS) in 10 control (left panel), 16 short/normal (middle panel) and 19 short/slowly growing children (right panel).

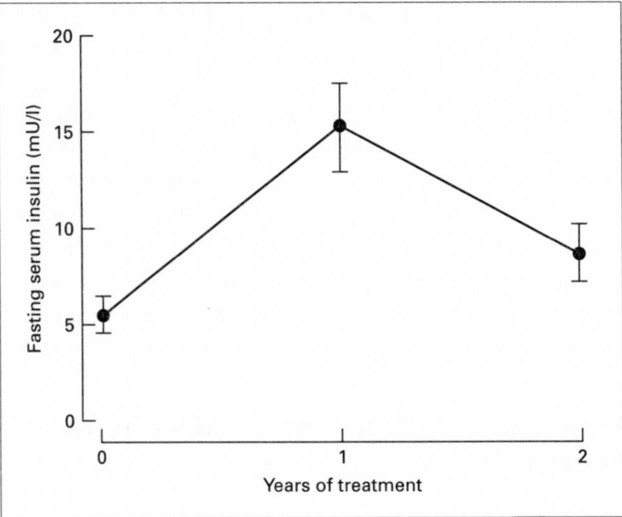

Fig. 62.8 Change in fasting serum insulin concentrations during the course of treatment with biosynthetic human growth hormone (hGH). Data shown as mean and SEM.

means that the height gain represented a true increment in predicted final height, which is approximately 6 cm for boys and 5 cm for girls. Follow-up of these children to final height demonstrated that treatment with exogenous GH for periods of up to 9 years made very little impact on final height. The net gain in stature was approximately 2.8 cm in boys and 2.5 cm in girls [83]. Similar results have been reported by Loche *et al.* [84].

Concern has been raised over the administration of GH to such individuals. Excessive GH secretion in adults leads to acromegaly with clearly defined metabolic and cardiovascular complications. The serum GH concentration profile following administration of a subcutaneous injection of biosynthetic GH has nothing in common with that observed in patients with acromegaly. Long-term treatment with GH had no effect on blood pressure [85]. Short-term studies showed no effect on the renin–angiotensin–aldosterone system [86]. Metabolic studies performed on these children during the course of GH administration demonstrated no abnormality in glucose tolerance over the study period. A transient increase in fasting serum insulin concentration has been observed over the first year of treatment, but this returned to pretreatment values by the end of the second year (Fig. 62.8). Glycated haemoglobin concentration did not change. Although a significant decrease in triceps and subscapular skinfold thicknesses during the first year of therapy was observed, the long-term effects suggested a gradual reaccumulation of subcutaneous fat with values at the end of therapy unchanged from those observed at the beginning. Echocardiographic studies of short normal children treated with GH for 4 years demonstrated no significant structural or functional changes to the heart [85].

Turner's syndrome

Children with Turner's syndrome have low birth weight, but their growth over the first 3 years of post-natal life is normal. After that period a gradual decrease in growth rate is observed which is responsible to a large extent for the final adult height observed in these patients. The lack of the pubertal growth spurt is also noticeable (Fig. 62.9), but is not the major cause of the short stature observed in adults with this condition.

Assessment of GH secretion in patients with Turner's syndrome has demonstrated that there is no difference in the amplitude or periodicity of GH secretion during childhood compared with controls [87]. During the time when the pubertal growth spurt might be expected, a decrease in GH secretion due to a diminution in GH pulse amplitude has been observed. Although the GH secretion in childhood is not different from controls, the rate of growth is. This could imply that there is 'end-organ resistance' in its broadest sense to the effects of endogenous GH in children with Turner's syndrome. The skeleton of girls with Turner's syndrome is abnormal, and the situation with respect to their

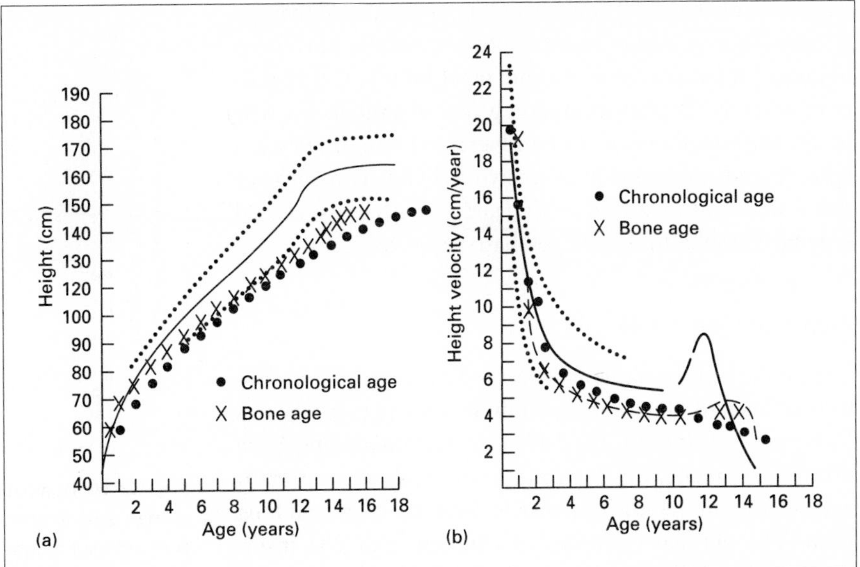

Fig. 62.9 Growth of children with Turner's syndrome. (a) Mean height; (b) mean height velocity. From [168], with permission.

growth begins to resemble that seen in patients with skeletal dysplasia.

In the original report of Tanner *et al.* [67], children with Turner's syndrome were given GH in the doses and at a frequency that was conventional at that time. The growth response was rather poor, probably reflecting the late age at which treatment was commenced. Long-term studies have demonstrated that treatment with GH alone or oxandrolone alone results in an increase in height relative to Turner standards and an increase in height prediction, but the actual improvement in final height is not yet known because the number of girls who have completed their growth remains small. Rosenfeld *et al.* [88,89] compared the effect of GH alone with GH and oxandrolone. While the combination treatments led in the short term to a further increase in growth rate over and above that obtained by either treatment modality alone, bone age advancement with oxandrolone was greater in the long term and final heights were not significantly different [88,89]. As with skeletal dysplasias, beneficial effects of GH treatment in children with Turner's syndrome requires doses in excess of 20 U/m^2/week, given in divided doses by daily injection [90].

These observations on the efficacy of GH should not lead the clinician to conclude that GH is the only form of therapy available for these individuals. Treatment combinations of oxandrolone and low-dose oestrogen provide excellent growth responses at a fraction of the cost of GH. Oestrogen therapy must be introduced in these girls to induce puberty at the correct age, not to mention its beneficial effects on the likely complication of osteoporosis in girls with Turner's syndrome. A fuller discussion of treatment options is given below in the section on steroid therapy.

Russell–Silver syndrome: intrauterine growth retardation

The children in this category display poor growth *in utero* yet normal growth once they escape from that environment. None the less, the end result of the severe intrauterine growth retardation is short stature. These children have lost their genetic potential. On conventional pharmacological testing they have normal GH secretion, but recent work has demonstrated clearly that the pattern of GH secretion is anything but normal [45]. The treatment of these children with GH increases their height velocity but results in no long-term improvement in height prediction [91]. Since these children have a tendency towards early pubertal development and the actions of GH are known to accelerate pubertal progress [92], treatment with GH would decrease final height. High-dosage regimens of GH treatment using 30 U/m^2/week are most effective in the short term [93], but, for the reasons outlined above, children whose short stature is due to intrauterine growth retardation are unlikely to benefit from GH treatment in the long term.

GH and renal disease

The common feature emerging from all these studies is that recombinant human GH (rhGH) will promote growth acceleration in the short term. Renal disease is no exception, and whether rhGH has been used to accelerate growth in children with chronic renal failure or in children with poor growth post-renal transplantation, all short-term studies have documented improvement in stature. Longer-term studies need evaluation because after 2 years therapy with a functioning allograft children are gaining <1 cm on their huge deficit in height. The effect of long-term steroid therapy is an important factor. More impressive results have been obtained in patients with chronic renal failure. Care needs to be taken in the post-transplant group of patients because of circumstantial evidence of an increased rate of rejection episodes in those individuals receiving rhGH. This suggests that it should be used with caution and perhaps its use should only be confined to trained paediatric nephrologists.

Administration of GH

The analysis of pulsatile GH secretion reveals that amplitude is the major factor in determining growth rate whereas frequency is relatively fixed [94]. In GH treatment, both dose and frequency of GH administration play an important role in determining the response in both the short and long term. The optimal treatment of children with GH insufficiency is still far from clear. Until recently, the generally accepted method has been to give GH by intramuscular injections two or three times a week to a total weekly dose of 0.5 U/kg or 12 U/m²/week. Animal experiments have demonstrated a clear dose–response curve for GH, and in particular the frequency of administration has been shown to have important effects on the pattern of growth.

Dose studies

There is a logarithmic dose–response relationship in GH-insufficient children between the amount of GH injected and the growth rate in the first year of treatment [95,96]. Despite the demonstration of this effect, the regimens used have represented a compromise between the growth response obtained and cost–benefit calculations because of the limited supplies of GH available. However, the impression that has been suggested is that for any individual the response is highly dependent on the rate at which the individual was growing before commencement of therapy [67,97]. The assessment of any of these reported dose–response relationships requires prior knowledge of the children's growth rates. The studies of Frasier *et al.* [96] are often quoted as being a definitive dose–response curve. Sadly, this study included a wide spectrum of children with varying pretreatment growth rates. The randomisation procedure ensured that children who were peripubertal and growing with a near-normal growth velocity received the smallest dose of GH whereas much younger children growing with the same growth velocity (and, therefore, growing extremely slowly) received higher doses.

For any range of pretreatment height velocity, a variable response to standard dose of GH will exist. This hypothesis has been explored recently. Figure 62.10 shows a family of dose–response curves for differing pretreatment height velocities for GH doses of between 10 and 25 U/m²/week.

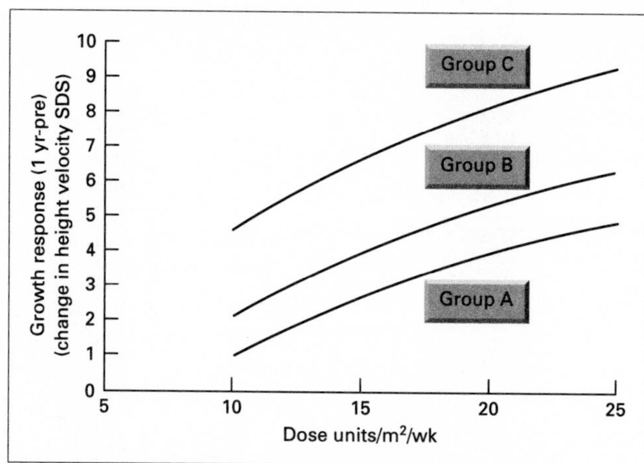

Fig. 62.10 Dose–response curves for treatment with biosynthetic human growth hormone (hGH). Group A children growing with a pretreatment height velocity standard deviation score (SDS) of zero to –0.8; group B, –0.9 to –2.0; group C, <–2.0.

Frequency of administration

In the 1979 report of the Medical Research Council working party, Milner *et al.* [98] demonstrated that intramuscular injections of 5 U GH three times a week gave a better growth response than 10 U twice a week. Kastrup *et al.* [99] showed a better growth rate on a regimen of injections six times a week rather than three times a week, although numbers in this study were small. In addition, these Scandinavian studies were performed on children who had received GH for a reasonable period of time such that their growth velocities were constant. Several other groups have confirmed these initial findings, and the daily injection of GH is now standard clinical practice [100–102].

Method of administration

The generally accepted route of administration in the past has been intramuscular injection. The reluctance to administer GH subcutaneously was based on experience with impure GH preparations which led to local reactions such as lipotrophy. Further, growth-attenuating antibodies were also demonstrated when impure preparations were administered by this route. Biosynthetic GH is less immunogenic than the original human pituitary-derived GH, and as a result no significant difference between the intramuscular and subcutaneous can be demonstrated. Neither method appears to have an advantage in terms of the growth rate obtained, but the subcutaneous route is preferred by patients [100].

Predictors of response

Auxology

Careful studies have been conducted to determine predictors of response to GH therapy. The rate at which the child grows before commencement of therapy has already been alluded to, and has been shown to be the most important factor in a large number of studies [67,97,102].

A growth response > 2 cm/year, irrespective of the pretreatment growth rate, dose or frequency of GH administration, has been used to decide whether a child should continue with GH therapy. This value was arrived at by considering what was the most likely variation in an individual's growth rate over a year that could occur by chance. In a sense, the value is arbitrary. Further, it does not take into account the condition being treated in the broadest sense. As mentioned already, several studies have demonstrated that children with Turner's syndrome can respond to GH if it is given in sufficient dosage [88]. The response of these individuals to a given dose was less than that of their peers. Applying similarly strict response criteria to children who have received craniospinal irradiation during the treatment of brain tumours is inappropriate. Their growth response is less than their similarly worse-off peers because the spinal component of growth has been lost due to radiation damage.

Biochemical factors

The peak serum GH concentration in response to pharmacological testing has been shown to be related to the growth response observed in some studies [67,98], whereas other groups have questioned the particular value of this measure [97]. Several factors probably operate to reduce the value of the GH response. First, a wide variation of response in the same child is often seen. Secondly, there are documented instances of discrepancies between physiological and pharmacological testing of GH secretion [48]. Thirdly, children can grow poorly with apparent 'normal' GH secretion, raising questions as to the biological activity of the GH molecule or variability in tissue sensitivity.

There have been several attempts to use the short term IGF-1 response to GH therapy to predict the long-term growth response. Although the IGF-1 response to 5 days' GH treatment correlated highly with IGF-1 levels for up to 6 months of treatment, neither value accurately predicted the 6-month growth response.

GHRH therapy

The identification of GHRH in 1982 led to an explosion in knowledge of the control of GH secretion and in the understanding of GH-insufficient states. In 1985, Thorner *et al.* [103] reported the successful acceleration of growth in two GH-insufficient children receiving pulsatile GHRH (1–40) every 3 hours throughout the 24-hour period. The observations of an improvement in growth rate set the scene for clinical studies using this peptide.

Pulsatile therapy

In 1986, Smith *et al.* [104] reported their initial findings in GH-insufficient children receiving pulsatile GHRH (1–40) every 3 hours at night, with three of five children demonstrating a significant growth response. Eleven children were

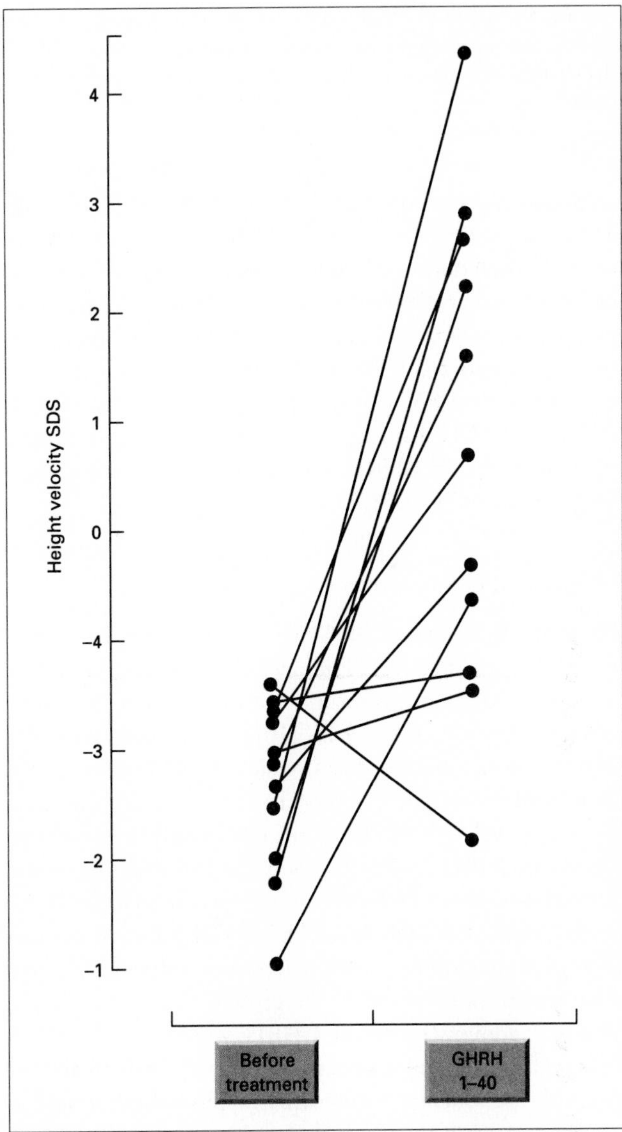

Fig. 62.11 Effect of treatment with growth hormone-releasing hormone (GHRH) (1–40) for 1 year on the height velocity standard deviation score (SDS) of 11 children with GH insufficiency.

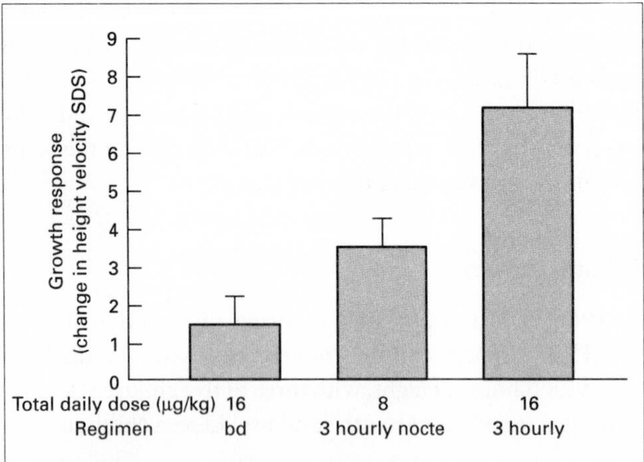

Fig. 62.12 Effects of differing growth hormone-releasing hormone (GHRH) treatment regimens on growth response in prepubertal GH-insufficient children. Data for the 3-hourly group are taken from [169].

subsequently treated with this form of therapy; the results are shown in Fig. 62.11. Pulsatile GH secretion was included in all children during GHRH treatment, although one child demonstrated progressive loss of GH secretion. A significant relationship was observed between the GH generated as the result of a pulsatile GHRH treatment and the growth rate induced. In the USA, Thorner *et al.* [169] performed similar studies in 10 GH-insufficient children but used a treatment regimen where the GHRH was administered over the whole 24-hour period (Fig. 62.12).

Intermittent injection regimen

Intermittent injections of GHRH (1–29) have been used by several investigators. Hummelink *et al.* [105] found a dose of 8–10 μg/kg was insufficient to achieve a significant growth response. Ross *et al.* [106], using approximately 25 μg/kg in two divided doses, achieved a 44% success rate. Smith and Brook. [107] observed a significant improvement in height velocity in 63% of GH-insufficient children receiving GHRH (1–29) in a daily dose of 16 μg/kg in two divided injections. Similar results were produced in the Dutch study [108]. Although much higher GH pulse amplitudes were observed following this twice-daily regimen compared with the pulsatile regimen, the growth rates were poorer. Pulsatile administration of GHRH would appear, therefore, to be important in generating maximal growth and the 3-hourly periodicity documented in physiological studies would appear to be necessary for this process (Fig. 62.6). Kirk *et al.* [109] showed that 12-month therapy with GHRH (1–29) 20 μg/kg given twice daily by subcutaneous injections promoted linear growth in short children who were not GH insufficient. This improvement in height velocity was followed by a catch-down growth and return to pre-treatment velocity after cessation of therapy.

The reason that twice-daily injections of GHRH are less effective in GH insufficient children may be related to the presentation of GH to the end organ, i.e. a signalling problem, but may also be related to the dual action of GHRH in not only releasing but synthesising adequate amounts of GH. It might be suggested that infrequent administration of GHRH does not lead to optimal synthesis of GH.

Continuous administration

A more practical long-term approach may be a GHRH depot preparation which would combine the advantages of several GH pulses per day with the convenience of infrequent administration. This assumes that SS tone is highly conserved in the patients being treated. This would be necessary to elicit pulsatile GH secretion in the face of continuous exposure of the pituitary gland to GHRH.

Twelve- to twenty-four-hour infusions of GHRH have demonstrated augmentation of naturally occurring GH pulses with no evidence of desensitisation, down-regulation or depletion of the GH pool in normal and GH-insufficient subjects [110–112]. Studies using the subcutaneous route have demonstrated a dose–response relationship between the amount of GHRH infused continuously and the amount of GH produced from the pituitary gland. Continuous subcutaneous GHRH (1–29) at a dose of 60 ng/kg/min has been shown to promote growth in short GH-insufficient children over a 12-month study period [113]. GHRH is more successful in children whose GH secretion is less impaired: GH treatment is better for the more severe cases [107,108,114].

Insulin-like growth factor 1

Experimental studies with the infusion of IGF-1 to promote growth in animals caused increases in bodyweight and body length. However, the growth of the animal is less than would be expected from the level of IGF-1 circulating in the blood, i.e. it is less than that which would be observed had GH treatment been used to produce the same serum IGF-1 level [115,116]. Further, the growth of the organs in the body is quite different in the IGF-1-treated animals.

Several studies have been conducted using IGF-1 in humans. A single intravenous injection of 100 μg/kg given to normal adult male volunteers resulted in hypoglycaemia within 15 min, reaching a nadir at 30 min and returning to normal within 2 hours [117]. Intravenous infusions of IGF-1 at continuous rates of 24 μg/kg/hour in normal men failed to produce significant hypoglycaemia [118]. A 250% increase in serum IGF-1 levels was observed following a 7 day subcutaneous administration of 100 μg/kg/day in healthy adults [119].

An obvious therapeutic use of recombinant IGF-1 therapy is in patients with GH insensitivity. An increase in growth rate in children with this condition has been reported by various workers [120–123].

Side-effects of IGF-1 include troublesome hypoglycaemia, headaches, convulsions and papilloedema. Until some way of preventing these side-effects is found, the use of this mode of treatment must remain limited.

Neurotransmitters

Pharmacological studies of GH secretion have demonstrated that many known neurotransmitters influence GH secretion. Two, dopamine and clonidine, have been studied for their therapeutic potential to promote growth. Huseman *et al.* [124] reported the effects of L-dopa and bromocriptine in children with severe GH insufficiency. A small increase in growth rate was observed, but this in no way equalled that seen with GH treatment in such individuals.

Administration of clonidine, an α_2-adrenoreceptor agonist, to short normal children in the short term resulted in an increase in GH secretion [125]. The effects of its long-term administration on growth have been studied, with confusing results. One group demonstrated an improvement in growth rate in the short term [126], and another, who used a double-blind placebo study, demonstrated no significant effect [127]. An increase in growth rate in children with constitutional delay and short stature treated with clonidine has been documented [128]. Clonidine failed to increase growth rate when administered to a group of short normal children [129]. The role of clonidine and the treatment of short children must at present remain open, and with its sedative and hypotensive effects this cannot be regarded as a useful therapeutic option.

Neuropeptides

In addition to GHRH and SS, the two main neuropeptides controlling GH secretion, several others such as thyrotrophin (TSH)-releasing hormone (TRH) and vasoactive intestinal polypeptide (VIP) are known to influence GH release, though their physiological role is unclear. Recent interest has been centred on a new group of synthetic peptides, known as GH-releasing peptides (GHRPs), capable of inducing massive GH release by an unknown mechanism [130]. GHRPs are synthetic six- or seven-amino-acid peptides which act on non-opiate, non-GHRH receptors on both the hypothalamus and pituitary [131,132]. A new G-protein-coupled receptor for GHRPs and other small GH secretagogues has been identified recently [133]. GHRPs are active following intravenous, subcutaneous, intranasal as well as oral administration. They act synergistically with GHRH [134] and enhance pulsatile GH secretion as demonstrated in the GHRP infusion studies by Huhn *et al.* [135], and remain active after repeated administration [136]. Although the bioavailability of orally and intranasally administered GHRP is only a minute fraction of that following the intravenous route, large doses are well tolerated and sufficient amounts are absorbed to bring about massive growth hormone release. The therapeutic advantage of an orally or intranasally administered GH secretagogue is obvious. Preliminary results in short normal and growth hormone insufficient children using intranasally or subcutaneously administered GHRP are promising [137,138]. No adverse effects of the treatment have been reported.

Anabolic steroids and sex steroids

The majority of children attending growth-disorder clinics are boys with delayed puberty. Following the observation that the growth acceleration seen with anabolic steroids was not dose related but that the advance in skeletal maturation was, the use of these agents to promote growth in such individuals has become established clinical practice.

Fluoxymesteone was one of the first products. Several studies have demonstrated stimulation of linear growth without an acceleration in bone age. The use of these agents in prepubertal children has not been clearly defined. In children with constitutional delay of growth and development, oxandrolone in doses of 1.25 or 2.5 mg/day produces a growth acceleration which is not at the expense of an inappropriate advance in skeletal maturity. In boys with a testicular volume > 5 ml, growth acceleration is maintained and blends with the onset of the spontaneous pubertal growth spurt. However, the acceleration of growth is mainly for psychosocial reasons, and final height does not appear to be enhanced. If the testicular volume is < 5 ml, the acceleration is not sustained, patients revert to their pretreatment growth rate, and several courses of treatment may be required [139–141].

Abnormal liver-function tests in patients treated with anabolic steroids have been reported but the abnormality seems to be benign and reversible on discontinuation of therapy. These effects were seen predominantly in patients treated with large doses of anabolic steroids for aplastic anaemia.

The use of sex steroids in the prepubertal child is not to be recommended. The one exception to this is the child with Turner's syndrome. The absence of the ovary, and with it the loss of oestrogen secretion, may leave these girls at risk of developing osteoporosis. By the age of 9 years osteoporosis can be clearly observed in radiographs of these children. As such, it has been suggested that oestrogen replacement should begin early to prevent bone-mineral loss, or rather, to allow bone-mineral accretion to occur. Introduction of oestrogen treatment at the age of 7 years in doses of 0.5 μg/day leads to a significant increase in growth rate without inducing pubertal changes. The growth rate induced by this low-dose oestrogen treatment is comparable with that observed with oxandrolone alone [87]. The advent of transdermal oestrogen preparations may facilitate the management of children with Turner's syndrome.

Tall stature

Definition

The problems encountered in defining short stature apply equally to tall stature. The height which may be acceptable in adult life must necessarily be a matter of opinion. For boys, heights up to 2 metres are probably acceptable, whereas, girls find a height in excess of 180 cm difficult to accommodate. Cultural background is, therefore, an important factor in determining who is going to require treatment.

The most comprehensive study of the auxology of tall stature has been provided by Dickerman *et al.* [142]. The mean birth length of tall girls and boys was on the 75th centile, and the maximal growth velocity was achieved from birth to 6 months of age. Although there was a gradual decrease in velocity after this time, it remained above the 50th centile until 9 years of age. The end-result was a stature above the 97th height centile in all cases. Like short children, the growth velocity of tall children is never normal, the height velocity centile being always greater than the 50th.

Tall stature is a familiar characteristic in the majority of cases. The diagnoses with which tall stature may be associated, although rare, are in several respects more sinister than those associated with short stature. Figure 62.13 shows a clinical algorithm for the management of tall stature. The principles of assessment differ little from that practised for the individual with short stature. Growth assessment is the key, and the height of the child should be compared with the measured height of the parents in exactly the same way as it is for short stature. Clinical examination will reveal answers to the question as to whether there is an underlying syndrome to be diagnosed, and additional clues may come from the child showing signs of puberty. Caution needs to be exercised with children who are growing fast and in whom

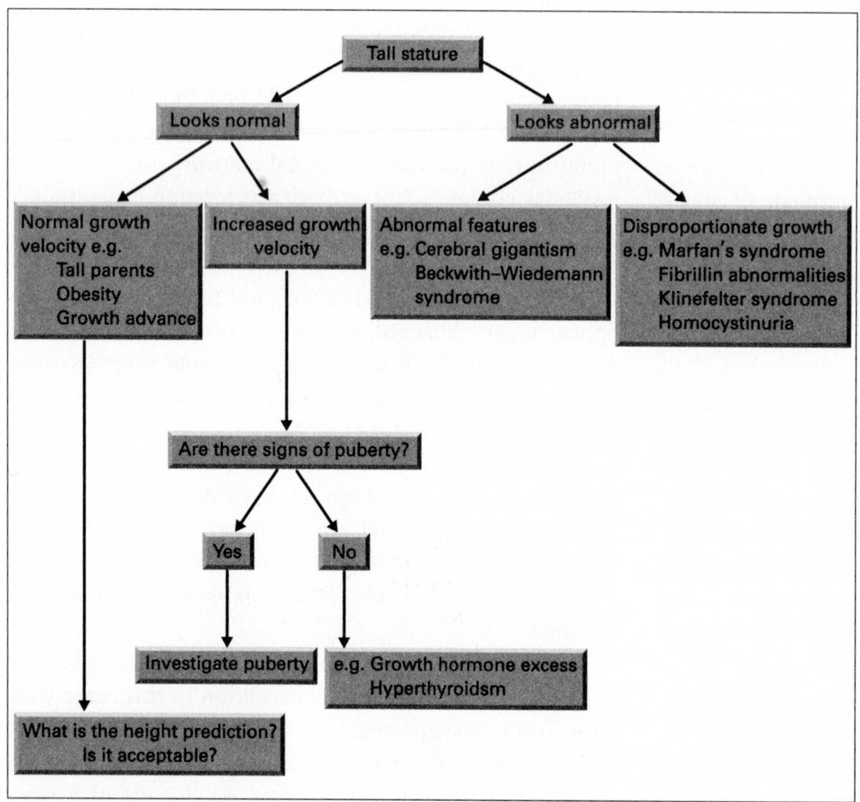

Fig. 62.13 Flow chart for use in the differential diagnosis of tall stature. From [167].

there are no signs of puberty. GH excess and hyperthyroidism are suggested diagnoses in the algorithm, but it is important to realise that although adrenal disease usually presents with the appearance of pubic hair and growth of the phallus, increased growth velocity may be the only complaint initially. Precocious puberty, either gonadotrophin dependent or gonadotrophin independent, is also an important diagnosis to consider, and this is discussed further in the section on puberty and its disorders.

Paediatric textbooks contain descriptions of many of the syndromes associated with tall stature, and the reader is referred to such a text for further information. However, it is worth mentioning the clinical and endocrine features of gigantism, as this helps in understanding the endocrinology of tall stature and how the two may be differentiated.

Gigantism

Acromegaly in adult patients was described by Marie in 1886, while Hutchinson, 14 years later, noted that acromegaly and gigantism were similar diseases occurring in different age groups. The experience of management of children with gigantism is limited, and few clinicians have extensive experience of the condition. Endocrine investigations reveal features characteristic of acromegaly, elevated unstimulated serum GH concentrations, paradoxical GH responses to exogenous administration of thyrotrophin-releasing hormone (TRH), and failure to suppress serum GH concentrations with oral glucose loading. The 24-hour GH secretion in such individuals is very similar to that seen in acromegaly, and this can be a most helpful investigation, particularly when the child is in the pubertal years. Figure 62.14 shows a 24-hour GH profile from a boy with gigantism compared with that obtained from a boy with tall stature of a similar age. It should be noted that the height velocities of these patients were similar but the giant secreted far more GH to achieve this, thus re-emphasising the importance of pulsatility in the attainment of normal growth.

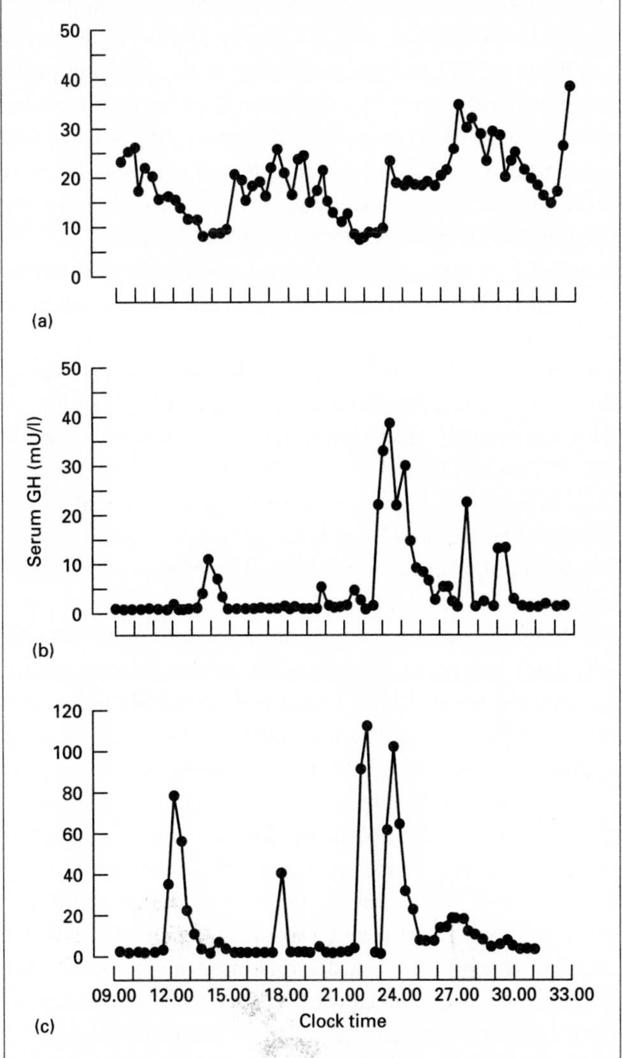

Fig. 62.14 Twenty-four-hour serum growth hormone (GH) concentration profiles in: (a) a 7-year-old boy with pituitary gigantism; (b) a 7-year-old prepubertal tall boy; and (c) a 14-year-old pubertal tall boy.

Endocrinology of tall stature

The investigation of children growing rapidly requires answers to the question of whether the hypothalamo-pituitary–adrenal, –thyroid or –GH axis is involved. Hyperthyroidism is relatively unusual in countries with low iodine intake, and is easily identified by measuring free levels of triiodothyronine (T_3) and thyroxine (T_4). Adrenal disorders, such as congenital or acquired adrenal hyperplasia, a functioning adrenal tumour or Cushing's syndrome, need to be excluded, and a useful screening test is the analysis of a 24–hour urine sample for steroid metabolites (where available). The tall stature and rapid growth of precocious puberty are detailed in Chapter 63.

Growth hormone

As stated above, mid-childhood growth is GH dependent, and during this period, tall children grow with a height velocity greater than their peers by secreting a greater concentration of GH over a 24-hour period. The majority of this secretion occurs during the night, but as age advances secretory episodes can also be observed during the day. Figure 62.14 shows the 24-hour GH secretory profiles from a boy who was prepubertal compared with another tall boy who was at the point of his pubertal growth spurt. It is important to realise that daytime GH secretion is more marked in tall than in small children, and in 13 of the 14 tall children who had 24-hour GH profiles performed by us, morning peaks could be detected, the exception being the youngest patient at 4.5 years [143]. As well as demonstrating greater GH concentrations on a 24-hour profile, tall children also have greater GH response to exercise [144], and to GH-releasing hormone [145], than controls of normal stature.

Because of these observations, it is difficult to interpret the results of pharmacological tests of GH secretion in tall children, as they are performed against a background of endogenous GH secretory activity. This may partly explain the poor association between measures of physiological secretion (stage 4 sleep) and pharmacological tests seen in tall children [143], and why tall children often have elevated unstimulated GH levels. In the study quoted, five of 38 tall children had elevated basal fasting serum GH levels, but all five were pubertal when daytime GH secretion had become most marked.

It has been observed that some constitutionally tall children have biochemical findings reminiscent of acromegaly. In tall children who have frequent daytime GH pulses it is difficult to separate abnormal responses from their normal endogenous secretory patterns. It is likely, therefore, that the paradoxical GH response to TRH is not a pathological disturbance in tall adolescents. In fact, this abnormality lacks specificity; it is seen in acromegaly, anorexia nervosa, chronic renal failure and diabetes mellitus, all conditions associated with elevated GH concentrations. The work of Edge *et al.* [146] has demonstrated quite clearly that 'paradoxical' responses can be predicted from simple analysis of the patient's own endogenous hormonal secretion.

A similar case can be advanced against the likelihood that the failure to suppress GH secretion by glucose administration is abnormal in these tall children. Paradoxical GH responses to oral glucose loading occur in adolescents and in tall pubertal girls, but return to normal in adult life. This could simply be an effect of puberty.

IGF-1 and insulin

Gourmelin *et al.* [147] had demonstrated that serum IGF-1 concentrations rise with age in a manner similar to that in normal subjects, although values are higher in tall children. These values are still elevated in puberty, where tall children have much higher values than controls. Values only return to within the normal range following epiphysial fusion.

Insulin is implicated in the biosynthesis of IGF-1 and is also important in regulating the circulating concentration of IGFBP-1 [148]. Insulin may also act independently of IGF-1; patients with diffuse idiopathic skeletal hyperostosis have normal serum IGF-1 and GH concentrations but display significant elevations of insulin concentrations after a glucose load.

Treatment regimens

As indicated above, the answer to the question 'Who needs treatment?' is highly dependent on the culture that the individual comes from. There are several reasons for treatment. Psychological problems expressed by tall children include difficulty with self-image and rejection by their peer group. A considerable number, particularly girls, express concern about how a tall person is treated by the opposite sex. Tall children may experience problems at school, as it is difficult for many to remember that a 6-year-old child with the stature of a 9-year-old is actually only 6. From the practical point of view, tall children find that they are unable to wear current fashion in clothes and shoes, which further exacerbates the problem. From a medical point of view, a common problem in tall children is that of kyphoscoliosis. In our experience approximately 15% of tall adolescents have some degree of kyphoscoliosis. Since the pubertal growth spurt is likely to make kyphoscoliosis worse, these children deserve consideration for medical treatment.

Height prediction

The measurement of skeletal maturity to predict height is important in the management of tall stature. It bears on the decision of whether or when to embark on therapy, and how to assess the effects. The prediction depends on the adequacy of the assessment of skeletal maturation which is best performed by the clinician. Overall, there is no superiority in any method.

The accuracy of prediction is judged by the size of the residual standard deviation. The standard deviation for a height prediction of girls at a bone age of 12 years is approximately 2.5 cm according to the method of Bayley and Pinneau [149]. The Tanner–Whitehouse method has a standard deviation of 3.5 cm for a 12-year-old boy, and 2.7 cm for a premenarcheal and 2.1 cm for a post-menarcheal 12-year-old girl. The newer Tanner–Whitehouse mark 2 method includes bone age assessment and height predictions of tall and very short individuals, reducing the error in the case of a 12-year-old boy to 3.2 and in the postmenarcheal girl to 1.1 cm [150]. These findings are important to take into account when assessing treatment regimens.

Once height prediction is known then it can be used to determine the timing of pubertal induction. The gain in height during puberty is relatively fixed at 20–30 cm. Therefore, if a final height of 180 cm is desired, puberty needs to be induced at 150 cm. In other words, sex steroid therapy for tall stature simply superimposes the pubertal growth spurt at an earlier time point.

Sex steroids

Oestrogen therapy for tall girls was based on the observation that children with precocious puberty did not become tall adults because premature epiphysial closure occurred. Although the basic tenet was that oestrogen slows growth due to the epiphysial closure, it is more likely that the oestrogen effect on growth is mediated by inhibition of IGF production. Oestrogen in low concentrations augments GH secretion, which may account for the initial spurt of growth seen on the commencement of therapy.

Various oestrogen preparations are available and many clinicians use ethinyl oestradiol continuously, together with a progestogen for 5–7 days every 3 weeks to promote endometrial shedding. Doses of up to 300 μg ethinyl oestradiol per day can be used although recent work suggests that low doses (100 μg/day) are as effective in final height reduction [151–153]. Simply inducing puberty and maintaining on a 20- or 30-μg pill is just as effective. The major factor affecting response is the chronological or skeletal age. The earlier treatment is started, the greater the reduction in final height [154].

Each patient requires regular assessment from the point of view of auxological measurement and also blood-pressure recording. When the height has remained unchanged for two successive measurements, radiography can be performed to check epiphysial fusion. This should include not only hand radiography but also an anteroposterior view of the iliac crests to check for fusion of the ilial apophyses. Unless these have fused, cessation of therapy will lead to a further increase in spinal height.

It is in the area of side-effects of oestrogen therapy that most concern lies. The reported side-effects are low but the long-term effects are difficult to assess. Headaches and nausea, particularly on starting treatment, have frequently been observed. Post-therapeutic amenorrhoea is less common than it is following withdrawal of the contraceptive pill. Fertility has been assessed in a detailed fashion in a large Australian study, and the high dose of oestrogen does not seem to affect reproductive function [155]. De Waal *et al.* showed that pharmacological doses of sex hormones had no long-term effect on reproductive function at a mean follow-up period of 10 years [156].

Thromboembolism, which is a source of concern in patients receiving the contraceptive pill, has only been reported occasionally, but can be devastating when it happens [157].

Long-term side-effects, such as diabetes mellitus, hyperlipidaemia, hypertension and carcinoma, are more difficult to assess. It is in the area of increased risk of gynaecological carcinoma that there is least information and most concern. The recent reports highlighting a 1.4–1.7-fold increased risk of breast cancer by the age of 35 in young girls who have received the oral contraceptive pill for between 5 and 10 years, respectively, is of great concern. Many of the tall children receive higher doses of oestrogen than are contained in the oral contraceptive pill, for periods of up to 5 years. These questions over the safety of oestrogens, and in particular the unanswered question of what may happen with high doses of oestrogen, has led many paediatric endocrinologists to consider other therapeutic options for tall stature.

Experience with testosterone therapy in boys is limited because fewer boys complain of tall stature than girls. Intramuscular injections of testosterone enanthate, 250 mg every 2 weeks, produced a mean reduction in height of 5.7 cm in one study [158]. There is the theoretical hazard of long-term impairment of Leydig-cell function although, practically, this does not seem to be the case.

Bromocriptine

Bromocriptine decreases serum GH levels in the majority of patients with acromegaly, and thus bromocriptine therapy (5 mg/day) has been used in tall children. When the error on height prediction is taken into account, there is little difference between pretreatment and treatment height predictions [159]. Placebo-controlled studies have failed to show a convincing role for bromocriptine in the management of tall stature [160].

Anticholinergic therapy

Acetylcholine is a neurotransmitter involved in the control of GH secretion. The precise mechanism of action is unclear, although evidence is accumulating to support the notion that muscarinic cholinergic antagonists modulate GHRH-induced GH release through changes in SS secretion.

Because the growth spurt of puberty has two endocrine components, sex steroids and GH, a logical approach to the treatment of tall stature would be to abolish the GH secretion, thereby reducing growth velocity and leave the sex steroids free to advance skeletal maturation. The advantage of this mode of therapy would be that prepubertal children could be treated, and as the effect on height reduction is ultimately dependent on how early therapy is commenced, this provides such individuals with a major advantage. It also offers an opportunity to diminish the school problems of tall children. The disadvantages of this approach would be that although long-term growth would be attenuated, spinal growth, which is predominantly sex steroid-dependent, would remain unaffected and maximal height limitation might not be realised.

One of the main problems with anticholinergic therapy is that rebound GH secretion takes place once the half-life of the drug has been exceeded. In addition, when agents such as atropine are used, impairment of short-term memory can result. These problems can be overcome to some extent by using preparations with a longer half-life, such as pirenzepine. Doses of 50 mg twice or three times daily were well tolerated and resulted in a mean reduction in final height of 0.5–1.5 cm, depending on the height prediction method used [161]. The clinical relevance of such a reduction is questionable.

Somatostatin

Intravenous infusion of native SS suppresses GH secretion in normal humans and in patients with acromegaly. Cessation of the infusion induces rebound GH secretion; furthermore, the short half-life limits the use of native SS for the treatment of patients with acromegaly. The development of octreotide, a long acting analogue of SS, has made possible the administration of this medication as a subcutaneous injection which suppresses GH secretion with no rebound secretion. Somatostatin analogues have been used by many groups to reduce the excessive GH secretion seen in acromegaly with the resolution of some of the clinical features. Octreotide also suppresses the 24-hour serum GH concentrations in tall children [162].

The role of subcutaneous administration of SS analogues in the management of children with tall stature has been investigated by Tauber *et al.* Using a regimen of twice-daily subcutaneous injections of 240 µg SS analogue they observed a mean reduction in height prediction over a period of 1 year of 4.9 cm [163]. A reduction in height prediction of between 3 and 5 cm has been observed following the treatment of seven tall children with octreotide using doses of 37.5–50 µg once or twice daily [164]. Octreotide appeared to suppress both GH and insulin secretion, but with the major effect observed on GH. Growth velocity decreases during treatment with octreotide and there are minimal effects on fasting blood glucose and glycated haemoglobin concentrations.

Single nocturnal subcutaneous injections of octreotide, although capable of suppressing GH secretion for some 8 hours, are probably not sufficient to suppress GH secretion during a 24-hour period in pubertal children. For this reason, several of the children have required a twice-daily treatment regimen of 50 µg per injection. Because of the need to give more frequent injections of octreotide during the pubertal growth spurt, a continuous infusion of the analogue seemed a logical alternative. Figure 62.15 shows the effect of an overnight 12-hour injection (50 µg per 12-hour period) on the serum GH concentration profile in an 8-year-old boy. On this treatment regimen his growth rate fell from 8.4 cm/year to 5 cm/year. Two-year follow-up of eight tall children treated with a 12-hour nocturnal infusion of octreotide in a dose of 1–1.5 µg/kg given subcutaneously showed a significant reduction in height prediction in seven subjects

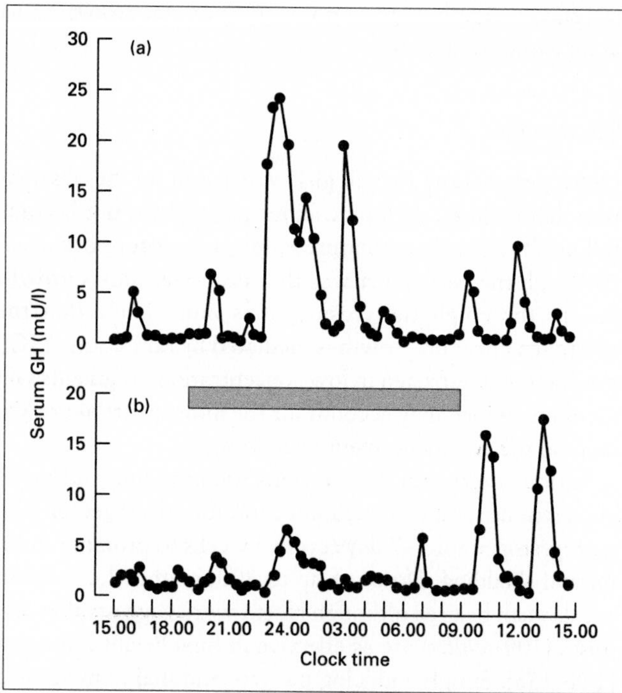

Fig. 62.15 Effect of a continuous infusion of octreotide (SMS 201-995) on growth hormone (GH) secretion in a 8.5-year-old boy: (a) pretreatment; (b) during a 12-hour infusion of 50 µg octreotide.

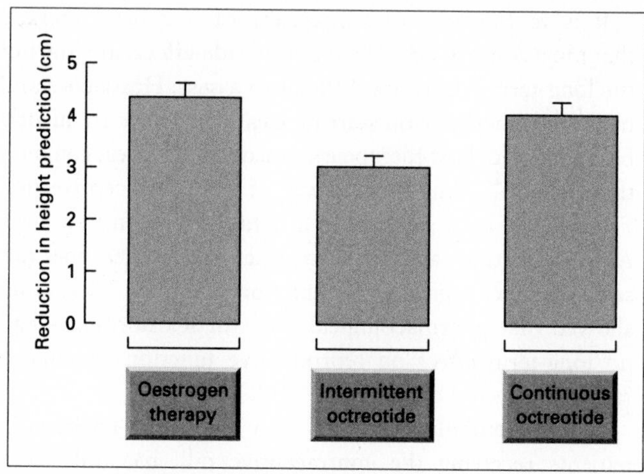

Fig. 62.16 Effects of treating tall girls with octreotide given as a once or twice daily subcutaneous injection compared with a 12-hour overnight infusion. Standard treatment with oestrogens is shown for comparison. Data shown as mean and SEM.

[162]. However, effects of the continuous infusion did not appear to lead a greater reduction in final height than that observed using the subcutaneous injection method given once or twice daily (Fig. 62.16).

It is important to realise when using GH-suppressing agents that growth velocity will not be reduced to zero. This is because of the nature of the asymptotic relationship described earlier in this chapter. The prediction from the asymptote is that as GH secretion approaches or reaches zero, growth is still possible, albeit at a reduced rate. We would predict that in the absence of any GH secretion at all, a growth rate of between 2.8 and 3.8 cm/year would still be observed in prepubertal tall children and a reduction of approximately 50% in pubertal children. A reduction of growth rate of this magnitude, however, would be sufficient to transfer the child from their previous growth centile to one close to the average.

Conclusions

Postnatal growth can be divided into three components: infancy, childhood and puberty. The first component of growth is almost entirely nutrition dependent, the second is GH dependent, and the third is a combination of GH and sex steroids. Therefore, the aetiology of disorders of stature and the investigation and treatment to be recommended depends on the age of the child.

The key to identifying growth disorders, whether resulting in tall or short stature, is careful measurement of height and calculation of growth rate. Departure from height velocities between the 25th and 75th centiles requires an explanation. Growth disorders in childhood leading to poor growth rates will nearly always be due to a disorder of GH secretion, and treatment with GH in the appropriate dose given by daily subcutaneous injection is the recommended approach. It is important to realise that other short children may also benefit in terms of an acceleration of growth rate by treatment with GH, for example girls with Turner's syndrome.

Tall stature can be as disadvantageous as short stature. Care must be taken in investigating such individuals, particularly if they are pubertal, as the endocrinology can resemble that observed in acromegaly. Sex steroids are probably no longer the first line of treatment, and manipulation of the endocrine system may prove to be more acceptable.

References

1 Gordon M, Crouthamel C, Post EM, Richman RA. Psychosocial aspects of constitutional short stature: social competence, behaviour problems, self-esteem and family functioning. *J Pediatr* 1982; **101**: 477–80.

2 Skuse D, Gilmour J, Tian CS, Hindmarsh PC. Psychosocial assessment of children with short stature. *Acta Paediatr Scand* 1994; **406** (Suppl.): 11–16.

3 Hindmarsh PC, Smith PJ, Brook CGD, Matthews DR. The relationship between height velocity and GH secretion in short prepubertal children. *Clin Endocrinol* 1987; **27**: 581–91.

4 Marshall WA. The relationship of variations in children's growth rates to seasonal climatic variations. *Ann Hum Biol* 1975; **2**: 243–50.

5 Russell A. A syndrome of intrauterine dwarfism recognisable at birth with craniofacial dysostosis, disproportionately short arms and other abnormalities. *Proc Roy Soc Med* 1954; **47**: 1040–4.

6 Silver HK. Asymmetry, short stature and variations of sexual development: a syndrome of congenital malformation. *Am J Dis Child* 1964; **107**: 495–515.

7 Duncan PA, Hall JG, Shapiro LP, Vibert BK. Three generation dominant inheritance of the Silver–Russell syndrome. *Am J Med Genet* 1990; **35**: 245–50.

8 Patton MA. Russell–Silver syndrome. *J Med Genet* 1988; **25**: 557–60.

9 Cattanach BM. Parental origin effects in mice. *J Embryol Exp Morphol* 1986; **97**: (Suppl.): 137–50.

10 Hall JG. Unilateral disomy as a possible explanation for Russell–Silver syndrome (letter; comment). *J Med Genet* 1990; **27**: 141–2.

11 Kotzot D, Schmitt S, Bernasconi F *et al.* Uniparental disomy 7 in Silver–Russell syndrome and primordial growth retardation. *Hum Mol Genet* 1995; **4**: 583–7.

12 Turner HH. A syndrome of infantilism, congenital webbed neck and cubitus valgus. *Endocrinology* 1938; **23**: 566–74.

13 Brook CGD, Murset G, Zachmann M, Prader A. Growth in children with 45,XO Turner's syndrome. *Arch Dis Child* 1974; **49**: 789–95.

14 Milner RDG, Burns EC. Investigation of suspected growth hormone deficiency. *Arch Dis Child* 1982; **57**: 944–7.

15 Rose SR, Municchi G, Barnes KM *et al.* Spontaneous growth hormone secretion increases during puberty in normal girls and boys. *J Clin Endocrinol Metab* 1991; **73**: 428–35.

16 Dattani MT, Pringle PJ, Hindmarsh PC, Brook CGD. What is a normal stimulated growth hormone concentration? *J Endocrinol* 1992; **133**: 447–50.

17 Celniker AC, Chen AB, Wert RM, Jr, Sherman BM. Variability in the quantitation of circulating growth hormone using commercial immunoassays. *J Clin Endocrinol Metab* 1989; **68**: 469–76.

18 Goossens M, Brauner R, Czernichow P, Duquesnoy P, Rappaport R. Isolated growth hormone (GH) deficiency type 1A associated with a double deletion in the human GH gene cluster. *J Clin Endocrinol Metab* 1986; **62**: 712–16.

19 Brewer DB. Congenital absence of the pituitary gland and its consequences. *J Pathol Bacteriol* 1957; **73**: 59–67.

20 Stanhope R, Hindmarsh P, Kendall B, Brook CGD. High resolution CT scanning of the pituitary gland in growth disorders. *Acta Paediatr Scand* 1986; **75**: 779–86.

21 Barinaga M, Yamonoto G, Rivier C, Vale W, Evans R, Rosenfeld MG. Transcriptional regulation of growth hormone gene expression by growth hormone-releasing factor. *Nature* 1983; **306**: 84–5.

22 Mayo KE, Hammer RE, Swanson LW, Brinster RL, Rosenfeld MG, Evans RM. Dramatic pituitary hyperplasia in transgenic mice expressing a human growth hormone-releasing factor gene. *Mol Endocrinol* 1988; **2**: 606–12.

23 Eicher EM, Beamer WG. Inherited ateliotic dwarfism in mice.

Characteristics of the mutation, little, on chromosome 6. *J Hered* 1976; **67**: 87–91.
24 Godfrey P, Rahal JO, Beamer WG, Copeland NG, Jenkins NA, Mayo KE. GHRH receptor of little mice contains a missense mutation in the extracellular domain that disrupts receptor function. *Nature Genet* 1993; **4**: 227–32.
25 Lin SC, Lin CR, Gukovsky I, Lusis AJ, Sawchenko PE, Rosenfeld MG. Molecular basis of the little mouse phenotype and implications for cell-specific growth. *Nature* 1993; **364**: 208–13.
26 Snell GD. Dwarf, a new mendelian recessive character of the house mouse. *Proc Natl Acad Sci USA* 1929; **15**: 733–4.
27 Schaible R, Gowen JW. A new dwarf mouse. *Genetics* 1961; **46**: 896.
28 Green McIn, Lyon M, Searly A, eds. *Genetic Variants and Strains of the Laboratory Mouse*. Oxford: Oxford University Press, 1989: 12–403.
29 Yoshimoto M, Kinoshita E, Baba T *et al.* A case of severe pituitary dwarfism associated with prolactin and thyroid stimulating hormone deficiencies. *Acta Paediatr Scand* 1990; **79**: 1247–51.
30 Wit JM, Drayer NM, Jansen M *et al.* Total deficiency of growth hormone and prolactin, and partial deficiency of thyroid stimulating hormone in two Dutch families: a new variant of hereditary pituitary deficiency. *Horm Res* 1989; **32**: 170–7.
31 Zhou X, Benson KF, Ashar HR, Chada K. Mutation responsible for the mouse pygmy phenotype in the developmentally regulated factor HMGI-C. *Nature* 1995; **376**: 771–4.
32 Hayek A, Peake GT, Greenberg RE. A new syndrome of short stature due to biologically inactive but immunoreactive growth hormone. *Pediatr Res* 1978; **12**: 413.
33 Valenta LJ, Sigel MB, Lesniak MA *et al.* Pituitary dwarfism in a patient with circulating abnormal growth hormone polymers. *N Engl J Med* 1985; **312**: 214–17.
34 Illig R, Prader A, Ferrandez A, Zachmann M. Hereditary prenatal growth hormone deficiency with increased tendency to growth hormone antibody formation. *Symp Deutsches Gesellschaft Endokrinol* 1970; **16**: 246–7.
35 Amselem S, Duquesnoy P, Goossens M. Molecular basis of Laron dwarfism. *Trends Endocrinol Metab* 1991; **2**: 35–40.
36 Johnson RJ. Diminution of pulsatile growth hormone secretion in the domestic fowl (*Gallus domesticus*): evidence of sexual dimorphism. *J Endocrinol* 1988; **119**: 101–9.
37 Hindmarsh PC, Matthews DR, Brook CGD. Growth hormone secretion in children determined by time series analysis. *Clin Endocrinol* 1988; **29**: 35–44.
38 Mauras N, Blizzard RM, Link K, Johnson ML, Rogol AD, Veldhuis JD. Augmentation of growth hormone secretion during puberty: evidence for a pulse amplitude-modulated phenomenon. *J Clin Endocrinol Metab* 1987; **64**: 596–601.
39 Sun Y, Xi Y, Fenogio CM *et al.* The effect of age on the number of pituitary cells immunoreactive to growth hormone and prolactin. *Hum Pathol* 1984; **15**: 169–80.
40 Schriock EA, Lustig RH, Rosenthal SM, Kaplan SL, Grumbach MM. Effect of growth hormone (GH)-releasing hormone (GHRH) on plasma GH in relation to magnitude and duration of GH deficiency in 26 children and adults with isolated GH deficiency or multiple pituitary hormone deficiencies: evidence for hypothalamic GHRH deficiency. *J Clin Endocrinol Metab* 1984; **58**: 1043–9.
41 Kajiwara S, Igarashi N, Imura E, Sato T. Correlation between pituitary growth hormone reserve and degree of growth failure in children with short stature. *Eur J Pediatr* 1988; **147**: 584–7.
42 Silbergeld A, Litwin A, Bruchis S, Varsano I, Laron Z. Insulin-like growth factor I (IGF-I) in healthy children, adolescents and adults as determined by a radioimmunoassay specific for the synthetic 53–70 peptide region. *Clin Endocrinol* 1986; **25**: 67–74.
43 Migeon CJ, Keller AR, Lawrence B, Shepard TH. Dehydroepiandrosterone and androsterone levels in human plasma. *J Clin Endocrinol Metab* 1957; **17**: 1051–61.
44 Faiman C, Winter JSD. Gonadotrophins and sex hormone patterns in pubescence: clinical data. In: Grumbach MM, Grove GD, Mayer FE, eds. *Control of the Onset of Puberty*. New York: Wiley, 1974: 126–35.
45 Ackland FM, Stanhope R, Eyre C, Hamill G, Jones J, Preece MA. Physiological growth hormone secretion in children with short stature and intra-uterine growth retardation. *Horm Res* 1988; **30**: 241–5.
46 Sukegawa I, Hizuka N, Takano K *et al.* Measurement of nocturnal urinary growth hormone values. *Acta Endocrinol* 1989; **121**: 290–6.
47 Wise PH, Burnet RB, Geary TD, Berriman H. Selective impairment of growth hormone response to physiological stimuli. *Arch Dis Child* 1975; **50**: 210–14.
48 Spiliotis BE, August GP, Hung W, Sonis W, Mendelson W, Bercu BB. Growth hormone neurosecretory dysfunction. A treatable cause of short stature. *JAMA* 1984; **251**: 2223–30.
49 Bercu BB, Root AW, Shulman DI. Preservation of dopaminergic and alpha-adrenergic function in children with growth hormone neurosecretory dysfunction. *J Clin Endocrinol Metab* 1986; **63**: 968–73.
50 Miller JD, Tannenbaum GS, Colle E, Guyda HJ. Daytime pulsatile growth hormone secretion during childhood and adolescence. *J Clin Endocrinol Metab* 1982; **55**: 989–4.
51 Devesa J, Lima L, Lois N *et al.* Reasons for the variability in growth hormone (GH) responses to GHRH challenge: the endogenous hypothalamic-somatotroph rhythm (HSR). *Clin Endocrinol* 1989; **30**: 367–77.
52 Veldhuis JD, Johnson ML. Cluster analysis: a simple versatile and robust algorithm for endocrine pulse detection. *Am J Physiol* 1986; **250**: E486–93.
53 Turner RC, Grayburn JA, Newman GB, Nabarro JDN. Measurement of the insulin delivery rate in man. *J Clin Endocrinol Metab* 1971; **33**: 279–86.
54 Veldhuis JD, Carlson ML, Johnson ML. The pituitary gland secretes in bursts: Appraising the nature of glandular secretory impulses by simultaneous multiple-parameter deconvolution of plasma hormone concentrations. *Proc Nat Acad Sci USA* 1987; **84**: 7686–90.
55 Matthews DR, Hindmarsh PC, Pringle PJ, Brook CGD. A distribution method for analysing the baseline of pulsatile endocrine signals as exemplified by the 24 hour growth hormone profiles. *Clin Endocrinol* 1991; **35**: 245–52.
56 Pincus SM, Cummins TR, Haddad GG. Heart rate control in normal and aborted SIDS infants. *Am J Physiol* 1993; **264**: R638–46.
57 Pincus SM, Goldberger AL. Physiological time-series analysis: What does regularity quantify? *Am J Physiol* 1994; **266**: H1643–56.
58 Prank K, Harms H, Dammig M, Brabant G, Mitschke F, Hesch R-F. Is there low-dimensional chaos in pulsatile secretion of parathyroid hormone in normal human subjects? *Am J Physiol*

1994; **266**: E653–8.

59 Mandelbrot BB. *The Fractal Geometry of Nature*. New York: Freeman, 1983.

60 Katz MJ, George EB. Fractals and the analysis of growth paths. *Bull Math Biol* 1985; **47**: 273–86.

61 Glenny RW, Robertson HT. Fractal properties of pulmonary blood flow heterogeneity. *J Appl Physiol* 1991; **70**: 1024–30.

62 Yeragani VK, Srinivasan K, Vempati S, Pohl R, Balon R. Fractal dimension of heart rate time series in an effective measure of autonomic function. *J Appl Physiol* 1993; **75**: 2429–38.

63 White P. *Diabetes in Childhood and Adolescence*. Philadelphia: Lea and Febiger, 1932.

64 Raben MS. Treatment of a pituitary dwarf with human growth hormone. *J Clin Endocrinol Metab* 1958; **18**: 901–3.

65 Soyka ZF, Ziskind A, Crawford JD. Treatment of short stature in children and adolescents with human pituitary growth hormone (Raben). *N Engl J Med* 1964; **271**: 754–64.

66 Prader A, Zachmann M, Poley JR, Illig R, Szeky J. Long-term treatment with human growth hormone (Raben) in small doses. Evaluation of 18 hypopituitary patients. *Helv Paediatr Acta* 1967; **22**: 423–40.

67 Tanner JM, Whitehouse RH, Hughes PCR, Vince FP. Effect of human growth hormone treatment for 1 to 7 years on growth of 100 children with growth hormone deficiency, low birth weight, inherited smallness, Turner's syndrome and other complaints. *Arch Dis Child* 1971; **46**: 746–82.

68 Milner RD, Preece MA, Tanner JM. Growth in height compared with advancement in skeletal maturity in patients treated with human growth hormone. *Arch Dis Child* 1980; **55**: 461–6.

69 Burns EC, Tanner JM, Preece MA, Cameron N. Final height and pubertal development in 55 children with idiopathic growth hormone deficiency, treated for between 2 and 25 years with human growth hormone. *Eur J Pediatr* 1981; **137**: 155–64.

70 Kowarski AA, Schneider J, Ben Galim E, Weldon VV, Daughaday WH. Growth failure with normal serum RIA-GH and low somatomedin activity: somatomedin restoration and growth acceleration after exogenous GH. *J Clin Endocrinol Metab* 1978; **47**: 461–4.

71 Grunt JA, Howard CP, Daughaday WH. Comparison of growth and somatomedin C responses following growth hormone treatment in children with small-for-date short stature, significant idiopathic short stature and hypopituitarism. *Acta Endocrinol (Copenh)* 1984; **106**: 168–74.

72 Bierich JR, Potthoff K. Die Spontansekretion bei der konstitutionellen Entwicklungsverzögerung und der frühnormalen Pubertät. *Monatsschr Kinderheilkd* 1979; **127**: 561–5.

73 Rudman D, Kurtner MH, Blackston RD, Jansen RD, Patterson JD. Normal variant short stature: subclassification based on response to exogenous growth hormone. *J Clin Endocrinol Metab* 1979; **49**: 92–9.

74 Dattani MT, Hindmarsh PC, Pringle PJ, Brook CGD, Marshall NJ. Measurement of growth hormone bioactivity in patient serum using an eluted stain bioassay. *J Clin Endocrinol Metab* 1995; **80**: 2675–83.

75 Foster CM, Borondy M, Padmanabhan V *et al.* Bioactivity of human growth hormone in serum: validation of an in vitro bioassay. *Endocrinology* 1993; **132**: 2073–82.

76 Frazer T, Gavin JR, Daughaday WH, Hillman RE, Weldon VV. Growth hormone dependent growth failure. *J Pediatr* 1982; **101**: 12–15.

77 Van Vliet G, Styne DM, Kaplan SL, Grumbach MM. Growth hormone treatment for short stature. *N Engl J Med* 1983; **309**: 1016–22.

78 Gertner JM, Genel M, Gianfredi SP *et al.* Prospective clinical trial of human growth hormone in short children without growth hormone deficiency. *J Pediatr* 1984; **104**: 172–6.

79 Carracosa A, Vincens-Calvet E, Audi L, Gusinye M, Albisu M, Potau N. Chronic growth retardation with normal growth hormone response to provocative stimuli and low somatomedin activity: long-term therapy with human growth hormone. *Acta Paediatr Scand* 1987; **76**: 489–94.

80 Wit JM, Rietveld DH, Drop SL *et al.* A controlled trial of methionyl growth hormone therapy in prepubertal children with short stature, subnormal growth rate and normal growth hormone response to secretagogues. Dutch Growth Hormone Working Group. *Acta Paediatr Scand* 1989; **78**: 426–35.

81 Rudman D, Kutner MH, Blackston RD, Cushman RA, Bain RP. Children with normal variant short stature: treatment with human growth hormone for six months. *J Clin Endocrinol Metab* 1982; **35**: 665–70.

82 Hindmarsh PC, Brook CGD. Effect of growth hormone on short normal children. *Br Med J* 1987; **295**: 573–7.

83 Hindmarsh PC, Brook CGD. Final height in short normal children treated with growth hormone. *Lancet* 1996; **348**: 13–16.

84 Loche S, Cambiaso P, Setzu S *et al.* Final height after growth hormone therapy in non-growth-hormone-deficient children with short stature. *J Pediatr* 1994; **125**: 196–200.

85 Daubeney PEF, McCaughey ES, Chase C *et al.* Cardiac effects of growth hormone in short normal children: results after four years of treatment. *Arch Dis Child* 1995; **72**: 337–9.

86 Barton JS, Hindmarsh PC, Preece MA, Brook CGD. Blood pressure and the renin–angiotensin–aldosterone system in children receiving recombinant human growth hormone. *Clin Endocrinol* 1993; **38**: 245–51.

87 Ross JL, Long LM, Loriaux DL, Cutler GB. Growth hormone secretory dynamics in Turner syndrome. *J Pediatr* 1985; **106**: 202–6.

88 Rosenfeld RG, Frane J, Attie KM *et al.* Six-year results of a randomized, prospective trial of human growth hormone and oxandrolone in Turner syndrome. *J Pediatr* 1992; **121**: 49–55.

89 Rosenfeld RG. Growth hormone therapy in Turner's syndrome: an update on final height. Genentech National Cooperative Study Group. *Acta Paediatr* 1992; **383**(Suppl.): 3–6.

90 Rongen Westerlaken C, Wit JM, Drop SL *et al.* Methionyl human growth hormone in Turner's syndrome. *Arch Dis Child* 1988; **63**: 1211–17.

91 Stanhope R, Preece MA, Hamill G. Does growth hormone treatment improve final height attainment of children with intrauterine growth retardation? *Arch Dis Child* 1991; **66**: 1180–3.

92 Darendeliler F, Hindmarsh PC, Preece MA, Coz L, Brook CGD. Growth hormone increases rate of pubertal maturation. *Acta Endocrinol* 1990; **122**: 414–16.

93 Stanhope R, Ackland F, Hamill G, Clayton J, Jones J, Preece MA. Physiological growth hormone secretion and response to growth hormone treatment in children with short stature and intrauterine growth retardation. *Acta Paediatr Scand* 1989; **349** (Suppl.): 47–52.

94 Jansson J-O, Albertsson-Wikland K, Eden S, Thorngren K-G, Isaksson O. Circumstantial evidence for a role of the secretory pattern of growth hormone in control of body growth. *Acta*

Endocrinol (Copenh) 1982; **99**: 24–30.

95 Preece MA, Tanner JM, Whitehouse RH, Cameron N. Dose dependence of growth response to human growth hormone in growth hormone deficiency. *J Clin Endocrinol Metab* 1976; **42**: 477–83.

96 Frasier SD, Costin G, Lippe BM, Aceto T, Bunger PF. A dose–response curve for human growth hormone. *J Clin Endocrinol Metab* 1981; **53**: 1213–17.

97 Wit JM, Faber JA, Van den Brande JL. Growth response to human growth hormone treatment in children with partial and total growth hormone deficiency. *Acta Paediatr Scand* 1986; **75**: 767–73.

98 Milner RD, Russell Fraser T, Brook CGD *et al.* Experience with human growth hormone in Great Britain: the report of the MRC Working Party. *Clin Endocrinol* 1979; **11**: 15–38.

99 Kastrup KW, Christiansen JS, Andersen JK, Orskov H. Increased growth rate following transfer to daily sc administration from three weekly im injections of hGH in growth hormone deficient children. *Acta Endocrinol (Copenh)* 1983; **104**: 148-52.

100 Albertsson-Wikland K, Westphal O, Westgren U. Daily subcutaneous administration of human growth hormone in growth hormone deficient children. *Acta Paediatr Scand* 1986; **75**: 89–97.

101 Moore WV, Kaplan S, Raiti S. Comparison of dose frequency of human growth hormone in treatment of organic and idiopathic hypopituitarism. *J Pediatr* 1987; **110**: 144–8.

102 Smith PJ, Hindmarsh PC, Brook CGD. The contribution of dose and frequency of administration to the therapeutic effect of growth hormone. *Arch Dis Child* 1988; **63**: 491–4.

103 Thorner MO, Reschke J, Chitwood J *et al.* Acceleration of growth in two children treated with human growth hormone-releasing factor. *N Engl J Med* 1985; **312**: 4–9.

104 Smith PJ, Brook CGD, Rivier J, Vale W, Thorner MO. Nocturnal pulsatile growth hormone releasing hormone treatment in growth hormone deficiency. *Clin Endocrinol* 1986; **25**: 35–44.

105 Hummelink R, Rohwedder R, Sippell WG. Nine months' subcutaneous therapy with synthetic growth hormone releasing factor in children with short stature. *Acta Paediatr Scand* 1987; **331** (Suppl.): 48–52.

106 Ross RJ, Rodda C, Tsagarakis S *et al.* Treatment of growth-hormone deficiency with growth-hormone-releasing hormone. *Lancet* 1987; **1**: 5–8.

107 Smith PJ, Brook CGD. GHRH or GH treatment in GH insufficient children. *Arch Dis Child* 1988; **63**: 629–34.

108 Wit JM, Otten BJ, Waelkens JJ *et al.* Short-term effect on growth of two doses of GRF 1–44 in children with growth hormone deficiency: comparison with growth induced by methionyl-GH administration. *Horm Res* 1987; **27**: 181–9.

109 Kirk JMW, Trainer PJ, Majrowski WH, Murphy J, Savage MO, Besser GM. Treatment with GHRH (1–29)NH_2 in children with idiopathic short stature induces a sustained increase in growth velocity. *Clin Endocrinol* 1994; **41**: 487–93.

110 Hulse JA, Rosenthal SM, Cuttler L, Kaplan SL, Grumbach MM. The effect of pulsatile administration, continuous infusion, and diurnal variation on the growth hormone (GH) response to GH-releasing hormone in normal men. *J Clin Endocrinol Metab* 1986; **63**: 872–8.

111 Rochiccioli PE, Tauber MT, Uboldi F, Coude FX, Morre M. Effect of overnight constant infusion of human growth hormone (GH)-releasing hormone-(1–44) on 24-hour GH secretion in children with partial GH deficiency. *J Clin Endocrinol Metab* 1986; **63**: 1100–5.

112 Brain C, Hindmarsh PC, Brook CGD, Matthews DR. Continuous subcutaneous growth hormone releasing factor analogue augments growth hormone secretion in normal male subjects with no desensitisation of the somatotroph. *Clin Endocrinol* 1988; **28**: 543–9.

113 Brain CE, Hindmarsh PC, Brook CGD. Continuous subcutaneous GHRH (1–29) NH2 promotes growth over 1 year in short slowly growing children. *Clin Endocrinol* 1990; **32**: 153–63.

114 Butenandt O, Staudt B. Comparison of growth hormone releasing hormone therapy and growth hormone therapy in growth hormone deficiency. *Eur J Pediatr* 1989; **148**: 393–5.

115 Isgaard J, Nilsson A, Lindahl A, Jansson JO, Isaksson OG. Effects of local administration of GH and IGF-1 on longitudinal bone growth in rats. *Am J Physiol* 1986; **250**: E367–72.

116 Skottner A, Clark RG, Robinson IC, Fryklund L. Recombinant human insulin-like growth factor: testing the somatomedin hypothesis in hypophysectomized rats. *J Endocrinol* 1987; **112**: 123–32.

117 Guler H-P, Zapf J, Froesch ER. Short-term metabolic effects of recombinant human insulin-like growth factor 1 in healthy adults. *N Engl J Med* 1987; **317**: 137–40.

118 Guler HP, Schmid C, Zapf J, Froesch ER. Effects of recombinant insulin-like growth factor I on insulin secretion and renal function in normal human subjects. *Proc Natl Acad Sci USA* 1989; **86**: 2868–72.

119 Takano K, Hizuka N, Shizume K, Asakawa K, Fukuda I, Demura H. Repeated sc administration of recombinant human insulin-like growth factor I (IGF-I) to human subjects for 7 days. *Growth Regul* 1991; **1**: 23–8.

120 Walker JL, Van Wyk JJ, Underwood LE. Stimulation of statural growth by recombinant insulin-like growth factor I in a child with growth hormone insensitivity syndrome (Laron type). *J Pediatr* 1992; **121**: 641–6.

121 Laron Z, Anin S, Klipper-aurbach Y, Klinger B. Effects of insulin-like growth factor on linear growth, head circumference, and body fat in patients with Laron-type dwarfism. *Lancet* 1992; **339**: 1258–61.

122 Savage MO, Wilton P, Ranke MB *et al.* Therapeutic response to recombinant IGF-1 in thirty two patients with growth hormone insensitivity. *Pediatr Res* 1993; **33**: (Suppl. abstract 17).

123 Wilton P. Treatment with recombinant human insulin-like growth factor I of children with growth hormone receptor deficiency (Laron syndrome). Kabi Pharmacia Study Group on Insulin-like Growth Factor I Treatment in Growth Hormone Insensitivity Syndromes. *Acta Paediatr* 1992; **383** (Suppl.): 137–42.

124 Huseman CA, Hassing JM, Sibilia MG. Endogenous dopaminergic dysfunction: a novel form of human growth hormone deficiency and short stature. *J Clin Endocrinol Metab* 1986; **62**: 484–90.

125 Ghigo E, Arvat E, Nicolosi M *et al.* Acute clonidine administration potentiates spontaneous diurnal, but not nocturnal, growth hormone secretion in normal short children. *J Clin Endocrinol Metab* 1990; **71**: 433–5.

126 Pintor C, Cella SG, Loche S *et al.* Clonidine treatment for short stature. *Lancet* 1987; **1**: 1226–30.

127 Pescovitz OH, Tan E. Lack of benefit of clonidine treatment for short stature in a double-blind, placebo-controlled trial. *Lancet* 1988; **2**: 874–7.

128 Castro Magana M, Angulo M, Fuentes B, Castelar ME, Canas A, Espinoza B. Effect of prolonged clonidine administration on growth

hormone concentrations and rate of linear growth in children with constitutional growth delay. *J Pediatr* 1986; **109**: 784–7.

129 Allen DB. Effects of nightly clonidine administration on growth velocity in short children without growth hormone deficiency: a double-blind, placebo-controlled study. *J Pediatr* 1993; **122**: 32–6.

130 Bowers CY, Momany FA, Reynolds GA, Hong A. On the *in vitro* and *in vivo* activity of a new synthetic hexapeptide that acts on the pituitary to specifically release growth hormone. *Endocrinology* 1984; **114**: 1537–45.

131 Bowers CY, Sartor AO, Reynolds GA, Badger TM. On the actions of the growth hormone-releasing hexapeptide, GHRP. *Endocrinology* 1991; **128**: 2027–35.

132 Bowers CY. GH releasing peptides—structure and kinetics. *J Pediatr Endocrinol* 1993; **6**: 21–31.

133 Pong S-S, Chaung L-YP, Dean DC, Nargund RP, Patchett AA, Smith RG. Identification of a new G-protein-linked receptor for growth hormone secretagogues. *Mol Endocrinol* 1996; **10**: 57–61.

134 Bowers CY, Reynolds GA, Durham D, Barrera CM, Pezzoli SS, Thorner MO. Growth hormone (GH)-releasing peptide stimulates GH release in normal men and acts synergistically with GH-releasing hormone. *J Clin Endocrinol Metab* 1990; **70**: 975–82.

135 Huhn WC, Hartman ML, Pezzoli SS, Thorner MO. Twenty-four-hour growth hormone (GH)-releasing peptide (GHRH) infusion enhances pulsatile GH secretion and specifically attenuates the response to a subsequent GHRP bolus. *J Clin Endocrinol Metab* 1993; **76**: 1202–8.

136 Massoud AF, Hindmarsh PC, Brook CGD. The effect of repeated administration of hexarelin, a growth hormone releasing peptide, and growth hormone releasing hormone responsivity. *Clin Endocrinol* 1996; **44**: 555–62.

137 Laron Z, FRenkel J, Deghenghi R, Snin S, Klinger B, Silbergeld A. Intranasal administration of the GHRP hexarelin accelerates growth in short children. *Clin Endocrinol* 1995; **43**: 631–5.

138 Mericq V, Cassorta F, Salazar T *et al.* Increased growth velocity during prolonged GHRP-2 administration to growth hormone deficient children. *Proceedings of the 77th Annual Meeting of the American Endocrine Society.* Washington DC: The Endocrine Society Press, 1995: 85.

139 Stanhope R, Brook CGD. Oxandrolone in low dose for constitutional delay of growth and puberty in boys. *Arch Dis Child* 1985; **60**: 379–81.

140 Hochberg Z, Korman S. Oxandrolone therapy in boys of short stature. *J Pediatr Endocrinol* 1987; **2**: 115–20.

141 Clayton PE, Shalet SM, Price DA, Addison GM. Growth and growth hormone responses to oxandrolone in boys with constitutional delay of growth and puberty (CDGP). *Clin Endocrinol* 1988; **29**: 123–30.

142 Dickerman Z, Loewinger J, Laron Z. The pattern of growth in children with constitutional tall stature from birth. *Acta Paediatr Scand* 1984; **73**: 530–6.

143 Hindmarsh PC, Stanhope R, Kendall BE, Brook CGD. Tall stature: a clinical, endocrinological and radiological study. *Clin Endocrinol* 1986; **25**: 223–31.

144 Greene SA, Torresani T, Prader A. Growth hormone response to a standardised exercise test in relation to puberty and stature. *Arch Dis Child* 1987; **62**: 53–6.

145 Batrinos M, Georgiadis E, Panitsa Faflia C, Stratigopoulos S. Increased GH response to GHRH in normal tall men. *Clin Endocrinol (Oxf)* 1989; **30**: 13–17.

146 Edge JA, Human DH, Matthews DR, Dunger DB. Spontaneous growth hormone (GH) pulsatility is the major determinant of GH release after thyrotrophin-releasing hormone in adolescent diabetics. *Clin Endocrinol* 1989; **30**: 397–404.

147 Gourmelin M, Le Bouc Y, Girard F, Binoux M. Serum levels of insulin-like growth factor (IGF) and IGF binding protein in constitutionally tall children and adolescents. *J Clin Endocrinol Metab* 1984; **59**: 1197–203.

148 Suikkari AM, Koivisto VA, Rutanen EM, Yki-Jarvinen H, Koronen SL, Seppala M. Insulin regulates the serum levels of low molecular weight insulin-like growth factor-binding protein. *J Clin Endocrinol Metab* 1984; **66**: 266–72.

149 Bayley N, Pinneau SR. Tables for predicting adult height from skeletal age. Revised for use with the Greulich–Lyle hand standards. *J Pediatr* 1952; **40**: 423–41.

150 Tanner JM, Whitehouse RH, Cameron N *et al.* Assessment of skeletal maturity and prediction of adult height (TW2 method). London: Academic Press, 1983.

151 Bierich JD, Schoenberg D. Hormonal treatment of familial tall stature. *Acta Paediatr Scand* 1973; **62**: 90–5.

152 Crawford JD. Treatment of tall girls with estrogen. *Pediatrics* 1978; **62**: 1189–201.

153 Sorgo W, Scholler K, Heinze F, Heinze E, Teller WM. Critical analysis of height reduction in oestrogen-treated tall girls. *Eur J Pediatr* 1984; **142**: 260–5.

154 Ignatius A, Lenko HL, Perheentupa J. Oestrogen treatment of tall girls: effect decreases with age. *Acta Paediatr Scand* 1991; **80**: 712–17.

155 Wettenhall HNB. The tall child. In: Brook CGD, ed. *Clinical Paediatric Endocrinology*. Oxford: Blackwell Scientific Publications, 1981: 134–40.

156 de Waal WJ, Torn M, de Muinck Keizer-Schrama SMPF, Aarsen RSR, Drop SLS. Long term sequelae of sex steroid treatment in the management of constitutionally tall stature. *Arch Dis Child* 1995; **73**: 311–15.

157 Werder EA, Waibel P, Sege D, Flüry R. Severe thrombosis during oestrogen treatment for tall stature. *Eur J Pediatr* 1990; **149**: 389–90.

158 Prader A, Zachmann M. Treatment of excessively tall girls and boys with sex hormones. *Pediatrics* 1978; **62**: 1202–10.

159 Schwarz HP, Joss EE, Zuppinger KA. Bromocriptine treatment in adolescent boys with familial tall stature: a pair-matched controlled study. *J Clin Endocrinol Metab* 1987; **65**: 136–40.

160 Schoenle EJ, Theintz G, Torresani T, Prader A, Illig R, Sizonenko PC. Lack of bromocriptine-induced reduction of predicted height in tall adolescents. *J Clin Endocrinol Metab* 1987; **65**: 355–8.

161 Hindmarsh PC, Pringle PJ, Brook CGD. Cholinergic muscarinic blockade produces short-term suppression of growth hormone secretion in children with tall stature. *Clin Endocrinol* 1988; **29**: 289–96.

162 Hindmarsh PC, Pringle PJ, Stanhope R, Brook CGD. The effect of a continuous infusion of a somatostatin analogue (octreotide) for two years on growth hormone secretion and height prediction in tall children. *Clin Endocrinol* 1995; **42**: 509–15.

163 Tauber MT, Tauber JP, Vigoni F, Harris AG, Rochicchioli P. Effect of the long-acting somatostatin analogue SMS 201–995 on growth rate and reduction of predicted adult height in ten tall adolescents. *Acta Paediatr Scand* 1990; **79**: 176–81.

164 Hindmarsh PC, Pringle PJ, Di Silvio L, Brook CGD. A preliminary

report on the role of somatostatin analogue (SMS 201–995) in the management of children with tall stature. *Clin Endocrinol* 1990; **32**: 83–91.

165 Hindmarsh PC, Brook CGD. Short stature and growth hormone deficiency. *Clin Endocrinol* 1995; **43**: 133–42.

166 Brook CGD. *Growth Assessment in Childhood and Adolescence.* Oxford: Blackwell Scientific Publications, 1982: 54.

167 Brook CGD (ed.) *Clinical Paediatric Endocrinology*, 2nd edn. Oxford: Blackwell Scientific Publications, 1989: 70–130.

168 Ranke MB, Stubbe P, Majewski F, Bierich JR. Spontaneous growth in Turner's syndrome. *Acta Paediatr Scand* 1988; **343** (Suppl.): 22–30.

169 Thorner MO, Rogol AD, Blizzard RM. Acceleration of growth rate in growth hormone-deficient children treated with human growth hormone-releasing hormone. *Pediatr Res* 1988; **24**: 145–51.

170 Tanner JM, Whitehouse RH. Clinical longitudinal standards for height, weight, height velocity, weight velocity and stages of puberty. *Arch Dis Child* 1976; **51**(3): 170–9.

CHAPTER 63

Premature sexual development

N.A. Bridges and C.G.D. Brook

The physiology of normal puberty

At the start of the second decade of life most children develop secondary sexual characteristics and attain reproductive capability. This is accompanied by a period of rapid growth and skeletal maturation, the pubertal growth spurt. The first sign of puberty in a girl is usually breast development and in boys an increase in testicular volume. Three per cent of normal girls have breast development associated with the onset of puberty before the age of 9 years, and 3% of normal boys acquire a testicular volume of 4 ml before their 10th birthday.

The activity of the hypothalamo-pituitary–gonadal axis changes with age (see also Chapter 48). Gonadotrophin secretion has been demonstrated in the fetus in the 17th week of gestation [1]. In the neonatal period there is pulsatile gonadotrophin secretion [2] followed by a fall in secretion with age. The nadir is reached at about 7 years of age, although some pulsatile gonadotrophin secretion can be demonstrated in children at all ages [3]. Prior to the physical changes of puberty there is an increase in the nocturnal pulsatile secretion of gonadotrophins with luteinising hormone (LH) predominating (4]. Gonadotrophin and sex steroid secretion increase with pubertal progress [5,6], but pulsatile gonadotrophin secretion throughout the 24 hours is required for the attainment of reproductive capability (Fig. 63.1).

Sex steroids have a direct effect in stimulating skeletal growth and a central action in stimulating increased growth hormone (GH) secretion [7]. The highest levels of GH are found at the time of the pubertal growth spurt in both sexes [8]. In girls, growth is fastest between breast stages 2 and 3 and is slowing down at the time of menarche. In boys, the fastest growth does not occur until a testicular volume of 10 ml has been reached.

The endocrine events of normal puberty are consistent between individuals and this results in a relatively constant pattern of physical development and growth. Loss of this normal pattern of development, or *consonance*, indicates that the underlying endocrine events are not the same as those of normal puberty (Fig. 63.2). If the pattern of premature sexual development is consonant, it is likely that the hypothalamo-pituitary–gonadal axis is activated in the same manner as in normally timed puberty.

Sexual precocity is defined as the development of any secondary sexual characteristic before 8 years in a girl and 9 years in a boy. The term precocious puberty should be reserved for consonant pubertal development before these ages. We have not used the term precocious pseudo-puberty, which has been applied to a number of different disorders in the past. Table 63.1 shows the causes of sexual precocity.

Causes of sexual precocity

Sexual precocity secondary to gonadotrophin-releasing hormone secretion

Idiopathic central precocious puberty

In idiopathic central precocious puberty, consonant pubertal development occurs in response to endocrine changes that are the same as those of normal puberty (Fig. 63.3). Idiopathic central precocious puberty is a disorder almost exclusively of girls [9]. This may be because the female and male pituitary glands differ in their sensitivity to gonadotrophin-releasing hormone (GnRH). Girls require smaller doses of exogenous GnRH to stimulate pubertal development [10], while conversely boys require smaller doses of GnRH analogues to suppress puberty [11].

In a study of patients presenting with sexual precocity to the Middlesex Hospital over a 15-year period, there were no boys with idiopathic central precocious puberty, compared with 85 girls. There were no girls in whom central

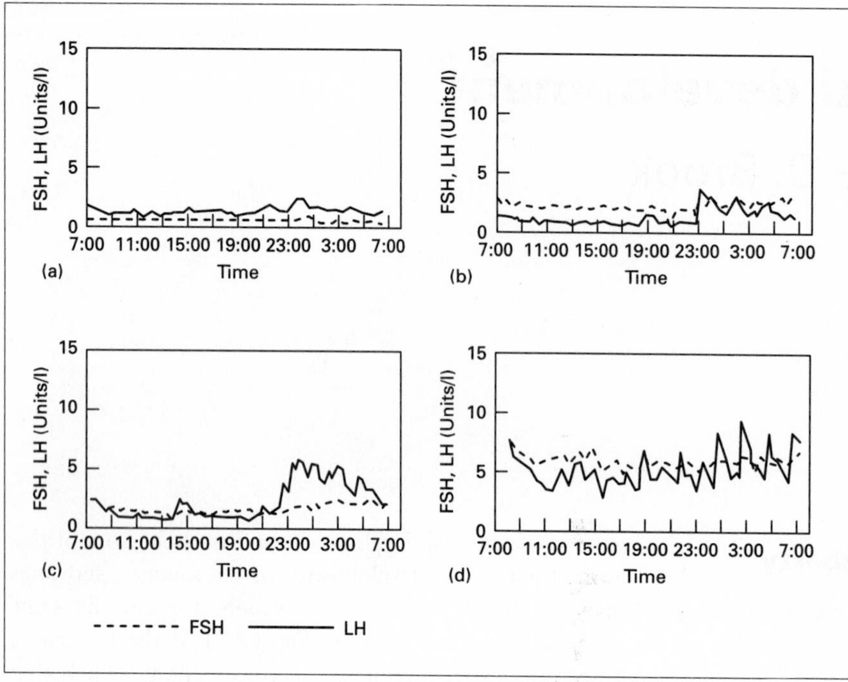

Fig. 63.1 Changes in gonadotrophin secretion throughout childhood. Twenty-four-hour profiles taken with 20-min sampling of luteinising hormone (LH) (solid line) and follicle-stimulating hormone (FSH), in four boys investigated for tall stature. (a) Age 5 years, (b) age 7 years, (c) age 12 years, (d) age 13 years. (a), (b) and (c) are prepubertal; (d) is in early puberty. Pulses of gonadotrophin can be detected at night in children as young as 5 years. The number and amplitude of pulse increase with age. By the onset of puberty there is overnight pulsatility with LH predominating.

precocious puberty was the sole presenting symptom of a central lesion [9]. While it is not necessary to scan all girls with central precocious puberty, a high index of suspicion must be maintained and all girls with neurological signs, or a suggestive history, should be scanned. Although other investigators have found males with central precocious puberty and no central lesion, we suggest that all boys with central precocious puberty should have appropriate imaging (computed tomography (CT) or magnetic resonance imaging (MRI)) [12,13]. All studies show that central precocious puberty secondary to tumours and cerebral lesions has an equal sex incidence.

Secondary central precocious puberty

Central lesions can provoke premature activation of the hypothalamo-pituitary–gonadal axis, even if not in the region of the hypothalamus. Tumours (particularly optic gliomas and pineal tumours), hydrocephalus, trauma and radiotherapy (see Chapter 18) have all been described as causes of central precocious puberty [14].

Hypothalamic hamartomas are associated with central precocious puberty and may also present with gelastic epilepsy and developmental delay [15]. It has been suggested that the tumour secretes GnRH rather than stimulating secretion from a normal hypothalamus [16].

Large doses of cranial irradiation are associated with loss of hypothalamic function, but the lower doses given as prophylaxis in acute lymphoblastic leukaemia are associated with early pubertal development in girls [17]. Children adopted from developing countries and moved to a more affluent environment have an increased incidence of early and precocious puberty [18]. Precocious puberty has been reported as a consequence of sexual abuse [19]. Sex steroid exposure has a direct maturational effect on the hypothalamus and can accelerate the onset of centrally mediated puberty. In congenital adrenal hyperplasia, poor control with elevated androgens can stimulate central precocious puberty which progresses even if control is subsequently improved [20].

Premature thelarche

Isolated breast development occurs in premature thelarche in response to pulsatile gonadotrophin secretion, with follicle-stimulating hormone (FSH) predominating [21] (Fig. 63.3). There is no pubertal progression and growth velocity remains normal. This is most common in girls below the age of 5 years. There may be a history of fluctuating breast size [22], or the development may be one-sided. Ultrasound may demonstrate ovarian cysts [23]. Uterine bleeding is exceptional in this situation. There appears to be no male equivalent of this condition. The cause of premature thelarche is unknown—presumably there is GnRH secretion underlying the gonadotrophin secretion, but this has not been demonstrated.

Slowly progressing central precocious puberty and thelarche variant

There is a clinical spectrum of sexual precocity between

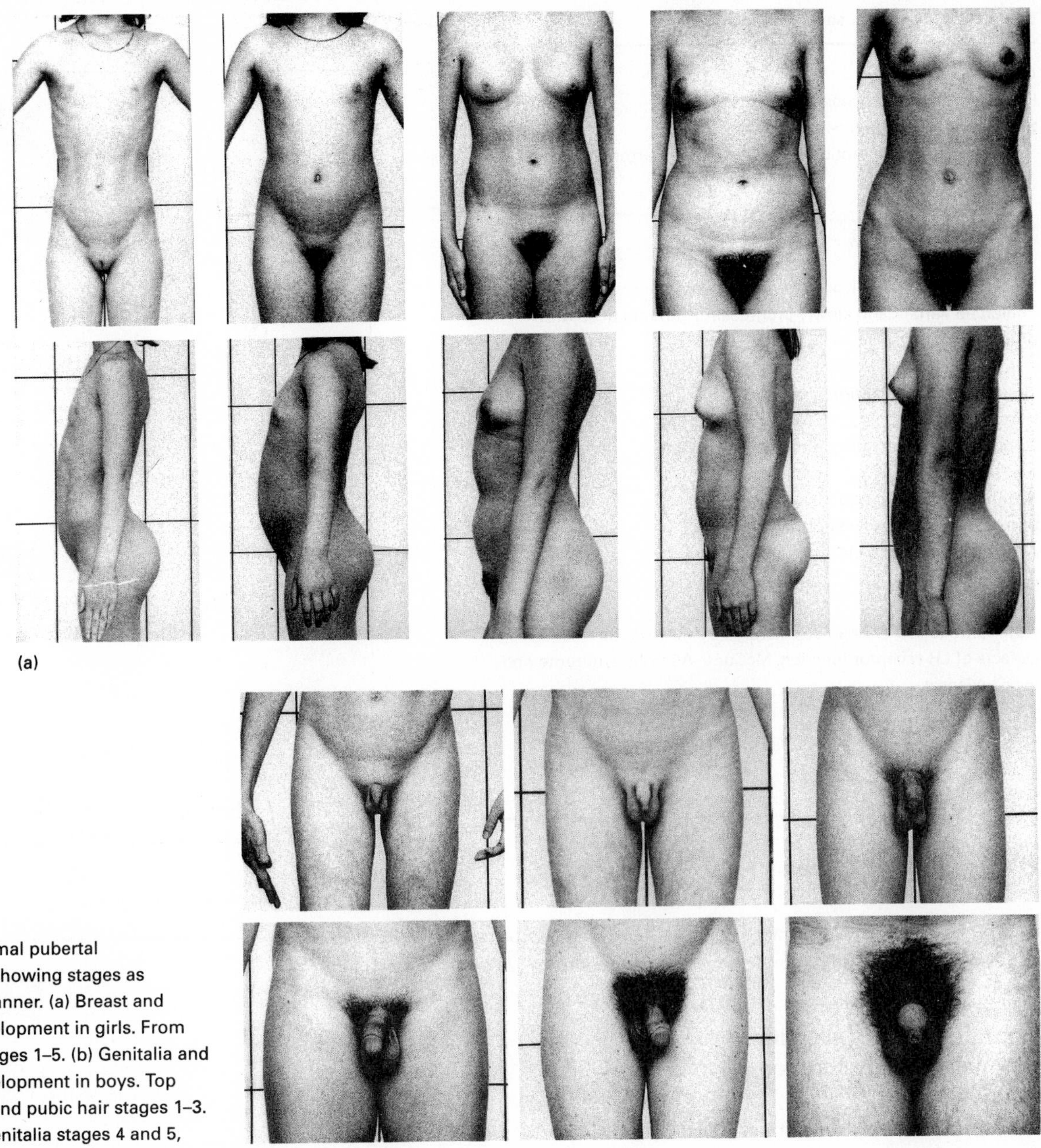

Fig. 63.2 Normal pubertal development, showing stages as described by Tanner. (a) Breast and pubic hair development in girls. From left to right, stages 1–5. (b) Genitalia and pubic hair development in boys. Top row, genitalia and pubic hair stages 1–3. Bottom row, genitalia stages 4 and 5, pubic hair stages 4–6.

premature thelarche and central precocious puberty with some girls having physical signs intermediate between the two, described as thelarche variant, or slowly progressing variants of precocious puberty. The endocrine changes are also intermediate between premature thelarche and central precocious puberty [24,25] (Fig. 63.3).

Sexual precocity secondary to gonadotrophin secretion

Hypothyroidism

Children presenting with untreated primary hypothyroidism have grossly elevated FSH levels as well as thyroid-stimulating hormone (TSH) (Fig. 63.4), which can result in abnormal pubertal development. The endocrine basis of the FSH secretion in hypothyroidism is not known—it may be secreted in response to thyrotrophin-releasing hormone (TRH). Boys may have enlarged testes without pubic hair growth, and girls breast development in advance of pubic hair growth. Girls have enlarged ovaries at ultrasound [26].

Gonadotrophin-releasing tumours

Gonadotrophin-releasing tumours are an extremely rare cause of sexual precocity; these are mostly hCG-secreting

Table 63.1 Causes of sexual precocity.

GnRH secretion
Idiopathic central precocious puberty
Secondary central precocious puberty
Cerebral tumours (optic nerve gliomas, hamartomas, etc.)
Hydrocephalus
Trauma
Radiotherapy
Adoption
Premature thelarche (isolated breast development)
Thelarche variant and slowly progressing variants of central precocious puberty
Gonadotrophin secretion
Hypothyroidism
Gonadotrophin-secreting tumours
Adrenal steroid secretion
Steroid secretion by the normal adrenal
Adrenal enzyme defects
Adrenal tumours
Autonomous secretion of sex steroids by the gonads
Defects of LH-receptor function: McCune–Albright syndrome and testotoxicosis
Gonadal tumours secreting sex steroids
Exogenous sex steroids

LH, luteinising hormone.

tumours of the liver or pineal [27,28]. Pituitary tumours secreting FSH and LH have been described in children [29].

Sexual precocity secondary to adrenal steroid secretion

Steroid secretion by the normal adrenal

The fetal adrenal secretes dehydroepiandrosterone sulphate (DHEAS), and this occasionally manifests as pubic hair or clitoromegaly in infancy, especially in premature babies [30]. Adrenal tumour and congenital adrenal hyperplasia must be excluded. The urine steroid profile is normal, and suppressibility by dexamethasone is helpful in excluding an adrenal tumour. Adrenal androgen levels diminish as the fetal adrenal zone regresses, and appearances return to normal.

In middle childhood, the adrenal gland starts to secrete increased amounts of adrenal androgens (DHEAS and androstenedione); this process is called adrenarche [31]. In a proportion of children, adrenarche is associated with a range of physical manifestations. There is an increase

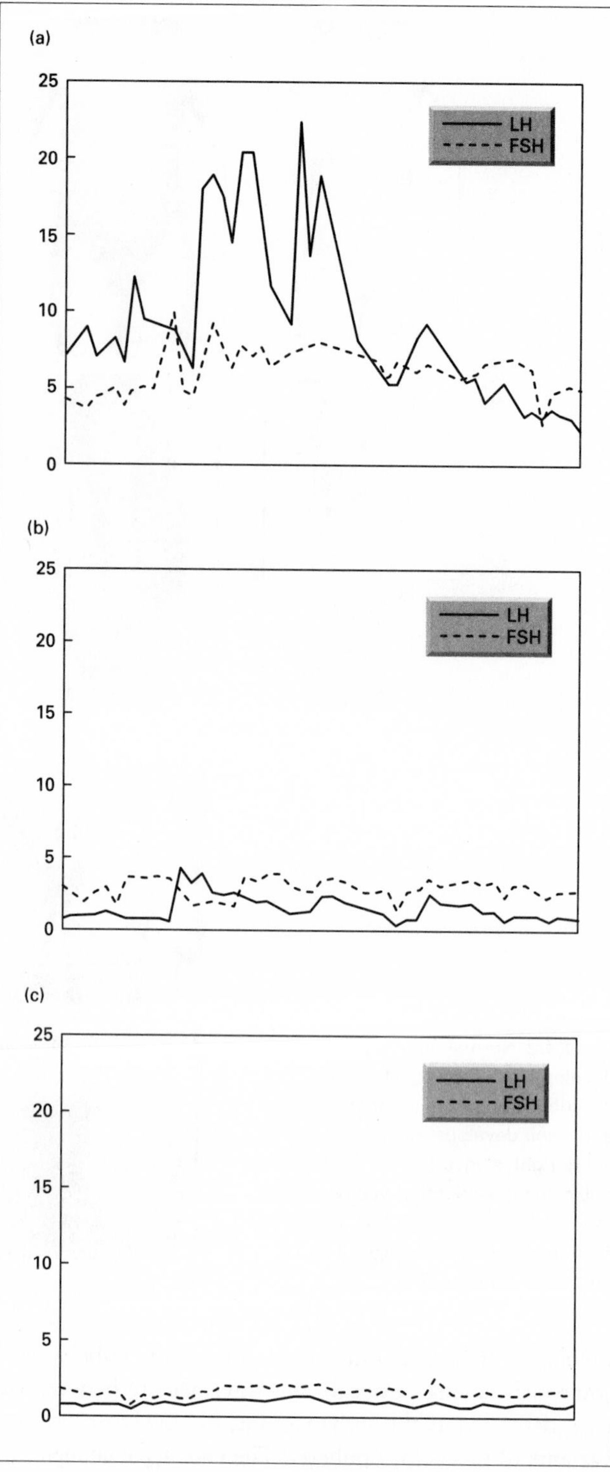

Fig. 63.3 Twenty-four-hour gonadotrophin profiles of three girls, taken by 20-min sampling, showing luteinising hormone (LH) and follicle-stimulating hormone (FSH). All are at Tanner breast stage 3. (a) Idiopathic central precocious puberty. There is nocturnal secretion of gonadotrophins with LH predominating. The pattern of gonadotrophin secretion is the same as that seen in normally timed puberty at the same stage. (b) and (c) show thelarche variant and premature thelarche. In premature thelarche, FSH secretion predominates; the pattern in thelarche variant is intermediate between (a) and (c).

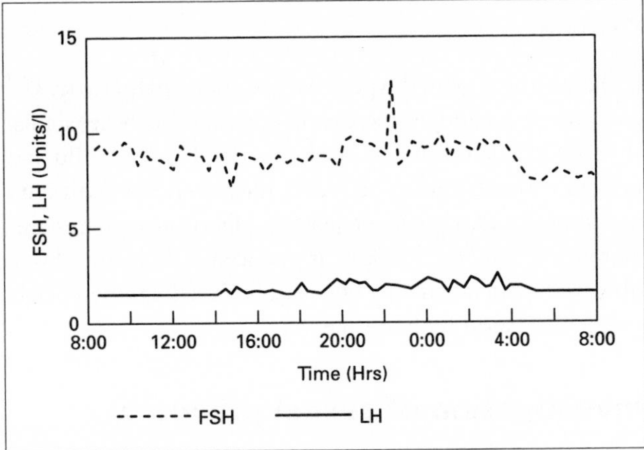

Fig. 63.4 Gonadotrophin profile in a 10-year-old girl with untreated hypothyroidism, showing elevated follicle-stimulating hormone (FSH) levels. LH, luteinising hormone.

in growth rate in all children (the mid-childhood growth spurt) which can be exaggerated in some, with an advance in bone age. Some children develop pubic and axillary hair with apocrine sweat at adrenarche. This is called premature adrenarche or premature pubarche (a misnomer because it is not premature). This finding is uncommon in white children. In non-white children the manifestations of adrenarche can be very marked, with rapid growth and bone age advance, but even in these cases the condition is benign and final height is not affected [32]. Investigation may be required to distinguish adrenarche from adrenal tumours or adrenal enzyme defects. Some investigators have proposed that a significant proportion of children presenting with signs of adrenarche have adrenal enzyme defects [33]. It is not clear if these abnormalities, revealed by supraphysiological doses of adrenocorticotrophic hormone (ACTH), are relevant to the activity of the adrenal gland under physiological conditions. There is no evidence that the long-term outcome in these individuals is different from those with no detectable abnormality.

Adrenal enzyme defects

Congenital adrenal hyperplasia may not be diagnosed at birth in boys who do not have the salt-losing form (some very virilised girls are also not diagnosed because they are raised as boys). High levels of adrenal androgens result in virilisation, with rapid growth, bone age advance, development of pubic and axillary hair and genital maturation without testicular enlargement. High levels of ACTH may result in pigmentation, especially of scars and flexures (typically the child appears suntanned but there are no lines from clothing). Virilisation also occurs in children with congenital adrenal hyperplasia who are undertreated, with pubic and axillary hair, enlargement of the penis or clitoris and increased pigmentation.

Adrenal tumours

Adrenal tumours are a rare cause of virilisation in children, and can be associated with syndromes of increased cancer risk [34]. The clinical course is more rapid and the clinical signs are more extreme than are seen in other causes of virilisation. The prognosis of malignant adrenal tumours is poor [35], and so any child in whom this is a possibility should be thoroughly investigated.

Autonomous secretion of sex steroids by the gonads

In testotoxicosis and the McCune–Albright syndrome there is autonomous secretion of sex steroids without gonadotrophin secretion—so-called gonadotrophin-independent precocious puberty. There is loss of normal feedback control and sex steroid concentrations can be very high. These disorders are associated with abnormalities in the function of the LH receptor. The LH receptor is bound to an associated G-protein, which is vital for the intracellular action of the hormone. Binding of LH to the receptor results in activation of the G-protein, and the conversion of guanosine diphosphate (GDP) to guanosine triphosphate (GTP). This starts the intracellular train of events which results in sex steroid synthesis. Phosphorylase activity of the G-protein converts the GTP to GDP and terminates the action of LH. Testotoxicosis is a dominantly inherited disorder associated with a number of mutations in the transmembrane domain of the LH receptor which affect the phosphorylation of GTP [36]. Virilisation occurs with very high levels of testosterone, and some testicular enlargement.

The McCune–Albright syndrome occurs in both sexes. Sexual precocity may be associated with other syndromes of hormonal hypersecretion. Pubertal development is not consonant, and menstrual bleeding can occur with relatively little breast development. In the McCune–Albright syndrome there is a mutation of the α-chain of the G-protein associated with LH, which results in failure of phosphorylation of GTP to GDP [37]. LH is one of a 'family' of similar membrane bound receptors which utilise the same G-protein system. These receptors can be affected by the same mutation, and the McCune–Albright syndrome can be associated with hypersecretion of other hormones, such as ACTH, growth hormone (GH), parathyroid hormone (PTH) and TSH [38]. The occurrence of the mutation in every cell of the body would probably not be compatible with life and the G-protein mutation is thought to be a somatic cell-line mutation, with affected individuals chimaeric for the condition [39]. The variable clinical picture depends on the cell lines affected, and it seems likely that individuals who have gonadotrophin-independent precocious puberty without any other signs of the McCune–Albright syndrome have only gonadal tissues affected. The syndrome has been found in only one of identical twins [40].

The McCune–Albright syndrome is associated with characteristic skin pigmentation (Plate 63.1, opposite p. 332) [41] and polyostotic fibrous dysplasia of bone. The G-protein mutation has been demonstrated in affected bone but not in adjacent normal bone [42]. G-protein mutation abnormalities are found in a number of other endocrine conditions: mutations of the α-chain of the G-protein resulting in hormonal resistance are seen in pseudo-hypoparathyroidism [43]. Cell lines with G-protein mutations resulting in autonomous hormone secretion have been demonstrated in some tumours, such as GH-secreting pituitary adenomas and thyroid adenomas [39].

Gonadal tumours secreting sex steroids

Gonadal tumours secreting sex steroids have been described in a very few cases of sexual precocity [44]. Development is not consonant and sex steroid concentrations are above the normal adult range.

Exogenous sex steroids

Exogenous sex steroids can occasionally be the cause of sexual precocity. Hormones used in chicken rearing have been implicated as a cause of 'epidemics' of premature thelarche, although the relationship remains unproven [45].

The problems associated with sexual precocity

Social and psychological

These problems are often the major consideration for families of children with sexual precocity [46]. The child may feel (and be made to feel) self-conscious about his or her appearance. Pubertal levels of sex steroids in a young child may result in behaviour problems; these children are often described as disruptive and difficult to control at school. The child may appear much older than they are capable of acting. Girls may be the object of sexual advances that they cannot deal with. In boys, erections may be an embarrassment. There can be particular problems for children with special educational needs, who can have disinhibited sexual behaviour.

Growth

If the pubertal growth spurt occurs abnormally early, GH concentrations and the increase in growth velocity are similar to those seen in normally timed puberty [47]. The child may present with tall stature. However, the pubertal growth spurt has commenced when inadequate childhood growth has been completed and final height is reduced. Clinically, this is observed as an advancing bone age with reduction in height prediction based on bone age.

Investigation of sexual precocity

Pubertal staging and height measurement should be carried out in all children presenting with sexual precocity. Bone age estimation is required where there is concern about loss of height potential. Follow-up of height velocity and pubertal progress is of value in confirming the diagnosis, for example in distinguishing girls with premature thelarche from those presenting with breast development at the start of central precocious puberty [48].

Sinister underlying causes for sexual precocity, such as tumours, should be considered and excluded, but extensive investigation of children with benign conditions should be avoided. Parents and patients who are persuaded to regard sexual development as a pathological process can find it very difficult to deal with subsequent normal puberty and adolescence.

Imaging

Boys with central precocious puberty should have a CT or an MRI scan (MRI scanning gives better views of the hypothalamo-pituitary area), for the reasons explained above. CT or MRI is of value in imaging adrenal tumours (CT usually produces better resolution). The adrenal is a difficult organ to image by ultrasound unless it is markedly enlarged.

Pelvic ultrasound is a valuable investigation in girls. During puberty the ovaries increase in volume [49] and the uterus changes from a tubular organ to a pear-shaped one (Fig. 63.5) [74]. Menstruation does not occur until at least 5 mm of endometrium is present. These uterine changes are not seen in premature thelarche [50] although ovarian cysts may be visualised [23].

Hormonal studies

'One-off' assays of gonadotrophins or sex steroids may not be of much help. Gonadotrophins are produced in a pulsatile manner, and in early puberty gonadotrophins and sex steroids are at prepubertal levels during most of the day. Gonadotrophin and sex steroid concentrations

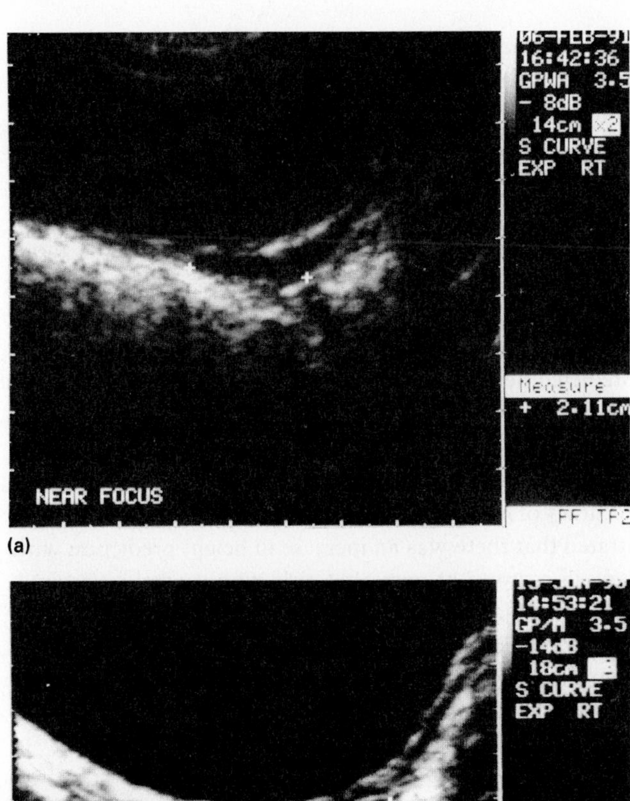

(a)

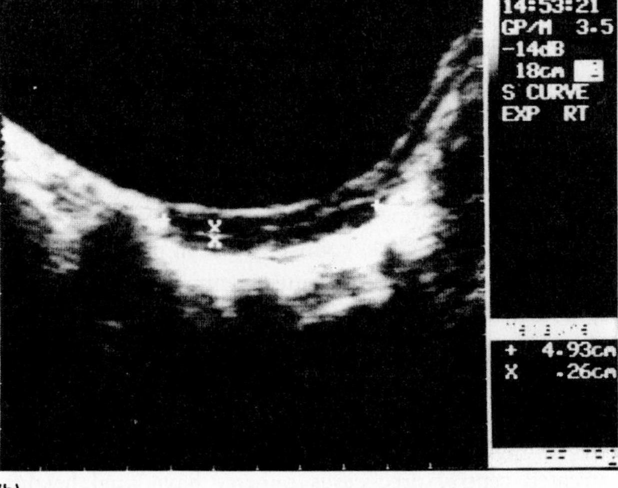

(b)

Fig. 63.5 Pelvic ultrasonography. (a) Prepubertal uterus. The fundus is narrower than the cervix and there is no endometrial echo. (b) Uterus of a girl in early puberty. There is an endometrial echo and the fundus has attained a greater diameter than the cervix.

will be low in most individuals with sexual precocity. Concentrations of sex steroids above the adult range with low gonadotrophins are found in the McCune–Albright syndrome and testotoxicosis.

In central precocious puberty the GnRH-stimulation test will have a pubertal response (peak LH concentration over 5 U/l [51]). In the McCune–Albright syndrome and testotoxicosis the gonadotrophin response will be suppressed by the high concentrations of sex steroids.

The normal suppression of adrenal secretion by dexamethasone is of value in excluding adrenal tumours. Plasma levels of adrenal steroids (DHEAS and androstenedione) may be elevated in adrenal tumours, and plasma 17α-hydroxyprogesterone is elevated in 21-hydroxylase deficiency. Urinary steroid profiles provide a non-invasive method of identifying abnormal secretion due to adrenal tumours and enzyme defects [52].

Treatment of sexual precocity

Treatment is indicated where there are advancing physical signs of puberty which would result in psychological harm. It may be important to halt menstruation in very young girls. Many children with precocious puberty are sufficiently mature to deal with their development, and should not be treated. Treatment will halt pubertal progress but significant regression of the signs of sexual precocity does not usually occur (there is some softening of breast tissue in girls, and reduction in testicular volume in boys). Treatment will halt the pubertal growth spurt but, for the reasons outlined below, treatment should not be initiated in the hope of significantly increasing final height.

For those with premature thelarche and the physical manifestations of adrenarche, breast and pubic hair development may be an embarrassment but unfortunately little can be done to regress this.

Cyproterone acetate and medroxyprogesterone

Cyproterone acetate is a peripherally acting antiandrogen, with some progestogenic and glucocorticoid actions, suppressing both gonadotrophin and gonadal steroid secretion [53]. It is effective in halting the progress of the physical features of puberty and useful in suppressing menstruation. GnRH analogues are ineffective in the McCune–Albright syndrome and testotoxicosis and cyproterone acetate remains the drug of choice for these children. Cyproterone is useful in suppressing the initial stimulatory effects of GnRH analogues. Medroxyprogesterone is a progestogenic agent which, like cyproterone acetate, is effective in halting the gonadal steroid-mediated events of puberty [54].

Ketoconazole and testolactone

Ketoconazole acts as an inhibitor of steroid synthesis, including that of testosterone [55]. Testolactone inhibits some of the actions of testosterone by inhibiting its aromatisation to oestradiol [56].

GnRH analogues

FSH and LH are produced in a pulsatile manner by the pituitary in response to pulsatile GnRH production by the hypothalamus. In order to induce puberty using exogenous GnRH, the drug must be given in a similar pulsatile manner commencing with a low dose. If GnRH is given continuously or in too high a dose, there is down-regulation of the GnRH receptors and gonadotrophin production is suppressed [57]. The analogues of GnRH used to suppress precocious puberty are much more active and long lasting than native GnRH.

When treatment is initiated, there is a period of stimulation, during which puberty may advance, but then gonadotrophin production falls because of the down-regulation of receptors (the initial stimulatory action of GnRH analogues may be suppressed with cyproterone acetate). Girls who have already developed significant endometrial thickening may have vaginal bleeding after commencing GnRH analogues. GnRH analogues have been produced as nasal sprays, daily injections and as depot preparations. For practical reasons depot preparations may be preferable in children.

Side-effects of treatment

Cyproterone commonly causes tiredness and lethargy and can be associated with profound ACTH and adrenal suppression [58]. Hepatocellular carcinoma has been reported in patients treated with cyproterone acetate, although there have been no reports of this with treatment for precocious puberty [59,60]. The high doses of ketoconazole required for suppression of pubertal progress (much greater than those required for an antifungal action) can result in deranged liver function [61]. Ketoconazole also carries the risk of adrenal suppression.

Withdrawal of sex steroids in adults results in loss of bone density, and this is a side-effect of GnRH analogue treatment in adults. Treatment with GnRH analogues for precocious puberty results in loss of bone density [62], and there is a theoretical risk that peak bone mineral density may be impaired, although there are no long-term data. Sex steroid withdrawal in children can result in 'menopausal' symptoms (hot flushes and/or mood swings). An increased prevalence of obesity has been reported in girls treated with GnRH analogues [63].

Outcome of treatment

Pubertal progress

Cyproterone acetate and GnRH analogues are both effective in halting the progress of puberty. GnRH analogues have fewer side-effects and are the treatment of choice for central precocious puberty.

Final height

Treatment to halt pubertal progress results in a fall in sex steroid concentrations and both the direct effect of sex steroids on growth, and the effect of sex steroids in stimulating growth hormone secretion, are lost. Treatment to halt puberty results in a fall in growth velocity.

Cyproterone was demonstrated to have no effect on final height in central precocious puberty [64]. When GnRH analogues were introduced, it was hoped that the more effective suppression of pubertal progress achieved would result in increased final height. The results of long-term studies have demonstrated an increase in final height over predicted height at the start of treatment [65] and in final height over untreated controls [66,67]. Assessment of the effect of treatment on final height must take into account the natural history of precocious puberty, and the potential accuracy of height-prediction methods. Werder *et al.* demonstrated that there was an increase in height prediction with time in a group of untreated girls with central precocious puberty [64]. Zachmann *et al.* demonstrated that the accuracy of predictions of final height was poor in children with abnormal growth patterns, including untreated precocious puberty [68]. Bayley–Pinneau predictions are more accurate than other methods in precocious puberty [69].

Outcome of long-term GnRH treatment was better for those starting treatment earlier and with younger bone ages. In clinical practice, younger children presenting with central precocious puberty require treatment for social and psychological reasons, apart from any considerations of height prognosis—older children with relatively mature bone ages will not get any useful improvement in final height and the decision to treat should be based on assessment of the psychological maturity of the child. Most girls with untreated central precocious puberty have final heights within the normal range [69]. The addition of GH to GnRH analogues has not been demonstrated to improve final height (N.A. Bridges, C.G.D. Brook, unpublished data).

Long-term follow up

Increased prevalence of polycystic ovarian appearance at ultrasound has been demonstrated in girls treated with a combination of GnRH analogue and GH after stopping treatment [70]. It is impossible to say if this finding is secondary to the treatment, or to central precocious puberty itself.

Fertility is normal in adults who have had centrally mediated precocious puberty [71]. There is no evidence that early menarche results in early menopause, but there is a relationship between early menarche and increased breast cancer risk [72]. In the McCune–Albright syndrome, the abnormal gonadal activation continues into adult life and may result in irregular menses and fertility problems [73].

References

1 Beck Peccoz P, Padmanabhan V, Baggiani AM *et al.* Maturation of the hypothalamic pituitary gonadal function in normal human fetuses: circulating levels of gonadotrophins, their common alpha subunit and discrepancy between immunological and biological activities of circulating FSH. *J Clin Endocrinol Metab* 1991; **73**: 525–32.

2 De Zegher F, Devlieger H, Veldhuis JD. Pulsatile and sexually dimorphic secretion of luteinising hormone in the human infant on the day of birth. *Pediatr Res* 1992; **32**: 605–7.

3 Bridges NA, Matthews DR, Hindmarsh PC, Brook CGD. Changes in gonadotrophin secretion during childhood and puberty. *J Endocrinol* 1994; **141**: 169–76.

4 Jackacki RI, Kelch RP, Sauder SE, Lloyd JS, Hopwood NJ, Marshall JC. Pulsatile secretion of luteinising hormone in children. *J Clin Endocrinol Metab* 1982; **55**: 453–8.

5 Wennink JMB, Delamarre Vandewaal HA, Schoemaker R, Schoemaker H, Schoemaker J. Luteinising hormone and follicle stimulating hormone secretion in girls through puberty measured using highly sensitive immunoradiometric assays. *Clin Endocrinol* 1990; **33**: 333–4.

6 Wennink JMB, Delamarre Vandewaal HA, Schoemaker R, Schoemaker H, Schoemaker J. Luteinising hormone and follicle stimulating hormone secretion in boys through puberty mesured using highly sensitive immunoradiometric assays. *Clin Endocrinol* 1989; **31**: 551–64.

7 Moll GW, Rosenfeld RL, Fang VS. Administration of low dose estrogen rapidly and directly stimulates growth hormone production. *Am J Dis Child* 1986; **140**: 124–7.

8 Stanhope R, Pringle PJ, Brook CGD. The mechanisms of the adolescent growth spurt induced by low dose pulsatle GnRH treatment. *Clin Endocrinol (Oxf)* 1988; **28**: 83–9.

9 Bridges NA, Christopher JA, Hindmarsh PC, Brook CGD. Sexual precocity: sex incidence and aetiology. *Arch Dis Child* 1994; **70**: 116–18.

10 Stanhope R, Brook CGD, Pringle PJ, Adams J, Jacobs HS. Induction of puberty by pulsatile GnRH. *Lancet* 1987; **2**: 522–5.

11 Donaldson MDC, Stanhope R, Lee TJ, Price DA, Brook CGD, Savage DCL. Gonadotrophin responses to GnRH in precocious puberty treated with GnRH analogues. *Clin Endocrinol (Oxf)* 1984; **21**: 499–503.

12 Robben SG, Oostdijk W, Drop SL, Tanghe HL, Veilvoye GJ, Meradji M. Idiopathic isosexual precocious puberty: magnetic resonance findings in 30 patients. *Br J Radiol* 1995; **68**: 34–8.

13 Kornreich L, Horev G, Blaser S, Daneman D, Kauli R, Grunebaum M. Central precocious puberty: evaluation by neuroimaging. *Pediatr Radiol* 1995; **25**: 7–11.

14 Blendonohy PM, Philip PA. Precocious puberty in children after traumatic brain injury. *Brain Injury* 1991; **5**: 63–8.

15 Boyko OB, Curnes JT, Oakes WJ, Burger PC. Hamartomas of the tuber cinereum: CT, MR and pathologic findings. *Am J Neuroradiology* 1991; **12**: 309–14.

16 Mahachoklertwattana P, Kaplan SL, Grumbach MM. The luteinising hormone releasing hormone secreting hypothalamic hamartoma is a congenital malformation; natural history. *J Clin Endocrinol Metab* 1993; **77**: 118–24.

17 Ogilvy Stuart AL, Clayton PE, Shalet SM. Cranial irradiation and early puberty. *J Clin Endocrinol Metab* 1994; **78**: 1282–6.

18 Proos LA, Hofvander Y, Tuvemo T. Menarcheal age and growth pattern of Indian girls adopted in Sweden. I. Menarcheal age. *Acta Paediatr Scand* 1991; **80**: 852–8.

19 Herman ME, Giddens AD, Sandler NE, Freidman NE. Sexual precocity in girls: an association with sexual abuse? *Am J Dis Child* 1988; **142**: 431–3.

20 Dacou-Voutetakis C, Karidis N. Congenital adrenal hyperplasia complicated by central precocious puberty: treatment with LHRH agonist analogue. *Ann NY Acad Sci USA* 1993; **687**: 250–4.

21 Stanhope R, Abdulwahid NA, Adams J, Brook CGD. Studies of gonadotrophin pulsatility and pelvic ultrasound distinguish between isolated premature thelarche and central precocious puberty. *Eur J Pediatr* 1986; **145**: 190–4.

22 Stanhope R, Adams J, Brook CGD. Fluctuation of breast size in premature thelarche. *Acta Paed Scand* 1985; **74**: 454–5.

23 Freedman SM, Kreitzer PM, Elkowitz SS, Saberman N, Leonidas JC. Ovarian microcysts in girls with isolated premature thelarche. *Pediatrics* 1993; **122**: 246–9.

24 Stanhope R, Brook CGD. Thelarche variant: a new syndrome of sexual maturation? *Acta Endocrinol (Copenh)* 1990; **123**: 481–6.

25 Fontoura M, Brauner R, Prevot C, Rappaport R. Precocious puberty in girls: early diagnosis of a slowly progressing variant. *Arch Dis Child* 1989; **64**: 1170–6.

26 Pringle PJ, Stanhope R, Hindmarsh P, Brook CGD. Abnormal sexual development in primary hypothyroidism. *Clin Endocrinol (Oxf)* 1988; **28**: 479–86.

27 Cohen AR, Wilson JA, Sedeghi-Nejad A. Gonadotrophin secreting pineal teratoma causing precocious puberty. *Neurosurgery* 1991; **28**: 597–603.

28 Perilongo G, Rigon F, Murgia A. Oncologic cases of precocious puberty. *Pediatr Hematol Oncol* 1989; **6**: 331–40.

29 Ambrosi B, Bassetti M, Ferrario R. Precocious puberty in a boy with a PRL LH and FSH secreting pituitary tumour: hormonal and immunocytochemical studies. *Acta Endocrinol (Copenh)* 1990; **122**: 569–76.

30 Adams DM, Young PC, Copeland KC. Pubic hair in infancy. *Am J Dis Child* 1992; **146**: 149–51.

31 Parker LN. Adrenarche. *Endocrinol Metab Clin North Am* 1991; **20**: 71–83.

32 Ibanez L, Virdis R, Potau N *et al.* Natural history of premature pubarche: an auxological study. *J Clin Endocrinol Metab* 1992; **74**: 254–8.

33 Del Balzo P, Borelli P, Cambiaso P, Danielli E, Cappa M. Adrenal steroidogenic defects in children with precocious pubarche. *Horm Res* 1992; **37**: 180–4.

34 Carson DA, Lois A. Cancer progression and p53. *Lancet* 1995; **346**: 1009–11.

35 Pommier RF, Brennan MF. An eleven-year experience with adrenocortical carcinoma. *Surgery* 1992; **112**: 963–70.

36 Yano K, Saji M, Hidaka A *et al.* A new constitutively activating point mutation in the luteinizing hormone/chorionic gonadotrophin receptor gene in cases of male limited precocious puberty. *J Clin Endocrinol Metab* 1995; 80: 1162–8.

37 Weinstein LS, Shenker A, Gejman PV, Merino MJ, Freidman E, Speigel AM. Activating mutations of the stimulatory G protein in the McCune Albright syndrome. *N Engl J Med* 1991; **325**: 1688–95.

38 Cremonini N, Graziano E, Chiarini V, Sforza A, Zampa GA. Atypical McCune Albright syndrome associated with growth hormone prolactin pituitary adenoma: natural history, long term follow up and SMS 201–995–bromocriptine combined treatment results. *J Clin Endocrinol Metab* 1992; **75**: 1166–9.

39 Weinstein LS, Shenker LA. G protein mutations in human disease. *Clin Biochem* 1993; **26**: 333–8.

40 Endo M, Yamada Y, Matsuura N, Niikawa N. Monozygotic twins discordant for the major signs of McCune Albright syndrome. *Am J Med Genet* 1991; **41**: 216–20.

41 Reiger E, Kofler R, Borkensein M, Schwingshandl J, Soyer HP, Kerl H. Melanotic macules following Blaschko's lines in McCune Albright syndrome. *Br J Dermatol* 1994; 130: 215–20.

42 Shenker A, Weinstein LS, Sweet DE, Speigel AM. An activating Gs alpha mutation is present in fibrous dysplasia of bone in the McCune Albright syndrome. *J Clin Endocrinol Metab* 1994; **79**: 750–5.

43 Miric A, Vechio JD, Levine MA. Heterogeneous mutations in the gene encoding the alpha subunit of the stimulatory G protein of adenyl cyclase in Albright hereditary osteodystrophy. *J Clin Endocrinol Metab* 1993; **76**: 156–8.

44 Dengg K, Fink FM, Heitger A *et al.* Precocious puberty due to a lipid cell tumour of the ovary. *Eur J Pediatr* 1993; **152**: 12–14.

45 Freni-Titulaer LW, Cordero JF, Haddock L, Lebron G, Martinez R, Mills JL. Premature thelarche in Puerto Rico. A search for environmental factors. *Am J Dis Child* 1986; **140**: 1263–7.

46 Ehrhardt AA, Meyer-Bahlburg HF. Psychosocial aspects of precocious puberty. *Horm Res* 1994; **41** (Suppl. 2): 30–5.

47 Ross JL, Pecovitz OH, Barnes K, Loriaux DL, Cutler GB. Growth hormone secretory dynamics in children with precocious puberty. *J Pediatr* 1987; **110**: 369–72.

48 Pasquino AM, Pucarelli I, Passeri F, Segni M, Mancini MA, Municchi G. Progression of premature thelarche to central precocious puberty. *J Pediatr* 1995; **126**: 11–14.

49 Bridges NA, Cooke A, Healy MJR, Hindmarsh PC, Brook CGD. Standards for ovarian volume in childhood and puberty. *Fertil Steril* 1993; **60**: 456–60.

50 Haber HP, Wollman HA, Ranke MB. Pelvic ultrasonography: early differentiation between isolated premature thelarche and central precocious puberty. *Eur J Pediatr* 1995; **154**: 182–6.

51 Hughes IA. *Handbook of Endocrine Investigations in Children.* London: Wright, 1986: 18.

52 Honour JW, Price DA, Taylor NF *et al.* Steroid biochemistry of virilising adrenal tumours in childhood. *Eur J Pediatr* 1984; **142**: 165–9.

53 Mcleod DG. Antiandrogenic drugs. *Cancer* 1993; **71**: 1046–9.

54 Perilongo G, Rigon F, Murgia A. Oncologic causes of precocious puberty. *Pediatr Hematol Oncol* 1989; **6**: 331–40.

55 Sonino N. The use of ketoconazole as an inhibitor of steroid production. *N Engl J Med* 1987; **317**: 812–18.

56 Feuillan PP, Foster CM, Pescovitz OH *et al.* Treatment of precocious puberty in the McCune Albright syndrome with the aromatase inhibitor testolactone. *N Engl J Med* 1986; **315**: 1115–19.

57 Stanhope R, Abdulwahid NA, Adams J, Jacobs HS, Brook CDG. Problems in the use of pulsatile GnRH for the induction of puberty. *Horm Res* 1985; **22**: 74–7.

58 Savage DCL, Swift PGF. Effect of cyproterone acetate on adrenocortical function in children with precocious puberty. *Arch Dis Child* 1981; **56**: 218–22.

59 Rudiger T, Beckmann J, Queisser W. Hepatocellular carcinoma after treatment with cyproterone acetate combined with ethinyloestradiol (letter). *Lancet* 1995; **345**: 452–3.

60 Kattan J, Spatz A, Culine S *et al.* Hepatocellular carcinoma during hormonotherapy for prostatic cancer. *Am J Clin Oncol* 1994; **17**: 390–2.

61 Babovic Vuksanovic D, Donaldson MD, Gibson NA, Wallace AM. Hazards of ketoconazole therapy in testotoxicosis. *Acta Paediatr* 1994; **83**: 994–7.

62 Saggese G, Bertelloni S, Baroncelli GI, Battini R, Franchi G. Reduction in bone density: an effect of gonadotrophin releasing hormone treatment in central precocious puberty. *Fertil Steril* 1993; **152**: 717–20.

63 Kamp GA, Manasco PK, Barnes KM *et al.* Low growth hormone levels are related to increased body mass and do not reflect impaired growth in LHRH agonist treated children with precocious puberty. *J Clin Endocrinol Metab* 1991; **72**: 301–7.

64 Werder EA, Murset G, Zachmann M, Brook CGD, Prader A. Treatment of precocious puberty with cyproterone acetate. *Pediatr Res* 1974; **8**: 248–56.

65 Sippell WG. Diagnosis and treatment of central precocious puberty—can final height be improved? German/Dutch precocious puberty study group. *Horm Res* 1994; **41**(Suppl. 2): 14–15.

66 Paul D, Conte FA, Grumbach MM, Kaplan SL. Long term effect of gonadotrophin releasing hormone agonist therapy on final and near final height in 26 children with true precocious puberty treated at a median age of less than 5 years. *J Clin Endocrinol Metab* 1995; **80**: 546–51.

67 Brauner R, Adan L, Malandry F, Zantleifer D. Adult height in girls with idiopathic true precocious puberty. *J Clin Endocrinol Metab* 1994; **79**: 415–20.

68 Zachmann M, Sobradillo B, Frank M, Frisch H, Prader A. Bayley Pinneau, Roche Wainer Thissen, and Tanner height predictions in normal children and in patients with various pathological conditions. *J Pediatr* 1978; **93**: 749–55.

69 Bar A, Linder B, Sobel EH, Saenger P, Di Martino Nardi J. Bayley Pinneau method of height prediction in girls with central precocious puberty: correlation with adult height. *J Pediatr* 1995; **126**: 955–8.

70 Bridges NA, Cooke A, Healy MJR, Hindmarsh PC, Brook CGD. Ovaries in sexual precocity. *Clin Endocrinol* 1995; **42**: 135–40.

71 Jay N, Mansfield MJ, Blizzard RM *et al.* Ovulation and menstrual function of adolescent girls with central precocious puberty after therapy with gonadotrophin releasing hormone agonists. *J Clin Endocrinol Metab* 1992; **75**: 890–4.

72 Apter D, Vihko R. Early menarche, a risk factor for breast cancer, indicates early onset of ovulatory cycles. *J Clin Endocrinol Metab* 1983; **57**: 82–6.

73 Boepple PA, Frisch LS, Weirman ME, Hoffman WH, Crowley WF. The natural history of autonomous gonadal function, adrenarche and central puberty in gonadotrophin independent precocious puberty. *J Clin Endocrinol Metab* 1992; **75**: 1550–5.

74 Bridges NA, Cooke A, Healy MJR, Hindmarsh PC, Brook CGD, Growth of the uterus. *Arch Dis Child* 1996; **75**: 330–1.

CHAPTER 64

Delayed puberty: diagnosis and management

J.-P. Bourguignon

Definition and aetiological classification

Puberty is delayed when no increase in testicular volume (<4 ml) has occurred at 14 years in a boy, or when breast development has not started at 13.5 years in a girl. Delayed adolescence also involves conditions with incomplete development of puberty such as primary amenorrhoea (no menarche at 16 years) or arrest of puberty (no progression from an intermediate pubertal stage for 2 years).

The causes of delayed adolescence in the male (Table 64.1) and in the female (Table 64.2) can be classified in three groups:

1 temporary impairment of gonadotrophin and sex steroid secretion—the most frequent situation is constitutional delay of puberty;

2 permanent hypothalamo-pituitary failure with deficient secretion of the gonadotrophins (hypogonadotrophic hypogonadism);

3 permanent primary gonadal failure resulting in increased plasma concentrations of the gonadotrophins (hypergonadotrophic hypogonadism).

In Table 64.1 are listed the various aetiologies of hypogonadism in phenotypic males. In some congenital conditions with hyper- or hypogonadotrophic hypogonadism, cryptorchidism and micropenis may be associated with delayed puberty. In some conditions with hypergonadotrophic hypogonadism, ambiguous genitalia may result from partial virilisation. In female subjects, hypogonadism may occur either as sexual infantilism (few or no signs of pubertal development) or primary amenorrhoea (absence of menarche in a subject having otherwise completed puberty). The aetiologies of female hypogonadism are listed in Tables 64.2 and 64.3.

Temporary delay of puberty

A number of different conditions result in a temporary delay of sexual maturation (Table 64.1).

Constitutional delay of puberty (and growth) is by far the most common cause of delayed adolescence [1]. This condition is consistent with an extreme physiological variant in the timing of onset of puberty. While a similar incidence would be expected in both sexes, about nine boys to one girl are referred for delayed puberty. Such a gender difference in incidence of delayed puberty may not simply result from a referral bias. The neuroendocrine clock which controls puberty can be prone to late onset in boys and early onset in girls, since idiopathic sexual precocity is much more common in girls than in boys. A familial tendency to constitutional delay of puberty can exist as shown by the late menarcheal age of the mother and sisters, and by a delayed growth spurt in the father. However, sporadic forms are also seen.

The clinical manifestations of delayed puberty are variable. Some patients with constitutional delay, as well as some with gonadotrophin deficiency, may show evidence of partial spontaneous pubertal development. In patients with constitutional delay of puberty, the degree of short stature is also variable on account of several factors including parents' height, and possible association with intrauterine growth retardation. The age at onset of growth failure may play a role. While some patients show reduced growth velocity starting around 12 years as a presumable consequence of delayed puberty, others show a slow growth velocity from early childhood. In the latter patients, delayed puberty may result from delayed growth, a pattern suggestive of isolated growth hormone (GH) deficiency though GH secretion may not be deficient. Attention should be paid to body proportions since pubertal growth involves spine and limbs equally while limbs are predominantly involved

Table 64.1 Causes of hypogonadism in phenotypic males.

Temporary delay of puberty

- Constitutional delay of puberty
  - Sporadic
  - Familial
- Chronic illnesses
  - Digestive tract (inflammatory bowel diseases)
  - Urinary tract (chronic renal failure)
  - Debilitating diseases (haemolytic anaemia, haemochromatosis)
- Nutritional disorders
  - Malnutrition
  - Malabsorptive states (coeliac disease, cystic fibrosis)
  - Debilitating diseases (malignancies, etc.)
  - High energy expenditure (e.g. young gymnasts)
- Hormonal disturbances
  - Hypothyroidism
  - Isolated growth hormone deficiency
  - Excess of glucocorticoids (Cushing's disease, corticotherapy)

Hypogonadotrophic hypogonadism

- Congenital
  - Isolated
    - Isolated gonadotrophin deficiency (sporadic or familial)
    - Luteinising hormone deficiency (fertile eunuch syndrome)
  - Polymalformative syndromes
    - With anosmia (Kallmann's syndrome, etc.)
    - With other features (Prader-Willi syndrome)
  - Pan-hypopituitarism or multiple pituitary hormone deficiences (idiopathic, empty sella syndrome)
- Acquired
  - Suprasellar tumours (craniopharyngioma, etc.)
  - Pituitary destruction (adenomas, surgical, traumatic)
  - Hyperprolactinaemia (adenomas)

Hypergonadotrophic hypogonadism

- Congenital
  - Anomalies of sex chromosomes
    - Klinefelter's syndrome (XXY and variants)
    - Gonadal dysgenesis*(XO/XY and variants)
  - Anomalies of hormone biosynthesis and receptivity
    - Enzymatic defects in testosterone biosynthesis*
    - 5α-reductase deficiency*
    - Partial insensitivity to androgens*
    - Mutation in β-luteinising hormone gene
    - Carbohydrate-deficient glycoprotein syndrome type 1
  - Polymalformative syndromes (Noonan's syndrome, etc.)
  - Syndromes of testicular regression
    - Anorchia (complete)
    - Rudimentary testes* (partial)
    - Leydig-cell agenesis or hypoplasia*
- Acquired
  - Known pathogenesis
    - Surgical or traumatic castration
    - Bilateral orchitis
    - Immunosuppressive or cytotoxic chemotherapy, radiotherapy
  - Unknown mechanism
    - Idiopathic oligo- or azoospermia
    - Sertoli cell-only syndrome

* With possible partial virilisation, ambiguous genitalia.

in prepubertal growth. This accounts for the eunuchoid appearance of patients with delayed puberty.

Chronic systemic diseases, either previously diagnosed or otherwise symptomless, may cause delayed growth and puberty. These include Crohn's disease, coeliac disease, chronic renal failure, severe cardiopathies and any debilitating disorder. Chronic inflammatory bowel diseases involve different pathophysiological mechanisms including the inflammatory process, undernutrition or malabsorption, and the side-effects of therapies such as corticosteroids. Surgical management results in a dramatic catch-up growth in such patients [2].

Nutritional disorders resulting in a chronic impairment of metabolic fuel availability may contribute to the delay of growth and puberty in systemic diseases [3]. Anorexia nervosa is a particular condition involving a primary central nervous system (CNS) alteration in the regulation of food intake as well as the neuroendocrine control of GH and the gonadotrophins (see Chapter 70). The delayed puberty or primary amenorrhoea seen in young gymnasts and long-distance runners may also involve interactions between energy intake, expenditure and the CNS, although the exact mechanisms remain to be elucidated. Quite remarkably, pubertal growth is not only delayed in gymnasts but a markedly reduced limb growth spurt is seen resulting in adult height below the genetic target [4].

Isolated GH deficiency may result in a clinical presentation similar to constitutional delay of puberty since some patients with constitutional delay can show early growth failure starting before 10 years with an important retardation in bone age. The differential diagnosis from isolated GH deficiency can be difficult, since a blunted GH response to provocative tests can result from the lack of physiological priming of GH secretion by sex steroids [5]. This might explain why 25–50% of patients previously diagnosed as idiopathic isolated GH deficiency are no longer found to be deficient when retested after stopping GH therapy [6,7]. In a recent study of 27 boys with pubertal delay and GH

Table 64.2 Causes of sexual infantilism in phenotypic females.

Temporary hypogonadism
Same causes as in males (see Table 64.1)

Permanent hypogonadotrophic conditions
Congenital
  Isolated gonadotrophin deficiency (sporadic or familial)
  Polydysmorphic syndromes
    With anosmia (Kallmann's syndrome etc.)
    With other features (Prader–Willi syndrome etc.)
  Pan-hypopituitarism or multiple pituitary hormone deficiencies (idiopathic, empty sella syndrome)
Acquired
  Suprasellar tumours (craniopharyngiomas etc.)
  Pituitary destruction (adenomas, surgical, traumatic, Sheehan's syndrome)
  Hyperprolactinaemia (adenomas)

Permanent hypergonadotrophic conditions
Congenital
  Anomalies of sex chromosomes
    Turner's syndrome (XO and variants)
    Gonadal dysgenesis (XO/XY, variants)
  Polymalformative syndromes
  Ovarian agenesis with XX karyotype
  Carbohydrate-deficient glycoprotein syndrome type 1
Acquired
  Known pathogenesis
    Surgical or traumatic castration
    Autoimmune ovaritis (+ thyroiditis or Addison's disease)
    Cytotoxic chemotherapy, radiotherapy
    Chronic infections (tuberculosis)
  Unknown mechanism
    Premature ovarian failure

peak responses to arginine–insulin < 10 ng/ml, 23 showed a response above that limit after four intramuscular injections of 100 mg long-acting testosterone at 15-day-intervals [8]. While this observation indicates the usefulness of sex-steroid priming before GH testing, the optimal modalities of such priming are unknown.

Other hormonal disorders such as acquired thyroid hormone deficiency or hyperprolactinaemia may temporarily delay sexual development [9]. Chronic therapy using corticosteroids may also delay growth and puberty; Cushing's disease will result in a similar picture, although increased secretion of adrenal androgens may cause the development of sexual hair and some penile growth while testicular size remains prepubertal.

Hypogonadotrophic hypogonadism

Kallmann's syndrome (De Morsier–Gauthier syndrome or hypogonadotrophic eunuchoidism) is an inherited condition with gonadotrophin deficiency of hypothalamic origin. The genetic transmission is either autosomal dominant (and relatively more frequent in males with a variable degree of expressivity [10]) or X-linked autosomal recessive [11].

Kallmann's patients have an impaired sense of smell related to agenesis or dysgenesis of the olfactory lobes in the CNS. In some kindreds, anosmia can be the only manifestation of the syndrome [10]. Kallman's syndrome has been shown to result from deletion of a gene localised to the terminal part of the short arm of the X chromosome (Xp22.3) and encoding for an adhesion molecule [12]. This factor is involved in migration of olfactory neurons and gonadotrophin-releasing hormone (GnRH) neurons from the olfactory placode where they originate during embryonic life. The failure of this migratory process to occur explains the association of hypogonadism and anosmia. Anomalies possibly associated with Kallmann's syndrome include cryptorchidism, micropenis, congenital deafness, mid-line defects such as cleft palate or harelip, colour blindness, renal malformations, and bone malformations such as congenital hip dislocation. Some patients may have obesity and mild mental retardation, but this is not usual.

Table 64.3 Causes of primary amenorrhoea.

Genital tract structural abnormalities
Vaginal anomalies (imperforate hymen)
Congenital absence of uterus or cervix (Rokitansky's syndrome)

Disorders of sex steroid effects
Testicular feminisation (complete insensitivity to androgens)

Gonadal disorders
Congenital
  Gonadal dysgenesis (pure, XO and variants)
  Defect in biosynthesis of testosterone
Acquired
  Premature ovarian failure
  Resistant ovary syndrome
  Polycystic ovary syndrome
  Androgen excess of ovarian (or adrenal) origin

Hypothalamopituitary disorders
Structural
  Pituitary adenomas or suprasellar tumours
  Sheehan's syndrome
Functional
  Weight loss (fear of obesity, anorexia nervosa)
  Psychological stress
  Exercise (e.g. long-distance runners)
  Debilitating diseases
  Drugs
  Hyperprolactinaemia

Hypogonadotrophic hypogonadism and anosmia are found in other syndromes than Kallmann's with distinctive features such as congenital ichthyosis (in Lynch's syndrome) and alopecia (in Johnson's syndrome).

Isolated gonadotrophin deficiency may occur sporadically or as an inherited disorder.

The *fertile eunuch syndrome* results from deficient luteinising hormone (LH) secretion while follicle-stimulating hormone (FSH) is normal, possibly reflecting partial GnRH deficiency. These patients show low androgens and incomplete spermatogenesis, both restored during therapy using human chorionic gonadotrophin (hCG).

In pan-hypopituitarism, gonadotrophin deficiency may be associated with GH, thyroid-stimulating hormone (TSH) and adrenocorticotrophic hormone (ACTH) deficiency, in order of decreasing frequency. This condition may be idiopathic or organic, such as long-term survivors of malignancies treated with irradiation of the CNS (see Chapter 75) or patients with tumours or inflammatory hypothalamo-pituitary lesions. The impairment of growth may be more pronounced in patients with idiopathic hypopituitarism than in those suffering from recent organic lesions, who may present without obvious growth retardation.

Hypergonadotrophic hypogonadism

Turner's syndrome is a major cause of hypogonadism in girls, with an incidence of about one in 2500 live female newborns. This syndrome is discussed in detail in Chapter 51. Of note is the fact that the diagnosis may only be made after several years despite the typical clinical features of the syndrome.

Klinefelter's syndrome does not usually present as delayed puberty. As discussed in Chapter 49, this syndrome is a cause of male infertility and a variable deficit in androgen secretion.

Congenital defects in sex steroid biosynthesis and peripheral effects result in delayed puberty together with anomalies of sex differentiation. Typical examples are the XY patients with 17-hydroxylase deficiency or complete insensitivity to androgens. The latter present as phenotypic females with normal breast development but an absence of pubic hair and primary amenorrhoea.

Recently, new congenital syndromes of hypogonadism have been recognised through increased secretion of immunoreactive gonadotrophins measured in the commonly used radioimmunoassays while bioactivity is altered. This may result from a single amino-acid substitution in the β-subunit of LH [13] or hypoglycosylation of the gonadotrophins in the carbohydrate-deficient glycoprotein syndrome type 1 [14].

Several *polydysmorphic syndromes* may involve primary hypogonadism (Steinert myotonic dystrophy, Lundberg, Bloom, Smith–Lemli–Opitz, Weinstein, Alström and Börjeson–Forssman–Lehmann syndromes). Short stature, mental retardation and ocular anomalies are common features of most dysmorphic syndromes with hypogonadism. In some conditions, such as the Prader–Willi–Labhart syndrome, hypogonadism may result from primary gonadal failure as well as from gonadotrophin deficiency.

Gonadal agenesis is uncommon and more frequent in boys than in girls as a result of a putative regression of the testes, presumably caused by testicular torsion during intrauterine life. *Gonadal hypoplasia* may also result from a failure to synthesise normally gonadotrophin receptors, which might also be the mechanism for the 'resistant ovary syndrome'.

Acquired primary gonadal deficiency may occur following trauma, chemotherapy using gonadotoxic drugs, irradiation, infections (mumps, tuberculosis) or autoimmune processes. Testicular atrophy can occur following surgical orchidopexy for bilateral cryptorchidism. In these disorders, gametogenesis is impaired more frequently and to a greater extent than sex steroid biosynthesis.

Diagnosis

While some patients seen for delayed puberty appear, on physical examination, with early signs of pubertal development, others do not. Thus, the reality of delayed puberty must be initially assessed via the rating of stages of pubertal development according to Tanner's classification [15] and accurate evaluation of penile, mammary or testicular size. The clinical keys to the aetiological diagnosis of delayed puberty are height and height velocity (growth curves drawn using the data obtained from family physician or school records), body proportions and dysmorphic features, as well as weight relative to height. Bone age and serum gonadotrophin levels should then be obtained and further assessment will be required for confirmation of diagnosis in some instances. Follow-up of the patient will finally be helpful to ascertain progression or arrest of pubertal development. We propose algorithms for the diagnosis of delayed puberty in a boy (Fig. 64.1), delayed puberty in a girl (Fig. 64.2) and primary amenorrhoea (Fig. 64.3).

Delayed puberty in a boy

Firstly, boys with small testes and absent virilisation should be managed differently from those with partial or adult virilisation. In the absence of virilisation, normal height and normal growth rate are suggestive of either primary testicular failure with high serum levels of gonadotrophins or isolated gonadotrophin deficiency with prepubertal or low serum levels of gonadotrophins. In the latter case, family

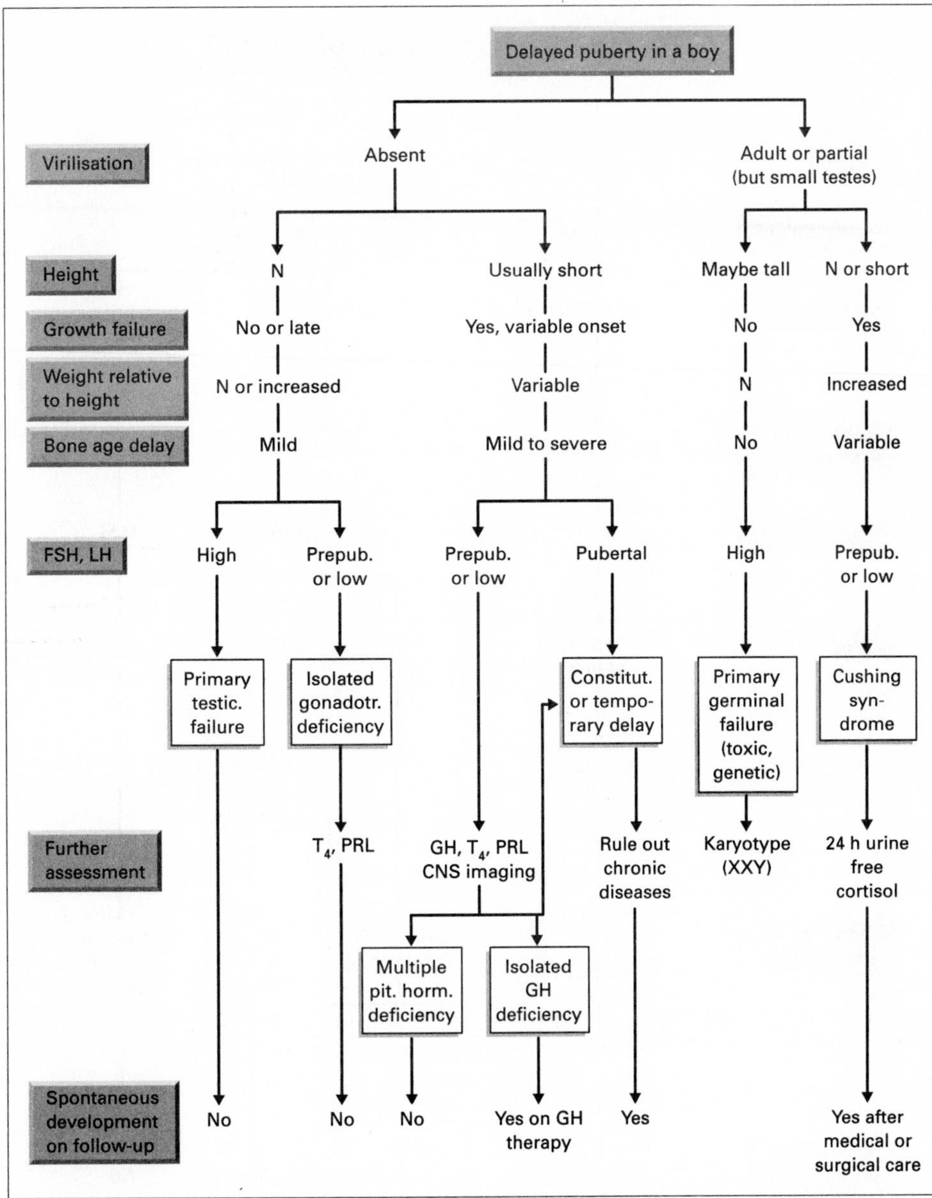

Fig. 64.1 Algorithm for the diagnosis of delayed puberty in a boy.

history may reveal hypogonadism. When taking a personal history, impairment of smell or colour blindness as well as cryptorchidism or micropenis are additional suggestive findings. Excess weight is commonly found in several syndromes. Thyroxine and prolactin levels should be assessed, and follow-up will show no spontaneous pubertal development.

In boys with absent virilisation, short stature and reduced growth velocity, the diagnosis of constitutional delay or temporary delay secondary to chronic diseases should be considered as well as isolated GH or multiple pituitary hormone deficiencies including GH and the gonadotrophins. Such a differential diagnosis may be particularly difficult. In constitutional delay, the family history may reveal late pubertal growth or late menarche in the parents or in siblings. A review of systems and current or previous therapies may indicate a disease or medication possibly accounting for the temporary delay of puberty. The history may also reveal a previous CNS disorder or a therapy such as irradiation which may cause hypothalamo-pituitary deficiency. Weight relative to height may be mildly increased in thyroid or GH deficiency, while it is variable in constitutional delay. Reduced weight is commonly seen in chronic diseases or nutritional defects. In some boys with constitutional delay of puberty, obesity may contribute to the physical disability. The patients with isolated gonadotrophin deficiency usually show slightly delayed bone age and they attain pubertal bone

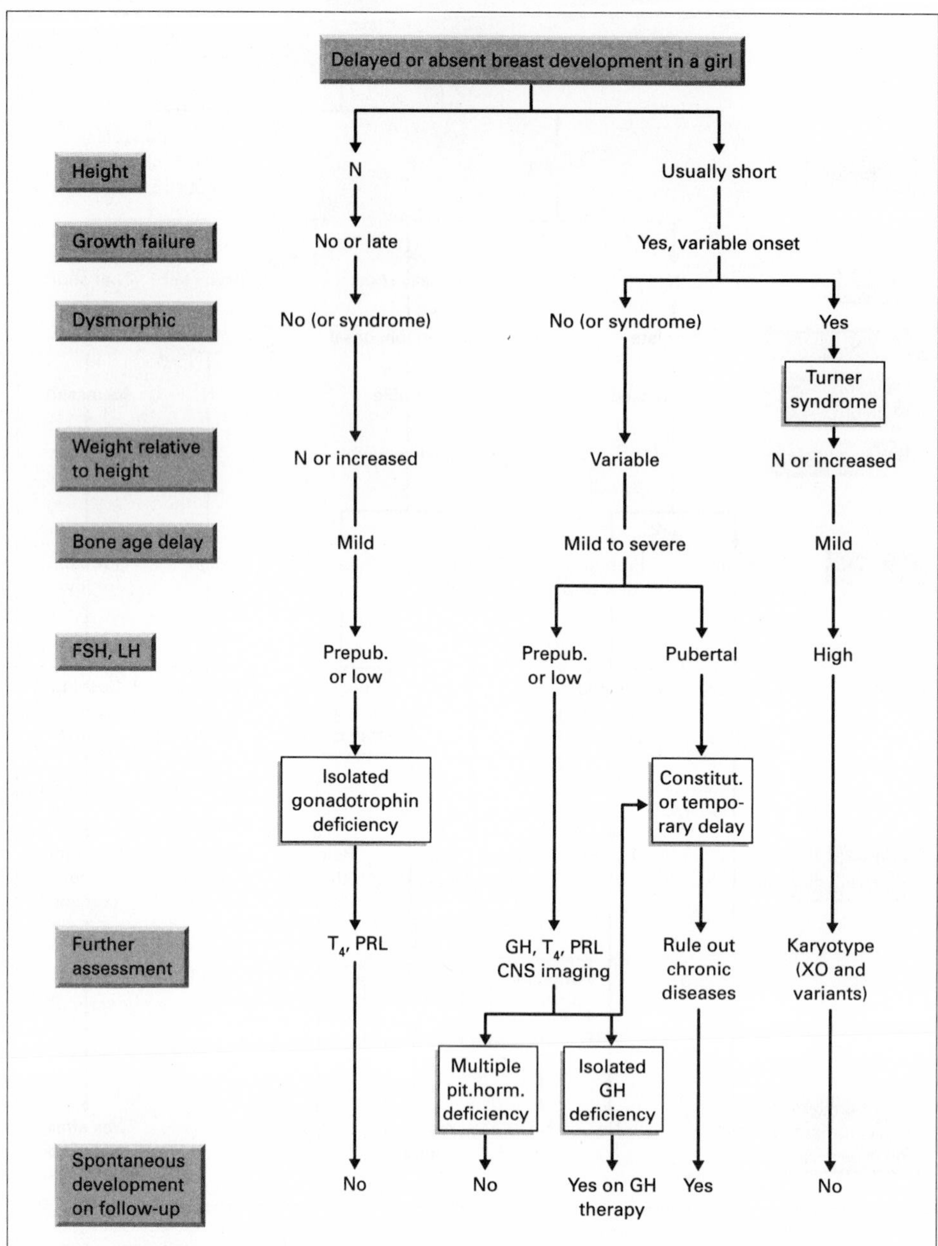

Fig. 64.2 Algorithm for the diagnosis of delayed puberty in a girl.

ages (12–13 years) without evidence of puberty. In patients with constitutional delay, bone age is often more retarded and is consistent with the degree of pubertal development. A severely retarded bone maturation is often seen in patients with multiple pituitary hormone deficiencies, depending on the time when replacement therapies have been started.

The differential diagnosis between multiple pituitary hormone deficiency, isolated GH deficiency and constitutional or temporary delay may not be possible without further diagnostic assessment which includes endocrine and anatomical studies (see below). The observation of a pubertal pattern of gonadotrophin secretion suggests constitutional delay. A chronic disorder such as coeliac disease should then be ruled out when there are any indications suggested by the history or physical examination. A prepubertal pattern of gonadotrophin secretion can be consistent with either diagnosis. In such situations, further endocrine and anatomical studies as well as the follow-up demonstration of progression or arrest of pubertal development will be critical.

In the less common situation of absent testicular development with partial or normal adult virilisation (Fig. 64.1), normal or even tall stature associated with a normal growth

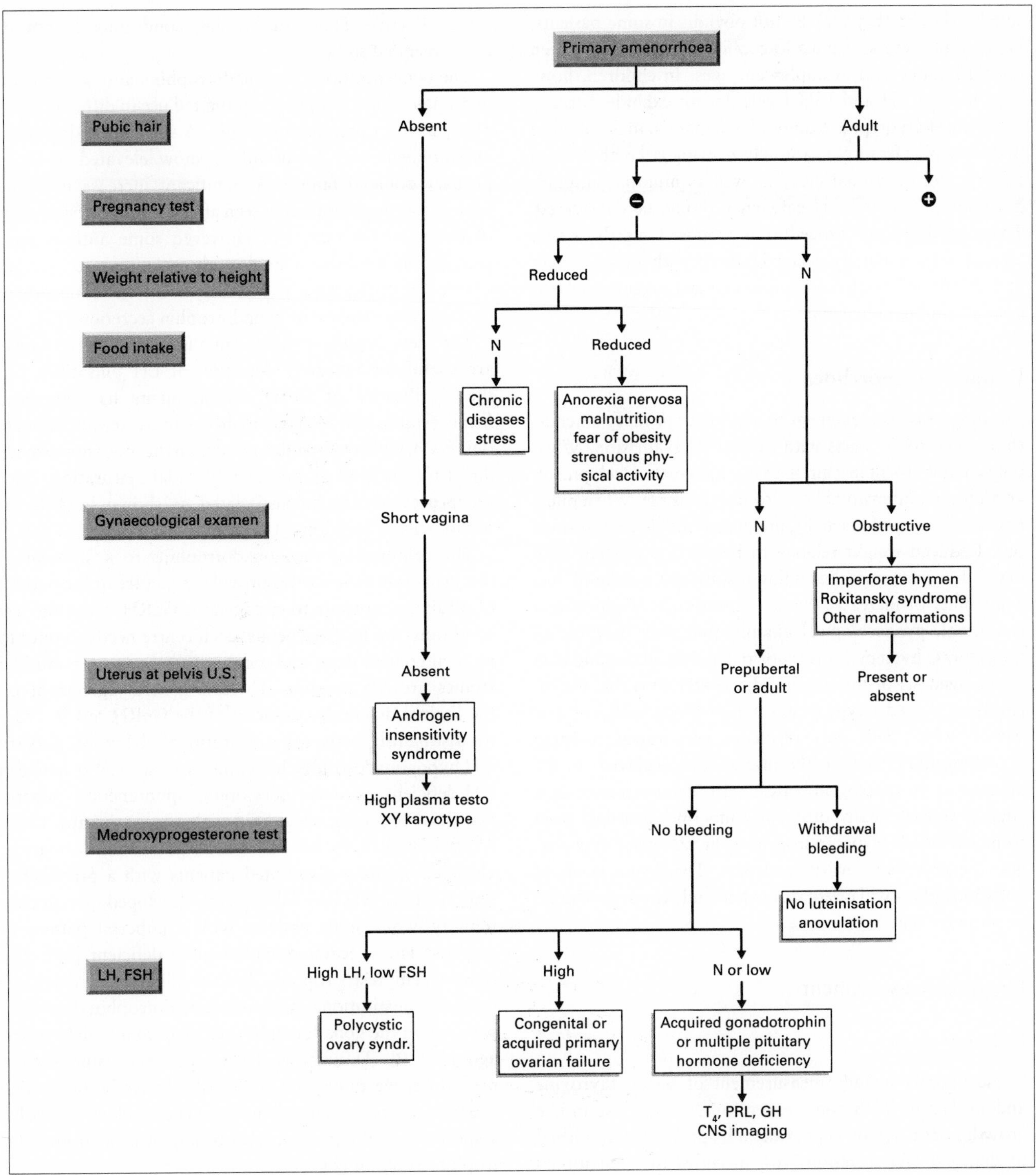

Fig. 64.3 Algorithm for the diagnosis of primary amenorrhoea.

rate, weight and bone age may indicate primary failure of spermatogenesis as in Klinefelter's syndrome (see Chapter 49). In contrast, reduced growth velocity with marked obesity may less commonly indicate Cushing's syndrome (see Chapter 33).

Delayed puberty in a girl

When a girl seen for delayed puberty shows short stature and early growth failure (Fig. 64.2), the typical dysmorphic features of Turner's syndrome (see Chapter 51) should be sought, though they may be not obvious in some patients. High serum levels of gonadotrophins are commonly seen during infancy and at adolescent ages. In children, however, normal LH and FSH levels do not exclude Turner's syndrome: karyotype is required for diagnosis. In the absence of dysmorphic features in a slowly growing girl with delayed puberty, constitutional delay as well as multiple pituitary hormone or isolated GH deficiency should be considered. The same diagnostic procedure is proposed in girls as seen already in boys. Finally, delayed puberty with normal height and absent or late growth failure in a girl suggests isolated gonadotrophin deficiency.

Primary amenorrhoea

The diagnostic management of a girl with primary amenorrhoea (Fig. 64.3) starts with pubic hair evaluation. When pubic hair is absent in a girl with normal breast development, an androgen-insensitivity syndrome is possible. When pubic hair has developed normally, pregnancy should first be ruled out. Reduced weight relative to height is consistent with many different causes including insufficient metabolic fuel availability or increased energy expenditure. When weight is normal, gynaecological examination may indicate an imperforate hymen; if this is normal, pelvic ultrasound may reveal agenesis of the uterus. The next step is the administration of medroxyprogesterone (5–10 mg daily for 1–2 weeks) which will only result in withdrawal bleeding if oestrogenic effects on the uterus have occurred. In the absence of an oestrogenic effect (also demonstrable via a vaginal smear), many different endocrine disorders need to be excluded. Hyperandrogenism or hirsutism may suggest the polycystic ovary syndrome. The serum levels of gonadotrophins will orientate further study towards ovarian or pituitary failure.

Diagnostic assessment

Endocrine studies

These initially include measurement of serum thyroxine and prolactin. With some exceptions, serum insulin-like growth factor 1 (IGF-1) provides a helpful index of normal or deficient GH secretion [16], provided that nutritional disorders have been ruled out. When GH-stimulation tests are performed, priming with sex steroids is required in order to rule out a deficient GH response caused by the absence of puberty [5]. We previously used testosterone propionate (50 mg i.m.) 3 days before testing in boys and 50 μg of ethinyl oestradiol per day orally for 3 days before testing in girls. To date, we feel that such priming may not be long enough and smaller doses given for a longer period of time might be more effective. Standard priming conditions cannot be recommended so far.

The concentrations of gonadotrophins and sex steroids in a single blood sample are of limited use in differentiating pubertal from prepubertal values. A single gonadotrophin measurement may be useful to show elevated levels in primary gonadal failure. A significant increase in serum testosterone levels is usually seen after obvious physical signs of puberty have occurred. However, some authors have recently reported that a single early morning measurement of serum testosterone is particularly useful as a reflection of the nightime increase of gonadotrophin secretion [17].

The new highly sensitive immunoradiometric assays are useful for the early detection of LH pulsatility, but the significance of single measurements has not been firmly established. Serum dehydroepiandrosterone sulphate (DHEAS), which is an index of adrenarche, does not provide direct information on pituitary–gonadal maturation, since the processes may be dissociated as shown in different pathological conditions [18].

The response of the gonadotrophins to a stimulation test using synthetic GnRH provides a picture of the pattern of pituitary exposure to endogenous GnRH. Since the test conditions are heterogeneous, each centre needs to refer to its own control data, and comparisons between published studies are not possible. There is general agreement on the limited diagnostic capacity of the GnRH test in order to distinguish between constitutional delay of puberty and hypogonadotrophic hypogonadism, as well as between GH-deficient patients developing spontaneous puberty and those requiring sex steroid replacement therapy. Using 25 μg/m^2 GnRH, we have obtained significant information, although we have also noted patients with a prepubertal response to GnRH who subsequently developed spontaneous puberty, while some patients with a pubertal pattern of response later became gonadotrophin deficient [19]. The most recent test proposed for the differential diagnosis between constitutional delay and gonadotrophin deficiency is based on the gonadotrophin response to a GnRH superagonist [20]. Though we lack experience using such a procedure, we think that there will always be borderline situations since gonadotrophin deficiency is likely to involve a spectrum of different degrees of impairment of gonadotrophin secretion [21].

A number of different protocols have been used to investigate the response of testosterone to hCG in male patients with delayed puberty: this test also provides interesting but not definitive information. It has been suggested that the study of both GnRH and hCG tests could be of greater diagnostic significance than a single test in isolation [22]. Indirectly, the reduced response of prolactin to thyrotrophin-releasing hormone (TRH) may be an index of deficient gonadotrophin secretion [23]. Using 24-hour study of pulsatile LH secretion, the degree of LH (and presumably of GnRH) deficiency can be estimated: such studies emphasise the heterogeneity of the biological expression of the disorder [21]. This variability is a major reason why there is no optimal procedure for the certain diagnosis of gonadotrophin deficiency. Thus, clinical follow-up of the patient will be required in order to ascertain the diagnosis of gonadotrophin deficiency.

Anatomical studies

These are particularly important when the clinical picture suggests an organic hypothalamo-pituitary or gonadal disorder. The standard radiograph of the sella turcica is only of limited utility. Most lesions can be demonstrated using computed tomography (CT) or magnetic resonance imaging (MRI) scans. The visual field has to be carefully evaluated. In order to study the gonadal structures in girls, pelvic ultrasonography may be performed initially, while CT or MRI scans are required for the diagnosis of gonadal or adrenal tumours.

Therapy

Objectives and modalities

The treatment of hypogonadism or delayed puberty aims: (1) to develop normal sex characteristics; (2) to accelerate growth rate; (3) to optimise adult stature; (4) to achieve normal libido and sexual activity; and (5) to obtain fertility. The first three objectives are predominant in the care of younger patients with delayed puberty. A new therapeutic objective has arisen during recent years since bone mineral density has been shown to increase during the pubertal growth spurt [24]. This appears to be critical for later life since osteopenia has been observed in men with a history of delayed puberty [25]. This observation, together with the psychological correlates of delayed puberty, emphasises the importance of appropriate management as early as possible. Such management includes therapy orientated to the cause of the condition whenever possible, psychological counselling (clear explanations with sometimes a more specific psychological guidance), adjuvant hormonal therapy using anabolic or sex steroids, and replacement hormonal therapy which may differ according to the aetiology of the hypogonadism.

Hormonal therapy in constitutional delay of puberty

Table 64.4 summarises the therapeutic alternatives in patients with delayed puberty or hypogonadism. Constitutional delay of puberty deserves special attention, since this is the most common situation, particularly in boys.

For many years, no hormonal treatment was proposed for constitutional delay of puberty. The patient was reassured and followed up. The psychological consequences of delayed sexual development [26] may have been underestimated by the physicians who were more concerned with the risk of increased bone maturation and reduced adult stature following sex steroid therapy. Retrospective studies have recently shown that adult stature is similar in patients with delayed puberty following adjuvant androgen therapy or without treatment [5,27]. Thus, it seems reasonable to propose androgens (testosterone oenanthate 50 mg/month) for 3–9 months as adjuvant therapy in boys with constitutional delay of puberty. Very recently, transdermal testosterone patches have been made available and offer a convenient and more physiological treatment alternative. However, no experience using such a new preparation has been reported as yet. We do not recommend the use of testosterone undecanoate since individual variations in testosterone bioavailability make dosage adjustment difficult. Testicular growth may occur during therapy, indicating progression of spontaneous puberty concomitant with, but not subsequent to, testosterone administration [28].

Anabolic steroids provide a means of stimulating growth without concomitant induction of sexual development. Oral administration of oxandrolone has been used by some groups at daily dosages of 0.05–0.1 mg/kg without significant adverse effects [29]. However, in some patients with delayed puberty, development of sex characteristics may also be a concern of the patient, in which case it may be preferable to use sex steroids.

Hormonal therapy of permanent hypogonadism

Androgens can effectively induce pubertal development (except testicular growth) and stimulate linear growth in boys. Only few or preliminary data have been reported using the transdermal delivery of testosterone. Long-acting esters such as testosterone oenanthate have been widely used as an intramuscular injection every 2–4 weeks. As substitution therapy, a monthly dosage of 50, 100 and 200 mg can be recommended for the first, second and third years of therapy, respectively [5]. The available data do not support the concept that late puberty prolongs active growth and increases final height [5]. Adult height is only very slightly increased in adults with hypogonadotrophic hypogonadism [30]. Though there are on-going studies on the effect of artificial postponement of puberty using GnRH agonists in short-stature patients, there is no clear reason to expect that final height will be increased. Thus,

Table 64.4 Hormonal therapies for delayed puberty or hypogonadism.

Hormone	Commonly used forms	Route of administration	Dosage	Frequency	Primary indications
Androgens	Long-acting esters of testosterone	i.m.	25–200 mg	1 every 2–4 weeks	Secondary sexual characteristics and linear growth
Oestrogens	Ethinyl oestradiol Conjugated oestrogens	Oral Oral	0.05–0.3 μg/kg 0.15–0.3 mg	1 per day 1 per day	Secondary sexual characteristics and linear growth
Anabolic steroids	Oxandrolone	Oral	0.05–0.1 mg/kg	1 per day	Constitutional growth delay
Gonadotrophin releasing hormone	Synthetic decapeptide	i.v./s.c. (pump)	25–250 ng/kg	60–120 min	Ovulation and spermatogenesis in hypothalamic deficiency, testicular growth
Human chorionic gonadotrophin	Urinary gonadotrophin extracts	i.m.	1500–2000 iu	1 per week	Ovulation and spermatogenesis in hypothalamopituitary deficiency, testicular growth
Human menopausal gonadotrophin		i.m.	150 iu	2 per week	

such treatment cannot be recommended and there is no reason for delaying onset of testosterone therapy. On the contrary, the psychological disturbances associated with delayed sexual maturation [26] may possibly be prevented by starting therapy at a chronological age as close to normal as possible.

Oestrogens are effective promoters of growth and sexual development in girls. The most commonly used forms are ethinyl oestradiol or conjugated oestrogens, given orally. The appropriate dose for stimulation of linear growth without excessive acceleration of bone maturation has yet to be determined. In Turner patients, short-term studies have indicated the biphasic relationship between oestrogen dosage and growth response, a daily dose of 0.1 μg/kg ethinyl oestradiol being optimal [31]. It is possible that even lower dosages of 0.05 μg/kg may be adequate for the initial induction of puberty in girls. Our current recommendation is to maintain such a dose on a continuous basis for the first year of therapy, while double this dose is given for the second year. Later on, considering the possibly increased risk of endometrial or breast cancer with oestrogens alone and the requirement for menarche, ethinyl oestradiol 0.2–0.3 μg/kg can be given for 3 weeks out of 4, together with a progestogen such as didrogesterone, 5–10 mg, from day 15 to day 25 of the cycle. Alternatively, a low dosage combined oestrogen–progestogen preparation can be used.

The time when oestrogen therapy should be initiated is not well defined. In girls with hypopituitarism and in Turner patients [5], the potential for a growth response to oestrogens decreases with age, whereas bone age at the onset of oestrogen therapy does not seem to affect final height [5]. There is thus no rationale for beginning oestrogen therapy at a bone age of 13 years, as has been previously recommended [5]. While it is obvious that initiation of therapy at earlier bone ages (around 11 years) will result in a better growth response, we do not yet know what the final height will be. Based on the recent observation that oestrogens are responsible for the promotion of bone maturation and mineralization [32], it is likely that the dose of oestrogen is critical for bone maturation and, thus, final height.

Pulsatile GnRH administration using a portable intravenous or subcutaneous infusion minipump is conceptually the most 'physiological' procedure that can be used in patients with intact functional capacity of the pituitary gland and the gonads. Considering the practical aspects of such a procedure, it seems reasonable to propose pulsatile GnRH therapy only for the induction of fertility. Pursuing a similar objective, gonadotrophins can be administered one to three times a week in men with hypogonadotrophic hypogonadism. hCG is usually given alone for 6 months at a dosage varying between 1500 and 5000 iu per injection. By using hCG alone for one to several years, a full therapeutic response including spermatogenesis can be achieved in men with partial gonadotrophin deficiency, who have shown some testicular growth before therapy [33]. In the remaining patients, hCG therapy is combined with the administration of human menopausal gonadotrophin (hMG), 75–150 iu In boys with hypopituitarism treated after completion of GH therapy and testosterone-induced puberty, satisfactory results were obtained using 1500 iu once a week, and hMG 150 iu twice a week [34]. An alternative regimen is to use hMG 300 iu three times a week, plus hCG 1000 iu twice-weekly. Recombinant gonadotrophin preparations are used more extensively, but experience in adolescent patients is lacking.

References

1 Prader A. Delayed adolescence. *Clin Endocrinol Metab* 1975; **4**: 143–55.

2 Lipson AB, Savage MO, Davies PSW, Bassett K, Shand WS, Walker-Smith JA. Acceleration of linear growth following intestinal resection for Crohn's disease *Eur J Pediatr* 1990; **149**: 687–90.

3 Warren PW. Effects of undernutrition on reproductive function in the human. *Endocr Rev* 1983; **4**: 363–77.

4 Theintz GE, Howald H, Weiss U, Sizonenko PC. Evidence for a reduction of growth potential in adolescent female gymnasts. *J Pediatr* 1993; **122**: 306–13.

5 Bourguignon JP. Linear growth as function of age of onset of puberty and sex steroid dosage: therapeutic implications. *Endocr Rev* 1988; **9**: 467–88.

6 Cacciari E, Tassoni P, Parisi G *et al.* Pitfalls in diagnosing impaired growth hormone (GH) secretion: retesting after replacement therapy of 63 patients defined as GH deficient. *J Clin Endocrinol Metab* 1992; **74**: 1284–9.

7 Nicolson A, Toogood AA, Rahim A, Shalet SM. The prevalence of severe growth hormone deficiency in adults who received growth hormone replacement in childhood. *Clin Endocrinol* 1996; **44**: 311–16.

8 Adan L, Souberbielle JC, Brauner R. Management of the short stature due to pubertal delay in boys. *J Clin Endocrinol Metab* 1994; **78**: 478–82.

9 Grossman A, Besser GM. Regular view: prolactinomas. *Br Med J* 1985; **290**: 182–4.

10 Santen RJ, Paulsen CA. Hypogonadotropic eunuchoidism. I: Clinical study of the mode of inheritance. *J Clin Endocrinol Metab* 1973; **36**: 47–54.

11 Leiblish JM, Rogol AD, White BJ, Rosen SW. Syndrome of anosmia with hypogonadotrophic hypogonadism (Kallmann syndrome). *Am J Med* 1982; **73**: 506–20.

12 Hardelin JP, Levilliers J, Young J *et al.* Xp 22.3 deletions in isolated familial Kallman's syndrome. *J Clin Endocrinol Metab* 1993; **76**: 827–31.

13 Weiss J, Axelrod L, Whitcomb RW, Harris PE, Crowley WF, Jameson JL. Hypogonadism caused by a single amino-acid substitution in the beta subunit of luteinizing hormone. *N Engl J Med* 1992; **326**: 179–83.

14 De Zegher F, Jaeken J. Endocrinology of the carbohydrate-deficient glycoprotein syndrome type 1 from birth through adolescence. *Pediatr Res* 1995; **37**: 395–401.

15 Tanner JM. Normal growth and growth assessment. *Clin Endocrinol Metab* 1986; **15**: 411–51.

16 Rosenfeld RG, Wilson DM, Lee PDK, Hintz RL. Insulin-like growth factors I and II in evaluation of growth retardation. *J Pediatr* 1986; **103**: 428–33.

17 Wu FCW, Brown DC, Butler GE, Stirling HF, Kelnar CJH. Early morning plasma testosterone is an accurate predictor of imminent pubertal development in prepubertal boys. *J Clin Endocrinol Metab* 1993; **76**: 26–31.

18 Sklar CA, Kaplan SL, Grumbach MM. Evidence for dissociation between adrenarche and gonadarche: studies in patients with idiopathic precocious upberty, gonadal dysgenesis, isolated gonadotrophin deficiency and constitutionally delayed growth and adolescence. *J Clin Endocrinol Metab* 1980; **51**: 548–56.

19 Bourguignon JP, Vanderschueren-Lodeweyckx M, Wolter R *et al.* Hypopituitarism and idiopathic delayed puberty: a longitudinal study in an attempt to diagnose gonadotrophin deficiency before puberty. *J Clin Endocrinol Metab* 1982; **54**: 733–44.

20 Ghai K, Cara JF, Rosenfield RL. Gonadotropin releasing hormone agonist (Nafarelin) test to differentiate gonadotropin deficiency from constitutionally delayed puberty in teenage boys. A clinical research center study. *J Clin Endocrinol Metab* 1995; **80**: 2980–6.

21 Spratt DI, Carr DB, Merriam GR, Scully RE, Narasimha RAO, Crowley WF. The spectrum of abnormal patterns of gonadotropin-releasing hormone secretion in men with idiopathic hypogonadotrophic hypogonadism: clinical and laboratory correlations. *J Clin Endocrinol Metab* 1987; **64**: 283–91.

22 Dunkel L, Perheentupa J, Virtanen M, Mäenpää J. GnRH and HCG tests are both necessary in differential diagnosis of male delayed puberty. *Am J Dis Child* 1985; **139**: 494–8.

23 Spitz IM, Hirsch HJ, Trestian S. The prolactin response to thyrotropin-releasing hormone differentiales isolated gonadotropin deficiency from delayed puberty. *N Engl J Med* 1983; **308**: 575–9.

24 Theintz G, Buchs B, Rizzoli R, Slosman D, Clavien H, Sizonenko P, Bonjour JPH. Longitudinal monitoring of bone mass accumulation in healthy adolescents: evidence for a marked reduction after 16 years of age at the levels of lumbar spine and femoral neck in female subjects. *J Clin Endocrinol Metab* 1992; **75**: 1060–5.

25 Finkelstein JS, Neer RM, Biller BMK, Crawford JD, Klibanski A. Osteopenia in men with a history of delayed puberty. *N Engl J Med* 1992; **326**: 600–4.

26 Dean HJ, McTaggart TL, Fish DG, Friesen HG. The educational, vocational and marital status of growth hormone-deficient adults treated with growth hormone during childhood. *Am J Dis Child* 1985; **139**: 1105–10.

27 Bourguignon JP. Growth and timing of puberty : reciprocal effects. *Horm Res* 1991; **36**: 131–5.

28 Uruena M, Pantsiotou S, Preece MA, Stanhope R. Is testosterone therapy for boys with constitutional delay of growth and puberty associated with impaired final height and suppression of the hypothalamo-pituitary-gonadal axis? *Eur J Pediatr* 1992; **151**: 15–18.

29 Clayton PE, Shalet SM, Price DA, Addison GM. Growth and growth hormone responses to oxandrolone in boys with constitutional delay of growth and puberty (CDGP). *Clin Endocrinol* 1988; **29**: 123–30.

30 Uriarte MM, Baron J, Garcia HB, Barnes KM, Loriaux DL, Cutler GB. The effect of pubertal delay on adult height in men with isolated hypogonadotropic hypogonadism. *J Clin Endocrinol Metab* 1992; **74**: 436–40.

31 Ross IL, Long LM, Skerda M, Cassorla F, Kurtz D, Loriaux DL, Cutler GB. Effects of low doses of estradiol on 6-month growth rates and predicted height in patients with Turner syndrome. *J Pediatr* 1987; **109**: 950–3.

32 Smith EP, Boyd J, Franck GR, Takahashi H, Cohen RM, Specker B, Williams TC, Lubahn DB, Korach KS. Estrogen resistance caused by a mutation in the estrogen-receptor gene in a man. *N Engl J Med* 1994; **331**: 1056–61.

33 Burris AS, Rodbard HW, Winters SJ, Sherins RJ. Gonadotropin therapy in men with isolated hypogonadotropic hypogonadism: the response to human chorionic gonadotropin is predicted by initial testicular size. *J Clin Endocrinol Metab* 1988; **66**: 1144–51.

34 Vandeweghe M. Complete virilization and spermatogenesis with combined HCG/HMG treatment in gonadotropin and growth-hormone deficient patients. In: Frish H, Thorner MO, eds. *Hormone Regulation of Growth*. New York: Raven Press, 1989; **58**: 283–7.

Part 14
Imaging in Endocrinology

CHAPTER 65

Endocrine imaging techniques

R.H. Reznek and P. Armstrong

Thyroid

Several modalities are available to image the thyroid gland. Functional imaging is performed by scintigraphy with a variety of radionuclides (see Chapter 25). Duplex and colour-flow Doppler (CFD) sonography, computed tomography (CT) and magnetic resonance imaging (MRI) are used to define anatomy and determine blood flow of the thyroid gland. These tests are used to:

1 detect a space-occupying lesion (SOL) when clinical suspicion is high;

2 detect other SOLs when one is palpable;

3 characterise a lesion as solid, cystic, calcified, or cystic degeneration within a solid lesion;

4 evaluate the trapping and organification activity of a thyroid nodule (hyper-, hypo-, autonomous or non-functioning);

5 detect cervical lymph-node metastases;

6 detect local recurrence of tumour after thyroid excision.

Thyroid masses

Ultrasound

Ultrasound provides the best anatomical representation of the thyroid gland. Modern machines, which use high-resolution 7.5–10 MHz probes, provide excellent spatial resolution which allows nodules as small as 2 mm to be detected. Ultrasound is of value in establishing whether a palpable nodule is solitary or part of a multinodular process as multinodular goitres have been said to have a lower incidence of malignancy (1–6%) than is associated with a single 'cold' nodule which is malignant in 15–25% of cases [1] although this has been disputed. In about 25% of patients, palpable nodules which appear on clinical examination to be solitary are shown by ultrasound to be multiple [2]. Ultrasound is also used to detect thyroid tumours in those patients at a high risk of developing thyroid carcinoma [3] and to determine whether a known mass is cystic or solid.

Ultrasound cannot reliably distinguish between benign and malignant thyroid masses. Benign follicular adenomas most commonly show decreased reflectivity compared with the surrounding tissue, but may show increased reflectivity or be isoechoic. A surrounding lucent 'halo' is often seen in benign disease, but may also be seen in malignant nodules. Ultrasound is also very effective in distinguishing between solid and cystic lesions. Purely cystic lesions with no soft-tissue component are virtually never cancers and in most institutions are managed with fine-needle aspiration [2]. However, cystic masses within a soft-tissue nodule cannot be used to predict histology as 86% will be degenerating benign adenomas, but 14% will be malignant [4] (Fig. 65.1). Twenty-three per cent of purely solid masses are malignant [2].

Certain ultrasound features increase the likelihood of malignancy of a thyroid nodule, notably, invasion into surrounding tissues results in loss of clear definition of the tissue planes [5]. Ultrasound is more sensitive than clinical examination in the detection of enlarged cervical nodes: nodes infiltrated with tumour tend to exceed 8 mm in their short axis [3]. Cervical lymph nodes, infiltrated by papillary carcinoma of the thyroid, may be entirely cystic and mimic other cystic masses of the neck such as a bronchial cyst, while calcification may be seen within nodes involved by medullary carcinoma (Fig. 65.2). Microcalcification smaller than 2 mm in diameter with acoustic shadowing favours malignancy as it is observed in about 60% of carcinomas but only 2% of benign nodules [3].

Radionuclide imaging

Radionuclide imaging of thyroid masses provides functional information which complements the anatomical information

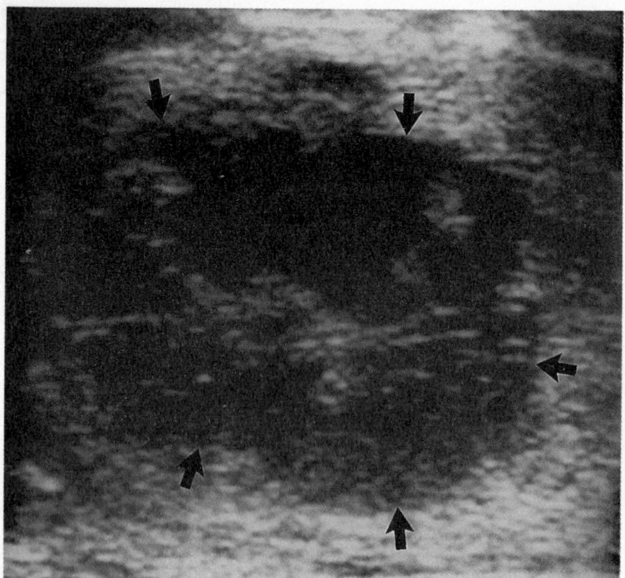

Fig. 65.1 Papillary carcinoma of the thyroid. Longitudinal scan through the right lobe of the thyroid showing a mixed cystic and solid thyroid mass (arrowed). The black areas represent anechoic fluid.

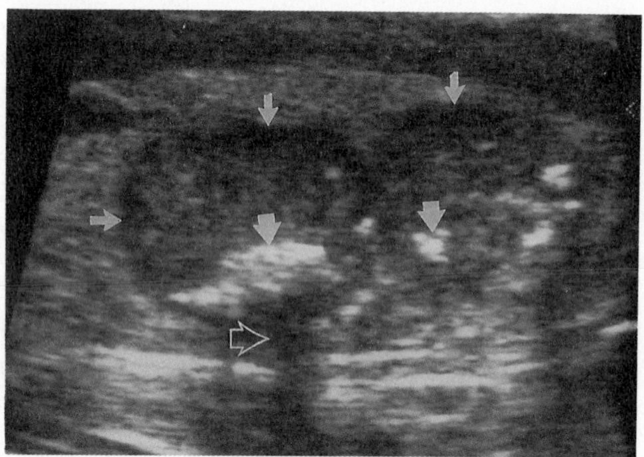

Fig. 65.2 Medullary carcinoma of the thyroid. A longitudinal scan through the thyroid gland showing a well-defined mass (arrowed) within mormal thyroid tissue. Highly echogenic material (thick arrowheads) casting an acoustic shadow (open arrow) is due to calcification.

obtained from ultrasound. The commonly used radiopharmaceuticals are ^{123}I, ^{99m}Tc-pertechnetate ($^{99m}TcO_4$) and ^{131}I. ^{123}I has a short half-life γ emission which gives one-hundredth of the thyroid radiation dose compared with ^{131}I making it the preferred isotope for functional assesment [6]. $^{99m}TcO_4$ is used for purely anatomical thyroid evaluation, since it gives excellent images but may fail to demonstrate hypofunction in some nodules that appear 'cold' on ^{123}I scans. Oral iodides, radiographic contrast media and iodine-containing drugs all compete with the radioisotopes and should be avoided before the imaging studies (see also Chapters 25 and 28).

Approximately 10–25 of non-functioning ('cold') solitary nodules are malignant, whereas functioning ('hot') nodules are almost always thyroid-stimulating hormone (TSH)-dependent adenomas [5]. Focal 'hot' nodules on thyroid scintigrams are very rarely malignant. Some authors describe a 'warm' nodule which carries a 7% incidence of carcinoma. Rarely, well-differentiated thyroid cancers have preserved trapping function, giving the appearance of function on a 24-hour scan but becoming 'cold' on delayed scans. This unusual pitfall can be overcome by doing delayed images on functioning nodules. Even though almost all thyroid cancers are non-functioning, most 'cold' nodules are adenomas, colloid nodules or foci of thyroiditis. Rarely, 'cold' nodules can be due to intrathyroidal lymph nodes, lymphoma or metastases in the thyroid gland. 'Cold' nodules always need further assesment, usually by fine-needle aspiration cytology, needle biopsy and/or excision biopsy. This combined imaging approach greatly reduces the rate of unnecessary surgery for benign non-functioning nodes [7].

Ultrasound-guided fine-needle aspiration for cytology

Fine needle aspiration for cytology (FNAC) is the most reliable non-operative method for obtaining a definitive diagnosis and has become a mainstay in the selection of patients for surgery [2]. Overall, the sensitivity of FNAC for the detection of malignancy in both cystic and solid lesions is high, ranging between 90 and 100% [7]. However, false positives occur quite frequently so that the specificity is only 55% for solid nodules and 52% for cystic lesions [4]. Another drawback is that FNAC may be less sensitive in cystic papillary carcinomas [4], and deciding between follicular adenoma and adenocarcinoma is often impossible because the pathologist relies on documenting capsular or venous invasion to make the distinction.

Computed tomography

CT scanning is seldom used in the detection and evaluation of thyroid tumours, but is occasionally used specifically to demonstrate the extent of local invasion, the presence of retrosternal and retrotracheal extension and to detect local recurrence.

Magnetic resonance imaging

As with CT, MRI may be useful in the staging of a known malignant tumour, to show local invasion and regional lymph-node metastases or to determine whether there is recurrence following thyroidectomy. A positive predictive value of 82% and a negative predictive value of 86% in the detection of recurrent disease in the neck has been achieved using MRI [8]. As with CT, false-positive results can be caused by inflammatory lymphatic hyperplasia and granulation tissue. Nevertheless, the results show a distinct advantage for MRI compared with ultrasound or CT in the detection of recurrent disease [8].

Scintigraphy in tumour follow-up
(see also Chapters 25 and 28)

^{131}I scanning with serum thyroglobulin measurement is the most appropriate technique for the detection of recurrence in patients who have undergone surgery for a well-differentiated thyroid carcinoma. The scans require induction of endogenous TSH to stimulate ^{131}I uptake, achieved by discontinuing triiodothyronine (T_3) for 2 weeks prior to scanning [9]. Occasionally, when the scan is equivocal in the presence of an elevated thyroglobulin level, ^{201}Tl whole-body imaging may be helpful, because it is very sensitive, albeit non-specific, for detecting tumour tissue. Following removal of medullary carcinoma, serum calcitonin levels are used to diagnose recurrence. When elevated, ^{99}Tc-DMSA (pentavalent dimercaptosuccinic acid) or ^{111}In-pentatreotide and ^{123}I-MIBG (metaiodobenzylguanidine) have been used for the detection and documentation of recurrent or residual disease [10,11].

Screening of the thyroid by ultrasound

Following radiation therapy there is an increased risk of papillary and follicular carcinoma. For example, in patients who have received radiotherapy for Hodgkin's disease, the risk of developing thyroid cancer is about 15% [12,13]. The carcinoma is unlikely to develop in under 5 years following exposure to radiation; thus, beyond 5 years, ultrasound provides a useful, sensitive and relatively inexpensive means of screening an at-risk population for thyroid cancer [13].

Thyroiditis

Acute thyroiditis

Acute thyroiditis typically appears as focal or diffuse hypoechoic enlargement of the gland on ultrasound. ^{131}I uptake is usually normal or diminished and scintigraphy reveals 'cold' nodules corresponding to the site of tenderness.

Subacute (de Quervain's) thyroiditis

Subacute thyroiditis also results in multiple hypoechoic areas in the thyroid with atrophy over time.

Hashimoto's thyroiditis

Hashimoto's thyroiditis shows a dramatic, diffuse inhomogenous hypoechoic ultrasound pattern (Fig. 65.3). Thyroid volume diminishes along with reduced function as the disease progresses. Patients with Hashimoto's thyroiditis are at slightly increased risk for the development of thyroid lymphoma, leukaemia and papillary and Hürthle cell neoplasms. These patients, therefore, can be followed closely and non-invasively with ultrasound.

Parathyroid gland imaging (see also Chapter 41)

About 80% of patients who present with primary hyperparathyroidism have a single parathyroid adenoma, 12–15% have primary parathyroid hyperplasia, 3–5% have multiple parathyroid adenomas and a small percentage have parathyroid carcinomas or cysts [5]. Secondary hyperparathyroidism produces hyperplasia of all parathyroid glands. About 80% of abnormal parathyroid glands are situated in and immediately adjacent to the thyroid. Ectopic glands may be found anywhere from the level of the third pharyngeal pouch, just behind the angle of the mandible at the level of the hyoid bone, down to the aortic root. Up to 5% may be in the posterior mediastinum [5,14].

The diagnosis of hyperparathyroidism is based on biochemical findings. Imaging is performed purely to localise parathyroid tumours and abnormal glands prior to surgery.

Localisation of abnormal parathyroid glands

The extent to which preoperative imaging is undertaken

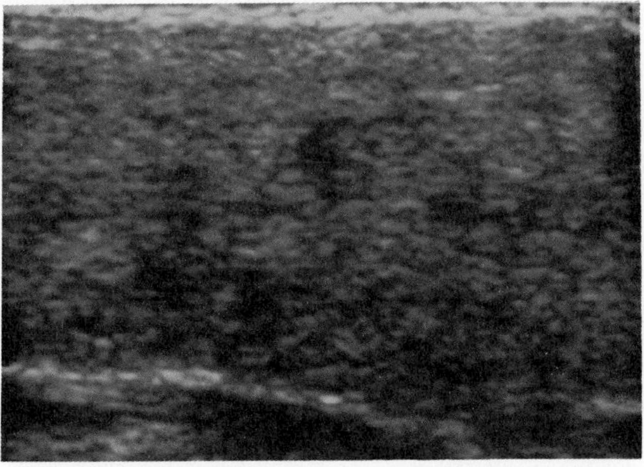

Fig. 65.3 Hashimoto's thyroiditis. A longitudinal scan through the thyroid gland showing an enlarged lobe with a diffuse, inhomogeneous decrease in the normal reflectivity of the thyroid gland. The appearance of normal thyroid tissue is seen in Figs 65.4a and b.

for preoperative localisation depends on the policy of the individual surgeon. In the hands of an experienced surgeon, a cure rate of approximately 95% can be expected in primary hyperparathyroidism following the initial exploration of the neck [15,16]. Preoperative localisation is unlikely to add significantly to the surgical success rate, nor to reduce the operation time for experienced surgeons [16–18]. Some authors, however, recommend unilateral neck dissection if one abnormal gland is demonstrated on preoperative imaging, only proceeding to bilateral exploration if the second ipsilateral gland appears abnormal at the time of operation [19,20]. A unilateral neck dissection saves a considerable amount of operating time. All authors advocate the use of a localisation study prior to reoperation, when surgical cure rate without preoperative localisation is 30–40% lower than in patients being operated on for the first time. Even though an increased proportion of pathological glands will lie in an ectopic site, the pathological gland is still most likely to be located in the neck. In these patients, imaging prior to surgery improves surgical results by demonstrating the location of a parathyroid tumour [7,21].

Localisation techniques

Radionuclide imaging. Both thallium-201 and ^{99m}Tc-sestamibi are taken up by parathyroid glands and are the agents of choice for imaging. In those centres which have reported results with both techniques, ^{99m}Tc-sestamibi appears to have a slightly higher sensitivity and lower radiation dose than ^{201}Tl, and the two are similar in cost. This would indicate that ^{99m}Tc-sestamibi should be regarded as the radiopharmaceutical of choice [22,23]. ^{201}Tl-chloride and ^{99m}Tc-sestamibi are taken up by both the parathyroid and thyroid glands; a subtraction technique is usually employed in order to identify abnormal parathyroid tissue (Fig. 65.4), for which a thyroid imaging agent (^{99m}Tc-pertechnetate or iodide) is given. The thyroid uptake is then subtracted from the ^{201}Tl or ^{99m}Tc-sestamibi image, allowing localisation of parathyroid tissue. Normal parathyroid glands are not seen since they are smaller and less metabolically active than adenomas or hyperplastic glands.

Ultrasound. Typically, parathyroid adenomas appear as oval, well-defined anechoic or hypoechoic masses posterior to the thyroid gland, and anterior to the longus colli muscle (Fig. 65.4) They tend to be of the order of 10 mm in diameter but can grow to a very large size (40–50 mm) [5]. As glands become larger, they are more likely to be multilobulated and to contain areas of echogenicity, cysts and calcifications. There are several problems inherent to ultrasound localisation of parathyroid adenomas. Retropharyngeal, retro-oesophageal and mediastinal parathyroid glands, which account for 5–15% of all glands, are inaccessible by ultrasound. Occasionally, in primary hyperplasia, one gland may predominate, leading to an erroneous conclusion that there is a solitary parathyroid adenoma. Other false-positive diagnoses can result when thyroid nodules, on the periphery of the gland, hyperplastic lymph nodes, prominent longus colli muscles and sympathetic ganglia are misinterpreted as parathyroid adenomas. Intraoperative ultrasound has been shown to be of value during reoperation for primary hyperparathyroidism, assisting the surgeon in localising the abnormal glands and reducing the operating time [24].

Computed tomography. CT does not have any advantage over ultrasound in detecting an adenoma located in a normal parathyroid site (Fig. 65.4), but it is very useful for detecting abnormalities lying in sites inaccessible to ultrasound such as behind the trachea, in the mediastinum, or in an undescended inferior parathyroid gland in the carotid sheath [25]. These are all common sites for adenomas to be missed at initial neck exploration. CT is therefore a very useful localisation procedure to perform before reoperation for primary hyperparathyroidism.

Magnetic resonance imaging. Excellent images of the neck can be obtained with high-field strength magnets and a small surface coil. The ability of MRI to localise parathyroid pathology appears to be at least comparable with the other imaging modalities. MRI has some advantages over CT for imaging the neck in that the bone artifact across the root of the neck arising from the shoulders is avoided with MRI, and vascular structures are visualised without the need for intravenous injection of contrast medium, which is essential for the interpretation of CT. Uncomplicated parathyroid adenomas typically show medium signal intensity on T1-weighted images, equivalent to muscle, and high signal on T2-weighted images, similar to fat.

The accuracy of imaging techniques in localising parathyroid disease

There is a great variation in the reported success of all imaging techniques in the localisation of parathyroid disease. The overall sensitivity for nuclear medicine techniques in identifying parathyroid adenomas (^{201}Tl and ^{99m}Tc-sestamibi) ranges from 27 to 95% with that of ^{99m}Tc-sestamibi slightly higher than that of ^{201}Tl [15,21,26,27]. The specificity is higher at 91–98%. The sensitivity of radiopharmaceutical techniques in demonstrating hyperplasia is lower than that for the detection of parathyroid adenoma, only about 45% [6], and similar to the sensitivity for detection of pathology at reoperation [6]. Modern

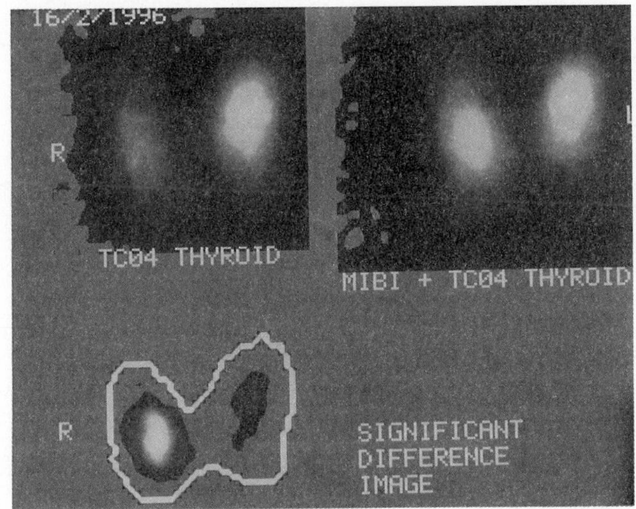

(a)

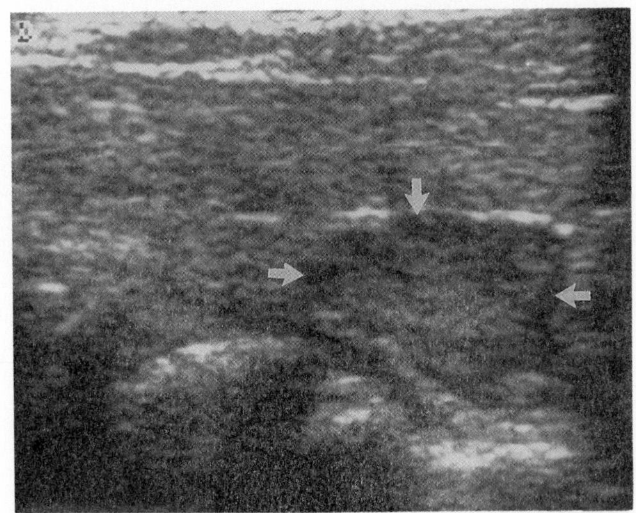

(b)

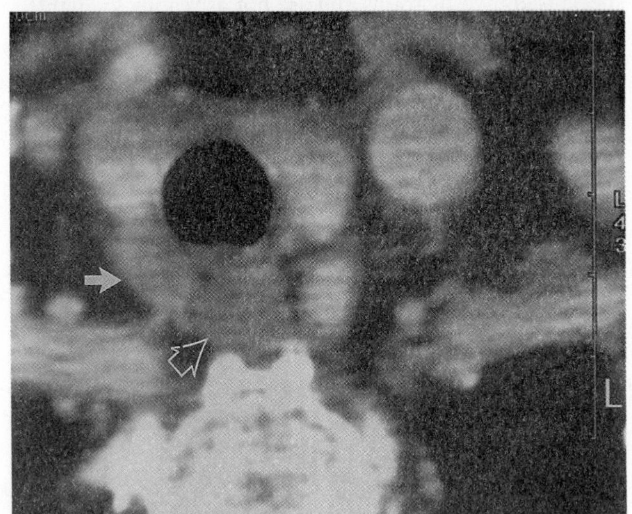

(c)

Fig. 65.4 Parathyroid adenoma. (a) ^{99m}Tc-sestamibi scan with a subtraction technique showing markedly increased activity on the right side after subtraction of the thyroid uptake. (b) Longitudinal ultrasound scan through the normal right lobe of the thyroid showing a small parathyroid mass lying posterior to the lower pole of the thyroid (arrows). (c) Computed tomography scan in the same patient showing the parathyroid tumour (arrowed) lying posterior to the thyroid gland. The oesophagus lies closely to the left of the tumour (open arrow).

ultrasound using 7.5 or 10 MHz high-resolution probes is only slightly less sensitive than nuclear medicine; the highest reported sensitivity for identifying an adenoma being 82% [8,28]. The specificity, however, is high, ranging from 78 to 100% [6]. As with all imaging techniques, the sensitivity of ultrasound drops to about 60% when identifying hyperplastic glands and about 50% when localising parathyroid pathology following a previous operation [6,15,17,28].

The sensitivity of CT in identifying parathyroid adenomas is similar to that of ultrasound with the best results to date being about 80% with specificities ranging from 92 to 95% [17,27]. After failed exploration of the neck, a sensitivity of 44–50% can be expected [25,28].

The results for MRI do not differ significantly from those for CT [6,17,27].

Gastrointestinal endocrine tumours

Islet-cell tumours

Insulinomas and gastrinomas account for over 78% of all islet-cell tumours. Confident localisation of functioning islet-cell tumours often requires the correlation of the findings of a number of investigations; the tumours are usually extremely small and to be confident of the diagnosis often requires support from more than one test. Ninety per cent of insulinomas are < 20 mm in diameter and 50% are < 13 mm [29]. Gastrinomas are equally difficult to detect as their mean size is only 22 mm [30] and may be anywhere within the 'gastrinoma triangle' which covers the stomach or duodenal wall, lymph nodes, peripancreatic tissue or even in the mesentery. Duodenal wall gastrinomas have an average size of 6 mm [31]. Thus, careful attention to technique is required and it has to be accepted that many islet-cell tumours will not be detected by any current imaging modality [32].

Glucagonomas, vasoactive intestinal polypeptide (VIP)-secreting tumours (VIPomas), somatostatinomas and non-functioning islet-cell tumours all tend to be large at the time of diagnosis, measuring several centimetres [33]. Carcinoid tumours, secreting 5-hydroxytryptamine or related compounds resulting in the carcinoid syndrome, vary in size [34] (see Chapter 45).

Ultrasound

Transabdominal ultrasound will usually be the first imaging investigation for localisation of islet-cell tumours since it is relatively inexpensive and readily available. Endoscopic and intraoperative ultrasound are more sensitive but more specialised investigations and are not as readily available.

Transabdominal ultrasound

Although visualisation of the entire pancreas is often possible on ultrasound, in about one-quarter of all patients, part or all of the pancreas is obscured by overlying gas in the stomach or colon. An islet-cell tumour is usually seen as a small area of reduced echogenicity (Fig. 65.5). There may be a hypoechoic rim, necrosis or calcification. Some tumours, especially gastrinomas, may be hyperechoic (Fig. 65.6), whereas others may be isoechoic, rendering them invisible unless anatomical distortion is present. The sensitivity of transabdominal ultrasound for the detection of primary islet-cell tumours ranges from only 30% to 61% [35,36], but falls to about 15% for the detection of multiple insulinomas [36].

Endoscopic ultrasound

A high-frequency ultrasound probe (10 MHz), when passed through an endoscope to lie in close proximity to the pancreas, provides high-resolution images and improves the sensitivity for the detection of islet-cell tumours (Fig. 65.7). Although data are still sparse, sensitivities of approximately 80% have been reported [37,38]. However, endoscopic

(a)
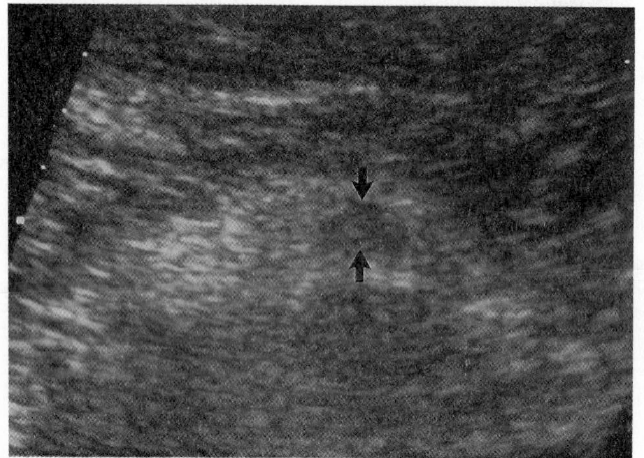

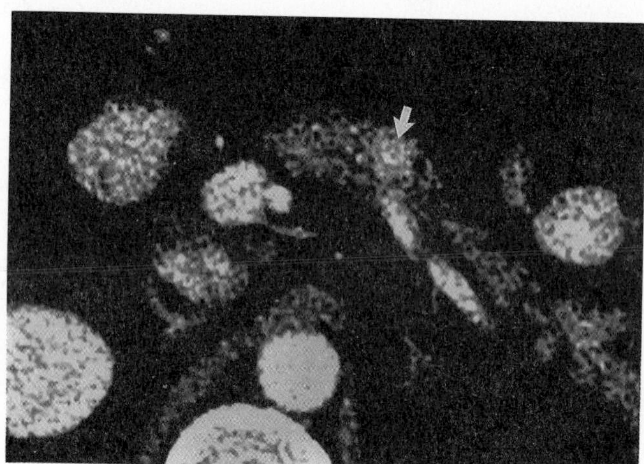
(b)

(c)
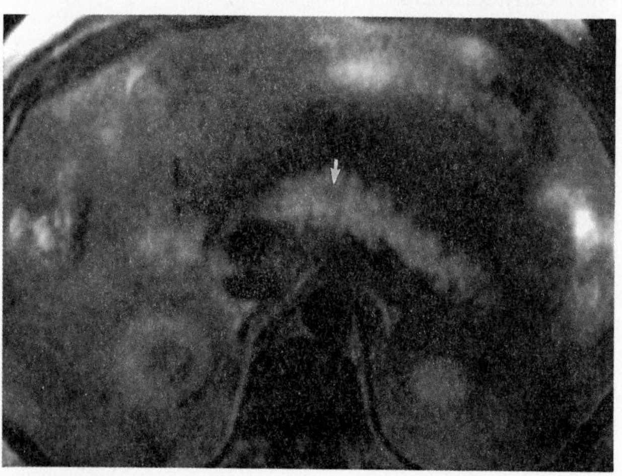

Fig. 65.5 Insulinoma. (a) Transverse, transabdominal ultrasound showing an 8-mm area of decreased echogenicity (arrowed) within the pancreas due to the presence of an insulinoma. (b) Computed tomography scan on the same patient, taken after intravenous injection of contrast medium showing an area of increased enhancement due to the insulinoma. (c) T1-weighted magnetic resonance imaging scan with fat suppression showing the typical appearance of decreased signal intensity corresponding to the insulinoma (arrowed).

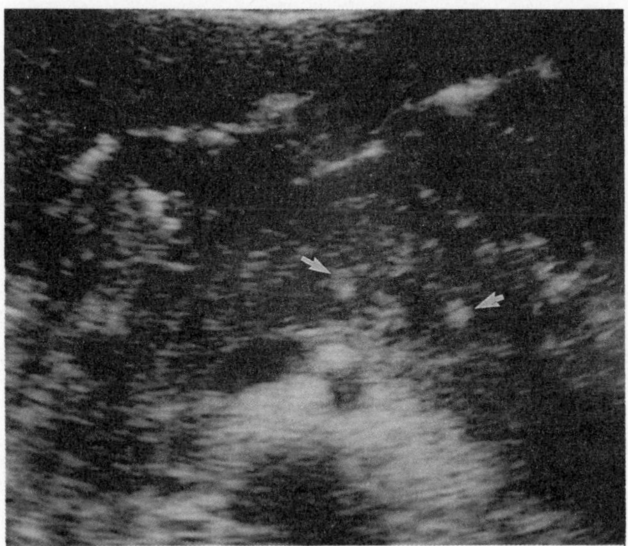

Fig. 65.6 Zollinger–Ellison syndrome. Transabdominal ultrasound showing multiple hyperechoic lesions (arrowed) within the pancreas due to the presence of multiple granulomas.

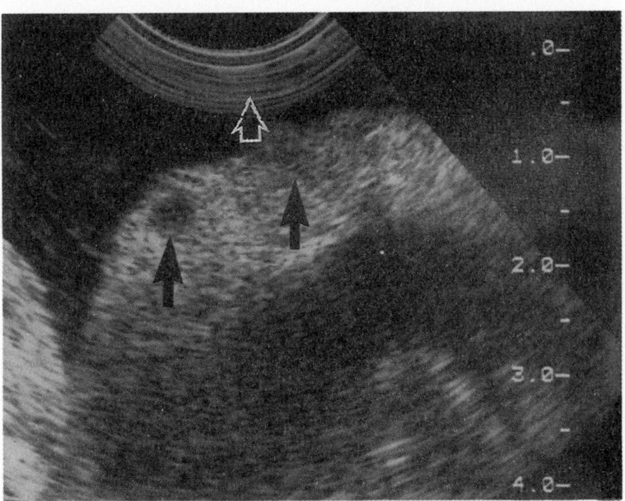

Fig. 65.7 Multiple insulinomas. Endoscopic ultrasound showing multiple hypoechoic lesions within the pancreas (arrowed). The transducer (open arrow) lies within fluid within the stomach.

ultrasound still requires very special expertise and specialised equipment, and is currently only available in a few institutions.

Intraoperative ultrasound

A high-frequency transducer applied directly to the pancreas during surgery can increase the sensitivity of detection of insulinomas to about 90% [32]. Intraoperative ultrasound and palpation are complementary, and a combination of the two techniques has led to correct localisation of solitary insulinomas in over 90% of patients [36]. As expected, intraoperative ultrasound will not detect extrapancreatic gastrinomas located in the gastric or duodenal wall.

Computed tomography

CT is widely available and together with ultrasound forms the mainstay of pancreatic imaging. The recent development of spiral (helical) scanning allows the pancreas to be scanned using contiguous 3-mm collimation during a single breath-hold, thereby reducing respiratory artifact, and improving vascular opacification and spatial resolution. After intravenous injection of contrast medium, islet-cell tumours typically enhance more than surrounding pancreatic tissue (Figs 65.5 and 65.8). Hypodense lesions are rare. Calcification, best demonstrated on the precontrast scans, is present in approximately 10% of islet-cell tumours, tends to be discrete and nodular, and is associated with malignancy in 70% of cases. The sensitivity of CT in detecting islet-cell tumours varies greatly, but should exceed 70% [36]. However, with significant advances in scanner technology, and using careful technique, the sensitivity of CT in the detection of insulinomas should exceed even this figure. The excellent enhancement of small tumours which can be achieved using spiral CT following intravenous injection of contrast medium has obviated the need for CT scanning during intra-arterial injection of contrast medium through the coeliac axis or superior mesenteric artery.

Magnetic resonance imaging

Following the development of rapid imaging sequences and respiratory gating, MRI has become an important modality in the imaging of islet-cell tumours. The appearance of the tumour depends on the imaging sequence used. Most islet-cell tumours are low signal intensity on T1-weighted images, and are particularly well seen on fat-suppressed T1-weighted scans (Figs 65.5 and 65.9). On T2-weighted images, the tumours are usually hyperintense compared with the normal pancreas, particularly gastrinomas. As with contrast-enhanced CT, insulinomas enhance markedly after intravenous injection of gadolinium, reflecting their vascularity. Early results on the use of MRI in detecting islet-cell tumours have been discouraging with sensitivities beween 20 and 25% for the detection of gastrinomas [39,40], substantially less than that for contrast-enhanced CT. However, in two smaller studies using gradient-echo T1-weighted sequences, which allowed acquisition of all the pancreatic images on a single breath-hold, better results were obtained [41,42]. Out of a total of 18 islet-cell tumours studied, only two were not identified. Our experience, using high-field strength MRI with conventional T1-weighted spin-echo and gradient-echo

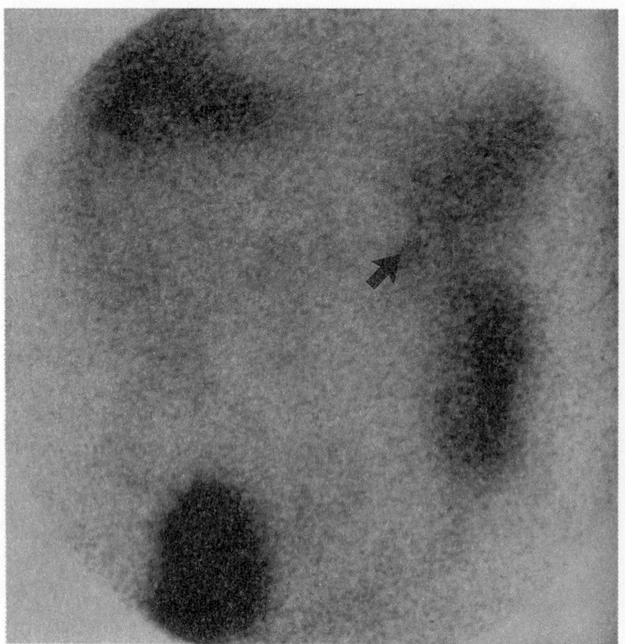
(a)

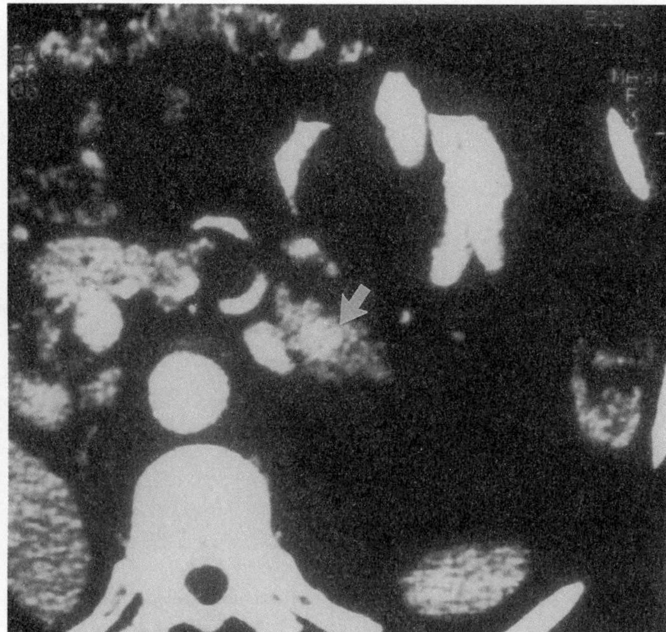
(b)

Fig. 65.8 Insulinoma. (a) Octreotide scan showing increased uptake (arrowed) corresponding to an insulinoma. (b) Computed tomography scan following intravenous administration of contrast medium showing a vascular insulinoma (arrowed). A right sided pelvic kidney is noted.

breath-hold techniques suggests that MRI is as sensitive as CT in the detection of small islet-cell tumours.

Radionuclide imaging (see also Chapter 66)

Many pancreatic endocrine tumours have somatostatin receptors of their cell membranes. Octreotide is a synthetic somatostatin analogue and a radiolabelled derivative, ^{111}In-pentatreotide binds to somatostatin receptors and can be used to localise islet-cell tumours which have such receptors. Fifty-five to sixty-six per cent of insulinomas and 65–90% of other islet-cell tumours can be localised using somatostatin-receptor scintigraphy [43,44] (Fig. 65.8). In our experience, ^{111}In-pentatreotide should not be used as a first-line investigation in patients with pancreatic endocrine tumours, but is extremely helpful in patients with disseminated disease or in those lesions regarded as equivocal on CT.

Arteriography

With the development of cross-sectional imaging techniques, arteriography is usually only needed when the initial investigations fail to demonstrate the suspected tumour or are equivocal. Selective injections of contrast medium are made into the coeliac axis and superior mesenteric artery, demonstrating the arterial anatomy of the pancreas and the portal vein. Many pancreatic lesions will be missed, however, unless super-selective studies are performed in the splenic, dorsal, pancreatic, gastroduodenal and pancreaticoduodenal arteries [45]. The typical appearance of an islet-cell tumour is a dense, circumscribed, homogeneous capillary blush appearing at 2–4 seconds following injection and persisting for 12–16 seconds (Fig. 65.9). Hepatic and nodal deposits have similar angiographic appearances to the primary lesion. In most studies, where angiography is compared with ultrasound, CT and MRI, the accuracy of angiography is equal to that or better than the other modalities individually [35,39,46,55].

Transhepatic portal venous sampling

This is a sensitive but invasive method of localising small functioning tumours with a significant complication rate of 9.2% and a mortality rate of 0.7% [47,48]. Reported complications include pneumothorax, haemorrhage, biliary peritonitis, inadvertent puncture of the gallbladder and other adjacent viscera. Briefly, the technique involves transhepatic catheterisation of the right portal vein under ultrasound or fluoroscopic guidance, and after performing portography, serial samples are taken peripherally from the splenic vein, superior mesenteric vein and portal confluence at 10-mm intervals. A localised 'step-up' in hormone concentration is found in the peripancreatic veins draining most tumours. The sensitivity for insulinomas is high (up to 92%) with few false positives, although lower for gastrinomas (73%) [49], with many more false positives. Transhepatic portal

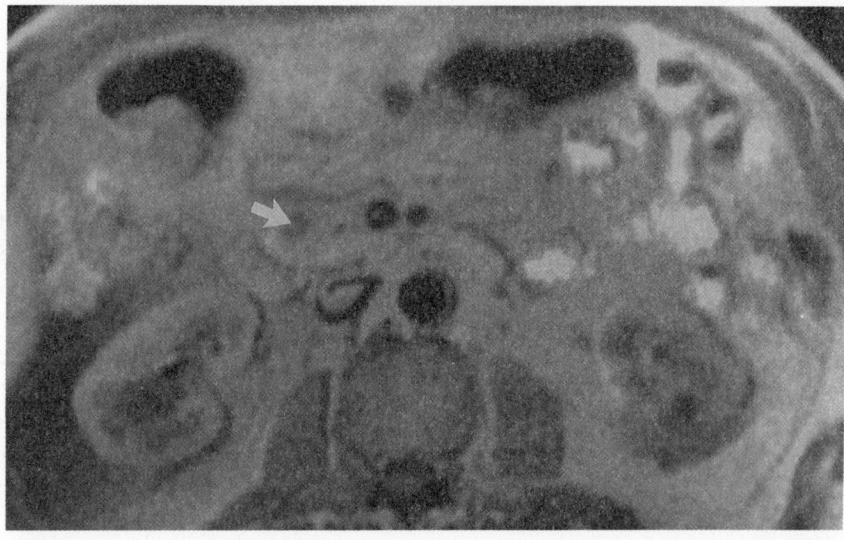

(a)

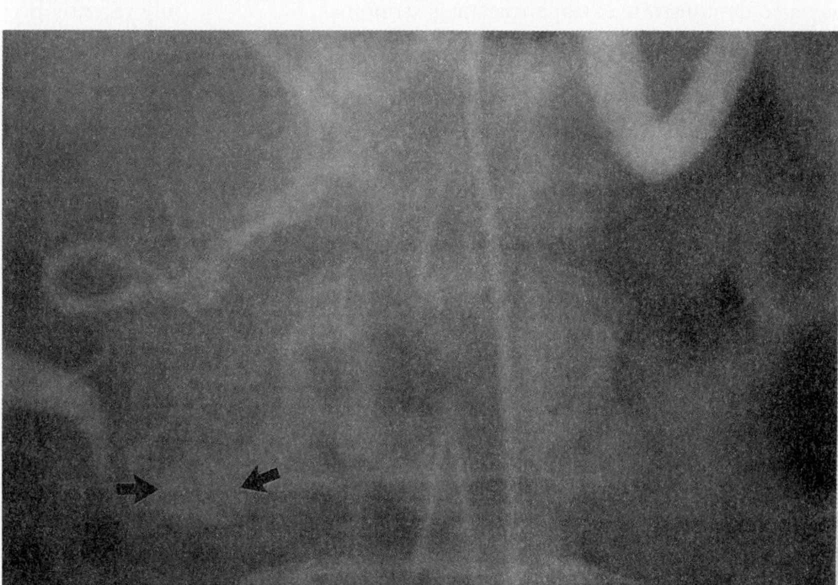

(b)

Fig. 65.9 Insulinoma. (a) Fat-suppressed T1-weighted magnetic resonance imaging scan showing a 6-mm insulinoma within the head of the pancreas (arrowed). (b) Coeliac arteriography in the same patient showing a vascular 'blush' (arrowed) corresponding to the insulinoma demonstrated in (a).

venous sampling cannot pinpoint a tumour in the same way as an imaging study but can localise it to a region of the pancreas. In addition, the venous drainage of the pancreas is variable with multiple collateral channels which may lead to false localisation. False negative results may also occur if hormone secretion is intermittent.

Arterial stimulation venous sampling

This technique involves selective, intra-arterial injection of a secretagogue producing a detectable rise of hormone in the hepatic venous effluent when the branch supplying the tumour is injected. The secretagogue is calcium gluconate for localising insulinomas and secretin for gastrinomas [40,50]. Arterial stimulation venous sampling can be performed at the time of diagnostic arteriography with little additional morbidity [50]. Initial results are encouraging and the technique does overcome some of the problems of transhepatic portal venous sampling as only the hepatic veins need to be cannulated.

Summary

As several imaging techniques are capable of demonstrating islet-cell tumours and none is absolutely accurate, a rational approach to the localisation of these tumours requires a careful consideration of cost, availability, local expertise and accuracy. In most institutions initial imaging is performed with a combination of transabdominal ultrasound and CT. This will demonstrate the tumour, and any hepatic metastases, in about 40% of gastrinomas, 80% of insulinomas and almost all other functioning tumours. MRI may prove to be at least as accurate as CT and will then be used instead of rather than in conjunction with CT. Where these tests are negative or equivocal, arteriography (which may be combined with arterial stimulation venous sampling) is the next line of investigation. Further investigation is dependent on local practice, availability of expertise and the tumour type. Transhepatic portal venous sampling is invasive, and while sensitive for insulinomas is frequently unhelpful in gastrinomas. Somatostatin-receptor scintigraphy, on the other hand, is more sensitive for gastrinomas. Both have the advantage that they are not directly dependent on tumour size. Endoscopic ultrasound is rapidly emerging as a technique of high sensitivity in detecting small pancreatic tumours and may also demonstrate extrapancreatic gastrinomas.

The adrenal glands

Introduction

CT has over the past decade made an enormous impact on the ease of detection of adrenal pathology, and modern scanners can detect masses as small as 5 mm in diameter. MRI may become the modality of choice. Currently, it plays an important role in the management of the indeterminate adrenal mass. Other techniques such as ultrasound, scintigraphy and venous sampling, although used less frequently still have a role in the investigation of patients with adrenal pathology.

Adrenal hyperfunction

Adrenal cortical hyperfunction

Cushing's syndrome

The diagnosis of the cause of Cushing's syndrome is made predominantly on clinical and biochemical findings. Nevertheless, difficulties in the biochemical differentiation between the causes of Cushing's syndrome are encountered and the main roles of diagnostic imaging are: (i) the localisation or exclusion of a unilateral adrenal mass; and (ii) the identification of an ectopic source of excess ACTH in those patients where an ectopic source is believed to be responsible.

Adrenocorticotrophic hormone-dependent Cushing's syndrome. Two types of hyperplasia are recognised pathologically in response to excess adrenocorticotrophic hormone (ACTH): smooth and nodular [51]. In smooth hyperplasia, the gland may appear normal on CT or it may appear enlarged but smooth in outline. The gland appears largest in patients with occult ectopic ACTH production.The less common nodular hyperplasia can be: (i) micronodular, in which case the gland often appears normal on CT, or (ii) macronodular, in which the gland appears enlarged with a lobular outline due to nodules of varying size, in some instances, due to a single nodule [52,53]. When macronodular hyperplasia is characterised by a single dominant nodule, it may be misdiagnosed radiologically as a unilateral adenoma [52]. However, additional smaller nodules or overall enlargement of both glands are usually present, which allows the correct diagnosis to be made [53]. It is uncertain how frequently the adrenal gland appears normal in ACTH-dependent Cushing's syndrome. Although the gland has been reported to be normal in 31% of patients with Cushing's syndrome [54], specific criteria for normal adrenal size on CT have only recently been documented [55].

Ectopic ACTH production. The investigation of patients with 'occult' ectopic ACTH production represents a major challenge as the clinical, biochemical and radiological features are often indistinguishable from pituitary-dependent Cushing's syndrome [56]. The radiological investigation requires special attention to detail since the responsible tumours are often extremely small. The commonest site of the source of 'occult' ACTH production is in the chest, accounting for 80% of cases [56]. The most common cause is a bronchial carcinoid [56,57]; other sources include thymic carcinoid, medullary carcinoma of the thyroid, pancreatic islet-cell tumours and phaeochromocytoma [56,57]. Bronchial carcinoids responsible for ACTH production tend to be small, ranging in size between 3 and 15 mm, and these can be impossible to distinguish from granulomas or hamartomas. CT is the most sensitive technique for detecting small nodules, but it is relatively non-specific and even the smallest of lesions should not be dismissed as a potential source of ACTH in patients with ACTH-dependent Cushing's disease. CT studies should always include images of the liver for metastases and the pancreas for islet-cell tumours.

Systemic venous sampling is frequently performed in difficult cases. Even if it does not demonstrate the source of the ACTH, the information is often useful because in patients shown to have a small intrapulmonary lesion, negative systemic venous sampling focuses attention on the intrapulmonary lesion as the potential source [56]. It should be noted that elevated ACTH levels in the thymic vein may be due to hormone production by a bronchial carcinoid, mediastinal metastases, a thymic carcinoid or diffuse thymic hyperplasia.

ACTH-independent Cushing's syndrome. Cushing's disease

not caused by excessive ACTH productions may be due to excess steroid production by adrenal pathology: adreno-cortical adenoma, adrenal carcinoma, primary pigmented adrenocortical hyperplasia and macronodular hyperplasia.

Adrenocortical adenomas account for 10–20% of cases of Cushing's syndrome and when responsible for Cushing's syndrome are usually larger than 20 mm [58]. On CT, they are usually of soft tissue or lower density, and often enhance slightly after intravenous injection of contrast medium. The contralateral gland tends to appear normal, but on occasion may look atrophic due to low circulating ACTH levels.

MRI readily demonstrates adrenal adenomas which tend to have homogeneous low signal intensity on T1-weighted sequences and signal intensity similar to or lower than liver on T2-weighted sequences [59,60], but some hyperfunctioning adenomas have higher intensity on T2-weighted signals [61]. After intravenous gadolinium, over 90% of adenomas demonstrate a thin hyperintense rim [62].

Imaging with cholesterol-based radiopharmaceuticals (^{75}seleno-cholesterol or NP_{59}) shows unilateral activity in functioning adnomas with virtual absence of radiopharmaceutical in the contralateral gland.

The detection of an adrenal mass in a patient with Cushing's syndrome does not necessarily indicate an adenoma as the cause; the differential diagnosis includes a phaeochromocytoma producing ACTH, a non-hyperfunctioning adrenal adenoma, a metastasis from an occult or known primary tumour or an adrenal carcinoma.

Adrenal carcinoma accounts for Cushing's syndrome in 10–15% of patients. Adrenal carcinoma is a rare tumour. At the time of diagnosis, 50–68% of patients have endocrine symptoms and 30% have distant metastases [63]. Cushing's syndrome is the most common endocrine presentation; androgen and oestrogen secretion are less common and pure hyperaldosteronism is very rare at initial presentation [63]. As corticosteroid production is low in malignant adrenocortical tissue, most carcinomas are large at the time of discovery and usually exceed 60 mm, and are often larger than 90 mm [64] (Fig. 65.10). On CT, these tumours are heterogeneous with areas of necrosis and calcification in 25% [64]. Only about 16% of carcinomas are < 60 mm in diameter and may resemble adenomas on CT. Adrenal carcinoma shows lower signal intensity than liver on T1-weighted MRI and higher signal on T2-weighted sequences [63] (Fig. 65.10). The tumours spread to regional lymph nodes, liver, lungs or bone. Direct growth along the adrenal vein into the inferior vena cava and right atrium is well-documented [65] (Fig. 65.10). All of these features are demonstrable on ultrasound, CT or MRI. Ultrasound or MRI best determine the upper extent of the thrombus, but neither will distinguish between tumour and blood clot. CT is currently the most sensitive method of detecting pulmonary metastases.

Adrenal cortical carcinoma causing Cushing's syndrome usually shows no uptake of cholesterol-based radiopharmaceutical but, very rarely, a well-differentiated carcinoma will show uptake.

Primary adrenocortical disease includes primary pigmented nodular adrenocortical disease (PPNAD), which is a rare cause of Cushing's syndrome. The adrenal gland contains multiple, unencapsulated cortical nodules which function autonomously, the intervening cortex being atrophic due to low ACTH levels [66]. The condition occurs in younger patients, does not have the strong female predisposition seen in classical pituitary-driven Cushing's syndrome, and may be associated with cardiac myxomas, skin tumours and testicular tumours (Carney's complex). CT and MRI show nodular hyperplasia bilaterally which is often asymmetrical [66].

Primary macronodular hyperplasia tends to occur in an older age group and usually produces massive hyperplasia of the gland (Fig. 65.11). The gland is usually nodular with nodules ranging from very small to 40 mm in diameter. Diffuse enlagement on CT or MRI is less frequent.

Primary aldosteronism (Conn's syndrome)

Imaging plays an important role in distinguishing between benign adrenocortical adenoma, responsible for Conn's syndrome in 79% of cases, and benign adrenocortical hyperplasia, the cause in 20% of cases [67]. In only 1% of cases is hyperaldosteronism due to an adrenocortical carcinoma [58]. On CT, Conn's adenomas tend to be of low density (0–10 Hounsfield units) [51] with a mean size of 16–18 mm [68] (Fig. 65.12). About 15–20% of aldosteronomas are < 10 mm and may, therefore, be overlooked on imaging examinations. With narrow collimation (30–50 mm) most adenomas between 5 and 10 mm will be detected on CT [69]. The reported sensitivity of CT for the detection of adenomas ranges between 70% [70] and 90% [68,71], with a positive predictive value of about 85% [69,70].

Experience to date indicates that the sensitivity of MRI in the detection of aldosteronomas is slightly less than that of CT. It is possible, however, that with the development of better techniques, the sensitivity of MRI will become at least comparable to that of CT.

On CT or MRI, a functioning adenoma may be overlooked when small incidental non-functioning adenomas are present in the ipsilateral or contralateral gland because the appearance is misinterpreted as hyperplasia, resulting in a false-negative diagnosis for adrenal adenoma. Conversely, a macronodule in nodular hyperplasia can very occasionally result in misinterpretation as a solitary adenoma [69]. Otherwise, a false-positive diagnosis of adrencortical adenoma is unusual [68,70].

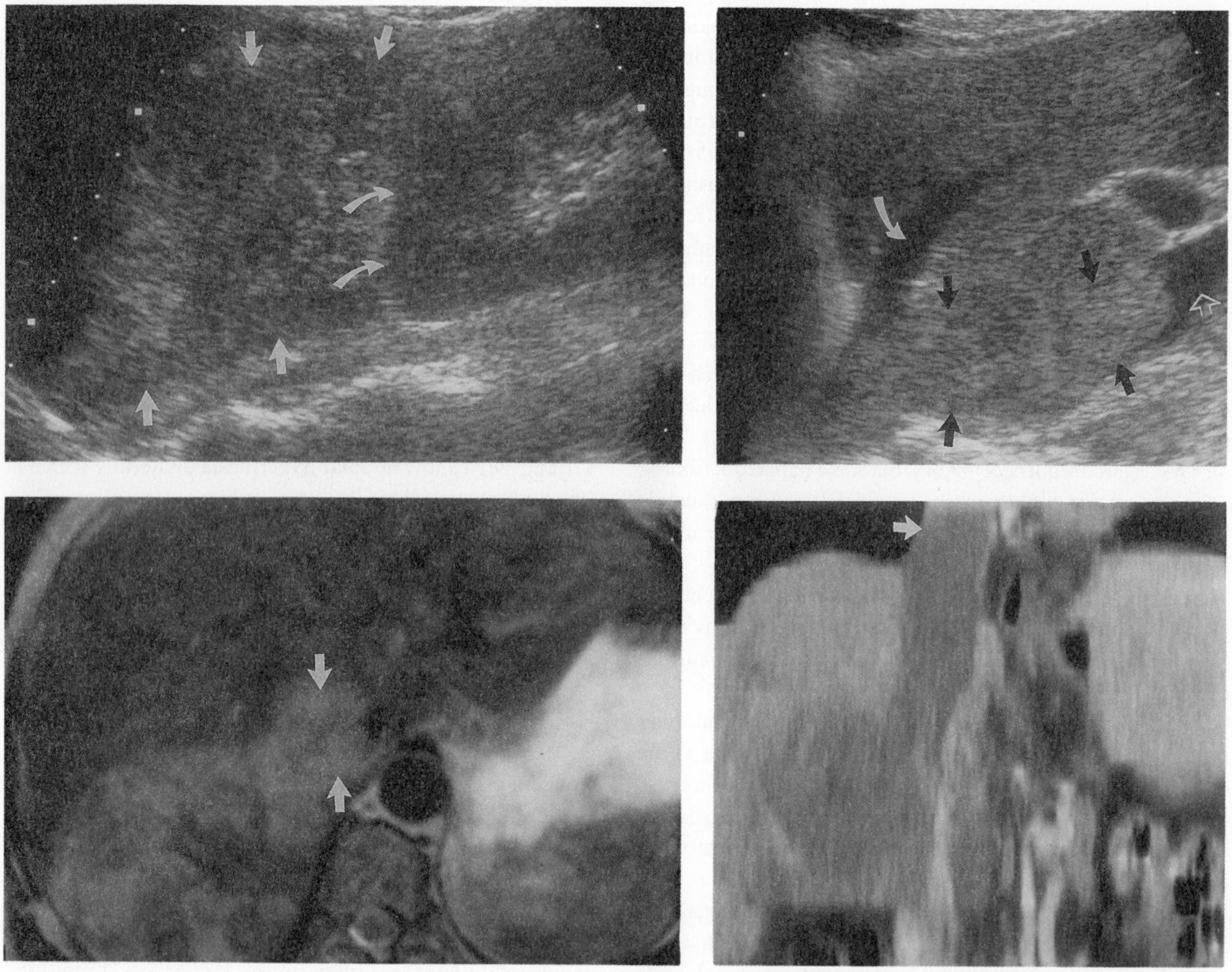

(a) (b)

(c) (d)

Fig. 65.10 Adrenal carcinoma. (a) Longitudinal ultrasound scan through the right upper quadrant showing a large inhomogeneous mass (arrowed), closely related to but separate from the upper pole of the right kidney (curved arrows). (b) Longitudinal ultrasound scan showing tumour infiltrating the inferior vena cava (arrows). The patent inferior vena cava is seen inferiorly (open arrow). The thrombus extends above the level of the patent hepatic vein (curved arrow). (c) T2-weighted magnetic resonance imaging scan showing tumour in the right adrenal region, of inhomogeneous signal intensity but higher than that of the adjacent liver. The tumour can be seen extending into the inferior vena cava (arrows). (d) Coronal reconstruction of a spiral computed tomography scan showing the right adrenal tumour extending into the inferior vena cava to a level above the diaphragm (arrow).

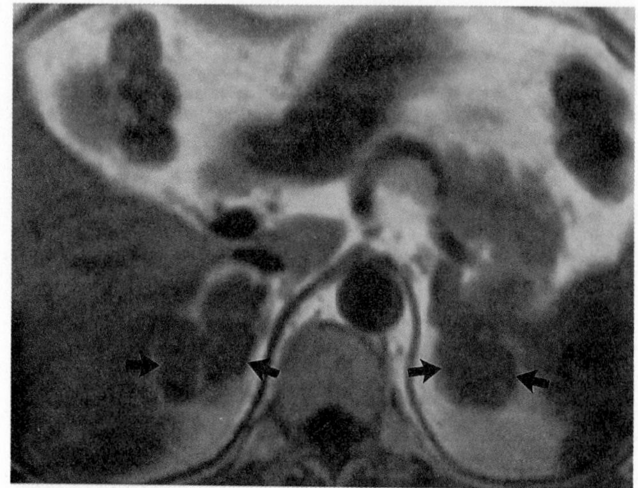

Fig. 65.11 Primary macronodular hyperplasia of the adrenal gland in a patient with Cushing's syndrome. T1-weighted magnetic resonance imaging scan through the adrenal gland showing massive nodular enlargement of both glands (arrowed).

Adrenal venous sampling for differential aldosterone levels is extremely accurate in the preoperative evaluation of primary aldosteronism [61,72] where a sensitivity of 100% [70] and a positive predictive value of 90% have been achieved [69]. However, complications of the procedure

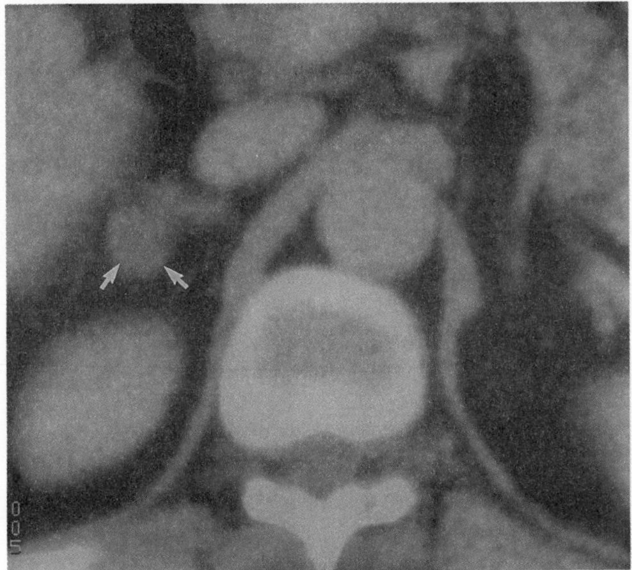

(a)

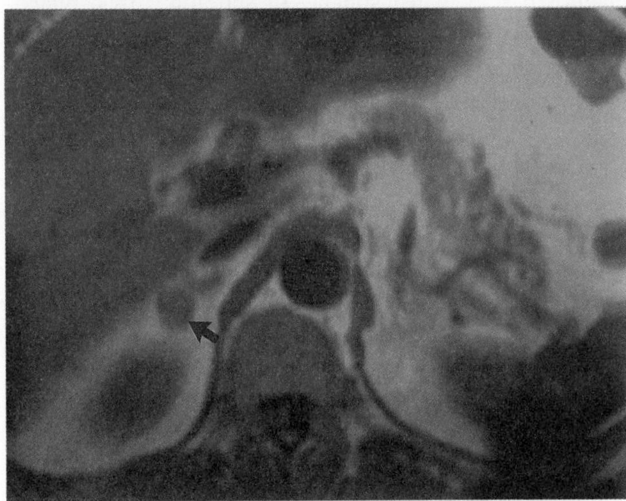

(b)

Fig. 65.12 Aldosteronoma. (a) Contrast-enhanced computed tomography (CT) scan showing a typical, small, low-density tumour of the right adrenal gland (arrowed). (b) T1-weighted magnetic resonance imaging scan in the same patient showing the typical appearance of a small mass of intermediate signal intensity (arrowed) corresponding to the CT appearance.

such as intra-adrenal haematoma, adrenal infarction, adrenal vein thrombosis and adrenal vein perforation are not infrequent, and may result in hypertensive crisis and adrenal insufficiency. Even in experienced hands, failure to catheterise the right adrenal vein occurs in 10–30% of cases [70].

In clinical practice, CT is considered in most institutions a sufficiently accurate test for the detection of cortical adenomas when the CT appearances are clear-cut and correlate with the biochemistry. Venous sampling is usually reserved for patients who show bilaterally normal glands on both sides, bilateral nodules on CT scans, or the CT and biochemical results are in conflict [68-70].

Adrenal causes of excess androgen production

The commonest adrenal cause of virilising states or precocious puberty in childhood is congenital adrenal hyperplasia (CAH). Androgen-secreting tumours of the adrenal gland are far less common; when seen they are usually malignant. Prolonged stimulation of the zona fasciculata and reticularis by excessive ACTH results in gross bilateral enlargement of the adrenal glands, easily recognisable on CT or MRI. On CT, these often enhance inhomogeneously after intravenous injection of contrast medium and can be mass-like, indistinguishable from a carcinoma (Fig. 65.13). Follow-up imaging after treatment shows return to normality of the adrenal glands. Rarely, long-term ACTH stimulation in CAH may lead to transformation of the adrenal hyperplasia into an adenoma or carcinoma [73].

Adenomas or carcinomas responsible for virilisation are usually greater than 20 mm in size and thus easily detectable by ultrasound, CT or MRI (Fig. 65.13). MRI has recently been shown to be accurate in the detection of these tumours and as the condition mostly occurs in young patients, in whom it is preferable to avoid CT, it may well become the initial imaging investigation of choice [74].

Adrenal medullary hyperfunction

Phaeochromocytoma and paragangliomas

Phaeochromocytomas can arise from paraganglion cells anywhere in the autonomic nervous system, but 90% arise in the adrenal medulla. Most extra-adrenal phaeochromocytomas are associated with the paravertebral sympathetic ganglia or the organ of Zuckerkandl, and rarely the urinary bladder. Only 2% of phaeochromocytomas occur outside the abdomen. About 10% of functioning paraganglionomas are malignant but this incidence is higher in extra-adrenal masses and in tumours larger than 60 mm [75]. Malignancy can often only be established by the presence of metastases rather than by the histological appearances. The majority, about 80–90%, are sporadic; the remainder are inherited either as an isolated disorder or as part of a systemic disorder, such as multiple endocrine neoplasia syndrome (MEN-2A or 2B), neurofibromatosis or von-Hippel–Lindau (VHL) syndrome. Phaeochromocytomas are multiple in up to 10% of sporadic cases. This figure rises to approximately 30% when part of a syndrome [76]. Ninety per cent of sporadic adrenal phaeochromocytomas are hormonally active and in addition to catecholamines may secrete parathyroid hormone, calcitonin, gastrin, serotonin and/or ACTH [76].

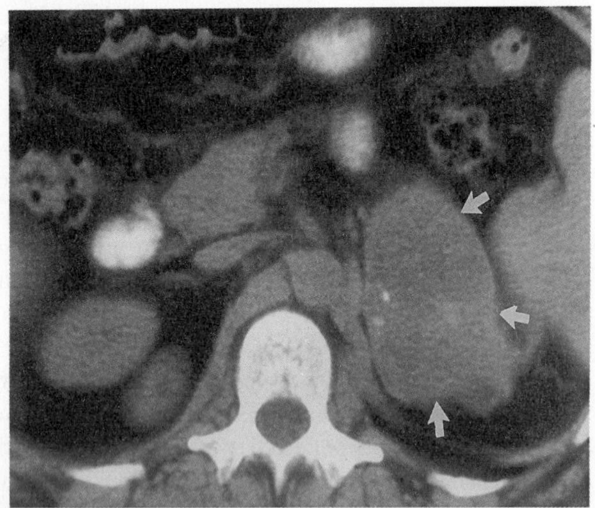
(a)

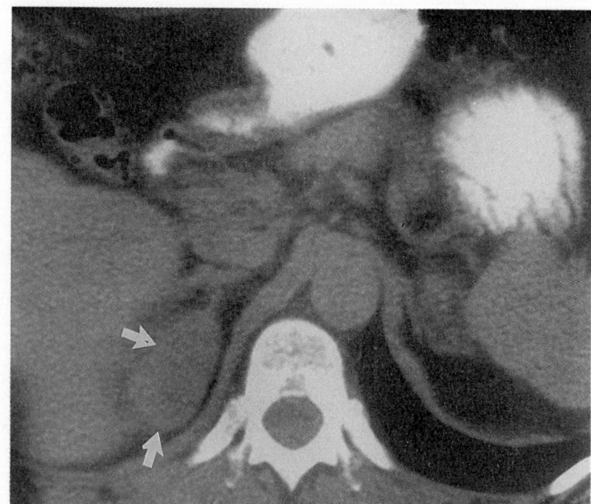
(b)

Fig. 65.13 Congenital adrenal hyperplasia in a 50-year-old patient. (a, b) Computed tomography scans in the same patient showing large inhomogeneous masses bilaterally (arrowed).

Phaeochromocytomas associated with MEN-2 are hormonally inactive in about half the patients and are often diagnosed only when sought. In sporadic cases, phaeochromocytomas do not usually present until they are large (average size 50 mm), although the lesions are usually smaller in patients with MEN or VHL [51].

Computed tomography. On precontrast CT, tumours are usually of soft-tissue attenuation, similar to liver, sometimes with central low attenuation due to necrosis or cystic change (Fig. 65.14). Calcification within the tumour occurs but is uncommon. These tumours enhance markedly after intravenous injection of contrast medium (Fig. 65.15). Intravenous injection of ionic contrast media can precipitate a hypertensive crisis in some patients who have not received α-adrenoceptor blockade [77]. Initial investigation suggests that this complication does not occur in patients receiving non-ionic contrast medium [78].

As most tumours are relatively large, especially in sporadic cases, CT is very accurate in the detection of adrenal phaeochromocytomas with reported sensitivities between 90 and 100% [51,75]. False positives are extremely unusual and thus the specificity is extremely high. The sensitivity is equal to that of MRI and scintigraphy. However, in the detection of extra-adrenal phaeochromocytomas and recurrent tumours, CT is not as sensitive s MRI or scintigraphy [79]. Quint *et al.* reported CT to have a sensitivity of 57% and MRI 80% in the detection of recurrent tumour [79].

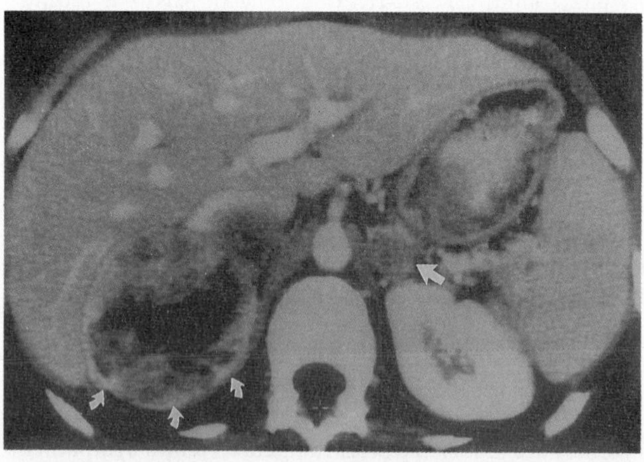
(a)

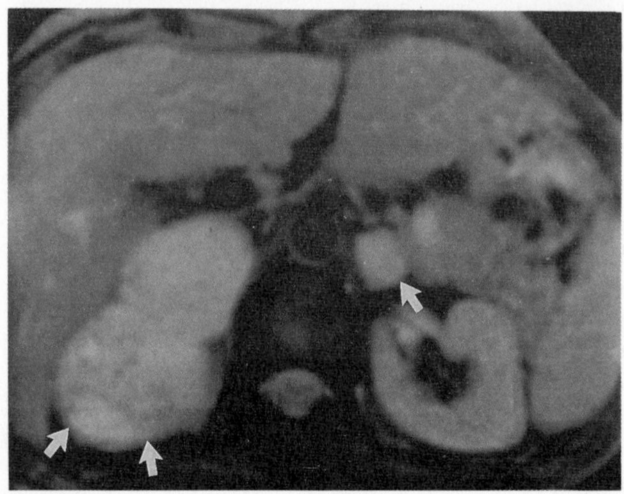
(b)

Fig. 65.14 Bilateral phaeochromocytoma. (a) Contrast-enhanced computed tomography showing bilateral phaeochromocytoma larger on the right than the left (arrowed). There is extensive central necrosis on the right, with only a thin rim of active tissue extending (curved arrow). (b) T2-weighted image on same patient, showing the typical very high signal intensity of both phaeochromocytomas (arrowed).

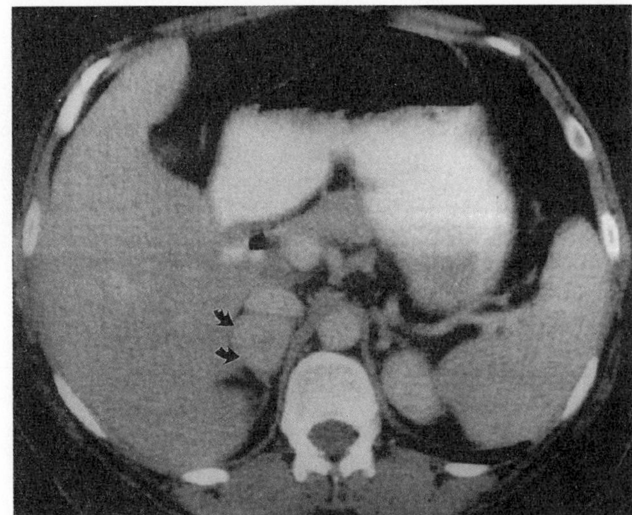

(a)

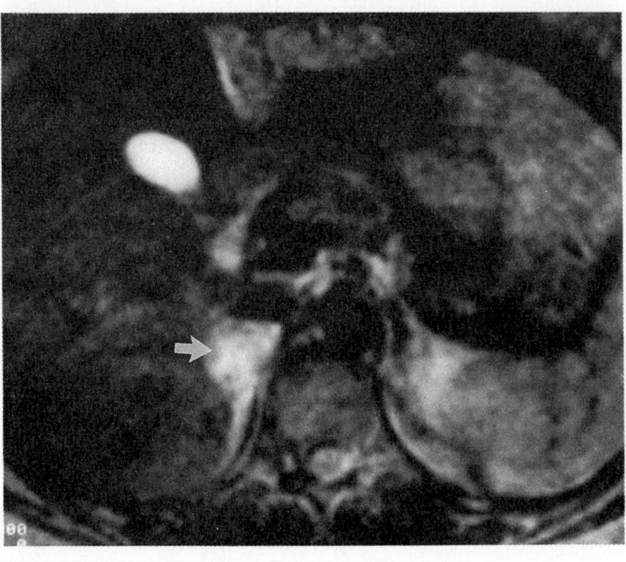

(b)

Fig. 65.15 Phaeochromocytoma. (a) Post-contrast computed tomography scan showing a 30-mm right-sided phaeochromocytoma (curved arrow). Enhancement is of similar intensity to that of adjacent major vessels. Note the normal left adrenal gland. (b) T2-weighted image of the same patient showing the typical high signal intensity of the phaeochromocytoma (arrowed).

Magnetic resonance imaging. On T1-weighted images, phaeochromocytomas show signal intensity similar to or slightly lower than that of the liver, but the tumours are fairly consistently hyperintense on T2-weighted sequences [51,79,80] (Figs 65.14 and 65.15). This pattern, on T2-weighted images, does, when present, have a high specificity as the signal intensity is very rarely as high on T2-weighting in other causes of adrenal masses. Only a few cases have been described that are not of very high signal intensity on T2-weighted images [60]. As expected, phaeochromocytomas show substantial enhancement after intravenous injection of contrast medium. Several studies using high- and mid-field strength magnets show that MRI is at least equivalent to CT in diagnosing adrenal phaeochromocytoma, but slightly more accurate than CT in detecting extra-adrenal tumours [79,81] (Fig. 65.16).

Metaiodobenzylguanidine. Sympathoadrenal imaging with ^{131}I (or ^{123}I) MIBG is particularly useful for the detection of extra-adrenal and metastatic disease, because unlike ultrasound, CT or MRI, MIBG is inherently a whole-body

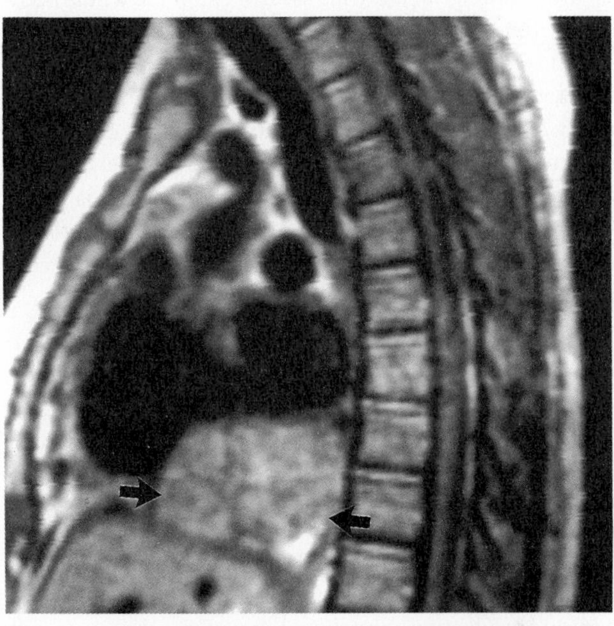

(a)

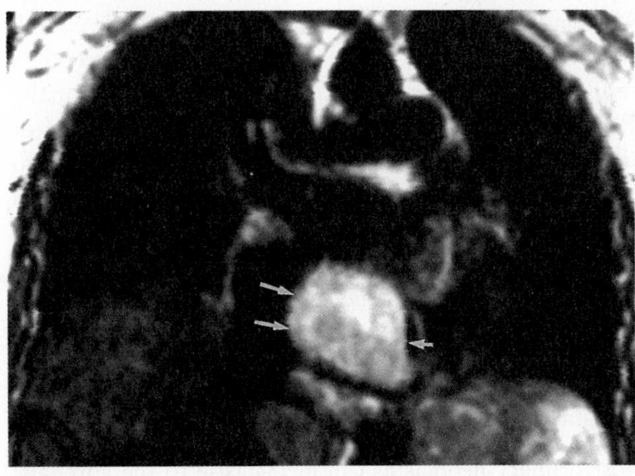

(b)

Fig. 65.16 Intracardiac phaeochromocytoma. (a) Sagittal T1-weighted image showing the phaeochromocytoma lying within the left atrium (arrowed). (b) Coronal T2-weighted image showing the typical high signal intensity of the phaeochromocytoma (arrowed).

imaging technique. The sensitivity of MIBG in detecting functioning phaeochromocytomas is slightly less than 90% and the specificity slightly greater than 90% [82,83].

Choice of technique. CT, MRI and MIBG are of roughly equal accuracy in the detection of adrenal phaeochromocytomas. Thus, the choice of initial investigation depends on several factors other than accuracy. Patients with known associated syndromes may have other tumours such as renal carcinoma, islet-cell tumours, neurofibromas or tumours associated with the MEN syndrome that cannot be detected on MIBG, and in these cases, CT or MRI will be essential. Conversely, MIBG has the advantage of allowing assessment of the whole body despite the disadvantage of poor anatomical resolution. Currently, MRI has several advantages over CT: it is more accurate in detecting extra-adrenal phaeochromocytomas, largely due to its multiplanar display; it does not expose the patient to ionising radiation; and does not routinely require intravenous administration of contrast medium. It is likely, therefore, that MRI will replace CT as the cross-sectional imaging technique of choice for the investigation of patients with biochemically proven phaeochromocytomas.

Adrenal disorders not resulting in increased hormonal activity

Adenoma

Adrenocortical adenomas are encountered in 0.6–1% of abdominal CT examinations [84]. These 'silent' adenomas consist of cholesterol-laden clear cells and contribute little to steroid production, even though they retain their potential to accumulate cholesterol esters and synthesise cholesterol [85]. On CT, these adenomas are characteristically round, <30 mm in diameter, well-defined without a perceptible wall, of homogeneous density, and enhance only minimally after intravenous injection of contrast medium [61,86]. Most will be of low density (–10 to 0 Hounsfield units) prior to intravenous contrast medium due to relatively large amounts of lipid [87]. On MRI, non-functioning adenomas are of low signal intensity on both T1- and T2-weighted sequences (although hypointense adenomas on T2-weighted sequences have been reported) [88].

Metastases

Most primary neoplasms can metastasise to the adrenals; the most common primaries are tumours of the lung, kidney, breast and digestive tract. Adrenal metastates may be of any size or configuration, and are more often unilateral than bilateral. Even in a patient with a known primary neoplasm, an adrenal mass of <30 mm is more likely to represent an adenoma than a deposit. For example, in a large series of 330 patients with small-cell lung cancer, adrenal adenomas were shown to be twice as frequent as metastases [89]. However, an adrenal mass of >30 mm, in a patient with a known primary malignancy, is more likely to represent a deposit [58,89]. On MRI, metastases tend to have a higher signal than adenomas on T2-weighted images and show thick, irregular, rim enhancement after intravenous injection of contrast medium on both MRI and CT [62,86].

Adrenal hyperplasia occurs in the presence of malignancy of many types and is detectable on CT [90]. The degree of hyperplasia is not linked to the stage of tumour and is not thought to be due to the presence of metastases. The mechanism of this phenomenon is not well understood, but it may be due to factors produced by the tumour [90].

Primary adrenal lymphoma without evidence of lymphomatous disease elsewhere is extremely rare. Secondary involvement of adrenals in widespread non-Hodgkin's lymphoma is relatively common, detected on CT in approximately 4% of cases and in up to 20% of cases at autopsy [91]. On CT there is usually bilateral involvement of the adrenals with masses of soft tissue attenuation that enhance slightly and inhomogeneously after intravenous contrast medium.

Adrenal myelolipoma (Fig. 65.17)

Adrenal myelolipoma is a rare benign neoplasm composed of adipose and bone-marrow elements in various proportions. The tumour is usually discovered incidentally, on cross-sectional imaging. Pain due to haemorrhage or necrosis within the tumour is occasionally the presenting feature [92]. Myelolipomas are usually non-functioning, but endocrine abnormalities have been reported, including Cushing's syndrome, Conn's syndrome and intersex [93]. Ultrasound, CT and MRI all usually show the presence of fat, the amount depending on the fat content relative to the presence of other soft tissue. Those tumours with only a small proportion of fat may be defficult to differentiate from other adrenal masses. The appearance on cross-sectional imaging may also be altered by previous haemorrhage, resulting in increased density or calcification. Usually, however, narrow collimated CT will almost always show the presence of fat, establishing the diagnosis (Fig. 65.17).

Adrenal infection

Acute adrenal infection is now most frequently seen in acquired immune deficiency syndrome (AIDS) patients with extrapulmonary cytomegalovirus or *Pneumocystis carinii* infection. The adrenals initially show diffuse bilateral low attenuation enlargement on CT before atrophying and

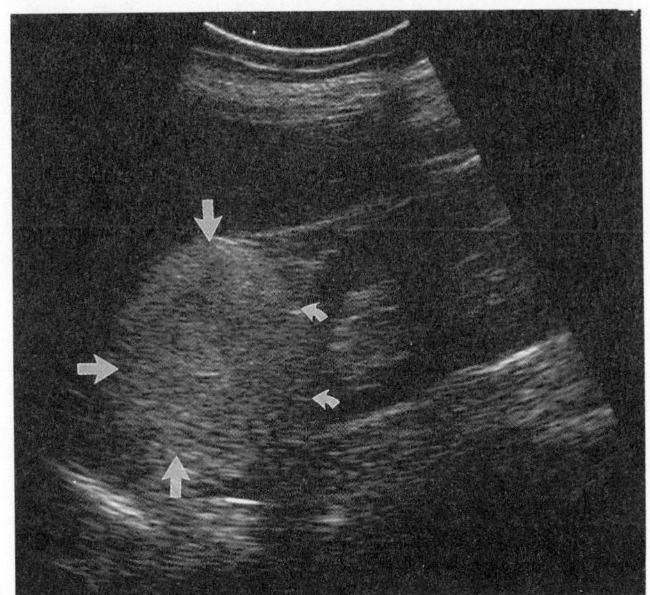

(a)

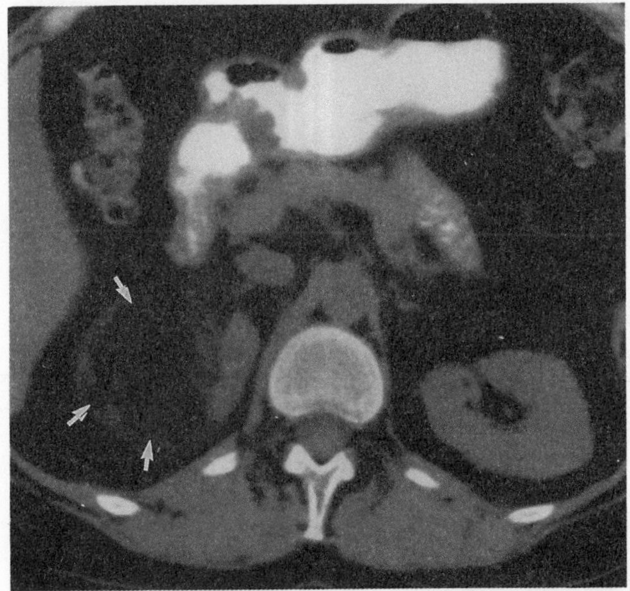

(b)

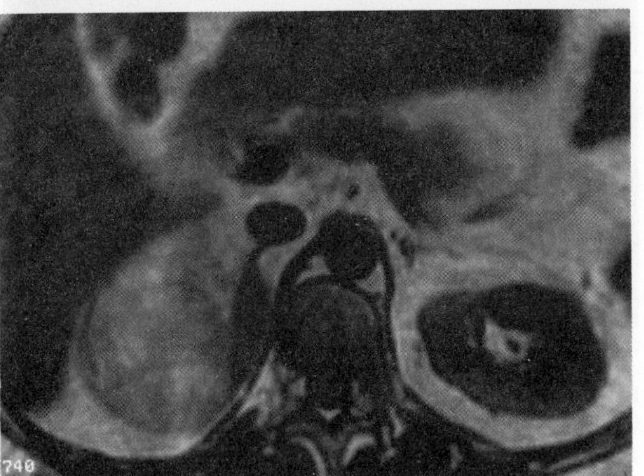

(c)

Fig. 65.17 Adrenal myelolipoma. (a) Longitudinal ultrasound scan showing a 50-mm mass (arrowed) of uniform high signal intensity consistent with fat. The mass is clearly separable from the upper pole of the right kidney (curved arrows). (b) Unenhanced computed tomography scan showing the large amount of fat (arrowed) within the right adrenal mass. (c) T1-weighted magnetic resonance imaging scan corresponding to (b) showing its contents of similar signal intensity to the surrounding fat.

eventually, on occasion, calcifying [94]. Also, acute adrenal abscesses may, rarely, complicate adrenal haemorrhage in childhood.

The appearance of tuberculosis on cross-sectional imaging varies depending on the stage of infection. During active infection, the glands are usually bilaterally enlarged and on CT are inhomogeneous in density, typically with punctate calcification (Fig. 65.18). After intravenous contrast medium injection, numerous small non-enhancing areas, representing caseating necrosis, can be identified (Fig. 65.18). Long-standing tuberculosis results in atrophic glands, which are often calcified.

Adrenal cysts

Endothelial cysts, which account for 45% of adrenal cysts, may be lymphatic or angiomatous, the former arising from blocked lymphatic ducts. The remaining adrenal cysts are epithelial, parasitic or pseudo-cysts presumed to result from haemorrhage [61]. They are almost always unilateral and detected incidentally. Ultrasound, CT and MRI all show the usual imaging characteristics of cysts anywhere in the body (Fig. 65.19).

On CT, adrenal cysts are of fluid density, have a clearly defined margin and a very thin wall, and no enhancement after intravenous contrast enhancement. A benign cortical adenoma, due to partial volume averaging of its lipid and soft tissue contents, may occcasionally appear of fluid density and simulate a cyst. Ultrasound or MRI allows ready distinction between these two possibilities.

Haemorrhage

Spontaneous adrenal haemorrhage in the acute or subacute phase results in marked bilateral enlargement and on CT the haemorrhage can be seen as increased density in the

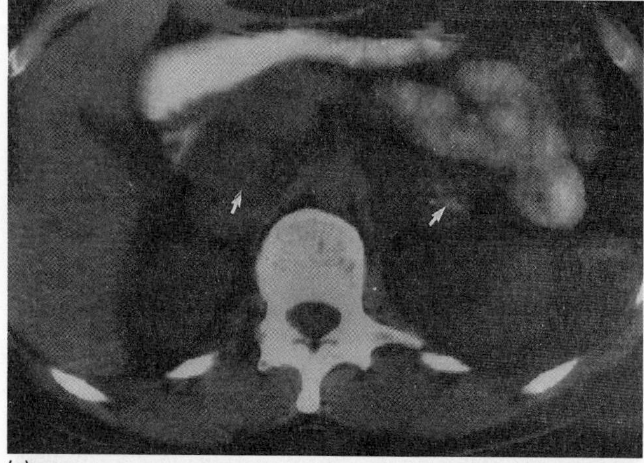

(a)

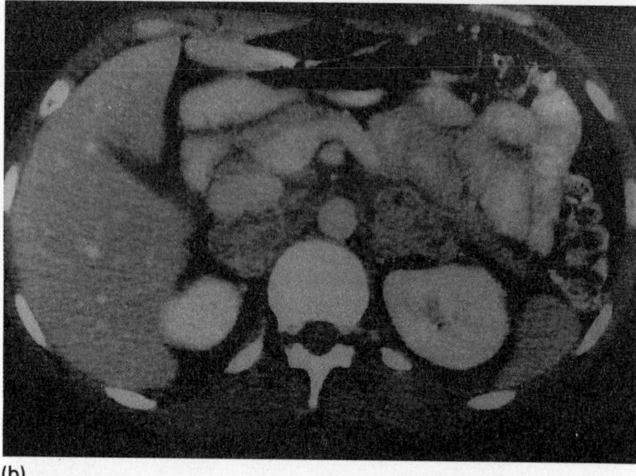

(b)

Fig. 65.18 Adrenal tuberculosis. (a) Unenhanced computed tomography (CT) scans showing bilateral adrenal masses with punctate calcification bilaterally (arrowed). (b) Enhanced CT showing bilateral adrenal masses with numerous small, non-enhancing areas typical of tuberculosis.

central part of enlarged adrenals (Fig. 65.20). As spontaneous haemorrhage, which is associated with bleeding disorders or stress caused by surgery or trauma, seldom results in clinically obvious hypoadrenalism, haematomas are usually detected incidentally on imaging. Blunt adrenal trauma is extremely unusual; it was seen in only 3% of children who had CT after sustaining blunt trauma to the abdomen [95]. It results from injuries to the right side of the abdomen, is usually unilateral and is associated with ipsilateral visceral injury [95]. In the elderly, anticoagulation may be associated with bilateral adrenal haemorrhage.

Evaluation of the incidentally discovered adrenal mass

(See also Chapter 37)

On CT adrenal masses of at least 10 mm in diameter are discovered incidentally in 0.6–1.5% of the population [84]. The management of such masses depends on whether they function and on their imaging characterictics. If biochemical analysis shows the mass to be non-functioning, the factors influencing further management include lesion size, composition and the clinical setting in which the adrenal lesion is discovered. The *size* of a lesion is important in predicting its nature. Seventy-eight to eighty-seven per cent of masses < 30 mm have been shown to be benign, whereas 91–95% of lesions > 50 mm are malignant [90]. Thus, lesions larger than 50-60 mm are so likely to be malignant that they should be removed without any further diagnostic test [97]. The *composition* of the adrenal lesion is another important factor. Adrenal adenomas contain much more intracellular lipid than metastases because they are composed of lipid-laden adrenocortical cells. Because CT attenuation is directly related to lipid content, low attenuation measurements imply the presence of lipid and therefore suggest the diagnosis of an adenoma. If masses below 10 Hounsfield units in CT density are called adenomas, a sensitivity of 79% and a specificity of 96% can be achieved [98]. The technique of chemical-shift imaging on MRI also exploits the lipid content of adenomas (Fig. 65.21). This technique relies on the observation that lipid protons precess at a different frequency than water protons within a magnetic field, so that lipid and water protons cycle in and out of phase with respect to one another every 2–3 msec. By selecting appropriate sequences, MRIs can be acquired timed to coincide with the in-phase and out-of-phase cycles. When in phase, fat and water will both contribute to the signal intensity; when out of phase, the net signal intensity is the difference between the signal intensities of fat and water, and is consequently diminished (Fig. 65.21). If there is no intracellular lipid, there will be no difference in signal intensities between the in-phase and out-of-phase images (Fig. 65.22). Several studies have suggested that this test can be close to 100% reliable in distinguishing between adenomas and non-adenomas [94–101]. Other magnetic resonance techniques such as calculated T2 measurements, and scanning after contrast enhancement, have been less discriminating [101]. Because adenomas are composed of functioning adrenocortical cells, one would expect the uptake of iodocholesterol-based radiopharmaceuticals by an adenoma, but not by metastases. Unfortunately, some adrenal carcinomas take up the agent, but carcinomas account for less than 5% of incidental lesions. Iodocholesterol scintigraphy is not as widely available as CT and is more time consuming and expensive to perform. The ability to easily direct a needle into an adrenal lesion would appear to provide an accurate method of determining whether a lesion is benign or malignant. However, the results can be misleading because although a specificity and a positive predictive value of over 95% can be achieved,

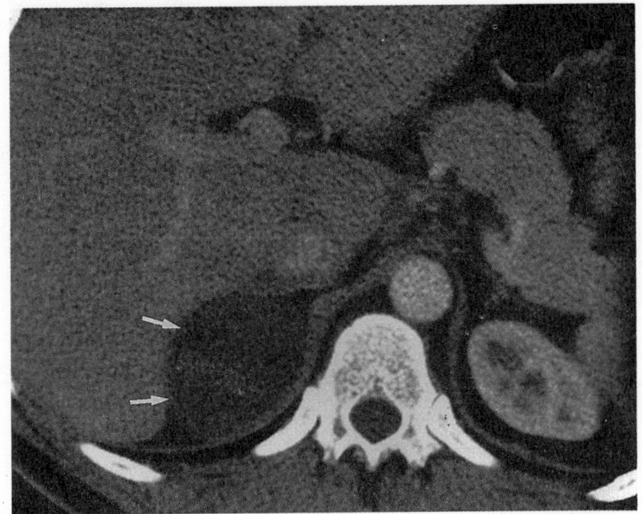
(a)

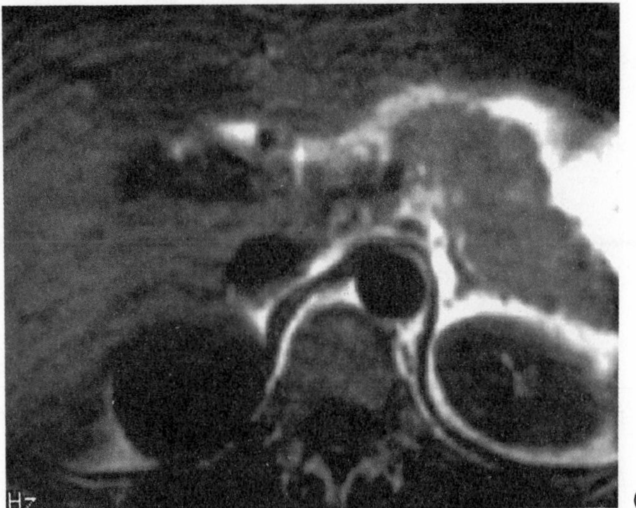

(b)

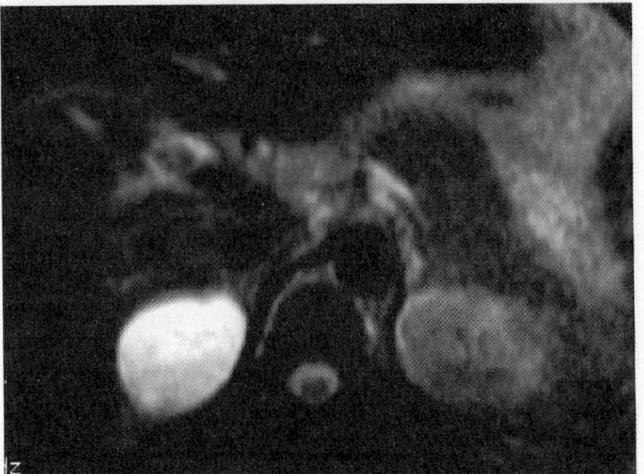

(c)

Fig. 65.19 Adrenal cyst. (a) Unenhanced computed tomography scan showing well-defined, non-enhancing, uniformly fluid-filled right adrenal cyst without discernible wall (arrowed). (b) T1-weighted magnetic resonance imaging (MRI) scan corresponding to (a) showing fluid-filled cyst. (c) T2-weighted MRI scan showing the typical appearance of a cyst with uniform high signal intensity.

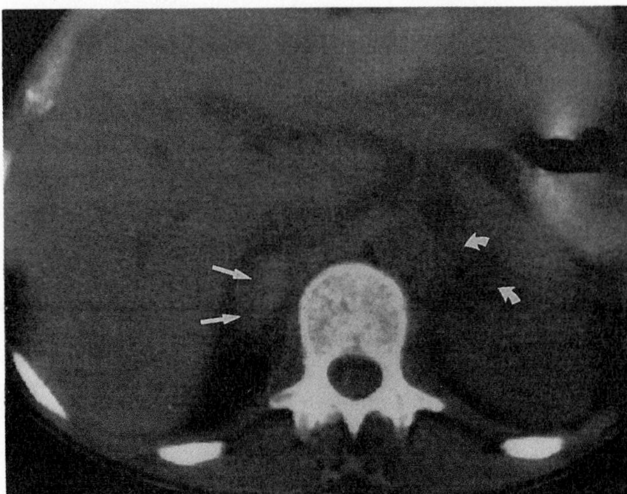

Fig. 65.20 Adrenal haemorrhage in a patient with myelofibrosis following splenectomy. Unenhanced computed tomography scan showing uniform high signal intensity due to haemorrhage (arrowed) in the enlarged right adrenal gland. The left adrenal gland is also enlarged (curved arrows).

the overall accuracy is usually only about 85%, partly due to the low sensitivity. Thus, fine-needle aspiration cannot be used to exclude a diagnosis of cancer [102]. Complications are relatively frequent, occurring in 10% of biopsies and include pneumothorax, pain and bleeding.

Hypoadrenalism

Imaging of the adrenals is seldom undertaken in patients presenting with hypoadrenalism because in western countries the condition is usually due to primary idiopathic atrophy [103]. However, imaging may be of value in identifying a potentially treatable cause. Enlarged adrenals resulting in hypoadrenalism are most commonly due to tuberculosis but may occasionally be due to other causes such as amyloid, sarcoidosis, metastatic disease, fungi or acute haemorrhage. When the adrenal glands are small, the differential diagnosis is usually between primary atrophy and chronic tuberculosis. Adrenal calcification, when present, excludes primary atrophy [103].

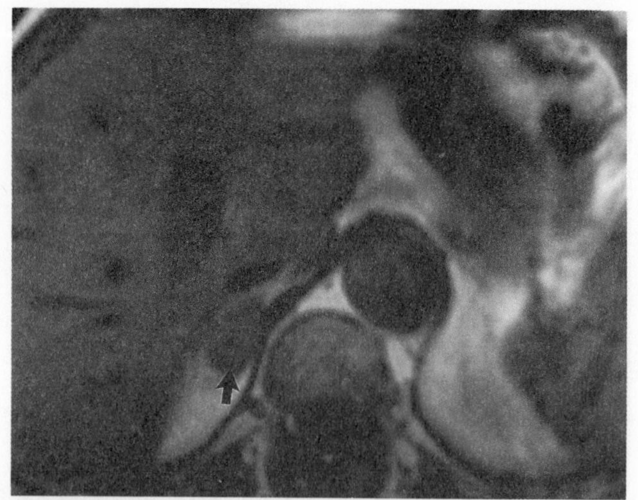
(a)

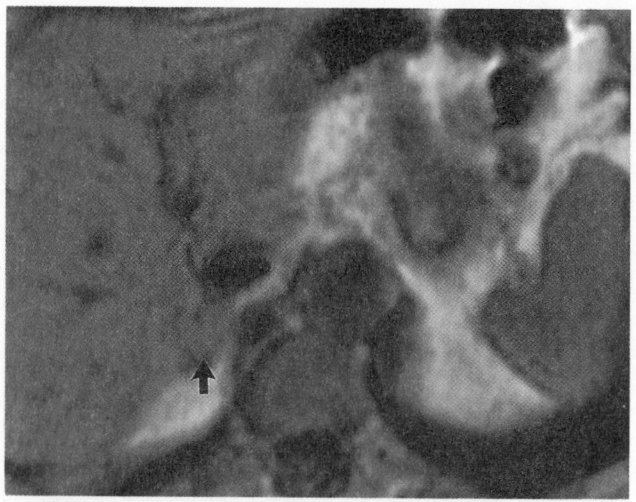
(b)

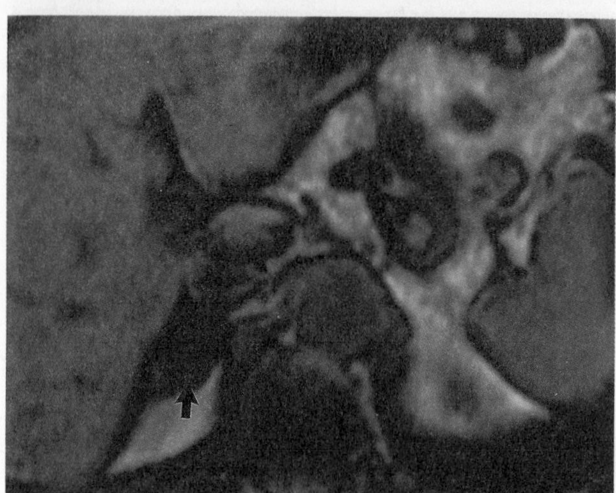
(c)

Fig. 65.21 In-phase and out-of-phase magnetic resonance imaging (MRI) scan to distinguish lipid-containing adenoma. (a) T1-weighted MRI scan showing an incidentally discovered adenoma (arrowed) in a patient with lung cancer. (b) 'In-phase' T1-weighted image showing the expected signal intensity of the mass (arrowed). (c) 'Out-of-phase' T1-weighted image showing marked decrease in signal intensity confirming the presence of fat.

Imaging of functioning gonadal disorders

The ovary

Ultrasound remains the examination of choice for screening for ovarian pathology and can detect a wide spectrum of ovarian pathology from simple ovarian cysts to complex ovarian masses. CT is the modality of choice to stage ovarian carcinoma but is otherwise usually only used to characterise suspected benign teratoma by demonstrating fat or calcium. Similarly, MRI is increasingly being used to characterise masses by demonstrating fat or haemorrhage.

Functioning ovarian pathology

Tumours

Ovarian tumours that cause virilisation and menstrual irregularities include Sertoli/Leydig-cell tumours, the rare lipoid cell tumours and Brenner tumours. Granulosa–theca tumours, the most common oestrogen-producing tumours, may also release testosterone. Ultrasound, CT and MRI all demonstrate solid unilateral ovarian masses, but there are no specific features to distinguish one type of tumour from another. Although MRI does not have an established role in the management of ovarian neoplasms, some workers claim that MRI is more accurate than ultrasound in distinguishing benign from malignant ovarian neoplasms [104].

Polycystic ovary syndrome (see also Chapter 54)

Polycystic ovary syndrome comprises a spectrum of abnormalities. Around 22% of the normal adult female population and 80% of women with a history of recurrent miscarriage in early pregnancy exhibit ultrasound features of polycystic ovaries [104]. At the extreme end of the spectrum is the syndrome of amenorrhoea, infertility and hirsutism, also known as the Stein–Leventhal syndrome.

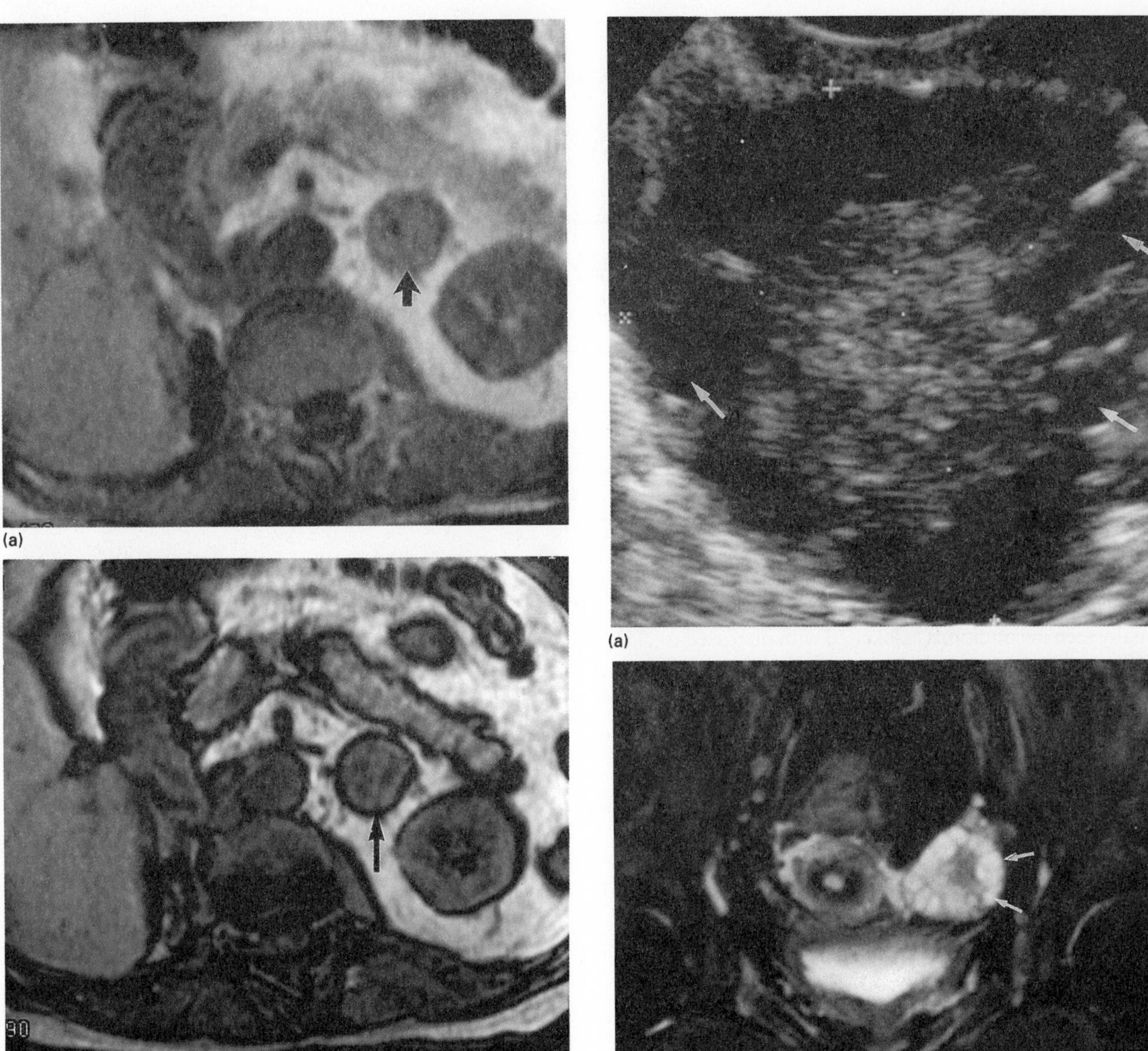

Fig. 65.22 In-phase and out-of-phase magnetic resonance imaging in patient with left adrenal metastasis. (a) In-phase T1-weighted image showing left adrenal mass (arrow). (b) Out-of-phase T1-weighted image showing that the signal intensity has not diminished (arrow).

Fig. 65.23 Polycystic ovary syndrome. (a) Transvaginal ultrasound showing marked enlargement of the left ovary with multiple cysts < 10 mm in diameter arranged peripherally (arrows). (b) T2-weighted MRI image showing the enlarged left ovary with high intensity cysts arranged peripherally (arrows). On both techniques, the appearances were identical bilaterally.

The imaging diagnosis is made using ultrasound, either transabdominally or, with greater accuracy, transvaginally. The classical appearance is bilateral enlargement of the ovaries which may be two or three times their normal volume, with multiple cysts of < 10 mm located subcortically (Fig. 65.23). However, up to 30% of women with the clinical syndrome have normal ovaries on ultrasound [105]. MRI is also very effective in the demonstration of polcystic ovary syndrome. On T2-weighted images, the peripherally situated cysts show as well-defined spheres of high signal in enlarged ovaries (Fig. 65.23). The cysts are of low signal intensity on T1-weighted images. The uterus may also be hypoplastic with reduced signal on T2-weighted images [106]. CT is of little diagnostic value because the cysts are shown less clearly and the investigation causes a significant radiation dose.

Stromal hyperthecosis

Stromal hyperthecosis is a hyperplastic abnormality of the ovary that shares many of the clinical features of polycystic ovary syndrome. The ultrasound and MRI appearances may mimic those of polycystic ovary syndrome. The diagnosis of hyperthecosis is made by histological examination. Differentiation is important because bilateral oophorectomy may be necessary to halt the syndrome caused by stromal hyperthecosis, whereas polycystic ovary syndrome responds to clomiphene, wedge resection or laser diathermy.

Testicular tumours

Ninety-five per cent of testicular tumours arise from germ cells and are almost always malignant. The remaining lesions arise from interstitial cells and are benign in 90% of cases. These non-germ-cell tumours arise from Sertoli cells, Leydig cells or cells of mesenchymal origin, may elaborate steroids and may cause endocrinopathies. Adrenal rest tumours are usually seen in conditions associated with increased ACTH, such as Addison's disease, Cushing's syndrome and CAH.

High-resolution scrotal ultrasound is the first and most reliable investigation in patients with suspected scrotal pathology, as the sensitivity for the detection of testicular tumours is greater than 95% [107]. In over 90% of cases scrotal pathology can be classified into intra- or extratesticular [107]. In general, testicular neoplasms are hypoechoic compared with the normal testis, but occasionally, highly reflective focal masses are seen. Adrenal rest tumours are often bilateral and multifocal, are frequently hypoechoic, and are usually impalpable, especially in CAH.

References

1 Godden AW. Tests of thyroid function *in vivo*. *J Clin Pathol* 1975; 28: 244–51.

2 Clark OH, Duh Q-Y. Thyroid cancer. *Med Clin North Am* 1991; 75: 211–34.

3 Solbiati L, Cioffi V, Ballaratti E. Ultrasonography of the neck. *Radiol Clin North Am* 1992; 30: 941–54.

4 de los Santos ET, Keyhani-Rofagha S, Cunningham JJ, Mzzaferri EL. Cystic thyroid nodules. *Arch Intern Med* 1990; **150**: 1422–7.

5 Gooding C. Sonography of the thyroid and parathyroid. *Radiol Clin North Am* 1993; **31**: 967–89.

6 Price D. Radioisotopic evaluation of the thyroid and the parathyroids. *Radiol Clin North Am* 1993; **31**: 991–1015.

7 Al-Sayer HM, Krukowski ZH, Williams VMM, Matheson NA. Fine needle aspiration cytology in isolated thyroid swellings: a prospective two year evaluation. *Br Med J* 1985; **290**: 1490–2.

8 Aufferman W, Clark OH, Thurnher S, Galante M, Higgins CB. Recurrent thyroid carcinoma: characteristics on MR images. *Radiology* 1988; **168**: 753–7.

9 Sandler MP, Delbeke D. Radionuclides in endocrine imaging. *Radiol Clin North Am* 1993; **31**: 909–21.

10 Talpos GB, Jackson CE, Froelich JW, Kambouris AA, Block MA, Tashjian AH. Localization of residual medullary thyroid cancer by thallium/technetium scintigraphy. *Surgery* 1985; **98**: 1189–95.

11 Ohta H, Yamamoto K, Endo K *et al.* A new imaging agent for medullary carcinoma of the thyroid. *J Nucl Med* 1984; **25**: 323–5.

12 Hancock SL, Cox RS, McDougall IR. Thyroid masses after treatment of Hodgkin's disease. *N Eng J Med* 1991; **325**: 599–605.

13 Healy JC, Reznek RH, Shafford EA *et al.* Sonographic abnormalities of the thyroid gland following radiotherapy in survivors of childhood Hodgkin's disease. *Br J Radiol* 1996; **69**: 617–23.

14 Lloyd MNH, Lees WR, Milroy EJG. Pre-operative localisation in primary hyperparathyroidism. *Clin Radiol* 1990; **41**: 233–43.

15 Gooding GAW, Okerlund MD, Stark DD, Clark OH. Parathyroid imaging: comparison of double-tracer (Tl-201, Tc-99m) scintigraphy and high-resolution US. *Radiology* 1986; **161**: 57–64.

16 van Heerden JA, James EM, Karsell PR, Charboneau JW, Grant CS, Purnell DC. Small-part ultrasonography in primary hyperparathyroidism. *Ann Surg* 1982; **195**: 774–9.

17 Krubsack AJ, Wilson SD, Lawson TL *et al.* Prospective comparison of radionuclide, computed tomographic, sonographic, and magnetic resonance localization of parathyroid tumors. *Surgery* 1989; **106**: 639–44.

18 Miller DL. Pre-operative localization and interventional treatment of parathyroid tumors: when and how? *World J Surg* 1991; **15**: 706–15.

19 Davidson J, Noyek AM, Gottesman I *et al.* The parathyroid adenoma: an imaging/surgical perspective. *J Otolaryngol* 1988; **17**: 282–7.

20 Lucas RJ, Welsh RJ, Glover JL. Unilateral neck exploration for primary hyperparathyroidism. *Arch Surg* 1990; **125**: 982–5.

21 Levin KE, Gooding GAW, Okerlund M *et al.* Localizing studies in patients with persistent or recurrent hyperparathyroidism. *Surgery* 1987; **102**: 917–25.

22 Coakley AJ. Parathyroid imaging. *Nucl Med Commun* 1995; **16**: 522–33.

23 Coakley AJ. Parathyroid localization—how and when? *Med Clin North Am* 1991; **75**: 211–34.

24 Freitas JE, Gross MD, Ripley S *et al.* Radionuclide diagnosis and therapy of thyroid cancer. Current Status Report. *Semin Nucl Med* 1985; **15**: 106–31.

25 Doppman J, Shawker TH, Krudy AG *et al.* Parathymic parathyroid: CT, US, and angiographic findings. *Radiology* 1985; **157**: 419–23.

26 Attie JN, Khan A, Rumancik WM, Moskowitz GW, Hirsch MA, Herman PG. Preoperative localization of parathyroid adenomas. *Am J Surg* 1988; **156**: 323–6.

27 Kohri K, Ishikawa Y, Kodama M *et al.* Comparison of imaging methods for localization of parathyroid tumours. *Am J Surg* 1992; **164**: 140–5.

28 Miller DL, Doppman JL, Shawker TH *et al.* Localization of parathyroid adenomas in patients who have undergone surgery. *Radiology* 1987; **162**: 133–7.

29 Service FJ, Dale AJD, Elveback LR, Jiang N-S. Insulinoma. Clinical and diagnostic features of 60 consecutive cases. *Mayo Clin Proc* 1976; **51**: 417–29.

30 Howard TJ, Zinner MJ, Stabile BE, Passaro E. Gastrinoma excision for cure. *Ann Surg* 1990; **211**: 9–14.

31 Thom AK, Norton JA, Axiotis CA, Jensen RT. Location, incidence, and malignant potential of duodenal gastrinomas. *Surgery* 1991; **110**: 1086–91.

32 Gooding GAW. Adrenal, pancreatic, and scrotal ultrasound in endocrine disease. *Radiol Clin North Am* 1993; **31**: 1069–83.

33 Rossi P, Allison DJ, Bezzi M. Endocrine tumors of the pancreas. *Radiol Clin North Am* 1989; **27**: 129–61.

34 King CMP, Reznek RH, Dacie JE, Wass JAH. Imaging islet cell tumours. *Clin Radiol* 1994; **49**: 295–303.

35 London JF, Shawker TH, Doppman JL *et al.* Zollinger–Ellison syndrome: prospective assessment of abdominal US in the localization of gastrinomas. *Radiology* 1991; **178**: 763–7.

36 Galiber AK, Reading CC, Charboneau JW *et al.* Localization of pancreatic insulinoma: comparison of pre- and intraoperative US with CT and angiography. *Radiology* 1988; **166**: 405–8.

37 Glover JR, Shorvon PJ, Lees WR. Endoscopic ultrasound for localisation of islet cell tumours. *Gut* 1992; **33**: 108–10.

38 Rosch T, Lightdale CJ, Botet JF *et al.* Localisation of pancreatic endocrine tumors by endoscopic ultrasonography. *N Engl J Med* 1992; **326**: 1721–6.

39 Frucht H, Doppman JL, Norton JA, *et al.* Gastrinomas: comparison of MR imaging with CT, angiography, and US. *Radiology* 1989; **171**: 713–17.

40 Pisegna JR, Doppman J, Norton JA, Metz DC, Jensen RT. Prospective comparative study of ablility of MR imaging and other imaging modalities to localize tumors in patients with Zollinger–Ellison syndrome. *Digest Dis Sci* 1993; **38**: 1318–28.

41 Semelka RC, Cumming MJ, Shoenut JP, *et al.* Islet cell tumors: comparison of dynamic contrast-enhanced CT and MR imaging with dynamic gadolinium enhancement and fat suppression. *Radiology* 1993; **186**: 799–802.

42 Moore N. Magnetic resonance imaging of endocrine tumours of the pancreas. *Br J Radiol* 1995; **68**: 3341–7.

43 King CMP, Reznek RH, Bomanji J, Ur E, Britton KE, Grossman AB, Besser GM. Imaging neuroendocrine tumours with radiolabelled somatostatin analogues and X-ray computed tomography: a comparative study. *Clin Radiol* 1993; **48**: 386–91.

44 Lamberts SWJ, Bakker WH, Reubi J-C *et al.* Somatostatin-receptor imaging in the localization of endocrine tumours. *N Engl J Med* 1990; **323**: 1246–9.

45 Clouse ME, Costello P, Legg MA *et al.* Subselective angiography in localizing insulinomas of the pancreas. *Am J Roentgenol* 1977; **128**: 741–6.

46 Fraker DL, Norton JA. Localization and resection of insulinomas and gastrinomas. *JAMA* 1988; **259**: 3601–5.

47 Hoevels J, Lunderquist A, Owman T. Complications of percutaneous transhepatic catheterization of the portal vein and its tributaries. *Acta Radiol Diagnost* 1980; **21**: 593–601.

48 Pedrazolli S, Pasquali C, Miotto D, Feltrin G-P, Petrin P. Transhepatic portal sampling for preoperative localization of insulinomas. *Surg Gynaecol Obstet* 1987; **165**: 101–6.

49 Doppman JF, Miller DL, Chang R *et al.* Gastrinomas: localization by means of selective intra-arterial injection of secretin. *Radiology* 1990; **174**: 25–9.

50 Doppman J, Miller DL, Chang R , Shawker TH, Gorden P, Norton JA. Insulinomas: localization with selective intraarterial injection of calcium. *Radiology* 1991; **178**: 237–41.

51 Francis IR, Gross MD, Shapiro B, Korobkin M, Quint LE. Integrated imaging of adrenal disease. *Radiology* 1992; **184**: 1–13.

52 Aron DC, Findling JW, Fitzgerald PA *et al.* Pituitary ACTH dependency of nodular adrenal hyperplasia in Cushing's syndrome. *Am J Med* 1981; **71**: 3020–3026.

53 Doppman JL, Miller DL, Dwyer AJ *et al.* Macronodular adrenal hyperplasia in Cushing's disease. *Radiology* 1988; **166**: 347–52.

54 Falke THM, van Seters AP. Adrenal imaging. In: Husband JES, ed. *CT Review*. London: Churchill Livingstone, 1989: 151–63.

55 Vincent JM, Morrison ID, Armstrong P, Reznek RH. The size of normal adrenal glands of computed tomography. *Clin Radiol* 1994; **50**: 202.

56 Vincent JM, Trainer PJ, Reznek RH *et al.* The radiological investigation of occult ectopic ACTH-dependent Cushing's syndrome. *Clin Radiol* 1993; 48: 11–17.

57 Doppman J, Nieman L, Miller DL *et al.* Ectopic adrenocorticotrophic hormone syndrome: localization studies in 28 patients. *Radiology* 1989; **172**: 115–24.

58 Moulton JS, Moulton JS. CT of the adrenal glands. *Semin Roentgenol* 1988; 28: 288–303.

59 Chang A, Glazer HS, Lee JKT, Ling D, Heiken JP. Adrenal gland: MR imaging. *Radiology* 1987; **163**: 123–8.

60 Kier R, McCarthy S. MR characterization of adrenal masses: field strength and pulse sequence considerations. *Radiology* 1989; **171**: 671–4.

61 Dunnick NR. Adrenal imaging: current status. *Am J Roentgenol* 1990; **154**: 927–36.

62 Ichikawa T, Ohmoto K, Uchiyama G *et al.* Adrenal adenomas: characteristic hyperintense rim sign on fat-saturated spin-echo MR images. *Radiology* 1994; **193**: 247–50.

63 Luton J-P, Cerdas S, Billaud L *et al.* Clinical features of adrenocortical carcinoma, prognostic factors, and the effect of Mitotane therapy. *N Engl J Med* 1990; **322**: 1195–201.

64 Dunnick NR, Heaston D, Halvorsen R, Moore AV, Korobkin M. CT appearance of adrenal cortical carcinoma. *J Comp Assist Tomog* 1982; **6**: 978–82.

65 Dunnick NR, Doppman J, Geelhoed GW. Intravenous extension of endocrine tumors. *Am J Roentgenol* 1980; **135**: 471–6.

66 Doppman JL, Travis WD, Nieman L *et al.* Cushing syndrome due to primary pigmented nodular adrenocortical disease: findings at CT and MR imaging. *Radiology* 1989; **172**: 415–20.

67 Weinberger MH, Drim CE, Hollifield JW *et al.* Primary aldosteronism: diagnosis, localization, and treatment. *Ann Intern Med* 1979; **90**: 386–95.

68 Dunnick NR, Leight GS, Roubidoux MA, Leder RA, Paulson E, Kurylo L. CT in the diagnosis of primary aldosteronism: sensitivity in 29 patients. *Am J Roentgenol* 1993; **160**: 321–4.

69 Goldin J, Sheaves R, RezneK RH, Dacie JE, Grossman A, Besser GM. The role of computed tomography and venous sampling in the investigation of hyperaldosteronism (Conn's syndrome). *Clin Radiol* 1993; **48**: 357.

70 Doppman JL, Gill JR, Miller DL *et al.* Distinction between hyperaldosteronism due to bilateral hyperplasia and unilateral aldosteronoma: reliability of CT. *Radiology* 1992; **184**: 677–82.

71 Ikeda DM, Francis IR, Glazer GM, Amendola MA, Gross MD, Aisen AM. The detection of adrenal tumors and hyperplasia in patients with primary aldosteronism: comparison of scintigraphy, CT, and MR imaging. *Am J Roentgenol* 1989; **153**: 301–6.

72 Young WF, Hogan MJ, Kee GG, Grant CS, van Heerden JA. Primary aldosteronism: diagnosis and treatment. *Mayo Clin Proc* 1990; **65**: 96–110.

73 Pang S, Becker D, Cotelingam J, Foley TP, Drash AL. Adrenocortical tumor in a patient with congenital adrenal hyperplasia due to 21-hydroxylase deficiency. *Pediatrics* 1981; **68**: 242–6.

74 Hanson JA, Weber A, Reznek RH *et al.* MR imaging of adrenocortical tumours in childhood: correlation with computed tomography and ultrasound. *Paediat Radiol* 1996; **26**: 794–9.

75 van Heerden JA, Sheps SG, Hamberger B, Sheedy PF, Poston JG, ReMine WH. Phaeochromocytoma: current status and changing trends. *Surgery* 1982; **91**: 367–73.

76 White MC, Hickson BR. Multiple paragangliomas secreting catecholamines and calcitonin with intermittent hypercalcaemia. *J Roy Soc Med* 1979; **72**: 525–31.

77 Raisanen J, Shapiro B, Glazer GM, Desai S, Sisson JC. Plasma catecholamines in phaeochromocytoma: effect of urographic contrast media. *Am J Roentgenol* 1984; **13**: 43–6.

78 Peppercorn PD, Kaltas G, Reznek RH, Mukerjee JJ, Besser GM, Grossman AB. Does intravenous injection of nonionic contrast medium result in elevation of plasma catecholamine levels in patients with pheochromocytoma? *Radiology* 1995; **197** (Suppl.) 422.

79 Quint LE, Glazer GM, Francis IR, Shapiro B, Chenevert TL. Phaeochromocytoma and paraganglionoma: comparison of MR imaging with CT and I-131 MIBG scintigraphy. *Radiology* 1987; **16**: 89–93.

80 Falke THM, te Strake L, Shaff MI *et al.* MR imaging of the adrenals: correlation with computed tomography. *J Comp Assist Tomog* 1986; **10**: 242–53.

81 Velchik MS, Alavi A, Kressel HY, Engelman K. Localization of phaeochromocytomas: MIBG, CT and MRI correlation. *J Nucl Med* 1989; **30**: 328–36.

82 Ackery DM, Tippett PA, Condon BR, Sutton HE, Wyeth P. New approach to the localisation of phaeochromocytoma: imaging with iodine-131-meta-iodobenzylguanidine. *Br Med J* 1984; **288**: 1587–91.

83 Bomanji J, Conry BG, Britton KE, Reznek RH. Imaging neural crest tumours with ^{123}I-metaiodobenzylguanidine and X-ray computed tomography: a comparative study. *Clin Radiol* 1988; **39**: 5002–6.

84 Glazer HS, Weyman PJ, Sagel SS, Levitt RG, McClennan BL. Nonfunctioning adrenal masses: incidental discovery on computed tomography. *Am J Roentgenol* 1982; **139**: 81–5.

85 Gross MD, Wilton GP, Shaprio B *et al.* Functional scintigraphic evaluation of the silent adrenal mass. *J Nucl Med* 1987; 28: 1401–7.

86 Berland LL, Koslin DB, Kenney PJ, Stanley RJ, Lee JY. Differentiation between small benign and malignant adrenal masses with dynamic incremented CT. *Am J Roentgenol* 1988; **151**: 95–101.

87 Miyake H, Maeda H, Tashiro M *et al.* CT of adrenal tumors: frequency and clinical significance of low-attenuation lesions. *Am J Roentgenol* 1989; **152**: 1005–7.

88 Smith J, Patel SK, Turner DA, Matalon DAS. Magnetic resonance imaging of adrenal cortical carcinoma. *Urolog Radiol* 1989; **11**: 1–6.

89 Oliver TW, Bernardino ME, Miller JI, Mansour K, Greene D, Davis WA. Isolated adrenal masses in nonsmall-cell bronchogenic carcinoma. *Radiology* 1984; **153**: 217–18.

90 Vincent JM, Morrison ID, Armstrong P, Reznek RH. Computed tomography of diffuse, non-metastatic enlargement of the adrenal glands in patients with malignant disease. *Clin Radiol* 1994; **49**: 456–60.

91 Paling MR, Williamson BRJ. Adrenal involvement in non-Hodgkin's lymphoma. *Am J Roentgenol* 1983; **141**: 303–15.

92 Fink DW, Wurtzebach LR. Symptomatic myelolipoma of the adrenal. Report of a case with computed tomographic evaluation. *Radiology* 1980; **134**: 451–2.

93 Jenkins P, Reznek RH, Lowe DG, Chew SL, Wass JAH. Adrenocorticotrophin-independent unilateral macronodular adrenal hyperplasia occurring with myelolipoma: an unusual cause of Cushing's syndrome.*Clin Endocrinol* 1994; **41**: 827–30.

94 Lubat E, Megibow AF, Balthazar EJ, Goldenberg AS, Birnbaum BA, Bosniak MA. Extrapulmonary pneumocystis carinii infection in AIDS: CT findings. *Radiology* 1990; **174**: 157–60.

95 Sivit CJ, Ingram JD, Taylor GA, Bulas DI, Kushner DC, Eichelberger MR. Posttraumatic adrenal hemorrhage in children: CT findings in 34 patients. *Am J Roentgenol* 1992; **158**: 1299–302.

96 Candel AG, Gattuso P, Reyes CV, Prinz RA, Castelli MJ. Fine needle aspiration biopsy of adrenal masses in patients with extraadrenal malignancy. *Surgery* 1993; **114**: 1132–7.

97 Gajraj H, Young AE. Adrenal incidentaloma. *Br J Surg* 1993; **80**: 422–6.

98 Lee MJ, Hahn PF, Papanicolaou N, Egglin TK, Saini S, Mueller PR, Simeone JF. Benign and malignant adrenal masses: CT distinction with attenuation coefficients, size, and observer analysis. *Radiology* 1991; **179**: 415–18.

99 Mitchell DG, Crovello M, Matteucci T, Peterson RO, Miettinen MM. Benign adrenocortical masses: diagnosis with chemical shift MR imaging. *Radiology* 1992; **185**: 345–51.

100 Tsushima Y, Ishizaka H, Matsumoto M. Adrenal masses: differentiation with chemical shift, fast low-angle shot MR imaging. *Radiology* 1993; **186**: 705–9.

101 Reinig JW, Stutley JE, Leonhardt CM, Spicer KM, Margolis M, Caldwell CB. Differentiation of adrenal masses with MR imaging: comparison of techniques. *Radiology* 1994; **192**: 41–6.

102 Tikkakoski T, Taavitsainen M, Paivansalo M, Lahde S, Apaja-Sarkkinen M. Accuracy of adrenal biopsy guided by ultrasound and CT. *Acta Radiolog* 1991; **32**: 371–4.

103 Vita JA, Silverburg SJ, Goland RS, Austin JHM, Knowlton AI. Clinical clues to the cause of Addison's disease. *Am J Med* 1985; **78**: 461–5.

104 Outwater EK, Dunton CJ. Imaging of the ovary and adnexa: clinical issues and applications of MR imaging. *Radiology* 1995; **194**: 1–18.

105 Yeh HC, Futterweit W, Thornton JC. Polycystic ovarian disease: US features in 104 patients. *Radiology* 1987; **163**: 111.

106 Occhipinti KA, Frankel SD, Hricak H. The ovary. Computed tomography and magnetic resonance imaging. *Radiol Clin North Am* 1993; **31**: 1115–32.

107 Feld R, Middleton WD. Recent advances in sonography of the testis and scrotum. *Radiol Clin North Am* 1992; **30**: 1033–51.

CHAPTER 66

New applications of radioisotopic scanning in neuroendocrinology

P.D. Hollett and E. Ur

Introduction

The last decade has seen important developments in the application of nuclear medicine to the identification and localisation of neuroendocrine pathology. More recent work utilising the novel approach of radioisotopic labelling of neuropeptide molecules and their analogues has enhanced our ability to identify a number of neuroendocrine lesions and has opened up wider clinical vistas.

Radioiodinated metaiodobenzylguanidine (MIBG) is the most widely used adrenosympathetic marker in nuclear medicine today. Since the first reports of uptake in human phaeochromocytomas with ^{131}I-MIBG, numerous studies have been published demonstrating its utility in identifying a variety of tumours originating from the same embryonic site, the neural crest.

In the last 5 years, the technique of receptor detection through the use of radiolabelled ligand has found important clinical application. A wide variety of neoplasms have been reported to have high-affinity binding sites for the peptide hormone somatostatin: these include gastroenteropancreatic (GEP) neuroendocrine tumours, pituitary adenomas, meningiomas, astrocytomas and neuroblastomas, as well as oat-cell carcinomas of the bronchus, breast cancers and lymphomas. These receptors are thought to mediate the inhibition of hormonal secretion from some of these tumours, and may also mediate the inhibition of tumour growth. A number of synthetic analogues of somatostatin have been developed for the purpose of radioisotopic labelling. These derivatives are actively taken up at somatostatin binding sites and have been used for *in vivo* localisation of tumours with great success. More recent work has looked at the possibilities of using other neuropeptides in a similar manner.

In recent years experience has accrued at a number of specialised centres in the use of MIBG coupled with more toxic radiopharmaceuticals for targeted delivery of therapeutic doses. Similar work with somatostatin remains a theoretical potential.

Metaiodobenzylguanidine

Distal neural crest tumours such as phaeochromocytoma, neuroblastoma, carcinoid, paraganglioma, chemodectoma and medullary carcinoma of the thyroid have been detected with varying sensitivity using radiolabelled MIBG. Cells of neural crest origin stain darkly with dichromate salts and are therefore called 'chromaffin' cells. Most of these APUD (amine precursor uptake and decarboxylation) tumours are metabolically active and secrete a wide variety of biogenic amines including dopamine, noradrenaline, adrenaline and calcitonin, as well as peptides including somatostatin, substance P, insulin and glucagon. These agents serve as a wide variety of chemical mediators and have an extensive effect on biological systems. They are also responsible for the characteristic symptomatology that can occur in these patients. Uptake of MIBG into these tumours is by an active, sodium- and energy-dependent uptake mechanism, with a lesser fraction entering by passive diffusion. Once inside there is a rapid concentration in vesicles and neurosecretory granules in the cytoplasm although this is by a different active mechanism than in the cell membrane.

After intravenous injection into humans, MIBG is distributed rapidly throughout the body and cleared by a wide variety of mechanisms. Since it is a polar compound, MIBG cannot cross the blood–brain barrier and therefore does not enter the central nervous system. A significant fraction enters red blood cells by passive diffusion while platelets actively concentrate MIBG. The principal route of excretion from the body is via the kidneys: in a normal individual 55% of the injected activity is excreted within 24 hours.

A number of familial diseases present with active APUD cell lines. They include neurofibromatosis type 1, von Hippel–

Lindau disease, multiple endocrine neoplasia (MEN) types 2A and 2B, as well as familial syndromes of bilateral carotid body tumours and familial phaeochromocytomas. An unusual syndrome called Carney's triad consists of gastric leiomyosarcomas, pulmonary hamartomas and multiple extra-adrenal phaeochromocytomas [1].

Radiopharmacy

MIBG can be labelled with various isotopes, commonly ^{131}I and ^{123}I for imaging, as well as ^{125}I for therapy uses. ^{123}I has a near ideal energy emission of 159 keV but has a shorter physical half-life of 13 hours. This allows a relatively large dose of about 200–370 MBq to be given intravenously for scanning. The target organ is the liver with a mean effective dose equivalent of 7.4 mSv or about twice that from a typical isotope bone scan. ^{131}I-MIBG, because of a β-emission, is associated with a higher radiation burden. The dose therefore is reduced 10-fold from ^{123}I to 10–37 MBq i.v. It also has a less desirable photon energy of 364 keV and a much longer physical half-life of 8 days. While heavier and less efficient collimation has to be used, this allows delayed imaging at 72 hours or more and greater flexibility in shipping and ordering (Fig. 66.1).

The majority of injected ^{131}I-MIBG is excreted unchanged into the urine (90% by 4 days), but some of it is metabolised and, in particular, the iodine label can be cleared and trapped by the thyroid. It is therefore important to treat patients with cold iodine blockade such as potassium iodine (100–200 mg/day for adults) starting at least 24 hours before injection and continuing daily for 4–5 days. For therapeutic administration of MIBG this iodine blockade should be continued for 4–5 weeks.

Many compounds can interfere with the uptake and retention of MIBG in APUD cell lines (Table 66.1). Although in theory large amounts of MIBG may trigger hormone release from an APUD tumour, this has not been shown to occur with slow injection of the tracer amounts used for scanning. Even in therapeutic doses, slow intravenous administration does not seem to cause a hormone surge from the tumour, although it is still often advisable to pretreat with adrenoceptor blockade. Imaging is generally performed at 24 and 48 hours post-injection of ^{131}I-MIBG. For ^{123}I early 4-hour and 24-hour imaging is most popular. Single photon emission computed tomography (SPECT) can be quite helpful in some cases.

Phaeochromocytoma (see also Chapter 38)

MIBG scintigraphy identifies the vast majority of phaeochromocytomas of all types and provides a single, safe, non-invasive whole-body screening procedure for this condition. The incidence of these catecholamine-secreting tumours is between 0.01% and 0.001%, but may increase in a hypertensive population to one in 1000. The diagnosis is important as it is a treatable and potentially surgically curable cause of high blood pressure. Unfortunately most phaeochromocytomas are not diagnosed during life and are first identified at autopsy.

Tumour uptake of MIBG does not directly correlate with noradrenaline/adrenaline concentrations. In a recent meta-analysis of 1396 patients suspected of phaeochromocytoma MIBG scanning had an overall sensitivity of 88% and a specificity of greater than 95%. This is clearly superior to results obtained to date with ultrasound, CT or MRI modalities, although this is not uniformly accepted [2] (Fig. 66.2).

Neuroblastomas

Neuroblastoma is the third most common solid tumour of childhood accounting for 7–14% of malignancies in this age group. It is certainly the most common solid non-central nervous system (CNS) malignancy with a peak incidence at 2 years of age. Neuroblastomas generally occur in the same locations as phaeochromocytomas but tend to be more malignant and aggressive, spreading early to bone marrow and bone as well as to regional lymph nodes and then to the liver, lung and skin [3]. In neuroblastoma the major clinical symptoms are from structural and expansion abnormalities as a result of metastases. The primary symptoms are therefore those of bone pain, bruising, anaemia and occasionally painful movement. Symptoms from elevated hormone levels are unusual but occasionally patients can suffer diarrhoea due to excess secretion of vasoactive intestinal polypeptide (VIP).

Bone lesions are found at presentation in at least half of patients, particularly so in older children. MIBG scanning has clearly been demonstrated to be the principal imaging modality in this condition. In 779 children scanned with ^{131}I-MIBG the cumulative sensitivity was 92% with a specificity of nearly 100% [2]. Despite this, some skeletal metastases are better visualised by diphosphonate bone scanning which is felt to be complementary [4]. MIBG has also proved to be superior to bone scanning when following lesion-by-lesion responses to chemotherapy as compared with specific markers for tumour growth such as urinary homovanillic and vanillylmandelic acids, serum ferritin, neuron-specific enolase and lactic dehydrogenase [5].

Carcinoid (see also Chapter 45)

Carcinoid tumours arise from Kulchitsky cells and are most commonly found in the gut or lungs. They can be classified

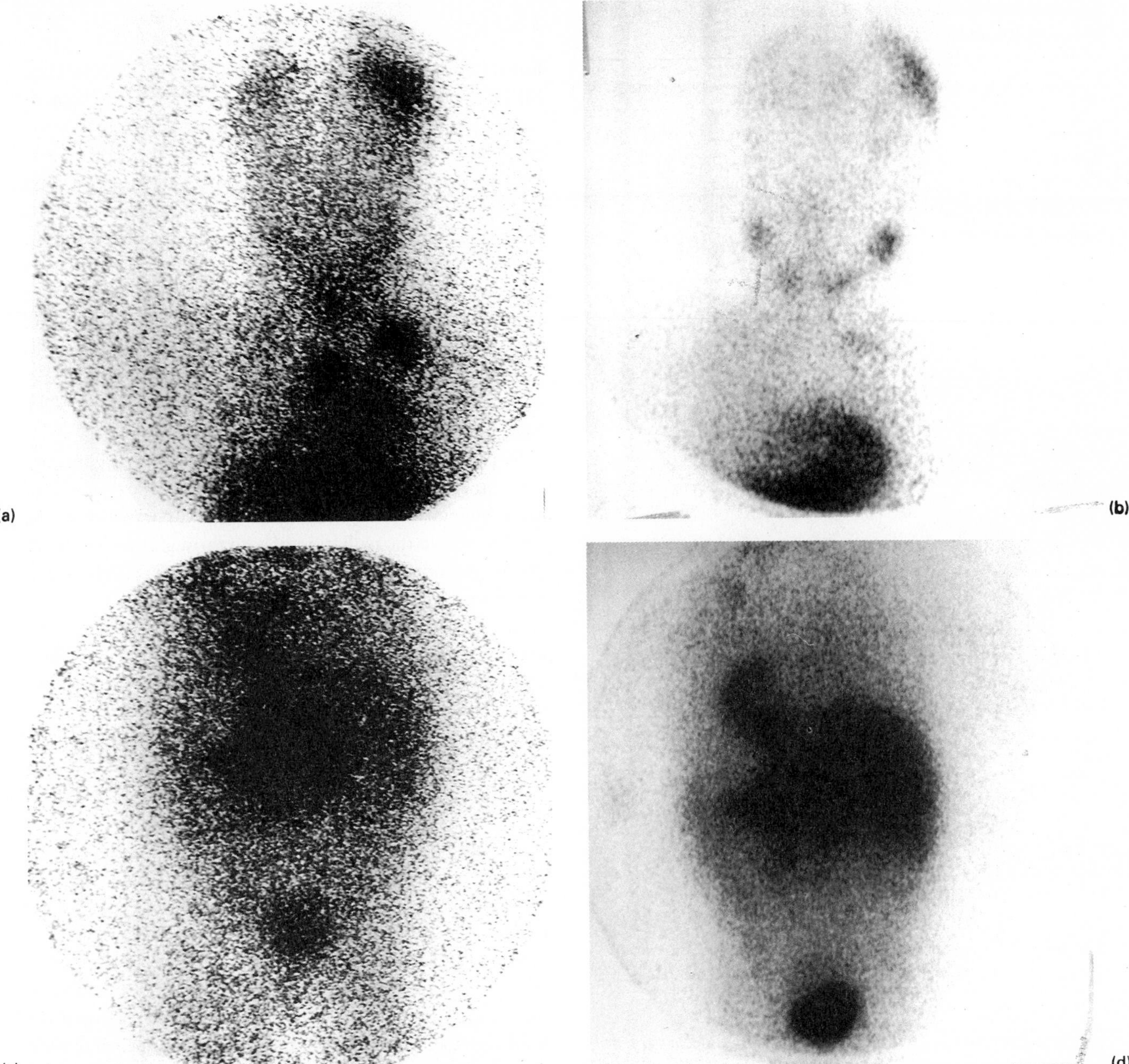

Fig. 66.1 (a,b) Anterior head images of a young girl with known metastatic neuroblastoma. Although performed at different times, note the image quality changes with ^{131}I-metaiodobenzylguanidine (MIBG) (a) and ^{123}I-MIBG (b). (c,d) Posterior abdomen images of a neuroblastoma with ^{131}I-MIBG (c) and ^{123}I-MIBG (d).

as foregut, midgut or hindgut tumours depending on where they arise. The biochemical diagnosis rests on elevated urinary 5-HIAA or increased serum levels of serotonin, 5-hydroxytryptophan and substance P. Identification of the primary tumour is generally not difficult, but a surgical cure depends on the absence of local invasion and distant metastases. Bone scanning typically identifies all bony metastases but combined series show that only 70% of carcinoids concentrate ^{131}I-MIBG [2]. Higher sensitivities could be expected in the more metabolically active midgut tumours or in those with elevated urinary 5-HIAA levels [6]. There appears to be no relationship between MIBG concentration and the presence of the carcinoid syndrome of facial flushing, diarrhoea and/or cardiac valvular disease.

Miscellaneous conditions

MIBG has been useful for the detection of other APUD

Table 66.1 Drugs that may interfere with the uptake, retention, or both, of metaiodobenzylguanidine. Modified from [23].

Drugs known to interfere	Drugs expected to interfere
Labetalol	Adrenergic blocking agents
Reserpine	Phenothiazines
Calcium-channel blockers	Butyrophenones
Tricyclic antidepressants	Thioxanthines
Sympathicomimetics	
Cocaine	

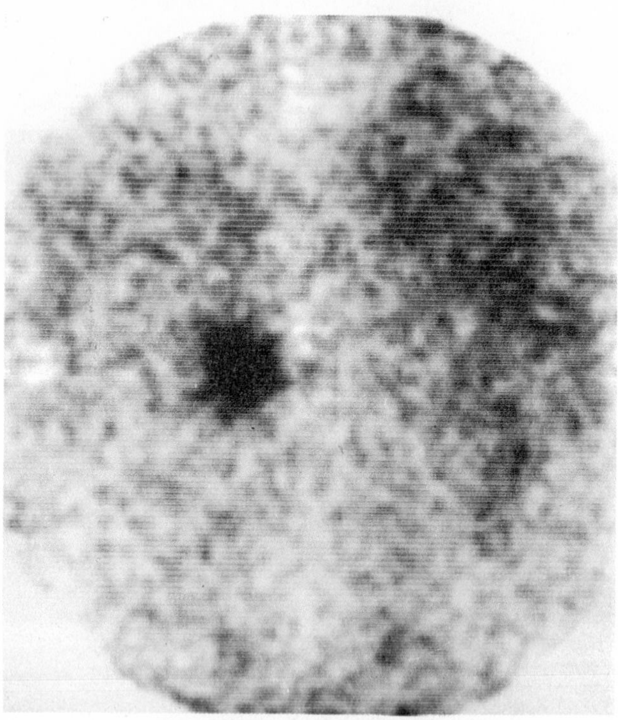

Fig. 66.2 ^{131}I-metaiodobenzylguanidine posterior abdominal image of a 40-year-old man with a proven left phaeochromocytoma.

cell-line tumours such as ganglioneuromas, secretory and non-secretory paragangliomas and chemodectomas. Less success has been found with pancreatic islet-cell tumours, retinoblastoma, Schwannomas and Merkel cell skin neoplasia. Results in imaging small-cell lung cancer and melanoma have been disappointing.

Interestingly, MIBG has proved useful in identifying adrenergic function in a number of non-tumorous conditions. Cardiac imaging has been done with idiopathic, hypertrophic or drug-induced cardiomyopathies,ischaemic heart disease, diabetic autonomic neuropathy, Friedrich's ataxia and even cardiac transplantation. Lack of normal sympathetic innervation causes decreased MIBG uptake, and this has been demonstrated in Horner's syndrome with decreased salivary gland accumulation on the affected side.

Therapy

Neural crest malignancies have been treated with labelled MIBG for about 10 years, and there is extensive experience at certain centres both with ^{131}I- and ^{125}I-MIBG. While the ^{125}I label does deliver relatively large local doses and may be best suited for the treatment of smaller tumours and micrometastases, it is unfortunately unsuitable for imaging.

The majority of experience lies in the treatment of extensive malignant phaeochromocytomas and neuroblastomas in children. Some therapies have been attempted in carcinoid with varying results, and very rarely in medullary carcinoma of the thyroid. In phaeochromocytoma, only patients with unresectable tumors are candidates for therapy, and these malignant tumours may or may not originate within the adrenal glands.

In the treatment of neuroblastoma initial surgery and chemotherapy remain the mainstays of therapy. Because of rapid bone invasion and spread, MIBG can nevertheless be very helpful in the palliation of pain through the slowing of the progression of bony spread. ^{131}I-MIBG has been used in three ways in the treatment of neuroblastoma:

1 as a primary radiation treatment directed at cure or preparation of the patient for surgical resection of the tumour;

2 for radiation therapy after chemotherapy has failed to cure the disease;

3 as a therapy that is part of the preparation of a patient for bone marrow transplantation.

Dosing regimens vary but are typically 3.7–11.1 GBq of highly specific ^{131}-I-MIBG slowly infused whilst using a lead-shielded system. Symptoms during infusion are limited and rare but might be related to the pharmacological action of MIBG itself in causing mild hypertension. Consecutive therapies are separated by at least 4 weeks and more typically 8 weeks. Dosing using ^{125}I is generally higher; typically 10–30 GBq, but both are targeted to deliver at least 150 Sv to the tumour. Pretherapy scans are useful for estimating the total body exposure as well as the dose to the principal tumour masses, but are notoriously inaccurate when compared with post-therapy examinations. The most frequent form of toxicity is thrombocytopaenia which generally occurs around 2 weeks after treatment. Sisson *et al.* [7] showed that the best predictors for low platelet counts are activity divided by surface area for ^{131}I and by activity divided by bodyweight for ^{125}I. Combined series for therapeutic effectiveness show that an objective response can be identified in 56% of patients, and that there is a higher rate of improvement with regard to symptoms and pain relief [2,8]. In 276 patients with neuroblastoma, mostly children with stage IV progressive disease and in whom other therapies had failed, there was a 35% objective response rate. In some centres ^{131}I-MIBG therapy has replaced chemotherapy for the preoperative shrinkage of tumour, and chemotherapy is reserved for the treatment of residual tumour [9]. ^{125}I-MIBG has been used in a limited number of centres for bone-marrow infiltration and when micrometastases are suspected. There are very few reports on the treatment of paragangliomas, but most have described some degree of pain relief. While palliation rates are above 50%, objective improvement rates in metastatic carcinoid have not met expectations.

Both the patient and anyone who is to provide intimate and prolonged care should receive cold iodine to protect thyroidal uptake of radioiodine. Either Lugol's solution or potassium iodide capsules at a dose of at least 100 mg of iodide a day should be maintained for 4–6 weeks after the therapy has been administered.

Somatostatin-receptor scanning

Somatostatin is a cyclic tetradecapeptide which exerts a widespread inhibitory effect at a number of sites including the hypothalamus, other parts of the brain and the pituitary gland, as well as the gut, the endocrine and the exocrine pancreas. A wide variety of neoplasms have been reported to have high-affinity binding sites for somatostatin: these include growth-hormone secreting pituitary adenomas, meningiomas, astrocytomas, neuroblastomas, small-cell carcinomas of the bronchus and breast cancers, as well as pancreatic and carcinoid tumours. These receptors are thought to mediate the inhibition of hormonal secretion from some of these tumours, and may also mediate the inhibition of tumour growth. Somatostatin has a very short half-life in plasma, and for this reason a biologically active analogue, octreotide, was developed for clinical use. Other analogues have been labelled with ^{125}I,^{123}I and ^{111}In for the *in vitro* and *in vivo* detection of somatostatin-receptor-positive tumours. Specifically ^{123}I-^{3}Tyr-octreotide and ^{111}In-DTPA-octreotide have been used in order to visualise a variety of somatostatin-receptor-positive tumour by γ-camera scintigraphy.

Radiopharmacy

Somatostatin analogues have been labelled with ^{123}I and with ^{111}In. For scanning, ^{123}I is given at a dose of up to 250 MBq, which results in an effective dose equivalent of 4.4 mSv. However, *in vivo* receptor imaging with ^{123}I-^{3}Tyr has some drawbacks. In the first place, the availability of chemically pure ^{123}I is limited, it has a relatively short half-life, and most importantly its predominant hepatobiliary clearance makes the identification of abdominal tumours difficult. Most of these problems are overcome by using ^{111}In-DTPA-D-^{1}Phe-octreotide, the dose of which ranges between 200 and 300 MBq. Images from this are generally obtained after 4 and 24 hours.

GEP tumours

GEP neuroendocrine tumours are often difficult to localise. However, many contain high-affinity binding sites for somatostatin and as a consequence a number of groups have looked at the value of receptor scintigraphy in the visualisation of these lesions. Meta-analysis of 451 patient studies reveals a sensitivity of 86% in all published carcinoid series [2]. Recently Scherubl *et al.* [10] studying 40 patients subdivided an overall sensitivity of 80% according to tumour location as: 87.5% in midgut GEP tumours, 64.7% in foregut lesions and 100% in metastatic tumours of unknown primary. In 40% of their patients scintigraphy revealed tumour not localised by ultrasonography, computed tomography (CT) scanning or magnetic resonance imaging (MRI). Conversely 20% of tumours visualised by conventional means were missed by somatostatin scintigraphy. King *et al.* [11] identified 73% of lesions using ^{111}In-DTPA-D-^{1}Phe-octreotide scintigraphy, in comparison with 93% using conventional CT. There were six out of 45 false positives using CT and none with scintigraphy. The authors concluded that while CT was more sensitive, the techiques were complementary, especially in patients with disseminated pathology, equivocal lesions on CT or a negative CT and strong clinical or biochemical evidence of a neuroendocrine tumour. Scintigraphic comparison of MIBG and somatostatin-receptor scanning showed a varying spectrum of uptake for both radiopharmaceuticals, and suggests that they represent complementary imaging techniques for detecting carcinoid tumours and their metastases [12].

Phaeochromocytoma

Although a high proportion of phaeochromocytomas appear to possess somatostatin receptors, the renal accumulation of ^{111}In-labelled somatostatin analogue is a major drawback in the identification of these tumours and MIBG scanning remains the preferred modality.

Neuroblastoma

Similarly, although ^{111}In-DTPA-D-^{1}Phe-octreotide scintigraphy has a sensitivity of almost 80% in such lesions, this modality offers no advantages over MIBG.

Insulinomas

β-Cell tumours of the pancreas secreting insulin are notoriously difficult to identify using conventional imaging modalities. Somatostatin-receptor scanning appears to have a sensitivity of about 50% in such cases. Moreover, a positive scan appears to be predictive of a therapeutic effect with octreotide [13].

Pituitary tumours

Both functioning and non-functioning pituitary tumours have been imaged with radiolabelled somatostatin analogues. None of the series is particularly large, but it is evident that activity cannot be used to be distinguish between tumours. In the case of GH-secreting tumours, however, Ur *et al.* [14] have shown that activity does correlate with the tumour's biochemical responsiveness to octreotide. In a recent study looking at the prediction of efficacy of octreotide therapy in patients with acromegaly the positive predictive value of acute testing with cold octreotide, short-term octreotide administration, and ^{111}In-pentetreotide scintigraphy was 53%, 70%, and 73%, respectively, when GH normalisation (< 5mg/l) after 3 months of therapy was considered [15].

Medullary carcinoma of the thyroid

Medullary carcinoma of the thyroid (MTC) arises from the parafollicular cells of the thyroid, which are neural crest derivatives. *In vitro* visualisation of somatostatin receptors is found in just over one-third of such tumours, but surprisingly meta-analysis of published data on somatostatin scintigraphy in these tumours reveals a sensitivity of 66% [2]. Higher serum calcitonin over carcino-embryonic antigen ratios in patients whose MTC is visualised with octreotide scintigraphy suggests that somatostatin receptors are present on more differentiated MTC [16].

Cushing's syndrome

Localisation of occult tumours underlying a Cushing's syndrome remains one of the most challenging scenarios in diagnostic medicine. De Herder *et al.*[17] studied 10 patients with Cushing's syndrome, nine with the ectopic adrenocorticotrophic hormone (ACTH) syndrome and one with a corticotrophin-releasing hormone (CRH)-secreting tumour. For comparison, eight ACTH-secreting pituitary tumours and one adrenal adenoma were scanned. Although somatostatin-analogue scintigraphy successfully identified the primary ectopic ACTH-secreting and CRH-secreting tumours or their metastases, or both, in eight of 10 patients, most were large lesions which were not truly occult. The usefulness of somatostatin-receptor imaging in the diagnostic work-up for Cushing's needs to be determined in lesions such as bronchial microcarcinoids (< 10 mm) which continue to elude detection with state-of-the-art cross-sectional imaging [18].

Breast cancer

Somatostatin receptors have been demonstrated in breast cancers, and van Eijck *et al.* [19] have recently reported positive ^{111}In-DTPA-D-^{1}Phe-octreotide scans in 39 of 52 primary breast cancers. These findings correlate with the presence of somatostatin receptors on these tumours as determined by tissue autoradiography. Significantly, more invasive ductal cancers could be shown than invasive lobular carcinomas (85% versus 56%). Since antiproliferative effects of somatostatin analogues have been reported in breast-cancer cell lines, they suggest that the technique may be of value in selecting patients for clinical trials with somatostatin analogues.

Lymphomas

Normal as well as activated lymphocytes, macrophages and leukaemic cells are known to possess somatostatin receptors. Vanhagen *et al.* [20] investigated 10 consecutive patients with malignant lymphomas (Hodgkin's disease and non-Hodgkin's lymphomas). In all of their patients lymphoma deposits were visualised using the ^{111}In-labelled somatostatin analogue. In four of the patients additional tumour localisations were observed as compared with conventional imaging modalities. They suggest that somatostatin receptor scintigraphy is of value in lymphoma staging. Clearly, further studies are needed in order to precisely define the value and limitations of this approach in lymphoma patients.

Therapy

The biodistribution of ^{111}In-DTPA-D-^{1}Phe-octreotide, in particular its renal excretion, and the generalised distribution of somatostatin-receptor activity throughout the body does not lend itself to radionuclide therapy using this agent with a β-emitting radionuclide currently. Limited reports of its therapeutic use have not been encouraging.

Other agents

Newer agents such as ^{123}I-labelled vasoactive intestinal polypeptide (VIP), currently being evaluated for carcinoid and gastrointestinal tumours [21] and ^{131}I-labelled –3F8 (monoclonal antibody for ganglioside 6_{D2}) [22] for neural crest tumours will add to our ability to image and treat these difficult lesions.

Conclusion

MIBG and somatostatin scintigraphy are important additions to the imaging armoury. For imaging tumours of neural crest origin the procedures are undoubtedly complementary. ^{111}In-DTPA-D-^{1}Phe-octreotide scanning is probably the best initial procedure in carcinoid and endocrine GEP tumours whilst ^{131}I-MIBG can be used for evaluation of the feasibility of therapy and for radionuclide therapy itself. ^{123}I-MIBG scintigraphy is an important imaging procedure in patients with phaeochromocytoma, neuroblastoma and malignant paraganglioma. In addition to structural information about a wide range of tumours, somatostatin receptor scintigraphy also provides useful information about function and may be a predictor of response to treatment with unlabelled octreotide.

References

1 Margulies KB, Sheps SG.Carney's triad: guidelines for management. *Mayo Clin Proc* 1988; **63**: 496–502.

2 Hoefnagel CA. Metiodobenzylguanidine and somatostatin in oncology: role in the management of neural crest tumours. *Eur J Nucl Med* 1994; **21**: 561–81.

3 Evans AE, D'Angio GJ, Propert K, Anderson J, Hann HW. Prognostic factors in neuroblastoma. *Cancer* 1987; **59**: 1853–9.

4 Gilday DL, Grenberg M. The controversy about the nuclear medicine investigation of neuroblastoma. *J Nucl Med* 1990; **31**: 135.

5 Maurea S, Lastoria S, Caraco C, Indolfi P, Casale F, di Tullio MT, Salvatore M. Iodine-131-MIBG imaging to monitor chemotherapy response in advanced neuroblastoma: comparison with laboratory analysis. *J Nucl Med* 1994; **35**: 1429–135.

6 Hanson MW, Feldman JM, Blinder RA, Moore JO, Coleman RF. Carcinoid tumours: iodine-131 MIBG scintigraphy. *Radiology* 1989; **172**: 699–703.

7 Sisson JC, Shapiro B, Hutchinson RJ, Carey JE, Zasadny KR, Zempel SA, Normolle DP. Predictors of toxicity in treating patients with neuroblastoma by radiolabelled metaiodobenzylguanidine. *Eur J Nucl Med* 1994; **21**: 46–52.

8 Troncone L, Galli G. Proceedings of the International Workshop on the role of I-131 metaiodobenzylguanidine in the treatment of neural crest tumours. *J Nucl Biol Med* 1991; **35**: 248–51.

9 Hoefnegel CA. Radionucleide therapy revisited *Eur J Nucl Med* 1991; **18**: 408–31.

10 Scherubl H, Bader M, Fett U *et al.* Somatostatin-receptor imaging of neuroendocrine gastroenteropancreatic tumours. *Gastroenterology* 1993; **105**: 1705–9.

11 King CMP, Bomanji J, Ur E *et al.* Imaging neuroendocrine tumours with radiolabelled somatostatin analogues and X-ray computed tomography: a comparative study. *Clin Radiol* 1993; **48**: 386–91.

12 Bomanji J, Ur E, Mather S *et al.* A scintigraphic comparison of 123-I-meta-iodobenzylguanidine (MIBG) and an 123-I labeled somatostatin analogue (Tyr-3-octreotide) in metastatic carcinoid tumours. *J Nucl Med* 1992; **33**: 1121–4.

13 Ur E, Bomanji J, Mather SJ *et al.* Localisation of neuroendocrine tumours of the carcinoid type and insulinomas using radiolabelled somatostatin analogues:^{123}I-TOCT and ^{111}In-DOCT. *Clin Endocrinol* 1993; **38**: 501–6.

14 Ur E, Mather SJ, Bomanji *et al.* Pituitary imaging using an 123-I labelled analogue of somatostatin in acromegaly. *Clin Endocrinol* 1992; **36**: 147–50.

15 Colao A, Ferone D, Lastoria S *et al.* Prediction of efficacy of octreotide therapy in patients with acromegaly. *J Clin Endocrinol Metab* 1996; **81**: 2356–62.

16 Kwekkeboom DJ, Reubi JC, Lamberts SWJ *et al. In vivo* somatostatin receptor imaging in medullary thyroid carcinoma. *J Clin Endocrinol Metab* 1993; 76: 1413–17.

17 de Herder WW, Krenning EP, Malchoff CD *et al.* Somatostatin receptor scintigraphy: its value in tumor localization in patients with Cushing's syndrome caused by ectopic corticotropin or corticotropin-releasing hormone secretion. *Am J Med* 1994; **96**: 305–12.

18 Doppmann JL. Somatostatin receptor scintigraphy and the ectopic ACTH syndrome—the solution or just another test? *Am J Med* 1994; **96**: 303–4.

19 van Eijck CH, Krenning EP, Bootsma A *et al.* Somatostatin-receptor scintigraphy in primary breast cancer. *Lancet* 1994; **343**: 640–3.

20 Vanhagen PM, Krenning EP, Reubi JC *et al.* Somatostatin analogue scintigraphy of malignant lymphomas. *Br J Haematol* 1993; **83**: 75–9.

21 Virgolini I, Raderer M, Kurtaran A *et al.* Vasoactive intestinal polypeptide-receptor imaging for the localization of intestinal adenocarcinomas and endocrine tumors. *N Engl J Med* 1994; **331**: 1116–21.

22 Yeh SD, Larson SM, Burch L et al. Radioimmunodetection of neuroblastoma with iodine-131-3F8: correlation with biopsy, iodine-131-metaiodobenzylguanidine and standard diagnostic modalities. *J Nucl Med* 1991; **32**: 769–76.

23 Hoefnagel CA, Metaiodobenzylguanidine and somatostatin in oncology: role in the management of neural crest tumours. *Eur J Nucl Med* 1994; **21**: 561–81.

Part 15
Disorders of Weight: Obesity and Anorexia

CHAPTER 67

Obesity: definition, assessment and dietary management

J.S. Garrow

Relation of fatness to mortality and morbidity

Obesity is a major public health problem in the developed world. Fig. 67.1 summarises the experience of life insurance companies concerning the relation of weight-for-height to all-cause mortality ratio among young adult men. To adjust for differences in stature the weight-for-height axis is shown as Quetelet's index (QI, also known as body-mass index, BMI), which is calculated from weight (kg) divided by the square of height (m). Quetelet, a Belgian astronomer, was the first to note that the weight of adults of normal build was proportional to their height squared [1], so the index (kg/m^2) is a convenient measure of obesity. Its validity as a measure of fatness is considered below. People who take out life insurance may not be representative of the general population, but the curve shown in Fig. 67.1 also fits the observed relation of bodyweight to all-cause mortality among 750 000 men and women monitored by the American Cancer Society [2].

The curve is J-shaped, with the minimum mortality rates observed in the range 20–25 kg/m^2. Below 20, and above 25, the mortality ratio increases, and doubles at 38 kg/m^2. Thereafter the curve rises even more steeply, but becomes more unreliable, since only a relatively small number of people have been studied (and even fewer have been insured) at values above 40 kg/m^2. However, it is evident that the curve in Fig. 67.1 is influenced by other factors as well as obesity; notably, the effect of cigarette smoking and pre-existing disease. For example, in a study of 115 000 white female nurses aged 30–55 years there were 4726 deaths during 16 years of follow-up [3], and these were related to QI as in Fig. 67.1. However, when data from those women who had never smoked, and who were of constant weight, were analysed separately, the mortality ratio was lowest in the leanest women (QI 19), and increased steadily to double the lowest rate by 30 kg/m^2.

Among non-smoking men aged 50 years, without evidence of disease at study entry and followed for 30 years, the minimum mortality is in the range 22–27 kg/m^2, with the mortality risk doubling the minimum level at QI 20 and again at QI 30 [4]. It appears, therefore, that although Fig. 67.1 serves well to help insurance companies to identify young adults who are liable to die young (and hence who are unprofitable to insure), the increase in mortality below 20 kg/m^2 in women probably shows the effect of cigarette smoking and pre-existing disease.

QI and body fat

The use of QI as a measure of fatness implies that lean body mass is constantly related to height squared, so any increase in QI reflects added fat, not added lean tissue. This assumption is not true in some instances; for example, certain types of athletes, such as weightlifters, build large muscles without increasing in height. Conversely, old people lose lean tissue faster than they lose height. However, for clinical purposes, QI serves very well, since the management of obesity is much more important in young people than old ones, and elite athletes in training are unlikely to become obese. Measurements in 104 women aged 14–60 years showed that the correlation between total body fat and QI was 0.955, and the slope of the regression line was 1.28, indicating that, for an increase of body fat by 1 kg, bodyweight increased by 1.28 kg, so the extra weight in obese people is about 75% fat and 25% fat-free mass [5].

A working definition of obesity

There are several reasons why it is not helpful to try to set a

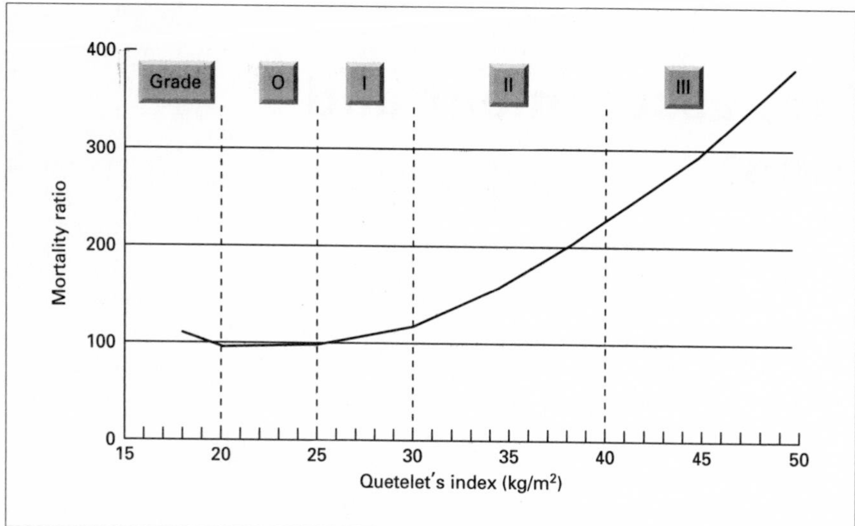

Fig. 67.1 The relationship between weight/height and mortality in young adult men. From [42].

single threshold of weight-for-height, or percentage body fat, at which a person switches from normality to obesity. First, a given percentage body fat has different health consequences for people who differ in age or gender. Secondly, the mortality risk and health penalties of obesity increase with increasing fatness, as shown in Fig. 67.1, so the best we can do is to assign zones of weight-for-height, as indicated in Fig. 67.2. Given the limitations of weight–height indices discussed above, it is clinically useful to assume, other things being equal, that an individual in zone 0 (QI 20–24.9) is of desirable weight, and that obesity of grades I,II and III indicates overweight, obesity and severe obesity, respectively [6].

Influence of fat distribution on mortality and morbidity

A major disadvantage in defining obesity by weight-for-height is that it does not take into consideration the distribution of fat in the body. Intra-abdominal fat causes a greater risk of cardiovascular disease than an equal weight of fat situated subcutaneously, and waist circumference is a good measure of intra-abdominal fat [7]. Indeed, a waist circumference of >94 cm in men, or >80 cm in women, is strongly associated with cardiovascular risk factors [8]. However, the disadvantages of relying solely on waist circumference for diagnosis of obesity are that some health consequences of obesity (e.g. osteoarthritis of weight-bearing joints) probably do not relate specifically to intra-abdominal fat, and also it is difficult to measure waist circumference precisely for an obese subject with a pendulous abdomen. With weight loss the ratio of intra-abdominal to total fat, and the waist/hip ratio, decreases. However, there is no evidence that fat distribution predicts the success of weight loss achieved by dietary therapy [9].

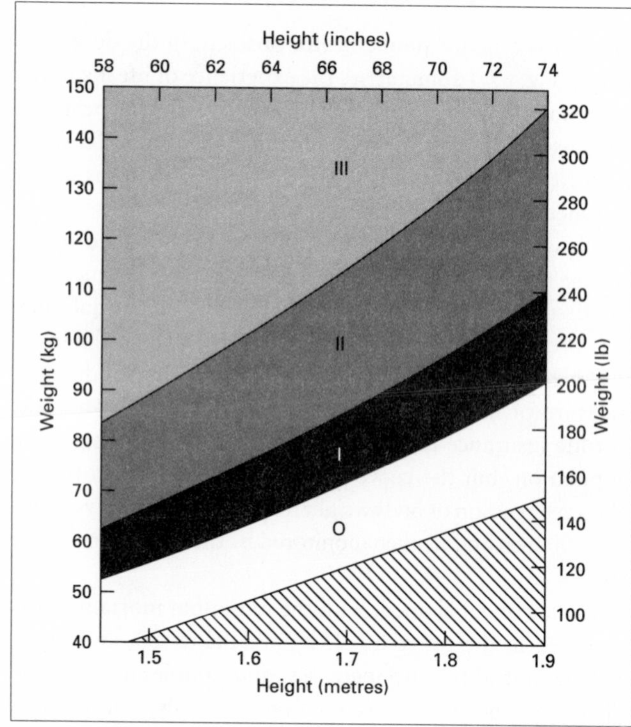

Fig. 67.2 Relationships of height to weight defining the desirable range (0), and grade I, II and III obesity, marked by the boundaries of W/H^2 = 25–29.9, 30–40- and >40, respectively. From [6].

Influence of age, sex and frame size on desirable weight-for-height

Total fat mass tends to increase with age. The 1990 US weight guidelines suggest that a gain in weight after the age of 35 years is consistent with good health, but data from the Nurses Health Study show that gain of more than 5 kg after the age of 18 years is associated with a significantly increased risk of coronary heart disease [10].

For a given weight and height women contain more fat than men, but for a given percentage body fat the health risks are greater in men than in women. These two tendencies cancel out, so the ranges of weight and height shown in Fig. 67.2 apply equally well to men and women.

Attempts have been made to 'correct' weight and height standards for frame size, as indicated by measures such as chest breadth, but this does not improve the accuracy by which QI predicts body fat [11].

Influence of prenatal growth on adult disease risk

A rapidly developing area of research suggests that diseases in adult life which are commonly associated with obesity, such as coronary heart disease and diabetes, may have their origins in fetal undernutrition during the second and third trimester of pregnancy [12]. Although severe obesity in children predicts obesity in adult life, longitudinal studies in defined populations show that only a small minority of obese adults were obese before the age of 7 years [13], and studies of monozygotic twins do not show that differences in birth weight relate to differences in adult obesity [14].

Prevalence of obesity in developed countries

In the UK the prevalence of obesity (>30 kg/m^2) among men aged 16–64 years increased from 6% in 1980 to 8% in 1987, and among women the increase was from 8 to 12%. In 1991 the Department of Health set a target of reducing the prevalence back to the 1980 levels, but in fact a survey in 1991 showed that the increase had continued to 13% in men and 16% in women. This rapid increase is mirrored in data from many European countries, and from Australia, Brazil, Canada, and among both black and white people in the USA [15]. Also, in less developed countries, modernisation of lifestyle is associated with a dramatic increase in obesity [16,17].

Metabolic control of energy balance

In the laboratory rat fed a monotonous laboratory chow, it is easy to demonstrate physiological mechanisms regulating energy intake and expenditure, and thus maintaining constant energy stores. In humans, with access to virtually unlimited quantities of palatable food, these mechanisms exist, but are easily overwhelmed by other factors. Many attempts have been made to demonstrate that obese subjects differ from lean controls in their perception of changes in the energy density of food, or in the magnitude of their thermic response to over- or under-feeding [18]. However, differences observed by some workers have not been confirmed by others who have attempted to replicate the experiments.

There is general agreement that resting metabolic rate (RMR) accounts for about 70% of energy expenditure in typical non-athletes, and the main determinant of RMR is fat-free mass (FFM). As noted above, FFM is proportional to height squared, so we might expect a person of normal body composition who was 6 feet (1.83 m) tall to expend 1.44 times as much energy as a person of the same age and sex who was 5 feet (1.52 m) tall. However, obesity is not inversely elated to stature because (usually) short people eat less than tall people. To what extent this adjustment of energy intake is achieved by cognitive or physiological control is not clear: probably both apply, but to different degrees in different people.

When obese people lose weight their energy expenditure decreases by several mechanisms [19]: the net effect is a decrease of about 16 kcal/kg weight lost in men, and about 12 kcal/kg in women. For example, a woman who was initially 100 kg and expended 10 MJ (2400 kcal) per day would, after reducing her weight to 70 kg, require only 8.5 MJ (2040 kcal) daily to maintain weight at 70 kg [19]. If she regarded 2400 kcal as a 'normal' diet, then by eating 'normally' she would eventually return to 100 kg. When subjects previously in energy balance on a defined diet are offered a varied diet ad libitum they tend to overeat, and to increase oxidation of carbohydrate but not fat, thus predisposing to the deposition of excess fat. However, these reactions occur to a similar extent in both lean and obese subjects [20].

Genetic factors in the aetiology of obesity

In 1995 it was shown that a gene product 'leptin' was missing in genetically obese mice, and if leptin was given to *ob/ob* mice they decreased their food intake, increased locomotor activity, and lost weight [21]. However, there is no evidence that leptin deficiency is a cause of obesity in humans; indeed, higher-than-normal leptin levels have been found in obese human subjects [47]. There are genetically determined syndromes in humans which are associated with obesity, such as the Prader–Willi syndrome, but human obesity does not segregate with these chromosomal regions [22]. There is now consensus that the heritability of human obesity is about 0.34, leaving more than half of the variability associated with non-heritable factors [23]. In a 6-year study of adult twin pairs, weight changes reflected environmental rather than genetic influences [24].

What a heritability of 0.34 means in practice is shown in Table 67.1 [25]. From a large series of adoptees, for whom the build of their biological parents was known, there were

Table 67.1 Percentage of obese, or overweight biological parents of adult Danish adoptees who were themselves thin, medium, or obese/overweight. Data from [25].

Adoptee status	Thin	Medium	Obese/overweight
Biological mother			
Obese	6	8	14
Overweight	12	27	27
Biological father			
Obese	3	9	10
Overweight	33	29	39

540 chosen for study who were thin (QI <20), medium (QI 21–25), overweight (QI 27–30) and obese (QI >30). The adoptees who were obese or overweight had a higher proportion obese or overweight mothers or fathers than adoptees who were thin or of medium build, and this difference was statistically significant. However, if an attempt had been made to forecast which adoptees would be obese or overweight on the basis of the weight status of their biological parents this forecast would have been more often wrong than correct.

Socio-economic predictors of obesity and rapid weight gain

Studies in Europe and North America have shown a remarkably consistent pattern of social and economic factors which identify those individuals who are at increased risk of obesity, or of rapid weight gain (>5 kg in 5 years). These are set out in Table 67.2. Some of the items on this table have a plausible explanation; for example, energy requirements for weight maintenance are lower in old, female and inactive people than in young, male and active ones, so it is tempting to conclude that decreased energy expenditure is the common aetiological factor. However, short people have lower energy requirements than tall ones, but the prevalence of obesity is not strongly related to stature.

Table 67.2 Social and economic factors associated with an increased risk of obesity, or of rapid weight gain, in affluent countries.

Age	Obesity increases with age up to age 55 in men and 70 in women
Gender	More women than men are obese over age 50
Educational level	Inversely related to prevalence of obesity
Income	Inversely related to prevalence of obesity
Parity (in women)	Positively associated with prevalence of obesity
Cigarette smoking	Inversely related to weight, weight gain on stopping
Physical activity	Inversely related to weight, weight gain on stopping
Alcohol intake	High intake related to obesity in some populations

The inverse relation between obesity and educational or economic status is strong and repeated in many surveys, yet hard to explain. Interactions between factors in Table 67.2 may provide important clues, for example higher parity in women of lower educational level is a strong predictor of rapid weight gain, but higher parity in women of high educational level is not [26]. Since the hormonal effects of parity are presumably not influenced by level of education, this suggests that the avoidance of weight gain in parous highly educated women is a result of cognitive control of bodyweight, which the equally parous but less educated women do not exercise.

Similarly, there is an interaction between level of education and the well-known association between smoking and relative body weight in men. Heavy smokers of high educational level are heavier than never-smokers, while in less educated men (and in women) this association is reversed [48]. Again, this argues for the importance of cognitive control of body weight [6].

Sociology of the anti-diet movement

In 1978 Susie Orbach published an important book entitled *Fat is a Feminist Issue* [27]. Its main (and true) message was that many young women, even including university students [28], were trying to be unreasonably thin to conform to a social stereotype of what a woman should be. They should escape from this form of oppression, and assert their own individuality. At about the same time the Metropolitan Insurance weight tables for women were revised, since the previous tables required lower weights for women than subsequent actuarial data justified. For the following two decades popular feminist authors have been claiming that the health risks of obesity have been exaggerated, and that any morbidity associated with obesity arises from the social stigmatisation of obese people, which is the factor which should be altered. There is truth in this view, but unfortunately many health writers have failed to distinguish between the situation in zone 0 of Fig. 67.1 (in which Orbach's views are to be endorsed) and grade III obesity, in which the health hazards are all too clear, and not explicable by social stigmata.

Effects of therapeutic weight loss on mortality and morbidity

When obese people lose weight the risk factors associated

with obesity (with the exception of gallstone formation) improve [6,49]. However, when longitudinal epidemiological data are examined it is clear that individuals who have a constant weight are less liable to death (especially from heart disease) than individuals who vary in weight [29], and that even among overweight people those who maintained weight lived longer than those who lost weight [30]. These observations threw doubt on the health benefit of weight loss among overweight people. However, more recent studies have been able to distinguish between intentional and unintentional weight loss [31,32,50]. These show a significantly decreased mortality and morbidity from intentional weight loss.

Assessment of the obese patient

A typical grade II obese patient (weight 100 kg, height 1.7 m, QI 34.6) is about 28 kg overweight, since at 72 kg QI would be 25 kg/m^2. Since excess weight has an energy value of 29 MJ (7000 kcal)/kg [5] the problem is to burn off the excess 820 MJ (196 000 kcal). If the patient's energy expenditure was constant at 8.4 MJ (2000 kcal)/day, then a diet supplying half this amount would generate the required energy deficit in about 7 months. In fact, a diet supplying 4.2 MJ (1000 kcal)/day would take longer than 7 months to reduce the patient from 100 kg to 72 kg, because with weight loss the requirements for weight maintenance decrease, as described above.

In practice, the best rate of weight loss is shown in Fig. 67.3. The upper limit is achieved by a daily energy deficit of 1000 kcal /day, and the lower limit by half this deficit. The rapid weight loss in the first month of dieting reflects the loss of glycogen with associated water, as well as adipose tissue.

Conditions through which obesity causes mortality and morbidity

A decade ago epidemiologists believed that obesity was not a threat to health, because if age, blood pressure, cigarette smoking and cholesterol concentration were taken into consideration, the addition of weight to the regression equation did not improve the accuracy with which heart attacks could be predicted in middle-aged men [33]. In fact, obesity is a risk factor for heart disease (and other causes of mortality and mortality) through the effects of other obesity-related conditions, such as hypertension and dyslipidaemia, as illustrated in Fig. 67.4. The evidence for a causal relationship indicated by the arrows is discussed elsewhere [34].

Investigation of 'refractory' obesity

The hospital specialist investigating a 'refractory' obese patient needs to find the answers to two questions. First, is the obesity in this patient a significant danger to health? As a first step, consult Fig. 67.2 and establish the zone of QI in which the patient falls. The other factors which influence the risk associated with a given degree of obesity are age (risks are greater in younger people [35]), the distribution of fat (risks are greater for a higher waist/hip ratio [36]), and presence of, or family history of, heart disease, hypertension and non-insulin-dependent diabetes mellitus.

Second, if so, is there any reason why normal dietary therapy should not be an appropriate line of treatment? There are two possible reasons: either that normal dietary treatment has been tried and failed to produce normal weight loss, or that normal dietary treatment is unacceptable to the patient. Often both objections to dietary treatment

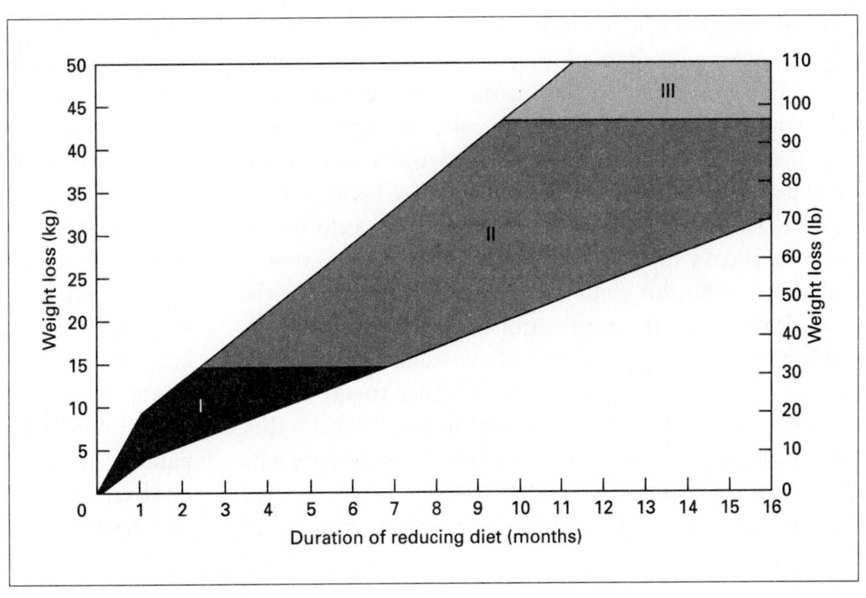

Fig. 67.3 Range of desirable rate of weight loss in obese patients. Younger, taller patients may achieve the rates at the upper limit of the range; older, shorter patients will be nearer the lower limit. The shaded areas indicate the time taken to reach normal weight for patients in grade I, II or III (see Fig. 67.2 for an explanation of these grades). From [6].

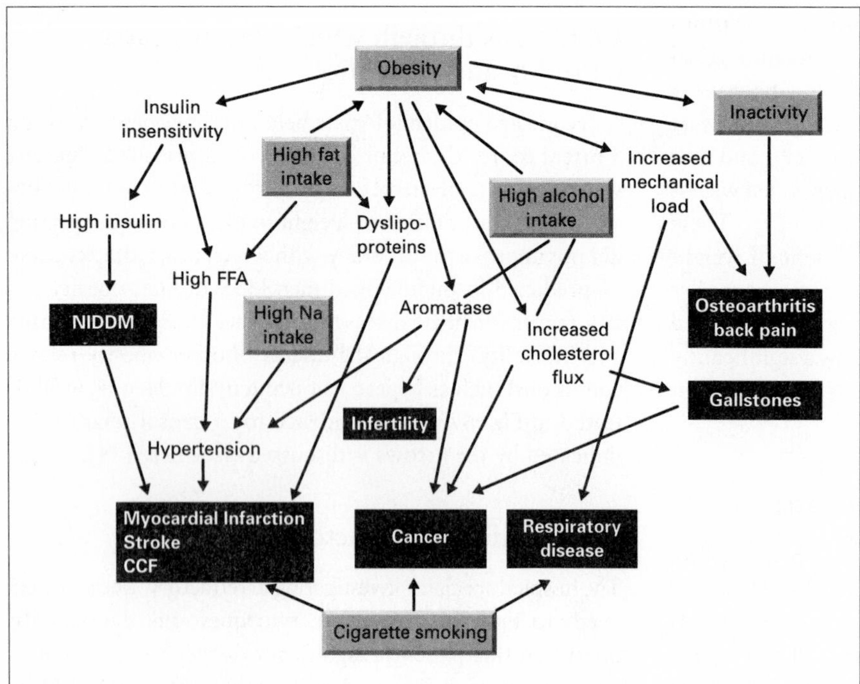

Fig. 67.4 Important diseases are shown in black boxes, and some alterable lifestyle factors which predispose to these diseases are shown in grey boxes. Mechanisms that link lifestyle factors to disease risk are discussed in the text. NIDDM, non-insulin-dependent diabetes mellitus. From [34].

are advanced. The 'failure' of dietary treatment is usually accounted for by non-compliance with the diet, or by an excessively optimistic expectation of the weight loss which should be achieved. Figure 67.3 should be helpful in establishing the long-term rate of weight loss to be associated with a given energy deficit. The acceptability of the diet can then be assessed against the health risk posed by the obesity: every patient is entiltled to judge (given accurate guidance) if the cure is worse than the disease.

A common problem among patients at a tertiary referral centre, which is more difficult to resolve, concerns the obese patient who fervently and sincerely believes that he or she maintains bodyweight on a low-energy intake (say, 1000 kcal/day). Patients who are not losing weight will not be willing to adopt a conventional reducing diet if they consider that is what they are already taking. In part, the explanation is that the period of monitored diet which the patient recalls is atypical [37], but this is not the whole story, because obese patients who have been confined in a chamber calorimeter for several days still recall their intake as much less than it really was [38]; this cannot be an attempt to deceive the investigator, since the investigator knows exactly what the subject in the calorimeter ate. Many studies have shown that obese adults or children have a higher energy output than lean ones [6,39,40], so to maintain energy balance they must have a higher energy intake. Paradoxically, women who perceive themselves to be 'small eaters' have a higher energy output than 'large eaters' [41]: this merely illustrates the unreliability of dietary histories as a means of investigating 'refractory' obesity.

Dietary management of obesity

The alleged inefficacy of dietary treatment is largely based on the non-success of a policy in which medical staff with no knowledge of dietetics offer general advice (which the patient has already had many times) in the expectation that they will return in 3 months having lost 20 kg. Of course this does not happen. Obese patients seen in a tertiary referral centre will have tried to diet, and have failed. The management of an obese out-patient is therefore an iterative process, for which a flow chart is shown in Fig. 67.5 [42]. The degree of obesity is assessed, and if it presents a significant health hazard (see above) the patient takes the 'treatment' route to the right of the diagram; if not, then the 'reassurance' route to the left.

The first step in the treatment route is to ask a competent dietitian to review the diet which the patient is taking, revise the advice if necessary, and agree to meet again in about 4 weeks to review progress. Very-low-calorie diets (<800 kcal/d) cause more side effects, and cause no greater weight loss in the long term, than conventional diets (900–1200 kcal/d). Initial losses which are not maintained undermine patients' morale [51]. If progress is good this loop is continued until target weight is reached, when a policy for weight maintenance is adopted (see below). If for three visits (i.e.

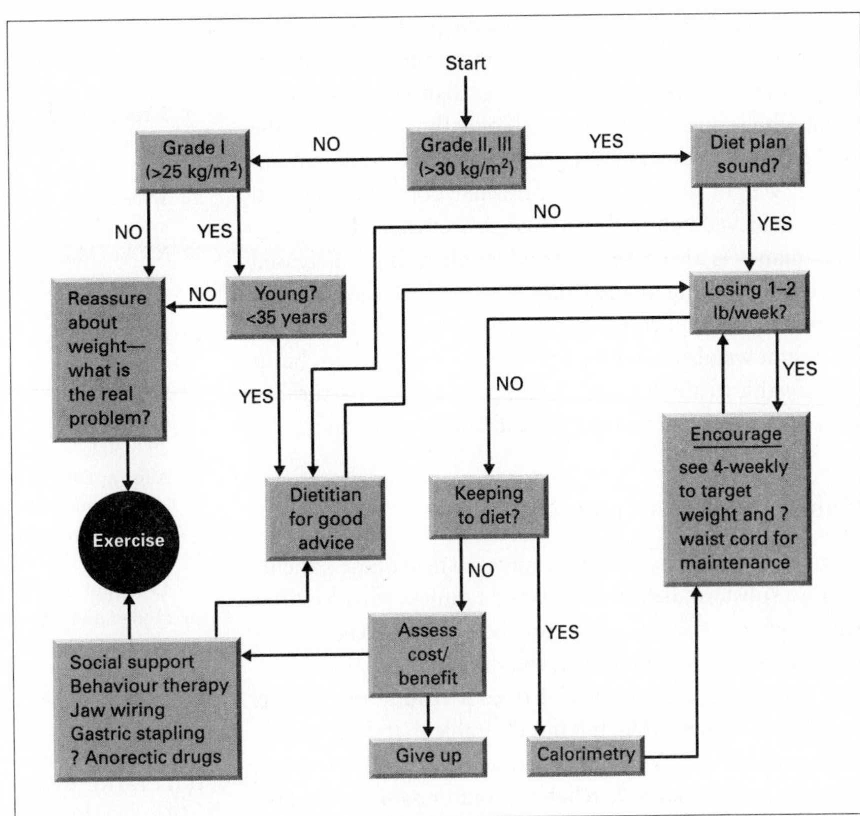

Fig. 67.5 Flow chart by which an obese patient may be matched to the appropriate treatment strategy. From [42].

over 2 months) no weight has been lost, it is necessary to find the reason for this. Ideally, the patient could be studied in a chamber calorimeter, which would provide reliable information about energy expenditure under conditions of known energy intake [6], but this facility is rarely available. It is sometimes helpful to ask the patient who apparently does not lose weight on a diet of (say) 1000 kcal/day to adopt for 3 weeks a diet in which the sole source of energy is 1800 ml (three pints) of whole cow's milk daily, which supplies 1200 kcal, with a careful measurement of weight at the start and end of this period. Everyone does, in fact, lose weight on this regimen, and this is sometimes sufficient to persuade the patient to try again with a conventional diet, although the milk diet is itself perfectly safe and effective [43]. It is not satisfactory to appeal to the large literature which says that obese people have high energy requirements, since refractory obese patients believe that they are different, and will only be convinced by data derived from themselves.

Ultimately, having carried out the above assessment, it may emerge that the cost–benefit of dietary treatment does not justify further investment, and a better option is to switch to drug or surgical treatment (see Chapter 69), or to give up. In all cases it is a good plan to encourage patients to take more exercise, but this will not, on its own, cause significant weight loss [44].

Roles of endocrinologist and dietitian

It surprises me that medical doctors, who would not consider taking over the work of a radiographer, or speech therapist, often feel quite comfortable about giving dietary advice. Therapeutic dietetics requires a fluent knowledge of the principles of energy balance and the nutrient content of food, patience, a persuasive personality, and a willingness to increase (rather than destroy) the self-esteem of the obese patient. This constellation of qualities is rarely found in doctors.

The role of the endocrinologist (or other medical specialist) in the dietary treatment of obesity is to assess the health risks arising from obesity and associated conditions, to exclude treatable endocrine causes, and to support the work of the dietitian in the manner indicated in Fig. 67.5.

Management of obesity in children and pregnant women

Particular problems arise when loss of excess fat in the patient has to be balanced against the need to maintain adequate growth in a child, or in the fetus of a pregnant woman. In children the best chance to treat obesity is between the ages of 5 and 12 years, since this is a period at which growth in both weight and height is rapid, and the diet of the child is (or should be) largely controllable by the parents and school authorities. A child who is on the 95th centile of weight-for-height at age 5 years is only 4 kg heavier than a child of similar height who is on the 50th centile. If over the next 7 years the child achieves normal height growth, but slightly-less-than-normal weight growth, then a normal body composition can be achieved before the teen years are reached.

Pregnancy is also a period at which there is an increased risk of developing obesity, and overweight significantly increases the complications of childbearing [45]. It is unwise to attempt weight loss during pregnancy or lactation, but it is reasonable to aim for zero weight gain, so after parturition the woman weighs less than she did before pregnancy.

Maintenance of weight loss

It is unethical and a waste of resources to help obese patients to lose a substantial amount of weight, unless you also offer help to enable them to maintain the reduced weight. This will not happen automatically: the stomach does not shrink after prolonged dieting, or if it does it readily re-expands when more food is eaten. It is not desirable that the formerly obese person should become addicted to self-weighing, so what is required is a reliable monitor which will give unmistakable warning of unwanted substantial weight gain. This may be achieved by a spouse, or a vigilant practice nurse in primary care, or by a local slimming club. The problem about all these monitors is that they can often be avoided or ignored. A nylon cord fitted round the waist is a reliable indicator which can neither be avoided nor ignored [46]; these have served to help many patients to maintain substantial weight loss over many years.

References

1 Quetelet LAJ. *Physique Sociale*. Brussels: C. Muquardt, 1869.

2 Lew EA, Garfinkel L. Variations in mortality by weight among 750000 men and women. *J Chron Dis* 1979; **32**: 563–76.

3 Manson JE, Willet WC, Stamfer MJ et al. Body weight and mortality among women. *N Engl J Med* 1995; **333**: 677–85.

4 Troiano RP, Frongillo EA, Sobal J, Levitsky DA. The relationship between body weight and mortality: a quantitative analysis of combined information from existing studies. *Int J Obes* 1996; **20**: 63–75.

5 Webster JD, Hesp R, Garrow JS. The composition of excess weight in obese women estimated by body density, total body water and total potassium. *Hum Nutr Clin Nutr* 1984; **38C**: 299–306.

6 Garrow JS. *Obesity and related diseases*. Edinburgh: Churchill-Livingstone, 1988.

7 Pouliot M-C, Deprés J-P, Lemiux S *et al.* Waist circumference and abdominal sagittal diameter: best anthropometric indexes of abdominal visceral adipose tissue accumulation and related cardio-vascular risk in men and women. *Am J Cardiol* 1994; **73**: 460–8.

8 Han TS, van Leer EM, Seidell JC, Lean MEJ. Waist circumference action levels in the identification of cardiovascular risk factors: prevalence study in a random sample. *Br Med J* 1995; **311**: 1401–5.

9 Svendsen OL, Hassager C, Christiansen C. The response to treatment of overweight in post-menopausal women is not related to fat distribution. *Int J Obes* 1995; **19**: 496–502.

10 Willett WC, Manson JE, Stampfer MJ *et al.* Weight, weight change and coronary heart disease in women. *JAMA* 1995; **273**: 461–5.

11 Rookus MA, Burema J, Deurenberg P, Van der Wiel-Wetzels WAM. The impact of adjustment of a weight–height index (W/H^2) for frame size on the prediction of body fatness. *Br J Nutr* 1985; **54**: 335–42.

12 Barker DJP. Fetal origins of coronary heart disease. *Br Med J* 1995; **311**: 171–4.

13 Braddon FEM, Rodgers B, Wadsworth MEJ, Davies JMC. Onset of obesity in a 36 year birth cohort study. *Br Med J* 1986; **293**: 299–302.

14 Allison DB, Paultre F, Heymsfield SB, Pi-Sunyer FX. Is the intrauterine period really a critical period for the development of obesity? *Int J Obes* 1995; **19**: 397–402.

15 Seidell JC. Obesity in Europe: scaling an epidemic. *Int J Obes* 1995; **19** (Suppl. 3): S1–4.

16 Hodge AM, Dowse GK, Koki G, Mavo B, Alpers MP, Zimmet PZ, Modernity and obesity in coastal and highland Papua New Guinea. *Int J Obes* 1995; **19**: 154–61.

17 Rode A, Shephard RJ. Modernisation of lifestyle, body fat content and body fat distribution: a comparison of Igloolik Inuit and Volochanka nGanasan. *Int J Obes* 1995; **19**: 709–16.

18 Leibel RL, Rosenbaum M, Hirsch J. Changes in energy expenditure resulting from altered body weight. *N Engl J Med* 1995; **332**: 621–8.

19 Garrow JS, Webster JD. Effect on weight and metabolic rate of obese women of a 3.4 MJ (800 kcal) diet. *Lancet* 1989; i: 31.

20 Larson DE, Rising R, Ferraro RT, Ravussin E. Spontaneous overfeeding with a 'cafeteria diet' in men: effects on 24-hour energy expenditure and substrate oxidation. *Int J Obes* 1995; **19**: 331–7.

21 Pelleymounter MA, Cullen MJ, Baker MB *et al.* Effect of the *obese* gene product on body weight regulation in *ob/ob* mice. *Science* 1995; **269**: 540–3.

22 Reed DR, Ding Y, Xu W, Cather C, Price RA. Human obesity does not segregate with the chromosomal regions of Prader–Willi, Bardet–Biedl, Cohen, Borjeson or Wilson–Turner syndromes. *Int J Obes* 1995; **19**: 599–603.

23 Vogler GP, Sørensen TI, Stunkard AJ, Srinivasan MR, Rao DC. Influences of genes and shared family environment on adult body mass index assessed in an adoption study by a comprehensive path model. *Int J Obs* 1995; **19**: 40–5.

24 Korkeila M, Kaprio J, Rissanen A, Kosenvuo M. Consistency and change of body mass index and weight. A study on 5967 adult Finnish twin pairs. *Int J Obes* 1995; **19**: 310–17.

25 Stunkard AJ, Sørensen TI, Hanis C et al. An adoption study of human obesity. *N Engl J Med* 1986; **314**: 193–8.

26 Rissanen A, Heliövaara M, Knekt P, Reuanen A, Aromaa A. Determinants of weight gain and overweight in Finns. *Eur J Clin Nutr* 1991; **45**: 419–30.

27 Orbach S. *Fat is a Feminist Issue*. London: Hamlyn, 1978.

28 Bellisle F, Monneuse M-O, Steptoe A, Wardle J. Weight concerns and eating patterns: a survey of university students in Europe. *Int J Obes* 1995; **19**: 723–30.

29 Wannameethee G, Shaper AG. Weight change in middle-aged British men: implications for health. *Eur J Clin Nutr* 1990; **44**: 133–42.

30 Higgins M, D'Agostino R, Kannel W, Cobb J. Benefits and adverse

effects of weight loss. *Ann Intern Med* 1993; **119**: 758–63.

31 Iribarren C, Sharp DS, Burchfiel CM, Petrovitch H. Association of weight loss and weight fluctuation with mortality among Japanese American men. *N Engl J Med* 1995; **333**: 686–92.

32 Williamson DF, Pamuk E, Thun M, Flanders D, Byers T, Heath C. Prospective study of intentional weight loss and mortality in never-smoking overweight US white women aged 40–64 years. *Am J Epidemiol* 1995; **141**: 1128–41.

33 Keys A, Menotti A, Aravanis C *et al.* The seven countries study: 2289 deaths in 15 years. *Prev Med* 1984; **13**: 141–54.

34 Garrow JS. Importance of obesity. *Br Med J* 1991; **303**: 704–6.

35 Chen Y, Rennie DC, Reeder BA. Age-related association between body mass index and blood pressure: the Humbolt study. *Int J Obes* 1995; **19**: 825–31.

36 Richelsen B, Pedersen SB. Associations between different anthropometric measurements of fatness and metabolic risk parameters in non-obese, healthy, middle-aged men. *Int J Obes* 1995; **19**: 169–74.

37 Ballard-Barbash R, Graubard I, Krebs-Smith SM, Schatzkin A, Thompson FE. Contribution of dieting to the inverse association between energy intake and body mass index. *Eur J Clin Nutr* 1996; **50**: 98–106.

38 Taylor MA. *Meal pattern and obesity*. PhD thesis, University of London, 1995.

39 Prentice AM, Black AE, Coward WA, Cole TJ. Energy expenditure in overweight and obese adults in affluent societies: an analysis of 319 doubly-labelled water measurements. *Eur J Clin Nutr* 1996; **50**: 93–7.

40 Maffeis C, Pinelli L, Zaffanello M, Schena F, Iacumin P, Schutz Y. Daily energy expenditure in free-living conditions in obese and non-obese children: comparison of doubly-labelled water method and heart rate monitoring. *Int J Obes* 1995; **19**: 671–7.

41 Clark DC, Thomas FM, Withers RT *et al.* Differences in substrate metabolism between self-perceived 'large-eating' and 'small-eating' women. *Int J Obes* 1995; **19**: 245–52.

42 Garrow JS. Obesity. In: Weatherall DJ, Ledingham JCG, Warrell DA, eds. *Oxford Textbook of Medicine*, 3rd edn, Vol. 1. Oxford: Oxford University Press, 1996: 1301–14.

43 Garrow JS, Webster JD, Pearson M, Pacy PJ, Harpin G. Inpatient–outpatient randomised comparison of Cambridge Diet versus milk diet in 17 women over 24 weeks. *Int J Obes* 1989; **13**: 521–9.

44 Garrow JS, Summerbell CD. Meta-analysis: effect of exercise, with or without dieting, on the body composition of overweight subjects. *Eur J Clin Nutr* 1995; **49**: 1–10.

45 Galtier-Dereure F, Montpeyroux F, Boulot P, Bringr J, Jaffiol C. Weight excess before pregnancy: complications and costs. *Int J Obes* 1995; **19**: 443–8.

46 Garrow JS. The management of obesity. Another view. *Int J Obes* 1992; **16** (suppl. 2): S59–63.

47 Niskanen L, Haffner S, Karhunen LJ *et al.* Serum leptin in relation to resting energy expenditure and fuel metabolism in obese subjects. *Int J Obes* 1997; **21**: 309–13.

48 Molarius A, Seidell JC. Differences in the association between smoking and relative body weight by level of education. *Int J Obes* 1997; **21**: 189–96.

49 Pasquali R, Vicennati V, Marinari G *et al.* Achievement of near-normal body weight as the prerequisite to normalise sex hormone-binding globulin concentrations in massively obese men. *Int J Obes* 1997; **21**: 1–5.

50 Williamson DF. Intentional weight loss: patterns in the general population and its association with mortality and morbidity. *Int J Obes* 1997; **21** (Suppl 1): S14–S19.

51 Rössner S, Flaten H. VLCD versus LCD in long-term treatment of obesity. *Int J Obes* 1997; **21**: 22–6.

CHAPTER 68

Neuroendocrine function in obesity

P.G. Kopelman

Introduction

In adult humans, weight does not change appreciably over long periods, which suggests that food intake is adjusted to the metabolic activity of the body. It is not surprising, therefore, that extremely obese patients are commonly referred to endocrinologists because the patient or their family has questioned a possible hormonal basis for their obesity. Alterations in neuroendocrine function are, indeed, found in association with increasing bodyweight, but it seems probable that these changes are a *consequence* rather than the *cause* of corpulence. Nevertheless, it is important for these alterations to be recognised in order to avoid unnecessary investigations and the raising of false hopes for a 'quick cure' by the patient. This chapter reviews changes in hypothalamo-pituitary function which frequently accompany extreme obesity, and includes a brief discussion of the possible aetiological factors.

Adrenocortical function

In animal models of obesity adrenal glucocorticoids appear to play an important role in regulating body fat: these obese animals have elevated serum cortisol levels associated with increased fat storage and protein metabolism. Obese humans have normal circulating serum cortisol levels with a normal circadian rhythm and normal urinary free cortisol [1], but have an accelerated degradation of cortisol which is compensated by an increased cortisol production rate [2]. This increased turnover of cortisol in obesity is reflected by an increased level of urinary 17-hydroxycorticosteroids. It has been suggested that enhanced cortisol metabolism by adipose tissue is the primary mechanism behind the changes. If the metabolism of cortisol is increased by adipose tissue in obesity, plasma cortisol will tend to fall resulting in an increase in pituitary secretion of adrenocorticotrophic hormone (ACTH); this in turn causes an increase in adrenal cortisol output to restore plasma cortisol levels to normal [3]. The increase in ACTH secretion will also stimulate adrenal androgen output and perhaps account for the enhanced urinary 17-ketosteroid excretion, which measures various androgen metabolites including etiocholanolone, androsterone, dehydroepiandrosterone (DHEA) and its sulphate conjugate (DHEAS), often found in obesity [4]. A correlation has been reported between the metabolic clearance of DHEA, androstenedione and the distribution of fat tissue in the upper body which suggests that DHEA may have a role in determining adipose tissue deposition [5]. Furthermore, a positive correlation between bodyweight and changes in DHEA and the DHEA/17-hydroxyprogesterone ratio after the exogenous administration of ACTH has been described [6]. This is suggestive of hyperresponsiveness of adrenal androgens in obesity. A moderate elevation of plasma ACTH has been reported in obesity, and Weaver *et al.* [7] have also provided evidence for increased release by reporting an association between the ACTH response to insulin-induced hypoglycaemia and increasing bodyweight.

In a preliminary study, a small group of obese subjects were found to have a normal ACTH response to corticotrophin-releasing hormone (CRH) and a slightly, but significantly, diminished change in serum cortisol [8]. This difference has not been confirmed by subsequent studies of larger numbers of obese and normal-weight subjects with almost identical responses of ACTH and cortisol being seen in the two groups. It is possible that a subgroup of obese subjects exists who respond less to CRH than normal-weight subjects, but the minor differences in pituitary–adrenal axis responses to insulin-induced hypoglycaemia reported in obese subjects suggest such differences may be ascribed to changes in cortisol metabolism in obesity [9]. However, specific investigation of CRH responsiveness in patients selected for central-type obesity would be of considerable interest.

A common clinical problem is excluding Cushing's syndrome in patients with obesity. CRH has been demonstrated to stimulate ACTH secretion in normal-weight human subjects and most patients with Cushing's disease, but not generally in the ectopic ACTH syndrome. In obesity, the cortisol and ACTH release after CRH are comparable with that seen in normal-weight subjects, which contrasts with the generally excessive rise seen in pituitary-dependent Cushing's or the absence of a response found in an adrenal adenoma or ectopic ACTH. Thus, a combination of low-dose dexamethasone suppression with CRH test may provide the most sensitive and specific method for differentiating Cushing's syndrome from obesity in those patients where clinical stigmata of the former condition are equivocal [9].

Prolactin secretion

Prolactin secretion is dependent on many factors but those most studied in human subjects are the effects of the time of day, certain chemical stimuli and diet [10]. Prolactin secretion is pulsatile throughout the day and night, and the hypothalamus is probably important for the regulation of this release. A circadian rhythm for prolactin secretion has been shown to exist with an increasing number of pulses during the night. This nocturnal rise generally occurs between 0300 and 0400 hours but is delayed in obesity [11]. Evidence for an abnormality in the hypothalamo-pituitary regulation of prolactin secretion comes from the finding of impaired responses to a variety of pharmacological stimuli.

Two distinct patterns of release to insulin-induced hypoglycaemia may be seen in obesity [12]. In some obese subjects there is no prolactin response to symptomatic hypoglycaemia (prolactin 'non-responders') while in other equally obese subjects a normal response is seen (prolactin 'responders') (Fig. 68.1). It has been suggested that the impaired prolactin response results from a primary disorder of hypothalamic function because an impaired prolactin response persists in such women despite their subsequent attainment of nearly normal weight [13]. Furthermore, some obese children have been reported to show no prolactin response of hypoglycaemia [14]. Jung *et al.* [15] found no significant rise of plasma noradrenaline to hypoglycaemia in obese subjects with an impaired prolactin response, although the adrenaline response remained unimpaired. This suggests that the hypothalamic alteration, which may occur in those with a propensity for obesity, not only involves the control of the pituitary but also affects the control of the sympathetic nervous system. Additional evidence for a broader alteration in the hypothalamic regulation of prolactin is provided by the finding of a decreased prolactin response to pituitary stimulation by thyrotrophin-releasing hormone (TRH) but an increased thyroid-stimulating hormone (TSH) response

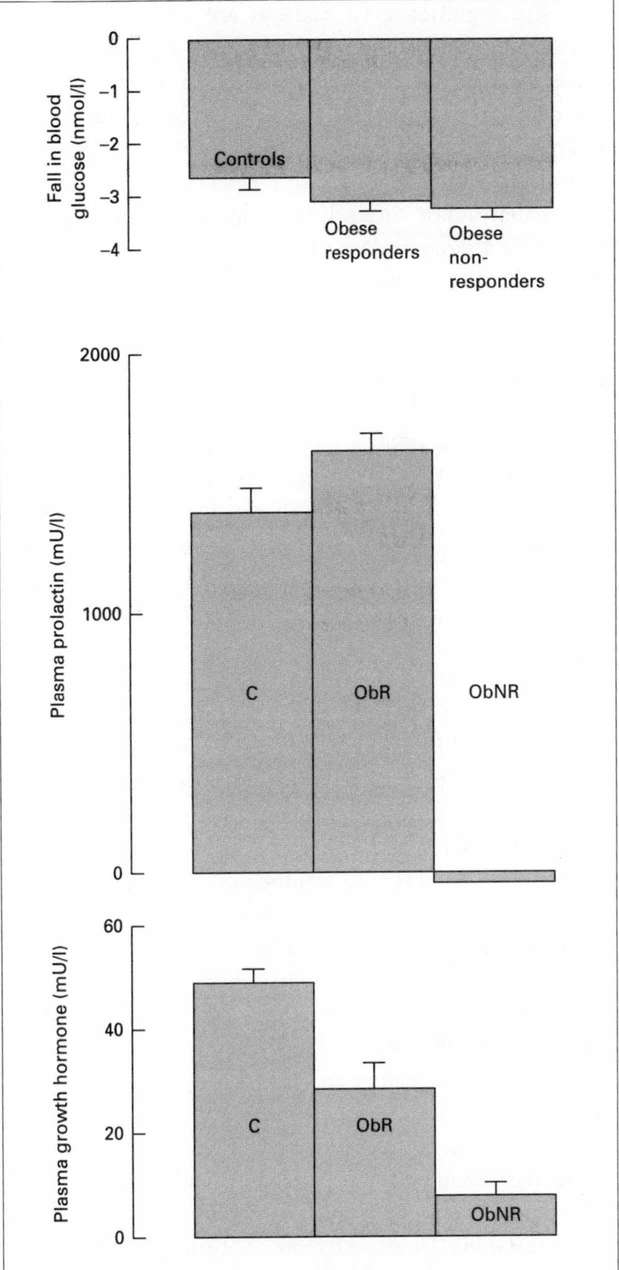

Fig. 68.1 Maximum alteration ± SEM in blood glucose, plasma prolactin and growth hormone (GH) concentrations from basal values (0) during symptomatic insulin-induced hypoglycaemia in six normal-weight controls and 14 obese women. The obese women have been divided on the basis of their prolactin response: seven obese responders (ObR) and seven obese non-responders (ObNR). There was no significant difference in basal glucose, prolactin or GH levels between the three groups.

[16]. It has been suggested that a central deficiency of serotonin may account for the disparity between the two responses.

More recent evidence suggests that hyperinsulinaemia may be the explanation for the impaired prolactin responses seen in obesity. Significant associations are observed between increased insulin secretion and resistance and the prolactin release to insulin hypoglycaemia [17]. In addition, an inverse correlation is observed between increasing upper body obesity (as measured by an increasing waist/hip ratio) and the prolactin response to hypoglycaemia [18]. These findings suggest that subtle alterations in hypothalamic function account for altered prolactin secretion found in some obese subjects but the situation is compounded by the metabolic alterations associated with regional fat distribution.

Growth hormone secretion

Growth hormone (GH) is an important regulator of body mass throughout life: subcutaneous fat is markedly increased in GH -deficient children as well as in GH-deficient adults [19]. Moreover, hypopituitary patients have abnormally high amounts of intra-abdominal fat which may be decreased by 30% after 6 months' treatment with GH [20]. Such evidence suggests that relative GH deficiency or insensitivity could play a role in the perpetuation of the obesity.

An impaired GH response to insulin-induced hypoglycaemia is found in association with obesity but this seems likely to be a consequence rather than a cause of extreme obesity. Sims *et al.* [21] have confirmed that weight gain decreases the GH response to all types of provocative stimuli whereas the GH response significantly increases in obese subjects following weight loss. An input of food in excess of energy expenditure appears to be important because impaired GH responsiveness is not a characteristic of subjects who are overweight as the result of increased musculature induced by vigorous exercise [22]. In this situation, energy expenditure is balanced by an increase in appropriate protein and energy intake whereas 10 days of overfeeding with carbohydrate can produce impaired GH responsiveness without an increase in bodyweight [23]. A significantly reduced GH response to an intravenous bolus of GH-releasing hormone (GHRH) is also a feature of obesity [24] (Fig. 68.2). This impairment is not dose dependent because doubling the dose of GHRH in obese subjects does not alter the GH release [25]. Repeated low doses of GHRH will, however, induce improved (but subnormal) GH release in some obese subjects, but do not lead to an enhanced response to further bolus doses of GHRH after 3 hours [26]. The explanation for the decreased GH output in obesity has not been fully elucidated. It is not due to an absolute deficiency because the impaired GH response to L-dopa or arginine may be augmented by propranolol or pharmacological doses of triiodothyronine [27]. Furthermore, in adult obese subjects a comparable rise of free fatty acids to that seen in lean individuals is found after the administration of GH in doses related to bodyweight; obese subjects eating a calorie-restricted diet, but treated with injections of GH, show raised oxygen consumption, increased weight loss and reduced nitrogen excretion [28]. The evidence suggests a combination of altered central cholinergic and somatostatinergic tone which influence GH release in obesity. An oral dose of pyridostigmine, an inhibitor of acetylcholinesterase , increases the GH response to GHRH in obese subjects although this still remains attenuated compared with controls [29].

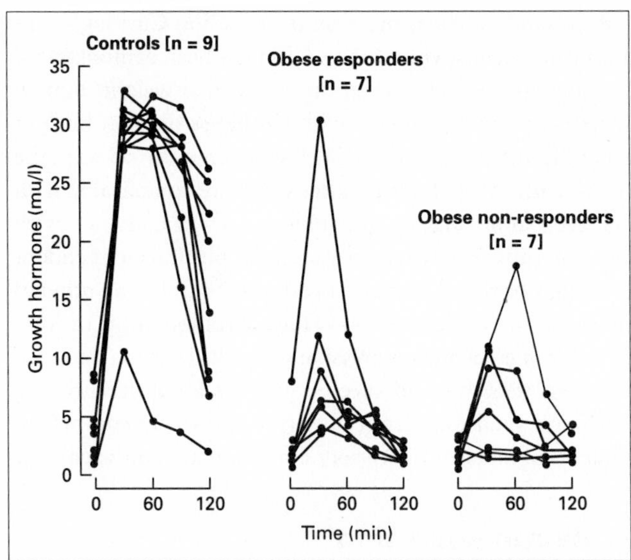

Fig. 68.2 Growth hormone response to i.v. growth hormone-releasing hormone (GHRH(1–29) NH_2) in normal-weight and obese women. The obese women are divided into responders and non-responders on the basis of their prolactin response to hypoglycaemia.

It is suggested that altered GH secretion results from alterations in insulin-like growth factor 1 (IGF-1) and its binding proteins. Synthesis of IGF-1 is stimulated by insulin and the hyperinsulinaemia of obesity could directly enhance IGF-1 production and suppress the production of GH from the pituitary by a negative-feedback mechanism. A negative-feedback effect of IGF-1 has been demonstrated in pituitary cells in culture [30]. However, several authors have reported that circulating levels of IGF-1 in obese adults are normal [31]. By contrast, IGF binding proteins 1 and 3 (IGFBP-1, IGFBP-3) are both reduced in obesity with decreased plasma concentrations of IGFBP-1 being inversely related to fasting plasma insulin and increasing upper body obesity [32,33]. A reduced level of IGFBP-1 suggests enhanced biological activity of IGF-1 which in turn may feedback via central pathways on the hypothalamo-pituitary axis to suppress GH release.

TSH and posterior pituitary function

There is no substantial evidence for any clinically significant defect in hypothalamo-pituitary–thyroid function in obesity. Plasma TSH, free thyroxine and free triiodothyronine are normal in obese subjects although a subnormal TSH response to TRH has been reported in some obese subjects [16]. Starvation or semi-starvation will decrease the TSH response to TRH; this underlines the importance of evaluating hypothalamo-pituitary function when subjects are eating adequate amounts of calories. Similarly, basal plasma arginine vasopressin (AVP) levels are normal in obesity although after water loading AVP levels do not suppress normally in obese subjects and water excretion is impaired [34]. Conversely, plasma AVP increases erratically after hypertonic saline administration. The AVP response to insulin hypoglycaemia is normal when adequate symptomatic neuroglycaemia occurs. It seems likely that any abnormalities of AVP secretion in obesity are minor and of no clinical significance [7].

Gonadotrophins

The association between obesity and abnormalities of reproductive function is well recognised, with decreased libido and impotence commonly seen in extremely overweight men, and an increased incidence of dysfunctional uterine bleeding and amenorrhoea being reported in obese women [35]. Subnormal plasma testosterone concentrations and reduced sex hormone-binding globulin (SHBG) levels occur in massively obese men, with an inverse relationship between plasma testosterone and bodyweight. In these men it has been proposed that elevated plasma oestrogens, which result from increased aromatisation of androgen precursors by adipose tissue, results in a negative feedback on the hypothalamo-pituitary axis with subnormal luteinising hormone (LH) and follicle-stimulating hormone (FSH) levels. Partial support for this hypothesis is the reversal of the reduced gonadotrophin levels following pituitary–adrenal suppressive doses of dexamethasone, but this was not accompanied by a change in testosterone [36].

In obese women, raised plasma testosterone and androstenedione concentrations are found with a reduced SHBG and increased ratio of oestrone to oestradiol; it is of interest that a similar pattern of changes of sex steroid concentration and binding are found in women with the polycystic ovary syndrome (PCOS), many of whom are obese [37]. In contrast to the women with PCOS, obese women have a normal LH and FSH response to direct stimulation by gonadotrophin-releasing hormone (GnRH) and normal gonadotrophin release following the administration of clomiphene, which acts through the hypothalamus. In obese subjects weight loss not only reverses the biochemical changes but frequently results in the reappearance of menses. The precise aetiology of these changes is unclear, but evidence points to a peripheral effect of adipose tissue on steroid secretion and binding in obesity which, in turn, influences the release of gonadotrophins from the pituitary [38].

Summary

Obesity may be characterised by changes in neuroendocrine function. The distinctive patterns of changes are related both to the degree of obesity and the distribution of fat tissue. Upper-body fat distribution may influence peripheral insulin sensitivity and insulin secretion; hyperinsulinaemia appears to alter both GH and prolactin release in obesity. Moreover, adipose tissue affects peripheral metabolism of sex steroids and their binding proteins which in turn may alter hypothalamo-pituitary function. Although the majority of these changes are reversed by substantial weight loss, it is possible that some of them, particularly abnormalities of the pituitary–adrenal axis, may play a role in the perpetuation of corpulence by influencing both appetite regulation and peripheral metabolism.

References

1 Galvo-Tales A, Graves L, Burke CW *et al.* Free cortisol in obesity: effect of fasting. *Acta Endocrinol* 1976; **81**: 321–9.

2 Migeon CJ, Green OC, Eckert JP. Study of adrenocortical function in obesity. *Metabolism* 1963; **12**: 718–30.

3 Slavnov VN, Epshtein EV. Somatotrophic, thyrotrophic and adrenotrophic functions of the anterior pituitary in obesity. *Endocrinologie* 1977; **15**: 213–18.

4 Simkin B. Urinary 17-ketogenic steroid excretion in obese patients. *N Engl J Med* 1961; **264**: 974–7.

5 Kurtz BR, Givens JR, Kominder S *et al.* Maintenance of normal circulating levels of Δ-androstenedione and dehydroepiandrosterone in simple obesity despite increased metabolic clearance rates: evidence for a servo-controlled mechanism. *J Clin Endocrinol Metab* 1987; **64**: 1261–7.

6 Brody S, Carlstrom K, Lagrelius A *et al.* Adrenal steroids in postmenopausal women: relation to obesity and bone mineral content. *Maturitas* 1987; **9**: 25–32.

7 Weaver JU, Kopelman PG, McLoughlin L *et al.* Hyperactivity of the hypothalamo-pituitary axis in obesity: a study of ACTH, AVP, β-lipoprotein and cortisol response to insulin-induced hypoglycaemia. *Clin Endocrinol* 1993; **39**: 345–50.

8 Kopelman PG, Grossman A, Lavender P *et al.* The cortisol response to corticotrophin-releasing factor is blunted in obesity. *Clin Endocrinol* 1988; **28**: 15–18.

9 Trainer PJ, Faria M, Newell-Price P *et al.* A comparison of the effects of human and ovine corticotrophin-releasing hormone on the pituitary–adrenal axis. *J Clin Endocrinol Metab* 1995; **80**: 412–17.

10 Kopelman PG. Neuroendocrine function in obesity. *Clin Endocrinol* 1988; **28**: 675–89.

11 Copinschi G, Dehaet MH, Brian JP *et al.* Simultaneous study of cortisol, growth hormone and prolactin nycthemeral variations in normal and obese subjects. Influence of prolonged fasting in obesity. *Clin Endocrinol* 1978; **9**: 15–23.

12 Kopelman PG, Pilkington TRE, White N, Jeffcoate SL. Impaired

hypothalamic control of prolactin secretion in massive obesity. *Lancet* 1979; i: 747–9.

13 Kopelman PG, Pilkington TRE, Wite N, Jeffcoate SL. Persistence of abnormal hypothalamic control of prolactin secretion in some obese women after weight reduction. *Br Med J* 1980; **281**: 358–9.

14 AvRuskin TW, Pillai S, Kasi K *et al.* Decreased prolactin secretion in childhood obesity. *J Paediatr* 1985; **106**: 373–8.

15 Jung RT, Campbell RG, James WPT, Callingham BA. Altered hypothalamic sympathetic responses to hypoglycaemia in familial obesity. *Lancet* 1982; i: 1043–6.

16 Donders SHJ, Pieters GF, Heeval JG *et al.* Disparity of thyrotrophin (TSH) and prolactin responses to TSH-releasing hormone in obesity. *J Clin Endocrinol Metab* 1985; **61**: 56–9.

17 Weaver JU, Noonan K, Kopelman PG. An association between hypothalamic-pituitary dysfunction and peripheral endocrine function in obesity. *Clin Endocrinol* 1991; **35**: 97–102.

18 Weaver JU, Noonan K, Kopelman PG, Coste M. Impaired prolactin secretion and body fat distribution in obesity. *Clin Endocrinol* 1990; **32**: 641–6.

19 Tanner JM, Whitehouse RH. The effect of human growth hormone on subcutaneous fat thickness in hyposomatotrophic and hypopituitary dwarfs. *J Endocrinol* 1967; **39**: 263–75.

20 Bengtsson BA, Eden S, Lonn L *et al.* Treatment of adults with growth hormone deficiency with recombinant GH. *J Clin Endocrinol Metab* 1994; **78**: 960–7.

21 Sims EAH, Danforth EH, Horton ES *et al.* Endocrine and metabolic effects of experimental obesity in man. *Rec Prog Horm Res* 1973; **29**: 457–87.

22 Kalkhoff R, Ferrow C. Metabolic differences between obese overweight and muscular overweight men. *N Engl J Med* 1971; **284**: 1236–9.

23 Merimee TJ, Fineberg SE. Dietary regulation of human growth hormone secretion. *Metabolism* 1973; **22**: 1491–7.

24 Williams ST, Berelowitz M, Joffe SN *et al.* Impaired growth hormone response to growth hormone releasing factor in obesity. *N Engl J Med* 1984; **311**: 1403–7.

25 Kopelman PG, Noonan K, Goulton R, Forrest AJ. Impaired growth hormone response to growth hormone releasing factor and insulin hypoglycaemia in obesity. *Clin Endocrinol* 1985; **23**: 87–94.

26 Kopelman PG, Noonan K. Growth hormone response to low dose intravenous injections of growth hormone releasing factor in obese and normal weight women. *Clin Endocrinol* 1986; **24**: 157–64.

27 Barbarino A, De Marinis L, Troncome L. Growth hormone response to propranolol and L-dopa in obese subjects. *Metabolism* 1978; **27**: 275–8.

28 Clemmons DR, Snyder DK, Williams R, Underwood LE. Growth hormone administration conserved lean body mass during dietary restriction in obese subjects. *J Endocrinol Metab* 1987; **64**: 878–83.

29 De Marinis L, Mancini A, Zuppi P *et al.* Influence of pyridostigmine on growth hormone (GH) response to GH-releasing hormone pre- and postprandially in normal and obese subjects. *J Clin Endocrinol Metab* 1992; **74**: 1253–7.

30 Glass AR. Endocrine aspects of obesity. *Med Clin North Am* 1989; **73**: 139–60.

31 Rasmussen MH, Juul A, Kjems LL *et al.* Lack of stimulation of 24 hour growth hormone release by hypocaloric diets in obesity. *J Clin Endocrinol Metab* 1995; **80**: 796–801.

32 Weaver JU, Kopelman PG, Holly JMP *et al.* Decreased sex hormone binding globulin (SHBG) and insulin-like growth factor binding protein (IGFBP-1) in extreme obesity. *Clin Endocrinol* 1990; **32**: 641–6.

33 Bang P, Brismar K, Rosenfeld RG, Hall K. Fasting affects serum insulin-like growth factor (IGFs) and IGF-binding proteins differently in patients with non-insulin-dependent diabetes versus healthy non-obese and obese subjects. *J Endocrinol Metab* 1994; **78**: 960–7.

34 Drenick EJ, Carlson HE, Robertson GL *et al.* The role of vasopressin and prolactin in abnormal salt and water metabolism of obese patients before and after fasting and during refeeding. *Metabolism* 1977; **26**: 309–17.

35 Glass AR, Burman KD, Dahms WT, Boehm TM. Endocrine function in human obesity. *Metabolism* 1981; **30**: 89–104.

36 Zumoff B, Strain GW, Miller LK *et al.* Partial reversal of the hypogonadotrophic hypogonadism of obese men by administration of corticosuppressive doses of dexamethasone. *Int J Obesity* 1988; **12**: 525–31.

37 Kopelman PG, Pilkington TRE, White N, Jeffcoate SL. Abnormal sex steroid secretion and binding in massively obese women. *Clin Endocrinol* 1980; **14**: 113–16.

38 Longcope C, Layne DS, Tait JF. Metabolic clearance rates and interconversions of oestrone and 17-β-oestradiol in normal males and females. *J Clin Invest* 1986; **47**: 93–106.

CHAPTER 69

Drugs and surgery in the treatment of obesity

R.T. Jung

Drug treatment

Drugs for the treatment of obesity can be classified into three major groups: appetite suppressants, thermogenic drugs and agents acting on the gastrointestinal tract.

Appetite suppressants (Table 69.1)

The currently available anorectic drugs belong to one of two groups, namely those that act on the catecholaminergic pathway and those that act on the serotoninergic system. In a review of about 7000 subjects who took part in 170 controlled trials, it was found that the anorectic agents resulted in a mean additional weight loss of 0.23 kg/week compared with placebo [1]. Currently, most attention is focused on the newer drugs which act on the serotoninergic system.

Dexfenfluramine

Dexflenfluramine is the active serotoninergic dextero-isomer of the racemix compound DL-fenfluramine, and has a selective action on carbohydrate consumption. In a 1-year trial of dexfenfluramine (30 mg/day), the average weight loss was 9.82 kg (in 256 subjects) compared with 7.15 kg ($n = 227$) in the placebo group, both groups being on similar weight-reducing diets [2].

Twice as many of those on dexfenfluramine (34.9%) lost more than 10% of their initial weight as compared with those on placebo (17%). Those with abdominal-type obesity appear to lose more weight on dexfenfluramine (13.7 kg) than those with gluteal–femoral obesity (8.4 kg) in a 6-month trial. Another use for dexfenfluramine has been to maintain a reduced weight once rapid weight loss has been achieved using very-low-calorie diets. Over 6 months' surveillance, those on the drug lost an average 5.9 kg, whereas those on placebo gained 3 kg [3].

Dexfenfluramine would also appear beneficial in diabetic patients, a group who find it difficult to lose weight except possibly in the immediate post-diagnostic period. In a 3-month trial of dexfenfluramine (30 mg/day) in obese long-standing diabetic patients, weight loss was 3.4 kg, compared with 1.6 kg on diet alone [4]. Smoking suppresses appetite and stimulates energy expenditure; one cigarette produces 3.7 kJ (9 kcal) of energy [5]. In a study of 768 smokers who quit for a year or more, weight gain averaged 2.8 kg in men and 3.8 kg in women, with 10% of men and 13.4% of women gaining more than 13 kg [6]. On average, cessation of smoking is associated with an increase in food intake of 1.24 MJ (300 kcal) per day [7]. Dexfenfluramine has been used to try and curtail this weight gain associated with smoking cessation. Those untreated gained 1.6 kg/week, whereas those given the drug lost 0.8 kg/week [8].

The use of anorectic agents in obesity has been subject to controversy due to worries regarding dependency, abuse and side-effects. The clinical use of centrally-acting catecholamine influencing drugs such as mazindol and diethylpropion have been curtailed in the UK by the General Medical Council due to this potential for abuse. Dexfenfluramine has been endorsed by the UN Commission on Narcotic Drugs as a drug that does not have amphetamine-like abuse potential. Many, however, would limit usage to those with a body-mass index >30 kg/m^2 where excessive appetite has seriously limited the action of a properly instructed diet and where weight loss is essential for health.

Depression may be a problem if dexfenfluramine is stopped suddenly, and rare cases of mainly reversible pulmonary hypertension have been reported with prolonged use. Dexfenfluramine is not recommended for those with depression. The treatment of the depressed obese patient

Table 69.1 Major appetite suppressants.

Affect catecholamine system
Phentermine
Mazindol
Diethylpropion
Affect serotoninergic system
DL-fenfluramine
Dexfenfluramine
Fluoxetine
Fluvoxamine
Affect both systems
Sibutramine

has been fraught with difficulties, as tricyclic antidepressants often produce weight gain which results in non-compliance. Lately, a new class of antidepressant which inhibits serotoninergic uptake has become available. Two of this family, fluoxetine and fluvoxamine, also reduce weight, possibly by suppressing appetite.

Fluoxetine

Weight loss on fluoxetine is dose dependent. In short-term trials (8 weeks) involving 754 subjects given fluoxetine, weight loss averaged 0.5 kg/week compared with 0.1 kg on placebo [9]. In another study comparing fluoxetine with benzphetamine or placebo, weight loss in 150 non-depressed subjects over an 8-week period was on average 4.8 kg on fluoxetine, 4.0 kg on benzphetamine and 1.7 kg on placebo. Subjects who reported carbohydrate craving lost more weight (5.5 kg) than those who did not (3.2 kg), suggesting that fluoxetine suppresses carbohydrate intake. Long-term trial of fluoxetine over 1 year produced a weight loss of 8.5 kg compared with 4.5 kg on placebo [10]. This drug has resulted in improvements of 8% against placebo for body-mass index and 10% for reduction in systolic blood pressure, total cholesterol and fasting blood glucose [11]. Fluoxetine may also have a role in the obese non-insulin-dependent diabetic patient by not only increasing weight loss but also modestly improving glycaemic control. Weight loss of 4.3 kg compared with 0.8 kg on placebo has been reported in diabetic patients [12].

Sibutramine

Sibutramine is both a serotonin- and noradrenaline-uptake inhibitor found to have weight-reduction potential. In a recent 12-week trial, sibutramine (30 mg/day) achieved a weight loss of 6.1 kg whereas on placebo subjects lost only 0.9 kg [13]. The side-effects of a dry mouth, headaches and dizziness were not a limitation.

New developments of peptide analogues of cholecystokinin, a potential inhibitor of appetite in animals and possibly humans, hold promise as potential anorectic agents, whereas the discovery that neuropeptide Y markedly increased appetite suggests that an inhibitor of this peptide might be a most effective method of appetite supression. The discovery of leptin, a 167 amino acid produced in mammalian white adipose tissue by the *ob* gene, and which alters appetite and thermogenesis in rodents, may result in a radical new approach to appetite control in humans [14].

Thermogenic drugs (Table 69.2)

Thyroid hormones

In pharmaceutical dosages thyroid hormones have the disadvantage of rapidly reducing lean body mass and hence their use is not recommended. Many obese patients are under the misapprehension that thyroxine-replacement therapy for hypothyroidism will result in significant weight loss. A recent study of 28 treated hypothyroid patients showed an average weight loss of only 0.6 kg after 1 year of treatment [15]. The other thermogenic drugs about to be discussed are still experimental and should be viewed as such.

Ephedrine

Chronic administration of ephedrine (60 mg/day) over 3 months has been reported to produce weight loss (5.5 kg) and a sustained 10% elevation of metabolic rate [16]. Acute ephedrine administration has the disadvantage of raising mean arterial blood pressure, on average 23 mmHg after the ingestion of 20 mg. However, with chronic therapy this rise in mean arterial pressure is reduced to 5 mmHg. Transient tremor and glucose intolerance are minor disadvantages, whereas its protein-sparing action is an important advantage compared with thyroid hormone. In rodents, aspirin, caffeine or theophylline administered with ephedrine increased its thermogenic and weight-reducing potency. In humans, those few trials done using such combinations have been

Table 69.2 Possible thermogenic agents

Thyroxine, triidothyronine
Ephedrine
Methylxanthines
Atypical β-adrenergic agonists
α_2-Adrenergic antagonists
Growth hormone

disappointing, though one such trial reported a weight loss over 24 weeks of 16.6 kg on a combination of ephedrine and caffeine, compared with 13.2 kg with placebo [16].

Atypical β-adrenergic agonists

In 1984 a new family of thermogenic atypical β-adrenergic agonists was reported [17]. In genetic obese rodents, this type of drug produced marked weight loss, without compromising muscle mass, by stimulating preferentially brown fat thermogenesis. Trials in humans have involved one of the less potent members, namely BRL 26830A [18]. Acute ingestion of 100 mg raised metabolic rate by an average 11.5% in obese women. Weight loss over 18 weeks averaged 15.4 kg on BRL 26830A compared with 10 kg on placebo, both groups taking a 3.3 MJ (800 kcal) diet. Nitrogen balance studies confirmed that, like ephedrine, BRL 26830A also had a protein-sparing action. However, an advantage over ephedrine was the finding that BRL 26830A did not alter the expected reduction in pulse rate and blood pressure that one observes upon dieting. Also, BRL 26830A enhanced insulin sensitivity and high-density lipoprotein (HDL) cholesterol to a slight degree. Tremor has been observed with BRL 26830A, but this can be obviated by altering the chemical structure. As this unique family of drugs also improves insulin sensitivity it has been tested in non-insulin-dependent diabetic patients but with only modest improvements in glycaemic control.

α_2-Adrenoceptor antagonists

Another experimental approach is the use of α_2-adrenoceptor antagonists. Cyclic adenosine monophosphate (cAMP) mediated lipolysis in adipose tissue of humans is regulated by the interplay of α- and β-adrenoceptors modulating adenyl cyclase activity; whereas β-adrenoceptors activate lipolysis, α_2-antagonists inhibit. Hence the possibility of blocking α_2-adrenoceptors, thus potentiating lipolysis and hopefully weight loss [19]. The difficulty with this approach is that this would also induce insulin release at the pancreatic islet which, of course, would then inhibit lipolysis. Research is therefore in progress to discover α_2-antagonists with differing potency for adipose tissue and pancreatic β-cells. Existing α_2-antagonists include yohimbine and idazoxan and new agents include a primidyl-piperazine agent, RP 55462. Yohimbine does increase lipolysis in humans and in conjunction with diet has been reported to have a 1 kg weight loss advantage compared with placebo over a 3-week trial [20].

Growth hormone

The recent advent of genetically engineered supplies of growth hormone has stimulated interest in its possible use for obesity [21]. Growth hormone accelerates lipolysis in lean and obese humans, enhances fat oxidation during caloric restriction and also promotes nitrogen conservation. However, an 11-week study in dieting obese subjects did not show any increased weight loss compared with placebo injections. As has been reported with its use in children, nitrogen conservation in the obese was markedly improved by growth hormone only for the initial 33 days of the trial. Serum triiodothyronine also increased during the first 45 days despite energy restriction, but thereafter declined to levels below that observed at the outset. Increases in energy expenditure of as much as 25% have been reported during the first month of therapy in growth hormone-treated hypopituitary adult patients [22]. This work has also indicated that after 6 months' treatment weight remained unchanged although fat mass decreased by, on average, 5.8 kg, whereas lean mass increased by 6.2 kg [23]. Such an increase in lean body mass should have increased energy expenditure in the long term and it is, therefore, surprising that growth hormone is not beneficial in obesity. At present the cost of growth hormone and the dangers involved of inducing acromegaly make this therapy unfeasible.

Gastrointestinal acting agents

Attempts have been made to reduce caloric intake by producing feelings of satiety with the use of bulk-forming agents such as bran or methylcellulose. There is little evidence to support this claim.

Cimetidine has been reported to promote weight loss. In one trial of cimetidine 200 mg or placebo with a 5 MJ (1200 kcal/day) diet, weight loss was reported 7.3 kg greater on the drug than on placebo [24]. Waist/hip ratio and perceived hunger were reduced on cimetidine. The mechanism of action is speculative but suggested as a reduction in hunger brought about by a decrease in gastric acid output. Nevertheless, another trial similarly conducted failed to confirm these findings, with no significant difference in weight loss on cimetidine versus placebo [25]. The use of this drug for weight loss remains speculative.

Another strategy is to restrict the bioavailability of dietary energy intake. Cholestyramine has been used but gastrointestinal side-effects made it unpopular. Diethyl aminoethyl dextran (DEAED), which acts in a similar fashion to cholestyramine by binding bile acids, has been tried in obese humans. Weight loss over 6 weeks averaged 0.83 kg/week compared with 0.41 kg/week on placebo [26]. Side effects of flatulence, loose stools and abdominal borborygmus and fullness are disadvantages.

Tetrahydrolipistatin is a chemically synthesised hydrogenated derivative of lipistatin, itself produced by *Streptomyces toxytricini*. This substance is a potent inhibitor of gastric, pancreatic and carboxylester lipase [27]. Given orally it operates within the lumen of the gut and is minimally absorbed. In short-term trials in humans the aim has been to increase faecal fat excretion by up to 50 g/day, which in theory should produce an energy loss of about 1.65 MJ (400 kcal) per 24 hours. In a 12-week double-blind, placebo-controlled trial using 150 mg/day of tetrahydrolipistatin, weight loss was moderate (4.3 kg) but more than placebo (2.1 kg). In another five-centre trial weight loss was dose dependent [28]. After 12 weeks, additional weight loss compared with placebo was 0.63 kg with 30 mg, 0.71 kg with 180 mg and 1.75 kg on 360 mg, per day [29]. Total and low-density-lipoprotein (LDL) cholesterol decreased slightly but significantly on the 180 and 360 mg dosages, whereas the LDL to HDL cholesterol only fell on the highest dosage. Mild, mostly gastrointestinal side-effects (loose stools, steatorrhoea, oily spotting, abdominal pains) were observed on tetrahydrolipistatin but caused premature withdrawal from the trial in only four out of the 188 subjects tested. Also, no laboratory abnormalities or significant reductions in the lipid-soluble vitamins A, D and E were reported after 12 weeks' usage. This latter observation is important as a potential problem of long-term usage might be eventual reduction in absorption of fat-soluble vitamins (which could be supplemented) and the possibility of colonic bacterial overgrowth limiting its use. It may also have a use in the maintenance of reduced weight in the hyperlipidaemic patient.

Acarbose is an α-glucosidase inhibitor used in diabetes mellitus to reduce carbohydrate absorption. Chronic usage indicates that it does not have any significant weight-reducing potential, although it may have a role in maintaining a reduced weight, especially in diabetic patients. Side-effects may limit its acceptibility for some.

Surgical treatments

Jaw wiring

Jaw wiring is certainly efficacious. In one trial of 101 patients, the average weight lost over 1 year averaged 52.6 kg. However, once the wires were removed, weight was rapidly regained. One method of limiting weight regain is by use of a nylon cord applied around the waist. As weight is regained, the cord tightens, reminding the patient to eat less. In one trial of this waist cord following weight loss with jaw wiring, the weight regained was on average 5.6 kg compared with 17.8 kg with no cord applied [30]. A 'waist line' is required for cord usage, and this is not always achieved. Teeth are required for wiring and the patient is usually given a liquid diet. A patient with an alcoholic tendency can, of course, overcome this therapy, and it is not to be recommended for such patients unless they can abstain from alcohol for at least 4 weeks before wiring. Some advocate that all patients considered for jaw wiring should be tried on a milk diet for some weeks or even months beforehand to assess dietary acceptability. Regular follow-up is mandatory and must be adhered to and agreed beforehand by the patient.

Jejuno-ileal bypass

This procedure has unacceptable mortality (5%) and morbidity (60%) and its use for the treatment of obesity has all but disappeared [31].

Vertical banded gastroplasty and gastric bypass

These two procedures now dominate surgical practice.

Vertical banded gastroplasty

This procedure involves the construction of a small stomach pouch fashioned by vertical stapling to restrict the volume to as low as 10–15 ml. The outlet is restricted to just 9–12 mm diameter, reinforced with non-absorbable mesh (Fig. 69.1). Another modification is gastric banding which involves pinching off a small part of the upper stomach with a Dacron type band, but is less popular than stapling. Weight loss over 1 year after vertical banded gastroscopy can average 36 kg with only 5 kg regained by 3 years.

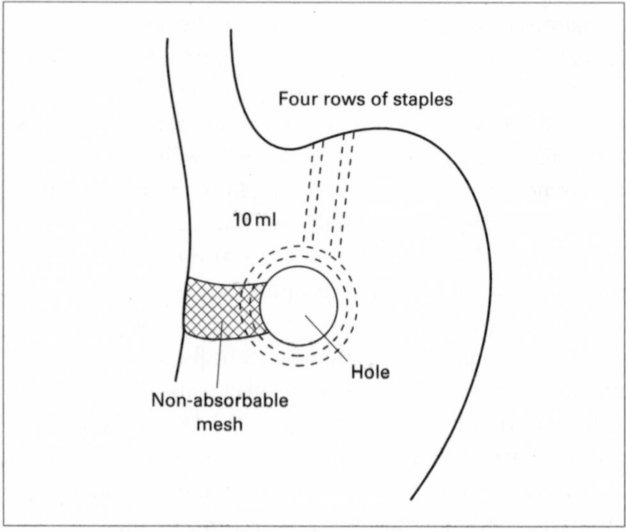

Fig. 69.1 Vertical banded gastroplasty. One method is to make a proximal pouch as small as 10 ml volume by the use of rows of staples applied as shown. Stoma is 9–12 mm diameter reinforced with non-absorbable mesh.

Gastric bypass (Roux-en-Y)

Gastric bypass involves fashioning a pouch of low volume (< 30 ml) by stapling across the stomach and then connecting a limb of small intestine as a conduit for food, hence bypassing the distal stomach, duodenum and upper jejunum (Fig. 69.2). Trials suggest that gastric bypass in experienced hands is more successful than gastroplasty with up to 92% of excess weight lost at 18 months after operation and 63% at 72 months [32]. Irrespective of the type of surgery, often 60% of excess weight may be lost, the weight loss nadir occuring in 18–24 months with some regain by 2–5 years after operation [33]. Often the choice of operation involves both the surgeon's preference and consideration of the patient's eating habits. The greater weight loss after gastric bypass has to be balanced against this operation's higher risk of nutritional deficiencies.

Surgical outcome

Surgery requires a multidisciplinary team including surgeon, physician, nutritionist and clinical psychologist. Preoperative psychological assessment is essential and the patient and family must be aware of the postoperative limitations, possible complications, the need for strict adherence to a gastroplasty diet and life-long follow-up. Postoperative respiratory problems usually make 24 hours in high-dependency care desirable, and should be available in those centres providing barometric surgery. A new laparoscopic approach may reduce this need, but its use is still experimental. Available publications suggest that the immediate operative mortality rate for the above two types of operation in experienced operators is relatively low.

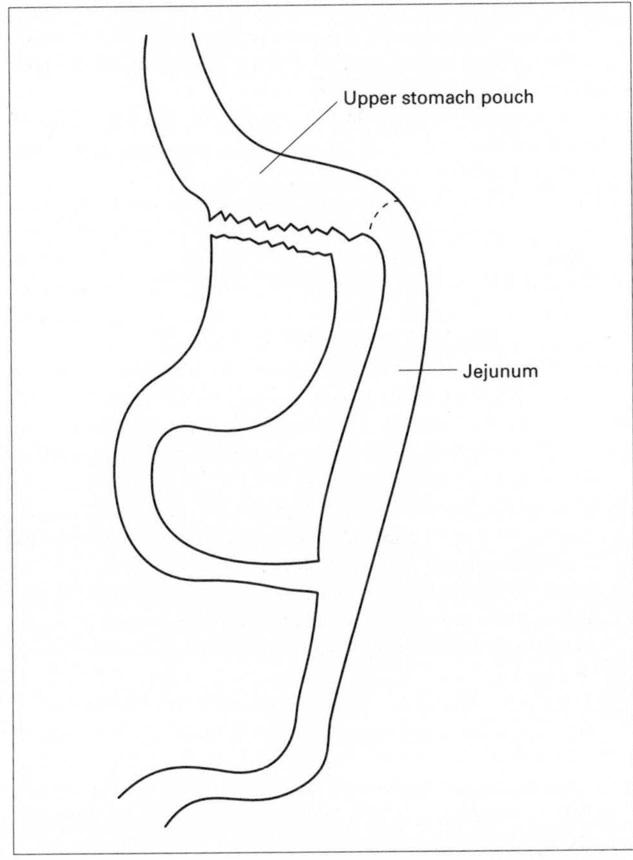

Fig. 69.2 Gastric bypass (Roux-en-Y gastrojejunostomy). A pouch of upper stomach, of volume usually <30 ml is constructed and then connected to a limb of jejunum, with a 'Y' loop connection draining the remaining gastric remnant.

Morbidity, however, in the early postoperative period from wound infection, dehiscence, staple leaks, stomal stenosis, marginal ulcers, pulmonary problems and venous thrombosis may be as high as 10% or more [33]. In the later postoperative period, other problems may arise such as pouch and distal oesophageal dilatation, persistent vomiting and cholecystitis, some requiring reoperation. The latter is associated with a higher morbidity and mortality than the primary operation. Later, micronutrient deficiencies, particularly of folate, B_{12} and iron are common, especially after gastric bypass, as is dumping syndrome. The major worry concerning the micronutrient deficiencies arises in those patients who subsequently become pregnant, for this can result in fetal damage. In North America some 80% of patients having barometric surgery are women of childbearing age [33]. Contraceptive advice is necessary during the phase of weight loss and the patient and health-care teams should be aware that maternal malnutrition may impair fetal development in any future pregnancy. Finally, the euphoria of weight loss can be followed by marked depression, and not all depression is relieved by surgery.

Overall, such surgery is widely used, and is *the* most effective method of weight reduction with the greatest benefits for patients with the greatest health risks. In some cases surgery may be life-saving, particularly in hypoventilation disorders and obstructive sleep apnoea syndrome. Hypertension, hyperlipidaemia and diabetic glycaemic control are markedly improved, with one report indicating that 80% of 163 subjects with impaired glucose tolerance achieved normoglycaemia [34]. Whether beneficial effects in the various metabolic disorders are maintained long enough to prevent end-organ damage is not known. Also, it is not clear whether the reported improvements in mood and psychosocial function are sustained.

The Swedish Obesity Study is now analysing the impact on health and quality of life of gastroplication with early results confirming improved outcomes compared with conventional dietary approaches [35]. Interestingly, obese subjects who were incapable of adherence to dietary restrictions prior to surgery seem to adapt rapidly to the enforced dietary restrictions after surgery. Also, one must consider the cost of surgery with immediate and long-term aftercare estimated at £5000 in UK or $10 000 in North America [32]. Some consider surgery worth the cost if it transforms an otherwise doomed life into an active person able to seek employment and benefit from social rehabilitation and reduced comorbidity.

The National Institute of Health has published a consensus statement after a thorough review of surgery for obesity and made five recommendations [33]. The *first* is that patients seeking therapy for severe obesity should be considered for non-surgical treatment in a programme with integrated components of a dietary regimen, appropriate exercise, behavioural modification and support. *Secondly*, the consensus agreed that gastric restriction and bypass procedures could be considered for well-informed and motivated patients with acceptable operative risks. Most would be patients with a body-mass index (BMI) exceeding 40, but in some cases those with less severe obesity (BMI 35–40) may also be considered for surgery if there is a high risk, comorbid life-threatening condition or severe physical problems considerably interfering with lifestyle. A *third* recommendation is that all patients are selected carefully after evaluation by a multidisciplinary team with medical, surgical, psychiatric and nutritional expertise. *Fourthly*, the operation must be performed by an experienced surgeon in the chosen technique with the appropriate procedures and working in a clinical setting with adequate support for all aspects of management and assessment. *Finally*, medical surveillance after surgical therapy is a necessity.

Intragastric balloon

The use of an intragastric balloon appears to be of little value in obesity treatment. The balloon in a collapsed state is inserted into the stomach using an endoscope and then inflated. Short-term trial over 3 months showed weight loss averaging 7 kg with the balloon compared with 3.3 kg with sham therapy [36]. After insertion side-effects include inability to sleep on the left side, abdominal cramps, fullness and vomiting. In those where perception of the balloon continues, weight loss is greater, but long-term results are disappointing as the balloon often deflates with only 20% maintaining their initial weight loss long term. Peptic ulcers, haemorrhage and intestinal obstruction are more serious disadvantages [37].

Apronectomy

Apronectomy is used to remove a large overhang of subcutaneous abdominal fat. This technique reduces weight only by the weight of the mass removed and is of no use as regards long-term weight control, for the fat mass redevelops if appetite is unrestricted. Its use should be confined to where the apron is infected, ulcerated or is a distinct nuisance.

Fat liposuction

Liposuction is a cosmetic operation which is not without risk, for fat emboli have been reported.

Acupuncture

Acupuncture as a technique to promote weight loss has been used for centuries by the Chinese. If used by the so-called 'auricular retention method' it may work by stimulation of the vagus nerve (via its auricular branch). Evidence of efficacy is subject to criticism. In one trial of 38 subjects, treatment for 1–6 months combined with diet resulted in an average weight loss of 5.5 kg [38].

References

1 Scoville BA. Review of amphetamine-like drugs by the Food and Drug Administration; clinical data and value judgements. In *Obesity in Perspective*. Proceedings of the Fogarty Conference. Washington DC: US Government, 1973: 441–3.

2 Guy-Grand B, Apfelbraum M, Crepaldi G, Cries A, Levebre P, Turner P. International trial of long-term dexfenfluramine in obesity. *Lancet* 1989; **2**: 1142–5.

3 Finer N, Finer S. Dexfenfluramine after successful weight reduction in a very low calorie diet. *Int J Obes* 1989; **13** (Suppl. 1, abstract 130).

4 Manning RM, Jung RT, Leese GP, Newton RW. The comparison of four weight-reducing strategies aimed at overweight diabetic patients. *Diabet Med* 1995;12: 409–15.

5 Hoffstetter A, Shutz Y, Jequier E, Wahren J. Increased 24 hour energy expenditure in cigarette smokers. *N Engl J Med* 1986; **413**: 79–82.

6 Williamson DF, Madans J, Anda RF, Kleinman JC, Giovino JC, Byers T. Smoking cessation and severity of weight gain in a national cohort. *N Engl J Med* 1991; **324**: 739–45.

7 Stamford BA, Matter S, Fell RD, Papanek P. Effects of smoking cessation on weight gain, metabolic rate, calorie consumption and blood lipids. *Am J Clin Nutr* 1986; **43**: 486–94.

8 Spring B, Wurtman J, Gleason R, Wurtman R, Kessler K. Weight gain and withdrawal symptoms after smoking cessation; a preventative intervention using D-fenfluramine. *Health Psychiatr* 1991; **10**: 216–23.

9 Levine LR, Thompson RG, Bosomworth JC. Fluoxetine, a serotonergic for drug obesity control. In Bjorntorp P, Rossner S eds. *Obesity in Europe 88*. London: John Libbey, 1989: 319–22.

10 Darga LL, Carroll-Micheals L, Borsford SJ, Lucas CP. Fluoxetine's effect on weight loss in obese subjects. *Am J Clin Nutr* 1991; **54**: 321–5.

11 Sayler ME, Goldstein DJ, Roback PJ, Atkinson RL. Evaluating success of weight loss programs worth, on application to fluoxetine weight reduction clinical trial data. *Int J Obes* 1994; **18**: 742–51.

12 O'Kane M, Wiles PG, Wiles JK. Fluoxetine in the treatment of obese

type 2 diabetic patients. *Diabet Med* 1993; **11**: 105–10.

13 Bray GA, Ryan DH, Gordon D, Heidingsfelder S, Macchiavelli R, Wilson K. Double blind randomised trial of sibutramine in overweight subjects. *Int J Obes* 1995; **19**(Suppl. 2): 393.

14 Zhang T, Proenca R, Maffei M, Barone M, Leopold L, Friedman JM. Positional cloning of the mouse obese gene and its human homologue. *Nature* 1994; **372**: 425–31.

15 Jung RT. *Colour Atlas of Obesity.* London: Wolfe Medical Publications, 1990.

16 Astrup A, Lunsgaard C, Madsen J, Christensen NJ. Enhanced thermogenic responsiveness during chronic ephedrine treatment in man. *Am J Clin Nutr* 1985; **42**: 83–94.

17 Arch JRS, Ainsworth AT, Cawthorne MA *et al.* Atypical beta adrenoceptor on brown adipocytes as target for anti-obesity drugs. *Nature* 1984; **309**: 163–5.

18 Connacher AA, Jung RT, Mitchell PEG. Weight loss in obese subjects in a restricted diet given BRL 26830A, a new atypical beta adrenoceptor agonist. *Br Med J* 1988; **296**: 1217–20.

19 Curtis-Prior PB, Tan S. Application of agents active at the alpha 2 adrenoceptor of fat cells to the treatment of obesity—a critical appraisal. *Int J Obes* 1984; **8**(Suppl. 1): 201–13.

20 Kocio C, Joanderko K, Piskorska D. Does yohimbine act as a slimming drug? *Isr J Med Sci* 1991; **27**: 550–6.

21 Synder DK, Clemmons DR, Underwood LE. Treatment of obese, diet restricted subjects with growth hormone for 11 weeks. Effects on anabolism lipolysis and body composition. *J Clin Endocrinol Metab* 1988; **67**: 54–61.

22 Chong PKK, Jung RT, Scrimgeour CM, Rennie MJ, Paterson CR. Energy expenditure and body composition in growth hormone deficient adults on exogenous growth hormone. *Clin Endocrinol* 1994; **40**: 103–10.

23 Salomon F, Cuneo RC, Hesp R, Sonksen PH. Effect on body composition of six months replacement treatment with recombinant human growth hormone in adults with growth hormone deficiency. *J Endocrinol* 1989; **321**: 1797–1803.

24 Stoa-Birketvedt G. Effect of cimetidine suspension on appetite and weight in overweight subjects. *Br Med J* 1993; **306**: 1091–3.

25 Rasmussen MH, Anderson T, Breum L, Gotzche PC, Hilsted J. Cimetidine suspension as adjuvant to energy restricted diet in treating obesity. *Br Med J* 1993; **306**: 1093–6.

26 Hogan S, Fileury A, Hadvary P, Lengsfeld M, Meier MK, Triscari J, Sullivan AC. Studies on the anti-obesity activity of tetrahydrolipstatin, a potent and delective inhibitor of pancreatic lipase. *Int J Obes* 1987; **11**(Suppl. 3): 35–42.

27 Hadvary P, Lengsfield H, Wolfer H. Inhibition of pancreatic lipase in-vitro by the covalent inhibitor tetrahydrolipstatin. *Biochem J* 1988; **256**: 357–61.

28 Drent M, Van der Veen E. Lipase inhibition: a novel concept in the treatment of obesity. *Int J Obes* 1993; **17**: 241–4.

29 Drent ML, Larsson I, William-Olsson T *et al.* Orlistat (RO-18-0647), a lipase inhibitor in the treatment of human obesity; a multiple dose study. *Int J Obes Relat Metab Disord* 1995; **19**: 221–6.

30 Garrow JJ, Gardiner GT. Maintenance of weight loss in obese patients after jaw wiring. *Br Med J* 1981; **282**: 858–60.

31 McFarland RJ, Gazet JC, Pilkington TRE. A 13 year review of jejunoilial bypass. *Br J Surg* 1985; **72**: 81–7.

32 Beales PL, Kopelman PG. Options for the management of obesity. In: Bjornthorp P, Vantallie TB, eds. *The Cost of Obesity*, Vol. 5 (Suppl. 1). Pharmacoeconomics, 1994: 18–32.

33 National Institute of Health. Gastro-intestinal surgery for severe obesity. National Institute of Health Consensus Development Conference Statement. *Am J Clin Nutr* 1992; **55**: 615S–19.

34 Pories WJ, MacDonald KG, Morgan E, *et al.* Surgical treatment of obesity and its effect on diabetes; 10 year follow-up. *Am J Clin Nutr* 1992; **55**: 582S–5.

35 Sjostrom L, Lissner L, Backman L, *et al.* SOS—Swedish Obesity Subjects. An intervention study of obesity. *Int J Obes* 1994: **18** (Suppl. 2): 14.

36 Ramhamadary EM, Baird IM. Effect of the gastric balloon versus sham procedure on weight loss in obese subjects. *First European Congress on Obesity*, 1988: Abstract 247.

37 Durrans D, Taylor TV, Pullan BR, Rose P. Intra-gastric balloons. *J Roy Coll Surg Edin* 1985; **30**: 369–71.

38 Alkaysi G, Leindler L, Bajusz H, Szervas F, Koracsonyi S. The treatment of pathological obesity by a new auricular acupuncture method; a five year clinical experience. *Am J Acupuncture* 1991; **19**: 323–8.

CHAPTER 70

Anorexia nervosa and bulimia nervosa

N. Joughin

Classification

The most widely used system of classifying these so-called 'eating disorders' is the fourth edition of *Diagnostic and Statistical Manual of Mental Disorders* (DSM-IV) of the American Psychiatric Association [1]. This manual offers diagnostic criteria for the disorders (see Table 70.1) but a significant proportion of patients who clearly need treatment do not meet the main criteria. Many therefore fall into a category of 'eating disorder not otherwise specified' which is unhelpful in guiding treatment. A high proportion of such patients have binge-eating behaviour, but without compensatory behaviours such as vomiting. A new diagnostic categorisation of 'binge-eating disorder' is being considered for this group. The principles of treating this disorder are largely similar to those for treating bulimia nervosa.

Anorexia nervosa

Theories of aetiology and psychopathology

Whilst some confusion continues, research into the aetiology of anorexia nervosa has matured in distinguishing the causes and consequences of the condition. Its nature as a unitary disorder must be open to question, but in any one patient it seems certain that a variety of factors will be relevant in explaining such extreme behaviour.

The most accepted diagnostic criteria for the disorder are given in Table 70.1, although recently there has been some question regarding the appropriateness of including amenorrhea among the criteria [2]. The criteria indicate some of the key elements of psychopathology in anorexia nervosa. The clinical picture is of a conflict imposed by the starving, foraging impulse on the one hand and the need to resist eating because of the terror of weight gain on the other. To avoid weight gain patients use restriction of diet, vomiting, laxatives, diuretics, fluid restriction and exercise. However, despite the name of the disorder, patients are usually hungry (although this is often denied) and to avoid hunger patients may use appetite-suppressant drugs, low-calorie drinks and diversionary activity. Not all patients are able to successfully deny their hunger, and fasting may break down into 'dietary chaos' with alternating periods of abstinence and bingeing. Behavioural consequences of the battle between foraging and restraint include a preoccupation with food and weight, ritualistic behaviour, cooking, work connected with food, shoplifting, hoarding of food, social isolation and arguments within the family.

The reported incidence of anorexia nervosa varies, perhaps because patients do not always present to doctors or are misdiagnosed. Case-register studies of the general population have suggested a prevalence as low as one in 100 000 in the general population. Studies of ballet students have suggested prevalence figures as high as 8%. The disorder is more common in higher social classes, virtually only occurs in developed countries and, at most, 5% of patients are male. The peak incidence occurs in late teens [3], but earlier [4] and later onset cases with a fairly classic syndrome have been reported. It remains unclear as to whether the general disorder is becoming more common, although the incidence of the earlier onset cases is almost certainly rising. For the endocrinologist, early-onset anorexia nervosa is an important differential diagnosis in patients with short stature or primary amenorrhea.

Genetics

Mounting evidence of a genetic component suggests the need for a diathesis/stress paradigm [5] for understanding the aetiology of anorexia nervosa. The most significant genetic studies use twin data, and the best study so far reported [6] showed a concordance rate for anorexia nervosa of 55%

Table 70.1 Diagnostic criteria from the fourth edition of *Diagnostic and Statistical Manual of Mental Disorders* (DSM-IV) [1].

Anorexia nervosa

A Refusal to maintain bodyweight at or above a minimally normal weight for age and height (e.g., weight loss leading to maintenance of bodyweight <85% of that expected; or failure to make expected weight gain during period of growth, leading to bodyweight <85% of that expected)

B Intense fear of gaining weight or becoming fat, even though underweight

C Disturbance in the way in which one's bodyweight or shape is experienced, undue influence of bodyweight or shape on self-evaluation, or denial of the seriousness of the current low bodyweight

D In post-menarcheal females, amenorrhea, i.e. the absence of at least three consecutive menstrual cycles. (A woman is considered to have amenorrhea if her periods occur only following hormone, e.g. estrogen administration)

The disorder can be sub-classified into restricting type or binge-eating/purging type.

Bulimia nervosa

A Recurrent episodes of binge eating. An episode of binge eating is characterised by both of the following:
(1) eating, in a discrete period of time (e.g. within any 2-hour period), an amount of food that is definitely larger than most people would eat during a similar period of time and under similar circumstances)
(2) a sense of lack of control over eating during the episode (e.g. a feeling that one cannot stop eating or control what or how much one is eating)

B Recurrent inappropriate compensatory behaviour in order to prevent weight gain, such as self-induced vomiting; misuse of laxatives, diuretics, enemas, or other medications; fasting; or excessive exercise

C The binge eating and inappropriate compensatory behaviour both occur, on average, at least twice a week for 3 months.

D Self-evaluation is unduly influenced by body shape and weight

E The disturbance does not occur exclusively during episodes of anorexia nervosa.

The disorder can be subclassified into purging type and non-purging type.

among 16 female monozygotic twin pairs and 7% amongst 14 dizygotic twin pairs. This finding must be interpreted with care. The patient series is highly selected, and the history of twin studies in other psychiatric disorders has suggested low reliability of the findings. Other putative evidence comes from other consanguinity studies, the finding of an unexpectedly high incidence of anorexia nervosa in patients with gonadal dysgenesis, and a possible human leucocyte antigen (HLA) association. If the genetic findings are substantiated, we still do not know how the genetic contribution is mediated or what environmental factors might explain the variable concordance in monozygotic twins.

Hunger/satiety

The perceived intensity of hunger in the human has been reported to reach a plateau after 2 days of total fasting and then to decrease. However, other reports indicate that severe restriction, contrary to the total fasting situation, maintains a continuous highly painful sensation of hunger. In anorexic subjects, the reporting of hunger and satiety is unreliable. In general, anorexics are hungry, although there may be stages in the disorder when hunger perception is distorted. Anorexics probably have normal gastric contractions, but have delayed gastric emptying (even after weight gain) and are less accurate in perceiving the amount of food introduced into their stomachs. Garfinkel [7] found normal hunger in anorexics, but they expressed their reasons for stopping eating as related to 'diet-limit set for figure or health', rather than 'feeling satisfied'. This effect survived weight gain, and those patients who did well learned to rely on external validators of meal size. Anorexics do not respond normally to glucose preloads in producing 'sucrose satiety', and this abnormality does not respond to weight restoration. Similarly, 'restrained eaters' (not anorexic subjects) seem to respond to glucose preloads by eating more subsequently. It has been suggested that in anorexics this unreliable satiety leads them to under-eat for fear of over-eating. This is in keeping with their expressed fear of weight gain if they start to eat.

Body-image abnormalities

Body-image disturbances in anorexia nervosa have been much publicised, but for a variety of reasons the findings of earlier studies need to be interpreted with care. First, it is clear that normal women misjudge their size. Secondly, the tendency of anorexic females to overestimate their body widths has not been found to extend to their perceptions of blocks of wood or to their own height. However, they do overestimate the size of other females, but to a lesser extent than their own body widths. Thirdly, reviews of the literature [8] and newer research [9] indicate that in anorexic subjects size-estimation and image-distortion techniques yield different results. Image-distortion techniques seem to reflect a relatively fixed, cognitive attitude to body size. By contrast, size-estimation error seems to reflect a fluid state of body-size sensitivity, which is strongly influenced by affective/emotional factors responsive to changes in both the external and the internal environment. The problem in patients with eating disorders seems centrally to be one of attitude to body image rather than a genuine perceptual disturbance.

Auto-opioid hypothesis

It is hard not to notice a similarity between anorexia nervosa and addictions to alcohol or opiates, and the possibility of an 'auto-addiction' has been considered [10]. Opiates and opiate antagonists are known to modify eating behaviour, and it is thought that opioids are mobilised in states of prolonged food deprivation. One study has shown increased endogenous opioid activity in the cerebrospinal fluid (CSF) of anorexics, and auto-opiates have been implicated in exercise addiction, which has parallels and a cross-over with anorexia nervosa. The effect of opiate antagonists in anorexia nervosa is as yet unclear.

Social factors

The epidemiology of anorexia nervosa strongly suggests the relevance of social factors in the origin of the condition. Social pressures emphasising the desirability of thinness have led to anorexia nervosa being labelled the 'golden girl illness'. Changes in perceived desirable female form have been used to explain possible changes in the incidence of anorexia nervosa over the last century. Similar factors have suggested the importance of changes in social mores ('sexual liberation'), changes in dietary habits and earlier physical maturity. There is no doubt that at least mild anorexic thinking about weight and shape is now common or normal in teenage girls in westernised societies. The reason for this being a predominantly female problem cannot be said to have been adequately explained.

Psychological mechanisms

Despite the above factors and a lack of substantiating scientific evidence, anorexia nervosa is seen by the majority of commentators as a disorder of predominantly psychological origin. The behaviour of anorexia nervosa is seen as either an expression of emotion, or a way of dealing with emotions.

The families of patients with anorexia nervosa have been said to demonstrate enmeshment, conflict avoidance, over-protectiveness and rigidity. Patients emerging from these families are seen as having 'ego deficits in autonomy' or 'ineffectiveness' [11]. They can be seen as ill-prepared for tackling the turmoil of adolescence concerning sexuality, examinations, leaving home, developing an identity and (possibly) offending their parents. It is suggested that patients are left with conflicting emotions without the skills to deal with them. Such theories of family functioning have led to the blaming of parents. There is little research evidence to substantiate this, although families are often disrupted (perhaps by the disorder) at the time of presentation, and involvement of the family can be vital in treatment.

Anorexia nervosa has been explained as a maladaptive expression of anger or a display of control in an individual otherwise rendered powerless by their background. However, perhaps more important is the use of anorexic behaviour to control emotions. Thus, significant weight loss seems to have a modifying effect on a variety of emotions patients find intolerable in themselves. Crisp [12] is more specific, and suggests that the psychobiological regression which results from weight loss is a particular strategy to abort developing sexuality (Fig. 70.1). Evidence to support this hypothesis comes from the difficulties of anorexic families in dealing with sexuality, and the coincidence of the chosen weights

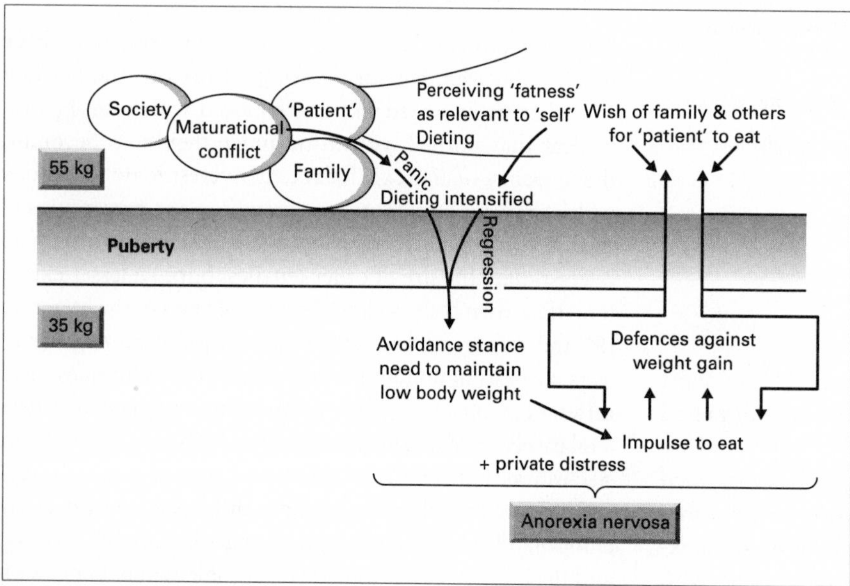

Fig. 70.1 Typical evolution of anorexia nervosa. (Courtesy of Professor A.H. Crisp St George's Hospital Medical School.)

of teenage girls and anorexics with weights at which luteinising hormone (LH) responsivity to gonadotrophin-releasing hormone (GnRH) will usually be poor, and typical of prepuberty. Possible support for the importance of sexuality in the development of anorexia nervosa comes from reports of sexual abuse preceding anorexia, although recent studies suggest that sexual abuse is a vulnerability factor for psychiatric disorder in general rather than eating disorders in particular [13].

There is abundant evidence of obsessive–compulsive behaviour in patients with anorexia nervosa, and an increased risk of developing anorexia nervosa in patients with obsessive–compulsive disorder. It is unclear as to how the disorders are related, but abnormalities in serotonin regulation might be one link.

Medical and neuroendocrine manifestations

The medical complications of anorexia nervosa are manifold [14] and consequent upon starvation and behaviours such as vomiting or laxative misuse. Patients frequently show bradycardia, hypotension, cardiac arrhythmias and electrocardiogram (ECG) abnormalities. Cardiac failure can be consequent upon cardiomyopathy and can be precipitated by overly fast refeeding or rehydration regimes. Dental erosion follows vomiting. Benign parotid enlargement can occur. Oesophageal complications can be a consequence of vomiting. Acute gastric dilatation has been reported during rapid refeeding of patients with preceeding low food intakes leading to decreased gastic volume and slow gastric emptying. Complex pictures of diarrhoea and constipation can result from poor food intake and chronic laxative misuse. Hypokalaemia, hyponatraemia and hypochloraemia are common. Phosphate abnormalities are common, with marked changes occurring during refeeding. Glomerular filtration rates are often decreased. Spectacular fluid retention can be seen during refeeding/rehydration in low-weight patients or those who have abused laxatives. A diuresis usually follows within 2 weeks, but the patient will be markedly psychologically distressed and the condition needs careful monitoring for possible cardiac failure. Newer scanning techniques indicate enlargement of the lateral ventricles and dilated sulci in the brain related to low weight rather than duration of illness.

The neuroendocrine abnormalities in anorexia nervosa may be misleading, and should not be seen as likely to be of aetiological significance. Most abnormalities are secondary to the physical condition and, even if apparently corrected, factors such as dehydration can radically alter the neuroendocrine implications in different patients. Dehydration can, for instance, explain the phenomenon of a patient menstruating at a weight of 40 kg.

Plasma cortisol levels are elevated in anorexia nervosa, apparently because of decreased clearance (possibly related to low triidothyronine (T_3)) and an increased rate of production relative to body size [15]. In addition, patients may show non-suppression of cortisol during the dexamethasone-suppression test, but similar findings are seen in patients with non-psychiatric malnutrition. In low-weight anorexia nervosa the level of corticotrophin-releasing hormone (CRH) in the CSF has been found to be increased, whilst the adrenocorticotrophic hormone (ACTH) response to CRH was found to be decreased. Many of these abnormalities are also seen in patients with depressive illness (see also Chapter 82).

Despite recent reservations [2], amenorrhoea is an important sign in anorexia nervosa. With weight loss reproductive hormones return to a prepubertal pattern [16]. Studies in markedly underweight patients with anorexia nervosa demonstrate low plasma gonadotrophins, particularly LH, with both LH and follicle-stimulating hormone (FSH) normalising as weight is regained. The 24-hour pattern of LH secretion resembles that found in normal prepubertal girls or early pubertal girls. These 'immature' patterns are found in both restricting and bulimic groups of patients. LH responses to GnRH are usually greatly reduced in patients with anorexia nervosa (in proportion to weight loss), and, in some subjects, hyperresponsiveness of FSH to GnRH has been observed during weight gain. Even in low-weight anorexics, the repeated pulsatile administration of GnRH causes a return of the LH response to normal; this supports the concept of a deficiency of endogenous GnRH secretion in low-weight anorexia nervosa patients. However, amenorrhoea can occur at relatively high weights suggesting additional causes, such as continued dietary chaos, which have not been adequately explored. Serum testosterone levels are normal in women with anorexia nervosa, but lowered in male anorexics at low weights.

In low-weight anorexia nervosa patients, thyroxine (T_4) levels may be low, but are usually still in the normal range. Serum T_3 levels are low, although there are increased levels of reverse T_3 and probably normal levels of thyroid-stimulating hormone (TSH). The TSH response to thryrotrophin-releasing hormone (TRH) is usually normal, but may be blunted. This pattern is found in other states of malnutrition [17].

The relationship between weight and melatonin is unclear, and the situation in anorexia nervosa even less clear. Studies of low-weight patients have shown nocturnal levels to be low, high and normal, although most studies suggest elevated levels, particularly in the binge-eating/purging subgroup. It has also been shown that most such patients do not have normal circadian rhythms of melatonin.

It is unclear whether eating disorders are over-represented in women with insulin-dependent diabetes mellitus [18,19].

The disorders are associated with high HbA_1 levels and retinopathy. It is thought that the weight and psychological effects of diabetes are of aetiological importance in these disturbances. However, glucose regulation is itself abnormal in anorexia nervosa. In low-weight anorexics plasma insulin levels are probably in the low range, while insulin binding to monocytes and *in vivo* sensitivity to insulin (measured by the insulin tolerance test) are probably increased. This is probably due to an increase in receptor numbers rather than receptor affinity [20]. Earlier authors had concluded that these patients are insulin resistant on the basis of glucose tolerance tests which show a delay in the clearing of blood glucose and prolonged elevation of plasma insulin. This has been confirmed by a recent study [21] which also examined other gastrointestinal hormones in anorexia nervosa. Whether or not there is an over-representation of eating disorders among diabetic patients, considering possible eating-disordered pathology is important in the care of diabetic patients. Insulin omission is clearly used by patients to achieve weight loss [22].

Various neurotransmitter systems, particularly those thought to be involved in the regulation of hunger and satiety, have been studied in eating disorders [23]. Noradrenaline turnover is reduced in low-weight anorexia nervosa, but corrects with weight restoration. Studies of serotoninergic and dopaminergic systems show normal activity. However, a recent intriguing finding suggests that dieting decreases plasma tryptophan and increases the prolactin response to L-tryptophan and D-fenfluramine in women but not in men. These results were not mirrored in a comparison of patients with anorexia nervosa and a control group. However, the latter work did show marked blunting of the growth hormone (GH) response to L-trytophan infusion in patients compared with controls. Opioid systems are of particular interest and are generating continuing research, but no consensus as yet exists as to their precise importance.

Bone mineral density is known to be decreased in anorexia nervosa. There is disagreement as to whether this should be termed osteoporosis. A review of published studies [24] concludes that low nutrient intake, low bodyweight, early onset and long duration of amenorrhoea, low calcium intake, reduced physical activity, and hypercortisolaemia are related to the degree of decrease in bone mineral density. The reversibility of the condition is unclear, as is the optimal management. Correction of the dietary inadequacies and low weight are obvious interventions. In the absence of successful treatment of the anorexia nervosa, i.e. the patient remaining at a low weight, it is possible that hormone replacement prevents deterioration. The role of dietary supplements is unknown. In all cases the benefits of moderate exercise seem likely to outweigh the risks of stress fractures (see also Chapter 71 for further discussion of dietary aspects).

Modes of therapy

The treatment of anorexia nervosa starts with an assessment and an attempt to engage the patient. This requires a diagnosis to be made on three levels [25]. First, at a behavioural level: how is weight lost? Often this level of diagnosis is as far as assessment goes, but it is inadequate to facilitate subsequent treatment. The second level of diagnosis attempts to elicit the weight phobia and avoidance stance. Patients will often deny a fear of gaining weight. For example, they may argue that the principal motivation relates to attractiveness. The terror of weight gain may only become manifest within treatment. The third level of diagnosis attempts to elicit an explanation for the fear of normal bodyweight, and here theoretical models differ. The model of Crisp [12] would look for an explanatory 'maturational crisis', but eliciting this crisis is difficult. Weight loss may resolve the problems being avoided (although bringing new problems). Thus, for example, the fear of one's own libido is not an active issue at low weight. At all three levels the patient or family may express ignorance as to 'why', and thus a high level of suspicion and understanding (derived from theories of aetiology) is essential. The diagnosis of anorexia nervosa is often unpopular with patient, family and carers. It is important not to accept that patients find anorexia a fulfilling way of life. If offered, this attitude is usually a defensive strategy for a patient who does not believe that others understand and sees no alternative defence strategy other than weight loss.

Assessment should try to avoid 'secrets', should involve the family and should involve the patient being weighed and height measured. Secrets will greatly hamper subsequent communication. The family usually constitute a potential therapeutic resource. Weight and height are essential in both initial and continuous assessments. Physical examination and investigations are important, but should not be overemphasised. For instance, after the diagnosis of low-weight anorexia nervosa, the discovery of low LH levels is inevitable and not informative. Dietary assessment is dealt with in Chapter 71.

Decisions about how to treat follow on from a decision about the aim of treatment: correcting the weight loss to keep the patient alive, treating the problems underlying weight loss, or supporting the patient within chronic anorexia nervosa. Whilst not exclusive, these aims should not be confused.

Simple correction of weight loss should rarely be appropriate given an adequate assessment and engagement with the patient. At very low weights admission to hospital may be necessary. Medical and psychiatric beds have different advantages. To an insightless patient a medical bed is often more acceptable, but a psychiatric bed may offer the opportunity to staff to engage the patient in treatment which leads beyond weight gain. Patients will often eat after admission to get themselves out of hospital. Whether the patient has been legally enforced to hospitalisation or not, the admission has usually occurred under duress. Parenteral or nasogastric feeding and the use of legal procedures are extremely distressing, and are usually counterproductive to subsequent therapeutic engagement. They should only be considered in immediately life-threatening situations, and can usually be avoided by adequate assessment and engagement of the patient and family.

Modes of therapy for the underlying disorder can be examined on two dimensions: the type of therapy and the setting for therapy. Medication has a very limited role. Antidepressants are tempting because patients can often describe a depressive syndrome, but have not proved useful, and may be counterproductive if they promote appetite. One exception to this is fluoxetine, which has shown some usefulness and is not associated with weight gain when prescribed to patients without eating disorders. Major tranquillisers such as chlorpromazine have been used, but without great success. They are sometimes still prescribed for their sedative properties or to treat a patient who has become psychotic during the process of weight gain. The risk of serious side-effects, particularly tardive dyskinesia, must render their routine use questionable. Benzodiazepines are contraindicated in this essentially addictive illness. Appetite stimulants are theoretically, and in practise, unjustified. Prokinetic agents, clonidine, zinc sulphate, delta 9-tetrahydrocannabinol and lithium have all been used in the treatment of anorexia nervosa, but are without proven efficacy.

Most proven treatment approaches utilise combinations of dietary, behavioural and psychotherapeutic interventions. Refeeding/weight gain is necessary, although it will distress the patient. Weight gain must be controlled, and one must recognise the patient's fear of overeating (dietary issues are dealt with in Chapter 71). Increased diet may lead to the use of compensatory mechanisms such as increased exercise, and the use or abuse of these will need to be addressed. A 'target weight' should be prescribed. One method of deriving this weight uses the normal weight for the patient's height at the age of onset of the disorder. Other authors have argued for aiming to achieve sufficient weight gain to establish or re-establish menstruation.

The psychological support which makes weight gain possible can take a number of forms. Family therapy, individual therapy and group therapy have all been used. A recent study suggests that family intervention is most appropriate in younger patients, and an individual approach for older patients [26]. Prolonged follow-up of the patients in this study clearly underlines family therapy as the treatment of choice in this younger group. The results are surprisingly good in this hard to treat disorder. Self-help groups, organisations and literature can all be useful if more intensive interventions are not possible, or to supplement the above treatments. Without adequate psychological help weight gain is unlikely to be sustained.

In-patient treatment [27] is most commonly used for patients at low weights, but should perhaps be used for particularly difficult problems and where the patient is in need of the security of external control. An appropriate rate of weight gain (after any period of rehydration) is in the region of 1–1.5 kg per week. Out-patient treatment is often slower in achieving overt change, but may achieve more stable change because the patient does not have to adjust to discharge from the supportive hospital environment. Day-clinic approaches [28] are increasingly popular and may represent an appropriate compromise of the benefits of in- and out-patient treatment.

All of these approaches should aim at weight gain as above, but treatment should not stop when the 'target weight' is reached. It is often at this point that the patient is most intensely distressed, but equally the psychological issues become more possible to understand. Target weight thus represents an opportunity for patient and parents to examine their difficulties and develop new coping strategies. As below, the immediate consequence of 'recovery' from anorexia nervosa may be depression or agoraphobia. It may be some years before the patient can expect to live a normal life. Symptoms such as depression emerging after weight gain need to be reassessed, and may be tackled within psychotherapy, using cognitive behavioural techniques or antidepressant medication.

Not all patients are treatable. Some will reject all help, others can only accept support which allows them to live within stable anorexia nervosa. In some such patients the caring clinician can be destructive in pushing a 'cure' model of therapy. After years within anorexia nervosa the patient may have very little alternative life, and the opportunities for a change of direction are increasingly curtailed. To get such patients to a normal weight can be to expose them to what they have lost, and this can be intolerable.

The prognosis of anorexia nervosa underlines the seriousness of this underestimated disorder [29]; at least 3% of patients will be dead within 10 years, 25% will still have severe problems after 4 years, and another 25% will have made partial recoveries although high rates of depression and psychosocial disturbance have been found at follow-up. Poor prognosis is suggested by lowest weight, chronicity, late onset, male sex, lower social class, premorbid obesity, dietary chaos and poor peer relationships.

Bulimia nervosa

Theories of aetiology and psychopathology

As for anorexia nervosa, the most accepted diagnostic criteria for bulimia nervosa come from DSM-IV [1] (Table 70.1). The weight of patients with bulimia nervosa varies, both within individual patients and between patients. With these criteria patients can be in any weight range, unless they met the criteria for anorexia nervosa. In this sense the diagnosis of anorexia nervosa 'trumps' that of bulimia nervosa, and if bulimic symptoms are present in combination with those of anorexia nervosa the diagnosis is anorexia nervosa of the binge-eating/purging type.

The DSM-IV criteria give a brief description of the clinical syndrome. The onset of binge eating is often associated with dieting and the desire to lose weight, and it has been suggested that the resultant hunger contributes to triggering the binge eating. Other important triggers of the binge-eating behaviour are emotional. Patients often report feelings of boredom, loneliness, and stress prior to a binge. For them, binge eating acts as a tranquilliser and suppresses these feelings. In other patients food binges are a stimulant, the bulimic attack being associated with excitement and expectation at the craving about to be fulfilled. The initial stages of a binge are often not distressing, but as the bulimic becomes more out of control, more unpleasant feelings of guilt and shame at the behaviour become prominent. Because of this shame, binge eating is invariably a secretive habit. Mean daily intake has been reported to be 6000 kcals, and self-induced vomiting is the most common method of avoiding weight gain. Laxatives are also commonly used, and diuretics less commonly.

Patients often give the impression of being coping and resourceful, but in treatment declare a very low self-esteem with exaggerated guilt and sadness. They are abnormally concerned with their body image, predominantly on an attitudinal and emotional level.

The syndrome affects predominantly women and, as in anorexia nervosa, seems uncommon in non-white patients although social class shows a greater heterogeneity in bulimia nervosa. The low levels of reporting in non-white patients are likely to be caused by women not presenting for help. Prevalence in the community is much higher than anorexia nervosa; possibly around 2–3% of young women meet the DSM-IV criteria. Patients seek help in their mid-20s, with an onset slightly later than for anorexia nervosa.

The aetiology of bulimia nervosa is very unclear, and must have a multidetermined origin. Predisposing factors include sociocultural pressures relating to 'femininity', parental marital conflict, the relationship of patient and parents and premorbid weight and food problems. Precipitants include 'loss' experiences, sexual conflicts and moves of location or occupation [30]. The mechanism by which the disorder is maintained is less well understood. The above factors may lead the patient to diet, and the dieting breaks down into the bulimic syndrome. An alternative hypothesis would suggest that the bulimic eating behaviour itself has a mood-modifying effect. The mechanism of this modification is unknown but it is possible that the binges modify serotonin transmission.

Studies have documented a high incidence of eating disorders in female relatives of women with eating disorders, but no twin studies exist. It has been suggested that bulimia nervosa is closely related to affective disorders, and this link may be genetic [31]. Serotonin metabolism has been proposed as one neurochemical link between the disorders.

Medical and neuroendocrine manifestations

Vomiting and laxative abuse produce dehydration, hypokalaemia, hyponatraemia and hypochloraemia. The loss of stomach acid through vomiting may produce a metabolic alkalosis and laxative abuse can induce metabolic acidosis. Serum amylase levels are often elevated, probably reflecting an increase in the salivary isoenzyme. Measurement of serum or salivary amylase has been suggested as one method for monitoring treatment response, but early results do not justify this in routine use. Physical complications of bulimia nervosa include dental erosion, parotid gland enlargement, oedema, and (rarely) gastric dilatation. The dorsal surface of the knuckles may develop calluses consequent upon friction with the teeth in attempts to induce vomiting.

In bulimia nervosa neuroendocrine studies have been carried out for a variety of reasons, but in particular have been used to investigate links to depressive disorders. The parallels to depressive disorders are not impressive, and a normal weight state of 'malnourishment' or intermittent starvation may be an important factor in the abnormalities seen [32]. In contrast to anorexia nervosa, patients with bulimia nervosa do not show elevated plasma cortisol levels, although they do show a higher than expected incidence of dexamethasone non-suppression. The latter finding may relate to low plasma dexamethasone levels due to inadequate absorption. Dexamethasone sensitivity seems to normalise with the discontinuation of bulimic behaviour [32]. Menstrual irregularity is common with abnormalities of ovarian morphology on ultrasound. Patients with bulimia nervosa do not have a serious weight deficit, but amenorrhoea still occurs in about half of these patients. LH and possibly FSH secretion are low but, in contrast to low-weight anorexia nervosa, LH may show an increased response to GnRH. Low gonadotrophin levels are probably secondary to increased activation of the hypothalamo-pituitary–adrenal axis and disrupted GnRH secretion, possibly caused by binge eating, episodic starvation, weight fluctuations, excessive exercise, stress and depression [32,33]. No consistent abnormalities in thyroid indices have been found in bulimia nervosa. It is possible that T_3 levels are slightly low, basal TSH levels seem to be normal and TRH-induced levels are normal, but often delayed [17,32,34]. As with diabetes there is some suggestion that thyroid disorders leading to weight-regulation problems can have an aetiological role in bulimia [35]. Melatonin has been studied in bulimia nervosa because of the possible relationship to affective disorders. Interest has been accentuated by the similarities between bulimia nervosa and seasonal affective disorder. Nevertheless, the limited current data suggest normal melatonin regulation in this condition [36]. Basal GH levels are elevated in some normal-weight bulimics, and the GH response to TRH appears to be increased. Some bulimics may have low basal prolactin levels and heightened responsivity to TRH. Different studies suggest that β-endorphin levels may be low or high, and an interesting finding shows that naloxone and naltrexone may attenuate binge-eating behaviour.

Glucose regulation in anorexia nervosa has been studied in detail. There are fewer studies in bulimia nervosa, but these suggest insulin secretion and glucose levels are relatively elevated after meals. This is a possible perpetuating factor for binge eating [37]. Much of what has been said about the relationship between anorexia nervosa and diabetes applies to bulimia nervosa. As for anorexia nervosa, bulimia nervosa possibly has an increased incidence among female patients with insulin-dependent diabetes mellitus [18,19]. Significant binge eating has also been found to be a common problem in obese type II diabetic patients, and seems to relate to depression [38]. Suggestions have been made about the management of patients with comorbidity for the two disorders [39].

Osteoporosis may occur in bulimia nervosa, but usually relates to a previous history of anorexia nervosa and similar risk factors and management issues apply.

Among the neurotransmitters, serotonin has proved to be of most interest. Normal-weight bulimic patients show blunted prolactin responses to L-tryptophan. Patients who satiate and stop binge eating have an increase in their plasma L-tryptophan/large neutral amino acids ratio. It is thought that this ratio determines transport of tryptophan into the central nervous system (CNS). Increased CNS L-tryptophan levels lead to increased serotonin synthesis, and it is proposed that this leads to satiety. It has thus been suggested that bulimia is a consequence of hyposerotoninergic activity. Binge eating may exaggerate diet-induced serotonin synthesis as a means of compensating for this underactivity. Thus, mood and neuroendocrine disturbances could either be due to the primary disturbance of serotonin or be secondary to binge-induced effects [23,32].

Modes of therapy

Much of what has been said about the assessment of anorexia nervosa applies to bulimia nervosa. Views of the subsequent management and treatment differ. One author has called the condition 'intractable', another author called it 'highly treatable'.

Because of the possible relationship to affective disorder the majority of antidepressants have been used in the treatment of bulimia nervosa. Most studies show antidepressants to have an effect superior to that of placebo, with short-term symptom relief relapsing on discontinuation of the drug [40]. Fluoxetine is licensed in the UK for the treatment of bulimia nervosa, but with a recommended dosage above that used in the treatment of depressive disorder. In view of the efficacy of psychological interventions, antidepressants cannot be recommended as first-line treatment, but further research is needed.

'Packages' of psychological treatment have been clearly described [41,42]; they utilise time-limited intervention, usually in an out-patient setting. The treatments have been well assessed and improvements achieved are maintained at follow-ups of at least 4 years. The packages of treatment have many factors in common. Patients are assessed, and screened to exclude those with anorexia nervosa. They then usually benefit from education about how their problem can be understood, and the physiological consequences of their weight-controlling strategies. They are then asked to modify their diet. To this end they are asked to keep a record of their eating and behaviours associated with it (such as vomiting). Whilst doing this they are asked to add structure to their diet, in particular to include foods which will reduce the likelihood of hunger shortly following food. This issue is discussed further below. Patients are weighed regularly, and it is important that they do not attempt to change their weight during this treatment phase. Most patients consider themselves overweight, and some actually are. Suggesting to such patients that they maintain their current weight usually meets with active resistance, but is essential. If patients are determined to change their weight it is appropriate to ask them to return for treatment when they are stabilised at a weight they can tolerate (provided they have not developed anorexia nervosa). As dietary chaos comes under control it becomes possible for patients to identify the emotional precipitants of their binge eating. This can be facilitated by asking patients to include information about events and feelings in their record of eating. Patients can then be helped to examine the train of thoughts that may lead from a small event into a major emotional trauma, and to develop alternative coping strategies to that of binge eating. Treatment can be either individual or in groups. Group treatment is obviously economically attractive, but needs to be supplemented by some individual work. There is increasing evidence that a significantly number of patients will respond to very limited interventions, including self-help books [43,44]. Most patients believe that if they can give up their eating disorder that life will be transformed. This is usually true, but the change is not always simply for the better. On giving up their obvious behaviour patients can become depressed [41], and their established relationships need to adapt, or may come under threat.

When impulsive eating is complicated by other impulsive behaviour such as stealing, overdosing or substance abuse, the prognosis is much worse and may call for in-patient treatment [45].

References

1 American Psychiatric Association. *Diagnostic and Statistical Manual of Mental Disorders*, 4th edn. Washington D.C: American Psychiatric Association, 1994.

2 Garfinkel PE, Lin E, Goering P *et al.* Should amenorrhoea be necessary for the diagnosis of anorexia nervosa? Evidence from a Canadian community sample. *Br J Psychiatr* 1996; **168**: 500–6.

3 Jones DJ, Fox MM, Babigian HM, Hutton HE. Epidemiology of anorexia nervosa in Monroe Country, New York: 1960–1976. *Psychosom Med* 1980; **42**: 551–8.

4 Lask B, Bryant-Waugh R. Early-onset anorexia nervosa and related eating disorders. *J Child Psychol Psychiatr* 1992; **33**: 281–300.

5 Scott DW. Anorexia nervosa: a review of possible genetic factors. *Int J Eating Disord* 1986; **5**: 1–20.

6 Holland AJ, Hall A, Murray R, Russel GFM, Crisp AH. Anorexia nervosa: a study of 34 twin pairs and one set of triplets. *Br J Psychiatr* 1984; **145**: 414–19.

7 Garfinkel PE. Perception of hunger and satiety in anorexia nervosa. *Psycholog Med* 1974; **4**: 309–15.

8 Slade P. A review of body–image studies in anorexia nervosa and bulimia nervosa. *J Psychiatr Res* 1985; **19**: 255–65.

9 Bowden PK, Touyz SW, Rodriguez PJ, Hensley R, Beumont PJV. Distorting patient or distorting instrument? Body shape disturbance in patients with anorexia nervosa and bulimia. *Br J Psychiatr* 1989; **155**: 196–201.

10 Parrazzi M, Luby ED. An auto-addiction opioid model of chronic anorexia nervosa. *Int J Eating Disord* 1986; **5**: 191–208.

11 Palazzoli MS. *Self starvation. From the Intrapsychic to the Transpersonal Approach to Anorexia Nervosa.* London: Chaucer Publishing (Human Context Books), 1974.

12 Crisp AH. The psychopathology of anorexia nervosa: getting the 'heat' out of the system. In: Stunkard AJ & Stellar E, eds. *Eating and Its Disorders*. New York: Raven Press: 209–34.

13 Vize CM, Cooper P. Sexual abuse in patients with eating disorder, patients with depression and normal controls. A comparative study. *Br J Psychiatr* 1995; **167**: 80–5.

14 Sharp CW, Freeman CPL. The medical complications of anorexia nervosa. *Br J Psychiatr* 1993; **162**: 452–62.

15 Walsh BT. Hypothalamic–pituitary–adrenal axis in bulimia. In: Hudson JI, Pope HG, eds. *The Psychobiology of Bulimia.* Washington, DC: American Psychiatric Press, 1988.

16 Weiner H. The hypothalamic–pituitary–ovarian axis in anorexia nervosa and bulimia nervosa. An appraisal. *Int J Eating Disord* 1983; **2**: 109–16.

17 Kaplan AS. Thyroid function in bulimia. In: Hudson JI, Pope HG, eds. *The Psychobiology of Bulimia.* Washington, DC: American Psychiatric Press, 1988.

18 Steel JM, Young RJ, Lloyd GG, MacIntyre CCA. Abnormal eating attitudes in young insulin-dependent diabetics. *Br J Psychiatr* 1989; **155**: 515–21.

19 Rodin GM, Daneman D. Eating disorders and IDDM. A problematic association. *Diabetes Care* 1992; **15**: 1402–12.

20 Wachslicht-Rodbarb H, Gross HA, Rodbarb D, Ebert MH, Roth J. Increased insulin binding to erythrocytes in anorexia nervosa. Restoration to normal with refeeding. *N Engl J Med* 1979; **300**: 882–6.

21 Alderdice JT, Dinsmore WW, Buchanan KD, Adams C. Gastro-intestinal hormones in anorexia nervosa. *J Psychiatric Res* 1985; **19**: 207–13.

22 Polonsky WH, Anderson BJ, Lohrer PA, Aponte JE, Jacobson AM, Cole CF. Insulin omission in women with IDDM. *Diabetes Care* 1994; **17**: 1178–85.

23 Fava M, Copeland PM, Schweiger U, Herzog DB. Neurochemical abnormalities of anorexia nervosa and bulimia nervosa. *Am J Psychiatr* 1989; **146**: 963–71.

24 Salisbury JJ, Mitchell JE. Bone mineral density and anorexia nervosa in women. *Am J Psychiatr* 1991; **148**: 768–74.

25 Crisp AH. The differential diagnosis of anorexia nervosa. *Proc Roy Soc Med* 1977; **70**: 686–90.

26 Russell GFM, Szmukler GI, Dare C, Eisler I. An evaluation of family therapy in anorexia nervosa and bulimia nervosa. *Arch Gen Psychiatr* 1987; **44**: 1047–56.

27 Crisp AH, Norton KRS, Jurczak S, Bowyer R, Duncan S. A treatment approach to anorexia nervosa—25 years on. *J Psychiatr Res* 1985; **19**: 393–404.

28 Piran N, Kaplan A, Kerr A, *et al.* A day hospital program for anorexia nervosa and bulimia. *Int J Eating Disord* 1989; **8**: 511–21.

29 Patton G. The course of anorexia nervosa (Editorial). *Br Med J* 1989; **299**: 139–40.

30 Lacey JH, Coker S, Birtchnell SA. Bulimia: factors associated with its etiology and maintenance. *Int J Eating Disord* 1986; **5**: 475–87.

31 Swift WJ, Andrews D, Barklage NE. The relationship between affective disorder and eating disorders: a review of the literature. *Am J Psychiatr* 1986; **143**: 290–9.

32 Levy AB. Neuroendocrine profile in bulimia nervosa. *Biolog Psychiatr* 1989; **25**: 98–109.

33 Schweiger U, Pirke K–M, Laessle RG, Fichter MM. Gonadotrophin secretion in bulimia nervosa. *J Clin Endocrinol Metab* 1992; **74**: 1122–7.

34 Spalter AR, Gwirtsman HE, Demitrack MA, Gold PW. Thyroid function in bulimia nervosa. *Biolog Psychiatr* 1993; **33**: 408–14.

35 Schmidt U, O'Donoghue G. Bulimia nervosa in thyroid disorder. *Int J Eating disord* 1992; **12**: 93–6.

36 Mortola JF, Laughlin GA, Yen SS. Melatonin rhythms in women with anorexia nervosa and bulimia nervosa. *J Clin Endocrinol Metab* 1993; **77**: 1540–4.

37 Russell J, Hooper M, Storlien L, Smythe GA. Insulin, glucose, and cortisol levels in bulimia: effect of treatment. *Int J Eating Disord* 1989; **8**: 635–46.

38 Wing RR, Marcus MD, Epstein LH, Blair EH, Burton LR. Binge eating in obese patients with Type II diabetes. *Int J Eating Disord* 1989; 8: 671–9.

39 Peveler RC, Fairburn CG. The treatment of bulimia nervosa in patients with diabetes mellitus. *Int J Eating Disord* 1992; **11**: 45–53.

40 Mitchell JE, Raymond N, Specker S. A review of the controlled trials of pharmacotherapy and psychotherapy in the treatment of bulimia nervosa. *Int J Eating Disord* 1993; **14**: 229–47.

41 Lacey JH. Bulimia nervosa, binge-eating and psychogenic vomiting: a controlled treatment study and long-term outcome. *Br Med J* 1983; **286**: 1609–13.

42 Fairburn CG. Cognitive behavioural treatment for bulimia. In: Garner DM, Garfinkel PE, eds. *Handbook of Psychotherapy for Anorexia Nervosa and Bulimia*. New York: Guildford Press, 1985: 160–92.

43 Treasure J, Schmidt U, Troop N, Tiller J, Todd G, Turnbull S. Sequential treatment for bulimia nervosa incorporating a self–care manual. *Br J Psychiatr* 1996; **168**: 94–8.

44 Waller D. Fairburn CG, McPherson A, Kay R, Lee A, Nowell T. Treating bulimia nervosa in primary care—a pilot study. *Int J Eating Disord* 1996; **19**: 99–103.

45 Lacey JH, Evans CDH. The implusivist: a multi-impulsive personality disorder. *Br J Addict* 1986; **81**: 715–23.

CHAPTER 71

Dietary aspects of anorexia nervosa and bulimia nervosa

J.D. Challis

Dietetic involvement

Although patients with anorexia nervosa (AN) are not eating sufficient to maintain a healthy weight, the problem is not one of appetite, nor of eating *per se*. A denial of appetite and fear of gaining weight are fundamental problems in the disorder which cannot be solved by dietitians. Likewise in bulimia nervosa (BN), dietary advice in the absence of psychological support may be less than helpful. However, a dietitian can help in the areas of assessment and negotiation of an appropriate diet to either increase or maintain weight and, perhaps most importantly, in the teaching of more normal eating habits once the patient is recovering. Patients seen by non-specialist units may have a range of eating disorders, as many young women are overly concerned about weight gain and employ dietary strategies to avoid it [1,2].

Intervention and nutritional counselling at an early stage may avoid the onset of a severe long-term eating disorder. Beumont [3] provides considerable further detail regarding nutritional counselling for those with AN and BN.

Dietary assessment

Historically, the foods avoided by those with AN were those rich in carbohydrate (both sugar and starch) whilst protein-rich foods, often high in fat, for example cheese, were acceptable [4]. In 1981, Beumont *et al.* found that diets of patients with AN were proportionately higher in protein, lower in fat and provided the same proportion of carbohydrate as diets of controls [5]. Personal observation and discussion with other dietitians working with anorectics has led the author to conclude that the trend of diet selection in these people is an extreme version of the type of weight-reducing diet recommended for the obese in the general population: whilst once carbohydrates in all forms were perceived as 'bad', the 'healthy eating message' of reduced fat and sugar is now making a major impact on the food choices of many of those with AN. Simon *et al.* demonstrated a marked taste aversion to fat-rich foods amongst anorectics [6]. Misconceptions and fads gleaned from magazines and diet books may also influence food choices in anorectics [7]. Alcohol is also commonly avoided. This may be due to its high energy content, potential for appetite stimulation, or effects on self-control.

Although it is often difficult to determine what patients with eating disorders including AN are exactly eating, time spent establishing a working relationship with the patient and discussing the areas described below is well spent, especially if the patient is to be treated on an out-patient basis.

Out-patient assessment

Sufficient time must be allowed for the interview(s): a busy dietetic out-patient clinic rarely allows the patient enough time to build up trust in the interviewer, and this is vital if the patient is to be honest. Patients will tend to restrict their communication if they feel time is limited, and not fully explain their difficulties which may result in problems of communication from the start.

Areas that need exploring include:

1 weight history;

2 current eating pattern including use of vitamin/mineral supplements;

3 eating/dieting history;

4 current living situation with regard to shopping and food preparation;

5 foods classified by the patient as 'good' or 'bad';

6 any 'forbidden' foods, i.e. foods that patients will not allow themselves;

7 food likes and dislikes;

8 existence of any allergies/intolerances, and the source of these diagnoses;

9 patterns of bingeing behaviour which may be coupled with vomiting and/or purging—this information may be withheld by patients initially until they feel confident in the interviewer;
10 bizarre eating habits;
11 fluid intake.

Vegetarianism has been shown to be linked to more abstemious forms of AN, as opposed to bingeing/starving, and the families of such sufferers tend to be more overprotective and enmeshed [8]. Vegetarianism is now increasing particularly in the young female population [9] and thus it is important to establish whether or not vegetarianism predates the onset of an eating disorder. If patients are asked to keep a food record this must be interpreted with caution; patients may overstate the amount eaten either deliberately to try and make their intake appear adequate, or because of guilt and anxiety over eating. Despite this, a record can give useful information about eating patterns and indicate times of day/types of food patients find it easiest to allow themselves to eat.

In-patient assessment

A dietary assessment as described above is also appropriate for in-patients.

If food records are to be kept for patients, careful thought needs to be given as to whether these are to be kept without the patient knowing. It is extremely difficult to keep accurate records without the patient becoming aware of their existence, and if patients find out that 'secret records' are being kept their sense of trust in those treating them may be diminished.

It is not surprising that patients with AN have anormalities in vitamin status [10–12], as, in addition to abnormal intakes of many foods, patients may be using vitamin supplements. Both deficiencies and intoxications are possible, requiring monitoring.

Dietary plans/dietary treatment

It is vital that the entire team involved in the treatment of a patient with AN communicate well between themselves. If it is decided to embark upon active treatment patients need not only to gain weight, but also must be given simultaneous psychological help to deal both with the stress of weight gain and also the underlying causes of the anorexia, as these need to be resolved if the anorectic coping strategies are to be given up.

A contract system is often used in treatment programmes. Vandereycken [13] provides a detailed example of such a programme and the information provided both for patients and for their families.

Target weight

A realistic target weight helps the patient to have a physical goal to achieve, but it must be remembered that weight gain alone will not solve the problem of AN. Target weight may be based on a mean population matched weight for age of onset, or previous healthy weight as an adult, or as a particular body-mass index (BMI). Once the target has been set it should not be altered, and anorectics must be helped to stabilise at this weight once it has been reached. Touyz *et al.* compared the effects of weighing daily versus three times weekly; there was no significant difference in weight gain between the groups, and it was felt that less frequent weighing had advantages [14]. In practice, twice-weekly weighing allows monitoring of weight gain without stressing the patients any more than necessary as most find 'weigh days' upsetting.

Out-patient versus in-patient treatment

In-patient treatment is required at dangerously low body-weights. For other patients, whichever route is chosen, progress will depend to some extent on the amount of psychological support available. Weight gain for in-patients may be up to 1–1.5 kg/week; out-patients will rarely be able to achieve this and initial gains may be very small. If weight loss has been fast prior to treatment commencing, weight maintenance may be the initial target.

Energy requirements

Energy requirements for weight maintenance in AN have been documented by Gwirtsman [15] who found that subjects at 57% ideal bodyweight maintained their weight on 1017 ± 54 kcal/day, compared with 1651 ± 108 kcal/day for controls at 94% ideal bodyweight. Calculation of energy costs for weight gain are complicated by the facts that on commencing refeeding programmes many patients are dehydrated and may experience initial fluctuations in fluid balance, and that basal metabolic rate will increase as lean body mass increases. Russell and Mezey [16] and Walker *et al.* [17] both found an average 'cost' of 7500 kcal/kg weight gain whilst Dempsey *et al.* [18] calculated the mean excess calorie requirement for 1 kg weight gain to be 9768 (range 5569–15 619 kcal/kg). Activity level will obviously also influence the energy cost of weight gain: Kaye [19] found that patients with a lower activity level gained 1 kg every 5.1 ± 1.2 days compared with 1 kg every 7.2 ± 1.9 days at a mean cost of 8301 ± 2272 kcal/kg weight gain.

In a review of refeeding, metabolic rate and weight gain in AN, Salisbury *et al.* found the average excess number of kilocalories to gain 1 kg bodyweight was 7462, approximately the average of 9300 and 5300 (required for the gain of 1 kg fat and protein, respectively) [20]. Realistic energy intakes for a weight gain of 1–1.5 kg/week are thus in the region of 2500–3000 kcal/day. It must be remembered that even if a lower level is chosen initially, on the basis of lower requirements at a lower weight, patients will not necessarily find the regimen any easier. This is because any increase in intake will lead to feelings of being out of control with their eating, and this will not be directly related to weight gain *per se*.

Weight gain

Patients at 15–20 kg below ideal bodyweight are going to require lengthy periods of treatment for weight gain before discharge can be contemplated; weight gain will be slower as an out-patient, and patients discharged immediately target weight is reached will find it difficult to adjust their intake to maintain weight. This is further complicated by evidence that a greater than normal energy intake is required to maintain a stable weight in the period immediately after weight restoration [21], more specifically, in non-bulimic patients [22]. Furthermore, the sensations of hunger and satiety are initially dull, leaving the patient in need of guidance about their dietary intake for some time.

A high-protein diet does not seem to be indicated for adequate replenishment of lean body tissue [23]. Although there is no general agreement as to the exact proportions of lean tissue versus fat gained during refeeding [16,23–25], both are gained. The lack of consensus may be because more lean tissue than fat may be gained early in refeeding, with more fat than lean tissue gained as patients approach a more normal weight [20].

Activity levels

In the past, activity during weight gain has been severely limited, sometimes to strict bed rest. However, whilst weight gain may be slowed by activity, as described above, consideration must be made of the necessity of severely restricting activity in view of reports of vitamin D deficiency and low osteocalcin levels in AN [26], osteoporosis in AN [27–30], and the known protective effect of exercise [31]. It would seem reasonable to allow modest amounts of activity, for example movement around the ward, rather than prescribe bedrest, although to prevent patients from vomiting after meals it may be necessary to limit activity at these times. One solution is to limit activity only when weight gain is less than agreed and in severely ill patients. Beumont *et al.* report on a supervised exercise programme in which patients above BMI 14 without significant medical symptoms participate. This was felt to allow a more normal attitude to exercise to develop but still allow weight gain [32]. Out-patients will usually be more active than in-patients but again should be advised against intensive exercise.

There is a group of patients who present with amenorrhoea due to both low weight and intensive exercise who require particular consideration. This group, for professional reasons, aim to sustain a medically undesirable low weight (e.g. ballet-dancers, gymnasts, some athletes). Although there is undoubtedly a subsection of this group who have eating disorders, the majority pursue thinness as a professional necessity and they should be encouraged to maintain their weight at the maximum permissible level, and given appropriate nutritional advice to achieve this. Exercise should be limited to that required professionally. For those within this group who demonstrate an eating disorder and pursuit of excessive weight loss, decisions must be made as to whether a target weight compatible with continuation/resumption of career should be set. The alternative, setting the target weight at the usual level for age/height, will preclude rapid return to employment where a degree of thinness is a prerequisite. Most reputable dance schools/coaches react rapidly to students pursuing excessive thinness by limiting training until a more appropriate weight is reached. Failure to reach and maintain such a weight will result in exclusion, until improvement occurs. Unfortunately, with the professional athlete/dancer, intervention may occur later as both the performer and their employer/coach will be reluctant for them to miss performances. Whether it is wise or even possible for someone with a severe eating disorder to remain in these highly competitive fields must be questioned before treatment begins.

In-patient eating plans

Various issues need to be agreed by all treating the patient before a refeeding programme commences. These should be documented in the protocol and relevant issues discussed with the patient.

If alterations are permitted once the plan has started, it is important to decide who will take responsibility for this, for example nurse, dietitian, doctor, psychiatrist. For consistency, one person should be appointed. Generally, a meal plan should be prescribed, including quantities, so the patient knows exactly what is to be served. Adjustments should only be made if problems such as insufficient/excess weight gain arise. If weight gain is less than anticipated, all opportunities for disposing of food, such as out of windows, down sinks/toilets, in rubbish bags, under beds etc., should be excluded before increasing the diet. A weight chart plotted graphically may help both doctor and patient, assuming a realistic scale is used.

It is not advisable to start patients who are very emaciated on admission, or whose recent food intake has been minimal, on the full increasing diet. Half portions may be given for the first week, with a gradual increase after this to a diet of 2000–2500 kcal or more according to weight gain. Excesses of fibre should particularly be avoided. Patients should be monitored for refeeding syndrome as rapid hyperalimentation may result in pancreatitis and/or serious electrolyte disturbances, for example hypophosphataemia, hypomagnesaemia and hypokalaemia. Bed rest may be necessary and magnesium supplements may help if refractory hypocalcaemia or hypokalaemia are present. Hypophosphataemia is unlikely if refeeding is initiated gradually, but phosphate levels should be monitored and supplements may be necessary [33].

If patients are following a vegetarian diet on admission this will require reviewing; generally, if this has arisen before AN, it may be continued. If vegetarianism has arisen within AN, ideally it should be given up, in the same way that the anorectic's other imposed dietary restrictions are to be relinquished, but a policy on this should be decided on by the treatment team.

If the hospital menu includes salad meals and/or sandwiches as an alternative to cooked main courses, a decision must be reached as to whether these are permitted, and if so, how frequently. It is good practice to include cooked meals where possible, as these will often have been omitted by the patient in favour of salads. However, for in-patients on a general ward, it seems reasonable to give the same meals as the other patients receive, rather than further isolating the patient from everybody else at meal times. It should also be borne in mind that the satiety factor of hot meals is greater than for cold meals and patients may need reassurance about this.

Patients will often be constipated as a result of both a low intake of food/fluid and laxative withdrawal and may request bran/bran cereals to help this. If bran is taken this may be at the expense of other foods, as bran is both bulky with a low nutrient density and may actively inhibit mineral absorption. Provided adequate fluid is taken, and wholemeal bread and wholegrain breakfast cereals are allowed, together with normal portions of vegetables and some fruit (in puddings where appropriate), an adequate fibre intake will be achieved. Transit time may in any case be longer in AN [34] and complaints of feeling full for longer than is usual after meals (although these may be due to perception, and not reflect physiological reality [35]) should not be disregarded. Any patient who complains of severe pain after eating should receive appropriate medical examination.

Many patients will be concerned about including specific foods in their diet which they perceive as being particularly 'bad', i.e. 'fattening'. In addition to this, many anorectics will be concerned that they are including sugar-rich and fat-rich foods which are portrayed by the media as 'bad', for example biscuits, puddings, butter, cooked breakfasts. It is important to explain to this group that they need to include such foods to get used to incorporating a wide selection of foods into their diet. It is also important to stress that there is no absolute 'healthy' or 'unhealthy' food. From a practical point of view, the volume of food to be consumed to achieve an adequate energy intake if fat and sugar are totally avoided would be unrealistic, and patients would find it impossibly bulky.

It is accepted that many people have foods they do not like, for a variety of reasons. Similarly, some consideration should be made of the anorectic's likes and dislikes; Crisp [36] uses a 3000 kcal diet for all patients, with the option of three non-carbohydrate dislikes (e.g. curry, offal). An alternative is to offer two main-course choices with similar energy content.

The area of nasogastric feeding and the use of dietary supplements in AN has undergone revision in the last few years. Whilst nasogastric feeding has rarely been shown to be necessary, unless a patient is physically too weak to eat, the role of supplements requires more consideration. Supplying hidden supplements, for example glucose polymers, in drinking water is dishonest, and only serves to distort the patient's perceptions of the effect of food on their body still further, as they will appear to be gaining weight on a smaller intake than would be the case with 'real food'. Providing adequate support can be given to the patient, it should be possible to avoid the use of other supplements, and rely upon ordinary food and drink to meet the patient's requirements.

Total parenteral nutrition would normally only be used if the gut cannot be used to supply nutrition.

At present in the UK, policies on the inclusion of 'bad/forbidden' foods into patients' refeeding programmes varies widely. Some units permit patients to select their own meals from the menus provided, but this will tend to lead to a very restricted choice. Other units compromise and allow patients to select their own meals, but specify that foods currently avoided are to be reintroduced one at a time. If only limited food dislikes are allowed it is reasonable to expect in-patients to eat the meals provided on a refeeding/treatment programme within a week or so, providing psychological support is given.

Once issues such as those discussed above have been resolved, a meal plan can be devised. In general, on non-specialist units the patient with AN should be given the same meals as the other patients, although quantities will generally need to be specified. Other patients will often take an interest and care must be taken that the anorectic patient is not 'helped' by other patients disposing of food! A sample

Table 71.1 Meal plan (2500 kcal) for anorectic in-patients, with modifications for 3000 kcal.

Meal plan	Modifications
Breakfast	
Small glass of fruit juice	
Medium bowl of cereal with 1 cup milk and 2 teaspoons sugar	
1 poached egg on 1 medium slice buttered toast	
1 medium slice bread and butter	
Tea/coffee with milk	
Mid-morning	
Tea/coffee with milk	Milky coffee
2 sweet biscuits	Sandwich (2 slices bread)
Lunch	
Beef casserole (100 g meat)	
4 small potatoes	
100 g portion vegetables	
Fruit pie (90 g portion) and custard (100 mg)	
Mid-afternoon	
Tea/coffee with milk	
Sandwich (2 slices bread)	+ Cake (60 g slice)
Evening meal	
1 medium bowl soup	+ 1 roll & butter (10 g)
Roast lamb (100 g)	
4 small potatoes	
Vegetables (100 g)	
Small bowl fruit and 1 brickette ice-cream	
Bedtime	
Milky drink	
2 plain biscuits	

meal plan for in-patients is shown in Table 71.1: the meal plan provides about 2500 kcal, and the modifications would adjust this to about 3000 kcal.

To avoid head-on battles at meal times, it is essential to specify exact portion sizes, particularly if those serving meals are unused to patients with AN. Patients will feel very insecure if they are served varying portions by different members of nursing staff—an inevitable result if inadequate detail is provided. Furthermore, staff will be tempted to serve an overly large portion even if the patient is actually attempting to request the correct amount. Feelings of insecurity will be worsened by inexperienced staff who ask patients to specify their own meal portion sizes.

Out-patient advice

While attitudes to weight gain and dietary prescription vary widely for in-patients, the units dealing with AN in the UK that the author was able to speak to had a remarkably uniform treatment of out-patients. It is accepted that patients not receiving the intensity of psychological input available to in-patients will not be able to increase their food intake in the same way as these patients. Targets for increasing intake are small but reviewed regularly. If patients are taking less than three meals per day, the first aim is to eat something for each 'meal'. Once this has been achieved, increases of around 200 kcal/day are aimed for each week, with a progression from foods the patient finds easy to include in their diet, to those felt to be 'bad'. Carbohydrate should be included at each meal, the quantity being gradually increased, and protein should be included in normal amounts. These patients have little idea of normal portion sizes and frequently find shopping for food a frightening experience, as they find themselves confronted by so much choice. It is usually necessary to specify details of foods exactly, for example two slices of bread from a small loaf from a specific bakery with two teaspoons butter and one slice cheese from a specified brand. If patients present with weight-related amenorrhoea of short duration and/or weight loss with an inadequate but still reasonable energy intake, it is prudent to immediately prescribe a high-energy diet. Counselling will, however, often be required for the patient to be able to meet the prescription.

Weight maintenance

In-patients should ideally not be discharged immediately target weight is reached, although hospitals with long waiting lists may find themselves under pressure to do this. Patients with AN often find the period of establishing a level of intake to maintain their weight stressful, and it could be argued that using relatively moderate energy intakes for weight gain is beneficial, as weight gain will slow as requirements increase and fairly minor adjustments will permit weight maintenance. It is particularly at this stage of treatment that dietetic involvement is valuable [37]. If the anorectic has until now had no choice of meals, and all responsibility for meal provision has been with the treatment team, this responsibility and choice must be returned to the patient. If time permits this should be done gradually, i.e. one meal at a time. As eating patterns have usually been distorted for months, often years, re-education of patients regarding 'normal' meal patterns is required. The information required is often very basic, for example a snack meal alternative to a cooked meal and pudding, and guidance as to average portion sizes.

Bulimia nervosa

Patients with BN may be at or above ideal bodyweight, or may suffer from AN simultaneously. Patients presenting at or above ideal weight will often feel they need a strict reducing diet prescribed. In reality, the key to breaking a starve/binge/starve cycle (where a self-imposed drastic reducing diet proves unsustainable, leading to consumption of vast amounts of food resulting in extreme distress and subsequent return to the punitive reducing diet until this once more becomes unbearable), or a pattern of bingeing and vomiting, is to prescribe a diet providing adequate energy and carbohydrate and to stress to the patient that this is not the time to try and lose weight. This is to allow the patient time to learn to distinguish between physiological and emotional hunger. In practice, planned regular meals and snacks including at least 180–200 g carbohydrate per day, depending on predicted energy requirements, will release the patient from the stress of the deprivation and hunger normally experienced. Carbohydrate should come both from the dietary staples of cereals, bread, potatoes, rice, pasta and also from foods containing sugar such as cakes, biscuits and puddings. Patients will often find the idea of incorporating the latter group of foods extremely distressing as these have often only been consumed in binges. Patients are often terrified that they will be unable to stop after, for example, two biscuits or one slice of cake, and may initially only be able to include such foods under supervision. Laxative abusers need to know that their habit will not significantly affect their weight, as laxative use has little impact on energy balance [38]. For those initially overweight, following a diet that is far more than they would allow themselves on a 'good' day (but substantially less than on days when binges occur) will result in a gradual reduction of weight. This requires careful explanation to the patient as many find the prospect of a sustained 'normal' diet incompatible with weight control.

Long-term support

Many patients find it takes some months before the senses of hunger/satiety return sufficiently to be relied upon. During this time, review of the patient's diet and weight by the dietitian allows the patient to explore meal patterns and relearn about 'normal' eating. Crises in the patient's life provide a temptation to revert to their anorectic/bulimic behaviour, hence the need for long-term psychological support.

Additional help

In the UK, the major organisation providing help and support for both sufferers and their families is the Eating Disorders Association (EDA). The EDA can give guidance towards appropriate counsellors in particular geographic areas and also supply a list of relevant literature for patients and their families (Eating Disorders Association, Sackville Place, 44 Magdalen Street, Norwich, Norfolk NR3 1JE).

References

1 Bailey S, Goldberg J. Eating patterns and weight concerns of college women. *J Am Dietet Ass* 1989; 1: 95–6.

2 Ash JB, Piazza E. Changing symptomatology in eating disorders. *Int J Eating Disord* 1995; **18**: 27–38.

3 Beumont PJV, O'Connor M, Touyz SW, Williams H. Nutritional counselling in the treatment of anorexia and bulimia nervosa. In: Beumont PJV, Burrows GD, Caspar R, eds. *Handbook of Eating Disorders*, Part 1. Amsterdam: Elsevier Science Publishers, 1987.

4 Russell GFM. The nutritional disorder in anorexia nervosa. *J Psychosom Res* 1967; **11**: 141–9.

5 Beumont PJV, Chambers TL. The diet composition and nutritional knowledge of patients with anorexia nervosa. *J Hum Nutr* 1981; **35**: 265–73.

6 Simon Y, Bellisle F, Monneuse M-O, Samuel-Lajeunesse B,

Drewnowski A. Taste responsiveness in anorexia nervosa. *Br J Psychiatr* 1993; **162**: 244–6.

7 Beumont P. The clinical presentation of anorexia and bulimia nervosa. In: Brownell KD, Fairburn C (eds). *Eating Disorders and Obesity: A Comprehensive Handbook*. New York: The Guildford Press, 1995.

8 Kadambari R, Gowers S, Crisp A. Some correlates of vegetarianism in anorexia nervosa. *Int J Eating Disord* 1986; **5**: 539–44.

9 Beardsworth AD, Keil ET. Vegetarianism, veganism and meat avoidance: recent trends and findings. *Br Food J* 1991; **93**: 19–24.

10 Philipp E, Pirke K-M, Seidl M *et al.* Vitamin status in patients with anorexia nervosa and bulimia nervosa. *Int J Eating Disord* 1988; **8**: 209–18.

11 Rock C, Vasantharajan S. Vitamin status of eating disorder patients: relationship to clinical indices and effect of treatment. *Int J Eating Disord* 1995; **18**: 257–62.

12 Woodruff P, Morton J, Russell G. Neuromyopathic complications in a patient with anorexia nervosa and vitamin C deficiency. *Int J Eating Disord* 1994; **16**: 205–9.

13 Vandereycken W, Meerman R. How should an inpatient treatment programme be structured? *Anorexia Nervosa: A Clinician's Guide to Treatment*. Berlin: de Gruyter, 1984.

14 Touyz SW, Lennerts W, Freeman RJ, Beumont PJ. To weigh or not to weigh? Frequency of weighing and rate of weight gain in patients with anorexia nervosa. *Br J Psychiatry* 1990; **157**: 752–4.

15 Gwirtsman H, Kaye W, Curtis S, Lyter L. Energy intake and dietary macronutrient content in women with anorexia nervosa and volunteers. *J Am Dietet Ass* 1989; **1**: 54–7.

16 Russell GFM, Mezey AG. An analysis of weight gain in patients with anorexia nervosa treated with high calorie diets. *Clin Sci* 1962; **23**: 449–61.

17 Walker J, Roberts S, Halmi K, Goldberg S. Caloric requirements for weight gain in anorexia nervosa. *Am J Clin Nutr* 1979; **32**: 1396–400.

18 Dempsey D, Crosby L, Pertschuk M, Feurer I, Buzby G, Mullen J. Weight gain and nutritional efficacy in anorexia nervosa. *Am J Clin Nutr* 1984; **39**: 236–42.

19 Kaye W, Gwirtsman H, Obarzanek E, George D. Relative importance of calorie intake needed to gain weight and level of physical activity in anorexia nervosa. *Am J Clin Nutr* 1988; **47**: 987–94.

20 Salisbury JJ, Levine AS, Crow SJ, Mitchell JE. Refeeding, metabolic rate, and weight gain in anorexia nervosa: a review. *Int J Eating Disord* 1995; **17**: 337–45.

21 Kaye W, Gwirtsman H, George T, Ebert M, Petersen R. Caloric consumption and activity levels after weight recovery in anorexia nervosa: a prolonged delay in normalization. *Int J Eating Disord* 1986; **5**: 489–502.

22 Kaye W, Gwirtsman H, Obarzanek E, George T, Jimerson D, Ebert M. Caloric intake necessary for weight maintenance in anorexia nervosa: nonbulimics require greater caloric intake than bulimics. *Am J Clin Nutr* 1986; **44**: 435–43.

23 Forbes G, Kreipe R, Lipinski B, Hodgman C. Body composition changes during recovery from anorexia nervosa: comparison of two dietary regimes. *Am J Clin Nutr* 1984; **40**: 1137–45.

24 Vaisman N, Corey M, Rossi M, Goldberg E, Pencharz P. Changes in body composition during refeeding of patients with anorexia nervosa. *J Pediatr* 1988; **113**: 925–9.

25 Pirke K, Pahl J, Schweiger U, Munzing W, Lang P, Bull U. Total body potassium, intracellular potassium and body composition in patients with anorexia nervosa during refeeding. *Int J Eating Disord* 1986; **5**: 347–54.

26 Fonseca V, D'Souza V, Houlder S, Thomas M, Wakeling A, Dandona F. Vitamin D deficiency and low osteocalcin concentrations in anorexia nervosa. *J Clin Pathol* 1988; **41**: 195–7.

27 Biller B, Saxe V, Herzog D, Rosenthal D, Holzman S, Klibanski A. Mechanisms of osteoporosis in adult and adolescent women with anorexia nervosa. *J Clin Endocrinol Metab* 1989; **68**: 548–54.

28 Rigotti N, Nussbaum S, Herzog D, Neer R. Osteoporosis in women with anorexia nervosa. *N Engl J Med* 1984; **311**: 1601–6.

29 Szmukler G, Brown S, Parsons V, Darby A. Premature loss of bone in chronic anorexia nervosa. *Br Med J* 1985; **290**: 26.

30 Kotler L, Katz L, Angan W, Comite F. Case study of the effects of prolonged and severe anorexia nervosa on bone mineral density. *Int J Eating Disord* 1994; **15**: 395–9.

31 Snow-Harter C, Bouxsein ML, Lewis BT, Carter DR, Marcus R. Effects of resistance and endurance exercise on bone mineral status of young women: a randomised exercise trial. *J Bone Miner Res* 1992; **7**: 761–9.

32 Beumont PJ, Arthur B, Russell JD, Touyz SW. Excessive physical activity in dieting disorder patients: proposals for a supervised exercise program. *Int J Eat Disord* 1994; **15**: 21–36.

33 Sharp CW, Freeman CP. The medical complications of anorexia nervosa. *Br J Psychiatr* 1993; **162**: 452–62.

34 Lautenbacher S, Galfe G, Hoelzl R, Pirke K. Gastrointestinal transit is delayed in patients with bulimia. *Int J Eating Disord* 1989; **8**: 203–8.

35 Robinson PH. Perceptivity and paraceptivity during measurement of gastric emptying in anorexia and bulimia nervosa. *Br J Psychiatr* 1989; **154**: 400–5.

36 Crisp A. *Anorexia Nervosa: Let Me Be*. London: Academic Press, 1980.

37 Bowyer C. Dietary factors in eating disorders. In: Scott D, ed. *Anorexia and Bulimia Nervosa: Practical Approaches*. London: Croom Helm, 1988.

38 Lacey JH, Gibson E. Does laxative abuse control body weight? A comparative study of purging and vomiting bulimics. *Hum Nutr Appl Nutr* 1985; **39**: 36–42.

Part 16
The Hyperlipidaemias: Diagnosis and Management

CHAPTER 72

The hyperlipidaemias: diagnosis and management

D.J. Galton and M.G. Baroni

Lipid physiology

Lipids as fuels: transport

In order to maintain the homeostatic mechanisms of the body, a constant and well-regulated supply of fuel is required. The basic elements of a simple fuel supply involve storage, transport and oxidation for release of energy [1]. Fats are excellent storage fuels, but are difficult to transport in plasma because of their insolubility in water [2]. Fatty acids circulate as a complex with albumin and constitute an important immediate supply of energy. Although their concentration is 10-fold lower than glucose in plasma (they were unrecognised for a long time as a circulating fuel), their turnover time is seven times greater than that of glucose; they can therefore provide calories in the same range as the fasting blood glucose. However, there is an upper limit set to their concentration in plasma because they are fatty acids and thus will cause a metabolic acidosis if their concentration rises too high. For this reason they circulate in esterified form as triglycerides, which in turn has led to the evolution of the lipoproteins. Lipoproteins are designed to transport triglyceride and cholesterol from the intestines and liver for use in peripheral tissues as an oxidisable fuel and supply of apolar molecules for the assembly and maintenance of cell membranes [3]. Lipoproteins are complex aggregates of lipid and protein molecules which are sufficiently stable to form particles (or micelles) for circulation in plasma [4]. A complicated set of proteins, enzymes and receptors has evolved to optimise the transport and delivery of fat to peripheral tissues. Unfortunately, this not infrequently breaks down and gives rise to the common disorders of lipid transport (the hyperlipidaemias) and disorders of lipid storage (particularly atherosclerosis [5]).

Lipoprotein structure

The lipoprotein particle consists of an outer shell of phospholipids and cholesterol in which are embedded various peptide components (the apolipoproteins). This outer shell stabilises the particle in the aqueous environment of the plasma (Fig. 72.1). Some of the peptides carry sites for receptor recognition to allow uptake of the particle into cells; others can activate enzymes involved in the breakdown of the particle for release of its lipid load. The core of the particle carries the lipid load: as triglyceride in the case of chylomicrons or very-low-density lipoprotein (VLDL); as cholesterol in the case of low-density lipoprotein (LDL); or as phospholipid in the case of high-density lipoprotein (HDL) (Fig. 72.1). The particle size will clearly vary depending on the nature and quantity of the lipid core, the triglyceride-rich particles (chylomicrons and VLDL) being larger than the cholesterol-rich particles (LDL). The size of the particle and its lipid composition will also affect its buoyant density or flotation rates, and this provides one way of separating the major lipoprotein classes into chylomicrons, VLDL, LDL and HDL by means of density-gradient centrifugation [6].

Lipoprotein(a) (Fig. 72.2)

One extraordinary lipoprotein has recently been analysed which consists of the cholesterol-rich lipoprotein LDL attached to a long repeated chain of a structure found in plasminogen called Kringle 4 (Kringle because of its supposed resemblance to a pastry, like a pretzel). Plasminogen is part of the fibrinolytic system, being converted to the enzyme plasmin which breaks down fibrin and assists in the dissolution of a thrombus. The reason why a component of plasminogen should be found attached to a cholesterol-rich lipoprotein at present defies explanation. However, elevated

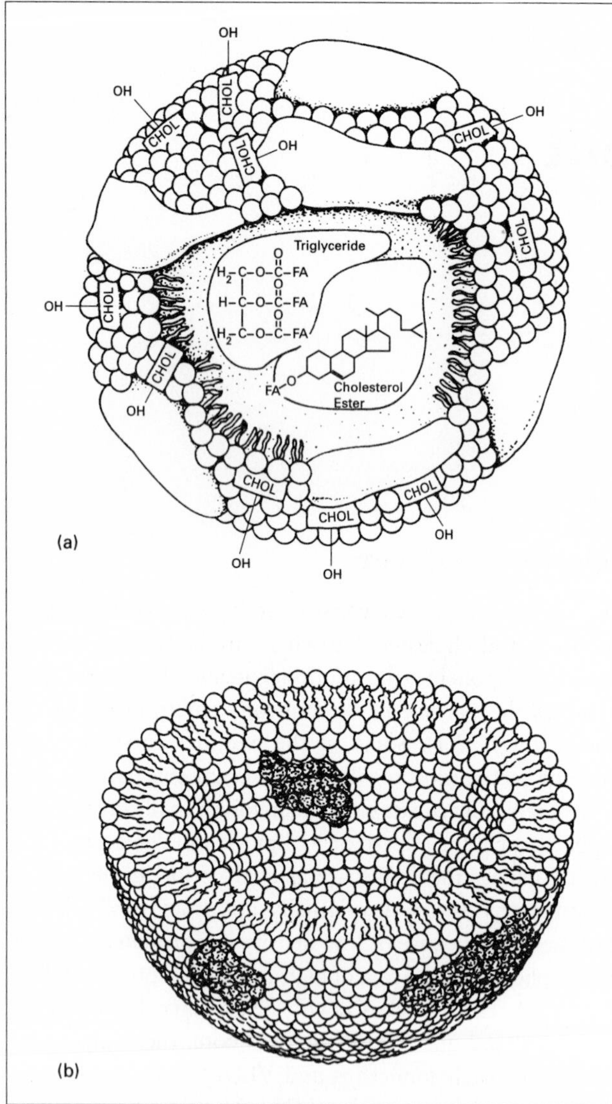

Fig. 72.1 (a) Schematic model for plasma lipoproteins. CHOL, cholesterol; OH, hydroxyl group; FA, fatty acid. (b) The outer shell of a lipoprotein particle carrying peptides and phospholipids.

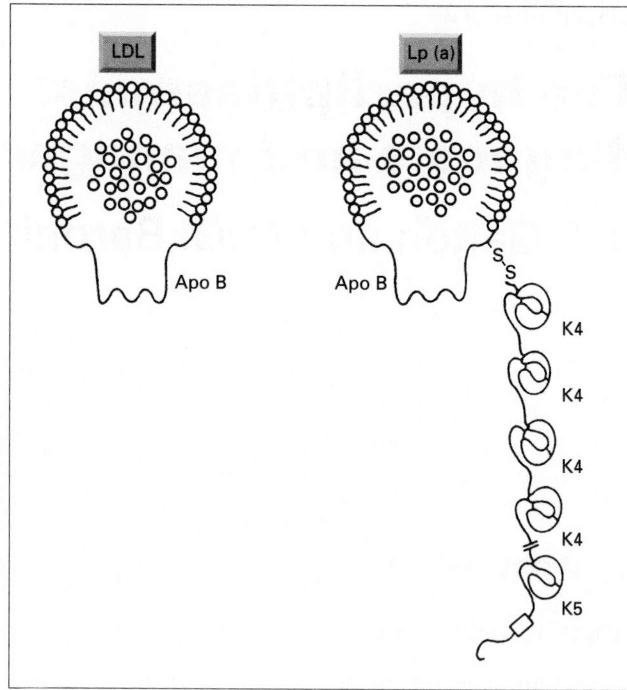

Fig. 72.2 Schematic representation of low-density lipoprotein (LDL) and lipoprotein(a) (Lp(a)). Note the apo(a) peptide linked by a disulphide bridge to apo B in the Lp(a) particle. K4 and K5 denote Kringles 4 and 5, respectively.

levels of lipoprotein(a) have been found in patients with premature coronary artery disease and in some way it may interfere with the normal function of plasminogen at the endothelial lining of arteries to remove small fibrin deposits and therefore promote thrombosis, particularly at the site of the atheromatous deposit.

Lipid composition of lipoproteins

As can be seen in Fig. 72.3, the triglyceride content of lipoproteins decreases steadily from chylomicrons at 90% to HDL at 3%. Conversely, the phospholipid content increases from 4% in chylomicrons to 27% in HDL. The decreasing content of triglyceride from chylomicrons to HDL largely accounts for the differences in buoyant densities of these lipoproteins.

The peptide composition of the lipoproteins also varies considerably amongst the classes, although in no regular way. Table 72.1 illustrates the main component peptides of each lipoprotein; it should be noted that LDL probably contains only one apolipoprotein B molecule per particle. Properties of the individual peptides and their possible functions are presented in Tables 72.1 and 72.2. Some notable features are the apo-B100 peptide, the most abundant protein in LDL, which contains a domain for binding to the LDL receptor on peripheral cells; mutations at this site can interfere with the removal of LDL cholesterol from plasma. The apo-CII peptide is an essential activator of the enzyme lipoprotein lipase, and defects of this peptide can interfere with the removal of triglyceride-rich lipoproteins from plasma.

Sources of lipoproteins

The triglyceride-rich lipoproteins originate from the intestines and liver. Dietary fat is broken down to fatty acids and partial glycerides in the small intestine by the action of pancreatic and intestinal lipases. During absorption in the

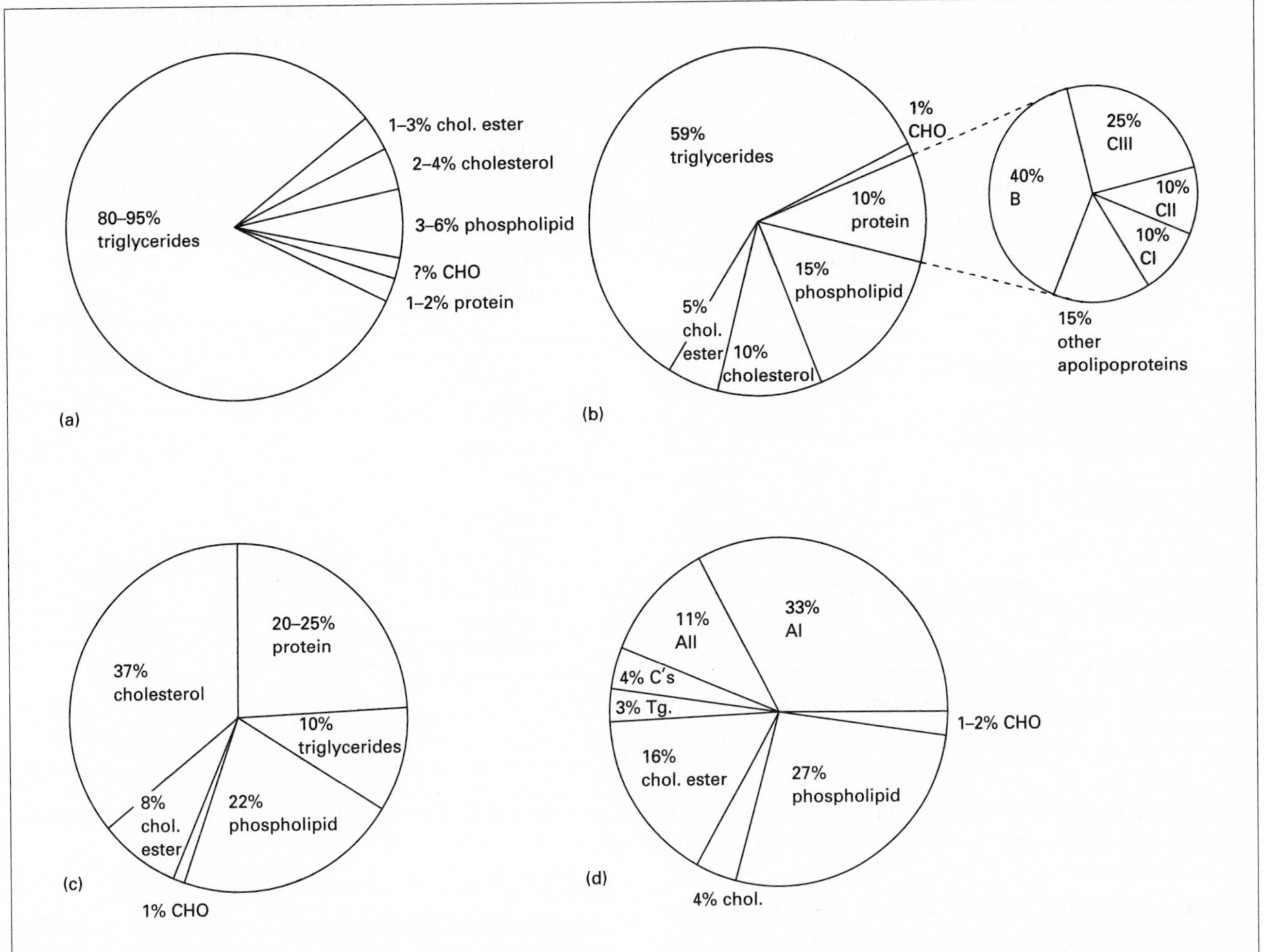

Fig. 72.3 Lipid and protein composition of the lipoproteins. (a) Chylomicron; (b) very-low-density lipoprotein (VLDL); (c) low-density lipoprotein (LDL) (the mass of apolipoprotein B remains constant in each lipoprotein particle, whereas apolipoprotein C is present in only the less dense LDL in the process of conversion from VLDL and intermediate-density lipoprotein (IDL)); (d) high-density lipoprotein (HDL).

Table 72.1 Apolipoproteins of human plasma. From [40].

Apolipoprotein	Density class	Function
AI	HDL	Activation of LCAT, transport of polar lipids
AII	HDL	Activation of hepatic lipase
B	VLDL, LDL, Lp(a)	Mediates receptor-mediated catabolism of LDL
CII	CYM, VLDL	Activates LPL
CIII	CYM, VLDL	Involved in triglyceride clearance
E	VLDL, IDL	Binds to specific E receptor, causes CYM remnant clearance
Lp(a)	HDL_1	Unknown

CYM, chylomicron; HDL, high-density lipoprotein; IDL, intermediate-density lipoprotein; LCAT, lecithin–cholesteryl acyltransferase; LDL, low-density lipoprotein; Lp(a), lipoprotein(a); LPL, lipoprotein lipase; VLDL, very-low-density lipoprotein.

mucosal wall of the gut they are resynthesised to triglyceride for packaging into chylomicrons for transport through the lymphatic ducts into the bloodstream. Endogenous fat synthesised in the liver from glucose and fatty acids is secreted into the bloodstream as VLDL. Small chylomicrons are virtually indistinguishable in their lipid composition from

Table 72.2 Properties of human apolipoproteins.

Apolipoproteins	Molecular weight	No. of residues	Site of synthesis	Function
AI	28300	243	Intestine, liver	Activates LCAT
AII	17000	154	Liver, intestine	–
B100	549000	4536	Liver	Binds LDL receptor
B48	246000	2152	Intestine	–
CI	6331	57	Liver	Activates LCAT
CII	8837	78	Liver	Activates LPL
CIII	8764	79	Liver	?Inhibits LPL
E2, E3, E4	33000	299	Liver, intestine	Binds to remnant receptors

LDL, low-density lipoprotein; LPL, lipoprotein lipase; LCAT, lecithin–cholesteryl acyltransferase.

large VLDL, the quantity of triglyceride per particle varying with the nutritional status at the time of synthesis. During the circulation of triglyceride-rich lipoproteins, they are gradually delipidated by the action of lipolytic enzymes (lipoprotein lipase and hepatic lipase) and converted by way of intermediate-density lipoprotein (IDL) into the cholesterol-rich lipoproteins (LDL). During the conversion of VLDL to LDL some particles can be removed directly by binding to cell receptors such as the LDL receptor or remnant receptors [7].

Circulation of lipoproteins

The circulation of endogenous (liver-derived) lipoproteins is shown in Fig. 72.4. The output of liver VLDL depends on the supply of free fatty acids from adipose tissue stores

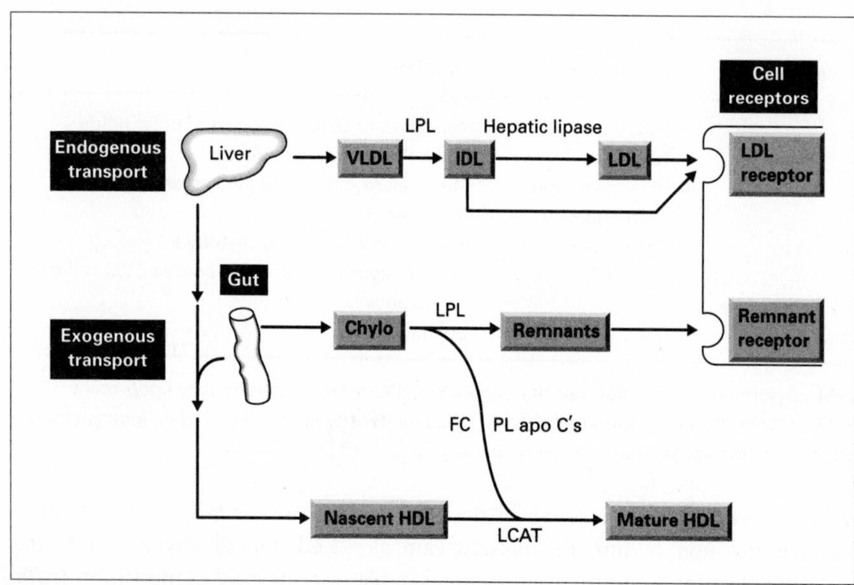

Fig. 72.4 Simplified scheme for lipid transport. Apo C, C apolipoproteins; Chylo, chylomicron; FC, free cholesterol; HDL, high-density lipoprotein; IDL, intermediate-density lipoprotein; LCAT, lecithin–cholesteryl acyltransferase; LDL, low-density lipoprotein; LPL, lipoprotein lipase; PL, phospholipids; VLDL, very-low-density lipoprotein.

and the supply of glucose to provide the glycerol. Under conditions of caloric excess the liver would be expected to synthesise and secrete large amounts of VLDL, but even in the fasting state the liver secretes VLDL from the influx of free fatty acids mobilised from adipose tissue and this maintains the fasting levels of plasma triglycerides. There are still many uncertainties in the circulation of lipoproteins; for example, what quantities of IDL are removed directly by cell receptors or metabolised through to LDL? Also, how many chylo-remnants are metabolised to LDL or removed directly by remnant receptors?

Source of HDL

HDL particles are secreted by the liver and intestines as disc-shaped structures where they are initially modified in the plasma by association with other apolipoproteins and enzymatic action (particularly the enzyme lecithin–cholesteryl acyltransferase, LCAT) converting them into spherical particles. They are further modified during the breakdown of VLDL into IDL where the small HDL_3 particle picks up surface components of VLDL, such as phospholipids and apolipoproteins C and E, to transform them into the larger HDL_2 particle. Another function of HDL may be in the reverse transport of cholesterol from peripheral tissues such as the arterial wall back to the liver for further metabolism, for example into bile salts [8]. HDL_3 would pick up cholesterol from the cell membrane, convert it to cholesteryl ester (by the action of LCAT) for transport in the core of the particle to the liver [9]. This is one mechanism whereby the body can deplete its peripheral stores of cholesterol and excrete it as bile salts into the intestines.

Enzymes involved in lipid transport

Lipoprotein lipase

This enzyme determines the rate of removal of triglyceride-rich lipoproteins derived from the liver and intestines from the bloodstream (Fig. 72.5). It catalyses the sequential hydrolysis of core triglyceride into di- and monoglycerides, and the final breakdown to free fatty acids and glycerol for uptake by peripheral tissues. The enzyme is synthesised in parenchymal cells such as heart, muscle and adipose tissue, and is then secreted by these cells into the capillary system for attachment to the luminal surface of endothelial cells; it binds circulating VLDL and chylomicrons for hydrolysis of their core lipid [10]. The particle is sequentially delipidated and eventually converted into a cholesterol-rich particle, LDL. Under fed conditions, lipoprotein lipase is induced in adipose tissue and diverts dietary fat for storage here. Under fasting conditions, the enzyme activity decreases in the capillary bed of adipose tissue and is induced in muscle and heart to divert VLDL to these sites for uptake of fatty acids as a fuel supply in addition to glucose. During lactation, there is a great increase of the enzyme activity in the capillary bed of the mammary gland to divert blood fat into the secreted milk.

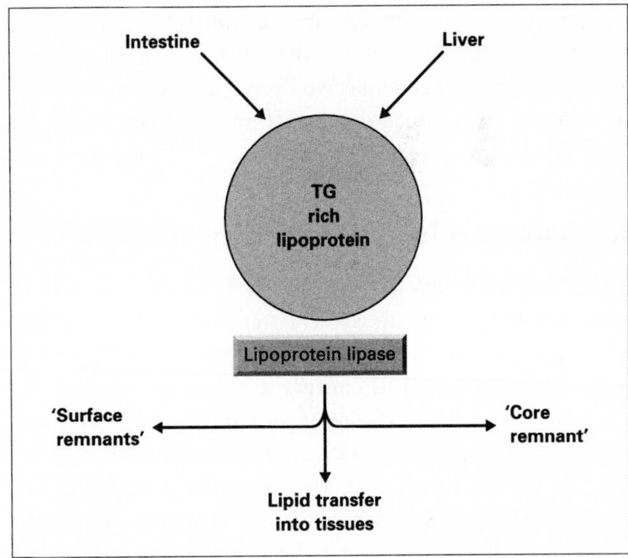

Fig. 72.5 Overview of the role of lipoprotein lipase in lipid transport and in the conversion of triglyceride (TG)-rich lipoproteins into other, denser lipoproteins.

Hepatic lipase

This enzyme is similar to lipoprotein lipase, except that it is made only in the liver and does not require apolipoprotein CII as activator. It too is involved in the sequential lipolytic breakdown of triglyceride-rich lipoproteins.

Lecithin–cholesteryl acyltransferase

This enzyme esterifies the reactive hydroxyl group of cholesterol with a fatty acid derived from lecithin, converting cholesterol into a more apolar (less electrically charged) molecule for transport in the core rather than shell of the lipoprotein particle. It is used in the maturation of HDL secreted by the liver, and probably also in the reverse transport of cholesterol from peripheral tissues by HDL back to the liver.

Cholesteryl ester transfer protein

There are other proteins involved in the exchange of cholesteryl esters amongst the different lipoproteins and between peripheral cells and lipoproteins. Cholesteryl ester transfer protein (CETP) acts mainly in the transfer of cholesteryl esters between HDL and trigylceride-rich lipoproteins. Mutants of these proteins have been recently found but do not appear to produce disease. If anything, they may be associated with increased longevity.

Receptors involved in lipoprotein catabolism

The delipidation of VLDL leads to LDL which now delivers cholesterol to peripheral cells. The steps in the cellular uptake of LDL are shown in Fig. 72.6. The particle binds to special LDL receptors found as clusters in the coated pits of the cell membrane. The LDL–receptor complex enters the cell as an endosome; the receptor is split off and possibly recycles back to the cell membrane. The endosome is acidified and converts to a lysosome where the apo-B peptide is digested and the cholesterol is liberated for use by the cell in the manufacture of cell membranes, at the same time switching off intracellular cholesterol synthesis by inhibiting the key enzyme in the pathway, hydroxymethylglutaryl coenzyme A (HMG-CoA) reductase. The structure of the LDL receptor has been worked out by the brilliant investigations of Brown and Goldstein (Nobel Prize winners for Medicine in 1985), and is shown in Fig. 72.7. It is divided into functional parts or domains with some of the key elements being the binding domain for LDL (the ligand), the membrane-spanning domain which anchors the receptor into the cell membrane, and the intracellular portion of the molecule which is involved in the formation of endosomes. Mutations at any of these sites can interfere with the function of the receptor leading to the genetic disease, familial hypercholesterolaemia [7].

The stages in the synthesis of the receptor involve its migration to the cell surface and eventual intracellular recycling. This complex regulation of the LDL receptor underlines the importance to the body of proper homeostatic mechanisms to maintain physiological tissue pools of cholesterol and prevent overloading of peripheral tissue sites [11].

Remnant receptor

During the circulation of lipoproteins chylomicrons are broken down to remnant particles which are thought to be removed by an additional receptor, the remnant receptor. A candidate has been recently discovered which bears some resemblance to the LDL receptor. Further work is still needed to prove whether this is in fact the receptor for the removal of remnants.

Epidemiology of blood lipid disorders and atherosclerosis

The size of the epidemiological problem is illustrated in Fig. 72.8, where the deaths from all the cancers are seen to be less than those from coronary heart disease in the UK. The difference is made even greater if stroke cases are added to the coronary heart disease group, as some of the former will arise on the basis of cerebrovascular atherosclerosis [12]. However, there is widespread variation in mortality rates from coronary heart disease among the various countries (Fig. 72.9), and this generally follows the order of mean blood cholesterol levels of the different populations (Fig. 72.10). If the two sets of data are put together (Fig. 72.11), there appears to be a good linear relationship between mean total blood cholesterol and relative incidence of coronary heart disease among world populations. Rural Chinese have

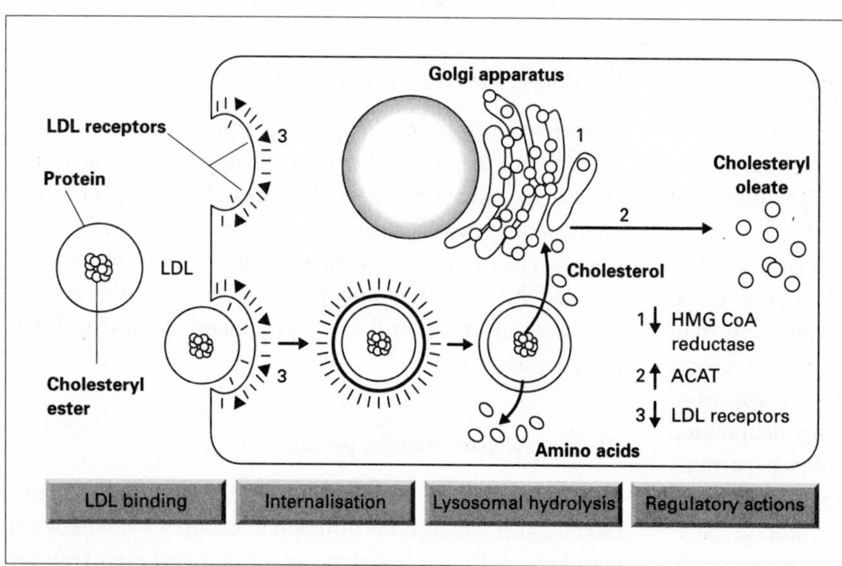

Fig. 72.6 Diagrammatic representation of a fibroblast showing uptake and partial degradation of low-density lipoprotein (LDL) via the LDL-receptor pathway. The resultant increase in free cholesterol down-regulates hydroxymethylglutaryl coenzyme A (HMG-CoA) reductase and LDL-receptor synthesis, and results in an increased rate of cholesterol esterification via acyl (ACAT). Adapted from [43].

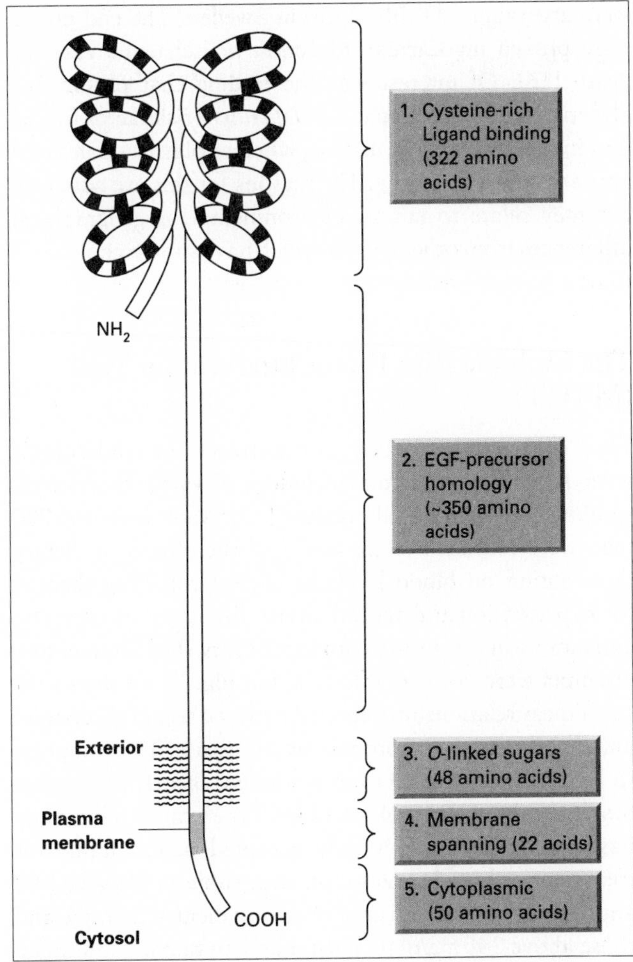

Fig. 72.7 The five domains in the structure of the human low-density lipoprotein (LDL) receptor. The sequence of the protein was deduced from the sequence of the cloned cDNA. The receptor is a dimer of two identical 839-residue polypeptides. From the amino-terminus, these domains are: (1) the ligand-binding site; (2) residues homologous to the precursor of the epidermal growth factor (EGF); (3) a region for O-linked glycosylation; (4) a membrane-spanning segment; (5) the COOH-terminal residue that projects into the cytoplasm. Adapted from [44].

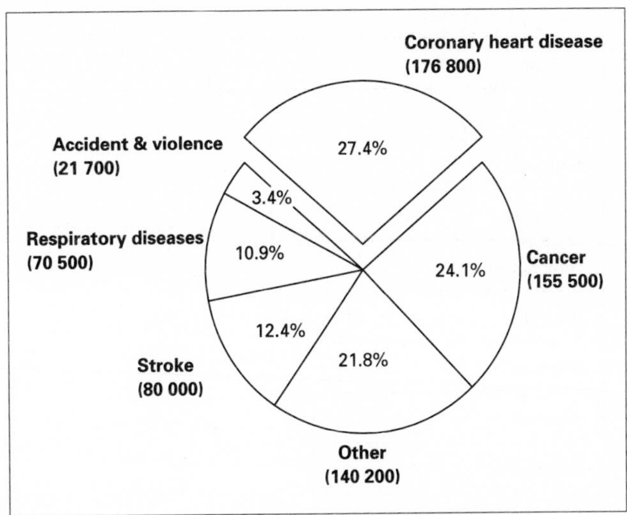

Fig. 72.8 Total deaths in the UK analysed by cause. From [45].

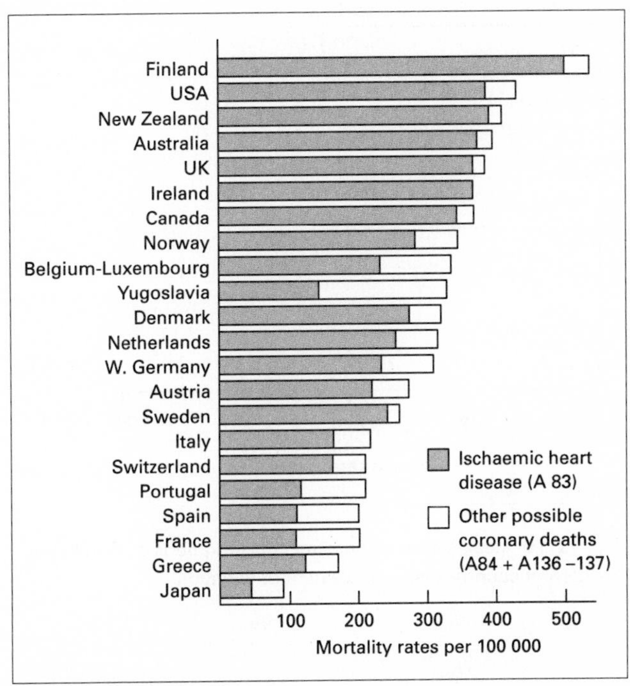

Fig. 72.9 Estimation of mortality rates from coronary heart disease among the 22 countries of the Organisation for Economic Cooperation and Development (OECD). Age-standardised rates for men aged 35–64 years. Adapted from [44].

the lowest mean blood cholesterol of 125 mg/dl (3.2 mM), and a mean coronary heart disease mortality rate in middle-age of only about 5% of those in the UK.

Many population studies have confirmed the relationship between the level of blood lipids and the incidence of coronary artery disease [13,14]. Three of these studies are reviewed briefly below.

The Framingham study

This was one of the earliest studies that followed prospectively the town members of Framingham just north of Boston, Massachusetts, for over 20 years [15]. The study revealed strong relationships between the level of total serum cholesterol and the risk of coronary heart disease (Fig. 72.12). The ratio of either total cholesterol/HDL cholesterol or LDL cholesterol/HDL cholesterol was strongly related to the risk of coronary heart disease, and there was also a strong relationship between triglyceride level and coronary heart disease in subjects with low levels of HDL (Fig. 72.13).

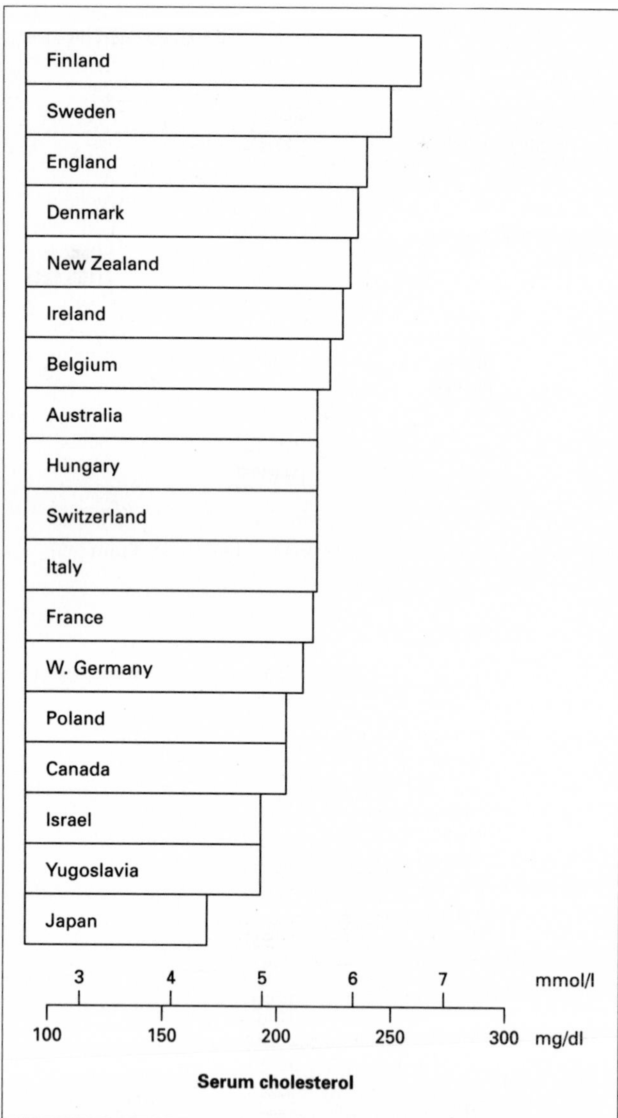

Fig. 72.10 Mean serum cholesterol concentrations of men living in different countries, showing extent of variation.

Many other epidemiological studies have confirmed and extended these observations. The Framingham study did not initially find that triglyceride-rich lipoproteins were an independent risk factor for coronary heart disease, but others such as the Stockholm prospective study did observe this. Subsequently the epidemiologists at Framingham have reconsidered the role of plasma triglycerides as a risk factor for atherosclerosis.

The Stockholm prospective study

This studied 3486 men prospectively for 14.5 years who were attending a health centre in Sweden. The end points were proven myocardial infarction or ischaemic vascular death [16]. Of interest was the finding that plasma triglycerides constitute a major *independent* risk factor for the development of arterial disease, whereas plasma cholesterol appears to be less strong. The reasons for this are not clear, but may relate to ethnic, environmental or geographical differences from other studies which have shown cholesterol to be a stronger risk factor.

The Multiple Risk Factor Intervention Trial (MRFIT)

This often-quoted study concentrated on individuals with several risk factors including elevated cholesterol, smoking and high blood pressure [17]. More than 300 000 men were recruited in the study of the effects of dietary intervention on blood levels of cholesterol, drug therapy for hypertension and special advice for stopping cigarette consumption, on future coronary events. The intervention attempts were not very effective, but Fig. 72.14 shows the curvilinear relationship obtained between serum cholesterol and death rates from coronary heart disease. There appears to be no threshold effect but a gradient of risk which rises more steeply as the cholesterol level is elevated. This study has given rise to the widely accepted action limits for treatment of blood cholesterol, with subjects between 200 and 240 mg/dl (5.2–6.5 mM) requiring dietary therapy, and those above 240 mg/dl (6.5 mM) likely to require additional drug therapy.

Disorders of lipid transport: the hyperlipidaemias

There are five main disorders of lipid transport which were initially classified by Fredrickson according to the lipoprotein that accumulates in plasma. The plasma appearance of the Fredrickson types are illustrated in Plate 72.1 (opposite p. 332), and the diagnosis in some cases can be made by simple visual inspection of a fasting plasma sample, for example for type I or type V hyperlipidaemia, where a creamy layer floats to the top of the tube with either a clear or turbid infranatant. However, this is a classification of greatest use to pathologists, while for clinicians a more aetiological classification is helpful, since this suggests treatments for possible causes.

A simple way to consider the origin of the hyperlipidaemias is to use the pool concepts of input and output from the plasma compartment (Fig. 72.15). Thus, an increased inflow of triglyceride from the liver, or a decreased output into peripheral tissues, will result in a hypertriglyceridae-

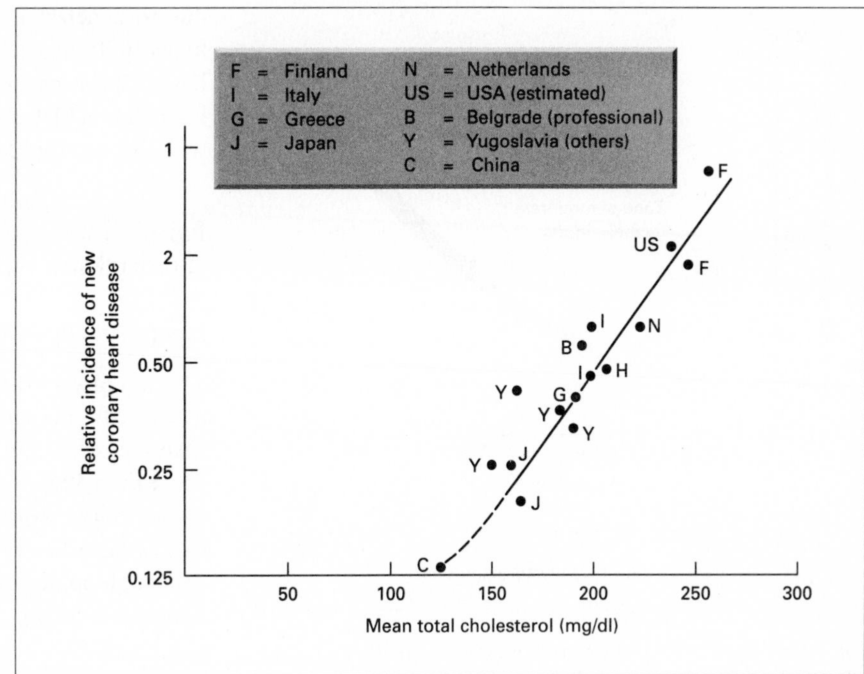

Fig. 72.11 Incidence of new coronary heart disease (any type) in different populations. (A recent survey in rural China has revealed a mean cholesterol level of 125 mg/dl, and mean coronary heart disease certification rates in middle age that are only 4% of those in the UK.)

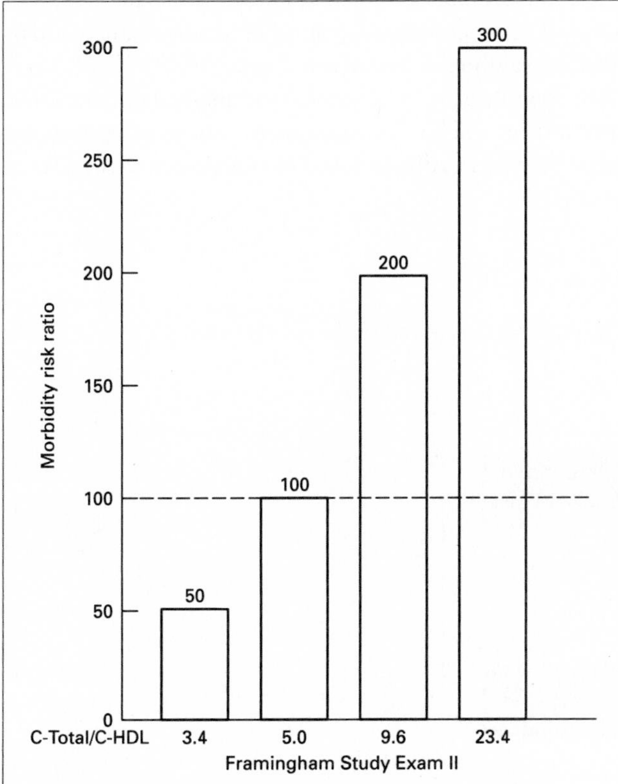

Fig. 72.12 Four-year risk of coronary heart disease according to the ratio of cholesterol/lipoprotein fractions. C-total, total cholesterol; C-HDL, high-density lipoprotein cholesterol. Adapted from [45].

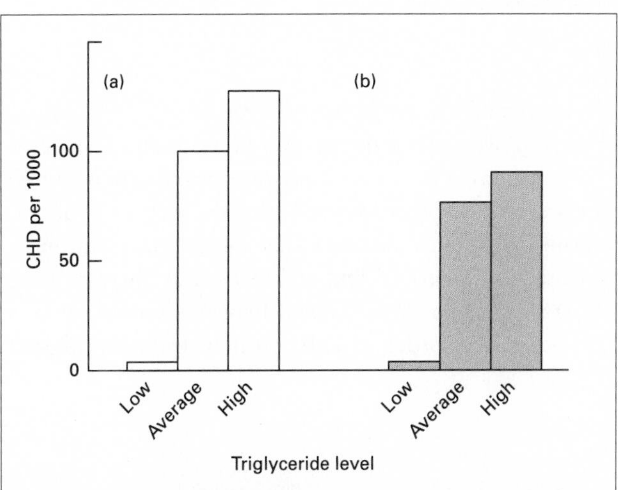

Fig. 72.13 Relationship between serum triglyceride level and incidence of coronary heart disease (CHD) in men and women with low levels of high-density lipoprotein (HDL) cholesterol in the Framingham study. (a) Men, HDL cholesterol < 40 mg/dl (< 1.04 mmol/l): low triglyceride < 94 mg/dl (< 1.1 mmol/l); average triglyceride 94–144 mg/dl (1.1–1.6 mmol/l); high triglyceride ⩾ 145 mg/dl (> 1.6 mmol/l). (b) Women, HDL cholesterol < 50 mg/dl (< 1.30 mmol/l): low triglyceride < 88 mg/dl (< 1.0 mmol/l); average triglyceride 88–135 mg/dl (1.0–1.5 mmol/l); high triglyceride 136 mg/dl (> 1.5 mmol/l). Eighty-five individuals per group. Adapted from [23].

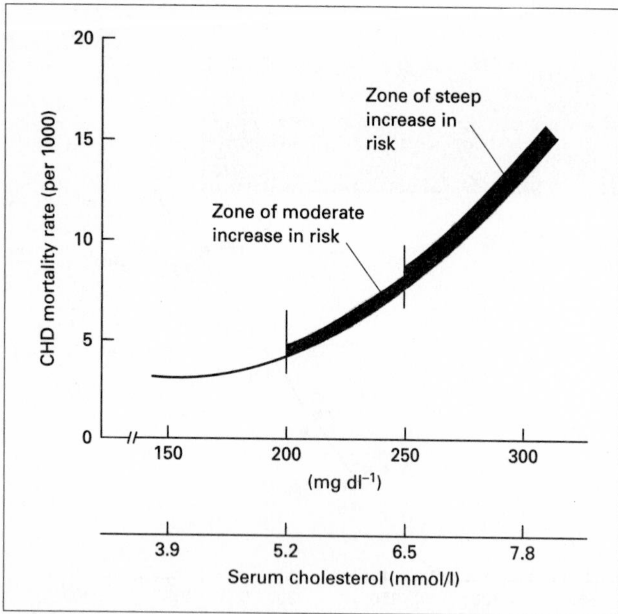

Fig. 72.14 Relationship between serum cholesterol level and risk of fatal coronary heart disease (CHD) in a longitudinal study of more than 361 000 men screened for entry into the Multiple Risk Factor Intervention Trial.

mia, and similarly for hypercholesterolaemia. The causes of the inflow–outflow defects can be primarily genetic or environmental (with a genetic predisposition). The acquired causes are often other systemic diseases such as hypothyroidism or diabetes mellitus. This clinical classification is presented in Table 72.3 and will be used in the rest of the text [18]. On this basis, familial hypercholesterolaemia is a monogenic disorder of LDL outflow from the plasma due to a defect in the LDL receptor. Familial combined hyperlipidaemia is a polygenic disorder (the genetic basis has not yet been elucidated) which gives rise to elevation of both plasma LDL and VLDL. The common hyperlipidaemias will now be considered.

Familial hypertriglyceridaemia (Fredrickson type IV)

Lipoprotein lipase defects

This is a rare autosomal recessive disorder in which there is a defect of the enzyme lipoprotein lipase which impairs clearance of VLDL and/or chylomicrons from the plasma. More than 39 different mutations have now been identified in the coding sequence of lipoprotein lipase that gives rise to this disorder. Very rarely it can be secondary to a dysgammaglobulinaemia which interferes with the function of lipoprotein lipase.

Diagnosis

The condition appears in childhood or adult life with episodes of acute abdominal pain (due to acute pancreatitis), eruptive xanthomas and lipaemia retinalis (Plates 72.2 and 72.3, opposite p. 332). Diagnosis is established by the plasma appearances and lipid measurements. Assays of lipoprotein lipase activity in adipose tissue or muscle define the nature of the lesion.

Treatment [19]

The major aim is to reduce blood fats as quickly as possible

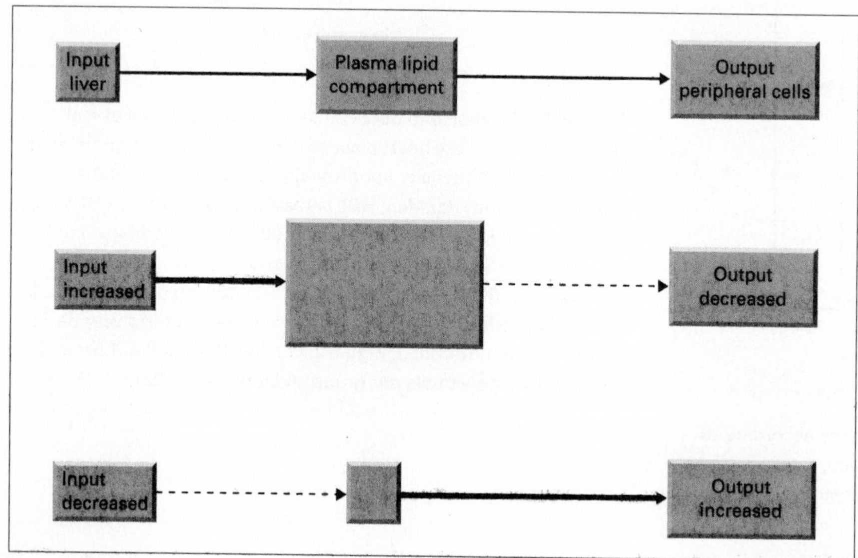

Fig. 72.15 Pool concept for origin of hyperlipidaemia.

Table 72.3 Classification of the hyperlipidaemias.

Disease	Elevated plasma cholesterol	Elevated plasma triglyceride
Familial (or primary)	Monogenic (LDL receptor and apolipoprotein B100 mutations) Polygenic	Monogenic (lipoprotein lipase and apolipoprotein CII mutations) Polygenic
Secondary	Hypothyroidism Nephrotic syndrome Diabetes mellitus [41,42] Biliary cirrhosis	Alcohol abuse Carbohydrate-induced Diabetes mellitus Obesity

to prevent further attacks of acute pancreatitis or retinal vascular thrombosis. A strict dietary reduction of long-chain triglycerides to < 0.29 g/kg bodyweight/day and substitution with medium-chain triglycerides to make a total daily intake of < 25 g/day will reduce the chylomicronaemia. Life-long adherence to this diet is required.

This condition is not characteristically associated with premature atherosclerosis; chylomicrons are not atherogenic, perhaps because their size excludes them from entry into the subendothelial space of the arterial wall.

Polygenic familial hypertriglyceridaemia [20]

This is a common heterogeneous group of disorders in which a genetic predisposition interacts with environmental factors such as dietary intake of fat or carbohydrate to produce a hypertriglyceridaemia. The possible causative factors are an increased synthesis of VLDL by the liver and/or an impaired clearance of VLDL by peripheral tissues. This hyperlipidaemia can present with ectopic lipid deposition at the corneal–scleral junction and eruptive xanthomas over the skin. The condition is atherogenic and should be actively treated. The major guidelines are reduction of bodyweight, reduction of animal fats in the diet and administration of hypolipidaemic drugs such as fibrates, nicotinates or marine oils if the plasma triglyceride levels fail to respond to simple dietary measures. Fuller details of treatment are given below.

Severe hypertriglyceridaemia (Fredrickson type V)

This forms a spectrum with the polygenic hypertriglyceridaemias and is characterised by a gross accumulation of triglyceride-rich lipoproteins in plasma, both of VLDL and chylomicrons. Uncontrolled diabetes mellitus is often the precipitating environmental factor in an individual who is already predisposed to develop a hypertriglyceridaemia [21,22]. The diagnostic features are profuse eruptive xanthomas, recurrent bouts of acute pancreatitis, lipaemia retinalis and retinal vascular occlusions [23–26].

The major guidelines of treatment are to bring the secondary conditions (such as diabetes mellitus) under control; to commence a low animal fat diet (< 15 g/day); to use hypolipidaemic drugs (fibrates or nicotinates); and in severe cases to perform plasma exchange.

Familial dyslipoproteinaemia ('broad-J' disease; remnant disease; Fredrickson type III)

In this polygenic disorder an abnormal IDL accumulates in plasma due to a defect in the VLDL lipolytic cascade. As a result a 'broad-J', lipoprotein accumulates which carries equal amounts of cholesterol and triglyceride.

Diagnostic features are:

1 a broad J-migrating band on electrophoresis;

2 a 'floating' LDL-like band on ultracentrifugation (floating because of its triglyceride content);

3 95% of cases are E2.E2. homozygous for the apoprotein;

4 tendinous and planar xanthomas, particularly in the skin creases of the hands.

Since this hyperlipidaemia is very atherogenic, it is important to treat it promptly; most cases respond well to the administration of fibrates.

Familial combined hyperlipidaemia (Fredrickson type IIb)

This is a fairly common hyperlipidaemia in which both plasma LDL and/or VLDL are elevated in many individuals of a pedigree, and there is overproduction of apolipoprotein B-100 by the liver. All the different types of hyperlipidaemia occur in the family members, and the lipoprotein phenotypes can be very variable in the same individual depending on nutritional status. It has been found as the commonest genetic form of hyperlipidaemia in relatives of survivors of myocardial infarction, occurring in up to 30% of the survivors. However, the genetics of the condition have not been elucidated, and it could be either due to the variable expression of a single autosomal dominant gene or to the segregation of two or more separate genes.

Familial combined hyperlipidaemia is clearly atherogenic and should be treated actively on the following lines:

1 reduction of bodyweight if obese;
2 a low animal fat/low cholesterol diet;
3 hypolipidaemic drugs (fibrates, nicotinates, statins);
4 regular monitoring of plasma lipids.

Familial hypercholesterolaemia (Fredrickson type IIa)

This has been the most intensively studied hyperlipidaemia following the discovery of the LDL receptor which plays a major role in the removal of LDL cholesterol from the blood. It is an autosomal dominant disorder occurring at a frequency of about 0.2% in Caucasian populations, and is due to a family of mutations occurring in the LDL-receptor gene on chromosome 19. These mutations involve deletions of part of the gene (e.g. the French-Canadian mutation deletes exon 1 and regulatory sequences close to it) or point mutations which may alter the structure of the LDL-receptor protein, and so interfere with LDL clearance from the blood. One reason why so many deletional mutants may occur in the LDL-receptor gene is the presence of numerous repeat sequences (the *Alu* repeats) which makes unequal recombination between parental genes more likely to occur.

The plasma abnormality of an elevation of LDL cholesterol, usually much higher than that found in polygenic hypercholesterolaemia, combined with ectopic cholesterol deposits in the cornea and in the extensor tendons of the hands or legs, and a positive family history of early arterial disease, establishes the diagnosis.

Treatment is aimed at reducing the blood cholesterol to <6.5 mmol/l (or to <4.5 mmol/l if arterial disease is already present) by the use of diet and drugs. Other procedures such as partial ileal bypass or LDL plasmapheresis can be helpful in the more severe cases. For the future, gene-replacement therapy of the LDL receptor is now feasible and has been performed in selected cases of homozygous familial hypercholesterolaemia with partial success. Regular follow-up is essential to ensure the blood cholesterol is maintained within normal limits, and to monitor the onset and progress of any signs of arterial disease.

Summary of defects in the lipoprotein cascade

A simple way to summarise the defects in lipoprotein breakdown is illustrated in Fig. 72.16. Considering the transformation of VLDL into LDL and then subsequent receptor-mediated clearance by peripheral cells, then:

1 defects at (a) (either of lipoprotein lipase or apo-CII) give rise to hypertriglyceridaemia;
2 defects at (b) (hepatic lipase) cause accumulation of IDL, for example broad-β, or remnant disease.
3 defects at (c) (at the receptor-binding domain of the B-apolipoprotein, such as the B-3500 mutation) lead to accumulation of LDL and a disease resembling familial hypercholesterolaemia;
4 defects of the LDL-receptor (d) give rise to familial hypercholesterolaemia.

Lipid-lowering therapy

When to treat

Cholesterol

The problem here is to know what is a 'normal' level of blood cholesterol [27,28]. Figure 72.10 shows that there is wide variation in the mean blood cholesterol among different countries [29]. Should we all try to maintain our blood cholesterol at the level of the rural Japanese? They have a comparably low incidence of coronary artery disease: what accounts for this variation? Partly it may be genetic, and partly environmental, depending on the amount of animal fats the population consumes. Classic dietary studies have shown a striking relationship between the percentage of calories derived from dietary fats and levels of blood cholesterol among groups as diverse as Japanese farmers and Europeans from Cape Town, South Africa (Fig. 72.17).

To eliminate the genetic component, one can study only Japanese men consuming traditional Japanese diets in southern Japan as compared with those on more Europeanised diets in Los Angeles, and again the consumption of animal fats bears a striking relationship with blood cholesterol levels (Fig. 72.18). So the problem of when to treat depends on which group of people one is considering, and where they live. One way to simplify this is to consider the curvilinear relationship of blood cholesterol to coronary heart disease, as found in the MRFIT study (Fig. 72.14).

Individuals with a blood cholesterol of <5.2 mmol/l (200 mg/dl) have a very low risk of coronary heart disease, which rises moderately between 5.2 and 6.5 mmol/l (200–250 mg/dl), and becomes steeper after 6.5 mmol/l (250 mg/dl). It seems reasonable therefore to treat individuals who have a high risk profile, for example family history of coronary artery disease, diabetes, previous angina or infarction, if their blood cholesterol is above 5.2 mmol/l (200 mg/dl). If they have a low-risk profile then only treat them if their blood cholesterol is above 6.5 mmol/l (250 mg/dl). Cholesterol levels requiring treatment as related to age groups as recommended by a USA consensus conference are given in

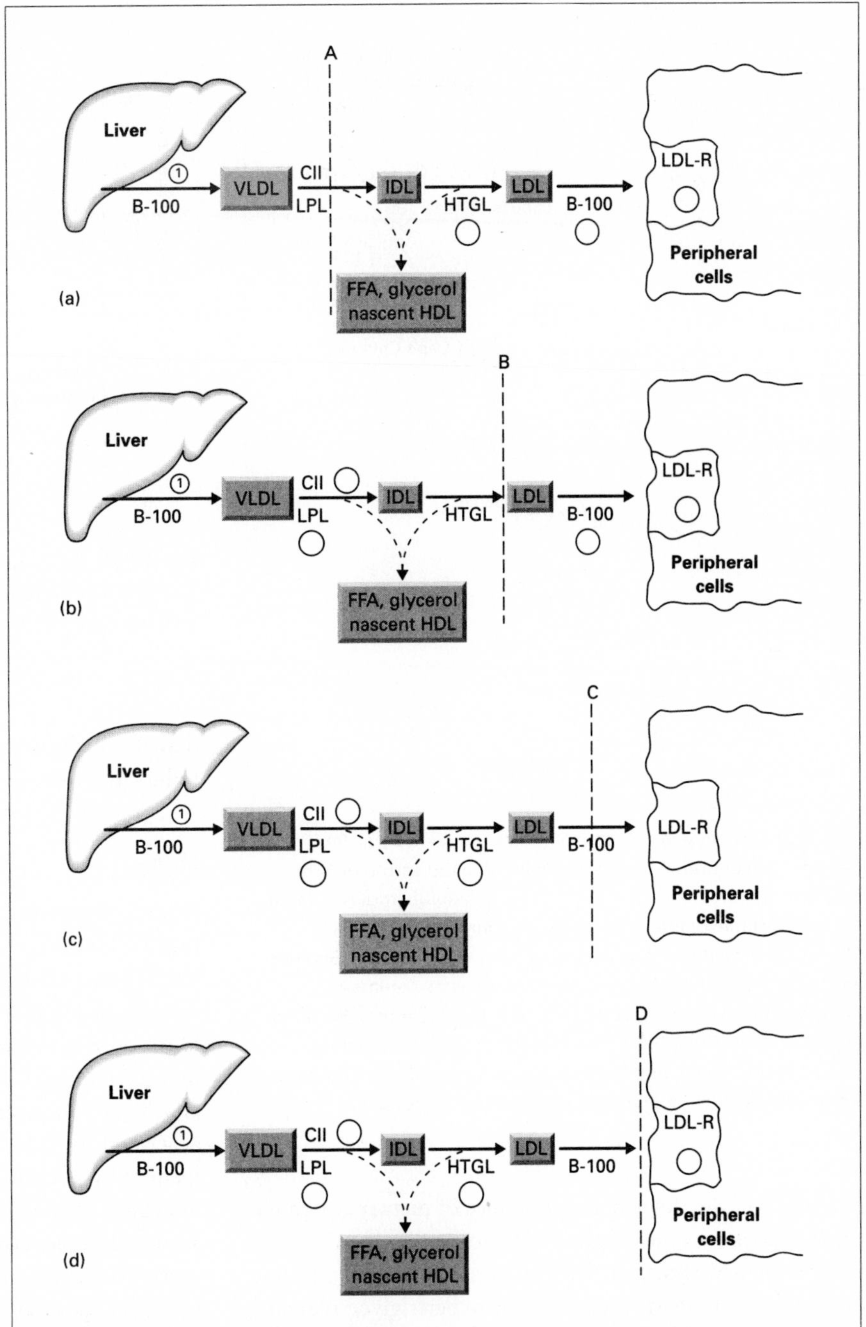

Fig. 72.16 Summary of defects in lipoprotein breakdown. FFA, free fatty acids; HDL, high-density lipoproteins; HTGL, hepatic triglyceride lipase; IDL, intermediate-density lipoprotein; LDL, low-density lipoprotein; LDL-R, LDL receptor; LPL, lipoprotein lipase; VLDL, very-low-density lipoprotein. See text for further explanation.

Table 72.4. Other consensus conferences have been formed, and have give broadly similar values of blood cholesterol at which treatment is desirable.

Triglycerides

The levels to treat are easier to establish since there are normal ranges (as for blood glucose) holding throughout world populations which are age and sex related. For middle-aged men, levels > 2.0 mmol/l (180 mg/dl) can be considered for dietary therapy, and > 4 mmol/l (360 mg/dl) for diet and drug therapy. If the hypertriglyceridaemia is accompanied by low HDL levels, it becomes more important to treat actively since this combination is known to be potently atherogenic.

How to treat

Diets

In view of the strong dietary influence on blood cholesterol

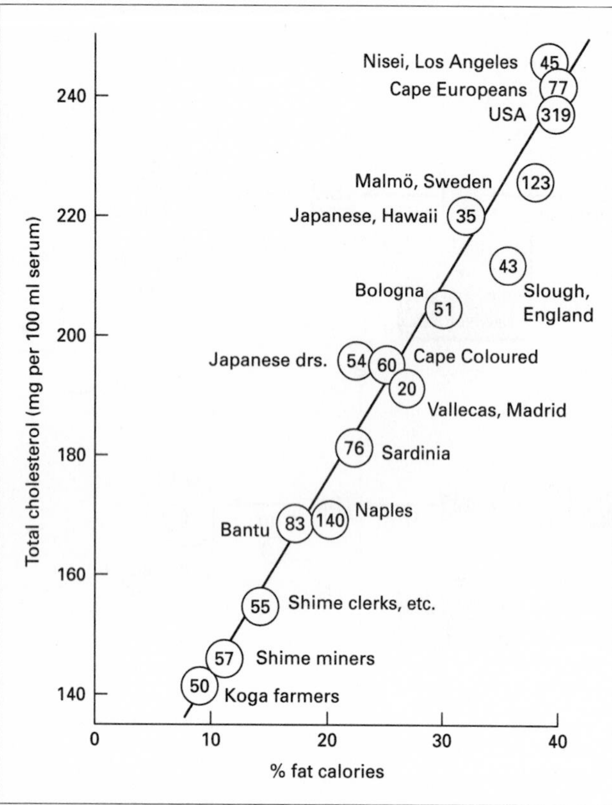

Fig. 72.17 Mean percentage of calories provided by all fats in the diet and concentration of total cholesterol in the serum of 1288 clinically healthy men aged 40–49 years in gainful employment in the USA (Minnesota railroad clerks, switchmen, dispatchers; Minnesota firefighters; Los Angeles Caucasians), Malmö, Sweden (shipyard workers, firefighters, clerks, engineers, foremen), Bologna (police officers, factory workers, businessmen), Sardinia (police officers, firefighters, coal miners), Naples (firefighters, steelworkers, clerks), and in other groups as indicated. Numbers within circles show the number of men in each group.

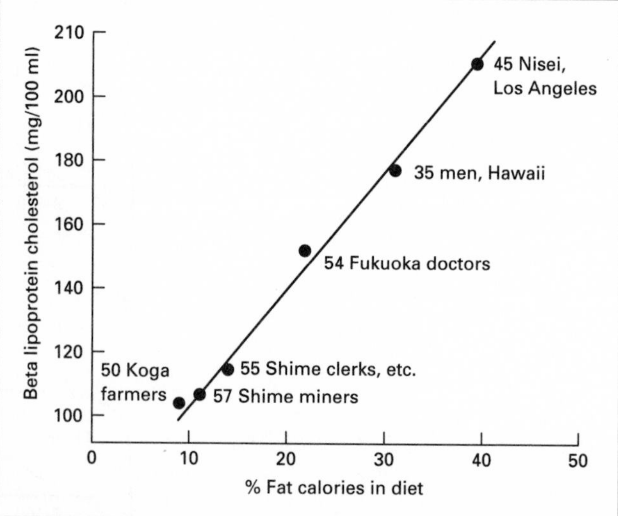

Fig. 72.18 Mean percentage of calories provided by all fats in the diet, and concentration of LDL cholesterol in the serum of Japanese men aged 40–49 years in Japan, Hawaii and Los Angeles.

and triglyceride, the general principles of dietary treatment are to reduce the consumption of the offending nutrient, i.e. reduce dietary cholesterol for hypercholesterolaemia and reduce neutral fats (triglyceride) for hypertriglyceridaemia. For the hyperlipidaemias with a strong environmental (as opposed to genetic) component, this form of treatment can often work very effectively [30].

The general principles of such diets are shown in Table 72.5. The patient needs to spend at least a half hour with a sympathetic dietitian to go through his or her current diet and assess what changes need to be made for it to become therapeutic. To be given a diet sheet by a doctor with a brief explanation would in most cases prove ineffective. Follow-up by the dietitian is also required to encourage and to ensure compliance with the diet. Obviously, all the additional factors, such as hypertension, obesity, smoking, diabetes mellitus' etc., must be treated in their own right to reduce the risks of developing atherosclerosis.

Drugs

After 2–3 months' trial of dietary therapy, the blood fats may still fail to return to desirable levels, particularly if the initial levels are high, so the use of drugs must then be considered. In 1970, when the Lipid Clinic at St Bartholomew's Hospital was opened, there were only three classes of drugs in use: bile-acid resins (cholestyramine), nicotinates and clofibrate. There are now seven classes of drug, which are described in Table 72.6. Their general uses for the treatment of hypercholesterolaemia or hypertriglyceridaemia are indicated. The use of hypolipidaemic drugs varies widely among different countries, and the UK is one of the minimal users. Prescription of hypolipidaemic drugs bears no relation to the incidence of hyperlipidaemias in the population, and within the UK drugs to lower blood fats are the least-used

Table 72.4 Cholesterol values requiring treatment according to the recommendations of the USA consensus conference.

Age (years)	Moderate risk mg/dl	Moderate risk mmol	High risk mg/dl	High risk mmol
20–29	>200	5.17	>220	5.69
30–39	>220	5.69	>240	6.21
>40	>240	6.21	>260	6.72

Table 72.5 The general lipid-lowering diet: principles, nutrient composition and sources.

Principle	Sources
Decreased total fat intake and reduction of saturated fats	Butter, hard margarine, whole milk, cream, ice cream, hard cheese, cream cheese, visible meat fat, usual cuts of red meat and pork, duck, goose, usual sausage, pastry, usual coffee whiteners, coconut, coconut oil and palm oil-containing foods
Increased use of high protein, low saturated fat foods	Fish, chicken, turkey, game, veal
Increased complex carbohydrate and fruit, vegetable and cereal fibre, with some emphasis on legumes	All fresh and frozen vegetables, all fresh fruit, all unrefined cereal foods, lentils, dried beans, rice
Moderately increased use of polyunsaturated and monounsaturated fats	Sunflower oil, corn oil, soybean oil and products unless hardened (hydrogenated), olive oil
Decreased dietary cholesterol	Brain, sweetbreads, kidneys, tongue; eggs (limit to 1–2 yolks per week); liver (limit to twice per month)
Moderately decreased sodium intake	Salt, sodium glutamate, cheese, tinned vegetables and meats, salt-preserved foods (ham, bacon, kippers), high-salt mineral waters, many convenience foods

72.6 Drugs used in the treatment of hypercholesterolaemia and hypertriglyceridaemia.

Hypercholesterolaemia	Hypertriglyceridaemia
Resins	*Fibrates*
Cholestyramine	Ciprofibrate
Colestipol	Bezafibrate
'Fibre'	Fenofibrate
	Gemfibrozil
Fibrates	*Nicotinic acids*
Ciprofibrate	Acipimox
Bezafibrate	Nicofuranose
Gemfibrozil	
Statins	*Marine oils*
Simvastatin	Omega-3 marine oils
Lovastatin	Maxepa
Pravastatin	
Fluvastatin	
Rivastatin	
Antioxidants	
Probucol	

compared with agents used to treat other, equally common, disorders such as diabetes or hypertension.

Bile-acid resins

The two common bile-acid resins in use for treatment of hypercholesterolaemia are cholestyramine and colestipol. Their polymeric structures are shown in Fig. 72.19. They bind bile acids in the small intestine and interrupt the enterohepatic circulation of bile acids, so promoting their excretion in the faeces (Fig. 72.20). Bile acids are derived directly from cholesterol, so this is one way of excreting cholesterol from the body; up to 15 g steroid per day may be eliminated in this way. The drug is not absorbed into the body, so systemic side-effects do not occur. The bile acid–resin complex may cause mild constipation or sometimes may irritate the colon and produce loose motions or even a mucous diarrhoea, but adjustment of the dosage usually can minimise this. The drug should be taken just before the major meals of the day, timed to reach the duodenum when the maximum flow of bile acid is likely to occur. There is obviously no point in taking the drug under fasting conditions, when it will be excreted having bound no bile acids. Because of the lack of absorption and systemic side-effects of the drug, it is suitable for children and teenagers with hypercholesterolaemia and can be used during pregnancy. The dosage is up to two or three sachets of resin three times daily, depending on the severity of the hypercholesterolaemia and associated clinical features which may relate to the development of coronary atherosclerosis [31]. During use of the drug the plasma triglycerides may rise slightly for as yet unexplained reasons, but this is usually not serious. Resins may also interfere with the absorption of other drugs such as digoxin, warfarin, thiazide diuretics, etc., so it is advisable to take other medications at least 1 hour before or 3 hours after the resin.

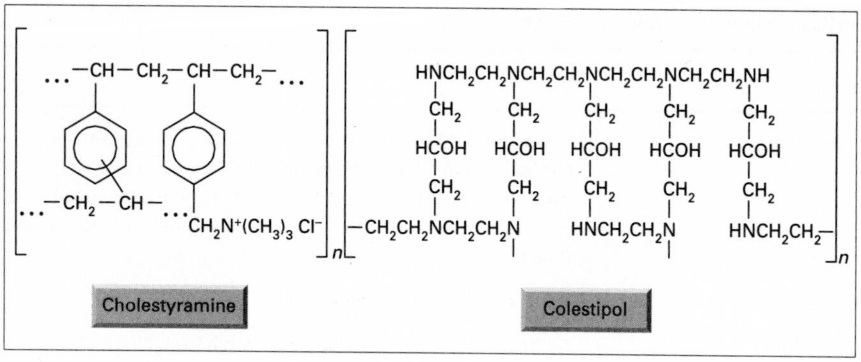

Cholestyramine

Colestipol

Fig. 72.19 Structure of two commonly used bile-acid resins.

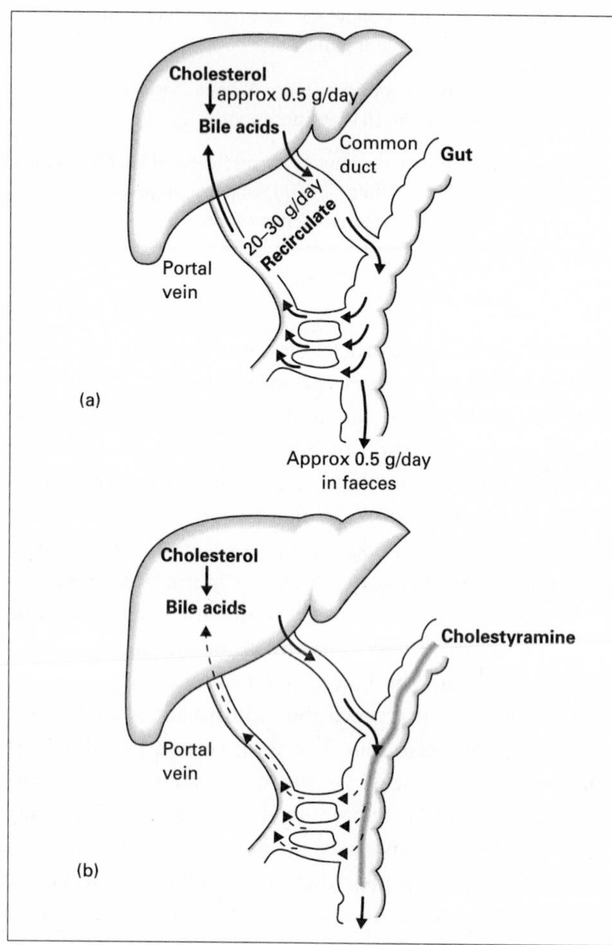

Fig. 72.20 Postulated effect of cholestyramine on the enterohepatic cycle of bile aids. (a) Enterohepatic cycle of bile acids; (b) effect of bile-acid sequestrant on cycle.

Plant fibres such as guar gum may have a similar action to the resins by binding (more loosely) bile acids in the intestine and promoting their excretion in the faeces.

The fibrates

The compound initially used was clofibrate, and some of its clinically useful derivatives are shown in Fig. 72.21. Their mechanism of action is ill-understood, but they can induce lipases which clear lipoproteins from the bloodstream (Fig. 72.5), as well as possibly inhibiting lipid synthesis in the liver. They are very safe compounds with only minimal side-effects, the most common being skin rashes and marrow dysplasias. Gemfibrozil was used in the Helsinki Heart Study and was shown to lower LDL cholesterol, raise HDL cholesterol, and reduce the incidence of coronary events over a 5-year trial period. They act synergistically with the bile-acid resins and are frequently used in such combinations before attempting to use the stronger drugs.

Nicotinates

The active drug is shown in Fig. 72.22. One of its mechanisms of action is to inhibit the breakdown of intracellular triglycerides to free fatty acids (i.e. an antilipolytic action) and so reduce the flux of free fatty acids in plasma to the liver. This impairs hepatic triglyceride synthesis and reduces the levels of plasma triglycerides. However, the therapeutic dose of the drug (up to 3–5 g/day) is close to the dosage that produces side-effects, making the use of the drug difficult. The dose should be built up slowly, starting with as little as 100 mg daily. Vasomotor effects leading to skin flushing, sunburn-like rashes and feelings of prickly heat are signs to reduce the drug dosage. Some of these symptoms can be alleviated by aspirin. The drug was used in the cholesterol-lowering atherosclerosis (CLAS) trial in combination with colestipol, and was shown to be effective in reducing the number of adverse coronary events [32].

Acipimox (Fig. 72.22) is a derivative of nicotinic acid which appears to have fewer side-effects, but still retains a strong antilipolytic action. Its use in the hypertriglyceridaemias is under clinical evaluation.

Probucol

This drug lowers plasma cholesterol by a mechanism that is not well established, and it may also have independent

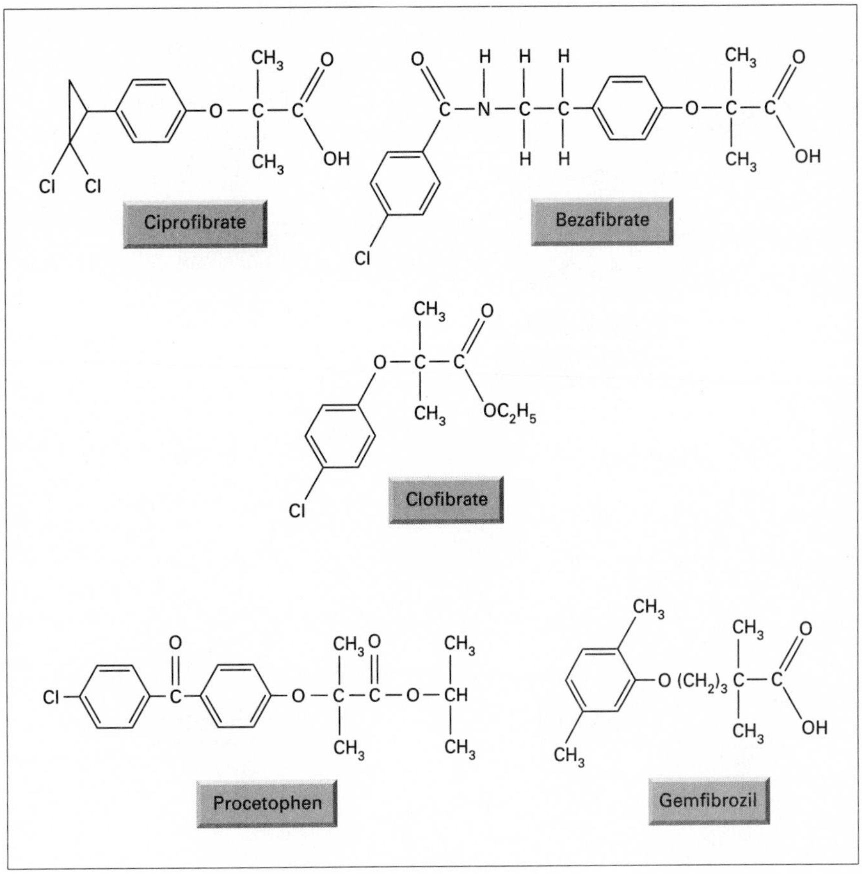

Fig. 72.21 Clofibrate and some of its clinically used derivatives.

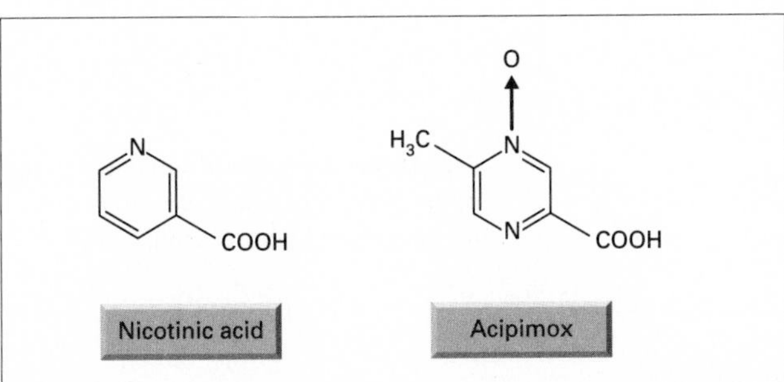

Fig. 72.22 Structure of nicotinic acid (niacin) and one of its derivatives.

antiatherogenic properties. These may be related to its antioxidant properties, which prevent the oxidative modification of lipoproteins before their incorporation into foam cells as the fatty streak of the arterial wall. The drug appears to be quite safe and it is worthwhile if more conventional therapies (fibrates and bile-acid resins) have failed.

The statins

This is a very effective group of drugs which directly inhibit cholesterol synthesis in the liver and peripheral tissues. The parent compound (Fig. 72.23) was a fungal metabolite initially tested for antibacterial activity but found to possess cholesterol-lowering properties. Derivatives such as lovastatin, pravastatin, simvastatin, fluvastatin and rivastatin are shown in Fig. 72.23. They all act by competitive inhibition of the rate-determining enzyme of HMG-CoA reductase, and directly inhibit intracellular pathways of cholesterol synthesis (Fig. 72.24). The rationale for their use is shown in Fig. 72.24, where it is seen that inhibition of cholesterol synthesis (Fig. 72.24b) induces formation of the LDL receptor on the liver-cell membrane and promotes cholesterol clearance from the bloodstream. Synergistic effects can be obtained with bile-acid resins (Fig. 72.24c) which deplete intracellular bile acids and induce still more LDL-receptor activity on the cell membrane for removal of LDL cholesterol from the blood. The drug is ineffective in patients with homozygous familial hypercholesterolaemia because such patients cannot respond by increasing the synthesis and numbers of LDL receptors in the liver-cell membrane.

The drug can be taken after the evening meal at doses of up to 40 mg daily. Side-effects include myopathies and a rise in liver enzymes, in which case the drug should be reduced or stopped altogether, depending on the severity of the

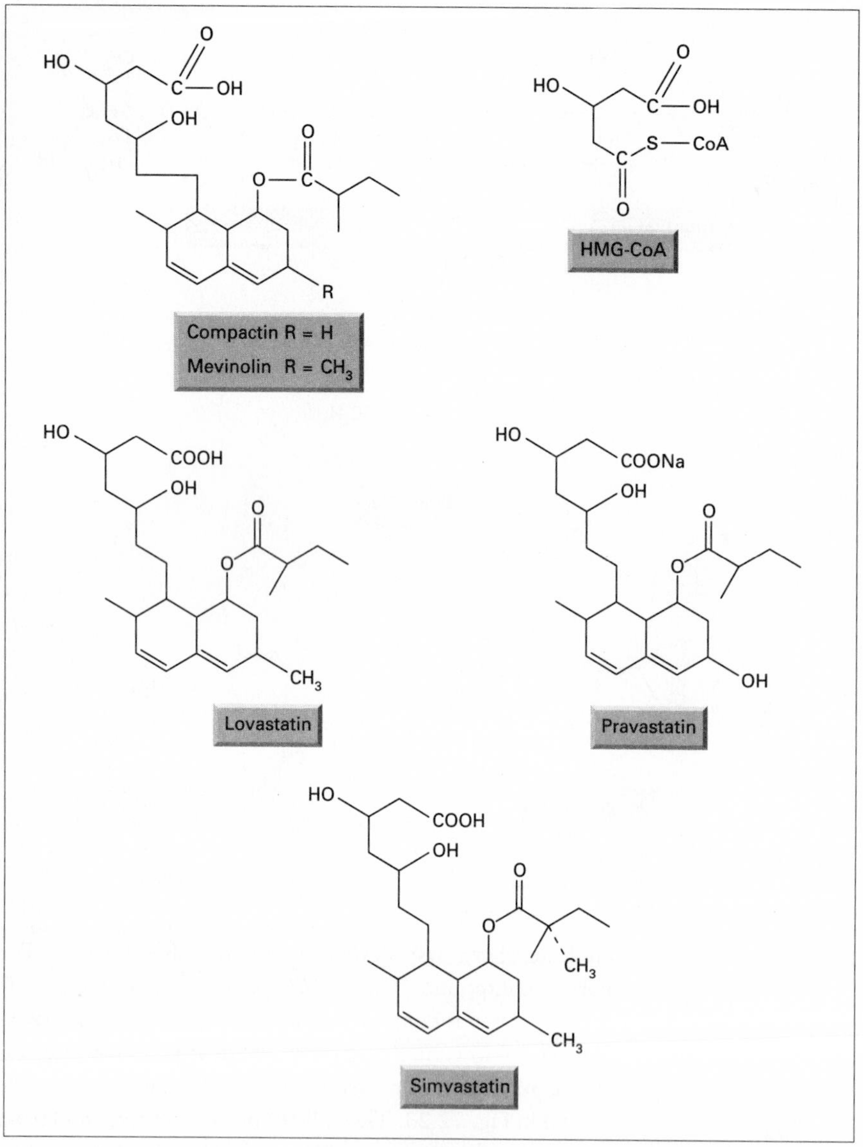

HMG-CoA

Compactin R = H
Mevinolin R = CH_3

Lovastatin

Pravastatin

Simvastatin

Fig. 72.23 Structure of some members of the statin group of drugs. HMG-CoA, hydroxymethylglutaryl coenzyme A.

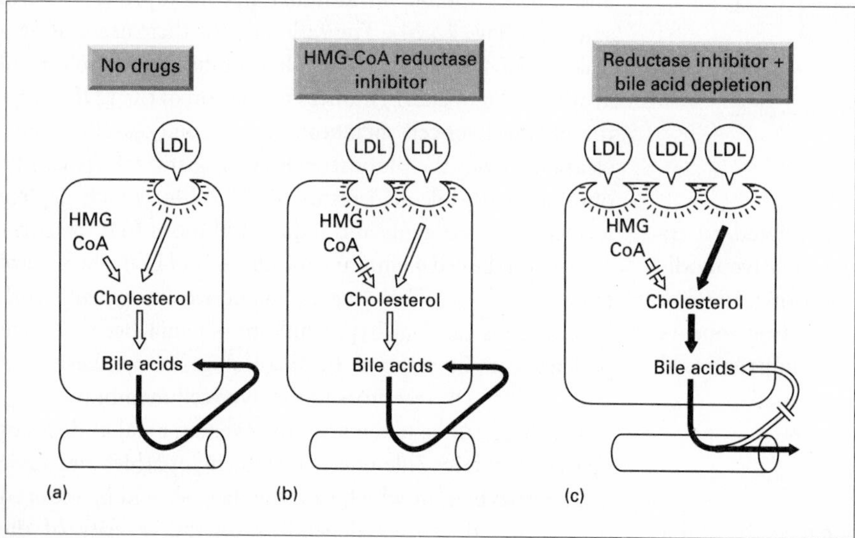

Fig. 72.24 Rationale for the use of an inhibitor of hydroxymethylglutaryl coenzyme A (HMG-CoA) reductase alone or in combination with bile-acid depletion to stimulate increased hepatic low-density lipoprotein (LDL)-receptor expression and to lower plasma LDL levels. See text for further explanation. Adapted from [43].

condition. The drug may be cautiously used in combination with fibrates but side-effects are then more likely to occur and careful monitoring is required.

Marine oils (eicosapentanoic acids)

These are polyunsaturated fatty acids which are found in high concentrations in fish oils, and the structures of two of them are shown in Fig. 72.25. For reasons that are not clear, they reduce the plasma levels of triglycerides and can be quite useful in the treatment of moderate to severe hypertriglyceridaemia; sometimes plasma cholesterol is lowered as well. The dosage is between 4 and 8 g/day. They are naturally occurring fatty acids and are generally non-toxic. Changes in platelet aggregation or bleeding time may be observed, but this may be beneficial in that intravascular thrombosis may thus be impaired. Marine oils are currently under trial to see if they can prevent coronary artery thrombosis.

Summary of drugs

A summary of the properties of some of the more commonly used drugs in the treatment of the hyperlipidaemias are presented in Table 72.7. In terms of practice, the steps used in the Bart's Lipid Clinic to manage a patient with hyperlipidaemia are shown in Fig. 72.26.

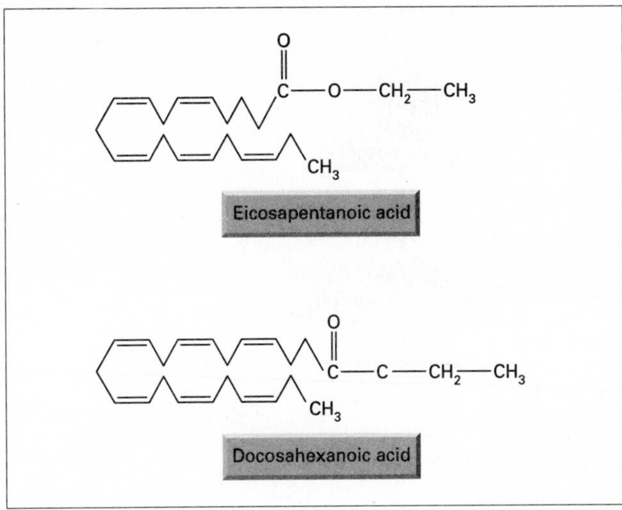

Fig. 72.25 Structure of two polyunsaturated fatty acids found in high concentrations in fish oil.

Other measures

Ileal bypass surgery

For severe hypercholesterolaemia resistant to drug action, or for patients who cannot tolerate large amounts of hypolipidaemic drugs, partial ileal bypass can be a useful procedure. This is a type of surgical interruption of the

Table 72.7 Summary of the major drugs used in hyperlipidaemia.

Drugs	Reduces CHD risk	Long-term safety	Maintaining adherence	LDL-cholesterol lowering (%)	Special precautions
Cholestyramine, colestipol	Yes	Yes	Requires considerable education	15–30	Can alter absorption of other drugs; can increase triglyceride levels and should not be used in patients with hypertriglyceridaemia
Nicotinic acid	Yes	Yes	Requires considerable education	15–30	Test for hyperuricaemia, hyperglycaemia and liver function abnormalities
Lovastatin	Not proven	Not established	Relatively easy	25–45	Monitor for liver function abnormalities and possible lens opacities
Gemfibrozil	Yes	Preliminary evidence satisfactory	Relatively easy	5–15	May increase LDL cholesterol in hypertriglyceridaemic patients; should not be used in patients with gallbladder disease
Probucol	Not proven	Yes	Relatively easy	10–15	Lowers HDL cholesterol; significance of this has not been established; prolongs QT interval
Fish oils	Not proven	Not established	Relatively easy	10–15	Can prolong bleeding time

CHD, coronary heart disease; LDL, low-density lipoprotein.

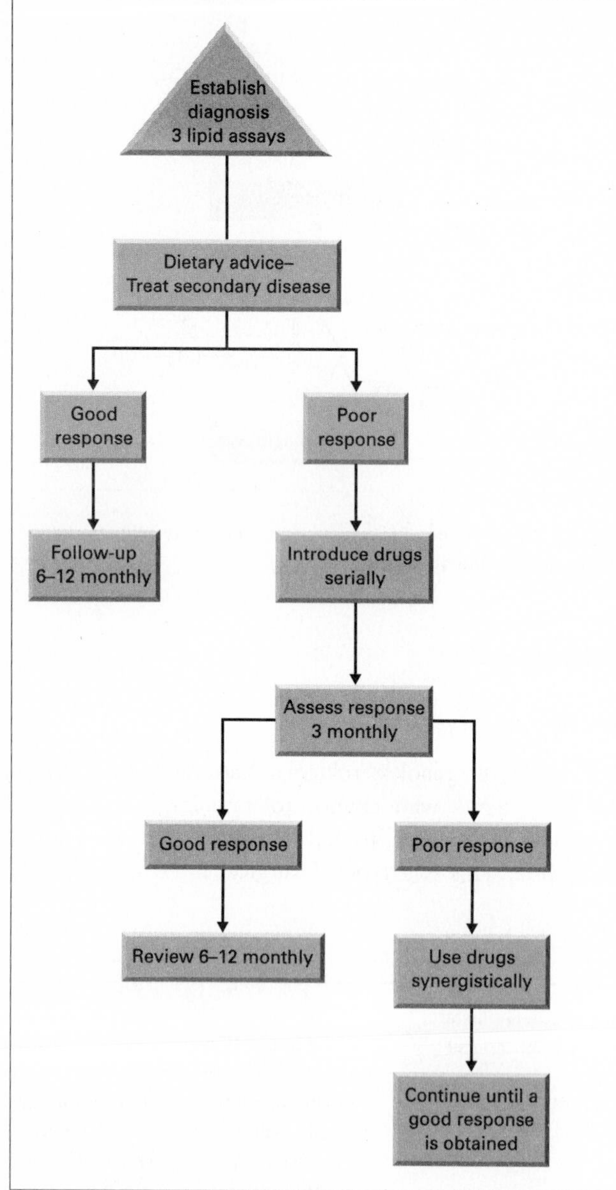

Fig. 72.26 Steps used in the management of patients with hyperlipidaemia at the Lipid Clinic, St Bartholomew's Hospital, London.

enterohepatic circulation of bile acids (Fig. 72.20b), and up to 15 g/day of steroids can be excreted in the faeces. Unfortunately, the fall in plasma cholesterol is not always maintained because the liver starts to augment its cholesterol synthetic activity, which tends to restore plasma levels of cholesterol. However, ileal bypass can reduce the amount of drugs that a heterozygous hypercholesterolaemic patient needs to take. The major side-effects of the operation are watery diarrhoea, due to irritation by the bile-salt load that passes through the colon.

Obviously, if this becomes too severe (which is rare), the bypass can be restored to normal.

Plasma exchange and LDL apheresis [33]

These are hospital procedures to reduce the circulatory levels of LDLs in severe hypercholesterolaemia by either plasma exchange or binding of LDLs to solid-support materials in columns. They are primarily used in the rarer forms of homozygous familial hypercholesterolaemia.

Gene therapy

Several cases of homozygous familial hypercholesterolaemia have been treated by *ex vivo* gene-replacement therapy of the LDL receptor. Blood cholesterol levels have initially fallen but the response appears to be short-lived. This may perhaps be due to poor integration of the receptor DNA into the host genome [34], or production of antibodies against the receptor.

Is treatment effective?

Intervention trials (primary or secondary)

Does the treatment for hyperlipidaemia work? Many clinical trials, both on subjects with no previous arterial disease (primary trials) or on patients with established arterial disease (secondary prevention trials), have addressed this issue, and they almost all show the same trend—lowering blood cholesterol by whatever means also lowers rates of coronary artery disease. Of these trials, the Lipid Research Clinics, the Helsinki Heart Study and the Cholesterol-Lowering Atherosclerosis Study (CLAS) are some of the most persuasive.

The Lipid Research Clinics Study

This study was conducted for 7 years on 3800 middle-aged men attending 10 North American lipid clinics using cholestyramine (8 g t.d.s.) as the active agent [35,36]. The results in Fig. 72.27 show an approximate 20% fall in total cholesterol, very little change in HDL cholesterol or plasma triglyceride, and about a 20% reduction in coronary events (defined as fatal or non-fatal infarction, new angina, or development of an abnormal exercise electrocardiogram in the drug-treated group).

The Helsinki Heart Study [37]

This was conducted at lipid clinics in Finland, using gemfibrozil as the active agent in approximately 2000 men compared with placebo in a further 2000 men over 6

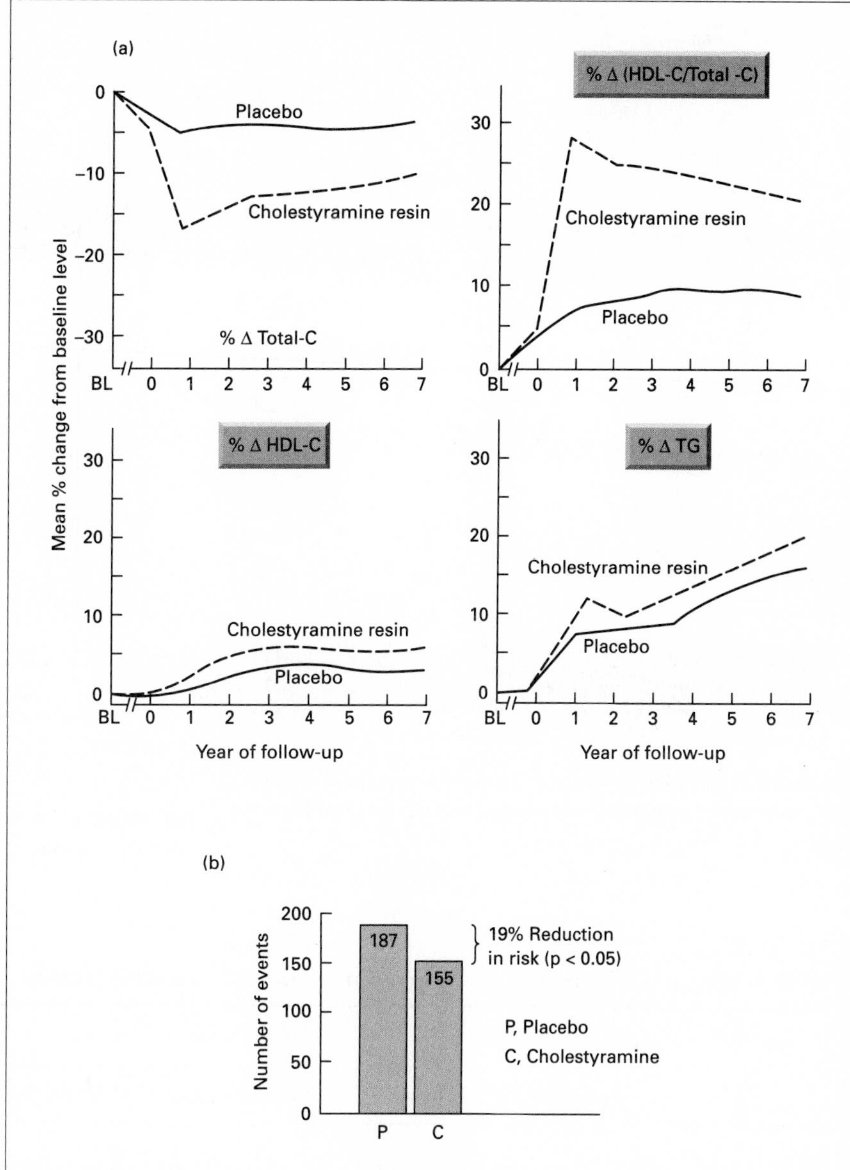

Fig. 72.27 (a) Mean yearly plasma lipid levels for cholestyramine and placebo-treated men. On abscissa, BL represents baseline (prediet) period and 0 years represents the 3-month interval between initiation of the Lipid Research Clinic's diet and study medication. Year 1 is the average of visits 7–13, and each year thereafter represents an average of six visits. Δ indicates change from baseline level; Total-C, plasma total-cholesterol levels; TG, triglyceride levels; HDL-C, high-density lipoprotein cholesterol. (b) Comparison of primary endpoints occurring in the cholestyramine (C) and placebo (P) groups. Adapted from [36].

years. The results showed an 11% fall in LDL cholesterol, a 10% rise in HDL cholesterol and a 35% fall in plasma triglycerides. The cumulative incidence of coronary events (defined as fatal or non-fatal infarction) showed a significant difference between gemfibrozil and placebo-treated groups (Fig. 72.28), with an overall 34% reduction in ischaemic heart disease rates.

The Cholesterol-Lowering Atherosclerosis Study

This was a placebo-controlled trial using colestipol and nicotinic acid therapy in 162 non-smoking men aged 40–59 years who had undergone coronary bypass surgery. The end points were coronary angiographic appearances assessed objectively after 2 years of treatment. They found a 26% reduction in total cholesterol, a 43% reduction in LDL cholesterol and a 37% increase in HDL cholesterol. This was associated with a significant reduction in the average number of atherosclerotic lesions per subject that progressed ($P < 0.03$), and in the percentage of subjects with new atheroma formation in native coronary arteries ($P < 0.03$). Deterioration in overall coronary status was significantly less in drug-treated subjects than in the placebo group ($P < 0.001$).

More than nine other angiographically controlled trials of lipid-lowering therapy have shown unequivocally beneficial effects on the incidence of clinical events or structural changes in the arterial wall. The beneficial effects of lipid lowering for primary prevention of coronary artery disease are more controversial.

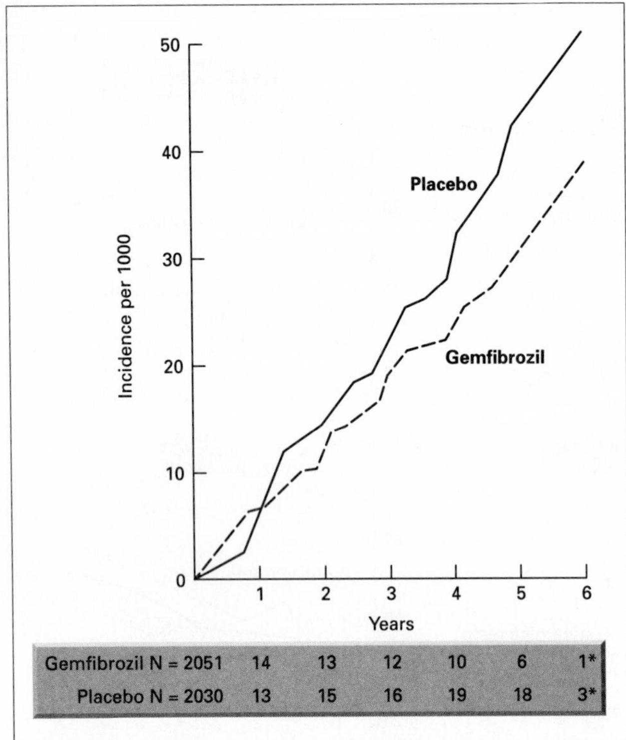

Fig. 72.28 Cumulative incidence of coronary events (fatal or non-fatal infarction) in gemfibrozil and placebo groups. Adapted from [46].

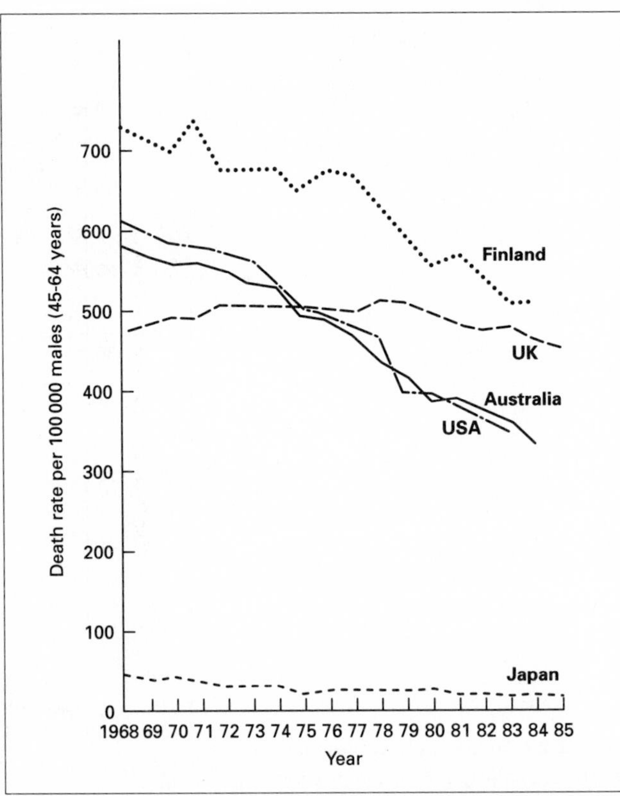

Fig. 72.29 Death rates from ischaemic heart disease among males aged 45–64 years.

Table 72.8 Major lipid-lowering trials of coronary heart disease (CHD) prevention, 1978–88.

Trial	Treatment	Duration (years)	Change in serum lipids (%)			Outcome
			Total cholesterol	Triglycerides	HDL cholesterol	
Primary						
Oslo	Diet and anti-smoking	5	−20	−29	–	45% ↓ all CHD
World Health Organization	Clofibrate	5.3	−9	–	–	25% ↓ non-fatal CHD 25% ↑ total mortality
LRC-CPPT	Cholestyramine	7	−12	+17	+6	19% ↓ all CHD
Helsinki Heart Study	Gemfibrozil	5	−9	−35	+9	34% ↓ all CHD
Secondary						
Coronary Drug Project	Nicotinic acid	6.2	−9	−27	–	12% ↓ fatal CHD* 11% ↓ total mortality†
Stockholm trial	Clofibrate + nicotinic acid	5	−13	−19	–	36% ↓ fatal CHD 26% ↓ total mortality
Mean change			−12	−19	+7.5	29% ↓ CHD

* After 15 years. † After 9.6 years.
LRC-CPPT, Lipid Research Clinic's Coronary Primary Prevention Trial.

Summary

A brief summary of some of the other trials is presented in Table 72.8. Although there is widespread variation, it appears that most trials show that a reduction in blood cholesterol by whatever means is accompanied by a reduction in coronary events, which strongly supports the rationale of lipid-lowering treatment to prevent coronary artery disease [10,38]. A strategy to aid prevention of atherosclerosis might be expected to yield the results of a decline in coronary mortality rate [30,39], as shown in Fig. 72.29 for such countries as the USA or Australia. In the UK, 20 million working days are lost each year due to ischaemic heart disease, more than for influenza or arthritis, making an impressive case for reduction of blood lipids to prevent coronary disease.

References

1 Hanawalt PC, Hayes RH. The chemical basis of life. In: Hanawalt PC, Haynes RH, eds. *Readings from Scientific American*. San Francisco: WH Freeman & Co, 1978: 241–55.

2 Durrington PN. *Hyperlipidaemia: Diagnosis and Management*. London: Wright, 1989.

3 Bloomfield VA, Harrington RE. Biophysical chemistry. In: Bloomfield VA, Harrington RE, eds. *Readings from Scientific American*. San Francisco: WH Freeman & Co, 1974: 90–9.

4 Galton DJ, Thompson GR. Lipids and cardiovascular disease. In: Galton DJ, Thompson GR, eds. *British Medical Bulletin*, Vol. 46. Edinburgh: Churchill Livingstone, 1990: 873–959.

5 Stanbury JB, Wyngaarden JB, Fredrickson DS, Goldstein JL, Brown MS. *The Metabolic Basis of Inherited Disease*. New York: McGraw-Hill, 1983.

6 Suckling KE, Groot PHE. *Hyperlipidaemia and Atherosclerosis*. London: Academic Press, 1988.

7 Brown MS, Goldstein JL. A receptor mediated pathway for cholesterol homeostasis. *Science* 1986; **232**: 34–7.

8 Bierman EL, Oram JF. The interaction of high density lipoproteins with extrahepatic cells. *Am Heart J* 1987; **113**: 549–50.

9 Reichl D, Miller NE. The anatomy and physiology of reverse cholesterol transport. *Clin Sci* 1986; **70**: 221–31.

10 Schlierf G, Morl H. *Expanding Horizons in Atherosclerosis Research*. Berlin: Springer-Verlag, 1987.

11 Darnell J, Lodish H, Baltimore D. *Molecular Cell Biology*. San Francisco: WH Freeman & Co, 1988.

12 Fuller JH, Shipley KJ, Rose G, Jarrett RJ, Keen H. Coronary heart disease risk and impaired glucose tolerance: The Whitehall Study. *Lancet* 1980; **i**: 1373–6.

13 Reckless JPD, Betteridge DJ, Wu P, Galton DJ. High-density and low-density lipoproteins and prevalence of vascular disease in diabetes mellitus. *Br Med J* 1978; **1**: 883–6.

14 Ross R. The pathogenesis of atherosclerosis. An update. *N Engl J Med* 1986; **341**: 488–500.

15 Castelli WP, Garrison RJ, Wilson RWF, Abbott RD, Kannel WB. Incidence of coronary heart disease and lipoprotein cholesterol levels. The Framingham Study. *JAMA* 1986; **256**: 2835–8.

16 Carlson LA, Bottiger LE. Serum triglycerides, to be or not to be a risk factor for ischaemic heart disease? (The Stockholm Prospective Study). *Atherosclerosis* 1981; **39**: 287–91.

17 Stamler J, Wentworth D, Neaton JD. Is relationship between serum cholesterol and risk of premature death from coronary heart disease continuous or graded? Findings in 356 222 primary screenees of the Multiple Risk Factor Intervention Trial (MRFIT). *JAMA* 1986; **256**: 2823–8.

18 Galton DJ. *Molecular Genetics of Common Metabolic Disease*. London: Edward Arnold, 1985.

19 Rifkind BM, Levy RI. Hyperlipidaenia: Diagnosis and therapy. New York: Grune & Stratton, 1977.

20 Lusis AJ, Sparkes RS. *Genetic Factors in Atherosclerosis*. Basle: Karger, 1989.

21 Keen H, Jarrett J. *Complications of Diabetes*. London: Edward Arnold, 1982.

22 Reaven GM, Greenfield MS. Diabetic hypertriglyceridaemia. Evidence for three clinical syndromes. *Diabetes* 1981; **30**: 66–75.

23 Castelli WP. The triglyceride issue: A view from Framingham. *Am Heart J* 1986; **112**: 432–7.

24 Dodson PM, Galton DJ, Hamilton AM, Blach RK. Retinal vein occlusion and the prevalence of lipoprotein abnormalities. *Br J Opthal* 1981; **66**: 161–4.

25 Dodson PM, Galton DJ, Winder AF. Retinal vascular abnormalities in the hyperlipidaemias. *Trans Opthal Soc UK* 1981; **101**: 17–21.

26 Monsolf FA. The eye and systemic disease. Saint Louis: CV Mosby Co, 1975.

27 Lewis B, Chait AI, Wootton IDP *et al*. Frequency of risk factors for ischaemic heart disease in a healthy British population with particular reference to serum lipoprotein levels. *Lancet* 1974; **i**: 141–6.

28 LaRosa JC, Hunninghake D, Bush D *et al*. The cholesterol facts: a summary of evidence relating dietary fats, serum cholesterol and coronary heart disease. *Circulation* 1990; **81**: 1721–33.

29 Myant NB. *The Biology of Cholesterol and Related Steroids*. London: Heinemann Medical, 1981.

30 Hjermann I, Byre K, Holme I, Leren P. Effect of diet and smoking intervention on the incidence of coronary heart disease; report from the Oslo Study Group. *Lancet* 1981; **11**: 303–10.

31 Shepherd J, Packard CJ, Bicker S, Lawrie TDV, Morgan HG. Cholestyramine promotes receptor mediated low density lipoprotein catabolism. *N Engl J Med* 1980; **302**: 1219–22.

32 Blankenhorn DH, Nessim SA, Johnson RL, Sammarco ME, Azen SP, Cashin-Hemphill L. Beneficial effects of combined colistipol and niacin therapy on coronary atherosclerosis and coronary vein bypass grafts. *JAMA* 1987; **257**: 3233–40.

33 Thompson GR, Barbir M, Michishita I, Larkin S. Comparison of plasma exchange and LDL aperesis in the treatment of hypercholesterolaemia. In: Crepaldi G, Gotto AM, Manzato E, Baggio G, eds. *Atherosclerosis VIII*. Amsterdam: Excerpta Medica, 1989: 815–18.

34 Alberts B, Bray D, Lewis J, Raff M, Roberts K, Watson JD. Molecular biology of the cell. New York: Garland, 1989.

35 Lipid Research Clinics Programme Epidemiology Committee. Plasma lipid distributions in selected North American populations: The Lipid Research Clinics Programme Prevalence Study. *Circulation* 1979; **60**: 427–39.

36 Lipid Research Clinics Programme. The Lipid Research Clinics Coronary Primary Prevention Trial Results. The relationship of reduction in incidence of coronary heart disease to cholesterol lowering. *JAMA* 1984; **251**: 365–74.

37 Manninen V, Elo O, Frick H *et al*. Lipid alterations and decline in the incidence of coronary heart disease in the Helsinki Heart Study. *JAMA* 1988; **260**: 641–51.

38 Steinberg D. Lipoproteins and atherosclerosis. A look ahead. *Arteriosclerosis* 1983; **3**: 283–301.

39 Keys A. *Seven Countries: A Multivariate Analysis of Death and Coronary Heart Disease*. Cambridge, MA: Harvard University Press, 1980.
40 Utermann G. Apolipoprotein E polymorphisms in health and disease. *Am Heart J* 1987; **113**: 433–40.
41 Belfiore F, Galton DJ, Reaven GM. *Diabetes Mellitus: Etiopathogenesis and Metabolic Aspects*. Basle: Karger, 1984.
42 Crepaldi G, Tiengo A, Baggio G. Diabetes, obesity and hyperlipidaemias. Amsterdam: Excerpta Medica, 1985.
43 Brown MS, Goldstein JL. How LDL receptors influence cholesterol and atherosclerosis. *Sci Am* 1984; **251**: 58–66.
44 Richard JL. Peculiarities of coronary heart disease in the French population. *Atherosclerosis* 1984; **iv**: 821.
45 Kannel WB. Nutrition and the occurrence and prevention of cardiovascular disease in the elderly. *Nutr Rev* 1988; **46**: 68–78.
46 Frick MH, Elo O, Haapa K *et al.* Helsinki Heart Study: primary prevention trial with gemfibrozil in middle-aged men with dyslipidemia. *N Engl J Med* 1987; **317**: 1237–45.

Part 17
The Endocrinology of Cancer

CHAPTER 73

Ectopic hormone production

A.J.L. Clark and J. Newell-Price

Introduction

Some of the most dramatic manifestations of endocrine disease are caused by the ectopic production of a hormone by a benign or malignant tumour. These uncommon occurrences may be remarkable because of the severity of the clinical manifestations or the biochemical disturbances, and because of the response to complete removal of the tumour when this can be achieved.

Such cases are, of course rare, and may often be overshadowed clinically by the underlying neoplasm. Nevertheless, ectopic hormone secretion remains important in clinical endocrinology because:

1 it is part of the differential diagnosis of many endocrine diseases, for example hypercalcaemia and Cushing's syndrome;

2 hormone secretion can lead to the early detection of cancer, and act as a marker of that tumour's response to treatment, for example human chorionic gonadotrophin (hCG) production by various neoplasms including bladder tumours;

3 it can lead to new insights and discoveries in endocrinology, for example growth hormone (GH)-releasing hormone (GHRH) was first identified in ectopically secreting carcinoid tumours, and parathyroid hormone-related protein (PTHrP) was discovered through the study of the humoral hypercalcaemia of malignancy.

This chapter is divided into two main sections. In the first, we try to define the phenomenon of ectopic hormone production, and describe its essential characteristics which should be accounted for by any explanatory theory. In the second section we discuss the various theories that have been proposed, and the problems with each of them.

Features of ectopic hormones

The phenomenon can be described as the synthesis (and usually the secretion) of a hormone by a neoplastic lesion that has arisen from a tissue that is not normally considered to be the source of that hormone.

The term 'neoplastic lesion' includes both benign and malignant tumours. There are rare cases of hyperplastic lesions that have been associated with hormone production, and although infrequently studied it seems probable that many of the conclusions and hypotheses that relate to neoplasia may also be applicable to this group.

The phrase 'a tissue that is not normally considered to be the source of the hormone' is vague, but since there is now evidence that many genes are expressed in most tissues at very low levels [1,2] it becomes very difficult to be more precise than this. In some cases no single tissue is recognised as the normal source of the peptide in question (e.g. PTHrP), and in such situations it is very obvious that the term 'ectopic' is inappropriate. However, since the concept of 'ectopic hormones' is now well entrenched in medical terminology, it would seem more likely to confuse the issue to attempt to use alternative expressions.

While ectopic hormone production and secretion is relatively commonplace, ectopic hormone syndromes—the clinical conditions listed in Table 73.1—are rare. This is presumably because tumour output to active hormone is usually insufficient to cause clinical sequelae, or for them to be recognised as such in the presence of more obvious symptoms resulting from the direct physical effects of the primary tumour or its metastases.

Criteria of ectopic hormone production

In order to conclude that a hormone source is ectopic, one or more of the features listed in Table 73.2 need to be established. These comprise definite criteria—demonstration of hormone synthesis and secretion by the tumour, and suggestive criteria—findings which are usually typical of an

Table 73.1 The principal clinical syndromes caused by ectopic hormone production.

Hormone	Clinical syndrome
Adrenocorticotrophic hormone	Cushing's syndrome
Vasopressin	Syndrome of inappropriate antidiuretic hormone
Parathyroid hormone	Hypercalcaemia
Human chorionic gonadotrophin	Gynaecomastia/loss of libido (hyperthyroidism)
Corticotrophin-releasing hormone	Cushing's syndrome
Growth hormone-releasing hormone	Acromegaly
Erythropoietin	Polycythaemia
Insulin-like growth factor 2	Hypoglycaemia

Table 73.2 Criteria of ectopic hormone production.

Firm criteria
Hormone messenger RNA in tumour
Immunocytochemical demonstration of peptide in tumour
In vitro hormone secretion in primary culture
Arteriovenous gradient across tumour *in vivo*
Suggestive criteria
Fall in hormone levels after removal/treatment of tumour
Persistence of hormone levels despite removal of normal source
Molecular forms of peptide typical of ectopic source
Clinical biochemistry typical of ectopic source
Dynamic endocrine tests typical of ectopic source

ectopic tumour, and which can be applied before any major invasive procedure is undertaken. A description of these points in relation to each hormone is found in the appropriate chapters. Although it is not common practice to measure hormone levels in the blood supply to and from a tumour, the process of tumour localisation by venous catheterisation and blood sampling for hormone assay effectively achieves the same result as measuring an arteriovenous difference.

Any theory that attempts to explain the phenomenon of ectopic hormones has to account for a number of general observations, as well as specific examples, as outlined below.

Hormone type

Ectopic hormones are peptide or glycoprotein hormones. Thyroid, steroid hormones or catecholamines are not widely recognised as being secreted ectopically. This is because peptide hormones are the product of a single gene. Many of the processing steps subsequent to the synthesis of a peptide chain (e.g. glycosylation and proteolytic processing) are common to many cell types. In contrast, synthesis of a steroid, thyroid or catecholamine hormone requires a complex and highly specific enzyme chain.

Some peptide hormones are very infrequently found as ectopic tumour products. Table 73.3 lists many of the potential ectopic hormones in groups that suggest which are common and which are rare tumour products. It is striking to compare these peptides with the list of peptides in groups that indicate their prevalence in non-tumorous normal tissues. The two sets of groupings completely agree, a comparison which must surely tell us something about the origin of the condition.

Tumour type

Although almost all non-endocrine tumour histologies have been associated with ectopic hormone production, certain tumours are more frequently associated with the condition than others. Indeed, it is impressive that there exists such a close relationship between tumour type and clinically apparent hormone secretion. Some of these associations are illustrated in Fig. 73.1.

Mutant peptides do not occur

There is no clearly proven case of an ectopic hormone having an abnormal peptide (or DNA) sequence. These peptides are the products of the same genes that are responsible for their normal production. There are, however, many examples of variation at a post-translational stage, in, for example, abnormal proteolytic cleavage [3], or abnormal glycosylation [4].

Multiple hormones

If one looks hard enough, many, if not most, ectopic hormone-producing tumours express the genes for more than one hormone. Less frequently, evidence for the secretion of more than one peptide can be found *in vivo*, and much less frequently does a second secretory product cause a clinically apparent syndrome.

Absence of regulation

Ectopic hormone production would not cause a clinical problem if the hormones concerned were under the same

Table 73.3 Comparison of the frequency with which certain hormones are produced ectopically by tumours and the frequency with which the peptides are found in normal non-endocrine tissues.

Prevalence in normal tissues	Prevalence in tumours
Widespread	*Common*
Pro-opiomelanocortin	Pro-opiomelanocortin
Parathyroid hormone-related protein	Parathyroid hormone-related protein
Vasopressin	Vasopressin
Calcitonin	Calcitonin
GRP (bombesin)	GRP
Growth hormone-releasing hormone	Growth hormone-releasing hormone
Restricted	*Rare*
Growth hormone	Growth hormone
Prolactin	Prolactin
Insulin	Insulin
Thyroid-stimulating hormone	Thyroid-stimulating hormone
Luteinising hormone	Luteinising hormone
Follicle-stimulating hormone	Follicle-stimulating hormone
Oxytocin	Oxytocin
Parathyroid hormone	Parathyroid hormone

GRP, Gastrin-releasing peptide.

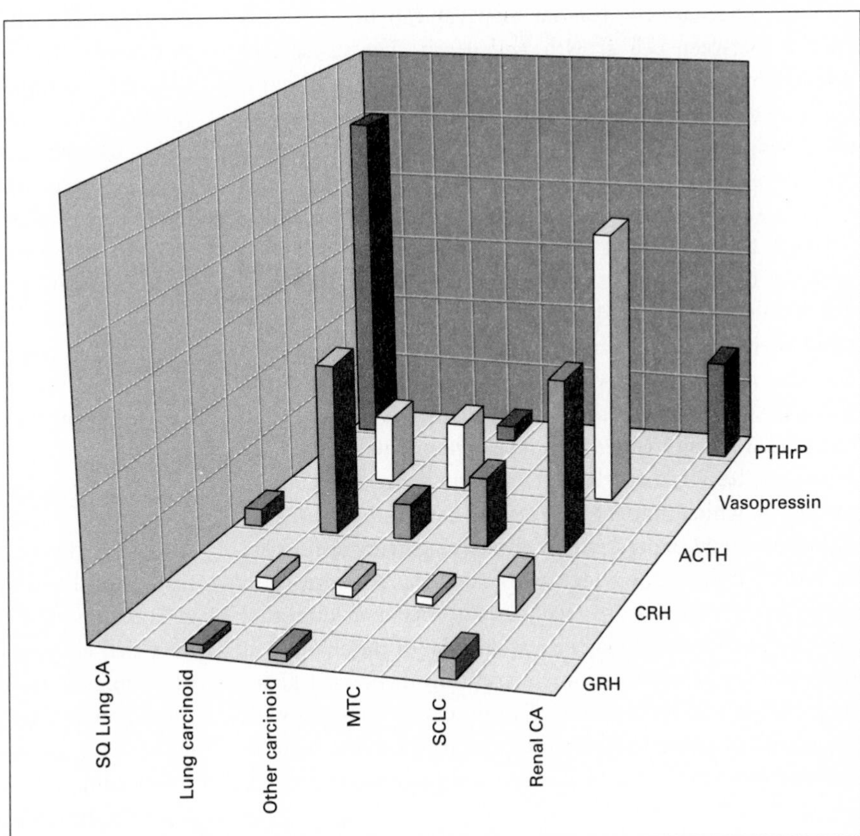

Fig. 73.1 Histogram depicting the typical associations of some ectopic hormones with certain tumour types. SQ Lung CA, squamous cell carcinoma of the lung; MTC, medullary carcinoma of the thyroid; SCLC, small-cell carcinoma of the lung; renal CA, renal carcinoma.

regulatory controls as their normal counterparts. This loss of regulation seems to be one of the most important prerequisites for ectopic hormone production. In some cases regulatory influences could not be exercised simply because of the anatomical distancing of the tumour from the normal regulatory processes, for example the absence of neuronal connections, or the absence of a locally acting endocrine modulator. In other cases it seems that a more fundamental defect in regulation has occurred. This is probably most clearly exemplified by the ectopic adrenocorticotrophic hormone (ACTH) syndrome. In this situation the pro-opiomelanocortin (POMC) gene, from which ACTH and β-endorphin are derived, loses its normal negative regulation by glucocorticoids which is normally only exercised in the corticotroph cells of the pituitary. It has been demonstrated that this is indicative of a global failure of glucocorticoid signalling in the cell, which can be restored by introduction of normal glucocorticoid receptors [5]. The defect may result from a mutation of the glucocorticoid receptor [6], or may be more complex in origin [7]. These findings imply that secretion of ACTH or related peptides may be of survival advantage to the tumour cell, or that some other aspect of defective glucocorticoid signalling may be advantageous. For example, there is evidence that β-endorphin may be trophic to certain lung tumours in culture, and thus persistent expression of the POMC gene, the precursor for β-endorphin, may have an autocrine role enhancing tumour growth. Alternatively, tumour survival can be seen as a balance between cell growth and death. The process of programmed cell death or apoptosis is liable to be a major factor determining the growth rate of the tumour. In many cell types glucocorticoids act as a stimulus to apoptosis, and thus development of glucocorticoid resistance may have considerable selective advantage for the tumour cell.

Other aspects of this loss of regulation may relate to genomic modifications that are typical of many tumours. For example, there is good evidence for alterations in DNA methylation in tumours. DNA methylation involves the addition of a methyl group to cytosine residues that precede a guanosine residue—a so-called CpG dinucleotide. Genes that are not expressed in certain normal tissues are frequently heavily methylated, but are unmethylated in those tissues in which they are expressed. Methylation probably influences gene expression by interfering with the access of certain transcription factors to the gene. Alterations in methylation patterns are recognised to occur in tumours, and this phenomenon may be responsible for the changes in promoter usage seen in some ectopically expressed genes (e.g. POMC, PTHrP) or conceivably could interfere with the access of some regulatory factors to the gene. A more detailed discussion of gene methylation can be found in [8].

Theories of the origin of ectopic hormones

As is so often the case in science, the large number of theories and their various elaborations belie the fact that we do not know why ectopic hormone production occurs. Recent developments in molecular and developmental biology may help our understanding, and will be discussed. All the major theories of the origins of ectopic hormones assume, reasonably enough, that this is a single phenomenon that may be manifest in different types of tumour with different hormones. This simplification may be wrong, but at present we are not in a position to be able to show this.

A second important assumption that we make is that of the clonal nature of tumours. It is usually considered that all tumours develop from a single cell in which some fundamental and irreversible change has occurred that gives it imperfectly regulated growth potential. There is good evidence supporting this concept.

It seems probable that multiple genes other than those for hormones are expressed 'ectopically', but because their products are not secreted, and because we do not have sensitive assays for them, we usually remain unaware of their existence. In some cases such molecules have been identified, for example α-fetoprotein or carcinoembryonic antigen, but they probably represent the tip of the iceberg of these non-hormonal proteins. Ectopic expression of non-hormone genes is compatible with all of the theories which are to be discussed.

So far as ectopic hormone-secreting tumours are concerned, the first vital question we need to know of its progenitor cell is whether it expressed the gene or had the capacity to express the gene for the hormone(s) in question prior to neoplastic change? The comparison in Table 73.3 might suggest this was likely. If it did, then hormone expression by the resulting tumour is not truly 'ectopic,' although the definition stated earlier may still be applicable. If the cell did not express the hormone concerned prior to transformation, then the study of this phenomenon should throw important light on the biology of cancer.

The de-repression hypothesis

This hypothesis, generally attributed to Gelhorn [9] and further outlined by Odell [10], takes note of the fact that all cells contain the same genetic information, only a fraction of which is expressed, and suggests that in the catastrophe of neoplastic transformation any number of genes can be turned on or off at random. In this form this proposal would make some incorrect predictions. It would imply:

1 any tumour could produce ectopic hormones;

2 a tumour could produce any ectopic hormone.

This is clearly not the case. However, it would also predict accurately that:

3 regulated expression of these hormones may be lost;

4 normal gene products would be made.

One might imagine that this very broad hypothesis could be refined in order to comply more accurately with observed fact. In some respects this is what has happened in the formulation of the de-differentiation hypothesis.

The de-differentiation hypothesis

The main difference between this hypothesis and the last is that in this case the de-repression process that leads to hormone gene expression is not random but rather retraces the development of that cell, to arrive at a precursor that normally expressed the hormone in question [11]. Our concepts of the development and differentiation of normal tissues are inextricably tied up with most theories of ectopic hormone production, and it would therefore be useful to discuss these now.

The only mammalian cell system in which we have any real understanding of the differentiation process is the haemopoietic system. Work in the early 1960s using irradiated mice identified the presence of the stem cell, a cell type that was capable of self-replication to produce more stem cells, or differentiation and division to produce so-called progenitor cells [10]. These progenitor cells could in turn differentiate and divide to give rise to each of the major cell types derived from the bone marrow: erythrocytes, platelets, macrophages, neutrophils, T cells, B cells, eosinophils and mast cells. From these early progenitor cells, differentiation proceeds in a stepwise fashion to give rise to the terminally differentiated cell types that are found in the peripheral blood.

In more recent years an understanding of the factors that regulate this process has been acquired, with the discovery of a number of differentiation factors that can act at the cell surface of certain incompletely differentiated cell types, and stimulate the proliferation and further differentiation of those cells in a certain direction [12]. This hormonal milieu can therefore shift the number and types of differentiated cell that are produced. At present the main sources for these differentiation factors are not well defined. For a more detailed discussion of this fascinating area the reader is referred to texts on haematology, immunology and developmental biology.

Our understanding of development and differentiation of solid tissues, such as those that give rise to most ectopic hormone-secreting tumours, is mainly by analogy with the haemopoietic system. Thus, it is suggested that epithelial surfaces which contain a variety of differential cell types contain a small population of stem cells which can give rise to progenitor cells, which in turn differentiate and proliferate in a series of usually unidentified stages to generate mature cell types. The factors that regulate these processes are poorly defined, but in various tissues they include growth factors such as epidermal growth factor (EGF), nerve growth factor (NGF), platelet-derived growth factor (PDGF) and transforming growth factor-β (TGF-β) and other molecules such as retinoic acid and 9-*cis*-retinoic acid.

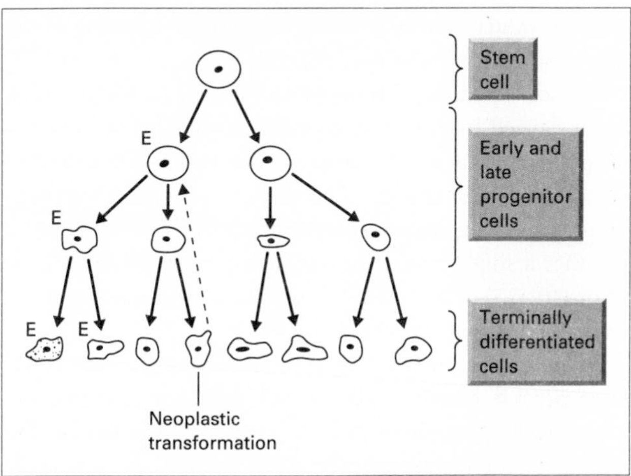

Fig. 73.2 The de-differentiation hypothesis suggests that endocrine cells develop by differentiation from a pluripotent stem cell. The endocrine cell lineage is indicated by the letter E beside some cells. Neoplastic transformation occurring in a non-endocrine cell may result in de-differentiation to a common progenitor cell (indicated by the dashed line), with the result that the tumour derived from this will have endocrine characteristics.

Thus, the de-differentiation process, represented diagrammatically in Fig. 73.2, must imply that this process could go into reverse. It is well established that neoplastic transformation is accompanied by a loss of differentiated function. For example, it can be shown using a cell line infected with a temperature-sensitive mutant of a transforming virus such as SV40, that when transformed by being grown at the permissive temperature, certain non-essential gene expression is lost in comparison with the controls grown at a non-permissive temperature, or uninfected with the virus. However, there is little or no evidence that this de-differentiation is an ordered process, and that it can lead to the switching on of new genes characteristic of the developmental precursor. This is unfortunate, since the theory correctly predicts that:

1 only certain tumours would be associated with certain ectopic hormones;

2 regulated expression of the ectopic hormone may differ;

3 normal gene products would result;

4 expression of characteristically fetal proteins and hormones could occur.

The oncogene hypothesis

This hypothesis has never really been defined, or championed by a single author or group of authors, but it has emerged as a byproduct of the explosion in the understanding of the causes of cancer in the past decade.

It is now apparent that neoplastic change is closely linked to, or caused by, alterations in the expression or function of certain cellular genes whose normal function was that of regulation of cell growth. The types of alteration that may occur include overexpression, underexpression or mutation at either a single residue or over a large stretch of the gene in question. For a detailed description of this subject the reader is referred elsewhere [13,14].

One obvious method by which these processes could alter peptide hormone gene expression is as a byproduct of oncogene overexpression. This may occur either by amplification of the oncogene or by placing the oncogene under the control of alternative regulatory elements, such as can occur following chromosomal translocation. Gene amplification signifies the generation of multiple repeats of a chromosomal segment, which contains the proto-oncogene in question, but also a significant amount of the flanking chromosomal DNA. Amplification, up to 50- to 100-fold, is often seen in tumours, or cell lines derived from tumours, as chromosomal homogeneously staining regions or as extrachromosomal fragments of DNA. Since many peptide hormone genes are in fairly close chromosomal proximity to known oncogenes [15], it is reasonable to propose that these genes could be included in the amplification segment. However, amplification of hormone genes has not yet been shown in any secreting tumour.

Thus, although these oncogene-related alterations of gene expression might provide a feasible explanation for the ectopic hormone phenomenon, there is no evidence of this as yet, and it is clearly not a unifying hypothesis. Proponents of this hypothesis could argue that although the hormone genes are intact, it could be the genes for the proteins that regulate the expression of these hormone genes that are altered, and since these factors are only just beginning to be identified, it will be some time before we know if they are perturbed in ectopic hormone-producing tumours. Taken to this level, the hypothesis becomes yet a further variation on the de-repression hypothesis, and as such is open to some of the criticisms of this hypothesis described previously.

The APUD/neuroendocrine cell hypothesis

The APUD (amine precursor uptake and decarboxylase) hypothesis is a theory of the development of endocrine cells, and not primarily a theory for the development of hormone-secreting tumours. This hypothesis, largely championed by Pearse [16,17], recognises that there are a number of morphological and cytochemical characteristics of normal peptide hormone-secreting cells including the presence of large numbers of secretory vesicles. These features are listed in Table 73.4. Such cells exist not only in the classical endocrine organs, but also widely dispersed in many other tissues, including the gut, pancreas and bronchi. Figure 73.3 shows the presence of two cells with APUD-type characteristics found in normal human small intestine. These APUD characteristics are well recognised and accepted features of many endocrine cells.

Table 73.4 APUD (amine precursor uptake and decarboxylase) characteristics.

5-Hydroxytryptophan uptake
Fluorogenic amine content
α-Glycerophosphate
Esterase and/or cholinesterase
Amino-acid decarboxylase present
Chromogranin present
Dense core secretory vesicles
Membrane-bound secretory vesicles
Rough endoplasmic reticulum
Smooth endoplasmic reticulum
Free ribosomes

Pearse and others have argued that all these cells derived developmentally by migration from the neural crest. Techniques such as the use of quail/chick early embryo chimaeras have provided good and widely accepted evidence that this is the case for certain types of cells including the calcitonin-secreting C-cells of the thyroid [18], but many authorities would now dispute that this was the case for most cells with APUD characteristics. The existence of these features is after all only a manifestation of the expression of a group of genes, and this does not necessarily imply that all these cells had a common embryological origin.

Many ectopic hormone-secreting tumour cells also have APUD characteristics suggesting that the tumour is derived from normal dispersed APUD cells (see for example Fig. 73.4). That this is the case cannot easily be demonstrated, and it could be that these characteristics are acquired by the tumour cell by the same processes that lead to the expression of peptide hormone genes. Thus, the relationship between the APUD tumour cell and the fully differentiated peripheral APUD cell is as tenuous as the relationship between that normal cell and its neural crest counterpart. Tumour cells with easily demonstrable APUD features appear to be highly active peptide secretors, and they often have a greater ability to process hormones derived from larger precursors such as POMC. Nevertheless, tumours completely lacking APUD features, which are often the more malignant undifferentiated tumours, can be high-level hormone producers.

As has been mentioned, if one looks hard enough with sensitive techniques, many, if not most, solid tumours can be shown to express one or more peptide hormone genes to

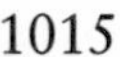

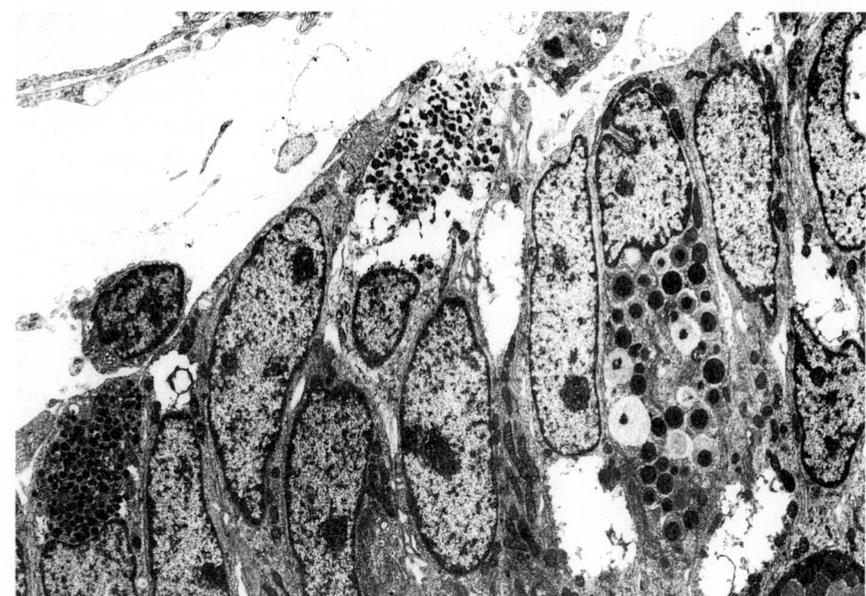

Fig. 73.3 Electron micrograph of human (fetal) small intestine. Two neuroendocrine cells are present, containing small electron-dense granules (left and top centre). These cells are surrounded by non-endocrine cell types, including a Paneth cell (right of centre) and a mucin-containing cell (bottom right). Magnification × 3920.

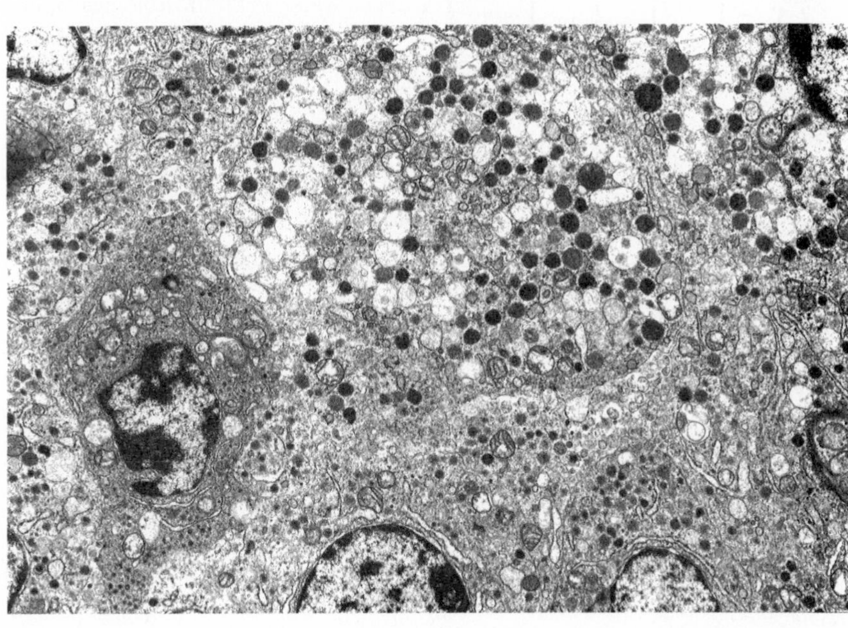

Fig. 73.4 Electron micrograph of carcinoid tumour of the lung removed from a patient with Cushing's syndrome. Immunocytochemistry revealed the presence of adrenocorticotrophic hormone in the cells of this tumour. The electron micrograph shows the presence of neurosecretory granules within the tumour cells. Note that the size of the granules is highly variable, a common feature of such tumours. Magnification × 8400.

some extent without necessarily exhibiting classical APUD features. It is not clear that the APUD hypothesis can be considered a unifying hypothesis in such cases, unless one implies a degree of associated de-differentiation.

The dys-differentiation hypothesis

The problems with the foregoing theories led Baylin and Mendelsohn to put forward a new hypothesis in 1980 [19] that took into account a large range of studies of gene expression and hormone secretion in developing and neoplastic tissue. This dys-differentiation hypothesis leaves several questions open to further research, but it is nevertheless the most complete proposal that has yet been put forward.

They envisioned the development of a normal epithelial surface, such as the bronchial mucosa or the gastrointestinal tract mucosa, to progress from a pluripotential stem cell through a series of progenitor cell stages to a mature, terminally differentiated cell.

Neoplastic change, it was suggested, occurred in a cell at an early stage of this differentiation process, a proposal supported by analogy to neoplastic change in the haemopoietic system. The resulting tumour, depicted in Fig. 73.5, is still capable, at least at this early stage, of all the subsequent steps of maturation and differentiation, although the neoplastic process is accompanied by a variable block in differentiation. As a result the relative cell numbers at each stage of differentiation will be distorted, with a preponderance of incompletely differentiated cells. Histological and immunocytochemical analysis of many different types of tumour is consistent with this view. The mean level of differentiation may be early or late. Cells at a variety of stages of differentiation may be present, as well as cells apparently differentiating in different directions. Predictably, a few scattered endocrine type cells containing secretory vesicles and perhaps immunostaining for one or more peptide hormones may be present in a typical carcinoma not associated with ectopic hormone production. Furthermore, extraction of peptide for assay or messenger RNA (mRNA) analysis would probably suggest a low level of hormone gene expression.

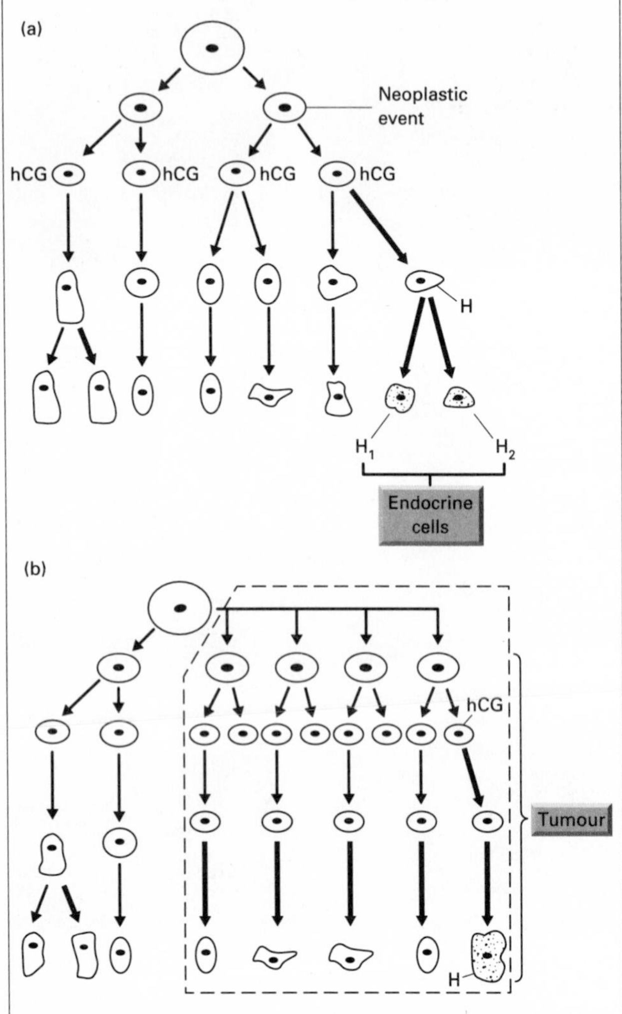

Fig. 73.5 The dys-differentiation hypothesis. Cells differentiate from a common stem cell in a hypothetical epithelial surface to produce a variety of mature, terminally differentiated cell types. The activity of each pathway is indicated by the thickness of the arrow, and the development of endocrine cells secreting peptide hormones H_1 and H_2 is a minor part of this. Early progenitor cells are depicted as secreting human chorionic gonadotrophin (hCG) (and probably also α-fetoprotein—not shown). A neoplastic event occurs in the cell indicated in (a), resulting in the proliferation of cells at this and subsequent stages of differentiation (b). Only a relatively small proportion of cells are fully differentiated, and the composition of the resulting tumour might be as shown within the dashed line.

According to the original proposal, development of a predominantly hormone-producing tumour required a second neoplastic event, or possibly an initial event, occurring at a stage of differentiation that only permitted an endocrine cell lineage to develop. Such occurrences are shown in Fig. 73.6. Unfortunately, our understanding of endocrine cell development is still so rudimentary that this suggestion remains a hypothesis. Second neoplastic events are certainly within the realms of possibility, and it is not unusual to find tumours that contain a variety of different histological appearances. Baylin and Mendelsohn proposed that such a clone might, in some situations, have a survival advantage over the other cells of varying degrees and directions of differentiation in the tumour, and that this would explain why, for example, the primary tumour may have hormone-secreting characteristics, whereas metastases

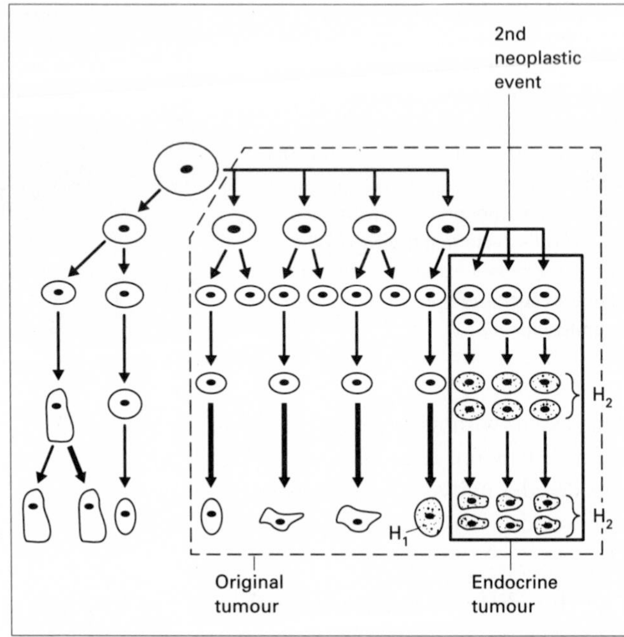

Fig. 73.6 A second neoplastic event, or possibly a primary event, occurs as indicated in the model described in Fig. 73.5. Proliferation of cells derived from this transformed cell now give rise to a typically endocrine type tumour, enclosed within the continuous line, capable of secreting one or more peptides.

which are selected for by the acquisition of other properties might lack the endocrine phenotype.

As suggested in Fig. 73.6, they also proposed that predominantly poorly differentiated tumours would be more likely to secrete 'developmental' hormones such as hCG, human placental lactogen (HPL) and α-fetoprotein, a further suggestion which seems compatible with many observations.

This model is attractive in that it predicts the association of certain hormones with certain tumours and tissues, since the tumour is essentially an amplification of the phenotype of a normal cell type. It also makes the finding of multiple hormones in individual tumours more probable, and would explain the widespread finding of very low level hormone production. It also exploits the observation that any differentiation in tumours is in a forward direction, and thus the coordinate expression of the multiple genes that give rise to APUD characteristics is reasonable.

Summary

Clinically significant ectopic hormone syndromes are uncommon, but nevertheless are extremely important because of the diagnostic and therapeutic challenges that they pose. Years after the first recognition of their existence we still do not understand why these conditions occur, although it is to be hoped that recent advances in developmental biology, cancer biology and in the techniques of molecular biology will soon resolve this. Study of these conditions may elucidate the causes of many tumour-associated phenomena, including pyrexia, weight loss and neurological manifestations of cancer. At a more fundamental level, ectopic hormone production is representative of the altered gene expression that characterises the tumour cell, and a complete understanding of this phenomenon should tell us why cancer is the disease it is, and perhaps what we can do about it.

References

1 Sarkar G, Sommer SS. Access to a messenger RNA sequence or its protein product is not limited by tissue or species specificity. *Science* 1989; **244**: 331–4.

2 Chelly J, Concordet J-P, Caplan J-C, Kahn A. Illegitimate transcription: transcription of any gene in any cell type. *Proc Natl Acad Sci USA* 1989; **86**: 2617–21.

3 Hale AC, Besser GM, Rees LH. Characterization of pro-opiomelanocortin-derived peptides in pituitary and ectopic adrenocorticotrophin-secreting tumours. *J Endocrinol* 1986; **108**: 49–56.

4 Ashitaka Y, Mochizuki M, Tojo S. Purification and properties of chorionic gonadotropin from the trophoblastic tissue of hydatidiform mole. *Endocrinology* 1972; **90**: 609–17.

5 Ray DW, Littlewood AC, Clark AJL, Davis JRE, White A. Human small cell lung cancer cell lines expressing the POMC gene have aberrant glucocorticoid receptor function. *J Clin Invest* 1994; **93**: 1625–30.

6 Gaitan D, DeBold CR, Turney MK, Zhou P, Orth DN, Kovacs WJ. Glucocorticoid receptor structure and function in an adrenocorticotropin-secreting small cell lung cancer. *Mol Endocrinol* 1995; **9**: 1193–201.

7 Ray DW, Davis JRE, White A, Clark AJL. Glucocorticoid receptor structure and function in glucocorticoid resistant small cell lung carcinoma cells. *Cancer Res* 1996; **56**: 3276–80.

8 Tate PH, Bird AP. Effects of DNA methylation on DNA binding proteins and gene expression. *Curr Opin Genet Dev* 1993; **3**: 226–31.

9 Gelhorn A. The unifying thread. *Cancer Res* 1963; **23**: 961–70.

10 Odell W. Glycoprotein hormones and neoplasms. *N Engl J Med* 1977; **297**: 609–10.

11 Shields R. Gene derepression in tumours. *Nature* 1977; **269**: 752–3.

12 Till JE, McCulloch EA. A direct measurement of the radiation sensitivity of normal bone marrow stem cells. *Radiation Res* 1961; **14**: 213–22.

13 Teich NM. Oncogenes and cancer. In: Franks LM, Teich NM, eds. *Introduction to the Cellular and Molecular Biology of Cancer.* Oxford: Oxford University Press, 1986: 200–28.

14 Pitot HC. The molecular biology of carcinogenesis. *Cancer* 1993; **72**: 962–70.

15 Hozier JC, Mass MJ, Siegfried JM. Genes for tumour markers are clustered with cellular protooncogenes on human chromosomes. *Cancer Lett* 1987; **36**: 235–45.

16 Pearse AGE. Common cytochemical and ultrastructural characteristics of cells producing peptide hormones (the APUD) series and their relevance to thyroid and ultimobranchial C-cells and calcitonin. *Proc Roy Soc Lond* 1968; **B170**: 71–80.

17 Pearse AGE. The cytochemistry and ultrastructure of polypeptide hormone-producing cells of the APUD series and the embryologic, physiologic, and pathologic implications of the concept. *J Histochem Cytochem* 1969; **17**: 303–13.

18 Le Douarin NM, Fontaine J, LeLievre C. New studies on the neural crest origin of the avian ultimobranchial glandular cells—interspecific combinations and cytochemical characteristics of C-cells based on the uptake of biogenic amine precursors. *Histochemistry* 1974; **38**: 297–305.

19 Baylin SB, Mendelsohn G. Ectopic hormone production by tumours: mechanisms involved and the biological and clinical implications. *Endocr Rev* 1980; **1**: 45–77.

CHAPTER 74

Hypercalcaemia of malignancy

V. Grill and T.J. Martin

Introduction

The calcium ion (Ca^{2+}) is an essential regulator of many body processes, including muscle contraction, many secretory mechanisms and neuronal excitation. Plasma calcium level is regulated within very narrow limits in healthy individuals, through the actions of parathyroid hormone (PTH) on bone resorption and the renal excretion of calcium, with dietary calcium provided chiefly through the action of 1,25-dihydroxyvitamin D on the intestine. Hypercalcaemia can result from excessive bone resorption, renal retention of calcium, excessive intestinal absorption or combinations of these.

Hypercalcaemia complicates many cancers, especially squamous cell cancer of the lung and other sites, breast cancer, renal cortical carcinoma and a number of haematological malignancies. The term humoral hypercalcaemia of malignancy (HHM) describes a clinical syndrome caused by secretion by a tumour of a calcaemic factor acting on the skeleton to increase bone resorption and on the kidney to increase conservation of calcium. This syndrome has now been explained, with the isolation, complementary DNA (cDNA) cloning and expression of PTH-related protein (PTHrP).

Primary hyperparathyroidism is the commonest cause of hypercalcaemia in the community with a prevalence of between five and 50 per 10 000. Among hospitalised subjects hypercalcaemia most frequently occurs as a complication of malignancy. Parathyroid disease and malignancy account for more than 80% of cases of hypercalcaemia. Other less common causes are listed in Table 74.1.

Differential diagnosis

The diagnosis of hypercalcaemia is made by the unequivocal demonstration of a plasma calcium level above the limit of the reference range for the testing laboratory. The concentration of Ca^{2+}, the fraction important in physiological processes, can be readily measured. The total serum calcium can be 'corrected' for changes in albumin concentration.

Primary hyperparathyroidism is such a common condition, and so readily treatable, that it needs to be excluded in all hypercalcaemic subjects, even in the presence of coexistent malignancy. Hypercalcaemia in cancer can occur even when the cancer is clinically occult.

The following laboratory tests are helpful to establish the cause of hypercalcaemia from the list of several possible differential diagnoses (Table 74.1). Plasma phosphate is usually below the normal range in primary hyperparathyroidism and in HHM because of the phosphaturic effects of PTH and PTHrP (Table 74.2). If renal function is significantly impaired, this lowering of phosphate is not seen. Plasma phosphate is not decreased in the other conditions listed in Table 74.1. In distinguishing between primary hyperparathyroidism and HHM, plasma bicarbonate and chloride can provide useful information, in that a mild hyperchloraemic acidosis often accompanies primary hyperparathyroidism, whereas a mild hypokalaemic, hypochloraemic alkalosis can accompany the humoral hypercalcaemia of malignancy syndrome (Table 74.2). Hypercalcaemia, alkalosis and renal impairment remain the hallmark of the milk-alkali syndrome which can occur in acute and chronic forms.

Plasma assay for PTH has reached a level of sensitivity that makes it the single most important measurement in the differential diagnosis of hypercalcaemia: there are now widely available two-site assays which detect full-length PTH. A non-suppressed level in the presence of an elevated plasma calcium concentration points to primary hyperparathyroidism as the diagnosis. The sensitivity of the two-site assays is such that in non-parathyroid hypercalcaemia the PTH level is usually suppressed below the normal range.

Table 74.1 Causes of hypercalcaemia.

Primary hyperparathyroidism
Malignancy
  Humoral hypercalcaemia of malignancy
  Solid tumours with bone metastases
  Haematological malignancy
Sarcoidosis and other granulomatous disorders
Endocrine causes
  Thyrotoxicosis
  Addison's disease
  Phaeochromocytoma
Milk-alkali syndrome
Immobilisation
Chronic renal failure
Medications
  Vitamin A and D analogues
  Oestrogens and antioestrogens
  Lithium
  Theophylline
  Thiazide diuretics
Familial hypocalciuric hypercalcaemia

Table 74.2 Biochemical features of primary hyperparathyroidism and humoral hypercalcaemia of malignancy (HHM).

	HHM	Primary hyperparathyroidism
Serum calcium	High	High
Serum phosphorus	Low	Low
Serum chloride	Low	High
Serum bicarbonate	High	Low
NcAMP	High	High
Steroid suppression	Variable	Rare

NcAMP, nephrogenous cyclic adenosine monophosphate.

Tests of stimulation or suppression of PTH have not proved to be helpful.

Although there is no existing assay which convincingly measures PTHrP in the plasma of normal adults, assays detect PTHrP in 90–100% of patients with the HHM, and in 50–70% of subjects with breast cancer-associated hypercalcaemia. The use of this assay is often to confirm a diagnosis which is suspected, or to monitor cancer treatment. However, the PTHrP levels are so invariably elevated in patients with HHM that in a given patient, suspected on clinical grounds to have HHM, failure to measure PTHrP would raise the possibility of primary hyperparathyroidism coexistent with the cancer.

Plasma assay of 25-hydroxyvitamin D (normal range 25–200 nmol/l) is essential to the diagnosis of vitamin D intoxication. Elevated levels of 1,25-dihydroxyvitamin D ($1,25\text{-}(OH)_2D$) may be found in patients with hypercalcaemia due to sarcoidosis, and in some cases of hypercalcaemia associated with lymphoma.

The tubular maximum for phosphorus (T_mP/GFR) is generally low and the fasting urinary cyclic adenosine monophosphate (cAMP)/creatinine ratio is elevated in both HHM and primary hyperparathyroidism, but not in other conditions. These tests are not of sufficient discriminatory value to be of use in the investigation of the hypercalcaemic patient.

Bone scintigraphy is useful in the evaluation of metastatic bone disease as a possible cause of hypercalcaemia.

A full-blood examination, erythrocyte-sedimentation rate (ESR), serum and urine protein electrophoresis and angiotensin-converting enzyme activity are other adjunctive tests of value in establishing the cause of the hypercalcaemia.

A prednisolone suppression test might rarely be carried out if the cause of hypercalcaemia cannot be resolved by other means. Prednisolone (60 mg/day) is administered for 10 days with daily fasting plasma calcium measurements. Significant lowering of plasma calcium occurs in sarcoidosis, vitamin D intoxication, lymphoma, multiple myeloma and in some cases of malignancy with solid cancers, but not in primary hyperparathyroidism.

Clinical features

Hypercalcaemia may present with symptoms referable to almost any organ system (Table 74.3) [1]. The severity of the symptoms in the individual patient depends on the level of the plasma calcium, on how rapidly it rose and on the general medical condition of the patient. The clinical features of hypercalcaemia are the same regardless of the aetiology, although patients with malignant disease and hypercalcaemia usually have a significant tumour burden, sometimes with widespread metastases, and are often symptomatic from the disease process itself. Because symptoms are non-specific they may be confused with features of malignant disease. It is important to recognise those symptoms and signs which may be due to hypercalcaemia because these are potentially reversible with appropriate treatment.

The gastrointestinal symptoms of hypercalcaemia are constipation, nausea and vomiting, and abdominal pain. Nausea and vomiting are early and frequent features in hypercalcaemia associated with malignancy, but they may be due to the disease process itself, to the cytotoxic therapy, or to the radiation therapy administered as treatment of the malignancy. In older patients, gastrointestinal symptoms are infrequent. A presentation with acute confusion and volume depletion is much more common in the elderly [2].

The major renal manifestations of hypercalcaemia are polyuria and polydipsia. Hypercalcaemia interferes with

Table 74.3 Symptoms and signs of hypercalcaemia.

Renal
Polyuria and thirst
Dehydration
Gastrointestinal
Nausea and anorexia
Vomiting
Constipation
Abdominal pain
Neurological
Headache
Confusion
Psychosis
Drowsiness
Coma

antidiuretic hormone action at the distal nephron causing a syndrome like diabetes insipidus. The resulting dehydration further exacerbates the hypercalcaemia.

Cardiovascular manifestations are related to effects of hypercalcaemia on cardiac repolarisation. Electrocardiographic abnormalities in hypercalcaemic patients include mild prolongation of atrioventricular (AV) conduction, prolongation of the QRS interval, shortening of the ST segment, and decrease in amplitude of the T waves [3]. The most consistent of these features is the shortening of the ST segment, most often described as shortening of the QTc interval. The amplitude of the T wave is also decreased in hypercalcaemia, with development of inverted, biphasic or notched T waves in severe cases, even in the absence of coexistent ischaemic heart disease [3,4]. These changes in T-wave morphology, polarity and amplitude disappear with normalisation of plasma calcium. Arrhythmias are an uncommon manifestation of hypercalcaemia [5], but an acute elevation of the plasma calcium may cause bradycardia and first-degree heart block.

Neurological manifestations of hypercalcaemia occur in over 50% of patients [6]. They consist of cognitive and behavioural changes, alteration in the level of consciousness and neuromuscular disturbances. Mild mental disturbances consist of fatigue, difficulty concentrating and a neurasthenic personality change characterised by lack of initiative, and depression [7–9]. Severe psychiatric symptoms may resemble mania, schizophrenia, acute confusion and even catatonic stupor. Whilst there is no correlation between psychiatric and cognitive changes and plasma calcium levels, the level of alertness does decrease with increased calcium concentrations culminating in coma. The main evidence that hypercalcaemia causes mental disturbances stems from the improvement that follows restoration of normal plasma calcium levels [10]. Electroencephalographic (EEG) tracings display several characteristic features even though they are not specific for hypercalcaemia. EEG abnormalities include slowing of the post-central rhythm, excess θ and δ activity, prominent λ waves and marked photic responses even in non-alert patients [11–13]. Lowering of plasma calcium is followed by an improvement of the EEG tracing with a delay of days or weeks.

Mechanisms of hypercalcaemia of malignancy

The hypercalcaemia of cancer has been traditionally considered as three separate syndromes:

1 the humoral hypercalcaemia of malignancy;

2 hypercalcaemia associated with localised osteolysis due to bone metastases;

3 hypercalcaemia associated with myeloma and other haematological malignancies.

Our understanding of the ways in which various tumours induce hypercalcaemia has increased rapidly in the last few years with the identification of several tumour-derived factors that elevate plasma calcium. The discovery of PTHrP, followed by the establishment of assays that enable its detection in the circulation, has provided new insights into the mechanisms for the hypercalcaemia in these three syndrome classes. It has become clear that this classification does not reflect distinct pathophysiological mechanisms, and the reasons for this will be expanded in the following discussion.

Humoral hypercalcaemia of malignancy

The term humoral hypercalcaemia of malignancy was introduced to describe patients with certain cancers in whom the blood calcium is elevated in the absence of skeletal metastases [14]. The commonest cause of this is squamous cell carcinoma of the lung. Squamous cell cancers at other sites, including skin, oesophagus, and head and neck may also be associated with humoral hypercalcaemia. Renal cortical carcinoma, primary liver cancer, breast cancer, pancreatic cancer, bladder and prostatic carcinoma, and melanoma may all be associated with humoral hypercalcaemia. In the absence of secondary lesions, removal of the primary tumour results in resolution of the hypercalcaemia [15]. Tumour factors are secreted that act on the skeleton generally to increase bone resorption, and on the kidney to reduce calcium excretion and increase phosphorus excretion [14]. Nephrogenous cAMP excretion (NcAMP) is also increased [16–18] and there is often a mild hypokalaemic, hypochloraemic alkalosis. The degree of hypercalcaemia can remain constant for many months; sometimes it progresses steadily and is associated with a mild hypokalaemic hypochloraemic alkalosis, and sometimes apparently stable hypercalcaemia can progress rapidly to severe, and even life-threatening forms. This may occur without any obvious explanation, or be associated with rapid progression of tumour. Alternatively, it may be a consequence of dehydration in the patient in association with treatment or coexistent infection. It is clear that patients with HHM resemble those with primary hyperparathyroidism in their main biochemical features (Table 74.3), a similarity which has been recognised for many years.

Hypercalcaemia associated with bone metastases

Despite many improvements in early cancer detection and more effective treatment, metastatic disease remains the leading cause of cancer-related deaths. Bone is the most common site of metastasis in breast cancer and 25% of early-stage patients will develop this complication. This figure increases to 75% in patients with advanced disease [19]. Currently, there is no single, accurate predictor to identify which patients will develop this complication. In the clinical follow-up of patients with breast cancer especially, bone scanning at regular intervals is important in the detection of bone metastases. Recognition of the symptoms of early hypercalcaemia is of the utmost importance, since further progression can be prevented by appropriate measures, including increased fluid intake, and anti-tumour therapy. A 'flare' of hypercalcaemia can accompany the use of anti-oestrogen therapy in some patients with breast cancer [20].

Although for many years it was considered that the main mechanism of hypercalcaemia in patients with breast cancer was the release of calcium from bone by osteolytic deposits [1], there is now evidence for a humoral contribution in these patients also. The extent of metastatic bone disease correlates poorly with both the occurrence and the degree of hypercalcaemia in malignancy [21]. In 80–90% of cases of unselected solid tumour patients with hypercalcaemia, irrespective of whether bone metastases are present, there is evidence of an underlying humoral mechanism [21]. The putative humoral mediator produces hypercalcaemia both by stimulating generalised osteolysis and, in most cases, by impairing the renal excretion of the resultant increase in filtered calcium load. A reduced renal phosphate threshold and increased tubular calcium reabsorption were observed in hypercalcaemic patients when compared with their normocalcaemic counterparts, emphasising the importance of renal mechanisms in mediating the hypercalcaemia. It is now well established that a high proportion of patients with hypercalcaemia and skeletal metastases have high circulating levels of PTHrP.

Hypercalcaemia in haematological malignancy

Haematological malignancies may be associated with osteolytic bone destruction and with hypercalcaemia. The overall incidence of hypercalcaemia in patients with lymphoma in the western world is relatively low when compared with that in patients with solid tumours or with multiple myeloma [22], accounting for approximately 5% of cases of hypercalcaemia in malignancy. There are case reports of hypercalcaemia associated with chronic myeloid leukaemia [23] and acute lymphoblastic leukaemia [24]. Hypercalcaemia is relatively uncommon in both non-Hodgkin's and Hodgkin's lymphoma, as shown by a series in which only one of 190 cases of Hodgkin's disease was associated with hypercalcaemia, and only three of 104 cases of non-Hodgkin's lymphoma [25]. In our series of 165 consecutive patients admitted to a haematology unit we documented hypercalcaemia in 18. It was due to primary hyperparathyroidism in three cases. In the remainder it was associated with multiple myeloma in nine, high-grade B-cell non-Hodgkin's lymphoma in five and with myeloid neoplasia in one [26]. A number of case reports have documented hypercalcaemia without lytic bone lesions in both Hodgkin's and non-Hodgkin's lymphoma which was associated with elevated 1,25-$(OH)_2D$ levels and low PTH levels in plasma [27–33]. In our patients with hypercalcaemia associated with haematological malignancy, plasma levels of PTHrP comparable with those in HHM were present in two of four patients with non-Hodgkin's lymphoma and in three of nine patients with multiple myeloma [26].

Although hypercalcaemia is an infrequent complication of lymphoma, a particular diagnostic subgroup of patients with adult T-cell lymphoma/leukaemia has a very high incidence of hypercalcaemia, varying from 26 to 100% in different reports [34–36]. 1,25-$(OH)_2D$ levels in this group of patients are uniformly suppressed [37]. This disease, with predominant geographic distribution in Japan and a small cluster in the West Indies, is strongly associated with a retrovirus, human T-cell lymphotrophic virus type I (HTLV-I) [38–40]. Hypercalcaemia is the most important prognostic determinant in this disease and also a frequent cause of death. Hypercalcaemia in these patients is associated with elevated NcAMP levels, low-normal immunoreactive PTH levels, and reduced serum 1,25–$(OH)_2D$ concentrations [41], in the absence of lytic lesions in bone. These features are similar to those seen in HHM and it is now well established that the hypercalcaemia in these patients is mediated by PTHrP.

Hypercalcaemia occurs in approximately one-third of all patients with multiple myeloma [1,42], a disease resulting from uncontrolled proliferation of plasma cells derived from a single clone. Bone involvement in myeloma is characterised by extensive bone destruction accompanied by pain and susceptibility to fracture. Skeletal X-rays reveal abnormalities in 79% of patients [42]. These consist of osteoporosis, lytic lesions and fractures, with over half of the patients having a combination of all three. The characteristic skeletal lesions of myeloma are the so-called punched-out lytic areas which are sharply circumscribed. The vertebrae, skull, thoracic cage, pelvis, and proximal portions of humerus and femur are the most common sites of bone involvement in multiple myeloma. Pathological fractures are common and should always suggest the possibility of myeloma. In contrast to patients with metastatic carcinoma, the vertebral pedicles are rarely involved in myeloma. Quantitative histological evaluation of myeloma-induced bone changes reveals increased osteoclastic resorption surfaces and increased numbers of osteoclasts in areas of bone invaded by plasma cells. Reduced thickness of osteoid seams and a low calcification rate are consistent with reduced osteoblastic activity [43]. This is reflected by significantly reduced levels of bone Gla protein (osteocalcin) which are low in advanced disease [44]. Bone Gla protein, a sensitive marker of osteoblastic bone formation, is *not* elevated in 80% of patients with this disease despite evidence of increased osteoclastic bone resorption [45]. This suggests an uncoupling of bone resorption and bone formation. The osteoblastic inhibition would also explain the negative isotopic bone scan observed in multiple myeloma [46]. Histomorphometric parameters are not changed by chemotherapy [43], highlighting the requirement for specific inhibitors of osteoclastic bone resorption in the treatment of the hypercalcaemia and the skeletal complications of this disease. Monthly infusions of pamidronate, a second-generation bisphosphonate have been shown to provide significant protection against skeletal complications in patients with advanced multiple myeloma [47]. The increased bone resorption leading to hypercalcaemia in myeloma is due to the secretion by myeloma cells of bone-resorbing cytokines which stimulate osteoclasts. A number of cytokines previously described by the generic name 'osteoclast-activating factor' [48–50] have been identified in activated leucocyte cultures: interleukin 1, tumour-necrosis factor-α (TNF-α) or cachectin, and TNF-β or lymphotoxin. It is not yet certain whether one or more of these cytokines are responsible for the stimulation of osteoclastic bone resorption in multiple myeloma. The bone-resorbing activity from human myeloma cell lines has been attributed mostly to lymphotoxin (TNF-β) by some workers [51], and to interleukin 1 by others [52]. Although production of these bone-resorbing cytokines may be related to osteoclastic bone destruction and hypercalcaemia in patients with myeloma, other cytokines may also be involved. A subset of patients with multiple myeloma do not exhibit either fragments or intact monoclonal immunoglobulins in their circulation [42,53,54]. This plasma-cell dyscrasia first identified in 1958 [55] is termed non-secretory myeloma. Although it is rare, accounting for approximately 1% of patients with multiple myeloma, bone loss [56] and hypercalcaemia may be the presenting features [57]. Therefore, this diagnosis must be considered in a patient in whom no other cause for the hypercalcaemia has been found. In patients with non-secretory myeloma, clinical and laboratory findings related to renal tubular complications, plasma expansion or hyperviscosity do not occur, and the diagnosis under these circumstances is obscure until suggested by skeletal pain, pathologic fractures or bony disruption. Screening a hypercalcaemic patient for the presence of multiple myeloma by immunoelectrophoresis of serum and urine alone does not exclude the diagnosis. Atypical clinical features seen in cases of non-secretory myeloma may be a normal or only slightly low haemoglobin level, absence of rouleaux formation in the peripheral blood smear and relatively normal ESR. In addition, low normal or depressed immunoglobulin values may be found for the three major fractions, and proteinuria is absent. The diagnosis in such cases is made by bone-marrow biopsy. Under these circumstances the clinician's awareness of the potential significance of mild elevations of plasma calcium, and a prompt bone-marrow examination if other causes have been excluded, is indicated to avoid delay in making the diagnosis.

Discovery of PTHrP

Hypercalcaemia as a complication of malignancy has been recognised since the 1920s [58]. In 1941, Fuller Albright discussed a patient in whom hypercalcaemia and hypophosphataemia resolved after the irradiation of a single bone metastasis from a renal carcinoma [59]. Albright proposed that the hypercalcaemia might be due to production of PTH by the cancer. In succeeding years this idea gained acceptance, and the term, 'ectopic PTH syndrome', was widely applied to patients with cancer who had a high plasma calcium, low phosphorus, and minimal or no bony metastases [60]. Support for this came in 1966 when Berson and Yalow [61] published results with the first radioimmunoassay for PTH, in which they found significant elevations of the PTH level in a number of unselected patients with lung cancer. Over the next several years until the early 1970s, several reports were published of measurable PTH (by radioimmunoassay) in extracts of cancer from such patients [1,14]. There was one report of an arteriovenous gradient across a tumour bed, indicating release of PTH from tumour [62], and production of immunoreactive PTH was shown by a cell culture established from a renal cortical carcinoma of a hypercalcaemic patient [63]. Throughout this time it was evident, however, that the radioimmunoassay of PTH presented technical problems, and in none of the above instances was the circulating level of PTH convincingly very high—certainly not at the levels frequently found with corresponding degrees of elevation of plasma calcium in patients with primary hyperparathyroidism. Two groups of workers in the early 1970s published results indicating that the circulating immunoreactive PTH in the cancer patients differed from 'authentic' PTH [64–66]. The levels in plasma were in these cases lower than in primary hyperparathyroidism; in one series the cancer immunoreactivity was significantly non-parallel to PTH standards [66] and in another it was of higher molecular weight than PTH [65]. Thus, the early 1970s saw some doubt arising that PTH itself was a major contributor to the clinical and biochemical features of this cancer syndrome. This doubt became more firmly based when Powell *et al.* [15] showed in studies of several patients with humoral hypercalcaemia that PTH could not be detected in plasma or in tumour extracts, despite their use of a wide range of PTH antisera directed against different parts of the molecule.

The more comprehensive clinical and biochemical investigations that followed [16–18] indicated that the manifestations of HHM were mediated via PTH receptors in kidney and bone [1], and the development of sensitive bioassays for PTH led to exciting developments in understanding of the syndrome. The bioassays revealed that these tumour extracts could stimulate adenylate cyclase in PTH-responsive renal cortical membranes [67,68]. A sensitive cytochemical assay for PTH in kidney cells could detect PTH-like bioactivity in the serum of patients in whom immunoreactive PTH was undetectable [69]. Studies in PTH-responsive osteogenic sarcoma cells showed that tumour extracts of rat and human origin could also stimulate adenylate cyclase in this system [70]. Peptide antagonists of PTH blocked biological activity but preincubation with PTH antisera was ineffective in blocking biological activity [70], indicating that the active material acted on PTH receptors but was immunologically distinct from PTH. Messenger RNA (mRNA) for PTH could not be detected in any of a series of tumours associated with the HHM syndrome [71]. These observations led to the identification and isolation of the factor responsible for the syndrome of HHM. Experimental animal models were developed and cell cultures established from animal and human tumours [72–75]. Purification of the active factor to homogeneity on gels was reported [76,77], and PTHrP was finally purified, sequenced and cloned from a cultured human lung cancer cell line (BEN) [76,78] and from other sources [79,80].

The amino-acid sequence of PTHrP bears 60% homology with that of PTH over the first 13 amino acids (Fig. 74.1). The gene codes for a protein of 141, 139 or 173 amino acids determined by alternate 3′ splicing of mRNA. A pre pro sequence of 36 amino acids contains potential cleavage points at residues 8 or 6 leaving a short pro sequence. The PTH-like biological activity of PTHrP is contained within the first 34 amino acids. Beyond this region the two molecules have unique sequences.

The limited homology at the amino-terminal region of the mature protein between PTHrP and PTH seemed sufficient to account for the similar actions of PTHrP and PTH. PTHrP mimics the actions of PTH *in vitro* and *in vivo* [81–87]. Immunohistochemical analyses of tumour sections using specific antibodies predominantly raised to PTHrP(1–34), but also to unique mid-molecule PTHrP(50–69) and C-terminal PTHrP(106–141) epitopes, have shown that PTHrP is present in the cells of all squamous cell cancers investigated [88], indicating the potential of these tumours to produce HHM. In a nude mouse model of HHM, both the hypercalcaemia and the bone abnormalities are effectively attenuated by treatment with neutralising antisera against PTHrP [89,90]. These passive immunisation experiments established that PTHrP was at least a major, if not the sole, mediator of hypercalcaemia in these models of HHM, even if they did not exclude the possibility that there could be other contributing factors. There are some discrepancies between the features of HHM and hyperparathyroidism [1] which may relate either to interactions with other tumour factors which may be cosecreted with PTHrP, or possibly to actions mediated via regions of the PTHrP molecule beyond the first 34 amino acids. An example is the hypokalaemic alkalosis seen in hypercalcaemia of cancer, whereas mild hyperchloraemic acidosis is more commonly

Fig. 74.1 Amino-acid sequences of parathyroid hormone (PTH)(1–34) and PTH-related protein (PTHrP)(1–34).

	1									10										20										30				
PTHrP	A	V	S	E	H	Q	L	L	H	D	K	G	K	S	I	Q	D	L	R	R	R	F	F	L	H	H	L	I	A	E	I	H	T	A
PTH	S	V	S	E	I	Q	L	M	H	F	L	G	K	H	L	N	S	M	E	R	V	E	W	L	R	K	K	L	Q	D	V	H	N	F

noted in primary hyperparathyroidism (Table 74.3). As a possible explanation for this, altered renal handling of bicarbonate by the rat kidney perfused with PTHrP(1–141) has been found as compared with PTHrP(1–34) [91]. Prolonged infusion with PTHrP(1–141) resulted in restricted bicarbonate excretion, after the initial increased excretion noted in response to both forms of PTHrP and to PTH itself.

As is the case with PTH, N-terminal fragments of PTHrP promote renal 1-α hydroxylation of vitamin D *in vitro* and *in vivo* [82,92]. Early clinical observations indicated that in contrast to primary hyperparathyroidism, low levels of 1,25-$(OH)_2D$ are present in most patients with HHM [16]. This is not true in all cases [93], and in a more recent study, serum 1,25-$(OH)_2D$ levels were not found to be generally suppressed in HHM, with a significant relation between plasma PTHrP and serum 1,25-$(OH)_2D$ in the absence of demonstrable bone metastases [94]. It is possible that, in some cases, factors other than PTHrP released by tumours causing hypercalcaemia may modify the capacity of the amino-terminal portion of PTHrP to stimulate the 1α-hydroxylase enzyme [95]. Alternatively, the suppression of 1α-hydroxylase may be mediated by another region of the PTHrP molecule. The controversy over vitamin D metabolism in HHM is yet to be resolved.

There is little doubt that PTHrP is the major, if not the sole, mediator of hypercalcaemia in patients with the HHM syndrome. It is still possible that in some cases other bone-resorbing factors could contribute to the development of hypercalcaemia on a humoral basis. A number of tumour-derived factors have been identified to be potent resorbers of bone: interleukin 1, TNF-α and -β, transforming growth factor-α. PTHrP and interleukin 1 can synergistically stimulate bone resorption *in vitro* and increase the serum calcium concentration in mice *in vivo* [96]. Production of interleukin 1 has been identified in clonal cell lines established from squamous cell cancers associated with hypercalcaemia and leucocytosis [97–99]. The significance of these factors and their possible interplay with PTHrP should become clear as our knowledge of the role of cytokines in bone metabolism is increased.

Role of PTHrP in the hypercalcaemia of cancer

Further confirmation of the aetiological link between elevated levels of PTHrP and hypercalcaemia associated with malignancy has been achieved by measurement of circulating levels by radioimmunoassay. Assays for PTHrP have provided further insight into the prevalence of PTHrP as a cause of hypercalcaemia of cancer and have the potential to become useful diagnostically.

Despite their 60% homology over the first 13 amino acids, PTH and PTHrP are immunologically distinct. Radioimmunoassays (RIAs) and two-site immunoradiometric assays (IRMAs) have documented circulating levels of PTHrP in high proportions of subjects with malignancy-associated hypercalcaemia [100–108]. These assays detect circulating levels of PTHrP with detection limits varying from 0.1 pmol/l to 20 pmol/l. In a sensitive two-site IRMA with a detection limit of 0.1 pmol/l [106], PTHrP levels were reported in some normal subjects with levels close to assay detection, not higher than 1.5 pmol/l. Other assays report higher levels of PTHrP in normal subjects [101,103]. This variability results from differences in sample handling, lack of knowledge of the circulating forms of PTHrP, and lack of an appropriate technique for correcting for non-specific protein effects on antibody binding to antigen, making interpretation of these data difficult. Without an adequate control matrix known to contain no PTHrP, such as the use of serum or plasma from patients with hypoparathyroidism to validate PTH measurements, these results are difficult to validate. Results so far suggest that PTHrP circulates at extremely low levels in healthy subjects, if at all, and may only rarely be detected by N-terminal radioimmunoassays.

The possibility that PTHrP might circulate and contribute to hypercalcaemia in primary hyperparathyroidism is raised by the demonstration of PTHrP mRNA in parathyroid adenomas [109] and the demonstration of PTHrP by immunohistochemistry and Western blotting in parathyroid adenomas [110] and also in hyperplastic parathyroid tissue associated with chronic renal failure [110]. However, circulating levels of PTHrP are not generally elevated in primary hyperparathyroidism. Burtis *et al.* [102] measured PTHrP in blood samples from draining neck veins obtained during parathyroid surgery in two patients using a two-site IRMA against PTHrP(1–74). No gradient between neck veins and peripheral levels was seen. In any event, it is clear that circulating levels of PTHrP in cancer-associated hypercalcaemia are very much higher than those in hyperparathyroidism.

Applying strict validation procedures to samples giving results near the assay detection limit (2 pmol/l), we have detected circulating PTHrP levels in 100% of patients with hypercalcaemia associated with malignancy without bone metastases, and in only one of 38 normal subjects by RIA using an antiserum against PTHrP(1–40) [105] (Fig. 74.2). We have analysed hypercalcaemic patients with solid tumours other than breast in two groups, according to the presence or absence of bone metastases, as demonstrated by isotope scanning. Breast cancer patients with hypercalcaemia were analysed separately. In patients with hypercalcaemia associated with solid tumours, and with no evidence of bone metastases, PTHrP was always detected in plasma (Fig. 74.2). PTHrP levels above those of normal subjects were also found

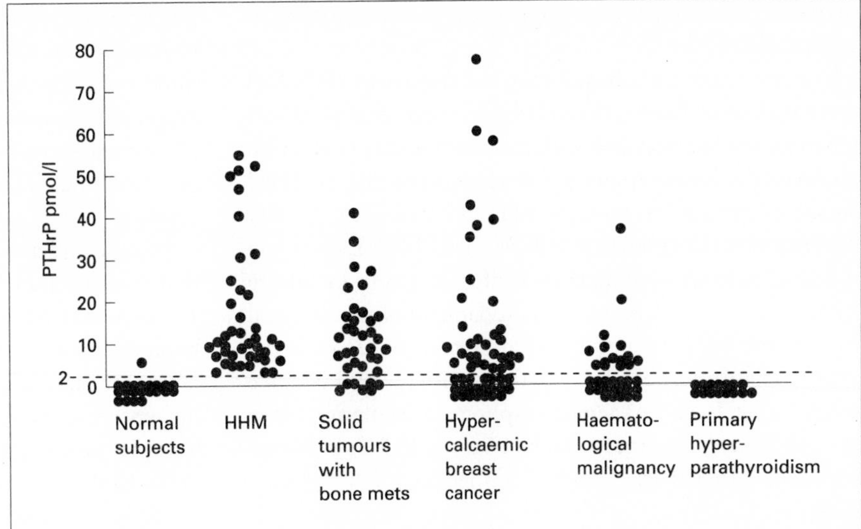

Fig. 74.2 Plasma parathyroid hormone-related protein (PTHrP) levels by N-terminal radioimmunoassay in different clinical groups. The dotted line indicates the assay detection limit.

in 64% of patients with hypercalcaemia and metastatic malignancy to bone, from primary sources other than breast (Fig. 74.2). This latter group included several patients in whom the mechanism of hypercalcaemia was likely to be humoral. Consistent with this is the finding that in the metastatic group, all squamous cell cancer patients had elevated PTHrP levels, as did one patient with a pancreatic neuroendocrine tumour in this group.

As previously indicated in clinical studies [16,21], the presence or absence of bone metastases, a feature that was used to distinguish between humoral and osteolytic mechanisms of hypercalcaemia, can no longer be used to define the syndrome of HHM. A humoral mechanism for the hypercalcaemia may still exist with metastatic bone disease. Of particular interest is the finding of elevated plasma levels of PTHrP in patients with hypercalcaemia associated with breast cancer and bone metastases [101,105,111] (Fig. 74.2). The hypercalcaemia in this situation had not generally been considered to have a humoral basis [1]. Patients with hypercalcaemia of breast cancer have been identified [112–115] with biochemical features of HHM. PTHrP has been purified from a breast cancer [77], and we have found evidence by immunohistology and *in situ* hybridisation for the presence of PTHrP in 60% of cases from an unselected series of breast cancers [116,117]. We have also found an increased incidence of positive localisation of PTHrP by immunohistochemistry in breast cancer metastases to bone compared with other sites [19]. A clinical study demonstrated a positive correlation between PTHrP expression in primary breast cancers and subsequent development of bone metastases [118]. All of these observations focus on a likely role for PTHrP in malignant breast disease. One possibility which is of particular interest is that PTHrP production might contribute to the ability of breast cancers to erode bone and establish there as metastases. The clinical observations have been extended by using a mouse model of bone metastases in which inoculation of a human cancer cell line into the left ventricle of the mouse reliably produces osteolytic metastases [119]. When the malignant cells were engineered to overexpress PTHrP (by transfection with the cDNA for preproPTHrP), an increase in the number of osteolytic metastases was observed [120]. These data strongly suggest that PTHrP expression by breast cancer cells enhances their metastatic potential to bone.

In some normocalcaemic patients with malignancy, levels close to the detection limit of various assays have been reported [100,102,108,111]. We have shown by immunohistology that PTHrP is present in 100% of a series of squamous cell cancers of various origins [88]. This suggests that further sensitivity is needed for PTHrP assays to be applied to the early identification of those patients with cancer, in whom circulating PTHrP levels are rising, and who are therefore at risk for the development of hypercalcaemia.

The development of RIAs that measure PTHrP in plasma has also resulted in the finding of elevated PTHrP levels in a proportion of patients with haematological malignancies and hypercalcaemia [100–102] (Fig. 74.2). We have detected circulating levels of PTHrP of the order of those associated with HHM in cases of non-Hodgkin's lymphoma of B-cell lineage and in cases of multiple myeloma [26]. Immunohistochemical staining demonstrated intracellular PTHrP in some of the neoplastic cells from a lymph-node section in one of the cases. In another case of blastic transformation of chronic myeloid leukemia, elevated plasma levels of PTHrP were temporally related to the development of hypercalcaemia, and a fall in PTHrP concentrations was associated with regression of disease following chemotherapy [121].

It is now well established that the retrovirus (HTLV-I) associated adult T-cell leukaemia/lymphoma often produces hypercalcaemia associated with increased urinary excretion of cAMP and low-normal PTH levels as is the case in HHM associated with solid tumours. PTH-like biological activity is secreted by the neoplastic cells *in vitro* [122]. Expression of PTHrP mRNA within HTLV-I-infected T cells in culture [123] has also been demonstrated, and immunohistochemical staining for PTHrP found in cells in lymph nodes involved with neoplastic tissue [124] in patients with HTLV-I positive human adult T-cell leukaemia/lymphoma. Circulating levels of PTHrP have been measured by two-site IRMA in hypercalcaemic patients with adult T-cell leukaemia/lymphoma [108].

These observations indicate that PTHrP-mediated hypercalcaemia not only occurs in association with solid tumours with or without skeletal metastases, but it can also occur in association with haematological malignancies. In the latter, PTHrP-mediated hypercalcaemia can extend not only to malignant processes involving the T-lymphocyte series but also to those involving the B-lymphocyte series and the myeloid series. It is possible that PTHrP has a role as local mediator of increased bone resorption in multiple myeloma, and that it is at times produced in sufficient quantities to reach the circulation and produce an endocrine effect. Such a process could contribute to the osteoporosis in multiple myeloma as well as to the hypercalcaemia.

The development of sensitive PTHrP assays has allowed a better understanding of its importance in hypercalcaemia associated with different malignancies. Breast cancer almost universally is associated with bone metastases when hypercalcaemia develops and a high proportion of patients with hypercalcaemia associated with this tumour have elevated PTHrP levels. PTHrP is produced by many tumour types and a role in the development of bone metastases in breast cancer has been suggested. Other tumours not traditionally associated with humoral factor production such as bowel cancer [125] can have elevated PTHrP levels. All patients with hypercalcaemia and squamous cell cancers have elevated levels of PTHrP regardless of whether or not bone metastases are present [105]. Although less frequently than is the case for solid tumours, PTHrP also has a role in the hypercalcaemia of haematological malignancy. It is now clear that the classification of hypercalcaemia of malignancy in three syndrome classes no longer reflects distinct pathophysiological mechanisms.

In contrast to assays directed against the amino-terminal portion of PTHrP, assays directed against the carboxy-terminal portion of the PTHrP molecule [102,126] measure markedly elevated levels in patients with renal failure. This points out the similarity of PTHrP to native PTH with respect to metabolism of carboxy-terminal fragments that depend upon renal mechanisms for their clearance. The accumulation of C-terminal fragments in renal failure suggests that PTHrP also originates in non-malignant tissues. The source of circulating PTHrP in the absence of malignancy remains unclear.

Specific and sensitive two-site, non-competitive methods that measure intact PTH do not detect PTHrP [127–129]. These assays have found PTH levels in tumour-induced hypercalcaemia to be suppressed below the normal range in most patients, consistent with the inhibition of PTH secretion by hypercalcaemia. Only five well-documented cases of true 'ectopic' production of authentic PTH have been reported [130–134].

Treatment

Severe symptomatic hypercalcaemia is a metabolic emergency requiring immediate treatment (see also Chapter 41). Continuous administration of intravenous isotonic saline (0.9% NaCl solution) will result in a modest decrease in the plasma calcium concentration due to a dilutional effect and enhanced calciuresis, and is the first step in the management of severe hypercalcaemia. The rate of administration is based on the severity of the hypercalcaemia, the degree of dehydration and the ability of the patient's cardiovascular system to tolerate volume expansion. Clinical improvement usually occurs after rehydration over 24–48 hours, but normalisation of plasma calcium rarely occurs except in very mild hypercalcaemia and other treatments are needed.

Although frusemide and ethacrynic acid inhibit calcium and sodium reabsorption in the ascending limb of the loop of Henle, loop diuretics should not be used routinely since they may exacerbate fluid loss and dehydration with consequent increase in hypercalcaemia. Intensive administration of frusemide in very large doses of 80–100 mg every 2 hours is effective in lowering plasma calcium [135] but requires an intensive-care unit to monitor electrolytes and central venous pressures at frequent intervals. This form of treatment can be dangerous in patients with myocardial dysfunction and is not necessary today with the availability of potent antiresorptive agents.

Calcitonin administered subcutaneously or intramuscularly in doses of 4–8 U/kg bodyweight every 6–12 hours can rapidly lower the plasma calcium, but the effect is brief with most patients showing only a transient response. This escape phenomenon may be decreased with concomitant administration of glucocorticoids [136,137]. However, the present role of calcitonin in the treatment of hypercalcaemia is that of an adjunctive drug in patients with severe hypercalcaemia while waiting for the effect of slower-acting agents with longer duration of action like the bisphosphonates.

The bisphosphonates are a class of drug developed over the past three decades for use in various diseases of bone and calcium metabolism [138]. Several are commercially available today and the availability and indications for which they are registered vary from country to country. Bisphosphonates are potent inhibitors of bone resorption. Their mode of action is not yet fully understood. Mechanisms other than their well-known physicochemical property of inhibition of crystal dissolution result in inhibition of the activity of the osteoclast. This effect appears to be at least in part mediated by an inhibitor of osteoclast survival or recruitment [139] secreted by osteoblasts in response to bisphosphonates. Bisphosphonates are very poorly absorbed from the gut. They have a very short plasma half-life, depositing rapidly into bone, in areas both of bone formation and destruction. Renal clearance is very high and skeletal retention is very long, possibly lifelong. Bisphosphonates have been used in a variety of schedules and dosages. Pamidronate disodium (PD) has been used successfully in the treatment of hypercalcaemia associated with cancer [140–142]. Pamidronate disodium given intravenously as a single dose of 15–90 mg according to the severity of the hypercalcaemia can result in normalisation of plasma calcium in the majority of patients. The duration of the response is variable lasting up to 3 or 4 weeks.

The most important adverse effect of bisphosphonates is their potential nephrotoxicity mediated by the precipitation of bisphosphonate–calcium complexes in the kidney [143]. This can be prevented by administering the drug by slow intravenous infusion over one to several hours depending on the dose given. A transient febrile reaction may occur within 24 hours.

In addition to their short-term efficacy in the treatment of the hypercalcaemia of malignancy, long-term studies have shown that bisphosphonates are effective in the long-term control of osteolysis [144,145]. Recent trials have examined the efficacy of oral bisphosphonates as adjuvant therapy showing encouraging results in patients at risk of developing bone metastases [173] and in reducing the skeletal complications in patients with advanced multiple myeloma [47].

Mithramycin, an inhibitor of DNA-directed RNA synthesis, exerts a hypocalcaemic effect by damaging the osteoclast [146]. Doses of 1.5–2.0 mg given as intravenous infusion over 4 hours result in lowering of plasma calcium after 24–48 hours. Its administration can be complicated by nausea, vomiting, thrombocytopoenia, hepatic, renal and neurotoxicity. It should only be considered if treatment with maximally tolerated doses of bisphosphonates fail to normalise the plasma calcium [147]. Clinical experience with gallium nitrate, another inhibitor of bone resorption is still limited. It is administered by continuous intravenous infusion for 5 days in a dose of 200 mg/m^2 daily. Nephrotoxicity is a potential adverse effect.

These agents are effective against the bone-resorptive component of tumour-induced hypercalcaemia, without influencing the increased renal tubular calcium reabsorption which PTHrP produces. Calcitonin and perhaps mithramycin have a weak calciuric effect but the main effect of these agents is also on bone.

Significance of PTHrP as a predictor of response to treatment of hypercalcaemia of malignancy with bisphosphonates

PTHrP has potent effects on the renal tubule and on bone resorption. These actions are detected by a rise in the tubular calcium threshold and nephrogenous cAMP and a fall in the tubular phosphate threshold. Despite PTHrP having a dual action on bone and kidney, the agents available for the treatment of hypercalcaemia in cancer are primarily aimed at reducing bone resorption and no agent has a substantial effect on calcium excretion. A poor response to pamidronate disodium occurs in cases of hypercalcaemia of malignancy that have evidence of renal tubular stimulation as indicated by a low tubular threshold for phosphate or high threshold for calcium [148]. It is therefore not surprising that in studies of patients with tumour-induced hypercalcaemia, the PTHrP level was the best determinant for the calcaemic response to pamidronate, with high levels correlating with poor response and vice versa [149]. Other parameters which indirectly indicated the presence of a humoral mechanism for the hypercalcaemia also correlated with response. The presence of bone metastases, on the other hand, predicted a good response to treatment [149].

Currently, the prediction of a poor response will not change clinical practice because agents are not available that conveniently increase calcium excretion. The development of drugs that inhibit the tubular reabsorption of calcium [150], specific inhibitors of PTH or PTHrP action [151], antibodies to PTHrP [89], or inhibitors of PTHrP production may allow better control of hypercalcaemia in these patients when used in combination with the available inhibitors of osteolysis. Of particular interest are the new analogues of vitamin D which have low calcaemic activity yet retain the property of inhibition of PTH gene expression. The first reported analogue of this type was 22-oxa-1,25-$(OH)_2D$, or 22-oxacalcitriol (OCT) [152], a non-calcaemic analogue of calcitriol which has been shown to inhibit expression of the PTH gene *in vitro* and *in vivo* [153], and is currently under investigation in the treatment of secondary hyperparathyroidism associated with chronic renal failure. 1,25-$(OH)_2D$ is also known to inhibit PTHrP gene expression [154], and 22-oxacalcitriol has now been shown to inhibit PTHrP gene expression *in vitro* in a human HTLV-I infected T-cell line [155]. These analogues may well offer a valuable option in addition to bisphosphonates in the treatment of PTHrP-mediated hypercalcaemia.

Plasma calcium concentrations do not influence tumour production of PTHrP

The factors which regulate the expression of the PTHrP gene are currently the subject of much interest. Consensus regulatory motifs for cAMP, 1,25-$(OH)_2D$ and glucocorticoids have been identified. Northern blot analysis of mRNA from control or cells treated with 1,25-$(OH)_2D$ or dexamethasone, or by transfection experiments using chimaeric constructs, indicate that these agents decrease gene transcription [154,156]. In contrast, agents which stimulate intracellular cAMP levels, such as calcitonin, increase mRNA levels for PTHrP [157] acting at the level of gene transcription. Both TGF-β and oestrogen have been shown to enhance PTHrP gene expression [158,159].

Ca^{2+} in extracellular fluid is known to be the main physiological regulator of PTH secretion [160,161]. In addition to the rapid effects of Ca^{2+} on PTH secretion, hypercalcaemia has been shown to reduce PTH mRNA levels, presumably reducing the long-term rate of hormone synthesis [162,163,164]. Extracellular Ca^{2+} concentrations have been varied over a wide range in animal studies [161] or using parathyroid cells in culture [165], demonstrating a sigmoidal relationship between PTH and Ca^{2+} concentrations. This raises the question of whether Ca^{2+} concentrations regulate PTHrP production by tumours. The effect of lowering Ca^{2+} on circulating PTH and PTHrP was assessed in hypercalcaemia of malignancy following treatment with pamidronate in patients with PTHrP-mediated hypercalcaemia [166]. A rapid rise in PTH concentrations was seen in most patients after lowering Ca^{2+} (Fig. 74.3a). In these patients with chronic hypercalcaemia, PTH levels increased within 6 days, demonstrating a rapid recovery of parathyroid gland secretion of intact PTH, even following prolonged suppression. This is consistent with the observed rapid recovery of secretion of PTH following surgical excision of a parathyroid adenoma [167]. Post-treatment PTH levels rose above the upper limit of the normal range in some patients even in the presence of normal Ca^{2+} concentrations. This is consistent with a rebound increase in PTH secretion in some patients. These findings may be explained by an increased responsiveness to a fall in calcium of parathyroid tissue which has been exposed to chronic hypercalcaemia, with a shift in the 'set-point' (calcium concentration at which PTH secretion is half-maximal). In the clinical setting it is important to measure PTH levels in patients with hypercalcaemia of malignancy prior to treatment with bisphosphonates since the results after lowering plasma calcium could be misleading.

In our hypercalcaemic patients with elevated PTHrP, levels did not change significantly following successful lowering

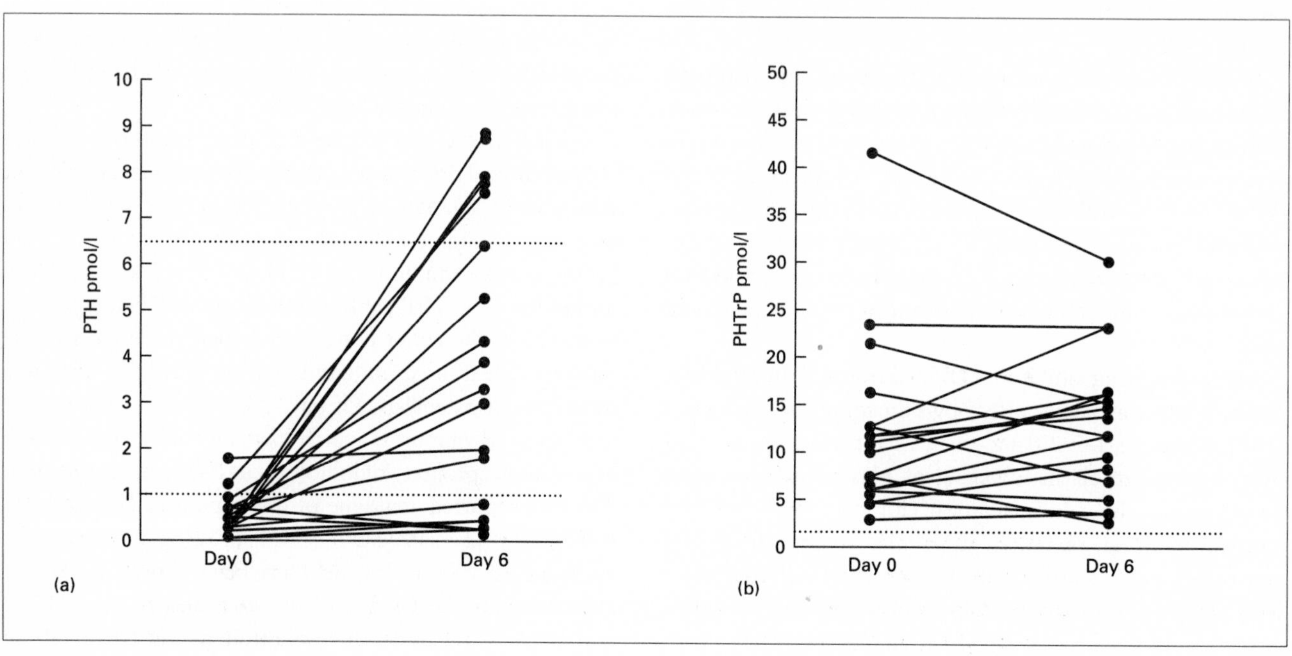

Fig. 74.3 Parathyroid hormone (PTH) (a) and PTH-related protein (PTHrP) (b) before and after treatment of hypercalcaemia of malignancy with pamidronate. The dotted lines indicate the reference range.

of Ca^{2+} concentration after treatment with pamidronate (Fig. 74.3b). An increase in PTHrP secretion has been reported in a PTHrP-secreting rat parathyroid cell line with fetal cell characteristics, in response to lowering calcium concentrations in culture medium [168]. This would be consistent with current evidence for PTHrP as a fetal hormone of the parathyroid gland [169,170], active in the regulation of fetal plasma calcium concentrations [171,172]. A calcium-regulatory effect does not appear to be present in PTHrP-secreting tumours within the range of calcium concentrations which are found in hypercalcaemia of malignancy.

References

1 Mundy GR, Martin TJ. The hypercalcemia of malignancy: pathogenesis and treatment. *Metabolism* 1982; **31**: 1247–77.

2 Gambert SR, Escher JE. Atypical presentation of endocrine disorders in the elderly. *Geriatrics* 1988; **43**: 69–71.

3 Douglas PS, Carmichael KA, Palevski PM. Extreme hypercalcaemia and electrocardiographic changes. *Am J Cardiol* 1984; **54**: 674–5.

4 Ahmed R, Yano K, Mitsuoka T, Ikeda S, Ichimaru M, Hashiba K. Changes in T wave morphology during hypercalcaemia and its relation to the severity of the hypercalcaemia. *J Electrocardiol* 1989; **22**: 125–32.

5 Chadli MC, Chaieb L, Jemni L *et al.* Bigeminal arrhythmia associated with hyperparathyroid crisis. *Can Med Ass J* 1988; **138**: 1115–16.

6 Kaminski HJ, Ruff RL. Neurologic complications of endocrine diseases. *Clin Neurol* 1989; **7**: 493–5.

7 Petersen P. Psychiatric disorders in primary hyperparathyroidism. *J Clin Endocrinol Metab* 1968; **28**: 1491–5.

8 Gatewood KW, Organ CH, Mead BT. Mental changes associated with hyperparathyroidism. *Am J Psychiatr* 1975; **132**: 131–4.

9 Keddie KMG. Case report. Severe depressive illness in the context of hypervitaminosis D. *Br J Psychiatr* 1987; **150**: 394–6.

10 Henson RA. The neurological aspects of hypercalcaemia: with special reference to primary hyperparathyroidism. *J Roy Coll Phys Lond* 1968; **1**: 41–9.

11 Lehrer GM, Levitt MF. Neuropsychiatric presentation of hypercalcaemia. *J Mount Sinai Hosp* 1960; **27**: 10–18.

12 Moure JMB. The encephologram in hypercalcaemia. *Arch Neurol* 1967; **17**: 34–51.

13 Allen EM, Singer FR, Melamed D. Electroencephalographic abnormalities in hypercalcaemia. *Neurology* 1970; **20**: 15–22.

14 Martin TJ, Atkins D. Biochemical regulators of bone resorption and their significance in cancer. *Essays Med Biochem* 1979; **4**: 49–82.

15 Powell D, Singer FR, Murray TM, Minkin C, Potts JT. Non-parathyroid humoral hypercalcemia in patients with neoplastic disease. *N Engl J Med* 1973; **289**: 176–81.

16 Stewart AF, Horst R, Deftos LJ, Cadman EC, Lang R, Broadus AE. Biochemical evaluation of patients with cancer-associated hypercalcemia. Evidence for humoral and non-humoral groups. *N Engl J Med* 1980; **303**: 1377–81.

17 Kukreja SC, Shermerdiak WP, Lad TE, Johnson PA. Elevated nephrogenous cyclic AMP with normal serum parathyroid hormone levels in patients with lung cancer. *J Clin Endocrinol Metab* 1980; **51**: 167–9.

18 Rude RK, Sharp CF, Jr, Fredericks RS *et al.* Urinary and nephrogenous adenosine 3′5′-monophosphate in the hypercalcemia of malignancy. *J Clin Invest* 1981; **52**: 765–71.

19 Powell GJ, Southby J, Danks JA *et al.* Localization of parathyroid hormone-related protein in breast cancer metastases: increased incidence in bone compared with other sites. *Cancer Res* 1991; **51**: 3059–61.

20 Legha SS, Powell K, Buzdar AU, Blumen-Schein GR. Tamoxifen-induced hypercalcemia in breast cancer. *Cancer* 1981; **47**: 2803–6.

21 Ralston SH, Fogelman I, Gardiner MD, Boyle IT. Relative contribution of humoral and metastatic factors to the pathogenesis of hypercalcaemia in malignancy. *Br Med J* 1984; **288**: 1405–8.

22 Burt ME, Brennan MF. Incidence of hypercalcaemia and malignant neoplasm. *Arch Surg* 1980; **115**: 704–7.

23 Kubota K, Yanagisawa T, Kurabayashi H, *et al.* Hypercalcaemia associated with osteolytic lesions in the extramedullary blastic crisis of chronic myelogenous leukaemia: report of a case. *Blut* 1989; **59**: 458–9.

24 Cohn SL, Morgan ER, Mallette LE. The spectrum of metabolic bone disease in lymphoblastic leukemia. *Cancer* 1987; **59**: 346–50.

25 Canellos GP. Hypercalcemia in malignant lymphoma and leukemia. *Ann NY Acad Sci* 1974; **230**: 240–6.

26 Firkin F, Seymour JF, Watson A-M, Grill V, Martin TJ. Circulating parathyroid hormone related protein in hypercalcaemia associated with haematological malignancy. *Brit J Haematol* 1996; **94**: 486–92.

27 Breslau NA, McGuire JL, Zerwekh JE, Frenkel EP, Pak CYC. Hypercalcaemia associated with increased serum calcitriol levels in three patients with lymphoma. *Ann Intern Med* 1984; **100**: 1–7.

28 Rosenthal N, Insogna KL, Godsall JW, Smaldone L, Waldron JA, Stewart AF. Elevations in circulating 1,25-dihydroxyvitamin D in three patients with lymphoma-associated hypercalcaemia. *J Clin Endocrinol Metab* 1985; **60**: 29–33.

29 Davies M, Mawer EB. Pathogenesis of hypercalcaemia in vitamin D poisoning. In: Norman AW, Schaeffer K, Grigoleit H-G, Herrath D (eds). *Vitamin D: A Chemical, Biochemical and Clinical Update.* Berlin: Walter de Gruyter, 1985: 57–8.

30 Mudde AH, Van den Berg H, Boshuis PG *et al.* Ectopic production of 1,25-dihydroxyvitamin D by B-cell lymphoma as a cause of hypercalcaemia. *Cancer* 1987; **59**: 1543–6.

31 Mercier RJ, Thompson JM, Herman GS, Messerschmidt GL. Recurrent hypercalcaemia and elevated 1,25–dihydroxyvitamin D levels in Hodgkin's disease. *Am J Med* 1988; **84**: 165–8.

32 Jacobson JO, Bringhurst FR, Harris NL, Weitzman SA, Aisenberg AC. Humoral hypercalcaemia in Hodgkin's disease. Clinical and laboratory evaluation. *Cancer* 1989; **63**: 917–23.

33 Adams JS, Fernandez M, Gacad MA *et al.* Vitamin D metabolite mediated hypercalcemia and hypercalcemia in patients with AIDS and non-AIDS associated lymphoma. *Blood* 1989; **73**: 235–9.

34 Bunn PA, Schechter GP, Jaffe E *et al.* Clinical course of retrovirus associated adult T-cell lymphoma in the United States. *N Engl J Med* 1983; **309**: 257–64.

35 Kinoshita K, Kamihira S, Ikeda S *et al.* Clinical, hematologic and pathologic features of leukemia T-cell lymphoma. *Cancer* 1982; **50**: 1554–62.

36 Grossman B, Schechter GP, Horton JE, Pierce L, Jaffe E, Wahl L. Hypercalcaemia associated with T cell lymphoma–leukemia. *Am J Clin Pathol* 1981; **75**: 149–55.

37 Dodd RC, Winkler CF, Williams ME *et al.* Calcitriol levels in

hypercalcaemic patients with adult T-cell lymphoma. *Arch Intern Med* 1981; **146**: 1971–2.

38 Poiesz BJ, Ruscetti FW, Gazdar AF, Bunn PA, Minna JD, Gallo RC. Detection and isolation of type C retrovirus particles form fresh and cultured lymphocytes of a patient with cutaneous T-cell lymphoma. *Proc Natl Acad Sci USA* 1980; **77**: 7415–19.

39 Yoshida M, Miyoshi I, Hinuma Y. Isolation and characterisation of retrovirus from cell lines of human adult T-cell leukemia and its implication in the disease. *Proc Natl Acad Sci USA* 1982; **79**: 2031–5.

40 Clark JW, Gurgo C, Franchini G *et al.* Molecular epidemiology of HTLVI-associated non-Hodgkin's lymphomas in Jamaica. *Cancer* 1988; **61**: 1477–82.

41 Fukumoto S, Matsumoto T, Ikeda K *et al.* Clinical evaluation of calcium metabolism in adult T-cell leukemia/lymphoma. *Arch Intern Med* 1988; **148**: 921–5.

42 Kyle RA. Multiple myeloma: Review of 869 cases. *Mayo Clin Proc* 1975; **50**: 29–40.

43 Valentin-Opran A, Charhon SA, Meunier PJ, Arlot CME, Arlot ME. Quantitative histology of myeloma-induced bone changes. *Br J Haematol* 1982; **52**: 601–10.

44 Bataille R, Delmas PD, Chappard D, Sany J. Abnormal serum bone gla protein levels in multiple myeloma. Crucial role of bone formation and prognostic implications. *Cancer* 1990; **66**: 167–72.

45 Bataille R, Chappard D, Marcelli C *et al.* Mechanisms of bone destruction in multiple myeloma: the importance of an unbalanced process in determining the severity of lytic bone disease. *J Clin Oncol* 1989; **7**: 1909–14.

46 Bataille R, Chevalier J, Rossi M, Sany J. Bone scintigraphy in plasma-cell myeloma: A prospective study of 70 patients. *Radiology* 1982; **145**: 801–14.

47 Berenson JR, Lichtenstein A, Porter L *et al.* Efficacy of Pamidronate in reducing skeletal events in patients with advanced multiple myeloma. *N Engl J Med* 1996; **334**: 488–93.

48 Mundy GR, Raisz LG, Cooper RA, Schechter GP, Salmon SE. Evidence for the secretion of an osteoclast stimulating factor in myeloma. *N Engl J Med* 1974; **291**: 1041–6.

49 Raisz LG, Luben RA, Mundy GR, Dietrich JW, Horton JE, Trummel CL. Effect of osteoclast activating factor from human leukocytes on bone metabolism. *J Clin Invest* 1975; **56**: 408–13.

50 Josse RG, Murray TM, Mundy GR, Jez D, Heersche JNM. Observations on the mechanism of bone resorption induced by multiple myeloma marrow culture fluids and partially purified osteoclast-activating factor. *J Clin Invest* 1981; **67**: 1472–81.

51 Garret IR, Durie BGM, Nedwin GE *et al.* Production of lymphotoxin, a bone-resorbing cytokine, by cultured human myeloma cells. *N Engl J Med* 1987; **317**: 526–32.

52 Kawano M, Yamamoto I, Iwato K *et al.* Interleukin-I-beta rather than lymphotoxin as the major bone resorbing activity in human multiple myeloma. *Blood* 1989; **73**: 1646–9.

53 Osserman EF, Takatsuki K. Plasma cell myeloma: Gamma globulin synthesis and structure. *Medicine* 1963; **42**: 357–84.

54 Rubio-Felix D, Girlalt M, Giraldo MP *et al.* Non-secretory multiple myeloma. *Cancer* 1987; **59**: 1847–52.

55 Sere H. Plasmacytome multiple et une forme osseuse pure sans protéinémie et sans protéinurie. *Bull Soc Méd Hôp (Paris)* 1958; **74**: 191–6.

56 Van Slyck EJ, Kleerekoper M, Abraham JP, Deegan MJ. Case report: non-secretory multiple myeloma with osteoporosis: immunocytologic and bone resorptive studies. *Am J Med Sci* 1986; **291**: 347–51.

57 Chew D, Playfel JR. Hypercalcaemia in a patient with non-secretory myeloma. *Postgrad Med J* 1988; **64**: 438–40.

58 Zondek H, Petrow H, Siebert W. Die Bedeutung der Calciumbestimmung im Blute fur die Diagnose der Niereninsuffizienz. *Z Klin Med* 1924; **99**: 129–32.

59 Albright F. Case records of the Massachusetts General Hospital (Case 27401). *N Engl J Med* 1941; **225**: 789–91.

60 Lafferty FW. Pseudohyperparathyroidism. *Medicine* 1966; **45**: 247–60.

61 Berson SA, Yalow RS. Parathyroid hormone in plasma in adenomatous hyperparathyroidism, uremia and bronchogenic sarcoma. *Science* 1966; **154**: 907–9.

62 Knill-Jones RP, Buckle RM, Parsons V, Caine RY, Williams R. Hypercalcaemia and increased parathyroid hormone activity in a primary hepatoma. Studies before and after hepatic transplantation. *N Engl J Med* 1970; **282**: 704–8.

63 Greenberg PB, Martin TJ, Sutcliffe HS. Synthesis and release of parathyroid hormone by a renal carcinoma in cell culture. *Clini Sci Mol Med* 1973; **45**: 183–7.

64 Riggs BL, Arnaud CD, Reynolds JC, Smith LH. Immunological differentiation of primary hyperparathyroidism from hyperparathyroidism due to non-parathyroid cancer. *J Clin Invest* 1971; **50**: 2079–83.

65 Benson RC, Riggs BL, Pickard BM, Arnaud CD. Immunoreactive forms of circulating parathyroid hormone in primary and ectopic hyperparathyroidism. *J Clin Invest* 1974; **54**: 175–81.

66 Roff BS, Carpenter B, Fink DJ, Gordan GS. Some thoughts on the nature of ectopic parathyroid hormones. *Am J Med* 1971; **50**: 686–91.

67 Stewart AF, Insogna KL, Goltzman D, Broadus AE. Identification of adenylate cyclase-stimulating activity and cytochemical glucose-6-phosphatedehydrogenase-stimulating activity in extracts of tumurs from patients with humoral hypercalcemia of malignancy. *Proc Natl Acad Sci USA* 1983; **80**: 1454–8.

68 Nissenson RA, Strewler GJ, Williams RD, Leung SC. Activation of the PTH receptor adenylate cyclase complex by human renal carcinoma factor. *Cancer Res* 1985; **45**: 5358–68.

69 Goltzman D, Stewart AF, Broaus AE. Malignancy-associated hypercalcemia evaluation with a cytochemical bioassay for parathyroid hormone. *J Clin Endocrinol Metab* 1981; **53**: 899–904.

70 Rodan SB, Insogna KL, Vignery AM-C *et al.* Factors associated with humoral hypercalcemia of malignancy stimulate adenylate cyclase in osteoblastic cells. *J Clin Invest* 1983; **72**: 1511–15.

71 Simpson EL, Mundy GR, D'Souza SM, Ibbotson KJ, Bockman R, Jacobs JW. Absence of parathyroid hormone messenger RNA in non-parathyroid tumors associated with hypercalcemia. *N Engl J Med* 1983; **309**: 325–30.

72 Strewler GJ, Williams RD, Nissenson RA. Human renal carcinoma cells produce hypercalcemia in the nude mouse and a novel protein recognized by parathyroid hormone receptors. *J Clin Invest* 1983; **71**: 769–74.

73 Gkonos PJ, Hayes T, Burtis W, Jacoby R, McGuire J, Baron R, Stewart AF. Squamous carcinoma model of humoral hypercalcemia of malignancy. *Endocrinology* 1984; **115**: 2384–90.

74 Rosol TJ, Capen CC, Brooks CP. Bone and kidney adenylate cyclase-stimulating activity produced by a hypercalcemia can ine adenocarcinoma line (CAC-8) maintained in nude mice. *Cancer Res* 1987; **47**: 690–5.

75 Ikeda K, Matsumoto F, Fukumoto S *et al.* A hypercalcemic nude rat model that completely mimics the human syndrome of

humoral hypercalcemia of malignancy. *Calcif Tiss Int* 1988; **43**: 97–102.

76 Moseley JM, Kubota M, Diefenbach-Jagger H *et al.* Parathyroid hormone-related protein purified from a human lung cancer cell line. *Proc Natl Acad Sci USA* 1987; **84**: 5048–52.

77 Burtis WJ, Wu J, Bunch CM *et al.* Identification of a novel 17,000-dalton parathyroid hormone-like adenylate cyclase-stimulating protein from a tumor associated with humoral hypercalcemia of malignancy. *J Biol Chem* 1987; **262**: 7151–6.

78 Suva LJ, Winslow GA, Wettenhall REH. A parathyroid hormone-related protein implicated in malignant hypercalcemia: cloning and expression. *Science* 1987; **237**: 893–6.

79 Mangin W, Webb AC, Dreyer BE *et al.* Identification of a cDNA encoding a parathyroid hormone-like peptide from a human tumor associated with humoral hypercalcemia of malignancy. *Proc Natl Acad Sci USA* 1988; **85**: 597–601.

80 Thiede MA, Strewler GA, Nissenson RA, Rosenblatt M, Rodan GA. Human renal carcinoma expresses to messages encoding a parathyroid hormone like peptide: evidence for the alterate splicing of a single copy gene. *Proc Natl Acad Sci USA* 1988; **85**: 4605–8.

81 Kemp BE, Moseley JM, Rodda CP *et al.* Parathyroid hormone-related protein of malignancy: active synthetic fragments. *Science* 1987; **238**: 1568–70.

82 Horiuchi N, Caulfield MP, Fisher JE *et al.* Similarity of synthetic peptide from human tumor to parathyroid hormone *in vivo* and *in vitro*. *Science* 1987; **238**: 1566.

83 Rodan SB, Noda M, Wesolowski G, Rosenblatt M, Rodan GA. Comparison of postreceptor effects of 1–34 human hypercalcemic factor and 1–34 human parathyroid hormone in rat osteosarcoma cells. *J Clin Invest* 1988; **81**: 924–7.

84 Stewart AF, Mangin M, Wu T *et al.* Synthetic human parathyroid hormone-like protein stimulates bone resorption and causes hypercalcemia in rats. *J Clin Invest* 1988; **81**: 596–600.

85 Yates AJP, Gutierrez GE, Smoleus P *et al.* Effects of a synthetic peptide of a parathyroid hormone-related protein on calcium homeostasis, renal tubular calcium reabsorption and bone metabolism *in vivo* and *in vitro* in rodents. *J Clin Invest* 1988; **81**: 932–8.

86 Ebeling PR, Adam WR, Moseley JM, Martin TJ. Actions of parathyroid hormone-related protein on the isolated rat kidney. *J Endocrinol* 1988; **12**: 45–52.

87 Zhou H, Leaver DD, Moseley JM, Kemp BE, Ebeling PR, Martin TJ. Actions of parathyroid hormone-related protein on the rat kidney *in vivo*. *J Endocrinol* 1989; **122**: 227–35.

88 Danks JA, Ebeling PR, Hayman J *et al.* Parathyroid hormone-related protein: immunohistochemical localization in cancers and in normal skin. *J Bone Miner Res* 1989; **4**: 273–8.

89 Kukreja SC, Shevrin DH, Wimbiscus SA *et al.* Antibodies to parathyroid hormone-related protein lower serum calcium in athymic mouse models of malignancy-associated hypercalcemia due to human tumors. *J Clin Invest* 1988; **82**: 1798–802.

90 Kukreja SC, Rosol TJ, Winbiscus SA *et al.* Tumor resection and antibodies to parathyroid hormone-related protein cause similar changes on bone histomorphometry in hypercalcemia of cancer. *Endocrinology* 1990; **127**: 305–10.

91 Ellis AG, Adam WR, Martin TJ. Comparison of the effects of parathyroid hormone (PTH) and recombinant PTH-related protein on bicarbonate excretion by the isolated perfused rat kidney. *J Endocrinol* 1990; **126**: 403–8.

92 Fraher LJ, Hodsman AB, Jonas K *et al.* A comparison of the *in vivo* biochemical responses to exogenous parathyroid hormone (1–34) [PTH(1–34)] and PTH-related peptide (1–34) in man. *J Clin Endocrinol Metab* 1992; **75**: 417–23.

93 Yamamoto I, Kitamura N, Aoki J *et al.* Circulating 1,25-dihydroxyvitamin D concentrations in patients with renal cell carcinoma-associated hypercalcemia are rarely suppressed. *J Clin Endocrinol Metab* 1987; **64**: 175–9.

94 Schweitzer DH, Hamdy NA, Frohlich M, Zwinderman AH, Papapoulos SE. Malignancy-associated hypercalcaemia: resolution of controversies over vitamin D metabolism by a pathophysiological approach to the syndrome. *Clin Endocrinol* 1994; **41**: 251–6.

95 Fukumoto S, Matsumoto T, Yamamoto H *et al.* Suppression of serum 1,25 dihydroxyvitamin D in humoral hypercalcemia of malignancy is caused by elaboration of a factor that inhibits renal 1,25 dihydroxyvitamin D production. *Endocrinology* 1989; **124**: 2057–62.

96 Sato K, Fujii Y, Kasono K *et al.* Parathyroid hormone-related protein and interleukin-1 alpha synergistically stimulate bone resorption *in vitro* and increase serum calcium concentration in mice *in vivo*. *Endocrinology* 1989; **124**: 2172–8.

97 Sato K, Fujii Y, Ono M, Nomura H, Shizume K. Production of interleukin 1-alpha like factor an colony-stimulating factor by a squamous cell carcinoma of the thyroid (T3M-5) derived from a patient with hypercalcemia and leukocytosis. *Cancer Res* 1987; **47**: 6474–80.

98 Sato K, Fujii Y, Kasono K, Tsishima T, Shizume K. Production of interleukin-1 alpha and parathyroid hormone-like factor by a squamous cell carcinoma of the esophagus (EC-GI) derived from a patient with hypercalcemia. *J Clin Endocrinol Metab* 1988; **67**: 592–601.

99 Sato K, Fujii Y, Kakiuchi T *et al.* Paraneoplastic syndrome of hypercalcemia and leukocytosis caused by squamous carcinoma cells (T3M-1) producing parathyroid hormone-related protein, interleukin 1 alpha, and granulocyte colony-stimulating factor. *Cancer Res* 1989; **49**: 4740–6.

100 Budayr A, Nissenson RA, Klein RF *et al.* Increased serum levels of a parathyroid hormone-like protein in malignancy-associated hypercalcemia. *Ann Intern Med* 1989; **111**: 807–12.

101 Henderson JR, Shustik C, Kremer R, Rabbani SA, Hendy GN, Goltzman D. Circulating concentrations of parathyroid hormone-like peptide in malignancy and hyperparathyroidism. *J Bone Miner Res* 1990; **5**: 105–13.

102 Burtis WJ, Brady TG, Orloff JJ *et al.* Immunochemical characterization of circulating parathyroid hormone-related protein in patients with humoral hypercalcemia of cancer. *N Engl J Med* 1990; **322**: 1106–12.

103 Kao CK, Klee GG, Taylor RL, Health H. Parathyroid hormone related peptide in plasma from patients with hypercalcemia and malignant lesions. *Mayo Clin Proc* 1990; **65**: 1399–406.

104 Ratcliffe WA, Norbury S, Heath DA, Ratcliffe JG. Development and validation of an immunoradiometric assay of parathyrin-related protein in unextracted plasma. *Clin Chem* 1991; **37**: 678–85.

105 Grill V, Ho P, Body JJ *et al.* Parathyroid hormone-related protein: elevated levels both in humoral hypercalcemia of malignancy and in hypercalcemia complicating metastatic breast cancer. *J Clin Endocrinol Metab* 1991; **73**: 1309–15.

106 Pandian MR, Morgan CH, Carlton E, Segre V. Modified immunoradiometric assay of parathyroid hormone-related protein: clinical application in the differential diagnosis of hypercalcemia. *Clin Chem* 1992; **38**: 282–8.

107 Fraser WD, Robinson J, Lawton R *et al.* Clinical and laboratory studies of a new immunoradiometric assay of parathyroid hormone-related protein. *Clin Chem* 1993; **39**: 414–19.

108 Ikeda K, Ohno H, Hane M *et al.* Development of a sensitive two-site assay for parathyroid hormone-related peptide: evidence for elevated levels in plasma from patients with adult T-cell leukaemia/lymphoma and B-cell lymphoma. *J Clin Endocrinol Metab* 1994; **79**: 1322–7.

109 Ikeda K, Weir E, Mangin M *et al.* Expression of messenger ribonucleic acids encoding a parathyroid hormone-like peptide in normal human and animal tissues with abnormal expression in human parathyroid adenomas. *Mol Endocrinol* 1989; **2**: 1230–5.

110 Danks JA, Ebeling PR, Hayman JA *et al.* Immunohistochemical localization of parathyroid hormone-related protein in parathyroid adenoma and hyperplasia. *J Pathol* 1990; **161**: 27–33.

111 Bundred NJ, Ratcliffe WA, Walker RA, Coley S, Morrison JM, Ratcliffe JG. Parathyroid hormone related protein and hypercalcemia in breast cancer. *Br Med J* 1991; **303**: 1506–9.

112 Percival RC, Yates AJP, Gray RE *et al.* Mechanisms of malignant hypercalcaemia in carcinoma of the breast. *Br Med J* 1985; **2**: 7766–9.

113 Kimura S, Adchi I, Yamaguchi K *et al.* Stimulation of calcium reabsorption observed in advanced breast cancer patients with hypercalcemia and multiple bone metastases. *Jpn Cancer Res* 1985; **76**: 308–14.

114 Isales C, Carangiu ML, Stewart AF. Hypercalcemia in breast cancer: reassessment of the mechanism. *Am J Med* 1987; **82**: 1143–7.

115 Gallacher SJ, Fraser WD, Patel U *et al.* Breast cancer associated hypercalcemia: a reassessment of renal calcium and phosphate handling. *Ann Clin Biochem* 1990; **27**: 551–6.

116 Southby J, Kissin MW, Danks JA *et al.* Immunohistochemical localization of parathyroid hormone-related protein in human breast cancer. *Cancer Res* 1990; **50**: 7710–16.

117 Vargas SJ, Powell GJ, Gillespie MT *et al.* Localization of parathyroid hormone-related protein mRNA expression in breast cancer and metastatic lesions by *in situ* hybridization. *J Bone Miner Res* 1992; **7**: 971–9.

118 Kohno N, Kitazawa S, Fukaze M *et al.* The expression of parathyroid hormone-related protein in human breast cancer with skeletal metastases. *Surg Today* 1994; **24**: 215–20.

119 Arguello F, Baggs RB, Frantz CN. A murine model of experimental metastasis to bone and bone marrow. *Cancer Res* 1988; **48**: 6878–81.

120 Guise TA, Yin JJ, Taylor SD *et al.* Evidence for a causal role of parathyroid hormone-related protein in the pathogenesis of human breast cancer-mediated osteolysis. *J Clin Invest* 1996; **98**: 1544–9.

121 Seymour J, Grill V, Lee N, Martin TJ, Firkin F. Hypercalcemia in the blastic phase of chronic myeloid leukemia associated with parathyroid hormone related protein. *Leukemia* 1993; **10**: 1672–5.

122 Fukumoto S, Matsumoto T, Watanabe T, Takahashi H, Miyoshi I, Ogata E. Secretion of parathyroid hormone-like activity from human T-cell lymphotropic virus type I-infected lymphocytes. *Cancer Res* 1989; **49**: 3849–52.

123 Motokura T, Fukumoto S, Takahashi S *et al.* Expression of parathyroid hormone-related protein in a human T cell lymphotrophic virus type 1-infected T cell line. *Biochem Biophys Res Commun* 1988; **154**: 1182–8.

124 Moseley JM, Danks JA, Grill V, Lister TA, Horton MA. Immunocytochemical demonstration of PTHrP protein in neoplastic tissue of HTLV-1 positive human adult T cell leukaemia/lymphoma: implications for the mechanism of hypercalcemia. *Br J Cancer* 1991; **64**: 745–8.

125 de Souza PL, Friedlander ML. Humoral hypercalcemia associated with adenocarcinoma of the rectum. A case report and review of the literature. *Am J Clin Oncol* 1995; **18**: 126–9.

126 Kashara H, Tsuchiya M, Adachi R, Horikawa S, Tanaka S, Tachibana S. Development of a C-terminal region specific radioimmunoassay of parathyroid hormone-related protein. *Biomed Res* 1992; **13**: 155–61.

127 Brown RC, Aston JP, Weekes I, Woodhead JS. Circulating intact parathyroid measured by a two-site immunochemiluminometric assay. *J Clin Endocrinol Metab* 1987; **65**: 407–14.

128 Nussbaum SR, Zahradnik RJ, Lavigne JR *et al.* Highly sensitive two-size immunoradiometric assay of parathyrin, and its clinical utility in evaluating patients with hypercalcemia. *Clin Chem* 1987; **33**: 1364–7.

129 Blind E, Schmidt-Gayk H, Scharla S, *et al.* Two-site assay of intact parathyroid in the investigation of primary hyperparathyroidism and other disorders of calcium metabolism compared with a mid-region assay. *J Clin Endocrinol Metab* 1988; **67**: 353–60.

130 Schmelzer HJ, Hersch RD, Mayer H. Parathyroid hormone in a human small cell lung cancer. In: Haveman K, Sorensen G, Gropp C, eds. *Peptide Hormones in Lung Cancer*. Berlin: Springer-Verlag, 1985: 83–93.

131 Yoshimoto K, Yamasaki R, Sakai H *et al.* Ectopic production of parathyroid hormone by small cell lung cancer in a patient with hypercalcemia. *J Clin Endocrinol Metab* 1989; **68**: 976–81.

132 Nussbaum SR, Gaz RD, Arnold A. Hypercalcemia and ectopic secretion of parathyroid hormone by an ovarian carcinoma with rearrangement of the gene for parathyroid hormone. *N Engl J Med* 1990; **323**: 1324–8.

133 Strewler GJ, Budayr AA, Clark OH, Nissenson RA. Production of parathyroid hormone by a malignant non parathyroid tumor in a hypercalcemic patient. *J Clin Endocrinol Metab* 1993; **76**: 1373–5.

134 Rizzoli R, Pache J-C, Didierjean L, Burger A, Bonjour J-P. A thymoma as a cause of true ectopic hyperparathyroidism. *J Clin Endocrinol Metab* 1994; **79**: 912–15.

135 Suki WN, Yium JJ, von Minden M, Saller-Herbert C, Eknovan G, Martinez-Maldonado M. Acute treatment of hypercalcemia with furosemide. *N Engl J Med* 1970; **283**: 836–40.

136 Ralston SH, Gardner MD, Dryburgh FJ, Jenkins AS, Cowan RA, Boyle IT. Comparison of aminohydroxypropylidene diphosphonate, mithramycin and corticosteroids/calcitonin in the treatment of cancer-associated hypercalcemia. *Lancet* 1985; **2**: 907–10.

137 Hosking DJ, Stone MD, Foote JW. Potentiation of calcitonin by corticoteroids during the treatment of hypercalcemia of malignancy. *Eur J Clin Pharmacol* 1990; **38**: 37–41.

138 Fleisch H. *Bisphosphonates in Bone Disease. From the Laboratory to the Patient*. London: The Parthenon Publishing Group, 1995.

139 Sahni M, Guenther HL, Fleisch H, Collin P, Martin TJ. Bisphosphonates act on rat bone resorption through the mediation of osteoblasts. *J Clin Invest* 1993; **91**: 2004–11.

140 Body JJ, Borkowski A, Cleeren A, Bijvoet OLM. Treatment of malignancy-associated hypercalcemia with intravenous aminohydroxypropylidenediphosphonate. *J Clin Oncol* 1986; **8**: 1177–83.

141 Thiebaud D, Jaeger B, Burckhard P. A single day treatment of tumor-induced hypercalcemia by intravenous APD. *J Bone Miner Res* 1986; **1**: 555–62.

142 Yates AJP, Murray RML, Jerums G, Martin TJ. A comparison of single and multiple intravenous infusions of APD in the treatment of hypercalcemia of malignancy. *Aust NZ J Med* 1987; **17**: 387–91.

143 Bounameaux HM, Schifferli J, Jung A, Chatelant F. Renal failure with intravenous bisphosphonates. *Lancet* 1983; **1**: 471.

144 Lahtinen R, Laasko M, Palva I *et al.* Randomised, placebo-controlled multicentre trial of clodronate in multiple myeloma. *Lancet* 1992; **340**: 1049–52.

145 Paterson AHG, Powles TJ, Kanis JA *et al.* Double-blind controlled trial of oral clodronate in patients with bone metastases from breast cancer. *J Clin Oncol* 1993; **11**: 59–65.

146 Brown JH, Kennedy BJ. Mithramycin in the treatment of testicular cancer. *N Engl J Med* 1965; **272**: 111–18.

147 Bonjour JP, Rizzoli R. Antiosteolytic agents in the management of hypercalcemia. *Ann Oncol* 1992; **3**: 589–90.

148 Gurney H, Kefford R, Stuart HR. Renal phosphate threshold and response to pamidronate in humoral hypercalcaemia of malignancy: see comments. *Lancet* 1989; **2**: 241–4.

149 Gurney H, Grill V, Martin TJ. Parathyroid hormone-related protein level predicts response to Pamidronate in the treatment of tumour-induced hypercalcemia. *Lancet* 1993; **341**: 1611–13.

150 Hirschel SS, Caverzasio J, Bonjour JP. Inhibition of parathyroid hormone secretion and parathyroid hormone-independent diminution of tubular calcium reabsorption by WR-2721, a unique hypocalcemic agent. *J Clin Invest* 1985; **76**: 1851–6.

151 Goldman ME, McKee RL, Caulfield MP *et al.* A new highly potent parathyroid hormone antagonist: D-Trp12,Tyr34:bPTH-(7–34)NH2. *Endocrinology* 1988; **123**: 2597–9.

152 Murayama E, Miyamoto K, Kubodera N, Mori T, Matsunaga I. Synthetic studies of Vitamin D3 analogues. VIII. Synthesis of 22-oxavitamin D3 analogues. *Chem Pharm Bull (Tokyo)* 1986; **34**: 4410–13.

153 Brown AJ, Ritter CR, Finch JL *et al.* The noncalcemic analogue of vitamin D, 22-oxacalcitriol, suppresses parathyroid hormone synthesis and secretion. *J Clin Invest* 1989; **84**: 728–32.

154 Ikeda K, Lu C, Weir EC, Mangin M, Broadus AE. Transcriptional regulation of the parathyroid hormone-related protein gene by glucocorticoids and vitamin D in a human C-cell lime. *J Biol Chem* 1989; **264**: 15743–6.

155 Inoue D, Matsumoto T, Ogata E, Ikeda K. 22-oxacalcitriol, a noncalcemic analogue of calcitriol, suppresses both cell proliferation and parathyroid hormone-related peptide gene expression in human T cell lymphotrophic virus, type I-infected T cells. *J Biol Chem* 1993; **268**: 16730–6.

156 Lu C, Ikeda K, Deftos LJ, Gazdar AF, Mangin M, Broadus AE. Glucocorticoid regulation of parathyroid hormone-related protein gene transcription in a human neuroendocrine cell line. *Mol Endocrinol* 1989; **3**: 2034–9.

157 Chilco PJ, Gerardi JM, Kaczmarczyk SJ, Chu S, Leopold V, Zajae JD. Calcitonin increases transcription of parathyroid hormone-related protein via cAMP. *Mol Cell Endocrinol* 1993; **94**: 1–7.

158 Kiriyama T, Gillespie MT, Glatz JA, Fukumoto S, Moseley JM, Martin TJ. TGFβ stimulation of parathyroid hormone-related protein: a paracrine regulator? *Mol Cell Endocrinol* 1993; **92**: 55–62.

159 Thiede MA, Harm SC, Hasson DM, Gardner RM. *In vivo* regulation of parathyroid hormone-related peptide messenger ribonucleic acid in the rat uterus by 17 β estradiol. *Endocrinology* 1991; **28**: 2317–23.

160 Sherwood LM, Potts JT, Jr, Care AD *et al.* Evaluation by radio-immunoassay of factors controlling the secretion of parathyroid hormone. Intravenous infusions of calcium and ethylenediamine tetraacetic acid in the cow and goat. *Nature* 1966; **209**: 52–5.

161 Mayer GP, Hurst JG. Sigmoidal relationship between parathyroid hormone secretion rate and plasma concentrations in calves. *Endocrinology* 1978; **102**: 1036–42.

162 Russell J, Lettieri D, Sherwood LM. Direct regulation by calcium of cytoplasmic messenger ribonucleic acid coding for pre-proparathyroid hormone in isolated bovine parathyroid cells. *J Clin Invest* 1983; **72**: 1851–5.

163 Farrow SM, Karmali R, Gleed JH, Hendy GN, O'Riordan JLH. Regulation of pre prohormone messenger RNA and hormone synthesis in human parathyroid adenomata. *J Endocrinol* 1988; **117**: 133–8.

164 Yamamoto M, Igarashi T, Murumatsu M, Fukagawa M, Motokura T, Ogata E. Hypocalcemia increases and hypercalcemia decreases the steady-state level of parathyroid hormone messenger RNA in the rat. *J Clin Invest* 1989; **83**: 1053–956.

165 Brown EM. Four-parameter model of the sigmoidal relationship between parathyroid hormone release and extracellular calcium concentration in normal and abnormal parathyroid tissue. *J Clin Endocrinol Metab* 1983; **56**: 572–81.

166 Grill V, Murray RML, Ho PMV *et al.* Circulating levels of PTH and PTHrP before and after treatment of tumor-induced hypercalcemia with Pamidronate Disodium. *J Clin Endocrinol Metab* 1992; **76**: 1468–70.

167 Brasier AR, Wang CA, Nussbaum SR. Recovery of parathyroid hormone secretion after parathyroid adenomectomy. *J Clin Endocrinol Metab* 1988; **66**: 495–500.

168 Zajac JD, Callaghan J, Eldridge C *et al.* Production of parathyroid hormone-related protein by a rat parathyroid cell line. *J Mol Endocrinol Metab* 1989; **67**: 107–12.

169 Abbas SK, Pickard DW, Illingworth D *et al.* Measurement of parathyroid hormone-related protein in extracts of fetal parathyroid glands and placental membranes. *J Endocrinol* 1990; **124**: 319–25.

170 McIsaac RJ, Caple IW, Danks JA *et al.* Ontogeny of parathyroid hormone-related protein in the ovine parathyroid gland. *Endocrinology* 1991; **129**: 757–64.

171 Rodda CP, Kubota M, Health JA *et al.* Evidence for a novel parathyroid hormone-related protein in fetal lamb parathyroid glands and sheep placenta: comparisons with a similar protein implicated in humoral hypercalcemia of malignancy. *J Endocrinol* 1988; **117**: 261–71.

172 Abbas SK, Pickard DW, Rodda CP *et al.* Stimulation of placental calcium transport by certain parathyroid hormone-related proteins. *Q J Exp Physiol* 1989; **74**: 549–52.

173 Kanis JA, Powles T, Paterson AHG, McCloskey EV, Ashley S. Clodronate decreases the frequency of skeletal metastases in women with breast cancer. *Bone* 1996; **19**: 663–7.

CHAPTER 75

Endocrine morbidity of cancer therapy

S.M. Shalet

Introduction

Radiation may directly impair hypothalamic, pituitary, thyroid, pancreatic and gonadal function, or alternatively it may induce the development of hyperparathyroidism, thyroid adenomas or carcinomas. Cytotoxic chemotherapy may damage the gonad, and both irradiation and cytotoxic chemotherapy may interfere with the normal growth of bone. These complications of treatment may lead to various clinical presentations including infertility, gynaecomastia, hypogonadism, impaired growth leading to short stature, failure to undergo normal pubertal development, precocious puberty, hyperparathyroidism, hypothyroidism, thyroid tumours, diabetes mellitus [1] and varying degrees of hypopituitarism.

Hypothalamo-pituitary axis

Deficiency of one or more anterior pituitary hormones is now a well-recognised sequela of external radiotherapy to the hypothalamo-pituitary axis. This may occur in patients treated for non-functioning pituitary adenomas, hormone-secreting pituitary adenomas and craniopharyngiomas. Anterior pituitary hormone deficiencies have also been reported when the hypothalamo-pituitary axis falls within the radiation field during the treatment of nasopharyngeal cancer and intracranial tumours distant from the pituitary fossa. Children at risk [2] include those irradiated for brain tumours, retinoblastoma, acute lymphoblastic leukaemia (ALL) or those who receive total-body irradiation [3] in preparation for a bone-marrow transplant. Growth hormone (GH) secretion is the most vulnerable of the anterior pituitary hormones following irradiation, irrespective of whether the damage is hypothalamic or pituitary in site.

In a large series [4] of adult patients with tumours of the pituitary, or closely related anatomical sites, pituitary function was studied annually for up to 10 years after external radiotherapy by a three-field technique, giving 3750–4250 cGy (rad) in 15 or 16 fractions over 20–22 days. Before radiotherapy 18% of patients had normal GH secretion, 21% had normal gonadotrophin secretion, 57% had normal corticotrophin reserve and 80% had normal thyrotrophin secretion. Life-table analysis demonstrated increasing incidences of all anterior pituitary hormone deficiencies with time: by 5 years all patients were GH deficient, 91% were gonadotrophin deficient, 77% were corticotrophin deficient and 42% were thyrotrophin deficient. At 8 years respective incidences of deficiencies were 100%, 96%, 84% and 49%. Although anterior pituitary hormone deficiencies most commonly developed in the order of GH, gonadotrophin, corticotrophin and thyrotrophin (61% of patients), other sequences were evident (Fig. 75.1). Most notably, adrenocorticotrophic hormone (ACTH) deficiency sometimes occurred before gonadotrophin deficiency. Radiation-induced hyperprolactinaemia was a common occurrence [4].

Early studies had suggested that the pituitary gland itself was resistant to the effects of radiotherapy. The endocrine tests used, however, were primitive by today's standards and the follow-up period was too short. Subsequently, in 1982, Samaan *et al.* [5] showed that in patients irradiated for nasopharyngeal carcinoma, the pituitary gland as well as the hypothalamus may be susceptible to radiation-induced damage. Other studies [6] have been reported in patients with pituitary adenomas treated by implantation of yttrium-90 seeds into the pituitary gland, with pituitary doses of between 50 000 and 150 000 cGy. These showed a combined incidence of thyroxine and cortisol deficiency of 39% at 14 years compared with over 90% at 10 years following conventional radiotherapy. The most likely explanation for the difference in the incidence of hypopituitarism after the two types of irradiation is that the fields for external

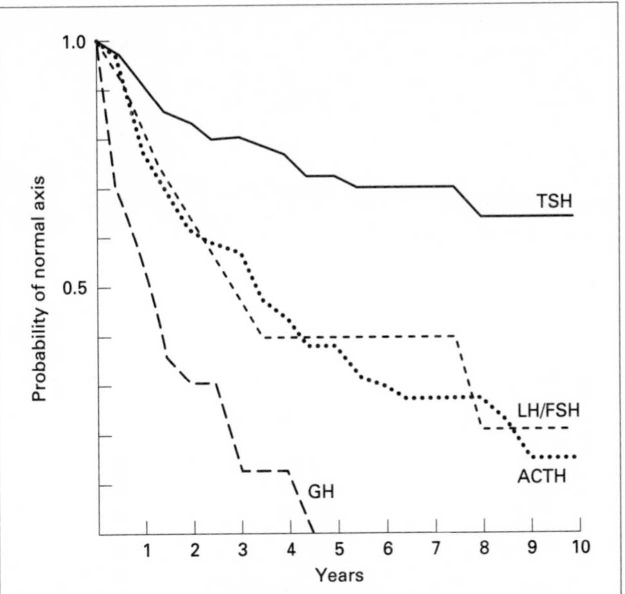

Fig. 75.1 Life-table analysis indicating probabilities of initially normal hypothalamo-pituitary–target gland axes remaining normal after radiotherapy.

radiotherapy include the hypothalamus which is relatively unaffected by the implantation of yttrium-90 seeds into the pituitary.

Site and nature of radiation damage

Despite the fact that diabetes insipidus has not been described following external irradiation to the hypothalamo-pituitary axis, there are a number of studies [2] which indicate that the hypothalamus is more vulnerable to radiation damage than the pituitary; discordant GH responses to arginine and to an insulin tolerance test (ITT) have been described in the monkey and in humans. In addition, normal GH responses to GH-releasing hormone (GHRH) in the presence of subnormal GH responses to an ITT may be seen.

Raised prolactin levels, subnormal thyroid function in the presence of a normal but delayed thyroid-stimulating hormone (TSH) rise after thyrotrophin-releasing hormone (TRH), subnormal gonadal function in the presence of a normal gonadotrophin response to gonadotrophin-releasing hormone (GnRH), and subnormal adrenocortical function in the presence of a normal ACTH response to corticotrophin-releasing hormone (CRH) have also been reported. Finally, the severe blunting of physiological GH secretion despite normal GH responses to pharmacological stimuli, both in the monkey and in humans, strongly suggests a hypothalamic locus for the defect.

The pathophysiology of the radiation-induced damage to the hypothalamus remains ill-understood; does it reflect vascular damage or direct neuronal damage? Chieng *et al.* [7] attempted to answer this question by studying regional cerebral blood flow with ^{99m}Tc-hexamethyl propyleneamine oxime (HMPAO) single-photon emission computed tomography (SPECT) in 34 patients with nasopharyngeal cancer. In cross-sectional endocrine and blood-flow studies performed before irradiation, 6 months, 1 year and more than 5 years after irradiation, regional hypothalamic blood flow was reduced after cranial irradiation but there was no significant difference in the hypothalamic/occipital blood flow ratio between 6 months and more than 5 years after irradiation. These observations were in stark contrast to the progressive endocrine dysfunction with time. These results [7] suggest that direct injury to hypothalamic neurons rather than reduced cerebral blood flow is the major cause of progressive hypothalamo-pituitary dysfunction after fractionated cranial irradiation.

Neuropharmacology has provided an additional tool to explore the pathophysiology of radiation injury. Ogilvy-Stuart *et al.* [8] investigated the impact of irradiation on the neuroregulatory control of GH secretion by manipulating cholinergic tone in young adults rendered GH deficient in childhood after cranial irradiation: this approach is based on the established contribution of cholinergic input in modifying somatostatin tone and thereby GH secretion. The number of patients studied was small but the results were consistent with dual sites of radiation damage. Somatostatin tone was reduced but not abolished and endogenous GHRH secretion was also reduced. Although somatostatin tone was reduced it could be increased by cholinergic manipulation and was not irreversibly fixed. This has possible implications if GHRH analogues or other GH-releasing peptides/non-peptides were used to treat patients with radiation-induced GH deficiency.

Radiation schedule and pituitary function

The total dose of radiation delivered to the hypothalamo-pituitary region is a major determinant of the incidence of anterior pituitary hormone deficiencies. This is illustrated by the increasing incidence of TSH deficiency [9] with increasing total radiation dose (Fig. 75.2). In the treatment of pituitary disease, the low-dose regimen of 2000 cGy in eight fractions over 11 days is associated with a significantly lower incidence of all deficiencies than the higher dose regimens of 3500–4500 cGy in 15 fractions over 21 days. The total dose of radiation directed at the hypothalamo-pituitary axis is not, however, the only factor determining the incidence of hypopituitarism. Our data indicate that a dose of 3000 cGy delivered in eight fractions over 11 days to the whole brain has a similar deleterious effect on gonadotrophin secretion as irradiation with 3700–4000 cGy

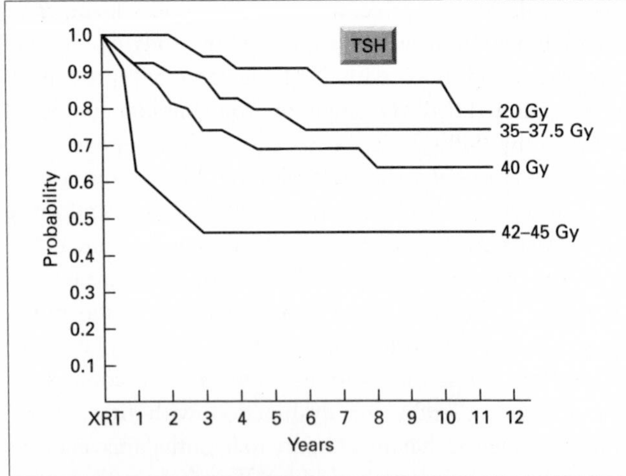

Fig. 75.2 Probability of thyroid-stimulating hormone (TSH) secretion remaining normal after radiotherapy for pituitary tumours using dose schedules of 2000cGy in eight fractions over 11 days and 3500–3700cGy, 4000cGy or 4200–4500cGy in 15 fractions over 21 days.

administered to the hypothalamo-pituitary region in 15 fractions over 21 days, which implies that fraction size is important; similarly, 14 out of 17 children who received cranial irradiation at a dose of 2500cGy in 10 fractions over 16 days had a subnormal GH response to an ITT, compared with one out of nine who received a dose of 2400cGy in 20 fractions over 4 weeks. Despite a nearly identical total radiation dose, the incidence of GH deficiency differed significantly due to the change in fraction size (Fig. 75.3).

The extent of hypothalamopituitary dysfunction is dose dependent, GH deficiency occurring at lower doses of irradiation and pan-hypopituitarism after higher doses. The speed with which individual pituitary hormone deficiencies occur is also dose dependent. The higher the radiation dose, the earlier the pituitary hormone deficit will develop after treatment.

Apart from radiation dose, the pre-irradiation pituitary hormone status influences the timing of onset of radiation-induced pituitary hormone deficit as illustrated by the evolution of radiation-induced GH deficiency [10]. This information may help the clinician to predict the frequency and timing of pituitary hormone deficits in patients receiving irradiation to the hypothalamo-pituitary region and the potential need for replacement therapy (Fig. 75.4).

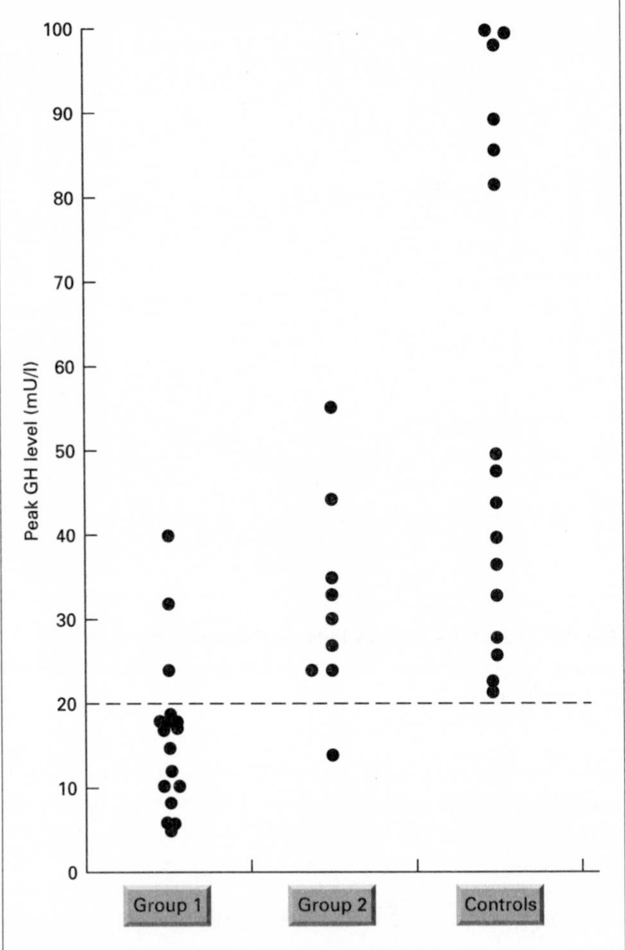

Fig. 75.3 Peak growth hormone (GH) responses to an insulin tolerance test (ITT) in children who received prophylactic cranial irradiation for acute lymphoblastic leukaemia (ALL) in a dose of 2500cGy in 10 fractions over 16 days (group 1) or 2400cGy in 20 fractions over 4 weeks versus controls. Fourteen out of 17 showed subnormal GH responses (<20mU/l) in group 1 and one out of nine in group 2.

Precocious puberty

Doses of cranial irradiation exceeding 5000cGy to the hypothalamo-pituitary axis may render a child gonadotrophin deficient. Paradoxically, lesser doses of irradiation may be associated with early puberty. This phenomenon has been demonstrated in both sexes in children irradiated with a dose of 2500–4750cGy for a brain tumour [11]. In 46 GH-deficient children previously irradiated for a brain tumour not involving the hypothalamo-pituitary axis there was a significant linear association between age at irradiation and age at onset of puberty (Fig. 75.5). The onset of puberty occurred at an early age in both sexes (mean 8.51 years in girls and 9.21 years in boys plus 0.29 years for every year of age at irradiation). For example, the estimated age at onset of puberty in a boy irradiated at 2 years of age would be 9.79 years and that for a boy irradiated at 9 years of age would be 11.82 years. In the context of GH deficiency, which is usually associated with a delay in the onset of puberty, this is abnormal.

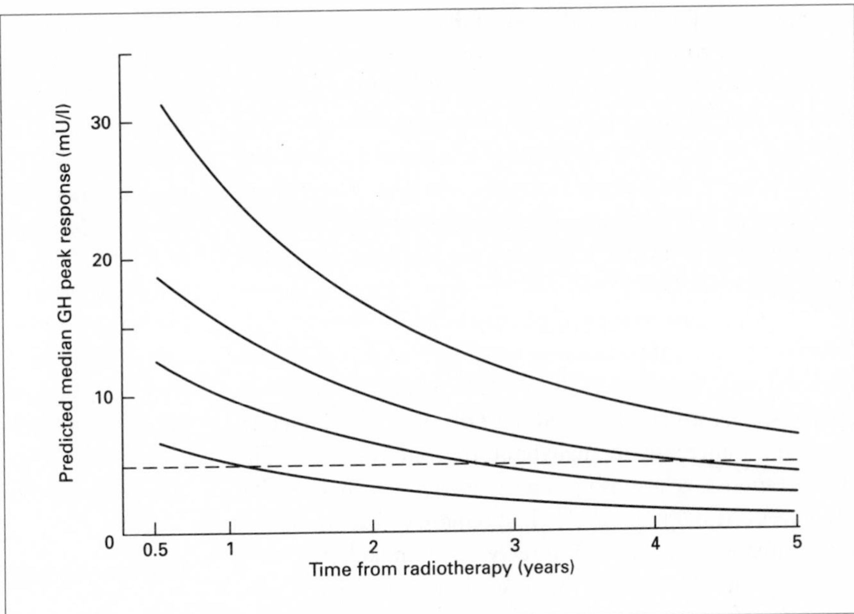

Fig. 75.4 The predicted median GH declines for baseline GH peaks of 50, 30, 20 and 10 mU/l over the first 5 years following radiotherapy. Dashed line at 5 mU/l, below which the degree of GH deficiency is considered to be severe.

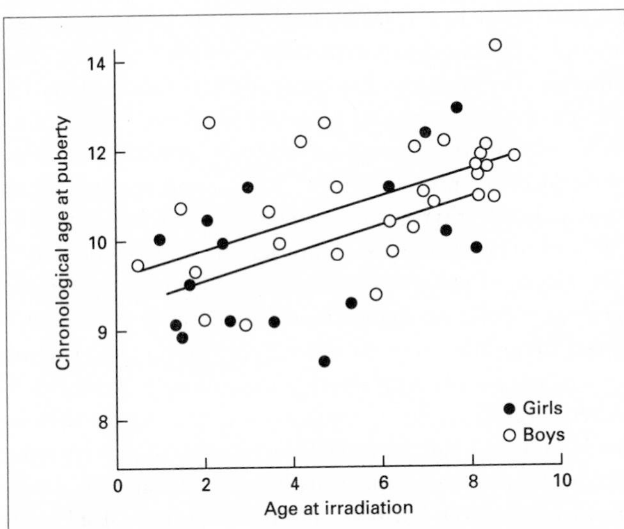

Fig. 75.5 Estimated and fitted chronological ages (years) at the onset of puberty for age at irradiation (years).

The largest number of children available for the study of pubertal timing after irradiation are those treated for childhood leukaemia (dose of irradiation 1800–2400 cGy). There is a high incidence of early puberty predominantly among girls. The number of boys entering puberty early is no greater than that anticipated in a normal population. This sexual dichotomy has been attributed to fundamental differences in the interaction between the central nervous system (CNS) and hypothalamic function. It has been postulated that the CNS restraint on the onset of puberty is more readily disrupted in girls than in boys by any insult, including irradiation. At the doses of irradiation employed in the treatment of brain tumours (2500–4700 cGy), however, radiation-induced early puberty is not restricted to girls.

The mechanism for early puberty after irradiation is likely to be related to disinhibition of cortical influences on the hypothalamus: puberty then proceeds through the increased frequency and amplitude of GnRH pulsatile secretion by the hypothalamus. The impact of early puberty in a child with radiation-induced growth failure is to foreshorten the time available for GH therapy. This has restricted the therapeutic efficacy of GH. Consequently, a number of these children are now treated with a combination of a GnRH analogue and GH therapy. It is relatively easy to halt the progression of puberty but there is limited information on the impact of this approach on final height.

Thyroid cancer

In 1950 Duffy and Fitzgerald [12] reported that nine of a series of 28 children with thyroid carcinoma had received irradiation for thymic enlargement previously, and raised the possibility that irradiation was an aetiological factor in the development of thyroid tumours. Subsequently, a number of large-scale surveys were undertaken, all of which confirmed unequivocally a causal relationship between external irradiation of the neck in childhood and thyroid cancer. Important determinants of cancer risk are radiation dose, age at exposure and length of time since exposure [13]. Thus, after neck irradiation, young children are more vulnerable to the subsequent development of thyroid cancer than older children, and all children are much more at risk than adults.

Within certain limitations, the risk of thyroid cancer appears proportional to the dose of radiation. After analysing the data from several large studies, Maxon *et al.* [14] concluded that the risk of developing thyroid cancer after receiving 600 and 1200 cGy was, respectively, almost 2.5-fold and 5-fold greater than after receiving 200 cGy. The risk of carcinogenesis is present over an extremely wide range of radiation doses and extends for at least 50 years. Thus, Ron *et al.* [15] identified 98 thyroid tumours during follow-up of 10 834 persons irradiated for tinea capitis during childhood compared with 57 among a population of 10 834 non-exposed matched individuals and 5392 sibling-comparison subjects. An estimated thyroid dose of 9 cGy was linked to a fourfold increase in malignant thyroid tumours. The dose–response relationship was consistent with linearity. However, Maxon *et al.* [14] speculated that radiation doses greater than 2000–3000 cGy were unlikely to prove carcinogenic, presumably because these doses were considered sufficient to ablate the thyroid. Nevertheless, it has since become apparent that thyroid cancer may occur even after considerably higher radiation doses. Thus, by 1986 a total of 21 patients with thyroid cancer following irradiation for Hodgkin's disease had been reported [16]. Seventy-four per cent of the patients received a radiation dose equal to or exceeding 2000 cGy. The latent periods spanned from 6 to 48 years. Histologically, the great majority of radiation-induced thyroid cancers are well-differentiated papillary carcinomas, but follicular tumours also occur. An important factor in the prognosis for spontaneously occurring thyroid cancer is the size of the lesion at diagnosis, those < 15 mm in diameter when detected having little or no effect on lifespan. Many radiation-induced tumours are small, but approximately half are greater than 15 mm in diameter and there is an increased incidence of multicentric disease, local invasion and distant metastases compared with tumours occurring in unirradiated patients. However, in thyroid cancer studies, when irradiated patients are matched for age, sex and extent of disease with unirradiated patients, there is no significant difference in disease-free interval or survival [17].

Large surveys conducted in the USA have shown that the risk of both spontaneous and radiation-induced thyroid cancer is increased among Jews. In Hawaii, the incidence of radiation-induced tumours in the Chinese is three or four times higher than in the Japanese or Caucasians. Women are at greater risk than men by a factor of 2–3.5 times, as they are also for spontaneously occurring thyroid cancer.

Further confirmation of the relationship between irradiation and thyroid cancer is provided by accidental irradiation exposure. During the initial period after the Chernobyl accident, large amounts of radioactive iodine were released in fallout, resulting in serious exposure to the thyroid gland in the residents of areas around the nuclear power station. Beginning in 1990, a definite increase in the incidence of thyroid cancer was noted in children of the Republic of Belarus [18]. Post-Chernobyl paediatric thyroid carcinoma is characterised by a short latency period, a higher proportion of tumours arising in young children and an almost equal sex ratio. Microscopically these tumours were usually aggressive, often demonstrating intraglandular tumour dissemination (92%), thyroid capsular and adjacent soft-tissue invasion (89%) and cervical lymph-node metastases (88%). Papillary carcinoma was diagnosed in 99% of cases, with a high frequency of solid growth patterns. Morphological changes in non-neoplastic thyroid tissue were present in 90% of the glands and the most specific findings were vascular changes and perifollicular fibrosis [18].

Benign nodules

Abnormalities of thyroid morphology, other than cancer, are frequently found in patients exposed to radiation. These include focal hyperplasia, single or multiple adenomas, chronic lymphocytic thyroiditis, colloid nodules and fibrosis. Investigators use many different definitions for benign thyroid tumours; some separate and others combine adenomas and colloid nodules, resulting in large differences in reported risk estimates. Certain studies suggest that palpable thyroid abnormalities occur in about 20–30% of an irradiated population as compared with a 1–5% prevalence of palpable nodular thyroid disease within the general population. Benign thyroid nodularity occurs much more frequently in an irradiated population than thyroid cancer, but the exact incidence is less precisely documented. After surgical removal, radiation-induced benign thyroid nodules have a high recurrence rate similar to that reported among unirradiated patients with similar lesions [19]. Treatment with thyroid hormone in order to suppress TSH levels after thyroid surgery decreases the incidence of recurrence of benign radiation-induced nodules [19].

Thyroid dysfunction

Most accumulated data about radiation-induced hypothyroidism are derived from studies performed in patients treated for lymphomas [20] or head and neck cancer. These individuals have generally received doses of irradiation in the range of 3000–5000 cGy given in multiple fractions over several weeks. Following a radiation dose to the neck of between 4000 and 5000 cGy over 4–5 weeks, approximately 25% of patients show an elevated TSH and low thyroxine concentration, whilst in a further 41% there is a raised TSH concentration in the presence of a normal thyroxine concentration [20]. The inclusion of a TRH test to amplify minor abnormalities in basal TSH secretion has revealed a further group of patients who show an exaggerated TSH response to TRH but normal basal TSH and thyroxine concentrations.

Various factors may influence the incidence of radiation-induced hypothyroidism in a particular study population. Previous hemithyroidectomy, lymphangiography or irradiation below the age of 20 years is claimed to be associated with a higher incidence, whilst lower radiation doses are associated with a lower incidence. Equally important is the time after irradiation at which the thyroid studies are carried out, as the time interval between irradiation and the peak incidence of thyroid dysfunction is unknown. Schimpff *et al.* [20] noted thyroid dysfunction in 14% of patients during the first year after irradiation, with the cumulative incidence rising to a maximum of 66% 6 years after irradiation. Alternatively, recovery of normal thyroid function several years after documented radiation-induced thyroid dysfunction may occur occasionally.

Apart from patients receiving neck irradiation for lymphoma or head and neck cancer, there are other groups of patients who are vulnerable to radiation-induced thyroid dysfunction or thyroid tumours. Direct irradiation is received by the thyroid gland during the spinal component of craniospinal irradiation administered to treat certain childhood brain tumours. Similarly at risk are children who receive total-body irradiation in preparation for bone-marrow transplantation. Total-body irradiation has been given in single dose exposures of 750–1000 cGy, and more recently in fractionated exposures of total doses ranging from 1200 to 1575 cGy given over 3–7 days [21]. In a series of 116 children who received transplants for malignancy after preparation with cyclophosphamide and total-body irradiation, 18% developed compensated thyroid dysfunction (raised TSH, normal thyroxine levels), 11% developed frank hypothyroidism, and two children developed thyroid tumours 4 and 8 years later [3]. The treatment of hypothyroidism (raised TSH, low thyroxine), whether it be due to radiation-induced thyroid damage or any other cause, is thyroxine. A similar therapeutic approach is justified for patients with compensated thyroid dysfunction (raised TSH, normal thyroxine) irrespective of whether or not the latter state represents a mild but significant form of hypothyroidism or merely a biochemical abnormality. Support for this view is derived from the observation following animal studies that an elevated TSH level in the presence of irradiation-damaged thyroid tissue is known to be carcinogenic.

Autoimmune thyroiditis

Apart from histological evidence of chronic lymphocytic thyroiditis, a greater proportion of irradiated patients screen positively for the presence of antimicrosomal and thyroglobulin antibodies than in the normal population. Thyroid dysfunction associated with either autoimmune thyroiditis, Graves' disease, atypical silent thyroiditis or exophthalmos, has been observed infrequently following neck irradiation for lymphoma.

Chemotherapy and thyroid function

Although there is no conclusive evidence that any cytotoxic drug alters thyroid function to the extent of causing clinical hypo- or hyperthyroidism, both 5-fluorouracil and L-asparaginase may modify circulating thyroid hormone levels. 5-Fluorouracil increases total thyroxine and triiodothyronine levels while L-asparaginase decreases the total thyroxine level. Patients receiving 5-fluorouracil are clinically euthyroid and have a normal free thyroxine index and TSH level. The drug either modifies the concentration of one or more thyroid hormone-binding proteins or causes a qualitative change in their binding capacity. L-Asparaginase has widespread effects on protein and DNA synthesis. It causes transient thyroxine-binding globulin (TBG) deficiency by diminishing hepatic synthesis of TBG, and appears to decrease free thyroxine concentrations into the hypothyroid range by inhibiting TSH secretion by the pituitary gland.

Atkins *et al.* [22] described hypothyroidism in 21% of 34 patients with advanced neoplasms who had received interleukin 2 (IL-2) and lymphokine-activated killer (LAK) cells. It was suggested that IL-2 and LAK cells exacerbate pre-existing autoimmune thyroiditis and thus cause hypothyroidism in susceptible individuals.

Chemotherapy may potentiate the adverse impact of radiation on thyroid function. Both Livesey and Brook [23] and Ogilvy-Stuart *et al.* [24] showed a higher incidence of thyroid dysfunction in children receiving adjuvant cytotoxic chemotherapy after craniospinal irradiation for a brain tumour compared with children receiving craniospinal irradiation alone.

Parathyroid gland

The results of several studies [25,26] have suggested a significantly increased risk of developing hyperparathyroidism in subjects who have received neck irradiation. The evidence for a causal relationship is predominantly based on retrospective studies which show that a significantly greater number of patients with hyperparathyroidism previously had received irradiation to the neck compared with normocalcaemic control subjects. The latency period between radiation exposure and the development of hyperparathyroidism appears to be very long, i.e. 25–47 years.

It has been difficult to establish with certainty that radiation exposure is a risk factor for developing hyperparathyroidism, partly because many cases of hyperparathyroidism remain asymptomatic and escape clinical detection. Recently, Schneider *et al.* [27] reviewed results from a study of 2555 subjects who received external irradiation to the head and neck area for benign conditions before their 16th birthday between 1939 and 1962. There were 36 confirmed cases of hyperparathyroidism. Based on a relative risk model the excess relative risk increased significantly by 0.11/cGy; the confidence interval however was wide (95% confidence interval 0.0–17.2). The demonstration of a dose–response relationship within an irradiated cohort supports the hypothesis of a causal association between radiation exposure and hyperparathyroidism. The clinical implication is that the calcium level of individuals who previously received neck irradiation should be monitored regularly.

Radiation-induced gonadal damage

Testis

Exposure to X-rays, neutrons and radioactive materials can cause germinal cell destruction. Under acute conditions of exposure, spermatogenesis may eventually recover, provided the dose is not excessive. Following graded single-dose irradiation (range 8–600 cGy) to the testes of adult men, spermatogonia were found to be the most radiosensitive cell type, with both morphological and quantitative changes at all dose levels except 8 cGy, at which no biopsies were taken. Spermatocytes were damaged at doses of 200–300 cGy as shown by their inability to complete maturation division which caused a decrease in resulting spermatid numbers. Spermatocytes were visibly damaged after 400–600 cGy. Spermatids showed no overt damage, but after 400–600 cGy the resultant spermatozoa were significantly decreased in number signifying covert spermatid damage [28].

At lower doses the decreased sperm count begins 60–80 days after exposure and its duration is dose dependent. Higher single doses cause a more rapid onset of oligospermia and azoospermia by their effect on the later as well as earlier stages of sperm production. With single-dose exposures, complete recovery, i.e. return to pre-irradiation sperm concentrations and germinal cell numbers, takes place within 9–18 months after < 100 cGy, 30 months for 200–300 cGy, and 5 or more years after 400–600 cGy.

Irradiation of the testis during radiotherapy usually involved fractionated exposures. Under certain conditions fractionation causes more stem-cell killing than does single treatments, although this has not been proven in humans. Hahn *et al.* [29] carried out serial semen examinations on 11 cancer patients who had received large pelvic field irradiation or interstitial ^{125}I seeds implanted in the prostate. The total calculated dose to the testes ranged from 118 to 228 cGy in 24–35 fractions. All patients suffered temporary aspermia beginning at about 3 months post-irradiation. Recovery of spermatogenesis was first noted between 10 and 18 months after irradiation in five patients. The same group [30] studied a cohort of patients who received total fractionated doses of 19–178 cGy to the remaining testis following unilateral orchidectomy for seminoma. Azoospermia occurred in 10 out of 14 patients who received > 65 cGy to the testis. Sperm reappeared in the semen within 30–80 weeks of the start of treatment.

Males in whom abdominal irradiation (inverted Y abdominal, pelvic and inguinal field) is given for Hodgkin's disease receive a scatter dose of irradiation to the testes. Speiser *et al.* [31] studied 10 such males who received an average daily dose of 12 cGy resulting in a total dose of 140–300 cGy. All were azoospermic, but only two patients were followed for longer than 16 months. Some 27.5% of the males studied retrospectively by Slanina *et al.* (32) were either oligospermic or had a normal sperm count following similar radiation treatment and scatter dosage to the testes. However, the follow-up period was longer in these patients.

Following fractionated courses of irradiation, azoospermia has been induced by a testicular dose as low as 35 cGy. After a radiation dose of between 200 and 300 cGy, the primary impact of the damage is on the germinal epithelium with recovery of spermatogenesis sometimes delayed for 10 years or more. Leydig-cell function is intact as judged by a normal serum testosterone concentration, although in some patients this may be maintained only by a minor rise in the circulating luteinising hormone (LH) concentration. As the testicular irradiation dose is increased to several thousand cGy [33], i.e. 3000 cGy, the serum testosterone often becomes frankly low and androgen-replacement therapy may be necessary.

Radiation-induced testicular damage is also a recognised complication following radioactive iodine therapy for thyroid cancer. Significant impairment of spermatogenesis appears to be restricted to men having multiple doses totalling over 100 mCi (equivalent to a testicular radiation dose of 50–100 cGy).

Men receiving total-body irradiation and high-dose chemotherapy in preparation for a bone marrow transplant all develop azoospermia. The total-body irradiation dose may range from 800 to 1400 cGy in total and may be given in a single or in multiple fractions. In some patients the azoospermia may reverse with time but the exact frequency of this phenomenon has not yet been documented [34].

Most boys with leukaemic relapse of the testes receive direct testicular irradiation with a total dose of between 2000 and 2400 cGy. The young prepubertal boy seems most vulnerable to the development of severe and persistent testicular dysfunction. The germinal epithelium is completely ablated in all, and Leydig-cell function seriously affected in most. However, gonadal damage in prepubertal life may not be associated with abnormal gonadotrophin concentrations, either basally or after GnRH stimulation (Fig. 75.6); these develop during the peripubertal years and will often first occur around the age of 9–10 years. The serum testosterone concentration is usually low, which is of course normal for a prepubertal boy, but there is an inadequate or absent testosterone response to an acute bolus of human chorionic gonadotrophin (hCG) (Fig. 75.7). Most boys require androgen replacement to enable normal pubertal development to occur. Initiation of androgen replacement should be considered at about 12–13 years of age: the requirement will be permanent [58].

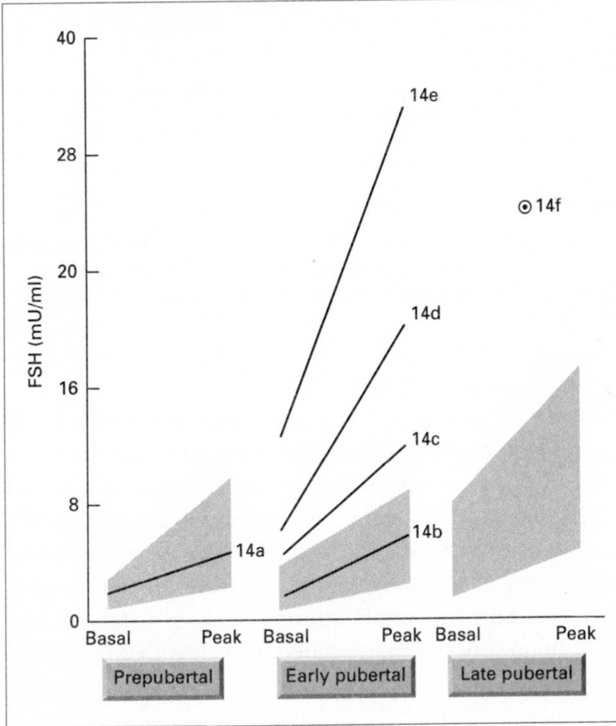

Fig. 75.6 Basal and peak follicle-stimulating hormone (FSH) concentrations after gonadotrophin-releasing hormone (GnRH) administration in a boy treated with multiple courses of MOPP for Hodgkin's disease between the ages of 6 and 9 years. The GnRH tests were performed at (a) 1 year; (b) 1.5 years; (c) 1.7 years; (d) 2 years; and (e) 3 years after completion of treatment; (f) is the basal FSH level 5 years after treatment. Normal ranges of values for each pubertal stage are shown (shaded areas). Note that basal and stimulated FSH levels remain normal until 1.7 years after completion of CT despite the fact that the testicular damage will have occurred at the time CT was administered. This illustrates the unreliability of FSH estimations in predicting such damage in prepubertal and peripubertal boys.

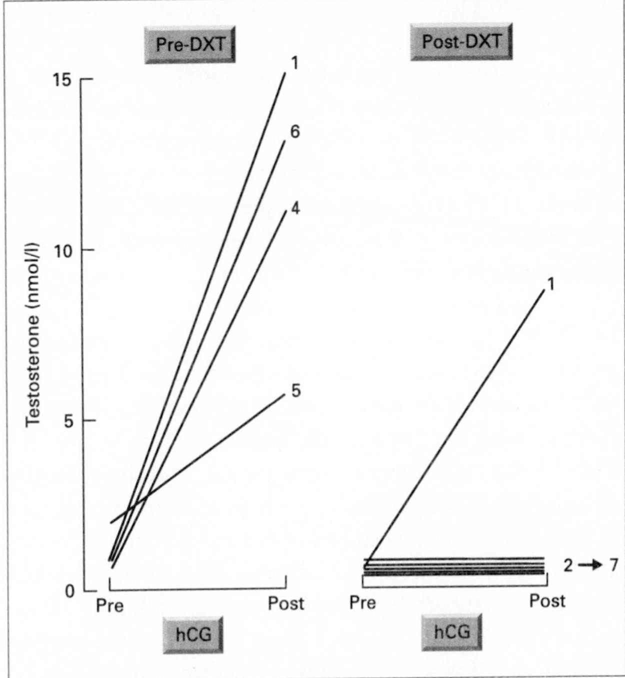

Fig. 75.7 Basal and post-hCG (human chorionic gonadotrophin) testosterone concentrations in seven prepubertal boys with acute lymphoblastic leukaemia (ALL) before (pre-DXT) and after testicular irradiation (post-DXT).

Lower doses of testicular irradiation are received by boys undergoing total-body irradiation for a bone-marrow transplant and those receiving spinal fields of irradiation as part of a craniospinal radiotherapy schedule for a brain tumour. The degree of damage inflicted by the testicular irradiation, i.e. germinal epithelial damage, with or without Leydig-cell dysfunction, is dependent on the radiation dose and the age and pubertal stage of the boy [21].

Ovary

When girls and adult women are irradiated, the response of the ovary involves a fixed population of cells which, once destroyed, cannot be replaced. Effects on fertility are most readily explained on the basis of a reduction in the fixed pool of oocytes. While a permanent menopause can be caused by a total radiation exposure of about 600 cGy in women aged 40 years or more, radiotherapists' estimates of the 50% probability level for permanent sterility are approximately 2000 cGy over a 6-week period in young women. If the radiation dose is delivered over a greater number of fractionated doses, the damage to the ovary and consequent chance of infertility is likely to be less. In agreement with this, Doll and Smith [35] found that 97% of 2068 women failed to menstruate again after two to four fractionated exposures to a total dose of 360–720 cGy (estimated ovarian dose).

The treatment of patients with Hodgkin's disease is influenced by the extent of the disease. Certain patients receive irradiation to the lymph nodes along the iliac vessels. Since the ovaries lie in this area, they receive a dose of about 3500 cGy, which inevitably causes ovarian failure.

Transposition of the ovaries (oophoropexy) before irradiation with a consequent reduction in the dose delivered to the shielded ovaries to a maximum of 600 cGy over 12–45 days has decreased the incidence of amenorrhoea by over 50%. None the less, the exact benefit to be derived from oophoropexy in women requiring inverted 'Y' therapy is controversial. The extent of the disease needs to be carefully staged before considering oophoropexy, and then the procedure needs to be performed with great accuracy and care.

There have been few studies of ovarian function following abdominal irradiation in childhood. After 2000–3000 cGy over 25–44 days to both ovaries, ovarian failure is almost universal. Morphological studies have revealed marked inhibition of follicular growth and severe reduction in the number of oocytes. Recent studies have indicated that the spinal component of craniospinal irradiation for the treatment of brain tumours and total-body irradiation for bone-marrow transplantation [3] may cause ovarian dysfunction due to radiation-induced ovarian damage. The patients present with either failure to undergo or to complete pubertal development, or later in adult life with a premature menopause. On occasions the ovarian failure may prove reversible. The LD_{50} for the human oocyte has been estimated [36] not to exceed 400 cGy and, in conjunction with information about the position of the ovaries in relation to the radiation field, the predicted age at ovarian failure can be calculated approximately. This may provide a factual basis for fertility counselling in such patients.

Uterus

In those women irradiated during childhood in whom ovarian function is preserved but in whom the uterus has been included in the radiation field, there is evidence that radiation changes to the uterus result in failure to carry a pregnancy. The risk of miscarriage or low-birthweight infants is greatly increased [37].

Following an irradiation dose in childhood of 2000–3000 cGy to the whole abdomen, these women have a significant reduction in uterine length (Fig. 75.8) and an endometrium which is unresponsive to physiological serum levels of oestradiol and progesterone attained by exogenous administration [38]. Doppler signals from the uterine arteries are absent in most. It is not yet clear whether this is a consequence of primary damage to the microvasculature of the uterus and associated blood supply. As appropriate vascularisation and subsequent growth of the endometrium are essential, however, for implantation and successful continuation of pregnancy, it is unlikely that women who have received a significant dose of abdominal irradiation in childhood will be able to sustain a pregnancy to term. This has implications for *in vitro* fertilisation with donor oocytes in irradiated women with concomitant ovarian failure.

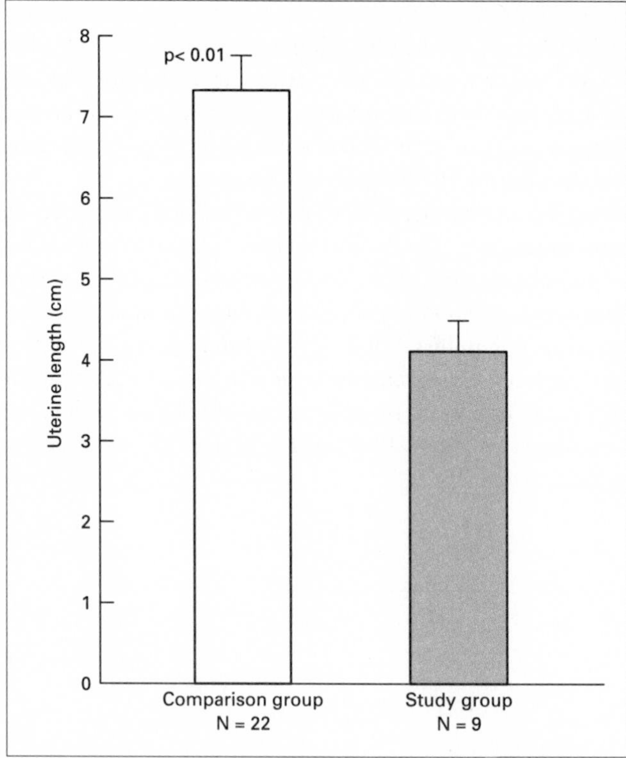

Fig. 75.8 Mean uterine length (±2 SE) in nine women exposed to whole abdominal irradiation in childhood compared with a control group of 22 women with premature ovarian failure who had not received whole abdominal irradiation (mean 4.0 versus 7.3 cm; $P < 0.01$).

Chemotherapy-induced gonadal damage

Testis

Gonadal damage by cytotoxic drugs was first described in humans by Spitz in 1948 [39]. At autopsy, the absence of spermatogenesis and the presence of tubules lined by Sertoli cells only was noted in the testes of 27 out of 30 men who had been treated with mechlorethamine (nitrogen mustard). In 1956, Louis *et al.* [40], reporting on the effects of busulphan in chronic myeloid leukaemia, were the first to comment upon the gonadal effects of cytotoxic chemotherapy in women. It has since become clear that a variety of cytotoxic drugs may damage the gonad. In humans gonadal damage has most frequently been described following the use of alkylating drugs such as cyclophosphamide and chlorambucil; however, nitrosoureas, procarbazine, vinblastine, cytosine arabinoside and *cis*-platinum have all been incriminated.

The extent of the damage and potential for recovery are dependent on the nature of the drugs received and the dosage. Watson *et al.* [41] have reported on the long-term outcome in a series of 30 males treated with cyclophosphamide during childhood in a dose of 2–3 mg/kg bodyweight/day for a mean of 280 (range 42–556) days. The mean age at evaluation was 22 (range 17–29.5) years, mean age at treatment was 9.4 (2.9–17.3) years, and the mean time from completion of treatment to study was 12.8 (range 6.7–15.8) years.

Of the 30 patients, four were azoospermic, nine were oligospermic (sperm count <20 million/ml) and 17 were normospermic (sperm count >20 million/ml). Although there was no significant correlation between total testicular volume and sperm density, the three groups of patients differed significantly in mean testicular volume, with the azoospermic group having a marked reduction in testicular size. A significant inverse correlation was evident between sperm density and cyclophosphamide dosage in terms of duration of treatment and total dosage.

Thirteen patients had undergone semen analysis 5.5–9 years previously. Nine of them remained in the same categories in the later study (four normospermic, three azoospermic and two oligospermic) but four who had previously been oligospermic ($n = 3$) or azoospermic ($n = 1$) were found to be normospermic after an average additional follow-up of 7.2 years. The impact of duration of treatment and total drug dosage on spermatogenesis could not be disentangled, but both appeared more important variables than the pubertal status of the subject. None of the patients who were treated for less than 112 days and received <10 g cyclophosphamide (or <300 mg/kg bodyweight) had a sperm count of <20 million/ml.

The reports of recovery of spermatogenesis in many of the patients previously treated with single cytotoxic drugs are encouraging. However, azoospermia appears to be permanent following certain combinations of cytotoxic drugs. Chapman *et al.* [42] studied a large group of men who had received MVPP (mustine, vinblastine, procarbazine and prednisolone) for advanced or recurrent Hodgkin's disease and had finished their chemotherapy between 1 and 62 months earlier. Of 64 men, only four showed any evidence of spermatogenesis.

Whitehead *et al.* [43] studied 74 men who were similarly treated for Hodgkin's disease. Out of the 49 men who received six or more courses of MVPP and provided a sperm count, 42 were azoospermic. Five of the seven who showed evidence of spermatogenesis had a sperm count of <1 million/ml. Furthermore, of 11 patients studied between 6 and 8 years after the end of chemotherapy, 10 were azoospermic. This strongly suggests that the chances of spermatogenesis recovering in the remaining patients must be extremely small. None the less well-documented but isolated reports of such recovery exist. Combination chemotherapy has been a major therapeutic advance in the treatment of metastatic testicular cancer. Regimens using *cis*-diamine-dichloroproplatinum (CDDP), vinblastine and bleomycin have been shown to be increasingly effective in the treatment of metastatic teratoma. Patients with testicular cancer are usually young, and azoospermia is a common finding after completion of chemotherapy. Fortunately, recovery of spermatogenesis after therapy with CDDP, vinblastine and bleomycin is more likely than after MVPP, as in 50% of patients the sperm count is normal at 3 years after completion of chemotherapy.

There is no doubt that the cytotoxic drugs which damage the testis predominantly affect the germinal epithelium. However, more recent studies in men treated with MVPP for Hodgkin's disease have suggested a subtle impairment of Leydig-cell function. The circulating testosterone concentration and the steroidogenic response to an acute bolus injection of hCG are normal. The basal LH concentration is frequently raised and the LH response to a GnRH test is exaggerated. The bioactive/immunoreactive LH ratio is normal and there is no disturbance of LH pulse frequency; however, the amplitude of the LH pulses is significantly elevated (Fig. 75.9). Due to this compensatory process, it has not usually been deemed necessary to offer androgen replacement therapy following chemotherapy induced testicular damage.

More recently, however, a significant reduction in bone mineral density (BMD) has been demonstrated in men who previously received chemotherapy for Hodgkin's disease [44]. The reduction in BMD affected both cortical bone, measured at the forearm by single-photon absorptiometry, and integral bone, measured at lumbar spine and femoral neck by dual-energy X-ray absorptiometry. Furthermore there was a significant positive correlation between the serum testosterone level and the BMD standard deviation score at the lumbar spine and femoral neck suggesting that a reduction in serum testosterone, as a consequence of chemotherapy-induced Leydig-cell damage, is associated with a reduction in integral BMD.

If confirmed by prospective studies, then these results have therapeutic implications. Androgen replacement therapy may be required for men with low normal testosterone and raised LH levels, even in the presence of normal sexual function.

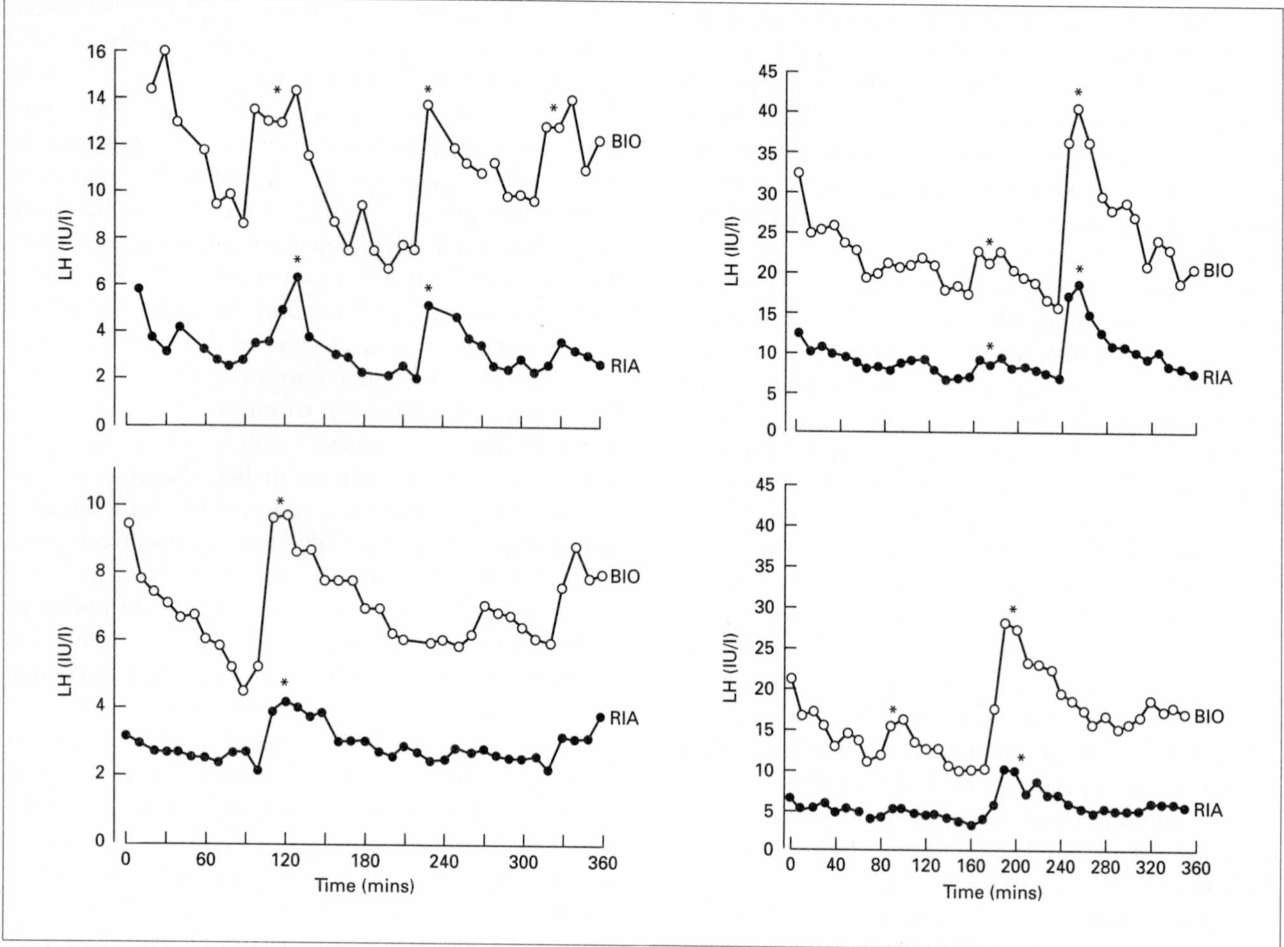

Fig. 75.9 The two graphs on the left show bioactive (o—o) and immunoreactive luteinising hormone (LH) (•—•) over 6h in two normal adult men. The two graphs on the right show bioactive (o—o) and immunoreactive LH (•—•) over 6 hours in two patients treated for Hodgkin's disease with six to nine courses of MVPP (mustine, vincristine, procarbazine, prednisolone) chemotherapy. Results represent the mean of quadruplicate measurements and duplicate measurements for bioactive and immunoreactive LH, respectively. An asterisk (*) represents a significant pulse. Note the different scales.

Gynaecomastia has been described as a complication of chemotherapy since it has been associated with the use of busulphan, vincristine, bischloronitrosourea as well as various combinations of cytotoxic drugs. It has been interpreted as a clinical manifestation of Leydig-cell dysfunction associated biochemically with a subtle alteration of the circulating oestrogen/androgen ratio. It may be transient and is more likely to occur in those prone to developing gynaecomastia such as the elderly.

Ovary

In the female, most information is available on the effects of cyclophosphamide on reproductive function. Uldall *et al.* [45] studied 34 women with glomerulonephritis treated with daily cyclophosphamide for an average of 18 months. Eighteen women developed amenorrhoea within an average time of 7 months from starting cyclophosphamide. Periods returned in only one out of nine patients who discontinued the drug 12 months (mean time) previously. Urinary oestrogens were low and urinary gonadotrophins elevated, suggesting that the amenorrhoea was due to cyclophosphamide-induced ovarian damage. The amenorrhoea may or may not be permanent. Furthermore, the total dose of the drug received will determine whether the amenorrhoea is reversible, and how soon after initiation of treatment the amenorrhoea will develop.

The susceptibility of women to develop cytotoxic-induced ovarian failure is age dependent. Koyama *et al.* [46] studied women with breast carcinoma who had been treated with different cytotoxic drugs including cyclophosphamide. The average dose of cyclophosphamide given before the onset of amenorrhoea in patients in their 40s, 30s and 20s was 5.2, 9.3 and 20.4g, respectively. It might be predicted that cytotoxic-induced ovarian failure would rarely occur in the prepubertal and pubertal female. However, clinical and morphological studies indicate that the young girl is not totally resistant to such damage.

Following the marked reduction in the mortality rate from gestational trophoblastic tumours and Hodgkin's disease, there has been increasing interest in the impact of chemotherapy on reproductive function. Walden and Bagshawe [47] analysed the reproductive performance of 314 women successfully treated for gestational trophoblastic tumours between 1962 and 1977; 159 of these patients had become pregnant despite previous treatment with methotrexate, 6-mercaptopurine, actinomycin D and 6-azauridine. A number of groups have studied the incidence of amenorrhoea after MOPP or MVPP (mustine, vincristine, procarbazine and prednisolone) therapy for Hodgkin's disease, and this has ranged from 15 to 62%. In some women the amenorrhoea is reversible [59], although the progression from regular menses to amenorrhoea is variable; in some it is abrupt, while in others there is a slow transition phase of oligomenorrhoea followed by a premature menopause (Fig. 75.10).

Chatterjee *et al.* [48] studied the acute effects of high-dose chemotherapy or total-body irradiation or both on ovarian function. All women showed subtle evidence of ovarian dysfunction before bone-marrow transplantation with lower basal and human menopausal gonadotrophin (hMG)-stimulated oestradiol levels, higher basal follicle-stimulating hormone (FSH) levels and exaggerated FSH responses to an acute bolus of GnRH than seen in controls. The conditioning regimens employed before bone-marrow transplantation caused further ovarian damage; gonadotrophin levels rose further into the menopausal range and basal oestradiol level fell and became unresponsive to hMG stimulation 3–4 months after bone-marrow transplantation. Contrary to expectation the hormonal changes occurring acutely were similar in patients undergoing radiation-based regimens and those conditioned with high-dose chemotherapy alone. In view of the differing prospects for recovery of ovarian function following chemotherapy versus total-body irradiation [49], it would imply that the severity of ovarian dysfunction occurring acutely after cytotoxic damage cannot be used to predict the long-term prospects of recovery of ovarian function.

Most women with chemotherapy-induced ovarian failure under the age of 50 years should receive sex steroid-replacement therapy with a preparation containing oestrogen and progestogen in order to prevent osteoporosis, reduce the mortality rate from ischaemic heart disease and to alleviate symptoms in the symptomatic. A minority of such women with a lesser degree of ovarian failure will produce sufficient oestrogen to avoid the need for replacement therapy.

Protection of gonadal function from cytotoxic damage

As a consequence of the high incidence of azoospermia following MVPP/MOPP therapy for Hodgkin's disease and CDDP, vinblastine and bleomycin for testicular teratoma, sperm-storage facilities have been offered to some male patients before they start chemotherapy. Sperm storage is

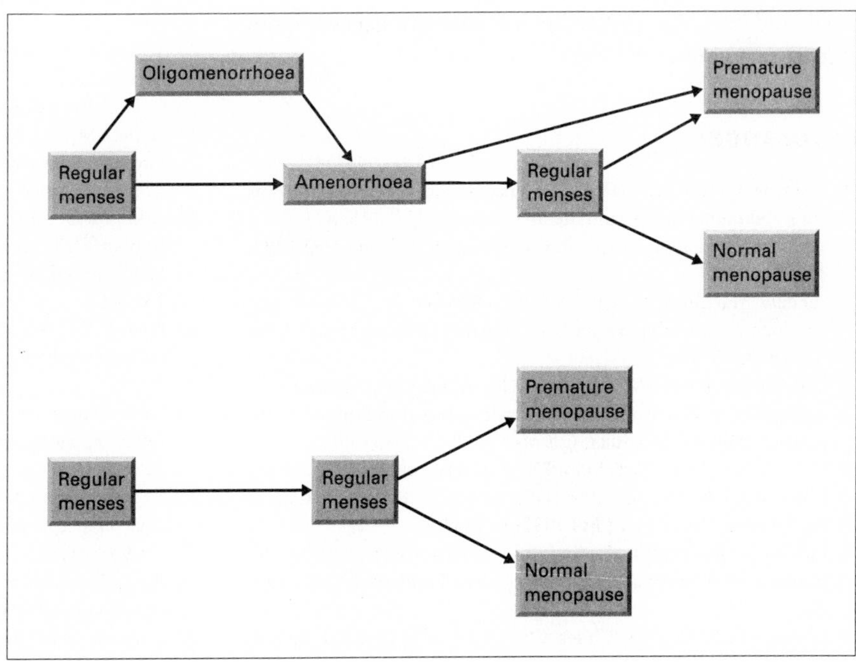

Fig. 75.10 Natural history and outcome in women with chemotherapy-induced ovarian damage.

likely to be most useful if the sperm concentration, morphology and motility are not severely affected by the disease process itself. This provides the only real possibility for fertility in a significant number of men with Hodgkin's disease or those who have had a hemicastration for testicular tumour [50]. Furthermore, with new advances in assisted reproductive techniques even the male who is oligospermic before chemotherapy has some chance of success subsequently [51,52]. Thus, sperm banking must be discussed with every male prior to potentially gonadotoxic chemotherapy being administered.

Alternative modalities of therapy are being sought to provide similar 'cure' rates to established regimens associated with a reduced incidence of gonadal toxicity; Viviani *et al.* [53] have proposed that ABVD (adriamycin, bleomycin, vinblastine and dacarbazine) chemotherapy fulfils this aim when compared with MOPP for the management of Hodgkin's disease in adults. Hybrid chemotherapy, however, proved no less gonadotoxic than conventional MVPP/MOPP chemotherapy [54].

More recently, there have been attempts to suppress hormonally the pituitary–gonadal axis to prevent chemotherapy-induced gonadal damage in humans. The attempts to achieve gonadotrophin suppression have been via GnRH agonist analogues in both sexes or oestrogen therapy in the female. In the human there has not been any convincing evidence of protection utilising this approach. However, in the rat model there is evidence that GnRH agonist and antagonist analogues or testosterone may protect, at least partially, the spermatogenic epithelium from cytotoxic damage [55]. Furthermore a combination of a GnRH antagonist analogue and an antiandrogen (flutamide) provides an even more rapid and efficient protection of spermatogenesis from procarbazine-induced damage in the rat [56].

References

1 Teinturier C, Tournade MF, Caillat-Zucman S *et al.* Diabetes mellitus after abdominal irradiation therapy. *Lancet* 1995; **346**: 633–4.

2 Shalet SM. Radiation and pituitary dysfunction. *N Engl J Med* 1993; **328**: 131–3.

3 Sanders JE, Buckner CD, Sullivan KM *et al.* Growth and development in children after bone marrow transplantation. *Horm Res* 1988; **30**: 92–7.

4 Littley MD, Shalet SM, Beardwell CG, Ahmed SR, Applegate G, Sutton ML. Hypopituitarism following external radiotherapy for pituitary tumours in adults. *Q J Med* 1989; **262**: 145–60.

5 Samaan NA, Vieto R, Schultz PN *et al.* Hypothalamic, pituitary and thyroid dysfunction after radiotherapy to the head and neck. *Int J Radiat Oncol Biol Phys* 1982; **8**: 1857–67.

6 Jadresic A, Jimenez LE, Joplin GF. Long-term effect of yttrium-90 pituitary implantation in acromegaly. *Acta Endocrinol* 1987; **115**: 301–6.

7 Chieng PU, Huang TS, Chang CC, Chong PN, Tien RD, Su CT. Reduced hypothalamic blood flow after radiation treatment of nasopharyngeal cancer: SPECT studies in 34 patients. *Am J Nucl Radiol* 1991; **12**: 661–5.

8 Ogilvy-Stuart AL, Wallace WHB, Shalet SM. Radiation and neuroregulatory control of growth hormone secretion. *Clin Endocrinol* 1994; **41**: 163–8.

9 Littley MD, Shalet SM, Beardwell CG, Robinson EL, Sutton ML. Radiation-induced hypopituitarism is dose-dependent. *Clin Endocrinol* 1989; **31**: 363–73.

10 Toogood AA, Ryder WDJ, Beardwell CG, Shalet SM. The evolution of radiation-induced growth hormone in adults is determined by the baseline growth hormone status. *Clin Endocrinol* 1995; **43**: 97–103.

11 Ogilvy-Stuart AL, Clayton PE, Shalet SM. Cranial irradiation and early puberty. *J Clin Endocrinol Metab* 1994; **78**: 1282–6.

12 Duffy BJ, Fitzgerald PJ. Thyroid cancer in childhood and adolescence. *Cancer* 1950; **3**: 1018–32.

13 De Groot LJ. Diagnostic approach and management of patients exposed to irradiation to the thyroid. *J Clin Endocrinol Metab* 1989; **69**: 925–8.

14 Maxon HR, Thomas SR, Saeger EL, Buncher CR, Kereiakes JG. Ionizing irradiation and the induction of clinically significant disease in the human thyroid gland. *Am J Med* 1977; **63**: 967–78.

15 Ron E, Modan B, Preston D, Alfandary E, Stovall M, Boice JD. Thyroid neoplasia following low-dose radiation in childhood. *Radiat Res* 1989; **120**: 516–31.

16 Moroff SV, Fuks JZ. Thyroid cancer following radiotherapy for Hodgkin's disease: a case report and review of the literature. *Med Pediatr Oncol* 1986; **14**: 216–20.

17 Samaan NA, Schultz PN, Ordonez NG, Hickey RC, Johnston DA. A comparison of thyroid carcinoma in those who have and have not had head and neck irradiation in childhood. *J Clin Endocrinol Metab* 1987; **64**: 219–23.

18 Nikiforov Y, Gnepp DR. Pediatric thyroid cancer after the Chernobyl disaster. *Cancer* 1994; **74**: 748–66.

19 Fogelfeld L, Wiviott MBT, Shore-Freedman E *et al.* Recurrence of thyroid nodules after surgical removal in patients irradiated in childhood for benign conditions. *N Engl J Med* 1989; **320**: 835–40.

20 Schimpff SC, Diggs CH, Wiswell JG, Salvatore PC, Wienik PH. Radiation-related thyroid dysfunction: implications for the treatment of Hodgkin's disease. *Ann Intern Med* 1980; **92**: 91–8.

21 Shalet SM, Didi M, Ogilvy-Stuart AL, Schulga J, Donaldson MDC. Growth and endocrine function after bone marrow transplantation. *Clin Endocrinol* 1995; **42**: 333–9.

22 Atkins MB, Mier JW, Parkinson DR, Gould JA, Berkman EM, Kaplan MM. Hypothyroidism after treatment with interleukin-2 and lymphokine-activated killer cells. *N Engl J Med* 1988; **318**: 1557–63.

23 Livesey EA, Brook CGD. Thyroid dysfunction after radiotherapy and chemotherapy of brain tumours. *Arch Dis Child* 1989; **64**: 593–5.

24 Ogilvy-Stuart AL, Shalet SM, Gattamaneni HRG. Thyroid function following the treatment of brain tumours in children. *J Pediatr* 1991; **119**: 733–7.

25 Rao SD, Frame B, Miller MJ, Kleerekoper M, Block MA, Parfitt, AM. Hyperparathyroidism following head and neck irradiation. *Arch Intern Med* 1980; **140**: 205–7.

26 Russ JE, Scanlon EF, Sener SF. Parathyroid adenomas following irradiation. *Cancer* 1979; **43**: 1078–83.

27 Schneider AB, Gierlowski TC, Shore-Freedman E, Stovall M, Ron

E, Lubin J. Dose–response relationships for radiation-induced hyperparathyroidism. *J Clin Endocrinol Metab* 1995; **80**: 254–7.

28 Rowley MJ, Leach DR, Warner GA, Heller CG. Effect of graded doses in ionising radiation on the human testis. *Radiat Res* 1974 **59**: 665–78.

29 Hahn EW, Feingold SM, Nisce L. Aspermia and recovery of spermatogenesis in cancer patients following incidental gonadal irradiation during treatment: a progress report. *Radiology* 1976; **119**: 223–5.

30 Hahn EW, Feingold SM, Simpson L, Batata M. Recovery from aspermia induced by low-dose radiation in seminoma patients. *Cancer* 1982; **50**: 337–40.

31 Speiser B, Rubin P, Casarett G. Aspermia following lower truncal irradiation in Hodgkin's disease. *Cancer* 1973; **32**: 692–8.

32 Slanina J, Musshoff K, Rahner T, Stiasny R. Long-term side effects in irradiated patients with Hodgkin's disease. *Int J Radiat Oncol Biol Phys* 1977; **2**: 1–19.

33 Shalet SM, Tsatsoulis A, Whitehead E, Read G. Vulnerability of the human Leydig cell to radiation damage is dose-dependent. *J Endocrinol* 1989; **120**: 161–5.

34 Littley MD, Shalet SM, Morgenstern GR, Deakin DP. Endocrine and reproductive dysfunction following fractionated total body irradiation in adults. *Q J Med* 1991; **287**: 265–74.

35 Doll R, Smith PG. The long-term effects of X-irradiation in patients treated for metropathia haemorrhagica. *Br J Radiol* 1968; **41**: 362–8.

36 Wallace WHB, Shalet SM, Hendry JH, Morris-Jones PH, Gattamaneni HR. Ovarian failure following abdominal irradiation in childhood: the radiosensitivity of the human oocyte. *Br Radiol* 1989; **62**: 995–8.

37 Li FP, Gimbrere K, Gelber RD *et al.* Outcome of pregnancy in survivors of Wilms' tumour. *JAMA* 1987; **257**: 216–19.

38 Critchley HOD, Wallace WHB, Shalet SM, Mamtora H, Higginson J, Anderson DC. Abdominal irradiation in childhood: The potential for pregnancy. *Br J Obstet Gynaecol* 1992; **99**: 392–4.

39 Spitz S. The histological effects of nitrogen mustard on human tumours and tissues. *Cancer* 1948; **1**: 383–98.

40 Louis J, Limarzi LR, Best WR. Treatment of chronic granulocytic leukaemia with Myleran. *Arch Intern Med* 1956; **97**: 299–308.

41 Watson AR, Rance CP, Bain J. Long-term effects of cyclophosphamide on testicular function *Br Med J* 1985; **291**: 1457–60.

42 Chapman RM, Sutcliffe SB, Rees LH, Edwards CRW, Malpas JC. Cyclical combination chemotherapy and gonadal function. *Lancet* 1979; **1**: 285–9.

43 Whitehead E, Shalet SM, Blackledge G, Todd I, Crowther D, Beardwell CG. The effects of Hodgkin's disease and combination chemotherapy on gonadal function in the adult male. *Cancer* 1982; **49**: 419–22.

44 Holmes SJ, Whitehouse RW, Clark ST, Crowther DC, Adams JE, Shalet SM. Reduced bone mineral density in men following chemotherapy for Hodgkin's disease. *Br J Cancer* 1994; **70**: 371–5.

45 Uldall PR, Kerr DNS, Tacchi D. Sterility and cyclophosphamide. *Lancet* 1972; **1**: 693–4.

46 Koyama H, Wada T, Nishizaw Y *et al.* Cyclophosphamide-induced ovarian failure and its therapeutic significance in patients with breast cancer. *Cancer* 1977; **39**: 1403–9.

47 Walden PAM, Bagshawe KD. Pregnancies after chemotherapy for gestational trophoblastic tumours. *Lancet* 1979; **11**: 1241.

48 Chatterjee R, Mills W, Katz M, McGarrigle HH, Goldstone AH. Prospective study of pituitary-gonadal function to evaluate short-term effects of ablative chemotherapy or total body irradiation with autologous or allogenic marrow transplantation post-menarchial female patients. *Bone Marrow Transpl* 1994; **13**: 511–17.

49 Sanders JE, Buckner CD, Amos D *et al.* Ovarian function following marrow transplantation for aplastic anaemia or leukaemia. *J Clin Oncol* 1988; **6**: 813–18.

50 Milligan DW, Hughes R, Lindsay KS. Semen cryopreservation in men undergoing cancer chemotherapy—a UK survey. *Br J Cancer* 1989; **60**: 966–7.

51 Tournaye H, Camus M, Bollen N, Wisanto A, Van Steirteghem A, Devroey P. *In vitro* fertilisation techniques with frozen-thawed sperm: a method for preserving the progenitive potential of Hodgkin patients. *Fertil Steril* 1991; **55**: 443–5.

52 Sanger WG, Olson JH, Sherman JK. Semen cryobanking for men with cancer—criteria change. *Fertil Steril* 1992; **58**: 1024–7.

53 Viviani S, Santoro A, Ragni G, Bonfante V, Beslett O, Bonnadonna G. Gonadal toxicity after combination chemotherapy for Hodgkin's disease. Comparative results of MOPP versus ABVD. *Eur J Cancer Clin Oncol* 1985; **21**: 601–5.

54 Clark ST, Radford JA, Crowther D, Swindell R, Shalet SM. Gonadal function following chemotherapy for Hodgkin's disease: a comparative study of MVPP and a seven-drug hybrid regimen. *J Clin Oncol* 1995; **13**: 134–9.

55 Morris ID, Shalet SM. Protection of gonadal function from cytotoxic chemotherapy and irradiation. *Clin Endocrinol Metab* 1990; **4**: 97–118.

56 Kangasniemi M, Wilson G, Parchuri N, Huhtaniemi I, Meistrich ML. Rapid protection of rat spermatogenic stem cells against procarbazine by treatment with a gonadotropin-releasing hormone antagonist (Nal-Glu) and an antiandrogen (Flutamide). *Endocrinology* 1995; **136**: 2881–8.

57 Adan L, Souberbielle JC, Zucker JM, Pierre-Kahn A, Kalifa C, Brauner R. Adult height in 24 patients treated for growth hormone deficiency and early puberty. *J Clin Endocrinol Metab* 1997; **82**: 229–33.

58 Grundy RG, Leiper AD, Stanhope R, Chessells JM. Survival and endocrine outcome after testicular relapse in acute lymphoblastic leukaemia. *Arch Dis Child* 1997; **76**: 190–6.

59 Nasir J, Walton C, Lindow SW, Masson EA. Spontaneous recovery of chemotherapy-induced primary ovarian failure: implications for management. *Clin Endocrinol* 1997; **46**: 217–19.

CHAPTER 76

The treatment of endocrine-responsive tumours

P. Savage and J. Waxman

Introduction

Despite the announcement in the 1970s of a war on cancer, and the diversion of an army's war chest of resources to basic scientific research and the development of new treatments, nearly 30 years on cancer remains the second leading cause of death in the western world and causes 160 000 deaths annually in the UK.

Hormone-sensitive cancers constitute approximately one-third of all malignancies. These tumours are unusual in that they are highly responsive to apparently simple, non-toxic therapies. The role of the sex hormones in cancer is of great interest. In addition to promoting normal development and maintaining tissue function, the sex hormones have a primary role in oncogenesis. This effect is clearly shown by the lower risks for prostate and breast cancer in groups with reduced sex hormone exposure.

It has become almost a truism to state that for most of the common malignancies there is no effective post-operative adjuvant treatment, and that the treatment of metastatic disease is limited. However, this is not the case for the endocrine-dependent tumours where there have been many spectacular advances in management.

These developments have resulted from the introduction of treatments which bring significant benefit as adjuvant therapies, are effective and minimally toxic in the management of metastatic disease, and may have potentially chemo-preventative actions in men and women at high risk of developing cancer.

Although some endocrine therapies may have additional actions, it is conventional to consider hormonal treatments as acting within the paradigm of limiting tumour growth by deprivation of the hormonal growth stimulus. The pharmacological agents currently used work at three main levels: by down-regulation of the hypothalamo-pituitary–gonadal axis: by inhibition of the production and peripheral conversion of adrenal sex hormone precursors; or by blockade of the cancer cells' hormone receptors. In this chapter we will review the sites of intervention, the agents in current and projected use and the mechanisms of hormone resistance and we aim to outline a consensus on the current preferred management of the hormone-sensitive malignancies.

The different levels of hormonal control of tumour growth

The hypothalamo-pituitary–gonadal axis

In health the pulsatile release of gonadotrophin-releasing hormone (GnRH) from the hypothalamus provides the stimulus to the pituitary gland for the release of luteinising hormone (LH) and follicle-stimulating hormone (FSH). Modification of the GnRH decapeptide results in the production of agonist analogues which are resistant to the pituitary aramylidases which provide the normal GnRH degradation pathway.

The enhanced stability of the analogues allows binding to the GnRH receptor to be greatly extended, with a consequent loss of the pulsatile signal. This results in an initial surge of gonadotrophin release which is followed by prolonged but reversible down-regulation of gonadotrophin release. The effect of this is to limit gonadal sex hormone production, which results in serum values falling to post-menopausal or castration levels [1].

The most frequent indication for GnRH-agonist treatment is in metastatic prostate cancer, where this therapy has been demonstrated to be equal in efficacy to either orchiectomy or oestrogen therapy but with improved patient acceptability and a safer side-effect profile [2,3]. The GnRH agonists in current use include goserilin, leuprorelin and buserelin which are administered as depot injections. These agents have virtually no side-effects beyond those of the initial androgen surge and subsequently those of androgen depletion.

The GnRH agonist-mediated hormone surge can lead to an episode of enhanced tumour growth termed 'tumour flare', which may result in potentially serious symptoms, in particular spinal cord compression and hypercalcaemia. When used in prostate cancer it is conventional to precede GnRH agonist administration with an antiandrogen to minimise this risk. The side-effects from androgen depletion include hot flushes, a decrease in muscle tone, gynaecomastia and impotence. Generally the symptoms are mild and few patients are significantly troubled; however, in younger patients who wish to maintain sexual function their use is contraindicated and optimum management can present a problem [4]. GnRH agonists also have an important role in the management of metastatic breast cancer in the premenopausal patient [5], where they produce oestrogen deprivation which may be further enhanced by the coadministration of an aromatase inhibitor [6]. Additionally, there is growing evidence that, in axillary lymph-node positive breast cancer in premenopausal women, ovarian ablation by GnRH agonist may produce benefits similar to those of adjuvant chemotherapy but with considerably less toxicity [7]. Whilst GnRH agonists have already proved to be of enormous value, it is possible that GnRH analogues with antagonist action could prove superior with a more rapid onset of action and by avoidance of the risk of tumour flare. The first generation of GnRH antagonists proved unsuitable for clinical use due to anaphylactoid reactions. However, more recent GnRH antagonists appear to have minimal side-effects and potentially high efficacy.

In a preliminary study, Cetrorelix appeared to be safe and effective in producing a 72% decrease in testosterone levels within 8 hours of the first administration [8]. On-going clinical trials will demonstrate if the theoretical benefits of GnRH antagonists will translate into worthwhile clinical benefits.

Extragonadal sex hormone production

In post-menopausal women the adrenal gland is the main source of oestrogenic steroids which are synthesised as precursors that are converted peripherally, using the aromatase and sulphatase systems, to give serum oestradiol levels of 10–30 pg/ml. The aromatase system is found in the skin, fat, muscle and gonads where it converts adrenal androstenedione into oestrone. Oestrone is then converted either to oestradiol by oestradiol dehydrogenase or into the large body pool of oestrone sulphate via the actions of sulphotransferase. In addition to producing serum levels which support proliferation, these enzymes can be overexpressed in the tumour, resulting in increased local conversion and enhanced tumour growth [9].

In men the adrenal glands procedure 10% of the 10 mg daily production of androgenic steroids. Testosterone is further metabolised by 5α-reductase to its metabolite, dihydrotestosterone, which is 10-fold more active.

Surgical adrenalectomy was first applied to the treatment of metastatic breast cancer and prostate cancer in the 1940s, but despite a significant response rate its use has obvious major drawbacks in this debilitated population. The understanding of the routes of production of sex steroids has allowed for the development of alternative medical therapies.

Over the last 15 years a number of agents have been investigated that block adrenal precursor production or inhibit the conversion of precursors by the sulphatase–aromatase system or 5α-reductase into the biologically more active oestradiol and dihydrotestosterone.

Adrenal steroidogenesis inhibition

The selective inhibition of production of the adrenal precursors, androstenedione and dehydroepiandrosterone, has proved difficult to achieve. Aminoglutethimide inhibits the action of the adrenal P-450 system, but this effect is only transient and the clinically significant effect of aminoglutethimide is inhibition of the peripheral aromatase system. The antifungal drug ketoconazole at high doses also inhibits adrenal steroid biosynthesis, but has only a limited role as a second-line agent in prostate cancer due to a poor side-effect profile [10]. Trilostane inhibits adrenal 3β-hydroxysteroid dehydrogenase activity, so reducing adrenal androgen production. Administration at doses of 240–720 mg/day together with hydrocortisone can produce a response rate of 30% in post-menopausal women with metastatic breast cancer. However, trilostane produces a high incidence of gastrointestinal symptoms, so only has a minor role in breast-cancer treatment [11].

Aromatase inhibition

In the past decade there have been important clinical advances following the introduction of aromatase inhibitors. Aminoglutethimide at doses of 250–500 mg produces a 70% reduction in serum oestradiol levels. In unselected post-menopausal patients with metastatic breast cancer it produces an overall response rate of 30% with a median response duration of 13 months. Unfortunately, at this dosage 40–60% of patients have significant side-effects particularly rashes, nausea and somnolence.

The addition of hydrocortisone to aminoglutethimide has been shown to be unnecessary in the treatment of breast cancer and may result in additional toxicity [12].

Historically, the combination of aminoglutethimide and hydrocortisone has been used as second-line treatment of advanced prostate cancer; however, it appears that hydrocortisone alone is the active agent with aminoglutethimide conferring no additional benefit [13]. Possibly the reason for the lack of effect of aminoglutethimide in men is the comparative insignificance of the aromatase system.

Currently, the most frequently used aromatase inhibitor is formestane or 4-hydroxyandrostenedione (4-OHA), which acts as a 'suicide inhibitor' of aromatase via the formation of a covalent bond. Due to poor oral availability and significant hepatic metabolism, 4-OHA is given as a 2-weekly depot injection. 4-OHA produces approximately 95% inhibition of the aromatase activity with serum oestrone levels declining by 80%. In first-line treatment of unselected post-menopausal patients with metastatic breast cancer, the overall response rate was 33% with a median response duration of 12 months, results which are very similar to those of tamoxifen [14]. 4-OHA has a good side-effect profile and is most commonly used as second-line treatment after the development of acquired tamoxifen resistance; in this situation an impressive response rate of 26% with disease stabilisation in a further 25% has been reported [15].

Anastrozole (Arimidex) is an orally active aromatase inhibitor that reduces serum oestradiol to 15% of pretreatment levels. In preliminary trials in 19 pretreated post-menopausal patients with metastatic breast cancer, seven patients achieved objective responses. During this study there were no significant side-effects, and anastrozole has now been licensed by the Committee of Medicines in the UK as the first orally active aromatase inhibitor [16].

A number of other aromatase inhibitors are currently being investigated; they may bring therapeutic advantages as a result of more effective enzyme inhibition and oral administration.

At a dose of 2.5–5 mg, vorazole is a potent inhibitor of the aromatase system producing a 90% reduction in serum oestradiol and a 70% fall in the levels of serum oestrone and oestrone sulphate. As a second-line agent in unselected patients it produces a response rate of 33% and disease stabilisation in a further 17%. In patients who had previously responded to tamoxifen the response rate is 66%. Vorazole is well tolerated without any unwanted endocrine actions and has an excellent side-effect profile [17]. Phase II and III clinical trials have been concluded and the manufacturers have applied to the UK Committee of Medicines for this product to be licensed.

Lentrozole (CGS 20267) is another orally active competitive non-steroidal aromatase inhibitor; it produces a 90% reduction in serum plasma oestrogen levels. In post-menopausal patients with hormone-resistant metastatic breast cancer it gives an overall response rate of 33% with disease stabilisation in a further 24% [18]. Data from this trial suggested that the higher level of aromatase inhibition produced by lentrozole could lead to important clinical advances, as a number of patients had previously failed with 4-OHA.

Sulphatase inhibitors

In post-menopausal women *de novo* oestrone formation occurs solely via the aromatase system. However, the action of sulphatase on the large pool of oestrone sulphate results in continued oestrone availability despite effective aromatase inhibition.

Selective inhibition of the sulphatase enzyme system has proved difficult to achieve. At present a number of agents including danazol, EMATE and the steroidal methylthiophosphonates are undergoing evaluation [19].

5α-reductase inhibition

In advanced prostate cancer GnRH agonists lead to a reduction in serum androgens by approximately 90%. However, 5α-reductase activity can produce intratumoral dihydrotestosterone levels up to 40% of the precastrate level which can result in on-going hormone-driven proliferation [20].

Finasteride is a 4-aza-steroid that inhibits the intracellular production of dihydrotestosterone by blocking the action of 5α-reductase. This drug has been extensively investigated in benign prostatic hypertrophy where it has established a good safety and side-effect profile. As a single agent in patients with metastatic prostate cancer, finasteride is only of limited value, producing 20% reductions in prostate specific antigen (PSA) levels, but with no significant clinical benefits. However, its use in combination with the antiandrogen flutamide to further limit tissue availability of androgens has led to reports of symptomatic benefits and PSA reduction with preservation of potency [21].

Hormone antagonists

Initially introduced in 1971 as a palliative agent for elderly patients with breast cancer [22], tamoxifen is now established as the first-choice hormonal agent in all stages of breast cancer. Within the framework of producing oestrogen deprivation tamoxifen functions as an anti-oestrogen to the tumour but exerts weak oestrogenic actions on other tissues.

Tamoxifen also has a number of possible non-hormonal mechanisms of action including interactions with protein kinase C and calmodulin, and immunostimulatory actions on natural killer (NK) cells and T cells. These additional effects may in part explain the responses seen in oestrogen receptor-negative breast cancers and other cancers which are not usually sensitive to hormonal manipulations [23].

The weak oestrogenic action of tamoxifen has a number

of important effects. An initial episode of enhanced tumour growth may occur which can be mistaken for tamoxifen resistance. The oestrogenic actions of tamoxifen produce important benefits in maintaining bone density and reducing cholesterol and low-density lipoprotein (LDL) levels. In short-term use tamoxifen is well tolerated with minimal side-effects and generally does not disturb the menstrual cycle in younger patients. However, with longer-term administration there is a 1.5–2-fold increased risk of invasive endometrial cancer and possibly an increased risk of gastrointestinal tract malignancies [24]. The concern over these risks has led to increasing caution over the long-term use of tamoxifen as an adjuvant or chemopreventative treatment [25].

After a period of response to tamoxifen, progression inevitably occurs through the molecular evolution of tumour resistance. Tamoxifen resistance is an important clinical problem which is not yet fully understood despite extensive investigation. Previously, loss of oestrogen receptor expression had been considered to be the most important mechanism; however, more recent immunohistochemical studies demonstrate that this is a very rare event. Other possible mechanisms of tumour resistance include alterations in tumour tamoxifen metabolism, which may result in up to a 10-fold reduction in intratumour drug concentrations at the time of relapse, compared with that at commencement of treatment [26]. The production of tamoxifen metabolites with agonist actions and so growth promoting-characteristics may occur, which could explain the occasional responses seen to tamoxifen withdrawal [27]. Alternatively, the response of the tumour to tamoxifen may alter as a result of the expression of oestrogen receptor-associated proteins, normally expressed in endometrial cells and osteoclasts. The result of tamoxifen binding to these altered receptors would be to transmit a stimulatory signal as it does in these tissues [23]. In clinical practice it is important to note that the development of acquired tamoxifen resistance does not equate to resistance to all other hormonal agents, as further oestrogen deprivation by aromatase inhibitions is associated with a significant response rate.

Tamoxifen is active in pre- and post-menopausal patients with metastatic breast cancer with an overall response rate in unselected patients of approximately 30%, and a 12–18 month median duration of response [28].

The risks of tamoxifen to the endometrium have spurred the development of antagonists with reduced oestrogenic activity. A number of other anti-oestrogens are in clinical evaluation. Droloxifene (3-OH-tamoxifen citrate) combines weaker oestrogenic actions with a 10–60-fold higher oestrogen-receptor binding affinity than tamoxifen. In phase II evaluation it produced a 45% response rate with minimal toxicity in patients with advanced metastatic breast cancer. An on-going phase III comparison with tamoxifen will help to clarify the future role for droloxifene [29]. Toremifene is a synthetic anti-oestrogen with only weak oestrogenic actions. In hormone-naive patients with metastatic breast cancer it produced a response rate of 20–30%, but it also appears to be cross-resistant with tamoxifen producing responses in just 5% of patients with tamoxifen resistance [30]. ICI 182780 is a steroidal anti-oestrogen given by depot injection. It acts by inhibition of oestrogen receptor dimerisation, and has no oestrogenic agonist activity. In a preliminary trial of 19 women with tamoxifen-resistant metastatic breast cancer it produced a response in seven (36.8%) and stabilisation in a further six (31.6%) with a median response duration in excess of 18 months. This combination of a high response rate, long response duration and minimal toxicity suggests that ICI 182780 may develop an important role in the first-line management of breast cancer [31].

Androgen antagonists have played a role in the management of advanced prostate cancer for over 30 years. When initially introduced they were used as monotherapy, but more recently their use is generally in combination with GnRH agonists to produce maximal androgen blockade.

The first agent used was cyproterone acetate, which has a number of actions including inhibition of gonadotrophin release and progesterone-like effects in addition to interfering with androgen-receptor binding and translocation. Whilst it is of value in reducing or preventing hot flushes, the increased risk of cardiovascular disease that occurs with cyproterone has led to it being superseded by newer antiandrogens [32].

Flutamide is the most commonly used antiandrogen; it is generally well tolerated with only mild side-effects of gastrointestinal disturbance. It has a 5-hour half-life that requires administration three times a day; when used in conjunction with GnRH agonists it effectively prevents tumour flare and produces an increased survival of 7 months compared with GnRH monotherapy.

The extensive use of flutamide has led to the clinical observation of responses that can lead to symptomatic benefits and falls in PSA levels in 30–40% of patients which, having become resistant to initial hormonal therapy, occurs when flutamide administration is withdrawn. The recognition of the flutamide withdrawal response has presented difficulties in the interpretation of previously observed responses to second-line hormonal strategies when their administration was combined with routine withdrawal of flutamide [33].

Nilutamide is structurally related to flutamide but has a long half-life allowing daily administration. It has a poorer side-effect profile than flutamide with decreased night vision, alcohol intolerance and interstitial pneumonitis reported.

Bicalutamide (Casodex) is a newer antiandrogen that may offer some important therapeutic advantages; it has more powerful antiandrogenic actions and the potential for effective monotherapy without producing impotence. In a preliminary study involving 23 hormone-naive prostate cancer patients, bicalutamide monotherapy produced a response in 22 with a mean 81% reduction in PSA value. The side-effects of bicalutamide include rises in LH, testosterone and oestradiol levels which can lead to mild gynaecomastia in up to 50% of patients. However, the benefits from this agent in monotherapy include the absence of hot flushes and the preservation of libido and potency in 75% of patients [34]. A phase III trial comparing bicalutamide and orchiectomy suggests that its efficacy may be lower than orchiectomy, with treatment failure in 53% on biclutamide as opposed to 42% with orchiectomy; however, the lack of significant side-effects at the doses investigated suggests that the efficacy of higher doses should be examined [35].

Oestrogens and androgens

Whilst current hormone therapy is centered around producing hormone deprivation, historically hormone agonist treatment with oestrogens has been used with considerable benefits in breast and prostate cancer.

Diethylstilboestrol produces an overall response rate of 44% and a median response duration of 20 weeks in post-menopausal patients with metastatic breast cancer. These results are broadly similar to those obtained with tamoxifen or other methods of hormone deprivation. However, the poorer side-effect profile of oestrogens has led to their use being generally superseded by the more modern treatments that produce hormone deprivation [36].

Androgenic steroids act via down-regulation of the hypothalamo-pituitary axis and by direct inhibition of tumour growth. However, these agents have low response rates and potentially unpleasant side-effects and have only limited application.

Historically, oestrogens played a major role in the management of advanced prostate cancer prior to the introduction of GnRH agonists. A number of studies have shown that the response rates to orchiectomy, GnRH agonists and oestrogens are all similar for patients with metastatic disease. The poorer side-effect profile of oestrogens, particularly in producing cardiovascular toxicity and feminisation, have resulted in their use declining substantially since the introduction of GnRH agonists [2].

The management of the hormone-sensitive malignancies

Breast cancer

Introduction

Breast cancer is the most common cause of cancer deaths in women, with death rates increasing by 1% each year over the last 50 years. Currently, there are 16 000 deaths annually in England and Wales. Hormonal intervention gives valuable clinical benefits in all stages of breast cancer. The most important predictor of response to hormonal therapy is the hormone receptor status of the tumour. For patients with oestrogen receptor-(ER) positive tumours the response rate in metastatic disease is approximately 40% and rises to 70% in those who also express the progestogen receptor. In these patients, after progression there is a 30–40% response rate to second-line hormonal treatment. Unfortunately, the receptor assays are often unavailable in routine clinical practice, although some clinical features, such as the patient's age, a long disease-free interval, and the presence of disease primarily in the bone or soft tissues, serve as useful predictors of a good response to hormonal treatment.

In patients with ER-negative metastatic breast cancer the response rate to hormonal therapy is approximately 10%. As chemotherapy is less well tolerated and offers only minimal survival advantages in metastatic disease, it is conventional to initiate a trial of hormonal therapy in the majority of patients.

Adjuvant treatment

The value of tamoxifen in the adjuvant treatment of breast cancer was clearly confirmed by the updated results of the Early Breast Cancer Trialists' Group which combined the results of 133 studies involving 75 000 patients [37]. Given at 20 mg/day for at least 2 years to patients with axillary nodal disease, tamoxifen led to an improvement in 10-year survival from 42.2 to 50.4%. The benefits were more marked in patients with ER-positive tumours who had a 19% reduction in annual risk, ER-negative patients having a 3% annual risk reduction. Patients who do not have axillary node involvement have a better overall prognosis but tamoxifen administration in this group also leads to an improvement in 10-year survival from 63.1 to 68.1%. The most appropriate duration for adjuvant tamoxifen administration is a subject of debate, the Early Trialists' study suggests an on-going benefit from prolonged treatment; however, this prolicy may result in increased risks of other malignancies. A number of ongoing trials are attempting to clarify this dilemma. In premenopausal patients with node-positive disease the use of adjuvant chemotherapy leads to a 10% improvement in 5-year survival. The addition of tamoxifen probably leads to increased efficacy, although the exact size of this benefit is unclear at present.

In post-menopausal patients with axillary lymph-node disease the benefits of adjuvant chemotherapy are not yet fully clarified, and in this situation many clinicians use tamoxifen alone [38]. In the patient group it gives a 28%

reduction in the annual risk of recurrence in all age ranges including the over-70s.

For premenopausal patients with axillary lymph-node disease, treatment with GnRH agonists can provide an effective alternative to chemotherapy in patients unfit or unwilling to receive it. Data from the Early Trialists' Group and randomised trials demonstrate that medical ovarian ablation produces results comparable with combination chemotherapy by increasing 10-year survival by 10% [7,37]. Preliminary data suggest that the addition of tamoxifen to medical ovarian ablation can lead to a further reduction in the risk of recurrence.

Metastatic disease

Metastatic breast cancer is at present an incurable condition in which the main aim of therapy is to prolong life and minimise symptoms, using treatments of low toxicity. It is conventional for patients to receive a trial of hormonal therapy before considering more toxic treatment with chemotherapy. There are exceptions to this, particularly in locally advanced disease, large liver metastases, marrow infiltration and lymphangitis, when rapid control of tumour growth is necessary. In these situations anthracycline-based chemotherapy is usually the treatment of choice.

As the use of adjuvant tamoxifen becomes more prevalent an increasing number of patients with metastatic disease will have had previous exposure. If the interval is greater than 2 years, tamoxifen rechallenge is frequently employed, but for shorter intervals an alternative drug is generally used.

At present hormonal agents are generally used sequentially with the introduction of a different agent when resistance becomes apparent; however, there is some evidence that combination hormonal therapy can lead to initial longer responses [39].

In premenopausal patients tamoxifen is the drug of choice for first-line treatment of metastatic disease where it gives an overall response rate of 30% and a 12-month median duration of response. An alternative method of hormonal treatment in this population is medical ovarian ablation using a GnRH agonist; this has the advantage over radiation or surgical ovarian ablations of reversibility so allowing the avoidance of menopausal symptoms in patients who fail to respond. The response rates to gonadotrophin-releasing hormone agonists are in the order of 30–40% with a median response duration of 9 months, and its use presents a valuable alternative to chemotherapy in this situation [40].

Progestogens such as medroxyprogesterone acetate and megestrol acetate have a response rate of 10–20% as third-line treatment where their administration combines the symptomatic benefits of increased appetite and weight gain.

In the face of primary hormonal resistance or later progression, the majority of premenopausal patients are offered treatment with chemotherapy which can result in significant symptom relief.

In post-menopausal patients with metastatic breast cancer, endocrine therapies give greater response rates and survival benefits than in the younger age group. This is thought to be due to the increased proportion of oestrogen receptor-positive tumours in this group of women.

Tamoxifen remains the first choice drug giving an overall response rate of 50% and a 12–15-month median duration of response.

The superior side-effect profit of the aromatase inhibitors has allowed them to replace aminoglutethimide as second-line treatments for patients with acquired resistance to tamoxifen where the response rate is 20–30% [15]. After progression or resistance to aromatase inhibitors the next step in management is either palliative chemotherapy or the use of a progestogen.

Chemoprevention

It is apparent that tamoxifen has a major impact on decreasing the development of a second primary breast cancer as shown by the Early Trialists' study which reported a 37% reduction in risk [37]. As a result the role of tamoxifen in chemoprevention of breast cancer in healthy but high-risk groups is being examined in major studies in Europe and the USA. However, this approach has to be viewed with caution as, paradoxically, tamoxifen has been shown to potentially act as a carcinogen by cross-linking DNA *in vitro*. Long-term administration causes a 1.5–2-fold increase in the risk of endometrial cancer and there are reports of a two- to three-fold increase in the risk of the more common stomach and colorectal cancers [24]. If these concerns are substantiated, the risk/benefits of tamoxifen chemoprevention will need to be very closely evaluated but will probably be only of limited application.

Prostate cancer

Prostate cancer is the most prevalent cancer of males, leading to nearly 8500 deaths annually in England and Wales. Deaths from prostate cancer have doubled over the last 20 years. Prostate cancer has a number of important characteristics, including a marked predilection for the elderly, a high response rate to hormonal therapy and frequently slow progression.

Localised prostate cancer

The optimum management policy for localised prostate cancer is currently unclear. In the older age group prostatectomy, radical radiotherapy and observation all appear to give similar survival figures, whilst in younger patients the survival benefits from aggressive management are at the most modest with frequent treatment-related toxicity [41]. The potential role for hormonal intervention at this early stage is also unclear: GnRH-agonist administration to patients with asymptomatic localised prostate cancer extends the average interval to progression from 43 months to 100 months, but at present it is not clear if this also produces a significant survival benefit [42]. These figures will be achieved at the expense of potentially causing hot flushes, decreasing muscle tone and producing impotence in an otherwise asymptomatic population. Recent studies of hormonal down-staging prior to radiation or surgery have shown no advantage to this approach.

Metastatic prostate cancer

In routine clinical practice hormonal therapy is the treatment of choice in patients with symptomatic locally advanced or metastatic disease.

GnRH agonists are equal in efficacy to orchiectomy or oestrogens but better tolerated without the psychological sequelae or cardiovascular risks of these older methods of treatment. As a result, GnRH agonists are the drug of choice giving a symptomatic benefit in up to 80% of patients and falls in PSA in 60%; the median duration of response in metastatic cancer is 14 months. The addition of anti-androgens plays an important role in preventing tumour flare, and it is suggested that their long-term combination with GnRH-agonist therapy to produce maximal androgen blockade may produce significant benefits with an increase in response duration to 16 months and of survival by 7 months [43]. An overview of 22 trials examining this question demonstrated that the addition of antiandrogens led to small reductions in the annual risk of death, with nilutamide producing a 6% decrease, cyproterone acetate 6.4% and flutamide 9% [44]. These figures do not reach statistical significance, but many clinicians feel that the addition of anti-androgens leads to worthwhile benefits in survival in addition to limiting tumour flare, and allowing the opportunity for further endocrine manipulation.

Relapsed prostate cancer

The management choices at relapse from first-line hormonal treatment are very limited, and patients at this point have a median survival of only 6 months. Patients on maximal androgen blockade can give a response rate of 30–40% to withdrawal of the antiandrogen, with some of these responses being prolonged [33]. It appears that, on occasion, reintroduction of the antiandrogen may produce a further response later in the disease course. In patients who develop clinical androgen independence it is conventional to continue GnRH agonist administration as this confers a modest survival advantage over GnRH withdrawal.

In androgen-independent disease hydrocortisone can give response rates of up to 20% which are usually of short duration. Progestogens can be used in progressive prostate cancer where they offer a low response rate but frequently valuable symptomatic benefits. At this stage of the disease symptom control, particularly that of bone pain, with effective analgesia and palliative radiotherapy is the main objective.

The close relationship between androgen exposure and the development of prostate cancer makes chemoprevention a theoretical possibility. Finasteride, which effectively inhibits the action of 5α-reductase and has a proven safety record in benign prostatic hypertrophy, is currently being investigated as a chemopreventative agent in a major trial being performed in the USA. The results of this study due soon should give valuable information on this exciting area [45].

Gynaecological malignancies

Ovarian cancer

Advanced ovarian cancer is treated with surgery and chemotherapy which produces response rates of up to 80% and a significant number of long-term survivors. *In vitro* studies show that 70% of ovarian tumours expressed oestrogen and progesterone receptors and that growth can be modulated by both tamoxifen and progestogens.

In clinical use tamoxifen can give response rates of 20% with some long-term survivors. However, direct oestrogen deprivation with aminoglutethimide is not effective, nor is the use of high dose megestrol acetate [46]. GnRH agonists are of value in this condition, and responses have been reported in 10–15% patients [47]. The role of hormonal therapy in recurrent ovarian cancer is still evolving, and as the response rates to hormonal agents are similar to those of third-line chemotherapy and achieved at minimal toxicity they represent an important alternative to chemotherapy in palliative treatment.

Endometrial cancer

Endometrial cancer is the fourth most common malignancy affecting women and has a strong causal link with oestrogen exposure. Whilst adjuvant hormonal treatment has not been demonstrated to produce a survival benefit, hormonal therapy is often the treatment of choice in metastatic disease. Historically, progestogens have been reported to give an overall response rate of approximately 30%, although more recent studies indicate the response rate to be lower (but still significant) at 10–20%. There appears to be no advantage in very-high-dose progestogen therapy over conventional doses.

The important indicators for response to hormonal treatment are high levels of expression of oestrogen and progestogen receptors which are closely linked to both good tumour grade and slowly developing disease.

A number of studies show tamoxifen to be active, with an overall response rate of approximately 22% and with responses more frequent in patients with well-differentiated tumours and previous responses to progestogens.

The combined use of tamoxifen and progestogens has been investigated and may give enhanced response rates, but serious side-effects such as thromboses and hepatic toxicity have precluded further work.

Preliminary data suggests that aromatase inhibition may be of value, as may GnRH-agonist administration, although it is unclear if this is due to down-regulation of the hypothalamo-pituitary system or due to the direct effects of tumour binding.

As endometrial cancer is relatively chemoresistant it is conventional to attempt a trial of hormonal therapy before considering the use of platinum-based chemotherapy [48].

Conclusion

The hormone-dependent cancers constitute a significant proportion of all malignancies. In the past decade there have been radical developments in the treatment of this tumour group, and new endocrine therapies that are specific and with minimal side-effects have been identified. In many instances it has been shown that these therapies act at the level of the tumour rather than by modulating paracrine loops. It is hoped that in the next decade the molecular basis of hormone independence will be more clearly understood such that the fundamental processes that control its evolution can be reprogrammed, and this group of cancers may eventually be cured rather than contained.

References

1 Waxman J. Gonadotrophin hormone releasing analogues open new doors in cancer treatment. *Br Med J Clin Res Ed* 1987; **295**: 1084–5.

2 Citrin DL, Resnick MI, Guinan P, al-Bussam N, Scott M, Gau TC. A comparison of zoladex and DES in the treatment of advanced prostate cancer: results of a randomized, multicenter trial. *Prostate* 1991; **18**: 139–46.

3 Vogelzand NJ, Chodak GW, Soloway MS *et al.* Goserelin versus orchiectomy in the treatment of advanced prostate cancer: final results of a randomized trial. *Urology* 1995; **46**: 220–6.

4 Denis L. Prostate cancer. Primary hormonal treatment. *Cancer* 1993; **71** (Suppl.): 1050–8.

5 Bajetta E, Zilembo N, Buzzoni R *et al.* Goserelin in premenopausal advanced breast cancer: clinical and endocrine evaluation of responsive patients. *Oncology* 1994; **51**: 262–9.

6 Dowsett M, Stein RC, Coombes RC. Aromatization inhibition alone or in combination with GnRH agonists for the treatment of premenopausal breast cancer patients. *J Steroid Biochem Mol Biol* 1992; **43**: 155–9.

7 Scottish Cancer Trials Breast Group and ICRF Breast Unit. Adjuvant ovarian ablation versus CMF chemotherapy in premenopausal women with pathological stage II breast carcinoma: the Scottish trial. *Lancet* 1993; **341**: 1293–8.

8 Klingmuller D, Schepke M, Enzweiler C, Bidlingmaier F. Hormonal responses to the new potent GnRH antagonist Cetrorelix. *Acta Endocrinol (Copenh)* 1993; **128**: 15–18.

9 Lipton A, Santner SJ, Santen RJ *et al.* Aromatase activity in primary and metastatic human breast cancer. *Cancer* 1987; **59**: 779–82.

10 Mahler C, Verhelst J, Denis L. Ketoconazole and liarozole in the treatment of advanced prostatic cancer. *Cancer* 1993; **71** (Suppl.): 1068–73.

11 Williams CJ, Barley VL, Blackledge GR, Rowland CG, Tyrrell CJ. Multicentre cross over study of aminoglutethimide and trilostane in advanced postmenopausal breast cancer. *Br J Cancer* 1993; **68**: 1210–15.

12 Cocconi G, Bisagni G, Ceci G *et al.* Low-dose aminoglutethimide with and without hydrocortisone replacement as a first-line endocrine treatment in advanced breast cancer: a prospective randomized trial of the Italian Oncology Group for Clinical Research. *J Clin Oncol* 1992; **10**: 984–9.

13 Plowman PN, Perry LA, Chard T. Androgen suppression by hydrocortisone without aminoglutethimide in orchiectomised men with prostatic cancer. *Br J Urol* 1987; **59**: 255–7.

14 Stein RC, Dowsett M, Hedley A *et al.* Treatment of advanced breast cancer in postmenopausal women with 4-hydroxyandrostenedione. *Cancer Chemother Pharmacol* 1990; **26**: 75–8.

15 Brodie AM. Aromatase inhibitors in the treatment of breast cancer. *J Steroid Biochem Mol Biol* 1994; **49**: 281–7.

16 Plourde PV, Dyroff M, Dowsett M, Demers L, Yates R, Webster A. Arimidex: a new oral, once-a-day aromatase inhibitor. *J Steroid Biochem Mol Biol* 1995; **53**: 175–9.

17 Johnston SR, Smith IE, Doody D, Jacobs S, Robertshaw H, Dowsett M. Clinical and endocrine effects of the oral aromatase inhibitor vorozole in postmenopausal patients with advanced breast cancer. *Cancer Res* 1994; **54**: 5875–81.

18 Iveson TJ, Smith IE, Ahern J, Smithers DA, Trunet PF, Dowsett M. Phase I study of the oral nonsteroidal aromatase inhibitor CGS 20267 in postmenopausal patients with advanced breast cancer. *Cancer Res* 1993; **53**: 266–70.

19 Purohit A, Howarth NM, Potter BV, Reed MJ. Inhibition of steroid sulphatase activity by steroidal methylthiophosphonates; potential therapeutic agents in breast cancer. *J Steroid Biochem Mol Biol* 1994; **48**: 523–7.

20 Geller J. Basis for hormonal management of advanced prostate cancer. *Cancer* 1993; **71** (Suppl.): 1039–45.

21 Fleshner NE, Trachtenberg J. Combination finasteride and flutamide in advanced carcinoma of the prostate; effective therapy with minimal side effects. *J Urol* 1995; **154**: 1642–5.

22 Cole MP, Jones CT, Todd ID. A new anti-oestrogenic agent in late breast cancer. An early clinical appraisal of ICI46474. *Br J Cancer* 1971; **25**: 270–5.

23 Wolf DM, Fuqua SA. Mechanisms of action of antiestrogens. *Cancer Treat Rev* 1995; **21**: 247–71.

24 Rutqvist LE, Johansson H, Signomklao T, Johansson U, Fornander T, Wilking N. Adjuvant tamoxifen therapy for early stage breast

cancer and second primary malignancies. Stockholm Breast Cancer Study Group. *J Natl Cancer Inst* 1995; **87**: 645–51.

25 Powles TJ, Hickish T. Tamoxifen therapy and carcinogenic risk. *J Natl Cancer Inst* 1995; **87**: 1343–5.

26 Johnston SR, Haynes BP, Smith IE *et al.* Acquired tamoxifen resistance in human breast cancer and reduced intra-tumoral drug concentration. *Lancet* 1993; **342**: 8886–7.

27 Howell A, Dodwell DJ, Anderson H, Redford J. Response after withdrawal of tamoxifen and progestogens in advanced breast cancer. *Ann Oncol* 1992; **3**: 587–8.

28 Litherland S, Jackson IM. Antioestrogens in the management of hormone-dependent cancer. *Cancer Treat Rev* 1988; **15**: 183–94.

29 Bruning PF. Droloxifene, a new anti-oestrogen in postmenopausal advanced breast cancer: preliminary results of a double-blind dose-finding phase II trial. *Eur J Cancer* 1992; **28A**: 1404–7.

30 Vogel CL, Shemano I, Schoenfelder J, Gams RA, Green MR. Multicenter phase II efficacy trial of toremifene in tamoxifen-refractory patients with advanced breast cancer. *J Clin Oncol* 1993; **11**: 345–50.

31 Howell A, DeFriend D, Robertson J, Blamey R, Walton P. Response to a specific antioestrogen (ICI 182780) in tamoxifen-resistant breast cancer. *Lancet* 1995; **345**: 29–30.

32 Schroder FH. Cyproterone acetate—mechanism of action and clinical effectiveness in prostate cancer treatment. *Cancer* 1993; **72** (Suppl.): 3810–15.

33 Scher HI, Kelly WK. Flutamide withdrawal syndrome: its impact on clinical trials in hormone-refractory prostate cancer. *J Clin Oncol* 1993; **11**: 1566–72.

34 Verhelst J, Denis L, Van-vliet P *et al.* Endocrine profiles during administration of the new non-steroidal anti-androgen Casodex in prostate cancer. *Clin Endocrinol (Oxf)* 1994; **41**: 525–30.

35 Chodak G, Sharifi R, Kasimis B, Block NL, Macramalla E, Kennealey GT. Single-agent therapy with bicalutamide: a comparison with medical or surgical castration in the treatment of advanced prostate carcinoma. *Urology* 1995; **46**: 849–55.

36 Ingle JN, Ahmann DL, Grees SJ *et al.* Randomized clinical trial of deithylstilbestrol versus tamoxifen in postmenopausal women with advanced breast cancer. *N Engl J Med* 1981; **304**: 16–21.

37 Early Breast Cancer Trialists' Collaborative Group. Systemic treatment of early breast cancer by hormonal, cytotoxic or immune therapy. 133 randomised trials involving 31 000 recurrences and 24 000 deaths among 75 000 women. *Lancet* 1992; **339**: 1–15, 71–85.

38 Gelber RD, Cole BF, Goldhirsch A *et al.* Adjuvant chemotherapy plus tamoxifen compared with tamoxifen alone for postmenopausal breast cancer: meta-analysis of quality-adjusted survival. *Lancet* 1996; **347**: 1066–71.

39 Ingle JN, Twito DI, Schaid DJ *et al.* Combination hormonal therapy with tamoxifen plus fluoxymesterone versus tamoxifen alone in postmenopausal women with metastatic breast cancer. An updated analysis. *Cancer* 1991; **67**: 886–91.

40 Kaufmann J, Jonat W, Schachner-Wunschmann E, Bastert G, Maass H. The depot GnRH analogue goserelin in the treatment of premenopausal patients with metastatic breast cancer—a 5 year experience and further endocrine therapies. Cooperative German Zoladex Study Group. *Onkologie* 1991; **14**: 22–4, 26–8.

41 Whitmore WF, Jr. Expectant management of clinically localized prostatic cancer. *Semin Oncol* 1994; **21**: 560–8.

42 Kramolowsky EV. The value of testosterone deprivation in stage D1 carcinoma of the prostate. *J Urol* 1988; **139**(6): 1242–4.

43 Crawford ED, Eisenberger MA, McLeod DG *et al.* A controlled trial of leuprolide with and without flutamide in prostatic carcinoma. *N Engl J Med* 1989; **321**: 419–24.

44 Prostate Cancer Trialists' Collaborative Group. Maximum androgen blockade in advanced prostate cancer; an overview of 22 randomised trials with 3283 deaths in 5710 patients. *Lancet* 1995; **346**: 265–9.

45 Feigl P, Blumenstein B, Thompson I *et al.* Design of the Prostate Cancer Prevention Trial (PCPT). *Control Clin Trials* 1995; **16**: 150–63.

46 Ahlgren JD, Ellison NM, Gottlieb RJ *et al.* Hormonal palliation of chemoresistant ovarian cancer: three consecutive phase II trials of the Mid-Atlantic Oncology Program. *J Clin Oncol* 1993; **11**: 1957–68.

47 Savino L, Baldini B, Susini T, Pulli F, Anignani L, Massi GB. GnRH analogs in gynecological oncology: a review. *J Chemother* 1992; **4**: 312–20.

48 Moore TD, Phillips PH, Nerenstone SR, Cheson BD. Systemic treatment of advanced and recurrent endometrial carcinoma: current status and future directions. *J Clin Oncol* 1991; **9**: 1071–88.

Part 18
Endocrine Manifestations of Systemic Disease

CHAPTER 77

Endocrine manifestations of systemic disease: the liver

E.M. Alstead and M.J.G. Farthing

Introduction

The liver is actively involved in the biotransformation of many steroids and other hormones. It is not surprising, therefore, that impairment of liver function by drugs or disease can have far-reaching effects on the endocrine axes and the action of their constituent hormones. The clinical observation that men with advanced liver disease are frequently impotent with associated testicular atrophy and feminisation was made in the time of Hippocrates, and during the past 100 years it has become generally accepted that these findings can be attributed to metabolic disturbances directly due to liver disease [1–3]. The development of methods for measuring hormone concentrations in urine and blood enabled the underlying biochemical mechanisms to be investigated [1]. There are a variety of endocrine manifestations of liver disease, while some endocrine diseases affect liver function. In liver disease, there may also be difficulty in interpreting the results of endocrine tests. Sex steroid changes are most marked in patients with liver disease and certain variables (gender, age, aetiology and severity of the liver disease) should be considered. The most profound disturbances of sex hormones are found in alcoholic liver disease, but although alcohol has specific toxic effects, there are many clinically relevant endocrine consequences of non-alcoholic liver disease, particularly those that influence gonadal function.

Sex hormones

Clinical and biochemical manifestations in men

Men with chronic liver disease are commonly hypogonadal and are feminised. These abnormalities have been attributed to metabolic imbalances occurring secondary to liver disease, based on the assumption that the liver plays a central role in the metabolism, detoxification and excretion of sex steroid hormones [3]. Liver disease itself causes hormone abnormalities and sexual dysfunction, and these abnormalities are amplified by alcohol [4,5]. The pathophysiological disturbances in men with chronic liver disease are complex and are difficult to separate from the effects of alcohol itself on the hypothalamo-pituitary–gonadal axis. Many studies are poorly controlled with regard to the aetiology and severity of liver disease.

Hypogonadism

Hypogonadism may be found in 70–80% of men with chronic liver disease, particularly when due to alcohol [4,6–8]. Impaired spermatogenesis as well as Leydig-cell failure is common in these men. In 70–80% of men with chronic liver disease, hypogonadism presents with loss of libido and impotence [5,9,10]. Testicular atrophy is found in 50–80% of male cirrhotics, especially those with alcohol-related liver disease. The pathogenesis of the hypogonadism of liver disease is partly due to primary testicular failure and partly to failure of hypothalamo-pituitary regulation. There has been confusion over the relative roles of chronic liver disease itself and alcohol, which is undoubtedly a contributory factor and may act independently to produce gonadal dysfunction [11,12]. There are, however, well-characterised endocrine abnormalities associated with non-alcoholic liver disease [13,14]. The changes vary with the severity of the liver disease, gonadal failure being more marked in advanced disease. Aetiology of the liver disease also plays a part; gonadal failure can be an early presenting feature in haemochromatosis but is rarely, if ever, associated with Wilson's disease [15]. Hypogonadism has also been related to the complications of chronic liver disease such as hepatic encephalopathy and portosystemic shunting [12]. In advanced, decompensated liver disease with shunting, relatively weak sex steroids and other compounds such as dietary phyto-oestrogens enter the systemic circulation through the intrahepatic shunt and are thus able to have a biological effect in the periphery [10]. Alterations in central nervous system dopaminergic activity may decrease gonadotrophin-releasing hormone (GnRH) secretion in advanced disease [12]. A blunted response to GnRH has been shown in some cirrhotics [16]. Direct gonadal damage by alcohol and impairment of testicular steroid hormone synthesis has been shown to be related to the testicular redox state, although other mechanisms of damage may also be involved [2].

Sex hormone changes seen in chronic liver disease in men are summarised in Table 77.1. Low or normal plasma testosterone concentrations are generally found. There is, however, no correlation between low serum free testosterone concentrations and impotence. In primary testicular atrophy, plasma testosterone and dehydroepiandrosterone sulphate concentrations are usually reduced [28]. The changes are more marked in alcoholic liver disease, presumably because of the combined effects of chronic liver disease itself in addition to the direct toxic effect of alcohol on the testes. Alcohol directly inhibits testosterone production by blocking 17β-hydroxylase and 17,20-desmolase activities which are key enzymes in the biosynthetic pathway [29].

Well-compensated cirrhotic patients may have no overt evidence of hypogonadism. Plasma sex hormone-binding globulin (SHBG) concentration is increased, but generally does not result in a reduction of free testosterone. Increased peripheral conversion of sex steroids towards androstenedione and oestrone already takes place at this stage. With deteriorating liver function, total and free testosterone and SHBG concentrations approach normal values.

Table 77.1 Sex steroid hormone changes in men with chronic liver disease.

Hormone	Total	Free	References
Testosterone	↓	↓	4,8,17,18
Dihydrotestosterone	↓		19
Dehydroepiandrosterone	↓↓	↓↓	11
Dehydroepiandrosterone sulphate	↓↓	↓↓	11
Androstenedione	↑↑		17,20,21
Oestrone	↑	↑→	20,22
Oestradiol	↑→		17,23
Oestradiol/testosterone ratio	↑		17,24
Oestriol	↑		
Progesterone	↑		25
Luteinising hormone	↑→		13,18
Follicle-stimulating hormone	↑→		13
Prolactin	↑→		26,27
Sex hormone-binding globulin	↑		7

↑, increased; ↓, decreased; →, unchanged.

Table 77.2 Sex hormones and severity of liver injury. Data from [13].

		Alcoholic cirrhotics*		
Hormone	Total ($n = 43$)	A ($n = 11$)	B ($n = 19$)	C ($n = 13$)
Testosterone	→	↑	↑	↓
Oestrone	↑	↑	↑↑	↑↑
Oestradiol	↑	↑	↑	↑
Follicle-stimulating hormone	↑	↑	↑	→
Luteinising hormone	↑	↑	↑	→
Sex hormone binding globulin	↑	↑	↑	↑

* Child's grades A, B, C.
↑, increased; ↓, decreased; →, unchanged.

Encephalopathic patients have severely impaired gonadal function and markedly reduced levels of total and free testosterone, and may have high plasma luteinising hormone and prolactin concentrations [30]. Sex hormone concentrations have been correlated with the severity of liver disease and are shown in Table 77.2.

Feminisation

The biochemical basis for feminisation is less well established than hypogonadism. Feminisation is characterised by a loss of the male escutcheon, loss of body hair and redistribution of body fat in 20–50% [9], palmar erythema in 50%, spider angiomas in 40% and gynaecomastia in 15–50% [15]. These changes are also more common in alcoholics, the direct toxic effect of alcohol and its metabolites accounting for much of the hypoandrogenisation.

Men are clinically feminised but have normal or minimally increased oestradiol levels. There is increased SHBG (which has a higher affinity for testosterone than oestrogens), increased oestrogen-sensitive neurophysin, prolactin, growth hormone, thyroid-stimulating hormone (TSH) and oestrone, all of which may contribute to feminisation [6,22,31]. Hypogonadism may be related to alcohol alone, whereas feminisation usually occurs only in the presence of cirrhosis although spider angiomas and gynaecomastia can appear in acute alcoholic hepatitis [2]. There is increased conversion of testosterone and androstenedione to oestrone, which has been attributed to portosystemic shunting. The substantial increase in SHBG concentration favours the increase of the oestrogen/testosterone ratio because testosterone has a higher affinity for SHBG. Other metabolites of oestradiol such as 16-hydroxyoestrone are increased in cirrhosis and may be biologically active. There is, however, a poor correlation between increased oestrogen concentration and gynaecomastia

[1], the best relationship being with oestrone [22]. There is no evidence that hyperprolactinaemia is causally related to gynaecomastia in chronic liver disease [25,26]. Spironolactone, which is a common cause of gynaecomastia in men with chronic liver disease [4], acts partly by reducing testosterone synthesis by inhibition of 17-hydroxylase [32]. The number of hepatic oestrogen receptors is increased in men with chronic alcoholic liver disease and this change in oestrogen receptor status may facilitate feminisation [33]. There is an increase in the ratio between free oestradiol and free testosterone (E_2/T ratio) [34].

In addition to deficiency of gonadal hormones there is a central hypothalamo-pituitary defect in the regulation of gonadotrophin secretion [6,12,23,35]. One study has suggested that testosterone treatment may improve prognosis in cirrhosis [36] but these findings have not been confirmed [37,38]. Oral testosterone therapy has *not* been shown to be beneficial in the treatment of sexual dysfunction in men with alcoholic liver disease, although there may be an improvement in free testosterone concentrations and some improvement in hypogonadal symptoms [37].

Clinical and biochemical manifestations in women

Premenopausal women

Sex hormone changes in women with liver disease, especially in premenopausal women who have normal changes relating to the menstrual cycle, are less well characterised than those in men. In premenopausal female alcoholics, alcohol consumption increases the frequency of menstrual disturbances and spontaneous abortion but possibly not infertility. Chronic alcohol abuse leads to reduced concentrations of sulphated steroids and these changes may be seen before severe liver dysfunction has appeared [39]. In women with liver disease, liver dysfunction is associated with an early menopause compared with normal controls. This observation is seen in both alcohol- and non-alcohol-related liver disease [40]. Women with liver disease, especially of alcoholic aetiology, have loss of libido and sexual dysfunction [41]. In addition, they may have oligomenorrhoea or amenorrhoea, loss of secondary sexual characteristics with decreased breast and pelvic fat and infertility [42]. Reproductive failure has been documented in premenopausal women who have died from alcoholic cirrhosis with a paucity of developing ovarian follicles and few corpora lutea [43]. Sex hormone changes in premenopausal women with alcoholic liver disease are summarised in Table 77.3.

Post-menopausal women

The majority of studies in women with liver disease have been performed in post-menopausal women with alcoholic liver disease (Table 77.3). Alcohol is the predominant cause of hypogonadism rather than liver disease itself. In women with non-alcoholic liver disease, hypogonadism usually occurs late in the course of their disease and is associated with encephalopathy and disturbance of GnRH secretion [12]. Changes in sex steroid hormones in a group of women with chronic liver disease are summarised in Table 77.4. There is a disturbed regulation of gonadotrophin secretion as well as a direct effect on ovarian function [41]. Plasma androstenedione concentration is increased while dehydroepiandrosterone and dehydroepiandrosterone sulphate are reduced. Plasma testosterone and oestrone concentrations are usually normal [45]. It is not clear whether the alteration of plasma androgen profile in women with chronic liver disease is due to hepatic or adrenocortical abnormalities. SHBG levels are increased in women with primary biliary cirrhosis but are normal in women with alcoholic liver disease [46]. 5α-dihydroxytestosterone levels are reduced

Table 77.3 Sex hormones in premenopausal women with alcoholic liver disease. Data from [41].

	Premenopausal alcoholic liver disease (n = 9)	Normal women	
		Premenopausal (n = 9)	Post-menopausal (n = 10)
Oestrone (pg/ml)	60 ± 10*	29 ± 3	15 ± 2
Oestradiol (pg/ml)	47 ± 8*	82 ± 14	26 ± 2
Progesterone (ng/ml)	0.28 ± 0.09†	1.2 ± 0.16	0.22 ± 0.01
Sex hormone-binding globulin (pg/ml)	235 ± 34	328 ± 59	298 ± 18
Luteinising hormone (mi.u./ml)	7.8 ± 2.0	7.1 ± 0.7	38.6 ± 4.7
Follicle-stimulating hormone (mi.u./ml)	11.4 ± 2.2	8.5 ± 0.6	206.7 ± 17.6

* $P < 0.05$ and † $P < 0.001$ compared with both pre- and post-menopausal women.

Table 77.4 Sex steroid hormones in women with chronic liver disease. Data from [44].

Hormone	Level
Testosterone	↓
Oestrone	↑
Oestradiol	→
Progesterone	→
Sex hormone-binding globulin	↑ or normal

↑, increased; ↓, decreased; →, unchanged.

and the degree of liver dysfunction is the major determinant for the observed disturbances [39]. The presence of high-affinity, low-capacity oestrogen receptors in the liver has been confirmed [39]; these are reduced in liver disease, in proportion to the extent of hepatic dysfunction. Alcohol is not an independent determinant of oestrogen receptor density in the liver. The importance of this observation has not yet been determined.

Thyroid hormones

The liver is involved in transport, storage, metabolism and excretion of thyroid hormones, and is an important target for their biological activity. The liver also synthesises plasma proteins that bind thyroid hormones such as albumin, thyroxine (T_4)-binding prealbumin (TBPA) and T_4-binding globulin (TBF), and therefore may influence the distribution of these hormones. Thus, in liver disease, there are marked alterations in 'thyroid function tests' which can complicate the biochemical diagnosis of thyroid disease.

Clinical and biochemical manifestations

Most patient with liver disease are clinically euthyroid although certain clinical features of cirrhosis, such as a hyperdynamic circulation, increased adrenergic tone and muscle wasting may resemble thyrotoxicosis. In addition, thyroid function tests must be interpreted with caution in patients with acute and chronic liver disease as total thyroid hormone concentrations may be abnormal despite the clinically euthyroid state. There are a number of mechanisms by which thyroid hormone status becomes disturbed in liver disease, including impaired hypothalamo-pituitary regulation with basal plasma TSH concentrations being commonly elevated in cirrhosis [19,31].

Binding and transport of thyroid hormones are also important, as in peripheral thyroid hormone metabolism. There are marked abnormalities of thyroid binding proteins in liver disease, which largely account for the increased total serum T_4 which is found in both acute and chronic liver disease. Both T_4 and triiodothyronine (T_3) circulate in association with plasma proteins (albumin, TBPA and TBG), binding covalently and reversibly [47,48]. In viral hepatitis, TBG is increased early in the infection, presumably because it is released from damaged hepatocytes; this results in increased total serum T_4 [48]. In cirrhosis and chronic active hepatitis, TBG is decreased in proportion to the severity of the liver damage. TBG may occasionally be raised in hepatocellular carcinoma [45,46]. Plasma TBG may, however, be increased in alcoholic cirrhosis, primary biliary cirrhosis, and liver tumours such as hepatocellular carcinoma [47,48].

Peripheral conversion of T_4 to T_3 is reduced in liver disease, with preferential conversion of T_4 to reverse T_3 (rT_3) [48,49]. The liver deiodinates T_4 to T_3 and in health is a major source of circulating T_3. The rT_3/T_3 ratio has been used in the assessment of hepatic impairment. Recently interest has focused on whether interleukin 6 may account in part for changes in thyroid economy found in non-thyroidal illnesses [50].

Thyroid function tests in liver disease

There have been attempts to utilise abnormal thyroid function tests as prognostic indices in liver disease. Whilst in general

Table 77.5 Alterations of serum thyroid function tests in liver disease.

Disease	Total T_4	Free T_4	Total T_3	Free T_3	Total reverse T_3	Thyroid-stimulating hormone	Thyroxine-binding globulin
Acute hepatitis	↓↑	↑	↓	↓	↑	↑	↑
CAH/PBC	↑	→	↑	↓	→	↑	↓
Cirrhosis	↓	↑	↓	↓	↓	↑→	↓

T_4, thyroxine; T_3, triiodothyronine; CAH, chronic active hepatitis; PBC, primary biliary cirrhosis.
↑, increased; ↓, decreased; →, unchanged.

the more abnormal the tests, the worst the prognosis, especially the rT_3/T_3 ratio, these tests are not reliably applicable to individual patients [51]. Table 77.5 summarises the changes in thyroid hormones in liver disease.

In acute viral hepatitis there is increased total T_4 and T_3 which return to normal on recovery. The free T_4 index, however, is normal, the apparently increased total T_4 being related to the raised TBG and to decreased peripheral conversion of T_4 to T_3. Cirrhosis is associated with an increased free T_4 index and a decreased total and free T_4 index. TSH is slightly increased although the TSH response to thyrotrophin-releasing hormone (TRH) is normal [52]. Abnormalities are likely to relate to decreased intrathyroidal conversion of T_4 to T_3 [48,49]. Caution is thus required in the interpretation of thyroid function tests in acute and chronic liver disease. Estimation of free T_4 and T_3 concentrations or their respectively free indices is essential for the accurate interpretation of thyroid function tests in patients with liver disease. The direct measurement of TBG and total T_4 is an alternative approach. However, all thyroid binding proteins may be affected and so TBG measurements may not be reliable (Table 77.5). Increases in T_3-receptor expression in non-thyroidal illnesses may be responsible for the maintenance of euthyroidism in the face of reduced levels of circulating thyroid hormones. Increased T_3-receptor messenger RNA (mRNA) has been shown in liver and polymorphonuclear leucocytes from patients with chronic liver disease [53].

Thyroid function tests have also been used to predict survival in patients undergoing liver transplantation. Increased total T_4 and decreased total T_3 and decreased T_3/T_4 ratio are reported to be good prognostic indicators [46,49,54]. The worst prognostic indicator is an increased rT_3/T_4 ratio and increased total rT_3 [51].

Adrenal hormones

Clinical and biochemical manifestations

In some patients with liver disease, Cushingoid facies, centripetal obesity, striae and loss of peripheral muscle mass may be related to increased plasma cortisol concentrations. The term 'pseudo-Cushing's syndrome' has been used to describe this clinical situation which occurs most commonly in alcohol abuse.

Chronic liver disease may lead to functional disturbances of the adrenal cortex. Serum cortisol is normal in chronic liver disease but serum albumin may be decreased and cortisol-binding globulin (CBG) increased [56]. Biochemical abnormalities suggestive of Cushing's syndrome with adreno-corticoid hyperresponsiveness [57] have been found in some alcoholics. These abnormalities are reversible on abstinence. The half-life of cortisol is also prolonged in patients with chronic liver disease [58], resulting in increased plasma cortisol and androstenedione concentrations, loss of normal variation of plasma cortisol and failure to suppress with dexamethasone [58]. Increased plasma aldosterone concentrations are also found in chronic liver disease, but this does not appear to be a major determinant of fluid retention in this condition [59].

Glucose metabolism

Clinical and biochemical manifestations

Although minor abnormalities of glucose intolerance are commonly found in patients with chronic liver disease, there are rarely any clinical sequelae, and overt diabetes mellitus is said to be uncommon. The only exception is in haemochromatosis, where 80% of individuals have impaired glucose tolerance and most patients with extensive iron overload and hepatic fibrosis have diabetes mellitus [60]. Hypoglycaemia is an infrequent complication of liver disease. It has been consistently documented only in acute fulminant hepatic failure, terminal hepatic failure and in association with hepatic neoplasms.

The liver is a major site for the degradation of insulin. Approximately 50% of the insulin secreted by the pancreas is cleared from the circulation by the first-pass effect. This is increased in chronic liver disease when there is portosystemic shunting. Increased fasting plasma insulin has been reported in patients with chronic liver disease. Despite this, the blood glucose of cirrhotics is generally higher than normal after glucose loading [61,62], implying insulin resistance [63,64]. Basal plasma glucagon and growth hormone levels are elevated [65]. Hypokalaemia, which inhibits pancreatic secretion of insulin, is also a factor in glucose intolerance in chronic liver disease. These minor abnormalities of glucose tolerance are relatively common but are not indicative of diabetes mellitus and do not require therapeutic intervention.

Tumours

Overt metabolic disturbance is a rare clinical presentation of hepatocellular carcinoma but laboratory investigations in these patients reveal extensive subclinical metabolic disturbances, many of which have been attributed to hormone synthesis by hepatic tumour cells [66,67] (Table 77.6). There is often little evidence of the precise mechanism for the endocrine abnormality, although a number of mechanisms have been implicated. These include the synthesis of hormones, hormone-releasing factors, precursors or hormone-like substances by neoplastic cells and the production of non-hormonal tumour substances which influence circulating

Table 77.6 Hormone production by primary hepatic tumours and the sequelae.

Hormone	Sequelae	References
Parathyroid hormone/parathyroid hormone-like substances	Hypercalcaemia	68
Gonadotrophins (mainly human chorionic gonadotrophin; luteinising hormone)		66
Erythropoietin	Erythrocytosis	69
5-hydroxyindolacetic acid; 5-hydroxytryptamine	Carcinoid syndrome; various syndromes	70
Thyroid-stimulating hormone-like substances	Hyperthyroidism	66
Adrenocorticotrophic hormone; renin	Cushing's syndrome	69
Insulin-like growth factor 2	Hypoglycaemia	70

levels of active hormone produced elsewhere. Abnormal hepatic handling of hormones may also occur, such as the conversion of androgens to oestrone and oestradiol within the tumour [73]. Fasting hypoglycaemia can occur in patients with hepatoma. Tumours may synthesise insulin-like growth factors, particularly insulin-like growth factor 2 [59,72]. Oestrogen receptor mRNA has been shown to be present in the majority of hepatocellular carcinomas [73]. Androgen receptors have been shown to have reduced activity in hepatic adenoma and carcinoma [74,75].

References

1 Edmondsson HA, Glass SJ, Sole SN. Gynecomastia associated with cirrhosis of the liver. *Proc Exp Biol Med* 1939; **42**: 97–9.

2 Gavaler JS, van Thiel DH. Gonadal dysfunction and inadequate sexual performance in alcoholic cirrhotic men. *Gastroenterology* 1988; **95**: 16880–4.

3 Lloyd CW, Williams RH. Endocrine changes associated with Laennec's cirrhosis of the liver. *Am J Med* 1948; **4**: 2315–30.

4 Bannister P, Oakes J, Sheridan P, Losowsky MS. Sex hormone changes in chronic liver disease: a matched study of alcoholic versus non-alcoholic liver disease. *Q J Med* 1987; **63**: 305–13.

5 Cornely CM, Schade RR, van Thiel DH, Gavaler JS. Chronic advanced liver disease and impotence: cause and effect? *Hepatology* 1984; **4**: 1227–30.

6 Green JRB. Progress report. Mechanism of hypogonadism in cirrhotic males. *Gut* 1977; **18**: 843–53.

7 Johnson PJ. Sex hormones and the liver. *Clin Sci* 1984; **66**: 369–76.

8 van Thiel DH, Lester R, Sherins RJ. Hypogonadism in alcoholic liver disease: evidence for a double defect. *Gastroenterology* 1974; **67**: 1188–99.

9 Kew MC. Sexual dysfunction in men with chronic liver disease. *Hepatology* 1988; **8**: 428–31.

10 van Thiel DH. Ethanol: its adverse effects upond the hypothalamic–pituitary gonadal axis. *J Lab Clin Med* 1983; **101**: 21–33.

11 Bahnsen M, Gluud C, Johnsen SG *et al.* Pituitary–testicular function in patients with alcoholic cirrhosis of the liver. *Eur J Clin Invest* 1981; **11**: 473–9.

12 van Thiel DH, Gavaler JS, Schade R. Liver disease and the hypothalamopituitary axis. *Semin Liver Dis* 1985; **5**: 35–45.

13 Gludd C, Bahnsen M, Bennet P *et al.* Hypothalamic–pituitary–gonadal function in relation to liver function in men with alcoholic cirrhosis. *Scand J Gastroenterol* 1983; **18**: 939–44.

14 van Thiel DH, Gavaler JS, Spero JA *et al.* Patterns of hypothalamic–pituitary gonadal dysfunction in men with liver disease due to differing etiologies. *Hepatology* 1981; **1**: 39–46.

15 van Thiel DH. Disorders of the hypothalamic–pituitary gonadal axis in patients with liver disease. In: Zakim D, Boyer TD, eds. *Hepatology: A Texbook of Liver Disease*. Philadelphia: WB Saunders Co., 1982: 516–28.

16 Mooradian AD, Shamma M, Salti AL, Cortas N. Hypophyseal–gonadal dysfunction in men with non-alcoholic liver cirrhosis. *Andrologia* 1985; **17**: 72–9.

17 Kley HK, Strohmeyer G, Kruskemper HL. Effect of testosterone application on hormone concentrations of androgens and estrogens in male patients with cirrhosis of the liver. *Gastroenterology* 1979; **76**: 235–41.

18 Mowatt NAG, Edwards CRW, Fisher R, McNeilly AS, Green JRB, Dawson AM. Hypothalamic–pituitary gonadal function in men with cirrhosis of the liver. *Gastroenterology*1979; **76**: 235–41.

19 Chopra IJ, Tulchinsky D, Greenway FL. Estrogen–androgen imbalance in hepatic cirrhosis: studies in 13 male patients. *Ann Intern Med* 1973; **79**: 198–203.

20 Kley HK, Keck E, Kruskemper HL. Esterone and estradiol in patients with cirrhosis of the liver: effects of ACTH and dexamethasone. *J Clin Endocrinol Metab* 1976; **433**: 557–60.

21 Valimaki M, Salaspuro M, Harkonen M, Yukahri R. Liver damage and sex hormones and chronic male alcoholics. *Clin Endocrinol* 1982; **17**: 469–77.

22 Green JRB, Mowatt NAG, Fisher RA, Anderson DC. Plasma oestrogen in men with chronic liver disease. *Gut* 1976; **17**: 426–440.

23 Baker HWG, Burger HG, Krester DM *et al.* A study of the endocrine manifestations of hepatic cirrhosis. *Q J Med* 1976; **177**: 145–78.

24 Lester R, Eagon PK, van Thiel DH. Feminisation of the alcoholic—the estrogen/testosterone ratio (E/T). *Gastroenterology* 1979; **76**: 415–17.

25 Farthing MJG, Green JRB, Edwards CRW, Dawson AW. Progesterone, prolactin and gynaecomastia in men with liver disease. *Gut* 1982; **23**: 276–9.

26 Morgan MY, Jakobovits AW, Gore MBR, Wills MR, Sherlock S. Serum prolactin in liver disease and its relationship to gynaecomastia. *Gut* 1978; **19**: 170–4.

27 Turkington RW. Serum prolactin levels in patients with gynaecomastia. *J Clin Endocrinol* 1972; **34**: 62–6.

28 Bannister P, Handley T, Chapman C, Losowsky MS. Hypogonadism

in chronic liver disease: impaired release of luteinising hormone. *Br Med J* 1986; **293**: 1191–3.
29 Lieber CS. The effects of alcohol and alcoholic liver disease on the endocrine system and intermediary metabolism. In: Lieber CS, ed. *Medical Disorders of Alcoholism, Pathogenesis and Treatment*. Philadelphia: W.B. Saunders, 1982: 65–141.
30 De Besi L, Zucchetta P, Zotli S, Mastrogiacomo I. Sex hormone and sex hormone binding globulin in males with compensated and decompensated cirrhosis of the liver. *Acta Endocrinol (Copenh)* 1989; **120**: 271–6.
31 Green JRB, Snitcher EJ, Mowat NAG, Ekins RP, Rees LH, Dawson AM. Thyroid function and thyroid regulation in euthyroid men with chronic liver disease: evidence of multiple abnormalities. *Clin Endocrinol* 1977; **7**: 453–61.
32 Rose LI, Underwood RH, Newmark SR, Kisch ES, Williams GH. Pathophysiology of spironolactone-induced gynaecomastia. *Ann Intern Med* 1977; **87**: 398–403.
33 Villa E, Baldini GM, Rossini GP *et al.* Ethanol-induced increase in cytosolic estrogen receptors in human male liver: a possible explanation for biochemical feminisation in chronic liver disease due to alcohol. *Hepatology* 1988; **8**: 1610–14.
34 Kley HK. E_2/T ratio. *Gastroenterology* 1979; **76**: 1079–80.
35 van Thiel DH, Gavaler JS. Hypothalamic pituitary gonadal function in liver disease with particular attention to the endocrine effect of chronic alcohol abuse. *Prog Liver Dis* 1986; **8**: 273–82.
36 Gluud C. Anabolic-androgenic steroid treatment of liver disease. *Liver* 1984; **4**: 159–69.
37 Gluud C, Wantzin P, Eriksen J. Copenhagen Study Group for Liver Diseases. No effect of oral testosterone treatment on sexual dysfunction in alcoholic cirrhotic men. *Gastroenterology* 1988; **95**: 1582–7.
38 Gluud C, Dejgaard A, Bennett P, Svenstrup B. Androgens and oestrogens before and following oral testosterone administration in male patients with and without alcoholic cirrhosis. *Acta Endocrinol (Copenh)* 1987; **115**: 385–91.
39 Becker U. The influence of ethanol and liver disease on sex hormones and hepatic oestrogen receptors in women. *Dan Med Bull* 1993; **40**: 447–59.
40 Becker U, Gluud C, Farholt S, Bennett P, Micic S, Svenstrup B, Hardt F. Menopausal age and sex hormones in post-menopausal women with alcoholic and non-alcoholic liver disease. *J Hepatol* 1991; **13**: 25–32.
41 Valimaki M, Pelkonen R, Salaspuro M, Harkonen M, Hirovnen E, Yukahri R. Sex hormone in amenorrhoeic women with alcoholic liver disease. *J Clin Endocrinol Metab* 1984; **59**: 133–8.
42 van Thiel DH, Lester R. Hypothalamic–pituitary gonadal function in liver disease. *Viewpoints Dig Dis* 1980; **12**: 13–16.
43 Jung Y, Russfield AB. Prolactin cells in the hypophysis of cirrhotic patients. *Arch Pathol* 1972; **94**: 265–70.
44 Shaaban MM, Ghaneimah SA, Hammad WA, El-Sharkawy MM, Elwan SI, Ahmed YA. Sex steroids in women with cirrhosis. *Int J Gynaecol Obstet* 1980; **18**: 181–4.
45 Carlstrom K, Eriksson S, Rannevik G. Sex steroids and steroid binding proteins in female alcoholic liver disease. *Acta Endocrinol (Copenh)* 1986; **111**: 75–9.
46 Becker V, Gluud C, Bennett P. Thyroid hormone and thyroxine-binding globulin in relation to liver function and serum testosterone in men with alcoholic cirrhosis. *Acta Med Scand* 1988; **224**: 367–73.
47 Ross DS, Daniels GH, Dienstag JL, Ridgway EC. Elevated thyroxine levels due to increased thyroxine-binding globulin in acute hepatitis. *Am J Med* 1983; **74**: 564–9.
48 Sheridan P. Thyroid hormones and the liver. *Clin Gastroenterol* 1983; **12**: 797–818.
49 Itoh S, Yamaba Y, Oda T, Kawagoe K. Serum thyroid hormone triiodothyronine, thyroxine and triiodothyronine/thyroxine ratio in patients with fulminant, acute and chronic hepatitis. *Am J Gastroenterol* 1986; **81**: 444–9.
50 Bartalena L, Brogioni S, Grasso L, Velluzzi F, Martino E. Relationship of the increased serum interleukin-6 concentration to changes of thyroid function in non-thyroidal illness. *J Endocrinol Invest* 1994; **17**: 269–74.
51 Kano T, Kojima T, Takahashi T, Muto Y. Serum thyroid hormone levels in patients with fulminant hepatitis: usefulness of rT_3 and the rT_3/T_3 ratio as prognostic indices. *Gastroenterol Jpn* 1987; **22**: 344–53.
52 van Thiel DH, Tarter R, Gavaler JS, Schade RR, Sanghri A. Thyroid and pituitary hormone responses to TRH in advanced non-alcoholic liver disease. *J Endocrinol Invest* 1986; **9**: 479–86.
53 Williams GR, Franklyn JA, Neuberger JM, Sheppard MC. Thyroid hormone receptor expression in the 'sick euthyroid' syndrome. *Lancet* 1989; **2**: 1477–81.
54 Pasqualini T, Feinstein-Day P, Gutman R, Balzaretti M, D'Agostino D. Thyroid function and serum IGF-1 in children before and after liver transplantation. *J Paediatr Endocrinol* 1994; **7**: 343–8.
55 van Thiel DH, Udani M, Schade RR, Sanghri A, Starzel TE. Prognostic value of thyroid hormone levels in patients evaluated for liver transplantation. *Hepatology* 1985; **5**: 862–6.
56 Kley HC, Both H, Kruskemper HL. Hypercortisolism in patients with cirrhosis of the liver due to decreased binding of plasma cortisol. *Horm Metab Res* 1978; **i**: 726–8.
57 Rees LH, Besser GM, Jeffcoate WJ. Alcohol-induced pseudo Cushing's syndrome. *Lancet* 1977; **i**: 726–8.
58 Hasselback H, Selmer J, Sestoft L, Kehlet H. Hypothalamic–pituitary–adrenocortical function in chronic alcoholism. *Clin Endocrinol* 1982; **16**: 73–6.
59 Gerdes H. Glucocorticoid and mineralcorticoid hormones in chronic liver disease. *Zeitschr Gastroenterol* 1979; **17**: 439–46.
60 Holland HK, Spivak JL. Haemochromatosis. *Med Clin North Am* 1989; **73**: 831–45.
61 Feingold KR, Siperstein MD. Abnormalities of glucose metabolism in liver disease: In: Zakim D, Boyer TD, eds. *Hepatology: A Textbook of Liver Disease*. Philadelphia: WB Saunders Co., 1982: 499–515.
62 Johnston DG, Alberti KGMM, Binder C, Faber OK, Wright R, Orskov H. Hormonal and metabolic changes in hepatic cirrhosis. *Horm Metab Res* 1982; **14**: 34–9.
63 Priovietto J, Dudley FJ, Aitken P, Alford FP. Hyperinsulinaemia and insulin resistance of cirrhosis: the importance of insulin hypersecretion. *Clin Endocrinol* 1984; **21**: 657–65.
64 Shankar TP, Fredi JL, Himmelstein S, Soloman SS, Duckworth WC. Elevated growth hormone levels and insulin resistance in patients with cirrhosis of the liver. *Am J Med Sci* 1986; **291**: 248–54.
65 Smith-Laing G, Orskov H, Gore MBR, Sherlock S. Hyperglucagonaemia in cirrhosis. Relationships to hepatocellular damage. *Diabetologia* 1980; **19**: 103–8.
66 Reeve NL, Fox H. Endocrine effects of tumours of the liver. *Invest Cell Pathol* 1980; **3**: 151–8.
67 Scheuer A, Griin R, Lehmann F-G. Peptide hormones in liver cirrhosis and hepatocellular carcinoma. *Oncodev Biol Med* 1981; **2**: 1–10.
68 Knill-Jones RP, Buckle RM, Parsons V, Calne RY, Williams R. Hypercalcaemia and increased parathyroid hormone activity in primary hepatoma. Studies before and after hepatic transplantation. *N Engl J Med* 1970; **282**: 704–8.

69 McFadzean AJS, Todd D, Tsang KC. Polycythaemia in primary carcinoma of the liver. *Blood* 1958; **13**: 427–35.
70 Primack A, Wilson J, O'Connor GT, Engelman K, Hull E, Canellos GP. Hepatocellular carcinoma with the carcinoid syndrome. *Cancer* 1971; **27**: 1182–9.
71 Burmeister P, Bianchi L, Klietmann W, Torhorst J. Paraneoplastisches Cushing-Syndrome bei primären Leberkarzinoma. *Deutsche Med Wochenschr* 1968; **93**: 164–5.
72 Fradkin JE, Eastman RC, Lesniak MA, Roth J. Specificity spillover at the hormone receptor—exploring its role in human disease. *N Engl J Med* 1989; **320**: 640–5.
73 Kew MC, Kirschner MA, Abrahams GE, Katz M. Mechanism of feminisation in primary liver cancer. *N Engl J Med* 1977; **296**: 1084–8.
74 Eagon PK, Elms MS, Stafford EA, Porter LE. Androgen receptors in human liver: characterisation and quantitation in normal and diseased liver. *Hepatology* 1994; **19**: 92–100.
75 Pacchioni D, Papotti M, Androno E *et al*. Expression of estrogen receptor mRNA in tumorous and non-tumorous liver tissue as detected by *in situ* hybridisation. *J Surg Oncology* 1993; **3**: 14–17.

CHAPTER 78

Endocrine manifestations of systemic disease: the kidney

I.G. Lawrence and T.A. Howlett

Introduction

The development of end-stage renal failure (ESRF) causes profound changes in the life of an individual. Life itself becomes no longer possible without complex replacement therapy; severe anaemia and general physical ill-health limit activity; job loss or reduced earnings often herald major social changes; and psychological problems are common. In this context it is perhaps not surprising that endocrine changes associated with ESRF may not have the highest priority in the immediate management of the patient. Endocrine abnormalities are common, however, in ESRF and are frequently causally related to clinically important complications of the disease. Changes occur at all levels of endocrine regulation and represent a combination of appropriate or exaggerated responses to metabolic change, changes in hormone clearance, hyper- and hyposecretion of renal and other hormones, and 'toxic' effects of azotaemia on endocrine organs [1]. Assessment of hormone levels is also subject to a number of methodological problems in ESRF, largely due to changes in protein binding and to changes in hormone metabolism.

Changes in renal hormones

Although the kidney is rarely considered as an endocrine organ in patients with normal renal function, changes in secretion of hormones by the kidney are responsible for some of the most important pathological changes in ESRF.

Erythropoietin

Serum erythropoietin levels in ESRF are within the normal range, but disproportionately low for the degree of anaemia, and hence this relative deficiency is the primary cause of the marked anaemia. Indeed, uraemic patients have been reported to produce substantial amounts of erythropoietin during acute hypoxia and blood loss, and post-parathyroidectomy. In the past, repeated blood transfusions have formed the mainstay of therapy, but in recent years treatment with recombinant human erythropoietin (rhEPO) has been shown to correct the anaemia and result in dramatic improvements in patient well-being. rhEPO is now widely used in both the dialysis and predialysis ESRF populations and subcutaneous administration, which is increasingly used, has enabled self-administration and often a reduction in dosage compared with the intravenous route. The main adverse side-effect of rhEPO has been the development of hypertension or aggravation of pre-existing hypertension, which has been particularly manifest in uraemic patients. Over recent years there have been a number of studies suggesting direct effects of rhEPO on endocrine function, with the strongest evidence favouring a pituitary or hypothalamic action in the production and secretion of GH and prolactin [2–4]. Interestingly, there is striking homology of the extracellular domains of receptors for erythropoietin, GH and prolactin [5], as well as for interleukin 2 and interleukin 3 [6].

Calcitriol

The kidney is responsible for the conversion of 25-hydroxyvitamin D_3 to the active hormone calcitriol (1,25–$(OH)_2D_3$), and therefore plays a major role in the endocrinology of calcium metabolism. Levels of calcitriol are low in ESRF, and this is an important contributor to renal osteodystrophy, and possibly to growth retardation, as discussed below.

Renin

Renin is secreted by the juxtaglomerular cells of the kidney, and clearly plays an important endocrine role. In ESRF plasma renin levels are usually high, and this is a major contributor to hypertension, which may be severe and difficult to control, occasionally leading to the need for nephrectomy.

Parathyroid hormone and renal osteodystrophy

Parathyroid hormone and calcitriol secretion

In the past, measurement of serum parathyroid hormone (PTH) in ESRF was complicated by the presence of immunoreactive, but non-bioactive, metabolites. Newer immunometric assays, however, appear to accurately reflect levels of biologically active intact PTH in serum of patients with ESRF [7]. Serum PTH rises steadily with progressive renal impairment due to at least two stimuli; decreased renal clearance of phosphate and decreased renal secretion of calcitriol, both of which result in lowering of serum calcium. As renal function deteriorates, a rise in PTH and fall in calcitriol is first detectable at a creatinine clearance as high as 50 ml/min, but initially the rise in PTH is sufficient for complete compensation and serum calcium and phosphate levels remain normal. In ESRF, however, most untreated patients are markedly hyperphosphataemic and hypocalcaemic. The degree of hyperparathyroidism increases with the severity and duration of renal impairment. Parathyroid function may become autonomous (tertiary hyperparathyroidism) and result in hypercalcaemia, and/or persistent elevation of PTH after successful transplantation.

Renal osteodystrophy

Renal osteodystrophy affects a majority of patients in ESRF, and includes a range of skeletal disorders from high-turnover to low-turnover lesions. The resulting bone disease is the sum of a variety of pathological processes, the relative contribution of which varies from patient to patient and from bone to bone. Hyperparathyroid bone disease and osteomalacia are usually the predominant factors and both result in bone pain, tenderness and deformity. However, the prevalence has changed over recent years, and adynamic renal osteodystrophy has increased substantially in both the adult and paediatric dialysis populations [8]. Avascular necrosis occurs less commonly, and is particularly associated with steroid therapy. Extraskeletal calcification is a frequent accompanying feature.

First-line treatment of renal osteodystrophy consists of the control of phosphate metabolism with phosphate binders and the treatment of the osteomalacia. Aluminium hydroxide was traditionally used as a phosphate binder, but is now rarely used in view of the established role of aluminium toxicity in adynamic bone disease and dialysis dementia, so that alternatives such as calcium carbonate are widely prescribed. Nevertheless, the use of large doses of calcium carbonate, as well as intensive vitamin D therapy and peritoneal dialysis, have also been implicated in the increased prevalence of adynamic renal osteodystrophy (other risk factors include diabetes, increasing age, parathyroidectomy, previous renal transplant and/or corticosteroid treatment) [9].

Osteomalacia is most conveniently treated with calcitriol or alfacalcidol, avoiding the need for 1α-hydroxylation by the kidney. Established renal osteodystrophy is treated with calcitriol 1–2 μg/day, which results in considerable, but usually incomplete, healing in the majority of patients. In addition, treatment with low doses of calcitriol (250–500 ng/day) has now been advocated from an early stage in ESRF to prevent the development of osteodystrophy and hyperparathyroidism [10]. Intermittent intravenous or large oral doses of calcitriol have also been used for mild to moderate secondary hyperparathyroidism, but a substantial proportion of paediatric patients develop adynamic (or aplastic) bone disease after 8–12 months of therapy. Parathyroidectomy, total or partial, has been a traditional treatment for severe osteodystrophy and is still required in many patients in spite of the treatments outlined above. Indications for parathyroidectomy include bone disease uncontrolled by vitamin D therapy, and the development of tertiary hyperparathyroidism with hypercalcaemia.

Other roles of PTH

In addition to its obvious role in calcium metabolism, high circulating levels of PTH have also been implicated, as a 'uraemic toxin', in the aetiology of many other complications of ESRF. Thus, PTH has been advocated as the inhibitor of erythropoiesis, and the cause of impaired glucose tolerance, goitre, hyperprolactinaemia, impotence and hypogonadism. In animals, for example, both infusions of PTH and experimental acute uraemia reduce testosterone secretion, and in the latter case this is prevented by prior parathyroidectomy. In patients with ESRF, workers have reported a good statistical correlation between serum levels of PTH, prolactin and testosterone, but all are clearly related to the degree of renal impairment, and well-controlled studies have, as yet, failed to demonstrate unequivocally a causal link [4,11]. Interestingly, parathyroidectomy has been shown to cause a striking increase in serum immunoreactive erythropoietin and blood reticulocytes in uraemic patients with secondary hyperparathyroidism, but only blood reticulocytes in patients with primary hyperparathyroidism [12], suggesting tissue resistance to erythropoietin in ESRF.

Gonadal function and prolactin

Prolactin secretion

Hyperprolactinaemia is a frequent finding in ESRF in both sexes, whether on conservative therapy, haemodialysis (HD) or continuous ambulatory peritoneal dialysis (CAPD). The precise incidence varies from study to study (from 50 to 100%), and with the definition of the upper limit of normal for serum prolactin. The degree of hyperprolactinaemia is usually mild; in most patients levels are below 1000 mU/l, although higher values (up to 5000 mU/l) are occasionally seen, and levels tend to be higher in females. Evidence favours increased secretion of prolactin as the main cause, although clearance is also decreased.

Hypothalamo-pituitary–gonadal axis

Clinical and biochemical hypogonadism is a frequent finding is ESRF, and abnormalities exist at all levels of the hypothalamo-pituitary–gonadal axis [13]. Basal luteinising hormone (LH) levels are usually elevated in both sexes, which might suggest end-organ failure, and LH responses to gonadotrophin-releasing hormone (GnRH) are often exaggerated and prolonged. However, detailed analysis of LH pulsatility in a group of male HD patients has demonstrated that the elevation in LH is primarily due to a prolongation of the LH half-life [14]; there is a shortening of the LH secretory burst duration and a consequent decrease in the amount of LH secreted at each burst, but no reduction in the LH secretory pulse frequency. Recently, a circulating inhibitor of human LH receptors has been demonstrated in boys with chronic renal failure; this factor appears to be a large protein with a molecular weight between 30 000 and 60 000 Da [56]. Serum FSH levels are normal or mildly elevated, except in men with severe testicular atrophy. In men, most studies agree that serum total testosterone levels are lower than in the normal control population. The degree of hypotestosteronaemia reported varies widely, however, and levels remain within the normal range in the majority of subjects. Mean levels of serum LH rise and testosterone fall progressively with progressive renal impairment. Alterations in protein binding associated with ESRF also play a role, and 'free' hormone levels are usually low. The testosterone response to the administration of human chorionic gonadotrophin (hCG) is also blunted, providing further evidence of a direct toxic effect of azotaemia on the testis, and testicular biopsy usually reveals arrest of spermatogenesis. Although serum testosterone levels are less reduced in CAPD compared with HD patients, there is no difference in the incidence of symptoms such as impotence. Reported levels of oestrogens vary; however, serum oestradiol, oestrone levels and 'total oestrogens' are often raised in men. In the female, levels of oestradiol, progesterone and follicle-stimulating hormone (FSH) are generally reported to be within the normal range for the early follicular phase, but fail to show the usual cyclical changes.

Clinical problems and their treatment

Symptoms of hypogonadism are a frequent problem for male patients in ESRF. In the largest reported survey of 100 uraemic men [11], 79% complained of sexual dysfunction, decreased libido was common and 61% had complete or partial impotence; on examination 78% were found to have testicular atrophy, and 14% gynaecomastia (more common in some other studies). Evidence suggests a significant hormonal contribution toward this high incidence of impotence; thus, in the same series only 6% of men had investigations compatible with a vascular cause, there was no evidence for neuropathy in most cases, and impotence was reversed by successful transplantation. Oligo- and azoospermia are also common. However, with the changing demography of the dialysis population (an older group of patients, in whom the most common cause of ESRF in the western world is now diabetic nephropathy, often being associated with widespread arteriopathic disease), it is likely that vascular disease will increasingly constitute the major component of uraemic impotence.

In women, menstrual disturbances are present in the majority of patients. Amenorrhoea or severe oligomenorrhoea are most common, but polymenorrhoea and menorrhagia can also occur on dialysis, and the latter is worsened by the anticoagulation during HD. Anovulation and infertility are almost universal, and reported conception on dialysis is rare.

Galactorrhoea can occur in both sexes, usually in patients with the highest prolactin levels, but the reported prevalence varies widely. Delayed puberty is common in adolescents of both sexes. All problems are most severe in the final stages of conservative therapy, and may improve slightly with the commencement of regular dialysis.

Treatment of the hypogonadism of ESRF remains problematical. In the male, replacement therapy with depot or oral testosterone has been advocated, but there is general agreement that this does not usually result in clinical improvement, except in a minority of patients with frankly low serum testosterone levels. There is no controlled trial of gonadal steroid replacement therapy in the female, but this may at least restore regular menstruation. Gonadal steroids have also been used in ESRF for reasons other than simple physiological replacement: prior to the widespread use of rhEPO, testosterone was used for the treatment of anaemia in ESRF, although its haematopoietic effect has been shown to be independent of its action on serum erythropoietin levels. Nevertheless, 60% male HD patients in one study had increased serum erythropoietin on testosterone treatment [15]. Transdermal 17β-oestradiol, meanwhile, has been recently advocated as a safe and effective way of reducing the prolonged bleeding time of uraemia in the context of patients requiring a renal biopsy or having recurrent gastrointestinal bleeding from telangiectasiae [16].

Clomiphene citrate (100 mg daily for 5–12 months) has been reported to restore serum testosterone to normal in men, with further elevation of LH and FSH, and to improve libido, potency and well-being, but without a consistent effect on spermatogenesis [17]. However, this therapy has not been widely adopted and long-term studies are required to establish the lowest effective dose and side-effect profile. A significant decrease in prolactin in male HD patients given clomiphene for 1 week has also been described, which was not found in normal controls [18], suggesting that the positive feedback of oestrogens on prolactin production is greater in uraemic males.

Zinc supplementation (50 mg Zn daily as acetate) has also been shown to improve testosterone and LH levels, sperm count, potency and libido in a double-blind study [19], although others have been unable to demonstrate an improvement in hormonal disturbances [20] or gonadal disorders [21]. Again, the potential effects of long term therapy in ESRF are unknown.

Since hyperprolactinaemia due to other causes frequently results in impotence and oligomenorrhoea, it is not surprising that attempts to lower prolactin levels and treat symptoms of hypogonadism with dopamine agonists have been reported. Studies report treatment of only relatively small numbers of patients, largely male, but both bromocriptine (1.25–2.5 mg, two to three times daily) and lisuride (75 μg daily) may result in considerable improvement in potency in the majority of men, and restoration of menstruation in some women [22–24]. Treatment may be limited by side-effects, particularly nausea and postural hypotension, which appear to occur more frequently in ESRF than in other patient groups, and treatment with newer, better tolerated, dopamine agonists has not yet been reported. A trial of dopamine-agonist therapy is therefore justified in any male patient with impotence due to ESRF who demonstrates a normal serum testosterone and hyperprolactinaemia. However, many will be unable to tolerate such treatment.

Little attention has been paid to the sexual disturbances of ESRF in the female dialysis population, and indeed anovulation and infertility could be viewed as protective. A survey of 99 female HD patients found 80% had reduced libido and decreased frequency of intercourse, with hyperprolactinaemia being correlated to lower frequency of having intercourse and achieving an orgasm [25]. Anecdotal evidence suggests a proportion of female dialysis patients with hyperprolactinaemia and menstrual disturbances would also benefit from dopamine agonist therapy, but this does not seem to have been subjected to a formal trial.

The recent availability of rhEPO has led to another fascinating observation. Treatment with rhEPO for anaemia in HD patients was reported to improve sexual function in four out of seven males, and restore regular menstruation in five out of nine females [4]; furthermore, therapy was associated with a dramatic normalisation of serum prolactin. A number of subsequent small studies, all in HD patients, have confirmed the improved sexual function, but conflict over the response of prolactin [2,26–28]. In normal subjects, the acute administration of therapeutic doses of rhEPO does not interfere with prolactin secretion both after a direct pituitary stimulus (thyrotrophin-releasing hormone (TRH)) and after stimuli involving dopaminergic and serotoninergic pathways [29]. LH pulsatility studies of seven haemodialysed men have demonstrated that rhEPO therapy causes a decrease in the plasma half-life of LH, but a quantitative and qualitative increase in LH signal strength [57]. Meanwhile, a recent large cross-sectional study of predominantly CAPD-treated men (attending an impotence clinic) has demonstrated higher serum testosterone and sex hormone binding globulin (SHBG) in the rhEPO recipients, but not suppression of hyperprolactinaemia or hyperoestrogenism [58]. A large prospective study in the predialysis chronic renal failure, HD and CAPD populations is still required to answer the question whether rhEPO ameliorates or normalises the endocrine disturbances of uraemia.

Our approach to impotence difficulties in the male dialysis population is to firstly optimise the patient's clinical state by the correction of anaemia (using rhEPO) and metabolic abnormalities (such as underdialysis or poor glycaemic control), as well as the substitution of any medications possibly contributing toward impotence (usually β-adrenoceptor blockers, but occasionally thiazides or antiemetic phenothiazines, the latter having a tendency to cause severe hyperprolactinaemia). However, these measures alone do not usually fully restore erectile difficulties. All patients with primary hypogonadism are treated with intramuscular depot testosterone (on non-dialysis days for the HD population), unless there is a contraindication (e.g. recurrent fluid overload or previous prostatic carcinoma). Again, the results have been disappointing, even in patients who initially seem to respond. In contrast, we have found vacuum tumescence devices to be effective (as well as acceptable) in most younger and middle-aged male dialysis patients [59], although the older population tend to be more reluctant to use them. Intracavernosal injection therapy with alprostadil is an alternative, but there has not been a published study in this group as yet: a potential problem is the risk of bleeding at the site of injection, and it would seem inadvisable in the HD patient on his dialysis day. Penile implants should be regarded as the last option, after all other therapies have been pursued, and only employed following careful patient selection, including psychological assessment. Clearly, psychotherapy is unlikely to be effective in most impotent dialysis patients in view of the invariable organic aetiologies.

Finally, symptoms of hypogonadism are often reversed by successful renal transplantation, including restoration of fertility, although some biochemical abnormalities may persist. Residual hypogonadism in patients with established good allograft function has been shown to correlate with the duration of HD pretransplantation, and is associated with elevated basal LH and excessive LH response to LHRH, presumably reflecting impaired Leydig-cell function. However, the main determinant of testicular endocrine function is allograft function, as plasma LH strongly correlates with urea and creatinine. No difference has been found between different immunosuppressive regimens.

Growth and growth hormone

Growth hormone secretion

Basal serum growth hormone (GH) levels are normal or slightly raised in ESRF, fail to suppress normally during a glucose tolerance test, and may show a paradoxical rise after TRH, but fail to suppress after bromocriptine therapy. Resistance to GH is described in uraemia, but with normal insulin-like growth factor 1 (IGF-1) and moderately elevated IGF-2 levels [30]; however, IGF-binding proteins (IGFBPs) are markedly raised [31] and thus there is reduced IGF bioactivity in ESRF.

There are many reports of diminished GH secretion in response to insulin-induced hypoglycaemia, but, in most studies, adequate hypoglycaemia was not consistently achieved. However, one well-controlled study [32] confirmed impaired GH secretion (peak <40 mU/l) in four out of 10 patients on HD and seven out of 10 on CAPD. In contrast, serum GH responses to GH-releasing hormone (GHRH) are increased in ESRF compared with normal controls, in both children and adults, and responses to arginine are normal. However, both a reduction in basal GH and GH response to GHRH have been demonstrated following HD, irrespective of the buffer used during dialysis.

Treatment with rhEPO has no effect on basal GH, but both unchanged and potentiated GH response to GHRH have been reported after partial correction of anaemia, as well as elimination of the paradoxical response to TRH [2]. The acute administration of rhEPO has also been demonstrated to potentiate the GH response to GHRH, and reduce the paradoxical GH response to TRH in patients with ESRF [3]. A direct effect of rhEPO at the hypothalamic or pituitary level thus seems likely.

Growth retardation and its treatment

Growth retardation has long been recognised as an important clinical problem in children with chronic renal insufficiency. Greatest disturbance occurs at the times of greatest growth velocity, in the first 2 years of life and during the normal pubertal growth spurt. In addition, pubertal delay due to the hypogonadism of ESRF may worsen the problems of short stature during adolescence. During renal replacement therapy with haemodialysis or peritoneal dialysis, impaired linear growth persists and the improvement post-renal transplantation is usually insufficient to correct pre-existing growth retardation.

Recombinant human growth hormone (rhGH) has been shown to be an effective treatment of growth retardation in children with stable chronic renal failure, ESRF requiring dialysis and successful renal transplantation. The doses of rhGH given are pharmacological, rather than physiological, presumably reflecting GH resistance of uraemia, and usually growth velocity doubles, with the effect being sustained for at least 3 years. However, the clinical responses differ, with a smaller increase in linear growth in children receiving dialysis than those with stable chronic renal failure [33]. Furthermore, during the second year of rhGH therapy, there is almost 50% reduction in height velocity in prepubertal children receiving dialysis [34].

A number of other, non-hormonal, factors also contribute to the growth retardation of ESRF and may require independent correction [35]. As part of their renal osteodystrophy children have hypomineralisation of the growth plate, with unmineralised woven bone and osteitis fibrosa, which can impede bone growth rate and ossification of normal maturation centres. An early study with calcitriol showed improved linear growth [36], but a subsequent larger trial has failed to demonstrate substantial differences between calcitriol and dihydrotachysterol (DHT) in the rate of linear growth in children with stable chronic renal failure [37]. Calcitriol is widely used in children and adolescents with renal failure, but its role is currently being reconsidered, and the previously reported beneficial effect may be limited to those with severe secondary hyperparathyroidism [38].

In addition, poor growth velocity in ESRF has been demonstrated to correlate with poor control of metabolic acidosis, and with protein and calorie malnutrition due to strict 'renal' diets. Every effort should be made in children with ESRF to control hyperparathyroidism and renal osteodystrophy, and to provide adequate protein and energy in the diet. However, it is clear that apparently optimum control of non-hormonal aspects of ESRF has, in the past, still resulted in poor final adult height, so that treatment with rhGH must always be considered.

GH and malnutrition

There is accumulating evidence for indices of malnutrition being predictive of morbidity and mortality in dialysis patients. An international study recently demonstrated a prevalence of 8% severe and 33% mild to moderate malnutrition in CAPD patients [39]. Given the known anabolic effects of GH therapy, there is increasing interest in the treatment of malnutrition of ESRF in adults with rhGH. A number of small, short-term studies have been undertaken in both HD and CAPD patients, and these have shown increased IGF-1, improved nitrogen balance, and reduced phosphate and PTH levels on GH therapy [40]. Preliminary studies using IGF-1 have also commenced, although side-effects may be limiting. This is clearly an area of great promise, and it will be interesting to see whether these early results are translated into reduced morbidity and mortality.

Thyroid axis

Thyroid function tests

In common with other severe non-thyroidal illness, ESRF is associated with a number of abnormalities in thyroid function tests in the absence of overt hypothyroidism. Many of the changes in both the HD and CAPD populations are similar to the 'sick-euthyroid syndrome' (Chapter 31) with low serum levels of thyroxine (T_4) and triiodothyronine (T_3) (total, free and indices), frequently entering the hypothyroid range, alterations in serum binding proteins and high levels of circulating thyroid hormone-binding inhibitors. In contrast to the sick-euthyroid syndrome, however, levels of reverse T_3 on dialysis are usually normal or low rather than elevated, with T_4 to reverse T_3 conversion being normal. Serum thyroid-stimulating hormone (TSH) assessed by sensitive immunometric assays is higher than the normal population, but within the normal range and thus inappropriate in the presence of reduced thyroidal hormones. Studies of TSH secretion have shown attenuation of the usual evening rise, and pulsatile secretion of shorter periodicity but decreased amplitude. The TSH response to TRH is also blunted, and frequently delayed.

Thus, changes differ from other types of non-thyroidal illness, and are consistent with impaired function at both the thyroid and hypothalamic–pituitary level. Changes may, however, still be adaptive and protective in most cases, since treatment with T_3 (50 μg/day) in one study was associated with impairment in nitrogen balance in all patients (who were on a low-protein diet), and conversion to negative nitrogen balance in many cases [41]. Erythropoietin does not appear to correct the thyroid abnormalities despite a partial correction of the anaemia [2,27,42].

Goitre and hypothyroidism

Goitre and hypothyroidism are both reported with increased frequency in ESRF. In the largest study [43], a visible or palpable goitre was found in over 40% of 306 patients with ESRF, compared with 7% of controls, and the incidence of goitre increased with time on dialysis. Goitre was more common in women, and was unrelated to the presence or absence of thyroid microsomal antibodies. Suggested goitrogens include TSH, PTH and altered iodide metabolism, but the precise cause remains to be defined. In the same study [43], 2.6% of patients in ESRF were frankly hypothyroid (low free thyroxine index (FT_4I) and high TSH), compared with a population incidence of 1%, while other studies have reported hypothyroidism in nearly 10% of patients. CAPD patients have significant peritoneal losses of T_4, T_3 and free T_3, and this presumably contributes to the development of hypothyroidism if there is a low thyroid reserve. There seems to be no change in the incidence of hyperthyroidism.

Screening for thyroid function is therefore advisable in all patients with ESRF, with institution of appropriate thyroxine replacement where required. Interpretation of T_4 and T_3 levels is clearly difficult in this regard, and a sensitive TSH assay would appear to be the most appropriate screening investigation.

Adrenal axis

Multiple, and inconsistent, abnormalities of the hypothalamo-pituitary–adrenal axis have been reported in ESRF. Basal cortisol levels are generally normal, with a normal circadian rhythm, but impaired or absent responses to stress, in particular hypoglycaemia, have been widely reported. However, it is clear that in the majority of studies conventionally adequate hypoglycaemia (< 2.2 mmol/l) had not been consistently achieved. In one well-controlled study [32], the cortisol response to hypoglycaemia was, in fact, normal in the majority of patients studied, both on HD and CAPD. Two of 20 patients studied did show, however, a subnormal response (peak cortisol < 550 nmol/l) and such a 10% incidence of hypoadrenalism could clearly represent an important clinical problem.

The clinical implication of this degree of adrenal insufficiency in ESRF is the additive susceptibility to the stresses of sepsis and surgery. Patients returning to dialysis after long-term steroids for renal transplantation are known to have adrenal insufficiency [44] and a particularly high-risk subgroup are patients with systemic amyloidosis and renal impairment: seven of 16 patients in one study [45] had an abnormal response to exogenous adrenocorticotrophic hormone (ACTH) and four of 12 deaths occurred in Addisonian crisis, with hypoadrenalism probably contributing to the deaths of a further two patients. It is thus recommended that all patients with renal amyloid should have their adrenal function assessed, and if abnormal, replacement steroid therapy commenced.

Plasma ACTH levels in ESRF remain the subject of controversy, and have been described as either high or normal. Adrenal responses to exogenous ACTH are agreed to be normal, although studies using physiological rather than pharmacological doses are required. Cortisol responses to corticotrophin-releasing hormone (CRH) are blunted in both HD and CAPD patients, whereas ACTH responses are normal; however, ACTH precursors are elevated throughout [46], and the earlier finding of increased ACTH may have been due to cross-reactivity with the precursors. An earlier study also found rhEPO treatment (with partial correction of anaemia) led to higher basal and CRH-stimulated ACTH levels, but normal plasma cortisol [27]. Impaired dexamethasone suppressibility of serum cortisol is well described, but is, at least in part, due to reduced absorption of oral dexamethasone in ESRF.

Other hormones

Vasopressin

Basal arginine vasopressin (AVP), adrenaline and noradrenaline are elevated in patients with refractory haemodialysis-induced hypotension. However, patients without nausea show absent or insufficient AVP and catecholamine stimulation during acute hypotension; in contrast, patients with nausea have a dramatic elevation of AVP [47]. Autonomic neuropathy is the probable aetiology, primarily involving the afferent limb of the reflex arc from baroceptors to the central nervous system. Lysine vasopressin has been shown to decrease the number of hypotensive episodes and the amount of fluid administered for symptomatic hypotension, with no side-effects, and should thus be considered for this HD subgroup when other correctable causes have been excluded [48].

Opioid peptides

ESRF is associated with markedly elevated plasma levels of Met-enkephalin and modest elevations of β-endorphin, but no change in plasma dynorphin. Since opioids are known to stimulate prolactin secretion and inhibit gonadotrophin secretion (see Chapter 6), it is tempting to speculate that they may mediate some of the endocrine changes described above. Evidence for this proposition is, however, hard to find: naloxone fails to suppress the hyperprolactinaemia of ESRF, and extensive studies on hormonal responses to dynamic tests have failed to demonstrate clinically significant differences between patients and controls [49]. The clinically most relevant experiment of long-term administration of an orally active opioid antagonist to patients in ESRF does not appear to have been performed.

One small study has shown naloxone causing an improved haemodynamic status in the context of septic shock and acute renal failure, allowing the instigation of haemodialysis and providing time to treat the underlying source of sepsis [50]. However, others have shown that naloxone prevents the renal vasodilatory response of head-out water immersion in normal volunteers, which would be detrimental in septicaemia, and its role, if any, remains uncertain.

Other peptides

A variety of pancreatic and gut hormones are moderately elevated in ESRF including pancreatic polypeptide, gastrin, glucagon, gastrointestinal polypeptide, somatostatin, secretin and the pituitary peptide 7B2. The clinical significance of these changes remains uncertain.

Endocrinology of transplantation

Organ recipients

Successful renal transplantation results in the reversal of the majority of the endocrine abnormalities of ESRF, in particular those affecting bone, prolactin, gonadal function and growth. Patients treated with cyclosporin for immunosuppression frequently develop marked hypertrichosis, but this change does not appear to have an endocrine basis, and is not androgen dependent clinically or biochemically. Concern has arisen over potential endocrinological side-effects of cyclosporin as it has been shown to induce a reversible dose-dependent inhibition of the hypothalamo-pituitary–gonadal axis of the rat, with low testosterone, increased gonadotrophins and hyperprolactinaemia; however, the doses were considerably higher than in transplant recipients, in whom normalisation of endocrinological disturbances has been shown to be independent of the type of immunosuppression [51].

Both 'true' and 'relative' polycythaemia are well recognised in 10–15% of renal transplant recipients, the aetiology being unknown, but associated with inappropriate erythropoietin production in many patients (often from a native kidney). However, studies have shown that between 40 and 57% of these patients have undetectable erythropoietin levels, and clearly there is a multifactorial pathogenesis. Nevertheless, angiotensin-converting enzyme (ACE)-inhibitor therapy has recently been found to be effective in almost all polycythaemic renal transplant recipients, whether they have 'true' or 'relative' polycythaemia and irrespective of their erythropoietin level. Recurrence of polycythaemia develops on withdrawal of ACE inhibition. Further studies are required to define the interaction between angiotensin II, erythropoietin and other potential mediators of erythropoiesis, such as IGF-1, cytokines and androgens [52].

Serum erythropoietin may also have prognostic value for rejection outcomes in renal transplant recipients with stable graft function. In chronic rejection associated with marked anaemia and acute rejection with poor response to immunosuppression or transplant failure, low erythropoietin levels are found, while acute rejection with good outcome is associated with higher erythropoietin levels [53].

Organ donors

Most kidneys for transplantation are obtained from donors with brainstem death resulting from a variety of pathological conditions. Since brainstem function is destroyed, and cerebral circulation is absent, it seemed reasonable to assume *a priori* that such donors be pan-hypopituitary; indeed, replacement with T_3 and cortisol has been advocated by some workers. Detailed studies have revealed, however, that the situation is more complex [54]. A majority of donors have diabetes insipidus which responds to treatment with desmopressin, although a recent study has suggested its use is associated with a higher rate of primary non-function of renal allografts [55]. Thyroid function is typical of the sick-euthyroid syndrome rather than hypothyroidism. Serum cortisol is rarely undetectable, and often exceeds 550 nmol/l, but is lower than might be expected in severe illness. Other pituitary hormones show variable responses, but again are rarely undetectable. In summary, therefore, desmopressin replacement of such donors is frequently adopted, while the use of cortisol can be theoretically justified but is not of proven benefit.

Conclusion

ESRF results in severe disruption of endocrine regulation. However, there is often disagreement in the literature regarding the precise nature of endocrine abnormalities present, their aetiology, and their response to therapeutic intervention. These differences partly relate to difficulties in measurement of hormone levels in ESRF, and may reflect improving technology and specificity of assay systems, but are also a reflection of patient heterogeneity, and the differing policies and continuing evolution of therapies for the treatment of ESRF. This remains a fruitful field for endocrine investigation and intervention.

References

1 Emmanouel DS, Lindheimer MD, Katz AI. Pathogenesis of endocrine abnormalities in uremia. *Endocr Rev* 1980; **1**: 28–44.

2 Ramirez G, Bittle PA, Sanders H, Bercu BB. Hypothalamo-hypophyseal thyroid and gonadal function before and after erythropoietin therapy in dialysis patients. *J Clin Endocrinol Metab* 1992; **74**: 517–524.

3 Díez JJ, Iglesias PL, Sastre J, Gómez-Pan A, Selgas R, Martínez-Ara J, Miguel JL, Méndez J. Influence of erythropoietin on paradoxical responses of growth hormone to thyrotropin-releasing hormone in uremic patients. *Kidney Int* 1994; **46**: 1387–91.

4 Schaefer RM, Kokot F, Wernze H, Geiger H, Heidland A. Improved sexual function in hemodialysis patients on recombinant erythropoietin: a possible role for prolactin. *Clin Nephrol* 1989; **31**: 1–5.

5 Bazan JF. A novel family of growth factor receptors. *Biochem Biophys Res Commun* 1989; **164**: 788–96.

6 D'Andrea AD, Zon LI. Erythropoietin receptor. Subunit structure and activation. *J Clin Invest* 1990; **86**: 681–7.

7 McCarthy JT, Klee GG, Kao PC, Hodgson SF. Serum bioactive parathyroid hormone in hemodialysis patients. *J Clin Endocrinol Metab* 1989; **68**: 340–5.

8 Hutchison AJ, Whitehouse RW, Boulton HF *et al.* Correlation of bone histology with parathyroid hormone, vitamin D_3, and radiology in end-stage renal disease. *Kidney Int* 1993; **44**: 1071–7.

9 Pei Y, Hercz G, Greenwood C *et al.* Risk factors for renal osteodystrophy: a multivariant analysis. *J Bone Miner Res* 1995; **10**: 149–56.

10 Editorial. Low-dose Vitamin D analogues for renal osteodystrophy. *Lancet* 1989; **i**: 1364–5.

11 Rodger RS, Fletcher K, Dewar JH *et al.* Prevalence and pathogenesis of impotence in one hundred uremic men. *Uremia Invest* 1984–85; **8**: 89–96.

12 Ureña P, Eckardt K-U, Sarfati E *et al.* Serum erythropoietin and erythropoiesis in primary and secondary hyperparathyroidism: effect of parathyroidectomy. *Nephron* 1991; **59**: 384–93.

13 Handelsman DJ. Hypothalamic–pituitary gonadal dysfunction in renal failure and renal transplantation. *Endocr Rev* 1985; **6**: 151–82.

14 Veldhuis JD, Wilkowski MJ, Zwart AD *et al.* Evidence for attenuation of hypothalamic gonadotrophin-releasing hormone (GnRH) impulse strength with preservation of GnRH pulse frequency in men with chronic renal failure. *J Clin Endocrinol Metab* 1993; **76**: 648–54.

15 Teruel JL, Marcén R, Navarro JF *et al.* Evolution of serum erythropoietin after androgen administration to hemodialysis patients: a prospective study. *Nephron* 1995; **70**: 282–6.

16 Sloand JA, Schiff MJ. Beneficial effect of low-dose transdermal estrogen on bleeding time and clinical bleeding in uremia. *Am J Kidney Dis* 1995; **26**: 22–6.

17 Lim VS, Fang VS. Restoration of plasma testosterone levels in uremic men with clomiphene citrate. *J Clin Endocrinol Metab* 1976; **43**: 1370–7.

18 Martin-Malo A, Benito P, Castillo D *et al.* Effect of clomiphene citrate on hormonal profile in male hemodialysis and kidney transplant patients. *Nephron* 1993; **63**: 390–4.

19 Mahajan SK, Abbasi AA, Prasad AS, Rabbani P, Briggs WA, McDonald FD. Effect of oral zinc therapy on gonadal function in hemodialysis patients: a double blind study. *Ann Intern Med* 1982; **97**: 357–61.

20 Bonomini M, Di Paolo B, De Risio F *et al.* Effects of zinc supplementation in chronic haemodialysis patients. *Nephrol Dial Transplant* 1993; **8**: 1166–8.

21 Brook AC, Ward MK, Cook DB, Johnston DG, Watson MJ, Kerr DNS. Absence of a therapeutic effect of zinc in the sexual dysfunction of haemodialysis patients. *Lancet* 1980; **2**: 618–20.

22 Wass VJ, Wass JAH, Rees L, Edwards CRW, Ogg CS. Sex hormone changes underlying menstrual disturbances on haemodialysis. *Proc Eur Dialysis Trans Assoc* 1978; **15**: 178–85.

23 Muir JW, Besser GM, Edwards CRW *et al.* Bromocriptine improves reduced libido and potency in men receiving maintenance hemodialysis. *Clin Nephrol* 1983; **20**: 308–14.

24 Ruilope L, Garcia-Robles R, Paya C *et al.* Influence of lisuride, a dopaminergic agonist, on the sexual function of male patients with chronic renal failure. *Am J Kidney Dis* 1985; **5**: 182–5.

25 Mastrogiacomo I, De Besi L, Serafini E *et al.* Hyperprolactinemia and sexual disturbances among uremic women on hemodialysis. *Nephron* 1984; **37**: 195–9.

26 Bommer J, Kugel M, Schwöbel B, Ritz E, Barth HP, Seelig R. Improved sexual function during recombinant human erythropoietin therapy. *Nephrol Dial Transplant* 1990; **5**: 204–7.

27 Watschinger B, Watzinger U, Templ H, Spona J, Graf H, Luger A. Effect of recombinant human erythropoietin on anterior pituitary function in patients on chronic hemodialysis. *Horm Res* 1991; **36**: 22–6.

28 Steffensen G, Aa Aunsholt N. Does erythropoietin cause hormonal changes in haemodialysis patients? *Nephrol Dial Transplant* 1993; **8**: 1215–18.

29 Bernini GP, Mariotti F, Brogi G *et al.* Effects of erythropoietin administration on prolactin secretion in normal subjects. *Nephron* 1993; **65**: 522–6.

30 Powell DR, Rosenfeld RG, Baker BK, Liu F, Hintz RL. Serum somatomedin levels in adults with chronic renal failure. The importance of measuring insulin-like growth factor I (IGF-I) and IGF-II in acid-chromatographed uremic serum. *J Clin Endocrinol Metab* 1986; **63**: 1186–92.

31 Blum WF, Ranke MB, Kietzmann K, Tönshoff B, Mehls O. Growth hormone resistance and inhibition of somatomedin activity by excess of insulin-like growth factor binding protein in uraemia. *Pediatr Nephrol* 1991; **5**: 539–44.

32 Rodger RSC, Dewar JH, Turner SJ, Watson MJ, Ward MK. Anterior pituitary dysfunction in patients with chronic renal failure treated by haemodialysis or continuous ambulatory peritoneal dialysis. *Nephron* 1986; **43**: 169–72.

33 Wühl E, Haffner D, Tönshoff B, Mehls O. German Study Group for Growth Hormone Treatment in Chronic Renal Failure: Predictors of growth response to rhGH in short children before and after renal transplantation. *Kidney Int* 1993; **44**(Suppl. 43): S76–82.

34 Schaefer F, Wühl E, Haffner D, Mehls O. German Study Group for Growth Hormone Treatment in Chronic Renal Failure: Stimulation of growth by recombinant human growth hormone in children undergoing peritoneal or hemodialysis treatment. *Adv Perit Dial* 1994; **10**: 321–6.

35 Chesney RW. Growth retardation in childhood renal disease: a hormonal or nutritional problem? *Am J Nephrol* 1987; **7**: 253–6.

36 Chesney RW, Moorthy AV, Eisman JA, Tax DK, Mazess RB, De Luca HF. Increased growth after long-term oral 1,25-dihydroxyvitamin D3 in childhood renal osteodystrophy. *N Engl J Med* 1978; **298**: 238–42.

37 Chan JCM, Mcenery PT, Chinchilli VM *et al.* A prospective, double-blind study of growth failure in children with chronic renal insufficiency and the effectiveness of treatment with calcitriol versus dihydrotachysterol. *J Pediatr* 1994; **124**: 520–8.

38 Salusky IB, Goodman WG. Growth hormone and calcitriol as modifiers of bone formation in renal osteodystrophy. *Kidney Int* 1995; **48**: 657–65.

39 Young GA, Kopple JD, Lindholm B *et al.* Nutritional assessment of continuous ambulatory peritoneal dialysis patients: an international study. *Am J Kidney Dis* 1991; **17**: 462–71.

40 Blake PG. Growth hormone and malnutrition in dialysis patients. *Perit Dial Int* 1995; **15**: 210–16.

41 Lim VS, Flanigan MJ, Zavala DC, Freeman RM. Protective adaptation of low serum triiodothyronine in patients with chronic renal failure. *Kidney Int* 1985; **28**: 541–9.

42 Goffin E, Oliveira DBG, Raggatt P, Evans DB. Assessment of the thyroid function of patients undergoing regular haemodialysis. *Nephron* 1993; **65**: 568–72.

43 Kaptein EM, Quion-Verde H, Chooljian CJ *et al.* The thyroid in end-stage renal disease. *Med Balt* 1988; **67**: 187–97.

44 Rodger RSC, Watson MT, Sellars L, Wilkinson R, Ward MK, Kerr DNS. Hypothalamic–pituitary–adrenocortical suppression and recovery in renal transplant patients returning to maintenance dialysis. *Q J Med* 1986; **61**: 1039–46.

45 Danby P, Harris KPG, Williams B, Feehally J, Walls J. Adrenal dysfunction in patients with renal amyloid. *Q J Med* 1990; **76**: 915–22.

46 Grant AC, Rodger RSC, Mitchell R, Gibson S, White A, Robertson WR. Hypothalamo-pituitary–adrenal axis in uraemia; evidence for primary adrenal dysfunction? *Nephrol Dial Transplant* 1993; **8**: 307–10.

47 Friess U, Rascher W, Ritz E, Gross P. Failure of arginine-vasopressin and other pressor hormones to increase in severe recurrent dialysis hypotension. *Nephrol Dial Transplant* 1995; **10**: 1421–7.

48 Lindberg JS, Copley JB, Melton K, Wade CE, Abrams J, Goode D. Lysine vasopressin in the treatment of refractory hemodialysis-induced hypotension. *Am J Nephrol* 1990; **10**: 269–75.

49 Grzeszczak W, Kokot F, Dulawa J. Effects of naloxone administration on endocrine abnormalities in chronic renal failure. *Am J Nephrol* 1987; **7**: 93–100.

50 Duarte RR, Ali MM, Sayegh NY, Nayak P, Grace BW. Effects of naloxone infusion in patients with septic shock and renal failure: a limited experience. *Am J Nephrol* 1992; **12**: 431–6.

51 Peces R, de la Torre M, Urra JM. Pituitary-testicular function in cyclosporin-treated renal transplant patients. *Nephrol Dial Transplant* 1994; **9**: 1453–5.

52 Gaston RS, Julian BA, Curtis JJ. Posttransplant erythrocytosis: an enigma revisited. *Am J Kidney Dis* 1994; **24**: 1–11.

53 Heidenreich S, Tepel M, Fahrenkamp A, Rahn KH. Prognostic value of serum erythropoietin levels in late acute rejection of renal transplants. *Am J Kidney Dis* 1995; **25**: 775–80.

54 Howlett TA, Keogh AM, Perry L, Touzel R, Rees LH. Anterior and posterior pituitary function in brain-stem-dead donors: a possible

role for hormonal replacement therapy. *Transplantation* 1989; **47**: 828–34.

55 Hirschl MM, Matzner MP, Huber WO *et al*. Effect of desmopressin substitution during organ procurement on early renal allograft function. *Nephrol Dial Transplant* 1996; **11**: 173–6.

56 Dunkel L, Raivio T, Laine J, Holmberg C. Circulating luteinising hormone receptor inhibitor(s) in boys with chronic renal failure. *Kidney Int* 1997; **51**: 777–84.

57 Schaefer F, van Kaick B, Veldhuis JD, Stein G, Schärer K, Robertson WR, Ritz E. Changes in the kinetics and biopotency of luteinising hormone in hemodialyzed men during treatment with recombinant human erythropoietin. *J Am Soc Nephrol* 1994; **5**: 1208–15.

58 Lawrence IG, Price DE, Howlett TA, Harris KPG, Feehally J, Walls J. Erythropoietin and sexual dysfunction. *Nephrol Dial Transplant* 1997; **12**: 741–7.

59 Lawrence IG, Price DE, Howlett TA, Harris KPG, Feehally J, Walls J. Correction of impotence in the male dialysis patient. *Nephrol Dial Transplant* 1996; **11**: A151.

CHAPTER 79

Endocrine manifestations of systemic disease: the heart

R.C. Thuraisingham and A.E.G. Raine

Introduction

Traditionally, a relatively limited interface has been recognised between disorders of the heart and cardiovascular system, and those of the endocrine systems. This view has been challenged in the last decade for several reasons. An important discovery was that of atrial natriuretic peptide (ANP) by de Bold *et al.* [1], with the consequent recognition that the heart itself is an endocrine gland. Equally, there has been a growing perception that endocrine responses play a central role on the pathophysiology of heart failure and other circulatory disorders.

Endocrine abnormalities in congestive cardiac failure

It is now clear that the status of several important hormonal systems is not only modified in cardiac failure, but that these modifications are a major cause of the sodium retention and oedema that characterise congestive cardiac failure. The main systems involved include the renin–angiotensin system, the sympatho-adrenal axis, arginine vasopressin (AVP) and ANP.

Classically, the sodium retention and extracellular volume expansion of heart failure is attributed to impaired cardiac pumping ability. Renal blood flow is reduced in heart failure, but glomerular filtration rate is relatively well preserved, and thus filtration fraction, the ratio of glomerular filtration to renal perfusion, is increased. Hence, a simple explanation of sodium retention is that increased loss of glomerular ultrafiltrate results in increased oncotic pressure of plasma leaving the glomerulus via the efferent arteriole, and entering the peritubular capillar network. This favours enhanced tubular sodium and water reabsorption.

However, animal studies have shown clearly that even when impairment of ventricular function is minimal in experimental heart failure, the inability to excrete a sodium load may be dramatic, and the likeliest explanation for this is the activation of neuroendocrine systems [2]. Observations in both animal models [3] and in humans [4] have shown that activation of the renin–angiotensin–aldosterone axis occurs in recent onset or decompensated heart failure. However, the activity of this system is also dependent on sodium intake and diuretic therapy, and levels return to normal in stable chronic heart failure [5]. Increase in renin release in heart failure is assumed to occur in response to reductions in renal perfusion pressure and filtered sodium, and enhanced renal sympathetic drive: all are known stimuli for renin secretion and all occur in heart failure. Activation of this system leads to increased systemic vascular resistance through the vasoconstrictor effects of circulating angiotensin II. Of particular importance, activation of the intrarenal renin–angiotensin system leads to efferent arteriolar vasoconstriction, maintaining glomerular capillary hydrostatic pressure and glomerular filtration rate when renal perfusion is impaired by poor cardiac output [6]. Both angiotensin II and aldosterone promote renal sodium reabsorption, thus augmenting sodium retention.

Activation of the sympatho-adrenal axis is also increased in patients with congestive heart failure. Plasma levels of adrenaline and noradrenaline are increased, reflecting both an enhanced rate of firing of sympathetic nerves [7] and catecholamine release from the adrenal medulla. Plasma catecholamine levels are directly related to the degree of left-ventricular dysfunction [8]. The mechanism of the increase in efferent sympathetic activity in heart failure is very probably a result of impaired mechanoreceptor function, leading to decreased inhibition of the vasomotor centre [9]. Consequently, sympathetic activation often is marked well before hypotension and is severe enough to cause increased sympathetic outflow by normal baroreflex mechanisms.

Increased sympatho-adrenal activation will, as with renin–aldosterone system stimulation, act to maintain arterial pressure by increasing systemic vascular resistance. Concomitantly, renal vascular resistance increases with a fall in renal plasma flow. Renal sympathetic activation also increases tubular sodium and water reabsorption, an additional mechanism leading to increased blood volume. Micropuncture studies in rats with experimental heart failure induced by coronary ligation have suggested that the role of the sympathetic nervous system in maintaining renal vasoconstriction and sodium retention predominates over that of the renin system, as inhibition of angiotensin II by saralasin adds little to the effects of sympatholytic procedures [10].

Close interaction between activation of the renin and sympatho-adrenal systems in heart failure is likely, moreover, since sympathetic activation is a potent stimulus for renin release, and equally angiotensin II facilitates noradrenaline release from adrenergic neurons. Release of the vasoconstrictor peptide endothelin is also stimulated by sympathetic activation [11], and there is now evidence that there is increased activity of this peptide in patients with severe heart failure [12] with elevated levels correlating with poor prognosis [13].

Unlike the renin system, whose activity returns to normal in stable heart failure [5], plasma AVP concentrations are consistently elevated in low-output heart failure [14]. Enhanced AVP release is non-osmotic, and is triggered by falls in cardiac output and blood pressure. It acts to augment vasoconstriction and to increase water reabsorption via aquaporin water channels in the collecting duct of the kidney, resulting in hyponatraemia. The degree of hyponatraemia in heart failure correlates also with activation of the renin–angiotensin and adrenergic systems [15]. Experimental evidence in rats also suggests upregulation of aquaporin expression in chronic heart failure [53]. In some series plasma sodium concentration has proven to be a prognostic indicator in patients with severe cardiac failure, being inversely related to survival [15].

Thus, there is in heart failure activation of several different and powerful pressor and vasoconstrictor systems. The primary goal is presumably adaptive, an attempt to maintain blood pressure and thus organ perfusion as cardiac function diminishes. Nevertheless, excessive vasoconstriction clearly may result in impaired perfusion of skeletal muscle, brain, kidney and other organs, accounting for many of the symptoms of heart failure. In addition, these vasoconstrictor hormonal systems all exert specific intrarenal actions, resulting in promotion of sodium and water retention and favouring the development of oedema.

Other hormonal systems are activated in heart failure which, to a degree, may counteract the effects of these vasoconstrictors. There is enhanced local production of vasodilator prostaglandins. Dzau *et al.* [16] demonstrated a direct relationship between circulating concentrations of metabolites of the vasodilator prostaglandin E_2 (PGE_2) and PGI_2, and plasma renin activity and angiotensin II concentrations. Moreover, an inverse relationship between serum sodium concentration and plasma PGE_2 metabolites was also observed. The functional importance of generation of vasodilator prostaglandins is emphasised by the marked decreases in renal blood flow and glomerular filtration which follow the administration of non-steroidal anti-inflammatory agents in patients with heart failure, whereas these drugs have little or no effect on renal function in normal subjects [2]. Recently, abnormalities of the nitric oxide (NO) system have also been demonstrated in cardiac failure. Levels of plasma nitrate, the stable breakdown product of NO, are elevated in patients with heart failure [17]. Moreover, administration of NO inhibitors results in larger rises in systemic vascular resistance in patients with cardiac failure compared with controls implying increased basal NO production [18], possibly to compensate for increased levels of vasoconstrictors.

Atrial natriuretic peptide

The classic studies of de Bold *et al.* [1] demonstrated the existence of a humoral natriuretic factor in atrial myocytes, and earlier work [19] had shown that the density of atrial granules, now known to store ANP, varies with salt and water intake. Proof that ANP was a circulating hormone and intimately involved in intravascular volume regulation came with the development of specific radioimmunoassays for tissue and plasma ANP [20]. The primary stimulus for atrial release of ANP is stretch of atrial myocytes, and in most instances increases in intravascular volume lead to increases in atrial pressure and distension of the atria, and thus to enhanced ANP release [21].

Atrial pressure is increased in heart failure in relation to its severity, leading to the expectation that activation of ANP will occur in this condition. In accordance, a direct relationship was found in patients with heart failure between both left and right atrial pressure and cardiac release of ANP [22], as illustrated in Fig. 79.1. Both left and right atrial myocytes make an independent contribution, via coronary venous drainage to circulating ANP, and hence it is also elevated in pure right or left heart failure.

In addition to atrial release of ANP in heart failure, it has been shown that ventricular tissue expresses messenger RNA (mRNA) for ANP, and that ventricular production of ANP becomes appreciable in congestive cardiac failure [23], although it is several orders of magnitude less than atrial synthesis. It is also known that, as well as the 28-amino-acid ANP, the heart and brain synthesise another 32-amino-acid natriuretic peptide, termed brain natriuretic peptide

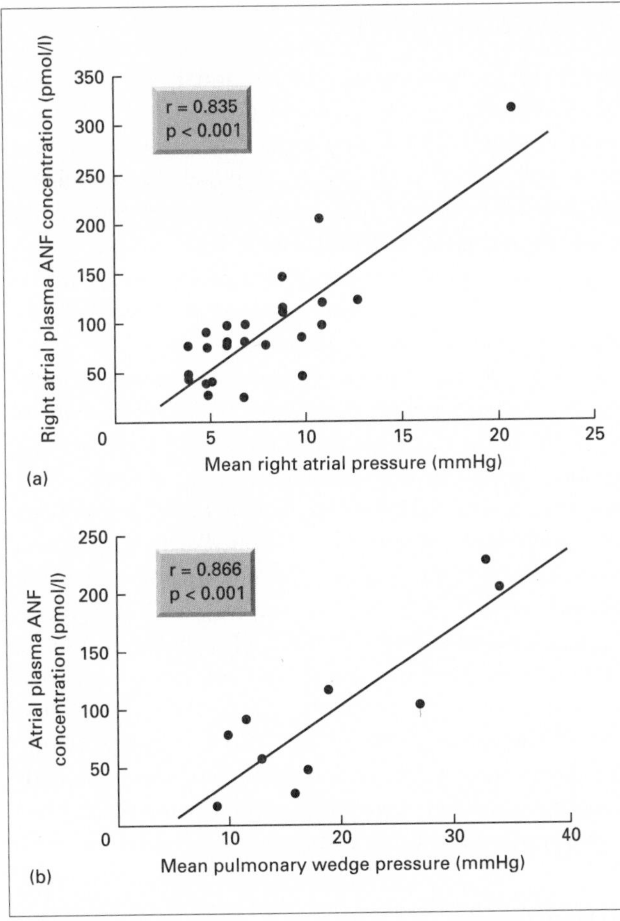

Fig. 79.1 (a) Relation between mean right atrial pressure and right atrial plasma ANF concentration in patients undergoing cardiac catheterisation. (b) Relation between mean pulmonary wedge pressure and systemic arterial plasma ANF concentration.

(BNP). The primary cardiac source of this peptide is the ventricles, contributing 60–80% of the cardiac BNP secretion [24]. Analogous to ANP, BNP secretion occurs with increased ventricular wall tension. Circulating levels of both these peptides tend to rise in parallel; however, in congestive cardiac failure BNP levels are increased some 200-fold as opposed to the 10–20 fold for ANP [25]. In hypertrophic cardiomyopathy circulating BNP levels are also elevated to a much higher degree than those of ANP [26]. More recently a further natriuretic peptide, CNP has been identified. In severe heart failure, CNP levels in the circulation are not elevated but there is increased immunohistochemical and immunoreactive CNP in the atria and ventricles of these patients, suggesting a possible paracrine role for this peptide [27]. Cytokines such as transforming growth factor-β (TGF-β), interleukin 1α (IL-1α) and tumour-necrosis factor-α (TNF-α) are known to stimulate CNP; however the significance of these findings in relation to heart failure is not known.

Enhanced ANP release appears to be an appropriate response in heart failure, the aim being to counteract sodium retention and promote sodium excretion, and to reduce vasoconstriction as ANP has direct vasorelaxant properties [28]. Despite high ANP and BNP concentrations, patients in heart failure develop sodium retention implying a blunted response to natriuretic peptides. This is borne out by clinical studies demonstrating greatly attenuated natriuretic effects of synthetic ANP when infused into patients with heart failure [29]. The explanation probably lies in the knowledge that many factors may modulate or even abolish the renal effects of ANP. Those factors impairing the renal responsiveness include activation of the renin–angiotensin and sympatho-adrenal systems, and reduction in renal perfusion pressure [30]. All of these are characteristic changes which typically accompany heart failure.

Complex interactions also exist between ANP and these other hormonal systems. For example, ANP inhibits aldosterone secretion from the zona glomerulosa and may also directly reduce renin release and inhibit central sympathetic outflow. *In vivo*, AVP, angiotensin II and adrenergic agonists have all been shown to increase plasma ANP levels, although enhanced ANP release here may well be secondary to the haemodynamic effects of these agents. In contrast, the vasoconstrictor peptide endothelin appears to stimulate the release of ANP directly, an action demonstrable in the cultured atrial myocyte [31]. This phenomenon may be explained by the ability of endothelin to increase intracellular free calcium concenration, a potent stimulus for ANP release.

ANP and other hormones in hypertension

No consistent pattern of hormonal change is seen in human essential hypertension, although many theories of the aetiology of hypertension have invoked subtle abnormalities of several hormonal systems. Laragh has advanced the hypothesis that inappropriately elevated plasma renin activity in relation to volume status underlies essential hypertension in at least a subset of patients, whereas other patients have volume-dependent hypertension with low plasma renin activity [32]. Others have, conversely, emphasised the possible role of inappropriately elevated activity of the sympatho-adrenal system in the pathogenesis of hypertension. They have shown that some young prehypertensive and early hypertensive subjects have evidence of enhanced sympathetic activation, with elevated cardiac output and raised plasma catecholamines [33]. However, in established essential hypertension there is no conclusive evidence for any consistent abnormalities of plasma catecholamines, AVP, or the renin–angiotensin aldosterone system.

There is controversy also as to whether plasma concentrations of ANP are abnormal in mild and moderate essential hypertension. In some cases, both elevated plasma ANP concentrations and a correlation of plasma ANP with systolic and diastolic blood pressure have been found [34], whereas others have observed no difference in plasma ANP levels between patients and matched normotensive controls [35,36]. However, with increasing severity of hypertension, and especially with the development of left-ventricular hypertrophy, there is a consensus that plasma ANP is elevated [37]. The likeliest explanation is a haemodynamic one; even in mild to moderate hypertension it is known that central blood volume may be increased, with accompanying small but significant increases in left and right atrial filling pressures [38]. Development of left-ventricular hypertrophy, with loss of ventricular compliance, results in more marked elevation of ventricular end-diastolic and hence atrial pressure, with a predictable increase in plasma ANP. Whether these alterations in plasma ANP are of functional significance remains unknown. However, enhanced ANP secretion may partly account for the phenomenon of 'exaggerated natriuresis' in hypertension, the enhanced sodium excretion which is known to occur when hypertensive subjects are given an intravenous sodium load. Saline challenge resulted in an exaggerated rise in plasma ANP in hyptertensives, together with augmented sodium excretion [39]. These two phenomena may be causally related, and explained by a greater elevation of atrial pressure in response to saline loading in hypertensive subjects.

In contrast to mild and moderate hypertension, there is no doubt that many hormonal systems are grossly disturbed in accelerated and malignant hypertension. It is well established that plasma concentrations of renin, angiotensin II, catecholamines and AVP may all be greatly elevated in malignant hypertension, and are restored to normal with successful treatment. The same is true of ANP, levels of which may be dramatically increased in the malignant phase, and fall with effective therapy [40]. In practice it is very difficult to dissociate these changes from those of heart failure as ventricular dysfunction is an almost automatic accompaniment of the accelerated and malignant phase. Intracellular tissue concentrations of hormones such as angiotensin II, however, may be more important in determining end-organ damage than circulating levels. Ramipril, an angiotensin-converting enzyme inhibitor with high tissue binding, protects against end-organ damage when given to a rat model of malignant hypertension at doses that do not alter systemic blood pressure or circulating angiotensin II levels [41]. This demonstrates that at least some of the pathological processes that occur in malignant hypertension may be related to hormonal derangement independent of blood pressure.

Bartter's syndrome

Bartter's syndrome is characterised by urinary potassium and chloride wasting, hypokalaemic alkalosis and normal or low blood pressure, with high plasma renin and aldosterone levels, and clinical evidence of low blood pressure. Thus, suppressed plasma ANP concentrations might be anticipated in this condition. In contrast, studies have indicated inappropriate elevations of plasma ANP in patients with Bartter's syndrome [42], together with hyporesposiveness of plasma ANP to intravenous saline challenge [43].

The pathogenesis of Bartter's syndrome remains unknown: possible causes include increased renal production of prostaglandins, and impaired sodium/potassium chloride cotransport in the thick ascending loop of Henle [44], but none is universally accepted. It is possible that inappropriately high secretion of ANP in Bartter's syndrome might in part account for some of its clinical features, including reduced pressor response to angiotensin II infusion—a known vascular effect of ANP [21] and reduction of intravascular volume. If this is the case, excessive cardiac release of ANP may be a primary event in Bartter's syndrome, contributing to its pathogenesis. This possibility remains speculative at present, and the cause of the apparently inappropriately high plasma ANP concentrations encountered in this syndrome remains unknown.

Nitric oxide

The presence of an endothelial-dependent relaxing factor was first demonstrated by Furchgott and Zawadzki in 1980 [45]. This substance was identified as NO or a closely related substance a few years later [46]. NO is produced during the conversion of L-arginine to L-citrulline in the presence of a family of enzymes (NO synthases (NOS)) present in many tissues including the vascular endothelium, where it plays an important role in the maintenance of vascular tone. When blocked with inhibitors of NOS, animals [47] and humans develop hypertension and more recently a mouse unable to express the endothelial isoform of NOS (eNOS) has been shown to be hypertensive [48]. Conversely, in hypertensive animal and human subjects impaired endothelium-dependent vasodilatation has been demonstrated [49] as has reduced total body NO production [54] but this may be a consequence and not a cause of elevated blood pressure.

Human and animal myocardium also express an isoform of NOS constitutively with similar characteristics to endothelial NOS. Its role in the heart is not clear, but there is some evidence to suggest that NO attenuates myocyte contractility [50]. In severe sepsis, the presence of lipopolysaccharide and cytokines such as TNF-α and γ-interferon result in the expression of inducible NOS (iNOS) [51], resulting in greatly increased quantities of NO in the vasculature and thus hypotension [55]. Furthermore, there is expression of iNOS in the heart in sepsis [56], which may explain the impaired cardiac function seen in septic shock. Biopsies from patients with idiopathic dilated cardiomyopathy have also shown evidence of the abnormal expression of iNOS [52].

Conclusion

The recognition that the heart is an endocrine gland, the source of natriuretic peptides, and increasing knowledge of the role of ANP in intravascular volume regulation have served to focus general attention on the humoral mechanisms in cardiovascular disease [39]. Most is known of the contribution of the hormonal systems intimately involved in fluid and electrolyte balance—the renin–aldosterone axis, AVP, the sympatho-adrenal axis and, latterly, the natriuretic peptides. It is clear now that the volume expansion and sodium retention that accompany heart failure are largely a result of activation of these hormonal systems.

No specific alteration of hormonal status characterises essential hypertension, but subtle modifications of activity of the renin–aldosterone system, the sympatho-adrenal axis, and of ANP release remain of potential interest in its pathogenesis. Of particular interest, there is the possibility that inappropriate secretion of ANP may be of relevance in specific and hitherto poorly understood conditions, such as Bartter's syndrome.

Finally, the discovery that NO plays an important role in the maintenance of cardiovascular integrity is of great interest, both in health and in diseases such as hypertension, heart failure and septic shock.

References

1 de Bold AJ, Borenstein HB, Veress AT, Sonnenberg H. A rapid and potent natriuretic response to intravenous injection of atrial myocardial extracts in rats. *Life Sci* 1981; **28**: 89–94.

2 Dzau VJ. Renal and circulatory mechanisms in congestive heart failure. *Kidney Int* 1987; **31**: 1402–15.

3 Watkins L, Jr, Burton JA, Haber E, Cant JR, Smith FW, Barger AC. The renin–angiotensin–aldosterone system in congestive failure in conscious dogs. *J Clin Invest* 1976; **57**: 1606–17.

4 Dzau VJ, Colucci WS, Hollenberg NK, Willimas GH. The relation of renin–angiotensin–aldosterone system to clinical state in congestive heart failure. *Circulation* 1981; **63**: 645–51.

5 Dzau VJ, Hollenberg NK, Willimas GH. Neurohormonal mechanisms in heart failure. Role in pathogenesis, therapy and drug tolerance. *Fed Proc* 1983; **42**: 3162–9.

6 Ichikawa I, Pfeffer JM, Pfeffer MA, Hostetter TH, Brenner BM. Role of angiotensin II in the altered renal function of congestive heart failure. *Circ Res* 1984; **55**: 669–75.

7 Leimbach WN, Wallin G, Victor RG, Aylward PE, Sundlof G, Mark AL. Direct evidence from intrarenal recordings for increased central sympathetic outflow in patients with heart failure. *Circulation* 1986; **73**: 913–19.

8 Levine TB, Francis GS, Goldsmith SR, Simon AB, Cohn JN. Activity of the sympathetic nervous system and renin–angiotensin system assessed by plasma hormone levels and their relationship to hemodynamic abnormalities in congestive heart failure. *Am J Cardiol* 1982; **49**: 1659–66.

9 Ferguson DW, Abboud FM, Marks AL. Selective impairment of baroreflex-mediated vasoconstrictor responses in patients with ventricular dysfunction. *Circulation* 1984; **69**: 451–60.

10 Kon V, Yared A, Ichikawa I. Role of renal sympathetic nerves in mediating hypoperfusion of renal cortical microcirculation in experimental congestive heart failure and acute extracellular fluid volume depletion. *J Clin Invest* 1985; **76**: 1913–20.

11 Knupfer MM, Han SP, Tropani AJ, Fok KF, Westfall TC. Regional haemodynamic and baroreflex effects of endothelin in rats. *Am J Physiol* 1989; **257**: H918–26.

12 Kiowski W, Sutsch G, Hunziker P *et al*. Evidence for endothelin-1-mediated vasoconstriction in severe chronic heart failure. *Lancet* 1995; **356**: 732–6.

13 Omland T, Bonarjee VVS, Terje Lie R, Caidahl K. Neurihumoral measurements as indicators of long-term prognosis after myocardial infarction. *Am J Cardiol* 1995; **76**: 230–5.

14 Riegger GAJ, Leibau G, Kochsiek K. Antidiuretic hormone in congestive heart failure. *Am J Med* 1982; **72**: 49–57.

15 Lee WH, Packer M. Congestive heart failure: prognostic importance of serum sodium concentration and its modification by converting-enzyme inhibition in patients with severe chronic heart failure. *Circulation* 1986; **73**: 257–67.

16 Dzau VJ, Packer M, Lilli LS, Swartz SL, Hollenberg NK, Williams GH. Prostaglandins in severe congestive heart failure: relation to activity of renin–angiotensin system and hyponatraemia. *N Engl J Med* 1984; **310**: 347–52.

17 Winlaw DS, Smythe GA, Keogh AM, Schyvens CG, Spratt PM, Macdonald PS. Increased nitric oxide production in heart failure. *Lancet* 1994; **344**: 373–4.

18 Habib F, Dutka D, Crossman D, Oakley CM, Cleland JGF. Enhanced basal nitric oxide production in heart failure: another counter-regulatory vasodilator mechanism? *Lancet* 1994; **344**: 371–3.

19 de Bold AJ. Heart atria granularity effects of changes in water–electrolyte balance. *Proc Soc Exp Biol Med* 1979; **161**: 508–11.

20 Lang RE, Tholken H, Ganten D, Luft FC, Ruskoaho H, Unger T. Atrial natriuretic factor—a circulating hormone stimulated by volume loading. *Nature* 1985; **314**: 264–6.

21 Raine AEG. Release of atrial natriuretic factor. In: Struthers AD, ed. *Atrial Natriuretic Factor*. Oxford: Blackwell Scientific Publications, 1990: 235–50.

22 Raine AEG, Erne P, Burgisser E *et al*. Atrial natriuretic peptide and atrial pressure in patients with congestive heart failure. *N Engl J Med* 1986; **315**: 533–7.

23 Franch HA, Dixon RAF, Blaine EH, Siegl PKS. Ventricular atrial natriuretic factor in the cardiomyopathic hamster model of congestive heart failure. *Circ Res* 1988; **62**: 31–6.

24 Hosoda K, Nakao K, Mukoyama M *et al*. Expression of brain natriuretic peptide gene in human heart—production in the ventricle. *Hypertension* 1991; **17**: 1152–6.

25 Mukoyama M, Nakao K, Saito Y *et al*. Human brain natriuretic peptide, a novel cardiac hormone. *Lancet* 1990; i: 801.

26 Yoshibayashi M, Kamiya T, Saito Y, Matsuo H. Increased plasma levels of brain natriuretic peptide in hypertrophic cardiomyopathy. *N Engl J Med* 1993; **329**: 433–4.

27 Wei C, Heublein D, Perrella M *et al.* Natriuretic peptide system in heart failure. *Circulation* 1993; **88**: 1004–9.
28 Bolli P, Muller FB, Linder L *et al.* The vasodilator potency of atrial natriuretic peptide in man. *Circulation* 1987; **75**: 221–8.
29 Cody RJ, Atlas SA, Laragh JH, Kubo SH *et al.* Atrial natriuretic factor in normal subjects and heart failure patients. Plasma levels and renal hormonal and hemodynamic responses to peptide infusion. *J Clin Invest* 1986; **78**: 1362–74.
30 Raine AEG, Firth JD, Ledingham JGG. Renal actions of atrial natriuretic factor. *Clin Sci* 1989; **76**: 1–8.
31 Fukuda Y, Hirata Y, Yoshimi H *et al.* Endothelin is a potent secretagogue for atrial natriuretic peptide in cultured rat atrial myocytes. *Biochem Biophys Res Commun* 1988; **115**: 167–72.
32 Laragh JH. Vasoconstriction volume analysis for understanding and treating hypertension: the use of renin and aldosterone profiles. *Am J Med* 1973; **55**: 261–74.
33 Julius S, Johnson EH. Stress, autonomic hyperactivity and essential hypertension: an enigma. *J Hypertens* 1985; **3** (Suppl. 4): S11-17.
34 Sagnella GA, Markandu ND, Shore AC, MacGregor GA. Raised circulating levels of atrial natriuretic peptides in essential hypertension. *Lancet* 1986; **i**: 179–81.
35 Larochelle P, Cussons JR, Gutkowska J *et al.* Plasma atrial natriuretic factor concentrations in essential and renovascular hypertension. *Br Med J* 1987; **294**: 1249–51.
36 Nilsson P, Lindholm L, Schersten B, Rudiger H, Melander A, Hesch RD. Atrial natriuretic peptide and blood pressure in a geographically defined population. *Lancet* 1987; **ii**: 883–5.
37 Montorsi P, Tonolo G, Polonia J, Hepburn D, Richards AM. Correlates of plasma atrial natriuretic factor in health and hypertension. *Hypertension* 1987; **10**: 570–6.
38 Tarazi RC. The role of the heart in hypertension. *Clin Sci* 1982; **63** (Suppl. 8): 347–58s.
39 Sorensen SS, Danielsen H, Amidsen A, Pedersen EB. Atrial natriuretic peptide and exaggerated natriuresis during acute hypertonic volume expansion in essential hypertension. *J Hypertens* 1989; **7**: 21–9.
40 Richards AM, Tonolo G, Tillman D, Connell JM, Hepburn D, Robertson JIS. Plasma atrial natriuretic peptide in stable and accelerated essential hypertension. *J Hypertens* 1986; **4**: 790–1.
41 Montgomery H, Whitworth C, Mullins J, McEwan J. Inhibition of angiotensin–converting enzyme prevents development of malignant hypertension at non-hypotensive doses: studies in the TGR (mRen-2d)27 rat. *Circulation* 1995; **92**: I553–4.
42 Yamada K, Tojima K, Moriwaki K *et al.* Atrial natriuretic peptide in Bartter's Syndrome. *Lancet* 1986; **i**: 273.
43 Tunny TJ, Gordon RD. Plasma atrial natriuretic peptide in primary aldosteronism (before and after treatment) in Bartter's and Gordon's syndrome. *Lancet* 1986; **i**: 272–3.
44 Bartter FC. On the pathogenesis of Bartter's syndrome. *Min Electrolyte Metab* 1980; **3**: 61–5.
45 Furchgott R, Zawadzki JV. The obligatory role of endothelial cells in the relaxation of arterial smooth muscle by acetylcholine. *Nature* 1980; **288**: 373–6.
46 Palmer RMJ, Ferrige AG, Moncada S. Nitric oxide release accounts for the biological activity of endothelium-derived relaxing factor. *Nature* 1987; **327**: 524–6.
47 Manning RD, Hu L, Mizelle HL, Montani J-P, Norton MW. Cardiovascular responses to long-term blockade of nitric oxide synthesis. *Hypertension* 1993; **22**: 40–8.
48 Huang PL, Huang Z, Mashimo H *et al.* Hypertension in mice lacking the gene for endothelial nitric oxide synthase. *Nature* 1995; **377**: 239–42.
49 Calver A, Collier J, Moncada S, Vallance P. Effect of local intra-arterial N^G-monomethyl-L-arginine in patients with hypertension: nitric oxide dilator mechanism appears abnormal. *J Hypertens* 1992; **10**: 1025–31.
50 Finkel MS, Oddis CV, Jacob TD, Watkins SC, Hattler BG, Simmons RL. Negative ionotropic effects of cytokines on the heart mediated by nitric oxide. *Science* 1992; **257**: 387–9.
51 Szabo C, Salzman AL, Ischiropolous H. Endotoxin triggers the expression of an inducible isoform of nitric oxide synthase and the formation of peroxynitrite in the rat *in vivo*. *FEBS Lett* 1995; **363**: 235–8.
52 de Belder AJ, Radomski MW, Why HJF *et al.* Nitric oxide synthase activities in human myocardium. *Lancet* 1993; **341**: 84–5.
53 Xu D-L, Martin P-Y, Ohara M *et al.* Up regulation of aquaporin-2 water channel expression in chronic heart failure rat. *J Clin Invest* 1997; **99**: 1500–5.
54 Forte P, Copland M, Smith LM *et al.* Basal nitric oxide synthesis in essential hypertension. *Lancet* 1997; **349**: 837–42.
55 Petros A, Bennet D, Vallance P. Effect of nitric oxide synthase inhibitors on hypotension in patients with septic shock. *Lancet* 1991; **338**: 1557–8.
56 Balligand J-L, Ungureanu D, Kelly RA *et al.* Abnormal contractile function due to induction of nitric oxide synthesis in rat cardiac myocytes follows exposure to activated macrophage-conditioned medium. *J Clin Invest* 1993; **91**: 2314–19.

CHAPTER 80

Endocrine manifestations of systemic disease: the lungs

J.C. Moore-Gillon

Introduction

The endocrine manifestations of respiratory tract malignancy are far more widely recognised than are endocrine problems occurring in association with non-malignant respiratory conditions. We expect, however, alterations in hormonal secretion in response to changes in the internal milieu, and it should thus be predictable and unsurprising if respiratory disturbance and its accompanying hypoxaemia and alterations in acid–base balance were to cause alterations in hormonal secretion.

With only one or two notable exceptions, research in this field has been relatively neglected. One particular difficulty is that people with chronic lung disease are in an extremely unstable state. They are subject to frequent exacerbations (often infective) of their condition. In addition to these 'macrodisturbances' of their respiratory status, they may have alterations in degree of oxygenation from hour to hour and, indeed, from minute to minute even when apparently clinically stable. In normal subjects, lung and arterial Po_2 are on the flat upper part of the haemoglobin/oxygen dissociation curve. Minor fluctuations in Po_2 thus make little difference to carriage of oxygen by haemoglobin, the largest determinant of blood oxygen content. By comparison, individuals with lung disease live on the steep and slippery slope of the oxygen/haemoglobin dissociation curve where very small—and short lived—changes in arterial Po_2 can make major changes to the amount of oxygen available for delivery to tissues, including endocrine sensors and effectors.

Perhaps because of these difficulties, much of our knowledge of the effects upon the endocrine system of hypoxia are derived from investigation of apparently healthy individuals at actual or stimulated high altitude, and from animal models of hypoxic disease using hypobaric chambers. Such studies are only approximations to the situation pertaining in chronic lung disease, the most obvious difference being that hypobaric human subjects and animals will be hypocapnic whilst many people with lung disease will be hypercapnic. It is only with the development of reliable oximeters, which can produce a continuous record of oxygen saturation, that real strides have been made in identifying and understanding the endocrine problems in such individuals. In this chapter, the principal respiratory disorders associated with endocrine disturbance are outlined, and the major endocrine systems where such effects have been found are then considered in turn.

Respiratory disorders

Chronic obstructive pulmonary disease

Description of the syndrome characterised by irreversible limitation of airflow within the lungs is hampered by semantic difficulties. Strictly, chronic bronchitis simply means chronic mucus hypersecretion, and may not be associated with airflow limitation. Emphysema is dilatation and destruction of airspaces beyond the terminal bronchioles. The most common cause of both chronic bronchitis and emphysema, smoking tobacco, also leads to narrowing and fibrotic changes in airways smaller than those affected by bronchitis and larger than those affected in emphysema. Chronic obstructive pulmonary disease (COPD) was introduced as a blanket term to describe individuals with largely irreversible limitation to airflow due to unspecified combinations of these conditions. Synonyms for COPD are chronic obstructive airways disease (COAD) and chronic airflow limitation.

In COPD there is mismatching between pulmonary ventilation and perfusion, which tends to disturb blood gases and acid–base balance. Individuals with COPD may have normal blood gases (albeit at the cost of increased respiratory effort), may have hypoxia with normal arterial Pco_2 (type I respiratory failure), or may have both hypoxia and hypercapnia (type II respiratory failure). It is in patients with type II respiratory failure that endocrine effects have been most studied.

Respiratory dysfunction due to musculoskeletal disorders

Subjects with muscular weakness or skeletal deformities such as kyphoscoliosis may develop type II respiratory failure. It is thought that hypoventilation during sleep leads to a progressive 'resetting' of the medullary receptors responsible for the maintenance of normocapnia. As in patients with type II failure due to COPD, these individuals rely largely upon stimulation of receptors sensitive to hypoxia (principally within the carotid body) to maintain their respiratory drive. Although little studied, endocrine disturbance is likely to be similar to that found in COPD.

Abnormalities of breathing during sleep

Sleep-disordered breathing has seen an explosion of research interest in the past 20 years. Even in normal individuals, a fall in the tone of pharyngeal dilator muscles accompanies sleep onset. The upper airway thus narrows during inspiration, when the luminal pressure is negative. As further narrowing occurs, vibrations start and snoring is heard. In individuals with sleep apnoea, there is further narrowing still, complete obstruction occurs and airflow stops despite continued respiratory effort (an 'obstructive apnoea'). Progressive hypoxia and hypercapnia develops, stimulating arousal mechanisms. As near-wakefulness is reached, pharyngeal dilator tone is restored, the obstruction stops, and breathing resumes. This restores normoxia and normocapnia, sleep supervenes, and the whole cycle is repeated, sometimes hundreds of times each night.

Subjects with obstructive sleep apnoea (OSA) are thus subject not only to any endocrine disturbance that might occur with repetitive hypoxia and hypercapnia, but also to the consequences of gross sleep fragmentation and of the very large intrathoracic pressure swings which accompany the frustrated respiratory effort. One factor complicating the interpretation of any endocrine abnormalities found in such individuals is that many OSA sufferers are morbidly obese, weight being the principal risk factor for the development of the syndrome.

Endocrine function in respiratory disorders

Gonadal function

The occurrence of erectile impotence in men with COPD has long been recognised. The attribution of this to decreased gonadal function specifically in response to hypoxia is not, however, straightforward. The COPD population is elderly, often has other medical problems (most particularly vascular disease), and some individuals may be receiving chronic glucocorticoid treatment. Semple *et al.* found serum testosterone levels lower in chronically hypoxic men with COPD than in age-matched controls, the levels being correlated with the degree of hypoxia [1,2]. Gosney reported Leydig-cell atrophy in the testes of men with COPD, but without information as to whether such individuals were hypoxic in life [3]. However, data as to whether this is a primarily hypothalamic, pituitary or gonadal disorder are few, and the locus of the disorder is thus unclear.

Aasebo *et al.* investigated 19 chronically hypoxic patients with impotence, giving seven of them oxygen for 24 hours and 12 of them oxygen for 1 month [4]. There was no control group. Five of the 12 individuals in the subjects treated for 1 month experienced a return of morning erections. In these five 'responders', there were significant rises in testosterone and falls in sex hormone-binding globulin (SHBG); no significant changes were seen in the seven 'non-responders' treated for 1 month, nor in any of the group treated for only 24 hours.

Testosterone levels are also depressed in patients with obstructive sleep apnoea, and may be improved by treatment with a continuous positive airways pressure (CPAP) mask, which prevents the apnoeic and hypopnoeic episodes and their accompanying arousals [5].

Growth hormone

In normal subjects the secretion of growth hormone is closely related to the sleep–wake cycle (see Chapter 6). In OSA, the disruption of normal sleep architecture, and the relative absence of slow-wave sleep, leads to decreased growth hormone (GH) secretion [6]. Treatment with CPAP restores normal patterns of GH secretion [7,8]. Impaired growth in children with adenotonsillar hypertrophy was, in the early and middle years of this century, attributed to 'chronic sepsis' and regarded as an indication for adenotonsillectomy. The demonstration of sleep apnoea in many such children, and the demonstration of 'catch-up' growth in them after operation, suggests that impaired GH secretion due to the sleep fragmentation may have been the responsible mechanism.

Unexpectedly high GH levels may occasionally be found in patients with OSA, because the macroglossia and increased pharyngeal soft tissue of acromegaly is a strong risk factor for OSA and the association between the two conditions is well recognised [9,28]. In one group of individuals with the two conditions, treatment with octreotide not only reduced GH levels but also improved measurements of oxygen saturation and sleep quality, and subjective daytime sleepiness [10].

Fluid and electrolyte balance

Fluid retention may occur in chronic lung disease, particularly where there is hypercapnia in association with hypoxia. It thus occurs in individuals with type II respiratory failure due to musculoskeletal deformity and weakness, as well as those with COPD. Impaired sodium and water homeostasis in COPD is multifactorial, and apart from strictly hormonal factors may involve autonomic dysfunction as well as changes in renal blood flow and glomerular filtration rate (GFR) [11,12]. The appearance and disappearance of oedema during and after exacerbations of the underlying lung disease may, in some cases, be due to a redistribution between intravascular and extravascular compartments rather than a change in whole-body water content [13]. In patients with obstructive sleep apnoea, there is increased salt and water excretion at night, and again this is likely to be multifactorial in origin [14].

Raised plasma atrial natriuretic peptide (ANP) levels are found in individuals with hypoxic COPD, more particularly when there is oedema present [15,16]. There is evidence that these raised ANP levels selectively reduce right-ventricular afterload, and thus may be beneficial in these patients [17]. In patients with obstructive sleep apnoea, the usual nadir of plasma ANP levels in the early hours of the morning is abolished. It is restored by CPAP [18] but not by overnight oxygen [19], suggesting that atrial distension by the high intrathoracic pressure swings in OSA may be at least as relevant as distension due to transient hypoxic pulmonary hypertension.

Secretion of vasopressin is depressed at night in patients with OSA [20] contributing to their nocturnal diuresis. In chronic hypoxic COPD, plasma levels may be inappropriately raised for osmolality [12]. Whilst the syndrome of inappropriate antidiuresis is most commonly recognised with malignant tumours of the lung, it has been reported in many other respiratory conditions, including pneumonia, tuberculosis and acute severe asthma [21]. The mechanisms influencing the renin–angiotensin–aldosterone system are considered in detail in Chapter 79. Although disturbance of this axis is undoubtedly present in COPD [11,22], such individuals appear in addition to have depressed renal function unrelated to its activation [12,23].

Calcium metabolism

The lungs are the most common organ to be affected by sarcoid, and even when plain radiography suggests that only hilar lymph-gland enlargement is present, more detailed investigation often demonstrates the typical non-caseating granulomas in the lung parenchyma. Hypercalciuria occurs at some stage in up to 50% of patients with sarcoid, and hypercalcaemia in up to 10% [24]. Alveolar pulmonary macrophages, and macrophages within the sarcoid granulomas produce 1,25-$(OH)_2D_3$ without the action of renal 1α-hydroxylase. The 1α-hydroxylation occurring in sarcoid is poorly inhibited by 1,25-$(OH)_2D_3$ itself, and apparently uninfluenced by parathyroid hormone (PTH), calcium or phosphate [25–27]. It is inhibited by glucocorticoids, which are the usual treatment for hypercalcaemia occurring in sarcoid. Rarely, similar abnormalities of calcium metabolism are seen in other pulmonary granulomatous disorders, including tuberculosis.

Conclusions

At least 5% of the general population has a significant long-term respiratory disorder. Respiratory abnormalities during sleep (a period occupying 25% of the life even of doctors!) are extremely common. The influences of respiratory function upon hormonal secretion, during both sleep and wakefulness, have been largely neglected. Enough, however, has been discovered to show that profound effects do occur and that this is an unjustifiably ignored area. Modern investigatory techniques, which enable non-invasive yet quantitative and continuous measurements of oxygenation, should ensure rapid advances in our understanding of this field.

References

1 Semple Pd'A, Beastall GH, Watson WS, Hume R. Serum testosterone depression associated with hypoxia in respiratory failure. *Clin Sci* 1980; **58**: 105–6.

2 Semple Pd'A, Beastall GH, Watson WS, Hume R. Hypothalamic–pituitary dysfunction in respiratory hypoxia. *Thorax* 1981; **36**: 605–9.

3 Gosney R. Atrophy of Leydig cells in the testes of men with longstanding chronic bronchitis and emphysema. *Thorax* 1987; **42**: 615–19.

4 Aasebo U, Gyltnes A, Bremnes R, Aakvaag A, Slordal L. Reversal of sexual impotence in male patients with chronic obstructive pulmonary disease and hypoxemia with long term oxygen therapy. *J Steroid Biochem Mol Biol* 1993; **46**: 799–803.

5 Santamaria JD, Prior JC, Fleetham JA. Reversible reproductive dysfunction in men with obstructive sleep apnoea. *Clin Endocrinol* 1988; **28**: 461–70.

6 Grunstein RR, Handelsman DJ, Lawrence SJ, Blackwell C, Caterson ID, Sullivan CE. Neuroendocrine dysfunction in sleep apnea: reversal by continuous positive airways pressure therapy. *J Clin Endocrinol Metab* 1989; **68**: 352–8.

7 Saini J, Krieger J, Blandenberger G, Wittersheim G, Simon C, Follenius H. Continuous positive airways pressure treatment. Effects

on growth hormone, insulin and glucose profiles in obstructive sleep apnea patients. *Horm Metab Res* 1993; **25**: 375–81.

8 Cooper BG, White JE, Ashworth LA, Alberti KG, Gibson GJ. Hormonal and metabolic profiles in subjects with obstructive sleep apnea syndrome and the acute effects of nasal continuous positive airway pressure (CPAP) treatment. *Sleep* 1995; **18**: 172–9.

9 Perks WH, Horrocks PM, Cooper RA *et al.* Sleep apnoea in acromegaly. *Br Med J* 1980; **280**: 894–7.

10 Grunstein RR, Ho KK, Sullivan CE. Effect of octreotide, a somatostatin analog, on sleep apnea in patients with acromegaly. *Ann Intern Med* 1994; **121**: 478–83.

11 Anand IS, Chandrashekhar Y, Ferrari R *et al.* Pathogenesis of congestive state in chronic obstructive pulmonary disease. Studies of body water and sodium, renal function, haemodynamics, and plasma hormones during oedema and after recovery. *Circulation* 1992; **86**: 12–21.

12 Stewart AG, Waterhouse JC, Billings CG, Baylis PH, Howard P. Hormonal, renal and autonomic nerve factors involved in the excretion of sodium and water during dynamic salt and water loading in hypoxaemic chronic obstructive pulmonary disease. *Thorax* 1995; **50**: 838–45.

13 Campbell RH, Brand HL, Cox JR. Howard P. Body weight and body water in chronic cor pulmonale. *Clin Sci* 1975; **49**: 323–5.

14 Warley AR, Stradling JR. Abnormal diurnal variation in salt and water excretion in patients with obstructive sleep apnoea. *Clin Sci* 1988; **74**: 183–5.

15 Skwarski K, Lee M, Turnbull L, MacNee W. Atrial natriuretic peptide in stable and decompensated chronic obstructive pulmonary disease. *Thorax* 1993; **48**: 730–5.

16 Nardini S. Atrial natriuretic peptide and COPD. *Monaldi Arch Chest Dis* 1995; **50**: 67–8.

17 Rogers TK, Sheedy W, Waterhouse J, Howard P, Morice AH. Haemodynamic effects of atrial natriuretic peptide in chronic obstructive pulmonary disease. *Thorax* 1994; **49**: 233–9.

18 Lin CC, Isan KW, Lin CY. Plasma levels of atrial natriuretic factor in moderate to severe obstructive sleep apnoea syndrome. *Sleep* 1993; **16**: 37–9.

19 Mackay TW, Fitzpatrick MF, Freestone S, Lee MR, Douglas NJ. Atrial natriuretic peptide levels in the sleep apnoea/hypopnoea syndrome. *Thorax* 1994; **49**: 920–1.

20 Ichioka M, Hirata Y, Inase N *et al.* Changes of circulating atrial natriuretic peptide and antidiuretic hormone in obstructive sleep apnoea syndrome. *Respiration* 1992; **53**: 164–8.

21 Dawson KP, Fergusson DM, West J, Wynne C, Sadler WA. Acute asthma and antidiuretic hormone secretion. *Thorax* 1983; **38**: 589–91.

22 Piperno D, Pacheco Y, Hosni R *et al.* Increased levels of atrial natriureteic factor, renin activity and leukotriene C4 in chronic obstructive pulmonary disease. *Chest* 1993; **104**: 454–9.

23 Adnot S, Sediame S, Defouilloy C *et al.* Role of atrial natriuretic factor in impaired sodium excretion of normocapnic and hypercapnic patients with chronic obstructive lung disease. *Am Rev Respir Dis* 1993; **148**: 1049–55.

24 Adams JS. Vitamin D metabolite-mediated hypercalcaemia. *Endocrinol Metab Clin North Am* 1989; **18**: 765–78.

25 Adams JS, Sharma OP, Diz MM, Endres DB. Ketoconazole decreases the serum 1,25 dihydroxyvitamin D and calcium concentration in sarcoidosis associated hypercalcaemia. *J Clin Endocrinol Metab* 1990; **70**: 1090–95.

26 Barbour GL, Coburn JW, Slatolpsky E, Norman AW, Horst RL. Hypercalcaemia in an anephric patient with sarcoidosis. Evidence for extrarenal generation of 1.25 hydroxy vitamin D. *N Engl J Med* 1981; **305**: 440–3.

27 Montagnani M, Gonnelli S, Zacchei F *et al.* Calcium–phosphorus metabolism in sarcoidosis. *Sarcoidosis* 1993; **10**: 150–1.

28 Rosenow F, Reuter S, Deuss U, Hilgers RD, Winkelman W, Heiss WD. Sleep apnoea in treated acromegaly: relative frequency and predisposing factors. *Clin Endocrinol* 1996; **45**: 563–9.

CHAPTER 81

Endocrine manifestations in haemoglobinopathies

B. Wonke and V. De Sanctis

Introduction

The haemoglobinopathies is the collective term for inherited disorders of haemoglobin, of which thalassaemias (β-thalassaemia major, intermedia and haemoglobin (Hb)E/β-thalassaemia) and sickle-cell syndrome (sickle-cell disease, sickle β-thalassaemia, sickle-cell C disease) are the commonest causes of clinical problems. 260 000 children are born yearly with a major haemoglobinopathy: 20% with thalassaemia and 80% with the sickle-cell syndrome [1]. In Europe (including the former Soviet Union) more than 1500 infants are born yearly with β-thalassaemia major. The number of patients surviving stands at over 11 000 and this number is increasing. The inheritance is through symptomless carriers (heterozygotes) in a Mendelian recessive manner.

Haemoglobinopathies are endemic in southern Europe, the Middle East, the Indian subcontinent and South-East Asia, but due to migration they are now common throughout the world and rank amongst the commonest inherited diseases in many urban areas.

β-Thalassaemia major

Patients with β-thalassaemia major are healthy at birth, but develop severe anaemia before the age of 2 years requiring regular monthly blood transfusions throughout their life to maintain a mean Hb concentration of about 12–12.5 g/dl. Without diagnosis and treatment most die from anaemia or infection before 2–5 years of age, although a few with a milder disease, thalassaemia intermedia, survive into adult life.

For the prevention and/or treatment of transfusional iron overload, intravenous intramuscular or subcutaneous iron chelation with desferrioxamine mesylate (DF) are given. This treatment is burdensome, expensive and life-long, and is only available in developed countries. To our knowledge not more than 15 000 thalassaemia patients are receiving this treatment modality. The major endocrine problem in these patients is due to iron overload secondary to the blood transfusions. The actuarial predicted survival of 239 thalassaemia major patients, most of whom began chelation with subcutaneous DF between 1977 and 1978 in London is 80% to 35 years of age (Fig. 81.1) (B. Wonke, personal data). Causes of death in 17 thalassaemia major patients were: cardiac failure 60%, infections 20%, bone-marrow transplantation-related complications 13% and liver failure in the others. The age distribution of the 222 currently surviving thalassaemia major patients in the Whittington hospital in London are shown in Fig. 81.2.

Most of the complications in thalassaemia major are attributable to tissue hypoxia (in the presence of anaemia), transfusional iron overload and transfusion-transmitted viral diseases.

In iron overload, excess iron may be deposited in all tissues [2] (Table 81.1). The toxicity of iron to the tissue cells is a complex process involving free-radical formation and lipid peroxidation resulting in mitochondrial, lysosomal and sarcolemmal membrane damage [3] (Fig. 81.3).

Endocrine abnormalities

Growth

The causes of short stature in patients with thalassaemia major are complex and multifactorial. Chronic hypoxia secondary to anaemia (when pretransfusion Hb level is <8.5 g/dl) [4], growth hormone (GH) insufficiency [5], defective hepatic biosynthesis of somatomedin (insulin-like growth factor 1 (IGF-1) [6] and sex steroid deficiency are the principal responsible factors. A list of the classifications of the GH–IGF-1 disorders is given in Table 81.2.

High doses or hypersensitivity to DF in therapeutic doses may also result in growth retardation. It is known that DF

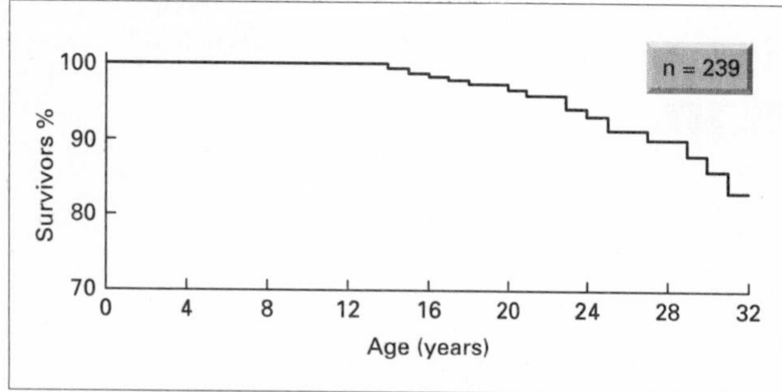

Fig. 81.1 Actuarial survival (Kaplan–Maier plot) of 239 thalassaemia major patients attending the Whittington and Royal Free Hospitals in London.

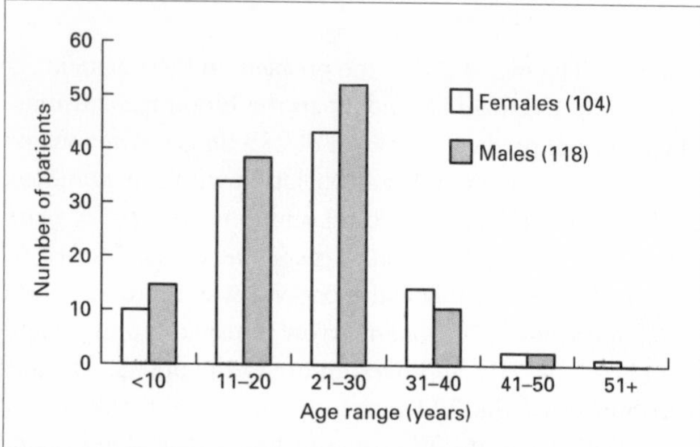

Fig. 81.2 Age distribution of 222 thalassaemic major patients in London.

Table 81.1 Iron concentration measured by atomic absorption spectrophotometry in tissue from a 42-year-old thalassaemia patient.

Tissue	Iron concentration (μg/100 mg dry tissue)
Pancreas	2860
Hypophysis	2070
Liver	1710
Myocardium	77
Duodenum	53
Testicle	46
Kidney	32
Skin	21

Table 81.2 Causes of short stature in thalassaemia major.

Chronic anaemia
Folate deficiency
Hypersplenism
Hypothyroidism
Delayed/arrested puberty
Growth hormone insufficiency
Growth hormone resistance
Chronic liver disease
Zinc deficiency
Desferrioxamine mesylate toxicity
Emotional (psychosocial) stress
Corticosteroid administration after bone-marrow transplantation

inhibits DNA synthesis, fibroblast proliferation, collagen formation and may also cause zinc deficiency [7]. The toxic effects of DF may result in painful hips, lower back and wrists, and sometimes walking difficulties.

The body measurements of both children and adults are disproportionate. Characteristically, they have a short trunk with discrepancy between pubis–heel and crown–pubis and span measurements [4]. Swelling of the wrists and knees and genu valgum of variable severity are often found. These

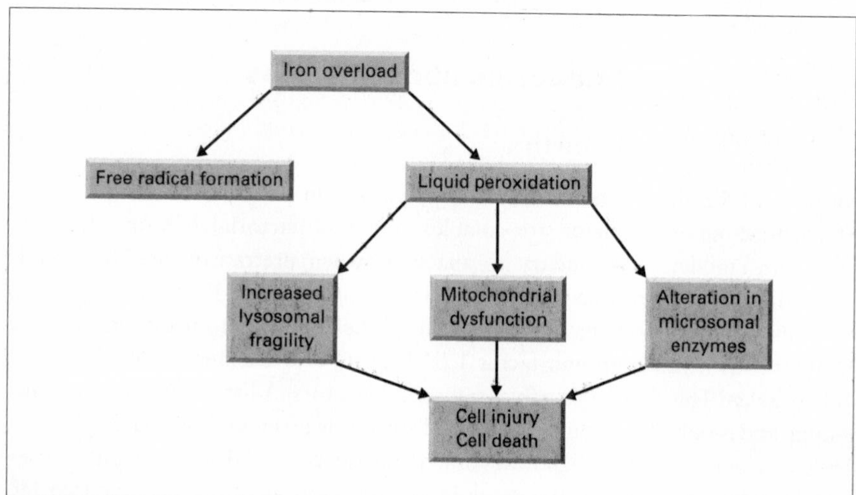

Fig. 81.3 Pathophysiological mechanism of cellular injury in thalassaemia.

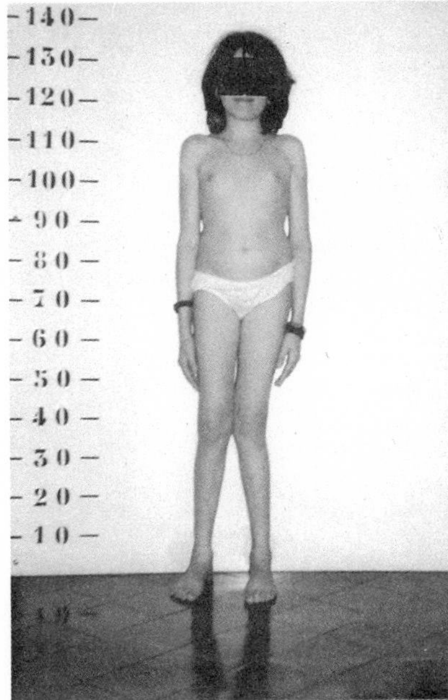

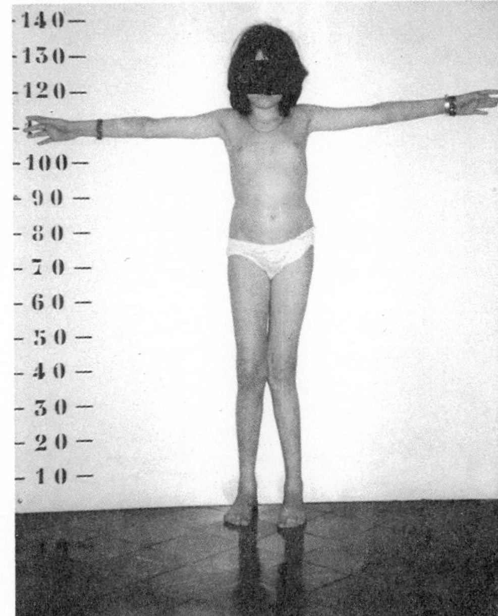

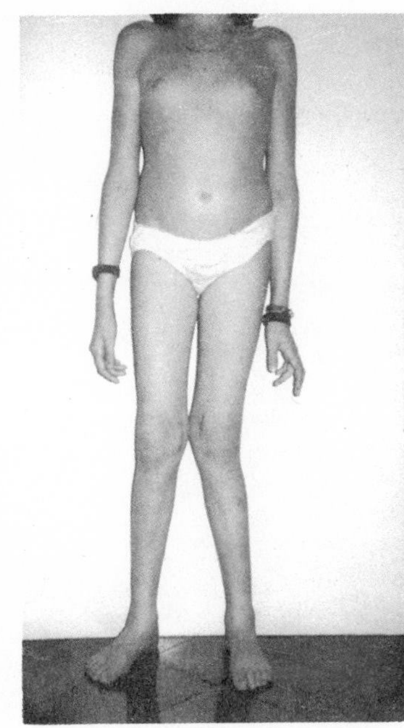

Fig. 81.4 A 12-year-old thalassaemic girl showing short trunk, disproportionately long arms and legs, genu valgum and short stature. Sexual development Tanner stage 3.

patients almost always have a normal onset of puberty and pubertal development (Fig. 81.4).

Investigation of a thalassaemic child with short stature is not different to that of a non-thalassaemic. In addition to the routine investigations for stunted growth we recommend assessment of serum ferritin, iron balance studies and overall mean Hb levels. In patients with DF toxicity serum ferritin levels are usually, but not invariably, below 1000 μg/l, the 24-hour urinary iron excretion is low, plasma zinc is low-normal, while granulocyte zinc and granulocyte alkaline phosphate activities are reduced [7]. Radiological changes are platyspondylosis of the vertebrae (Fig. 81.5a) and pseudo-rickets-like lesions of the extremities (Fig. 81.5b). Slipped femoral head, uni- or bilateral, and genu valgum (Fig. 81.5c) may also be present. Twenty per cent of these patients have neurosensorial high-tone deafness [7].

The treatment of anaemia consists of regular transfusions usually at 2–3 week intervals to maintain an overall mean Hb concentration of about 12 g/dl. GH insufficiency is treated with recombinant human GH (rhGH) given subcutaneously, self-administered daily, in doses varying from 0.6 to 0.9 iu/kg bodyweight/week. In our experience the response to treatment is variable. Less than half of patients have a good response to rhGH treatment while the remaining show poor or no response, suggesting some degree of GH resistance; chronic liver disease may contribute to this. These data also indicate that higher doses of rhGH may be required to obtain improvement in growth velocity. During treatment glucose tolerance must be controlled as thalassaemics are prone to develop an abnormality of glucose homeostasis.

In DF toxicity the drug can be replaced by deferiprone (L_1) an oral iron-chelating agent, which is licensed in India and is available in Europe and the USA on a named-patient basis or as an 'orphan' drug.

Hypothyroidism

Hypothyroidism is observed most commonly in iron-overloaded patients. In 1961 patients, the incidence of primary hypothyroidism was 6.2% [8]. Hypothyroidism develops earlier in females than in males. The female/male ratio is 1.4 : 1 and it occurs after the age of 10 years.

This endocrine complication is common in patients who are anaemic and/or poorly chelated but it is rare in patients who are well treated. In the last 9 years we have not observed any new cases of primary hypothyroidism among our group of patients.

Histologically, the thyroid gland contains large amounts of iron granules in follicular epithelium, and iron-laden macrophages can be seen in the interstitium. Fibrosis of the gland is moderate to marked.

Three types of thyroid dysfunction have been recognised in thalassaemics: preclinical, mild and overt hypothyroidism. The majority of patients have primary thyroid dysfunction; secondary hypothyroidism due to iron damage to the pituitary is very rare.

Classical symptoms of hypothyroidism in patients with preclinical or mild hypothyroidism are absent, whereas in overt hypothyroidism the whole spectrum of typical clinical features of hypothyroidism has been observed. These include

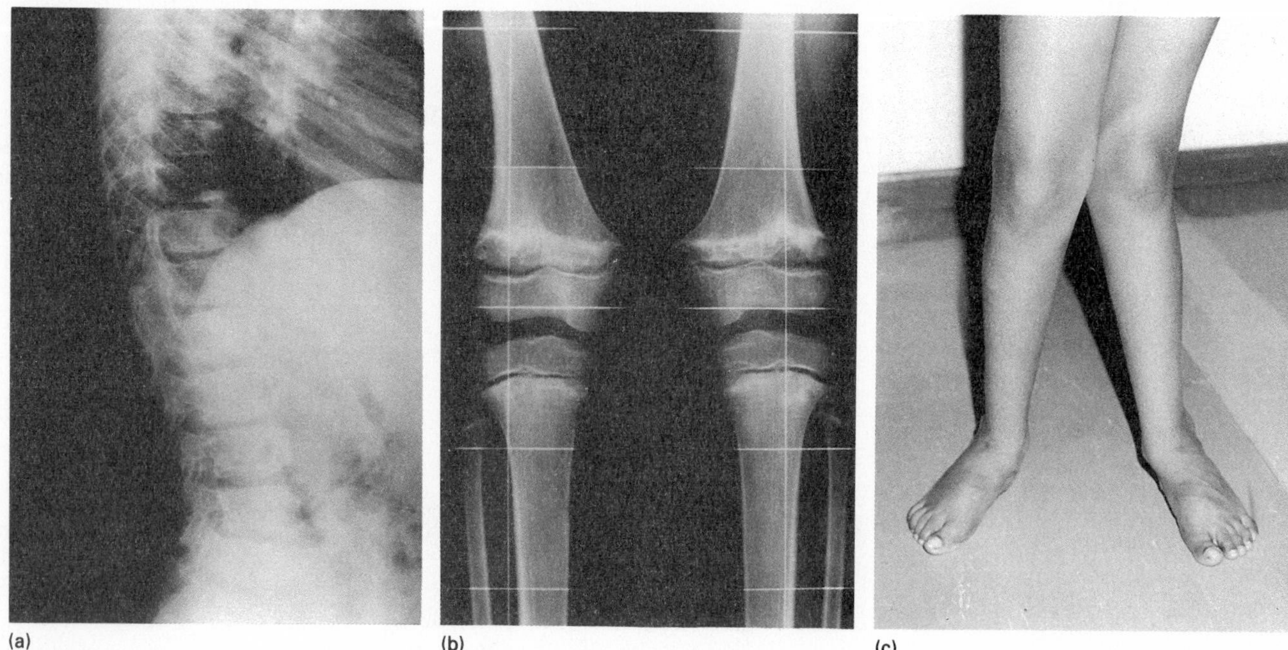

Fig. 81.5 Radiological changes found in patients with desferrioxamine toxicity. (a) Platyspondylosis of the vertebrae; (b) pseudo-rickets-like lesions of the lower extremities; (c) genu valgum.

growth retardation, decreased activity, dry skin, cardiac failure and pericardial effusion (Fig. 81.6). The thyroid gland is usually not enlarged.

Biochemically, serum thyroid-stimulating hormone (TSH) is elevated, and the TSH response to thyrotrophin-releasing hormone (TRH) is proportional to the baseline serum TSH concentration. Serum thyroglobulin estimation in conjunction with thyroxine (T_4) and TSH helps to detect preclinical or mild hypothyroidism (88% of patients have increased thyroglobulin levels). The increased thyroglobulin level could reflect the alteration of thyroid cell structure due to iron overload, which allows thyroglobulin to cross cell membranes and enter into the circulation. Classically, in thalassaemics with primary hypothyroidism antibodies against the thyroglobulin and microsomal components are absent. Thyroid ultrasonography shows a homogeneous echo pattern with thickening of the thyroid capsule. The electrocardiogram (ECG) shows a prolonged QT interval and in patients with pericardial effusion low ECG voltages are present.

In secondary hypothyroidism serum T_4 concentrations are low and a lack of TSH response to TRH stimulation is present.

Treatment depends on the severity of the organ failure. For the severely affected patients gradual replacement

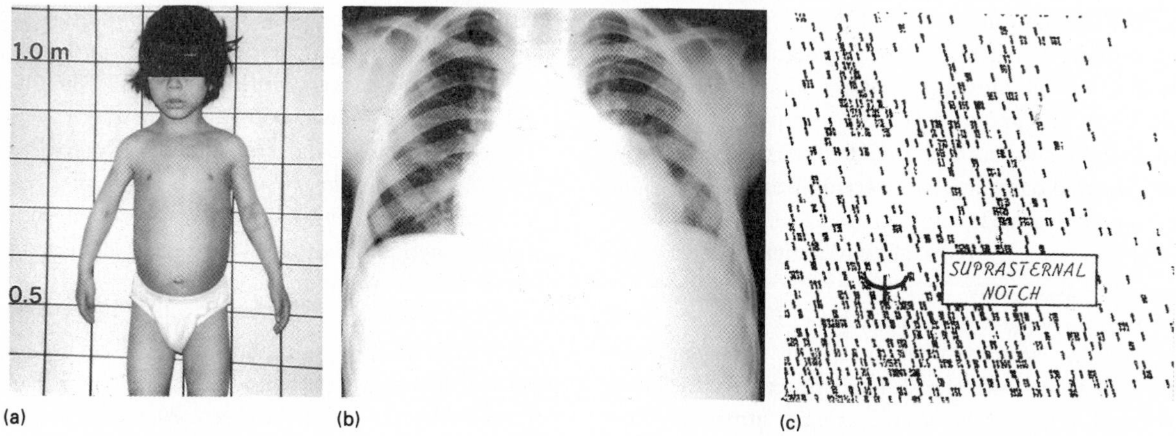

Fig. 81.6 (a) An 8-year-old iron-overloaded thalassaemic patient with primary hypothyroidism showing short stature. (b) Pericardial effusion. (c) Uneven uptake of ^{99}Tc in the thyroid gland.

therapy with L-T_4 is recommended. A starting dose of 25 µg/day L-T_4 is given for 2–3 weeks, with gradual increases of 25 µg until a maintenance dose is reached (100 µg/m²/day). In mild hypothyroidism the decision to treat depends on each individual case. In 52% of patients we have followed, intensification of iron-chelation therapy has eradicated the mild thyroid dysfunction. The remaining cases require treatment with low doses of L-T_4. Preclinical hypothyroidism requires only careful follow-up.

Low-triiodothyronine syndrome

The low-triiodothyronine (T_3) syndrome which is associated with chronic disorders (see also Chapter 31), also occurs in thalassaemics [9]. Decreased T_3 and decreased T_4 concentrations with normal TSH and normal response to TRH stimulation is the common finding. This condition does not require treatment.

Parathyroid

Hypoparathyroidism

Hypocalcaemia due to hypoparathyroidism is a recognised late complication of the iron overloaded and/or anaemic thalassaemic patient. In our experience the incidence of this complication is 3.6%. The majority present after the age of 16 years (mean age 18) and it may be associated with bone complications. Both sexes are equally affected.

Hypoparathyroidism is thought to be the consequence of iron deposition in the parathyroid glands or the suppression of parathyroid secretion induced by bone reabsorption resulting from increased haematopoiesis secondary to the chronic anaemia. Hypocalcaemia classified according to Parfitt's grading [10] showed that grade 4–5 was present in 59% of patients. This classification relates to the concentration of serum calcium values. The majority of patients have a mild disease with paraesthesiae only, while in the more severely affected tetany (Fig. 81.7) seizures or cardiac failure may occur. Spontaneous fractures due to osteoporosis, genu valgum of differing severity and short stature are the most commonly observed bone complications.

Laboratory findings are low serum calcium, increased serum phosphate, low or inappropriately normal parathyroid hormone for the serum calcium level and low levels of 1,25-dihydroxyvitamin D. Twenty-four-hour urinary calcium and phosphate excretions are reduced. Calcitonin has not been studied in this condition. Radiological changes in the bones include osteoporosis with trabecular destruction and 'cod-fish' deformities of the vertebrae.

Cardiac, hepatic and other endocrine complications are almost invariably present with hypoparathyroidism. In a large multicentre study conducted in Italy of 1861 patients, 70% had hypogonadism, 38.4% cardiac complications, 37% primary hypothyroidism and 18.4% insulin-dependent diabetes mellitus [8].

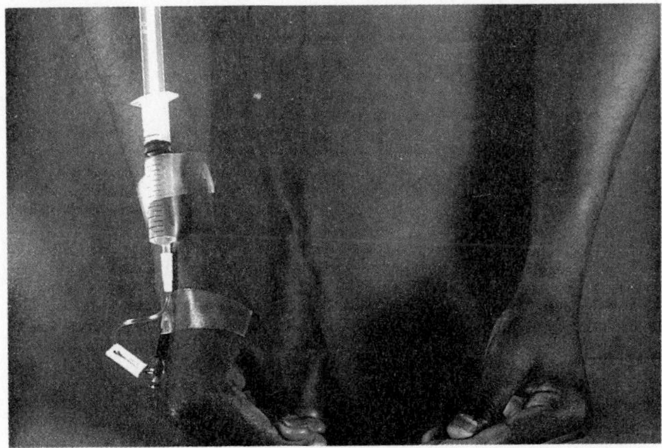

Fig. 81.7 Tetany in a 25-year-old thalassaemic man secondary to hypoparathyroidism treated with i.v. calcium.

Treatment is with oral vitamin D or one of its analogues. Some patients require high doses of vitamin D in order to normalise serum calcium levels. This should be carefully monitored as hypercalcaemia is a not uncommon complication of this treatment. Calcitriol, 0.25–1.0 µg twice daily, is usually sufficient to normalise plasma calcium and phosphate levels. At the start of treatment weekly blood tests are required, followed by 3-monthly plasma and 24-hour urinary calcium and phosphate estimations. In patients with persistently high serum phosphate levels a phosphate binder (not aluminium) should also be given. Tetany and cardiac failure due to severe hypocalcaemia require intravenous administration of calcium under careful cardiac monitoring, which is followed by oral vitamin D.

Pancreas

Carbohydrate metabolism

Impaired glucose tolerance and diabetes mellitus are frequently observed complications in patients with thalassaemia. The incidence of impaired glucose tolerance in thalassaemia major patients varies between 11 and 24%, and of diabetes mellitus 4.7–10.5% in the Mediterranean countries. In the UK the incidences are 33% and 24%, respectively [11]. There is no obvious difference between the sexes. The onset of diabetes in the majority of patients occurs after the age of 10 years.

Impaired glucose tolerance and diabetes mellitus may be the consequence of β-cell destruction secondary to iron overload, chronic liver disease, viral infection and/or genetic factors. The pathogenetic mechanism of this endocrinopathy is different compared with non-thalassaemic diabetic patients of the same age group. The difference lies in the initial disturbance of carbohydrate metabolism due to insulin resistance secondary to liver derangement leading to impaired glucose tolerance. Overt diabetes is a later event when sufficient damage to pancreatic cells has occurred and appropriate insulin secretion cannot be maintained (Fig. 81.8). In the pancreas iron deposition in the interstitial cells results in excessive collagen deposition and defective microcirculation. Impaired oxygen supply eventually leads to insulin deficiency [12]. Whilst impaired glucose tolerance is asymptomatic, diabetes mellitus itself presents with the classical symptoms, accompanied by ketosis and rarely ketoacidosis. Biochemical diabetes may be reversible with intensive iron chelation therapy, strict diabetic diet and weight reduction where applicable. In symptomatic patients insulin treatment is essential, but metabolic control can be difficult to achieve. In monitoring this group of patients fructosamine estimations are helpful, but glycosylated haemoglobin levels or urinary glucose are *un*helpful. The latter is unreliable due to increased renal glucose threshold, whilst the former is influenced by haemolysis interfering with the effect of glycosylation. The role of oral hypoglycaemic agents remains to be fully determined. Ten years ago the life expectancy of diabetic thalassaemic patients was short [13], death commonly occurred from heart failure or cirrhosis, and less frequently from acidosis or cerebral thromboembolism. At present the prognosis has improved, and 34% of diabetic thalassaemic patients are alive 8 years after the diagnosis of diabetes. Several factors have contributed to this: early identification of thalassaemic patients with impaired glucose tolerance, improvement in iron chelation therapy and early treatment of chronic liver disease. It is now recommended that oral glucose tolerance tests are performed yearly in all patients older than 10 years.

Adrenals

In iron overloaded patients a variety of abnormalities of the pituitary–adrenal axis have been reported with adreno-corticotrophic hormone (ACTH) deficiency and reduced adrenal cortical reserve [14]. Clinical adrenal deficiency is a very rare complication in well-chelated thalassaemic patients. Functional studies in a group of well-chelated and transfused thalassaemic patients have shown normal ACTH reserve as well as normal cortical responses to ACTH stimulation. It seems likely, therefore, that long-term chelation therapy protects both pituitary ACTH reserve and the capacity of the adrenal to synthesise cortisol [15].

Sexual maturation

Hypogonadism

The delayed puberty is *rare* in patients with thalassaemia major whilst hypogonadotrophic hypogonadism is the commonest endocrine complication (Table 81.3). In a recent study, failure of puberty was present in 51% of males and 47% of females over the age of 15 years [8]. Transfusional

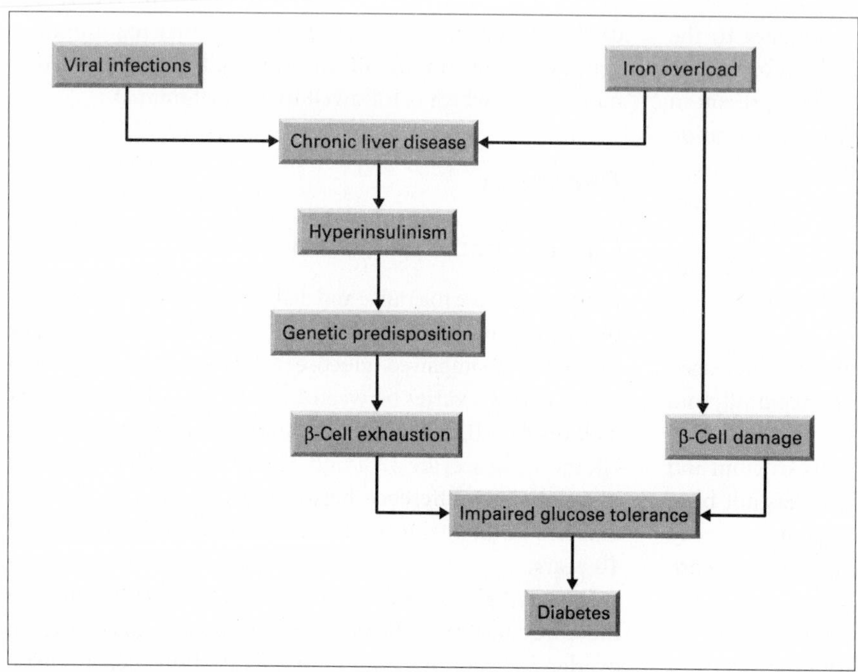

Fig. 81.8 Pathogenetic mechanisms of glucose intolerance and diabetes in thalassaemia major.

Table 81.3 Incidence of hypogonadism and primary/secondary amenorrhoea in thalassaemic female patients. Group A started desferrioxamine chelation therapy late in life; group B early in life.

Thalassaemic patients	Group A ($n = 85$)	Group B ($n = 45$)
Males	33	24
Females	52	21
Year of birth of patient	1956–73	1974–79
Primary amenorrhoea	26 (50%)	5 (23%)
Secondary amenorrhoea	13 (25%)	5 (23%)
Hypogonadism and arrested puberty (males)	22 (66.6%)	10 (41.6%)

haemosiderosis in the pituitary gonadotroph cells causing gonadotrophin deficiency is responsible for this endocrine dysfunction [16].

The anterior pituitary gland is particularly sensitive to free-radical-caused oxidative stresses, and exposure to this early in childhood results in pituitary damage. Iron deposition as measured by magnetic resonance imaging shows that even modest iron deposition within the anterior pituitary can interfere with its function.

Histological examination of the gonads shows minimal siderosis with occasional iron-containing macrophages in the ovaries and reduced number of primordial follicles (Plate 81.1, opposite p. 332). In the testes, most of the iron is deposited in the seminiferous tubules and in the interstitial tissue, and only a minimal amount in the Leydig cells (Plate 81.2). A reduction of Leydig cells and hyalinisation of basement membrane of the seminiferous tubules may also occur.

The clinical presentation of hypogonadism is variable in this patient group. Definition of delayed puberty is not different in the thalassaemic population from that of non-thalassaemics. Arrested puberty is characterised by lack of progression of puberty for 12 months or longer with reduced or absent growth velocity. In the majority of cases the testicular size remains between 6 and 8 ml and breast size is at Tanner's stage 3; pubic and axillary hair is scanty. In hypogonadotrophic hypogonadism there are no signs of puberty at the age of 16 years. Patients present with short stature and their weight corresponds to their height. If hypogonadism develops after complete pubertal maturation (secondary hypogonadism), in males this is manifested by impotence of varying degrees with absence of ejaculation and in females with secondary amenorrhoea, associated with weight gain, hot flushes, dry vagina and bone pain.

Another very characteristic clinical finding in male thalassaemic patients is the reduced beard growth that gives an immature facial appearance which has an important psychological impact on their body image.

Diagnostic findings in delayed or arrested puberty are basal plasma luteinising hormone (LH) and follicle-stimulating hormone (FSH) levels in the prepubertal range, and reduced responses of plasma gonadotrophins to gonadotrophin-releasing hormone (GnRH). Basal plasma sexual steroid levels (testosterone, 17β-oestradiol) are low. There is a normal response of plasma testosterone to human chorionic gonadotrophin (hCG) stimulation, and a normal 17β-oestradiol response to human menopausal gonadotrophin (hMG) (Pergonal) stimulation. In hypogonadotrophic hypogonadism the basal gonadotrophin responses to GnRH stimulation are reduced, and the response of plasma testosterone and 17β-oestradiol to hCG and hMG stimulation is normal or reduced. In hypogonadism the bone age is markedly delayed compared with the chronological age in both sexes. Pelvic ultrasonography shows a reduced number of ovarian follicles and reduction in the size of the uterus.

Thalassaemic patients with pubertal disorders frequently have other endocrine, hepatic and cardiac complications.

The treatment of delayed puberty, arrested puberty and hypogonadotrophic hypogonadism depends on many factors: age, severity of iron overload, damage to the hypothalamo-pituitary–gonadal axis, chronic liver disease and presence of psychological problems resulting from hypogonadism. Treatment should be withheld in the young well-chelated age group without emotional distress, but regular follow-up is essential. In teenagers with psychological problems treatment is recommended in order to minimise the risk of complete rejection of thalassaemia treatment. In girls, therapy may begin with oral ethinyl oestradiol (2.5–5 μg daily) continuously for 6 months followed by hormonal reassessment. If spontaneous puberty does not take place after months of stopping treatment, oral oestrogens are reintroduced with gradually increasing dosages (ethinyl oestradiol from 5–10 μg daily) for another 12 months. If breakthrough uterine bleeding does not occur, oral medroxyprogesterone acetate (5 mg daily) is added to the oestrogen treatment for 12 days. If bleeding occurs, this treatment may be maintained by transdermal oestrogen–progesterone patches. In males with delayed puberty, low dosages of intramuscular testosterone esters (25–50 mg) are given monthly for 6 months followed by hormonal reassessment. If no spontaneous progression has occurred, intramuscular depot-testosterone (25–50 mg) is given at shorter intervals. In patients with pubertal arrest and hypogonadotrophic hypogonadism the treatment consists of low doses of oral sex hormones as for delayed puberty. In secondary hypogonadism hormone-replacement therapy is indicated.

With the much improved survival of the thalassaemics the desire for a family is becoming an important issue. In the authors' experience, over 60 thalassaemic patients are married and of these 37 have one or more children. In 15 patients ovulation or spermatogenesis was induced by gonadotrophins [17,18]. This approach requires cooperation of haematologists, cardiologists and reproductive endocrinologists.

The treatment of pubertal disorders in thalassaemic patients is a complex issue due to the many associated complications from which these patients often suffer. Post-splenectomy, high platelet count, impaired glucose tolerance, or diabetes and chronic liver disease all may have a bearing on the decision-making process. Each patient has to be assessed individually.

Sickle-cell syndrome

Patients with sickle-cell disorders suffer from anaemia and sickling of deoxygenated red blood cells in various organs which leads to chronic organ damage and unpredictably severe morbidity and mortality. Management of sickle-cell disorders is non-specific in the majority of patients. However, a small minority require regular transfusion therapy and subcutaneous DF chelation similar to thalassaemic patients.

Diagnosis of the sickle-cell syndrome in the first few months of life, and regular medication with the appropriate education of the child's parents, have improved the overall survival. The probability of patients with sickle-cell disease surviving to the age of 20 years or more is now 85% [19].

In sickle-cell syndrome regular blood transfusions are only given to a small, select group of patients. These are children, adolescents or adults who have had strokes, women during pregnancy and patients of all ages with severe sickle-cell syndrome requiring frequent hospital admissions for life-threatening illness. A small minority of patients with this disorder suffer from endocrine complications secondary to a variety of causes.

Hypopituitarism and testicular dysfunction may be the result of vaso-occlusion. Iron overload can cause tissue damage similar to that seen in thalassaemic patients.

Growth

Growth impairment in sickle-cell patients is variable. In northern Europe and North America, due to the improved socioeconomic circumstances, medical care and nutrition, growth and development are by and large normal, whilst in Jamaica the aetiology of reduced growth in sickle-cell disease is multifactorial: delayed puberty, poor nutrition and reduced metabolic rate in response to anaemia all play an important role. The most obvious changes are reduced sitting height at the age of 16 years [20].

Sexual maturation and fertility

Delayed puberty in sickle-cell syndrome is not an uncommon finding. The mean age of menarche in a Jamaican cohort was 2.5 years delayed in sickle-cell patients compared with the controls [20]. The delayed puberty is thought to be due to constitutional delay in sexual maturation in adolescents. Zinc and folate deficiency may be contributory. Primary or secondary hypogonadism may be the result of vascular occlusion of either the central or the target organs [21]. Hormonal assessment reflects the extent and the location of the pathology. Hypothalamo-pituitary and gonadal damage may occur in the same patient.

Delayed puberty usually requires no treatment. Primary or secondary gonadal failure should be treated depending on the level of the lesion. A minority of patients are subfertile. Males with increasing age have low sperm count, subnormal sperm motility and abnormal sperm morphology [22]. Priapism is a major cause of impotence. Women may have fewer pregnancies and increased numbers of miscarriages and premature deliveries.

Blood transfusions or exchange transfusions from early pregnancy is a well-recognised treatment. There have been many trials evaluating the beneficial effects of blood transfusions during pregnancy. No universal approach has so far been adopted.

Bone-marrow transplantation in haemoglobinopathies

The only available cure for patients with thalassaemia major and sickle-cell disease is bone-marrow transplantation [23]. This treatment modality is now well established [24]. The preconditioning treatment regimen results in hypergonadotrophic hypogonadism in the majority of cases [25]. The ovarian dysfunction may be reversible [26,27]. The testicular damage affects spermatogenesis causing azoospermia or severe oligoasthenospermia.

References

1 Royal College of Physicians. *Prenatal Diagnosis and Genetic Screening* In Thalassaemia. *Community and Service Implications*. London: Royal College of Physicians, 1989.

2 Cacace E, Mela Q, Frigerio R, Sole G, Olla N, Carcassi U. Iron chelation therapy in β thalassaemia intermedia. In: Aksoy M, Birdwood GFB, eds. *Hypertransfusion and Iron Chelation in Thalassaemia*. Berne: Hans Huber Publishers, 1984: 48–61.

3 Hershko C. Biological models for studying iron chelating drugs. *Clin Haematol* 1989; **2**: 321.

4 de Sanctis V, Katz M, Vullo C, Bagni B, Ughi M, Wonke B. Effect of different treatment regimes on linear growth and final height in β-thalassaemia major. *Clin Endocrinol* 1994; **40**: 791–8.

5 Pintor C, Cella SG, Manso P *et al.* Impaired growth hormone (GH) response to GH-releasing hormone in thalassaemia major. *J Clin Endocrinol Metab* 1986; **62**: 263–7.

6 Saenger P, Schwartz E, Markenson AL *et al.* Depressed serum

somatomedin in B-thalassaemia. *J Pediatr* 1980; **96**: 214–18.

7 de Virgiliis S, Congia M, Frau F *et al*. Deferoxamine-induced growth retardation in patients with thalassaemia major. *J Pediatr* 1988; **113**: 661–9.

8 Italian Working Group on Endocrine Complications in Non-endocrine Diseases. Multicentre study on endocrine complications in thalassaemia major. *Clin Endocrinol* 1995; **42**: 581–6.

9 Sabato AR, De Sanctis V, Atti G, Capra L, Bagni B, Vullo C. Primary hypothyroidism and low T3 syndrome in thalassaemia major. *Arch Dis Child* 1983; **58**: 120–7.

10 Parfitt AM. The spectrum of hypoparathyroidism. *J Clin Endocrinol Metab* 1972; **34**: 152–6.

11 Wonke B, Hanslip JI. Glucose intolerance and diabetes in thalassaemia major. In: Ando S, Brancati C, eds. *Endocrine Disorders in Thalassaemia*. Berlin: Springer-Verlag, 1995: 65–7.

12 Iancu, TC. *Biological and Ultra Structural Aspects of Iron Overload; An Overview*. New York: Hemisphere, 1990: 251–95.

13 de Sanctis V, Zurlo MG, Senesi E, Boffa C, Cavallo L, DiGregorio F. Insulin dependent diabetes in thalassaemia. *Arch Dis Child* 1981; **63**: 58–62.

14 Costin G, Kogut MD, Hyman CB, Ortega JA. Endocrine abnormalities in thalassaemia major. *Am J Dis Child* 1979; **133**: 497–502.

15 Sklar CA, Lew LQ, Yoon DJ, David R. Adrenal function in thalassaemia major following long-term treatment with multiple transfusions and chelation therapy. *Am Dis Child* 1987; **141**: 327–30.

16 Bergeron C, Kovacs K. Pituitary siderosis. A histologic, immunocytologic and ultrastructural study. *Am J Pathol* 1978; **93**: 295–310.

17 de Sanctis V, Vullo C, Katz M, Wonke B, Nannetti C, Bagni B. Induction of spermatogenesis in thalassaemia. *Fertil Steril* 1988; 50: 969–75.

18 Jensen CE, Tuck SM, Wonke B. Fertility in β thalassaemia major: a report of 16 pregnancies, preconceptual evaluation and a review of the literature. *Br J Obstet Gynaecol* 1995; **102**: 625–9.

19 Leikin SL, Gallaher D, Kinney TR, Sloane D, Klug P, Rida W. Cooperative Study Group of Sickle Cell Disease. Mortality in children and adolescents with sickle cell disease. *Pediatrics* 1989; **84**: 500–8.

20 Singhal A, Thomas P, Cook R, Wierenga K, Serjant G. Delayed adolescent growth in homozygous sickle cell disease. *Arch Dis Child* 1994; **71**: 404–8.

21 Osegbe DN, Akinyanju OO. Testicular dysfunction in men with sickle cell disease. *Postgrad Med J* 1987; **63**: 95–8.

22 Osegbe, DN, Akinyanju OO, Amaku EO. Fertility in males with sickle cell disease. *Lancet* 1981; ii: 975–6.

23 Apperly JF. Bone marrow transplant for the haemoglobinopathies: past, present and future. *Ballière's Clin Haematol* 1993; **6**: 299–322.

24 Lucarelli G, Galimberti M, Polchi P *et al*. Marrow transplantation in patients with thalassaemia responsive to iron chelation therapy. *N Engl J Med* 1993; **329**: 840–4.

25 Manenti F, Galimberti M, Lucarelli G *et al*. Growth and endocrine function after bone marrow transplantation for thalassaemia major. *Prog Clin Biol Res* 1989; **309**: 273–80.

26 De Sanctis V, Galimberti M, Lucarelli G *et al*. Gonadal function after allogenic bone marrow transplantation for thalassaemia. *Arch Dis Child* 1991; **66**: 517–21.

27 De Sanctis V, Galimberti M, Lucarelli G *et al*. Pubertal development in thalassaemic patients after allogenic bone marrow transplantation. *Eur J Pediatr* 1993; **152**: 993–7.

CHAPTER 82

The endocrinology of mental disease

F. Holsboer

Introduction

Alterations of mood and behaviour have long been recognised as concomitant symptoms of many endocrine diseases. The association between hormones, mood and behaviour has occupied the central stage in psychiatric research, and Manfred Bleuler, after having been a research assistant of Harvey Cushing, established the concept of psychiatric endocrinology in clinical psychiatry. Since then a wealth of information has been gathered which leaves no doubt that hormones strongly influence neuronal function in the brain, which among other effects may result in a variety of behavioural changes including mood and cognition. While initially embraced with enthusiasm, the idea of treating psychiatric disorders with hormones waned after the introduction of psychotropic drugs. Over the past 20 years the focus of neuroendocrine research has moved from the psychopathology of endocrine diseases to neuroendocrine changes that concur with major psychiatric disorders. This development was enhanced by progress in all branches of neuroscience. In particular, the availability of specific probes for individual neuroendocrine systems and refinements of various bioanalytical techniques finally justified the use of peripherally available hormone data to develop an integrative model of neuroendocrine dysfunction linked to brain function, and specifically to psychopathology.

In this chapter the neuroendocrinology of affective disorders is reviewed by describing the observations in a series of neuroendocrine systems, and the pathophysiology involved in these findings. The neuroendocrine findings in several other selected psychiatric conditions will then be summarised, and attempts made to demonstrate that a neuroendocrine assessment not only provides insight into altered brain function, but may also be of potential value in predicting genetic proneness to psychiatric illness, in evaluating adequacy of treatment and in relapse prevention.

Depression

The hypothalamo-pituitary–adrenocortical system

Major depression is diagnostically delineated by a number of symptoms that are defined by interviewing patients. Identification of this syndrome allows one to predict with some confidence heritability, course and response to treatment. The cardinal symptoms of major depression encompass not only depressive mood and altered psychomotor activity, but also severe changes in sleep architecture as objectified by sleep polygraphy, altered eating behaviour, decreased libido, cardiovascular changes, profound cognitive deficits and changes in hormone secretion. These symptoms (which are mostly reversible) strongly point to involvement of the limbic-hypothalamic system as a relay station between central neural circuits and peripheral hormone and autonomic nervous function.

While objectifiable symptoms of depression, such as sleep changes or hormonal perturbations, are not used in current diagnostic algorithms, they provide the most straightforward basis for scientific research in depression. Considering the epidemiological data of depression and the associated risk of suicide, it becomes clear that identifying causal factors and the development of better treatment for this most disabling condition is an urgent public-health demand.

Baseline measures

Approximately 50-60% of patients presenting with major depressive disorder show distinct changes in their adrenocorticotrophic hormone (ACTH) and cortisol secretory activity, as demonstrated by measuring cortisol and ACTH levels in plasma and cerebrospinal fluid (CSF). Halbreich *et al.* [1] showed that cortisol secretory profiles of depressives resulted in mean 24-hour plasma cortisol levels which were significantly elevated when compared with controls. Deuschle *et al.* [2] and Mortola *et al.* [3] studied the pulsatile activity and circadian rhythmicity of ACTH in relation to cortisol; these studies demonstrated that in depression the number of ACTH pulses was increased, while for cortisol it was not the number, but the amount of cortisol released per burst, that was increased. The increase in 24-hour ACTH pulse frequency is of particular interest in these studies as it reflects an altered functional status of the hypothalamus resulting in enhanced corticotrophin-releasing hormone (CRH) pulse generator activity. More recent studies in controls have documented a linear relationship between the magnitudes of ACTH and cortisol pulses [4]. However, the degree of temporal coincidence between ACTH and cortisol pulses was found to be variable [4,5]. The occurrence of ACTH pulses without changes in plasma cortisol concentrations, and of cortisol peaks with no observable change in plasma ACTH, raises the possibility that mechanisms other than ACTH may be involved in regulating cortisol secretion [6]. Sympathetic innervation of the adrenal cortex and adrenogenic humoral factors, which act independently of the pituitary and are probably derived from the immune system, may also be involved [7]. The coincidence of increased ACTH burst frequency and enhanced cortisol secretory amplitude among depressives is probably a secondary consequence of the hypersensitivity of the adrenal glands which occurs in these patients [8]. This hypersensitivity may develop after prolonged overexposure to ACTH, which is a trophic hormone, and renders the gland hyperplastic. Two lines of research support this interpretation.

1 Following synthetic ACTH infusions to depressives with or without dexamethasone pretreatment, plasma cortisol surges have been found to be more pronounced among depressives and dexamethasone non-suppressors than in controls or dexamethasone suppressors [8-10].

2 Enlarged adrenal size has been demonstrated in a group of depressives by computed tomography [11]. These radiological data, which are supported by indications of pituitary enlargement in depression, were confirmed by Rubin *et al.* [12], who measured adrenal volumes by nuclear magnetic resonance imaging and found that patients with depression had larger adrenals during depressive episodes than after successful treatment.

Suppression of hypothalamo-pituitary–adrenocortical activity with dexamethasone

The dexamethasone suppression test (DST) has received considerable attention in psychiatric research because it is very easily conducted and had been advocated to be an ancillary diagnostic aid to identify patients with endogenous or melancholic depression. After administration of a small dose (1–2 mg) of the long-acting synthetic steroid dexamethasone at 2300 hours to normal subjects, plasma cortisol levels remain suppressed throughout the following day. A large number of studies has shown that depressives frequently escape from this suppressive effect of dexamethasone [13,14]. Regarding the physiological validity of the DST, some confusion arose after reports that non-suppressed plasma cortisol levels following dexamethasone were associated with lower plasma concentrations of the test drug [15–17]. However, studies of early biophase kinetics and studies comparing drug distribution after oral and intravenous dexamethasone administration among depressed suppressors and non-suppressors have shown that the outcome of the DST is not simply an artifact of the pharmacokinetics of the test drug [18,19]. To date, the DST is no longer considered as a diagnostic aid [20], which is not surprising since psychiatric diagnoses are not based on pathophysiology but on clinical conventions related to psychopathology and course.

Today, there is a trend to create an increasing number of diagnostic categories, which is reflected by the fact that the official diagnostic manual of the American Psychiatric Association for diagnoses released in the 1980s (DSM-III) contained 265 diagnostic categories, while the current version of this manual (DSM-IV) has been expanded to over 400 categories. In this light, any attempt to validate a psychiatric diagnosis with laboratory findings must be frustrating. Instead of syndromes or diagnoses being *contrasted* with hypothalamo-pituitary–adrenocortical (HPA) measures, the latter should be considered as one of the *features* of the clinical phenotype. Ideally, these abnormalities should be incorporated as signs and symptoms into a multi-axial diagnostic scheme.

To date, the most promising application of the DST remains its use as a state marker, which can be applied longitudinally to follow up treatment response. Depressives who intially have elevated plasma cortisol levels after dexamethasone gradually normalise on the test during successful antidepressant treatment. Those patients who remain dexamethasone non-suppressors despite improvement of the psychopathology are at risk of relapse into depression [9,15,21–25]. This time-course pattern, in which neuroendocrine alterations precede depressive psychopathology and normalise prior to full remission of psychopathology, strongly resembles the situation in patients with Cushing's syndrome [26].

The role of CRH and vasopressin

The presence of a hypothalamic neuropeptide controlling ACTH secretion was first predicted by Harris more than 40 years ago. However, it took until 1981 for CRH to be isolated from ovine hypothalami [27]. The detection and sequencing of the gene coding for human CRH on chromosome 8 [28] was immediately followed by many studies on human stress physiology and disorders associated with hypothalamo-pituitary–adrenal pathophysiology.

The first series of reports utilising human CRH (hCRH) in depressives revealed a blunted ACTH response after intravenous administration of a test dose of CRH [29–31]. Baseline cortisol secretion prior to CRH stimulation was significantly higher in depressives, and was inversely related to the amount of ACTH produced by stimulation. We further observed that the cortisol responses among depressives were indistinguishable from those of controls, despite significantly lower ACTH release. This again points toward a hypersensitive adrenal cortex resulting from long-term overexposure to ACTH, confirming conclusions drawn from ACTH and cortisol profiles at baseline and after ACTH challenges. Furthermore, pretreatment of depressives with metyrapone, which suppresses cortisol biosynthesis, was found to result in normalised ACTH release after CRH stimulation [32,33]. From these data we concluded that elevated circulating cortisol is the main but not sole abnormality preventing an adequate ACTH response via negative feedback. Therefore, exaggerated secretory activity of corticotrophic and adrenocortical cells appeared to be related to a suprapituitary abnormality. This interpretation was consistent with our earlier studies using ovine CRH [15,34,35] and similar studies using the ovine heterologue by Amsterdam *et al.* [11] and by Gold *et al.* [36,37]. In addition to baseline hypercortisolism, other mechanisms which might account for blunted ACTH responses to CRH must be considered: among these possibilities are altered processing and storage of ACTH precursors, desensitised CRH receptors on pituitary corticotrophs, and alternative processing of proopiomelanocortin (POMC), the precursor of ACTH and β-endorphin. For example, Rupprecht *et al.* [38] reported a dissociation of ACTH and β-endorphin responses after CRH stimulation in depression. Young *et al.* [39] applied a low-dose ovine CRH challenge to depressives and controls and measured β-endorphin, β-lipotropin and cortisol in order to obtain information on the acute feedback regulation and actual CRH-receptor sensitivity. They found a decreased total β-endorphin and β-lipotropin response and a normal cortisol response in depressives, which agrees with our original studies measuring ACTH and cortisol after human CRH. The β-endorphin response pattern was found to be biphasic, showing an initial rapid release of β-endorphin preceding the cortisol surge and a second period of β-endorphin increase, while cortisol was elevated but stable. This clinical study confirms conclusions drawn from animal investigations [40], and from our work on combined dexamethasone–CRH challenges among depressives. These studies suggest that, in addition to resting cortisol levels and adrenal hypersensitivity, it is also necessary to consider changes in corticosteroid receptor-mediated feedback mechanisms of the hypothalamo-pituitary system (see below).

In agreement with the notion that overactive central CRH neurons are involved in depression with hypercortisolism are the studies by Nemeroff and colleagues. These investigators measured CRH in the CSF and found elevated levels of this peptide in depression [41]. In this and other studies a large number of patients had normal CRH concentrations in the CSF, which is also in line with the view that CRH is centrally overproduced, because in these patients peripheral indices of hypothalamo-pituitary–adrenal function were elevated. In the presence of undisturbed interaction between glucocorticoid levels and central CRH, the latter peptide would be decreased in the presence of elevated cortisol levels. For example, patients with Cushing's syndrome have significantly lower CSF levels of CRH [42]. While it must be noted that CRH levels in the CSF do not necessarily reflect CRH in the pituitary portal system, this observation agrees with a study showing that CRH receptors were down-regulated in the frontal cortex of suicide victims (B_{max} in suicides, 521 ± 43 fmol/mg protein; B_{max} in controls, 680 ± 51 fmol/mg protein; $P < 0.02$), which is best explained by central overproduction of CRH [43].

Using hCRH and its ovine analogue, it has been demonstrated that receptor binding of CRH in the pituitary and in the brain stimulates activation of adenylate cyclase and the accumulation of cyclic adenosine monophosphate (cAMP). This action is thought to regulate biosynthesis and processing of POMC, the precursor of ACTH.

As illustrated in Fig. 82.1, CRH has been implicated not only in the mediation of neuroendocrine signs and symptoms of depression, but also in behavioural changes [44]. There are at least two receptors (CRH-R_1 and CRH-R_2), which convey the CRH signal [45]. Whereas the CRH-R_1 is more widely distributed, the CRH-R_2 is mainly expressed in the limbic brain, suggesting that the two receptors are differently involved in mediating central effects of CRH. Both receptors are potential targets for a new generation of antidepressants acting directly at CRH receptors by antagonising the effect of CRH. Suppressing the translation of CRH-R_1 mRNA by administration of a specific oligodeoxynucleotide antisense probe into the central amygdala or intracerebroventricularly produced anxiolysis in rats, whereas an antisense probe directed against CRH-R_2 mRNA was ineffective [46–48].

Whereas animal studies provide good evidence for an involvement of CRH in behavioural states and the results are consistent with an anxiogenic effect of CRH, the evidence that increased CRH secretion is also related to psychiatric morbidity is derived from correlations rather than from direct evidence. Only the availability of specific CRH-receptor

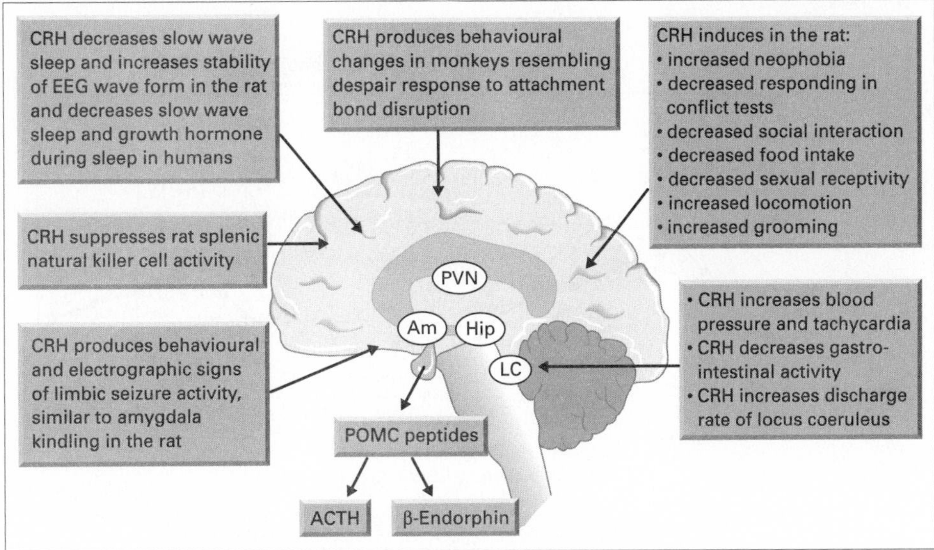

Fig. 82.1 Behavioural effects of central corticotrophin-releasing hormone (CRH). Behavioural effects mostly obtained from animal studies administering CRH or blocking CRH receptors agree that CRH is a key hormone to coordinate behavioural response to stress. ACTH, adrenocorticotrophic hormone; Am, amygdala; Hip, hypothalamus; LC, locus coeruleus; POMC, proopiomelanocortin; PVN, paraventricular nucleus.

subtype antagonists that can be administered therapeutically will provide a conclusive answer to the question of whether CRH is causally linked to the development and course of depression.

Certainly, CRH acts not alone but in concert with other neurotransmitters and neuropeptides. In dexamethasone-pretreated normal controls, ACTH and cortisol cannot be elevated by CRH infusions to the extent seen among depressives who are defined as DST non-suppressors. In contrast, dexamethasone-pretreated depressives have exaggerated ACTH and cortisol responses to CRH (see below). This led us to postulate that not only CRH, but also vasopressin, is hypersecreted from hypothalamic nuclei into the pituitary portal system [49–51]. Recently, studies have determined post-mortem the number of CRH- and vasopressin-immunoreactive neurons in the hypothalamic paraventricular nuclei of depressed patients [52,53]; this Dutch group, led by Swaab, found four times as many CRH-expressing neurons and three times as many CRH neurons coexpressing vasopressin as in the paraventricular nuclei (PVN) of controls. Moreover, the fact that the total number of vasopressin-immunoreactive neurons was also increased can be taken as a further indication of increased vasopressin activity in depression. The possibility that enhanced vasopressin secretory activity not only contributes to HPA hyperdrive in depression, but might also contribute to the behavioural changes seen in affective disorders has been documented by Landgraf *et al.* [54]. These investigators showed that decreasing the number and function of septal vasopressin receptors by local injection of antisense oligodeoxynucleotides to the V_1-receptor subtype mRNA reduces anxiety-related behaviour in rats.

Combined dexamethasone–CRH test

Since elevated plasma cortisol levels in depressed patients contribute to the blunted ACTH response following stimulation with CRH via negative feedback, one would expect that pretreatment with dexamethasone would even further suppress ACTH and cortisol release. However, as illustrated in Fig. 82.2, we found that unlike normal controls depressed patients respond with exaggerated ACTH and cortisol release after CRH if pretreated with dexamethasone [48,50,51,55, 56]. While this test is not specific for diagnostic categories [57–59], it is interesting that the ACTH and cortisol hyperresponse gradually disappears after successful treatment. Persisting high hormonal release is associated with less favourable clinical outcome [56,60–62]. It is noteworthy that the escape from dexamethasone-suppressed ACTH and cortisol secretion following CRH is more pronounced in aged individuals [51,63], particularly women [64].

Summarising broad clinical experience with the dexamethasone–CRH test, Heuser *et al.* [65] concluded that the sensitivity (i.e. the likelihood of differentiating normal from pathological state) of this test is about 80%, and greatly exceeds that of the standard DST (20–50%). Endocrine laboratory tests are usually interpreted in relation to the patient's age. If psychiatric patients are clustered into different age groups, the sensitivity of the dexamethasone–CRH test

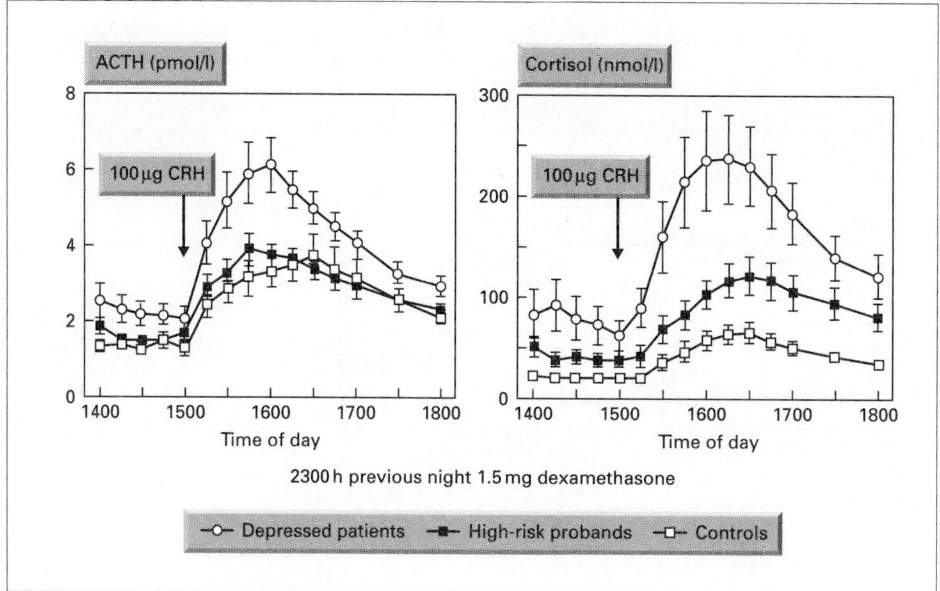

Fig. 82.2 Dexamethasone (DEX)–corticotrophin-releasing hormone (CRH) test in depressed patients and healthy controls from families with or without high genetic risk for depression. Plasma cortisol secretion in DEX-pretreated depressives is enhanced after CRH infusion in comparison to normal controls from unaffected families. Probands with high genetic risk have plasma cortisol responses that were higher among controls, but lower among depressives [67].

can be increased even further to above 90%, making this test a prime candidate for laboratory characterisation of mentally ill patients, worthy of inclusion in diagnostic schemes [65].

As illustrated in Fig. 82.3, dose–response curves established for depressed patients and controls revealed that patients need higher dexamethasone dosages to suppress ACTH and cortisol secretion after CRH infusion [174]. This finding points to decreased capacity and/or function of corticosteroid receptors to convey the glucocorticoid signal to regulatory systems that are involved in the production and release of CRH, vasopressin and ACTH. These studies, as well as studies using cortisol infusions that also found that the fast feedback component of pituitary response is insensitive in depression [66], do not reveal whether defective corticosteroid sensitivity is the primary *cause* of HPA hyperdrive. Likewise, primary hypersecretion of CRH and vasopressin and exaggerated ACTH secretion might have increased corticosteroid levels to a degree that consequently led to corticosteroid-receptor desensitisation in the limbic brain.

In studies on healthy subjects who had never suffered from minor or major psychiatric illness, but who were members of families highly 'loaded' with depression, several neurobiological signs of depression were found to be present including the response to the dexamethasone–CRH test [67]. In comparison to a control group, a much higher proportion of these subjects at genetic risk for depression showed an exaggerated cortisol response, but a normal ACTH response (Fig. 82.2). This finding supports the notion that in probands with increased genetic risk a functional defect at the corticosteroid receptor level is present, which is only disclosed by a neuroendocrine function test; thus, under baseline conditions plasma ACTH and cortisol in remitted patients and high-risk probands are indistinguishable from those of controls. The postulated defective corticosteroid receptor function results, in dexamethasone-pretreated patients, in decreased suppression of ACTH, CRH and vasopressin, the last being able to synergise with exogenously administered CRH resulting in enhanced elaboration of ACTH and cortisol. The relevance of this finding must await clarification of whether those individuals from a high genetic risk population, who present with abnormal dexamethasone–CRH test results, are indeed at higher risk for developing the disease than those who have normal test results. Importantly, the inappropriate cortisol response to the dexamethasone–CRH test remains stable over time in high-risk probands (S. Modell, unpublished results).

Neuroregulation of the HPA system by internal and external signals

The negative-feedback machinery preserves its flexibility by using a binary corticosteroid-receptor system, the mineralocorticoid and the glucocorticoid receptors (MRs or type I, and GRs or type II). This dual receptor system for a single class of hormones is advantageous in dealing with the manifold physiological functions of corticosteroids. Under

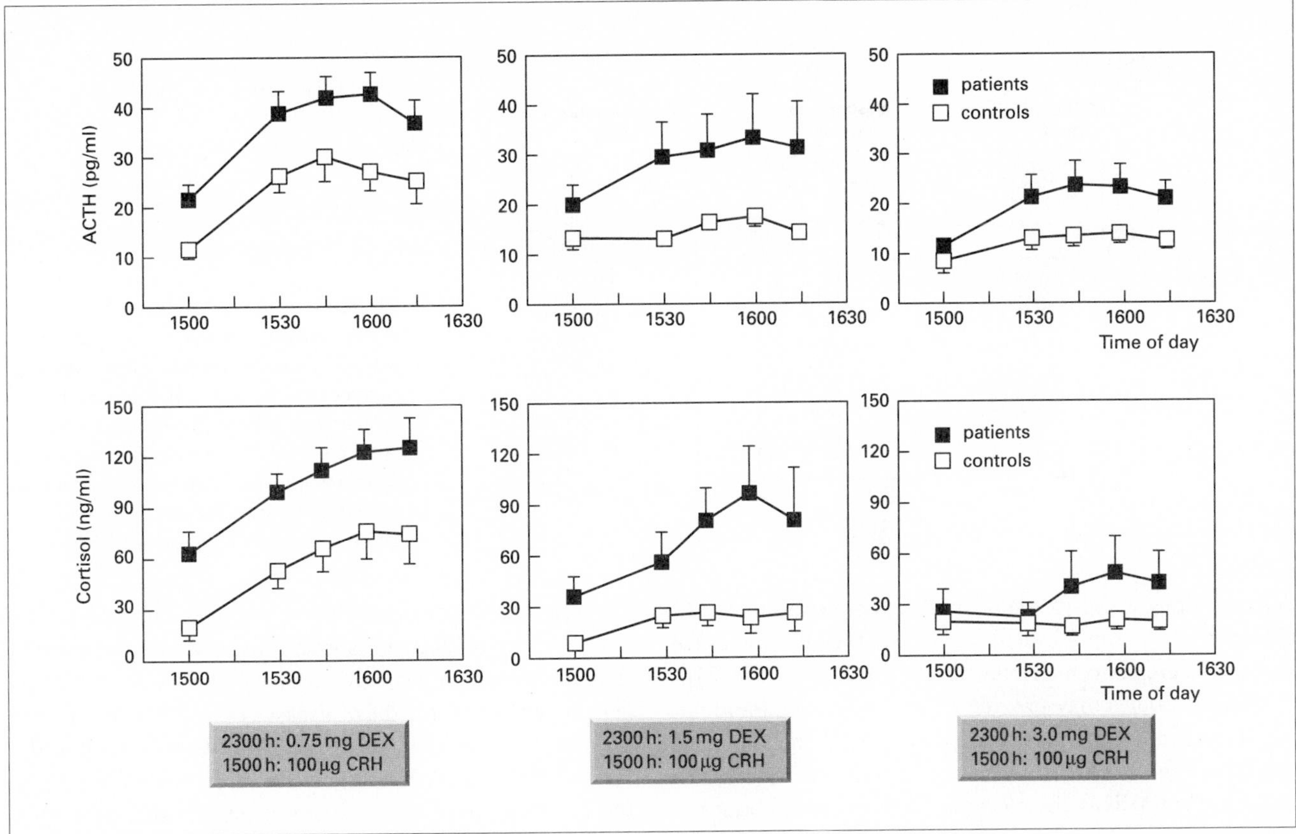

Fig. 82.3 Patients with depression have a shift of the dexamethasone (DEX) dose–response of adrenocorticotrophic hormone (ACTH) and cortisol to corticotrophin-releasing hormone (CRH) that indicates lowered glucocorticoid receptor function in depression when compared with controls. From [174].

resting conditions, plasma cortisol undergoes characteristic fluctuations ranging from about 0.5 to 50 nmol/l. Under very stressful conditions circulating levels of corticosteroids may rapidly exceed 100 nmol/l and a single receptor system would not be capable of translating this hormone signal into an adequate physiological response. This is particularly important in the hippocampus, which not only serves as an important structure to regulate HPA activity, but also plays a key role in memory consolidation. Because disturbances of memory and cognition are key symptoms across all diagnostic categories, functional studies of this structure are of foremost interest in psychiatric research. Interestingly, the hippocampus is richly endowed with both MRs and GRs. There, cortisol (in humans) and corticosterone (in rats) binds to MRs with a 10-fold higher affinity than to GRs. Therefore, it is believed that MRs primarily serve to mediate tonic effects such as sensitivity to stress and its behavioural reflexes and circadian fluctuations. In contrast, the main function of GRs seems to be curtailment of stress-elicited HPA hyperactivity and information storage [68]. Both receptors, GR and MR, act as dimers when activated by cognate ligands. In principle, homodimers (GR–GR; MR–MR) and heterodimers (GR–MR) can be formed if both receptors are present in the same cell. All three dimers have different DNA-binding and *trans*-activation properties [69,70]. Because dexamethasone activates GRs much more specifically than cortisol, the previously mentioned differences in CRH response to hypercortisolaemic depressives with or without dexamethasone pretreatment can be explained by activation of a different set of corticosteroid-receptor dimers. The potential clinical relevance of this concept has been recently underlined by Hassan *et al.* [71], who showed that high dosages of dexamethasone administered to rats induce apoptosis in the dentate gyrus of the hippocampus, whereas very high dosages of corticosterone are not apoptotic and may even prevent dexamethasone-induced cell death. Thus, formation of GR–MR heterodimers through corticosterone induces cell-protective mechanisms, while dexamethasone, mostly acting through GR–GR, does the opposite. The clinical relevance of these preclinical observations is apparent.

The view that corticosteroid-receptor function might be causally involved in the development and course of affective disorders is also indicated by the finding that initially abnormal DST or dexamethasone–CRH test results normalise along with amelioration of depressive psychopathology, and that, as shown in Fig. 82.4, CRH levels in the CSF

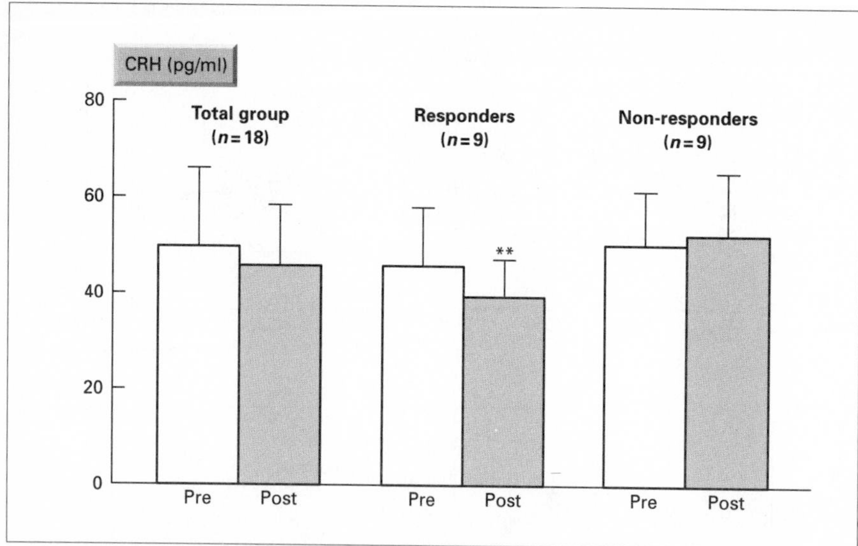

Fig 82.4 Long-term antidepressant administration reduces corticotrophin-releasing hormone (CRH) concentrations in the cerebrospinal fluid of treatment responders, but not of non-responders. After a 6-week treatment period with amitriptyline only those patients who favourably responded had decreased cerebrospinal fluid CRH concentrations.

decrease along with successful antidepressant treatment [72, IJ Heuser *et al.*, unpublished]. This raises the question as to how antidepressants interfere with the HPA system [73,74]. Preclinical studies may provide an in-depth understanding for these clinical findings. Peiffer *et al.* [75] showed that antidepressants are capable of enhancing GR gene expression in the rat brain. This effect is most likely brought about by a mechanism different from the noradrenaline re-uptake blockade, since desmethylimipramine (a specific noradrenaline re-uptake inhibitor) also induces GR expression in fibroblast cells, where catecholamines are absent [76]. In addition, a transgenic mouse which expresses antisense complementary to the GR mRNA was created by Pepin *et al.* [77]. This mouse has a GR deficit along with severe endocrine and cognitive disturbances which resemble the clinical condition in depression [78,79]. As shown by Montkowski *et al.* [79], treatment of these transgenic mice with antidepressants not only resolves the endocrine disturbance but also improves cognition. Finally, Reul *et al.* [80,81] administered amitriptyline (a very non-specific antidepressant) and moclobemide (a reversible inhibitor of monoamine oxidase type A) to rats and found that GR and MR capacity increased under the influence of long-term antidepressant treatment. Interestingly, MR induction precedes that of GR in almost all brain areas tested, which led W Hundt *et al.* (unpublished) to postulate that antagonism of MRs would impede the clinical effect of antidepressants. Therefore, in a double-blind controlled study, he administered either placebo or spironolactone (an MR antagonist) as an adjunct to amitriptyline in patients with major depression. Those cotreated with the MR antagonist indeed responded less favourably, which strongly supports the notion that functional MRs are necessary for successful initiation of antidepressant action.

Psychosocial stressors play a pre-eminent role in the development of affective disorders, and it is well documented that life events may trigger an affective episode in individuals genetically at risk for these diseases [82]. Early discoveries [83,84] showed that post-natal stimulation shapes the adrenocortical secretion response to stress in later life. More recent studies have also consistently shown that post-natal treatment of rats such as handling prevents excessive glucocorticoid release following a stressful experience even 1 or 2 years after birth [85,86].

Reul *et al.* [87] recently showed that prenatal immune challenge by human red blood cells injected into pregnant rats produced increased HPA responses in adult progeny, which is secondary to decreased GR and MR capacity in these animals. This finding may explain increased diathesis for mental illness as a consequence of prenatal infection, which alters fetal brain development leading—among other disturbances—to an inadequate response to stress. The group led by Nemeroff recently showed that early stress, such as maternal deprivation, produces long-term effects on CRH neural systems such as increases in CRH concentrations and CRH-binding sites in several hypothalamic and extrahypothalamic areas [88].

The fact that the early experiences of an animal, and most probably also of humans, affect not only behavioural response patterns but also hormonal response patterns throughout life, favours the concept that hormones are involved in the dialogue between the genetic blueprint carried in the chromosomes and experience-related changes in neural activity.

Pituitary-growth hormone system

The secretion of growth hormone (GH) has been subject

to considerable neuroendocrine investigation in affective disorders, and a number of alterations in its secretory pattern under baseline conditions and after pharmacological challenges have been identified. Plasma GH is secreted in a pulsatile and episodic fashion, resulting in plasma hormone levels that vary over a range of three orders of magnitude, with highly diverse amplitudes [89]. In adults, the largest portion of GH is secreted around the time of sleep onset, extending into the first non-REM (rapid eye movement) period of sleep [90] (see also Chapter 6)

Daytime GH hypersecretion has been reported to occur among unmedicated men with major depression [91]. In contrast, the sleep-related nocturnal GH surge is blunted during depression and also after remission of psychopathology [92,93]. GH secretion is under the dual control of GH-releasing hormone (GHRH) and somatostatin; these neuropeptides are regulated by a number of neurotransmitters and neuropeptides whose dysregulation is considered to be of aetiological importance in depression, and which are involved in the action of antidepressant drugs. Therefore, the GH response to pharmacological challenges has been used to identify altered neuroregulatory pathways in depression.

A large number of challenge tests have led to the assumption that acetylcholine, noradrenaline, serotonin, dopamine and histamine stimulate GH, while γ-aminobutyric acid (GABA) acts as an inhibitor. More specifically, the GH stimulatory effect of insulin-induced hypoglycaemia and amphetamine can be blocked by α_2-adrenergic antagonists. This finding and the blunted GH secretory response that follows infusion of clonidine (an α_2-adrenergic agonist) to depressives support the view that postsynaptic α_2-adrenergic receptors are subsensitive in depression [94–96].

These studies are in keeping with studies administering antidepressant drugs with varying neuroreceptor specificity. Laakmann *et al.* [97], for example, showed that the GH-elevating effect of desmethylimipramine is blocked by the mixed α_1-/α_2-antagonist phentolamine, but not by the specific α_1-antagonist prazosin or the 5-hydroxytryptamine antagonist methysergide. These observations and the decreased GH release following desmethylimipramine challenges in depressives further support the view of altered α_2-adrenergic-receptor dynamics in these patients. These conclusions, however, assume an undisturbed GHRH-receptor responsiveness at the pituitary somatotroph. A substantial number of reports measuring the GH response following GHRH administration have not fully clarified this issue. Several authors have reported that GH secretion after administration of GHRH is blunted [98–100]; others have found no change [101] or exaggerated responses [102]. The diminished GH response to GHRH in depression may be due to:

1 GHRH-receptor desensitisation, secondary to central GHRH hypersecretion, which would be consistent with the daytime, but not the sleep-associated GH secretory pattern;

2 enhanced insulin-like growth factor 1 (IGF-1) levels, which negatively feed back at the pituitary level and inhibit GH release from the pituitary;

3 direct inhibitory effects of GH on its own hypersecretion at the somatotroph, strongly underlining the need to take into account baseline GH status prior to pharmacological GH challenges.

As long as these effects are not fully understood, the conclusions drawn from centrally acting neurotropic drugs remain speculative.

Another serious confounder is the interaction between hormones of the HPA system and GH release. Glucocorticoids as well as thyroid hormones increase the rate of GH gene transcription *in vitro*, while long-term corticosteroid administration *in vivo* results in GH inhibition (e.g. decreased growth of children treated with corticosteroids for rheumatoid arthritis). Central administration of CRH to rats inhibits the pulsatile release of GH, possibly by increased release of somatostatin [103]. Also, peripheral administration of CRH is capable of blunting GHRH-induced GH release [104] or the spontaneous sleep-related GH surge [105]. A recent study, which administered minute dosages of ACTH and CRH during daytime to normal men, documented that activation of the pituitary–adrenocortical system or the adrenocortical gland alone results in daytime activation of GH release with a concurrent decrease of the nocturnal sleep-related GH surge [106].

Finally, gonadal function, frequently suppressed in depressives, plays an important role in the modulation of GH and IGF-1 concentrations. It is well known that, compared with men, women have higher 24-hour integrated GH concentrations and show more vigorous responses to pharmacological stimuli of GH secretion [107]. This gender difference gradually disappears with increasing age, pointing to oestrogens as important modulators of GH secretory activity. To what degree altered pituitary–gonadal and pituitary–adrenocortical status is responsible for changes in GH secretion among depressives needs clarification.

The behavioural sequelae of the suspected GHRH increase during the day followed by nocturnal decrease in the context of depression are not yet clear [108]. Ehlers *et al.* [109] showed that intraventricular administration of GHRH to rats increases slow-wave sleep and decreases locomotor activity, indicating a decrease in the arousal state. This observation is consistent with our finding of blunted GH release during sleep in depression [92], and the parallel decrease of slow-wave sleep and GH after CRH administration to normal controls [105]. Likewise, GHRH injections to humans increase slow-wave sleep [110], while somatostatin impairs sleep at least in elderly study subjects [175]. These findings are in keeping with the hypothesis by

Ehlers and Kupfer, who proposed a shift in the balance between the somatotrophic and the HPA systems. As a result, the GHRH/CRH ratio is decreased, which weakens mechanisms that activate slow-wave sleep [111,112].

The pituitary–thyroid system

Functional disturbances of the pituitary system have been observed in patients with major depression and in patients with thyroid disease, particularly primary hypothyroidism, frequently exhibiting prominent depressive symptoms. The obvious role for this endocrine system in influencing mood and behaviour led to studies exploring the effect of thyroid hormones on the acceleration or potentiation of the clinical effect of tricyclic antidepressants. The most frequently reported changes of pituitary–thyroid function are:

1 reduced thyroid stimulating hormone (TSH) and thyroid hormone concentrations [113];

2 a blunted TSH response to thyrotrophin-releasing hormone (TRH) [114];

3 an attenuated circadian rhythm of TSH secretion, which normally peaks at 2300 hours and reaches a minimum 12 hours later [115].

More recent studies, which carefully took the age-related changes of pituitary–thyroid regulation into account, reported that the main changes of this system among depressives are reductions of basal TSH and triiodothyronine (T_3) [116], reduced nocturnal rises in TSH and blunted TSH responses to TRH [117]. The latter stimulation response is higher in the evening than in the morning and this difference in responsiveness is attenuated among patients with major depression [118]. It needs to be pointed out that the likelihood of detecting manifest pituitary–thyroid suppression among depressives is rather low, while the percentage of subjects showing blunted TSH response to TRH, reportedly varying between 20 and 30%, depends largely on the criteria for defining the phenomenon. It is of note that the largest and most carefully designed study failed to detect statistically significant differences of TRH test results between depressives and controls [116]. In addition, as has been elaborated by Loosen *et al.* [119], TSH blunting is not limited to depression, but may occur also in alcoholism, schizophrenia, mania, panic disorders and anorexia nervosa.

Given the reciprocal interaction between thyroid function, mood and behaviour which is well known from clinical endocrinology, one might speculate whether the modest reduction of pituitary–thyroid function in depression has any metabolic significance for neuronal function. The occasional success of T_3 augmentation of tricyclic antidepressant therapy would suggest that it might. However, there are no studies that have correlated pituitary–thyroid function with the observed beneficial effects of T_3. Moreover, it remains unclear as to whether in depression there is a central hypo- or hyperthyroid state, since most of the intracellular T_3 in the brain derives from intracellular deiodination of thyroxine (T_4) while only a small amount is contributed by circulating T_3 [120,121].

One possible explanation for impaired TSH secretion at baseline or following TRH stimulation would be pituitary–thyrotroph desensitisation secondary to enhanced TRH release from the hypothalamus. This would be in keeping with reported reduction in the nocturnal TSH surge following low-dose TRH administration [122], and the finding of elevated TRH levels in the CSF of depressed patients [123].

Another possibility would be that the concomitant hyperactivity of the pituitary–adrenocortical system accounts for the reduced TSH secretion. Cortisol and other glucocorticoids are known to reduce TSH secretion [117,124]. However, among depressives this issue remains controversial, but studies opposing the view of HPA overactivity as the determining factor for TSH blunting are largely cross-sectional and therefore of limited value. Two studies comparing the functional TSH status, either by measuring nocturnal TSH rises or TSH rises after TRH, showed that TSH blunting is either negatively correlated with cortisol levels [117] or is positively correlated with the ACTH release following CRH administration [125]. Both studies strongly support the existence of a causal relationship between TSH secretory activity and HPA activity. However, longitudinal studies of the same patients before and after treatment are needed to ascertain clearly the relationship between these two endocrine systems and its physiological and clinical significance.

Of particular clinical interest are reports of depressed patients having a higher than expected occurrence of symptomless autoimmune thyroiditis, as defined by the abnormal presence of circulating antimicrosomal thyroid and/or antithyroglobulin antibodies. Here also, a relationship to the HPA activity has been shown as there is a higher incidence of symptomless autoimmune thyroiditis among DST non-suppressors.

Anxiety disorders

Anxiety is part of the symptom pattern present in many psychiatric illnesses. Anxiety disorders are defined as those in which excessive anxiety predominates in isolation. At the phenomenological level several subtypes have been defined, including generalised anxiety disorder, post-traumatic stress disorder, phobias or panic disorder. Results from a large number of animal behavioural studies are consistent with CRH having an anxiogenic effect (reviewed in [126]). These conclusions were based on studies with rats [127] and primates [128], applying intracerebral CRH injections, and manipulating the behavioural effects by CRH antagonists and benzodiazepine anxiolytics.

Under baseline conditions patients with anxiety disorders do not show signs of excessive HPA activation. However, anxiety fluctuates, and excessive states of anxiety are accompanied with elevation of HPA activity in humans and animals, suggesting a role for CRH also in the non-endocrine aspect of response to fear and anxiety.

This hypothesis is in line with the observation that benzodiazepines may reduce circulating levels of ACTH and cortisol, while inverse agonists stimulate them [129]. Recently, Kalogeras *et al.* [130] have reported that the triazolobenzodiazepine alprazolam attenuates stimulated CRH release from isolated rat hypothalami. Moreover, Owens *et al.* [131] have found that benzodiazepines prevent the release of CRH from the median eminence. Interestingly, the CRH content of the locus coeruleus (LC) decreased after treatment with benzodiazepines. This brainstem nucleus is of particular interest for two reasons:

1 its activity has repeatedly been implicated in stress responses, fear and arousal functions;

2 CRH-containing neurons are located in close proximity to noradrenergic neurons in the LC [132].

A strong functional interaction is also supported by the increases of LC firing rates observed after CRH injections into this area and the increases of CRH concentrations found in the LC in response to stress [133]. These stress-responsive CRH surges are reduced by the anxiolytic drug alprazolam. The effect of alprazolam in deactivating CRH neurons can be blocked by benzodiazepine antagonists [131]. All these data suggest that panic and anxiety disorders are precipitated by a rapidly progressing dysregulation between CRH neurons and noradrenergic neurons at the LC. This positive-feedback cascade would result temporarily in explosive neuronal LC–CRH disinhibition, mutually triggering panic anxiety and a variety of LC- and HPA-regulated autonomic and endocrine changes.

A recent study by Coplan *et al.* [134] used the α_2-adrenoceptor agonist clonidine and measured reductions of plasma 3-methoxy-4-hydroxyphenylglycol (MHPG) as an index of noradrenaline neuroactivity and plasma cortisol levels in patients with panic disorder. These investigators found a significant 'coupling' of several MHPG and cortisol measures in controls, whereas patients were 'uncoupled'. From a study by Abelson and Curtis [135] additional signs of HPA abnormality emerged. These authors found elevated cortisol secretion and increased activity in ultradian secondary episodes, while ACTH release was only elevated in those patients who had a lower frequency of panic attacks. Studies that employed CRH-stimulation tests [136–138] found blunted ACTH response despite normal cortisol levels prior to intravenous CRH administration, which suggests desensitised pituitary CRH-R_1 on anterior pituitary corticotrophs. These receptor changes are probably due to excessive exposure by hypothalamic CRH as part of the complex symptom pattern during recurrent panic attacks. These subtle HPA changes also involve changes in GR and MR capacity and function that can be corrected by antidepressant treatment. Whether or not such a mechanism is involved in antidepressant-induced recovery from panic disorder is still speculative.

Whereas under baseline conditions subtle HPA alterations are now well documented, the absence of profound HPA activation during experimentally induced panic attacks using lactate infusions or carbon dioxide inhalations is enigmatic [139,140]. However, the absence of peripherally demonstrable HPA overactivity does not automatically reject the possibility that the central motor of the HPA system has been activated. Kellner *et al.* [141] recently offered an explanation by showing that patients who panicked during lactate infusions had more pronounced surges of plasma atrial natriuretic peptide (ANP). Because these authors found that ANP also acts in humans at the pituitary as a CRH antagonist [142], they postulated that the immediate rise in ANP during panic attacks suppresses CRH-elicited ACTH and cortisol and would thus explain the reported lack of pituitary–adrenal activation during lactate-induced panic. Based on these clinical findings, animal studies were employed to investigate whether ANP secreted from heart atria may also be involved in muting or termination of excessive anxiety-related behaviour. Preliminary evidence supports such a possibility since cerebral as well as higher dosed peripheral administration of an ANP analogue was found to be anxiolytic [176]. Of course, anxiety and panic are regulated by extremely complex mechanisms, including other neuropeptides such as cholecystokinin [143] or GABA-receptor-mediated effects [144].

Relatively little neuroendocrine research has been done in other endocrine systems. Roy-Byrne *et al.* [145] have demonstrated that the TSH response to TRH is blunted, and following GHRH administration the GH release is reported to be decreased [146]. Both findings agree with the observations in depression, and it remains unresolved to what degree coexisting depression is responsible for the hormonal response to TRH and GHRH in anxiety disorders.

A special category of anxiety disorders was defined after patients were studied who had experienced extremely distressing psychological insults such as combat or the holocaust. Among populations that have experienced these 'human-made' emergencies it is not uncommon that the traumatic event is re-experienced in a variety of ways including recurrent intrusive thoughts, distressing dreams, 'flash-back', which are all precipitated by cues or symbols resembling the traumatic event. As demonstrated by the group of

Yehuda, these patients suffer from what is called post-traumatic stress disorder (PTSD) and present with several neuroendocrine signs that are surprising: compared with normal controls and in contrast to other psychiatric disorders, these patients have *lower* mean 24-hour urinary cortisol secretion [147], lower baseline plasma cortisol concentrations [148], increased glucocorticoid binding in lymphocytes [149] and increased sensitivity to the HPA-suppressive effect of dexamethasone [150,151], which taken together indicate *enhanced* negative-feedback capacity in these patients. The mechanisms accounting for these findings remain unknown. It appears that, unlike mild to moderate stressors which occur in a cumulative fashion according to life experience (e.g. loss of a partner, illness, extreme athletic activities, lifestyle, etc.) and that tend to weaken negative-feedback capacity, extreme life-threatening stressors that result in chronic psychopathology produce enhanced negative-feedback response. To what extent other factors in some of these PTSD patients (nutrition, substance abuse, etc.) may have confounded these neuroendocrine changes awaits further study.

Schizophrenia

The neuroendocrine changes observed in schizophrenia are much less consistent than among depressives. One reason is that the schizophrenic phenotype is extremely variable, ranging from an acute exacerbation with disturbed content and formal organisation of thought, hallucinations, arousal and inadequate affect, to a so-called 'negative symptom pattern' dominated by social withdrawal and loss of motivation, sometimes associated with a flattened affect. Frequently symptoms of severe anxiety and depression coexist, which further obscures neuroendocrine study results.

A residual form of schizophrenia is usually not associated with significant changes of the HPA system [41]. In a state of acute exacerbation, the pituitary–adrenocortical system is activated as shown by dexamethasone non-suppressed cortisol levels [152]. Patients with schizophrenia showed normal plasma ACTH and cortisol response to CRH [153]; however, if pretreated with a low dose of dexamethasone, a subtle disturbance of the HPA system became apparent as they responded with elevated plasma cortisol levels after CRH administration. If an activity score for these patients is taken into account, it became obvious that those who were less aroused also showed a lower HPA response, pointing to the possibility that acute exacerbation of illness or distress may confound the dexamethasone–CRH test result [57].

A study by Van Cauter *et al.* [154] measured 24-hour profiles of plasma ACTH, cortisol, GH and prolactin levels, and also performed polygraphic sleep recordings because nocturnal secretion of these hormones is profoundly modulated by sleep. The major abnormality observed in this study was an almost threefold increase in sleep-related plasma prolactin levels, associated with an increased number of nocturnal prolactin pulses. In contrast, plasma ACTH and cortisol concentrations were indistinguishable from controls with the only exception that immediately after sleep onset plasma cortisol, but not ACTH levels, were elevated. Moreover, GH secretion was found to be unaltered confirming studies obtained with GHRH that also found stimulated GH release to be normal in schizophrenia. Studies that measured the plasma GH response to apomorphine, a dopamine agonist, found increased GH levels and a correlation between thought disorder and the magnitude of hormonal response [155]. Although these findings would be in agreement with the 'dopamine hypothesis of schizophrenia', it is apparent that the regulation of GH is far more complex and does not allow for an extrapolation of GH secretion to dopaminergic neurotransmission.

Eating disorders (see also Chapter 70)

Anorexia nervosa and bulimia nervosa are syndromes that occur predominantly among adolescent girls and young women. These patients achieve a low bodyweight by restricting the food intake and increasing their physical activity. Bulimia nervosa is characterised by episodic binge eating and may exist separately or in combination with anorexia. Neuroendocrine research in eating disorders must consider the effects of weight changes, which result in adaptive endocrine changes. In particular, the pituitary–adrenocortical system is activated in the underweight phase, which is manifested by a high frequency of dexamethasone non-suppression, elevated CRH in the CSF and a blunted ACTH response after CRH [37,156,157]. Studies in rats and rhesus monkeys showed that CRH mediates anorectic behaviour, which allows one to speculate that anorexia is at least in part mediated by a central disturbance resulting in elevated secretion of CRH [158].

Recently, another member of the CRH family has been characterised that is related to urotensin (63% sequence identity) and CRH (45% sequence identity), and has thus been named urocortin. This peptide is a ligand for both CRH-R_1 and CRH-R_2 and has a strong anorectic effect [159]. Because urocortin is more potent than CRH at binding and activating CRH-R_2 located in the lateral septum, dorsal raphe and solitary tract nuclei, one might assume that a non-peptide agent antagonising specifically these CRH-R_2 would be a promising pharmaceutical tool to treat anorexia. Moreover, patients with bulimia nervosa show signs of HPA hyperactivation, which normalises after abstinence of bingeing in a similar way to the endocrine normalisation of weight.

In anorexia nervosa there is a change in thyroid hormone regulation, which is consistent with the pattern seen in starvation, particularly decreased T_3 levels, elevated reverse T_3 concentrations and delayed, sometimes blunted, TSH peak responses after TRH administration. Recently, Lesem *et al.* [160] measured TRH in the CSF of anorectic patients when both underweight and after attaining goal weight were studied. These investigators found reduced TRH concentrations in both cases, which is opposite to that seen among depressives [161].

Basal GH levels appear to be increased in anorexia nervosa, similar to major depression [162]. The GH response to GHRH is exaggerated and normalises with weight recovery. Similar GH changes are observed among bulimics. Because the weight changes and/or hypercortisolism in these conditions results in a decrease in IGF-1 production, it was speculated that the reduced restraint of IGF-1 upon somatotrophic cells would account for the enhanced GH response to GHRH. In addition, underweight anorectics have a negative correlation between somastostatin in their CSF and pituitary–adrenocortical activity measures.

From the animal studies it was concluded that intracerebroventricular administration, and, in higher dosages also intravenous administration, of GHRH stimulates food intake [163], whereas antagonism of endogenous GHRH activity might attenuate food intake [164]. Therefore, Vaccarino *et al.* [165] investigated whether infusion of GHRH to anorectic patients might affect food consumption. These authors found that GHRH indeed stimulates food intake in anorectic patients and attenuates the excessive food intake in bulimics. While these pilot data are intriguing, they await confirmation in more rigidly controlled studies before non-peptidergic GHRH analogues can enter clinical practice.

One of the early symptoms of anorexia nervosa is loss of menses, which frequently precedes weight loss. Several studies have agreed that attenuated pituitary–gonadal function in anorexia is secondary to increased CRH secretion which inhibits hypothalamic gonadotrophin-releasing hormone (GnRH) secretion via increased secretion of ß-endorphin from the arcuate nucleus [166]. However, this cannot be the entire explanation as naloxone fails to re-establish gonadotrophin pulsatility. In addition, excessive release of glucocorticosteroids can suppress gonadal function at central and peripheral levels. In patients with bulimia nervosa disturbances of menstrual function also occur, either secondary to decreased oestradiol levels impairing follicular development or after decreased progesterone secretion in the luteal phase. The possibility that disturbed melatonin secretion accounts for the frequent occurrence of amenorrhoea in these patients has also been ruled out [167]. In general, altered menstrual function returns to normal after correction of weight fluctuations and a return to physiological nourishment.

It was demonstrated that cholecystokinin (CCK), which is released after a meal, plays a central role not only for the passage of food through the gastrointestinal tract, but also for mediating satiety [115]. A clinical study showed that at baseline and after a test meal the plasma levels of this gastrointestinal peptide are significantly increased in patients with anorexia nervosa [168], pointing to disturbed satiety effects of CCK in these patients. Whether or not peripheral CCK is a physiological regulator of satiety in humans remains uncertain. It is of note, however, that CCK acts in the brain either by central receptors or via ascending vagal fibres. Recently, Rose *et al.* [169] purified a CCK-inactivating peptidase that was found in neurons responding to CCK, but also in non-neuronal cells. This peptidase could be inactivated by butabindide, thus prolonging the satiating effect of endogenous CCK-8, which is reflected by reduced food intake in rats and mice. Further studies applying drugs that increase or decrease actions of CCK will prove whether the neuroendocrine and preclinical studies can be translated into effective therapies for anorexia or bulimia nervosa.

Another compound which promises to be causally involved in eating disorders, is neuropeptide Y (NPY). Central administration of NPY to rats stimulates food intake, while antibodies and antisense oligonucleotides directed against NPY mRNA block normal onset of feeding. If administered chronically, NPY induces obesity and suppresses HPA activity in rats [170]. Interestingly, NPY suppresses HPA activity not only in rats but also in humans after nocturnal pulsatile administration [177].

The recent availability of obese mouse mutants demonstrated mRNAs that are differentially expressed in the hypothalami of control mice. One or more of these mRNAs may encode for a neuropeptide that is directly involved in regulation of food consumption. Qu *et al.* [171] applied this powerful technology and showed that obese mouse mutants overexpress melanin-concentrating hormone, which increases the food intake of rats after intraventricular injection. From these obese mouse mutants a gene encoding leptin was cloned and subsequent studies confirmed also its role in regulation of food intake [178]. Leptin is produced in adipose tissue and acts in part by inhibition of NPY biosynthesis and release [172], which further points to NPY as a key regulator of food intake. Indeed, Considine *et al.* [179] showed that serum leptin levels correlated with body mass and fasting insulin. Therefore, it came as a surprise when Erickson *et al.* [173] reported that NPY knockout mice maintained normal bodyweight and feeding behaviour. Future studies employing conditional knockout techniques that direct gene deletions in specific brain areas in a time-specific manner will provide more precise insights into the various regulatory levels of satiety, food consumption and eventually pathology underlying eating disorders.

Conclusion

Behaviour is the most complex form of biological organisation, and understanding the neural and endocrine mechanisms governing normal and abnormal behaviour is the key goal of neuroscience. In this effort neuroendocrinology will play a major role because hormones are used by the brain to respond to challenges from the outside world. These challenges comprise demands such as sensory stimuli or stored memories, which are promptly retrieved in response to specific situations. Apart from these cognitive demands, non-cognitive stressors such as infection also activate the endocrine system, often in conjunction with neuroimmune function. These hormonal responses to the outside world are used for appropriate adaptation to a demanding confrontation. If these neuroregulatory pathways are deranged, mechanisms come into action that lead to persistent changes of humoral homeostasis, precipitating a clinical phenotype that presents as psychopathology. Genetic research in affective disorders currently supports the view that several different major loci are responsible for familial transmission of disease susceptibility. In the presence of a certain set of genes carrying noxious information, additional external stimuli, for example psychosocial stressors, are needed to activate these genes. The neuroendocrine hypothesis suggests that hormones play a major role in this activating cascade and thus maintain the dialogue between external experience-related factors and the genetic blueprint.

In the past, the endocrinology of mental diseases has mainly served to provide laboratory data as additional characteristics of certain clinical conditions. With the advances of molecular and cellular biology, brain imaging and behavioural pharmacology, endocrine research now has the chance to provide leads for better treatments.

References

1 Halbreich U, Asnis GM, Shindledecker R. Cortisol secretion in endogenous depression. *Arch Gen Psychiatry* 1985; **42**: 904–8.

2 Deuschle M, Schweiger U, Weber B *et al.* Diurnal activity and pulsatility of the hypothalamus–pituitary–adrenal system in male depressed patients and healthy controls. *J Clin Endocrinol Metab* 1997; **82**: 234–8.

3 Mortola JF, Liu JH, Gillin JC, Rasmussen DD, Yen SSC. Pulsatile rhythms of adrenocorticotropin (ACTH) and cortisol in women with endogenous depression: evidence for increased ACTH pulse frequency. *J Clin Endocrinol Metab* 1987; **67**: 962–8.

4 Krishnan KRR, Ritchie JC, Saunders W, Wilson W, Nemeroff CB, Carroll BJ. Nocturnal and early morning secretion of ACTH and cortisol in humans. *Biol Psychiatry* 1990; **38**: 47–57.

5 Follenius M, Simon C, Brandenberger G, Lenzi P. Ultradian plasma corticotropin and cortisol rhythms. Time series analysis. *J Endocrinol Invest* 1987; **10**: 261–6.

6 Fehm HL, Klein E, Holl R, Voigt KH. Evidence for extrapituitary mechanisms in the regulation of cortisol secretion in man. *J Clin Endocrinol Metab* 1984; **58**: 410–14.

7 Holsboer F, Stalla GK, von Bardeleben U, Hammann K, Müller H, Müller OA. Acute adrenocortical stimulation by recombinant gamma interferon in human controls. *Life Sci* 1988; **42**: 1–5.

8 Amsterdam JD, Winokur A, Abelman E, Lucki J, Richels K. Cosyntropin (ACTH alpha 1–24) stimulation test in depressed patients and healthy subjects. *Am J Psychiatry* 1983; **140**: 907–12.

9 Gerken A, Holsboer F. Cortisol and corticosterone response after syn-corticotropin in relationship to dexamethasone suppressibility of cortisol. *Psychoneuroendocrinology* 1986; **11**: 185–94.

10 Jaeckle RS, Kathol RG, Lopez JF, Meller WH, Krummel SJ. Enhanced adrenal sensitivity to exogenous ACTH $_{1-24}$ stimulation in major depression: relationship to dexamethasone suppression test results. *Arch Gen Psychiatry* 1987; **44**: 233–40.

11 Amsterdam JD, Maislin G, Winokur A, Kling M, Gold P. Pituitary and adrenocortical responses to the ovine corticotropin-releasing hormone in depressed patients and healthy volunteers. *Arch Gen Psychiatry* 1987; **44**: 775–81.

12 Rubin RT, Phillips JJ, Sadow TF, McCracken JT. Adrenal gland volume in major depression. *Arch Gen Psychiatry* 1995; **52**: 213–18.

13 Rubin RT, Poland RE, Lesser IM, Winston RA, Blodgett ALN. Neuroendocrine aspects of primary endogenous depression. *Arch Gen Psychiatry* 1987; **44**: 328–36.

14 Carroll BJ, Feinberg M, Greden JF *et al.* A specific laboratory test for the diagnosis of melancholia. *Arch Gen Psychiatry* 1981; **38**: 15–22.

15 Holsboer F. Prediction of clinical course by dexamethasone suppression test (DST) response in depressed patients—physiological and clinical construct validity of the DST. *Pharmacopsychiatry* 1983; **16**: 186–91.

16 Holsboer F, Haack D, Gerken A, Vecsei P. Plasma dexamethasone concentrations and differential glucocorticoid suppression response of cortisol and corticosterone in depressives and controls. *Biol Psychiatry* 1984; **19**: 281–91.

17 Arana GW, Workman RJ, Baldessarini RJ. Association between low plasma levels of dexamethasone and elevated levels of cortisol in psychiatric patients given dexamethasone. *Am J Psychiatry* 1984; **141**: 1619–20.

18 Holsboer F, Wiedemann K, Boll E. Shortened dexamethasone half-life in depressed dexamethasone nonsuppressors. *Arch Gen Psychiatry* 1986; **43**: 813–15.

19 Wiedemann K, Holsboer, F. The effect of dexamethasone dosage upon plasma cortisol and dexamethasone during DST. *J Affective Disord* 1990; **19**: 133–7.

20 Holsboer F, Philipp M, Steiger A, Gerken A. Multisteroid analysis after DST in depressed patients—a controlled study. *J Affective Disord* 1986; **10**: 241–9.

21 Holsboer F, Liebl R, Hofschuster E. Repeated dexamethasone suppression test during depressive illness. Normalization of test result compared with clinical improvement. *J Affective Disord* 1982; **4**: 93–101.

22 Greden JF, Gardner R, King D. Grunhaus L, Carroll BJ, Kronfold Z. Dexamethasone suppression tests in antidepressant treatment of melancholia—the process of normalization and test–retest reproductibility. *Arch Gen Psychiatry* 1983; **40**: 493–500.

23 Grunhaus L, Zelnik T, Albala AA *et al.* Serial dexamethasone suppression test in depressed patients treated only with electroconvulsive therapy. *J Affective Disord* 1987; **13**: 233–40.

24 Charles GA, Schittecatte M, Rush AL, Panzer M, Wilmotte J.

Persistent cortisol non-suppression after clinical recovery predicts symptomatic relapse in unipolar depression. *J Affective Disord* 1989; **17**: 271–8.

25 Coryell W. DST abnormality as a predictor of course in major depression. *J Affective Disord* 1990; **19**: 163–9.

26 Haskett R. Diagnostic categorization of psychotic disturbance in Cushing's syndrome. *Am J Psychiatry* 1985; **142**: 911–16.

27 Vale W, Spiess J, Rivier C, Rivier J. Characterization of a 41-residue ovine hypothalamic peptide that stimulates secretion of corticotropin and β-endorphin. *Science* 1981; **213**: 1394–7.

28 Shibahara S, Morimoto Y, Furutani Y *et al.* Isolation and sequence analysis of the human corticotropin-releasing factor percursor gene. *EMBO J* 1983; **2**: 775–9.

29 Holsboer F, von Bardeleben U, Gerken A, Stalla GK, Müller OA. Blunted corticotropin and normal cortisol response to human corticotropin-releasing factor (h-CRF) in depression. *N Engl J Med* 1984; **311**: 1127.

30 Holsboer F, Gerken A, von Bardeleben U *et al.* Human corticotropin-releasing hormone in depression. *Biol Psychiatry* 1986; **21**: 601–11.

31 Holsboer F, Gerken A, Stalla GK, Müller OA. Blunted aldosterone and ACTH release after human CRH administration in depressed patients. *Am J Psychiatry* 1987; **144**: 229–31.

32 Von Bardeleben U, Stalla GK, Müller OA, Holsboer F. Blunting of ACTH response to human CRH in depressed patients is avoided by metyrapone pretreatment. *Biol Psychiatry* 1988; **24**: 782–6.

33 Lisansky J, Peake GT, Strassman RJ *et al.* Augmented pituitary corticotropin response to a threshold dosage of human corticotropin-releasing hormone in depressives pretreated with metyrapone. *Arch Gen Psychiatry* 1989; **46**: 641–9.

34 Holsboer F, Müller OA, Doerr HG *et al.* ACTH and multisteroid responses to corticotropin-releasing factor in depressive illness: relationship to multisteroid responses after ACTH stimulation and dexamethasone suppression. *Psychoneuroendocrinology* 1984; **9**: 147–60.

35 Holsboer F, Gerken A, Stalla GK, Müller OA. ACTH, cortisol and corticosterone output after ovine corticotropin-releasing factor challenge during depression and after recovery. *Biol Psychiatry* 1985; **20**: 276–86.

36 Gold PW, Chrousos G, Kellner C *et al.* Psychiatric implications of basic and clinical studies with corticotropin-releasing factor. *Am J Psychiatry* 1984; **141**: 619–27.

37 Gold PW, Loriaux DL, Roy A *et al.* Responses to corticotropin-releasing hormone in the hypercortisolism of depression and Cushing's disease. Pathophysiologic and diagnostic implications. *N Engl J Med* 1986; **314**: 1329–35.

38 Rupprecht R, Lesch KP, Müller U, Beck G, Beckmann H, Schulte HM. Blunted adrenocorticotropin but normal β-endorphin release after depression. *J Clin Endocrinol Metab* 1989; **69**: 600–3.

39 Young EA, Watson SJ, Kotun J *et al.* β-Lipotropin–β-endorphin response to low-dose ovine corticotropin releasing factor in endogenous depression. *Arch Gen Psychiatry* 1990; **47**: 449–57.

40 Young EA, Akil H. Corticotropin releasing factor stimulation of ACTH and β-endorphin release: effects of acute and chronic stress. *Endocrinology* 1985; **117**: 23–30.

41 Nemeroff CB, Widerlöv E, Bissette G *et al.* Elevated concentrations of CSF corticotropin-releasing factor-like immunoreactivity in depressed patients. *Science* 1984; **226**: 1342–4.

42 Kling MA, Roy A, Doran AR *et al.* Cerebrospinal fluid immunoreactive corticotropin-releasing hormone and adrenocorticotropin secretion in Cushing's disease and major depression: potential clinical implications. *J Clin Endocrinol Metab* 1991; **72**: 260–71.

43 Nemeroff CB, Owens MJ, Bissette G, Andorn AC, Stanley M. Reduced corticotropin releasing factor binding sites in the frontal cortex of suicide victims. *Arch Gen Psychiatry* 1988; **45**: 577–9.

44 Holsboer F, Spengler D, Heuser I. The role of corticotropin-releasing hormone in the pathogenesis of Cushing's disease, anorexia nervosa, alcoholism, affective disorders and dementia. *Prog Brain Res* 1992; **93**: 385–417.

45 De Souza EB. Corticotropin-releasing factor receptors: physiology, pharmacology, biochemistry and role in central nervous system and immune disorders. *Psychoneuroendocrinology* 1995; **20**: 789–819.

46 Skutella T, Behl C, Probst JC, Renner U, Nitsch R, Holsboer F. Modulation of corticotropin releasing hormone receptor in cell culture with antisense. *J Mol Med* 1995; **73**: B25.

47 Liebsch G, Landgraf R, Gerstberger R *et al.* Chronic infusion of a CRH_1 receptor antisense oligodeoxynucleotide into the central nucleus of the amygdala reduced anxiety-related behavior in socially defeated rats. *Regul Pept* 1995; **59**: 229–39.

48 Montkowski A, Skutella T, Liebsch G, Behl C, Landgraf R, Holsboer F. Antisense 'knockdown' of CRH_1- but not of CRH_2-receptors is anxiolytic in rats. *Biol Psychiatry* 1996; **39**: 566.

49 Von Bardeleben U, Holsboer F, Stalla GK, Müller OA. Combined administration of human corticotropin-releasing factor and lysine vasopressin induces cortisol escape from dexamethasone suppression in healthy subjects. *Life Sci* 1985; **37**: 1613–18.

50 Von Bardeleben U, Holsboer F. Cortisol response to a combined dexamethasone–human corticotropin-releasing hormone challenge in patients with depression. *J Neuroendocrinol* 1989; **1**: 485–8.

51 Heuser I, Wark HJ, Keul J, Holsboer F. Altered pituitary–adrenocortical function in elderly endurance athletes. *J Clin Endocrinol Metab* 1991; **73**: 485–8.

52 Raadsheer FC, Hoogendijk WJG, Stam FC, Tilders FJH, Swaab DF. Increased numbers of corticotropin-releasing hormone expressing neurons in the hypothalamic paraventricular nucleus of depressed patients. *Clin Neuroendocrinol* 1994; **60**: 436–44.

53 Purba JS, Hoogendijk WJG, Hofman MA, Swaab DF. Increased number of vasopressin and oxytocin expressing neurons in the paraventricular nucleus of the human hypothalamus in depression. *Arch Gen Psychiatry* 1996; **53**: 137–43.

54 Landgraf R, Gerstberger R, Montkowski A *et al.* V1 vasopressin receptor antisense oligodeoxynucleotide into septum reduces vasopressin binding, social discrimination abilities, and anxiety-related behavior in rats. *J Neurosci* 1995; **15**: 4250–8.

55 Holsboer F, von Bardeleben U, Wiedemann K, Müller OA, Stalla GK. Serial assessment of corticotropin-releasing hormone response after dexamethasone in depression—implications for pathophysiology of DST nonsuppression. *Biol Psychiatry* 1987; **22**: 228–34.

56 Holsboer-Trachsler E, Strohler R, Hatzinger M. Repeated administration of the combined dexamethasone–hCRH stimulation test during treatment of depression. *Psychiatry Res* 1991; **38**: 163–71.

57 Lammers CH, Garcia-Borreguero D, Schmider J *et al.* Combined dexamethasone/corticotropin-releasing hormone test in patients with schizophrenia and in normal controls II. *Biol Psychiatry* 1995; **38**: 803–7.

58 Schmider J, Lammers CH, Gotthardt U, Dettling M, Holsboer F, Heuser IJ. Combined dexamethasone/corticotropin-releasing hormone test in acute and remitted manic patients, in acute depression and in normal controls I. *Biol Psychiatry* 1995; **38**: 797–802.

59 Schreiber W, Lauer CJ, Krumrey K, Holsboer F, Krieg JC. Dysregulation of the hypothalamic–pituitary–adrenocortical system in panic disorder. *Neuropsychopharmacology* 1996; **15**: 7–15.

60 Holsboer-Trachsler E, Hemmeter U, Strohler R, Hatzinger M, Gerhard U, Hobi V. The dexamethasone–hCRH stimulation test and cognitive performance during antidepressant treatment with trimipramine. *Eur Neuropsychopharmacol* 1991; **1**: 338–40.

61 Holsboer-Trachsler E, Hemmeter U, Hatzinger M, Seifritz E, Gerhard U, Hobi V. Sleep deprivation and bright light as potential augmenters of antidepressant drug treatment—neurobiological and psychometric assessment of course. *J Psychiatr Res* 1994; **28**: 381–99.

62 Heuser IJE, Schweiger U, Gotthardt U *et al.* Pituitary–adrenal system regulation and psychopathology during amitriptyline treatment in elderly depressed patients and in normal controls. *Am J Psychiatry* 1996; **153**: 93–9.

63 Von Bardeleben U, Holsboer F. Effect of age on the cortisol response to human CRH in depressed patients pretreated with dexamethasone. *Biol Psychiatry* 1991; **29**: 1042–50.

64 Heuser IJ, Gotthardt U, Schweiger U *et al.* Age-associated changes of pituitary-adrenocortical hormone regulation in humans: importance of gender. *Neurobiol Aging* 1994; **15**: 227–31.

65 Heuser I, Yassouridis A, Holsboer F. The combined dexamethasone/CRH-test: a refined laboratory test for psychiatric disorders. *J Psychiatr Res* 1994; **28**: 341–56.

66 Young EA, Haskett RF, Murphy-Weinberg V, Watson S, Akil H. Loss of glucocorticoid fast feedback in depression. *Arch Gen Psychiatry* 1991; **48**: 693–9.

67 Holsboer F, Lauer CJ, Schreiber W, Krieg JC. Altered hypothalamic–pituitary–adrenocortical regulation in healthy subjects at high familial risk for depression. *Neuroendocrinology* 1995; **62**: 340–7.

68 de Kloet ER. Brain corticosteroid receptor balance and homeostatic control. *Front Neuroendocrinol* 1991; **12**: 95–164.

69 Trapp T, Rupprecht R, Castrén M, Reul JMHM, Holsboer F. Heterodimerization between mineralocorticoid and glucocorticoid receptor: a new principle of glucocorticoid action in the central nervous system. *Neuron* 1994; **13**: 1–6.

70 Trapp T, Holsboer F. Heterodimerization between mineralocorticoid and glucocorticoid receptor increases the functional diversity of corticosteroid action. *Trends Pharmacol Sci* 1996; **17**: 145–9.

71 Hassan AHS, von Rosenstiel P, Patchev VK, Holsboer F, Almeida OFX. Exacerbation of apoptosis in the dentate gyrus of the aged rat by dexamethasone and the protective role of corticosterone. *Exp Neurol* 1996; **140**: 43–52.

72 De Bellis MD, Gold PW, Geracioti TD, Jr, Listwak SJ, Kling MA. Association of fluoxetine treatment with reductions in CSF concentrations of corticotropin-releasing hormone and arginine vasopressin in patients with major depression. *Am J Psychiatry* 1993; **150**: 656–7.

73 Holsboer F, Barden N. Antidepressants and hypothalamic–pituitary–adrenocortical regulation. *Endocr Rev* 1996; **17**: 187–205.

74 Barden N, Reul JMHM, Holsboer F. Do antidepressants stabilize mood through actions on the hypothalamic–pituitary–adrenal system? *Trends Neurosci* 1995; **18**: 6–11.

75 Peiffer A, Veilleux S, Barden N. Antidepressant and other centrally acting drugs regulate glucocorticoid receptor messenger RNA levels in rat brain. *Psychoneuroendocrinology* 1991; **16**: 505–15.

76 Pepin MC, Govindan MV, Barden N. Increased glucocorticoid receptor gene promoter activity after antidepressant treatment. *Mol Pharmacol* 1992; **41**: 1016–22.

77 Pepin MC, Pothier F, Barden N. Impaired type II glucocorticoid receptor function in mice bearing antisense RNA transgene. *Nature* 1992; **335**: 725–8.

78 Stec I, Barden N, Reul JMHM, Holsboer F. Dexamethasone nonsuppression in transgenic mice expressing antisense RNA to the glucocorticoid receptor. *J Psychiatr Res* 1994; **28**: 1–5.

79 Montkowski A, Barden N, Wotjak C *et al.* Long-term antidepressant treatment reduces behavioural deficits in transgenic mice with impaired glucocorticoid receptor function. *J Neuroendocrinol* 1995; **7**: 841–5.

80 Reul JMHM, Stec I, Söder M, Holsboer F. Chronic treatment of rats with the antidepressant amitriptyline attenuates the activity of the hypothalamic–pituitary–adrenocortical system. *Endocrinology* 1993; **133**: 312–20.

81 Reul JMHM, Labeur MS, Grigoriadis DE, De Souza EB, Holsboer F. Hypothalamic–pituitary–adrenocortical axis changes in the rat after a long-term treatment with the reversible monoamine oxidase-A inhibitor moclobemide. *Neuroendocrinology* 1994; **60**: 509–19.

82 Brown GW, Bifulco A, Harris TO. Life events, vulnerability and onset of depression. *Br J Psychiatry* 1987; **150**: 508–11.

83 Levine S. Plasma-free corticosteroid response to electric shock in rats stimulated in infancy. *Science* 1962; **135**: 795–6.

84 Levine S, Mullins RF, Jr. Hormonal influences on brain organization in infant rats. *Science* 1966; **152**: 1585–92.

85 Meaney MJ, Aitken DH, van Berkel C, Bhatnagar S, Sapolsky RM. Effect of neonatal handling on age-related impairments associated with the hippocampus. *Science* 1988; **239**: 766–8.

86 Meaney MJ, Aitken DH, Bhatnagar S, Sapolsky RM. Postnatal handling attenuates certain neuroendocrine, anatomical, and cognitive dysfunctions associated with aging in female rats. *Neurobiol Aging* 1991; **12**: 31–8.

87 Reul JMHM, Stec I, Wiegers GJ *et al.* Prenatal immune challenge alters the hypothalamic–pituitary–adrenocortical axis in adult rats. *J Clin Invest* 1994; **93**: 2600–7.

88 Ladd CO, Owens MJ, Nemeroff CB. Persistent changes in corticotropin-releasing factor neuronal systems induced by maternal deprivation. *Endocrinology* 1996; **137**: 1212–18.

89 Winer LM, Shaw MA, Baumann G. Basal plasma growth hormone levels in man: new evidence for rhythmicity of growth hormone secretion. *J Clin Endocrinol Metab* 1990; **70**: 1678–86.

90 Steiger A, Herth T, Holsboer F. Sleep-EEG and the secretion of cortisol and human growth hormone in normal controls. *Acta Endocrinol* 1987; **116**: 36–42.

91 Mendlewicz J, Linkowski P, Kerkhofs M *et al.* Diurnal hypersecretion of growth hormone in depression. *J Clin Endocrinol Metab* 1985; **60**: 505–12.

92 Steiger A, von Bardeleben U, Herth T, Holsboer F. Sleep-EEG and nocturnal secretion of cortisol and growth hormone in male patients with endogenous depression before treatment and after recovery. *J Affective Disord* 1989; **16**: 189–95.

93 Jarrett DB, Miewald JM, Kupfer DJ. Recurrent depression is associated with a persistent reduction in sleep-related growth hormone secretion. *Arch Gen Psychiatry* 1990; **47**: 113–18.

94 Matussek N, Ackenheil M, Hippius H *et al.* Effects of clonidine on growth hormone release in psychiatric patients and controls. *Psychiatry Res* 1980; **2**: 25–36.

95 Checkley SA, Slade AP, Shur E. Growth hormone and other responses to clonidine in patients with endogenous depression. *Br J Psychiatry* 1984; **144**: 633–9.

96 Siever LJ, Uhde TW, Silberman EK *et al.* The growth hormone response to clonidine as a probe of noradrenergic receptor responsiveness in affective disorder patients and controls. *Psychiatry Res* 1982; **6**: 171–83.

97 Laakmann G, Zygan K, Schoen HW *et al.* Effect of receptor blockers (methysergide, propranolol, phentolamine, yohimbine and prazosin) on desipramine-induced pituitary hormone stimulation in humans. 1. Growth hormone. *Psychoneuroendocrinology* 1986; **11**: 447–61.

98 Lesch KP, Laux G, Erb A, Pfüller H, Beckmann H. Attenuated growth hormone response to growth hormone-releasing hormone in major depressive disorder. *Biol Psychiatry* 1987; **22**: 1495–9.

99 Risch SC, Ehlers C, Janowsky DS *et al.* Human growth hormone releasing factor infusion effects on plasma growth hormone in affective disorder patients and normal controls. *Peptides* 1988; **9**: 45–8.

100 Peabody CA, Warner MD, Markoff E, Hoffman AR, Wilson DM, Csernansky JG. Growth hormone response to growth hormone releasing hormone in depression and schizophrenia. *Psychiatry Res* 1990; **33**: 269–76.

101 Thomas R, Beer R, Harris B, John R, Scanlon M. GH responses to growth hormone releasing factor in depression. *J Affective Disord* 1989; **16**: 133–7.

102 Krishnan KR, Manepalli AN, Ritchie JC *et al.* Growth hormone releasing factor stimulation test in depression. *Am J Psychiatry* 1988; **145**: 90–2.

103 Rivier C, Vale V. Involvement of corticotropin-releasing factor and somatostatin in stress-induced inhibition of growth hormone secretion in the rat. *Endocrinology* 1985; **117**: 2478–82.

104 Barbarino A, Corsello SM, della Casa S *et al.* Corticotropin-releasing hormone inhibition of growth hormone-releasing hormone-induced growth hormone release in man. *J Clin Endocrinol Metab* 1990; **71**: 1368–74.

105 Holsboer F, von Bardeleben U, Steiger A. Effects of intravenous corticotropin-releasing hormone upon sleep-related growth hormone surge and sleep-EEG in man. *Neuroendocrinology* 1988; **48**: 62–8.

106 Wiedemann K, von Bardeleben U, Holsboer F. Influence of h-CRH and ACTH (1–24) upon spontaneous growth hormone secretion. *Neuroendocrinology* 1991; **54**: 462–8.

107 Ho KY, Evans WS, Blizzard RM *et al.* Effects of sex and age on the 24-hour profile of growth hormone secretion in man: importance of endogenous estradiol concentrations. *J Clin Endocrinol Metab* 1987; **64**: 52–8.

108 Wehrenberg WB, Ehlers CL. Effects of growth hormone-releasing factor in the brain. *Science* 1986; **232**: 1271–2.

109 Ehlers CL, Reed TK, Henriksen SJ. Effects of corticotropin-releasing factor and growth hormone-releasing factor on sleep and activity in rats. *Neuroendocrinology* 1986; **42**: 467–74.

110 Steiger A, Guldner J, Hemmeter U, Rothe B, Wiedemann K, Holsboer F. Effects of growth hormone-releasing hormone and somatostatin on sleep EEG and nocturnal hormone secretion in male controls. *Neuroendocrinology* 1992; **56**: 566–73.

111 Ehlers CL, Kupfer DJ. Hypothalamic peptide modulation of EEG sleep in depression: a further application of the S-process hypothesis. *Biol Psychiatry* 1987; **22**: 513–17.

112 Seifritz E, Müller MJ, Trachsel L *et al.* Revisiting the Ehlers and Kupfer hypothesis: the growth hormone cortisol secretion ratio during sleep is correlated with electroencephalographic slow wave activity in normal volunteers. *Biol Psychiatry* 1996; **39**: 139–42.

113 Rubin RT, Poland RE. The chronoendocrinology of endogenous depression. In: Müller EE, MacLeod RM, eds. *Neuroendocrine Perspectives*, Vol. 1. Amsterdam: Elsevier, 1982: 305–37.

114 Loosen PT, Prange AJ, Jr. Serum thyrotropin response to thyrotropin-releasing hormone in psychiatric patients: a review. *Am J Psychiatry* 1982; **139**: 405–16.

115 Morley JE. Neuropeptide regulation of appetite and weight. *Endocr Rev* 1987; **8**: 256–87.

116 Rubin RT, Poland RE, Lesser IM, Martin DJ. Neuroendocrine aspects of primary endogenous depression. IV. Pituitary-thyroid axis activity in patients and matched control subjects. *Psychoneuroendocrinology* 1987; **12**: 333–47.

117 Bartalena L, Placidi GF, Martino E *et al.* Nocturnal serum thyrotropin (TSH) surge and the TSH response to TSH-releasing hormone: dissociated behavior in untreated depressives. *J Clin Endocrinol Metab* 1990; **71**: 650–5.

118 Duval F, Macher JP, Mokrani MC. Difference between evening and morning thyrotropin responses to protirelin in major depressive episode. *Arch Gen Psychiatry* 1990; **47**: 443–8.

119 Loosen PT, Garbutt JC, Prange AJ. Evaluation of the diagnostic utility of the TRH-induced TSH responses in psychiatric disorders. *Pharmacopsychiatry* 1987; **20**: 90–5.

120 Joffe RT, Blank DW, Post RM, Uhde TW. Decreased triiodothyronines in depression: a preliminary report. *Biol Psychiatry* 1985; **20**: 922–5.

121 Larsen PR, Silva JE, Kaplan MM. Relationship between circulating and intracellular thyroid hormones: physiological and clinical implications. *Endocr Rev* 1981; **2**: 87–102.

122 Spencer CA, Greenstadt MA, Wheeler WS, Kletzky OA, Nicoloff JT. The influence of long term low dose thyrotropin-releasing hormone infusions on serum thyrotropin and prolactin concentration in man. *J Clin Endocrinol Metab* 1980; **51**: 771–5.

123 Banki CM, Bissette G, Arato M, Nemeroff CB. Elevation of immunoreactive CSF TRH in depressed patients. *Am J Psychiatry* 1988; **145**: 1526–31.

124 Kendler KS, Davis KL. Elevated corticosteroids as a possible cause of abnormal neuroendocrine function in depressive illness. *Commun Psychopharmacol* 1977; **1**: 183–94.

125 Holsboer F, Gerken A, von Bardeleben U, Grimm W, Stalla GK, Müller OA. Relationship between pituitary responses to human corticotropin-releasing factor and thyrotropin-releasing hormone in depressives and normal controls. *Eur J Pharmacol* 1985; **110**: 153–4.

126 Dunn AJ, Berridge CW. Physiological and behavioral responses to corticotropin-releasing factor administration: is CRF a mediator of anxiety or stress responses? *Brain Res Rev* 1990; **15**: 71–100.

127 Britton DR, Koob GF, Rivier J, Vale W. Intraventricular corticotropin-releasing factor enhances behavioral effects of novelty. *Life Sci* 1982; **31**: 363–7.

128 Kalin NH, Shelton SE, Barksdale CM. Behavioral and physiologic effects of CRH administered to infant primates undergoing maternal separation. *Neuropsychopharmacology* 1989; **2**: 97–104.

129 Insel TR, Ninan PT, Aloi J, Jimerson DC, Skolnick P, Paul SM. A benzodiazepine receptor-mediated model of anxiety. *Arch Gen Psychiatry* 1984; **41**: 741–50.

130 Kalogeras KT, Calogero AE, Kuribayiashi T *et al. In vitro* and *in vivo* effects of the triazolobenzodiazepine alprazolam on hypothalamic–pituitary–adrenal function: pharmacological and clinical implications. *J Clin Endocrinol Metab* 1990; **70**: 1462–71.

131 Owens MJ, Bissette G, Nemeroff CB. Acute effects of alprazolam and adinazolam on the concentrations of corticotropin-releasing

factor in rat brain. *Synapse* 1989; **4**: 196–202.
132 Swanson LW, Sawchenko PE, Rivier J, Vale WW. Organization of ovine corticotropin-releasing factor immunoreactive cells and fibers in the rat brain: an immunohistochemical study. *Neuroendocrinology* 1983; **36**: 165–86.
133 Butler PD, Weiss JM, Stout JC, Nemeroff CB. Corticotropin-releasing factor produces fear-enhancing and behavioral activating effects following infusion into the locus coeruleus. *J Neurosci* 1990; **10**: 176–83.
134 Coplan JD, Pine D, Papp L *et al.* Uncoupling of the noradrenergic–hypothalamic–pituitary–adrenal axis in panic disorder patients. *Neuropsychopharmacology* 1995; **13**: 65–73.
135 Abelson JL, Curtis GC. Hypothalamic–pituitary–adrenal axis activity in panic disorder. 24-hour secretion of corticotropin and cortisol. *Arch Gen Psychiatry* 1996; **53**: 321–31.
136 Roy-Byrne PP, Uhde TW, Post RM, Gallucci W, Chrousos GP, Gold PW. The corticotropin-releasing hormone stimulation test in patients with panic disorder. *Am J Psychiatry* 1986; **143**: 896–9.
137 Rapaport MH, Risch SC, Golshan S, Gillin JC. Neuroendocrine effects of ovine corticotropin-releasing hormone in panic disorder patients. *Biol Psychiatry* 1989; **26**: 344–8.
138 Holsboer F, von Bardeleben U, Buller R, Heuser I, Steiger A. Stimulation response to corticotropin-releasing hormone (CRH) in patients with depression, alcoholism and panic disorder. *Horm Metab Res* 1987; **16**: 80–8.
139 Klein DF. False suffocation alarms, spontaneous panics, and related conditions. *Arch Gen Psychiatry* 1993; **50**: 306–17.
140 Hollander E, Liebowitz MR, Gorman JM, Cohen B, Fyer A, Klein DF. Cortisol and sodium lactate-induced panic. *Arch Gen Psychiatry* 1989; **46**: 135–40.
141 Kellner M, Herzog L, Yassouridis A, Holsboer F, Wiedemann K. Possible role of atrial natriuretic hormone in pituitary–adrenocortical unresponsiveness in lactate–induced panic. *Am J Psychiatry* 1995; **152**: 1365–7.
142 Kellner M, Wiedemann K, Holsboer F. ANF inhibits the CRH-stimulated secretion of ACTH and cortisol in man. *Life Sci* 1992; **50**: 1835–42.
143 Abelson J. Cholecystokinin in psychiatric research: a time for cautious excitement. *J Psychiatr Res* 1995; **29**: 389–96.
144 Nutt DJ, Glue P, Lawson C, Wilson S. Flumazenil provocation of panic attacks. *Arch Gen Psychiatry* 1990; **47**: 917–25.
145 Roy–Byrne PP, Uhde TW, Rubinow DR, Post RM. Reduced TSH and prolactin responses to TRH inpatients with panic disorder. *Am J Psychiatry* 1986; **143**: 503–7.
146 Rapaport MH, Risch SC, Gillin JC, Golshan S, Janowsky DS. Blunted growth hormone response to peripheral infusion of human growth hormone-releasing factor in patients with panic disorder. *Am J Psychiatry* 1989; **146**: 92–5.
147 Yehuda R, Southwick SM, Nussbaum G, Giller EL, Mason JW. Low urinary cortisol excretion in PTSD. *J Nerv Ment Dis* 1991; **178**: 366–9.
148 Yehuda R, Reicher M, Trestman RL, Levengood RA, Siever LJ. Cortisol regulation in post-traumatic stress disorder: a chronobiological analysis. *Ann NY Acad Sci* 1994; **746**: 378–80.
149 Yehuda R, Lowy MT, Southwick SM, Shaffer D, Giller EL. Lymphocyte glucocorticoid receptor number in post-traumatic stress disorder. *Am J Psychiatry* 1991; **148**: 499–504.
150 Yehuda R, Southwick SM, Krystal JH, Charney DS, Mason JW. Enhanced suppression of cortisol following a low dose of dexamethasone in combat veterans with posttraumatic stress disorder. *Am J Psychiatry* 1993; **150**: 83–96.
151 Yehuda R, Boisoneau D, Lowy MT, Giller EL, Jr. Dose–response changes in plasma cortisol and lymphocyte glucocorticoid receptors following dexamethasone administration in combat veterans with and without posttraumatic stress disorder. *Arch Gen Psychiatry* 1995; **52**: 583–93.
152 Holsboer-Trachsler E, Buol C, Wiedemann K, Holsboer F. Dexamethasone suppression test in severe schizophrenic illness: effects of plasma dexamethasone and caffeine levels. *Acta Psychiatr Scand* 1987; **75**: 608–13.
153 Roy A, Pickar D, Doran A *et al.* The corticotropin releasing hormone stimulation test in chronic schizophrenia. *Am J Psychiatry* 1986; **143**: 1393–7.
154 Van Cauter E, Linkowski P, Kerkhofs M *et al.* Circadian and sleep-related endocrine rhythms in schizophrenia. *Arch Gen Psychiatry* 1991; **48**: 348–56.
155 Zemlan FP, Hirschowitz MD, Garver DL. Relation of clinical symptoms to apomorphine-stimulated growth hormone release in mood-incongruent psychotic patients. *Arch Gen Psychiatry* 1986; **43**: 1162–7.
156 Gold PW, Kaye W, Robertson GL, Ebert M. Abnormalities in plasma and cerebrospinal fluid arginine vasopressin in patients with anorexia nervosa. *N Engl J Med* 1983; **308**: 1117–23.
157 Gold PW, Gwirtsman H, Avgerinos PC *et al.* Abnormal hypothalamic–pituitary–adrenal function in anorexia nervosa. *N Engl J Med* 1986; **314**: 1335–42.
158 Glowa JR, Gold PW. Corticotropin releasing hormone produces profound anorexigenic effects in the rhesus monkey. *Neuropeptides* 1991; **18**: 55–61.
159 Vaughan J, Donaldson C, Bittencourt J *et al.* Urocortin, a mammalian neuropeptide related to fish urotensin I and to corticotropin-releasing factor. *Nature* 1995; **378**: 287–92.
160 Lesem MD, Kaye WH, Bissette G, Jimerson DC, Nemeroff CB. Cerebrospinal fluid TRH immunoreactivity in anorexia nervosa. *Biol Psychiatry* 1994; **35**: 48–53.
161 Banki CM, Bissette G, Arato M, Nemeroff CB. Elevation of immunoreactivity CSF TRH in depressed patients. *Am J Psychiatry* 1988; **145**: 1526–31.
162 Vigersky RA, Loriaux DL, Anderson AE, Lipsett MB. Anorexia nervosa: behavioral and hypothalamic aspects. *Clin Endocrinol Metab* 1976; **5**: 517–24.
163 Dickson PR, Vaccarino FJ. Characterization of feeding behavior induced by central injection of GRF. *Am J Physiol* 1990; **259**: R651–7.
164 Feifel D, Vaccarino FJ, Rivier J, Vale W. Evidence for a common neural mechanism mediating GRF-induced and somatostatin-induced feeding. *Neuroendocrinology* 1993; **57**: 299–305.
165 Vaccarino FJ, Kennedy SH, Ralevski E, Black R. The effects of growth hormone-releasing factor on food consumption in anorexia nervosa patients and normals. *Biol Psychiatry* 1994; **35**: 446–51.
166 Almeida OFX, Nikolarakis KE, Herz A. Evidence for the involvement of endogenous opioids in the inhibition of luteinizing hormone by corticotropin-releasing factor. *Endocrinology* 1988; **122**: 1034–41.
167 Mortola JF, Laughlin GA, Yen SSC. Melatonin rhythms in women with anorexia nervosa and bulimia nervosa. *J Clin Endocrinol Metab* 1993; **77**: 1540–44.
168 Philipp E, Pirke KM, Kellner MB, Krieg JC. Disturbed cholecystokinin secretion in patients with eating disorder. *Life Sci* 1991; **48**: 2443–50.
169 Rose C, Vargas F, Facchinetti P *et al.* Characterization and inhibition of a cholecystokinin-inactivating serine peptidase. *Nature* 1996; **380**: 403–9.

170 Davies L, Marks JL. Role of hypothalamic neuropeptide Y gene expression in body weight regulation. *Am J Physiol* 1994; **226**: R1687–91.

171 Qu D, Ludwig DS, Gammeltoft S *et al.* A role for melanin-concentrating hormone in the central regulation of feeding behaviour. *Nature* 1996; **380**: 243–6.

172 Stephens TW, Basinski M, Bristow PK *et al.* The role of neuropeptide Y in the antiobesity action of the obese gene product. *Nature* 1995; **377**: 530–2.

173 Erickson JC, Clegg KE, Palmiter RD. Sensitivity to leptin and susceptibility to seizures of mice lacking neuropeptide Y. *Nature* 1996; **381**: 415–8.

174 Modell S, Yassouridis A, Huber J, Holsboer F. Corticosteroid receptor function is decreased in depressed patients. *Neuroendocrinology* 1997; **65**: 216–22.

175 Frieboes RM, Murck H, Schier T, Holsboer F, Steiger A. Somatostatin impairs sleep in elderly human subjects. *Neuropsychopharmacology* 1997; **16**: 339–45.

176 Ströhle A, Jahn H, Montkowski A *et al.* Central and peripheral administration of atriopeptin is anxiolytic in rats. *Neuroendocrinology* 1997; **65**: 210–15.

177 Bohlhalter S, Murck H, Holsboer F, Steiger A. Cortisol enhances non-REM sleep and growth hormone secretion in elderly subjects. *Neurobiol Aging* (in press).

178 Lonnqvist F, Arner P, Nordfors L, Schalling M. Overexpression of the obese (*ob*) gene in adipose tissue of human obese subjects. *Nat Med* 1995; **1**: 950–3.

179 Considine RV, Sinha MK, Heiman ML *et al.* Serum immunoreactive-leptin concentrations in normal-weight and obese humans. *N Engl J Med* 1996; **334**: 292–5.

Part 19
Protocols for Common Endocrine Tests

CHAPTER 83

Protocols for common endocrine tests

R.C. Jenkins and R.J.M. Ross

Introduction

Endocrinology is sometimes viewed as an art form rather than a science. This is because endocrinologists often design complex and uninterpretable tests for rare and bizarre conditions. In truth, good practice of endocrinology requires the same principles of scientific logic as any branch of medicine.

Most hormones are secreted in pulses, frequently with circadian or ultradian rhythms, and their release controlled by negative feedback. The single measurement of a hormone, therefore, without reference to time or conditions, is of little value, and stimulation and suppression tests are frequently required. The interpretation of tests is dependent on their appropriate use, and the precise and careful planning of test protocols. It is essential to accurately record the timing of samples, administration of drugs, and any symptoms the patient experiences (see example record of insulin tolerance test, Fig. 83.1).

The present chapter aims to provide a 'recipe book' for the common and useful endocrine tests, and references are given for more detailed reviews. The format used to describe each test is similar, i.e. indications, precautions, procedure, normal response, interpretation. For many tests, although a normal response is described, absolute values are not given because the measurement of hormones is dependent on the assay used and the laboratory. In some instances, absolute values are given; this is either because there is little variation in the measurement between laboratories, for example plasma osmolality, or because most laboratories are unable to provide a normal range for that hormone, for example the cortisol response to corticotrophin-releasing hormone (CRH). In the latter group it is essential to exercise caution in interpreting the test and a reference is always given in the text for the origin of the data.

Assessment of anterior pituitary reserve

Introduction

The pituitary controls various target tissues through the secretion of six known hormones: growth hormone (GH), luteinising hormone (LH), follicle-stimulating hormone (FSH), adrenocorticotrophic hormone (ACTH), thyroid-stimulating hormone (TSH) and prolactin. If those target tissues are functioning normally then it is clear that the hypothalamo-pituitary axis is also functioning appropriately. Thus, a woman with regular menses who is ovulating must have a normal gonadotroph, and similarly a euthyroid patient will have a normal thyrotroph. The assessment of the gonadotroph and thyrotroph therefore predominantly requires basal hormone levels. For ACTH, GH and the gonadotrophins in some situations, however, 'stimulation tests' are required.

ACTH and GH are both 'stress hormones'; i.e. they rise in response to certain stressful situations such as illness and hypoglycaemia. This is the basis of the insulin tolerance or stress test (ITT or IST) and the glucagon test, both of which stimulate ACTH and GH release through the hypothalamus (Fig. 83.2). Clomiphene blocks oestrogen feedback at the pituitary and hypothalamus and can be used as a stimulation test of the gonadal axis.

Insulin tolerance test or stress test

Indications. Diagnosis of secondary adrenal failure. Diagnosis of growth hormone deficiency. Diagnosis of Cushing's syndrome.

Contraindications. Ischaemic heart disease, epilepsy,

Patient: Richards Ross No Consultant:
Address & Tel:

DIAGNOSIS AND REASON FOR REASSESSMENT:
? Hypopituitary

PRESENT TREATMENT: None

TESTS REQUESTED:
Insulin tolerance test

For IST: any. fits? No IHD? No ECG? ✓ FT4 14.5 Cortisol 320

PRESCRIPTIONS

Drug	Dose	Route
Insulin	0.5 units/kg	iv

SIGNATURE R Ross DATE 8.2.90

TEST ITT DATE 8.2.90

TIME	SAMPLE TIME	TREATMENT & COMMENTS	HORMONE RESULTS						
			Bm	BS	Cortisol	GH			
Cannulated	08.30								
0'	09.00	← Insulin 0.15 u/kg	4.0	3.9	220	<0.5			
30'	09.30	← Sweaty + tachycardia	2.0	1.9	210	10.0			
45'	09.45		3.0	3.0	300	40.0			
60'	10.00		3.4	3.3	600	35.0			
90'	10.30		3.5	3.2	660	15.0			
120	11.00		3.7	3.5	600	7.0			

INTERPRETATION: Normal cortisol and GH response to insulin hypoglycaemia

SIGNATURE DATE OUTPATIENT APPOINTMENT

Fig. 83.1 Example record of insulin tolerance test (ITT).

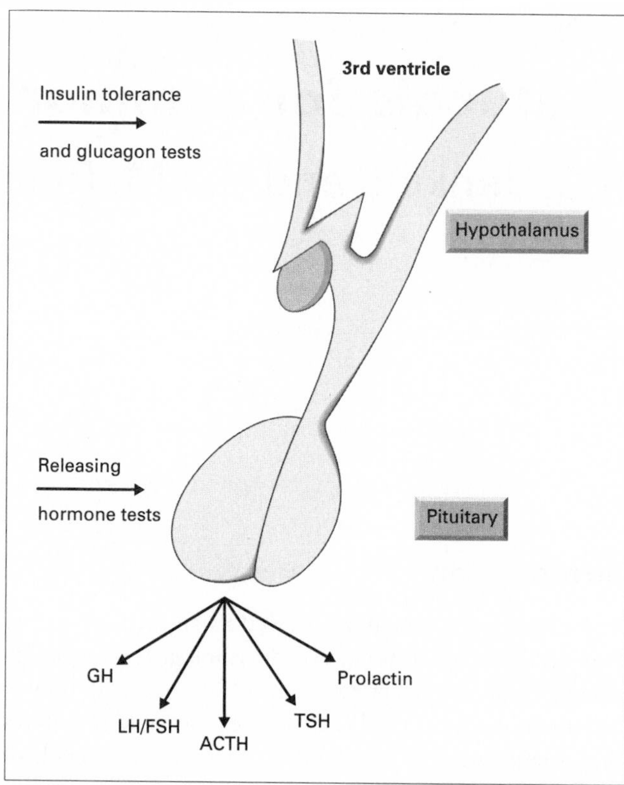

Fig. 83.2 Site of action for pituitary 'stimulation' and 'releasing hormone' tests: the insulin tolerance and glucagon tests act at the hypothalamus and therefore test the hypothalamo-pituitary axis, but the releasing hormone tests act only at the pituitary. ACTH, adrenocorticotrophic hormone; FSH, follicle-stimulating hormone; GH, growth hormone; LH, luteinising hormone; TSH, thyroid-stimulating hormone.

severe long-standing hypoadrenalism, age <2 years, glycogen storage diseases.

Precautions. A trained nurse and doctor *must* always be in attendance throughout the test. Electrocardiogram (ECG) must be normal; 0900 hours cortisol >100 nmol/l; and thyroxine (T_4) level normal. Intravenous dextrose and hydrocortisone should be readily available.

Procedure. Fast from midnight; at 0800–0900 hours weigh patient and place an intravenous cannula for sampling and giving insulin (this should be secure and preferably plastic rather than a 'butterfly'). At 0900 hours, give an intravenous bolus of soluble insulin: 0.15 U/kg to normal subjects and 0.3 U/kg to patients who are insulin resistant with severe Cushing's or acromegaly.

Observe for symptoms and signs of hypoglycaemia (sweating, tachycardia, neuroglycopenia) which should occur about 20–30 min after insulin administration. If the patient is not clinically or biochemically hypoglycaemic at 45 min (check with finger-prick glucose), then give a second dose of insulin equivalent to the first dose.

Once the patient has been symptomatically hypoglycaemic then an adequate 'stress' has been provided, and the hypoglycaemia may be reversed with intravenous or oral dextrose without altering the cortisol or GH responses. With severe and prolonged hypoglycaemia (>20 min), impending loss of consciousness or fits the test should be terminated by giving 25–50 ml 25% glucose i.v. followed by a 5% dextrose infusion. Continue sampling to the end of the test. Consider hydrocortisone 100 mg i.v. at the end of the test or during the test if the patient appears hypoadrenal. The patient should have a meal and be observed for 2 hours after the test. The test may be combined with gonadotrophin-releasing hormone (GnRH) and thyrotrophin-releasing hormone (TRH) tests.

Sampling. Blood glucose, serum cortisol, serum GH, at 0, 30, 45, 60, 90, 120 min. If insulin dose repeated: 0, 30, 45, 60, 75, 90, 120, 150 min. Bedside glucose monitoring at the same time-points is useful but can be misleading at low readings.

Normal response. Blood glucose must fall to <2.2 mmol/l. Plasma cortisol rises by >170 nmol/l to above 550 nmol/l. GH rises to >20 mU/l.

Interpretation. Inadequate hypoglycaemia and hypothyroidism result in subnormal cortisol and GH responses.

A normal cortisol response means the patient will withstand stress such as major surgery without corticosteroid replacement. Patients with a marginally subnormal response should have steroid cover for surgery or an illness and a repeat ITT in 6–12 months. If the peak cortisol is <300nmol/l consider starting hydrocortisone-replacement therapy.

Patients with Cushing's syndrome usually show no rise in cortisol with hypoglycaemia while depressed or alcoholic patients may have a normal rise.

GH deficiency, of sufficient severity for GH replacement to have been shown to be of benefit, is present in adults whose peak GH is <9 mU/l. An inadequate GH response may occur in obese patients, and those who have had a recent spontaneous pulse of GH (high GH level at the zero sample).

See [1,2,3].

Glucagon test

Indications. Diagnosis of secondary adrenal failure and diagnosis of GH deficiency in patients in whom the ITT is contraindicated.

Contraindications. Patients who have not eaten for 48 hours; glycogen storage diseases; severe cortisol deficiency (i.e. situations where glycogen stores are low).

Precautions. Cortisol at 0900 hours >100 nmol/l is preferable, and normal T_4 levels.

Procedures. Fast from midnight; weigh, and insert intravenous cannula at 0830 hours. Give glucagon 1 mg s.c. at 0900 hours (1.5 mg if >90 kg). Children's dose (15 μg/kg). Patients often feel nauseated after glucagon and may vomit, but other side-effects are rare.

Sampling. Blood glucose, serum cortisol, serum GH, at 0, 90, 120, 150, 180, 210, 240 min.

Normal response. Blood glucose usually rises then falls. Plasma cortisol rises by >170 nmol/l to >550 nmol/l. GH rises to >20 mU/l.

Interpretation. The interpretation is as for the ITT but the glucagon test is a less reliable test as some normal individuals do not respond. See [4,5].

Clomiphene test

Indications. To differentiate gonadotrophin deficiency from weight-related hypogonadism and idiopathic delayed puberty.

Side-effects. Depression, visual flickering or central haloes and symptoms of oestrogen deficiency. Depression may warrant discontinuation of the test.

Procedure. Clomiphene 3 mg/kg/day in divided doses (usually three doses, maximum 200 mg/day) for 7 days.

Sampling. Serum LH and FSH on days 0, 4, 7, 10. Serum progesterone on day 21 in females.

Normal response. LH and FSH show a definite rise to outside the normal range, or to double the basal value. Day 21 progesterone may confirm ovulation. Menstruation should occur.

Interpretation. Lack of response suggests gonadotrophin deficiency due to pituitary or hypothalamic disease. In females a normal response may be followed by menstruation. Patients with anorexia nervosa may show no response to clomiphene, but the response returns to normal as the patient regains weight, even before the onset of menstruation. Prepubertal children show no response to clomiphene and children in early puberty may show a fall in gonadotrophins during the test as clomiphene is a partial oestrogen agonist. See [6].

Releasing hormone tests

There are four hypothalamic releasing hormones which have been characterised, synthesised, and are available for use as clinical tests: TRH, GnRH, CRH and GH-releasing hormone (GHRH). All these releasing hormones act directly at the pituitary, and therefore test the 'readily releasable' pituitary pool; they do not test the intact hypothalamo-pituitary axis (Fig. 83.2). Releasing hormone tests have a limited role in investigating the hypothalamo-pituitary axis, although all may differentiate hypothalamic from pituitary hormone deficiencies. In the present chapter, only the indications considered clinically useful have been given. The TRH and GnRH tests may be performed in conjunction with the ITT. For a full review of releasing hormone tests, see [7].

TRH test

Indications. Diagnosis of thyrotoxicosis (when sensitive TSH assays are unavailable). Differentiation of pituitary TSH deficiency from hypothalamic TRH deficiency in secondary hypothyroidism. Assessment of acromegaly.

Side-effects. Usually mild and include nausea, flushing and a desire to micturate. Very occasionally, pituitary apoplexy has been recorded.

Procedure. Non-fasting. Insert intravenous cannula at 0830 hours then give TRH 200 µg i.v. at 0900 hours. Sample for serum TSH (and GH if assessing acromegaly) at 0, 20, 60 min and T_4 at 0 min. May be combined with ITT and GnRH tests.

Normal response. TSH rises by more than 2 mU/l to > 3.4 mU/l and the 20-min value is greater than the 60-min value. No rise in GH levels. A GH response is a rise to greater than 10 mU/l or more than 50% of the basal value.

Interpretation of TSH response. This is based largely on the results of basal tests. A delayed and exaggerated response (60-min value greater than 20-min value) is characteristic of hypothalamic disease, but may occur in pituitary disease, sick patients and renal failure. A flat response in the presence of raised T_4 or triiodothyronine (T_3) levels confirms thyrotoxicosis. A blunted TSH response occurs in Cushing's syndrome and an exaggerated response in primary hypothyroidism.

Interpretation of GH response. Occasional normal subjects show a response to TRH, and diabetic patients and those in renal failure may also show a response. In addition, spontaneous GH secretion may simulate a response to TRH. The TRH test is not useful in the diagnosis of acromegaly, but may be useful in determining whether a cure has been achieved after surgery. Some researchers claim that an absent GH response to TRH after surgery is the best predictor of a cure in acromegaly [8].

GnRH test

Indication. Investigation of gonadotrophin deficiency.

Side-effects. None, although pituitary apoplexy has been reported.

Procedure. Non-fasting. Insert cannula at 0830 hours and give 100 µg GnRH i.v. at 0900 hours. Sample for LH and FSH at 0, 20 and 60 min. May be combined with ITT and TRH tests.

Normal response. LH and FSH both rise, the precise threshold depending on individual laboratories. The peak response may be seen at either 20 or 60 min.

Interpretation. This is based largely on the basal tests. In a patient with delayed puberty a normal response or a response in which the LH peak is greater than that for FSH suggests that the patient is about to go into puberty and does not have gonadotrophin deficiency. The response to GnRH may be suppressed by intervening illness.

CRH test

Indications. Diagnosis and differential diagnosis of Cushing's syndrome. Differentiation of hypothalamic from pituitary causes of ACTH deficiency.

Side-effects. Many patients experience a facial flush that comes on 1 min after injection and lasts for about 2 min. Hypotension may occur.

Procedure. Fasting from midnight. Insert cannula at 0830 hours, and at 0900 hours give 100 µg (or 1 µg/kg) i.v. of either ovine or human CRH. Collect samples for plasma cortisol and ACTH at –15, 0, 15, 30, 45, 60, 90, 120 min.

Normal response. Cortisol rises to a peak of < 800 nmol/l.

Interpretation. The response to human CRH may be slightly less than that seen after ovine CRH. Eighty to ninety per cent of patients with Cushing's disease show a 20% rise in cortisol concentrations during the CRH test, whilst ectopic ACTH-secreting tumours and adrenal tumours rarely show a response [9]. Over 90% of patients with Cushing's disease have a greater than 35% rise in ACTH over basal compared with no response in patients with ectopic ACTH syndrome [10]. Patients with depression show a normal cortisol response but blunted ACTH response, and those with obesity show a normal or blunted response. See [11,12].

GHRH test

Indications. Differential diagnosis of isolated GH deficiency. Mainly used for research but could in the future provide a predictor of patients who will respond to GHRH therapy. There are three analogues that have been used but all are equipotent: GHRH(1–29)NH_2, GHRH(1–40)OH, GHRH(1–44)NH_2.

Side-effects. Most patients experience a facial flush 1 min after injection, lasting for 2 min.

Procedure. Fast from midnight. Insert intravenous cannula

at 0830 hours and give 100 μg GHRH i.v. at 0900 hours. Take serum for GH at time –15, 0, 15, 30, 45, 60, 90, 120 min.

Normal response. In the largest study reported, short children with a normal response to the ITT showed a peak GH level after GHRH from < 10 to > 100 mU/l; the mean ± SEM was 46.0 ± 5.0 [13]. In a study of normal adult subjects the peak serum GH was > 12 mU/l in all subjects [14].

Interpretation. There is considerable individual variation in GH response which declines with age and is influenced by weight and oestrogen status; a rise in GH suggests the presence of normal somatotrophs.

Tests of GH and prolactin secretion

Growth hormone

GH is secreted in a pulsatile fashion, with greatest release occurring at night. GH pulse amplitude and frequency increase at puberty and decline after the age of 40 years. Many of the metabolic effects of GH are mediated through insulin-like growth factor 1 (IGF-1), which probably acts both in an endocrine and paracrine fashion. GH levels are influenced by gender, weight, nutritional status and oestrogen levels. This pattern of hormone release makes it difficult to define normal values and single samples are of little value.

Tests of GH secretion can be broadly divided into physiological and pharmacological tests. As might be expected in an area of controversy, there are numerous tests and only the commonly used tests are given here.

Pharmacological tests for GH deficiency

The ITT and glucagon test are the most widely used and offer the advantage of also assessing ACTH reserve.

Normal response. GH rises to > 20 mU/l. In adults with a peak GH < 9 mU/l GH replacement is of proven benefit [3].

Interpretation. Inadequate hypoglycaemia, hypothyroidism, corticosteroids, obesity and recent spontaneous GH release may cause attenuated GH responses.

Sex steroid priming. Peripubertal subjects (bone age 10–15 years) may show subnormal GH secretion. Pretreatment with sex steroids (priming) may help differentiate this group from GH-deficient children. Stilboestrol 1 mg twice daily for 48 hours before the ITT or glucagon test provides adequate priming for both sexes. Stilboestrol treatment is usually without side-effects, although some children may feel nauseous. The interpretation of GH responses is as for an unprimed test, but cortisol levels are higher due to raised binding proteins [15].

GH profiles

GH has a half-life of approximately 20 min; therefore sampling should be done at least every 20 min. Profiles are usually done overnight or for a full 24-hour period.

Normal values. GH pulses should occur approximately every 3 hours with undetectable or very low values between pulses. In normal children, a peak GH value > 20 mU/l usually occurs during sleep, and the peak GH level seen during sleep correlates with the peak GH seen during hypoglycaemia. See [16,17].

Diagnosis of acromegaly

Acromegaly is characterised by persistent GH secretion and loss of GH suppression after a glucose load.

Glucose tolerance test

Procedure. Fasting from midnight. At time zero give 75 g glucose. Take blood for blood glucose and GH at –15, 0, 30, 60, 90, 120, 150 min.

Precautions. Care with known diabetics who frequently show elevated GH levels which do not suppress (the major problem would be the diagnosis of acromegaly complicated by mild diabetes).

Normal response. GH suppresses to < 2 mU/l [18].

Interpretation. Failure of GH to suppress is highly suggestive of acromegaly, although some tall children show a failure of suppression whilst growing. Some acromegalics show a paradoxical increase in GH concentrations.

Follow-up of acromegalic patients

Follow-up of acromegalic patients has a number of purposes: to assess the severity of the disease, the effect of treatment, and whether a patient is cured. The definition of a cure is almost impossible; however, a patient who shows some undetectable GH levels during a day curve and after glucose, has normal IGF-1 levels and an absent GH response to TRH is likely to be cured. A more pragmatic approach is to aim to control GH with the mean level during a day curve being < 5 mU/l; levels higher than this have been associated with excess mortality [19].

Day curves

Procedure. Fast from midnight. Sample for GH at 0900, 1200, 1500, 1700 hours (the times are arbitrary and chosen only to fit into the working day). After the first sample, subjects can eat and drink normally and take medication as required.

Interpretation. Normal subjects usually show undetectable GH levels at the majority of times sampled. The mean level of GH over the four time-points provides a useful biochemical assessment of the severity of acromegaly and the effect of treatment. It is currently a matter of controversy as to whether a single level is as useful a measure of control as the mean of a day curve.

IGF-1 levels

Single measurements of IGF-1 provide a useful marker of the severity of acromegaly and the effect of treatment. IGF-1 levels correlate well with the results of GH day curves, although there is a ceiling above which the levels do not rise despite a continuing rise in GH levels [20,21]. IGF-1 concentrations decrease with age and thus normal ranges should be age related.

TRH test

See pp. 1119–1120.

Prolactin secretion

Basal samples. A single sample of prolactin usually provides all the information required, although stress, and in particular, fainting or fits, will raise values. A moderately raised prolactin which is thought to be stress related may be followed up by measuring three prolactin levels at 30-min intervals through a venous cannula.

TRH test

Indication. Differential diagnosis of hyperprolactinaemia.

Procedure. Prolactin release is stimulated by TRH in normal subjects. The test should be performed separately from an ITT, which also stimulates prolactin release. Patients can eat normally. Give 200 μg TRH i.v. and sample for prolactin at 0, 20, 60 min.

Normal response. Basal prolactin levels are <360 mU/l (18 μg/l) and rise to greater than 100% of the basal value.

Interpretation. The value of the TRH test in assessing prolactin release is much disputed. Undetectable prolactin levels with no response to TRH are usually seen only in Sheehan's syndrome or during dopamine-agonist therapy. Some authors have argued that a lack of prolactin response to TRH suggests a prolactinoma; however, this remains a controversial issue [22,23].

Assessment of posterior pituitary function

Assessment of vasopressin secretion from the posterior pituitary is usually made indirectly through the measurement of plasma and urine osmolality. Although the test protocols are fairly simple, the patients require continuous observation; interpretation of the results is complex.

Basal investigations

Samples. Plasma (*P*) and urine (*U*) osmolality obtained simultaneously on rising, or as soon as possible thereafter.

Interpretation. In normal subjects the plasma osmolality will be in the normal range (280–295 mosmol/kg), and the urine will be concentrated. The *U/P* ratio is usually more than 2:1, and if the plasma osmolality is not raised this excludes diabetes insipidus (DI). If the plasma osmolality is >295 mosmol/kg and the *U/P* ratio is <2.0 then the patient may have DI. A raised glucose, urea, ethanol or recent mannitol administration raises the plasma osmolality, and makes interpretation difficult.

A plasma osmolality <280 mosmol/kg with a urine osmolality >100 mosmol/kg suggests the syndrome of inappropriate vasopressin secretion, assuming the patient is not dehydrated, but remember this picture may also complicate cortisol deficiency.

Water-deprivation test

Indications. Diagnosis of DI, and differential diagnosis of thirst, polyuria and nocturia.

Precautions. Care in patients with severe clinical DI. Thyroid and adrenal reserve must be normal or adequately replaced. Perform in a side room with no water available and tap handles removed under continuous observation.

Procedure. Stop desmopressin for at least 24 hours before the test. Patients should have: normal corticosteroid replacement on the day of the test; fluids *ad libitum* until 0730 hours on the morning of the test; a light breakfast at 0630 hours but no tea, coffee or smoking. From 0730 hours give no fluid or food for 8 hours.

Weigh the patient basally, calculate 97% of this weight and record on the chart. Weigh the patient at 4, 6, 7, 8 hours. If the patient loses more than 3% of bodyweight then measure the plasma osmolality urgently; if >305 mosmol/kg then give desmopressin and allow the patient to drink. If the plasma osmolality is lower than this then the patient may have been fluid overloaded before the test. The patient should be reviewed by a doctor experienced with the test.

After 8 hours give desmopressin 2 μg i.m. or 20 μg intranasally. Collect urine samples hourly for 4 hours but allow free fluids.

Sample record sheet. See Table 83.1.

Normal response. The plasma osmolality remains in the normal range (280–295 mosmol/kg), and the *U*/*P* ratio rises to >2.0.

Interpretation

1 Central DI. Urine osmolality fails to rise appropriately, and urine volumes remain inappropriately high in spite of rising plasma osmolality. Plasma osmolality rises to >295mosmol/kg by the end of the test but *U*/*P* ratio is <2.0. Urine concentrates normally after desmopressin.

If the plasma osmolality has not risen to >295 mosmol/kg then a *U*/*P* ratio of <2.0 is not diagnostic of DI as the patient has not been adequately fluid deprived. A prolonged water-deprivation test is then required.

If the plasma osmolality rises to >295 mosmol/kg and the *U*/*P* ratio is >2.0, the patient may have abnormal vasopressin secretion. Consider a prolonged water deprivation test and/or a hypertonic saline infusion.

2 *Primary polydipsia.* *U*/*P* ratio rises to >2.0, provided that adequate dehydration is achieved. A prolonged water-deprivation test is frequently required.

3 *Nephrogenic diabetes insipidus.* Plasma osmolality rises and urine osmolality fails to rise as for central DI but urine osmolality does not increase after desmopressin.

Note: with prolonged polyuria from any cause, the maximum urine concentrating power of the kidney is reduced. This is due to 'wash out' of the osmotic gradient within the renal medulla. Maximum urine osmolality obtained after desmopressin may therefore be less than that seen in normal subjects. See [24].

Prolonged water-deprivation test

Indications. Differential diagnosis of mild central DI from primary polydipsia and other causes of thirst/polyuria.

Contraindications. Severe clinical DI.

Precautions. Unless symptoms are very mild (objectively 24-hour urine volume <4 litres) and DI is clinically unlikely, a normal 8-hour water deprivation test should be performed first.

Procedure. The patient should be nil by mouth from 1800 hours on the day before the test, otherwise the general management is as for the normal water-deprivation test.

Table 83.1 Sample record sheet. Record 97% of weight = ?

Time (hours)	Hours	Weight	Urine volume	*U*	*P*
0730	0	+	+	Discard	
0800	0.5				P_1
0830	1		+	U_1	
1030	3		+	Discard	
1100	3.5				P_2
1130	4	+	+	U_2	
1330	6	+	+	Discard	
1400	6.5				P_3
1430	7	+	+	U_3	
1530	8	+	+	U_4	P_4
Give desmopressin 2 μg i.m. intranasally					
1630	9		+	U_5	
1730	10		+	U_6	
1830	11		+	U_7	
1930	12		+	U_8	

U, urine osmolality; *P*, plasma osmolality.

Start the test at 0800 hours, weigh patient and calculate 97% of this weight. Blood and urine sampling from 0800 hours.

Weigh the patient every 2 hours. If the patient loses more than 3% of bodyweight then measure the plasma osmolality urgently; if >305 mosmol/kg then give desmopressin and allow the patient to drink. If lower than this then the patient may have been fluid overloaded before the test. The patient should be reviewed by a doctor experienced with the test.

Urine and plasma osmolalities are measured immediately. Continue water deprivation until the urine osmolality reaches a plateau (<30 mosmol/kg increase between consecutive samples).

When a plateau is reached, give desmopressin 2 μg i.m. Patient is then allowed to drink.

Sampling. Collect urine for osmolality hourly from 0800 hours and plasma every 2 hours. Label as shown in Table 83.2.

Normal response. Urine osmolality rises to reach a plateau and there is no more than 5% further increase in urine osmolality after desmopressin. Plasma osmolality is maintained in the normal range. *U/P* ratio is >2.0 at the end of dehydration.

Interpretation. If maximum urine osmolality >290 mosmol/kg before desmopressin:

1 no further rise in urine osmolality after desmopressin in the presence of polydipsia and polyuria suggests primary polydipsia, plasma osmolality at P_1 is usually low;

2 a rise in urine osmolality of 9% or more after desmopressin suggests partial cranial DI, i.e. endogenous maximal vasopressin is insufficient to concentrate the urine maximally;

3 a 'normal' urine osmolality response in the presence of a high plasma osmolality (>295 mosmol/kg) is compatible with a subtle defect of vasopressin secretion or 'reset osmostat'.

If maximum urine osmolality <290 mosmol/kg before desmopressin:

1 this means the test should not have been performed;

2 a rise in urine osmolality of 50% or more after desmopressin suggests severe cranial DI, while less than 50% suggests nephrogenic DI.

See [25].

Table 83.2 Labelling of urine and plasma samples.

Time (hours)	Hours	Weight	*U*	*P*
0800	0	+	U_1	P_1
0900	1	+	U_2	
1000	2	+	U_3	P_2
1100				
1200				

U, urine osmolality; *P*, plasma osmolality

Hypertonic (5%) saline infusion

Indications. Assessment of possible mild DI, and other subtle effects of vasopressin secretion.

Contraindications. Severe DI, heart failure and oedematous states.

Procedure. Patient fasting from midnight, with water only until the time of the test and no smoking. Start the test at 0900 hours after checking urgent plasma osmolality or sodium concentration. Empty bladder; note volume and measure osmolality. Record volume and osmolality of any further urine passed. Record blood pressure at 5-min intervals.

Infuse 5% saline at 0.06 ml/kg/min for 2 hours from 0–120 min (use 0.04 ml/kg/min if severe DI suspected). After 135 min patient to void urine; record volume and osmolality.

Sampling. Heparinised blood 10 ml, cold spun within 30 min for plasma osmolality (2 ml) and vasopressin (3 ml, flash frozen) at −15, 0, 30, 60, 90, 120, 135 min. Record thirst on a visual analogue scale at each sampling time.

Normal response. Plasma osmolality rises during the infusion. Plasma vasopressin begins to rise at a plasma osmolality of about 285 mosmol/kg; the onset of thirst at a plasma osmolality of about 295 mosmol/kg.

Interpretation. The study may reveal a reset osmotic threshold for vasopressin secretion and/or reset onset of thirst compatible with the clinical findings. See [26].

Thyroid function

Accurate assessment of thyroid function can be made using basal tests as described in Chapter 24. Dynamic tests such as the TRH test are rarely required; the method for the TRH test is described above.

Hypercalcaemia

The investigation of hypercalcaemia is now much easier with the new assay for intact parathyroid hormone (PTH) which gives a clearer separation of normal patients from those with hyperparathyroidism or malignancy [27]. Occasionally, it is still useful to assess whether the high calcium is suppressible with corticosteroids. Measurement of the combined urinary calcium and creatinine clearance is important to define patients with familial hypocalciuric hypercalcaemia.

Hydrocortisone-suppression test

Indications. Differential diagnosis of hypercalcaemia.

Precautions. Care in patients with diabetes mellitus and dyspepsia.

Procedure. Hydrocortisone 40 mg orally, 8 hourly for 10 days commencing after the baseline sample.

Sampling. Measure serum calcium corrected for albumin on days 0, 4, 7 and 10.

Interpretation. Patients with primary hyperparathyroidism only very rarely show suppression of the calcium level. Significant suppression (a fall by 0.25 mmol/l or into the normal range) during the test is highly suggestive of other cause of hypercalcaemia especially malignancy, sarcoid, vitamin D excess and myeloma. See [28].

Combined urine calcium and creatinine clearance

Indications. Differentiation of familial hypocalciuric hypercalcaemia and primary hyperparathyroidism.

Procedures. Twenty-four-hour urine collection into boric acid for measurement of calcium and creatinine. Measure serum creatinine and obtain corrected calcium on the morning at the end of the urine collection.

Interpretation. It is most important that the measurements are made on the same collection. The calcium clearance is then corrected for the creatinine clearance.

In hyperparathyroidism, the ratio of the calcium clearance divided by the creatinine clearance is >0.01, and a ratio of <0.01 suggests familial hypocalciuric hypercalcaemia. Therefore, when assayed on the same 24-hour sample, the ratio can be calculated as follows:

$$\frac{\text{calcium}_{\text{urine}} \times \text{creatinine}_{\text{plasma}}}{\text{calcium}_{\text{plasma}} \times \text{creatinine}_{\text{urine}}}$$

See [29].

Pancreas

Glucose tolerance test

Indications. Diagnosis of diabetes mellitus.

Contraindications. None.

Procedure. Fasting from midnight. Seventy-five gram glucose orally at time zero. Sample for glucose at 0, 30, 60, 90 and 120 min.

Normal response. See Table 83.3. Thresholds are lower in pregnancy.

In the presence of classical symptoms one blood sugar in the diabetic range described in Table 83.3 is diagnostic. In the asymptomatic patient two abnormal values should be obtained. The finding of abnormal, but not diagnostic, glucose concentrations on fasting or random samples should lead to the patient having a glucose tolerance test.

Values for plasma glucose and capillary blood are 1.1 mmol/l higher.

Tests for hypoglycaemia

The clinical features of hypoglycaemia are often non-specific; to attribute symptoms to hypoglycaemia requires both unequivocal demonstration of hypoglycaemia whilst symptomatic, and the resolution of the symptoms by correction of hypoglycaemia [30]. Demonstration of a normal glucose concentration during a symptomatic episode excludes hypoglycaemia as a cause. In many cases, the cause for the

Table 83.3 Glucose responses in venous whole blood in mmol/l (World Health Organisation criteria).

	Normal	Impaired glucose tolerance	Abnormal but not diagnostic	Diagnostic of diabetes
Random blood glucose (mmol/l)	<6.7		6.7–9.9	≥10
Fasting blood glucose (mmol/l)	<5.0		5.0–6.6	≥6.7
Glucose tolerance test				
Fasting	<6.7	<6.7		≥6.7
2 hours	<6.7	6.7–10		≥10

hypoglycaemia is obvious, for example drugs, sepsis or liver failure, and no further investigation is needed [31].

Tests to provoke hypoglycaemia

Eighteen-hour overnight fast

Precautions. Patients with insulinomas or other causes of hypoglycaemia may die from hypoglycaemia. The patient should therefore have an indwelling venous cannula throughout the test and be under continuous observation. Twenty-five millilitres of 25% dextrose should be drawn up so it may be administered if required.

Procedure. The patient should fast from 1500 hours on the day preceding the test and then have blood taken at 0900 hours. Three overnight fasts are required and will give positive results in over 90% of insulinoma patients [32].

Samples. Blood for glucose and saved for plasma insulin, C-peptide and proinsulin.

Rigorous exercise

Procedure. Exercise the patient intensively for 30 min or until exhaustion on an exercise bicycle or treadmill.

Samples. Take samples before exercise and then every 5–10 min whilst exercising. Assay for glucose and save for plasma insulin, C-peptide and proinsulin.

Prolonged 72-hour fast

Indications. Investigation of hypoglycaemia which has not been demonstrated by simpler tests.

Precautions. As for 18-hour fast.

Procedure. Start the fast after an evening meal at 1800 hours. The patient should then receive only water or black coffee. Place an intravenous cannula for sampling.

The patient must be carefully monitored for symptoms; if these occur they should be recorded, and blood sampled as below. The test should be terminated if the patient's plasma glucose is persistently <2.2 mmol/l on laboratory samples, or if they become comatose. The test may be terminated by giving 25 ml 25% dextrose i.v. or oral glucose and a substantial meal. The test should be terminated after 72 hours. If the patient has not become hypoglycaemic by the end of the test they can be exercised vigorously for 2 hours before being given some food, as exercise will produce a further fall in blood glucose.

Sampling. Blood should be taken for glucose, insulin, C-peptide and proinsulin every 6 hours for the first 24 hours, then every 4 hours until the end of the test. If the patient has symptoms the blood should be taken at that time and this should be accurately recorded. Urinary ketones are a useful confirmation that the patient is fasting. Blood samples with glucose <2.5 mmol/l should be assayed for immunoreactive insulin (IRI), C-peptide and proinsulin.

Normal response. In men plasma glucose should not fall below 2.5 mmol/l; however, in normal women the plasma glucose has been observed to fall below 2.0 mmol/l during a prolonged fast.

Interpretation. Patients may be divided into two groups.

1 Blood glucose <2.5 mmol/l and IRI >30 pmol/l. If C-peptide is also raised then the hyperinsulinism is endogenous and if ingestion of sulphonylurea drugs is excluded by a drugs screen, the patient has an insulinoma or very rarely nesidioblastosis. Proinsulin should also be high and if not, the diagnosis should be revised. If C-peptide is low then the patient is taking exogenous insulin.

2 Blood glucose <2.5 mmol/l and IRI <25 pmol/l. The hypoglycaemia is not insulin mediated. If β-hydroxybutyrate levels are low (as would be the case if insulin were acting), then either the patient has liver disease or some other compound is mimicking insulin; IGF-1, IGF-2 and insulin-receptor antibodies should be assayed. IGF-2 mediates non-islet-cell tumour-induced hypoglycaemia. High β-hydroxybutyrate concentrations suggest an inborn error of metabolism or hypopituitarism [31].

Six-hour oral glucose tolerance test

Indications. Diagnosis of reactive hypoglycaemia. This diagnosis is now recognised to be very rare and the test is rarely indicated.

Precautions. Patients with insulinomas or other causes of hypoglycaemia may die from hypoglycaemia. The patient should therefore have an indwelling intravenous cannula throughout the test and be under continuous observation. 25 ml of 25% dextrose should be drawn up so it may be administered if required.

Procedure. The patient should fast from midnight; after obtaining a fasting sample at 0900 hours, 75 g glucose is administered orally. It is most important to record any symptoms and the time they occur. If symptoms occur take samples as below.

Samples. Blood should be taken for plasma glucose, insulin and C-peptide basally and every 30 min, or if symptoms occur, for 6 hours.

Normal response. The significance of hypoglycaemia is minimised by the observation that normal individuals may have plasma glucose levels of <2.5 mmol/l during the third to fifth hour of the test. Such values, however, are not usually associated with symptoms.

Interpretation. Patients with reactive hypoglycaemia become symptomatically hypoglycaemic, but almost always have spontaneous recovery of their plasma glucose from the lowest value by the end of the test. In contrast, patients with fasting hypoglycaemia do not show recovery of their blood glucose level until they have ingested carbohydrate. See [33].

Adrenal cortex

Investigation of cortisol excess

The investigation of Cushing's syndrome is divided into two parts: first, one has to establish that there is an abnormality of cortisol secretion such as loss of the normal circadian rhythm and cortisol feedback; secondly, the cause must be investigated.

Tests to diagnose Cushing's syndrome

Circadian rhythm study

Procedure. The patient should be acclimatised to hospital (admission of not less than 48 hours), and not be stressed during the study. Measure cortisol and ACTH at 0900, 1800, 2400 hours. The midnight sample should preferably be performed when the patient is asleep and the patient should not be warned that the sample is going to be taken.

Normal values. Cortisol at 0900 hours is usually >170 nmol/l and at midnight is <100 nmol/l. A recent study of 150 patients clearly showed that a sleeping midnight cortisol of >50 nmol/l was 100% sensitive for the diagnosis of Cushing's syndrome [34].

Interpretation. Loss of the circadian rhythm suggests Cushing's syndrome; however, this may also occur during stress, intervening illness, severe endogenous depression and alcoholic pseudo-Cushing's. An undetectable ACTH with loss of the cortisol circadian rhythm suggests an adrenal tumour; a detectable or elevated ACTH suggests ACTH-dependent Cushing's syndrome.

Overnight dexamethasone-suppression test

Indication. Screening for suspected Cushing's syndrome.

Procedure. Dexamethasone 1 mg (2 mg if obese) is taken at midnight and cortisol measured 8–9 hours later.

Normal response. Normals should suppress cortisol to <50 nmol/l.

Interpretation. A false-negative rate of <2% means that a normal response is strongly against the diagnosis of Cushing's syndrome. False positives occur commonly (12.5–30%) and an abnormal response may occur in obesity, depression, alcoholism, oestrogen therapy or severe illness [35].

Low-dose dexamethasone-suppression test

Indications. Diagnosis of Cushing's syndrome. Differential diagnosis of the polycystic ovary syndrome (PCOS) from autonomous androgen-secreting tumours.

Precautions. Care in diabetes mellitus and psychologically disturbed patients.

Procedure. Measure cortisol and ACTH at 0900 hours on day 0 (label DEX 2 + 0), then given dexamethasone 0.5 mg orally strictly 6-hourly at 0900, 1500, 2100, 0300 hours for 48 hours. Measure cortisol and ACTH again at 0900 hours 48 hours after the first dose of dexamethasone (label DEX 2 + 48). If measuring androgens, take samples for testosterone, dehydroepiandrosterone sulphate (DHEAS) and androstenedione at the same time-points as cortisol. The labelling of samples is a useful convention, and for DEX 2 + 0 means dexamethasone 2 mg daily, basal sample.

Normal response. Plasma cortisol is in the normal resting 0900 hours range (170–700 nmol/l) at DEX 2 + 0 and suppresses to <50 nmol/l at DEX 2 + 48.

Serum testosterone and other androgens (but not DHEAS because of its prolonged half-life) fall on dexamethasone in normals and patients with PCOS.

Interpretation. A plasma cortisol of <50 nmol/l excludes Cushing's syndrome, although exceptional cases may have 'cyclical' Cushing's.

A number of conditions may cause non-suppression of cortisol: severe endogenous depression, severe stressful illness, hepatic enzyme-inducing drugs and oestrogen therapy. Oestrogen therapy causes a rise in cortisol-binding globulin and therefore the basal cortisol may be high and not fully suppressed.

Cross-reactivity in cortisol radioimmunoassay. The above values are for an in-house assay which shows no cross-reactivity with dexamethasone. Knowledge of the assay is very important in interpreting the results of the dexamethasone test.

Androgens. The failure of serum testosterone or other androgens to show suppression to within the normal range after low-dose dexamethasone is suggestive of an autonomous androgen-secreting tumour, although this occasionally occurs in patients with PCOS in whom a significant proportion of the androgens are of ovarian origin.

Intravenous dexamethasone suppression test

Indication. Exclusion of Cushing's syndrome in obesity.

Procedure. Insert intravenous cannula at 0900 hours and weigh patient. Start infusion at 1000 hours of 50 ml 0.9% saline plus 25 μg/kg dexamethasone via a syringe driver at 10 ml/hour.

Samples. Take blood for cortisol at 0940, 1000, 1700 and 1900 hours.

Interpretation. Cortisol concentrations in obese patients are <48 nmol/l at 1700 hours and <37 nmol/l at 1900 hours. In Cushing's syndrome patients the corresponding values are >72 nmol/l at 1700 hours and >75 nmol/l at 1900 hours. See [36].

Tests to determine the cause of Cushing's syndrome

Measurement of ACTH with cortisol will allow the disease to be classified as ACTH independent or dependent [37]. The former category is synonymous with primary adrenal disease and the adrenal glands should be imaged. ACTH-dependent Cushing's syndrome is due to ACTH secretion by either the pituitary or an ectopic source, usually a tumour.

Differential diagnosis of ACTH-dependent Cushing's syndrome

High-dose dexamethasone suppression test

Indications. Differential diagnosis of ACTH-dependent Cushing's syndrome.

Precautions and procedure. These are the same as for the low-dose dexamethasone-suppression test, although 2 mg dexamethasone 6-hourly is used instead of 0.5 mg. The basal sample should be labelled DEX 8 + 0 and the second sample DEX 8 + 48 (8 as 8 mg dexamethasone given every 24 hours). This test may conveniently follow the low-dose dexamethasone-suppression tests. In this case, DEX 2 + 48 = DEX 8 + 0, and the basal value used for interpretation of the high dose test is the DEX 2 + 0 value.

Normal response. The test is not performed in normal individuals (who would suppress plasma cortisol to <50nmol/l).

Interpretation. Plasma cortisol classically suppresses to 50% or less of the basal value in Cushing's syndrome (pituitary-dependent Cushing's), but not in ectopic ACTH secretion or in adrenal tumours. There are, however, significant exceptions and about 20% of patients with Cushing's syndrome fail to suppress according to these criteria. See [38,39].

CRH test

See earlier.

Inferior petrosal sinus (IPS) sampling with CRH administration

Indication. Differential diagnosis of ACTH-dependent Cushing's syndrome—ectopic ACTH versus pituitary-derived ACTH.

Side-effects. Many patients experience a facial flush that comes on 1 min after injection of CRH and hypotension may occur. There may be complications related to the site of venous puncture, for example haematoma, thrombosis, and brainstem lesions have been induced by the petrosal catheter itself, although this is very rare in experienced hands.

Procedure. Insert a peripheral intravenous cannula and then cannulate both IPSs. At each sampling time take blood for ACTH from each IPS and peripherally and label appropriately. Samples should be cold spun and flash frozen immediately. Give 100 μg CRH i.v. peripherally after warning patient of possible flushing.

Sampling. Sample basally and then at 5, 10 and 15 min post-CRH for ACTH.

Normal response. The test should not be performed on normals.

Interpretation. A central/peripheral ACTH ratio of >2 at baseline or >3 post-CRH stimulation has been reported to be 100% sensitive and specific for pituitary-driven disease.

A gradient between left and right IPS provides a pointer to tumour lateralisation but cannot be relied upon. See [37].

Diagnosis of cure of Cushing's disease after pituitary surgery

Undetectable serum cortisol at 0900 hours postoperatively has been reported in one series to be 100% predictive of cure with a follow-up of 15–70 months. See [40].

Investigation of cortisol deficiency

Cortisol deficiency may be primary, due to adrenal failure, or secondary, due to ACTH deficiency or suppression. The investigation of secondary adrenal failure is described in the assessment of anterior pituitary function. This section describes the Synacthen test, which is the stimulation of the adrenal by synthetic ACTH. The hydrocortisone day curve is a useful method for assessing the adequacy of hydrocortisone replacement therapy.

Synacthen tests

Indications. Diagnosis of adrenocortical insufficiency—primary or secondary.

Precautions. Allergy to Synacthen. Synacthen is contraindicated in asthma and allergic disorders.

Procedure. Non-fasting. Begin test at 0900 hours.

Short Synacthen test. Plain Synacthen (tetracosactrin, CIBA Laboratories, Horsham, West Sussex, UK) 0.25 mg i.m. at time zero.

Long Synacthen test. Depot Synacthen 1mg i.m. at time zero.

Sampling. Short Synacthen test plasma cortisol 0, 30, 60 min; long Synacthen test 0, 30, 60, 90, 120 min, 4, 6, 8, 12, 24 hours.

Normal response. Plasma cortisol rises. Short Synacthen test: plasma cortisol >550 nmol/l at 30 min with an increment of at least 200 nmol/l (manufacturer's figures). The use of an incremental value is controversial, and some authorities advise a lower threshold of 500 nmol/l at 30 min. The 60-min value is usually above 550 nmol/l. See Table 83.4 for long Synachten test values.

Interpretation. A failure to respond to the short Synacthen test indicates adrenal failure; this may be primary, or secondary to ACTH deficiency which may be due to suppression by glucocorticoids or hypothalamo-pituitary disease. Primary adrenal failure—Addison's disease—can be confidently excluded only by a long Synacthen test, so that if this diagnosis seems likely do not perform a short Synacthen test first (the responses in the first hour are superimposable).

Table 83.4 Long Synacthen test values of normal plasma cortisol.

Time	95% confidence limits (nmol l^{-1})
60 min	605–1265
120 min	750–1520
4 hours	960–1650
8 hours	1025–1600
24 hours	609–1496

Addison's disease. Plasma cortisol is usually low or undetectable (<50 nmol/l) and fails to rise following depot Synacthen. Rarely, in cases investigated at an early stage, the plasma cortisol response may fall within the normal range at 60 min but then declines so that the 24-hour value is low.

Secondary adrenal atrophy. (ACTH deficiency or glucocorticoid treatment). The use of the short Synacthen test to screen for or diagnose secondary adrenal failure is controversial. The rationale for using a test of adrenal function to evaluate pituitary function derives from the adrenal atrophy that occurs in the lack of endogenous ACTH stimulation; for this reason the test should not be used within 6 weeks of pituitary surgery. When employed for this purpose the 0- and 30-min samples should be used alone as only these sampling times are validated against the 'gold standard' insulin stress test [41]. The results should be interpreted cautiously taking into account other indicators of cortisol deficiency, and if doubt exists an insulin stress test should be performed.

In response to depot Synacthen, plasma cortisol fails to rise normally in the first hour but slowly rises to reach a peak at 24 hours, instead of 4-8 hours as in normals. In prolonged adrenal atrophy, depot Synacthen may have to be given for a number of days before an adrenal response is seen. See [42].

Hydrocortisone day curve

The measurement of cortisol levels after hydrocortisone has provided a useful means for assessing hydrocortisone-replacement therapy. The test has not been fully evaluated, but the following is a protocol that has proved useful.

Precautions. Cannot interpret results in patients on oestrogens.

Procedure. Fasting from midnight, and the patient delays taking the morning dose of hydrocortisone until arriving on the ward. Document the times at which the patient usually takes hydrocortisone and then calculate the periods between doses. The patient should take the first dose of hydrocortisone as close to his or her normal time as possible and then subsequent doses at normal intervals as determined earlier. Take blood for cortisol immediately before and 60min after each dose to assess trough and peak concentrations.

Interpretation. The aim is to have adequate circulating levels of cortisol throughout the day (except for the time zero sample, which is usually <50 nmol/l), whilst avoiding excessive peaks after each dose. The peak level after a dose should not exceed 1200 nmol/l (usually 800–1200 nmol/l), and the trough level before the next dose should not be <100 nmol/l. Frequently, a midday dose is required to avoid excess levels after the morning dose but sufficient levels to provide adequate cover until the evening. Recent studies have suggested that a total daily dose of 10–20 mg hydrocortisone may be sufficient in most patients.

Endocrine hypertension

Hypertension due to endocrine causes is rare, but it is important to diagnose because it is potentially curable. Hypertension is commonly present in such endocrine conditions as acromegaly, Cushing's syndrome and thyrotoxicosis; this discussion will focus upon conditions with hypertension as the dominant feature. Investigation is frequently dictated by the tests available, but the following tests have proved clinically useful.

Phaeochromocytoma

Measurement of urinary catecholamine and metanephrine levels in 24-hour collections on at least two occasions is the most effective screening investigation. Vanillylmandelic acid (VMA) is still frequently assayed; however, it is noted in Chapter 38 that VMA is of low sensitivity and specificity, and metanephrines are only slightly better. Measurement of urinary catecholamine levels is clearly preferable where the assay is available, and can be carried out on the same acidified urine as for VMAs and metanephrines. Patients should be on a vanilla-free diet during the collection of VMAs, and for at least 3 days beforehand, although most healthy subjects will have normal values on a normal diet (no vanilla containing foods including ice-cream, cakes, biscuits, puddings, desserts, custard, bananas, nuts, chocolate drinks, coffee or 'cola' type drinks). No dietary restrictions are required for urinary catecholamines.

Measurement of plasma catecholamine levels is a sensitive screening test, but false negatives may occur where secretion from tumours is intermittent; stress also elevates catecholamines and will produce false-positive results. Nevertheless, grossly elevated levels may be diagnostic, and normal levels during a bout of hypertension and/or palpitations, are very much against the diagnosis. Very high levels of noradrenaline compared with adrenaline suggest either an extra-adrenal paraganglioma, or a very large adrenal tumour that has lost contact with the adrenal cortex. Various drugs, particularly labetalol, may interfere with catecholamine assays.

Pentolinium-suppression test

Indications. Diagnosis of phaeochromocytoma. This test is rarely required and should be reserved for cases with equivocal catecholamine levels possibly due to stress.

Precautions. Blood pressure may fall during the test and care should be taken when standing the patient up at the end of the test.

Procedure. Non-fasting at any time. Patient should be lying down for at least 30 min before the test with an intravenous cannula *in situ*. Give pentolinium 2.5 mg i.v. over 1 min.

Sampling. Blood pressure at 0, 10, 30 and 60 min. Plasma catecholamines at 0 and 10 min.

Normal response. Plasma adrenaline and noradrenaline levels fall to within the normal range.

Interpretation. Failure of catecholamines to suppress into the normal range after pentolinium administration is suggestive of a phaeochromocytoma, although patients with Cushing's syndrome may also show this lack of suppression. See [43].

Hypertension associated with hypokalaemia

(see also Chapter 34)

The investigation of hypertension associated with hypokalaemia involves establishing whether the aetiology is primary hyperaldosteronism or another cause. If the cause is primary hyperaldosteronism, then it is important to determine whether this is due to a unilateral aldosterone-producing adenoma (APA), bilateral idiopathic hyperaldosteronism (IHA), glucocorticoid-suppressible hyperaldosteronism, or the very rare aldosterone-producing adrenocortical carcinoma.

Establishing whether there is inappropriate kaliuresis is fundamental to the investigation of hypokalaemia. A variety of tests has been described, but the following is a practical protocol.

Diagnosis of primary hyperaldosteronism

Paired aldosterone and plasma renin activity

Indication. Diagnosis of primary hyperaldosteronism.

Precautions. All medication should, if possible, be stopped before investigation: spironolactone and oestrogens for 6 weeks; diuretics, prostaglandin synthetase inhibitors, cyproheptadine, angiotensin-converting enzyme inhibitors for 2 weeks; and vasodilators, calcium-channel antagonists, sympathomimetics and adrenergic inhibitors for 1 week before the study. If medication is required to control hypertension, then use prazosin or nifedipine.

Correct hypokalaemia with oral slow-release potassium before test as hypokalaemia will decrease aldosterone production.

Procedure. Admit to hospital.
Day 1 Give 120 mmol sodium chloride daily. Correct potassium deficit.
Day 2 At 0800 hours with patient in bed overnight and supine, take plasma for aldosterone, plasma renin activity and potassium. Patient should then get up and remain upright until 1200 hours when the aldosterone and plasma renin activity are repeated. Start 24-hour urine collection for aldosterone and tetrahydroaldosterone.
Day 3 Finish urine collection.

Interpretation. Elevated aldosterone in plasma and urine with suppressed plasma renin activity confirms primary hyperaldosteronism. If the plasma renin activity is not suppressed then there is secondary hyperaldosteronism which may be due to renal disease, essential hypertension, diuretic abuse, a renin-secreting tumour or heart failure. See [44].

Differential diagnosis of primary hyperaldosteronism

Sixty-five per cent of patients have an APA, 34% IHA and the remaining diagnoses of glucocorticoid-suppressible aldosteronism and adrenal carcinoma make up the remaining 1%.

Aldosterone levels in APA are partially under ACTH control and fall with the diurnal variation in ACTH, so that levels at 1200 hours are lower than at 0800 hours in 90% of cases [44]. In contrast, IHA is partially responsive to small increases in plasma renin activity, and aldosterone levels will rise following 4 hours in the upright posture. The adrenals should be imaged using CT or MRI, and adrenal iodoscintigraphy or adrenal vein sampling may also be indicated.

Glucocorticoid suppression of aldosterone

Indications. The diagnosis of glucocorticoid-suppressible hyperaldosteronism.

Precautions. Care in patients with diabetes mellitus or dyspepsia.

Procedure. Dexamethasone 2 mg/day for 3 weeks. Measure blood pressure, potassium and aldosterone weekly.

Interpretation. Serum potassium, blood pressure and aldosterone levels return to normal by 3 weeks in patients with glucocorticoid-suppressible hyperaldosteronism. See [45].

Renal

Renal tubular acidosis may present to the endocrinologist as a patient with unexplained hypokalaemia or growth failure.

Acid load test

Indications. Diagnosis of type 1 renal tubular acidosis.

Contraindications. None.

Precautions. None.

Procedure. Normal breakfast and meals thereafter. At 0800 hours empty bladder and start hourly urine collections for pH testing over 10 hours. At 1000 hours, give ammonium chloride 0.1g/kg orally (made into capsules in pharmacy), taken over 1 hour to avoid gastric irritation as this frequently causes nausea.

Sampling. Hourly urine for pH testing and blood for electrolytes and bicarbonate at 1000, 1400 and 1800 hours.

Interpretation. Urine pH level should fall to 5.3 or less. Plasma bicarbonate should fall to confirm absorption of ammonium chloride. See [46].

Gonadal function

In assessing gonadal function it is important to know whether there is any gonadal tissue present. The human chorionic gonadotrophin (hCG)-stimulation test and Pergonal test assess, respectively, testicular and ovarian function.

hCG-stimulation test

Indications. Differential diagnosis of male hypogonadism.

Precautions. None.

Procedure. hCG (Profasi, Pregnyl) 2000 iu i.m. on days 0 and 2.

Normal response. Serum testosterone level rises from a subnormal level to within the normal range.

Interpretation. In hypogonadism, a failure of testosterone levels to rise after hCG suggests the absence of functioning testicular tissue. Conversely, a rise shows that a testis is present, which may be intra-abdominal if none is palpable in the scrotum.

In gonadotrophin deficiency, without a primary testicular abnormality, the low basal testosterone value should triple after hCG. See [6].

Pergonal stimulation test

Indications. Differential diagnosis of female hypogonadism.

Precautions. None. The test should be done only if the patient is amenorrhoeic (and not pregnant).

Procedure. Pergonal (human menopausal gonadotrophin), three ampoules daily for 3 days (days, 0, 1, 2).

Sampling. Serum oestradiol on days 0, 1, 2 and 3.

Normal response. Serum oestradiol clearly rises.

Interpretation. Absence of a serum or urinary oestrogen response to Pergonal in this dose suggests premature ovarian failure. Resistant ovary syndrome also shows no response and can be distinguished only by full-thickness ovarian biopsy at laparotomy.

Miscellaneous

Pentagastrin-stimulation test

Indications. Screening for medullary carcinoma of the thyroid.

Contraindications. Hypocalcaemia.

Side-effects. Transient feelings of burning, flushing, numbness, nausea, abdominal discomfort and rarely hypotension.

Procedure. Check corrected plasma calcium level to exclude hypocalcaemia. Obtain basal calcitonin sample then give pentagastrin 0.5µg/kg as a rapid intravenous bolus (< 5 sec). Take blood samples for calcitonin at 1.5 and 5 min after administration of pentagastrin.

Normal response. Peak calcitonin levels are < 0.21 ng/ml for males and < 0.11 ng/ml for females.

Interpretation. An above-normal peak calcitonin level after pentagastrin administration is suggestive of C-cell hyperplasia and possibly a medullary carcinoma of the thyroid. See [47].

Gastric acid secretion studies

Indication. To diagnose Zollinger–Ellison syndrome in the presence of raised gastrin levels.

Procedure. Stop proton pump inhibitors 2 weeks before test and H_2 antagonists at least 3 days before test. Fast overnight and then insert nasogastric tube. Aspirate the stomach completely prior to test. Collect gastric secretions for 1–2 hours in 15-min aliquots. Records volume of secretion and assay for acid concentration.

Interpretation. Gastric acid secretion of over 20 mmol/hour is diagnositc whilst levels between 10 and 20 mmol/hour are suggestive of Zollinger–Ellison syndrome. Patients whose raised gastrin is due to achlorhydria will have acid secretion well below 10 mmol/hour.

Acknowledgement

Some of the material in this chapter is taken from the endocrine protocols of St. Bartholomew's Hospital, and has been reproduced by permission of the Department of Endocrinology at St Bartholomew's Hospital [48].

References

1 Landon J, Wynn V, James VHT. The adrenocortical response to insulin-induced hypoglycaemia. *J Endocrinol* 1963; **27**: 183–92.

2 Plumpton FS, Besser GM. The adrenocortical response to surgery and insulin-induced hypoglycaemia in corticosteroid-treated and normal subjects. *Br J Surg* 1969; **56**: 216–19.

3 Thorner MO, Bengtsson BA, Ho KY *et al.* The diagnosis of growth hormone deficiency (GHD) in adults (Letter). *J Clin Endocrinol Metab* 1995; **80**: 3097–8.

4 Editorial. Glucagon and growth hormone. *Br Med J* 1973; **1**: 188–9.

5 Littley MD, Gibson S, White A, Shalet SM. Comparison of the ACTH and cortisol responses to provocative testing with glucagon and insulin hypoglycaemia in normal subjects. *Clin Endocrinol* 1989; **31**: 527–33.

6 Anderson DC, Marshall JC, Young JL, Russell Fraser T. Stimulation tests of pituitary–Leydig cell function in normal male subjects and hypogonadal men. *Clin Endocrinol* 1972; **1**: 127–40.

7 Besser GM, Ross RJM. Are hypothalamic releasing hormones useful in the diagnosis of endocrine disorders? In: Edwards CRW, Lincoln DW, eds. *Recent Advances in Endocrinology and Metabolism*. London: Churchill Livingstone, 1989; **135–58**.

8 Arafah BM, Rozenweig JL, Fenstermaker R, Salazar R, McBride CE, Selman W. Value of growth hormone dynamics and somatomedin C (insulin-like growth factor 1) levels in predicting the long-term benefit after transsphenoidal surgery for acromegaly. *J Lab Clin Med* 1987; **109**: 346–54.

9 Trainer PJ, Grossman A. The diagnosis and differential diagnosis of Cushing's syndrome. *Clin Endocrinol* 1991; **34**: 317–30.

10 Nieman LK; Oldfield EH, Wesley R, Chrousos GP, Loriaux DL, Cutler GB. A simplified morning ovine corticotropin-releasing hormone stimulation test for the differential diagnosis of adrenocorticotropin-dependent Cushing's syndrome. *J Clin Endocrinol Metab* 1993; **77**: 1308–12.

11 Chrousos GP, Schuermeyer TH, Doppman J *et al.* Clinical applications of corticotrophin-releasing factor. *Ann Intern Med* 1985; **102**: 344–58.

12 Grossman A, Howlett TA, Perry L *et al.* CRF in the differential diagnosis of Cushing's syndrome: a comparison with the dexamethasone suppression test. *Clin Endocrinol* 1988; **29**: 167–78.

13 Chatelain P, Alamercery Y, Blanchart J *et al.* Growth hormone (GH) response to a single intravenous injection of synthetic GH-releasing hormone in prepubertal children with growth failure. *J Clin Endocrinol Metab* 1987; **65**: 387–93.

14 Grossman A, Savage MO, Lytras N *et al.* Responses to analogues of growth hormone-releasing hormone in normal subjects and in growth hormone deficient children and young adults. *Clin Endocrinol* 1984; **21**: 321–30.

15 Lippe B, Wong SR, Kaplan SA. Simultaneous assessment of growth hormone and ACTH reserve in children pretreated with diethylstilbestrol. *J Clin Endocrinol* 1971; **33**: 949–56.

16 Hindmarsh PC, Taylor BJ, Smith PJ, Pringle PJ, Brook CDG. Comparison between a physiological and a pharmacological stimulus of growth hormone secretion: response to stage 4 sleep and insulin-induced hypoglycaemia. *Lancet* 1985; **ii**: 1033–5.

17 Albertsson-Wikland K, Rosberg S. Analyses of 24 hour growth hormone profiles in children: relation to growth. *J Clin Endocrinol Metab* 1988; **67**: 493–500.

18 Stewart PM, Smith S, Seth J, Stewart SE, Cole D, Edwards CRW. Normal growth hormone response to the 75 g oral glucose tolerance test measured by immunoradiometric assay. *Ann Clin Biochem* 1989; **26**: 205–6.

19 Bates AS, Van't Hoff W, Jones JM, Clayton RN. An audit of outcome of treatment in acromegaly. *Q J Med* 1993; **86**: 293–9.

20 Lamberts SWJ, Uitterlinden P, Verleun T. Relationship between growth hormone and somatomedin-C levels in untreated acromegaly, after surgery and radiotherapy and during medical therapy with Sandostatin (SMS 201–995). *Eur J Clin Invest* 1987; **17**: 354–9.

21 Barkan AL, Beitins IZ, Kelch RP. Plasma insulin-like growth factor-I/somatomedin-C in acromegaly: correlation with the degree of growth hormone hypersecretion. *J Clin Endocrinol Metab* 1988; **67**: 69–73.

22 Kleinberg DL, Noel GL, Frantz AG. Galactorrhea: a study of 235 cases, including 48 with pituitary tumours. *N Engl J Med* 1977; **296**: 589–600.

23 Boyd AE, Reichlin S, Turksoy RN. Galactorrhea–amenorrhoea syndrome: diagnosis and therapy. *Ann Intern Med* 1977; **87**: 165–75.

24 Dashe AM, Cramm RE, Crist CA, Habener JF, Solomon DH. A water deprivation test for the differential diagnosis of polyuria. *JAMA* 1963; **185**: 699–703.

25 Miller M, Dalakos T, Moses AM, Fellerman H, Streeten DHP. Recognition of partial defects in antidiuretic hormone secretion. *Ann Intern Med* 1970; **73**: 721–9.

26 Baylis PH, Robertson GL. Plasma vasopressin response to hypertonic saline infusion to assess posterior pituitary function. *J Roy Soc Med* 1980; **73**: 255–60.

27 Logue FC, Beastall GH, Fraser WD, O'Reilly DS. Intact parathyroid hormone assays. *Br Med J* 1990; **300**: 210–11.

28 Dent CE, Watson L. The hydrocortisone test in primary and tertiary hyperparathyroidism. *Lancet* 1968; **ii**: 662–4.

29 Marx SJ, Stock JL, Attie MF *et al.* Familial hypercalcemia: recognition among patients referred after unsuccessful parathyroid exploration. *Ann Intern Med* 1980; **92**: 351–6.

30 Service FJ. Hypoglycaemic disorders. *N Engl J Med* 1995; **332**: 1144–52.

31 Marks V, Teale JD. Investigation of hypoglycaemia. *Clin Endocrinol* 1996, **44**: 133–6.

32 Marks V. Recognition and differential diagnosis of spontaneous hypoglycaemia. *Clin Endocrinol* 1992; **37**: 309–16.

33 Field JB. Hypoglycaemia: definition, clinical presentation, classification, and laboratory tests. *Endocrinol Metab Clin North Am* 1989; **18**: 27–44.

34 Newell-Price J, Trainer PJ, Perry L, Wass JA, Grossman A, Besser GM. A single sleeping midnight cortisol has 100% sensitivity for the diagnosis of Cushing's syndrome. *Clin Endocrinol* 1995; **43**: 545–50.

35 Cronin C, Igoe D, Duffy MJ, Cunningham SK, McKenna TJ. The overnight dexamethasone test is a worthwhile screening procedure. *Clin Endocrinol* 1990; **33**: 27–33.

36 Atkinson AB, McAteer EJ, Hadden DR, Kennedy L, Sheridan B, Traub AI. A weight-related intravenous dexamethasone suppression test distinguishes obese controls from patients with Cushing's syndrome. *Acta Endocrinol (Copenh)* 1989; **120**: 753–9.

37 Orth DN. Cushing's syndrome. *N Engl J Med* 1995; **332**: 791–803.

38 Liddle GW. Tests of pituitary–adrenal suppressibility in the diagnosis of Cushing's syndrome. *J Clin Endocrinol Metab* 1960; **20**: 1539–60.

39 Howlett TA, Drury PL, Perry L, Doniach I, Rees LH, Besser GM. Diagnosis and management of ACTH dependent Cushing's syndrome: comparison of the features in ectopic and pituitary ACTH production. *Clin Endocrinol* 1986; **24**: 699–713.

40 Trainer PJ, Lawrie HS, Verhelst J *et al.* Transphenoidal resection in Cushing's disease: undetectable serum cortisol as the definition of successful treatment. *Clin Endocrinol* 1993; **38**: 73–8.

41 Wang TWM, Wong MS, Falconer Smith J, Howlett TA. The use of the short tetracosactrin test for the investigation of suspected pituitary hypofunction. *Ann Clin Biochem* 1996; **33**: 112–18.

42 Galvao-Teles A, Burke CW, Fraser TR. Adrenal function tested with tetracosactrin depot. *Lancet* 1971; I: 557–60.
43 Brown MJ, Allison DJ, Jenner DA, Lewis PJ, Dollery CT. Increased sensitivity and accuracy of phaeochromocytoma diagnosis achieved by use of plasma-adrenaline estimations and a pentolinium-suppression test. *Lancet* 1981; I: 174–7.
44 Melby JC. Endocrine hypertension. *J Clin Endocrinol Metab* 1989; **69**: 4.697–703.
45 Young WF, Klee GG. Primary aldosteronism: diagnostic evaluation. *Endocrinol Metab Clin North Am* 1988; **17**: 367–96.
46 Wrong O, Davies HEF. The excretion of acid in renal diseaes. *Q J Med* 1959; **28**: 259–313.
47 Hennessy JF, Wells SA, Ontjes DA, Cooper CW. A comparison of pentagastrin injection and calcium infusion as provocative agents for the detection of medullary carcinoma of the thyroid. *J Clin Endocrinol Metab* 1974; **39**: 487–95.
48 Trainer PJ, Besser GM. *The Bart's Endocrine Protocols*. Edinburgh: Churchill-Livingstone, 1995.

Part 20
History of Endocrinology

CHAPTER 84

Notes on the history of endocrinology

V.C. Medvei

Introduction

The same rules apply to the writing of a history of endocrinology as to the writing of general history. The following principles must be understood.

1 Bertrand Russell, in his lecture on 'History as an Art'[1], gave his reasons for believing that the application of scientific laws to the writing of history is not as important as Hegel and his disciple, Marx, had suggested. They believed that the history of past events was subject to a logical scheme, enabling historians to foretell the future. Neither could foresee the hydrogen bomb and its effect. He maintained that historians should have feelings about the events they were telling about or the characters they were portraying. It was essential that they should not distort the facts, but it was not necessary that they should be neutral in the conflicts described in the narrative. Russell disliked the tendency of some modern historians to tone down everything dramatic, and pretend that heroes were not heroic and villains not so villainous. There seemed to be a current tendency to pay too little attention to the individual and too much to the multitude. We were so indoctrinated that we lived in the age of the common people that people became common even when they might be otherwise. What was dangerously false was the opinion that people who were regarded as heroes were merely representing forces, whose work could or would have been done by someone else if it had not been done by them. Heroic lives have always been inspired by heroic ambitions; the young person who thought there was nothing important to be done was pretty sure to do nothing important. This 'individualistic' view of history is thus opposed to more fashionable 'structuralist' interpretations.

2 History rarely occurs in a smooth chronological sequence, as some historians like to present it in school textbooks, or even in textbooks for more mature students. To quote only one example from the field of endocrinology: de Graaf produced in his short life (1641–73) an enormous wealth of important research on the sex glands and on the pancreas; this was followed by an arid desert of stagnation for many decades. A similar development occurred in the research leading to the discovery of insulin. Eventually, very many scientists worked on the problem simultaneously after years of little interest, most of them labouring independently. This progress simulates the method of discharge into the body of many hormones, which occurs in spurts rather than along a continuous smooth line. Accordingly, history may appear fragmented, uneven and unbalanced, as it really happens in nature.

3 For the reasons given above, it is not always possible to mention all the names of researchers involved in a major investigation. Those accredited are mainly the successful ones, especially those who first passed the goal-post. However, one should always try to mention those who worked along the correct lines, but were overlooked because of circumstances that prevented their work from being noticed, for example, because they published their findings in an unpopular language.

4 Finally, the writing of a history of a specialised field, such as endocrinology, is easier for someone who has been personally involved in the subject, who is a clinical endocrinologist, than it would be for an outsider or even a biochemist whose interest has been restricted to only a small part of the field. My own experience covers the years from 1928, when my first paper on an endocrine subject was published [2], to 1988, when my last paper on clinical endocrinology appeared [3]. My first chief, Julius Bauer (1887–1979), was a Professor of Medicine with a special interest in genetics, constitution and endocrinology. He had known a great number of endocrinologists in Austria, Hungary, Germany, France, the UK, Italy, Spain and the USA between 1910 and 1970, and handed down first-hand information. This personal involvement, however, may have

its drawbacks. 'The historian selects and evaluates events according to his own interpretation of the past. Especially is this true when the writer is a participant like myself,' said Alan Hill (in *Pursuit of Publishing*, Preface, page xi).

5 In the case of the history of scientific discoveries, there is also the vexed question of priority. A good example of such a problem, and pitfall, occurred fairly recently. In April 1886 a paper was published in '*Revue de Médecine*', volume VI, in Paris by Pierre Marie: 'Sur deux cas d'Acromégalie'. It was the first description of acromegaly under this name. At the end of the paper it was clearly stated: 'Ce mémoire a été remis à la Revue de médecine en Septembre 1885'. In spite of this, a centenary jubilee meeting commemorating the first description of acromegaly was held in the USA in April 1986. This implied that if somebody else had published a clinical description of acromegaly, say, in December 1885, they could have claimed priority and would have been accepted as such in the USA. As will be seen later, there did occur an overlooked case of priority in this particular instance. Similar problems of disputed priority of descriptions or discoveries in the endocrine field have occurred in several other cases, with the earliest notation not being duly accredited.

Some definitions

Endocrinology originally concerned the study of the glands of internal secretion and their role in the physiology of the body. The word 'endocrine' was devised to describe glands that poured their secretions directly into the bloodstream (from Greek words meaning 'within' and 'separate'). This is in contrast to 'exocrine' glands (Greek 'outside'), which issue their secretions through a duct to their site of action. The terms were first used officially in 1913. We now know that the situation is much more complex. The notion of internal secretion was first introduced in 1855 when Claude Bernard said that the liver has an external secretion of bile and an internal secretion in the form of sugar.

For the internal secretion or chemical messengers, the name 'hormone' (Greek 'to excite') was suggested by Sir William B. Hardy (1864–1934) of Cambridge based on advice from his classicist colleague, W.I. Vesey. The term was first used by Sir Ernest Starling in his Croonian Lecture to the Royal College of Physicians in London in June 1905. Today, we know that hormones are formed not only in the traditional endocrine glands, but in many other tissues, such as the kidneys, the gut and the brain. Observations which can now be seen to have endocrine connotations have been recorded throughout the centuries. In the 18th century, Albrecht von Haller grouped together the thymus, the thyroid gland and the spleen as glands which have no ducts. In 1775, the Frenchman de Bordeu declared that each organ gave off 'emanations', which were carried by the blood and were necessary to maintain the body's health. In 1836 King, at Guy's Hospital in London, described the colloid of the thyroid gland. He suggested that it entered the circulation through the lymphatic vessels. At the beginning of the present century, it was Sharpey-Schaefer in the UK who laid the physiological foundations of endocrinology.

In 1936, Edward Adelbert Doisy (b. 1893) of the St Louis University School of Medicine, USA, proposed four criteria required to establish endocrinology as an acceptable area for scientific study:

1 the gland must be identified as producing an internal secretion;

2 methods of detecting such an internal secretion must be available;

3 extracts must be produced from which a purified hormone can be obtained;

4 the pure hormone must be isolated, its structure determined, and its synthesis achieved.

Since Doisy's postulates, endocrinology has grown immensely. Early development of the field depended mainly on the recognition of clinical syndromes caused by excessive or inadequate activity of the individual endocrine glands. In the last decades, the many causes of glandular malfunction, the successful estimation of the level of circulating hormones in the blood, the complex mechanisms of interactions between hormones and their target organs, and hormone production by body tissues, not previously recognised as having endocrine activity, have all attracted attention.

The testicles

The earliest knowledge of endocrine function concerned the male sex glands or testicles. The results of castration had been known and connected with testicular function from the dawn of history. In the Bible, castrates and eunuchs were known. Eunuchoids were called 'sun castrates' (also by the Egyptians). In the Talmud, the same word was used for testicle and ovary. Hermaphrodites were known and described. Hippocrates (*c.* 460–400 BC) wrote on 'the Seed'. He knew that mumps could be followed by sterility. Aristotle (384–322 BC) wrote on sperm; he said that the semen was the formative, activating agent or 'soul'. Aretaeus (second century AD) taught that it is the semen that turns youths into men. In 1132 Hsu Shu-Wei in China was prescribing desiccated pig's testicle for impotence. The structure of the testicle was described in the 17th century. Jean Riolan the Younger described the seminiferous tubules in 1626. In 1668 de Graaf gave an accurate account of testicular structure and of the seminiferous tubes. He also practised ligation of the vas deferens.

During the 17th and 18th centuries, Chinese iatrochemists produced preparations of androgens from urine. In 1771 John Hunter in London mentioned his testicular transplant experiments, giving an accurate description of the testis in 1786. In the same year, Lazzaro Spallanzani proved in a brilliant filtration experiment in frogs that the spermatozoon is essential for fertilisation. He carried out artificial insemination in animals. This was also suggested in humans by John Hunter in 1790. (In husbandry, the effects of castration had been known from the earliest times.) In 1830 Astley Cooper in London published his *Observations on the Structure and Diseases of the Testis*. The cellular origin of the spermatozoon was demonstrated by Koelliker (Germany) in 1841.

Experimental evidence of testicular endocrine activity was provided by A.A. Berthold (Germany) in 1849, showing that transplantation of a cock's testis prevented atrophy of the comb after castration. In 1850 Franz Leydig (1821–1908) described the interstitial cells in animal testes; the Leydig cells in humans were described by Koelliker, 4 years later.

In 1889 Brown-Séquard, in Paris, reported on the effect of testicular extract on himself. However, it was not until 1911 that Pézard produced an effective testicular extract. In 1920 E. Steinach (Vienna) ligated the vas deferens to rejuvenate the ageing 'puberty gland'. Voronoff, in Algiers, carried out his rejuvenation experiments in 1923 by means of testicular implants into humans of monkey glands. In 1931 Adolf Butenandt (Germany) isolated androsterone in crystalline form. It was synthesised by Leopold Ruzicka in Switzerland in 1934. The following year, Ernst Laqueur's team in Amsterdam isolated testosterone from the testis. In 1973 Luiz de Lazerda and his colleagues at the Johns Hopkins Hospital studied circadian variations of plasma testosterone in normal men, while male infertility due to autoimmunity to sperm was reported in the late 1970s.

The ovaries

In ancient Egypt ovariotomy was performed on humans. Aristotle (384–322 BC) described ovariotomy in sows and camels as a means of increasing growth and strength. In the same century, Herophilus wrote about the 'female testicles'. In AD 1555 Vesalius described the 'female testicles'. In 1561 Fallopio gave a good description of the tubes, ovaries, the corpus luteum, hymen, clitoris and the round ligaments. Volcherus Coiter (1534–90), a pupil of Fallopio, discussed the corpus luteum in 1573, although the term 'corpus luteum' was coined by Malpighi in 1668. The word 'ovarium' was used by Fabricius in 1621, but it was Niels Stensen of Copenhagen who wrote that the female testes of mammals contained eggs and were analogous to the ovaries of oviparous species. William Harvey, who published in 1651 the '*Exercitationes de Generatione Animalium*', suggested the gradual building up of the embryo from the ovum. The next important contribution came in 1672 from Regnier de Graaf of Leyden, who described ovulation and the vesicles now known as the graafian follicles.

In the 17th century, Chinese iatrochemists also produced preparations of oestrogens from urine (see section on testicles). In 1773 Percival Pott in London noted cessation of menstruation and shrinking of the breasts in a young woman of 23 years from whom he had removed the herniated ovaries. From this, John Davidge, an American student in Edinburgh, concluded in his MD thesis in 1794, that 'menstruation attributable to a peculiar condition of the ovaries...'. Until 1872, this was the only scientific account of the effect of bilateral oophorectomy on the menses. In 1786 John Hunter in London reported on the effect on fertility after removing one ovary in a sow. In 1827 Prevost and Dumas described ovulation and the formation of corpus luteum in the bitch. In 1827 Carl Ernst von Baer, in Koenigsberg, discovered the human ovum. In 1896 Emil Knauer and Joseph Halban, both in Vienna, independently established the existence of ovarian hormones by implanting ovarian tissue into spayed rabbits. In 1889 F. Lataste, a zoologist in Bordeaux, discovered that female laboratory rodents had periods of sexual activity which were connected with the rhythms of the ovary. It was then found by Marshall and Jolly (1905) in the UK that ovarian extracts caused oestrus in castrated animals.

Within the next 20 years the ovarian hormones were isolated (oestrin by Allen and Doisy in 1923 in the USA). In 1926 Alan Parkes and Bellerby in London extracted oestrin. In 1927 Laqueur and his team discovered a female hormone (menformon) in male urine. A year later, Selmar Aschheim and Bernhard Zondek published their pregnancy test from female urine. Also during these amazingly productive 20 years, George Washington Corner in the USA discovered the structure of progesterone in 1929. This was followed by Guy Marrian (London, Toronto, Edinburgh) isolating pregnanediol (1929) and, in 1930, obtaining crystalline oestriol. In the same year, Doisy isolated crystalline oestrone from pregnancy urine. In 1934 Adolf Butenandt obtained crystalline progesterone, thus completing the search for the second ovarian hormone. Finally, in 1938, Charles Dodds and his colleagues in London presented the first synthetic oestrogen, stilboestrol.

No notes on the history of the testicles and the ovaries would be complete without some remarks on the history of hormonal contraception. Prolonged lactation by breast feeding was used by the ancient (and modern) Chinese, in ancient Egypt, but it is also recorded in Chesham, Buckinghamshire (England) between 1578 and 1601. Ludwig Haberlandt in Innsbruck (Austria) reported first 'On the hormonal (temporary) sterilisation of the female animal' (rabbit and guinea-pig) in 1921. He was followed, independently, by Otto Fellner, of Vienna, in 1922. The proper denomination of the new effective method of contraception in humans was given by Alan Guttmacher of Columbia University in 1961. This was followed by Gregory Pincus of Massachusetts, 'the father of the Pill', who published in 1965 *The Control of Fertility*. He was unaware of the work of Haberlandt and Fellner.

The thyroid

The thyroid also has an ancient history of investigation. In 1600 BC the Chinese used burnt sponge and seaweed for the treatment of goitre. Caesar spoke of 'big neck' as being a characteristic of the Gauls. Pliny and Juvenal (80 BC to AD 50) mentioned epidemics of goitre in the Alps and the use of burnt seaweed as treatment, as did Galen (AD 130–200). About AD 1050 Albucasis mentioned operation for 'elephantiasis' of the throat. In AD 1110, Jurjani of Persia connected exophthalmos with goitre. In 1530 Paracelsus noted the connection between endemic goitre and cretinism, while Shakespeare mentioned goitre in *The Tempest*. In 1659 Wharton used the term 'thyroid' in his *Adenographia*, while in 1769 Prosser in the UK mentioned treatment and cure of 'Derbyshire neck' with a powder of calcined sponge. In a posthumously published paper in 1825, Caleb Parry of Bath in England first described exophthalmic goitre (Parry's disease). Five years earlier, Coindet in Geneva first used iodine for the treatment of goitre. Iodine had been discovered in 1811 by Courtois in Paris in ashes of seaweed.

In 1835 Robert James Graves in Dublin published his description of exophthalmic goitre. Five years later (1840), Carl von Basedow in Merseburg, Germany, published his paper on 'the Merseburg triad', whereas in Italy the disease description 'morbo di Flajani' (1802) is preferred. In 1849 Dalrymple's eye sign was reported on by White Cooper and, in 1864, as von Graefe's sign. Conversely, Sir William Gull gave in 1873 an accurate account of hypothyroidism in women, while in 1878 Ord coined the actual term 'myxoedema'. Ludwig Rehn carried out the first thyroidectomy in exophthalmic goitre in 1880. Sir Felix Semon in London put forward in 1883 the view that myxoedema, the cachexia strumipriva of Emil Kocher (a surgeon in Berne), and cretinism were all caused by loss of thyroid function. This was at first ridiculed, but was fully confirmed by Sir Victor Horsley and his committee in 1886. In 1871 Charles Fagge of Guy's Hospital in London was able to report that endemic cretinism in Chiselborough in Somerset, described by H. Norris in 1848, had died out. Paul Moebius in Leipzig postulated in 1886 that exophthalmic goitre was due to hyperfunction of the thyroid (he later achieved notoriety by his monograph *On the Physiologic Mental Deficiency of Woman*.)

In 1891 George Murray of Newcastle reported on his successful treatment of myxoedema with extract of sheep thyroid by subcutaneous injection. In 1896 Vaughan Pendred (England) drew attention to the association of goitre with deaf-mutism. In the same year there occurred the description of Riedel's thyroiditis (Bernhard Riedel in Germany), although it had been described first by A.A. Bowlby in London in 1885. Charles Mayo in 1907 first used the term 'hyperthyroidism'. In the same year, David Marine, the 'Nestor of thyroidology' in New York, established that iodine was necessary for thyroid function. In 1911 he proposed the treatment of Graves' disease with iodine; this idea was taken up by Henry Plummer in 1923. In 1917, Marine suggested (with O. Kimball) goitre prevention with iodine; in 1932 he described cyanide goitre. In 1910, Kocher of Berne had coined the term 'iod-Basedow', while in 1912, Hakaru Hashimoto described struma lymphomatosa (Hashimoto's disease). In 1914, Edward C. Kendall (USA) isolated thyroxine in crystalline form while 10 years later in 1924 Plummer and Boothby reported on the preoperative use of iodine in exophthalmic goitre. Sir Charles Harington in London determined the chemical structure of thyroxine in 1926, and a year later it was synthesised by Harington and George Barger.

In 1943 Saul Hertz and Arthur Roberts at the Massachusetts General Hospital, and—independently—C.P. Leblond in Paris, introduced radioiodine in the assessment of Graves' disease and later for its treatment. In the same year, Edwin Astwood began to use thiourea and thiouracil successfully (as thyroid-blocking drugs) in the medical treatment of Graves' disease. In 1931, Naffziger (USA) introduced orbital decompression for the treatment of malignant exophthalmos. In 1951, A. Lawson, C. Rimington and C.E. Searle synthesised carbimazole.

In 1953, Jack Gross and Rosalind Pitt-Rivers in London isolated triiodothyronine from the thyroid gland and synthesised it. Three years later, Ivan Roitt and Deborah Doniach (London), together with P.N. Campbell and R.V. Hudson, demonstrated autoantibodies in Hashimoto's disease, pioneering the understanding of autoimmunity as one of the major causal factors in endocrine disorders. Adams, Purves and McKenzie in Otago, New Zealand, discovered long-acting thyroid stimulator (LATS) in the serum of thyrotoxic patients in 1956. In Switzerland mass neonatal screening programmes were soon after started for metabolic disorders. In 1972–78, screening began for neonatal (congenital) hypothyroidism in the USA, Canada, the UK, Japan and some other countries.

The parathyroids

The parathyroids were described much later than the thyroid gland. Sir Richard Owen noted animal parathyroid glands in 1852 when dissecting a rhinoceros at the London Zoological Gardens. The first description of these glands in humans was not until 1880, when Ivar Sandstroem in Uppsala was prosector in the Department of Anatomy. Eugene Gley in Paris demonstrated in 1891 that the parathyroids were essential for life. In 1895 A. Kohn in Germany proved the independence of the parathyroids from the thyroid. G. Vassale and F. Generali in Italy showed experimentally in 1896 that tetany follows removal of the parathyroids. Max Askanazy in Tuebingen connected osteitis fibrosa cystica with a parathyroid adenoma found at postmortem. In 1906 Jacob Erdheim in Vienna described hyperplasia of the parathyroids in osteomalacia in humans. W.G. MacCallum and Carl Voegtlin showed in 1909 that, following parathyroidectomy, tetany and hypocalcaemia could be controlled by calcium administration.

In the same year, the surgeon William S. Halstead in Baltimore attempted auto- and isotransplantation of parathyroid glands into thyroid tissue of dogs. In 1914, Jacob Erdheim (Vienna) described compensatory parathyroid hyperplasia in spontaneous rickets in rats (secondary hyperparathyroidism), but it was not until 1923 that Adolph Hanson in Washington reported, independently, the isolation of an effective parathyroid extract from cattle. Two years later, James B. Collip in Toronto, who had purified Banting and Best's insulin, partially purified parathormone and, with Douglas Leitch, used it successfully in the treatment of tetany. In the same year, 1925, the Viennese surgeon Felix Mandl achieved the first cure of primary hyperparathyroidism (osteitis fibrosa) by surgical removal of a parathyroid adenoma. Between 1934 and 1948 Fuller Albright (a pupil of Erdheim) at Harvard in Boston described the biochemistry of primary hyperparathyroidism, and kidney stones as one of the important features. It was not until 1959 that Rasmussen and L.C. Craig in the USA isolated parathyroid hormone and defined its structure as a polypeptide hormone.

In 1942, Fuller Albright and his group described 'pseudohypoparathyroidism', in which hypocalcaemia is not corrected by the administration of parathyroid hormone. In the 1960s S.A. Berson and R.S. Yalow (USA) introduced a radioimmunological method for the estimation of parathyroid hormone in serum.

The pancreas

The pancreas is another gland with an ancient history. Moreover, it has recently been proved that it is simply an anatomical marriage of an exocrine and endocrine gland. The present trend of endocrine search points towards integration in medicine rather than segregation (see below).

An Egyptian papyrus dating from *c.*1550 BC, discovered by Ebers in Thebes in 1862, described diabetic polyuria and its treatment. In the fourth century Susruta (India) mentioned 'sugarcream' urine which attracted ants. Around AD 30, Cornelius Celsus described a condition that sounded like diabetic polyuria. Aretaeus of Kappadokia (AD 81–136) gave the complete clinical description of diabetes mellitus and called it 'diabetes' (from the Greek 'to pass through'). Galen (AD 131–201) regarded diabetes as due to weakness of the kidneys. In 7th century China, Chen Chan recorded 'sweet urine' in diabetes mellitus. Rhazes (Al Razi) (AD 860–932) in Persia and Baghdad introduced a regimen of treatment in diabetes mellitus. In AD 1020, Avicenna mentioned the multitude of urine and the occurrence of impotence and furunculosis in diabetes. Paracelsus (*c.* 1530) thought diabetes was a generalised disease. It was Thomas Willis (1621–75), of Oxford and London, who described the sweet taste of urine in diabetes mellitus. In 1642 the Bavarian George Wirsung in Padova described the pancreatic duct in humans. His contemporary, Sylvius (Frans de la Boe) in Leyden, suspected that a juice was excreted from the pancreas into intestine, and in 1664 Regnier de Graaf, a pupil of Sylvius, published some of his brilliant experiments on obtaining pancreatic juice, similar to salivary gland secretion. Sganarelle, in Molière's 'Le médecin volant', tasted the urine for sweetness. Matthew Dobson in Liverpool proved in 1776 that the sweetness of urine in diabetes was caused by sugar, which was also present in the blood (hyperglycaemia), and in 1815 Michel Chevreul in Paris showed that the sugar in diabetic urine is glucose. William Prout (1785–1830) in England, first recognised diabetic coma. In 1841 Carl Trommer in Heidelberg published his test for glucose in the urine, followed in 1848 by Christian von Fehling.

In 1849 Claude Bernard in Paris discovered glycogen in the liver and quantitatively estimated sugar in the blood. He also described the piqûre diabétique in the brain of the dog. His observation that an organ can produce a substance and pass it directly into the blood has been stated as the official date of inception of the modern era of endocrinology. In 1857 Wilhelm Petters demonstrated the presence of acetone in the urine of diabetics. In 1869 Paul Langerhans in Berlin described the islet cells of the pancreas in his doctoral thesis, but he died in 1888, aged 41 years, without suggesting any function for these cells.

In 1874 Adolf Kussmaul in Germany explained diabetic coma as due to acetonaemia; he also described 'Kussmaul's respiration' in acidaemia. Three years later,

Étienne Lancereaux in Paris causally connected two cases of diabetes with pancreatic lesions (calculi). In 1886 Joseph von Mering (1849–1908) in Strasbourg produced experimental diabetes by means of phloridzin. He and Oscar Minkowski (1858–1931) produced diabetes in a dog by removal of the pancreas in 1890. Giulio Vassale (1862–1912) in Italy experimentally destroyed the pancreatic acini by ligation of the excretory duct without destruction of the islet cells (in 1891). Minkowski obtained temporary cure of diabetes in the pancreatectomised dog by subcutaneous reimplantation of the excised organ (1892).

In 1893 Gustave-Edouard Laguesse (1861–1927) suggested that the cells described by Langerhans should be called the 'islets of Langerhans', and suspected that they produced a hormone. In 1902 Sir William Bayliss and Ernest Starling discovered 'secretin'. In 1906 Ivar Bang published his method for the estimation of sugar in the blood. A year later, M.A. Lane in Chicago described oxyphil (α) and basophil (β) islet cells. In 1909 Jean de Meyer (Brussels) suggested the name 'insuline' for the hormone of the islet cells. In 1913 J. Homans (one of Cushing's original team) came to the conclusion that it is the β-cells that secrete the (then still hypothetical) insulin.

In June 1921 Nicolas Constantin Paulesco (Paris and Bucharest), a pupil of Lancereux (1869–1931), reported on 'pancreatine', a blood-sugar lowering extract from the pancreas, discovered by him between 1914 and 1916, and became the 'forgotten man of the discovery of insulin'. In November 1921 Frederick Grant Banting (1891–1941) and J.J.R Macleod, in Toronto, reported the discovery of insulin by Banting and Charles Herbert Best (1899–1978). The first clinical application occurred in 1922. James Bertrand Collip (1892–1965) of Toronto purified insulin which was crystallised by J.J. Abel in 1926.

In 1927 J. Wilder and colleagues reported the first case of hyperinsulinism due to carcinoma of the islands of the pancreas. Two years later, Howland, Campbell, Maltby and Robinson cured hyperinsulinism by surgical removal of an islet-cell tumour.

In 1937 alloxan hyperglycaemia was described by Jacobs. In 1942 M.J. Janbon in Montpellier noticed the hypoglycaemic effect of a sulphonamide product, which was then further investigated. Its mode of action was explained by his pupil, Auguste Loubatières. This led to the use of sulpha drugs for the oral treatment of diabetes. In 1952 Knud Hallas-Møller and his group introduced the insulin–zinc suspensions. In 1923 J.R. Murlin and his team in Rochester, Minnesota, discovered a hyperglycaemic substance, produced by the pancreas as a second hormone, which he named 'glucagon' (structure discovered in 1956).

In 1955, Frederic Sanger (Cambridge, UK) published the structure of the bovine insulin molecule. In 1957 S.A. Berson and Rosalyn Yalow described their radioimmunological method for the measurement of plasma insulin (see below). Between 1961 and 1968, glucagon was synthesised by E. Wuensch and his team in Munich, after Bromer, Sinn, Staub and Behrens in Indianapolis had synthesised porcine glucagon in 1956. Its isolation and crystallisation had been achieved in 1953 by A. Staub and his colleagues. Between 1964 and 1966, insulin was synthesised, independently, by P.G. Katsoyannis (USA).

M.H. McGarvan, R.H. Unger and their colleagues (USA) first described in 1966 'A glucagon-secreting alpha cell carcinoma of the pancreas'. In 1969 the drug company Boehringer introduced glibenclamide for the oral treatment of diabetes. In 1978 Deborah Doniach and G.F. Bottazzo (London) reported on autoimmunity in diabetes. Recently, evidence has been accumulating that the exocrine and the endocrine part of the pancreas are functionally related. Henderson, Daniel and Fraser (London) found in 1981 that there was a direct influence of the endocrine pancreas on its exocrine function.

Gut hormones

Next in line to the pancreas are perhaps the fairly recently discovered gut hormones. As mentioned above, Sir William Bayliss and Ernest Starling discovered in 1902 that a crude extract of duodenal mucosa injected into the bloodstream excited pancreatic secretion; they called the agent 'secretin'. Between 1903 and 1906 John Sidney Edkins described 'gastrin', which was isolated in 1966 and its structure defined by R. Gregory. It was, however, Frederick Feyrter in Danzig who from 1935 to 1953 made a special study of the peripheral (paracrine) endocrine glands in humans. In 1955 Robert M. Zollinger and Edwin H. Ellison described the syndrome, named after them, of islet-cell tumour of the pancreas, liberating a large amount of gastrin and causing peptic ulceration of the jejunum (the name of 'gastrinoma' was suggested). In 1969, A.G.E. Pearse introduced the APUD concept (*a*mine content, amine *p*recursor *u*ptake and amino *d*ecarboxylase content). From 1974 onwards, numerous peptides have been described, located in the islet organ, the stomach, duodenum, jejunum, ileum and colon. Many of these peptides are now known to be common to the brain and to the gastrointestinal tract.

The pituitary

In the 1930s it was customary to talk about the 'endocrine orchestra', and Sir Walter Langdon-Brown (1870–1946) of St Bartholomew's Hospital, London, was the first to coin the phrase in 1931: 'the pituitary is the leader of the endocrine orchestra'. Although this view has now been superseded, it is still true that the pituitary gland plays a major role in the control and direction of the endocrine band.

The adenohypophysis or anterior pituitary

Around 400 BC, in his *Aphorisms*, Hippocrates mentions amenorrhoea in women with galactorrhoea: if a woman, who is neither pregnant nor has given birth, produces milk, her menstruation has stopped (Aphorism No. 39, Section V). Giants were repeatedly mentioned in the Old Testament, where dwarfs were regarded as misfits. Galen (AD 129–201) thought that the pituitary drained the phlegm from the brain to the nasopharynx (refuted in 1660 by Conrad Victor Schneider (1614–80) of Wittenberg and by Richard Lower (1631–91) of Oxford). Lower thought that substances passed from the brain through the infundibulum and pituitary stalk to the gland, where they were distilled back in the blood. In 1543 Vesalius described the 'glandula pituitaria cerebri excipiens'. Joseph Lieutaud (1703–80) in Paris described in 1742 the pituitary stalk ('la tige'). Anton de Haën (1704–76) in Vienna mentioned amenorrhoea in connection with the finding of pituitary tumour.

In 1772 in Paris, Nicolas Saucerotte (1741–1812) described Sieur Mirbeck, who suffered from acromegaly; it seems that the Irish giants Cornelius Magrath (1742–68) and Charles Byrne or O'Brien (1761–83) were also acromegalic. Samuel Thomas von Soemmering (1755–1830) in Goettingen introduced the term 'hypophysis cerebri' in 1778. In 1786 John Hunter in London described 'pigeon's milk'. In 1822 Baron Jean Louis Alibert in Paris presented his 'Géant scrofuleux', who suffered from acromegaly and diabetes insipidus.

Giants

Giants were repeatedly mentioned in the Old Testament, not only as individuals (Goliath) but also in families and tribes (Joshua 14:15). Interestingly, there were tribes of giants described in Nordic Sagas. In many of these individuals there must have been pituitary dysfunction. If there were low gonadotrophin values, the chances of procreation must have also been diminished; thus, occurrence of families and tribes of giants in Nordic and Oriental folklore must have a different explanation.

In 1838 Martin Heinrich Rathke (1793–1860) described the formation of the pituitary gland. In 1840 Bernhard Mohr of Wuerzburg reported on an obese woman who was later described by Alfred Froehlich (1871–1953) of Vienna as dystrophia adiposogenitalis. In 1851 A. Nièpce in France noted enlargement of the pituitary in connection with parenchymatous goitre. Andrea Verga in Milan, published the first post-mortem report of a case of acromegaly in 1864, describing a pituitary tumour which had destroyed the sphenoid and pressed on the optic chiasm. He called the disease 'prosopectasia'. In 1877 Vincenzo Brigidi (Italy) found a pituitary tumour during the post-mortem examination of the actor Ghirlenzoni, whose skeleton had been preserved, including the histology of the pituitary tumour.

More importantly, Christian F. Fritsche (1851–1938) published in 1884 from Glarus in Switzerland (together with Theodor A.E. Klebs, a pathologist in Zurich) a 'contribution to the pathology of giantism', the long-term observation and post-mortem examination of a patient with a large thymus and a striking enlargement of the pituitary gland and the sella turcica. The Viennese anatomist Carl Langer (1819–87) had written in 1872 that enlargement of the sella was found only in giants with a 'monstrous lower jaw, thick lips and large nostrils'. All this was unknown to Pierre Marie in Paris when he submitted his two cases of acromegaly for publication in September 1885.

In 1887 Oscar Minkowski was the first to suspect a causal relation between pituitary enlargement and acromegaly. In 1893 Richard Caton and Frank Thomas Paul in Liverpool performed pituitary decompression in a woman aged 33 years with acromegaly to relieve cranial pressure. The first successful operation of a pituitary tumour by the nasal route was performed in 1906 by Hermann Schloffer (1868–1937) in Innsbruck, Austria; the method was later perfected, after 1911, by Oscar Hirsch in Vienna. In 1900 Carl Benda (1857–1933) demonstrated that the pituitary tumour of the anterior lobe in acromegaly consists of chromophil cells. In 1900 J.F. Babinski (France), in 1901 Alfred Froehlich (Vienna) and in 1906 Harvey Cushing all described dystrophia adiposogenitalis. In 1909 Bernhard Aschner of Vienna (1883–1960) showed that transbuccal hypophysectomy in a growing dog causes dwarfism.

In 1910 Harvey Cushing and his team presented the first experimental proof of the link between the anterior pituitary and the organs of reproduction. In 1913 L.K. Glinski described post-partum necrosis of the anterior pituitary, unfortunately in the Polish language. In 1914 Morris Simmonds of Hamburg described post-partum pituitary cachexia. In 1939 Harold L. Sheehan (Liverpool) described patients with 'Simmonds' disease'. From that time, however, this condition has been called in the English literature 'Sheehan's syndrome'! In 1915 Walter Lee Gaines (USA) demonstrated the action of the pituitary in lactation.

Jacob Erdheim in Vienna described pituitary dwarfism in 1916. In 1921 Herbert McLean Evans (1881–1971) and Joseph A. Long demonstrated the effect of anterior lobe extract on the growth of rats. In 1928 Bernhard Zondek and Selmar Aschheim in Berlin published their pregnancy test in urine. In the same year, they isolated the gonadotrophin hormones of the anterior pituitary, now known as follicle-stimulating hormone (FSH) and luteinising hormone (LH). In 1929 P. Stricker and F. Grueter in Paris discovered prolactin (but see Gaines in 1915). In the same year Aron (Strasbourg) and, independently, Loeb and Bassett, described the action of thyroid-stimulating hormone (TSH). Its structure was determined by Pierce, Liao and colleagues in 1971. In 1932 Cushing described pituitary basophilism. Since then 'Cushing's disease', first so-named by the late F.M.P. Bishop and R.G. Close of Guy's Hospital, London, has been intensively studied and discussed. In the same year, E.M. Anderson and James Collip gave an account of TSH, which was purified in 1937. Oscar Riddle (1877–1968) and colleagues in the USA identified and assayed prolactin in 1933. Three years later, Herbert M. Evans and his group at Berkeley isolated interstitial cell-stimulating hormone (ICSH) in the male, now known as LH. Between 1940 and 1949, Choh Hao Li (b. 1913), a pupil and collaborator of H.M. Evans at Berkeley, California, isolated LH, adrenocorticotrophic hormone (ACTH), growth hormone (GH) (in 1945) and FSH. In 1965, together with his group, he isolated β-lipotrophin, which is manufactured and released together with ACTH. Finally, between 1966 and 1971, he described the structure of human GH and synthesised it. From 1975, hyperprolactinaemia (the galactorrhoea–amenorrhoea syndrome) and its treatment has been described and studied by various groups, especially by G.M. Besser and his colleagues in London.

The neurohypophysis or posterior pituitary

The much-travelled scientist Johann Peter Frank (1745–1821) differentiated diabetes insipidus (or spurius, as he called it) from diabetes mellitus in 1794, probably when he was still working in Lombardy. It was his namesake, Alfred Erich Frank (1884–1957) who, in 1912, was the first to connect the posterior lobe with diabetes insipidus. In 1895 George Oliver (1841–1915) and Edward Schaefer (as he then was) published the vasopressor effect of pituitary gland extract in a number of exciting experiments. In 1906 Sir Henry Dale (1875–1968) in London described the oxytocic action of posterior pituitary extract. In 1908 Schaefer and Percy T. Herring (1872–1967) showed that there was a diuretic principle in the posterior pituitary.

In 1909 William Blair-Bell (1871–1936) used posterior pituitary extract in the treatment of shock, uterine atony and intestinal paresis. Aschner, Paulesco and Cushing (between 1908 and 1910) and Blair-Bell (in 1916) showed that apituitarism led to death, be it due to the removal of the anterior lobe or clamping of the pituitary stalk. Death was due to cachexia hypophysiopriva and to atrophy of the adrenal cortex, but isolated removal of the posterior lobe was not lethal. Foges and Hofstaetter in Vienna used pituitrin in the treatment of post-partum haemorrhage (1910). In 1911 I. Ott and J.C. Scott in Philadelphia recorded a galactokinetic (milk ejection) action of posterior pituitary extracts in mammals.

In 1913 Farini (Venice) and van den Velden (Duesseldorf) reported on the antidiuretic effect of posterior pituitary extracts. Ernest Starling and Verney demonstrated in 1924 the antidiuretic effect of posterior pituitary extracts on the isolated kidney. In 1928 O. Kamm and his team (USA) isolated vasopressin and oxytocin. Between 1940 and 1947 there were Hans Hellert's (1905–74) studies in Bristol of the antidiuretic principle in numerous non-mammalian species.

In 1947 Verney (UK) postulated the release of vasopressin in the anterior hypothalamus. In 1951, Bergmann and E. Scharrer (1905–65) described the site of origin of the posterior pituitary hormones in the nuclei of the hypothalamus. Analysis and synthesis of oxytocin and vasopressin was achieved in 1953–58 by V. du Vigneaud and his group in the USA. In 1966 Klein, Roth and Petersen described a radioimmunoassay for arginine vasopressin.

When in 1975 Peter M. Daniel and Marjorie Pritchard (London) published the result of their 25-year studies of the anatomy and histology of the hypothalamus and the pituitary with special reference to the portal system, it contained a correction of G.T. Popa and V. Fielding's reports in 1930 (London) on the portal circulation from the pituitary to the hypothalamic region; the blood flows, in fact, in the opposite direction. G.H. Friedman and M.H. Friedman in the USA had indicated in 1934 that the secretion of the posterior lobe is discharged into the blood and not into the cerebrospinal fluid (see below).

The hypothalamus

Pituitary function is mainly controlled by the hypothalamus. The pituitary portal system as the hypothalamo-hypophysial connection (in the pituitary stalk) was first described by Joseph Lieutaud (1703–80) in 1742 in Aix-en-Provence. In 1860 Hubert von Luschka (Germany) described the primary capillary loops of the pituitary portal vessels. In 1865 Jules B. Luys (1828–97) in Paris described the hypothalamus (nucleus of Luys). Johann P. Karplus (1866–1936) and Alois Kreidl (1864–1928) in Vienna reported in 1909 on the first experimental studies on the hypothalamus. Four years later, Jean Camus (1872–1924) and Gustave Roussy (1874–1948) in France produced experimental diabetes insipidus in dogs by injury to the hypothalamus.

In 1936 Hans Selye (1907–82) in Montreal described the 'stress–general adaptation syndrome', which is closely connected with the circadian secretion of ACTH generated by the hypothalamus. In 1944 Berta and Ernst Scharrer compared the intercerebral cardiacum-allatum system of insects with the hypothalamo-hypophysial system of vertebrates. In 1948 Geoffrey W. Harris (1913–72) in Cambridge published *Neural Control of the Pituitary*, and until 1951 carried out intensive experimental studies on hypothalamic control.

From then on until 1968 a number of hypothalamic releasing or inhibiting factors (hormones), originally forecast by Harris, were described by various researchers. Greenwood, Landon and Stamp (London 1966) introduced insulin-induced hypoglycaemia as a test to investigate adrenal insufficiency due to hypothalamic or pituitary disease. In 1971 Schally (New Orleans), Arimura and colleagues isolated LH/FSH-releasing hormone. In 1973 I. Brazeau, Roger Guillemin and collaborators defined somatostatin. Rosalyn Yalow described the heterogeneity of peptide hormones (1974).

In 1977 P.M. Daniel and C.S. Treip (London) published their definitive study of the pathology of the hypothalamus. A year later J.H. Henderson and P.M Daniel discussed portal circulations and their relation to countercurrent systems. In 1977 Dorothy Krieger (New York) suggested that the circadian variation of the pituitary–adrenal function reflects the circadian variation of the central nervous mechanism involved in the control of the corticotrophin-releasing hormone (CRH).

Anorexia nervosa

Pituitary deficiency has long been suspected in anorexia nervosa. Recent evidence suggests that the endocrine disturbance of this disorder, and of bulimia nervosa, is of hypothalamic origin. Soranos of Ephesos (AD 98–138) described amenorrhoea and anorexia in women. In *c.* AD 155 Galen mentioned a condition of emaciation because a patient could not (or would not) eat. In 1689 Richard Morton (1637–98) gave the first description of anorexia nervosa in England (including a 16-year-old boy). In 1873, Ernest Charles Lasègue (1816–83) in Paris described 'l'anorexie hystérique'. In the same year, Sir William W. Gull (1816–90) of Guy's Hospital, London, described the condition and named it 'anorexia nervosa' (he had given the classic description of myxoedema in women in the same year). In 1874, Joseph J. Déjérine (1849–1917) in Paris called it 'l'anorexie mentale'.

In 1934 Ernst von Bergmann (1836–1907) in Germany, and a year later E. Kylin (Germany), claimed successful treatment with transplants of animal anterior pituitary tissue. In 1937 Max Schur and V.C. Medvei called it pituitary insufficiency due to 'disturbance of correlation'. J.H. Sheldon (UK) in 1939 talked of anorexia nervosa as a functional Simmonds' disease.

In 1948 E.C. Jacobs (USA) studied the effects of starvation on sex hormone production in the male. In 1954 W.H. Perloff and colleagues (USA) reported on functional hypopituitarism induced by starvation. H.H. Srebnik and M.M. Nelson recorded in 1962 that pituitary LH concentration was reduced after malnutrition.

In 1969 Peter J. Dally in London suggested a three-scale classification: obsessional, hysterical and mixed; he and his co-workers said in 1979 'There is thus clear evidence of hypothalamic dysfunction in anorexia nervosa'. G.M. Besser (London) argued in 1973 that the endocrine dysfunction in anorexia nervosa originated in the hypothalamus and not in the anterior pituitary. P.V.J. Beumont and his group found, in 1976, that circulating LH levels were reduced in anorexia nervosa and so was the response to gonadotrophin-releasing hormone. Two years later, T.F. Davies and M. Lewis (London) thought that functional hypopituitarism may be explained by changes of oestrogen metabolism, associated with the loss of body fat, which alter the gonadotrophin dynamics and result in excessive LH suppression. Such a concept would also explain the close association between menarche and bodyweight and food intake and infertility, as detailed by the epidemiologist, Rose Frisch.

In 1979 the psychiatrist George F.M. Russell (London) described bulimia nervosa, an ominous variant of anorexia nervosa.

The brain

The gland that eventually emerged as the 'master gland' was the brain. Galen (AD 129–201) thought that the pituitary drained the phlegm from the brain to the nasopharynx (see section on the pituitary). The blood was thought to flow to and fro in the arteries carrying 'vital spirit' from the brain to various parts of the body. The waste products of this chemical reaction flow to the base of the brain, down the pituitary stalk and so to the pituitary gland, down to the sphenoid and ethmoid bones, emerging as the nasal mucus.

It took 1500 years before Conrad Victor Schneider of Wittenberg and Richard Lower of Oxford (in 1660 and 1670) disproved the existence of a communication between the ventricles of the brain and the nasopharynx (see also above). In 1543 Andreas Vesalius (1514–64) called the brain 'a glandular organ'. René Descartes (1596–1650) considered the brain as the organ integrating the functions of mind and body, with the pineal in a pivotal role (1637). In 1733 Giovanni Battista Morgagni (1681–1771) in Padova, in 1792 Samuel von Soemmering (1755–1830) in Goettingen, and in 1802 Johann F. Meckel the Younger (1781–1833) of Halle (the 'German Cuvier') all observed absence of the adrenal cortex in anencephaly.

In 1849–50, Claude Bernard (1813–78) in Paris demonstrated that 'piqûre diabétique' of the floor of the posterior part of the fourth ventricle in the dog causes temporary glycosuria. Piqûre a little anterior to the glycosuria centre causes polyuria. In 1870 C. Eckhard (1822–1915) in Giessen found that injury to certain other parts of the brain may also cause polyuria. In 1951 J. Lhermitte (France) stressed regulation of mental life by hormones in *Le Cerveau et la Pensée.*

Between 1971 and 1975, Hans W. Kosterlitz, J. Hughes and their colleagues in Aberdeen identified the pentapeptides in brain which possess potent opiate agonist activity. In 1973 Snyder and his group (Johns Hopkins), Eric Simon and colleagues (New York) and Lars Terenius and his team in Uppsala, had demonstrated that opiates attach themselves to specific receptor sites in the brain as their target cells. In 1975 A.F. Bradbury and his colleagues isolated β-endorphin and described its structure. In 1978 Wilhelm Feldberg (London) reported on the pharmacology of the central actions of endorphins. In 1979 Vicky Clement-Jones and her colleagues in London, together with Wen in Hong Kong found that during withdrawal of heroin addicts treated with acupuncture, the Met-enkephalin levels of the cerobrospinal fluid showed a clear rise. The same investigators demonstrated increased levels of β-endorphin, but not of Met-enkephalin, in human cerebrospinal fluid after acupuncture for treatment of recurrent pain. They concluded that β-endorphin may be released from the pituitary or from the brain (1980). It is now clear that the endogenous opioids, including the recently discovered dynorphins, are important neuronal and endocrine modulators, particularly of pain input.

Neuroendocrinology

It became clear that the role of the brain, the hypothalamus and of the anterior and posterior pituitary in the field of neuroendocrinology had to be explored. In fact, it turned out that knowledge of this relationship had existed for quite some time. In 1818 Franz Joseph Gall (1758–1828) in Paris, and in 1835 J. Vimont in Brussels, reported that unilateral castration causes atrophy of the contralateral hemisphere of the cerebellum in the rabbit. Arnold A. Berthold (1803–61) of Goettingen, in his celebrated experiment of testicular transplant, implicated the nervous system as a target organ (in 1849). In 1856 Maestre de San Juan (Spain) observed gonadal hypoplasia in men with agenesis of the olfactory lobes. This clinical observation was confirmed by several people between 1914 and 1960, and experimentally by Ernst and Berta Scharrer in 1963.

In 1877 Emil H. Du Bois Reymond (1818–96), the German physiologist, suggested a chemical transmission from motor nerve endings to striated muscle. In 1905 Schiefferdecker in Bonn described the secretion of endocrine substances by neurons as a means of communication between neurons or between a neuron and an effector cell in muscle or gland. This was based on some of the ideas of Robert A.A. Tigerstedt (1853–1923) of Leipzig and Helsinki, of 'automatic' irritation by metabolic products, and on Schiefferdecker's own observations. In 1908 Maxime P.M. Laignel-Lavastine (1875–1953) in Paris discussed the connection between psychiatry and internal secretions ('sécrétions internes et psychoses').

In 1913 Jean Camus (1872–1924) and Gustave Roussy (1874–1948) in France stressed the predominance of the hypothalamus. Déjérine and Roussy had published a paper 'Le syndrome thalamique' in 1906, investigating the effect of localized thalamic injury; but Roussy's magnum opus of this field was his publication with Michel Mosinger in 1946 of the great volume *Traité de Neuro-endocrinologie: Le Système Neuro-endocrinien; Le Complexe Hypothalamo-Hypophysaire; La Neuro-ergonologie et son Evolution Récente.*

Sir Henry H. Dale (1875–1968) in London published in 1914 'The action of certain esters and ethers of acetylcholine'. In the same year, T.R. Elliott (1877–1961) in London conceived the idea of chemical transmission in the autonomic nervous system. This prediction was realised when Wilhelm Feldberg and Fessard published in 1942: 'On the cholinergic nature of the nerves to the electric organ of Torpedo'. From 1921 to 1924, Otto Loewi (1873–1961) in Graz, Austria proved the theory of chemical intermediaries in nervous stimulation. Berta and Ernst Scharrer reported in 1928 (still from Germany) on the function of the hypothalamus in teleost fishes. F.H. Lewy (Germany) declared in 1929 that the vegetative nuclei of the central nervous system form with the posterior pituitary a single unified system.

Walter B. Cannon (1871–1945) at Harvard and Z.M. Bacq of Liège, Belgium, described in 1931 'sympathin', a hormone produced by sympathetic action on smooth muscle. Two years later, Wilhelm Feldberg and Sir John Gaddum produced evidence that acetylcholine acts in the transfer of nerve impulses from neuron to neuron in sympathetic ganglia. In 1934 Walter Cannon discussed the chemical mediation of nerve impulses. In 1936 Francis H.A. Marshall (1878–1944) in Cambridge referred in his Croonian lectures to the higher animals in whom 'the internal rhythm brought into relation with ... other external phenomena ... in part ... through the nervous system and probably through the hypothalamus upon the anterior pituitary and thence upon the testis and the ovary ...'. In 1949 R.G. Hoskins (USA) introduced Norbert Wiener's idea (1948) of the (servo-)feedback mechanism into the field of endocrinology. In 1951 Max Reiss (then in Bristol, UK) discussed the application of endocrine research methods to psychiatry. In 1954 M. Bleuler published his book (in German) on endocrine psychiatry.

The most prominent representative and brilliant experimenter in the field of neuroendocrinology was, however,

Geoffrey W. Harris (1913–72) of Cambridge, London and Oxford. His premature death was a great loss to modern endocrinology. One of his collaborators was G.T. Popa (from Romania). Highlights of his contributions to neuroendocrinology over many years were, in 1955, his discussion of the relationships between endocrine activity and the development of the nervous system, and especially his Dale lecture in 1971, given just a few months before his death, on 'humours and hormones'. He was certainly one of the founders of neuroendocrinology.

In 1966 A.G.E. Pearse (creator of the APUD concept) put forward the theory that the endocrine cells are all derivatives of the neural crest and thus neuroectodermal and, strictly speaking, neuroendocrine. In 1974 Z.M. Bacq published 'Les transmission chimiques de l'influx nerveux'. In 1968 P.W. P. Butler and G.M. Besser were the first to report on pituitary–adrenal function in severe depressive illness.

The adrenals

The adrenal glands are, like the pituitary, an anatomical mixture of two, functionally distinct, structures, which are developmentally and histologically quite separate. In 1563 Bartolomeo Eustachius (1520–74) in Rome described them as glands lying next to the kidneys. Adrianus Spigelius (Adriaan van den Spieghel, 1578–1625) talked in 1627 (published posthumously) of the 'capsulae renales'. Nathaniel Highmore (1613–85) in England agreed in 1651, but added that they might serve to absorb humid exudates from the large vessels nearby. It was George Frédéric Baron Cuvier (1769–1832) in Paris who, in 1805, defined the medulla and cortex of the adrenal gland. According to H.P. Schoenwetter, in his doctoral thesis in 1951, it was Emil Huschke (1797–1858), anatomist and embryologist in Jena, who first made a clear distinction between the adrenal cortex and medulla. Huschke, like Antonio Valsalva (1666–1723) before him, thought that there was a connection between the adrenals and the gonads.

Adrenal cortex

In 1855 Thomas Addison (1793–1860) of Guy's Hospital, London, published his book *On the Constitutional and Local Effects of Disease of the Suprarenal Capsules*. In it, he 'stumbled', as he said, on the bronzed disease (melasma suprarenale), while searching for the cause of pernicious anaemia. A year later, Charles E. Brown-Séquard (1817–94) of Paris proved in animal experiments that the adrenals were essential for the maintenance of life. In 1896 Sir William Osler, found that orally administered adrenal extract was temporarily effective in Addison's disease.

William Bulloch (1868–1941) and James H. Sequeira (1865–1948) in England described in 1905 patients with the adrenogenital syndrome, the first report made under that name. This was followed by E.E. Glynn's publication in England in 1911–12 *'The adrenal cortex, its rests and tumours, in relation to the other ductless glands and, especially, to sex'*. The earliest connection is the occurrence of a probable tumour in a virilised girl described by Henry Sampson in 1697 (but Michael Kelly in Australia made a similar claim in 1956 for two patients of Hippocrates).

In 1926 Philip E. Smith (1884–1970), then at Stanford University, showed that hypophysectomy caused atrophy of the adrenals, which Herbert Evans (1882–1971) prevented by administration of pituitary extracts. This was confirmed a year later by Frank A. Hartman (England) and Katherine A. Brownell. They also observed that liquid extracts of cortical tissue maintained adrenalectomised cats indefinitely, as did Joseph J. Pfiffner and Wilbur W. Swingle (USA) in 1929–32.

In 1932 Harvey Cushing connected 'the polyglandular syndrome' of pituitary basophilism (first described by him in 1912) with pituitary adrenal hyperactivity. In the same year, R.F. Loeb observed low serum sodium in patients with Addison's disease, which he then followed by treatment of such patients with sodium chloride. Between 1937 and 1952 the steroid hormones of the adrenal cortex were isolated and their structure was determined and synthesised by Edward C. Kendall (1886–1972) of the Mayo Foundation, Arthur Grollman (USA), Tadeus Reichstein (Zurich and, later, Basle) and J. von Euw, Oscar P. Wintersteiner and Joseph J. Pfiffner. In 1948 Philip S. Hench (1896–1965) of the Mayo Clinic and his colleagues discovered the anti-inflammatory effect of cortisone (Kendall's compound E). As mentioned before (in the section on the anterior pituitary), C. Ho Li, M.E. Simpson and Herbert Evans isolated ACTH from sheep pituitary in 1942–43, as did George Sayers and his colleagues at Yale from swine pituitaries.

In 1946 Hans Selye described the general adaptation syndrome. In 1949 Hench, Kendall, Slocumb and Polley of the Mayo Foundation described the effect of compound E and of adrenocorticotrophic hormone (ACTH) on rheumatoid arthritis. Between 1953 and 1955 there occurred the isolation and analysis of the structure of aldosterone (S.A. Simpson, J.F. Tait and P.G.G. Bush isolated 'electro cortin', aldosterone). In fact, a publication by Hilary M. Grundy, S.A. Simpson and J.F. Tait, 'Isolation of highly active mineralo-corticoid from beef adrenal extract' (in *Nature (London)* 1952; **169**: 795–6) is regarded as the first publication on the subject. Aldosterone was synthesised by Wettstein and Schmidlin. In 1955 Jerome W. Conn (b. 1907) of Ann Arbor, Michigan described 'Primary aldosteronism. A new syndrome'. In 1958 Jack Gross suggested that angiotensin controlled aldosterone secretion. In 1966 Schwyzer and Sieber synthesised corticotrophin.

The adrenal medulla

Whereas the adrenal cortex is of mesodermal origin, the medulla consists of cells of neural origin. After Cuvier and Huschke, there came in 1856 the staining method of Edme F.A. Vulpian of Paris, causing the emerald green colour which the medulla stains with perchloride of iron. A similar reaction is given by the blood in the adrenal veins, but nowhere else in the body.

In 1886 Felix Fraenkel in Freiburg im Breisgau described in his MD thesis the first patient with phaeochromocytoma. Post-mortem examination revealed tumours in both adrenals. Fraenkel's description was followed 6 years later by A. Berdez of Lausanne, and in 1914 by J. Orth (1847–1923) in Prussia. Next came Ernest M. Labbé (1870–1939), J. Tinel and E. Doumer in Paris in 1929, Charles Mayo in 1927, and a number of other authors. One case was observed, diagnosed and studied by V.C. Medvei in 1933 and published by Julius Baver (1887–1979) of Vienna and Reé Lériche (1879–1955) of Lyon.

In 1894 pressor substances in adrenal extract were discovered by George Oliver (1841–1915) and Sir Edward E. Schaefer in London. Independently, they were discovered and described in the same year by Szymonowicz and Cybulski at the Polish University at Cracow (then Austria), and were first published in Polish. Between 1898 and 1904, adrenaline was isolated; its structure was determined and synthesised by John Jacob Abel (1857–1938) and Albert Cornelius Crawford (1869–1921) of Johns Hopkins Hospital, Baltimore. Jôkicki Takamine (1834–1922) isolated adrenaline as 'the blood pressure-raising principle of the adrenal glands' in 1901 (Takamine had worked previously in J.J. Abel's laboratory). Independently of him, Thomas Bell Aldrich, in the same year, succeeded in isolating adrenaline in crystalline form; it was the first hormone to be isolated, fulfilling one of Edward Aldelbert Doisy's essential criteria of hormone investigation. Friedrich Stolz in Germany achieved its synthesis in 1904.

The granules in the cells of the adrenal medulla were, after Friedrich G.J. Henle (1809–85), Goettingen and Manasse's staining experiments in 1904, later called 'chromaffin', 'chromophil' or 'phaeochrome' cells, because they stained with chromaffin salts. In 1922, Ernest Marcel Labbé (1870–1939) with J. Tinel and E. Doumer in Paris (see also above) connected paroxysmal hypertension with chromaffinomas of the adrenal. In 1927 Charles Mayo first removed a phaeochromocytoma successfully.

In 1945 Holtz, Credner and Kronenberg discovered noradrenaline. A year later, Ulf Svante von Euler showed that noradrenaline is the predominant transmitter of the effects of sympathetic nerve impulses. As the adrenal medulla is of ectodermal origin, it responds mainly to nervous stimuli and is not under feedback control. The medullary hormones are called catecholamines because of their catechol nucleus and amine side chain. In 1957 vanillylmandelic acid (VMA) was found to be a metabolite of catecholamines (M.D. Armstrong and A. McMillan, USA). In 1988 V.C. Medvei and W. Cattell described psychiatric symptoms presenting in some cases of phaeochromocytoma.

The first kidney hormone—renin

In 1898 some observations of Robert A.A. Tigerstedt (1853–1923) of Leipzig and Helsinki suggested that the kidney formed a pressor agent which entered the circulation by the renal veins. This substance became known as 'renin' and, according to J.W. Fisher, it was A. Goormaghtigh who suggested in 1939 that renin, 'the first kidney hormone', might be secreted by the cells of the juxtaglomerular apparatus. It seems that it might also be produced in other cells of the vascular pole regions of the glomeruli. The actual discovery of 'haemopoietin' was made by P. Carnot and G. Déflandre of Paris in 1906. It was given the new name 'haemopoietin' by the Finnish researchers E. Bondsdorff and E. Jalavista in 1948; they felt that this name was more indicative of its effects on erythroid cells. In 1950 Kurt Reissmann confirmed the existence of an erythropoietic factor by an ingenious experiment.

Four years later, Fred Stohlman Jr and his colleagues showed convincingly the erythropoietic effect in plasma from a patient with regional hypoxia and polycythaemia, secondary to a patent ductus arteriosus. Renin is now known to be an enzyme which—on release into the circulation—acts upon a substrate called angiotensinogen which is present in the plasma.

Ectopic hormone production

Hormones secreted by tissues other than those normally responsible for their synthesis are called ectopic. The term was coined by G.W. Liddle (Ann Arbor) and his colleagues during their studies between 1962 and 1965. The existence of ectopic hormones may be the first indication of the presence of a tumour. Such tumours are not necessarily malignant, for example bronchial carcinoids. The most important is perhaps the ectopic ACTH syndrome. W.H. Brown described in 1928 a patient with Cushing's syndrome and bilateral cortical hyperplasia; after the patient's death an oat-cell carcinoma of the bronchus was found. F.C. Bartter and W.B. Schwartz (USA) described in 1967 bronchial carcinomas also producing excessive vasopressin, causing excretion of hypertonic urine (high rate of sodium excretion), in spite of hypotonic plasma and expanded extracellular fluid volume and water retention.

Infertility

Herodotus remarked on specialisation among the Egyptian doctors in the fifth century BC: they included experts in conception, infertility and contraception. In 1975 A. Preus wrote an important paper on 'Biomedical techniques for influencing human reproduction in the fourth century BC'. He stressed that Plato, Aristotle and other fourth century thinkers were concerned about the problem of controlling the size of human population in a well-ordered state. Medical knowledge was available from the Hippocratic treatises. Castration was one of the causes of male infertility, while if semen is put into water and it floats, it is infertile. Mumps followed by orchitis causes infertility. In the Hippocratic 'Airs, Waters, Places', there is a discussion on the infertility of the Scythians: climate, nutrition and the menstrual cycle are discussed. Surgical removal of the ovaries was known as a cause of infertility. The ancient Hindus quoted impotence and obesity (?polycystic ovaries) as causing infertility. The ancient Jews recognised infertility in men and women (Deuteronomy, 7: 14), but sterility of the man was no legal cause for divorce, in contrast to sterility in the woman. Diseases, permanent uterine bleeding, were known and treated.

In modern times, the role of the endocrine glands plays a large part in the study and treatment of infertility. The latest developments include the gonadotrophic hormones and also the immune reactions (autoimmunity) of the sperm. Sperm agglutinins in the serum, causing male infertility, were described by P. Ruemke in 1954 and by L. Wilson in the same year. Some women produce anti-sperm antibodies, especially some prostitutes, as mentioned by W.B. Schwimmer *et al.* in 1967. Finally, the studies of anatomists, animal breeders and physiologists have to be mentioned in the context of infertility. There were the transplant experiments of J. Hunter (1728–93) and A. A. Berthold's (1803–61) of Goettingen, and Hunter's interest in the bovine freemartin, later studied and discussed extensively by F. R. Lillie (1870–1947) in 1916 and, lately, by R.V. Short between 1969 and 1971. There are also the studies of the mule by Clarke and his group (1980); he uses the term 'uncertainty principle' for this complex situation (see *Lancet* 1980; **ii**: 784).

A hormone from the heart

Although it was suspected by Paul Wood (London) nearly 30 years ago, and by Gauerand Henry in 1963, that the cardiac atria could serve as sensors of blood volume, the idea of central volume receptors has been known for centuries, in the form of water immersion as a treatment for dropsy. In 1956 Kisch described secretory-like granules in the cardiac atria of guinea pigs. They were found in all mammals. In 1976 Marie Guillemot and Hatt suggested that these granules might be associated with changes in the body fluid volume. This led de Bold and colleagues in 1981 to show a potent natriuretic response to intravenous injection of atrial myocardiac extract in rats. The peptide sequence of an atrial peptide was established based on de Bold's work. Needleman and colleagues described 'atrial peptins' as cardiac hormones in 1985. Ruth Nutt and colleagues synthesised peptides with the atrial natriuretic factor sequence in 1984. In the same year M. A. Napier *et al.* established the existence of specific membrane receptors for atrial natriuretic factor in renal and vascular tissues. However, this factor may not be related to other natriuretic factors with Na^+/K^+- ATPase activity.

The pineal

A little understood gland until recently, the pineal, was mentioned in the Ayur-Veda medicine of the Hindus, by Herophilus of Alexandria (*c.* 300 BC) and by Galenus of Pergamon. It was described by Thomas Wharton (1614–73) of Oxbridge and Thomas's Hospital in London in 1659. René Descartes in 1662 thought the human body a material machine, controlled by a rational soul, seated in the pineal body. Thomas Willis in Oxford called it the 'pineal body' in his *Cerebri Anatome* in 1664 meaning little pine, because of its shape. In 1878, O. Huebner described a 4.5-year-old boy with precocious sexual development: at autopsy a teratoma of the pineal was found. By 1907, Otto Marburg of Austria had collected 40 similar cases which he called 'the macrogenitosomia praecox syndrome' which he ascribed to hypopinealism. However, removal of the pineal in animals and in man caused no detectable deficiency symptoms. J.I. and M.D. Altschule published their monumental review: *The Pineal Gland* (Harvard University Press). Their analysis of pineal tumours in the world literature concluded that destructive tumours of pineal origin (pineocytomas) cause delayed sexual development. In 1958, A.B. Lerner and his group isolated the pineal hormone, melatonin, a methoxy derivative of serotonin. They called it 'melatonin' because it is related to melanin and serotonin.

References

1 Russell B. *History as an Art.* 2nd Hermon Ould Memorial Lecture to the Members of the P.E.N. Club in London on 4 May 1954.

2 Kraus H, Medvei VC. The distribution of bloodgroups in hyperthyroidism. *Muench Wschr* 1929; **I**: 493.

3 Medvei VC, Cattell WR. Mental symptoms presenting in phaeochromocytomas: a case report and review. *J Roy Soc Med* 1988; 81: 550.

All other references can be found in Medvei VC. *The History of Clinical Endocrinology*. Parthenon Publishing Group, Lancaster, 1993.

Index

Note: Page numbers in *italic* refer to figures and/or tables. Numbers in **bold** refer to plates.

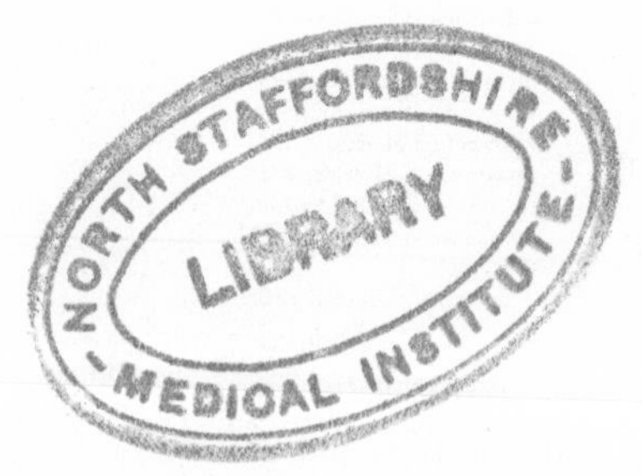